Operative Neurosurgical Techniques

Books edited by:

H. H. Schmidek

Schmidek HH (ed): Pineal Tumors. New York, Masson Publishing USA, Inc., 1977.

Schmidek HH, Sweet WH (eds): Current Techniques in Operative Neurosurgery. New York, Grune & Stratton, 1977.

Schmidek HH, Sweet WH (eds): Operative Neurosurgical Techniques: Indications, Methods, and Results, in Two Volumes. New York, Grune & Stratton 1982; 2nd Edition, 1988.

Kapp JB, Schmidek HH (eds): The Cerebral Venous System and its Disorders. New York, Grune & Stratton, 1984.

Dunsker SB, Schmidek HH, Frymoyer J, Kahn A (eds): The Unstable Spine: Thoracic, Lumbar and Sacral Regions. New York, Grune & Stratton, 1985.

Sundaresan N, Schmidek HH, Schiller A, Rosenthal D (eds): Tumors of the Spine: Diagnosis and Clinical Management. Philadelphia, WB Saunders Co, 1991.

Schmidek HH (ed): Meningiomas and Their Surgical Management. Philadelphia, WB Saunders Co, 1992.

Levine AJ, Schmidek HH (eds): Molecular Genetics of Nervous System Tumors. New York, Wiley, 1993.

W. H. Sweet

White JC, Sweet WH (eds): Pain: Its Mechanisms and Neurosurgical Control. Springfield, Illinois, Charles C Thomas, 1955.

Krayenbuhl H, Maspes P, Sweet W (eds): Progress in Neurological Surgery. Vols. 1–10. (Switzerland) and New York, S. Karger, 1966–1981.

White JC, Sweet WH (eds): Pain and the Neurosurgeon: A Forty Year Experience. Springfield, Charles C Thomas, 1969.

Fields WS, Sweet WH (eds): Neural Bases of Violence and Aggression. St. Louis, Warren H. Green, Inc., 1975.

Sweet WH, Obrador S, Martin-Rodriguez JG (eds): Neurosurgical Treatment in Psychiatry, Pain and Epilepsy. Baltimore, University Park Press, 1977. (Proceedings of the Fourth Congress of Psychiatric Surgery, Madrid, Spain, September 7–10, 1975.)

Gybels JM, Sweet WH (eds): Neurosurgical Treatment of Persistent Pain: Physiological and Pathological Mechanisms of Human Pain. Series edited by PL Gildenberg, Basel, S Karger, 1989.

Volume 2

Operative Neurosurgical Techniques

Indications, Methods, and Results

THIRD EDITION

Henry H. Schmidek, MD, FACS
Marion, Massachusetts

William H. Sweet, MD, DSc
Department of Neurosurgery
Massachusetts General Hospital
Harvard Medical School
Boston, Massachusetts

W.B. SAUNDERS COMPANY
A Division of Harcourt Brace & Company
Philadelphia   London   Toronto   Montreal   Sydney   Tokyo

W.B. SAUNDERS COMPANY
A Division of
Harcourt Brace & Company

The Curtis Center
Independence Square West
Philadelphia, Pennsylvania 19106

Library of Congress Cataloging-in-Publication Data

Operative neurosurgical techniques: indications, methods, and results / [edited by] Henry H. Schmidek, William H. Sweet. — 3rd ed.

    p.   cm.

Includes bibliographical references and index.

ISBN 0-7216-5541-6

1. Nervous system—Surgery.   I. Schmidek, Henry H. II. Sweet, William Herbert.   [DNLM: 1. Nervous System Diseases—surgery.   2. Neurosurgery—methods. WL 368 O61 1995]

RD593.O63 1995

617.4'8—dc20

DNLM/DLC   93-42522

Operative Neurosurgical Techniques, 3rd Edition   Volume 1 0-7216-5542-4
                                                                         Volume 2 0-7216-5543-2
                                                                     Two Volume Set 0-7216-5541-6

Copyright © 1995, 1988, 1982 by W.B. Saunders Company

All rights reserved. No part of this publication may be reproduced or transmitted in any form or by any means, electronic or mechanical, including photocopy, recording, or any information storage and retrieval system, without permission in writing from the publisher.

Printed in the United States of America.

Last digit is the print number: 9   8   7   6   5   4   3   2

Contributors

Adnan A. Abla, M.D.
Departments of Neurosurgery and Orthopedic Surgery, Medical College of Pennsylvania, Pittsburgh; Allegheny General Hospital; North Hills Passavant Hospital; Suburban General Hospital, Pittsburgh, Pennsylvania
Surgical Approach to Lesions of the Orbit

Phil A. Aitken, M.D.
Division of Ophthalmology, University of Vermont College of Medicine, Burlington, Vermont
Anterior and Lateral Approaches to Lesions of the Orbit

Melvin G. Alper, M.D.
Departments of Ophthalmology and Neurological Surgery, The George Washington University School of Medicine and the Washington Hospital Center, Washington, D.C.
Anterior and Lateral Approaches to Lesions of the Orbit

A. L. Amacher, M.D., F.R.C.S.(C)
Department of Neurosurgery, Geisinger Medical Center, Danville, Pennsylvania
Surgical Management of Meningoceles and Myelomeningoceles

Michael L. J. Apuzzo, M.D.
Department of Neurosurgery, University of Southern California School of Medicine; Kenneth R. Norris Cancer Center; University of Southern California Hospital; Los Angeles County–University of Southern California Medical Center, Los Angeles, California
Transcallosal Approach to the Third Ventricle

Takao Asano, M.D., D.M.Sc.
Department of Neurosurgery, Saitama Medical Center/School, Kawagoe, Saitama, Japan
Surgical Management of Ossification of the Posterior Longitudinal Ligament

Peter W. Ascher, M.D.
University Clinic for Neurosurgery, Karl-Franzens University of Graz, Graz, Austria
Percutaneous Lumbar Discectomy

Erik-Olof Backlund, M.D., Ph.D.
Linköping University Hospital, Linköping, Sweden
Stereotactic Radiosurgery for Pituitary Adenomas and Craniopharyngiomas

Roy A. E. Bakay, M.D.
Department of Neurological Surgery, Emory University School of Medicine; Emory University Hospital; Crawford Long Hospital; Grady Memorial Hospital; Veterans Administration Medical Center, Atlanta, Georgia
Transplantation in the Nervous System

H. Thomas Ballantine, Jr., M.D., F.A.C.S.
Department of Surgery, Harvard Medical School; Department of Neurological Surgery, Massachusetts General Hospital, Boston, Massachusetts
Surgical Treatment of Intractable Psychiatric Illness and Chronic Pain by Stereotactic Cingulotomy

Armando Basso, M.D., Ph.D.
Department of Neurosurgery, University of Buenos Aires School of Medicine, Buenos Aires, Argentina
Transcranial Approach to Lesions of the Orbit

H. Hunt Batjer, M.D.
Department of Neurological Surgery, The University of Texas Southwestern Medical School; Zale Lipshy University Hospital; Parkland Memorial Hospital; Veterans Administration Hospital–Dallas; St. Paul Medical Center, Dallas, Texas
Surgical Management of Intraoperative Aneurysmal Rupture

B. L. Bauer, M.D.
Department of Neurosurgery, Philipps University Hospital and Medical School, Marburg, Germany
Surgical Management of Intracranial Arachnoid, Suprasellar, and Rathke's Cleft Cysts; Intracranial and Intraspinal Endoscopy

Janet W. Bay, M.D.
Department of Surgery, Riverside Methodist Hospitals; Columbus Children's Hospital; Mt. Carmel Medical Center; Doctors Hospital West; University Hospital, Columbus, Ohio
Surgery of the Sympathetic Nervous System

Donald P. Becker, M.D.
Division of Neurosurgery, School of Medicine, University of California at Los Angeles; University of California at Los Angeles Health Sciences Center, Los Angeles, California
Surgical Management of Severe Closed Head Injury in Adults; Surgical Management of Traumatic Posterior Fossa Hematomas

A. L. Benabid, M.D., Ph.D.
J. Fourier University; Hospital of Grenoble, Grenoble, France
Multilobar Resections for the Control of Epilepsy

Vallo Benjamin, M.D.
Department of Neurosurgery, New York University Medical Center; Bellevue Hospital Center; Manhattan Veterans Administration Hospital, New York, New York
Surgical Management of Tuberculum Sellae and Sphenoid Ridge Meningiomas

Claude M. Bertrand, M.D., F.R.C.S.(C)
Division of Neurosurgery, University of Montreal; Hospital Notre Dame, Montreal, Quebec, Canada
Surgical Management of Spasmodic Torticollis and Adult-Onset Dystonia

Ravi Bhatia, M.S., M.Ch.
Department of Neurosurgery, All India Institute of Medical Sciences, New Delhi, India
Surgical Management of Tuberculous and Fungal Infections of the Nervous System

Don C. Bienfang, M.D.
Department of Ophthalmology, Harvard Medical School; Brigham and Women's Hospital, Boston, Massachusetts
Diagnosis and Investigation of Unilateral and Bilateral Exophthalmos

Jurij R. Bilyk, M.D.
Department of Ophthalmology, Harvard Medical School; Eye Plastics and Orbit Service, Massachusetts Eye and Ear Infirmary, Boston, Massachusetts
Optic Nerve Sheath Fenestration in the Management of Pseudotumor Cerebri

Perry Black, M.D.
Department of Neurosurgery, Hahnemann University; Hahnemann University Hospital; North Philadelphia Health System; Roxborough Memorial Hospital; St. Agnes Medical Center, Philadelphia, Pennsylvania
Surgical Management of Brain Metastasis

Peter McL. Black, M.D., Ph.D.
Department of Neurosurgery, Harvard Medical School; Children's Hospital, Boston, Massachusetts
Surgical Management of Endocrinologically Silent Pituitary Tumors

J. B. Blacklock, M.D.
Department of Neurosurgery, Baylor College of Medicine; Methodist Hospital; Ben Taub General Hospital; Veterans Affairs Medical Center; Texas Children's Hospital, Houston, Texas
Transcranial Resection of Tumors of the Anterior Skull Base

Lawrence F. Borges, M.D.
Department of Neurological Surgery, Massachusetts General Hospital; Harvard Medical School, Boston, Massachusetts
Surgical Approaches to the Thoracic and Thoracolumbar Spine for Decompression and Stabilization

James M. Borthwick, M.B., Ch.B., F.R.C.A.
Institute of Neurological Sciences, Southern General Hospital, Glasgow, Scotland
Surgical Management of the Rheumatoid Cervical Spine

Robert E. Breeze, M.D.
Division of Neurosurgery and Neural Transplantation Program for Parkinson's Disease, University of Colorado School of Medicine; Division of Neurosurgery, Denver General Hospital; St. Anthony Hospital Central; The Children's Hospital; University Hospital; Veterans Administration Medical Center, Denver, Colorado
Transplantation in the Nervous System

Jeffrey A. Brown, M.D.
Department of Neurological Surgery, Medical College of Ohio, Toledo, Ohio
Percutaneous Trigeminal Nerve Compression

Derek A. Bruce, M.D.
Department of Neurosurgery, The University of Texas Southwestern Medical School; Children's Medical Center of Dallas; Medical City Dallas, Dallas, Texas
Surgical Management of Spinal Injuries in Children

Jeffrey N. Bruce, M.D.
Departments of Neurological Surgery and Pathology, College of Physicians and Surgeons of Columbia University; Columbia–Presbyterian Medical Center, New York, New York
Supracerebellar Approach for Pineal Region Neoplasms

F. X. Brunner, M.D., D.D.S.
Department of Otolaryngology, University of Würzburg, Würzburg, Germany
Surgical Management of Trauma Involving the Skull Base and Paranasal Sinuses

John C. M. Brust, M.D.
Department of Neurology, Harlem Hospital Center, New York, New York
Surgical Management of Infected Intracranial Aneurysms

Michael Buchfelder, M.D.
Department of Neurosurgery, University of Erlangen-Nürnberg, Erlangen, Germany
Transsphenoidal Microsurgery for Craniopharyngioma

Alexa I. Canady, M.D.
Department of Neurosurgery, Wayne State University School of Medicine; Children's Hospital of Michigan, Detroit, Michigan
Surgical Management of Hydrocephalus in Children

Paolo Cappabianca, M.D.
Department of Systematic Pathology, Federico II University School of Medicine, Naples, Italy
Repair of the Sella Following Transsphenoidal Surgery

Antonio Carrizo, M.D.
Department of Neurosurgery, University of Buenos Aires School of Medicine; Hospital Santa Lucia, Buenos Aires, Argentina
Transcranial Approach to Lesions of the Orbit

Benjamin S. Carson, M.D.
Departments of Neurosurgery, Pediatrics, Oncology, and Plastic Surgery, The Johns Hopkins University School of Medicine; Department of Neurosurgery, The Johns Hopkins Hospital, Baltimore, Maryland
Management of Achondroplasia and Its Neurosurgical Complications

Paul H. Chapman, M.D.
Department of Surgery, Department of Neurological Surgery, Massachusetts General Hospital; Harvard Medical School, Boston, Massachusetts
Radiosurgery of Cranial Arteriovenous Malformations; Surgical Management of Occult Spinal Dysraphism

E. T. Chappell, M.D.
Department of Surgery, Division of Neurosurgery, University of California Davis–East Bay, Oakland, California
The Neurosurgical Management of HIV-Related Brain Lesions

In Sup Choi, M.D.
Department of Radiology, Harvard Medical School; Department of Neuroradiology, Massachusetts General Hospital, Boston, Massachusetts
Direct Brain Revascularization

W. Craig Clark, M.D., Ph.D.
Neurosurgery Center of North Georgia, Dalton, Georgia
Transtemporal Approaches to the Posterior Cranial Fossa; Surgical Management of Glomus Jugulare Tumors

Edwin W. Cocke, Jr., M.D.
Department of Otolaryngology—Head and Neck Surgery, University of Tennessee–Memphis; Baptist Memorial Hospital, Memphis, Tennessee
Surgical Management of Glomus Jugulare Tumors

Robert J. Coffey, M.D.
Department of Neurosurgery, Mayo Clinic, Mayo Medical School, Rochester, Minnesota
Surgical Management of Dural Arteriovenous Malformations

James C. Collias, M.D.
Division of Neurosurgery, University of Connecticut School of Medicine, Farmington, Connecticut; Department of Neurosurgery, Hartford Hospital, Hartford, Connecticut
Posterior Surgical Approaches for Cervical Disc Herniation and Spondylotic Myelopathy

Shlomo Constantini, M.D., M.Sc.
Department of Neurosurgery, Hebrew University; Hadassah University Hospital, Jerusalem, Israel
Surgical Management of Intramedullary Spinal Cord Tumors

G. Rees Cosgrove, M.D., F.R.C.S.(C)
Department of Surgery, Harvard Medical School; Department of Neurological Surgery, Massachusetts General Hospital, Boston, Massachusetts
Surgical Treatment of Intractable Psychiatric Illness and Chronic Pain by Stereotactic Cingulotomy

James B. Costales, M.D.
Radionics Software Applications, Inc., Burlington, Massachusetts
Radiosurgery of Cranial Arteriovenous Malformations

Paul R. Cosyns, M.D.
Department of Psychiatry, University of Antwerp; University Hospital Antwerp, Antwerp, Belgium
Cerebral Lesions for Psychiatric Disorders and Pain

William T. Couldwell, M.D., Ph.D.
Department of Neurosurgery, University of Southern California School of Medicine; USC University Hospital, Los Angeles, California
Surgical Management of Growth Hormone–Secreting and Prolactin-Secreting Pituitary Adenomas

Robert M. Crowell, M.D.
Department of Neurosurgery, Berkshire Medical Center, Pittsfield, Massachusetts
Direct Brain Revascularization; Surgical Management of Cavernous Angiomas of the Nervous System

T. Forcht Dagi, M.D., M.P.H., F.A.C.S.
Department of Surgery, The Uniformed Services University of the Health Sciences; Department of Neurosurgery, St. Joseph's Hospital; Scottish Rite Children's Medical Center; Northside Hospital, Atlanta, Georgia
Surgical Management of Penetrating Missile Injuries of the Head; Surgical Management of Cranial Cerebrospinal Fluid Fistulas

Lawrence W. Davis, M.D.
Emory University School of Medicine, Atlanta, Georgia
Implantation of Radionuclides in Brain Tumors

Arthur L. Day, M.D.
Department of Neurosurgery, University of Florida College of Medicine; Shands Hospital at the University of Florida; Veterans Administration Medical Center, Gainesville, Florida
Surgical Management of Aneurysms and Fistulas Involving the Cavernous Sinus

J. Diaz Day, M.D.
Department of Neurosurgery, University of Southern California School of Medicine; LAC/USC Medical Center, Los Angeles, California
Surgical Management of Tumors Involving the Cavernous Sinus; Surgical Management of Vertebro-PICA Aneurysms

Patrick J. Derome, M.D.
Department of Neurosurgery, Foch Hospital, Suresnes France
Transbasal Approach to Tumors Invading the Skull Base

Enrico de Divitiis, M.D.
Department of Systematic Pathology, Federico II University School of Medicine, Naples, Italy
Repair of the Sella Following Transsphenoidal Surgery

Jacquez Charl de Villiers, M.D., F.R.C.S.(Eng, Edin.) Sc. (h.c)
Department of Neurosurgery, University of Cape Town; Medical School of the University of Cape Town; Groote Schuur Hospital, Cape Town, Republic of South Africa
Neurosurgical Management of Sclerosteosis

P. C. Taylor Dickinson, M.D.
Department of Medicine, Columbia University College of Physicians and Surgeons, New York, New York; Nyack Hospital, Nyack, New York; Good Samaritan Hospital, Suffern, New York
Surgical Management of Infected Intracranial Aneurysms

Curtis A. Dickman, M.D.
Division of Neurological Surgery, Barrow Neurological Institute; Maricopa Medical Center, Phoenix, Arizona
Surgical Techniques for the Stabilization of the Cervical Spine

Donald D. Dietze, M.D.
Methodist Medical Center, Oak Ridge, Tennessee
Surgical Approaches to the Cervicothoracic Junction

George V. DiGiacinto, M.D.
St. Luke's–Roosevelt Hospital, New York, New York
Surgical Management of Primary and Metastatic Tumors of the Spine

Concezio Di Rocco, M.D.
Section of Pediatric Neurosurgery, Catholic University Medical School; Policlinico A. Gemelli, Catholic University, Rome, Italy
Surgical Management of Craniosynostosis and Craniofacial Deformities

Edward F. Downing, M.D.
Department of Neurosurgery, Memorial Medical Center; Candler Hospital; St. Joseph's Hospital, Savannah, Georgia
Surgical Management of Extracranial Lesions of the Vertebral Artery

Werner K. Doyle, M.D.
Department of Neurosurgery, New York University School of Medicine; Hospital for Joint Diseases, New York, New York
Temporal Lobe Operations for Epilepsy: Radical Hippocampectomy

Charles G. Drake, M.D., F.A.C.S., F.R.C.S.(C)
Division of Neurosurgery, University of Western Ontario Faculty of Medicine; University of Western Ontario Hospital, London, Ontario, Canada
Surgical Management of Terminal Basilar and Posterior Cerebral Artery Aneurysms

John C. Drummond, M.D., F.R.C.P.(C)
Department of Anesthesiology, University of California, San Diego, School of Medicine; Veterans Affairs Medical Center, San Diego, California
Anesthetic Management of Intracranial Aneurysm Surgery

Stewart B. Dunsker, M.D.
Department of Neurosurgery, University of Cincinnati College of Medicine; Mayfield Neurological Institute, Cincinnati, Ohio
Surgical Management of Thoracic Disc Herniations

Jacques J. du Plessis, M.B., Ch.B., M.Med., F.C.S. (S.A.) Neuro.
Department of Neurosurgery, University of Pretoria; Pretoria Academic Hospital, Pretoria, South Africa
Neurosurgical Management of Sclerosteosis

Fred Epstein, M.D.
   Division of Pediatric Neurosurgery, New York University Medical Center, New York, New York
   Surgical Management of Intramedullary Spinal Cord Tumors

Mel H. Epstein, M.D.
   Department of Clinical Neurosciences, Brown University School of Medicine; Department of Neurosurgery, Rhode Island Hospital, Providence, Rhode Island
   Surgical Management of Hydrocephalus in Adults

Calvin B. Ernst, M.D.
   Department of Surgery, University of Michigan Medical School, Ann Arbor, Michigan; Henry Ford Hospital, Detroit, Michigan
   Surgical Exposure of the Distal Internal Carotid Artery

Francisco Escobedo, M.D.
   Department of Neurosurgery, The National University of Mexico at the Neurological and Neurosurgical Institute, Mexico City, Mexico
   Neurosurgical Aspects of Neurocysticercosis

Rudolf Fahlbusch, M.D.
   Department of Neuosurgery, University of Erlangen-Nürnberg, Erlangen, Germany
   Transsphenoidal Microsurgery for Craniopharyngioma

Richard G. Fessler, M.D., Ph.D.
   Department of Neurological Surgery, University of Florida College of Medicine; Shands Hospital of the University of Florida; Veterans Administration Medical Center, Gainesville, Florida
   Surgical Approaches to the Cervicothoracic Junction

Bernard E. Finneson, M.D., F.A.C.S.
   Low Back Pain Center, Crozer–Chester Medical Center, Upland, Pennsylvania
   Lumbar Disc Excision

Edwin G. Fischer, M.D.
   Division of Neurosurgery, New England Deaconess Hospital, Boston, Massachusetts
   Spinal Deformities Following Neurosurgical Procedures in Children

S. Francione, M.D.
   Department of Neurology, University of Genoa, Genoa, Italy
   Multilobar Resections for the Control of Epilepsy

Clair Francomano, M.D.
   Departments of Medicine and Pediatrics, The Johns Hopkins University School of Medicine; The Johns Hopkins Hospital, Baltimore, Maryland; Medical Genetics Branch, National Center for Human Genome Research, National Institutes of Health, Bethesda, Maryland
   Managment of Achondroplasia and Its Neurosurgical Complications

Curt R. Freed, M.D.
   Division of Clinical Pharmacology and Toxicology, University of Colorado School of Medicine; Neurotransplantation Program for Parkinson's Disease, University of Colorado Hospital, Denver, Colorado
   Transplantation in the Nervous System

Stephen R. Freidberg, M.D.
   Department of Neurosurgery, Lahey Clinic, Burlington, Massachusetts; New England Deaconess Hospital (Courtesy Staff), Boston, Massachusetts; Atlanticare Medical Center, Lynn, Massachusetts
   Surgical Management of Cerebrospinal Fluid Leakage After Spinal Surgery

Arno H. Fried, M.D.
   Departments of Neurosurgery and Pediatrics, Brown University School of Medicine; Department of Pediatric Neurosurgery, Rhode Island Hospital/Hasbrow Children's Hospital, Providence, Rhode Island
   Surgical Management of Hydrocephalus in Adults

Takanori Fukushima, M.D., D.M.Sc.
   Department of Neurosurgery, Medical College of Pennsylvania, Pittsburgh; Allegheny General Hospital, Pittsburgh, Pennsylvania; University of Southern California, Los Angeles, California; Karolinska Institute, Stockholm, Sweden; Komonji Hospital, Kitakyushu City, Japan; St. Mary's Hospital, Kurume City, Japan; Nagasaki Morinoki Hospital, Nagasaki City, Japan; Kagoshima Atsuchi Hospital, Kagoshima City, Japan; Tokyo Nishikasai Moriyama Hospital, Tokyo, Japan; Honolulu Kaiser Permanente Hospital, Honolulu, Hawaii
   Surgical Management of Tumors Involving the Cavernous Sinus

Giuseppe Galli, M.D.
   Department of Neurosurgery, University of Brescia, Brescia, Italy
   Intraventricular Morphine in the Treatment of Pain Secondary to Cancer

Gale Gardner, M.D.
   Department of Otolaryngology–Head and Neck Surgery, University of Tennessee–Memphis; Baptist Memorial Hospital, Memphis, Tennessee
   Transtemporal Approaches to the Posterior Cranial Fossa; Surgical Management of Glomus Jugulare Tumors

Eugene D. George, M.D.
   Department of Neurosurgery, University of Rochester Medical Center; Strong Memorial Hospital, Rochester, New York
   Surgical Management of Penetrating Missile Injuries of the Head; Surgical Management of Cranial Cerebrospinal Fluid Fistulas

Steven L. Giannotta, M.D.
Department of Neurological Surgery and Neurovascular Surgery, University of Southern California School of Medicine; USC University Hospital; LAC/USC Medical Center, Los Angeles, California
Surgical Management of Vertebro-PICA Aneurysms

Ida E. Giriunas, R.N.
Department of Neurological Surgery, Massachusetts General Hospital, Boston, Massachusetts
Surgical Treatment of Intractable Psychiatric Illness and Chronic Pain by Stereotactic Cingulotomy

Renato Giuffrè, M.D.
Institute of Neurosurgery, Tor Vergata University Medical School of Rome, Rome, Italy
Surgical Management of Low-Grade Gliomas of the Cerebral Hemispheres

S. K. Gorelyshev, M.D.
Burdenko Institute of Neurosurgery, Moscow, Russia
Surgery of Diencephalic and Brainstem Tumors

Daryl R. Gress, M.D.
Department of Neurology, University of California, San Francisco, School of Medicine; Neurovascular Service, University of California, San Francisco, Medical Center, San Francisco, California
Direct Brain Revascularization

Robert G. Grossman, M.D.
Department of Neurosurgery, Baylor College of Medicine; Neurosurgical Services, The Methodist Hospital, Houston, Texas
Temporal Lobe Operations for Drug-Resistant Epilepsy

Robert L. Grubb, Jr., M.D.
Department of Neurology and Neurological Surgery, Washington University School of Medicine; Barnes Hospital; Jewish Hospital of St. Louis; Children's Hospital, St. Louis, Missouri
Surgical Therapy for Diseases of the Extracranial Carotid Artery

B. L. Guthrie, M.D.
Department of Neurosurgery, The University of Alabama Hospitals, Birmingham, Alabama
The Neurosurgical Management of HIV-Related Brain Lesions

Jan M. Gybels, M.D., Ph.D.
Department of Neurosurgery, University of Leuven; University Hospital of Leuven, Leuven, Belgium
Brain Stimulation in the Management of Persistent Pain; Cerebral Lesions for Psychiatric Disorders and Pain

Sten Håkanson, M.D., Ph.D.
Department of Neurosurgery, Karolinska Hospital, Stockholm, Sweden
Retrogasserian Glycerol Rhizolysis in Trigeminal Neuralgia

John E. Hall, M.D.
Department of Orthopedic Surgery, Children's Hospital Medical Center, Harvard Medical School, Boston, Massachusetts
Spinal Deformities Following Neurosurgical Procedures in Children

Steven D. Ham, D.O.
Department of Neurosurgery, Wayne State University School of Medicine; Children's Hospital of Michigan, Detroit, Michigan
Surgical Management of Hydrocephalus in Children

Mark G. Hamilton, M.D.C.M., F.R.C.S.(C)
Department of Neurosurgery, University of Calgary; Alberta Children's Hospital; Foothills Hospital; Tom Baker Cancer Center, Calgary, Alberta, Canada
Surgical Management of Midbasilar and Lower Basilar Aneurysms

Winifred J. Hamilton, Ph.D.
Department of Neurosurgery, Baylor College of Medicine, Houston, Texas
Temporal Lobe Operations for Drug-Resistant Epilepsy

Russell W. Hardy, Jr., M.D.
Professor, Neurological Surgery, University Hospital, Case Western Reserve University, Cleveland, Ohio
Surgery of the Sympathetic Nervous System

Griffith R. Harsh IV, M.D., M.A.
Department of Surgery, Harvard Medical School; Department of Neurological Surgery, Massachusetts General Hospital, Boston, Massachusetts
Surgical Management of Recurrent Gliomas

Carl B. Heilman, M.D.
Department of Neurosurgery, Tufts University School of Medicine; New England Medical Center, Boston, Massachusetts
Surgical Management of Glomus Jugulare Tumors; Surgical Management of Anterior Cerebral Artery Aneurysms Distal to the Anterior Communicating Artery

O. Heiskanen, M.D.
Neurosurgical Department, Helsinki University Central Hospital, Helsinki, Finland
Surgical Management of Unruptured Cerebral Aneurysms

Mark C. Held, M.D.
Department of Neurosurgery, Mayo Graduate School of Medicine, Rochester, Minnesota
Surgical Management of Dural Arteriovenous Malformations

Dieter Hellwig, M.D.
Department of Neurosurgery, Philipps University Hospital and Medical School, Marburg, Germany
Surgical Management of Intracranial Arachnoid, Suprasellar, and Rathke's Cleft Cysts; Intracranial and Intraspinal Endoscopy

Juha A. Hernesniemi, M.D., Ph.D.
Department of Neurosurgery, University of Kuopio; University Hospital of Kuopio, Kuopio, Finland
Surgical Management of Terminal Basilar and Posterior Cerebral Artery Aneurysms

Roberto C. Heros, M.D.
Department of Neurosurgery, University of Minnesota School of Medicine–Minneapolis; University of Minnesota Hospitals, Minneapolis, Minnesota
Surgical Management of Unclippable Intracranial Aneurysms

Alan Hirschfeld, M.D.
Department of Neurosurgery, New York Medical College, Valhalla, New York; St. Vincent's Hospital and Medical Center of New York, New York, New York
Implantation of Radionuclides in Brain Tumors

E. R. Hitchcock, M.D. (Deceased)
Midland Center for Neurosurgery, Birmingham, United Kingdom
Neural Transplantation

D. Hoffmann, M.D.
Hospital of Grenoble, Grenoble, France
Multilobar Resections for the Control of Epilepsy

Robert N. N. Holtzman, M.D.
Department of Neurological Surgery, Columbia University College of Physicians and Surgeons; Columbia–Presbyterian Medical Center; Lenox Hill Hospital; Beth Israel Medical Center; Harlem Hospital Center, New York, New York
Surgical Management of Infected Intracranial Aneurysms

Jürgen Honegger, M.D.
Department of Neurosurgery, University of Erlangen-Nürnberg, Erlangen, Germany
Transsphenoidal Microsurgery for Craniopharyngioma

Edgar M. Housepian, M.D.
Department of Neurosurgery, Columbia University College of Physicians and Surgeons; New York Neurological Institute; Columbia–Presbyterian Medical Center, New York, New York
Surgical Management of Intraorbital Tumors

Alan R. Hudson, M.B., Ch.B., F.R.C.S.(Edin), F.C.S. (SA) (Hon.)
Division of Neurosurgery, University of Toronto; The Toronto Hospital, Toronto, Ontario, Canada
Surgical Management of Peripheral Nerve Tumors

James E. O. Hughes, M.D.
Department of Neurosurgery, Columbia University College of Physicians and Surgeons; St. Luke's–Roosevelt Hospital Center; Harlem Hospital Center; Beth Israel Medical Center, New York, New York
Surgical Management of Infected Intracranial Aneurysms; Surgical Management of Primary and Metastatic Tumors of the Spine

Robin P. Humphreys, M.D., F.R.C.S.(C), F.A.C.S.
Department of Surgery, University of Toronto; Hospital for Sick Children; Women's College Hospital; Hugh Macmillan Rehabilitation Centre, Toronto, Ontario, Canada
Surgical Management of Arteriovenous Malformations in Children

Orest Hurko, M.D.
Departments of Neurology and Medicine, The Johns Hopkins University School of Medicine; Division of Neurogenetics, The Johns Hopkins Hospital, Baltimore, Maryland
Management of Achondroplasia and Its Neurosurgical Complications

Robin A. Johnston, M.D., F.R.C.S.
Department of Neurosurgery, Institute of Neurological Sciences, Southern General Hospital, Glasgow, Scotland
Surgical Management of the Rheumatoid Cervical Spine

Michael Joseph, M.D.
Departments of Otology and Laryngology, Harvard Medical School; Department of Otolaryngology, Massachusetts Eye and Ear Infirmary, Boston, Massachusetts
Pedicled Rhinotomy for Exposure of the Clivus

P. Kahane, M.D.
J. Fourier University; Hospital of Grenoble, Grenoble, France
Multilobar Resections for the Control of Epilepsy

John P. Kapp, M.D., Ph.D., J.D.
Galax, Virginia
Surgical Management of Dural Sinus Lacerations

B. Karlsson, M.D.
Department of Neurological Surgery, Karolinska Institute; Karolinska Hospital, Stockholm, Sweden
Gamma Knife Surgery in Vascular, Neoplastic, and Functional Disorders of the Nervous System

Howard H. Kaufman, M.D.
Department of Neurosurgery, West Virginia Medical Center, Morgantown, West Virginia
Surgical Management of Civilian Gunshot Wounds to the Head

xii / Contributors

Daniel F. Kelly, M.D.
Division of Neurosurgery, School of Medicine, University of California at Los Angeles; University of California at Los Angeles Health Sciences Center, Los Angeles, California; Harbor–U.C.L.A. Medical Center, Torrance, California
Surgical Management of Severe Closed Head Injury in Adults; Surgical Management of Traumatic Posterior Fossa Hematomas

Patrick J. Kelly, M.D.
Department of Neurological Surgery, New York University Medical Center; Tisch Hospital; Bellevue Hospital; Veterans Administration Medical Center, New York, New York
CT/MRI-Based Computer-Assisted Volumetric Stereotactic Resection of Intracranial Lesions

E. A. Khuhlaeva, M.D.
Burdenko Institute of Neurosurgery, Moscow, Russia
Surgery of Diencephalic and Brainstem Tumors

T. T. King, F.R.C.S.
Department of Neurologic Surgery, The Royal London Hospital, Whitechapel, London, England
Translabyrinthine Approach to Acoustic Neuromas

N. D. Kitchin, F.R.C.S.
The National Hospital for Neurology and Neurosurgery, London, England
Stereotactic Biopsy and Resection of Intracranial Lesions

David G. Kline, M.D.
Division of Neurosurgery, Louisiana State University, Baton Rouge, Louisiana
Surgical Management of Peripheral Nerve Tumors

Robert S. Knego, M.D.
Department of Neurosurgery, University of Florida College of Medicine; Shands Hospital at the University of Florida; Veterans Administration Medical Center, Gainesville, Florida
Surgical Management of Aneurysms and Fistulas Involving the Cavernous Sinus

A. N. Konovalov, M.D.
Burdenko Institute of Neurosurgery, Moscow, Russia
Surgery of Diencephalic and Brainstem Tumors

Thomas A. Kopitnik, Jr., M.D.
Department of Neurological Surgery, The University of Texas Southwestern Medical School; Zale Lipshy University Hospital; Parkland Memorial Hospital; Veterans Administration Hospital–Dallas; St. Paul Medical Center, Dallas, Texas
Surgical Management of Intraoperative Aneurysmal Rupture

Paul Kornblith, M.D.
Department of Neurosurgery, University of Pittsburgh School of Medicine, Pittsburgh, Pennsylvania
Implantation of Radionuclides in Brain Tumors

Alfredo Kreutel, M.D.
Department of Neurosurgery, Hospital Santa Lucia, Buenos Aires, Argentina
Transcranial Approach to Lesions of the Orbit

George Krol, M.D.
Department of Radiology, Memorial Sloan-Kettering Cancer Center and Cornell University Medical Center, New York, New York
Craniofacial Resection for Anterior Skull Base Tumors

Rakesh Kumar, M.D., F.R.C.S.(E.)
Department of Neurosurgery, University of Cincinnati College of Medicine; University of Cincinnati Hospital, Cincinnati, Ohio
Surgical Management of Thoracic Disc Herniations

Ron C. Kupers, Ph.D.
Department of Brain and Behaviour Research, Gasthuisberg (O & N), KUL University, Leuven, Belgium
Brain Stimulation in the Management of Persistent Pain

Alex M. Landolt, M.D.
Department of Neurosurgery, University of Zürich; Park Clinic, Zürich, Switzerland
Surgical Management of Recurrent Pituitary Tumors

Jeremy A. Lauer, M.A., M.S.
The Johns Hopkins University School of Medicine, Baltimore, Maryland
Management of Achondroplasia and Its Neurosurgical Complications

Edward R. Laws, Jr., M.D.
Departments of Neurosurgery and Medicine, University of Virginia; University of Virginia Hospital, Charlottesville, Virginia; George Washington University Hospital, Washington, D.C.
Transsphenoidal Approach to Pituitary Tumors

David W. Leitner, M.D.
Department of Surgery, University of Vermont College of Medicine; Medical Center Hospital of Vermont, Burlington, Vermont; Fanny Allen Hospital, Colchester, Vermont
Surgical Considerations in the Fashioning of Scalp Flaps; Surgical Correction of Facial Nerve Palsy

Alberto Lenzi, M.D.
Department of Neurosurgery, University of Brescia; Regional Hospital of Brescia, Brescia, Italy
Intraventricular Morphine in the Treatment of Pain Secondary to Cancer

Adam I. Lewis, M.D.
Department of Neurosurgery, University of Cincinnati Medical Center, Cincinnati, Ohio
Surgical Management of Brainstem Vascular Malformations; Surgical Management of Thalamic–Basal Ganglia Vascular Malformations

Bengt Linderoth, M.D., Ph.D.
Department of Neurological Surgery, Karolinska Institute, Stockholm, Sweden
Retrogasserian Glycerol Rhizolysis in Trigeminal Neuralgia

C. Lindquist, M.D., Ph.D.
Department of Neurological Surgery, Karolinska Institute; Karolinska Hospital, Stockholm, Sweden
Gamma Knife Surgery in Vascular, Neoplastic, and Functional Disorders of the Nervous System

Peter C. Linton, M.D.
Department of Surgery, University of Vermont College of Medicine; Medical Center Hospital of Vermont, Burlington, Vermont
Surgical Considerations in the Fashioning of Scalp Flaps

Ali Liu, M.D.
Beijing Neurosurgical Institute, Beijing, China
Surgical Management of Nonglomus Tumors of the Jugular Foramen

Don M. Long, M.D., Ph.D.
Department of Neurosurgery, The Johns Hopkins University School of Medicine; The Johns Hopkins Hospital, Baltimore, Maryland
Management of Persistent Symptoms Following Lumbar Disc Surgery

G. Lo Russo, M.D.
Department of Neurosurgery, Epilepsy Surgery Regional Center, Niguarda Hospital, Milan, Italy
Multilobar Resections for the Control of Epilepsy

R. Loch Macdonald, M.D.
Section of Neurosurgery, University of Chicago Medical Center, Chicago, Illinois
Perioperative Care Following Aneurysmal Subarachnoid Hemorrhage

Giovanni Marini, M.D.
Department of Neurosurgery, University of Brescia; Regional General Hospital, Brescia, Italy
Intraventricular Morphine in the Treatment of Pain Secondary to Cancer

Joseph C. Maroon, M.D.
Department of Neurosurgery, Allegheny General Hospital; Medical College of Pennsylvania, Pittsburgh, Pittsburgh, Pennsylvania
Surgical Approach to Lesions of the Orbit

Robert L. Masson, M.D.
Department of Neurosurgery, University of Florida College of Medicine; Shands Hospital at the University of Florida; Veterans Administration Medical Center, Gainesville, Florida
Surgical Management of Aneurysms and Fistulas Involving the Cavernous Sinus

Duncan Q. McBride, M.D.
Division of Neurosurgery, School of Medicine, University of California at Los Angeles, Los Angeles, California; Harbor–U.C.L.A. Medical Center, Torrance, California
Surgical Management of Severe Closed Head Injury in Adults; Surgical Management of Traumatic Posterior Fossa Hematomas

Bruce McCormack, M.D.
Department of Neurosurgery, University of California San Francisco, School of Medicine; Moffit–Long Hospital; Mount Zion Hospital and Medical Center; Veterans Administration Medical Center, San Francisco, California
Surgical Management of Tuberculum Sellae and Sphenoid Ridge Meningiomas

Thomas M. McCormack, M.D.
Department of Neurosurgery, Hahnemann University; Hahnemann University Hospital; North Philadelphia Health System; Roxborough Memorial Hospital; St. Agnes Medical Center, Philadelphia, Pennsylvania
Surgical Management of Brain Metastasis

Arnold H. Menezes, M.D., F.A.C.S.
Department of Neurosurgery, University of Iowa College of Medicine; University of Iowa Hospital and Clinics, Iowa City, Iowa
Craniovertebral Abnormalities and Their Neurosurgical Management

P. Mertens, M.D., M.S.
Department of Neurosurgery, University of Lyon; Pierre Wertheimer Neurological Hospital, Lyon, France
Neurosurgical Management of Spasticity

Frederic B. Meyer, M.D.
Department of Neurosurgery, Mayo Clinic, Mayo Medical School, Rochester, Minnesota
Surgical Management of Dural Arteriovenous Malformations

Björn A. Meyerson, M.D., Ph.D.
Department of Neurosurgery, Karolinska Institute; Karolinska Hospital, Stockholm, Sweden
Anterior Capsulotomy for Intractable Anxiety Disorders

J. Parker Mickle, M.D.
Department of Neurosurgery, University of Florida College of Medicine; Shands Hospital at the University of Florida, Gainesville, Florida
The Multidisciplinary Management of Vein of Galen Malformations

J. Douglas Miller, M.D., Ph.D., F.R.C.S.(Edin), F.R.S.(E)
Department of Clinical Neurosciences, University of Edinburgh; Western General Hospital, Edinburgh, Scotland
Surgical Management of Traumatic Intracranial Hematomas

H. Millesi, M.D.
Department of Plastic and Reconstructive Surgery, University of Vienna Medical School, Vienna, Austria
Surgical Management of Lesions of the Peripheral Nerves and Brachial Plexus

Per Mindus, M.D., Ph.D.
Department of Psychiatry, Karolinska Hospital, Stockholm, Sweden; University of Trondheim, Trondheim, Norway
Anterior Capsulotomy for Intractable Anxiety Disorders

Michael E. Miner, M.D., Ph.D.
The Ohio State University Hospitals, Columbus, Ohio
Neurosurgical Considerations in the Management of Ankylosing Spondylitis

Stuart Mirvis, M.D.
Department of Radiology, The University of Maryland School of Medicine; The University of Maryland Hospital, Baltimore, Maryland
Surgical Management of Injuries of the Cervical Spine and Spinal Cord

Kazuo Mizoi, M.D.
Department of Neurosurgery, Tohoku University School of Medicine, Sendai, Japan
Intraoperative Endovascular Techniques in the Management of Intracranial Aneurysms

Sean Mullan, M.D., D.Sc., F.R.C.S.
Division of Neurosurgery, The University of Chicago Medical Center, Chicago, Illinois
Percutaneous Trigeminal Nerve Compression

C. Munari, M.D.
Department of Neurosurgery, University of Genoa, Genoa, Italy; Hospital of Grenoble, Grenoble, France
Multilobar Resections for the Control of Epilepsy

F. Mundinger, Ph.D., M.D.
Albert Ludwig University; St. Joseph's Hospital, Freiburg, Germany
Sterotactic Biopsy and Implantation of Radionuclides Guided by Computed Tomography or Magnetic Resonance Imaging for Therapy of Brain Tumors

Cheryl A. Muszynski, M.D.
Department of Neurosurgery, Baylor College of Medicine, Ben Taub General Hospital, Houston, Texas
Surgical Management of Penetrating Injuries of the Spine

Raj K. Narayan, M.D.
Department of Neurosurgery, Baylor College of Medicine; Ben Taub General Hospital; The Methodist Hospital; Houston, Texas
Surgical Management of Penetrating Injuries of the Spine

Blaine S. Nashold, M.D.
Department of Neurosurgery, Duke University Medical Center, Durham, North Carolina
Microsurgical DREZotomy in Treatment of Deafferentation Pain

James R. B. Nashold, M.D.
Department of Neurosurgery, Duke University Medical Center, Durham, North Carolina
Microsurgical DREZotomy in Treatment of Deafferentation Pain

Douglas A. Nichols, M.D.
Department of Diagnostic Radiology, Mayo Clinic, Mayo Medical School, Rochester, Minnesota
Surgical Management of Dural Arteriovenous Malformation

Horace Norrell, M.D.
Department of Neurosurgery, Sarasota Memorial Hospital, Sarasota, Florida
Vestibular Nerve Section in the Management of Vertigo

Richard B. North, M.D.
Department of Neurosurgery, The Johns Hopkins Hospital, Baltimore, Maryland
Spinal Cord Stimulation for Chronic Intractable Pain

A. F. O'Connor, M.D.
St. Thomas Hospital, London, England
Translabyrinthine Approach to Acoustic Neuromas

Christopher S. Ogilvy, M.D.
Department of Neurosurgery, Massachusetts General Hospital; Harvard Medical School, Boston, Massachusetts
Direct Brain Revascularization; Surgical Management of Vascular Lesions and Tumors Associated with

Pregnancy; Surgical Management of Cavernous Angiomas of the Nervous System; Radiosurgery of Cranial Arteriovenous Malformations

George A. Ojemann, M.D.
Department of Neurological Surgery and The Epilepsy Center, University of Washington School of Medicine, Seattle, Washington
Awake Operations with Mapping in Epilepsy

Robert G. Ojemann, M.D.
Department of Neurosurgery, Massachusetts General Hospital; Harvard Medical School, Boston, Massachusetts
Surgical Management of Anterior Basal Meningiomas: Olfactory Groove; Suboccipital Transmeatal Approach to Vestibular Schwannomas; Surgical Management of Cavernous Angiomas of the Nervous System

Andre Olivier, M.D., Ph.D.
Division of Neurosurgery, McGill University; Montreal Neurological Hospital and Institute, Montreal, Quebec, Canada
Diagnostic Operative Techniques in the Treatment of Epilepsy: Depth Electrodes

Dwight Parkinson, M.D., F.R.C.S.(C), F.A.C.S.
Department of Neurosurgery, The University of Manitoba Faculty of Medicine; Health Sciences Centre; General Hospital; Children's Hospital, Winnipeg, Manitoba, Canada
Anatomy of the Lateral Sellar Compartment (Cavernous Sinus); Surgical Management of Traumatic Intracranial Aneurysms

Francesco S. Pastore, M.D.
Institute of Neurosurgery, Tor Vergata University Medical School of Rome, Rome, Italy
Surgical Management of Low-Grade Gliomas of the Cerebral Hemispheres

Rana Patir, M.S., M.Ch.
Department of Neurosurgery, All India Institute of Medical Sciences, New Delhi, India
Surgical Management of Tuberculous and Fungal Infections of the Nervous System

Russel H. Patterson, Jr., M.D.
Department of Neurosurgery, Cornell University Medical College; The New York Hospital, New York, New York
Surgical Management of Arteriovenous Malformations of the Brain

Sidney J. Peerless, M.D.
Department of Neurosurgery, University of Miami School of Medicine; Jackson Memorial Hospital; Neuroscience Institute, Mercy Hospital, Miami, Florida
Surgical Management of Terminal Basilar and Posterior Cerebral Artery Aneurysms

Keith R. Peters, M.D.
Department of Radiology, University of Florida College of Medicine, Gainesville, Florida
The Multidisciplinary Management of Vein of Galen Malformations

Joseph Petronio, M.D.
Departments of Neurosurgery and Pediatrics, Emory University School of Medicine, Atlanta, Georgia
Surgical Management of Cerebellar Tumors in Children

David G. Piepgras, M.D.
Department of Neurologic Surgery, Mayo Medical School; Mayo Clinic, Rochester, Minnesota
Surgical Management of Primary Intracerebral Hemorrhage; Surgical Management of Dural Arteriovenous Malformations

Joseph M. Piepmeier, M.D.
Section of Neurosurgery, Yale University School of Medicine; Yale–New Haven Hospital, New Haven, Connecticut
Surgical Management of Intraventricular Tumors of the Lateral Ventricles

Charles E. Poletti, M.D.
Hartford Hospital, Hartford, Connecticut
Complication of Percutaneous Rhizotomy and Microvascular Decompression Operations for Facial Pain; Open Cordotomy and Medullary Tractotomy

C. E. Polkey, M.D., F.R.C.S.
Department of Neurosurgery, Maudsley Hospital, London, England
Amygdalo-Hippocampectomy for Drug-Resistant Temporal Lobe Epilepsy

Kalmon D. Post, M.D.
Department of Neurosurgery, Mt. Sinai School of Medicine, New York, New York
Surgical Management of Spinal Cord Tumors and Arteriovenous Malformations

D. Prasad, M.D.
Department of Neurosurgery, University of Virginia Health Sciences Center, Charlottesville, Virginia
Gamma Knife Surgery in Vascular, Neoplastic, and Functional Disorders of the Nervous System

Ronald G. Quisling, M.D.
Department of Radiology, University of Florida College of Medicine, Gainesville, Florida
The Multidisciplinary Management of Vein of Galen Malformations

Craig H. Rabb, M.D.
Department of Neurosurgery, University of Southern California School of Medicine, Los Angeles, California
Transcallosal Approach to the Third Ventricle

Robert A. Ratcheson, M.D.
Department of Neurological Surgery, University Hospitals of Cleveland; Veterans Administration Medical Center; MetroHealth Medical Center, Cleveland, Ohio
Surgical Therapy for Diseases of the Extracranial Carotid Artery

Kenneth W. Reichert II, M.D.
Department of Neurosurgery, Medical College of Wisconsin; Froedtert Memorial Lutheran Hospital; Veterans Affairs Medical Center; John Doyne Hospital; Children's Hospital of Wisconsin, Milwaukee, Wisconsin
Surgical Management of Thalamic–Basal Ganglia Vascular Malformations

Albert L. Rhoton, Jr., M.D.
Department of Neurological Surgery, University of Florida College of Medicine; Shands Hospital at the University of Florida, Gainesville, Florida
Microsurgery of Syringomyelia and Syringomyelic Cord Syndrome

Daniele Rigamonti, M.D.
Department of Neurosurgery, The Johns Hopkins School of Medicine; The Johns Hopkins Center for the Treatment of Cerebrovascular Diseases and Stroke; The Johns Hopkins Hospital, Baltimore, Maryland
Surgical Management of Injuries of the Cervical Spine and Spinal Cord

David W. Roberts, M.D.
Department of Neurosurgery, Dartmouth Medical School, Hanover, New Hampshire; Dartmouth–Hitchcock Medical Center, Lebanon, New Hampshire
Section of the Corpus Callosum for Epilepsy

Melville P. Roberts, M.D.
Department of Neurosurgery, University of Connecticut School of Medicine; University of Connecticut Health Center, Farmington, Connecticut; Hartford Hospital, Hartford, Connecticut
Posterior Surgical Approaches for Cervical Disc Herniation and Spondylotic Myelopathy

Jon H. Robertson, M.D.
Department of Neurological Surgery, The University of Tennessee Center for the Health Sciences; Baptist Memorial Hospital; The University of Tennessee Hospital, Memphis, Tennessee
Transtemporal Approaches to the Posterior Cranial Fossa; Surgical Management of Glomus Jugulare Tumors

Franklin Robinson, M.D.
Department of Neurosurgery, Yale University School of Medicine; Yale–New Haven Hospital; Hospital of St. Raphael, New Haven, Connecticut
Dorsal Root Ganglionectomy for Intractable Monoradicular Sciatica

Maurice I. Saba, M.D.
Division of Neurosurgery, School of Medicine, American University of Beirut; American University of Beirut Medical Center, Beirut, Lebanon
Surgical Management of Missile Injuries of the Head

Ved Sachdev, M.D.
Department of Surgery, Mount Sinai Medical Center and Mount Sinai Medical School, New York, New York
Craniofacial Resection for Anterior Skull Base Tumors

Anthony Salerni, M.D.
Concord, New Hampshire
Brain Biopsy in Nonneoplastic Neurologic Disorders

Amir Samii, M.D., Ph.D.
Medical School Hannover; Neurosurgical Clinic, Norstadt Hospital, Hannover, Germany
Surgical Management of Craniopharyngiomas

Majdid Samii, M.D., Ph.D.
Medical School Hannover; Director of the Neurosurgical Clinic, Norstadt Hospital, Hannover, Germany
Surgical Management of Craniopharyngiomas

Duke S. Samson, M.D.
Department of Neurological Surgery, The University of Texas Southwestern Medical Center; Zale Lipshy University Hospital; Parkland Memorial Hospital; Veterans Administration Hospital–Dallas; St. Paul Medical Center, Dallas, Texas
Surgical Management of Intraoperative Aneurysmal Rupture

Robert A. Sanford, M.D.
Department of Neurosurgery, University of Tennessee–Memphis; St. Jude Children's Research Hospital; LeBonheur Children's Hospital; Semmes–Murphey Clinic, Memphis, Tennessee
Surgical Management of Supratentorial Tumors of Childhood

Keiji Sano, M.D., D.M.Sc.
Department of Neurosurgery, Teikyo University School of Medicine; Teikyo University Hospital; Fuji Brain Institute and Hospital, Tokyo, Japan
Alternate Surgical Approaches to Pineal Region Neoplasms

Kimberlee Sass, Ph.D.
Department of Neurosurgery, Yale University School of Medicine; Yale–New Haven Hospital, New Haven, Connecticut
Surgical Management of Intraventricular Tumors of the Lateral Ventricles

Henry H. Schmidek, M.D.
Marion, Massachusetts
Surgical Management of Supratentorial Gliomas; Surgical Management of Intracranial Arachnoid, Suprasellar, and Rathke's Cleft Cysts; Brain Biopsy in Nonneoplastic Neurologic Disorders; The Management of Pineal Region Neoplasms; Surgical Management of Cerebellar Tumors in Adults; Surgical Management of Aneurysms of the Internal Carotid Artery; Anterior Cervical Disc Excision in Cervical Spondylosis

Luis Schut, M.D.
Department of Neurosurgery and Pediatrics, University of Pennsylvania School of Medicine; Neurosurgical Services, Children's Hospital of Philadelphia, Philadelphia, Pennsylvania
Surgical Management of Encephaloceles

U. Schwab, M.D., D.D.S.
Department of Otorhinolaryngology, University of Würzburg, Würzburg, Germany
Surgical Management of Trauma Involving the Skull Base and Paranasal Sinuses

R. Michael Scott, M.D.
Department of Surgery, Harvard Medical School; Department of Pediatric Neurosurgery, The Children's Hospital, Harvard Medical School, Boston, Massachusetts
Management of Neurosurgical Problems in the Neonate

Volker Seifert, M.D., Ph.D.
Neurosurgical Clinic, University of Essen, Essen, Germany
Anterior Surgical Approaches in Multisegmental Cervical Spondylosis

Robin P. Sengupta, M.Sc., F.R.C.S.(Eng.), F.R.C.S. (Edin.)
Department of Neurosurgery, University of Newcastle upon Tyne; Regional Neurosciences Centre, Newcastle General Hospital, Newcastle upon Tyne, England
Surgical Management of Anterior Cerebral and Anterior Communicating Artery Aneurysms

Masato Shibuya, M.D.
Department of Neurosurgery, Nagoya University, Nagoya, Japan
Surgery of Paraclinoid Aneurysms

John W. Shore, M.D.
Department of Ophthalmology, Harvard Medical School; Eye Plastics and Orbit Service, Massachusetts Eye and Ear Infirmary, Boston, Massachusetts
Optic Nerve Sheath Fenestration in the Management of Pseudotumor Cerebri

William A. Shucart, M.D.
Department of Neurosurgery, Tufts University School of Medicine; New England Medical Center, Boston, Massachusetts
Surgical Management of Anterior Cerebral Artery Aneurysms Distal to the Anterior Communicating Artery

Tali Siegal, M.D.
Department of Neurology, Hebrew University Medical School; Neuro-Oncology Clinic, Hadassah University Hospital, Jerusalem, Israel
Surgical Management of Malignant Epidural Tumors Compressing the Spinal Cord

Tzony Siegal, M.D., D.M.D.
Spinal Surgery Unit, Chosen Specialties Clinics, Tel Aliv; Meuhedet and Leumit Sick Funds; Assuta Hospital, Tel Aviv, Israel
Surgical Management of Malignant Epidural Tumors Compressing the Spinal Cord

Herbert Silverstein, M.D.
Department of Surgery, University of South Florida College of Medicine, Tampa, Florida; Sarasota Memorial Hospital, Sarasota, Florida; Department of Otolaryngology, University of Pennsylvania School of Medicine, Philadelphia, Pennsylvania
Vestibular Nerve Section in the Management of Vertigo

Marie F. Simard, M.D.
Department of Endocrinology, University of Southern California School of Medicine; LAC/USC Medical Center, Los Angeles, California
Surgical Management of Growth Hormone–Secreting and Prolactin-Secreting Pituitary Adenomas

Marc P. Sindou, M.D., D.Sc.
Department of Neurosurgery, University of Lyon; Pierre Wertheimer Neurological Hospital, Lyon, France
Microsurgical DREZotomy; Neurosurgical Management of Spasticity

Donald A. Smith, M.D.
Department of Neurosurgery, University of Florida, Tampa, Florida
Anterior Cervical Disc Excision in Cervical Spondylosis

Robert R. Smith, M.D.
Mississippi Medical Center; Neuroscience Center, Methodist Hospital, Jackson, Mississippi
Surgical Management of Complex and Giant Anterior Circulation Aneurysms

Volker K. H. Sonntag, M.D., F.A.C.S.
Division of Neurosurgery, University of Arizona College of Medicine, Tucson, Arizona; Barrow Neurological Institute, Phoenix, Arizona
Surgical Techniques for the Stabilization of the Cervical Spine

Sandeep Sood, M.B., M.Ch.
Department of Neurosurgery, Sir Ganga Ram Hospital, New Delhi, India
Surgical Management of Hydrocephalus in Children

Renato Spaziante, M.D.
Department of Systematic Pathology, Federico II University School of Medicine, Naples, Italy
Repair of the Sella Following Transsphenoidal Surgery

Dennis D. Spencer, M.D.
Section of Neurosurgery, Yale University School of Medicine; Yale–New Haven Hospital, New Haven, Connecticut
Surgical Management of Intraventricular Tumors of the Lateral Ventricles; Temporal Lobe Operations for Epilepsy: Radical Hippocampectomy

Robert F. Spetzler, M.D., F.A.C.S.
Division of Neurosurgery, University of Arizona College of Medicine, Tucson, Arizona; St. Joseph's Hospital; Barrow Neurological Institute, Phoenix, Arizona
Surgical Management of Midbasilar and Lower Basilar Aneurysms

Patrick F. X. Statham, M.B., F.R.C.S.(Eng), F.R.C.S. (SN)
Department of Clinical Neurosciences, University of Edinburgh; Western General Hospital, Edinburgh, Scotland
Surgical Management of Traumatic Intracranial Hematomas

Bennett M. Stein, M.D.
Department of Neurosurgery, Columbia University College of Physicians and Surgeons; Columbia–Presbyterian Medical Center, New York, New York
Supracerebellar Approach for Pineal Region Neoplasms; Surgical Management of Spinal Cord Tumors and Arteriovenous Malformations

L. Steiner, M.D., Ph.D.
Lars Leksell Center for Gamma Knife Surgery and Department of Neurosurgery, University of Virginia School of Medicine, Charlottesville, Virginia
Gamma Knife Surgery in Vascular, Neoplastic, and Functional Disorders of the Nervous System

M. Steiner, M.D.
Department of Neurosurgery, University of Virginia School of Medicine, Charlottesville, Virginia
Gamma Knife Surgery in Vascular, Neoplastic, and Functional Disorders of the Nervous System

Kenichiro Sugita, M.D.
Department of Neurosurgery, Nagoya University, Nagoya, Japan
Surgery of Paraclinoid Aneurysms

Narayan Sundaresan, M.D.
Department of Neurosurgery, Mt. Sinai Hospital, New York, New York
Craniofacial Resection for Anterior Skull Base Tumors; Surgical Management of Primary and Metastatic Tumors of the Spine

Thoralf M. Sundt, Jr. (Deceased)
Department of Neurosurgery, The Mayo Clinic, Rochester, Minnesota
Surgical Management of Dural Arteriovenous Malformations

Charas Suwanwela, M.D.
Department of Neurosurgery, Chulalongkorn University; Chulalongkorn Hospital, Bangkok, Thailand
Surgical Management of Frontoethmoidal Encephalomeningoceles

Nitaya Suwanwela, M.D.
Department of Radiology, Faculty of Medicine, Chulalongkorn University; Chulalongkorn Hospital, Bangkok, Thailand
Surgical Management of Frontoethmoidal Encephalomeningoceles

Brooke Swearingen, M.D.
Department of Neurosurgery, Massachusetts General Hospital; Harvard Medical School, Boston, Massachusetts
Surgical Management of Cushing's Disease; Surgical Management of Falx and Parasagittal Tumors

William H. Sweet, M.D., D.Sc.
Department of Neurosurgery, Massachusetts General Hospital; Harvard Medical School, Boston, Massachusetts
Optic Gliomas: Their Diagnosis, Capacity for Spontaneous Regression, and Radical Surgical Treatment; Craniopharyngiomas: A Summary of Recent Data; Surgical Management of Intracranial Arachnoid, Suprasellar, and Rathke's Cleft Cysts; Complications of Percutaneous Rhizotomy and Microvascular Decompression Operations for Facial Pain; Cervicothoracic Ankylosing Spondylitis

Lindsay Symon, T.D., F.R.C.S., F.R.C.S.(Edin)
Gough-Cooper Department of Neurological Surgery, Institute of Neurology, University of London; Department of Neurosurgery, The National Hospital; St. Thomas' Hospital; The Royal National Nose, Throat and Ear Hospital, London, England
Surgical Management of Middle Cerebral Artery Aneurysms

Jamal M. Taha, M.D.
Department of Neurosurgery, University of Cincinnati College of Medicine, Cincinnati, Ohio
Percutaneous Rhizotomy in the Treatment of Intractable Facial Pain (Trigeminal, Glossopharyngeal, and Vagal Nerves)

Akira Takahashi, M.D.
Department of Neurosurgery, Division of Intravascular Neurosurgery, Kohnan Hospital, Sendai, Japan
Intraoperative Endovascular Techniques in the Management of Intracranial Aneurysms

Prakash Narain Tandon, M.S., F.R.C.S(Engl)
Department of Neurosurgery, All India Institute of Medical Sciences, New Delhi, India
Surgical Management of Tuberculous and Fungal Infections of the Nervous System

Edward C. Tarlov, M.D.
Department of Neurosurgery, Lahey Clinic, Burlington, Massachusetts
Surgical Management of Tumors of the Tentorium and Clivus; Surgical Management of Primary Lumbar Disc Herniaton—Commentary; Surgery of Ruptured Lumbar Intervertebral Disc

R. R. Tasker, M.D., F.R.C.S.(C)
Department of Surgery, University of Toronto Faculty of Medicine; The Toronto Hospital, Western Division, Toronto, Ontario, Canada
Percutaneous Cordotomy

L. Tassi, M.D.
Department of Neurology, Epilepsy Surgery Regional Center, Niguarda Hospital, Milan, Italy
Multilobar Resections for the Control of Epilepsy

Stephen B. Tatter, M.D., Ph.D.
Department of Surgery, Harvard Medical School; Department of Neurosurgery, Massachusetts General Hospital, Boston, Massachusetts
Surgical Management of Vascular Lesions and Tumors Associated with Pregnancy

Arthur Taub, M.D., Ph.D.
Departments of Anesthesiology and Neurology, Yale University School of Medicine; Department of Neurology, Yale–New Haven Hospital; Hospital of St. Raphael, New Haven, Connecticut
Dorsal Root Ganglionectomy for Intractable Monoradicular Sciatica

Ethan Taub, M.D.
Division of Neurosurgery, Department of Surgery, Cornell University Medical College; The New York Hospital, New York, New York
Dorsal Root Ganglionectomy for Intractable Monoradicular Sciatica

Juan M. Taveras, M.D.
Department of Radiology, Massachusetts General Hospital; Harvard Medical School, Boston, Massachusetts
Optic Gliomas: Their Diagnosis, Capacity for Spontaneous Regression, and Radical Surgical Treatment

John M. Tew, Jr., M.D.
Department of Neurosurgery, University of Cincinnati College of Medicine; The Christ Hospital; Good Samaritan Hospital; Children's Hospital Medical Center; Veterans Administration Medical Center; University of Cincinnati Hospital, Cincinnati, Ohio
Percutaneous Rhizotomy in the Treatment of Intractable Facial Pain (Trigeminal, Glossopharyngeal, and Vagal Nerves); Surgical Management of Brainstem Vascular Malformations; Surgical Management of Thalamic–Basal Ganglia Vascular Malformations

D. G. T. Thomas, F.R.C.P.(Glas), F.R.C.S.(Edin)
Department of Neurosurgery, The National Hospital for Neurology and Neurosurgery; Northwick Park Hospital, London, England
Stereotactic Biopsy and Resection of Intracranial Lesions

Suzie C. Tindall, M.D.
Department of Neurosurgery, Emory University School of Medicine, Atlanta, Georgia
Surgical Management of Thoracic Outlet Syndrome and of Peripheral Entrapment Neuropathies

Joseph Ting, Ph.D.
Department of Radiation Oncology, University of Miami School of Medicine; Baptist Hospital of Miami, Miami, Florida
Implantation of Radionuclides in Brain Tumors

Nobuyuki Tsuzuki, M.D., D.M.Sc.
Department of Orthopedics, Saitama Medical Center/School, Kawagoe, Saitama, Japan
Surgical Management of Ossification of the Posterior Longitudinal Ligament

John C. Van Gilder, M.D.
Department of Neurosurgery, University of Iowa School of Medicine; University of Iowa Hospitals and Clinics, Iowa City, Iowa
Craniovertebral Abnormalities and Their Neurosurgical Management

Jean-Guy Villemure, M.D., F.R.C.S.(C)
Department of Neurology and Neurosurgery, McGill University Faculty of Medicine; Montreal Neurological Hospital, Montreal, Quebec, Canada
Cerebral Hemispherectomy for Epilepsy

Marion L. Walker, M.D.
Departments of Neurosurgery and Pediatrics, University of Utah College of Medicine; Division of Pediatric Neurosurgery, Primary Children's Medical Center, Salt Lake City, Utah
Surgical Management of Cerebellar Tumors in Children

Chung-cheng Wang, M.D.
Capital Medical College; Beijing Neurosurgical Institute, Beijing, China
Surgical Management of Nonglomus Tumors of the Jugular Foramen

Mark A. Weiner, M.D.
Department of Neurologic Surgery, Mayo Clinic, Rochester, Minnesota
Surgical Management of Primary Intracerebral Hemorrhage

Philip R. Weinstein, M.D.
Department of Neurological Surgery, University of California, San Francisco, School of Medicine; University of California Hospitals, San Francisco, California
Surgical Management of Lumbar Spinal Stenosis

Bryce Weir, M.D., C.M., F.R.C.S.(C.)
Department of Neurosurgery, University of Chicago Medical Center, Chicago, Illinois
Perioperative Care Following Aneurysmal Subarachnoid Hemorrhage

Martin H. Weiss, M.D.
Department of Neurological Surgery, University of Southern California School of Medicine; LAC/USC Medical Center; USC University Hospital, Los Angeles, California
Surgical Management of Growth Hormone–Secreting and Prolactin-Secreting Pituitary Adenomas

Michael Westerveld, Ph.D.
Department of Neurosurgery, Yale University School of Medicine; Yale–New Haven Hospital, New Haven, Connecticut
Surgical Management of Intraventricular Tumors of the Lateral Ventricles

Richard M. Westmark, M.D.
Department of Neurological Surgery, University of California, San Francisco, School of Medicine, San Francisco, California
Surgical Management of Lumbar Spinal Stenosis

Robert H. Wilkins, M.D.
Division of Neurosurgery, Duke University Medical Center, Durham, North Carolina
Neurovascular Decompression Procedures in the Surgical Management of Disorders of Nerves V, VII, IX, and X

Harold A. Wilkinson, M.D., Ph.D.
Division of Neurosurgery, University of Massachusetts Medical School; University of Massachusetts Hospital; St. Vincent Hospital and Medical Center of Central Massachusetts, Worcester, Massachusetts
Surgery for Hyperhidrosis and Sympathetically Mediated Pain Syndromes

Bernard Williams, M.D.
Consultant Neurosurgery, Syringomyelia Clinic, The Midland Centre for Neurosurgery and Neurology, Warley, United Kingdom
Surgical Management of Non–Hindbrain-Related and Posttraumatic Syringomyelia

Aizik L. Wolf, M.D.
The Miami Neuroscience Center, Health South Doctors' Hospital, Miami, Florida
Surgical Management of Injuries of the Cervical Spine and Spinal Cord

R. Lewis Wright, M.D.
Department of Neurosurgery, Stuart Circle Hospital; St. Mary's Hospital, Richmond, Virginia
Surgical Management of Intracranial and Intraspinal Infections

Allen R. Wyler, M.D.
Epilepsy Center, Swedish Medical Center, Seattle, Washington
Diagnostic Operative Techniques in the Treatment of Epilepsy: Grids and Strip Electrodes

Michael J. Yaremchuk, M.D.
Department of Surgery, Massachusetts General Hospital; Harvard Medical School, Boston, Massachusetts
Surgical Repair of Major Defects of the Scalp and Skull

Takashi Yoshimoto, M.D.
Department of Neurosurgery, Tohoku University School of Medicine, Sendai, Japan
Intraoperative Endovascular Techniques in the Management of Intracranial Aneurysms

Ronald F. Young
Northwest Hospital, Gamma Knife Center, Seattle, Washington; Department of Neurological Surgery, University of California, Irvine Medical Center, College of Medicine, Orange, California
Commentary

Nicholas T. Zervas, M.D.
Department of Neurosurgery, Massachusetts General Hospital; Harvard Medical School, Boston, Massachusetts
Surgical Management of Cushing's Disease

Yuri N. Zubkov, M.D.
A. L. Polenov Research Institute, St. Petersburg, Russia
Surgical Management of Complex and Giant Anterior Circulation Aneurysms

Preface

Related works prior to this third edition in two volumes have involved the same editors, Henry Schmidek and William Sweet. These works were preceded in 1977 by a single volume entitled *Current Techniques in Operative Neurosurgery,* a 517-page, 33-chapter work dealing only with selected topics that seemed to us especially worthy. The reception accorded this publication led us to enlist the neurosurgical community's talents to produce by 1982 a much more comprehensive work, as indicated not only by its title *Operative Neurosurgical Techniques: Indications, Methods and Results* but as well by its 1550 pages of text, divided into 94 chapters with 116 authors.

Early in 1981, when nearly all of the chapters were written, two major improvements in the lives of neurosurgeons had evolved in the previous decade in terms of what we can fruitfully do for our patients. The first of these improvements was computerized tomography (CT), which was brought into clinical utility by Hounsfield, for which he became a Nobel Laureate. It was improved in successive technical leaps by industrial engineers so that the models of the third-stage devices could reveal in conjunction with myelography hitherto inscrutable details of disease, even in the spinal canal. This is but one example of the entirely new world of primary diagnosis of disease states and of the complications and successes attendant on their treatment. The virtually complete elimination of risk by CT because of the minimal dose of radiation has meant that we could document follow-up of our patients ad libitum. At the same time, the value of the double-binocular operating microscope for surgeon and assistant was becoming steadily more evident, and the ease of swinging the scope into action at the operating table was facilitated by design improvements. The net result of these two major aids to our efforts was to make a thorough rewrite of our entire neurosurgical texts a mandatory task. Although the latter half of the title of the book, *Indications, Methods and Results,* is printed in lower case type, the sections on INDICATIONS AND RESULTS (especially COMPLICATIONS), in our view, have assumed a steadily more important role in the field.

By the mid-1980s, the fruits of intensive application of the new tools were apparent as neurosurgeons all over the world eagerly moved into the ranks of medical writers and speakers to report the good news. Neurosurgical meetings all over the world attracted steadily larger numbers. The standard neurosurgical journals grew rapidly in size, and several new ones appeared. Two deficiencies became apparent: (1) Complications were likely to elicit but little attention from speakers and writers. Gone were the Cushing-like blow by blow accounts of "harrowing episodes" at the operating table. (2) Long-term critical detailed follow-ups were infrequent. The need for comprehensive analytical reviews emphasizing not only the good but also the bad results with tactics for decreasing these results and follow-ups of a decade and more seemed clear. This led to our specific citation of these objectives in our invitations to neurosurgeons to contribute chapters to what became the second two-volume edition in 1988.

For the 1982 edition, we used a double-column format for the index and a single-column format for text and citation of references, and the book was printed on slightly smaller pages than the 1988 two-volume second edition. By using double columns on each page for text and citation of references and triple columns for the index, we were astonished to find that we had 39 percent more space for information in a book that looked only a trifle larger and was only slightly more expensive to produce. Despite inflation, we were providing more facts per dollar.

Another factor that has given concern to all of us who edit these multi-volume compendia such as Youmans, Wilkins and Rengachary, and Apuzzo, has been the uneven merit of the contributions. Unfortunately, those who have the best and most comprehensive experience in any given area and have published excellent accounts documenting this fact are likely to have little time left for review articles. By subdividing each general domain into several subsections and urging the senior author to have one or more of the juniors work with him or her on the project, we have been able to minimize the number of declinations to participate in this work. Happily, this leads to overlap in the coverage, with useful presentation of differing points of view.

It has been progressively more obvious that the torch of innovation and superior performance in neurosurgery is being carried by enormous numbers of individuals from many parts of the world. Among other factors diminishing the number of torch-wielding leaders in the United States is the frightful black cloud of malpractice litigation. By far, the most important feature of patient management determining whether or not a lawsuit will ensue is the severity of disablement of the patient, regardless of the absence of any intimation whatsoever of negligence. Hence, it is to be expected that we are looking increasingly to neurosurgeons outside of the United States for advances. We recognized this fact but responded inadequately in our second edition, increasing the number of chapters written by authors outside of the United States from 12 of 94 (13 percent) in 1982, to 27 of 136 (20 percent) in 1988, and up to 52 of 175 (31 percent) of 175 chapters in the forthcoming edition. The total pagination in each of the three editions is 1604, 1635, and circa 2400 for the current volumes, respectively.

By early 1987, when the text of the second edition was in press, the most spectacular innovation of the century in medical diagnosis, nuclear magnetic resonance imaging (MRI), was in use with modestly effective units in only a few centers. The theoretical advantages of MRI over CT scanning are colossal. A fundamental feature of MRI behavior is related to the enormous inherent contrast that for two soft types of tissue can be several hundred percent. This contrast is vastly superior to all types of x-ray images, including CT, in which contrast is consequent on differences in the attenuation coefficients for two adjacent structures and is, at best, a few percent. Another feature of MRI that puts a special premium on a powerful magnetic field is that the resolution of the desired signal increases as the square of the magnetic field, whereas the noise level increases only linearly with increase in the magnetic field.

Developments in ultrapowerful magnets for the great superconducting magnets of the elementary particle physicists used in giant accelerators have yielded units a thousand of which work together in perfect unison in the Fermilab accelerator. (The magnetic field of the earth is < 1 gauss. 10,000 gauss = 1 Tesla.) The 10,000 magnets of the presently abandoned superconductivity supercollider consistently operate at 6.4 Tesla. The scores of millions of dollars that have gone into the development of these magnets have lighted the way for the related similar problems of a large single magnet for medicobiologic uses. The circa 1000 Fermilab magnets have operated for years at 4 Tesla. MRI units at this energy are now in operation in some hospitals.

In addition to imaging of static structures, fluid flow can also be imaged, as can blood vessels so that magnetic resonance angiography is now available and fat saturation techniques largely eliminate the obscuration by fat of other soft tissues. The unrealized potential of the method staggers the imagination inasmuch as potentially every odd-numbered isotope in the entire table of isotopes can be imaged by this tactic.

Any publication that discusses neurologic diagnosis without a major emphasis on MRI is obsolete. We had to publish a third edition that not only emphasizes the role of this modality but also includes more subjects dealt with more thoroughly covering 175 chapters with 284 authors. We were mindful also that many authors whose native tongue is not English may not be able to write in good, idiomatic English, although for all other purposes their command of the language is excellent. In fact, the task of converting a text into idiomatic medical English has devolved on the editors because a knowledge of neurosurgery may be required for understanding of the foreign author's intended meaning. We hope that such rewording has not changed the meaning intended by the author.

Our three editions prior to this were entrusted to the publisher Grune and Stratton, who merged in 1987 with W.B. Saunders Company, who is publishing the present edition. We are impressed by the thoroughness of their copy editors, especially with the careful check they have made on the galley proofs. If the publication is delayed beyond their promised date of the November 1994 meeting of the Congress of Neurological Surgeons, it will be attributable to the unconscionably delayed arrival of several chapters despite repeated reassurances from their senior authors that their manuscripts were virtually in the mail to us.

We wish to thank the overwhelming majority of the authors for sending their efforts reasonably close to the due date and hope that their treatment by W.B. Saunders Company and by the editors will yield two eminently satisfactory tomes. The number of neurosurgeons who actually lighten their pocketbooks for these printed books is the type of ballot that will provide the crucial data on the value of the combined efforts of all of us concerned.

H. H. SCHMIDEK, MD
W. H. SWEET, MD, DSc

Contents

VOLUME 1

SECTION I

SURGERY OF THE SCALP AND SKULL, 1

CHAPTER 1
Surgical Considerations in the Fashioning of Scalp Flaps, 3
Peter C. Linton and David W. Leitner

CHAPTER 2
Surgical Repair of Major Defects of the Scalp and Skull, 13
Michael J. Yaremchuk

CHAPTER 3
Surgical Management of Trauma Involving the Skull Base and Paranasal Sinuses, 27
F. X. Brunner and U. Schwab

SECTION II

HEAD INJURIES, 45

CHAPTER 4
Surgical Management of Severe Closed Head Injury in Adults, 47
Daniel F. Kelly, Duncan Q. McBride, and Donald P. Becker

CHAPTER 5
Surgical Management of Traumatic Posterior Fossa Hematomas, 69
Daniel F. Kelly, Duncan Q. McBride, and Donald P. Becker

CHAPTER 6
Surgical Management of Traumatic Intracranial Hematomas, 73
J. Douglas Miller and Patrick F. X. Statham

CHAPTER 7
Surgical Management of Penetrating Missile Injuries of the Head, 81
T. Forcht Dagi and Eugene D. George

CHAPTER 8
Surgical Management of Missile Injuries of the Head, 89
Maurice I. Saba

CHAPTER 9
Surgical Management of Civilian Gunshot Wounds to the Head, 105
Howard H. Kaufman

CHAPTER 10
Surgical Management of Dural Sinus Lacerations, 111
John P. Kapp

CHAPTER 11
Surgical Management of Cranial Cerebrospinal Fluid Fistulas, 117
T. Forcht Dagi and Eugene D. George

SECTION III

CRANIOFACIAL LESIONS, 133

CHAPTER 12
Surgical Management of Craniosynostosis and Craniofacial Deformities, 135
Concezio Di Rocco

CHAPTER 13
Surgical Management of Encephaloceles, 149
Luis Schut

CHAPTER 14
Surgical Management of Frontoethmoidal Encephalomeningoceles, 159
Charas Suwanwela and Nitaya Suwanwela

CHAPTER 15
Transcranial Resection of Tumors of the Anterior Skull Base, 167
J. B. Blacklock

SECTION IV
ORBIT, 175

CHAPTER 16
Diagnosis and Investigation of Unilateral and Bilateral Exophthalmos, 177
Don C. Bienfang

CHAPTER 17
Surgical Management of Intraorbital Tumors, 183
Edgar M. Housepian

CHAPTER 18
Surgical Approach to Lesions of the Orbit, 195
Joseph C. Maroon and Adnan A. Abla

CHAPTER 19
Transcranial Approach to Lesions of the Orbit, 205
Armando Basso, Antonio Carrizo, and Alfredo Kreutel

CHAPTER 20
Anterior and Lateral Approaches to Lesions of the Orbit, 213
Melvin G. Alper and Phil A. Aitken

CHAPTER 21
Optic Nerve Sheath Fenestration in the Management of Pseudotumor Cerebri, 237
John W. Shore and Jurij R. Bilyk

CHAPTER 22
Optic Gliomas: Their Diagnosis, Capacity for Spontaneous Regression, and Radical Surgical Treatment, 253
William H. Sweet and Juan M. Taveras

SECTION V
PITUITARY TUMORS, 281

CHAPTER 23
Transsphenoidal Approach to Pituitary Tumors, 283
Edward R. Laws, Jr.

CHAPTER 24
Surgical Management of Endocrinologically Silent Pituitary Tumors, 293
Peter McL. Black

CHAPTER 25
Surgical Management of Cushing's Disease, 301
Brooke Swearingen and Nicholas T. Zervas

CHAPTER 26
Surgical Management of Growth Hormone–Secreting and Prolactin-Secreting Pituitary Adenomas, 305
William T. Couldwell, Marie F. Simard, and Martin H. Weiss

CHAPTER 27
Surgical Management of Recurrent Pituitary Tumors, 315
Alex M. Landolt

CHAPTER 28
Repair of the Sella Following Transsphenoidal Surgery, 327
Renato Spaziante, Enrico de Divitiis, and Paolo Cappabianca

CHAPTER 29
Stereotactic Radiosurgery for Pituitary Adenomas and Craniopharyngiomas, 347
Erik-Olof Backlund

SECTION VI
CRANIOPHARYNGIOMAS, 355

CHAPTER 30
Surgical Management of Craniopharyngiomas, 357
Madjid Samii and Amir Samii

CHAPTER 31
Transsphenoidal Microsurgery for Craniopharyngioma, 371
Rudolf Fahlbusch, Jürgen Honegger, and Michael Buchfelder

CHAPTER 32
Craniopharyngiomas: A Summary of Recent Data, 381
William H. Sweet

SECTION VII
LESIONS OF THE SKULL BASE, 391

CHAPTER 33
Surgical Management of Anterior Basal Meningiomas: Olfactory Groove, 393
Robert G. Ojemann

CHAPTER 34
Surgical Management of Tuberculum Sellae and Sphenoid Ridge Meningiomas, 403
Vallo Benjamin and Bruce McCormack

CHAPTER 35
Craniofacial Resection for Anterior Skull Base Tumors, 415
Narayan Sundaresan, Ved Sachdev, and George Krol

CHAPTER 36
Transbasal Approach to Tumors Invading the Skull Base, 427
Patrick J. Derome

CHAPTER 37
Stereotactic Biopsy and Implantation of Radionuclides Guided by Computed Tomography or Magnetic Resonance Imaging for Therapy of Brain Tumors, 443
F. Mundinger

CHAPTER 38
Pedicled Rhinotomy for Exposure of the Clivus, 469
Michael Joseph

SECTION VIII
CAVERNOUS SINUS, 477

CHAPTER 39
Anatomy of the Lateral Sellar Compartment (Cavernous Sinus), 479
Dwight Parkinson

CHAPTER 40
Surgical Management of Tumors Involving the Cavernous Sinus, 493
Takanori Fukushima and J. Diaz Day

SECTION IX
INTRACRANIAL TUMORS ABOVE THE SKULL BASE, 511

CHAPTER 41
Surgical Management of Falx and Parasagittal Tumors, 513
Brooke Swearingen

CHAPTER 42
Surgical Management of Supratentorial Gliomas, 517
Henry H. Schmidek

CHAPTER 43
Surgical Management of Recurrent Gliomas, 535
Griffith R. Harsh IV

CHAPTER 44
Surgical Management of Low-Grade Gliomas of the Cerebral Hemispheres, 549
Renato Giuffrè and Francesco S. Pastore

CHAPTER 45
Surgical Management of Supratentorial Tumors of Childhood, 571
Robert A. Sanford

CHAPTER 46
Surgical Management of Intracranial Arachnoid, Suprasellar, and Rathke's Cleft Cysts, 579
B. L. Bauer, Dieter Hellwig, William H. Sweet, and Henry H. Schmidek

CHAPTER 47
Surgical Management of Brain Metastasis, 599
Perry Black and Thomas M. McCormack

CHAPTER 48
Brain Biopsy in Nonneoplastic Neurologic Disorders, 615
Anthony Salerni and Henry H. Schmidek

CHAPTER 49
CT/MRI-Based Computer-Assisted Volumetric Stereotactic Resection of Intracranial Lesions, 619
Patrick J. Kelly

CHAPTER 50
Sterotactic Biopsy and Resection of Intracranial Lesions, 637
D. G. T. Thomas and N. D. Kitchin

CHAPTER 51
Implantation of Radionuclides in Brain Tumors, 655
Paul Kornblith, Alan Hirschfeld, Joseph Ting, and Lawrence W. Davis

CHAPTER 52
Gamma Knife Surgery in Vascular, Neoplastic, and Functional Disorders of the Nervous System, 667
L. Steiner, D. Prasad, C. Lindquist, B. Karlsson, and M. Steiner

CHAPTER 53
Intracranial and Intraspinal Endoscopy, 695
B. L. Bauer and Dieter Hellwig

CHAPTER 54
Transcallosal Approach to the Third Ventricle, 715
Craig H. Rabb and Michael L. J. Apuzzo

CHAPTER 55
Surgical Management of Intraventricular Tumors of the Lateral Ventricles, 725
Joseph M. Piepmeier, Michael Westerveld, Dennis D. Spencer, and Kimberlee Sass

CHAPTER 56
The Management of Pineal Region Neoplasms, 739
Henry H. Schmidek

CHAPTER 57
Alternate Surgical Approaches to Pineal Region Neoplasms, 743
Keiji Sano

CHAPTER 58
Supracerebellar Approach for Pineal Region Neoplasms, 755
Jeffrey N. Bruce and Bennett M. Stein

CHAPTER 59
Surgery of Diencephalic and Brainstem Tumors, 765
A. N. Konovalov, S. K. Gorelyshev, and E. A. Khuhlaeva

CHAPTER 60
Surgical Management of Tumors of the Tentorium and Clivus, 783
Edward C. Tarlov

SECTION X
POSTERIOR FOSSA TUMORS, 789

CHAPTER 61
Surgical Management of Cerebellar Tumors in Adults, 791
Henry H. Schmidek

CHAPTER 62
Surgical Management of Cerebellar Tumors in Children, 801
Joseph Petronio and Marion L. Walker

CHAPTER 63
Translabyrinthine Approach to Acoustic Neuromas, 813
T. T. King and A. F. O'Connor

CHAPTER 64
Suboccipital Transmeatal Approach to Vestibular Schwannomas, 829
Robert G. Ojemann

CHAPTER 65
Transtemporal Approaches to the Posterior Cranial Fossa, 843
Gale Gardner, Jon H. Robertson, and W. Craig Clark

CHAPTER 66
Surgical Management of Glomus Jugulare Tumors, 851
Jon H. Robertson, Gale Gardner, Edwin W. Cocke, Jr., and Carl B. Heilman

CHAPTER 67
Surgical Management of Nonglomus Tumors of the Jugular Foramen, 865
Chung-cheng Wang and Ali Liu

SECTION XI
VASCULAR DISORDERS, 875

CHAPTER 68
Surgical Therapy for Diseases of the Extracranial Carotid Artery, 877
Robert A. Ratcheson and Robert L. Grubb, Jr.

CHAPTER 69
Surgical Exposure of the Distal Internal Carotid Artery, 891
Calvin B. Ernst

CHAPTER 70
Surgical Management of Extracranial Lesions of the Vertebral Artery, 897
Edward F. Downing

CHAPTER 71
Direct Brain Revascularization, 909
Robert M. Crowell, Christopher S. Ogilvy, In Sup Choi, and Daryl R. Gress

CHAPTER 72
Surgical Management of Primary Intracerebral Hemorrhage, 929
Mark A. Weiner and David G. Piepgras

SECTION XII
INTRACRANIAL ANEURYSMS, 935

CHAPTER 73
Perioperative Care Following Aneurysmal Subarachnoid Hemorrhage, 937
R. Loch Macdonald and Bryce Weir

CHAPTER 74

Anesthetic Management of Intracranial Aneurysm Surgery, 957

John C. Drummond

CHAPTER 75

Intraoperative Endovascular Techniques in the Management of Intracranial Aneurysms, 967

Kazuo Mizoi, Akira Takahashi, and Takashi Yoshimoto

CHAPTER 76

Surgical Management of Aneurysms and Fistulas Involving the Cavernous Sinus, 975

Arthur L. Day, Robert L. Masson, and Robert S. Knego

CHAPTER 77

Surgical Management of Intraoperative Aneurysmal Rupture, 985

Thomas A. Kopitnik, Jr., H. Hunt Batjer, and Duke S. Samson

CHAPTER 78

Surgery of Paraclinoid Aneurysms, 993

Masato Shibuya and Kenichiro Sugita

CHAPTER 79

Surgical Management of Aneurysms of the Internal Carotid Artery, 1003

Henry H. Schmidek

CHAPTER 80

Surgical Management of Anterior Cerebral and Anterior Communicating Artery Aneurysms, 1011

Robin P. Sengupta

CHAPTER 81

Surgical Management of Anterior Cerebral Artery Aneurysms Distal to the Anterior Communicating Artery, 1035

William A. Shucart and Carl B. Heilman

CHAPTER 82

Surgical Management of Complex and Giant Anterior Circulation Aneurysms, 1041

Yuri N. Zubkov and Robert R. Smith

CHAPTER 83

Surgical Management of Middle Cerebral Artery Aneurysms, 1055

Lindsay Symon

CHAPTER 84

Surgical Management of Terminal Basilar and Posterior Cerebral Artery Aneurysms, 1071

Sidney J. Peerless, Juha A. Hernesniemi, and Charles G. Drake

CHAPTER 85

Surgical Management of Midbasilar and Lower Basilar Aneurysms, 1087

Mark G. Hamilton and Robert F. Spetzler

CHAPTER 86

Surgical Management of Vertebro-PICA Aneurysms, 1103

J. Diaz Day and Steven L. Giannotta

CHAPTER 87

Surgical Management of Unclippable Intracranial Aneurysms, 1113

Roberto C. Heros

CHAPTER 88

Surgical Management of Traumatic Intracranial Aneurysms, 1127

Dwight Parkinson

CHAPTER 89

Surgical Management of Infected Intracranial Aneurysms, 1133

Robert N. N. Holtzman, John C. M. Brust, James E. O. Hughes, and P. C. Taylor Dickinson

CHAPTER 90

Surgical Management of Unruptured Cerebral Aneurysms, 1155

O. Heiskanen

CHAPTER 91

Surgical Management of Vascular Lesions and Tumors Associated with Pregnancy, 1163

Christopher S. Ogilvy and Stephen B. Tatter

VOLUME 2

SECTION XIII

ARTERIOVENOUS MALFORMATIONS, 1175

CHAPTER 92

Surgical Management of Arteriovenous Malformations of the Brain, 1177

Russel H. Patterson, Jr.

CHAPTER 93
Surgical Management of Cavernous Angiomas of the Nervous System, 1183
Robert G. Ojemann, Robert M. Crowell, and Christopher S. Ogilvy

CHAPTER 94
Surgical Management of Arteriovenous Malformations in Children, 1197
Robin P. Humphreys

CHAPTER 95
Radiosurgery of Cranial Arteriovenous Malformations, 1205
Christopher S. Ogilvy, Paul H. Chapman, and James B. Costales

CHAPTER 96
The Multidisciplinary Management of Vein of Galen Malformations, 1213
J. Parker Mickle, Ronald G. Quisling, and Keith R. Peters

CHAPTER 97
Surgical Management of Dural Arteriovenous Malformations, 1219
Mark C. Held, Thoralf M. Sundt, Jr., David G. Piepgras, Frederic B. Meyer, Robert J. Coffey, and Douglas A. Nichols

SECTION XIV
HYDROCEPHALUS AND NEONATAL SURGERY, 1229

CHAPTER 98
Surgical Management of Hydrocephalus in Children, 1231
Alexa I. Canady, Sandeep Sood, and Steven D. Ham

CHAPTER 99
Surgical Management of Hydrocephalus in Adults, 1245
Mel H. Epstein and Arno H. Fried

CHAPTER 100
Management of Neurosurgical Problems in the Neonate, 1255
R. Michael Scott

SECTION XV
EPILEPSY, 1263

CHAPTER 101
Diagnostic Operative Techniques in the Treatment of Epilepsy: Grids and Strip Electrodes, 1265
Allen R. Wyler

CHAPTER 102
Diagnostic Operative Techniques in the Treatment of Epilepsy: Depth Electrodes, 1271
Andre Olivier

CHAPTER 103
Temporal Lobe Operations for Drug-Resistant Epilepsy, 1287
Robert G. Grossman and Winifred J. Hamilton

CHAPTER 104
Amygdalo-Hippocampectomy for Drug-Resistant Temporal Lobe Epilepsy, 1295
C. E. Polkey

CHAPTER 105
Temporal Lobe Operations for Epilepsy: Radical Hippocampectomy, 1305
Dennis D. Spencer and Werner K. Doyle

CHAPTER 106
Awake Operations with Mapping in Epilepsy, 1317
George A. Ojemann

CHAPTER 107
Multilobar Resections for the Control of Epilepsy, 1323
C. Munari, S. Francione, P. Kahane, D. Hoffmann, L. Tassi, G. Lo Russo, and A. L. Benabid

CHAPTER 108
Cerebral Hemispherectomy for Epilepsy, 1341
Jean-Guy Villemure

CHAPTER 109
Section of the Corpus Callosum for Epilepsy, 1351
David W. Roberts

SECTION XVI
CNS TRANSPLANTATION, 1359

CHAPTER 110
Transplantation in the Nervous System, 1361
Roy A. E. Bakay, Robert E. Breeze, and Curt R. Freed

CHAPTER 111
Neural Transplantation, 1371
E. R. Hitchcock

SECTION XVII
FUNCTIONAL NEUROSURGERY, 1387

CHAPTER 112
Brain Stimulation in the Management of Persistent Pain, 1389
> Jan M. Gybels and Ron C. Kupers

CHAPTER 112A
Commentary, 1399
> Ronald F. Young

CHAPTER 113
Spinal Cord Stimulation for Chronic Intractable Pain, 1403
> Richard B. North

CHAPTER 114
Cerebral Lesions for Psychiatric Disorders and Pain, 1413
> Jan M. Gybels and Paul R. Cosyns

CHAPTER 115
Surgical Treatment of Intractable Psychiatric Illness and Chronic Pain by Stereotactic Cingulotomy, 1423
> H. Thomas Ballantine, Jr., G. Rees Cosgrove, and Ida E. Giriunas

CHAPTER 116
Intraventricular Morphine in the Treatment of Pain Secondary to Cancer, 1431
> Alberto Lenzi, Giuseppe Galli, and Giovanni Marini

CHAPTER 117
Anterior Capsulotomy for Intractable Anxiety Disorders, 1443
> Per Mindus and Björn A. Meyerson

CHAPTER 118
Neurovascular Decompression Procedures in the Surgical Management of Disorders of Nerves V, VII, IX and X, 1457
> Robert H. Wilkins

CHAPTER 119
Percutaneous Rhizotomy in the Treatment of Intractable Facial Pain (Trigeminal, Glossopharyngeal, and Vagal Nerves), 1469
> John M. Tew, Jr. and Jamal M. Taha

CHAPTER 120
Surgical Management of Brainstem Vascular Malformations, 1485
> John M. Tew, Jr. and Adam I. Lewis

CHAPTER 121
Surgical Management of Thalamic–Basal Ganglia Vascular Malformations, 1501
> Kenneth W. Reichert II, Adam I. Lewis, and John M. Tew, Jr.

CHAPTER 122
Retrogasserian Glycerol Rhizolysis in Trigeminal Neuralgia, 1523
> Bengt Linderoth and Sten Håkanson

CHAPTER 123
Percutaneous Trigeminal Nerve Compression, 1537
> Jeffrey A. Brown and Sean Mullan

CHAPTER 124
Complications of Percutaneous Rhizotomy and Microvascular Decompression Operations for Facial Pain, 1543
> William H. Sweet and Charles E. Poletti

CHAPTER 125
Vestibular Nerve Section in the Management of Vertigo, 1547
> Horace Norrell and Herbert Silverstein

CHAPTER 126
Open Cordotomy and Medullary Tractotomy, 1557
> Charles E. Poletti

CHAPTER 127
Surgery for Hyperhidrosis and Sympathetically Mediated Pain Syndromes, 1573
> Harold A. Wilkinson

CHAPTER 128
Dorsal Root Ganglionectomy for Intractable Monoradicular Sciatica, 1585
> Arthur Taub, Franklin Robinson, and Ethan Taub

CHAPTER 129
Percutaneous Cordotomy, 1595
> R. R. Tasker

CHAPTER 130
Microsurgical DREZotomy, 1613
> Marc P. Sindou

CHAPTER 131
Microsurgical DREZotomy in Treatment of Deafferentation Pain, 1623
> James R. B. Nashold and Blaine S. Nashold, Jr.

CHAPTER 132
Surgery of the Sympathetic Nervous System, 1637
> Russell W. Hardy, Jr. and Janet W. Bay

CHAPTER 133
Surgical Management of Spasmodic Torticollis and Adult-Onset Dystonia, 1649
> Claude M. Bertrand

CHAPTER 134
Neurosurgical Management of Spasticity, 1661
Marc P. Sindou and P. Mertens

SECTION XVIII
INTRACRANIAL INFECTIONS, 1671

CHAPTER 135
Surgical Management of Intracranial and Intraspinal Infections, 1673
R. Lewis Wright

CHAPTER 136
The Neurosurgical Management of HIV-Related Brain Lesions, 1681
E. T. Chappell and B. L. Guthrie

CHAPTER 137
Surgical Management of Tuberculous and Fungal Infections of the Nervous System, 1689
Ravi Bhatia, Rana Patir, and Prakash Narain Tandon

CHAPTER 138
Neurosurgical Aspects of Neurocysticercosis, 1705
Francisco Escobedo

SECTION XIX
SURGERY OF THE CRANIOVERTEBRAL JUNCTION AND SPINE, 1717

CHAPTER 139
Craniovertebral Abnormalities and Their Neurosurgical Management, 1719
John C. Van Gilder and Arnold H. Menezes

CHAPTER 140
Surgical Management of the Rheumatoid Cervical Spine, 1731
Robin A. Johnston and James M. Borthwick

CHAPTER 141
Microsurgery of Syringomyelia and Syringomyelic Cord Syndrome, 1745
Albert L. Rhoton, Jr.

CHAPTER 142
Cervicothoracic Ankylosing Spondylitis, 1765
William H. Sweet

CHAPTER 143
Neurosurgical Considerations in the Management of Ankylosing Spondylitis, 1775
Michael E. Miner

CHAPTER 144
Anterior Cervical Disc Excision in Cervical Spondylosis, 1783
Henry H. Schmidek and Donald A. Smith

CHAPTER 145
Anterior Surgical Approaches in Multisegmental Cervical Spondylosis, 1791
Volker Seifert

CHAPTER 146
Posterior Surgical Approaches for Cervical Disc Herniation and Spondylotic Myelopathy, 1805
James C. Collias and Melville P. Roberts

CHAPTER 147
Surgical Management of Ossification of the Posterior Longitudinal Ligament, 1817
Takao Asano and Nobuyuki Tsuzuki

CHAPTER 148
Surgical Management of Injuries of the Cervical Spine and Spinal Cord, 1831
Daniele Rigamonti, Aizik L. Wolf, and Stuart E. Mirvis

CHAPTER 149
Surgical Techniques for the Stabilization of the Cervical Spine, 1849
Curtis A. Dickman and Volker K. H. Sonntag

CHAPTER 150
Surgical Approaches to the Cervicothoracic Junction, 1875
Richard G. Fessler and Donald D. Dietze

CHAPTER 151
Surgical Approaches to the Thoracic and Thoracolumbar Spine for Decompression and Stabilization, 1887
Lawrence F. Borges

CHAPTER 152
Surgical Management of Thoracic Disc Herniations, 1895
Rakesh Kumar and Stewart B. Dunsker

CHAPTER 153
Lumbar Disc Excision, 1905
Bernard E. Finneson

CHAPTER 154
Surgical Management of Primary Lumbar Disc Herniation—Commentary, 1925
Edward C. Tarlov

CHAPTER 155
Percutaneous Lumbar Discectomy, 1927
Peter W. Ascher

CHAPTER 156
Management of Persistent Symptoms Following Lumbar Disc Surgery, 1935
Don M. Long

CHAPTER 157
Surgery of Ruptured Lumbar Intervertebral Disc, 1941
Edward C. Tarlov

CHAPTER 158
Surgical Management of Lumbar Spinal Stenosis, 1957
Richard M. Westmark and Philip R. Weinstein

CHAPTER 159
Spinal Deformities Following Neurosurgical Procedures in Children, 1965
Edwin G. Fischer and John E. Hall

CHAPTER 160
Surgical Management of Penetrating Injuries of the Spine, 1971
Cheryl A. Muszynski and Raj K. Narayan

CHAPTER 161
Surgical Management of Primary and Metastatic Tumors of the Spine, 1981
Narayan Sundaresan, James E. O. Hughes, and George V. DiGiacinto

CHAPTER 162
Surgical Management of Malignant Epidural Tumors Compressing the Spinal Cord, 1997
Tzony Siegal and Tali Siegal

CHAPTER 163
Surgical Management of Spinal Cord Tumors and Arteriovenous Malformations, 2027
Kalmon D. Post and Bennett M. Stein

CHAPTER 164
Surgical Management of Cerebrospinal Fluid Leakage After Spinal Surgery, 2049
Stephen R. Freidberg

CHAPTER 165
Surgical Management of Meningoceles and Myelomeningoceles, 2055
A. L. Amacher

CHAPTER 166
Surgical Management of Occult Spinal Dysraphism, 2069
Paul H. Chapman

CHAPTER 167
Surgical Management of Spinal Injuries in Children, 2081
Derek A. Bruce

CHAPTER 168
Surgical Management of Intramedullary Spinal Cord Tumors, 2095
Shlomo Constantini and Fred Epstein

CHAPTER 169
Management of Achondroplasia and Its Neurosurgical Complications, 2107
Benjamin S. Carson, Clair Francomano, Jeremy A. Lauer, and Orest Hurko

CHAPTER 170
Surgical Management of Non–Hindbrain-Related and Posttraumatic Syringomyelia, 2119
Bernard Williams

CHAPTER 171
Neurosurgical Management of Sclerosteosis, 2141
Jacquez Charl de Villiers and Jacques J. du Plessis

SECTION XX
CRANIAL AND PERIPHERAL NERVES, 2153

CHAPTER 172
Surgical Correction of Facial Nerve Palsy, 2155
David W. Leitner

CHAPTER 173
Surgical Management of Lesions of the Peripheral Nerves and Brachial Plexus, 2159
H. Millesi

CHAPTER 174
Surgical Management of Thoracic Outlet Syndrome and of Peripheral Entrapment Neuropathies, 2173
Suzie C. Tindall

CHAPTER 175
Surgical Management of Peripheral Nerve Tumors, 2183
David G. Kline and Alan R. Hudson

INDEX, I

SECTION XIII

Arteriovenous Malformations

CHAPTER 92

Surgical Management of Arteriovenous Malformations of the Brain

Russel H. Patterson, Jr.

INDICATIONS FOR TREATMENT

Arteriovenous malformations (AVMs) are generally detected because of a seizure, intracranial hemorrhage, or, occasionally, for having caused an ischemic neuropathic deficit. Sometimes, they are discovered on an image of the brain taken for other purposes. In any case, if the patient is well or perhaps has seizures but no other sequelae, the question of whether or not to treat the lesion arises. This decision depends on the risk of treatment versus nontreatment of the AVM. In addition, the patient's fear of a craniotomy, if craniotomy is an option, is also considered.

AVMs, even if asymptomatic when discovered, are likely to become symptomatic. Asymptomatic AVMs at autopsy are distinctly rare, and bleeding, which is the most devastating complication, occurs at a cumulative rate of 3 percent annually, regardless of whether the lesion has already bled.[1-3] Therefore, unless the lesion is hopelessly large and in a bad location, it probably should be treated. Fortunately, there is usually a way of treating the AVM that carries a lower risk than that of the natural history of the disease.[4-6]

METHODS OF MANAGEMENT

AVMs can be treated by embolization, radiation, surgery, or some combination of these modalities. Embolization is the first treatment considered because it makes the vascularized portion of the AVM smaller, and the smaller the AVM, the smaller the job for the surgeon or radiotherapist.

What can and cannot be embolized depends on the nature of the AVM and the skills of the interventionalist. Embolization is not free of risk, but fortunately, the frequency of serious complications is about 5 percent in large series. A patient with a small AVM probably does not have to accept even this risk, but if the AVM is large, surgery is greatly facilitated if much of the blood supply can be interrupted before the operation.[7-11]

Generally, the embolization is performed with N-butyl cyanoacrylate glue that is mixed with tantalum to make the material visible on scout films from the angiogram. Several sessions may be required to achieve the best results. Because the glue forms a cast in the blood vessels, the lesion need not be immediately excised after the embolization. Sometimes, the AVM can be completely obliterated solely by embolization, but this happy event occurs only in about 10 percent of cases. If even a bit of AVM remains after embolization, the risk of hemorrhage remains high, regardless of the treatment used.

STEREOTACTIC RADIATION

An AVM whose nidus is smaller than about 3 cm can be treated by stereotactic radiation, whether by gamma knife, a heavy particle source, or a linear accelerator. Larger AVMs are not suitable for stereotactic radiation because if a larger volume is irradiated, even through a large number of ports, the normal brain receives an excessive amount of radiation, and the advantage of any of the specialized machines over conventional radiation is lost.[12-15]

The outcome of radiation therapy is related to the size of the lesion. The chance of obliterating a lesion not larger than 1 cm is about 90 per cent; for a lesion of over 3 cm, it is about 30 per cent. The optimal lesion for such treatment is spherical, but unfortunately, most lesions are not spherical. However, with the gamma knife, by using several different isocenters in a pattern to cover the lesion (like piling up snowballs), this difficulty can be overcome. When a linear accelerator is used, the same effect is accomplished by using multiple arcs and turning the beam on and off at certain times in each arc.

Radiation therapy for AVMs is not without problems because it carries some risk to the brain; late neurologic complications are reported in approximately 5 percent of cases.[16] In additional, it may take a year or two or even longer for the effects of the radiation to obliterate the lesion, if this happens at all. Thus, the patient is at risk from a hemorrhage for that length of time. If some of the AVM still fills after 2 years, radiation may fail, and because of the continued risk of hemorrhage, the clinician must decide how next to proceed.

Radiosurgery is most effective when the AVM is small (< 3 cm in diameter). These small lesions are also the ones most readily treated by an experienced surgeon. Surgery, when properly performed on a suitable lesion, carries a low risk, has a high probability of cure, and is free of the delayed onset of effectiveness and possible failure of radiosurgery. In addition, surgery avoids the poorly understood long-term risks that must be considered with any kind of radiotherapy. For these reasons, radiotherapy is best reserved for small lesions in areas that carry prohibitive surgical risk (Fig. 92–1).[17]

SURGERY

The typical AVM of the cerebral hemispheres is wedge shaped, with a broad surface at or near the cortex and an apex that reaches the ventricle from where the AVM receives an important feeder (Fig. 92–2). Some AVMs do not reach the ventricle, but these are relatively few, and for planning purposes, the surgeon should anticipate that an important arterial feeder that arises from the ventricle and is difficult to occlude will be located deep in the brain underneath the AVM. This deep feeder is often poorly seen on preoperative angiograms because of the greater flow of blood contributed by more superficial arteries.

When an AVM is identified and surgery seems the proper course of action, an interventional neuroradiologist should be consulted (Fig. 92–3) to reduce blood flow, if possible. If, in the opinion of the interventionalist, the lesion is suitable for embolization, several sessions may be needed for the embolization to be completed (Fig. 92–4).

The surgery itself is performed through a suitable bone flap. Care must be taken when the dura is opened because about 15 percent of AVMs receive some of their blood supply via the dura. If the dura is lifted carelessly off the brain, one of these feeders may tear. After the dura is opened, the surgeon can operate sitting down, using a small instrument table both as an armrest and to hold instruments, and, of course, the microscope for its light and magnification.

The AVM may be quite obvious on the surface of the brain, but often the main feature is a large, red vein that serves as one of the principal draining veins. The AVM itself is not visible because it is entirely or partly covered by a thin layer of cerebral cortex. Because the cortex may be functional, it should be preserved, if possible.

If only the draining vein is visible, the vein should be freed up from the arachnoid and followed into the AVM. This process allows the surgeon to identify the top of the AVM, and from there, a plane may be slowly developed between the AVM and the brain all around the circumference of the lesion. This process is not always as simple as it sounds. A well-defined glial plane may exist around AVMs, but this area may be quite hard to identify, and frequently, the surgeon may find himself or herself working within the anomaly.

Bleeding from the small vessels in the lesion can be hard to control because the vessel wall may be composed of mostly endothelium with little substance. Bipolar coagulation does not seem to work very well, and, even if the bleeding can be slowed 90 percent, often a persistent 10 percent of ooze remains. Fortunately, tamponade for a short period seems to work. Topical absorbable gelatin sponge (Gelfoam) is not always the best choice for temporary tamponade, because it becomes very sticky and is hard to remove after the job is completed. Cotton pledgets seem to work better for this purpose. Optimally, the AVM is not entered, and the mass of embolization glue with its tantalum color helps define the proper plane.

In the course of dissection, the surgeon is sure to see several sizable arteries that appear to be supplying the AVM. These should be left intact until it is clear where the arteries go and what they supply. Some of them may, after sending a feeder to the AVM, continue on and supply normal brain distal to the lesion. Therefore, no large artery should be divided until the artery clearly terminates in the AVM. Otherwise, the taking of the artery may lead to an unwanted and unexpected cerebral infarction.

Some of the arteries on the surface of the cortex or in the sulci appear tortuous but not enlarged. These vessels are not necessarily a part of the nidus and probably should be left alone. Because veins that drain the nidus carry red blood, the color of the veins can sometimes be a useful guide to what is AVM and what is not.

As the lesion is slowly encircled, deeper and deeper, coagulating some of the mass and removing part of it may give better exposure. Partial removal is particularly feasible in the segments of the AVM that have been solidly embolized.

The principle problem usually comes at the end of the operation from deep arterial feeders coming up from the ventricle and the choroidal arteries. These can be difficult to control and may require an aneurysm clip to stop all the bleeding. The lesion commonly appears to have been all resected except for some small, pesky bleeders at the bottom of the hole that will not coagulate properly or that appear to retract into the white matter but continue to bleed. In such a case, suspect a large feeder coming in from the ventricle that has been overlooked. The best plan may be to continue down into the ventricle and thoroughly coagulate the choroid plexus and its arteries. This action can be the most expeditious solution to a vexing problem.[18–20]

After the AVM has been entirely resected, the blood pressure should be raised to about 150 mm Hg with a vasopressor. Phenylephrine, 50 µg, is useful for this purpose. If any residual AVM is present or if hemostasis is less than perfect, then the hypertension will probably provoke bleeding. Complete hemostasis is required at this point, not some hours later, when the patient has become stuporous and hemiplegic in the intensive care unit. If the patient withstands the challenge of a blood pressure of 150 mm Hg with the head open, the surgeon can feel reasonably confident that the patient will not develop a postoperative hematoma. If the patient fails the test and bleeding occurs, then hemostasis must be re-established and the test repeated as often as needed until the patient successfully withstands the challenge.

Many cases of postoperative hemorrhage that are attributed to breakthrough bleeding likely result from poor hemostasis at the time of surgery. Rough handling of the brain at surgery is the likeliest reason for excessive brain swelling postoperatively, not some poorly understood abnormality of vascular permeability. Gentleness with the brain and thoroughness in hemostasis help ensure a smooth postoperative course.[21, 22]

Some surgeons prefer to identify eloquent cortex during surgery through brain stimulation to identify motor cortex, and perform surgery with the patient under local anesthesia to evaluate speech, if speech is an issue. Although these efforts are reasonable, equally good results can be achieved if care is taken to preserve as much normal brain as possible around the AVM.

Soon after surgery, the patient should have a repeat angio-

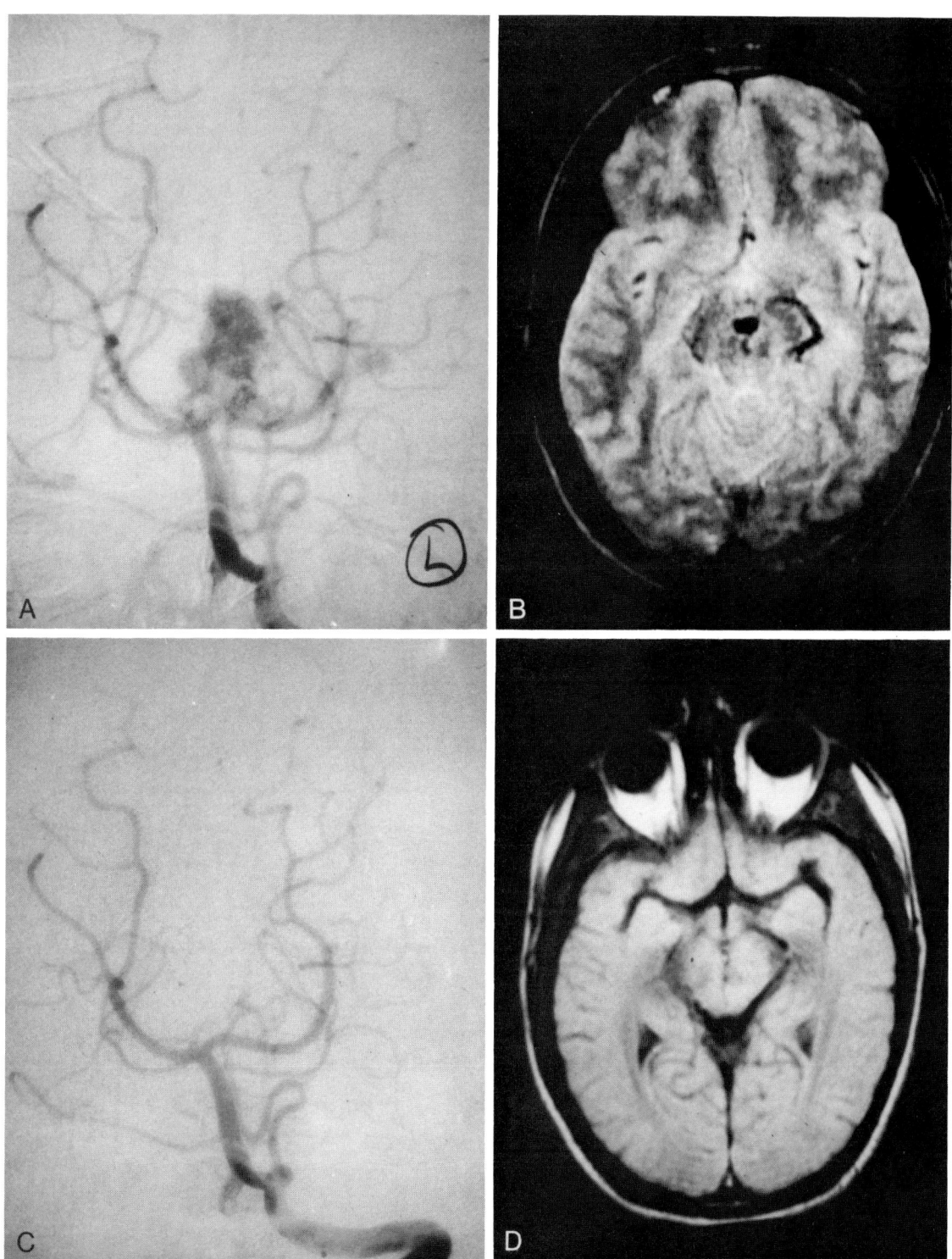

FIGURE 92–1. A 28-year-old fireman with a subarachnoid hemorrhage. (A and B) Angiogram and MRI pretreatment. (C and D) Angiogram and MRI 18 months after gamma knife surgery.

1180 | Arteriovenous Malformations

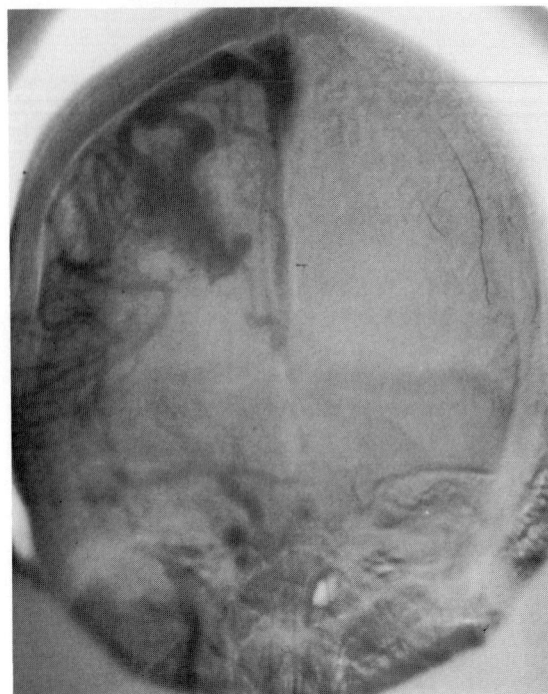

FIGURE 92–2. A frontoparietal AVM that shows the typical wedge-shaped configuration and feeding vessels derived from the ventricle.

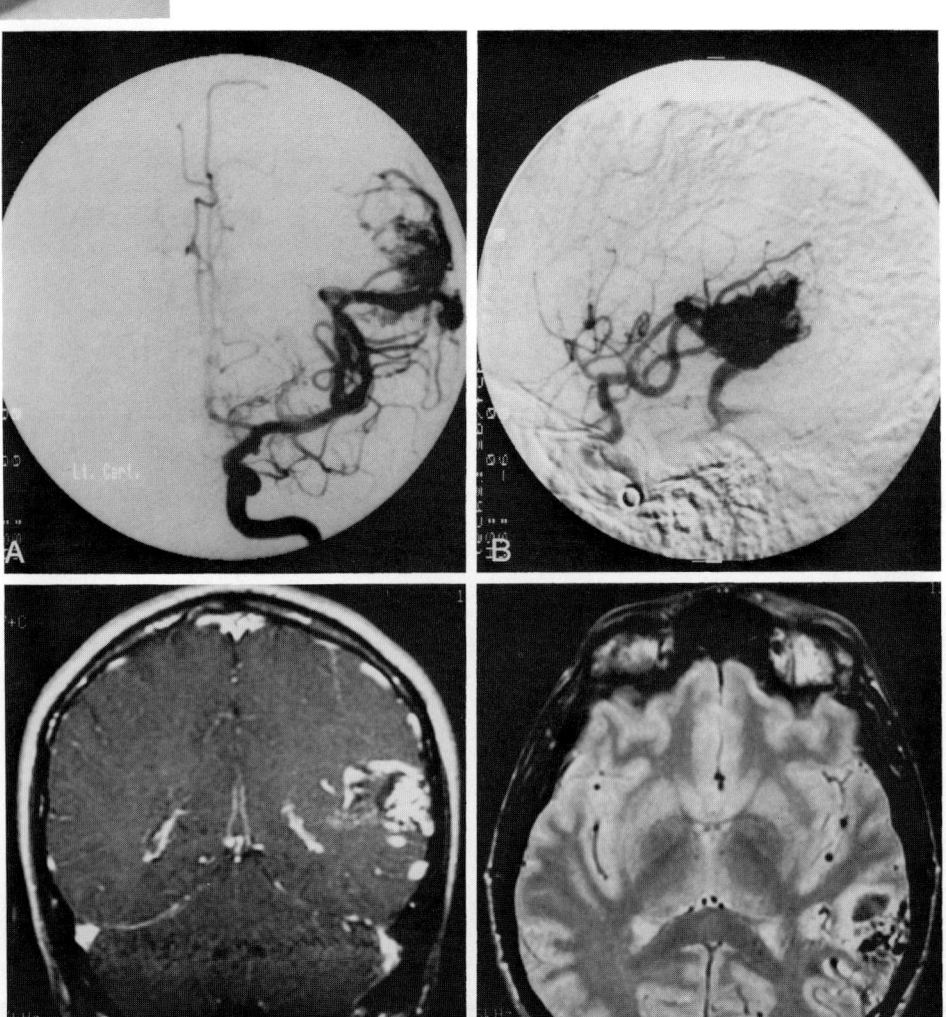

FIGURE 92–3. An AVM in the left sylvian fissure. (A and B) Frontal and lateral angiographic projection. (C and D) The MRIs show the extent of the AVM.

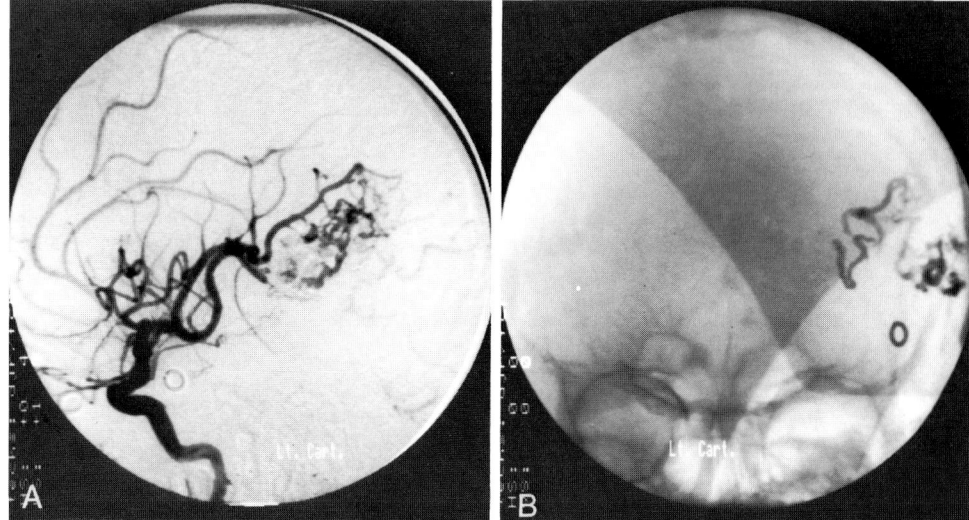

FIGURE 92-4. (A) Angiogram after the second session of embolization. (B) Plain AP film showing the embolic material in the AVM.

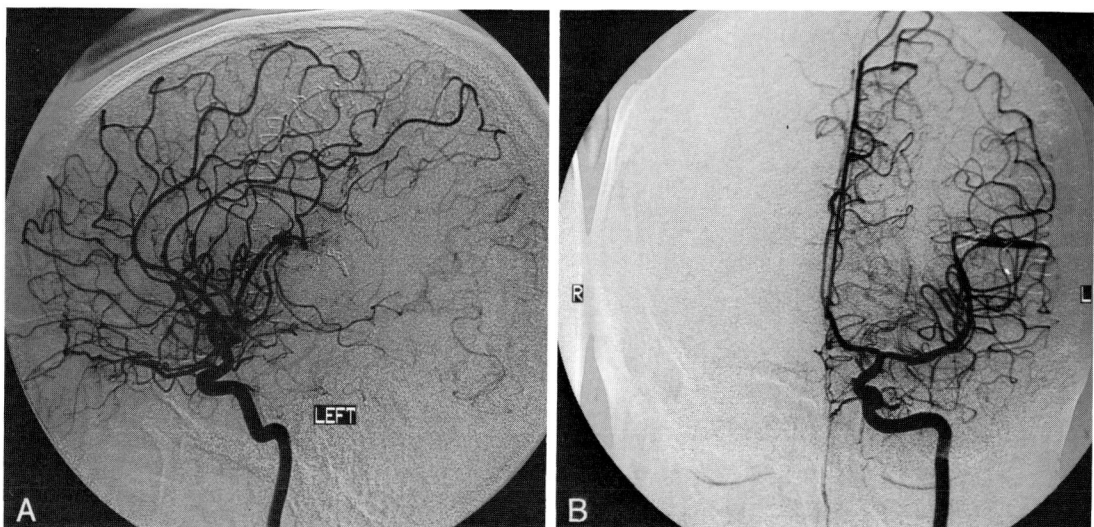

FIGURE 92-5. (A and B) Lateral and AP angiogram 6 days after surgical resection. The patient did well and had no deficits except for a mild dysphasia that dated from his last intracranial hemorrhage.

gram to determine that the lesion is gone. If some lesion remains, then this residual AVM should be excised in a second operation or possibly treated with focused radiation therapy. An angiogram may be obtained while the patient is on the operating table. Provided that the films are of good quality, this is a reasonable procedure to take to reduce the chances of leaving behind residual AVM (Fig. 92–5).[23–30]

REFERENCES

1. Ondra SL, Troupp H, George ED, Schwab K: The natural history of symptomatic arteriovenous malformations of the brain: A 24-year follow-up assessment. J Neurosurg 73(3):387–391, 1990; Comment in: J Neurosurg 75(2):338–339, 1991
2. Itoyama Y, Uemura S, Ushio Y, et al: Natural course of unoperated intracranial arteriovenous malformations: Study of 50 cases. J Neurosurg 71(6):805–809, 1989
3. Steinmeier R, Schramm J, Muller HG, Fahlbusch R: Evaluation of prognostic factors in cerebral arteriovenous malformations. Neurosurgery 24(2):193–200, 1989
4. Heros RC, Tu YK: Unruptured arteriovenous malformations: A dilemma in surgical decision making. Clin Neurosurg 33:187–236, 1986
5. Aminoff MJ: Management of unruptured cerebral arteriovenous malformations. Clin Neurosurg 33:177–185, 1986
6. Wilkins RH: Natural history of intracranial vascular malformations: A review. Neurosurgery 16(3):421–430, 1985
7. Schweitzer JS, Chang BS, Madsen P, et al: The pathology of arteriovenous malformations of the brain treated by embolotherapy: II. Results of embolization with multiple agents. Neuroradiology 35(6):468–474, 1993
8. Setton A, Berenstein A: Interventional neuroradiology. Curr Opin Neurol Neurosurg 5(6):870–880, 1992
9. Jafar JJ, Davis AJ, Berenstein A, et al: The effect of embolization with N-butyl cyanoacrylate prior to surgical resection of cerebral arteriovenous malformations. J Neurosurg 78(1):60–69, 1993
10. Livingston K, Hopkins LN: Endovascular treatment of intracerebral arteriovenous malformations. Clin Neurosurg 39:331–347, 1992
11. Fournier D, TerBrugge KG, Willinsky R, et al: Endovascular treatment of intracerebral arteriovenous malformations: Experience in 49 cases. J Neurosurg 75(2):228–233, 1991
12. Lunsford LD, Kondziolka D, Flickinger JC, et al: Stereotactic radiosurgery for arteriovenous malformations of the brain. J Neurosurg 75(4):512–524, 1991; Comment in: J Neurosurg 76(6):1045–1047, 1992
13. Marks LB, Spencer DP: The influence of volume on the tolerance of the brain to radiosurgery. J Neurosurg 75(2):177–180, 1991; Erratum in: J Neurosurg 76(2):343, 1992; Comment in: J Neurosurg 76(3):557–559; 559–560, 1992
14. Steiner L, Linquist C, Cail W, et al: Microsurgery and radiosurgery in brain arteriovenous malformations. J Neurosurg 79(5):647–652, 1993
15. Lunsford LD, Kondziolka D, Flickinger JC, et al: Stereotactic radiosurgery for arteriovenous malformations of the brain. J Neurosurg 75(4):512–524, 1991; Comment in: J Neurosurg 76(6):1045–1047, 1992
16. Statham P, Macpherson P, Johnston R, et al: Cerebral radiation necrosis complicating stereotactic radiosurgery for arteriovenous malformation. J Neurol Neurosurg Psychiatry 53(6):476–479, 1990
17. Sisti MB, Kader A, Stein BM: Microsurgery for 67 intracranial arteriovenous malformations less than 3 cm in diameter. J Neurosurg 79(5):653–660, 1993
18. Heros RC: Brain resection for exposure of deep extracerebral and paraventricular lesions. Surg Neurol 34(3):188–195, 1990
19. Sisti MB, Stein BM: Arteriovenous malformations of the brain stem. Neurosurg Clin North Am 4(3):497–505, 1993
20. Stein BM, Kader A: Intracranial arteriovenous malformations. Clin Neurosurg 39:76–113, 1992
21. Sakaki T, Tsujimoto S, Nishitani M, et al: Perfusion pressure breakthrough threshold of cerebral autoregulation in the chronically ischemic brain: An experimental study in cats. J Neurosurg 76(3):478–485, 1992
22. Spetzler RF, Hamilton MG: Pressure autoregulation is intact after arteriovenous malformation resection. Neurosurgery 33(4):772–774, 1993
23. Lee JP: Surgical treatment of thalamic arteriovenous malformations. Neurosurgery 32(4):498–503, 1993; Discussion, 503–504
24. Heros RC: Brain resection for exposure of deep extracerebral and paraventricular lesions. Surg Neurol 34(3):188–195, 1990
25. Kashiwagi S, van Loveren HR, Tew JM Jr, et al: Diagnosis and treatment of vascular brain-stem malformations. J Neurosurg 72(1):27–34, 1990
26. Deruty R, Pelissou-Guyotat I, Mottolese C, et al: The combined management of cerebral arteriovenous malformations. Experience with 100 cases and review of the literature. Acta Neurochir (Wien) 123(3–4):101–112, 1993
27. Grzyska U, Westphal M, Zanella F, et al: A joint protocol for the neurosurgical and neuroradiologic treatment of cerebral arteriovenous malformations: Indications, technique and results in 76 cases. Surg Neurol 40(6):476–484, 1993
28. Sisti MB, Stein BM: Arteriovenous malformations of the brain stem. Neurosurg Clin North Am 4(3):497–505, 1993
29. Gentili F, Schwartz M, TerBrugge K, et al: A multidisciplinary approach to the treatment of brain vascular malformations. Adv Tech Stand Neurosurg 19:179–207, 1992
30. Vinuela F, Dion JE, Duckwiler G, et al: Combined endovascular embolization and surgery in the management of cerebral arteriovenous malformations: Experience with 101 cases. J Neurosurg 75(6):856–864, 1991

CHAPTER 93

Surgical Management of Cavernous Angiomas of the Nervous System

Robert G. Ojemann
Robert M. Crowell
Christopher S. Ogilvy

Cavernous angiomas have long been recognized as one of the major clinicopathologic categories of vascular malformations of the nervous system.[1-3] Since no abnormal vascularity is seen on angiography, they have been included in the descriptions of cryptic or occult vascular malformations, a term that has been used to describe any vascular malformation that cannot be seen on angiography.[4-9] They have also been called cavernous hemangioma or cavernoma, but the term *cavernous angioma* was used by Russell and Rubinstein[3] in their excellent description of the pathology of these lesions.

Before computed tomography (CT), the diagnosis of this angioma was rarely made prior to operation or autopsy. CT suggested the diagnosis in some patients; however, when high-field magnetic resonance imaging (MRI) became available, a picture characteristic of cavernous angioma was defined, thereby allowing the diagnosis to be established in many cases.

The management of patients with cavernous angioma usually includes a consideration of surgical treatment or of observation. Rarely radiosurgery is considered, but in general the results have been disappointing. The indications and guidelines for management decisions continue to evolve.

This chapter reviews the surgical management of 62 cases of cavernous angiomas seen by the authors. From this information and a review of the literature, we make recommendations for treating patients with this disorder.

PATHOLOGIC FEATURES

Cavernous angiomas can occur throughout the brain or spinal cord parenchyma and on cranial and spinal nerves.[2,10] The lesions, which may be multiple, can range in size from a few millimeters to several centimeters. Occasionally, an associated venous angioma of the brain may be present, and, rarely, similar lesions in other parts of the body.[11]

How a cavernous angioma develops is unknown. In some groups of patients, the lesions are clearly acquired, appearing in areas of brain that were normal on prior MRI studies.[9] These groups include patients with familial lesions and those in whom the cavernous angioma has developed in an area of previously irradiated brain tissue. Wilson[9] has proposed a possible pathogenesis for the development of acquired lesions.

The lesion is well defined and usually has a lobulated appearance. There is often a very characteristic gross appearance that has been likened to a mulberry, characterized by a dark red or purple color. Inside the lesion is a honeycomb of thin-walled vascular spaces.[2] Small hemorrhages adjacent to or within the lesion may occur, but large hemorrhages are rare. A variable number of small blood vessels enter the lesion. Gliotic tissue surrounds the mass and it is usually stained yellow. In some patients, the lesion may gradually enlarge as a result of small hemorrhages, progressive hyalinization and thickening of the vascular walls, or gradual thrombosis.[10,12,13]

Irregular sinusoidal spaces are visible on microscopic examination, and many contain areas of thrombosis and organization with thin walls devoid of elastic tissue and muscle. These walls consist of a single layer of endothelium with varying amounts of extraluminal connective tissue. No intervening or neural tissue is present except at the periphery, a layer of gliotic tissue exists that contains hemosiderin-packed macrophages adjacent to the lesion. Hematomas of varying ages, extensive calcification, and on the surface, collections of capillaries, may be seen.

RADIOLOGIC FEATURES

High-quality CT scans suggest the diagnosis of cavernous angioma in some patients. The characteristic findings are a roughly circular or irregularly shaped lesion located in the brain parenchyma, which shows high density on the noncontrast scan and slight or no contrast enhancement. In some patients, extensive calcification is noted. However, other types of occult vascular malformations and some tumors associated with hemorrhage have the same CT appearance.

MRI accurately establishes the diagnosis in most cases and often is the only study needed. The criteria for MRI diagnosis

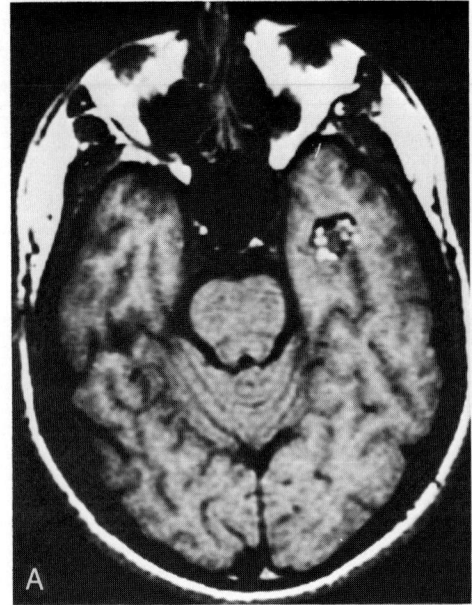
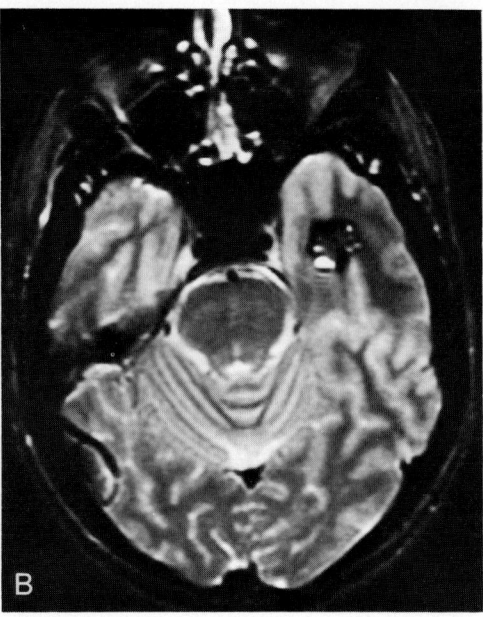

FIGURE 93–1. Temporal cavernous angioma in a 34-year-old man presenting with a seizure. Removal of the lesion was followed by a normal recovery. MRI axial T1- and T2-weighted images (A and B, respectively) show a well-circumscribed lesion in the left temporal lobe with a mottled core of mixed signal intensity and a surrounding rim of decreased signal intensity.

is a well-circumscribed lesion with a combination of a reticulated or mottled core of mixed signal intensity and a prominent surrounding rim of decreased signal intensity (Fig. 93–1).[14] Hemorrhages of different ages may be seen within or around the lesion, and rarely a draining vein may be seen. On T2-weighted images, an increased signal may be present in the adjacent brain as a result of edema. Usually little or no enhancement follows the administration of gadolinium. Although appearance on MRI has a high correlation with the diagnosis of cavernous angioma, occasionally, an occult arteriovenous malformation or a tumor can have a similar appearance.[9, 15] Significant enhancement suggests the possibility of a tumor.

The angiographic results are almost always normal because the lesion has small blood vessels with low flow and no hypertrophied feeding arteries or early draining veins. Since the development of MRI, angiography is rarely indicated. Occasionally, angiography is needed to give information regarding the vascular anatomy to help plan a surgical approach. If the MRI suggests an association with another vascular malformation or if the diagnosis is in doubt, angiography should be done.

FAMILIAL OCCURRENCE

Several cases of familial cavernous angiomas have been reported.[16–18] An autosomal dominant pattern of inheritance has been found with an incomplete penetrance. Rigamonti and colleagues[18] estimated a 73 percent familial incidence of multiple angiomas of the brain, compared with a 10 to 15 percent incidence in the sporadic form. In this series, three patients were members of one family, and two had multiple lesions.

Hayman and associates[16] reported on seven patients with familial cavernous angiomas who were followed up with CT over 5 years. In two patients, large new lesions appeared where the CT had previously shown normal tissue; in one, the pre-existing lesion was unchanged, and in the other it had bled. In one patient, a single lesion continued to bleed repeatedly over months while adjacent lesions remained unchanged. In four patients, no change occurred. The authors recommended that all first-degree relatives of a patient with familial cavernous angioma be evaluated with a CT scan. This approach can clarify the potential risks and the need for close radiographic and clinical follow-up and can give data regarding the natural history.

CLINICAL PRESENTATION

In 1976, Voigt and Yasargil[19] analyzed 163 cases reported up to 1974. They found that these lesions occurred in every age group and that the sex incidence was equal. In 1988, Simard and colleagues[20] reviewed 126 cases published since 1960 and added 12 of their own. The male:female ratio was 0.9:1, and the ages ranged from neonate to 75 years. In 1991, two publications were based on the analysis of consecutive MRI scans performed over several years.[11, 12] In the report by Robinson and coworkers,[11] of 68 patients, the male:female ratio was 1.2:1, and the age ranged from 4 months to 84 years (mean, 34.6 years). In the report of 32 patients by Curling and associates,[12] the male:female ratio was 1.1:1, the age ranged from 16 to 72 years (mean, 37.6 years), and multiple lesions were present in six patients (19 percent). Scott and colleagues[21] reported on 18 children ranging in age from 7 months to 17 years. In this series there were 29 males and 33 females. Three patients had multiple lesions, and two had associated venous angiomas.

Four general categories of clinical presentation are seizures, headache, neurologic deficit, and asymptomatic presentation.[11, 12, 19, 20] In many patients, more than one of the symptoms is present. Within each of the symptomatic categories, some patients have had a hemorrhage into the adjacent brain parenchyma. The hemorrhages are usually small, but on rare occasion can be large, with the patient having rapid deterioration. In some patients, the cavernous angioma gradually enlarges, and the lesion can act as a mass that causes a progressive neurologic deficit.

NATURAL HISTORY

In 1985, Wilkins[8] reviewed the natural history of vascular malformations. He concluded that not enough information was present in the literature to describe the natural history of cavernous angiomas. In 1991, two reports of cavernous angiomas diagnosed in large consecutive series of MRI scans gave some information about the short-term natural history,[11, 12] and data from familial cases have also contributed to our knowledge.

The long-term risk of recurrent hemorrhage or of hemorrhage from a lesion that has not bled is unknown. Most hemorrhages are small, but there are occasional exceptions. Zimmerman and coworkers[22] reported on one patient who died from rehemorrhage of a tectal cavernous angioma. In the short follow-up periods reported by Curling and colleagues[12] and Robinson and colleagues,[11] no new hemorrhages occurred in patients who presented with seizures. In the entire series of patients in these two reports, the risk of new hemorrhage was 0.25 percent and 0.81 percent, respectively, per person per year. Tung and coworkers[6] reported on recurrent hemorrhage occurring in seven patients whose diagnosis of cavernous angioma was confirmed at surgery. The interval from the initial hemorrhage to the recurrent hemorrhage ranged from 1 to 16 months, and a second rebleed occurred at a shorter interval. They found that as the number of hemorrhages increased, there was a higher incidence of lasting neurologic deficit. Pozzati and associates[13] reported on three patients in whom the cavernous angioma markedly enlarged over 2 months, 2 years, and 6 years because of small hemorrhages. Curling and colleagues[12] reported that in 35 patients, many of whom had been symptomatic and followed up with MRI over a period of 3 months to 4 years (mean, 11.7 months), three showed enlargement of the lesion, presumably because of small hemorrhages. Both Lunsford and associates[23] and Tung and associates[6] have suggested that the rehemorrhage rate is 2 percent per year, similar to that of true arteriovenous malformations. Little information is available about asymptomatic patients. In the report by Robinson and coworkers[11] four of nine asymptomatic patients developed symptoms related to the cavernous angioma over a relatively short follow-up period of 6 months to 2 years (mean, 18 months).

MANAGEMENT CONSIDERATIONS

Treatment for patients with cavernous angiomas is based on careful comparison of the benefits and risks associated with the treatment options, usually either surgery or observation. Occasionally, radiosurgery is used. The age and medical condition of the patient are considered in this decision. Because knowledge and experience are still in the accumulative stage, only guidelines can be offered.

SURGERY

The reports by Robinson and colleagues,[11, 24] Curling and colleagues,[12] and Golfinos and colleagues[25] recommend that surgical resection be considered for patients with recurrent hemorrhage, progressive neurologic deterioration, and intractable epilepsy unless the location is associated with an unacceptably high surgical risk. We agree that when the surgical risk is high, observation or radiosurgery should be considered. However, we also believe that because the risk of surgery is very low for lesions in many locations, there are other groups of patients, including those with cavernous angioma of the cerebrum or cerebellum with a single hemorrhage, those with the onset of a seizure disorder, and those who are worried about the presence of the lesion, in whom surgery should be considered. Robinson and associates[24] also recommend surgical excision of accessible cavernous angiomas that have "manifested an overt hemorrhage." In children, Scott and coworkers[21] have a "policy to recommend surgery for patients with cavernous angiomas if the lesion is safely accessible, is currently symptomatic either by mass effect and/or hemorrhage or seizure, or shows evidence of having bled in the past."

In a special category is the young woman who wants to become pregnant (Fig. 93–2). Robinson and colleagues[11] noted that two of their six patients with acute hemorrhage were in the first trimester of pregnancy. They suggested that in women contemplating pregnancy, one of the indications for surgical excision was an accessible lesion.

When surgical excision of a cavernous angioma is indicated, the lesion can usually be totally removed with low morbidity. This procedure is facilitated by microsurgical dissection in the gliotic tissue that surrounds the lesion, thereby allowing a distinct plane of cleavage to be developed through microsurgical techniques, bipolar coagulation, and the use of fine-regulated suction. When the lesion is exposed, internally decompressing the mass and retracting the capsule into the area of the decompression may help avoid pressure on the surrounding normal parenchyma. When the lesion is densely calcified, the Cavitron ultrasonic surgical aspirator may be used for debulking. Bleeding is usually not a significant problem.

In some patients, splitting a cortical fissure may be possible rather than performing a full corticectomy to approach the lesion. For lesions in critical areas, cortical mapping and stimulation may be used. When removal of a cavernous angioma in the deep portions of the cerebral hemispheres is indicated, the lesion is localized with stereotactic techniques and intraoperative ultrasound.[6] For brainstem lesions, special monitoring with evoked potentials may be helpful, and arrangements for temporary cardiac pacing may be prudent.

RADIOSURGERY

Stereotactic radiosurgery has been used to treat patients with cavernous angiomas thought to be inoperable and associated with progressive worsening of their neurologic symptoms because of mass effect or recurrent hemorrhage. Lunsford and associates[23] reported on the use of the gamma knife and noted the difficulty in analyzing the results in these patients. The natural history is poorly understood, complications can be related to either minor rebleeding or delayed, radiation-induced injury, and MRI results may not change significantly during the follow-up period. They noted that complications were somewhat higher in these patients than in those with arteriovenous malformations, possibly because of the fact that most of the lesions were in deep or critical

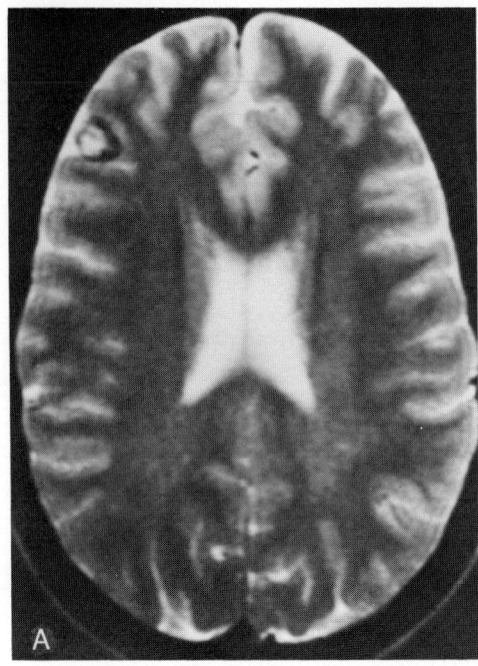 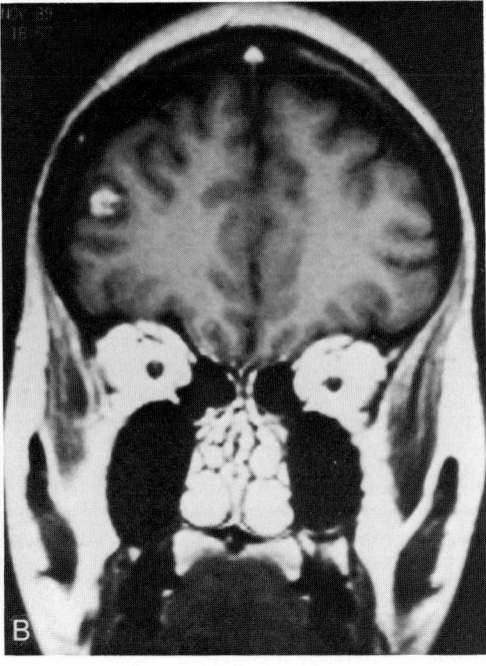

FIGURE 93–2. Frontal cavernous angioma in a 34-year-old physician presenting with seizures. The seizures were controlled with medication but she wanted to become pregnant and requested surgical excision. Removal of the lesion was followed by normal recovery. MRI axial T2- and coronal T1-weighted images (A and B, respectively) show a superficial right frontal lesion with no parenchymal hemorrhage.

brain regions. In patients treated more recently, the radiation dosage has been reduced, and guidelines for the dose to volume of the lesion have been developed.

Stereotactic charged-particle radiosurgery, both helium-ion radiosurgery and proton beam therapy, has also been used to treat cavernous angiomas. Fabrikant and associates[26] noted that the clinical results after helium-ion radiosurgery for cavernous angiomas were not as good as those for arteriovenous malformations. However, long-term follow-up results have not been reported.

Radiosurgery using a linear accelerator has also been reported.[27] The number of patients treated is small and no long-term data are available.

In summary, the results of radiosurgery have not been encouraging. This modality is presently recommended only rarely for deep, inaccessible lesions associated with repeated hemorrhage and progressive neurologic deficit.

OBSERVATION

Some patients with cavernous angiomas can be treated with observation only. Almost all asymptomatic lesions are observed because some lesions are asymptomatic indefinitely, and when there is a hemorrhage, it is usually small and is not associated with a major neurologic deficit. Another group that may be observed is those with symptomatic lesions in a deep or critical area when the risks of surgery are judged to be significant, and recurrent hemorrhage or an increasing neurologic deficit is not present. Some patients with seizures or headache in whom no hemorrhage has occurred have been observed, but some of these patients are now having surgery. The decision of which treatment is appropriate depends on a detailed evaluation of the clinical problem and discussion with the patient.

No clear guidelines exist on how often the MRI should be repeated. We generally perform MRI on the patient at 6-month intervals for 2 years, and if the lesion is stable, we repeat the scan once a year.

CAVERNOUS ANGIOMAS OF THE CEREBRUM

MANAGEMENT

Patients Presenting with Seizures

The treatment of patients with cavernous angioma presenting with seizures continues to evolve. With the good results of surgical removal, the indications for operation have enlarged beyond conditions in which medical control of seizures is difficult and in which the diagnosis is in question (which was more common before the advent of MRI). Surgery is recommended in most patients who have had a parenchymal hemorrhage and in many patients who have not had a hemorrhage when the surgical risk is low. These patients are usually in their third to fifth decade but are sometimes younger, and they are often concerned about the presence of the lesion. Although the seizures can often be controlled with medication, the removal of the cavernous angioma and the adjacent gliotic yellow-stained tissue may reduce the long-term frequency and severity of seizures and allow the patients to discontinue their medication.[2, 11, 12] Robinson and colleagues[11] reported that all 18 patients who did not have surgery continued to require medical control of their seizures. In the surgically treated group, 50 percent had no more seizures, and the others had a reduction in seizure frequency.

Rengachary and Kalyan-Raman[2] described a possible basis for recommending surgery. They suggest that slow lysis of red cells sequestrated in the cavernous spaces allows red cell pigment to diffuse out of the lesion into the adjacent tissue. This pigment seems to induce gliosis, which may contribute to the development of a seizure focus. The authors quote experimental studies that suggest that chemical compounds

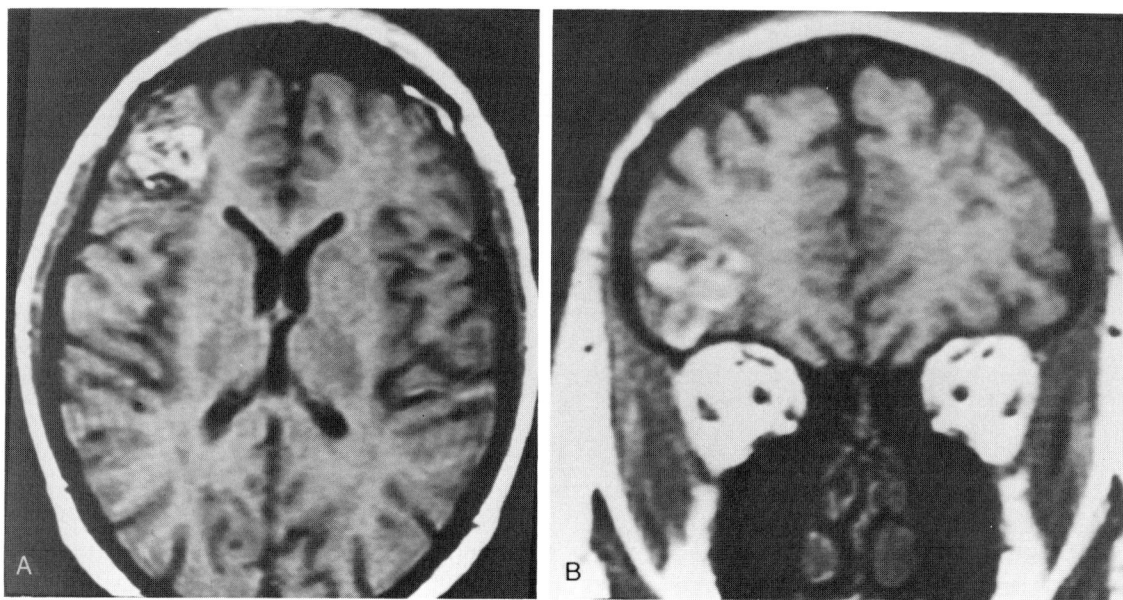

FIGURE 93-3. Frontal cavernous angioma in a 45-year-old man with a history of mild frontal headache for several weeks who then presented with a seizure. Removal was followed by a normal recovery. T1-weighted axial and coronal images (A and B, respectively) show findings consistent with a cavernous angioma but no hematoma in the adjacent parenchyma. These findings were confirmed at operation, but there was yellow staining in the adjacent cerebral tissue.

containing iron play important roles in inducing a seizure focus.

In our series, a seizure was the primary presenting symptom in 21 of 38 patients with lesions of the cerebrum (Table 93-1). Some of these patients also had other symptoms, usually headache, and almost half had an associated parenchymal hematoma. One patient was initially followed up by CT, and the lesion gradually enlarged. Patients with cavernous angiomas presenting with seizure are seen in Figures 93-1 (temporal), 93-2 and 93-3 (frontal), 93-4 (parietal), and 93-5 (motor-sensory cortex).

Patients Presenting with Headache

If the headache is a new symptom or is recurrent, it can often be related to the cavernous angioma. In these patients, MRI often shows a recent hemorrhage. In our series, seven of 10 patients had a parenchymal hemorrhage (Table 93-1). Surgery is indicated in most of these patients for reasons noted previously, except in patients with unacceptably high surgical risk because of a critical anatomic location. An example is illustrated in Figure 93-6.

Patients Presenting with Neurologic Deficit

In most patients with a progressive or acute neurologic deficit, there is an associated hematoma, and surgical removal of the lesion is indicated to prevent further neurologic damage and to help restore neurologic function. Some of these patients also have had headaches. In the patient whose

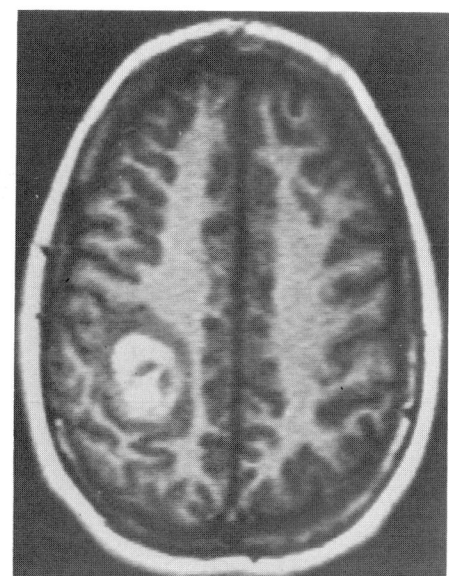

FIGURE 93-4. Parietal cavernous angioma in a 19-year-old man who presented with a seizure. Removal of the lesion was followed by full recovery of the patient. MRI axial T1-weighted image showed the circumscribed mottled core with adjacent hematoma and edema.

Table 93-1. LOCATION AND PRESENTING SYMPTOMS OF CAVERNOUS ANGIOMAS OF THE CEREBRUM

		Seizure		Headache		Neurologic Deficit	
	No.	Hem	No Hem	Hem	No Hem	Hem	No Hem
Frontal	16	3	6	4	2	1	0
Temporal	11	2	3	3	1	2	0
Parietal	10	4	2	0	0	4	0
Occipital	1	1	0	0	0	0	0
Total	38	10	11	7	3	7	0

Hem = hemorrhage into parenchyma.

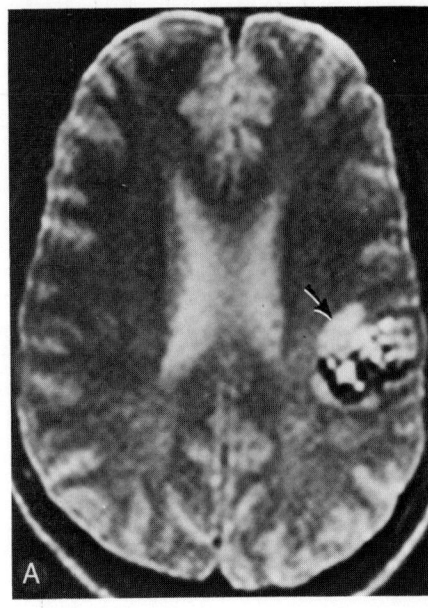
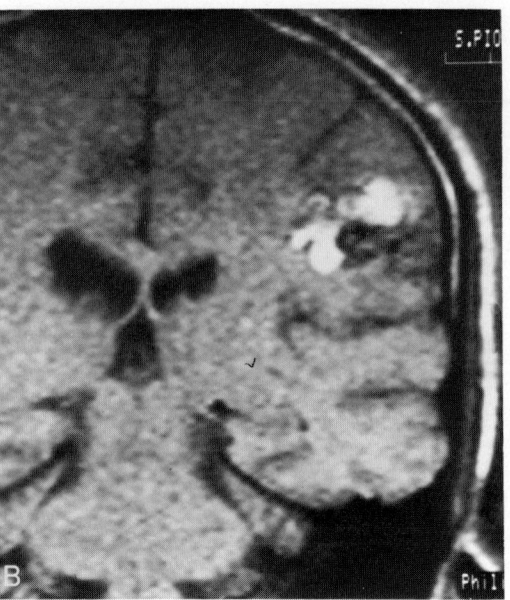

FIGURE 93–5. Frontoparietal cavernous angioma in a 36-year-old neurosurgeon who had a focal seizure involving the right face and hand. After another seizure occurred 4 months later, MRI axial T2-weighted and coronal T1-weighted images (A and B, respectively) show the cavernous angioma in the left inferior motor-sensory cortex and an area of new hemorrhage (arrow) that was not seen on the scan after the first seizure. The patient carefully considered the treatment options and concluded, as we had, that further hemorrhage entailed a risk of ending his career with damage to his dominant hand, and he wanted to reduce the probability of a seizure and end medication. Surgical removal was followed by full recovery, with no focal neurologic deficit and resumption of neurosurgical practice.

deficit is improving, observation can initially be done. However, if the surgical risks are judged to be relatively low, the lesion should be electively removed to prevent the effects of rehemorrhage. These patients are generally less than 60 years old and are at risk for repeat hemorrhages and neurologic deficits.[6] Involvement of the speech or motor-sensory cortex should not preclude the consideration of surgery, but a final decision should include an assessment of the surgical accessibility of the lesion.

All seven patients in our series presenting with a neurologic deficit had an associated hemorrhage. The indications for surgery were progressive neurologic deficit, sudden severe neurologic deficit, recurrent episodes of neurologic deficits lasting days to weeks, and history of a hemorrhage followed by recovery. An example is illustrated in Figure 93–7.

RESULTS

Several reports documented good results in the surgical treatment of cavernous angiomas of the cerebral hemispheres.[9, 19, 21, 28–33] With accessible lesions, surgical morbidity is minimal and mortality is almost zero. Chadduck and co-workers[34] reported a good outcome in patients with intraventricular cavernous hemangiomas.

The treatment of cavernous angiomas of the basal ganglia and thalamus has been controversial, and these lesions along with brainstem lesions may be considered dangerous to excise. Some practitioners suggest that surgery be considered when there are recurrent episodes of hemorrhage or progressive worsening neurologic deficit.[21] Lorenzana and associates[35] reported on a patient with a cavernous angioma that involved the anterior third of the lentiform nucleus and a

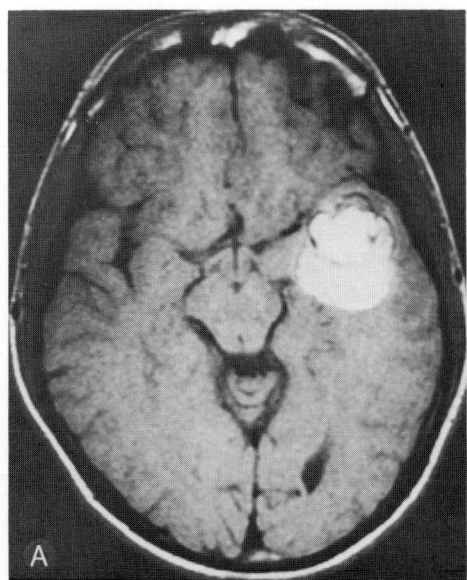
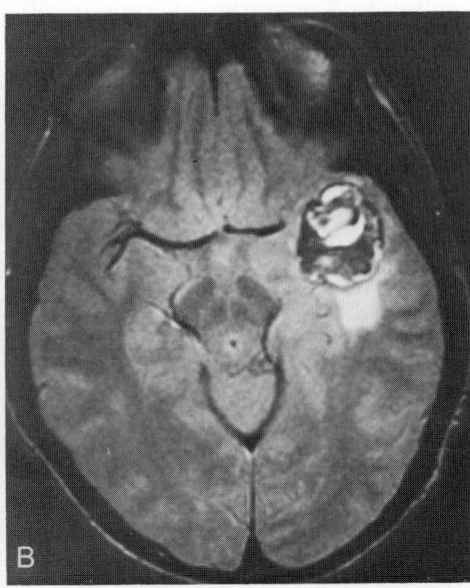

FIGURE 93–6. Temporal cavernous angioma in a 26-year-old man who had the onset of headache with weight lifting; the occurrence of the headaches increased. MRI showed a left temporal cavernous angioma with hemorrhage. Angiography showed no abnormal vascularity or stain. The patient was followed up, and his headaches persisted. Neurologic examination remained normal, but repeat MRI axial T1- and T2-weighted images (A and B, respectively) showed an increase in the size of the hematoma. Surgical removal of the left temporal cavernous angioma and hematoma was followed by a full recovery, with no speech difficulty.

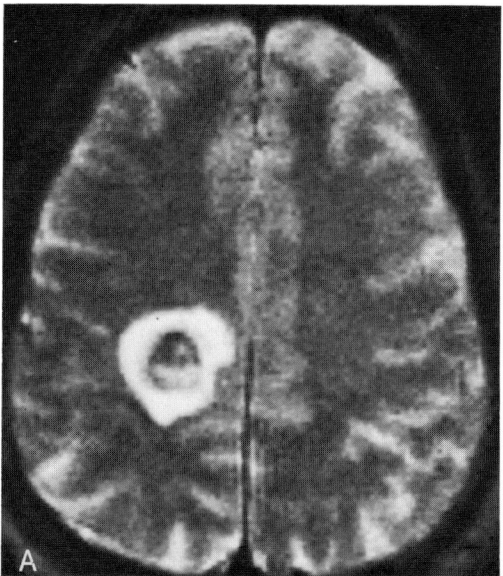
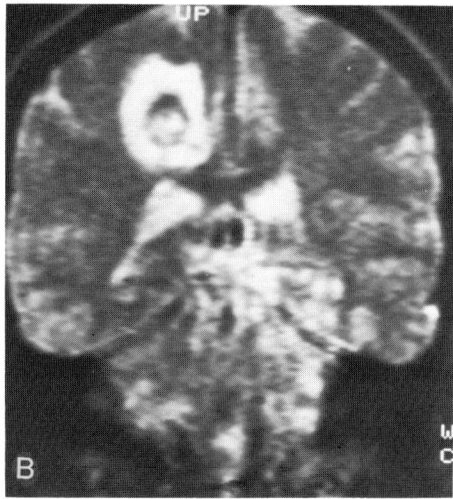

FIGURE 93–7. Parietal cavernous angioma in a 42-year-old man who had a brief episode of weakness in his left lower extremity 2 weeks before being seen. Nine days before admission, he developed a limp because of weakness in his left lower extremity. The next day, his foot became weaker and then he noted weakness in his left upper extremity. The progression of the weakness stopped when he was given steroids. MRI axial T2-weighted and coronal images (A and B, respectively) show a hemorrhage associated with a cavernous angioma deep in the right parietal region. Stereotactic localization was performed, and the lesion removed. Full recovery of the patient followed except for slight residual weakness in his foot.

large part of white matter anterior to the nucleus. The patient was cured by use of CT-assisted stereotactic craniotomy with an approach through the second frontal sulcus. However, in the report by Roda and colleagues[36] the results of treatment of cavernous angiomas in the thalamus were discouraging.

In our series of 38 patients with angiomas of the cerebrum outside the basal ganglia and thalamus, operative mortality was zero, and all patients had complete removal of the lesion (Table 93–2). One patient with a frontal cavernous angioma had an associated venous angioma that was not treated. All 38 patients were able to return to work. Thirty-six patients had a good outcome, were able to return to their previous level of activity, and in most cases, had normal results on neurologic examination. Two patients were classified as fair because of residual disability, one with persistence of a preoperative deficit and one with a new deficit, but both were able to work and carry on most of their previous activities.

Scott and colleagues[21] reported similar results in children. No patient presenting with seizure or headache worsened, and all but two patients who had cerebral hemisphere lesions made a good recovery.

CAVERNOUS ANGIOMAS OF THE CEREBELLUM

MANAGEMENT

The general management guidelines are similar to those outlined for the cerebral hemisphere. Surgery is indicated for most cerebellar cavernous angiomas because the patient has presented with a neurologic deficit, there is an associated hemorrhage, the morbidity of removal is low, and the risk of significant neurologic disability with repeat hemorrhage is high.

RESULTS

There were five patients with cavernous angiomas of the cerebellum in our series (Table 93–3). All made a good recovery. One patient, illustrated in Figure 93–8, had an associated venous angioma. At operation, a typical cavernous angioma was resected, and the large venous angioma was carefully preserved. The patient made an uneventful recovery.

CAVERNOUS ANGIOMAS OF THE BRAINSTEM

MANAGEMENT

Based on their experiences with eight patients (four had surgery), Falbusch and colleagues[37] recommended that cavernous angiomas of the brainstem that are associated with recurrent episodes of hemorrhage, MRI-confined diagnosis, negative angiographic results, and a progressive neurologic disability should have the lesion removed. Patients with recovery or stabilization of their neurologic deficit or those who are asymptomatic should be observed. The report by Zimmerman and associates[22] summarized 24 patients (16 who had surgery). They recommended that neurologically intact patients with cavernous angiomas that did not touch the pial surface should be observed. When the lesion was associated with repeated hemorrhages or progressive neurologic deficit and was close to the pial surface, surgery was

Table 93–2. RESULTS OF SURGICAL EXCISION OF CAVERNOUS ANGIOMAS OF THE CEREBRUM

	No.	Good†	Fair†	Poor†
Frontal	16	17	0	0
Temporal	11	10	1	0
Parietal	10	9	1*	0
Occipital	1	1	0	0
Total	38	36	2	0

*Persistent preoperative disability.
†Good, free of major neurologic deficit and able to return to previous activity; fair, independent but some neurologic disability; poor, dependent with significant neurologic disability.

Table 93-3. CAVERNOUS ANGIOMAS OF THE CEREBELLUM

Age/Sex	Location	Clinical Course	Outcome
53f	Vermis	Ataxia and headache	Good
47m	Medial cerebellar hemisphere (associated venous angioma)	Ataxia	Good
27f	Deep cerebellar hemisphere	Upper extremity incoordination	Good (mild residual effects)
35m	Medial cerebellar hemisphere	Gait instability	Good
30f	Deep cerebellar hemisphere; came to surface in cerebellopontine angle	Dizziness, nausea, and vomiting	Good

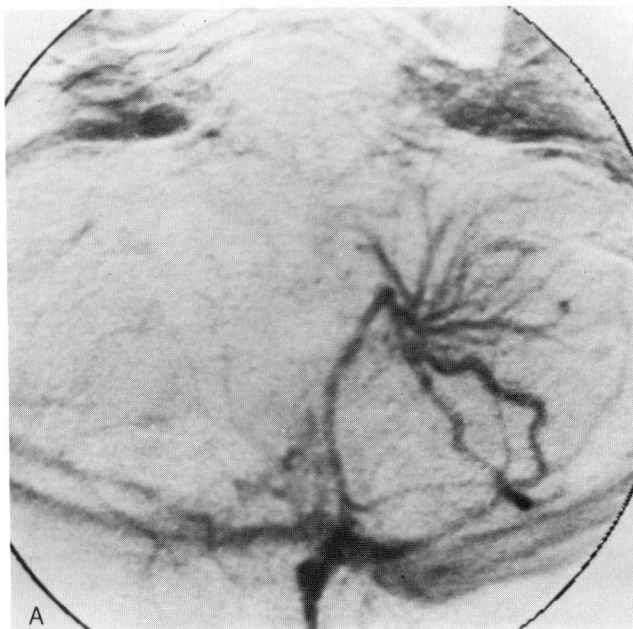
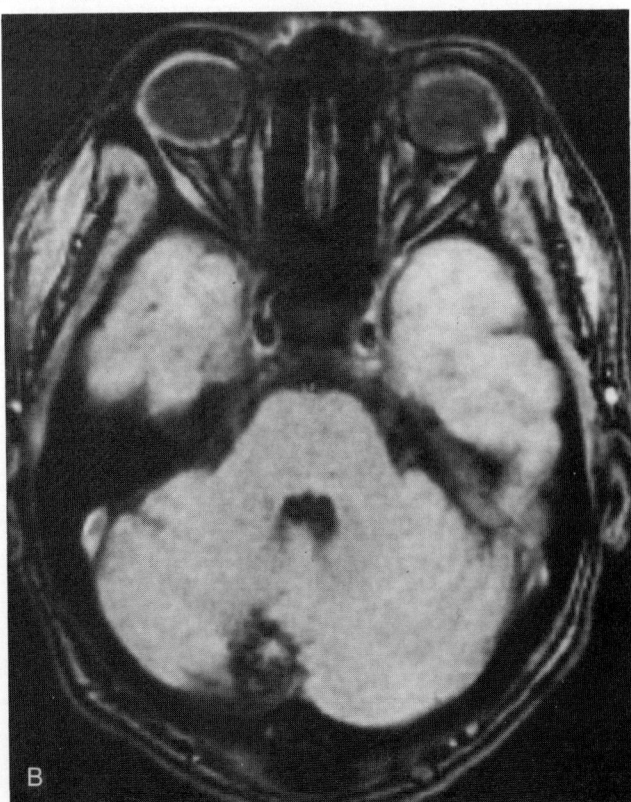
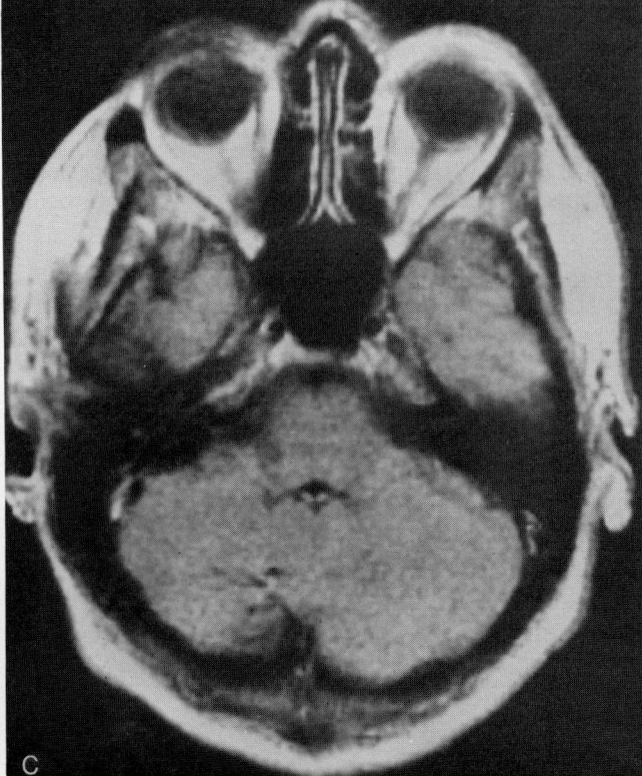

FIGURE 93-8. Cerebellar cavernous angioma in a 32-year-old woman who had sudden severe headache with nausea and vomiting and severe ataxia. At another hospital, a CT scan showed a right cerebellar hemorrhage, and angiography (A) showed no early-filling veins but a large venous angioma. The patient recovered, and her neurologic examination was normal.

Three months later, MRI axial T1-weighted images (B and C) showed evidence of the adjacent venous anomaly and the old hemorrhage with a mottled appearance within this area, supporting the diagnosis of cavernous angioma. Surgery was recommended because of the serious disability that resulted from the first hemorrhage. The venous angioma was not treated, and the patient had a good recovery.

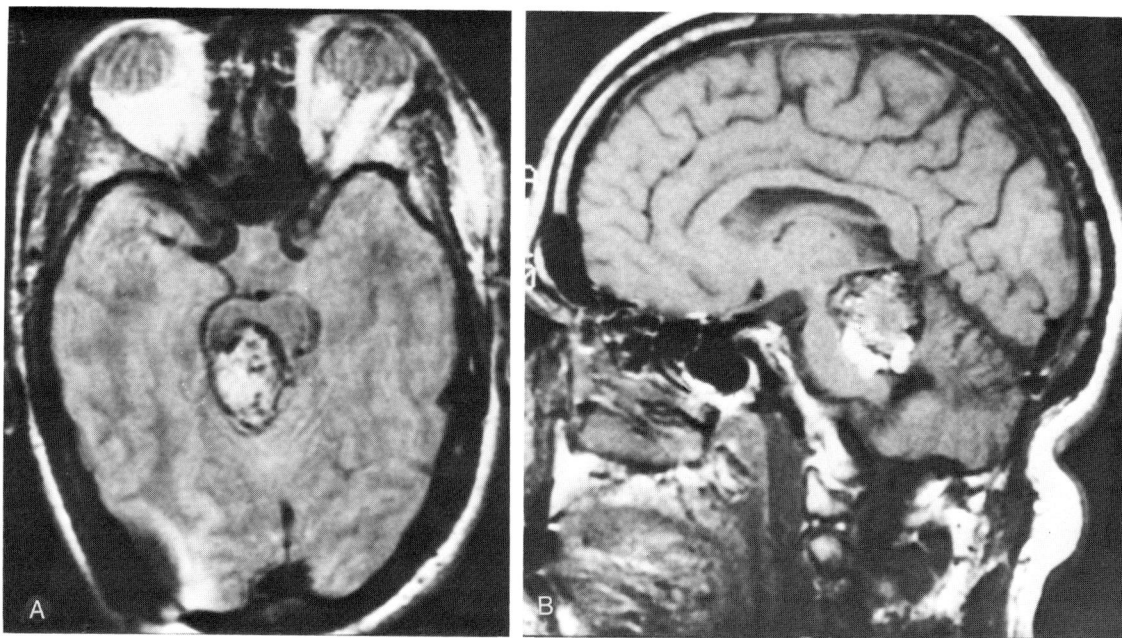

FIGURE 93–9. Brainstem cavernous angioma in a 27-year-old man treated with radiosurgery 4 years prior to presenting with increased dysarthria and ataxia. MRI T1-weighted axial (A) and sagittal (B) images show the lesion with new hemorrhage around the inferior margin. The patient declined to undergo surgery.

performed. They also suggested that any symptomatic lesion of the brainstem located superficially be considered for surgery if eloquent tissue could be spared.

In the past, some cavernous angiomas of the brainstem were treated with radiosurgery when recurrent hemorrhages and increased neurologic deficit were present. The patient whose MRI is illustrated in Figure 93–9 was treated for this reason several years ago. The lesion did not become smaller, and recurrent hemorrhage with worsening symptoms occurred. The patient declined surgical management.

The indication for operation in our patients was either progressive or recurrent neurologic symptoms (Table 93–4). The risk of surgery is probably lower when the lesion comes to the surface, obviating pial incision. The risk of surgery is probably higher when the lesion is large without associated hemorrhage or when it is densely calcified, making removal more difficult.

Careful study of the MRI aids in planning of the precise corridor of exposure and resection. Pontomedullary cavernous angiomas can be approached through a midline suboccipital craniotomy and exposure of the fourth ventricle. Lesions in the pontomesencephalic region are more difficult to manage but may be treated by a subtemporal or combined subtemporal-suboccipital approach. Falbusch and colleagues[37] used a supracerebellar infratentorial approach for midline pontomesencephalic lesions.

In our patients, three upper brainstem cavernous angiomas were removed by a subtemporal approach (Fig. 93–10); in one patient, a laterally placed brainstem lesion was approached through the cerebellopontine angle between the

Table 93–4. CAVERNOUS ANGIOMAS OF THE BRAINSTEM

Age/Sex	Location	Clinical Course	Outcome
37f	Pontomesencephalic	Two episodes of third and sixth nerve palsy, dysmetria, hemisensory loss, impaired walking with persistent disability	Slightly worse
34f	Pontomesencephalic	Acute hemiparesis, hemisensory loss, paresis of nerves IV, V, VI	Improved
34m	Upper pons	Sudden coma, decerebrate	Improved but disabled: ambulatory with help; hemiparesis, third nerve palsy
28m	Lateral pons	Headache, numbness and weakness in right extremities, facial anesthesia	Good: weakness gone, no change in facial sensation
50f	Pons	Progressive quadriparesis	Worse
16m	Pons	Hemiparesis, then coma	Improved but disabled: ambulatory with walker, paralysis of sixth through eighth nerves, dysarthria
55m	Pons	Mild hemiparesis, decreased sensation on face, ocular palsies	Improved: walks with care, facial numbness unchanged, ocular palsies resolved
49f	Obex	Ataxia and hiccups	Good: almost normal

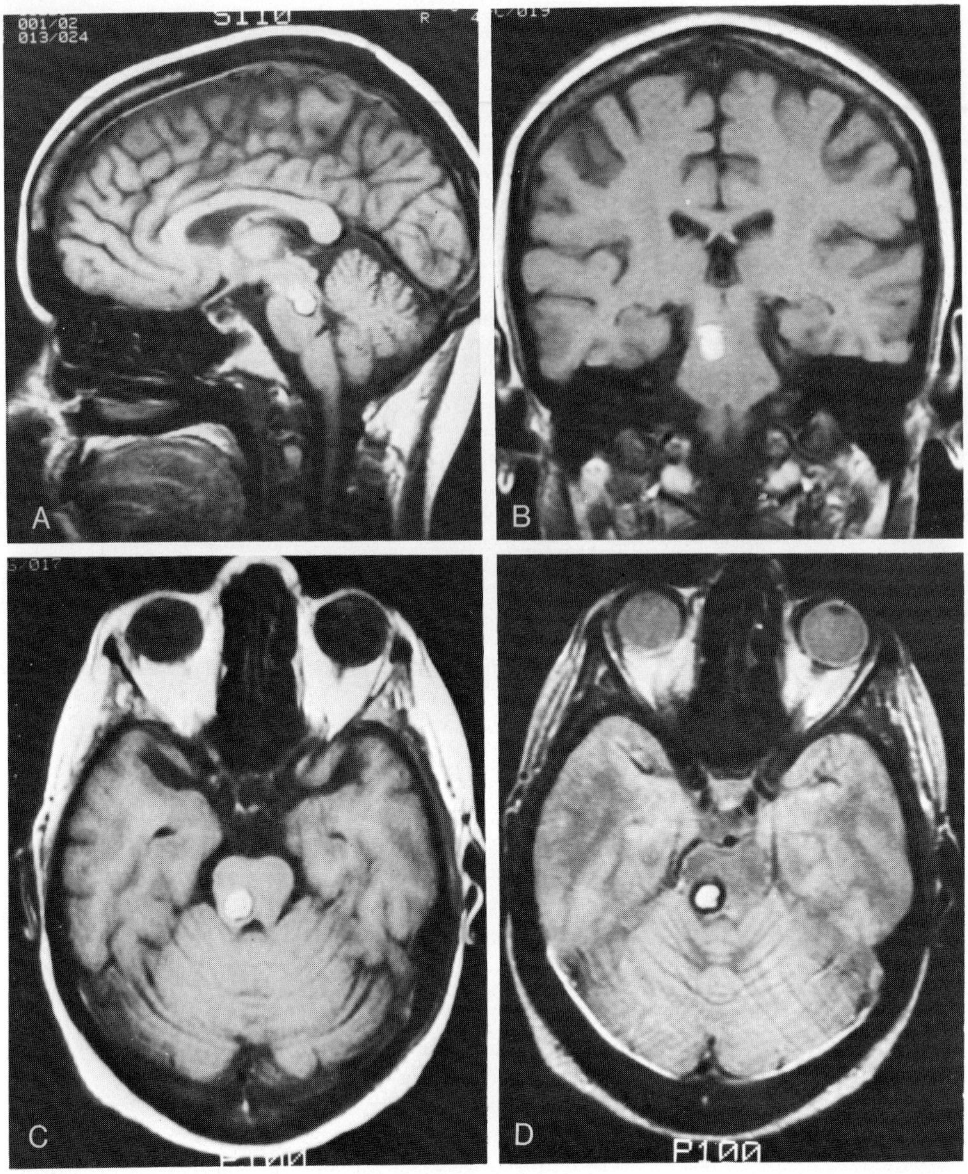

FIGURE 93–10. Upper brainstem cavernous angioma in a 37-year-old woman. Because of recurrent symptoms (second hemorrhage and inability to walk), the lesion was removed using a right subtemporal approach. MRI T1-weighted sagittal (A), coronal (B), and axial (C) and T2-weighted axial (D) images. Note that the lesion almost comes to the surface and is localized to one side.

fifth and seventh cranial nerves. In four patients with lesions in the pons or medulla, a midline exposure through the floor of the fourth ventricle was used.

RESULTS

Zimmerman and coworkers[22] reported that in 16 patients who underwent surgery, some had transient postoperative worsening, but the outcome in all except one was the same or improved. Isamat and Louesa[38] had six patients with cavernous angiomas in either the pons or medulla that were in contact with the floor of the fourth ventricle and were removed through the floor of the ventricle. All patients returned to their previous activities and had improvement in their neurologic deficits. Three other patients are being followed up because the lesion was completely surrounded by normal brainstem tissue. Falbusch and coworkers[37] noted improvement in preoperative symptoms after surgery in two patients with pontomedullary and two with pontomesencephalic cavernous angiomas. Kashiwagi and associates[39] reported on four patients treated surgically: all improved, as did the two patients reported on by Yoshimoto and Suzuki.[40] Other reports of single cases noted improvement, although temporary worsening can occur.[28, 41] However, not all reports have been so favorable.[21]

In our series of eight patients, six improved, but some residual neurologic deficits that had been present before surgery were usually present (Table 93–4). Two of these patients presented with a rapidly evolving neurologic deficit that led to coma. Both improved but still had disability. One patient presented with a progressive quadriparesis, and at operation, the large lesion was calcified and difficult to remove. She was much worse after operation, and she has a permanent disability. The other patient's gait was slightly worse than before surgery.

CAVERNOUS ANGIOMAS OF THE CRANIAL NERVES

MANAGEMENT

Cavernous angiomas have been reported to involve cranial nerves in the following locations: optic nerves and chiasm, third nerve, seventh nerve in the temporal bone, and seventh and eighth nerves in the internal auditory canal.[17, 42-46] The presenting symptoms relate to the nerve involved with the lesion. The MRI usually suggests the diagnosis, but in some patients, the pathology may not be evident until surgery. Surgery does not usually restore function in the involved nerve but is indicated to prevent hemorrhage into adjacent neural structures or, as in the patient with the facial nerve lesion, to remove the cavernous angioma and place a sural nerve graft, which may restore some function.

RESULTS

In this series of five patients (Table 93-5), one patient had a cavernous angioma in the optic chiasm. A field deficit developed during pregnancy as a result of hemorrhage and then improved, only to worsen after a second hemorrhage a few months after delivery. The field deficit improved somewhat after removal of the lesion. Malik and colleagues[17] reported on the partial removal of a cavernous angioma from the underside of the optic nerve and chiasm in one patient. Vision did not improve, but no further symptoms occurred.

Two patients in this series had lesions involving the seventh and eighth nerves in the internal auditory canal. Involvement in the internal auditory canal has been reported in five patients, including the two in our series.[43, 46] The eighth nerve could not be saved in any patient, but reasonable facial nerve function remained in three. When the facial nerve cannot be saved, a nerve graft is placed at operation. In one patient in our series, the angioma involved the seventh nerve in the temporal bone. The cavernous angioma and nerve were removed, and a sural nerve graft was placed.

The last patient had a lesion of the third cranial nerve,[44] which was extensively involved and was resected to remove the cavernous angioma. The case reported by Scott was treated in the same way.[45]

CAVERNOUS ANGIOMAS OF THE SPINAL CORD

CLINICAL PRESENTATION

Through 1991, 36 patients with 37 spinal lesions were reported, including six of our patients.[10] The series included 25 (69 percent) females and 11 (31 percent) males. The locations of the lesions along the spinal axis were cervical medullary junction in three (8 percent), cervical in 12 (32 percent), thoracic in 20 (54 percent), lumbar spinal cord in one (3 percent), and conus medullaris in one (3 percent). Two patients had a history of familial cavernous angioma, four had a cavernous angioma at some other site in the central nervous system, and one had a second spinal lesion.

The ages ranged from 12 to 62 years, and the most common age for the appearance of initial symptoms was in the fourth decade. Four clinical categories of symptoms were identified:

1. Thirteen patients presented with episodes of neurologic deterioration with variable degrees of neurologic recovery between episodes. The episodes lasted hours to days. The interval between events was often months to years.

2. Twelve patients had a clinical course characterized by slowly progressive neurologic deterioration. The duration of the progression was usually several years. Two patients had discrete episodes of gradual worsening separated by many years.

3. Eight patients had an acute onset of symptoms followed by neurologic worsening over several days.

4. Three patients had the acute onset of mild symptoms, followed by weeks or months of deterioration of neurologic function.

MANAGEMENT

The diagnosis of cavernous angiomas of the spinal cord is established by the characteristic MRI appearance (Fig. 93-11). There are no reports of long-term follow-up of untreated patients with cavernous angioma of the spinal cord. From the history obtained from symptomatic patients, it is evident that in some patients, there can be intervals of up to several years between episodes of recurrent neurologic problems that presumably result from hemorrhage. In these intervals, a neuro-

Table 93-5. CAVERNOUS ANGIOMAS OF THE CRANIAL NERVES

Age/Sex	Location	Clinical Course	Outcome
33f	Optic chiasm	Developed visual field deficit during pregnancy, second hemorrhage after delivery	Good: residual visual field deficit
25m	Third nerve	Progressive third nerve palsy	Good: third nerve palsy
53m	Seventh nerve	Progressive facial weakness	Good: seventh nerve paralysis
27f	Seventh and eighth nerves in internal auditory canal and posterior fossa	Fullness in ear, facial twitch	Good: loss of hearing, facial nerve graft placed with some recovery
42m	Seventh and eighth nerves in internal auditory canal	Decreased hearing, progressive facial weakness	Good: loss of hearing, facial nerve graft placed with some recovery

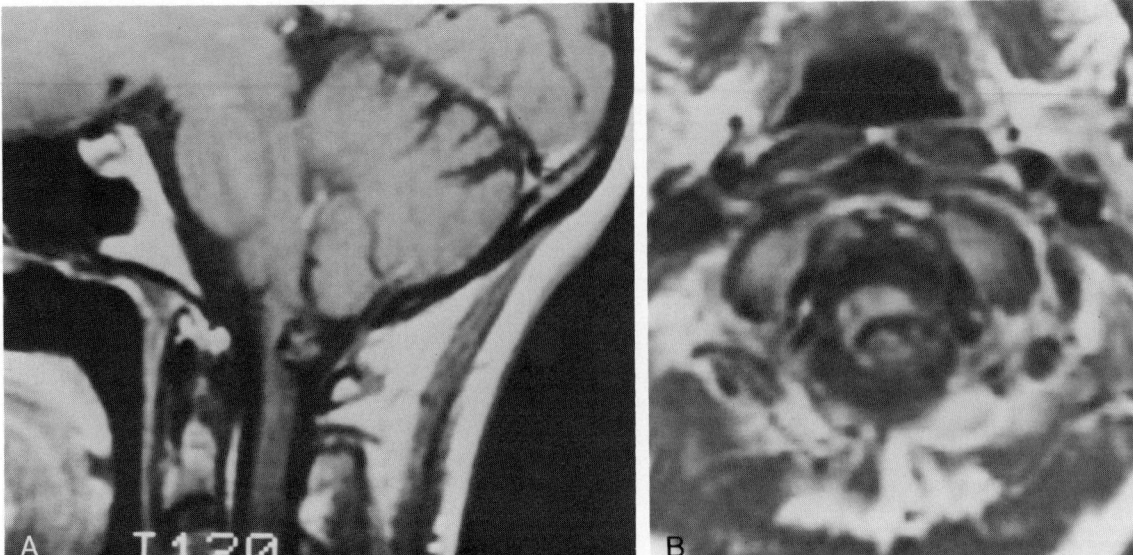

FIGURE 93–11. Cervical medullary junction cavernous angioma in a 36-year-old woman who had the onset of generalized headache 4 months before surgery. Twenty-four hours later, she noted numbness in the left lateral leg that progressed over the next week to involve the entire left lower extremity; this condition improved. CT scan of the head was normal. Two weeks later, she noted difficulty jogging because of discoordination in the left lower extremity. MRI T1-weighted sagittal (A) and axial (B) images show a posteriorly placed lesion involving the midline and left side of the cervical medullary junction consistent with a cavernous angioma; the patient was followed up. Ten days prior to admission, she had the onset of nausea and vomiting and increased numbness and weakness on the left side of her body. Complete excision of the lesion was followed by improvement in the left lower extremity function, temporary worsening of position sense in the left hand, and numbness in the left upper extremity. Subsequently, she had a good recovery, was able to jog, and returned to work.

logic deficit is stable or the patient is free of symptoms. Also, in recurrent hemorrhages, the neurologic deficit often increases and does not always fully recover.

In most patients, lesions present on the dorsal or dorsolateral aspect of the spinal cord. We usually recommend surgery. The findings at operation are similar to those found at operation in cavernous angioma of the brain. A well-defined gliotic plane exists around the lesion, which aids in the microsurgical removal. The use of fine sutures in the pia to retract the spinal cord when the lesion is deep, a fine-regu-

Table 93–6. CAVERNOUS ANGIOMA OF THE SPINAL CORD

Age/Sex	Location	Clinical Course	Outcome
36f	Cervicomedullary junction	Headache, acute left lower extremity numbness 4 months pta; improved; discoordination of left lower extremity while running; nausea and vomiting with left body numbness and weakness 10 days pta	Improved: increased loss of position sense in left hand, ambulating and returned to work
31f	C3-4	Acute pain, Brown-Séquard syndrome 16 months pta; subtotal removal 13 months; recurrent pain, weakness, spasticity 4 months pta	Improved: ambulatory, minimal numbness right hand
51f	C4	Acute weakness in right arm with Brown-Séquard 13 years pta; headache, dysesthesia in right side 5 months pta; acute right arm and leg weakness	Improved: fully functional at 2 years
43f	C5	Acute right arm pain and weakness 5 years pta with gradual recovery; recurrent episode of pain 2 years pta; acute numbness and weakness in right arm and leg	Improved: temporarily worse but ambulatory 2 weeks after surgery
52m	T3-4	Mild right foot weakness and numbness 9 years pta; progressive weakness and spasticity of both lower extremities, loss of posterior column function, bowel and bladder dysfunction 6 months pta	Improved: some residual posterior column dysfunction, walks with cane, working
38f	T12	Acute onset of foot numbness, progressive weakness and numbness 3 years pta; rapidly progressive Brown-Séquard 1 month pta	Improved: increased strength, ambulatory

pta = prior to admission.

lated suction, and microbipolar forceps facilitate the dissection. Gross total removal of the cavernous angioma should be the goal of surgical treatment.

RESULTS

In our series of cavernous angiomas of the spinal cord, there were six patients ranging in age from 31 to 52 years (Table 93-6).[10] The lesion was completely removed in all six patients. On follow-up, all patients were ambulatory, and their conditions were as good as or better than before the operation. One patient had a previous subtotal removal at another institution and had a further small hemorrhage with a neurologic deficit that did not fully recover. In two of our patients, the cavernous angioma protruded from the dorsal aspect of the spinal cord. In the other four, a myelotomy was required, and in three of these patients the lesion projected more to one side, and a myelotomy was placed in the dorsal root entry zone. Anson and Spetzler[47] also reported a good outcome in six patients with intramedullary spinal cord cavernous malformations.

SUMMARY

The management of patients with cavernous angioma continues to evolve. Our current recommendations for management are as follows:

Patients who are asymptomatic are observed.

Patients with acute severe or progressive neurologic deficits are operated on.

Patients presenting with a seizure are usually operated on, but some are observed, depending on the factors discussed in this chapter.

Patients with a single hemorrhage in the cerebrum, cerebellum, or spinal cord are usually operated on. When the hemorrhage is in the brainstem, thalamus, or basal ganglia, the patients are observed.

Patients with a recurrent hemorrhage are usually operated on, but there are exceptions when the lesion is in a deep area with high surgical risk.

Acknowledgment

Portions of this chapter are reproduced from Ojemann RG, Crowell RM, Ogilvy CS: Management of cranial and spinal cavernous angiomas. Clin Neurosurg 40:98–123, 1993.

REFERENCES

1. McCormick WF: The pathology of vascular ("arteriovenous") malformations. J Neurosurg 24:807–816, 1966
2. Rengachary SS, Kalyan-Raman UP: Other cranial intradural angiomas, in Wilkins RH, Rengachary SS (eds): Neurosurgery, vol 2. New York, McGraw-Hill, 1985, pp 1465–1472
3. Russell DS, Rubinstein LJ: Pathology of Tumors of the Nervous System. London, Edward Arnold, 1959, pp 79–83
4. Ogilvy CS, Heros RC, Ojemann RG, New PFJ: Angiographically occult arteriovenous malformations. J Neurosurg 69:350–355, 1988
5. Ojemann RG, Heros RG, Crowell RM: Surgical Management of Cerebrovascular Disease. Baltimore, Williams & Wilkins 1988, pp 401–403
6. Tung H, Giannotoa SL, Chandrasoma PT, et al: Recurrent intraparenchymal hemorrhage from angiographically occult vascular malformations. J Neurosurg 73:174–180, 1990
7. Wakai S, Ueda Y, Inoh S, et al: Angiographically occult angiomas: A report of thirteen cases with analysis of the cases documented in the literature. Neurosurgery 17:549–556, 1985
8. Wilkins RH: Natural history of intracranial vascular malformations: A review. Neurosurgery 16:421–430, 1985
9. Wilson CB: Cryptic vascular malformations. Clin Neurosurg 38:49–84, 1992
10. Ogilvy CS, Louis DN, Ojemann RG: Intramedullary cavernous angiomas of the spinal cord: Clinical presentation, pathologic features and surgical management. Neurosurgery 31:219–230, 1992
11. Robinson JR Jr, Awad IA, Little JR: Natural history of the cavernous angioma. J Neurosurg 75:709–719, 1991
12. Curling OD Jr, Kelly DL, Elster AD, Craven TE: An analysis of the natural history of cavernous angiomas. J Neurosurg 75:702–708, 1991
13. Pozzati E, Giuliani G, Nuzzo G, Poppi M: The growth of cerebral cavernous angiomas. Neurosurgery 25:92–97, 1989
14. Rigamonti D, Drayer BP, Johnson PC, et al: The MRI appearance of cavernous malformations (angiomas). J Neurosurg 67:518–524, 1987
15. Roda JM, Carceller F, Perez-Higueras A, et al: Encapsulated intracerebral hematoma: A defined entity. J Neurosurg 78:829–833, 1993
16. Hayman LA, Evans RA, Ferrell RE, et al: Familial cavernous angiomas: Natural history and genetic study over a 5-year period. Am J Med Genet 11:147–160, 1982
17. Malik S, Cohen BH, Robinson J, et al: Progressive vision loss. A rare manifestation of familial cavernous angiomas. Arch Neurol 49:170–173, 1992
18. Rigamonti D, Hadley MN, Drayer BP, et al: Cerebral cavernous malformations. Incidence and familial occurrence. N Engl J Med 319:343–347, 1988
19. Voigt K, Yasargil MG: Cerebral cavernous haemangiomas or cavernomas. Incidence, pathology, localization, diagnosis, clinical features and treatment. Review of the literature and report of an unusual case. Neurochirurgia (Stuttg) 19:59–68, 1976
20. Simard JM, Garcia-Bengochea F, Ballinger WE Jr, et al: Cavernous angioma: A review of 126 collected and 12 new clinical cases. Neurosurgery 18:162–172, 1986
21. Scott RM, Barnes P, Kupsky W, Adelman LS: Cavernous angiomas of the central nervous system in children. J Neurosurg 76:38–46, 1992
22. Zimmerman RS, Spetzler RF, Lee KS, et al: Cavernous malformations of the brain stem. J Neurosurg 75:32–39, 1991
23. Lunsford LD, Kondziolka D, Bissonette DJ, et al: Stereotactic radiosurgery of brain vascular malformations. Neurosurg Clin North Am 3:79–98, 1992
24. Robinson JR Sr, Awad IA, Magdinee M, Paranandi L: Factors predisposing to clinical disability in patients with cavernous malformations of the brain. Neurosurgery 32:730–736, 1993
25. Golfinos JG, Wascher TM, Zabramskik JM, et al: The management of unruptured intracranial vascular malformation. Barrow Neurol Inst Q 8:2–11, 1992
26. Fabrikant JI, Levy RP, Steinberg GK, et al: Charged-particle radiosurgery for intracranial vascular malformations. Neurosurg Clin North Am 3:99–139, 1992
27. Alexander E III, Loeffler SS: Radiosurgery using a modified linear accelerator. Neurosurg Clin North Am 3:167–190, 1992
28. Giombini S, Morello G: Cavernous angiomas of the brain. Account of fourteen personal cases and review of the literature. Acta Neurochir (Wien) 40:61–82, 1978
29. Little JR, Awad IA, Jones SC, Ebrahim ZY: Vascular pressures and cortical blood flow in cavernous angioma of the brain. J Neurosurg 73:555–559, 1990
30. Schneider RC, Liss L: Cavernous hemangiomas of the cerebral hemispheres. J Neurosurg 15:392–399, 1958
31. Tagle P, Huete I, Mendez J, Zee CS: Intracranial cavernous angioma: Presentation and management. J Neurosurg 64:720–723, 1986
32. Vaquero J, Leunda G, Martinez R, Bravo G: Cavernomas of the brain. Neurosurgery 12:208–210, 1983
33. Yamasaki T, Hande H, Yamashita J, et al: Intracranial and orbital cavernous angiomas. J Neurosurg 64:197–208, 1986
34. Chadduck WM, Binet EF, Farrell FW Jr, et al: Intraventricular cavernous hemangioma: Report of three cases and review of the literature. Neurosurgery 16:189–197, 1985

35. Lorenzana L, Cabezudo JM, Porras LF, et al: Focal dystonia secondary to cavernous angioma of the basal ganglia: Case report and review of the literature. Neurosurgery 31:1108–1112, 1992
36. Roda JM, Alvarez F, Isla A, Blazquez G: Thalamic cavernous malformations. J Neurosurg 72:642–649, 1990
37. Falbusch R, Strauss C, Huk W, et al: Surgical removal of pontomesencephalic cavernous hemangioma. Neurosurgery 26:449–457, 1990
38. Isamat F, Louesa G: Cavernous angioma of the brain stem. Neurosurg Clin North Am 4:507–518, 1993
39. Kashiwagi S, van Loveren HR, Tew JM Jr, et al: Diagnosis and treatment of vascular brain-stem malformations. J Neurosurg 72:27–34, 1990
40. Yoshimoto T, Suzuki J: Radical surgery on cavernous angioma of the brain stem. Surg Neurol 26:72–78, 1986
41. Seifert V, Gaab MR: Laser-assisted microsurgical extirpation of a brain stem cavernoma: Case report. Neurosurgery 25:986–990, 1989
42. Corboy JR, Galetta SL: Familial cavernous angiomas manifesting with an acute chiasmal syndrome. Am J Ophthalmol 108:245–250, 1989
43. Matias-Guiu X, Alejo M, Sole T, et al: Cavernous angiomas of the cranial nerves. J Neurosurg 73:620–622, 1990
44. Ogilvy CS, Pakzaban P, Lee JM: Oculomotor nerve cavernous angioma in a patient with Robert's syndrome. Surg Neurol 33:39–47, 1993
45. Scott RM: Third nerve palsy in a 14-year-old boy due to cavernous hemangioma of the third nerve, in Raimond AJ (ed): Concepts in Pediatric Neurosurgery. New York, Karger, 1983, pp 100–107
46. Sundaresan N, Ellen T, Civic I: Hemangiomas of the internal auditory canal. Surg Neurol 6:119–121, 1976
47. Anson JA, Spetzler RF: Surgical resection of intramedullary spinal cord cavernous malformations. J Neurosurg 78:446–451, 1993

CHAPTER 94

Surgical Management of Arteriovenous Malformations in Children

Robin P. Humphreys

The child's cerebral arteriovenous malformation (AVM) usually declares itself with a dramatic hemorrhagic ictus with no forewarning signals. At such a time, although the clinical profile may clearly suggest that the patient has suffered a spontaneous intracranial bleed, one must not conclude that it has occurred from an aneurysm rupture. In adults, a ruptured saccular aneurysm would be 6.5 times more likely than an AVM to account for that hemorrhage.[1] Whether the ratio is reversed in children is a moot point. Hourihan and colleagues,[2] in a review of 167 patients aged 20 years and younger, noted that subarachnoid hemorrhage (SAH) was caused by aneurysm twice as often as by AVM. Their paper includes the work of other authors studying the problem of pediatric SAH.[1, 3, 4] In a total review of 478 such patients, ruptured aneurysm accounted for 40 percent of children's SAHs and 26 percent of AVMs; no lesion was defined in 31 percent. This cumulative experience might appear to be at odds with the results of the Cooperative Study of Intracranial Aneurysms and Subarachnoid Hemorrhage, in which 33 percent of AVMs associated with hemorrhage occurred before the age of 20 years, in contrast with only 1.5 percent of intracranial aneurysms becoming symptomatic in that same period.[1, 5]

The material reviewed in this chapter is taken from the experience at The Hospital for Sick Children, Toronto.[6] This hospital serves as a widespread referral base exclusively for the care of children aged up to 18 years, and thus the intake of this particular problem reflects the general population's needs. In 26 children with ruptured intracranial aneurysm, SAH was the presenting symptom, whereas 104 children bled from their AVM and presented as subarachnoid or intraventricular hemorrhage (SAH/IVH). In our opinion, rupture of an AVM is almost four times more likely to be the cause of the SAH/IVH than is a burst aneurysm.[6]

CLASSIFICATION

This chapter considers only brain AVMs of the classical type, that is, those representing a structural defect in the formation of the primitive arteriolar-capillary network normally interposed between brain arteries and veins. Cavernous angioma, developmental venous anomalies, and the myriad of tortuous arteriovenous anomalies that accompany the Galen malformation are not discussed.

CLINICAL FEATURES

Matson declared the AVM "the most frequent abnormality of intracranial circulation in childhood" and reported on his experience with 34 patients.[7] Since then, numerous investigators have examined the problem of symptomatic AVMs in children under 19 years of age.[2, 4, 8–16] A greater percentage of children than adults experience hemorrhage as their first symptom, whereas relatively larger numbers of adults display the presumed ischemic symptoms of headache, dementia, and slowly progressive neurologic dysfunction. Neither surgery nor histopathologic examination of excised tissues can always reveal just where the hemorrhage originated. Certainly, deficiencies exist in some vessel walls, possibly making them liable to rupture, yet other abnormal channels are thickened.[17] The smaller AVMs bleed, and generally, less violent parenchymal disruption occurs after AVM hemorrhage than with burst aneurysms.[18]

Spontaneous subarachnoid or, more frequently, intracerebral-intraventricular bleeding is the most common cause of symptoms experienced by children. In our review, 79 percent of children experienced spontaneous intracranial hemorrhage, as determined by the syndrome of headache with bloody spinal fluid or blood clot recognized on computed tomography (CT) or recovered at operation or autopsy.[6] The ictus is often explosive, and the previously well child screams out about sudden headache. An unusual number of AVMs bleed during periods of quietude or even sleep.[1] Not surprisingly, therefore, subarachnoid grading reflects the critical nature of the child's condition at the time of first assessment (Table 94–1). Altered consciousness, meningism, and appropriate lateralized motor and sensory signs are present.

Epilepsy, which presumably results from gliosis of brain because of chronic ischemia adjacent to the arteriovenous shunt, occurs as a presenting symptom in 20 to 67 percent of adult patients with AVM.[5, 7, 19–21] Determining the proper treatment for a patient who has had one or two convulsions from an AVM exclusive of frank SAH is a challenge. Recent reports indicate, however, that more than 70 percent of patients with epilepsy related to AVM remain seizure free (or

Table 94–1. ADMISSION SUBARACHNOID HEMORRHAGE
GRADE VERSUS LONG-TERM CLINICAL OUTCOME
($n = 102$)

SAH Grade	Number of Patients Normal	Neurologic Deficit	Dead
I	11	3	1
II	15	4	2
III	22	5	1
IV	9	6	3
V	1	0	19

SAH = subarachnoid hemorrhage.

nearly so) when the associated epileptogenic tissue is excised.[20] A chronic seizure disorder associated with a subsequently defined AVM occurred in 12 percent of our patients.

The remaining children who had neither hemorrhage nor epilepsy in their profiles had presenting symptoms of delayed development or signs of cerebral ischemia, congestive heart failure, and chronic headache. Four children had an incidentally discovered malformation.

PREOPERATIVE EVALUATION AND MANAGEMENT

When a child is seen with a typical headache-hemorrhage ictus, the surgeon should proceed directly with CT and cerebral arteriography. The CT head scan outlines the blood clot and calcification, if present, and on enhanced study may detail the dilated feeding and draining vascular channels and large, blood-containing varices. It thus provides a clue to the site and side of the brain to be studied first with cerebral arteriography.

By means of selective internal carotid and vertebral artery injections, the numbers and locations of the arterial feeders can be examined by arteriography. The numbers of arterial contributors can be determined by properly timed sequential films processed with subtraction techniques. Seldom is a malformation served by only one arterial channel. There may be only one major artery contributing to the lesion, but the surgeon should anticipate any number of minor vessels coming from pial or deep perforating sources.

However, the venous drainage in a child's AVM is frequently through a solitary channel by either a large cortical vein or the deep venous system, and it is usually precisely defined on arteriography. The overall architecture of the lesion is carefully studied on the arteriogram, and its operability is thus determined.

Some vascular malformations are angiographically cryptic, that is, they are not demonstrated on angiography.[22] These lesions, often in the distribution of the middle cerebral artery, are usually small. Meticulous processing of the pathologic material uncovers the vascular malformation. Hence, close follow-up must be maintained for all children with an intracerebral hemorrhage small enough to be treated conservatively; these patients may harbor an occult malformation.

Whether or not the incidence of cryptic malformations will decline if all such patients are assessed also with magnetic resonance imaging (MRI) remains to be seen. The ability of this technique to detect small vascular anomalies almost reaches the intimidating. By the same token, the surgeon may have some difficulty correlating the MRI detail of an obvious AVM at operation with the exposed tissues. Hence, MRI examination is not mandatory in every circumstance, and indeed some patients are too desperately ill to have the procedure completed.

Ninety percent of the malformations are found supratentorially, most typically within the distribution of the middle cerebral artery.[5, 23] However, any intracranial artery can be associated with the malformation, and in our experience, 24 percent of the lesions were found below the tentorium.[24]

Inasmuch as the presenting symptom of 79 percent of the lesions in children is spontaneous intracranial hemorrhage, urgent neurodiagnostic assessments and operative care are usually undertaken to identify and release the associated clot. Because AVM surgery can be tedious and protracted, the malformation excision should be planned as an elective procedure whenever possible. Thus, if only SAH occurred, or if the intracerebral hemorrhage is small and the patient's condition is stable, interval surgery may be staged after a few days' wait. During that time, the child's condition is monitored appropriately. Cerebral vasospasm is seldom a problem in children with AVMs, but rebleeding during the interval often is. Thus, antispasm and antihypertensive pharmacologic measures are not required. If the operation can possibly be delayed for 3 to 7 days after the hemorrhage, then the surgeon will be rewarded with a properly prepared patient whose relaxed brain contains a liquefying hematoma.

A number of children's AVMs bleed into the ventricular system. Although this effect presents a dramatic CT appearance, the blood may actually be vented into that system. If draining the ventricular cerebrospinal fluid is deemed necessary, the inserted catheter for an external drainage device must be placed remote to the site of the malformation. The presence of ventricular blood usually occurs when the tail of the malformation extends into the choroid plexus and picks up choroidal arterial supply.

The same urgency is not present for the 21 percent of patients whose presenting symptom is something other than spontaneous hemorrhage. The children in this group have undergone a traditional assessment for headaches, seizures, and developmental delay, and the malformation has been discovered during the testing or even during elective surgery. The clinical challenge is to determine in advance whether surgical obliteration of the malformation will influence the headache, seizure, or developmental problem and whether, therefore, it should even be undertaken.[25, 26]

NATURAL HISTORY AND MANAGEMENT DECISIONS

The criteria for patient selection for AVM therapy are still controversial. Understandably, matched trials of nonsurgical and surgical management programs for patients with cerebral AVM have not been reported. Although certain conservatism has been expressed in earlier studies,[25, 27–31] it is now recognized that with advances in surgical and anesthetic technology, the indications for, and success with, surgery have broadened. Some argue that the current improved results depend more on the selection criteria than on surgical technique.[25] The matter is now further complicated by additional treatment options—proton-beam irradiation, stereotactic cryosurgery, and various forms of endovascular embolization.

The natural history of AVMs in children is not well understood. In our series, 79 percent of the lesions presented with hemorrhage, a rate that is higher than that reported for adults.[5, 32] By defining our population as patients aged up to 18 years, we do not imply that differences exist between AVMs in patients of 17 versus 20 years of age, but rather between the populations of children and adults. Celli and associates[18] reported a hemorrhage rate of over 80 percent for AVMs less than 2 cm in diameter. Mori and colleagues[14] concluded that the prognosis was less favorable in children with AVMs than in adults and described a higher mortality rate in younger patients that resulted from hemorrhage. Gerosa and colleagues[10] reported that the primary hemorrhage was fatal in 5.4 percent of their patients, but that rebleeding occurred in 29 percent, and it carried a grim prognosis.

The higher mortality rate from AVM hemorrhage in children (25 percent in our series; the Cooperative Study reported an adult mortality rate of between 6 and 10 percent[5]), may have several causes. First, there is a higher incidence of AVM in the posterior cranial fossa, where the effects of hemorrhage are more critical. A significant difference was found between the number of posterior fossa AVMs in our series of children[6] and that of the adult series of Jomin and coworkers.[33] Similarly, infratentorial AVMs were present in only 32 of 453 patients in the Cooperative Study; again, this difference was significant. We believe that the hemodynamic compressive or hemorrhagic effects of a critically located infratentorial AVM lead to an earlier symptomatic onset than do most supratentorial malformations. Second, hemorrhage from a pediatric AVM may be more severe than an adult AVM. Celli and colleagues[18] stated that cerebral hemorrhages in children show more violent and massive bleeding, demonstrated by a higher frequency of intraparenchymal and intraventricular hemorrhage. No evidence exists to suggest that the vessels of a "younger" AVM are more fragile than those in the adult. Finally, there is some evidence that smaller AVMs are more inclined to hemorrhage than are the larger ones.[19, 34] In fact, children's vascular malformations tend to be small rather than large and are secreted in unusual or awkward locations.

A large series of adult patients with AVM has indicated that the risk for rehemorrhage is 2 to 4 percent per year, independent of prior hemorrhage.[34–40] Risk estimates were provided by large series of patients treated conservatively. The lack of prior large pediatric AVM series and the small number of patients who did not have resection in our series prohibit a reasonable estimate of the rebleeding risk in children.

These treatment considerations in children clearly become academic when as many as 80 percent present with cerebral hemorrhage, and usually from a smaller rather than a larger lesion. For most children, the treatment decision is determined by the presence of a hematoma, its mass effect, and its relationship to, and the location of, the abnormal vascular channels. Very few such malformations are not explored.

REGIONAL SURGICAL ANATOMY

The conglomeration of turgid, tortuous vessels covered by opacified and thickened arachnoid on the brain's surface is easily recognizable as the classic AVM. Sometimes, the malformation is hidden in a sulcus or the subcortical tissue and is served by a dilated or unusually straightened artery running a nonanatomic course or by a red draining vein striking out toward an adjacent venous sinus. These manifestations may be its only surface hallmarks. The most reliable surface markings are the veins because, regardless of their origin, all cross the surface at some point.[41] The nearby cerebral convolutions show variable degrees of atrophy, and local rusty staining may be present from previous hemorrhage. The tough texture of the adjacent gray and white matter results from gliosis, which permits dissection of the lesion through this relatively inert tissue.

Although some malformations are globular in shape, most describe a course to the subjacent ventricle in an inverted wedge-shaped fashion. The component vessels show variation in their numbers, caliber, and the thickness of their walls. Venous tortuosity, intimal thickening, arteriolization of veins, and evidence of hemorrhage are indicative of the long-standing hemodynamic consequences within the malformation. Vessels with marked saccular dilatations are usually venous in origin.[42]

CHOICE OF SURGICAL APPROACH

The ideal treatment for a brain AVM is its total removal.[7, 43] Excision has now been achieved in almost all eloquent regions of brain (motor, basal ganglia, and brainstem) as well as in less critical areas. Thus, except for lesions that penetrate the brainstem or basal ganglia, it is not so much the anatomic location of the lesion in a child that restrains the surgeon as it is the lesion's size. Because large, lush, and thirsty AVMs are uncommon in children, and because the small malformations are usually those that produce hemorrhage, paradoxically, the small, awkwardly positioned AVM may present the greatest challenge to the surgeon.[19] Lesions that are about 1.0 cm across and located adjacent to or within a ventricle or positioned deeply along the medial face of the hemisphere can be difficult to isolate, particularly if the malformation lies between the surgical approach and the hemorrhage.

Under the best of circumstances, the AVM should be approached via the shortest route through noneloquent cortex. Planning for this route must also take into account the fact that the dissection is likely to proceed through to the underlying ventricle; therefore, the surgeon must not be restrained by superficial tissues from reaching that space. Occasionally, however, an indirect route is required, especially for small lesions that are seated beneath the midline cortical tissues, and for which on first inspection a transcortical approach direct from the hemispheric convexity may be considered. This strategy may place much uninvolved brain tissue at risk as well as in the surgeon's way, and it could first present the AVM's apex rather than base to the surgeon. A surgical attack through a midline craniotomy is a minimalist, noninvasive technique but could force the surgeon to work around a right angle from falx into cortex to secure the lesion. However, with the continuation of such dissection, the brain relaxes, and exposure becomes easier.

Perimeters are all-important, and the size of the craniotomy must take this into consideration so that the surgeon can always visualize the normal tissue surrounding the target, especially for malformations in the posterior fossa, where tissues are less mobile and may be more inclined to herniate into the dural wound. Although opening the dura widely over the entire extent of the craniotomy is unnecessary, the surgeon must have that option without removal of more bone, if circumstances subsequently dictate.

ANESTHETIC CONSIDERATIONS

The surgical treatment of a child with an AVM requires all of the major anesthetic and pharmacologic techniques currently available. Anesthesia is induced with thiopentone, followed by a muscle relaxant to facilitate intubation (with an armored orotracheal tube).[44] Anesthesia is maintained with nitrous oxide and oxygen, a muscle relaxant (*d*-tubocurarine or pancuronium), halothane and/or an intravenous narcotic, and positive-pressure ventilation. Mannitol, 20 percent, is usually given in a dose of 1.0 g/kg during the operative opening. If mannitol has been used as a diuretic, then intravenous fluid replacement consists of a solution of 5 percent dextrose and 0.2 percent saline, which is given only after the volume of urine exceeds 10 percent of the estimated blood volume plus the volume of mannitol infused.

Patient monitors consist of an esophageal stethoscope for breath and heart sounds; an electrocardiograph for cardiac rate, rhythm, and conduction; an appropriately sized blood pressure cuff and Doppler probe for blood pressure recording; an indwelling arterial cannula in the radial or dorsalis pedis artery for blood pressure and arterial blood gas analysis; and an indwelling urinary catheter and rectal thermistor probe. End-tidal carbon dioxide is also monitored. A central venous line, which can be difficult to insert in a small patient, is placed only if massive blood loss is anticipated. The head of the table is raised 15 degrees, and the ventilator is adjusted to give a $PaCO_2$ of 3.99 kPa (30 mm Hg), confirmed by blood gas analysis.

For patients in whom controlled hypotension is not required, systolic blood pressure is allowed to fall to 10.0 kPa (75 mm Hg). Thereafter, it is kept at this level with blood transfusions. Before closure, enough blood is transfused to return the systolic blood pressure to its preloss value, and then blood equal to 10 percent of the estimated blood volume is transfused during closure. Some patients do not require blood transfusion during operation, and they receive lactated Ringer's solution, 10 mg/kg, during closure instead.

The decision to induce controlled hypotension is based on results of the preoperative arteriogram. If the site and size of the AVM suggest that the operation will be facilitated by this measure, then pentolinium tartrate is administered after the procedure has started. If only a short period of hypotension is required, then halothane or sodium nitroprusside is chosen.

AIDS TO SURGERY

The operation for an AVM is approached as a traditional craniotomy, governed by standard techniques and instrumentation. Sometimes, finding a small lesion may be one of the initial major difficulties, as is often the circumstance with an occult malformation lying within the temporal lobe, especially if the malformation is not associated with a hematoma. CT and stereotactic guidance by either an applied frame or a hand-held wand can be of considerable assistance in directing the surgeon to the AVM, with minimal ablation of critical tissue.

The operating microscope is often an ally, although it may be a disadvantage to the surgeon dissecting around large-convexity or cerebellar lesions. In these circumstances, the surgeon may lose sight of the perimeter of the AVM when he or she works even with the lowest magnifications. Unbeknownst to the surgeon, malformation, bleeding, or brain swelling may exist beyond the microscopic field of vision. Meanwhile, the surgeon has become preoccupied with only the area that can be seen and is oblivious to what is going on around him or her. Certainly, the microscope has a vital role during excision of small or residual lesions, especially if they lie within basal ganglia or brainstem. Hence, magnifying loupes and a fiber-optic headlight can provide more mobility and permit the surgeon to stay at the margin of the malformation, in its glial plane.

SURGICAL TECHNIQUES

The ideal operation for a child's AVM should be a planned, elective procedure for which the entire operating team is fresh. Once the anesthetic and operative preparations are completed, then the generous craniotomy flap is turned. Fortunately, most children's AVMs do not sequester blood supply from the external carotid arterial system so that bone and dura are not unusually vascular. The dural opening, however, should be well planned in relation to the superficial draining veins from the malformation. If these veins are engorged, they may be adherent to the inner layer of dura and therefore must be directly teased from it. Once this is completed, the veins proceed in a characteristic fashion to the adjacent venous sinus.

The cortical topography may take on any of the features previously noted. The surgeon should be able to correlate this surface anatomy with the arteriographic features and then plan the malformation's margins to be excised. This planning may be accomplished by taking an obvious, central abnormal point and calculating multiple radii from it until the entire lesion is circumscribed. Bipolar forceps are used to coagulate the cortical surface, and from this point, the dissection proceeds with microinstruments in an organized circumferential fashion about the malformation, preserving one or two major draining veins until the end. Dual suctions and bipolar forceps should be available during the entire case so that the surgeon and assistant can work simultaneously with this equipment. In addition, clean forceps and suction tips should be ready as back-up. A parenchymal clot, if present, can create much autodissection of the AVM. After the clot is removed, the surgeon will recognize the AVM hanging like a chandelier from the wall or roof of the clot cavity. Sometimes, however, the clot can be located downstream from the AVM, which often is isolated before the hematoma is reached.

The feeding and draining vessels run a straight course to and from the malformation but become coiled within it. These vessels can be freed by dissection along their long axis and isolated with a blunt hook before application of the bipolar forceps. Curiously, AVMs are less likely to bleed spontaneously during surgery from their original site of hemorrhage than are aneurysms, and thus the various vascular coils and varices can be gently manipulated aside. When bleeding does occur, it tends to be less torrential than with aneurysm rupture, and the bleeding usually represents transgression into the malformation itself. This bleeding can be controlled with gentle packing while the dissection proceeds at a more remote site.

An accompanying artery or vein is sometimes hidden immediately deep to the vessel about to be severed, and manipulation with the blunt hook can bring this surreptitious neighbor into view for coagulation. This situation frequently arises with the major draining vein, which may obscure otherwise inconsequential arteries running beneath it or feeding it.[41] Most AVMs have a wedge or torpedo profile directed toward the adjacent ventricle, and the surgeon should not be content that a total excision has been achieved until the ventricular wall has been visualized and, if necessary, the choroid plexus detached from the choroidal feeders at the apex of the lesion. The protected major draining vein is now secured. Before doing so, the surgeon should be able to roll the AVM out on this venous pedicle, thus confirming that the lesion has been completely circumscribed. Even when this procedure is performed, this draining vein still appears red because an arterial feeder is lying on its deep surface. Both are clipped, coagulated, or both, simultaneously, and the lesion is lifted from its bed.

Once the malformation dissection is completed, bleeding ceases in its bed, and the brain is considerably relaxed. The AVM bed is pristine white matter of brain with no red coils poking through it, and the CSF or irrigating solution is free of evidence of continued bleeding. Under these circumstances, packing the bed with hemostatic gauze is not usually necessary. The wound is then closed as usual. An external ventricular drain is not usually required, even when the ventricle has been entered. That very act, with evacuation of the intraventricular clot, often re-establishes CSF circulation.

If operation has been decided on, then the surgeon should be satisfied with nothing less than total excision, even if two stages are necessary to achieve it. Proximal vessel ligation can be dangerous and is an inadequate solution; subtotal excision is messy, and the shunt remains served by newly recruited contributors.

AVOIDING INTRAOPERATIVE COMPLICATIONS

Angiographically occult AVMs usually lie within the middle cerebral artery territory but are not displayed on the arteriogram. They represent potential complications for two reasons: (1) An apparently simple operation for a clot or seizure focus may become a little more trying if a small tangle of vessels is encountered; and (2) even when an AVM is suspected and a hematoma is removed, the location of the AVM vessels may be quite uncertain, and their residua may trigger a subsequent delayed hemorrhage.[22, 45] The problem, if anticipated, may be resolved with preoperative MRI studies and intraoperative stereotactic localization.

The commonest complication arising during the management of the child's AVM is failure to recognize the choroidal contribution to the malformation. The posterior choroidal system in particular supplies many of these lesions, and it can be responsible for deep bleeding in the AVM bed at a time when it is thought that the malformation otherwise has been excised. The residual nidus of the malformation is the part glued onto the choroid plexus. The surgeon must not consider the lesion totally removed until the ventricular cavity, CSF, and choroid plexus have been visualized.

All neurosurgeons are aware of the hazards that arise if the venous drainage to an AVM is sacrificed before all of the arterial input has been obliterated. A conscious effort is thus made to protect at least one vein during the dissection around the malformation. This rule is paramount in the child because very frequently only one major draining vein is present from the entire lesion. Although minor exit routes may exist through the choroidal venous system, the surgeon should not rely on those and should instead protect the major superficial draining vein until the end of the surgery. The surgeon should not be disheartened if that vein remains "red" until the very end, even when all other deep connections have been severed. Characteristically, a small artery runs beneath the dilated vein, and both structures are thus clipped and divided simultaneously.

The experienced surgeon usually knows whether or not total removal of a cerebral AVM has been achieved by the conclusion of the surgery if a deliberate decision has not been made to stage the procedure. At other times, the mandatory postoperative arteriogram shows residual malformation, and reoperation becomes necessary to excise the residual lesion. Such malformation is also responsible for continued bleeding in the bed of the malformation, which tends to arise from tiny coils of vessels lying within the adjacent brain white matter. These must be circumscribed and excised.

The phenomenon of "breakthrough," as originally described, has not been encountered in our children,[46] possibly because of the combination of the small size of many pediatric AVMs and the protection that children have with regard to their cerebral circulation. Ischemic symptoms and evidence of poor filling of the normal hemispheric branches because of the sump effect of the AVM are not characteristic features seen in children's arteriograms.

POSTOPERATIVE CARE

The experienced surgeon who attempts total excision of the malformation usually knows if that goal has been achieved at the conclusion of the first craniotomy. If a deliberate decision has been made to stage the procedure, then the surgeon should discontinue the first procedure when the operative region is neither bleeding nor swelling. The child is then allowed to recover, and, if necessary, the situation is studied further with repeat arteriography. One or two strategically placed metallic hemostatic clips permit identification of the area of surgery and serve as coordinates for the further radiologic and surgical examination of the malformation that remains.

Regardless of whether one or two procedures are required to obliterate the lesion, the surgeon cannot be satisfied that total excision has been achieved until postoperative arteriography confirms it. The study also shows a diminished size of the proximal contributing arteries. If residual malformation is present, then reoperation becomes necessary to excise the remaining lesion. Such residual lesions can be responsible for continued bleeding in the bed of the malformation, which tends to arise from tiny coils of vessels lying within the adjacent brain white matter. These coils can usually be easily circumscribed and excised.

Thereafter, the child's convalescence depends only on his or her rehabilitation needs, if any. The degree of motor, speech, and cerebellar recovery can be remarkable. Prophylactic anticonvulsant medication is usually required for 6 to 24 months after AVM excision.

RESULTS

In the series from The Hospital for Sick Children, 128 patients were treated.[6] Twenty-three children received nonsurgical treatment, and 13 died from poor-grade hemorrhage. One hundred five patients were operated on, and any one or a combination of complete or incomplete AVM removal, obliteration of feeders, evacuation of hematoma, or shunting procedures was achieved. In 60 patients, the malformation was completely removed at the first operation, and in another 10 at a second procedure. Thirteen patients in the group treated by surgery died (12 percent mortality), all of whom were grade IV or V at the time of first assessment. All patients who died suffered hemorrhage; thus, the mortality from the bleed, regardless of the method of treatment, is 25 percent.[6]

A chronic seizure disorder was the reason for neurologic evaluation in 16 patients. All but one of these children were operated on, and three had lingering postoperative epilepsy. Fourteen patients had acute seizures, most related to their hemorrhages, and only one (7 percent) had lingering postoperative epilepsy. Paradoxically, six patients who had been operated on who did not have seizure disturbances before surgery were subject to this malady during the follow-up period. All these patients had intracerebral clots.

Except for patients who died, 103 children were available for follow-up examination 9 months to 30 years after treatment. One of these patients died suddenly at home 5 years after "total" resection of his AVM, but neither the completeness of resection nor the ultimate cause of death is known. Of the remaining 102 patients, 69 (67 percent) are neurologically normal. A fixed neurologic deficit persisted in 28 patients (27 percent). Progressive mental status deterioration occurred in another five, and one patient has had persistent chronic headache.

Nonoperative management was performed in 27 children. In 13 patients, death followed poor-grade hemorrhage, either before surgical intervention or in children in whom surgery offered no chance for clinical recovery. Of eight children still living who can be followed up and whose AVMs are intact, six are normal, one has a seizure disorder, and one has a persisting neurologic deficit.

SUMMARY

Hemorrhagic stroke in a child is more likely to result from bleeding from an AVM than a ruptured intracranial aneurysm. Certain distinguishing features are unique to children, vis-à-vis adults. More children bleed from their malformations, and fewer suffer chronic seizures than do adults. As many as 28 percent of children suffer overt repeat hemorrhage, and our studies show that the mortality rate from any hemorrhage is 25 percent. AVMs in children can be scattered throughout the brain, often in awkward locations, and an unusual number (24 percent) are located below the tentorium. Wherever possible, total excision of the malformation must be attempted, with the expectation that the child's brain vasculature may be resilient to operative intrusion. Seventy percent of children receiving surgical care can be expected to be neurologically intact after surgery. The surgical mortality of 4 percent is influenced by the severity of the SAH/IVH because all patients who died were clinical grades IV or V.

REFERENCES

1. Locksley HB: Report on the Cooperative Study of Intracranial Aneurysms and Subarachnoid Hemorrhage. Section V, Part I. Natural history of subarachnoid hemorrhage, intracranial aneurysms and arteriovenous malformations. Based on 6,368 cases in the Cooperative Study. J Neurosurg 25:219, 1966
2. Hourihan M, Gates PC, McAllister VL: Subarachnoid hemorrhage in childhood and adolescence. J Neurosurg 60:1163, 1984
3. Laitinen L: Arteriella aneuryusm med subarachnoidal-blodning hos barn. Nord Med 71:329, 1964
4. Sedzimir CB, Robinson J: Intracranial hemorrhage in children and adolescents. J Neurosurg 38:269, 1973
5. Perret G, Nishioka H: Report on the Cooperative Study of Intracranial Aneurysms and Subarachnoid Hemorrhage. Section VI. Arteriovenous malformations. An analysis of 545 cases of craniocerebral arteriovenous malformations and fistulae reported to the Cooperative Study. J Neurosurg 25:467, 1966
6. Kondziolka D, Humphreys RP, Hoffman HJ, et al: Arteriovenous malformations of the brain in children: A forty year experience. Can J Neurol Sci 19:40, 1992
7. Matson DD: Neurosurgery of Infancy and Childhood, 2nd ed. Springfield, IL, Charles C Thomas, 1969, pp 749–766
8. Amacher AL, Allcock JM, Drake CG: Cerebral angiomas: The sequelae of surgical treatment. J Neurosurg 37:571, 1972
9. Bruce DA, Schut L: Arteriovenous malformations in children. Childs Nerv Syst 8:232, 1981
10. Gerosa MA, Cappellotto P, Licata C, et al: Cerebral arteriovenous malformations in children (56 cases). Childs Nerv Syst 8:356, 1981
11. Kelly JJ Jr, Mellinger JF, Sundt TM Jr: Intracranial arteriovenous malformations in childhood. Ann Neurol 3:338, 1978
12. Laine E, Dhellemmes P, Clarisse C: Supratentorial arteriovenous malformations in children except aneurysm of the vein of Galen. Childs Nerv Syst 8:63, 1981
13. Monges J, Jaimovich R, Cragnaz RJ: Vascular malformations in children. Bol Asoc Argentina Neurocir 30:41, 1981
14. Mori K, Murata T, Hasimoto N, et al: Clinical analysis of arteriovenous malformations in children. Childs Nerv Syst 6:13, 1980
15. So SC: Cerebral arteriovenous malformations in children. Childs Nerv Syst 4:242, 1978
16. Tiyaworabun S, Kramer HH, Lim DP, et al: Cerebral arteriovenous malformations in children: Clinical analysis and followup results. Childs Nerv Syst 8:232, 1981
17. Takashima S, Becker LE: Neuropathology of cerebral arteriovenous malformations in children. J Neurol Neurosurg Psychiatry 43:380, 1980
18. Celli P, Ferrante L, Palma L, et al: Cerebral arteriovenous malformations in children. Clinical features and outcome of treatment in children and in adults. Surg Neurol 22:43, 1984
19. Waltimo O: The relationship of size, density and localization of intracranial arteriovenous malformations to the type of initial symptom. J Neurol Sci 19:13, 1973
20. LeBlanc R, Feindel W, Ethier R: Epilepsy from cerebral arteriovenous malformations. Can J Neurol Sci 10:91, 1983
21. Mohr JP: Neurological manifestations and factors related to the thera-

peutic decisions, in Wilson CB, Stein BM (eds): Intracranial Arteriovenous Malformations. Baltimore, Williams & Wilkins, 1984, pp 1–11
22. Cohen HCM, Tucker WS, Humphreys RP, et al: Angiographically cryptic histologically verified cerebrovascular malformations. Neurosurgery 10:704, 1982
23. Russel DS, Rubinstein LJ: Pathology of Tumors of the Nervous System, 4th ed. London, Edward Arnold Publishers, 1977, pp 136–138
24. Humphreys RP: Infratentorial arteriovenous malformations, in Edwards MSB, Hoffman HJ (eds): Cerebrovascular Disease in Childhood and Adolescence. Baltimore, Williams & Wilkins, 1988, pp 309–320
25. Troupp H: Arteriovenous malformations of the brain. What are the indications for operation? in Morley TP (ed): Current Controversies in Neurosurgery. Philadelphia, WB Saunders, 1967, pp 210–216
26. Wilson CB, Sang UH, Dominque J: Microsurgical treatment of intracranial vascular malformations. J Neurosurg 51:446, 1979
27. Forster DMC, Steiner L, Hakanson S: Arteriovenous malformations of the brain. A long-term clinical study. J Neurosurg 37:562, 1972
28. Schatz SW, Botterell EH: The natural history of arteriovenous malformations, in Milliken C (ed): Cerebrovascular Disease, Proceedings of the Association of Research in Nervous and Mental Diseases, vol 41. Baltimore, Williams & Wilkins, 1974, pp 180–187
29. Svien HJ, McRae JA: Arteriovenous anomalies of the brain. Fate of patients not having definitive surgery. J Neurosurg 23:23, 1965
30. Troupp H, Marttila I, Halonen V: Arteriovenous malformations of the brain: Prognosis without operation. Acta Neurochir (Wien) 22:125, 1970
31. Pellettieri L, Carlsson C-A, Grevsten S, et al: Surgical versus conservative treatment of intracranial arteriovenous malformations. Acta Neurochir Suppl (Wien) 29:1, 1980
32. Guidetti B, Delitala A: Intracranial arteriovenous malformations. Conservative and surgical treatment. J Neurosurg 53:149, 1980
33. Jomin M, Lesoin F, Lozes G: Prognosis for arteriovenous malformations of the brain in adults based on 150 cases. Surg Neurol 23:362, 1985
34. Graf CJ, Perret GE, Torner JC: Bleeding from cerebral arteriovenous malformations as part of their natural history. J Neurosurg 58:331, 1983
35. Heros RC, Korosue K, Diebold PM: Surgical excision of cerebral arteriovenous malformation: Late results. Neurosurgery 26:578, 1990
36. Itoyama Y, Uemura S, Ushio Y, et al: Natural course of unoperated intracranial arteriovenous malformations: Study of 50 cases. J Neurosurg 71:805, 1989
37. Fults D, Kelly DL: Natural history of arteriovenous malformations of the brain: A clinical study. Neurosurgery 15:658, 1984
38. Crawford PM, West CR, Chadwick DW, et al: Arteriovenous malformations of the brain: Natural history in unoperated patients. J Neurol Neurosurg Psychiatry 49:1, 1986
39. Ondra SL, Troupp H, George ED, et al: The natural history of symptomatic arteriovenous malformations of the brain: A 24-year follow-up assessment. J Neurosurg 73:387, 1990
40. Wilkins RH: Natural history of intracranial vascular malformations. A review. Neurosurgery 16:421, 1985
41. Stein BM: General techniques for the surgical removal of arteriovenous malformations, in Wilson CB, Stein BM (eds): Intracranial Arteriovenous Malformations. Baltimore, Williams & Wilkins, 1984, pp 143–155
42. McCormick WF: Pathology of vascular malformations of the brain, in Wilson CB, Stein BM (eds): Intracranial Arteriovenous Malformations. Baltimore, Williams & Wilkins, 1984, pp 44–63
43. Drake CG: Cerebral arteriovenous malformations: Considerations for and experience with surgical treatment in 166 cases. Clin Neurosurg 26:145, 1979
44. McLeod ME, Creighton RE, Humphreys RP: Anaesthesia for cerebral arteriovenous malformations in children. Can Anaesth Soc J, 29:299–306, 1982
45. Humphreys RP: Complications of hemorrhagic stroke in children. Pediatr Neurosurg 17:225–233, 1992
46. Spetzler RF, Wilson CB, Weinstein P, et al: Normal perfusion pressure breakthrough theory. Clin Neurosurg 25:651–672, 1977

CHAPTER 95

Radiosurgery of Cranial Arteriovenous Malformations

Christopher S. Ogilvy
Paul H. Chapman
James B. Costales

The use of radiation therapy to treat cerebral arteriovenous malformations (AVMs) is a concept that has been present for many years. Radiation in single, high-dose delivery or in fractionated delivery certainly has an effect on blood vessels. Standard techniques of external fractionated radiation therapy have been of limited success in the treatment of AVMs[1,2]; however, the use of single-dose, highly focused radiation (radiosurgery) has been proved effective in the management of certain carefully selected AVMs.

The overall effects of radiation and focused radiation on blood vessels are reviewed in this chapter, as is the proven efficacy of the various types of radiosurgery currently available. Finally, techniques that may enhance the abililty of radiosurgical techniques to achieve higher cure rates for AVMs are discussed.

THE EFFECT OF RADIATION ON NORMAL AND ABNORMAL BLOOD VESSELS

The presumed sequence of events that causes gradual occlusion of small vessels within an AVM and eventual angiographic obliteration over time has been reviewed previously.[1] The underlying goal in the use of radiation therapy, despite the mode of delivery, is to induce an inflammatory response in the vessel walls of the malformation that will result in permanent thickening of the abnormal vascular channels and ultimate occlusion and thrombosis. The rapidity at which pathologic changes occur within the walls of blood vessels depends on the total dose of radiation and the number of treatment fractions, yet qualitative changes are similar. The earliest changes occur in small vessels days to weeks after exposure to radiation. Endothelial cell swelling occurs with increased nuclear basophilia. With a low dose of radiation, the observed inflammatory changes are reversible, and the vascular wall returns to a normal appearance over time.[3] With large doses of radiation, or with repeated low doses, involvement of larger arterioles and associated breakdown of the blood-brain barrier occur. This phase occurs weeks to months after treatment and is thought to be the pathologic correlate of the low-density regions that are observed on computed tomographic (CT) scans. These changes in brain water content can also be observed on magnetic resonance imaging (MRI).[4] Endothelial cell degeneration progresses to necrosis in some areas, with an increase in interstitial exudate (increased colloids). Diapedesis of leukocytes into the interstitial space occurs, and fissuring of vessel walls and spot hemorrhages can also occur. In response to this injury, fibroblastic activity increases, and proliferation of the surviving endothelial cells occurs, along with increased deposition of collagen in the media of vessel walls. Fibrosis of the adventitia also occurs. Although this intimal lining proliferation continues as part of the inflammatory and reparative response, gradual vascular lumen narrowing and eventual obliteration occur.

A large amount of the data used to describe vascular changes after radiation have been obtained by histopathologic study of cerebral vasculature from animals exposed to whole-brain x-ray radiation[3] or high-energy protons.[5-7] The changes seen in animal and human pathology specimens after x-ray or gamma ray radiation are virtually identical to changes seen after exposure to a beam of high-energy protons.

Larger doses of radiation generally produce greater amounts of normal tissue necrosis, but in the treatment of AVMs, tissue necrosis is not the ultimate goal. As the dose of radiation is increased, however, one might expect to encounter a higher incidence of related complications. Complications can be reduced with lower radiation doses, yet in the case of AVMs, this reduction results in a lower rate of ultimate obliteration of the lesion.

Despite differences in doses, examination of tissue obtained at autopsy or after surgical removal of an AVM previously treated with x-ray, gamma radiation, or Bragg peak therapy reveals vascular wall morphology similar to changes described in animal studies.[5,8,9]

PATIENT SELECTION

Because several modalities are available to treat AVMs, including open microneurosurgical techniques, radiosurgery, and endovascular embolization, deciding which of these modalities is best for a given patient is sometimes difficult. We have used a team approach by reviewing available radiographs at a conference attended by vascular neurosurgeons, interventional radiologists, radiation therapists, and neurologists. The first consideration in the decision of whether or not a patient should be treated is the natural history of the AVM. Lesions are suspected to hemorrhage at a rate of approximately 4 percent per year, and over the course of a young patient's lifetime, this risk can be substantial.[10] The risk of disabling hemorrhage or death from hemorrhage has to be weighed against the risk of treating the AVM. At times, combined modality therapy that uses embolization techniques before radiosurgery or open surgery is often the best solution to treat larger AVMs. Although at first thought this approach seems to combine the risks of procedures, in fact, embolization may reduce risks of subsequent procedures. In addition to the annual risk of hemorrhage, certain features of a given AVM, such as a single draining vein, deep venous drainage, arterial or venous aneurysms, or venous outflow obstructions, have been identified as features that may increase the chance of hemorrhage from an AVM.[11]

The benefit of open surgery is that the risk of hemorrhage is removed with the AVM. For radiosurgery, regardless of the technique used, a risk of subsequent hemorrhage remains until the AVM is completely obliterated. This process can take 2 to 3 years to complete. Radiosurgery for AVMs should be considered when the risks of open surgery or embolization and combined modality therapy are higher than the risks of radiosurgery plus the risk of rehemorrhage after radiosurgery.

In addition to the risk factors of an AVM for hemorrhage and the risks of possible treatment, the patient's own concerns must enter into the treatment decision. Patients can have very strong feelings regarding the wish to avoid radiation or open surgery. These considerations must be taken into account when clinicians counsel a patient and decide on a final treatment option. Finally, in certain lesions, the risks of treatment are so high from any form of therapy that no treatment should be used.

RADIOSURGICAL TECHNIQUES

Three types of radiation sources are available to treat AVMs of the brain by use of stereotactic radiosurgery. Regardless of the type of technique used, the general concepts of treatment are the same. A high dose of energy (radiation) is delivered to the confines of the AVM nidus. By use of stereotactic techniques, the accuracy of the technique is maximized. With the confines of the target (AVM) known, the techniques described later are designed to deposit a high dose of radiation within the target volume, yet minimize the amount of radiation dose to adjacent and distant normal brain tissue. General features and potential advantages for the available techniques are discussed later.

Bragg Peak Therapy

Large-particle accelerators can be used to produce positively charged particles in the form of protons or helium ions. As these particles leave the accelerator, they carry energy with them. The point of particle deceleration gives rise to the Bragg peak, with a high amount of energy deposited at this point in space. The physical characteristics of the Bragg peak are such that the entry dose is low, and no exit dose exists.

Two main centers have reported results of Bragg peak therapy to treat AVMs. At Lawrence Berkeley Laboratory in California, a 230-MeV cyclotron provides a helium ion beam, and at Harvard a proton beam generated by a 160-MeV cyclotron is used. Bragg peak ionization theoretically allows little or no potential injury to adjacent vital structures because of a focused peak of particle delivery at a predetermined depth in brain tissue.

Linear Accelerator Radiosurgery

The linear accelerator in conjunction with stereotactic targeting techniques uses radiation fields that overlap at the AVM location, thereby producing a large dose of radiation to the target with relatively low doses to surrounding brain tissue.[12] By using overlapping beams, a low entry and exit dose can be obtained, and a high dose can be delivered to the AVM.

Gamma Radiosurgery (Gamma Knife)

Techniques for using stereotactically directed gamma radiation were pioneered by Leksell.[13–15] This technique makes use of gamma radiation emitted from approximately 200 small ^{60}Co sources located within a hemisphere that surrounds the patient's head. The isocenter of treatment is the stereotactic coordinate where the collimators from each source of cobalt are directed and overlap. Like linear accelerator radiosurgery, the overlap of separate sources of radiation gives rise to a high dose of radiation at the target and yields a low entry and exit dose to surrounding brain tissue.

Reports on the Gamma knife first appeared in the early 1970s.[16, 17] Follow-up results have been presented by Steiner.[8, 18] A recent report by Lunsford and associates[19] details the treatment of 227 patients treated with Gamma knife radiosurgery over a 3-year period (Table 95–1).[4, 5, 8, 16–26]

Results

A high efficacy of radiosurgery can be expected if the dose delivered to the AVM is sufficient, apparently regardless of the source of radiation (Table 95–1). The volume of tissue to be irradiated deeply affects exactly how much radiation dose will be tolerated by the patient without developing a complication. Smaller-volume lesions, those less than 4 cm³, can be covered adequately with a large enough dose of radiation to obliterate the lesion angiographically in 85 to 95 percent of patients. With larger lesions, (those greater than 4 cm³), the amount of radiation that can be delivered that has a 3- to 4-percent chance of radionecrosis is much less effective in obliterating the lesion (30- to 70-percent chance of obliteration). As noted earlier, the risk of radionecrosis and accompanying neurologic complications are related to the dose of radiation used.

Complications

Regardless of technique used, the expected complication rates are related to the dose delivered, which by design is related to the volume of the lesion.[27] The actual complication rates for representative reports from heavy ion beam treatment, the Gamma knife, and the linear accelerator are shown

Table 95-1. RESULTS AND COMPLICATIONS OF RADIOSURGERY OF ARTERIOVENOUS MALFORMATIONS*

Investigators	Therapy	No. of Patients	Results		Complications (%)		Rebleed Within 2 Years of Treatment
			Size of AVM (diameter)	Obliteration at 2 Years (%)	Reversible Worsening	Permanent Deficit	
Kjellberg and coworkers[5]	Proton beam	800	≤30 mm	42 (88% had >50% reduction)	n/a	0.96	5
			>30, ≤50 mm	6 (30% had >50% reduction)			
			>50 mm	1 (16% had >50% reduction)			
			Total	22			
			Size of AVM (volume)	Obliteration at 3 Years (%)			
Steinberg and coworkers[4]	Helium beam	426	<4 cm^3	100	10	11	12 (within 3 years)
			4–25 cm^3	95			
			>25 cm^3	73			
			Total	90			
			Size of AVM (volume)	Obliteration at 2 Years (%)			
Lansford and coworkers[19]	Gamma knife	227	≤1 cm^3	100	4.4	3.1	5.2
			1–4 cm^3	85			
			4–10 cm^3	58			
			Total	80			
			Size of AVM (diameter)	Obliteration at 2 Years (%)			
Colombo and coworkers[21]	Linear accelerator	180	<15 mm	96.5	5	2.2	12
			>15, ≤25 mm	73.9			
			>25%	33.3			
			Total	80			

AVM = arteriovenous malformation.
*This table is representative of results reported by several groups. For Gamma knife, other investigators making important contributions to the field with similar rates of obliteration and complications include Steiner and coworkers,[8, 16–18] Bunge and coworkers,[22] and Forster.[23] For linear accelerator data, similar results can be found in reports by Betti and coworkers,[24] Friedman and Bova,[25] and Oliver and coworkers.[26]

in Table 95–1. Reversible worsening is seen in 5 to 10 percent of the population treated and can occur 6 months to 2 years after treatment. Permanent deficit has been reported in 2 to 11 percent of patients treated (Table 95–1). As can be noted in Table 95–1, higher rates of obliteration were achieved with helium beam treatment; however, the complication rate was also higher in this group of patients.

Rehemorrhage

The effects of radiosurgery are not immediate, but generally, the interval from treatment to time of AVM obliteration is about 2 years. However, lesions that are decreasing in size by the second year after treatment may continue to be reduced in size and may totally obliterate by the third year after treatment. If the AVM remains patent on angiography or MRI, the risk of hemorrhage remains. The exact rate of hemorrhage reported from different series ranges between 5 and 12 percent per year during the interval it takes for the lesion to obliterate (Table 95–1). This rehemorrhage rate must be included in discussions with patients and their families as well as in the overall estimated risk of radiosurgery for AVMs.

SUMMARY

Radiosurgery is proving to be a useful and effective means of treating some carefully selected AVMs of the brain. We limit the use of this technique to small AVMs in locations that carry with them a high risk from standard microsurgical techniques. Although larger lesions can be treated with radiosurgery, the proven efficacy of AVM obliteration while the treatment is kept safe is higher. Future developments of fractionated stereotactic radiosurgery may help to keep the risk low yet increase the chance of obliteration in larger-sized AVMs. In addition, treatment strategies that use combined endovascular embolization of an AVM with radiosurgery may prove useful. The embolic agent used must be a permanent one and is usually glue material, such as N-butyl-cyanoacrylate. Particle embolization carries with it the possibility of vessel recanalization. When embolization is considered as an adjunct to radiosurgery, the risk of embolization must be factored into the total risk of treating the AVM. Often, embolization techniques can obliterate part of an AVM such that the vascular density of the lesion is decreased but the lesion is not decreased in its total volume. The effect on the dose in subsequent radiosurgery of a lesion that has decreased density of vasculature yet a similar pretreatment profile remains an unanswered question. If the endovascular techniques can be used to produce a volumetric decrease in the size of the AVM nidus, radiosurgery can apparently be used on the remaining nidus, with dosimetry applied as if the visible nidus is the only component of the AVM. This technique should increase the efficacy of radiosurgery.

ADVANCED CONCEPTS IN PROTON RADIOSURGERY: TREATMENT PLANNING

The recent availability of affordable powerful graphics workstations has greatly affected proton radiosurgery treatment planning. For many brain lesions, it is now possible to complete the entire treatment process as described later (from image acquisition to treatment planning to actual treatment) in a single day. Planning programs that use the full potential of these workstations are not only three dimensional, permitting the treatment planner full visual information on the precise stereotactic location of the target volume relative to the rest of the patient anatomy, but also truly interactive, allowing the planner to reconfigure beams and isocenters with relative ease and recalculate dose distributions in a short period of time. In addition, with such computers, the treatment planning process can be automated to a large extent and yet allow the process to remain interactive.

In this section, general features of treatment planning are discussed. Most treatment planning systems currently in clinical use are frame based (i.e., a stereotactic head frame is placed on the patient during image acquisition and actual treatment), and the discussions are limited to such frame-based systems. A sample treatment plan exemplifies the current range of possibilities. For a recent review of proton therapy, see the article by Bonnett.[28]

IMAGE ACQUISITION

The first step in treatment planning is the acquisition of stereotactic images of the treatment volume and relevant patient anatomy. The coordinate system is generally defined by a stereotactic head frame, which is attached to the patient's head. Such fixation is achieved by various means including pins surgically implanted into the skull while the patient is under local anesthetic, as well as facial masks and denture molds.[29] In some cases, the head frames permit repeat localization, thereby allowing fractionation of the treatment plan.

Depending on the exact design of the stereotactic reference system, attachments (localizers) to the head frame serve to place fiducials, such as rods or other markers, at precisely known locations in the reference system. The detection of such fiducials in the images registers, that is, permits the transcription of, the images to the planning and treatment coordinate system.

Depending on the type of lesion to be treated, such image modalities as CT, MRI of varying orientations, and angiography (normal, digitally subtracted, or MR angiography) may be necessary to fully determine the relation of the target volume relative to critically sensitive structures. Each of these image modalities has its strengths and weaknesses. For example, CT images are spatially exact and are subject to the pixel size and slice spacing but do not always afford clear outlines of the patient anatomy. MR images often afford such clear outlines, but often at the expense of spatial accuracy. Shifts in anatomic locations of up to 3 to 5 mm are typical of the amounts of distortion seen in MR images.[30, 31] Normal and digitized angiography can provide very good spatial accuracy but lack detailed three-dimensional information concerning the nidus shape and location of the AVM relative to other critical structures.

For ultimate versatility, a treatment planning program should permit the simultaneous use of multiple image modalities to plan cases. Because of their exact spatial accuracy, the stereotactically registered CT images can provide the best measure of anatomic location. The spatial accuracy requirements of radiosurgery depend on the location of the lesion. Current state-of-the-art spatial accuracy, considering all sources of error (including treatment volume definition and patient positioning during treatment), is approximately 1 to 2 mm. During image acquisition, sufficient quality assurance controls must be in place for the exact placement of the head frame to be monitored. Any shift of the head frame after or during the image acquisition relative to the patient's skull could lead to the degradation of spatial accuracy. In addition, to provide maximum spatial accuracy by restricting patient movement during image acquisition, the patient should be secured to the couch by use of tape or clamps.

Image acquisition and treatment planning are generally performed with different computers. Transfer of the image information from one computer to another can be performed electronically through computer networks or physically through media such as floppy disks, magnetic tape, film, or optical disks.

LOCALIZATION

Once the images are loaded into the treatment planning computer, the first step in treatment planning is the registration of images in stereotactic coordinate space. The determination of the localizer fiducials on the image slices or films provides this registration. In the case of CT- or MRI-derived images, such registration should be performed slice by slice to achieve the greatest accuracy.

Figures 95–1 to 95–4 in this section have been generated by a program called ProtonKnife (Radionics Software Applications, Burlington, MA). The program being developed in collaboration with Chapman, Koehler, and Cascio shows an example of the type of image data acquired by CT for a radiosurgery candidate. This particular patient had a low-grade astrocytoma, located inferior to and just to the right of

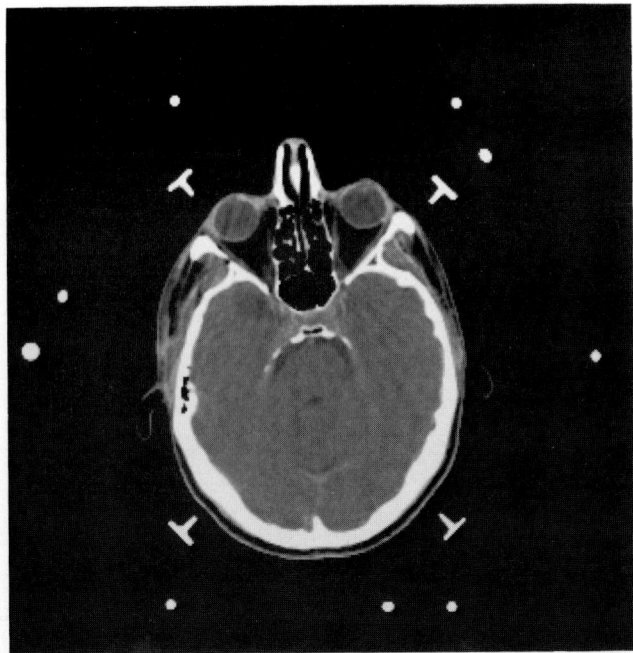

FIGURE 95–1. CT image of patient with partially resected low-grade astrocytoma. Note the presence of the nine rods used to register the image to BRW stereotactic coordinate space.

the right optic nerve, which has been partially resected. Figure 95–1 is an inferior axial view of the patient so that right and left sides are interchanged. Also visible in Figure 95–1 are nine fiducial rods and four posts of the Radionics Brown-Roberts-Wells head ring and CT localizer frame.[32] The location of these nine rods on the image slice contains information detailing the exact orientation and location of this plane in the Brown-Roberts-Wells coordinate system.

The stereotactically determined locations of image planes relative to one another should be compared with the scan slice spacing as a quality assurance control. Other quality assurance measures are often adopted to check that the image data were not corrupted during the transfer process.

IMAGE SEGMENTATION

Two- and three-dimensional representations of the target volume and critical structures can then be determined from the imaging data. On the simplest level, image segmentation can be performed manually by tracing around structures to form bounding contours. A stereotactically located three-dimensional volume representing an anatomic structure is generated from such contours. More complicated segmentation methods use sophisticated algorithms and/or anatomic atlases to automate this procedure. The use of such algorithms and atlases must take into account patient-to-patient variations. Whether the segmentation is performed manually or automatically, all spatial and dosimetric information determined subsequently relates to the exact determination of these anatomic structures.

TREATMENT PLAN PARAMETERS

A treatment plan consists of a set of entrance angles; target depths and doses; and beam collimator shapes, sizes, and

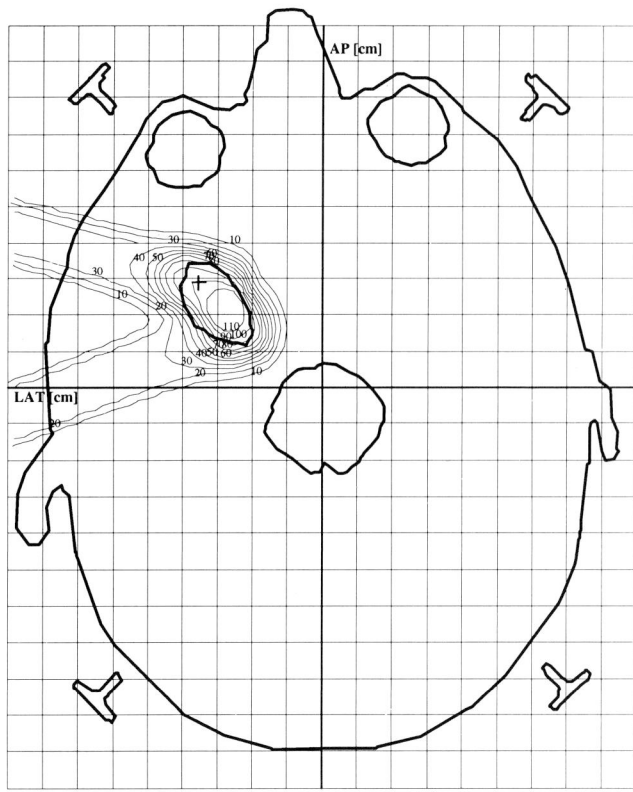

FIGURE 95–3. Isodose contours (arbitrary units) for an axial slice containing one of the treatment isocenters (indicated by a + sign) shown in Figure 95–2. The dose distribution reflects the summed contributions from all four portals and was generated using a ray-trace–based dose algorithm. Also indicated in the figure are outlines of various patient anatomic structures (eyes, brainstem, skin and tumor) and BRW posts. (Copyright © 1993, RSA, Inc.)

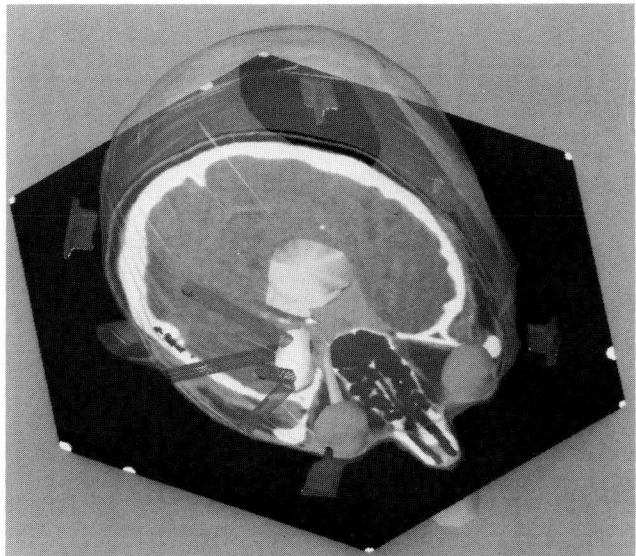

FIGURE 95–2. Three-dimension rendering of patient critical structures, tumor volume, and skin. Also displayed in the figure are the posts, treatment ports, and a CT image containing the center of the tumor volume.

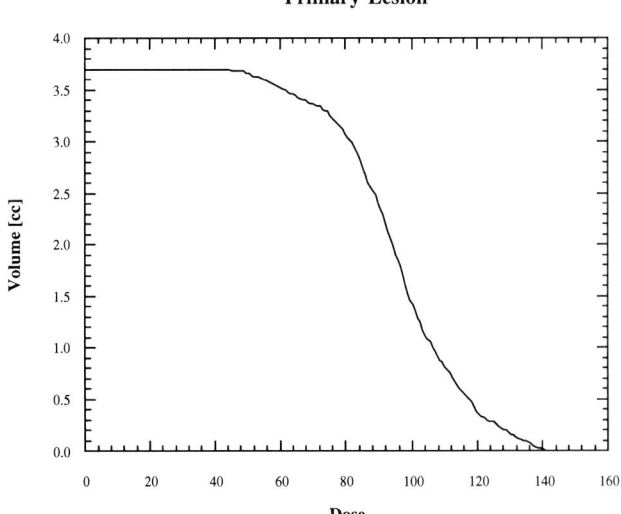

FIGURE 95–4. Integral dose-volume histogram for tumor volume. The units of dose are arbitrary but are the same as those used for Figure 95–3. In these units, the minimum and maximum doses to the tumor volume are 42 and 141, respectively, with the mean dose being 98. (Copyright © 1993, RSA, Inc.)

longitudinal (depth) profiles. A good treatment planning program design and layout (i.e., the user interface) permits the user to determine and manipulate these quantities with ease. The implementation of target isocenters and beam's-eye view coupled with three-dimensional graphics can greatly simplify the treatment planning process.

An isocenter is a three-dimensional point in stereotactic space through which a beam passes independent of its approach angles. Once an isocenter has been defined, all beams associated with that isocenter automatically intersect the target volume at the desired location. The isocenter concept is most useful when the treatment plans are limited to circular or symmetrically shaped apertures because in such cases, the center of the beam is well defined. Treatment plans need not necessarily be confined to a single isocenter, especially in cases of multiple or irregularly shaped target volumes.

In Figure 95–2, a three-dimensional graphic representation of the patient's anatomy and a proposed treatment plan are shown. The three-dimensional representations of critical structures (the brain stem, the eyes, the right optic nerve and optic chiasm, the brain tumor, and the patient's skin) have been generated from two-dimensional contours determined from CT data. A CT slice containing the center of the tumor has been texture mapped (superimposed) onto the three-dimensional display. The proposed treatment plan in this case consists of two isocenters, each having two associated beam portals. The diameters of the cylinders have been chosen to be the 90-percent isodose level (relative to the centerline value) for each beam portal. The head-ring posts are also rendered so that the treatment plan can avoid beam portals that would be obstructed by the posts. This figure exemplifies the tremendous amount of information that can be obtained from such graphic representations.

Beam's-eye view treatment planning refers to the ability to graphically view down the beam's line of sight to determine whether or not critical structures lie in the path of the beam. Moderately priced graphics workstations permit real-time rotations while in beam's-eye view or other arbitrary three-dimensional views. Such real-time graphic visualization is a very powerful tool that permits the planner to easily reject or select various approaches.

Besides the relative location of the critical structures to the beam, another important consideration may be the amount of inhomogenous material (bone or air, compared with soft tissue) through which the beam traverses on its way to the target volume. Such inhomogeneities can be monitored by digitally reconstructed radiograms or other similar means. A digitally reconstructed radiogram is generated by ray tracing from a point source through the CT volume and by use of the CT intensities along a given line of sight to determine the radiographic intensity. Such inhomogeneities can also be represented in other graphic manners, such as one-dimensional or multidimensional histograms.

The size and shape of the energy-deposition distributions can be modified in many ways.[33,34] Often, a set of circularly collimated beams centered around one or two isocenters can generate energy distributions that conform to the irregular shape of the target volume and avoid critical structures. To take maximal advantage of the inherent Bragg peak of the proton beam, beams are longitudinally adjusted such that the Bragg peak falls in or near the target volume. The longitudinal or depth profile of the relatively narrow Bragg peak can be modified in several ways. For example, an appropriately stepped absorber rotating through the beam can be used to spread out the longitudinal profile of the beam Bragg peak. Alternatively, discrete Bragg peaks of varying depths and dose normalization can also be used to shape the longitudinal profile.[33]

For very large irregular shapes (e.g., large AVMs) or for target volumes very close to critical structures, noncircular apertures and other means may be necessary. For example, a computer-controlled system can be used to selectively steer the beam to desired locations. Such systems are beyond the scope of this discussion but the article by Bonnett outlines further details for the shaping of the beam.[28] A collimator size and shape can be chosen to conform to the transverse outline of the tumor in the beam's-eye view. In addition, a compensating bolus (a block of material of varied thickness placed in the beam) can be employed to conform the back (distal) edge of the beam to the shape of the back edge of the target volume.

Such conformal apertures and compensating boluses reduce the amount of healthy tissue irradiated by the beam. In all cases, the computer can automatically determine the appropriate wedge, discrete beams, conformal aperture, or compensating bolus for a given view. However, whenever automation is used in the treatment planning process, direct user modification of the automated result must be permitted.

DOSE CALCULATIONS

Most often, when a treatment plan is evaluated, various dose (energy-deposition) distributions are studied. Such dose distributions can be calculated in many ways. The sophistication with which the dose calculations must be performed depends on the amount and shape of the inhomogeneities (i.e., soft tissue, air, bone, and cerebrospinal fluid) the beams traverse on their way to the target volume. The greater the inhomogeneities, the more sophisticated and computationally intensive the algorithms must be to properly calculate the energy-deposition distributions. The most sophisticated algorithms consist of detailed Monte Carlo (i.e., statistical) calculations that attempt to model the most important physical processes that govern energy deposition. These models are often computationally impractical for most clinical uses.

The simplest practical calculational method employs a ray-trace algorithm to determine the amount of matter the beam traverses to reach a certain calculational point. By finding the CT scan intensity values along the beam's path, this amount of matter is converted into an equivalent water depth. (Such ray-trace calculations can be used to determine the water-equivalent depth of the isocenter from the patient's skin, a quantity that is often used in the implementation of a plan). By use of measured longitudinal and transverse energy-deposition profiles obtained from water-based phantom studies, the program determines the energy deposition for that calculational point. Inherently one-dimensional, ray-tracing algorithms are often sufficient for most brain tumors and AVMs, provided that the beam does not traverse thick or highly irregular areas of bone or air. If such inhomogenous regions are encountered by the beams in the treatment plan, then other approaches, such as the differential pencil beam model, that are inherently two- or three-dimensional, must be employed. For further information regarding dose calculations, see the article by Petti for a detailed description of the differential pencil beam model as well as calculational comparisons with other models.[35]

To be fully understood and exploited, even the best dose calculational methods require two- and three-dimensional graphic displays whose views can be varied in position, perspective, and dosimetric isolevels in real time. For example, by studying the size and shape of a volume that receives a certain dose, the treatment planner can instantly understand the impact that the proposed beam portals have on the target volume and surrounding tissue. Graphic summaries and displays of the amount of dose administered to the surfaces of tumor and critical structures provide other powerful means by which the relationship between a given beam and the total dose distribution can be understood. In addition, the superposition of dose directly onto the two-dimensional image data allows the user to evaluate the plan as it relates directly to patient anatomy. The judicious use of color in all of these displays greatly enhances their interpretation.

As an example of a graphic representation of dose calculations, Figure 95–3 displays contours of constant energy deposition (in arbitrary units) for an axial plane passing through the center of the tumor. These isodose contours are superimposed on outlines of the patient anatomy. The axial plane represented in Figure 95–3 is adjacent to the one shown in Figure 95–1, and the calculations are for the treatment plan graphically represented in Figure 95–2. Note how the distal edge of the beams conform to the back edge of the tumor, thereby minimizing the dose to the right optic nerve. This plan used only circularly collimated beam apertures and no back-edge compensating boluses. The dose calculation was generated by a ray trace–based algorithm.

From a clinical standpoint, integral dose-volume histograms play a crucial role in the evaluation of a plan. For a given anatomic structure, dose-volume histograms relate the amount of volume (ordinate in ml) receiving at least a certain level of dose (abscissa in cGy) or greater. An ideal but physically unattainable dose distribution could be defined as one in which every point in the target volume receives exactly a certain level of dose, and everything outside the target volume receives zero dose. The dose-volume histogram for the target volume in such an ideal case would be characterized by a volume equal to the total target volume for dose values ranging from zero to the dose value in the target volume. At the target dose-volume value, the curve would drop to zero volume and remain there for larger values of dose. A dose-volume histogram for any structure outside the target volume in such a case would have a single point at a volume equal to the volume of the structure for a dose value of zero. For nonzero dose values, the volume would be zero; i.e., all of the volume has at least a zero dose, and no part of the volume receives any dose.

The tumor dose-volume histogram for the treatment plan represented in Figure 95–2 is shown in Figure 95–4. This dose-volume histogram deviates from a perfect one because the fall-off at large dose values (in the same arbitrary units as those in Figure 95–3) is gradual and not steep. The irregular shape of the tumor combined with the close proximity of critical structures keeps the energy deposition to the tumor from reflecting a perfect distribution. Note that the use of noncircular apertures and back-edge compensation would invariably lead to a better dose distribution.

If the treatment plan is found to be insufficient in any regard, the program must allow the user to easily modify the treatment plan accordingly and quickly re-evaluate the dose distributions. More sophisticated programs automatically attempt to determine a treatment plan based on dosimetric constraints supplied by the user. In most cases, the dosimetric results relate directly back to the exact definition of the target volume and critical structures.

SUMMARY

Given current computer technology, the factor limiting whether or not the patient is treated during the same day as the stereotactic image acquisition is the time required to manufacture any necessary irregularly shaped apertures or compensating boluses. In cases in which fractionated stereotactic treatments are to be performed, most of the treatment planning remains the same. A thorough understanding of the entire treatment planning process is vital for the establishment of a protocol that has sufficient quality assurance measures to address all hazards not explicitly handled by the planning software or hardware. Detailed and well-designed printouts can greatly assist in the administration of the quality assurance protocol.

REFERENCES

1. Ogilvy CS: Radiation therapy for arteriovenous malformations: A review. Neurosurgery 26:725–735, 1990
2. Redekop GJ, Elisevich KV, Gaspar LE, et al: Conventional radiation therapy of intracranial arteriovenous malformations: Long-term results. J Neurosurg 78:413–422, 1993
3. Clemente CD, Richardson ME: Some observations of radiation effects of the blood-brain barrier and cerebral blood vessels, in Haley TJ, Snider RS (eds): Response of the Nervous System to Ionizing Radiation. New York, Academic Press, 1962, pp 411–428
4. Steinberg GK, Levy RP, Marks MP, Fabrikant JI: Charged-particle radiosurgery, in Alexander E III, Loeffler JS, Lunsford LD (eds): Stereotactic Radiosurgery. New York, McGraw-Hill, 1993, pp 122–135
5. Kjellberg RN, Davis KR, Lyons S, et al: Bragg peak proton beam therapy for arteriovenous malformation of the brain. Clin Neurosurg 31:248–290, 1984
6. Larson B, Leksell L, Rexed B, Sourander P: Effect of high energy protons on the spinal cord. Acta Radiol 51:52–64, 1958
7. Rexed B, Mail W, Sourander P, et al: Effect of high energy protons on the brain of the rabbit. Acta Radiol 53:289–299, 1959
8. Steiner L: Treatment of arteriovenous malformations by radiosurgery, in Wilson CB, Stein BM (eds): Intracranial Arteriovenous Malformations. Baltimore, Williams & Wilkins, 1984, pp 295–313
9. Nielson SL, Kjellberg RN, Asbury AK, Koehler AM: Neuropathologic effects of proton-beam irradiation in man. Acta Neuropathol (Berl) 21:76–82, 1972
10. Ondra SL, Troupp H, George ED, et al: The natural history of symptomatic arteriovenous malformations of the brain: A 24-year follow-up assessment. J Neurosurg 73:387–391, 1990
11. Albert P, Salgado H, Polaina M, et al: A study on the venous drainage of 150 cerebral arteriovenous malformations as related to haemorrhagic risk and size of the lesion. Acta Neurochir (Wien) 103:30–34, 1990
12. Hartmen GH, Schlegel W, Sturm V, et al: Cerebral radiation surgery using moving field irradiation at a linear accelerator facility. Int J Radiat Oncol Biol Phys 11:1185–1192, 1985
13. Leksell L: Stereotaxis and Radiosurgery. An Operative System. Springfield, IL, Charles C Thomas, 1971
14. Leksell L: The stereotaxic method and radiosurgery of the brain. Acta Chir Scand 102:316–319, 1951
15. Leksell L: Stereotactic radiosurgery. J Neurol Neurosurg Psychiatry 46:797–803, 1983

16. Steiner L, Leksell L, Greitz T, et al: Stereotaxic radiosurgery for cerebral arteriovenous malformation. Report of a case. Acta Chir Scand 138:459–464, 1972
17. Steiner L, Leksell L, Foster DMC, et al: Stereotactic radiosurgery in intracranial arteriovenous malformations. Acta Neurochir Suppl (Wien) 21:195–209, 1974
18. Steiner L: Radiosurgery in cerebral arteriovenous malformations, in Fein JM, Flamm ES (eds): Cerebrovascular Surgery, vol 4. New York, Springer-Verlag, 1985, pp 1161–1215
19. Lunsford LD, Kondziolka D, Flickinger JC, et al: Stereotactic radiosurgery for arteriovenous malformations of the brain. J Neurosurg 75:512–524, 1991
20. Lunsford LD: The role of stereotactic radiosurgery in the management of brain vascular malformations, in Alexander E III, Loeffler JS, Lunsford LD (eds): Stereotactic Radiosurgery. New York, McGraw-Hill, 1993, pp 111–121
21. Colombo F, Pozza F, Chierego G, et al: Linear accelerator radiosurgery of cerebral arteriovenous malformations: An update. Neurosurgery 34:14–20, 1994
22. Bunge HJ, Chinela AB, Guevera JA, et al: Infratentorial arteriovenous malformations: Radiosurgical treatment, in Lunsford LD (ed): Stereotactic Radiosurgery Update. New York, Elsevier, 1992, pp 169–176
23. Forster DE: The Sheffield "gamma knife" experience: Results in arteriovenous malformation radiosurgery in 507 patients, in Lunsford LD (ed): Stereotactic Radiosurgery Update. New York, Elsevier, 1992, pp 113–115
24. Betti OO, Munari C, Rosler R: Stereotactic radiosurgery with the linear accelerator: Treatment of arteriovenous malformations. Neurosurgery 24:311–321, 1989
25. Friedman WA, Bova FJ: Linear accelerator radiosurgery for arteriovenous malformations. J Neurosurg 77:832–841, 1992
26. Olivier A, Sadikot AF, Leblanc R, et al: Stereotactic radiosurgery for cerebral arteriovenous malformations with linear accelerator, in Lunsford LD (ed): Stereotactic Radiosurgery Update. New York, Elsevier, 1992, pp 123–127
27. Flickinger JC, Lunsford LD, Kondziolka D: Dose prescription and dose-volume effects in radiosurgery. Neurosurg Clin North Am 3:51–59, 1991
28. Bonnett DE: Current developments in proton therapy: A review. Phys Med Biol 38:1371–1392, 1993
29. Gill SS, Thomas DGT, Warrington AP, et al: Relocatable frame for stereotactic external beam radiotherapy. Int J Radiat Oncol Biol Phys 20:599–603, 1991
30. Schad L, Lott S, Schmitt F, et al: Correction of spatial distortion in MR imaging: A prerequisite for accurate stereotaxy. J Comput Assist Tomogr 11:499–505, 1987
31. Sumanaweera TS, Glover GH, Song S, et al: Quantifying MRI geometric distortion in tissue. Magn Reson Med, in press
32. Heilbrun MP, Roberts TS, Wells TH, et al: Instruction Manual for the BRW Brown-Roberts-Wells CT Stereotaxic System, Burlington, MA, Radionics, 1983
33. Koehler AM, Schneider RJ, Sisteron JM: Range modulators for protons and heavy ions. Nucl Instrum Methods 131:437–440, 1975
34. Blattmann H: Beam delivery systems for charged particles. Radiat Environ Biophys 31:219–231, 1992
35. Petti PL: Differential-pencil-beam dose calculations for charged particles. Med Phys 19:137–149, 1992

CHAPTER 96

The Multidisciplinary Management of Vein of Galen Malformations

J. Parker Mickle
Ronald G. Quisling
Keith R. Peters

The group of deep high-flow fistulas constituting vein of Galen malformations presents an array of clinical problems early in life. Fortunately, these complex shunts deep within the midline structures of the brain are rare. The general practicing neurosurgeon occasionally is asked to see and care for one of these patients. The pediatric neurosurgeon confronts this difficult clinical problem more frequently but still does not develop a comfortable expertise in this area because of the rarity of the disease. Categorized within the spectrum of arteriovenous malformations involving the brain, these lesions remained primarily a surgical challenge until innovative and successful endovascular therapies were introduced in the 1980s (Fig. 96–1). Because of the rarity of this lesion, the clinical presentation, natural history, and therapeutic outcomes were poorly understood until the review of Hoffman[12] and the report of surgical results obtained by Yasargil were published.[29] Until these reports were available, this medical oddity remained nothing more than case report material or anecdotal reviews of small series. These high-flow central shunts pose a significant threat to survival and normal development in all children harboring them. The therapeutic goal is to effect a cure that is seldom ever achieved with a direct surgical approach. Use of this therapeutic option is usually successful in the infant with the simplest of malformations consisting of one or two feeders entering directly into the dilated venous sac. Even in this situation, direct surgical attack is difficult and fraught with many potential complications associated with retracting the poorly myelinated brain in a effort to reach the vein of Galen aneurysm on the surface of the midbrain. Too rapid elimination of the high-flow shunts in these malformations can result in acute venous outlet obstruction with neural edema, venous infarction, and ventricular hemorrhage. As a result of a better understanding of the venous contributions to the pathologic features of these malformations,[24] graded endovascular therapies are now the first choice in the treatment of these dangerous lesions. In all patients harboring vein of Galen malformations, the therapeutic goal today is to reduce the central shunt in a graded fashion to effect a cure. This entails an intelligent use of modern endovascular therapies both on the venous and arterial sides (Fig. 96–1).[3, 10, 11, 21, 22] Occasionally, an open operation is required, but this occurrence is rare. The great challenge today is the development of new embolic materials for the safe elimination of these lesions in a more controlled fashion.

CLASSIFICATION, CLINICAL FEATURES, AND PREOPERATIVE EVALUATION

The first clinical and pathologic classification of vein of Galen malformations was made by Jaeger and colleagues in 1937.[14] Litvak and associates[19] in 1960 and Norman and

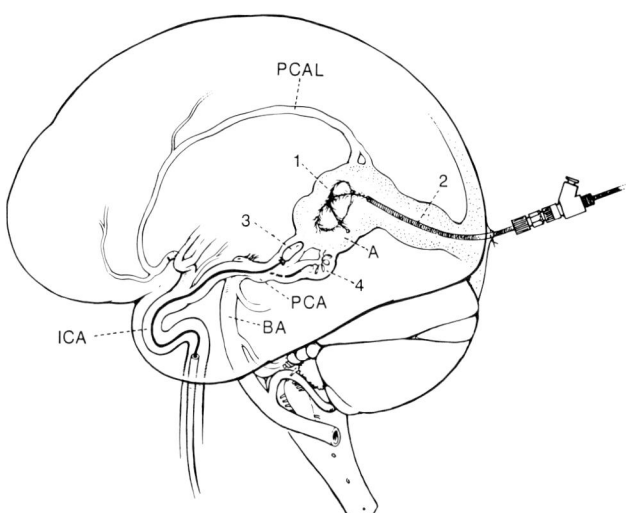

FIGURE 96–1. The usual major blood supply of a typical neonatal vein of Galen malformation and its endovascular treatment. The dilated venous sac (A) is catheterized through the torcular approach with a short angiography catheter. Embolic coils (1 and 2) can be deposited to reduce flow and begin the gradual elimination of the malformation through thrombosis. Fistulous connections through the pericallosal (PCAL), basilar (BA), internal carotid (ICA), and posterior cerebral arteries (PCA) can be approached transarterially for elimination with balloons (3) or microcoils (4). Gradual thrombosis must be used in order to eliminate many of the complications associated with venous outlet obstruction and normal perfusion breakthrough.

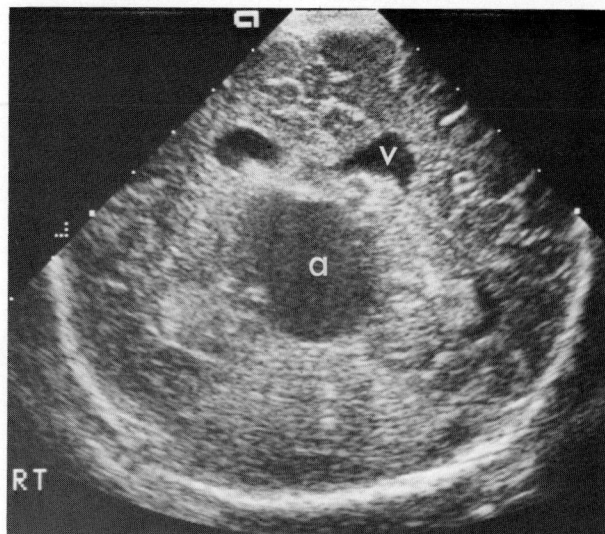

FIGURE 96–2. Postnatal ultrasound of the head of a neonate suffering from vein of Galen malformation with heart failure. The hypoechoic aneurysm (a) is clearly seen, and the minimally dilated ventricles are apparent (V). This technology is useful prenatally, and many more of these lesions are being defined during this early period, aiding in planned therapy.

Becker[23] expanded this classification and pointed out the fact that associated brain injury is common, especially in the neonate. Amacher and Shillito[1] and, subsequently, Hoffman and coworkers[12] looked at these lesions in detail and defined the importance of age of presentation in relation to clinical presentation and survival. Clinically, these patients present with three well-defined syndromes. These syndromes are age related and help define survival therapeutically. Although somewhat arbitrary, the classification of age of presentation is very useful in projecting the natural history and survival after therapy. The neonate with a symptomatic vein of Galen malformation most commonly presents with severe progressive and medically unresponsive high-output cardiac failure. Although most patients with vein of Galen malformations have some degree of cardiac involvement, in about a third of patients, this problem represents the greatest threat to survival. These patients usually look well at birth but have a hyperactive precordium with tachycardia and a rapidly progressive high-output cardiac failure that develops hours to days after birth. These babies have a machine-like murmur over the chest, neck, and head, with palpable thrills over the same regions. Prenatal diagnosis is becoming more common with the use of ultrasonography, especially with transvaginal ultrasonography (Fig. 96–2).[15, 16, 20] A clear picture of the offending lesion is obtained with this modality, and early treatment can be anticipated as a result of this early diagnosis. If the heart failure is medically refractory, which is often the case, then intervention and selective surgical procedures are required for survival. The only chance these neonates have is the aggressive but graded reduction of the central low-resistance shunt to allow cardiac survival. The infant harboring a more subtle lesion constitutes about another third of the individuals with vein of Galen malformations. These children often have mild enlargement of the heart at the time of birth but present after a month or so with progressive enlargement of the head as a result of hydrocephalus secondary to aqueductal stenosis or venous hypertension. Most of these patients have small lesions as far as the volume of shunted blood is concerned and commonly have venous anomalies representing some venous outlet obstruction at diagnosis.[18, 24] The therapeutic question remains the same in this group of individuals; that is, how to reduce and subsequently cure the fistula while maintaining integrity of the brain? There have been reports of spontaneous thromboses in this group of individuals, but these thromboses are rare.[5, 9, 13] The infant group has a much better prognosis than the neonate group, but as demonstrated by Hoffman and colleagues,[12] these lesions deteriorate progressively and still result in high morbidity and mortality when they are approached surgically. Children over 2 years of age tend to present with progressive neurologic deficit, seizures, and subarachnoid hemorrhage. Most of these patients have delayed development with motor deficits and hydrocephalus. Although this group has a better prognosis than the neonatal group, they tend to have more complex lesions than the infant group and, therefore, these lesions are much more difficult to eliminate therapeutically.

Anatomically, these central high-flow shunts are classified as type I and type II.[2, 26] The type I lesions consist principally of direct fistulous communications between terminal branches of the pericallosal and posterior cerebral arteries into the dilated vein of Galen (Fig. 96–3A). These tremendous shunts result in cardiac failure early in life and are primarily seen in the neonatal group. If these direct connections are small or few in number, then the clinical presentation is much less dramatic, and the lesion may go undetected until later in life. The so-called type II lesion more accurately represents a true arteriovenous malformation with a nidus being fed principally by posterior choroidal arteries and the postnidus veins draining into a secondarily dilated vein of

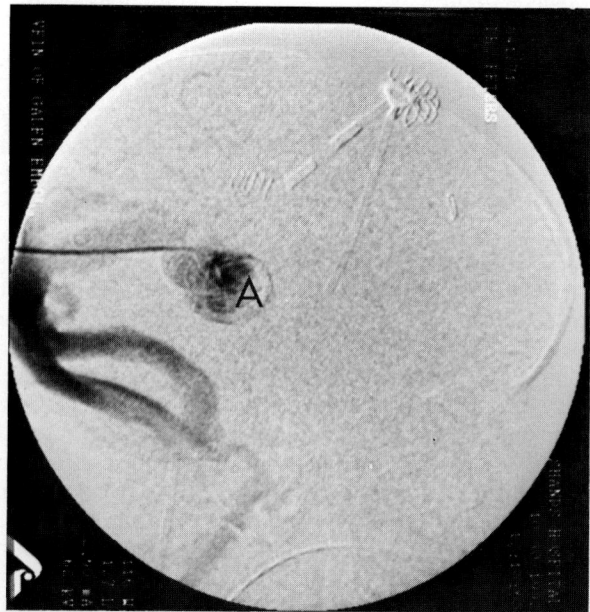

FIGURE 96–3. (A) This is a lateral carotid angiogram of a patient harboring a type I vein of Galen malformation consisting principally of direct high-flow arteriovenous fistulas into the dilated vein of Galen. (B) This is the venous phase of a more complex lesion representing a type II malformation with a complex arteriovenous nidus around the midbrain.

Galen (Fig. 96–3B). There are variations in this pathologic classification, and the pure types are rare. Therapeutically, the type II lesions are much more difficult to eliminate and are much more dangerous for the patient. High-quality, four-vessel angiography is required to define the anatomic substrate of these lesions and becomes critical in therapeutic planning.

The important concept in the therapeutic planning for vein of Galen malformation is the appreciation that these lesions represent a progressive threat to the patients harboring them.[8] Therefore, when the diagnosis is made, some form of therapeutic intervention is indicated. Before such a decision can be made, however, the patient must be in optimum clinical condition and the anatomic definition of the lesion clearly understood by the treating physician. These goals are most difficult in the neonate, and require a team consisting of the pediatric neurosurgeon, the neonatal specialist, and interventional neuroradiologist. The clinical classification discussed earlier dictates the urgency of radiologic evaluation and therapy. High-quality, four-vessel cranial angiography remains the gold standard of diagnosis and therapy. Computed tomography (CT) and ultrasonography[7] of the head are very useful technologies in defining the presence of hydrocephalus, the basic structure of the vascular malformation, and the presence or absence of any major brain insult. Magnetic resonance imaging (MRI) of the brain is helpful in defining central nervous system injury, but this study can be difficult to obtain in the neonate. Preoperative angiography is essential in defining the most efficacious endovascular route by which to administer to therapy in these lesions.

PATIENT SELECTION

Although in the past the authors have elected to treat all vein of Galen malformations aggressively, the neonate or infant presenting with major central nervous system insult as a result of these lesions should probably be treated conservatively.[23] If radiologic evaluation demonstrates major loss of brain substance, then the outlook for these patients, even with successful elimination of the fistula, is bleak. Major injury to the brain can be anticipated when the CT or MRI scan demonstrates marked atrophy, infarction, and calcification. One such patient that the authors successfully treated remains virtually vegetative with severe seizure disorder. Most patients with vein of Galen malformations however, have minimal injury to the brain and should be treated very aggressively. Today, there is almost no indication for direct surgical attack on these lesions, and endovascular therapy is becoming the treatment of choice. The therapeutic philosophy must be one of gradual reduction in the flow of these lesions with the attempt to effect a cure through graded thrombosis via the transarterial and transvenous routes (Fig. 96–4).[29] Neurosurgical intervention in these cases consists principally of the treatment of hydrocephalus with various shunting procedures and dealing with the lesion through the use of embolization technologies.

ANESTHETIC CONSIDERATION AND AIDS TO SURGERY

The neonate with massive unresponsive cardiac failure is a major anesthetic challenge.[25] Either in the operating room

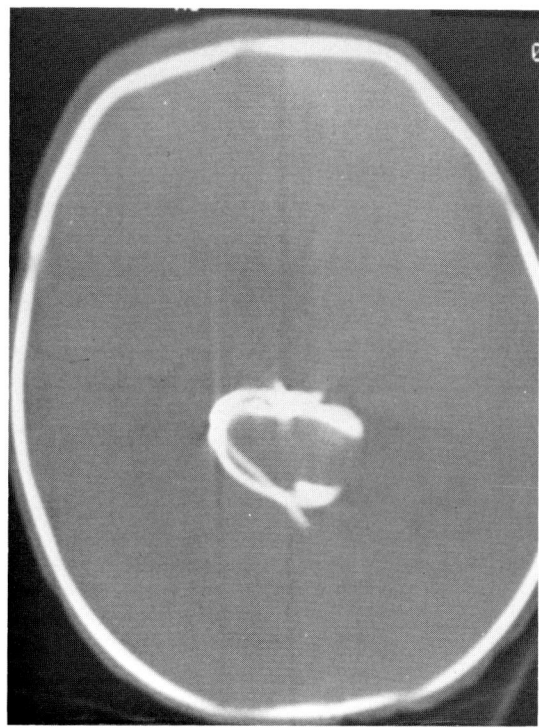

FIGURE 96–4. This is a photograph of a venogram obtained in a neonate suffering from cardiac failure as a result of vein of Galen malformation. The child has undergone placement of a VP shunt and the initial placement of multiple coils within the aneurysm. An excellent view of flow is obtained with this modality, and pressures within the aneurysm can be used to gauge the endpoint of therapy.

or in the neuroradiology suite, these unstable babies require careful monitoring and are at great risk for fluid overload and electrolyte imbalance. These babies have severe end-organ failure, especially involving the heart and kidneys. They are commonly acidotic, hyperkalemic, and hypotensive, even with the most aggressive medical therapy. This sets the stage anesthetically for major disaster as a result of fluid overload, angiographic dye toxicity, and too-rapid elimination of the central shunt. This anesthetic scenario exists in both the neuroradiology suite or the operating room. Any therapy administered to these patients must be rapid and effective because they are so unstable. In the infant and older child, these metabolic threats do not exist to the same degree and, therefore, the patient does not face as great a risk.

SURGICAL TECHNIQUES

Endovascular technologies have gradually replaced standard surgical approaches to vein of Galen malformations. The surgical attack described here is used rarely today. The feeders enter the dilated vein of Galen anterolaterally and ventrally. These arterial feeders can be approached through a paramedian occipital craniotomy via the supratentorial approach. This approach is similar to the supratentorial occipital approach to pineal region tumors, and retraction on the occipital lobe is minimized by positioning the patient so as to allow the occipital lobe to fall away from the midline as a result of the effects of gravity. In the neonate, this surgical exposure is extremely difficult to achieve because the poorly

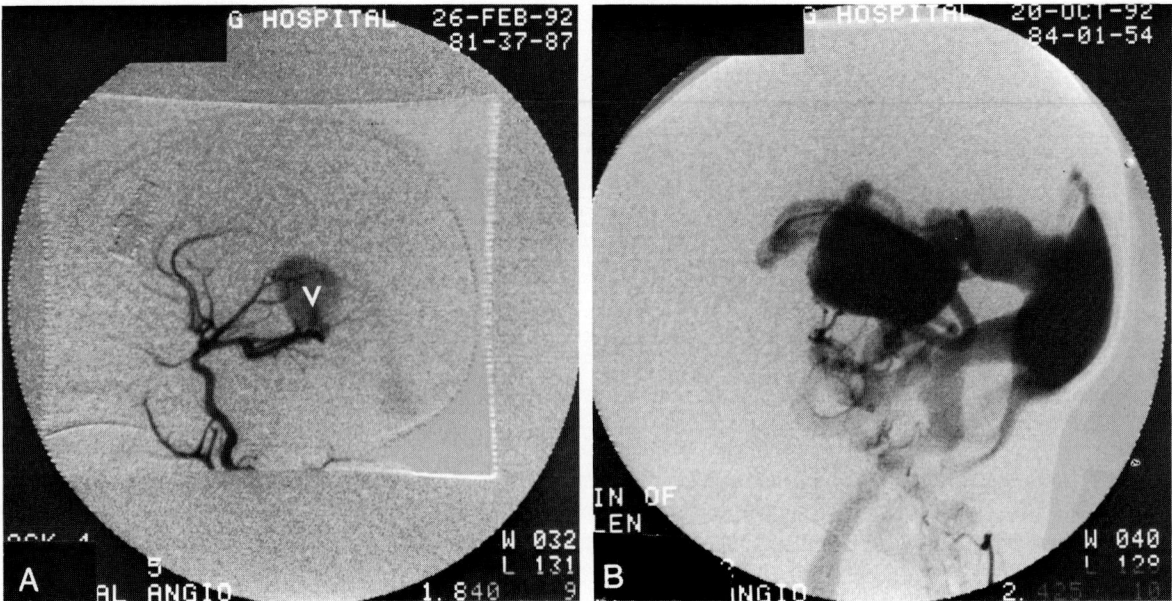

FIGURE 96–5. The CT scan in this patient shows a well-seated guidewire lattice without thrombosis in a vein of Galen aneurysm. This partially occluding lattice reduces flow within the vein of Galen malformation and also allows safer transvenous and transarterial therapies subsequently.

myelinated brain tends to tear easily. Multiple dilated arterialized sinuses and veins entering the superior sagittal sinus can impede this exposure. The dorsal surface of the vein of Galen is often tough and can be manipulated to some degree to reach feeders that must be doubly clipped or ligated and sectioned. The most ventral part of the malformation is usually paper thin, and any manipulation results in hemorrhage. Exposure can be aided by the placement of a ventriculostomy or with the use of dehydrating agents such as mannitol. Hydrocephalus is a frequent complication of vein of Galen malformations and often requires the placement of a ventriculoperitoneal shunt.[27] This procedure should be performed carefully when progressive hydrocephalus is present because dilated subependymal veins are also often present in these individuals, especially after transvenous therapy. The placement of a ventriculostomy can be extremely hazardous in these individuals and should be performed in the operating room under optimum conditions.

The goal of interventional therapy in these patients differs according to the clinical classification of each lesion. The neonate suffering from massive heart failure must have early and effective reduction of the shunt in order to achieve cardiac survival. The neonate with metabolic acidosis and falling urinary output cannot be stabilized or retrieved with medical therapy. Flow in the central fistula must be reduced so that cardiac performance is improved and peripheral perfusion is enhanced. As mentioned earlier, this is rarely accomplished with direct surgical attack or aggressive medical management. Angiography is performed and can be accomplished either by the femoral route or through an indwelling umbilical artery catheter placed at the time of delivery. Transarterial embolizations are time consuming and difficult to perform in the neonate, and these efforts often result in the overuse of fluids and toxic dyes in their evaluation and treatment. However, if the transarterial route can be used effectively and rapidly, and one or two large feeders can be eliminated, this will help the overall effort to eliminate these lesions (see Fig. 96–1). More commonly, the area of the aneurysm can be approached transvenously either via the femoral route or more directly through a transtorcular approach through the posterior fontanelle or a small craniectomy placed over the torcula.[4, 6, 17, 22] If because of venous obstruction, which is common in some of these lesions, the vein of Galen aneurysm cannot be reached via these techniques, then a direct approach for the deposition of embolic materials can be used through a small paramedian craniotomy similar to that used in the supratentorial approach. The transtorcular approach is rapid and simple. Use of ultrasound in the operating room or in the neuroradiology suite can identify the torcula, straight sinus, and aneurysm very nicely through either a craniectomy or an open posterior fontanelle (see Fig. 96–2). The torcula is punctured with an angiocatheter, and a soft, short guidewire is advanced through the straight sinus into the vein of Galen aneurysm. Over this, a short, soft, standard angiography catheter is advanced into the aneurysm and the guidewire removed. Venography is performed with a small amount of contrast, and intra-aneurysmal pressures are measured and compared with mean arterial pressure (see Fig. 96–4). The goal here is to reduce flow so that there is an immediate improvement in cardiac function. This goal can be accomplished with the deposition of various coils, balloons, and other embolic materials until a reduction of pressure is obtained within the aneurysm or a substantial change in flow characteristics is noted on venography. It is important never to force a wire in this situation because puncture of the aneurysm and hemorrhage will be disastrous. Also, too-aggressive deposition of the embolic agents can result in acute thrombosis with resulting venous infarction and hemorrhage.[29] In anticipation of the need for both transvenous and transarterial treatments of these lesions, we initially place a soft basket within the aneurysm constructed from a standard angiography guidewire, varying in length from 45 to 150 cm (Fig. 96–5). This Teflon-coated lattice is folded into the aneurysm without forcing its place-

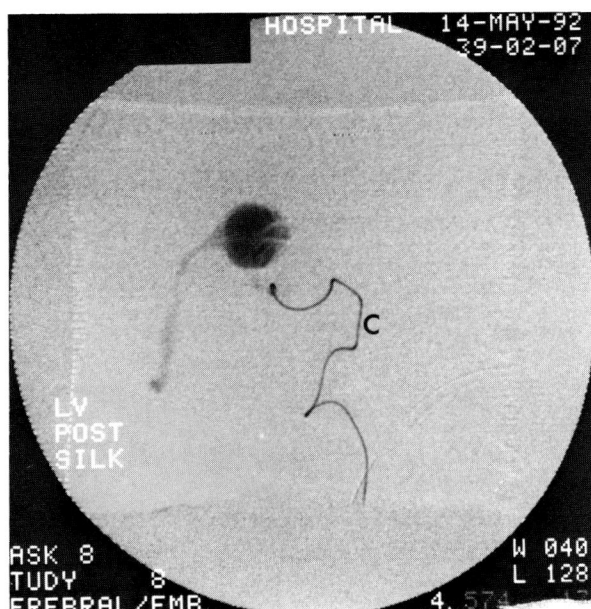

FIGURE 96-6. This patient with a vein of Galen malformation is undergoing the final stage of elimination of the lesion with transarterial embolization. The patient had previously been treated with a transvenous deposition of embolic wires, and the small persistent posterior cerebral feeder was catheterized with the microcatheter (C). Small pieces of 4-0 silk were used as the embolic agent to eliminate this lesion completely.

ment. This basket then acts as a lattice onto which, or within which, various embolic coils and balloons can be placed without the threat of peripheral embolization. Transarterial embolizations are then made safe because embolic agents such as silk thread and glues are less likely to traverse the complex. The neonate who is improving but does not have a persistent fistula after this initial embolization is allowed to stabilize and return for angiographic evaluation at 1 month of age. The initial improvement is usually short lived, and in hours to days, the patient again develops progressive high-output cardiac failure with increasing acidosis and falling urinary output. It is essential that the child be returned to the neuroradiology suite early and repeat embolization performed either transarterially or transvenously. The authors have preferred to use the transvenous approach because it is quicker and easier and requires less fluid and angiographic evaluation. This scenario may have to be repeated three to four times in order to ensure cardiac survival. In the neonate diagnosed with a vein of Galen malformation as a result of hydrocephalus or in the neonate successfully treated at birth who returns for further therapy in the infantile period, transarterial or transvenous therapy is again chosen in an effort to obtain a cure.

It would appear from the authors' initial results that progressive thrombosis is possible in certain lesions following initial treatment with endovascular therapies. Several patients the authors have re-admitted for angiography in anticipation of further therapy have demonstrated total obliteration of their shunts after multiple-staged procedures. If the infant has hydrocephalus, then we recommend an initial VP shunt, because following endovascular therapy, this simple procedure may become dangerous.[27] At this point in the development of therapy for infantile vein of Galen malformations, the authors perform an angiogram intraoperatively and, if hydrocephalus is present, perform a VP shunt. If appropriate, the authors then place a guidewire basket within the vein of Galen malformation but are very careful to avoid complete and rapid thrombosis of the lesion in this setting. The child is seen again in 1 month for an angiogram and a decision is made then concerning further use of embolization therapy, either transarterially or transvenously. In the authors' experience, large arterial shunts that are easily catheterized transarterially are eliminated with microcoils, balloons, or silk suture embolization (Fig. 96-6). This approach reduces the risk of transvenous embolization in an effort to eliminate the lesion completely. As in the infant, the older child and young adult are treated essentially in a similar fashion, but these lesions tend to be more complex and are categorized as arteriovenous malformations with less of a chance of cure. These patients often have major venous occlusion already with anomalous venous drainage of the lesion, and transarterial embolization of these lesions is attempted first. If a transvenous route is possible, then a guidewire basket is delivered into the aneurysm to act as a lattice, onto which other embolic agents can be deposited. Although to date we have not treated any persistent fistula with other adjunctive therapies such as stereotactic radiosurgery, it is anticipated that this new technology will be useful in certain patients to eliminate their lesions when no other embolization is appropriate or possible.

POSTOPERATIVE CARE

After surgery, all patients are returned to the intensive care unit and carefully monitored. Any change in neurologic status must be evaluated with emergency CT scan for the early diagnosis and management of complications. Progressive heart failure must be treated with further embolization. Acute and disastrous neurologic deterioration can result from acute thrombosis of the arteriovenous malformation complex with venous infarction or hemorrhage. The CT scan is the most rapid way of diagnosing this complication, and in the two instances in which this has occurred in the authors' series, we have performed ventriculostomies and placed the patient into pentobarbital coma. This is continued for at least 3 days, and the intracranial pressure is carefully monitored. Postoperative seizures are treated aggressively with antiepileptic medications. The deposition of thrombogenic coils within the vein of Galen malformation complex can result in thrombosis with consumption of red cells and also clotting factors, resulting in a rapidly dropping hematocrit and bleeding disorder. This problem is watched carefully, and the child is transfused when appropriate. Postembolization fevers are common for the first 2 to 3 days but have not persisted in any of the patients who were treated successfully.

RESULTS

The published results in 24 of the authors' patients treated with transvenous embolization are available for review.[21] In the past, virtually 100 percent of the neonates suffering from heart failure died.[14] Today with aggressive neonatal intensive care and endovascular therapy, a 40-percent survival rate can be expected in this high-risk group. About half of these patients can be expected to have good-to-excellent survival times, but the other half can be expected to demonstrate significant neurologic deficit as a result of their high-flow lesions. The report by Hoffman and coworkers defined a 17-percent mortality rate in the infant group, and this would appear to be similar after endovascular therapy.[12] The authors have lost two patients in this group in our series—one from a malfunctioning shunt and the other from a postembolization hemorrhage as a result of too-rapid occlusion of the vein of Galen malformation. Most of the patients successfully treated with whatever technique usually have some discernible deficits. In patients who have recovered, this usually expresses itself as mild spasticity and minimal learning disabilities. Seizures occur in about 50 percent of successfully treated patients.

DISCUSSION AND SUMMARY

Vein of Galen malformations represent a spectrum of high-flow fistulous connections between the deep central arteries of the carotid and vertebral circulations to the vein of Galen and its tributaries. These high-flow shunts can produce progressive high-output cardiac failure, cerebral ischemia, hydrocephalus, venous hypertension, and hemorrhage. The natural history of this disease is progressive and carries a very poor prognosis. There is a tendency today not to use direct surgical attack because the mortality rate that results from this procedure remains high and the cure rate is low. The transarterial interruption of some of the feeders is efficacious in reducing some of the complications of venous embolization. A reduction in the arterial supply can be expected to reduce the likelihood of normal profusion breakthrough if it is performed in a graded fashion.[29] The transvenous approach seems to offer the best chance for effective and lasting cure in this disease, but the ideal formula for achieving this goal in many of the patients has not been perfected yet. However, progress is being made and the exploding technology in endovascular therapy should improve the rate of survival in patients with vein of Galen aneurysms. The future is better now for the patient harboring a vein of Galen malformation, but the entity remains a great challenge to a multidisciplinary team committed to understanding and eliminating these dangerous lesions.

REFERENCES

1. Amacher AL, Shillito J Jr: The syndromes and surgical treatment of aneurysms of the great vein of Galen. J Neurosurg 39:89–98, 1973
2. Bartal AD: Classifications of aneurysms of the great vein of Galen [Letter]. J Neurosurg 42:617–619, 1975
3. Berenstein A, Epstein F: Vein of Galen malformations: Combined neurosurgical and neuroradiologic intervention, in American Association of Neurological Surgeons (eds): Pediatric Neurosurgery: Surgery of the Developing Nervous System. New York, Grune & Stratton, 1982, pp 638–647
4. Casasco A, Lylyk P, Hodes JE, et al: Percutaneous transvenous catheterization and embolization of vein of Galen aneurysms. Neurosurgery 28:260–265, 1991
5. Copty M, Bedard F, Turcotte JF: Successful removal of an entirely calcified aneurysm of the vein of Galen. Surg Neurol 14:396–400, 1980
6. Dowd CF, Halbach W, Barnwell SL, et al: Transfemoral venous embolization of vein of Galen malformations. AJNR 11:643–648, 1990
7. Deeg KH, Scarf J: Colour Doppler imaging of arteriovenous malformation of the vein of Galen in a newborn. Neuroradiology 32:50–63, 1990
8. Diebler C, Dulac O, Renier D, et al: Aneurysms of the vein of Galen in infants aged 2 to 15 months: Diagnosis and natural evolution. Neuroradiology 21:185–187, 1981
9. DiRocco C, Iannelli A, Puca A, Colosimo C Jr: Spontaneous thrombosis of an aneurysm of the Great Vein of Galen. Eur Neurol 22:529–532, 1983
10. Hanner JS, Quisling RG, Mickle JP, Hawkins IF: Retrievable Gianturco-Coil introducer. Radiology 158:262–264, 1986
11. Hawkins J, Quisling RG, Mickle JP, Hawkins IF: Retrievable Gianturco-Coil introducer. Radiology 41:424–428, 1986
12. Hoffman HJ, Chuang S, Hendrick EB, Humphreys RP: Aneurysms of the vein of Galen: Experience at the Hospital for Sick Children, Toronto. J Neurosurg 57:316–322, 1982
13. Hurst RW, Kagetsu NJ, Berenstein A: Angiographic findings in the two cases of aneurysmal malformation of vein of Galen prior to spontaneous thrombosis: Therapeutic implications. AJNR 13:1446–1450, 1992
14. Jaeger JR, Forbes RP, Dandy WE: Bilateral congenital cerebral arteriovenous communication aneurysm. Trans Am Neurol Assoc 63:173–176, 1937
15. Jeanty P, Kepple D, Roussis P, Shah D: In utero detection of cardiac failure from an aneurysm of the vein of Galen. Am J Obstet Gynecol 163:50–51, 1990
16. Johnston IH, Whittle IR, Besser M, Morgan MK: Vein of Galen malformation: Diagnosis and management. Neurosurgery 20:747–758, 1987
17. Lasjaunias P, Rodesch G, Terbrugge K, et al: Vein of Galen aneurysmal malformations: Report of 36 cases managed between 1982–1988. Acta Neurochir (Wien) 99:26–37, 1989
18. Lasjaunias P, Terbrugge K, Lopez Ibor L, et al: The role of dural anomalies in vein of Galen aneurysms: Report of six cases and review of the literature. AJNR 8:185–192, 1987
19. Litvak J, Yahr MD, Ransohoff J: Aneurysms of great vein of Galen and midline cerebral arteriovenous anomalies. J Neurosurg 17:945–954, 1960
20. Mendelsohn DB, Hertzanu Y, Butterworth A: In utero diagnosis of a vein of Galen aneurysm by ultrasound. Neuroradiology 26:417–418, 1984
21. Mickle JP: The transtorcular embolization of Vein of Galen aneurysms: An update of the use of this technique in 24 patients. Concepts in Pediatric Neurosurgery II, 1991
22. Mickle JP, Quisling RG: The transtorcular embolization of vein of Galen aneurysms. J Neurosurg 64:731–735, 1986
23. Norman MG, Becker LE: Cerebral damage in neonates resulting from arteriovenous malformation of the vein of Galen. J Neurol Neurosurg Psychiatry 37:252–258, 1974
24. Quisling RG, Mickle JP: Venous pressure measurements in vein of Galen aneurysms. AJNR 10:411–417, 1989
25. Rasch DK, Webster DB, Hutyra J, et al: Anesthetic management of hemodynamic changes during vein of Galen aneurysm clipping. Anesthesiology 69:993–995, 1988
26. Raybaud CA, Strother CM, Hald JK: Aneurysms of the Vein of Galen: Embryonic considerations and anatomical features relating to the pathogenesis of the malformation. Neuroradiology 31:109–128, 1989
27. Schneider SJ, Wisoff JS, Epstein FJ: Complications of ventriculoperitoneal shunt procedures or hydrocephalus associated with vein of Galen malformations in childhood. Neurosurgery 30(5):706–708, 1992
28. Spetzler RF, Wilson CB, Weinstein P, et al: Normal perfusion pressure breakthrough theory. Clin Neurosurg 25:651–672, 1978
29. Yasargil MG: Microsurgery, IIIB. New York, Theme Medical Publishers Inc, 1988, pp 323–357

CHAPTER 97

Surgical Management of Dural Arteriovenous Malformations

Mark C. Held
Thoralf M. Sundt, Jr.
David G. Piepgras
Fredric B. Meyer
Robert J. Coffey
Douglas A. Nichols

Arteriovenous fistulae (AVFs) of the lateral and dural sinuses are uniquely interesting because they have been proved to be acquired lesions that develop from a previously thrombosed sinus and the resultant venous hypertension.[1] Although dural AVFs represent between 6 and 15 percent of all intracranial vascular malformations, they generally have a more benign course than their intraparenchymal counterparts, presenting with hemorrhage only 10 percent of the time, versus 50 percent for the intraparenchymal variety.[2, 3] Dural AVFs are direct shunts between a dural arterial supply and a dural venous drainage system. Approximately two-thirds occur at the junction of the transverse and sigmoid sinuses, and one-third occur, in decreasing frequency, in the cavernous sinus, in the tentorial incisura, juxtaposed to sagittal sinus, and finally, in the anterior fossa. Although previously described as arteriovenous malformations, dural AVFs do not have the capillary nidus so familiar in arteriovenous malformations, and thus they lend themselves to a separate radiologic classification. It is not our purpose here to discuss the pathogenesis, symptomatology, or natural history of these lesions; these aspects of the illness have been discussed and reported previously.[2, 4–13]

In this chapter, we focus on the surgical approaches and techniques for the obliteration of AVFs. These approaches were originally reported in the *Journal of Neurosurgery* in 1983.[13] Our experience is based on 73 cases collected over 23 years that were limited to the transverse-sigmoid sinuses.

RADIOSURGERY AND PREOPERATIVE EMBOLIZATION

Significant advances in preoperative embolization techniques as an adjunct to open surgery deserve special mention. We diminish blood flow through these very vascular lesions by preoperative embolization 1 to 2 days before the anticipated date of surgery. This procedure has resulted in a dramatic reduction in the amount of bleeding during the operative procedure. There is obviously an inherent risk with this technique, but in the hands of skillful angiographers and with careful monitoring, it has proved in our experience to be amazingly safe.

It is beyond the scope of this chapter to discuss, the techniques for embolization of these malformations. Such a discussion requires careful analysis of the preoperative angiograms is necessary, including assessment of the size and number of feeding vessels, the routes of access for therapeutic catheterization; the degree of flow through the shunt, which determines the type of occlusive agent to be used; and potential patent communications between the external carotid and vertebral basilar systems. Good communication between surgeon and angiographer is mandatory in weighing the risks versus the benefits for different embolization methods for the overall treatment of the patient.

Pre-embolization and postembolization angiograms of a patient undergoing embolization before surgery are illustrated in Figures 97–1 and 97–2. Although the malformation appears to be well obliterated from embolization alone, we are reluctant to accept this as a treatment per se because our experience is that large malformations recur after embolization alone. When the malformation recurs, the circulation has been driven into the internal structures of the brain and dura, making excision extraordinarily difficult.

In patients considered to be poor surgical risks, preoperative embolization followed by stereotactic radiosurgery has recently become part of the modern neurosurgeon's armamentarium. Since October 1990, we have treated 19 patients with dural AVFs by use of the radiosurgical gamma knife at the Mayo Clinic. Twelve of these patients, who had prominent cortical or deep venous drainage associated with the lesion, underwent embolization of all accessible external carotid feeding vessels within 1 to 3 days after radiosurgery. Although radiosurgery can cause complete obliteration of dural AVFs, this effect occurs after a latency period of 2 years or longer. Performing embolization shortly after radiosurgery allows the entire nidus to remain angiographically visible for radiosurgical dosimetry and planning. Irradiation of the small nidus should cause long-term obliteration, and embolization should provide protection against early hemorrhage during the latency period as well as immediate symptomatic relief. We use particulate emboli in these cases to avoid the potential risks associated with glue passing into the venous circulation. A further rationale for this approach is that even if the embolized portion of the AVF were to undergo late recanalization, the entire nidus has been irradiated and simultaneously is undergoing occlusion.

PATIENTS AND METHODS

Eight patients were male, and 11 were female. Symptoms included headache ($n = 16$), hemorrhage ($n = 3$), seizures ($n = 2$), and neurologic deficits ($n = 10$). Eight AVFs involved the cavernous sinus, seven lesions involved the transverse or petrosial sinuses, one involved the tentorium, and three involved the supratentorial or suboccipital convexity dura. Two of the three patients underwent embolization, as did five patients with transverse or petrosal sinus AVFs and with five patients harboring cavernous sinus malformations.

All radiosurgical procedures were performed with the patient under local anesthesia, selective angiography was used for target-coordinate determination and dose planning. Complete coverage of each dural AVF nidus was accomplished with a single-fraction dose of 18 to 20 Gy (at the 50- to 55-percent isodose line). The mean nidus volume was 2900 mm^3 (2.9 ml). The embolization procedures were carried out in one to two stages, and polyvinyl alcohol particles, silk suture material, or both, were used.

RESULTS

Patients have been followed up for up to 36 months. To date, no dural AVF has hemorrhaged after treatment, and all patients are neurologically stable. The cortical venous drainage was reduced or eliminated immediately after postradiosurgical embolization in all patients in whom embolization was performed. Follow-up angiography in ten patients 12 to 36 months after treatment showed that the remaining nidus or fistula has disappeared ($n = 5$) or remained smaller ($n = 5$) in all cases. One patient developed mild, temporary dysphasia due to acute thrombosis of a small cortical vein after embolization of a cavernous sinus dural AVF. Another patient suddenly became vertiginous and lost hearing ipsilateral to a transverse sinus AVF 1 year after radiosurgery and embolization. The eighth nerve and cochlea were well outside the field of irradiation. The cause of this patient's hearing loss remains unknown, although the clinical history strongly suggests a vascular etiology. Figure 97–3 shows the pretreatment and posttreatment angiograms of another patient who underwent radiosurgery and embolization of a right transverse sinus dural AVF. Before referral, this patient had experienced the onset of left hemibody seizures and hemiparesis due to venous infarction in the right frontal and parietal lobes. We believe that radiosurgery, followed in selected cases by particulate embolization, is a safe and rational approach to certain high-risk dural AVFs.

SURGICAL TECHNIQUES

POSITIONING THE PATIENT

The patient can be positioned semiprone, as was the patient in the illustrative case (Fig. 97–4). Alternatively, the

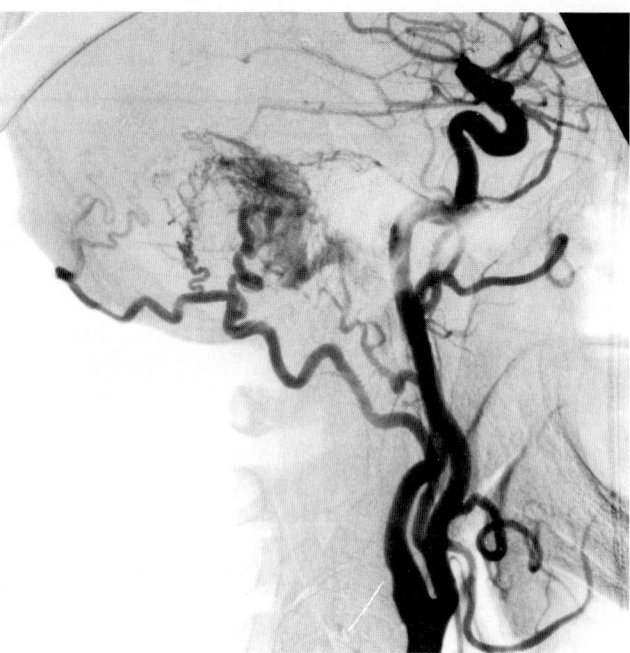

FIGURE 97–2. Postoperative angiogram demonstrating (1) occlusion of the arteriovenous fistula at the capillary shunting level, with preservation of the normal occipital artery; (2) closure of the shunting component of the posterior branch of the middle meningeal artery from occlusion at the capillary level (this would not happen if the occipital artery were ligated proximal to the shunt; in that case, the collateral supply from the meningeal circulation would continue); and (3) maintenance of the normal remaining external carotid artery and internal carotid artery branches.

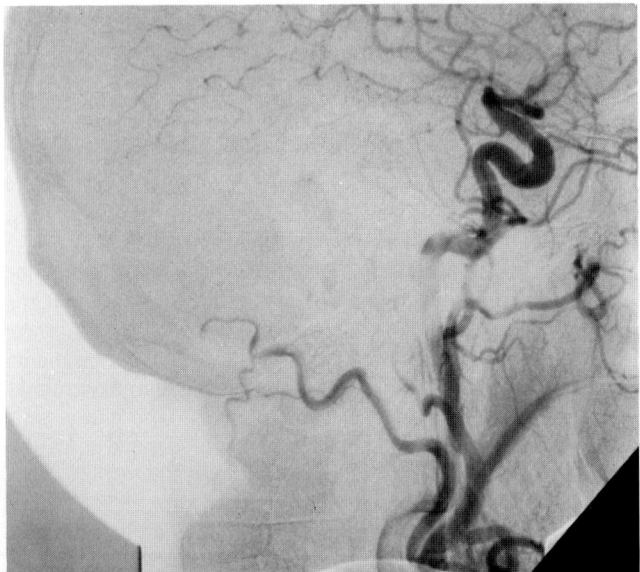

FIGURE 97–1. A preoperative lateral angiogram demonstrating a dural arteriovenous fistula involving the right lateral sinus. The primary blood supply to the malformation is derived from branches of the occipital artery.

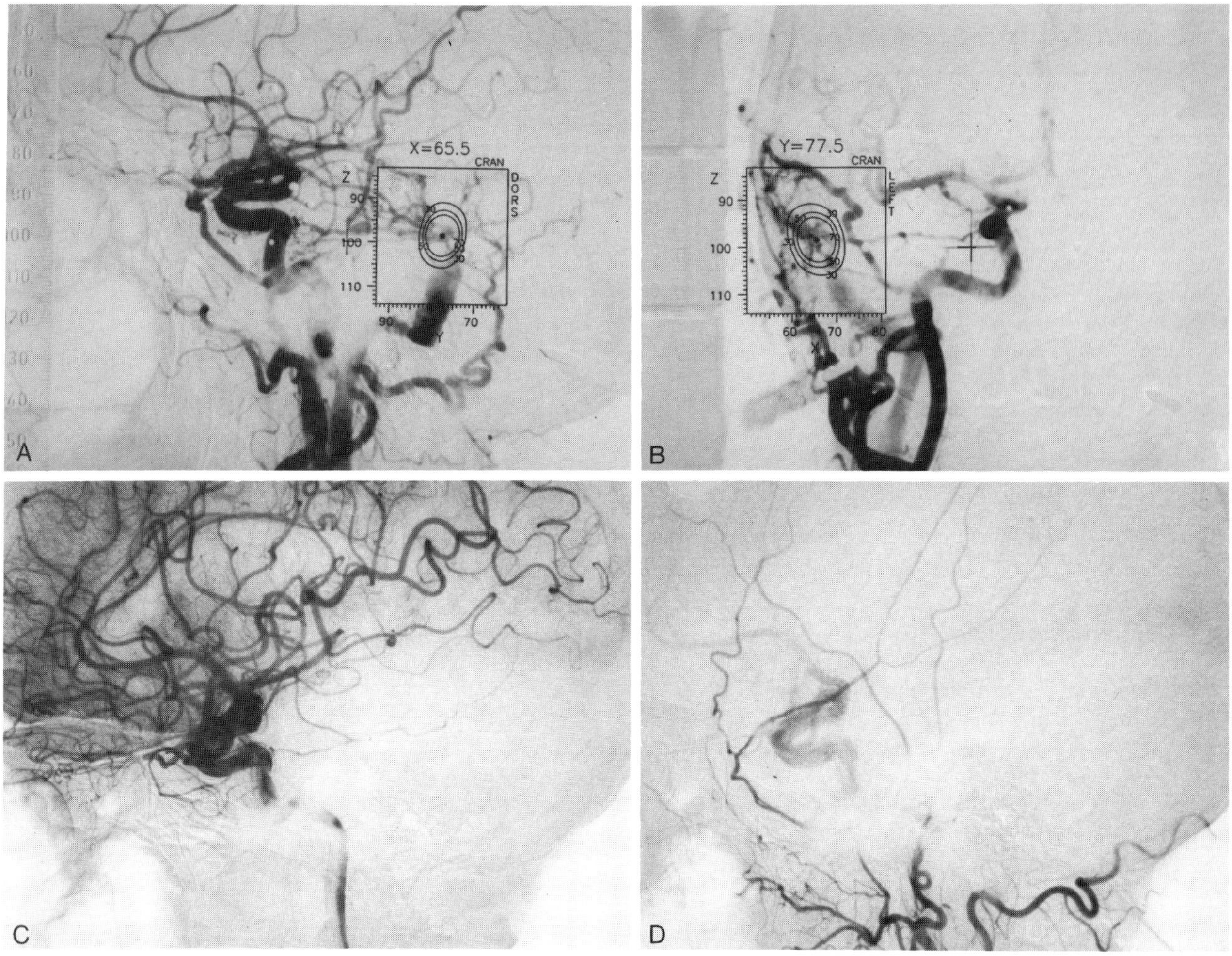

Surgical Management of Dural Arteriovenous Malformations | 1221

FIGURE 97-3. (A, B) AP and lateral common carotid angiogram films with superimposed isodose distributions during radiosurgical treatment of a right-sided transverse sinus dural AVM and fistula. Both external carotid and internal carotid artery branches feed the AVM. Follow-up selective internal (C) and external (D) carotid angiogram films 1 year after radiosurgery show complete obliteration of the AVF and fistula. The patient's neurologic condition had improved and her seizures had ceased since treatment.

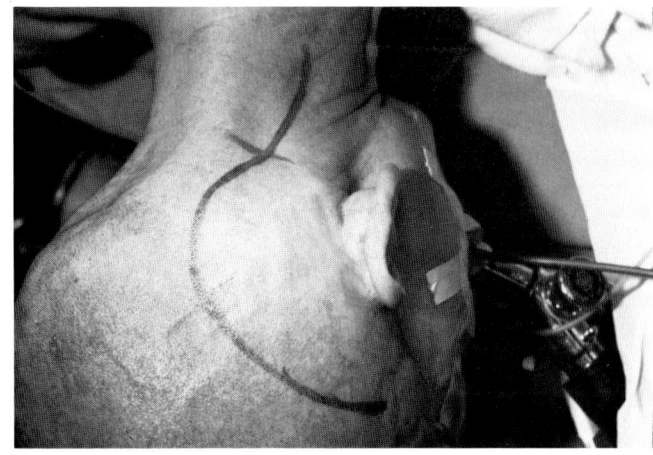

FIGURE 97-4. A curvilinear scalp incision extending inferior to the lateral sinus. It is shaped so that this structure can be exposed, with retraction, from the petrous bone to the torcular.

patient can be placed supine with the head turned sharply (see Fig. 97–6A). In either case, the surgeon must have ready access to the region between the inion and the mastoid. A malleable lumbar spinal needle is placed for later drainage of cerebrospinal fluid (CSF).

SCALP FLAP

The incision used is shaped much like a question mark (see Figs. 97–4 and 97–6A). For malformations involving the entire length of the transverse sinus, a U-shaped incision extending across the torcula is best. More than average bleeding occurs from the scalp margins that must be controlled and well secured to prevent troublesome or unnoticed blood loss during the remainder of the case. The scalp flap is reflected to its base, exposing the mastoid process, and the occipital margin is retracted to the inion. In so doing, a greatly enlarged occipital artery and posterior auricular artery are doubly ligated and divided, along with many of their branches. In some instances, the major blood supply to the malformation has thereby been interrupted.

SOFT-TISSUE DISSECTION

After the scalp flap is reflected, the deep cervical fascia and nuchal musculature are incised with a cutting current just below their insertion onto the occipital bone. Invariably, many large feeding and draining vessels are encountered here, and these vessels require coagulation or even clipping. The pericranium is now incised and stripped away from the bone along the path for the craniotomy (see Fig. 97–6B).

CRANIOTOMY

A wide bone flap is fashioned to extend both above and below the sinus. The craniotomy is effected by use of the cutting bit of the air drill (Figs. 97–5 and 97–6B). This step is very important, and considerable care and thought are required to avoid potentially catastrophic bleeding. The craniotome should not be used here, because a laceration of the highly vascular dura or sinus (both of which are quite adherent to the bone) could produce a fatal hemorrhage, which is analogous to the rupture of an intracranial aneurysm before the bone plate is elevated. The air drill must be held at an angle of approximately 30 degrees to the bone; if it is held vertically, it tends to drill through the bone. As the craniotomy is deepened, the drill bit is switched for a smaller one that allows better visualization in the depth of the cut and lessens the risk of a dural tear. The dura can be visualized through a thin layer of bone when the craniotomy has been carried to sufficient depth. The surgeon is now in position to elevate the bone plate.

Before the bone is removed, preparations should be made for the possibility of a major loss of blood in a very short time. Such loss is variable and is seemingly related to the amount of venous drainage that has developed from the AVF through the diploë of the bone. We have found it helpful to lower the blood pressure and to start a rapid transfusion of blood at the time the bone plate is elevated. In spite of these measures, the rapid loss of blood can be shocking to the patient and staggering to the surgeon. We have calculated blood loss to approach 300 ml/minute on several occasions. Although the loss is great, it can usually be slowed and controlled by digital compression of a large piece of thrombin-soaked Surgicel, reinforced with a surgical sponge packing, over the entire expanse of the exposed dura. The margins are then gradually enlarged as the pack is withdrawn, and bleeding points are individually arrested with bipolar coagulation until the pack is removed (Figs. 97–6C and D). As indicated, preoperative embolization greatly reduces this bleeding.

SINUS LIGATION

After good hemostasis is achieved, the margins of the dura are firmly affixed to the margins of the craniotomy with tacking sutures placed about 2 cm apart. These numerous sutures are required to obliterate the epidural space, which is more vascular than normal because of its participation in the drainage pattern of the AVF. Care should be taken to avoid drilling tack holes through the mastoid so as to prevent possible CSF leaks.

The lateral sinus lies in the middle area of the craniotomy (Fig. 97–6E). Two dural incisions are made parallel to the long axis of the sinus, one superior to and the other inferior to the sinus. These incisions are enlarged by secondary incisions vertical to them, so that two Ts are created above and below the sinus (Fig. 97–6E). Then, 30 to 40 ml of CSF is withdrawn through the malleable needle previously placed in the lumbar spinal space. Bridging veins off the occipital pole and superior cerebellum are coagulated with the bipolar coagulator and are divided.

Two curved hemostats are next placed with an intervening distance of at least 1.5 cm across the sinus, followed by two more if necessary, lateral and medial, respectively, to the first pair (Fig. 97–6F). The sinus is now cut with curved scissors (Fig. 97–6F). The medial sinus is closed with a running suture, and these hemostats are removed.

RESECTION OF THE ARTERIOVENOUS FISTULA

The lateral hemostats are used to elevate the sinus and its AVF from the wound (Fig. 97–6G). With minimal retraction of the occipital lobe and superior cerebellum, the tentorium is exposed, coagulated, and incised bit by bit with curved scissors laterally toward the petrous ridge. The traction applied to the hemostats securing the cut edge of the lateral sinus places tension on the tentorium. Large feeding dural vessels are best controlled with small hemostatic clips. In this manner, the sinus is isolated from the dura overlying the cerebellum and the occipital lobe, and from the tentorium (Fig. 97–6G).

This step brings us to the epicenter of the AVF, which is invariably located at the junction point between the lateral and sigmoid sinuses. The chief source of bleeding now seems to be the petrous bone itself from large feeding arteries con-

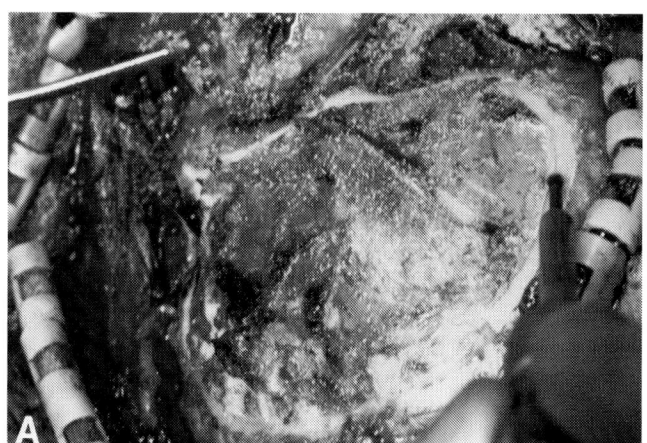
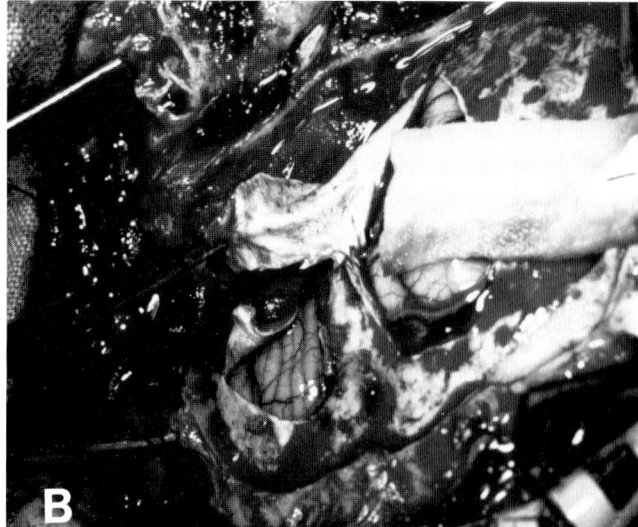

FIGURE 97–5. (A) Craniotomy is performed using a high-speed air drill. It extends above and below the lateral sinus and from the petrous bone almost to the midline. The proximal portion of the sigmoid sinus is visible through this craniotomy. (B) The dura is opened above and below the lateral sinus to facilitate resection of this structure.

tained in it. Some of these bleeding points can be arrested with the cutting current of the Bovie unit, but others are best handled with Surgicel or Avitene packed firmly into the vascular channels. In spite of the major bleeding that continues to develop as the bone is removed, it is necessary to resect the margins of petrous bone adjacent to the anterior surface of the proximal one-third of the sigmoid sinus to ensure that the arterial supply to the AVF has been interrupted. This goal is best accomplished with a diamond burr on the air drill (Fig. 97–6H).

Earlier in our experience, we attempted to resect the sigmoid sinus, but later we found this measure to be unnecessary if we opened it and securely occluded it by packing it tightly with Surgicel (Fig. 97–6I). This method has the distinct advantage of leaving a cuff of dura, which allows sufficient purchase for a tight homologous dural or fascia lata graft closure, which is important for avoiding the possibility of CSF leakage through resected mastoid air cells (Fig. 97–6I).

VEIN OF LABBÉ

Bridging veins that are red can be divided with relative impunity because they are draining the AVF rather than the brain. Those that are black must be respected, particularly the vein of Labbé, which fortunately rarely interferes (see Discussion). In most instances, the vein of Labbé drains through the deep petrosal sinus but may occasionally course through distal sigmoid sinus. Resection or packing of the sigmoid must not interfere with drainage of Labbé.

CLOSURE

The dura is replaced with a homologous dural graft or a piece of fascia lata. The bone plate is wired to the skull with four or five wires, and the scalp is closed with a single layer of vertical mattress sutures.

OPERATIVE RESULTS

There were 62 excellent, three good, and five poor results in the group, along with three deaths. Two poor results were in patients who did not recover the use of their vision, both having been legally blind from chronic papilledema before surgery. One of three deaths resulted from cardiac arrest related to blood loss; this occurred in the only infant in the series. The infant had a torcular malformation that was different from the other malformations in both its pathogenesis and magnitude. It was the only congenital malformation in the series. Another death occurred in a patient with a high-flow AVF that produced a progressing deficit and had been operated on and embolized previously. The usual external carotid system supply was replaced with multiple dural vessels arising from the internal carotid and vertebral arteries. When the bone plate was elevated, a torrent of blood followed, and the patient exsanguinated. Compression of the convexity dura was of no avail because the entire dura overlying the posterior aspect of the petrous bone was simply a pulsating arterial sinus. The third death in our series occurred in a patient who presented with occipital hemorrhage and bifrontal subdural hematomas—most likely secondary to venous hypertension. Despite operative excision of the fistula and evacuation of the clot, the patient succumbed to brainstem compression (Table 97–1).

Table 97–1. SURGICAL COMPLICATIONS IN THE TREATMENT OF ARTERIOVENOUS FISTULAE

Complication	Incidence
Venous hemorrhage	12
Seizure	4
Cerebrospinal fluid leak	1

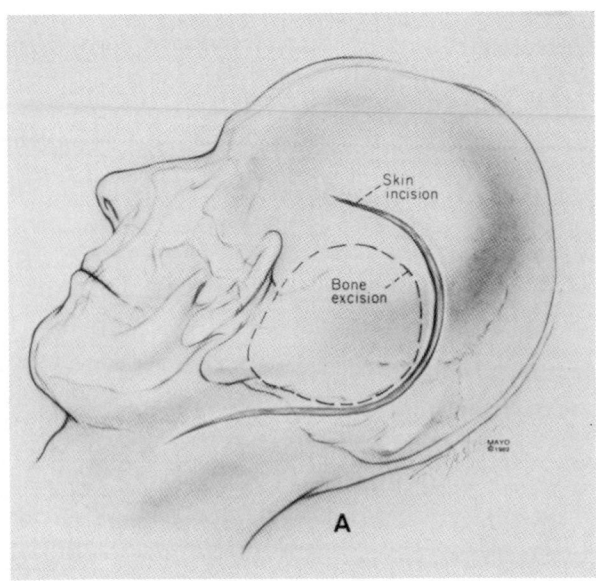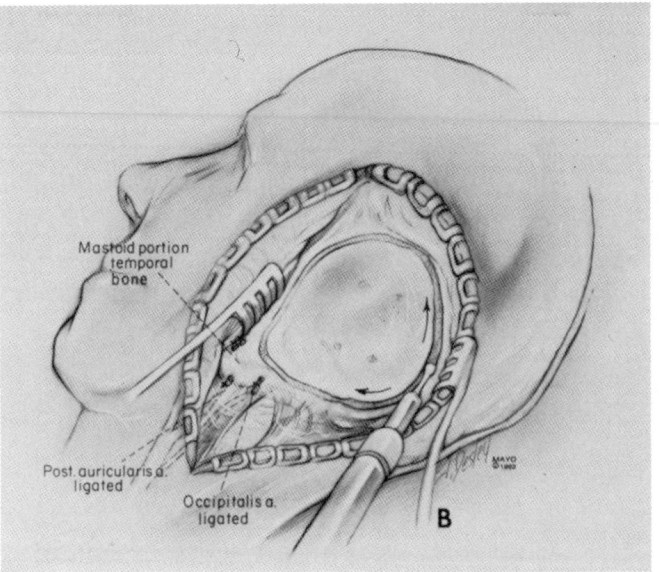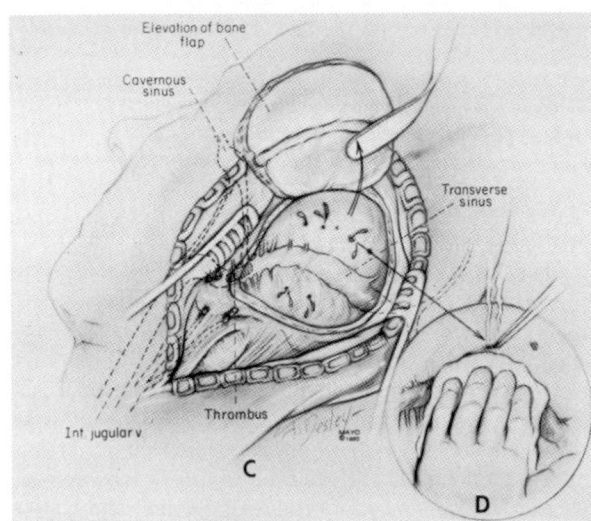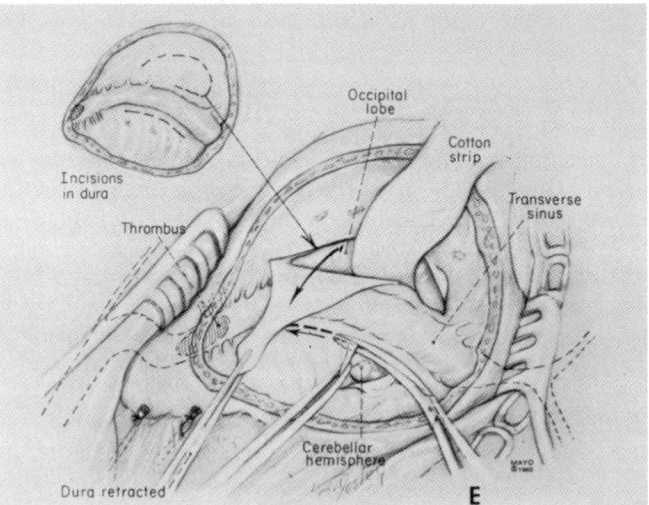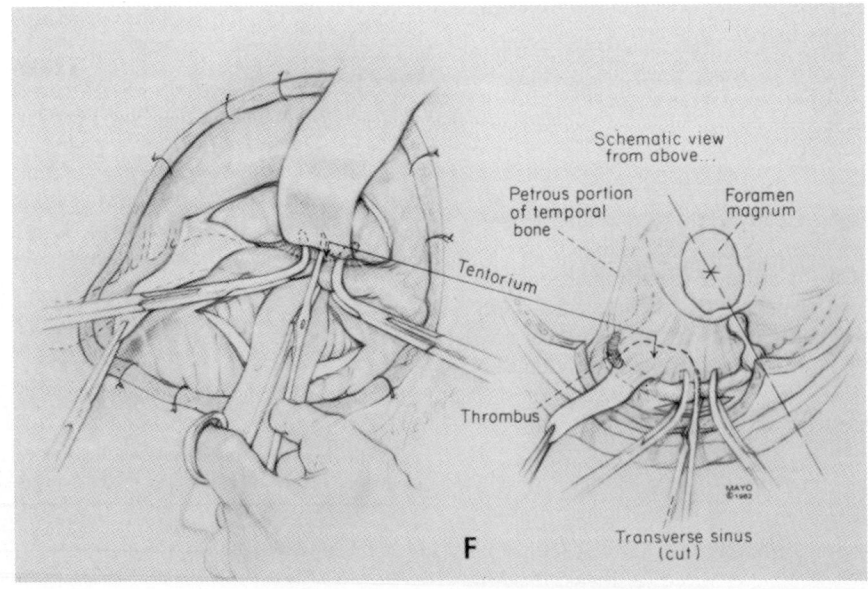

FIGURE 97–6. *See legend on opposite page*

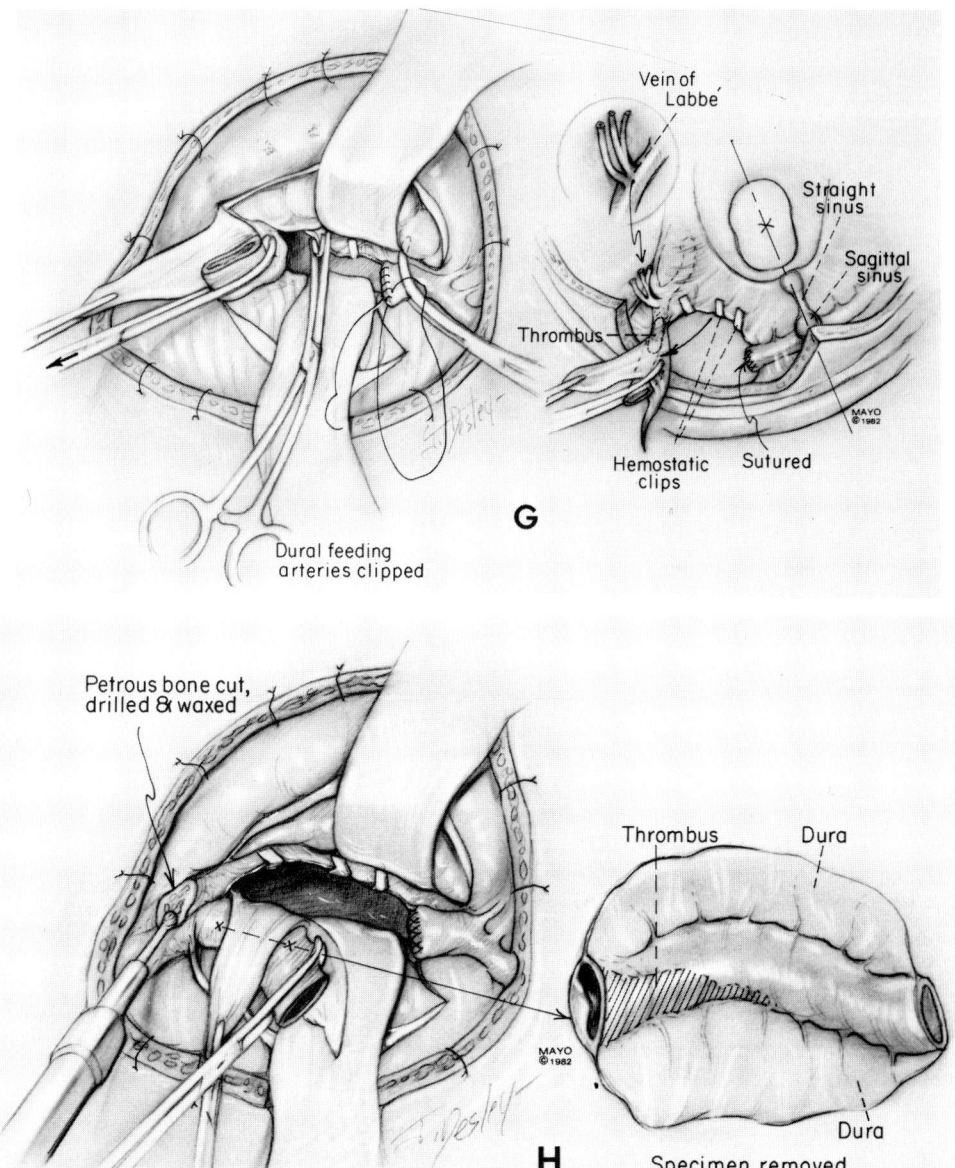

FIGURE 97–6. (A) Schematic representation of the skin incision and area of bone to be excised. (B) The bone plate is elevated using an air drill that is held at a 30-degree angle to prevent perforation of the dura. The area of osteotomy is gradually increased peripherally around the margin of the bone plate until the dura is just barely visible through a thin layer of cortical bone. The bone plate is then elevated using a periosteal elevator. (C and D) After removal of the bone plate, dural bleeding can be profuse. This is controlled with bipolar coagulation of bleeding points and a large piece of Gelfoam that is placed over the entire expanse of exposed dura and held in place with uniform digital compression. The margins of the dura are then gradually exposed, as the packing is retracted and bleeding points individually coagulated. (E) Preparations are made for excision of the lateral sinus by opening the dura above and below the lateral sinus with incisions that parallel the long axis of the sinus. (F) After the dura has been opened, it is tacked up to the margins of the craniotomy securely with multiple, closely placed, dural tacking sutures. The sinus is then incised between 2 hemostats occluding the sinus proximally and distally. (G) The medial portion of the sinus is closed with a running dural suture. The lateral portion of the sinus containing the arteriovenous fistula is elevated from the wound using a hemostat and is excised from the tentorium. Major bleeding points on the tentorium are best controlled with hemostatic clips. In patients with a large vein of Labbé, it is occasionally possible to save this vein by carrying the incision directly into the sinus itself and then closing the sinus with a running suture so that the vein of Labbé can drain into the superior petrosal sinus. (H) The AVF is excised as far lateral as the petrosal bone, and a considerable portion of the petrosal bone is removed with a high-speed air drill. Bleeding from this area can be profuse, but is controlled with cauterization of the bone using the cutting current of the Bovie coagulator and bone wax. Examination of the excised specimen will often reveal a thrombus in situ.

Illustration continued on following page

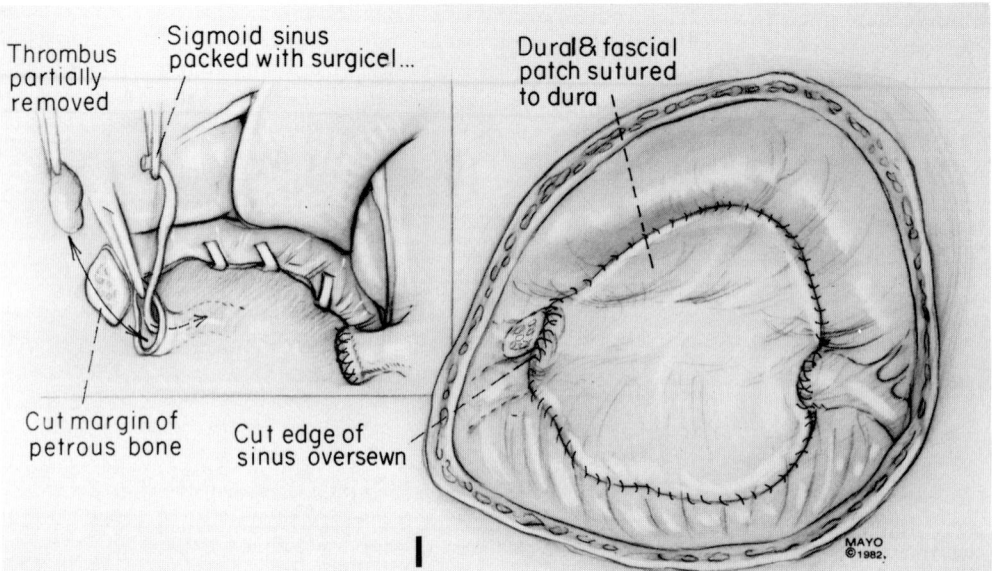

FIGURE 97-6. *Continued* (I) Following excision of the lateral sinus at its junction point with the sigmoid sinus, the sigmoid sinus is packed with Surgicel and then closed with a running suture to the dural or fascial patch. (Copyright © 1982 by the Mayo Clinic.)

DISCUSSION

SYMPTOMATOLOGY

Although symptomatology has been reviewed previously, and the purpose of this chapter is not to discuss the clinical presentation of these cases, a few brief comments are necessary for completeness. The commonest symptom encountered is pulsatile tinnitus. A bruit that is annoying to some patients and incapacitating to others, although usually present, is not, however, invariable, and some report no noise. Headaches are the next commonest complaint. These are relatively nonspecific in character and may be caused by intracranial hypertension. Other symptoms of increased intracranial pressure (ICP) include visual obscurations, dimness in vision, and blindness. Papilledema may also be present on examination. Two primary causes for symptoms of increased ICP and the findings of papilledema should be considered: (1) the impairment of venous run-off because of associated major sinus occlusion, and (2) an increase in ICP as a result of high flow into the draining sinuses, with an elevation in the intrasinus pressure. Retrograde flow was a common finding in patients with AVFs of the lateral sinus. A retrospective analysis of the case material has revealed that, invariably, patients with papilledema either had associated sinus occlusions or an AVF of a magnitude sufficient to produce retrograde flow with or without an occluded sinus.

Focal neurologic symptoms have included classic transient ischemic attacks and seizures, both of which have been attributed to increased venous pressure in the area of the AVF. Spontaneous subarachnoid hemorrhage has not occurred in patients without evidence of pial venous drainage, but it is a common occurrence in those with this angiographic sign (Tables 97–2 and 97–3).

PATHOGENESIS AND PATHOPHYSIOLOGY

Houser and associates[1] presented convincing evidence that AVFs are acquired lesions evolving from organization and vascularization of a previously thrombosed sinus. According to this hypothesis, the sinus thrombosis is the primary event. The mechanism of sinus occlusion may be idiopathic, secondary to infection, dehydration, puerperium, coagulopathy; it may be posttraumatic; or it may occur postoperatively. Subsequently, the clot in the sinus undergoes organization and, in the process, develops a dural blood supply with the potential for communicating with the patent portion of the sinus. The gradual hypertrophy of these vessels ultimately results in a dural AVF. Sequential angiograms have documented the

Table 97–2. INDICATIONS FOR SURGERY IN 73 PATIENTS WITH ARTERIOVENOUS FISTULAE

Indication	Incidence
Pulsatile tinnitus	30
Increased intracranial pressure	9
Headache	8
Increase in size of arteriovenous malformation	8
Visual obscuration	7
Hemorrhage	6
Spinal cord myelopathy	2
Seizures	1
Chronic thrombophlebitis, requiring anticoagulants	1
Congestive heart failure	1

Table 97–3. FREQUENCY OF SYMPTOMS IN 73 PATIENTS WITH ARTERIOVENOUS FISTULAE

Symptom	Incidence
Pulsatile tinnitus	57
Headache	32
Visual obscuration/papilledema	14
Hemorrhage	10
Seizures	9
Ataxia	6
Decreased memory, difficulty thinking	5
Transient ischemic attack	2

progression of a thrombosed sinus to a dural AVF, and the concurrence of an occluded sinus and dural AVF in our experience is common.

Nishijima and colleagues[14] recently described the fistula as being located within the sinus walls themselves. As sinus pressures increase with progressive occlusion or stenosis, they postulated that pre-existing physiologic arteriovenous shunts then become patent.[14]

If these theories are correct, and we believe that they are, then surgery will ultimately be required in most cases, because the AVF will continue to enlarge and progressively increase the intracranial venous pressure, producing the symptomatology discussed briefly earlier. Nevertheless, those affected are often elderly patients with other ailments, and a delay in surgery with a period of observation to follow the progression of the illness is acceptable. Insofar as subarachnoid hemorrhages are uncommon, they do not create emergency situations. If the signs of increased ICP appear, surgical intervention is mandatory.

DIAGNOSTIC STUDIES

Before the development of more modern imaging modalities, Aminoff[4] described the abnormalities associated with dural AVFs with respect to skull radiographs. Patients were frequently noted to have an enlarged foramen spinosum, widened meningeal arterial markings, or both.[4] Computed tomographic (CT) scans may also reveal bony changes, and more importantly, vermiform enhancement representing dilated vessels may be demonstrated.[15] Cerebral edema secondary to venous congestion is often obvious on CT or magnetic resonance imaging (MRI). MRI may prove to be more useful than CT because abnormal flow phenomena in venous channels can be resolved. MRI, however, has relatively low sensitivity in screening for dural AVFs. Three-dimensional time-of-flight sequences significantly increase sensitivity in detection of fistulae, but along with low resolution, saturation artifacts, and restricted fields of coverage, there is an inability to assess flow dynamics.[16] Angiography performed specifically for the purpose of evaluating a possible AVF clearly establishes the diagnosis. This angiography may include delayed venous-phase filming, superselective catheterization of potential feeders, vertebral as well as carotid injections, and contralateral vessel study to assess potential collateral supply.

RISK FACTORS FOR HEMORRHAGE

As might be expected, symptoms of hemorrhage in AVF are quite similar to those of aneurysmal subarachnoid hemorrhage; however, mortality is significantly lower: 10 versus 50 percent.[3] Intracerebral hemorrhage in AVF is significantly less apoplectic than that associated with intracerebral hemorrhage associated with intracranial aneurysms because the blood is under venous pressure.

Hemorrhage, of course, is a major concern. The primary risk factor to be considered is the venous drainage pattern, which is ultimately related to location (Table 97–4). Factors that do not correlate with risk include arterial supply, size, contralateral supply, or high flow shunting.

Table 97–4. RISK FACTORS FOR HEMORRHAGE IN ARTERIOVENOUS FISTULAE

Venous Drainage Area	Incidence n/n(%)
Dural sinus only	0/40(0)
Pial component	7/25(28)
Venous varix	4/8(50)

ARTERIAL SUPPLY

In primary (unoperated or untreated) AVFs, the arterial blood supply is derived from five general sources:
1. The occipital artery and its major branches.
2. In large or recurrent cases, perforating branches arising from the ascending pharyngeal or posterior auricular artery are often present. These result in a vascularized petrous bone.
3. Meningeal arteries in the dura overlying the cerebellum.
4. Branches of the middle meningeal artery in the dura of the temporal and occipital lobes.
5. Branches of the meningohypophyseal artery in the tentorium.

The occipital artery is usually the dominant feeder.

In recurrent cases, the occipital and more superficial dural arteries have been ligated, and the blood supply has been driven deeper, much as it is in parenchymal AVFs that have had partial and inadequate resection. The dura overlying the posterior aspect of the petrous bone seems to have a particular propensity for becoming the primary zone of supply, which creates a very dangerous situation because control of this bleeding is extraordinarily difficult. It may represent an indication for profound hypothermia (Table 97–5).

VENOUS DRAINAGE AND BRIDGING VEINS

Dural AVFs often drain primarily through the opposite lateral sinus if the sigmoid sinus is occluded (although sometimes both sigmoid sinuses are occluded). In other instances, the exact source of drainage is not clear from the angiogram, and in these cases, one should expect the drainage to be via the diploë of the overlying bone, making bone removal hazardous.

The secondary run-off can be composed of various routes involving the superior petrosal sinus; the epidural space, and hence flow to the diploë; and bridging veins. Thus, with removal of the bone plate and ligation of the medial portion of the lateral sinus, the venous drainage has in many instances been largely compromised. Although this reduced drainage increases bleeding from the AVF, it is unavoidable. By this point in the procedure, in unoperated (but not recur-

Table 97–5. ANGIOGRAPHIC FEATURES OF ARTERIOVENOUS FISTULAE

Arterial Supply	Number
External carotid	22
Internal carotid	3
Vertebral	4
Combination	44

rent) cases of AVFs, the major blood supply has been interrupted.

Before the operation, the surgeon should examine in great detail the venous drainage of the temporal and occipital lobes. It is virtually impossible to preserve major perforating veins from the lateral occipital pole or the posterior temporal lobe. Fortunately, however, the occlusion of the sigmoid sinus followed by the development of the AVF has interfered with normal venous drainage, and major functional bridging veins are uncommon, because the venous drainage has sought and found other avenues of escape. The reverse is, in fact, often the case with reversal of flow and presence of red veins. These, as indicated previously, can be severed with impunity.

The vein of Labbé is a vessel of special importance. In aneurysm surgery, this vein should be preserved if at all possible.

In dural AVF cases, Labbé is usually not prominent, perhaps because it never was large, explaining in part the low flow through the nondominant sinus (thought to be a major factor in cases of spontaneous occlusion of a lateral sinus). If the vein of Labbé is prominent, it should be preserved, if possible, and allowed to drain into the superior petrosal sinus. Obviously, in this situation, a radical resection of the sinus must be substituted by a less ambitious undertaking in which the dural supply and petrous bone are still resected, but in which a total resection of the sinus is replaced by a subtotal resection (see Fig. 97–6G). In these cases, the margin of the sinus serving the superior petrosal sinus is preserved, allowing a reversal of flow and thus drainage from the vein of Labbé through the petrosal sinus (Table 97–6).

TECHNICAL NOTES

The notorious vascularity of these malformations leads one to consider the possibility of placing the patient in a sitting position. In our judgment, this position is ill advised because the wide-open venous channels in the diploë make a major air embolism almost a certainty.

The second temptation is to attempt a piecemeal resection of the bone (in effect, making a craniectomy), using rongeurs, rather than to elevate the bone as a single plate. Not only does this method result in a less satisfactory cosmetic result, but, more importantly, the bleeding is greater because the exposure and isolation of the arterial inflow and venous run-off are more difficult to control.

Embolization through the external carotid artery may be a definitive form of treatment in patients with exclusively external carotid artery feeders. Embolization, however, may provide only transient improvement and ultimately compound the problem for the reasons cited earlier. It should be undertaken cautiously and the patients followed up closely thereafter. In cases in which the age of the patient or other medical conditions militate against excision of the lesion, embolization with or without radiosurgery is a reasonable approach. Fine particulate emboli or perhaps even tissue adhesives are useful in these cases because it is necessary to occlude the finest distal branches of the lesion rather than simply to obstruct the major feeding arteries. Embolization may be a consideration in selected, extremely vascular lesions as a preoperative treatment in an attempt to reduce some of the blood supply immediately before the operation.

Every attempt should be made to excise the malformation as completely as possible with the initial procedure. The surgeries for the five cases with recurrence were technically a great deal more difficult than those for the primary lesions, and two deaths occurred in this group. In our experience, recurrent lesions are more difficult to operate on because the primary blood supply to the malformation is no longer from the external carotid artery but rather from deep branches originating from the internal carotid artery.

We have not found the operating microscope to be particularly helpful in this procedure because of the extraordinary vascularity of the lesions and the size of the operative field. Magnification loupes have, however, been most helpful.

REFERENCES

1. Houser OW, Campbell JK, Campbell RJ, et al: Arteriovenous malformation affecting the transverse dural venous sinus—An acquired lesion. Mayo Clin Proc 54:651, 1979
2. Newton TH, Cronqvist S: Involvement of dural arteries in intracranial arteriovenous malformations. Radiology 93:1071, 1969
3. King WA, Martin NA: Intracerebral hemorrhage due to arteriovenous malformations and fistulae. Neurosurg Clin N Am 3(3):577, 1992
4. Aminoff MJ: Vascular anomalies in the intracranial dura mater. Brain 96:601, 1973
5. Handa J, Yoneda S, Handa H: Venous sinus occlusion with a dural arteriovenous malformation of the posterior fossa. Surg Neurol 4:433, 1975
6. Hugosson R, Bergstrom K: Surgical treatment of dural arteriovenous malformation in the region of the sigmoid sinus. J Neurol Neurosurg Psychiatry 37:97, 1974
7. Kosnik EJ, Hunt WE, Miller CA: Dural arteriovenous malformations. J Neurosurg 40:322, 1974
8. Kuhner A, Krastel A, Stoll W: Arteriovenous malformations of the transverse dural sinus. J Neurosurg 45:12, 1976
9. Lamas E, Lobato RD, Esparza J, et al: Dural posterior fossa AVM producing raised sagittal sinus pressure. Case report. J Neurosurg 46:804, 1977
10. Magidson MA, Weinberg PE: Spontaneous closure of a dural arteriovenous malformation. Surg Neurol 6:107, 1976
11. Nicola GC, Nizzoli V: Dural arteriovenous malformations of the posterior fossa. J Neurol Neurosurg Psychiatry 31:514, 1968
12. Obrador S, Soto M, Silvela J: Clinical syndromes of arteriovenous malformations of the transverse-sigmoid sinus. J Neurol Neurosurg Psychiatry 38:436, 1975
13. Sundt TM Jr, Piepgras DG: The surgical approach to arteriovenous malformations of the lateral and sigmoid dural sinuses. J Neurosurg 59:32, 1983
14. Nishijima M, Takaku A, Endo S, et al: Etiology evaluation of dural arteriovenous malformations of the lateral and sigmoid sinuses based on histopathological examinations. J Neurosurg 76:600, 1992
15. Chiros J, Bories J, Leger JM, et al: CT scan of dural arteriovenous fistulae. Neuroradiology 23:185, 1982
16. Chen J, Tsuruda JS, Halbach VV: Suspected dural arteriovenous fistulae. Results with screening MR angiography in 7 patients. Radiology 183:265, 1992

Table 97–6. ANGIOGRAPHIC FEATURES OF ARTERIOVENOUS FISTULAE

Venous Outflow Area	Number
Dural sinus only	40
Pial component	25
Pial component and venous varix	8

SECTION XIV

Hydrocephalus and Neonatal Surgery

CHAPTER 98

Surgical Management of Hydrocephalus in Children

Alexa I. Canady
Sandeep Sood
Steven D. Ham

Shunting is the commonest surgical procedure in a pediatric neurosurgical practice. The long-held principles on which shunting is based are undergoing scientific scrutiny, including the nature and design of valves, and nonshunt treatments of hydrocephalus, which have become more attractive with technologic advances, are being re-evaluated. Many assumptions about ventricular shunting (including such apparently straightforward items as the proper placement of the shunt catheter) have not been established in randomized surgical trials but are the result of an accumulation of experience. This chapter discusses the diagnosis of hydrocephalus, outlines the common surgical treatments, and discusses the complications that may occur.

EPIDEMIOLOGY

The occurrence of congenital hydrocephalus without spina bifida in the United States is approximately 3.18 to 5.2/10,000 live births. In 45 states and the District of Columbia, this condition occurred in 845 children in 1989.[1, 2] Glasgow, Scotland had a 5/10,000 live birth congenital hydrocephalus rate.[3] In 1988, 171 children in the United States with congenital hydrocephalus died in their first year of life, and one half of these children were in their first month of life.[4] In the United States, the rate of congenital hydrocephalus has remained reasonably stable throughout the 1970s and 1980s, whereas others have reported a decreased incidence during the same period in England and in Scotland.[1, 3, 5]

Hydrocephalus secondary to intraventricular hemorrhage in premature infants has increased the incidence of hydrocephalus. In Sweden, from 1967 to 1982, infantile hydrocephalus increased from 4.8 to 6.3/10,000 live births, an increase attributed to the number of preterm infants. Twenty-six percent of patients with infantile hydrocephalus died before the age of 2.[6] When compared with the survival of nonshunted children with infantile hydrocephalus in Sweden in the 1950s, the survival in children with shunting has considerably increased.[7]

A sample from Olmsted County, Minnesota is indicative of the age distribution of cerebrospinal fluid (CSF) shunt placement. Between 1956 and 1981, 64 percent of the initial shunts were placed before patients reached the age of twenty. From 1956 to 1981, the number of shunts increased, and the incidence of communicating and normal-pressure hydrocephalus treated by shunting also increased during that interval.[8]

The rate of hydrocephalus occurring among twins at birth has also been analyzed. From 1969 to 1985, in a Japanese study, this incidence was 15 percent, with a slightly higher rate in same-sex male twins (28 percent) than in same-sex female twins (14 percent). The rates were 21 percent in same-sex and zero percent in non–same-sex pairs. Two twin pairs had one anencephalic twin and one hydrocephalic twin.[9]

ETIOLOGY

Hydrocephalus is a clinical state in which disruption in normal CSF dynamics occurs. The disruption may be in production, absorption, or mechanical obstruction to the flow of CSF and is usually associated with an increase of ventricular size (Fig. 98–1). The changes in CSF dynamics may be caused by congenital brain malformations or by many disease processes occurring within the ventricle, the brain parenchyma, or the subarachnoid spaces.[10] Although classification systems for this state have some academic usefulness, hydrocephalus must be paired with some other diagnosis, for example, ''this patient has hydrocephalus secondary to meningitis or intraventricular hemorrhage.'' If conceptualized in this way, the treatment modalities available to that patient can be more easily formulated.

In a representative series of 107 children, the causes for hydrocephalus were myelomeningocele (54 percent), idiopathic (13 percent), posthemorrhagic (13 percent), postmeningitic (10 percent), aqueductal stenosis (7.5 percent), hydranencephaly (0.1 percent), and congenital toxoplasmosis (0.1 percent).[11] When Foltz and Shurtleff[12] looked at the diagnoses established by air studies and ventriculography in a series of 112 patients, there were 49 patients with communicating hydrocephalus, presumably from basilar arachnoiditis caused by infection, blood or both; 27 with aqueductal stenosis; eight with Dandy-Walker malformation; eight with Chiari malformation; seven with encephalocele; seven with multiple anomalies; three with cystic brain disease; and three in whom the condition was undiagnosed. Similar etiologies

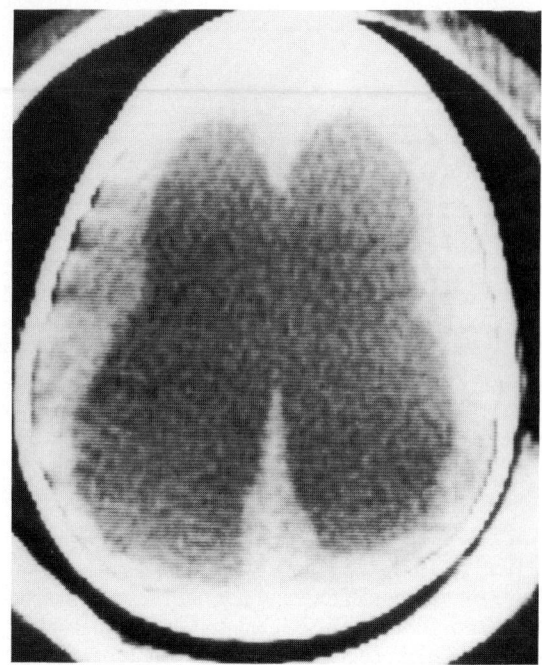

FIGURE 98–1. CT scan of hydrocephalus showing enlarged ventricular size.

were noted by Keucher and Mealey[13] in a series of 228 patients with infantile nonneoplastic hydrocephalus: 56 percent had hydrocephalus caused by myelomeningocele, 17 percent had aqueductal stenosis, 13.5 percent had communicating hydrocephalus, 9 percent had a postinfectious cause, 7 percent had Dandy-Walker malformation, and 7 percent had other causes.

Unusual causes of hydrocephalus include the association with syndromic craniosynostosis[14] and cranial base abnormalities, such as achondroplasia.[15] Venous hypertension may be the cause of the hydrocephalus in this population.[16]

DIAGNOSIS AND CLINICAL FEATURES

The identification of hydrocephalus begins with clinical suspicion based on history and physical examination. The clinical presentation depends on whether or not the cranial sutures are open and on the rate of progression of the hydrocephalus. In infants, the signs include enlarging head size (the growth rate being more important than the absolute size), split cranial sutures, sunset eye appearance from the midbrain effects of the hydrocephalus causing an inability to gaze upward, pupillary abnormalities, convergence abnormalities and nystagmus,[17] and scalp vein enlargement. In children with closed sutures, headache, irritability, vomiting, lethargy, and in late cases, papilledema and nuchal rigidity are more prominent. In children with chronic hydrocephalus, the complaints are more likely to relate to poor school performance and a decreased energy level.[18]

In a series of 51 patients with progressive hydrocephalus, 86 percent of whom were infants, the symptoms of hydrocephalus were as follows: asymptomatic (49 percent), headache and or irritability (33 percent), and vomiting (16 percent) (Table 98–1). The signs in the same population were increased head circumference (75 percent), tense anterior fontanel (65 percent), split sutures (39 percent), scalp vein distension (33 percent), sun-setting eye appearance (22 percent), and neck retraction or rigidity (14 percent).[11] These figures compare to the clinical presentation in a series of 33 patients with aqueductal stenosis in whom the mean age was 18.4 years. In this series, 78 percent presented with headache, 42 percent with decreased vision, 24 percent with gait disturbance, 24 percent with nausea and vomiting, 18 percent with endocrine dysfunction, 15 percent with epilepsy, 15 percent with diplopia, 12 percent with tinnitus, 9 percent with ataxia, 6 percent with weakness of the legs, and 3.1 percent with partial deafness and upward gaze limitation. The commonest ocular motility abnormality in hydrocephalus is abducens (cranial nerve VI) palsy with limited lateral movement. Trochlear (cranial nerve IV) nerve palsy may also be seen secondary to compression of the nerve as it crosses to become embedded in the tentorial edge. Third nerve dysfunction from hydrocephalus is rare.[19]

Imaging studies often determine the etiology and extent of the hydrocephalus. Ultrasound is useful in the child with an open fontanel, particularly the premature child with intraventricular hemorrhage, because it can be performed at the bedside without sedation.[20, 21] Computed tomography (CT) is superior to ultrasound in demonstrating parenchymal lesions, lesions of the posterior fossa, and some subdural lesions.[21]

CT is the commonest imaging procedure used to detect hydrocephalus. Ventricular size can be identified with CT, as can causative intracranial lesions. Although some clinicians favor qualitative assessment of ventricular size, others have identified ratios of ventricular width to various landmarks to diagnose ventricular enlargement.[22] Although the presence of a small fourth ventricle and large lateral and third ventricles has been interpreted as aqueductal stenosis, 20 to 35 percent of patients with communicating hydrocephalus have a small fourth ventricle.[23] CT is less effective at demonstrating the cause of functional versus anatomic causes of hydrocephalus.

Magnetic resonance imaging (MRI) has added to the accuracy of diagnosis in hydrocephalus, identifying sites of obstruction as well as small lesions not seen on CT (Fig. 98–2).[24, 25] Special MRI sequences also allow assessment of CSF flow, including flow through the aqueduct.[26, 27] Currently, MRI in the newborn can be frustrating to perform, and in the newborn period, the clinician might make the tentative diagnosis based on ultrasound or CT and delay MRI until the patient is 3 or 4 months of age, when images are better.

In addition to the anatomic images, functional measures are being explored to distinguish enlarged ventricles from hydrocephalus. Ultrasound and the resistive index (obtained by dividing the difference between the peak systolic and end-diastolic frequencies by the systolic frequency) can be used

Table 98–1. SYMPTOMS OF HYDROCEPHALUS

Symptom	Incidence (%)
Asymptomatic	49
Headache and irritability	33
Vomiting	16

(From Kirkpatrick M, Engleman H, Minns RA: Symptoms and signs of progressive hydrocephaly. Arch Dis Child 64:124–128, 1989.)

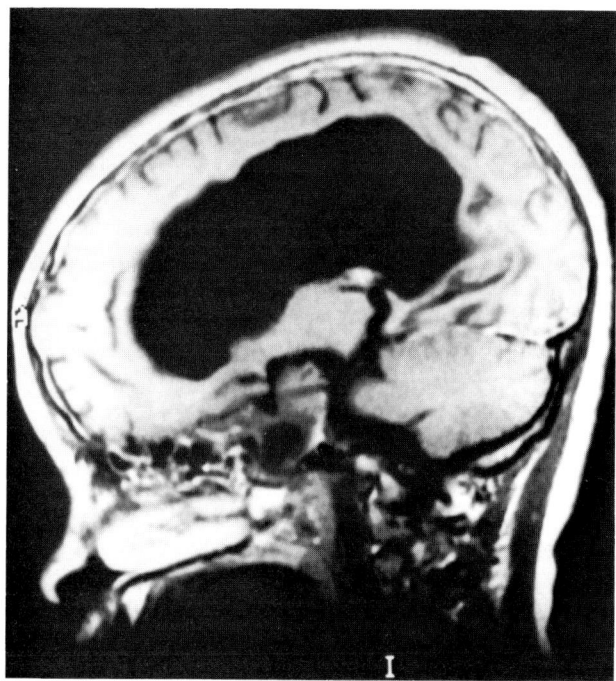

FIGURE 98-2. MRI with collicular lesion causing hydrocephalus.

to diagnose hydrocephalus, but because the index is age dependent and has overlapping ranges of normal and abnormal, it may be most helpful in comparing a patient's values over time.[28] Another functional method to distinguish ventriculomegaly from hydrocephalus is transcranial Doppler. The pulsatility index (peak systolic velocity minus end-diastolic velocity divided by mean velocity) was increased with hydrocephalus.[29]

Measurement of intracranial pressure plays a significant role in questionable cases of hydrocephalus, either by invasive or noninvasive techniques.[18] Infusion studies and their effect on intracranial pressure (ICP) have also been used to diagnose hydrocephalus,[30, 31] and lumbar cisternography has also been used to assess CSF dynamics.[32]

REGIONAL SURGICAL ANATOMY

Development of hydrocephalus usually results in expansion of all the components of the lateral ventricles. However, in children with congenital hydrocephalus, preferential enlargement of the frontal horns occurs with bulging of their superolateral angles,[33] whereas in those with posthemorrhagic hydrocephalus, enlargement of the occipital horns occurs.[34] Usually, the catheter tip in ventricular shunts is placed in the frontal horn because the absence of choroid plexus in this location may prevent obstruction of the catheter. The frontal horn may be cannulated through an anterior approach, or the lateral ventricle may be cannulated posteriorly and the catheter advanced into the frontal horn.

Kocher's point 1 cm anterior to the coronal suture and 3 cm from the midline is a reliable site for burr hole placement for direct cannulation of the frontal horn[35] in children with small ventricles or a preferentially large frontal horn. In children with macrocephaly or an abnormal head shape, the burr hole is positioned 1 cm in front of the coronal suture and in line with the ipsilateral pupil. The catheter is then directed parallel to the coronal plane and angled medially toward the nasion. A second pass may be attempted toward the ipsilateral pupil; however, a more lateral pass may injure the internal capsule. After the ventricle is entered, the catheter should be passed to a depth less than half the distance of the bregma to the external auditory meatus so as not to enter the third ventricle through the foramen of Monro.

Landmarks for cannulation of the lateral ventricle from a posterior approach are less consistent and depend on the preference of the neurosurgeon. Keen's point is a landmark for parietotemporal burr holes. Although originally described in children as lying 3 cm above and behind the external auditory meatus,[36] it is often measured from the highest point of the pinna.[37] In children with an abnormal shape of the head or macrocephaly, absolute measurements are less reliable, and proportions are preferred. The burr hole may be made just anterior to the lambdoid suture, medial to the midpoint of a line from the external auditory meatus to the sagittal suture,[38] or it may be positioned two thirds of the distance posteriorly on a line joining the inion with a point one third of the distance from the external auditory meatus to the vertex.[39] These landmarks ensure that the entry is made through the superior parietal lobule. Also, in this position, the burr hole does not migrate laterally with growth, which would make subsequent revisions difficult. The catheter is directed in the sagittal plane toward the midforehead.[38] The catheter length required to reach into the frontal horn varies with age and head circumference. The ratio of the head circumference to the optimum catheter length is 5.0 for neonates, 4.5 for children aged 1 month to 5 years, and 4.0 for children older than 5 years.[40]

SURGICAL TECHNIQUES AND INTRAOPERATIVE MANAGEMENT

EXTRACRANIAL VENTRICULAR SHUNTS

Ventriculoperitoneal Shunt

After anesthesia, the child is positioned supine with head turned to the opposite side to expose the parietal or the frontal region. Care is taken to adequately cushion the head to avoid decubitus ulceration. We prefer to use a soft foam ring or a silicone headrest. Because of the large head-to-body ratio in children, placing a roll below the shoulder may be necessary to extend the neck and straighten the neck folds. In infants with marked hydrocephalus and head circumference of more than 40 cm, elevating the body on a foam rest may be necessary to allow for the extension of the head.

The hair is shaved over the parietal or the frontal region extending to the side of the neck. The curvilinear incision, based anteroinferiorly and about 1.5 to 2 cm in length, is marked for parietotemporal (3 cm above and behind the highest point of the pinna) or for parieto-occipital (4 cm lateral and 6 cm above the inion) placement. Alternatively, the incision is marked 1 cm anterior to the coronal suture and 2 cm from the midline, with the base posterolaterally for a frontal placement. The incision is made so that the tubing does not pass directly under it. For the distal catheter, we prefer to use an abdominal incision over the rectus muscle because this incision involves dissection through one layer of muscle and hence minimizes the risk of incisional hernia. A subxiphoid incision is preferred by some surgeons; however, it tends to leave a wider scar. Alternatively, a trocar may be used for placement of the distal catheter intraperitoneally.[41]

A thorough surgical scrub is performed with povidone-iodine (Betadine) soap, and povidone-iodine paint is applied. We have found a single application of DuraPrep to be as effective. Sterile surgical drapes are placed, and a plastic Steri-Drape is applied over the field to minimize skin contamination. The incision site is infiltrated with 0.5-percent lidocaine in adrenaline diluted to 1:200,000 strength. No more than 7 mg/kg (i.e., 1.5 ml/kg of 0.5-percent lidocaine) should be used. Local infiltration reduces bleeding from the scalp edges.

The scalp incision is made first, and a retractor is placed. The scalp bleeders are controlled with bipolar cautery. Pericranium is incised anterior to the scalp incision and gently elevated from the bone. Scraping of the outer table while elevating the pericranium in small children may cause troublesome bone bleeding, which can be controlled with bone wax. Direct coagulation of the bone with unipolar cautery should be avoided because we have seen the cautery perforate the thin skull in children. A burr hole is made by use of a hand-held perforator in children younger than 2 years, and a regular Hudson perforator is used with care in older children. Bleeding from the bone is controlled with bone wax. With a curved hemostat, a subgaleal pocket is made for the valve assembly, and gentle pressure is applied to minimize bleeding. Even if brisk bleeding occurs from the subgaleal pocket, external pressure is preferred to exploration because significant blood loss may occur during exploration. At this stage, the scalp wound is covered with a sterile drape, and the paramedian abdominal incision is made. The anterior rectus sheath is opened either vertically or horizontally, and the rectus abdomen muscle is split vertically with a hemostat. The posterior rectus sheath is grasped with two hemostats, and a pursestring suture is placed around the intended site of opening and left loose. We have found paramedian umbilical exposure easy and convenient, even in obese children.

A subcutaneous tunnel is made from the scalp to the abdominal incision by use of a blunt Salmon passer. An intervening passing incision is rarely required in children and may be a source of shunt tethering, causing shunt malfunction as the growth of the child pulls on the shunt. It is therefore important that no connector be under the passing incision. Care should be taken to tunnel the skin under direct vision because the tunneler can perforate the thin skin of the neonate very easily. The distal catheter is passed through the subcutaneous tunnel. All exposed shunt parts must be covered with sterile drapes, and instruments must be used to handle the drapes. A special instrument set has been recently designed to assemble shunts with "no-touch" technique.[42]

The dura is then opened with a crucial incision. Using the landmarks mentioned earlier, the ventricle is cannulated with the proximal catheter on a stylet. The stylet is withdrawn as soon as the ventricle is entered, and the catheter is pushed in about 1 cm more than the distance of the parietal burr hole from the coronal suture. This action usually places the catheter in the frontal horn. Through a frontal burr hole, the catheter should be introduced to a depth no more than half the distance between the bregma and the external auditory meatus. In infants with an open fontanelle, the position of the catheter can be confirmed with ultrasonography.[43–45] Alternatively, endoscopically the catheter may be placed in the frontal horn.[46, 47] In patients with small ventricles in whom difficult cannulation is anticipated, the catheter may be stereotactically placed.[46, 48] If ventricular hemorrhage is encountered, the catheter is irrigated until it is clear. If it does not clear, it is left as an external drain, and a CT scan is obtained if the patient is stable. If the patient is not stable, a craniotomy must be performed to identify the source of the hemorrhage. This measure is rarely necessary. If the brain seems tense after cannulation obtains good CSF flow, a subdural or epidural hematoma may be present, and a CT scan should be obtained.

The opening pressure is recorded with a manometer. A medium-pressure valve is chosen for opening pressures of more than 10 cm, and a low-pressure valve is used when the opening pressure is less than 10 cm. We rarely use a high-pressure valve. The closing pressure of the valve is checked with a manometer before it is connected to the distal shunt system and is placed in the subgaleal pocket. A low-profile valve is used in neonates and infants. The valve is connected to the proximal catheter and secured with sutures in the subgaleal pocket. The CSF specimen is obtained from the distal catheter, and good flow is confirmed. At this stage, the posterior rectus sheath is opened, the peritoneum is identified, and the distal catheter is placed intraperitoneally under direct vision. The pursestring suture is gently tied, with the surgeon ensuring that the catheter is not strangulated. We leave 90 to 120 cm of tubing in the abdomen, which may be sufficient for life in some patients. The anterior rectus sheath is closed with absorbable suture, and subcuticular abdominal sutures are placed for good cosmesis. The scalp wound is closed with absorbable galeal sutures and running nylon on the skin.

Ventriculoatrial Shunt

All patients in whom a ventriculoatrial shunt is planned should have a preoperative Doppler study of the major neck veins to rule out any anomalies and thrombosis from previous cannulations if their history suggests possible problems.

The patient is positioned in fashion similar to that used for a ventriculoperitoneal shunt except there is no need for hyperextension at the neck and a 10 to 15 degree Trendelenburg's tilt of the table. A soft radiolucent bolster is placed between the shoulder blades.

The lateral ventricle is cannulated above, and the proximal catheter is kept clamped. An incision is made along the anterior border of the sternocleidomastoid muscle at the angle of the jaw. The platysma is incised, and the common facial vein is located and traced to its entry into the internal jugular vein. The common facial vein is tied proximally, and 2–0 Nurulon loops are placed on the internal jugular vein proximal and distal to the entry of the facial vein. This method gives good control of the internal jugular vein in case of tear. The loops are stretched to occlude the internal jugular vein, and a small longitudinal incision is made in the facial vein. A distal shunt catheter is filled with heparinized saline and is clamped, and the slit valve is cut off. The facial vein is then cannulated with the distal shunt catheter, which is passed into the jugular vein and, under fluoroscopic vision, is passed into the right superior vena cava. A small amount of meglumine diatrizoate (Angiografin) is injected into the distal catheter, and the position of its tip at the T4 vertebral body level is confirmed under fluoroscopy. This placement approximately corresponds to the cavostrial junction. Alternatively, the position may be confirmed by checking the venous pressure waves or by using electrocardiography through the catheter. Recently, esophageal echocardiography has been used to document the position of the catheter.[49] The catheter is then heparinized and clamped. The proximal shunt is completed, and the catheter distal to the valve is brought subcutaneously to the neck incision, where it is joined to the distal catheter with a connector. This connector is firmly secured to the soft tissue to prevent distal migration of the atrial catheter.

In some children, the facial vein is small, and an atrial catheter may need to be placed directly through the internal jugular vein. A pursestring suture is placed on one side of the jugular vein. After proximal and distal control, a small incision is made, and the atrial catheter is cannulated through it. After its approximate placement, the pursestring suture is tied.

A retrograde ventriculojugular shunt placed against the direction of the flow of blood has been recently described.[50] It is believed to offer the advantage of minimal siphon action and lack of need for replacement as the child grows.[50] We have no experience with this kind of shunt.

Percutaneous Placement of the Atrial Catheter

The right side is usually chosen for catheter placement because the internal jugular vein on this side is straight and provides the shortest route to the superior vena cava.[51] The internal jugular vein may be entered in the midneck at the level of the cricoid cartilage, lateral to the carotid artery and medial to the sternocleidomastoid muscle or between the two heads of the sternocleidomastoid. The needle is directed toward the ipsilateral nipple while a negative pressure is constantly maintained on the syringe. As the vein is entered, a guidewire is passed through the needle, and its position in the superior vena cava is confirmed under fluoroscopy before the Cook dilator with the peel-away sheath is passed. Again, before the dilator is withdrawn, its position in the superior vena cava is confirmed. The distal shunt catheter is then threaded through the peel-away sheath and appropriately positioned. The sheath is peeled off, and the catheter is joined to the proximal shunt system with a connector, which is firmly secured.

Sometimes, cannulation of the internal jugular vein is not possible because of thrombosis or anomalies. In these cases, we use percutaneous cannulation of the subclavian vein performed using Seldinger's technique, as described earlier, for internal jugular cannulation. Care should be taken to ensure that the shunt catheter does not kink as it angles at the clavicle to enter the subclavian vein; a right-angled connector may be used for this purpose. A postoperative chest x-ray study is performed to check for pneumothorax and confirm adequate shunt placement.

Ventriculopleural Shunt

A ventriculopleural shunt is placed only if ventriculoatrial or ventriculoperitoneal sites for distal shunt placement have been exhausted. Even so, the procedure is not performed in children below the age of 5 years because of the high incidence of pleural effusion.[52]

The proximal shunt is performed as discussed earlier. The distal catheter is brought out of the subcutaneous tunnel through a 1-cm incision at the upper surface of the second rib in boys and the fourth or fifth rib in girls. With a hemostat, the intercostal muscles are split, and in a single move, with the distal catheter tip grasped in the hemostat, the pleura is entered. The anesthetist is asked to hold the respiration in inspiration when the pleural entry is being made. We generally leave about 15 to 20 cm of tubing in the pleural cavity. The wound is closed in two layers, and a postoperative chest x-ray study is taken to check for pneumothorax.

SHUNT LENGTHENING

Shunt lengthening is usually required when the child is around 8 or 10 years of age unless a long peritoneal catheter was placed initially. The elective revision is performed when less than 10 cm of the distal catheter is left in the peritoneal cavity or when the distal atrial catheter of the ventriculoatrial shunt lies above the level of the T4 vertebral body.

PERITONEAL SHUNTS

If the results of the shunt tap suggest a functioning proximal catheter, we prepare and drape only the abdomen. The previous incision is opened, and the skin edges are retracted. With a combination of blunt and sharp dissection, the distal catheter and its sheath are isolated. Unipolar cautery is used to make a nick in the sheath. The distal catheter is retrieved, and the edges of the sheath are carefully held with an artery forceps. CSF is obtained for routine studies. An additional length of catheter is attached to the previous catheter and introduced through the previous sheath into the peritoneum. We prefer not to place the connector inside the abdomen because this position makes subsequent revisions difficult. The wound is then closed in the standard fashion. Some surgeons prefer to replace the entire catheter to avoid the possibility of tethering at the connector. Using the previous abdominal incision scar reduces the number of scars and gives as good a result as making a fresh intraperitoneal entry.

We do not attempt to remove disconnected or fractured shunt catheters that may be lying free in the peritoneum, unless the shunt is infected, although some surgeons prefer to remove them either laparoscopically or using a bidigital technique.[53]

ATRIAL SHUNTS

The neck is prepared and draped. The old incision is opened, and after clamping the distal catheter to prevent air embolism, the distal catheter is disconnected from the connector. A guidewire is passed through the distal catheter, which is removed. A new catheter is passed over the guidewire to the T4 level, and its position is confirmed on fluoroscope. It is then connected to the proximal shunt system.

SHUNT REVISION

The patient is positioned and draped as described earlier for shunt placement. The scalp incision is opened first, and by use of a combination of sharp dissection and unipolar cautery shunt, the junction of the proximal catheter with the valve is identified. The proximal catheter is disconnected from the valve. When there is absence of flow or poor flow of CSF from the catheter, the proximal catheter is removed and replaced along the same tract with a fresh catheter. If the catheter is firmly stuck and cannot easily be removed, gentle traction is applied to the catheter with gradual twisting. Often the catheter releases with a strand of choroid plexus attached to it, which must be coagulated before cutting; otherwise troublesome intraventricular hemorrhage may occur (Fig. 98–3). Alternatively, a stylet may be passed through the catheter, and low-voltage unipolar coagulation may be applied to it.[54, 55] A small amount of hemorrhage can be easily controlled with repeated flushing until returns are clear. If bleeding persists, the shunt is converted to an external drain, and a CT scan is obtained.

The distal shunt is then checked with a manometer placed proximal to the valve. If the CSF run-off is not satisfactory, it is checked distal to the valve to identify the site of the malfunction. If investigation suggests a valve malfunction, the valve is replaced; otherwise, the distal shunt catheter is retrieved and replaced after cleaning, just as for shunt lengthening.

STEREOTACTIC AND/OR ENDOSCOPIC THIRD VENTRICULOSTOMY

Stereotactic or endoscopic third ventriculostomy, or both, can be successfully used in patients with obstructive hydrocephalus. Concern has always been present about an underdeveloped subarachnoid space in these patients, but in one series of adolescents and adults, only one of 16 patients undergoing a third ventriculostomy subsequently required a shunt.[56]

POSTOPERATIVE COMPLICATIONS

SHUNT INFECTION

Shunt infection is a significant complication of shunt placement in children that has been recognized for many years.[57, 58] The rate of infection is evaluated in two ways: per procedure, dividing the number of infections by the number of procedures, and per patient, obtaining the incidence of infections in a specific patient, including revisions at different times. Although the per-procedure figure is the commonest figure given to patients by surgeons, the per-patient statistics may have greater relevance to the patient. This relevance is seen clearly in the retrospective review of shunt infections at the Hospital for Sick Children in Toronto. The review covered 20 years, from 1960 to 1979, and evaluated over 5000 shunt procedures: the shunt infection rate per procedure was 5 percent, but the infection rate per patient was 18 percent.[59] The infection rates per procedure ranged from 2 percent to more than 20 percent, the higher incidences occurring in children younger than 6 months of age, with a general range of 5 to 10 percent. The per patient rates were significantly higher and ranged from 17 to 27 percent (Fig. 98–4).[59–66] The infection rates per procedure have generally fallen over time. In addition to the obvious significance of acute illness, additional surgical procedures, prolonged hospitalization, and suggestions of cognitive damage,[67] shunt infection affects patient mortality, ranging from 18 percent in patients without shunt infection to 34 percent in patients who had shunt infection in the Sick Children's series,[59] and from 17 to 40 percent in the series reported by Schoenbaum and coworkers.[66]

Organisms responsible for shunt infections in children have been consistent over time and from series to series (Table 98–2). *Staphylococcus epidermidis* is the commonest, and more than 40 percent of the positive cultures with *Staphylococcus aureus* are approximately 20 percent. Gram-negative organisms are the next commonest group, with *Escherichia* sp., *Klebsiella* sp., and *Pseudomonas* sp. being the organisms specified.[59] Various other gram-positive organisms, such as *Corynebacterium*, *Streptococcus faecalis*, *Micrococcus*, *H. influenzae*, and *Propionibacterium* also appear.[63, 65, 66] Multiple organisms were present in 30.5 percent of shunt infections in Odio and colleagues' series but in only 10 percent in Schoenbaum and colleagues' series. The source of organisms remains unclear; only 20 percent in one series were identical to skin organisms in those patients, suggesting that perioperative contamination from patient skin may not be the only etiologic mechanism.[65]

Diagnosis of shunt infection in children can be frustrating because of the frequency of febrile illness in this population. A combination of clinical suspicion and laboratory testing, primarily analysis of the CSF, aid in the identification of shunt infection. In the 18 to 23 percent of shunt infections associated with wound infection, the diagnosis is more easily made.[59, 63, 68] Most infections present in the early postoperative period. In one series, the median onset was 8 days

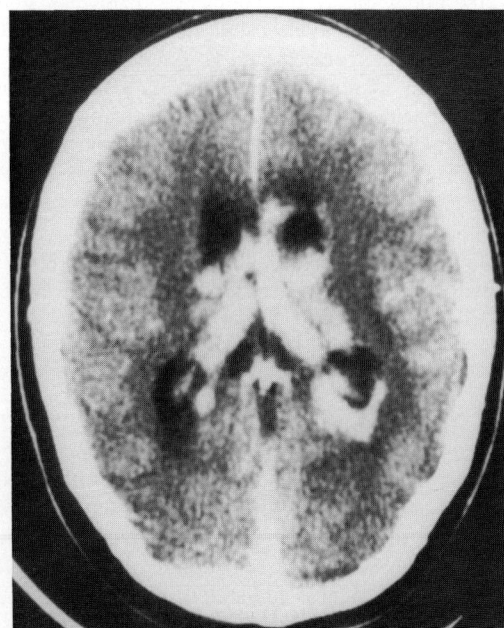

FIGURE 98–3. CT showing intraventricular blood.

SHUNT INFECTIONS
5000 PROCEDURES

FIGURE 98–4. Pie chart of shunt infections. (J Neurosurg 60:1911–1921, 1984.)

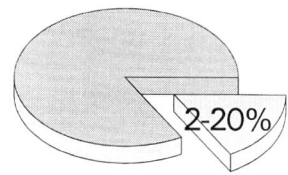
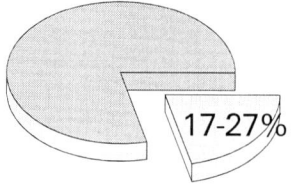

PER PROCEDURE RANGE   PER PERSON RANGE

postoperatively.[63, 66, 68] In some series, fever is present more than 90 percent of the time in patients with shunt infection. Caution is suggested by one series, in which fever was present in only 42 percent of infection cases and was the only symptom in 18 percent.[59] More than 80 percent of children with shunt infections had altered sensorium and irritability. Abdominal complaints were present in 19 to 36 percent of the cases, but frank peritonitis was uncommon.[63, 68] Primary peritonitis can ascend the shunt and cause meningitis, brain abscess, or both.[69] Abdominal pseudocysts occur in 37 percent of patients with shunt infection, and ultrasonography is the procedure of choice for identifying them.[70, 71] Twenty-three to sixty-five percent of infected shunts are also malfunctioning.[59, 63, 68]

Once the suspicion of shunt infection is raised, a shunt tap is the next step (Fig. 98–5). Peripheral white blood cell counts are not specific, and 25 percent are less than 10,000/mm^3 in patients with infected shunts.[66] Blood culture results are reliable in ventriculoatrial shunts but not in ventriculoperitoneal shunts, in which the positive rate was as low as 29 percent in one series.[59, 66, 68] CSF pleocytosis is strongly suggestive of shunt infection. A CSF white cell count of greater than 100/mm^3 is associated with an 89 percent positive culture rate, and a cell count of less than 20/mm^3 is associated with 47 percent positive CSF culture rate.[66] A CSF white cell count of greater than 6/mm^3 is associated with an increased incidence of shunt malfunction, as is recurrent distal peritoneal obstruction, both of which have been interpreted as possible subclinical shunt infections.[72, 73] The gold standard for shunt infection is not clearly established. Some clinicians use positive CSF culture results, but others note than 20 percent of the positive shunt apparatus culture results corresponded to negative CSF culture results.[59] Positive culture results from either the CSF or the shunt apparatus provide a reasonable working diagnosis for shunt infection. Gram stains are highly positive in *S. aureus* and gram-negative infections (82 and 91 percent, respectively) but may be misleading in *S. epidermidis* infection, in which gram stains may be positive in as few as 4 percent of shunt infections.[68]

Table 98–2. ORGANISMS CULTURED*

Organism	Shunt Infections, n(%)
Staphylococcus epidermidis	11(55)
S. aureus	4(20)
Corynebacterium	1(5)
α-Streptococcus	1(5)
Micrococcus	1(5)
Gram-negative bacilli	4(20)

(From Shapiro S, Boaz J, Kleinman M, et al: Origin of organisms infecting ventricular shunts. Neurosurgery 22(5):868–872, 1988.)

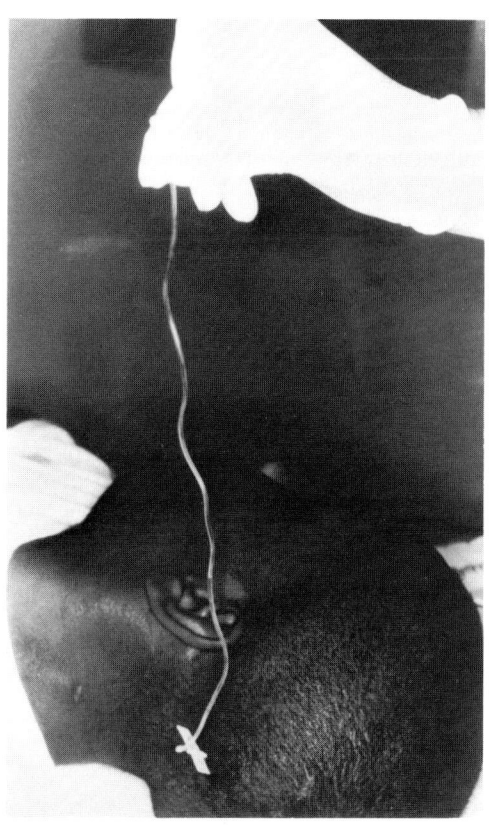

FIGURE 98–5. Shunt tap.

CSF eosinophilia has been associated with drug reactions, especially intraventricular gentamycin; fungal infection; and foreign body reaction to the shunt, but it may also signal bacterial infection.[68, 74-77] Low glucose and elevated protein levels may also be associated with shunt malfunction.[68]

Of all the factors that have been reported to predict an increased risk of shunt infection (time of surgery, etiology of hydrocephalus, use of prophylactic antibiotics, number of revisions, site of shunt placement, type of revision, age of patient, surgeon), only poor skin condition and age are clear predisposing factors.* Most series identify infants as children younger than 6 months of age. The reason for increased shunt infection in infants is not clear, but immaturity in the immune system and possible increased colonization of the skin have been postulated. An increased risk of gram-negative infections also exists in this population.[61, 62, 79] The value of prophylactic antibiotic administration in the prevention of shunt infection remains unproved. Efficacy and no efficacy have been alternately demonstrated in many studies with different study designs that tested various antibiotics and antibiotic regimens and different routes of administration (intraventricular, systemic, or intrashunt).[72, 80-87]

Treatment of shunt infection has been more difficult than expected, given the low virulence of the organisms in shunt infection. This difficulty has been attributed to the foreign body and its interaction with the host. Bacteria has increased adherence to shunt material, perhaps because of mucoid substance produced by *S. epidermidis*.[88] This adherence has been seen by others and is associated with irregularities on the shunt surface that increase with time.[89] Soaking the shunt preoperatively in bacitracin solution has been suggested as a way to reduce this bacterial adherence.[90] The presence of the catheter may also interfere with the phagocytic ability of the cells by stimulating exocytosis of intracellular myeloperoxidase before the cells contact the bacteria on the surface.[91]

All treatments for shunt infection fall into two categories: medical treatment alone or medical treatment with surgery. Information on antibiotic choice and mode of delivery is not well controlled in most treatment reports, despite the demonstration that variable pharmacokinetics occur with antibiotic regimens that affect both route of delivery (oral, intravenous, or intraventricular) and dosing. The studies also do not control for antibiotic levels.[85, 92-94] (Medical treatment has been successful, most often in patients with functioning shunts.)

Bayston reported on 11 of 17 shunt infections treated successfully with intraventricular gentamycin, intravenous trimethoprim, and oral rifampicin.[95] Mates and colleagues described successful medical treatment in seven of eight shunts treated medically only from a series of 48 shunt infections in which various intraventricular and systemic antibiotics were used. These patients had shunt infections within 2 weeks of surgery.[96] Frame and McLaurin described successful treatment in 11 of 12 shunt infections with oral trimethoprim-sulfamethoxazole and daily intrashunt vancomycin.[97] These are selected patients, however, and not randomized series. A prospective randomized series, with only 10 patients per group, showed only a 30 percent cure from medical therapy, as compared with a 90 percent cure from medical and surgical treatment.[98] In other series, antibiotic treatment alone is consistently less successful than that combined with surgical treatment consisting of shunt removal and immediate replacement, shunt removal and delayed replacement, or shunt removal with intermittent ventricular drain and shunt replacement.[59, 63] The last approach (interval drainage) is the commonest, although concern exists about secondary infection of the external drain.[99, 100]

In a nonrandomized series, medical treatment with systemic antibiotics alone was effective in 9 percent of patients, and systemic and intraventricular antibiotics, in 43 percent of patients. The combination of systemic antibiotics and immediate shunt placement succeeded in 56 percent of patients, shunt removal with delayed shunt replacement in 56 percent of patients, and shunt removal and external drainage in 58 percent of patients. Delayed shunt placement is applicable only to patients tolerating no shunt. Interestingly in the same series, the mortality from shunt infection was higher in those receiving medical treatment without intraventricular antibiotics.[59] In another series, length of hospitalization was twice as high in medically treated shunt infections.[68] Patients who have primary meningitis, such as *H. influenzae* meningitis, do not always require shunt removal.[101]

SHUNT COMPLICATIONS INCLUDING MALFUNCTION

Shunt malfunctions and complications are a significant problem in patients with hydrocephalus, as is demonstrated by the fact that 201 shunt procedures were performed in only 114 patients in one series.[102] In a series of 228 patients who received shunts at younger than 2 months of age that had an average follow-up of 7 years, there was a 16.2 percent death rate, 2.2 percent per year for both ventriculoperitoneal and ventriculoatrial shunts.[13] The symptoms of shunt malfunction are the same as seen with the initial hydrocephalus. Additionally, shunt specific findings, such as fluid around the shunt, abdominal pain, or distention and symptoms referable to infection may be seen.[102] Visual symptoms are prominent in shunt malfunction, those from the sixth cranial nerve being the commonest and the fourth cranial nerve less so.[19, 103] Visual loss may also occur, secondary to papilledema or to injury to the posterior cerebral artery.[104] Particularly in cases with a long history of papilledema, abrupt visual loss can occur after decompression of the ventricular system.[105] The signs of shunt malfunction may be stereotypic and easily recognized by the family in some patients. In addition, 23 to 65 percent of shunt infections present as shunt malfunction.[59, 63, 68]

Palpating the shunt valve has some value in detecting shunt malfunction; it has an 18- to 20-percent sensitivity in detecting shunt obstruction, and the predictive value of a negative shunt tap (indicating shunt patency) is 65 to 81 percent.[106] The most useful finding is the shunt valve that will not refill in over 10 minutes, suggesting proximal malfunction.

Imaging studies, ultrasound in children with open fontanelles, and CT can be used to assess ventricular size and exclude other causes of clinical symptoms, such as subdural collections or other intracranial lesions. Most often, CT demonstrates some evidence of shunt failure: bulging fontanelle, split sutures, periventricular edema, fullness of the previously slack ventricular contours, or increased size of part or all of

---

*See references 59, 61, 62, 64, 68, 72, and 78.

the ventricular system.²² Children younger than 2 years of age may have little reduction in ventricular size in the postoperative period despite resolution of symptoms and functioning shunt.¹⁰⁷ Older children and young adults, however, show a greater resistance to ventricular dilatation.¹⁰⁸, ¹⁰⁹ Periventricular edema may take 1 to several weeks to resolve but may resolve faster in acute than chronic hydrocephalus, again causing the radiographic appearance to lag behind the clinical picture.¹¹⁰ Because of these difficulties in assessing shunt function based on ventricular size alone, including patients with small-ventricle shunt malfunction, other strategies have been developed.

Shunt taps are useful in evaluating shunt malfunction. Performed with a small-gauge butterfly needle, and using the open end as a manometer to measure pressure, the tap can be performed at the patient's bedside. Concern about introducing infection is present, but a study has shown that this is not a major risk. The procedure correctly diagnosed 70 to 72 proximal shunt obstructions and 12 of 13 shunt infections.¹¹¹ Increased valve or reservoir pressure and easy aspiration suggest distal occlusion, and very low ICP with poor aspiration suggests proximal obstruction.¹¹² When the imaging studies and shunt taps still do not clarify the situation, shunt clearance studies can be performed in which the shunt is injected with contrast, usually water-soluble, and x-ray studies are taken, or the shunt is injected with ¹¹¹In–diethylenetriamine penta-acetic acid (DTPA) or ⁹⁹ᵐTc-DTPA and nuclear imaging is performed.¹¹³⁻¹¹⁵ Metrizamide ventriculography combined with CT scanning can identify proximal shunt problems and be useful when loculated collections are present.¹¹⁶ Measurement of ICP independent from the shunt may provide additional useful information.¹¹⁷

Shunt malfunctions result from proximal obstruction or malpositioning; valve malfunction or an inappropriate match between the patient's ICP and valve; or distal malfunction secondary to obstruction, malpositioning, or decreased absorption. Discontinuity of the shunt can also occur. Shunt infection seems to predispose to later obstruction.¹³, ¹¹⁸ Comparisons of ventriculoatrial and ventriculoperitoneal shunts suggest that ventriculoperitoneal shunts have less severe problems and decreased revision rates, especially because elective lengthening is less frequent.¹¹⁹ Others feel that the incidences of complications are similar in both types of shunts, but that the complications are more severe in ventriculoatrial shunts, for example, shunt nephritis, pulmonary emboli, perforation of the heart, and cor pulmonale.¹³, ¹²⁰ Ventriculopleural shunts are associated with pleural effusion.⁵²

In 186 shunt revisions, 73 were proximal. The histopathology, in the absence of infection, was most often glial tissue and choroid plexus obstructing the catheter.¹⁰² In the acute postoperative period, blood clots may obstruct the catheter, and 10 percent of CT scans performed on the second or third day after the shunt has been placed show blood in the occipital horns.¹²¹

Direct valve problems compose a small number of shunt malfunctions.¹³, ¹⁰² Recently, however, the question has been raised as to whether or not the valves directly influence the rate of proximal shunt malfunction. In an upright position, either sitting or standing, patients may develop a negative ICP with differential pressure valves, including slit valves, such as the Holter (Codman and Shurtleff) and the Holter-Hausner (Holter-Hausner International); ball valves, such as the Hakim (Cordis Corporation); programmable ball valves, such as the Sophy (Cordis Corporation) and the Medos Hakim (Cordis Corporation); and diaphragm valves, such as the PS Medical (PS Medical). The Cordis Orbis-Sigma valve functions differentially by maintaining flows of 20 to 30 ml/hour even when the differential pressure would promote greater flow rates.¹²²⁻¹²⁴ These design factors seem to influence the frequency and type of complications as well as the flow characteristics.¹²⁵⁻¹²⁷ The Orbis-Sigma valve in one series is associated with 18.4 percent proximal obstruction, compared with 24.1 percent for the standard differential pressure valve, but there was also an 18.3 percent valve obstruction in the Orbis-Sigma valve, compared with 9.7 percent in differential pressure valves.¹²⁸

Antisiphon devices, usually added in series with low-pressure differential pressure valves,¹²⁹ are also designed to prevent overdrainage of CSF. These devices may decrease shunt malfunctions,¹³⁰ but controversy exists regarding their function¹³¹ and proper location. According to the developers, the devices should be placed under free-floating scalp, and others advocate for placement 10 cm below the differential pressure valve.¹³², ¹³³

Distal shunt malfunctions were the reason for 62 of 163 (38 percent) revisions in intact shunts.¹⁰² Obstruction was the commonest cause of distal obstruction but connectors along the distal shunt tract may tether the shunt and cause functional shunt obstruction. Rarely, the catheter may erode a viscus or enter the scrotum through a patent processus vaginalis (Fig. 98–6).¹³⁴

Visual complications are significant. In a series of 50 children who received shunts at 5 to 17 years of age, only 36 of 100 eyes had normal optic discs. Corrected vision was ab-

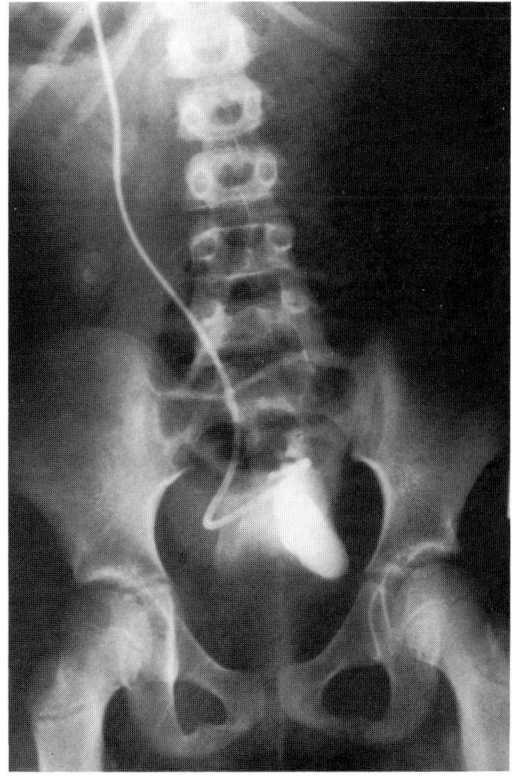

FIGURE 98–6. Shunt injection filling the rectum.

normal in 52 of 100 eyes. Nystagmus was also present in 18 percent of the patients. These findings strongly suggest the need for ongoing ophthalmologic evaluation in children with shunts.[135]

Endocrine history must be obtained as part of the routine follow-up of children with ventricular shunts. Both precocious and delayed puberty have been described in hydrocephalic children. In one series, 10.8 percent of a 37-patient series of patients with functioning shunts for nontumoral hydrocephalus developed precocious puberty with onset at an age range of 7.5 to 8.6 years. (Fig. 98–7) This condition resulted in a decreased adult height.[136] In a Swedish series of 68 children without tumor or myelomeningocele, eleven children (16 percent), five girls and six boys, developed precocious puberty.[137] Primary and secondary amenorrhea have also been described in association with hydrocephalus, some of which reverse with placement of ventricular shunting.[138–140] Hypothalamic hypopituitarism has also been seen in patients with hydrocephalus. The deficit is not necessarily corrected by shunt placement.[141]

MANAGEMENT OF FETAL HYDROCEPHALUS

With the rapid development of in utero diagnosis and treatment, the neurosurgeon has been increasingly involved in counseling mothers who carry a fetus diagnosed as having enlarged ventricles. The important questions are whether in utero treatment is desirable or possible should the infant be delivered early, should the obstetrical management be altered, and what is the expected outcome for the child. Experimental studies have not clearly answered the question of whether or not early intervention is desirable. In a lamb model, in utero decompression improved ventricular size but did not alter histologic damage and was associated with significant complications.[142] Some data suggest that brain regeneration may occur in certain circumstances of early intervention.[143] In utero interventions have been tried and are technically feasible: the report of the voluntary registry showed 44 drainage procedures for hydrocephalus from 1982 to 1985. There was 83 percent survival and a 10 percent procedure-related death rate. Of the 34 survivors, 53 percent were severely handicapped, 11.8 percent were less severely handicapped, and only 35.3 percent developed normally.[144] In a small series of four patients with in utero hydrocephalus, three of four were developmentally appropriate at 3.5 to 5.5 years of age. All received shunts at birth.[145] The outcome in this population, like in other hydrocephalic populations, is probably related to the specific cause of the hydrocephalus. The poor outcome in the patients with in utero shunts may be related to the 84 percent incidence of one or more central nervous system malformations in a series of 61 cases of in utero hydrocephalus, in which only 10 children had no concurrent anomalies.[146] Early delivery has been recommended if isolated ventriculomegaly is present.[147] How many of the in utero ventriculomegaly patients will even require shunting is unclear. In the San Francisco series of 24 patients, 10 had associated anomalies, and the pregnancies were terminated. Three patients were severely affected and underwent routine obstetrical management; all three died. Eleven of 24 had no associated abnormalities, and 9 of the 11 had stable ventricles throughout gestation, one had gradual resolution of ventricular enlargement, and one had progression of ventricular size but no signs of increased ICP at birth. Three of the eleven patients received shunts in the neonatal period, and an additional two patients received shunts by 5 months of age. The investigators concluded that most fetuses with ventriculomegaly do not require intervention before birth.[148]

Acknowledgments

We would like to acknowledge the help of Marilyn Keuning, Kanop Metriyakool, Srinlvasan Rajagopal, and Nancy Greninger in the preparation of this manuscript.

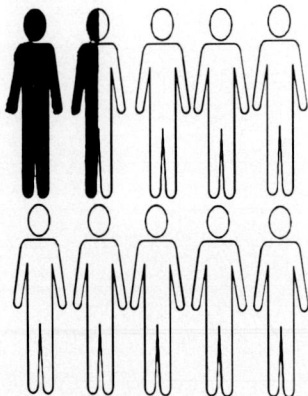

FIGURE 98–7. Incidence of precocious puberty. (Data from Helv Paediatr Acta 40:467–472, 1985.)

REFERENCES

1. Centers for Disease Control: Congenital Malformations Surveillance Report, January 1982–December 1985, page 19, issued March 1988
2. National Center for Health Statistics: Monthly Vital Statistics Report 40, No. 12(S):27, 1992
3. Stone DH, Womersley J, Sinclair T, Evans L: Declining prevalence of hydrocephalus. Eur J Epidemiol 5(3):398–399, 1989
4. National Vital Statistics System: Trends in infant mortality, cause of death, and other characteristics. 1960–1988; Series 20: Number 20. Report of HHS Publication No (PHS) 93–1857
5. Office of population censuses and surveys (1983): Congenital Malformation Statistics 1971–1980. Her Majesty's Statistical Office, London
6. Fernell E, Hagberg G, Wendt L: Epidemiology of infantile hydrocephalus in Sweden 1: Birth prevalences and general data. Acta Paediatr. Scand 75:975–891, 1986
7. Fernell E, Hagberg B, Hult G, Wendt L: Epidemiology of infantile hydrocephalus in Sweden: A clinical follow-up study in children born at term. Neuropediatrics 19:135–142, 1989
8. Hardie NA, Molgaard CA, Lawrs ER, et al: Incidence and effectiveness of cerebrospinal fluid shunts in Olmsted County, Minnesota, 1956–1981. Neuroepidemiology 5:95–104, 1986
9. Imaizumi Y: Concordance and discordance of congenital hydrocephalus in 107 twin pairs in Japan. Teratology 40:101–103, 1989
10. Mori K: Hydrocephalus—revision of its definition and classification with special reference to intractable infantile hydrocephalus. Childs Nerv Syst 6:198–204, 1990

11. Kirkpatrick M, Engleman H, Minns RA: Symptoms and signs of progressive hydrocephalus. Arch Dis Child 64:124–128, 1989
12. Foltz EL, Shurtleff AB: Five-year comparative study of hydrocephalus in children with and without operation. J Neurosurg 20:1064–1079, 1963
13. Kuetcher TR, Mealey J: Long-term results after ventriculoatrial and ventriculoperitoneal shunting for infantile hydrocephalus. J Neurosurg 50:179–186, 1979
14. Collmann H, Sorensen N, Karub J, Mehling J: Hydrocephalus in craniosynostosis. Childs Nerv Syst 4:279–285, 1988
15. Steinbok P, Hall J, Floodmand O: Hydrocephalus in achondroplasia: The possible role of intracranial venous hypertension. J Neurosurg 71:42–48, 1989
16. Sainte-Rose C, LaCombe J, Pierre-Kahn A, et al: Intracranial venous sinus hypertension: Cause or consequence of hydrocephalus in infants? J Neurosurg 60:727–736, 1984
17. Chattha AS, DeLong GR: Sylvian aqueduct syndrome is a sign of acute obstructive hydrocephalus in children. J Neurol Neurosurg Psychiatry 38:288–296, 1975
18. Gaab MR, Koos WT: Hydrocephalus in infancy and childhood: Diagnosis and indication for operation. Neuropediatrics 15:173–179, 1984
19. Corbett JJ: Neuro-ophthalmologic complications of hydrocephalus and shunting procedures. Semin Neurol 6:111–123, 1986
20. Blumhahagen JD, Mach LA: Abnormalities of the neonatal cerebral ventricles. Radiol Clin North Am 23:13–26, 1985
21. Volpe JJ. Anterior fontanel: Window to the neonatal brain. J Pediatr 100:395–397, 1982
22. Naidich TP, Schott LH, Baron RL: Computed tomography in evaluation of hydrocephalus. Radiol Clin North Am 20:143–167, 1982
23. Naidich TP, Gado MG: The small fourth ventricle in communicating hydrocephalus, Presented to the Annual Meeting of the Newport Western Neuroradiological Society of Los Angeles, 1978
24. Britton J, Marsh H, Kendall B, Kingsley D: MRI and hydrocephalus in childhood. Neuroradiology 30:310–314, 1988
25. Gammal T, Allen MB Jr, Brooks BS, Mark EK: MR evaluation of hydrocephalus. AJR 149:807–813, 1987
26. Quencer RM: Intracranial CSF flow in pediatric hydrocephalus evaluation with cine-MR imaging. AJNR 13:601–608, 1992
27. Mascalchi M, Ciraolo L, Bucciolini M, et al: Fast multiphase MR imaging of aqueductal CSF flow: II. Study in patients with hydrocephalus. AJNR 11:597–603, 1990
28. Chaddack WM, Siebert JJ, Adametz J, et al: Cranial Doppler ultrasonography correlated with criteria for ventriculoperitoneal shunting. Surg Neurol 31:122–128, 1989
29. Norelle A, Fischer AG, Flannery AM: Transcranial Doppler: A noninvasive method to monitor hydrocephalus. J Child Neurol 4:587–590, 1989
30. Sklar FH, Bever CW, Ramanthan M, Clark WK: Servo-controlled lumbar infusions in children: A quantitative approach to the problem of arrested hydrocephalus. J Neurosurg 52:87–98, 1980
31. DiRocco C, Caldarelli M, Magida A, Milani A: The lumbar subarachnoid infusion test in infants. Childs Nerv Syst 4:16–21, 1988
32. Donn SW, Roloff DW, Keyes JW: Lumbar cisternography in evaluation of hydrocephalus in the preterm infant. Pediatrics 72:670–676, 1983
33. Shackelford GD: Neurosonography of hydrocephalus in infants. Neuroradiology 28:452–462, 1986
34. Brann BS, Qualls C, Wells I, Papile L: Asymmetric growth of lateral cerebral ventricles in infants with post hemorrhagic ventricular dilation. J Pediatr 118(1):108–112, 1991
35. Krausse F: Puncturing the lateral ventricles. Surgery of the Brain and Spinal Cord, Vol 1. New York, Rebman & Comp, 1909, pp 254–256.39
36. Keen WW: Surgery of the lateral ventricles of the brain. Med News 57:275–278, 1980
37. Nulsen FE, Becker DP: Control of hydrocephalus by valve regulated shunt. J Neurosurg 26:231, 1967
38. Schott RM: Management of neurosurgical problems in neonates, in Schmidek HH, Sweet WH (ed): Operative Neurosurgery, Vol 1. San Diego, CA, Grune and Stratton, Inc., 1988, p 118
39. Epstein MH: Surgical management of hydrocephalus. In Schmidek HH, Sweet WH (ed): Operative Neurosurgery, Vol 1. San Diego, CA, Grune and Stratton, Inc., 1988, pp 141–150
40. Semik IK, Ceviker N, Baykaner K, Alp H: Index for optimum ventricular catheter length. Technical note. J Neurosurg 75:152–153, 1991
41. Mittal P, Chabbra DK: A modified technique for placement of the peritoneal end of a shunt system. Technical note. Br J Neurosurg 5(6):581–583, 1991
42. Ashpole RD: New instrumentation for the assembly of shunt systems by a non touch technique. Br J Neurosurg 6:237–242, 1992
43. Shkolnik A, Mclone DG: Intraoperative real time ultrasonic guidance of ventricular placement in infants. Radiology 141:515–517, 1981
44. Rubin JM, Dorhmann GJ: Use of ultrasonically guided probes and catheters in neurosurgery. Surg Neurol 18:143–148, 1991
45. Afschrift M, Jeannin P, Praeter CD, et al: Ventricular taps in the neonates under ultrasonic guidance. 59:1100–1101, 1983
46. Vries JK: Endoscopy as an adjunct to shunting for hydrocephalus. Surg Neurol 13:69–72, 1980
47. Hellwig D, Bauer BL: Minimally invasive neurosurgery by means of ultrathin endoscopes. Acta Neurochir (Wien) 54(suppl):63–68, 1992
48. Frank EH, Quattrochi KB, Hein L: An adapter for stereotactic insertion of unitized shunt systems. Surg Neurol 35(5):400–402, 1991
49. McGrail KM, Muzzi DA, Lossasso TJ, Meyer FB: Ventriculoatrial shunt distal catheter placement using transesophageal echocardiography. Technical note. Neurosurgery 30(5):747–749, 1992
50. Shafei IL: Ventriculojugular shunts against the direction of blood flow III. Operative techniques and results. Childs Nerv Syst 3:342–349, 1987
51. Kock-Jensen C, Clemmensen S, Andersen BB: Percutaneous insertion of CSF ventriculoatrial shunts—A new technique. Technical note. Acta Neurochirur 96(1–2):76–79, 1989
52. Venes JL, Shaw RK: Ventriculopleural shunting in management of hydrocephalus. Childs Brain 5:45–50, 1979
53. Pomeranz S, Rapaport HZ, Umansky F, Shalit NM: Technical note. The removal of free peritoneal catheters in the revision of ventriculoperitoneal shunts, Neurosurgery 22(2):436–438, 1988
54. Chambi I, Hendrick EB: A technique for removal of an adherent ventricular catheter. Pediatr Neurosurg 14:216–217, 1988
55. Steinbok P, Cochrane DD: Removal of adherent ventricular catheters. Pediatr Neurosurg 18:167–168, 1992
56. Kelly PJ: Stereotactic third ventriculostomy in patients with nontumoral adolescent/adult onset aqueductal stenosis and symptomatic hydrocephalus. J Neurosurg 75:865–873, 1991
57. Schmike RT, Black PB, Mark VH, Swartz MN: Indolent *Staphylococcus albus* or *aureus* bacteremia after ventriculoatriostomy. N Engl J Med 6:264–270, 1961
58. Bruce AM, Lorber J, Shedden WIH, Zachary RB. Persistent bacteremia following ventriculo-caval shunt operations for hydrocephalus in infants. Develop Med Child Neurol 5:461–470, 1963
59. Walters BC, Hoffman HJ, Hendrick EB, Humphreys RP. Cerebrospinal fluid shunt infection. J Neurosurg 60:1014–1021, 1984
60. James HE, Bejar R, Merritt A, et al: Management of hydrocephalus secondary to intracranial hemorrhage in the high-risk newborn. Neurosurgery 14:612–618, 1984
61. Pople IK, Bayston R, Hayward RD: Infection of cerebrospinal fluid shunts in infants: A study of etiological factors. J Neurosurg 77:29–36, 1992
62. Renier D, Lacombe J, Pierre-Kahn A, et al: Factors causing acute shunt infection. J Neurosurg 61:1072–1078, 1984
63. Odio C, McCracken GH, Nelson JD: CSF shunt infections in pediatrics. Am J Dis Children 138:1103–1108, 1984
64. Ammirati M, Raimondi AJ: Cerebrospinal fluid shunt infections in children. Childs Nerv Syst 3:106–119, 1987
65. Shapiro S, Boaz J, Kleinman M, et al: Origin of organisms infecting ventricular shunts. Neurosurgery 22(5):868–872, 1988
66. Schoenbaum SC, Gardner P, Shillito J: Infections of cerebrospinal fluid shunts: Epidemiology, clinical manifestations, and therapy. J Infect Dis 131(5):543–551, 1975
67. McClone DG, Czyzewski D, Raimondi AJ, Sommers R: Central nervous system infections as a limiting factor in the intelligence of children with myelomeningocele. Pediatrics 70:338–382, 1982
68. Nelson D. Cerebrospinal fluid shunt infections. Pediatr Infect Dis J 3(3):830–832, 1984
69. Gower DJ, Horton D, Pollay M: Shunt-related brain abscess and ascending shunt infection. J Child Neurol 5:318–320, 1990
70. Hahn YS, Engelhard H, McLone DG: Abdominal CSF pseudocyst. Pediatr Neurosci 12:75–79, 1985
71. Egelhoff J, Babcock DS, McLaurin R: Cerebrospinal fluid pseudocysts: Sonographic appearance and clinical management. Pediatr Neurosci 12:80–86, 1985
72. Hains SJ, Taylor F: Prophylactic methicillin for shunt operations:

Effects on incidence of shunt malfunction and infection. Childs Brain. 9:10–22, 1982
73. Frykberg T, Olsen L: Infection as a cause of peritoneal catheter dysfunction in ventriculoperitoneal shunting in children. Z Kinderchir 38(II):84–86, 1983
74. Tung H, Raffel C, McComb JG: Ventricular cerebrospinal fluid eosinophilia in children with ventriculoperitoneal shunts. J Neurosurg 75:541–544, 1991
75. Tzvetanova EM, Tzekov CT: Eosinophilia in the cerebrospinal fluid of children with shunts implanted for the treatment of internal hydrocephalus. Acta Cytol. 30(3):277–280, 1986
76. Traynelis VC, Powell RG, Koss W, et al: Cerebrospinal fluid eosinophilia and sterile shunt malfunction. Neurosurgery 23(4):645–649, 1988
77. Duhaime AC: Letter to the editor. J Neurosurg 76:724, 1992
78. Bierbrauer KS, Storrs BB, McLone DG, et al: Prospective, randomized study of shunt function and infections as a function of shunt placement. Pediatr Neurosurg 16:287–291, 1990
79. Lawton AR, Cooper MD: in Steihm ER, Fulginiti VA (eds): Immunologic Disorders in Infants and Children, 2nd ed. Philadelphia, WB Saunders Company, 1980 pp 36–51
80. Blum J, Schwarz M, Voth D: Antibiotic single-dose prophylaxis of shunt infections. Neurosurg Rev 12:239–244, 1989
81. Walter BC, Hoffman HJ, Hendrick EB, Humphreys RP: Decreased risk of infection in cerebrospinal fluid shunt surgery using prophylactic antibiotics: A case-control study. Z Kinderchir 40(I):15–18, 1985
82. Schmidt K, Gjerris F, Osgaard O: Antibiotic prophylaxis in cerebrospinal fluid shunting: A prospective randomized trial in 152 hydrocephalic patients. Neurosurgery 17(1):1–5, 1985
83. Bayston R, Bannister C, Boston V, et al: A prospective randomized controlled trial of antimicrobial prophylaxis in hydrocephalus shunt surgery. Z Kinderchir 45(I):5–7, 1990
84. Wang EL, Prober CG, Hendrick BE, et al: Prophylactic sulfamethoxazole and trimethoprim in ventriculoperitoneal shunt surgery. JAMA 251(9):1174–1177, 1984
85. LeRoux P, Howard MA III, Winn HR: Vancomycin pharmacokinetics in hydrocephalic shunt prophylaxis and relationship to ventricular volume. Surg Neurol 34:366–372, 1990
86. James HE, Wilson HD, Connor JD, Walsh JW: Intraventricular cerebrospinal fluid antibiotic concentration in patients with intraventricular infections. Neurosurgery 10:50–54, 1982
87. Bayston R, Grove N, Lawellin D, Barsham S: Prevention of hydrocephalus shunt catheter colonization in vitro by impregnation with antimicrobials. J Neurol Neurosurg Psychiatry 52:605–609, 1989
88. Bayston R, Penny SR: Excessive production of mucoid substance in Staphylococcus SHA: A possible factor in colonization in Holter shunts. Dev Med Child Neurol 14(27):25–28, 1972
89. Guevara JA, Zuccaro G, Treisan A, Denoya CD: Bacterial adhesion to cerebrospinal fluid shunts. J Neurosurg 67:438–445, 1987
90. Gower DJ, Gower VC, Richardson SH, Kelly DL Jr: Reduced bacterial adherence to silicone plastic neurosurgical prosthesis. Pediatr Neurosci 12:127–133, 1985
91. Borges LF: Cerebrospinal fluid shunts interfere with host defenses. Neurosurgery 10(1):55–60, 1982
92. Swayne R, Rampling A, Newsom SWB: Intraventricular vancomycin for treatment of shunt-associated ventriculitis. J Antimicrob Chemother 19:249–253, 1987
93. Pau AK, Smego RA Jr, Fisher MA: Intraventricular vancomycin: Observations of tolerance and pharmacokinetics in two infants with ventricular shunt infections. Pediatr Infect Dis J 5:93–96, 1986
94. Wilson HD, Bean JR, James HE, Pendley MM: Cerebrospinal fluid antibiotic concentrations in ventricular shunt infections. Childs Brain 4:74–82, 1978
95. Bayston RJ: Hydrocephalus shunt infections and their treatment. J. Antimicrob Chemother 15:239–261, 1985
96. Mates S, Glaser J, Shapiro K: Treatment of cerebrospinal fluid shunt infections with medical therapy alone. Neurosurgery 11:781–783, 1982
97. Frame PT, McLaurin RL: Treatment of CSF shunt infections with intrashunt plus oral antibiotic therapy. J Neurosurg 60:354–360, 1984
98. James HE, Walsh JW, Wilson HD, et al: Prospective randomized study of therapy in cerebrospinal fluid shunt infection. Neurosurgery 74:459–463, 1980
99. Smith RW, Alksne JF: Infections complicating the use of external ventriculostomy. J Neurosurg 44:567–570, 1976
100. Mayhall CG, Archer NH, Lamb VA, et al: Ventriculostomy-related infections: A prospective epidemiologic study. N Engl J Med 310:553–555, 1984
101. Petrak RM, Pottage JC, Harris AA, Levin S: *Hemophilus influenzae* meningitis in the presence of a cerebrospinal fluid shunt. Neurosurgery 18:79–81, 1986
102. Sehkar LN, Moossy J, Guthkelch AN: Malfunctioning ventriculoperitoneal shunts clinical and pathological features. J Neurosurg 56:411–416, 1982
103. Zeiner H, Prigatano G, Pollay M, et al: Ocular motility, visual acuity, and dysfunction of neuropsychological impairment in children with shunted uncomplicated hydrocephalus. Childs Nerv Syst 1:115, 1985
104. Arroyo HA, Jan JE, McCormick AQ: Permanent visual loss after shunt malfunction. Neurology 35:25–30, 1986
105. Obenchain TG, Crandall PH, Hepler RS: Blindness following relief of increased intracranial pressure. A sequel to severe papilledema. Bull LA Neurol Soc 35:147–151, 1970
106. Piatt JH: Physical examination of patients with cerebrospinal fluid shunts: Is there useful information in pumping the shunt? Pediatrics 89:470–473, 1992
107. Cardoso ER, DelBigio MR: Age-related changes in ventricular size. Acta Neurochir (Wien) 97:137–148, 1989
108. Cardoso ER, DelBigio MR, Schroeder G: Age-dependent changes of cerebral ventricular size, Part 1: Review of intracranial fluid collections. Acta Neurochirur (Wien) 97:40–46, 1989
109. Drapkin AJ, Sahar A: Experimental hydrocephalus: Cerebrospinal fluid dynamics and ventricular distensibility during early stages. Childs Brain 4:278–288, 1978
110. Naidich TP: CT evaluation of hydrocephalus, in Moss AA, Goldberg HI (eds): Computed tomography, Ultrasound and X-ray: An Integrated Approach. San Francisco, University of California, Department of Radiology, 1980
111. Noetzel MJ, Baker RP: Shunt fluid examination: Risks and benefits in the evaluation of shunt malfunction and infection. J. Neurosurg 61:328–332, 1984
112. LaFerla GA, Fyfe AHB, Drainer IK. A simple method of assessing intracranial pressure in hydrocephalic patients with shunts. Dev Med Child Neurol 26:732–736, 1984
113. Uverbrant P, Sixt R, Bjure J, Roos A: Evaluation of cerebrospinal fluid shunt function in hydrocephalic children using ^{99m}Tc-DTPA. Childs Nerv Syst 8:76–80, 1992
114. Savoiardo M, Solero CL, Passerini A, Migliavacca F: Determination of cerebrospinal fluid shunt function with water-soluble contrast medium. J Neurosurg 49:398–407, 1978
115. Gilday DL, Kellan J: ^{111}In-DPTA evaluation of CSF diversionary shunts in children. J Nucl Med 14:920–923, 1973
116. Faria MA Jr. O'Brien MS, Tindall GT: A technique for evaluation of ventricular shunts using Amipaque and computerized tomography. J Neurosurg 53:92–96, 1980
117. Rekate HL: Shunt revision: Complications and their prevention. Pediatr Neurosurg 17:155–162, 1991
118. Shurtleff DB, Stuntz JT, Hayden PW: Experience with 1201 cerebrospinal fluid shunt procedures. Pediatr Neurosci 12:49–57, 1985
119. Olsen L, Frykberg T: Complications in the treatment of hydrocephalus in children. A comparison of ventriculoatrial and ventriculoperitoneal shunts in a 20-year material. Acta Paediatr Scan 72:385–390, 1983
120. Sleigh G, Dawson A. Penny NT: Cor pulmonale. Dev Med Child Neurol 35:65–78, 1993
121. Palmieri A, Pasquini U, Menichelli F: Cerebral damage following ventricular shunt or infantile hydrocephalus evaluated by computed tomography. Neuroradiology 21:33–35, 1981
122. Sainte-Rose C, Hooven MD, Hirsch JF: A new approach in the treatment of hydrocephalus. J Neurosurg 66:213–226, 1987
123. Post EM: Currently available shunt systems: A review. Neurosurgery 16:257–260, 1985
124. Trost HA, Heissler HE, Claussen G, Gaab MR: Testing the hydrocephalus shunt valve: Long-term bench test results of various new and explanted valves. The need for a model for testing valves under physiological conditions. Eur J Pediatr Surg 1(1):38–40, 1991
125. Matsumae M, Sato O, Itoh K, et al: Quantification of cerebrospinal fluid shunt flow rates. Childs Nerv Syst 5:356–360, 1989
126. Lumenta CB, Roosen N, Dietrich U: Clinical experience with a pressure-adjustable valve SOPHY in the management of hydrocephalus. Childs Nerv Syst 6:270–274, 1990
127. Watts C, Keith HD: Testing the hydrocephalus shunt valve. Childs Brain 10:217–228, 1983

128. Sainte-Rose C: Shunt obstruction: A preventable complication Pediatr Neurosurg 19:156–164, 1993
129. Portnoy HD: Letter. J Neurosurg 61:1158, 1984
130. Gruber R, Jenny P, Herzog B: Experiences with the antisiphon device (ASD) in shunt therapy of pediatric hydrocephalus. J Neurosurg 61:156–162, 1984
131. McCullough DC: Symptomatic progressive ventriculomegaly in hydrocephalics with patent shunts and antisiphon devices. Neurosurgery 19:617–621, 1986
132. Portnoy HD: Letter. J Neurosurg 63:819, 1985
133. Tokoro K, Chiba Y: Optimum position for an antisiphon device in a cerebrospinal fluid shunt system. Neurosurgery 29:519–525, 1991
134. Prabhu S, Cochran W, Azmy AF: Wandering distal ends of ventriculoperitoneal shunts. Z Kinderchir 40:80–81, 1985
135. Mankinen-Heikkinen A, Mustonen E: Ophthalmic changes in hydrocephalus. A follow-up examination of 50 patients treated with shunts. Acta Opthal 65:81–86, 1987
136. De Luca D, Muritano M, Rizzo, G, et al: True precocious puberty: A long-term complication in children with shunted nontumoral hydrocephalus. Helv Paediatr Acta 40:467–472, 1985
137. Fernell E, Hagberg B, Hagberg G, et al: Epidemiology of infantile hydrocephalus in Sweden: A clinical follow-up study in children born at term. Neuropediatrics 19:135–142, 1988
138. Phansey SA, Holtz GL, Tsai CC, Williamson HD: Chronic hydrocephalus and primary amenorrhea with partial deficiency of gonadotropin-releasing factor. Fertil Steril 42:137, 1984
139. Jawadi MH, Kirsch W, Lock JP, Betz G: Hydrocephalus and amenorrhea. Obstet Gynecol 53:263, 1979
140. Moeslein S, Dericks-Tan JSE, Lorenz R, Taubert HD: Double-stimulation with LH-RH in primary amenorrhea caused by chronic internal hydrocephalus: A case study. Gynecol Endocrinol 1(2):201–207, 1987
141. Fiedler R, Krieger DT: Endocrine disturbances in patients with congenital aqueductal stenosis. Acta Endocrinol 80:1–13, 1975
142. Glick PL, Harrison MR, Halks-Miller M, et al: Correction of congenital hydrocephalus in utero II: Efficacy of in utero shunting. J Pediatr Surg 19:870–881, 1984
143. Michejda M, McCullough D, Bacher J, Queenan JT: Investigational approaches in fetal neurosurgery, in Humphrey RP: Concepts in Pediatric Neurosurgery. Basel, Switzerland, Karger 1983
144. Manning FA, Harrison MR, Rodeck C and members of the International Fetal Medical and Surgery Society: Catheter shunts for fetal hydronephrosis and hydrocephalus. Report of the International Fetal Surgery Registry. N Engl J Med 351:336–340, 1986
145. Amacher AL, Reid WD: Hydrocephalus diagnosed prenatally: Outcome of surgical therapy. Childs Brain 11:119–125, 1984
146. Nyberg DA, Mack LA, Hirsch J, et al: Fetal hydrocephalus: Sonographic detection and clinical significance of associated anomalies. Radiol 163:187–191, 1987
147. Cochrane DD, Myles S: Management of intrauterine hydrocephalus. J Neurosurg 57:590–595, 1982
148. Glick PL, Harrison MR, Nakayama DK, et al: Management of ventriculomegaly in the fetus. J Pediatr 105:97–105, 1984

SELECTED READINGS

Dandy WE, Blackfan KD: Internal hydrocephalus: An experimental, clinical and pathological study. Am J Dis Child 8:406, 1914

Mori K: Hydrocephalus—revision of its definition and classification with special reference to ''Intractable infantile hydrocephalus.'' Childs Nerv Syst 6:198–204, 1990

Naidich TP, Schott LH, Baron RL: Computed tomography in evaluation of hydrocephalus. Radiol Clin North Am 20:143–167, 1982

Sainte-Rose C: Shunt obstruction: A preventable complication. Pediatr Neurosurg 19:156–164, 1993

Walters BC, Hoffman HJ, Hendrick EB, Humphreys RP: Cerebrospinal fluid infection. J Neurosurg 60:1014–1021, 1984

CHAPTER 99

Surgical Management of Hydrocephalus in Adults

Mel H. Epstein
Arno H. Fried

The use of cerebrospinal fluid (CSF) shunts to treat hydrocephalus in both children and adults has made hydrocephalus one of the most treatable neurologic conditions. Before the use of ventricular shunts, other neurosurgical procedures were used to attempt to control ventricular size, including choroid plexectomy, which could be performed endoscopically or as an open procedure, such as that described by Dandy.[1] Stookey and Scarff tried third ventriculostomy, which yielded somewhat better results until ventricular shunts became far more successful.[2, 3] Recently, however, third ventriculostomy has become another option in the treatment of hydrocephalus, especially when stereotactic techniques are used to facilitate this procedure.[4, 5] These older techniques, however, were not very successful in treating hydrocephalus, and older textbooks of obstetrics showed instruments designed to crush the head of a hydrocephalic baby in utero.

Ventricular shunts have obviously changed the prognosis for individuals with hydrocephalus, and most attain fairly normal intelligence. The improved survival and outcome has come, however, with the price of many new problems related to shunting and the creation of shunt dependency in these individuals. The natural history of untreated hydrocephalus by Lawrence and Coates showed a 46 percent 10-year survival and intellectual impairment in 62 percent.[6] After shunting, however, Foltz and Shurtleff demonstrated a 10-year survival of nearly 95 percent and with intellectual impairment in only 30 percent of shunted children.[7] Furthermore, the syndrome of occult or normal-pressure hydrocephalus (NPH) in adults is now a well-recognized cause of gait disturbance and dementia.[8–10] However, differentiating NPH from ventricular enlargement that results from atrophy and aging is still quite difficult. The ability to predict responses to shunting of adult hydrocephalus depends on clinical, radiologic, and CSF biomechanical studies to determine which adults will improve after a shunt is placed.

This chapter reviews the pathophysiology of hydrocephalus in adults. The indications and technical aspects of shunting and shunt revisions are reviewed, as well as problems that have been created by shunt dependency, such as the slit ventricle syndrome. Adult hydrocephalus and the treatment of NPH are also discussed.

ETIOLOGY AND PATHOPHYSIOLOGY

Hydrocephalus is excessive accumulation of CSF within the ventricles. Often, this ventricular enlargement is accompanied by elevation in intracranial pressure (ICP). However, in clinical practice, enlarged ventricles are not always associated with elevated ICP; therefore, these states must be differentiated because indications for shunting vary. Some conditions associated with normal- or low-pressure ventricular enlargement include low-pressure ventricular dilatation, cerebral atrophy, porencephalic cysts, and adult NPH.

Congenital malformations account for a large percentage of childhood hydrocephalus. Aqueductal stenosis is the most common type of congenital hydrocephalus and is the cause in roughly 40 percent of cases. The lateral and third ventricles are enlarged and the fourth ventricle is normal. In addition, the cerebral aqueduct can become secondarily stenotic in shunted hydrocephalus as a result of other causes, a condition that causes the fourth ventricle to become trapped because of blockage of its outflow and inability of fluid to flow upward into the shunt.[11] If symptomatic, the encysted trapped fourth ventricle requires a second ventricular catheter, which is connected to the existing shunt above the valve to ensure equal flow in both compartments.

Most cases of aqueductal stenosis causing hydrocephalus are diagnosed in the first year or two of life because they present with typical signs of elevated intracranial pressure. However, the first appearance of hydrocephalus due to aqueductal stenosis can be in the adult, who can present with chronic headaches and has a head that is on the large size of the growth chart. There may also be a history of school problems and learning disabilities throughout childhood. Sometimes, aqueductal stenosis is first diagnosed after a mild-to-moderate head injury that seems to precipitate new signs of elevated ICP. Because of the frequent use of in utero ultrasound during pregnancy, aqueductal stenosis can also be diagnosed before a child is born, and a planned shunt can be inserted after birth.

The Chiari malformations can cause both childhood and adult hydrocephalus. Type I Chiari malformation with cerebellar tonsillar ectopia is usually seen without spina bifida and myelomeningocele. The symptoms can be referable to compression of the lower medulla and upper cervical spine, or hydrocephalus can be the initial presenting symptom. If the hydrocephalus is not recognized before posterior fossa decompression for a Chiari I malformation, it can lead to complications, including pseudomeningocele and wound leakage. Similarly, in patients with a symptomatic syrinx and hydrocephalus, the hydrocephalus should be treated with a ventriculoperitoneal shunt before posterior fossa decompression.

The Chiari II malformation is usually a cause of hydrocephalus in children with spina bifida and myelomeningocele. In children with myelomeningocele, 90 percent have an associated Chiari II malformation, and 70 to 80 percent have hydrocephalus.

Hydrocephalus can be caused by cysts, either porencephalic cysts within the brain tissue adjacent to the ventricle or arachnoid cysts in the subarachnoid space. In particular, arachnoid cysts of the suprasellar region obstruct the third ventricle, causing hydrocephalus, and quadrigeminal cysts of the dorsal midbrain compress the posterior third ventricle and cerebral aqueduct, also causing hydrocephalus. The use of intraoperative ultrasound can direct shunt catheters into both the arachnoid cysts and the ventricles, thereby enabling shunting of both compartments. Recently, fiberoptic ventriculoscopy was used to visualize the tough capsule of these arachnoid cysts and to puncture them with laser or cautery. This procedure can communicate the arachnoid cysts with the ventricle, and then a single common compartment can be shunted. The Dandy-Walker cyst is a posterior fossa cyst in communication with an enlarged fourth ventricle that is associated with hypoplasia of the cerebellar vermis. When this cyst is symptomatic and exists with ventricular enlargement, a shunt must be placed. Our practice is to shunt both the ventricle and the posterior fossa cyst, connecting the catheters from these structures to a single distal shunt system. The results of direct shunting are superior to those of craniotomy and fenestration of the cyst.

Acquired hydrocephalus in adults has many causes. Tumor-related hydrocephalus is most common with posterior fossa tumors, suprasellar tumors, and third ventricle and pineal region tumors. Although controversial, our practice is to not perform a preoperative shunt, to temporize with preoperative dexamethasone (Decadron) and acetazolamide (Diamox), and in some cases, to use a temporary ventriculostomy. The major goal of the tumor surgery is to unblock the CSF pathways, frequently avoiding a shunt. With this strategy, a shunt is needed in only 20 to 30 percent of cases postoperatively.

Vascular causes of hydrocephalus include vascular malformations such as Galen vein arteriovenous malformations, giant midline aneurysms, and subarachnoid hemorrhages. Hydrocephalus follows subarachnoid hemorrhage in 25 percent of cases. Other vascular causes of hydrocephalus include thrombosis of the dural sinuses, bilateral jugular vein disruption, such as in radical neck surgery or in superior vena cava obstruction due to tumors or long-standing indwelling catheters.[15] These occlusive disorders, however, often produce a pseudotumor-like picture of a swollen brain and small ventricles. However, occasionally progressive ventricular enlargement is seen.

CEREBROSPINAL FLUID DYNAMIC TESTING

The measurement of the CSF hydrodynamic profile is often useful in the evaluation of syndromes. This form of testing can measure intracranial and intraventricular pressure acutely and over an extended period of time, measure CSF absorption through measurement of resistance to CSF absorption, R_o, and measure neural axis volume buffering capacity as an indication of brain compliance. The use of these techniques has several purposes. First, in some cases of ventricular enlargement, a shunt is not clearly required; some symptoms may not be classic, and clear-cut progressive ventricular enlargement may not be present. Measurement of ICP, CSF absorption as R_o, and pressure-volume index (PVI) as an indication of compliance allows the comparison of the measured results with normal values, and the analysis of the differences from biomechanical profiles in active hydrocephalic syndromes (Table 99–1).[16–19] The second purpose is unique to adults with NPH, in whom an abnormal biomechanical profile can predict a good response to shunting, as opposed to those with hydrocephalus ex vacuo, in whom shunting would not improve symptoms.[20, 21] These techniques involve the placement of a catheter into the CSF, usually intraventricular. The lumbar subarachnoid space can sometimes be used, if communicating hydrocephalus is present. Once a pressure tracing is obtained, the measurement of ICP is the first and most straightforward parameter. Normal ICP in children should not exceed 10 mm Hg in infants, 15 mm Hg in older children, and 20 mm of Hg after the age of 15 years (Table 99–1). Once an initial ICP is measured, a multiple-day continuous measurement of ICP is useful because it frequently discerns abnormal pressure phenomena, including Lundburg A waves, which can rise to 80 to 100 mm Hg, and Lundburg B waves, which can rise up to 40 to 50 mm Hg and can occur at a rate of one per minute. Several investigators have correlated better responses to shunting adults

Table 99–1. BIOMECHANICAL PROFILE OF THE VARIOUS CLINICAL GROUPS OF HYDROCEPHALUS

	Intracranial Pressure (mm Hg)	Pressure-Volume Index (ml)	Resistance to CSF Absorption (mm Hg/ml/min)
Normal child	3–12	8–22*	<3
Normal adult	10–15	25	<3
Childhood hydrocephalus	10–20	28.1	7.2
Shunted hydrocephalus	0–10	18.4	Range, 2–30**
Normal-pressure hydrocephalus	10–15	16	17

*Dependent on size of intracranial and intraspinal compartments (see normograms in references 18 and 19).
**Resistance to cerebrospinal fluid (CSF) absorption (R_o) becomes dependent on intracranial pressure and is not constant in shunted hydrocephalus.[17]

who have NPH with an increased frequency of observing B waves.[22, 23] In shunted children who are shunt dependent and may have intermittent signs of elevated ICP with headaches, ICP monitoring techniques can be useful in the identification of those with true pressure abnormalities versus chronic headaches, which are either psychological in origin or are unrelated to abnormal CSF pressure events.

Measuring resistance to the absorption of CSF (R_o) is a way of measuring CSF absorption of flow. CSF absorption is pressure dependent, and the higher the ICP, the greater the rate of CSF absorption.[24, 25] R_o can be measured either with the bolus injection technique, as described by Marmarou and colleagues and Shapiro, or with the constant infusion technique.[20, 21, 26, 27] In all forms of hydrocephalus, significant absorptive reserve exists, so that impairment of CSF absorption is not as great as one would predict (Table 99–1). In childhood hydrocephalus, the R_o is elevated to a mild-to-moderate degree,[18] and in adults with NPH, R_o is more significantly elevated. R_o is most elevated in pseudotumor cerebri, yet ventricles remain small, thereby demonstrating that progressive ventricular size is a factor of both an impairment of CSF absorption and a change in brain-buffering capacity, as measured by the PVI.

The PVI is a measure of neural axis volume-buffering capacity. It is a numeric representation of the entire pressure-volume curve and can be compared with normal values in children and adults. The PVI is defined as the theoretical volume necessary to raise ICP tenfold.[27] In adults, the normal PVI value is 25 ml; however, in children, normal PVI values vary with the size of the child. In normograms described by Shapiro and colleagues,[18] a normal PVI value for a child of any size can be determined by measuring head circumference and spinal length.[19] The PVI is measured through a CSF catheter by injecting a known volume of saline and recording the initial (P_o) and peak (P_p) ICP. When the logarithm of ICP is plotted against the volume, a straight-line relationship characteristic of the PVI is determined. In childhood hydrocephalus, PVI is markedly elevated, indicating a shift of the pressure-volume curve to the right, which is a very compliant system.[18] This phenomenon allows progressive ventricular enlargement to occur with intraventricular pressure that does not exceed a threshold above which CSF absorption would be initiated. Even though the R_o is only modestly elevated, the very compliant brain does not allow adequate CSF absorption. In adults with NPH, the PVI has been measured in 25 cases and has been found to be reduced past normal values. This effect produces a relatively tight CSF system in which ICP may be normal, but such patients are prone to fluctuations in ICP and pressure waves, as is often observed on the long-term ICP monitoring. This group all had the classic triad of gait disturbance, urinary incontinence, and dementia, with gait disturbance being the predominant sign.

NORMAL-PRESSURE HYDROCEPHALUS

NPH was described in 1965 by Adams and coworkers[8] as occult hydrocephalus associated with normal CSF pressure (180 mm H_2O or less). The clinical syndrome included gait disturbance, dementia, and urinary incontinence. Furthermore, CSF shunting reversed these symptoms to a variable extent. The obvious importance of recognizing NPH is in distinguishing this form of dementia and gait abnormalities from other forms of senile dementia as a treatable entity. Many studies have subsequently tried to predict the type of patient most likely to respond to shunting based on various parameters.[28–30] The gait disturbance is characterized by a ''magnetic'' gait, with small steps and minimal movement of the feet, sometimes called a gait apraxia. In patients who responded best to shunting, gait disturbance was the initial and most disabling of the three symptoms. A variable amount of dementia is present with NPH. In contrast to the findings with gait apraxia, when dementia was the predominant feature, the response to shunting was minimal. Urinary incontinence is the third feature of NPH and is usually a frontal release sign often associated with a general loss of accepted social behavior. This incontinence can respond to shunting, but the improvement in urinary function is less than the improvement in gait. The methods used to investigate NPH for possible shunting involve ICP and CSF dynamic measurements, imaging studies, radioisotope cisternography, and trial CSF drainage.

ICP measurements are often normal in NPH. However, long-term monitoring can show the presence of A waves or B waves. One of the early and still useful tests for evaluating NPH is the Katzman infusion test, in which a CSF catheter is placed in the lumbar space, and a constant infusion of fluid is performed to determine the rate of rise of CSF pressure and the time required to reach a new steady-state pressure.[20, 21] This test, therefore, depends on both pressure-volume characteristics and on CSF absorption factors to determine the rate at which ICP rises and reaches a new steady-state pressure, if at all. Coupling the ICP monitoring with determination of R_o by bolus or infusion techniques is an excellent way to obtain this information all in one monitoring period.

DiChiro and colleagues[31] introduced radioisotope cisternography to describe a characteristic pattern in NPH. Radioactive iodinated serum albumin is introduced into the lumbar subarachnoid space, and cerebral radioisotope scanning is performed at 6, 24, and 48 hours later. Normally, CSF should flow from the lumbar space up over the convexities of the hemispheres, and subsequently be absorbed into the sagittal sinus. The supposed characteristic pattern for NPH demonstrates failure of the isotope to ascend over the cerebral convexities as well as prolonged reflux of the isotope into the ventricles. When this pattern is seen, it is interpreted as a pattern typical for NPH, and shunting is often recommended. Multiple studies, however, have failed to demonstrate this as the best test, and patients with the typical syndrome who respond well to shunting can have negative results on radioisotope cisternography.

Occasionally, a determination of response to shunting is made by withdrawal of a large volume of CSF and observation of the clinical response of the patients. This procedure can be performed with a lumbar puncture in which CSF is removed until the opening pressure is reduced to half its original value, or it can be accomplished with continuous lumbar drainage. These techniques, however, are poor predictors of response to shunting and should be abandoned.

The results of ventricular shunting for NPH can be quite dramatic. Often, however, despite all of these predictive tests, one cannot accurately determine which patient will respond well to shunting. In addition, an initial excellent response with improvement of symptoms often gives way to a re-emergence of symptoms several months later. Stein and Langfitt[32] reported improvement in 64 percent of patients, which then decreased to 24 percent sustained improvements. Laws and Morki[33] found 50 percent improvement, with 67 percent improvement in patients with the classic triad of NPH. Black[39] reported a 47 percent overall improvement, with a 60 percent improvement in those with the triad. Patients with a predominance of gait apraxia generally respond best, and those with dementia respond least, to shunting. Although all of the screening tests have been used on many patients, our preference is to use 2 days of ICP monitoring through a ventriculostomy, plus CSF dynamic measurements of PVI and resistance to CSF absorption (R_o) during this monitoring period to determine a biomechanical profile of the patient. We then compare this profile to normal adult values. A shunt is performed if the classic clinical triad is present with a gait disturbance as the predominant finding, or if a triad is suggested in an adult with large ventricles, an abnormality on ICP monitoring of pressure waves, low PVI, or elevated R_o.

INDICATIONS FOR SURGERY

Adults can present with hydrocephalus caused by similar conditions as those seen in children, such as aqueductal stenosis. Young adults usually have clear-cut signs of elevated ICP, with severe headaches, papilledema, and vomiting. In this situation, the decision to proceed with a shunt is clear-cut. Shunting is considered to treat NPH in older adults with the triad of dementia, gait disturbance, and incontinence. The previous discussion outlines the decision of who receives a shunt. Despite the screening tests described in the previous section, if a patient has the triad of gait disturbance, incontinence, and dementia in the presence of enlarged ventricles, with little visible cortical atrophy on CT scan, the surgeon has sufficient grounds for offering a surgical shunt as treatment.

VENTRICULAR SHUNTING FOR HYDROCEPHALUS

The vast array of shunting devices has many similar features. Current shunt systems have a valve incorporated within the shunt with an opening and closing pressure, so that currently used shunts are pressure regulated. Given the fact that shunts all drain CSF relatively quickly when the patient is in the upright position as a result of siphoning, most of the flow characteristics of currently available shunts are relatively unimportant. However, other technical aspects of the initial shunting procedure and hardware affect the success of the shunt and decrease the incidence of shunt malfunction. Shunt valves can be located proximally and distally. Distal slit valves are now to be avoided because of the high frequency of distal shunt malfunction and unpredictable flow characteristics. The currently used valve mechanisms include slit valves, spring-ball valves, and diaphragm valves.[35] Siphoning occurs when the patient is in the upright position, in which a negative pressure is exerted that is related to the vertical distance between the inlet and the outlet of the shunt.[36,37]

Although siphoning is usually not a detrimental factor in childhood-shunted hydrocephalus, adults can have more problems related to siphoning because of the longer length of the shunt in the vertical position and the rigid skull that is present at the time that the shunt is initially placed. For this reason, siphoning can cause low-pressure symptoms and subdural hematoma more frequently in the adult shunted hydrocephalus population.[38]

Although the flow characteristics of the shunt may not be particularly important, a one-piece shunt system is advantageous because it is easier to insert, has a quicker operation, and avoids the possibility of shunt disconnection or disintegration associated with a connector. A connector also prevents extra tubing from elongating because the connector becomes fixed in its position subcutaneously as a result of ingrowth of scar tissue. Another useful feature of shunts is a right-angled ventricular catheter, which is bonded to the valve system. This feature enables the surgeon to have easy access to the shunt catheter, and it avoids the surgeon's having to work underneath a reservoir with a catheter that has become embedded in the brain. The valve system should have incorporated in it some sort of flushing or tapping chamber to enable access to tapping a shunt, as well as the ability to pump and test a shunt to assess its function. The pumping mechanism also should have a proximal and distal occluder system so that the proximal and distal portions of the shunt can be isolated and tested separately by the placement of percutaneous pressure on these occluders. In children and young adults, a low-pressure ventriculoperitoneal shunt is the initial shunt of choice in most circumstances.

The patient's position is important to the correct implantation of the shunt. The head is turned sharply to the left, and the shunt is placed initially in the right occipital area (Fig. 99-1). By use of a Hudson Brace and nonpower burr, a burr hole is placed approximately 4 cm up from the inion and 3 to 4 cm off the midline (Fig. 99-2). This occipital placement allows a relatively straight pass into the body of the ventricle, so that the shunt catheter is mostly within the ventricle. This trajectory avoids the risk of too low an entry through the internal capsule, which can happen with shunt placement sites that are more lateral and inferior, such as at Kean's point. An adequate length of ventricular catheter must be selected, so that the tip is anterior to the foramen of Monro, where there is less choroid plexus. Generally, a 6-cm catheter is used in a small newborn, an 8-cm catheter in an older infant and young child, and a 10-cm catheter is used in children over 18 months and in adults. We also routinely use perioperative antibiotics and believe that they play an important role in reducing shunt infections, although this is a controversial point in the literature.[39-42]

A rolled towel is placed across the shoulder blades to elevate the chest and neck and to allow for a straight passage of the shunt passer, with no secondary incisions between the head and the abdomen. The abdominal incision is a horizontal incision, just below the rib cage or lateral to the umbilicus. Once the shunt is laid in position, the dura is opened with a pinpoint cautery to cause an opening just big enough to allow the passing of the shunt catheter. A large dural opening allows CSF to flow around the shunt and cause a subcutaneous fluid collection. The ventricle is tapped with a rigid brain cannula (Fig. 99-3), and once a good flow of CSF is obtained the ventricular catheter is fed into the ventricle

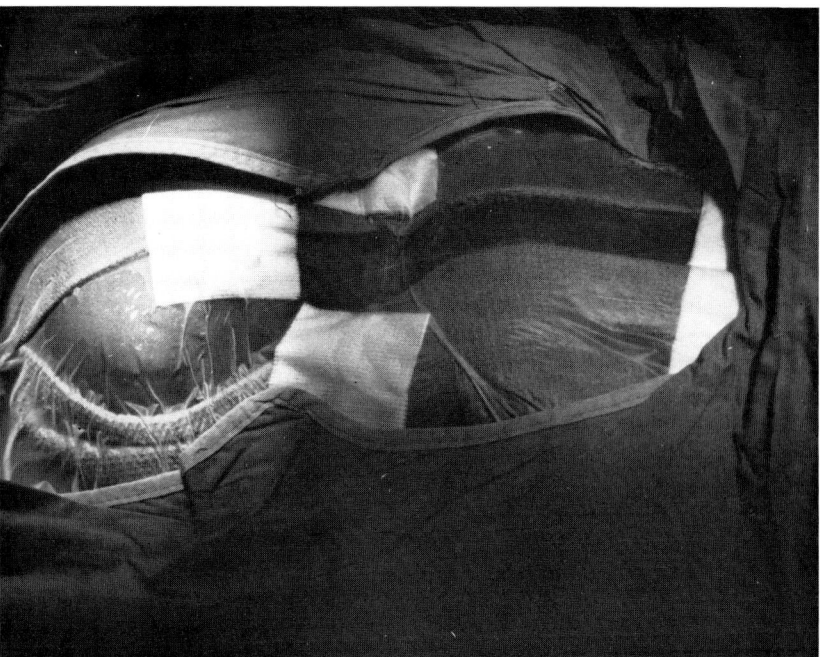

FIGURE 99-1. A plastic drape not only decreases skin contact but also helps maintain the body temperature of small children.

through this tract without a stylette (Fig. 99–4). Fluid should then be aspirated from the lower end of the shunt to ensure that the valve system is opened, and then it is placed into the peritoneal cavity. The full length of the peritoneal catheter can be placed to allow for subsequent growth.

A consideration that arises with growth of the child is whether or not the shunt needs to be lengthened. The first question to be asked in this situation is whether or not the child is shunt dependent and continues to need the shunt as it becomes short. Although most children are shunt dependent for life, elective shunt lengthening does not need to be performed, in all children, and we lengthen shunts only if the following conditions are present:

1. The child is shown to be shunt dependent from previous shunt malfunctions.
2. Neurosurgical care is not easily available.
3. A CT scan shows slit ventricles or a thick calvarium—both of these features are associated with shunt dependency.

If any of these criteria are met, then an elective lengthening is performed. However, the shunt must be lengthened just distal to the valve at the upper end of the shunt, so that a connector is not at the abdominal incision, which would prevent the elongation of the new tubing. A ventriculoperitoneal shunt is often the initial shunt of choice for adults with hydrocephalus. Because siphoning with subdural hematoma or low-pressure headaches may be a more common finding in adults with large ventricles and a rigid calvarium, a ventriculoatrial shunt may be a useful first option in adult hydrocephalus because the shorter shunt between the head and the heart provides less siphoning effect. A medium-pressure valve is usually chosen for shunting in adults.

To perform a ventriculoatrial shunt, the surgeon makes an incision across the anterior border of the sternomastoid muscle, and the jugular vein is identified. Our practice is to isolate the jugular vein both proximally and distally with ligatures, and to tie the vein off distally. A small opening is made into the jugular vein to pass the shunt down the jugular vein into the right atrium of the heart. On the right side, this step is easily performed with electrocardiographic control: An alligator clip is attached to the stylette of the distal tubing, and it is connected to lead II of the anesthesia electrocardiographic machine.[43] The atrium is indicated by the P-wave configuration becoming more and more upright, and when it becomes a biphasic P wave, the tip has entered the right atrium. A chest radiograph taken in the recovery room should confirm that the catheter is at the T6 level. On the left side, where there are more turns of the venous anatomy, fluoroscopic control with a flexible wire is useful for proper placement of the distal shunt in the right atrium. With ventriculoatrial shunts, lengthening should be considered when the shunt tip rises above the T4 level because above that, distal malfunction is significantly more common.

A pleural shunt is a very good option if the peritoneum cannot be used. This shunt is especially useful in patients older than age 8 years who cannot have a ventriculoperitoneal shunt.

SHUNT MALFUNCTION AND REVISION

Because ventricular shunting usually produces shunt dependency, the diagnosis of a shunt malfunction is usually obvious because of overt signs of elevated ICP, including headaches, vomiting, and lethargy. This mode of presentation occurs in approximately 70 percent of those who receive shunts.[17] In the other 30 percent of cases, however, signs of deterioration may be subtler and may include neuropsychological changes and cognitive and behavior symptoms.[16] In adults with NPH, a shunt malfunction may cause a re-emergence of the triad of symptoms. When a shunt malfunction is suspected, evaluation begins with a CT scan to compare ventricular sizes and look for interval enlargement of the ventricles. A shunt series can be performed to determine continuity of the shunt, shunt placement, or a distal shunt problem. In adults with NPH, the ventricles often do not change very much in size, so that a radionucleotide shunt

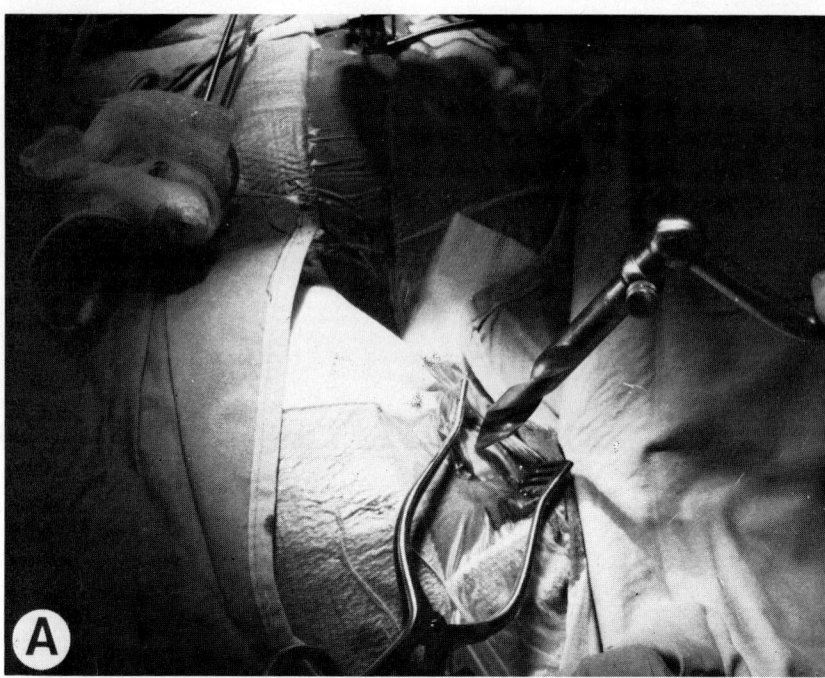
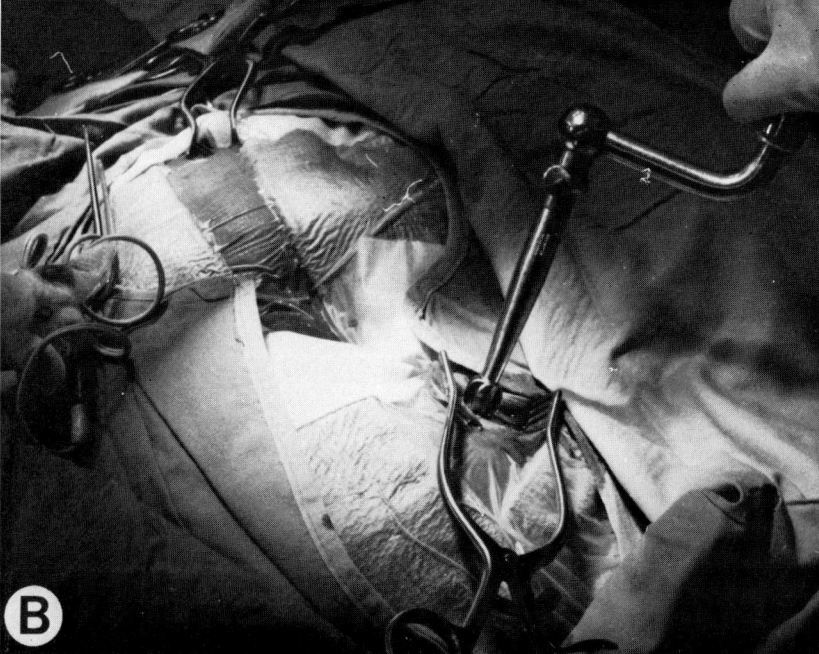

FIGURE 99–2. (A) The burr hole for the flushing device must be made carefully because the bit does not lock in the normal fashion within the skull of young children. (B) It is important that the burr hole be large enough to accommodate the flushing device if it is the type that is seated in the burr hole. This lowers the profile and decreases the risk of decubitus ulcer.

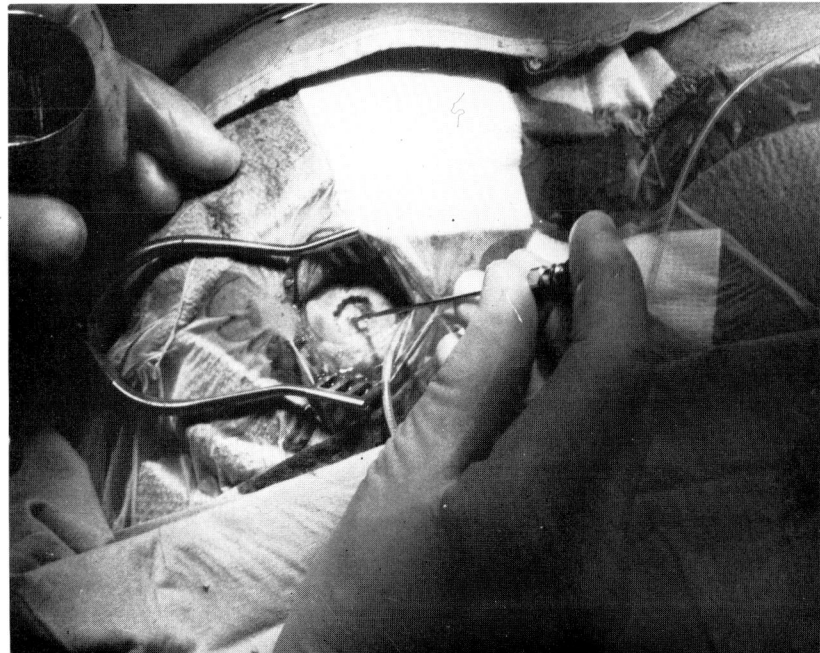

FIGURE 99–3. The needle is passed carefully using a CT scan as a guide for placement in the ventricle.

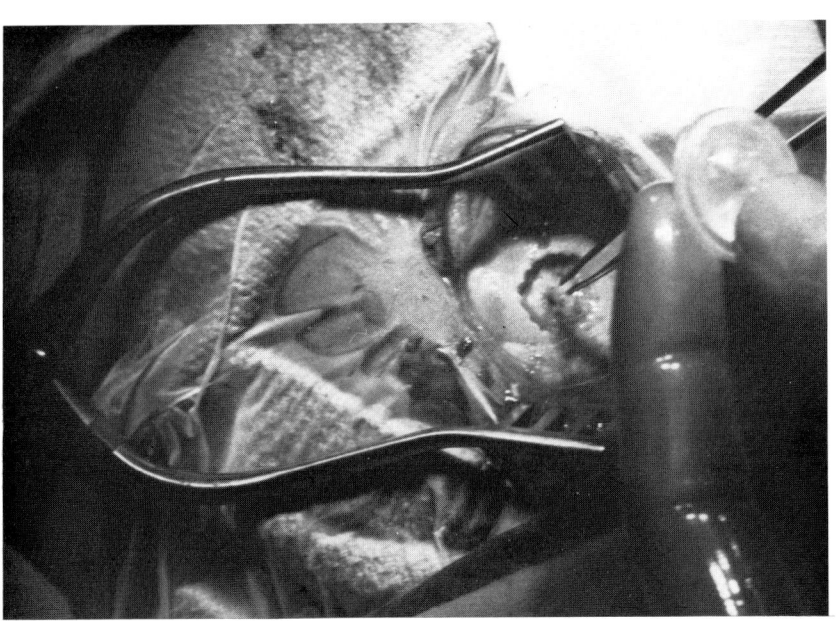

FIGURE 99–4. Immediately after the needle is withdrawn, the shunt tube is inserted along the needle track into the ventricular system.

flow study is often useful to establish the fact that the shunt is draining fluid from the ventricle into the peritoneum. With a suspected distal shunt malfunction, the surgeon should look carefully for signs of infection, which is a very common cause of distal shunt problems. A shunt tap is useful to measure ICP, to test both proximal and distal portions of the shunt, and to exclude a shunt infection. Table 99-2 gives the frequency of some common shunt complications. Interestingly, 58 percent of children with shunts have no complications.

The most common shunt malfunction is a proximal occlusion of the shunt. To try preventing proximal shunt problems, the surgeon should place the shunt catheter anterior to the foramen of Monro in the lateral ventricle, where there is less choroid plexus. This placement can be accomplished with an adequate length of ventricular catheter through an occipital placement, or with a 5- to 6-cm ventricular catheter in a frontal catheter placement with the burr hole at the coronal suture. The frontal route is especially useful when the ventricles are not particularly dilated. In a proximal revision, a ventricular catheter may be difficult to remove. In this revision, the occluded catheter is removed and replaced with a right-angled ventricular catheter, which is slid down the initial shunt tract and connected to the distal shunt assembly after distal shunt function is tested. When the ventricular catheter is stuck, several attempts can be made to relieve the adherence. First, the ventricular catheter can be grasped with a hemostat and rotated, which may free the catheter with a sudden give in the resistance. If twisting the catheter does not free it, the next step is to place the stylette down the shunt catheter and touch the Bovie cautery to the stylette. This procedure can sometimes coagulate the choroid plexus at the tip of the catheter, thereby releasing it. If resistance is still a problem, the catheter should be left in place, a new burr hole should be placed next to the existing one, and a new ventricular catheter should be used. Intraventricular endoscopy plays a more active role in the freeing of the adherent choroid plexus.

When more than one recent proximal shunt occlusion has occurred, different steps must be taken to prevent further occlusions. Endoscopy has shown that often a new catheter is placed into a sheath of scar tissue that is prone to occlude within the next several days to weeks. We therefore use a different site for placement, which is often the frontal route, with recurrent proximal occlusions.

When a proximal revision must be performed in the setting of relatively small ventricles, certain steps are taken. It is frequently wise to place a tube at a frontal site, leaving a blocked occipital catheter in place. A second alternative is to attempt to slide a new ventricular catheter down the same tract after the removal of the old ventricular catheter. No attempt should be made to place the catheter by use of a stylette or brain needle, because it may veer off the existing tract and into the ventricle. If the catheter does not find its way into the ventricle, then a single attempt with a brain needle can be made to try to cannulate the small ventricle. If this attempt is unsuccessful, repeated attempts should not be made, and the operation should be aborted. The patient should be watched closely for signs of elevated ICP, and serial CT scans and the proximal shunt revision should be subsequently performed when the ventricle has dilated.

In proximal revision in patients who have blood-tinged CSF after the new ventricular catheter is placed, an effort should be made to clear the ventricular system of this bleeding. The new catheter is attached to a three-way stopcock and is irrigated with saline until it begins to clear. This process often requires patience because up to 20 minutes of gentle irrigation of saline may be needed. Once the CSF clears, a new ventricular catheter should replace the catheter through which irrigation was being performed. If the blood does not clear, it may be wise to place a temporary ventriculostomy for several days until the CSF is clear.

DISTAL SHUNT MALFUNCTION AND REVISIONS

Distal shunt malfunctions are related to a short ventricular catheter and shunt occlusions. Distal shunt occlusions are most often seen in shunt infections, which can lead to impaired CSF absorption from the peritoneum and the formation of an abdominal pseudocyst. CSF should be sampled in patients with distal shunt problems to exclude infection and to allow the fluid to be analyzed in the laboratory for a long period of time because diphtheroids may not grow in culture media in the first 2 days. Distal shunts have been known to erode into various abdominal viscera,[44] and some shunts have eroded into the intestine, bladder, and vagina, and have even protruded from the anus. Most of these complications were seen with the spring-loaded distal shunt tubing, which is now avoided.

SHUNT INFECTIONS

Despite efforts to avoid infection with preoperative antibiotics and special routines for preparing and draping a patient for a shunt operation, each shunt operation is associated with a 2- to 8-percent rate of postoperative shunt infection.[39, 41, 42] Overall, between 5 and 15 percent of shunts can be expected to become infected over the life of the shunt. Roughly 66 percent of shunt infections are diagnosed within 1 month after surgery, and close to 80 percent manifest by 6 months.[39] Shunt infections can cause signs of meningitis, as well as external signs, such as redness along the path of the shunt. The most common agents are staphylococci, but gram-positive bacilli and enterobacilli can also infect shunts. The methods of treating shunt infections include

1. Antibiotics alone, both intravenous and intrathecal
2. Shunt removal with delayed reinsertion

Table 99-2. COMPLICATIONS OF SHUNTS AND THEIR FREQUENCY IN 380 CHILDREN WITH SHUNTS

Complication	Number/%
Infection	41/11.0*
Seizures	55/14.5
Subdural hematoma	12/3.0
Loculated ventricles	26/7.0
No complications	220/58.0
Slit ventricle syndrome	43/11.5

*Infection rate per shunt operation is 5.0%.

3. Antibiotics, shunt removal, and immediate shunt replacement
4. External ventricular drainage with delayed shunt reinsertion

Because most individuals with shunts are shunt dependent, shunt removal alone often does not allow adequate treatment of the hydrocephalus. The most successful and predictable treatment of a shunt infection is administration of intravenous antibiotics, removal of all shunt hardware, and placement of a temporary ventriculostomy for approximately 1 week. Once the infection is cleared, a new ventriculoperitoneal shunt is placed, either on the same side or at a different site. Antibiotics are continued for an additional several days and then discontinued. If signs of peritonitis or distal shunt failure are present, the shunt may need to be removed emergently. However, an individual with sepsis may be too great an anesthetic risk and may be best treated with antibiotics until vital signs have stabilized.

In cases in which a nonfulminating shunt infection is present without signs of sepsis, an attempt can be made to treat the shunt by leaving it in situ and using intravenous and intrathecal antibiotics alone.[45, 46] However, the families must understand that this treatment may fail in approximately 40 percent of cases. We believe that antibiotics alone are most likely to work when the infection is diagnosed just after a shunt operation has been performed.

In patients with ventriculoatrial shunts, shunt nephritis is a unique complication.[47] This condition presents with proteinuria, hematuria, and progressive decline in kidney function. Shunt nephritis should be considered diagnostic of a shunt infection. Often, the only positive culture results are obtained with culture of the shunt hardware.

REFERENCES

1. Dandy WE: The diagnosis and treatment of hydrocephalus resulting from strictures of the aqueduct of Sylvius. Surg Gynecol Obstet 31:340–358, 1920
2. Becker DP, Nulsen FE: Control of hydrocephalus by valve-regulated venous shunt: Avoidance of complications in prolonged shunt maintenance. Neurosurg 28:215–226, 1968
3. Stookey B, Scarff J: Occlusion of the aqueduct of Sylvius by neoplastic and non-neoplastic processes with a rational surgical treatment for relief of the resultant obstructive hydrocephalus. Bull Neurol Inst N Y 5:348–377, 1936
4. Hoffman HJ, Harwood-Nash D, Gilday DL: Percutaneous third ventriculostomy in the management of noncommunicating hydrocephalus. Neurosurgery 7:313–321, 1980
5. Kelly P: Stereotactic third ventriculostomy in patients with nontumoral adolescent/adult onset aqueductal stenosis and symptomatic hydrocephalus. J Neurosurg 75:865–873, 1991
6. Lawrence KM, Coates S: The natural history of hydrocephalus. Detailed analysis of 182 unoperated cases. Arch Dis Child 37:345–362, 1962
7. Foltz EL, Shurtleff DB: Five year comparative study of hydrocephalus in children with and without operation. Neurosurg 20:1064–1079, 1963
8. Adams RD, Fisher CM, Hakim S, et al: Symptomatic occult hydrocephalus with normal cerebrospinal fluid pressure. N Engl J Med 273:117–126, 1965
9. Hammock MK, Milhorat TH, Baron IS: Normal pressure hydrocephalus in patients with myelomeningocele. Dev Med Child Neurol 18(suppl 37):55–68, 1976
10. Ojemann RG, Fisher CM, Adams MD, et al: Further experience with the syndrome of normal pressure hydrocephalus. J Neurosurg 31:279–294, 1969
11. Foltz EL, Shurtleff DB: Conversion of communicating hydrocephalus to stenosis or occlusion of the aqueduct during ventricular shunt. J Neurosurg 24:520–524, 1966
12. Fraser RAR, Patterson RH: Intracranial hemorrhage in selected premature infants. Childs Nerv Syst 5:574, 1979
13. James HE, Bejar R, Merritt A, et al: Management of hydrocephalus secondary to intracranial hemorrhage in the high-risk newborn. Neurosurgery 14:612–617, 1984
14. McComb JG, Ramos AD, Platzker AC, et al: Management of hydrocephalus secondary to intraventricular hemorrhage in the preterm infant with a subcutaneous ventricular catheter reservoir. Neurosurgery 13:295–300, 1983
15. Symonds CP: Thrombophlebitis of the dural sinuses and cerebral veins. Brain 60:531–533, 1937
16. Fried A, Shapiro K: Subtle deterioration in shunted childhood hydrocephalus: A biomechanical and clinical profile. J Neurosurg 65:211–216, 1986
17. Shapiro K, Fried A: Pressure-volume relationships in shunt-dependent childhood hydrocephalus: The zone of pressure instability in children with acute deterioration. J Neurosurg 64:390–396, 1986
18. Shapiro K, Fried A, Marmarou A: Biomechanical and hydrodynamic characterization of the hydrocephalic infant. J Neurosurg 63:69–75, 1985
19. Shapiro K, Marmarou A, Shulman K: Characterization of clinical CSF dynamics and neural axis compliance using the pressure-volume index. The normal PVI. Am Neurol 7:508–514, 1980
20. Hussey F, Shanzer B, Katzman R: A simple constant infusion manometric test for measurement of CSF absorption: II. Clinical studies. Neurology 20:665–680, 1970
21. Katzman R, Hussey F: A simple constant-infusion manometric test for measurement of CSF absorption. Rationale and method. Neurology 20:534–544, 1970
22. Martin G: Lundberg's B waves as a feature of normal pressure hydrocephalus. Surg Neurol 8:247–249, 1978
23. Symon L, Dorsch NWC: Use of long-term intracranial pressure measurements to assess hydrocephalic patients prior to shunt surgery. J Neurosurg 42:258–273, 1975
24. Cutler RWP, Page L, Galicich J: Formation and absorption of cerebrospinal fluid in man. Brain 91:707–720, 1968
25. Sklar FH, Beyer CW Jr, Diehl JT, et al: Significance of the so-called absorptive reserve in communicating hydrocephalus: A preliminary report. Neurosurgery 8:525–530, 1981
26. Marmarou A, Shulman K, LaMorgese J: Compartmental analysis of compliance and outflow resistance of the cerebrospinal fluid system. J Neurosurg 43:523–534, 1975
27. Marmarou A, Shulman K, Rosende RM: A nonlinear analysis of the cerebrospinal fluid system and intracranial pressure dynamics. J Neurosurg 48:332–344, 1978
28. DiRocco C, DiTrapani G, Maira G, et al: Anatomical-clinical correlations in normotensive hydrocephalus. J Neurol Sci 33:437–452, 1977
29. Huckman MS: Normal pressure hydrocephalus: Evaluation of diagnostic and prognostic tests. Am J Neuroradiol 2:385–395, 1981
30. Salmon JH: Adult hydrocephalus—Evaluation of shunt therapy in 80 patients. J Neurosurg 37:423–428, 1972
31. DiChiro G, Reames PM, Matthews WB: RISA ventriculography and RISA-cisternography. Neurology 14:185–191, 1964
32. Stein SC, Langfitt TW: Normal pressure hydrocephalus. J Neurosurg 41:463–470, 1974
33. Laws ER, Morki B: Occult hydrocephalus: Results of shunting correlated with diagnostic tests. Clin Neurosurg 24:316–333, 1977
34. Black P: Idiopathic normal pressure hydrocephalus. J Neurosurg 52:371–377, 1980
35. Portnoy HD, Tripp L, Croissant PD: Hydrodynamics of shunt values. Childs Nerv Syst 2:242–256, 1976
36. McCullough DC: Symptomatic progressive ventriculomegaly in hydrocephalics with patent shunt and antisiphon devices. Neurosurgery 19:617–621, 1986
37. Portnoy HD, Schutte RR, Fox JL, et al: Antisiphon and reversible occlusion values for shunting in hydrocephalus and preventing post shunt subdural hematomas. J Neurosurg 38:729–737, 1973
38. Samuelson S, Long DM, Chou SN: Subdural hematomas as a complication of shunting procedures for normal pressure hydrocephalus. J Neurosurg 37:548–551, 1972
39. Choux M, Genitori L, Lang D, Lena G: Shunt implantation: Reducing the incidence of shunt infection. J Neurosurg 77:875–880, 1992
40. George R, Leibrock L, Epstein MH: Long-term analysis of cerebrospinal fluid shunt infections. J Neurosurg 51:804, 1979
41. Haines S, Taylor F: Prophylactic methicillin for shunt operations: Effect

on incidence of shunt malfunction and infection. Childs Nerv Syst 9:10–22, 1982
42. Walters BC, Hoffman HJ, Hendrick EB, et al: Cerebrospinal fluid shunt infection: Influences on initial management and subsequent outcome. J Neurosurg 60:1014–1021, 1984
43. McLaurin RL, Glass IH, Kaplan S: Ventriculoatrial shunt for hydrocephalus. Electrocardiographic control for accurate placement. Am J Dis Child 105:216–218, 1963
44. Grosfeld JL, Cooney DR, Smith J, Campbell RL: Intraabdominal complications following ventriculoperitoneal shunt procedures. Pediatrics 54:791–796, 1974
45. Mates S, Glaser J, Shapiro K: Treatment of CSF shunt infections with medical therapy alone. Neurosurgery 11:781–783, 1982
46. McLaurin RL, Frame PT: The role of shunt externalization in the management of shunt infections. Concepts Pediatr Neurosurg 6:133–146, 1985
47. Wald SL, McLaurin RL: Shunt associated glomerulonephritis. Neurosurgery 3:146–150, 1978

CHAPTER 100

Management of Neurosurgical Problems in the Neonate

R. Michael Scott

In planning a neurosurgical procedure for a premature or newborn baby, the neurosurgeon must be concerned not only with technical considerations related to the child's size but also with alterations in the routine neurosurgical protocol that must be made to protect the baby's fragile homeostatic mechanisms.

Hypothermia, because of its grave metabolic consequences in this age group, is an immediate risk when the child enters the operating room. Most neurosurgical cases require a relatively long period of preparation, and during this time, significant heat can be lost by the baby into the environment, particularly if the operative field involves a large surface area. To prevent this problem, the child must be transported to the operating room in an incubator, and the operating room temperature should be elevated before the child arrives. The baby must be kept covered during induction of anesthesia, and a temperature probe should be placed promptly. A heating blanket should be available on the operating table. An overhead radiant heating device is helpful during the time the intravenous lines are being placed and the child is being anesthetized, because a warm, vasodilated child makes placement of intravenous lines easier and observation of the child's entire body during induction is facilitated. Other aids in maintaining thermal regulation are the use of warmed humidified anesthetic gases and warmed blood, intravenous fluids, and irrigation and skin preparation solutions. Antiseptic solutions that evaporate rapidly and result in skin cooling such as alcohol should be avoided.

Although one expects minimal blood loss in most of the common neurosurgical procedures in the neonate, there are enough exceptions in even the most routine procedures that a good venous access route must be available to the anesthesiologist. One of the most frustrating preoperative delays in pediatric neurosurgery occurs when it is difficult to establish an intravenous line, and it is a good policy to limit this process to a time limit agreed on with the anesthesia team. Usable venipuncture sites in this age group include scalp veins (visualized with the aid of a circumferential rubber band tourniquet), an external jugular vein, and an almost constant but frequently invisible vein on the dorsum of the hand running parallel with the ring finger. Mild Trendelenburg positioning with fingertip pressure over the clavicle is a help in cannulating the external jugular vein. It is extremely rare for an experienced pediatric anesthesia team to be unable to place a percutaneous intravenous line, but if it cannot be placed rapidly, it is probably wise to proceed directly to a surgical exposure and cannulation of the greater saphenous or similar vein, rather than delay surgery longer.

As the child is positioned, care must be taken that all pressure points are completely padded and that the limbs are not so tightly restrained that traction is placed on the brachial plexus. This caveat applies particularly to a neonate being prepared for shunt surgery in whom the head is typically turned fully to the side for an occipital burr hole and the neck extended over a roll to aid in passing the shunt subcutaneously (Fig. 100–1). Pulling the arm firmly down and to the side and anchoring it can lead to traction palsies if care is not taken to avoid undue force. Pressure points can be protected with adhesive-backed foam cut to an appropriate size and fixed to the area of concern. In the neonate undergoing a posterior fossa procedure in the prone position, the foam can be placed over the entire face, with apertures cut for the esophageal stethoscope and endotracheal tube (Fig. 100–2).

INTRAOPERATIVE CONSIDERATIONS

Craniotomy techniques are modified when they are applied to the neonate. The skin is infiltrated with saline or a dilute solution of epinephrine (1:200,00) to aid in hemostasis when the skin flap is turned. In some children with relatively thick skin, the spring-loaded Children's Hospital (Cologne clips) or Raney clips can be used on the skin edges for hemostasis, but usually the limited bleeding that is encountered in younger children can be managed with bipolar cautery rather than skin clips. The Shaw scalpel, which uses a heated blade to effect hemostasis, dramatically reduces blood loss from the incision and eliminates the need for skin clips of any type, although some care must taken when the incision is made in order not to burn skin edges. The author has also used needle monopolar cautery after the superficial scalpel incision in order to limit blood loss. The flat blade of the monopolar cautery is used to incise the pericranium when necessary, but care must be taken not to penetrate the thin skull with the cautery tip. Venous bleeding from the bone can be extensive in the neonate, and meticulous hemostasis should be maintained with bone wax and the flat blade of the cautery. The skin flap is secured with a 3-0 suture placed through the base of the flap, which is, in turn, secured with a hemostat to the drapes. The bone flap can be elevated, often without burr holes, by curetting near the fontanelle or a

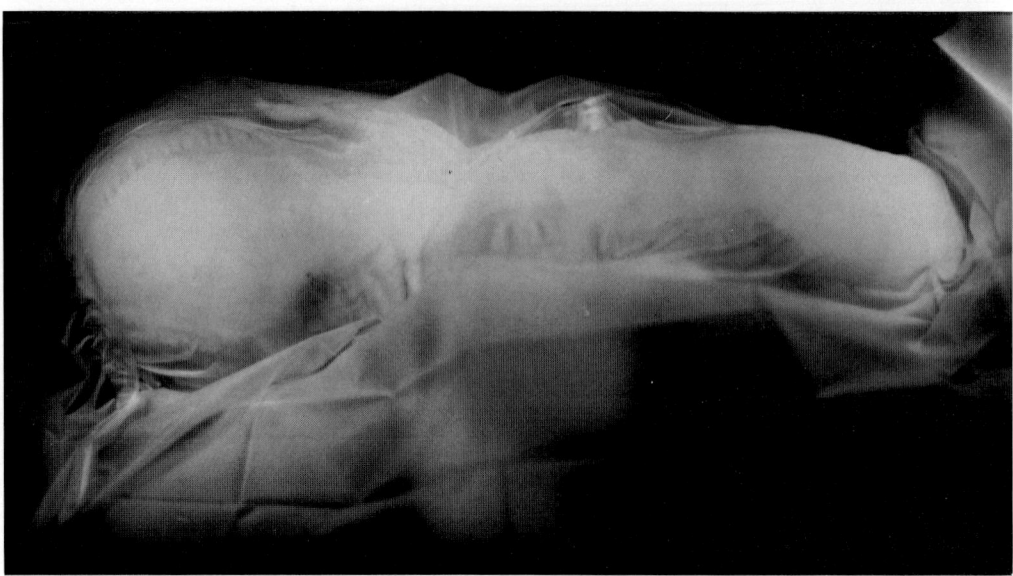

FIGURE 100–1. Positioning of a baby for a ventriculoperitoneal shunt using a right parieto-occipital burr hole. The head is turned fully to the left, a roll is placed under the shoulder to elevate the chest and extend the neck, and the entire field is draped with plastic drapes before skin preparation. The author uses a burr hole made just anterior to the lambdoid suture, medial to a point midway between the ear and the sagittal suture. The catheter is directed toward the midline of the forehead several centimeters above the glabella, placing the catheter along the long axis of the ventricle and much of its length within CSF. A more lateral burr hole will tend to migrate laterally on the skull as the child grows, making re-entry into small ventricles difficult if revision is subsequently necessary.

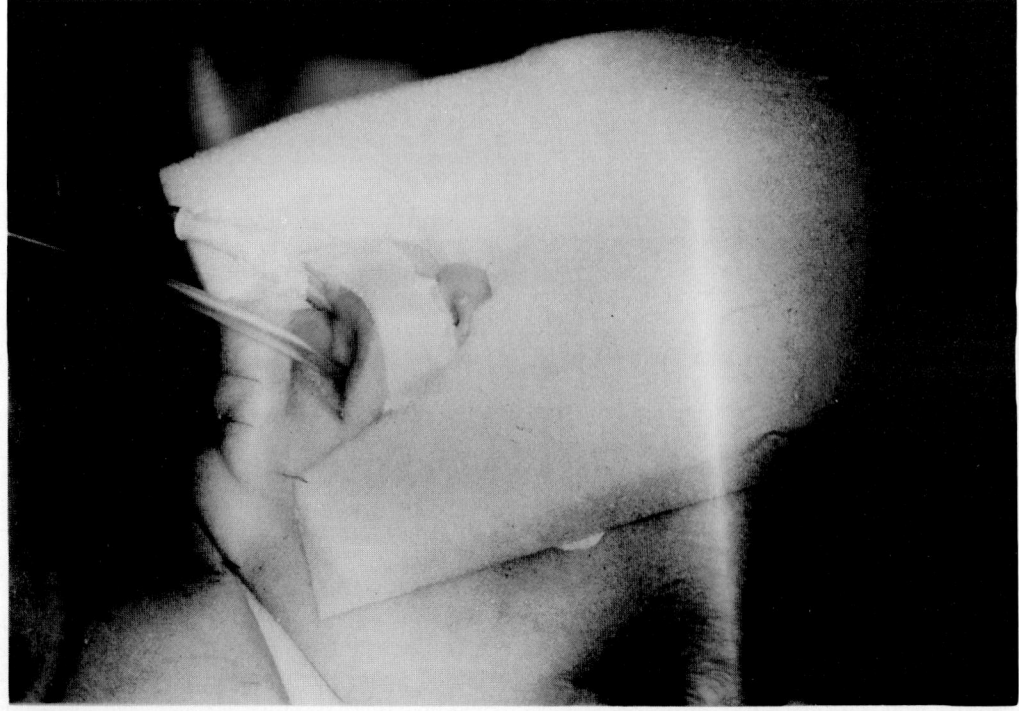

FIGURE 100–2. A baby prepared for prone positioning on the horseshoe headrest. An esophageal stethoscope is in place, the baby's eyes taped closed, and the entire face covered with adhesive-backed foam.

suture, identifying the epidural plane, and using a heavy scissors to cut a free flap. If necessary, a burr hole can be drilled in the pliable skull by rotating a perforator bit alone between the fingers while exerting gentle pressure. Care must be taken to replace blood as it is lost, particularly in operations in the posterior fossa, where the midline dura and dura at the craniospinal junction may contain large venous channels that can cause copious and rapid bleeding if opened inadvertently. Consideration of the child's limited blood volume must remain of foremost importance throughout every pediatric neurosurgical case. If bleeding is extensive, the surgeon should stop to allow the anesthesiologist to catch up on the blood replacement. If possible, the skin draping should allow for drainage of all wound effluent into a measurable container. Sponges should be weighed and irrigation and suction fluids carefully measured by the operating room nursing team to aid the anesthesiologist in the accurate assessment of blood loss.

At the close of the procedure, the bone flap can be secured with 3-0 absorbable or nonabsorbable suture material. A baby's skull is sufficiently thin that it may not be necessary to drill holes to secure the flap; the suture needle itself can be passed directly through the bone for this purpose.

Closure of the skin incision in the neonate can often be accomplished in two layers, if desired. At present, the author uses undyed 3-0 or 4-0 Dexon or Vicryl (polyglycolic acid suture) for the galea, because black silk or braided nylon or other synthetic sutures are often visible through the thin skin of the neonate and can spontaneously extrude from the wound weeks after closure. Certain pediatric neurosurgeons routinely use single-layered closures for their neonatal patients, and we also have noted no problems with wound healing with this technique.

The application of the dressing represents a final challenge to the healing process in neonates, because snug head wraps, which would be acceptable in a larger child, can cause skin and ear necrosis in a neonate. Dressings must be carefully applied, and pressure on the forehead and ears frequently checked, both during application of the dressing and subsequently.

HYDROCEPHALUS IN THE NEONATE

The ventricular shunt procedure is one of the most frequent neurosurgical operations performed on neonates. The major surgical hazards of this operation in this population are related to poor wound healing and cerebrospinal fluid (CSF) leak through skin that has been distended by a relatively bulky shunt apparatus. In a premature child with hydrocephalus requiring a shunt, the apparatus should have the lowest possible profile and minimum size. All incisions should be designed so that the tubing does not cross or run directly beneath them. Because the premature infant with hydrocephalus may be relatively immobile because of the use of a ventilator or other medical concerns, frontal burr hole catheter placement is usually preferable to an occipital site in order to avoid pressure necrosis over the shunt catheter simply due to the baby's recumbent position. In small premature babies with extremely thin and delicate skin, the valve and reservoir may need to be omitted, or a low-pressure distal slit valve used. In a valveless system, the intracranial pressure can be adjusted by raising and lowering the child's head relative to the abdomen, depending on the fontanelle tension. When the child is older, the shunt can be revised to include a valve and reservoir. A single layer of running locked 5-0 nylon is the usual closure technique for the scalp incisions in these children. The closure must be especially meticulous in these patients, because CSF can easily leak through any defects in the suture line.

INTRAVENTRICULAR HEMORRHAGE IN THE PREMATURE INFANT

In premature infants with intraventricular hemorrhage, the major neurosurgical problem is the management of increased intracranial pressure and progressive hydrocephalus in a child who is a significant anesthetic risk. Moreover, even if it is easily performed, standard ventricular shunting in this setting has a high likelihood of malfunction because of blood clots and debris in the ventricular CSF. In these babies, we prefer to deal with the increased pressure nonoperatively, including daily lumbar punctures and the use of medications such as acetazolamide (Diamox) to reduce CSF production. An ultrasound study after lumbar puncture that demonstrates reduction in ventricular size suggests that the hydrocephalus is of a communicating type and that further lumbar punctures will be helpful. If these techniques are not successful, the ventricles can be decompressed by placement (with the patient under local anesthesia) of a ventricular catheter with an attached subcutaneous reservoir. Percutaneous aspiration of the ventricular catheter reservoir using a small-gauge needle can then be carried out at the bedside to control intracranial pressure and remove CSF. Attempts can be made to reduce the frequency of the aspiration with the hope of promoting the re-establishment of the child's own CSF absorptive mechanisms. External ventricular drainage can also be instituted in this situation, although the risks of infection and subsequent ventriculitis are higher in these premature babies than in older children who are similarly treated, perhaps because of the extensive instrumentation and manipulation required as part of their daily care in the neonatal intensive care unit. A simple technique for the placement of external ventricular drainage in these babies is puncture of the skin and dura over the frontal or occipital bone with a 19-gauge needle-catheter assembly, threading the catheter into the ventricle, and connecting the opposite end to a standard external drainage system. Before the skin is punctured, the skin over the needle entry site is displaced laterally and the skin is entered at a slight angle so that leaking of CSF through the needle puncture site will be minimized when the needle is withdrawn. The catheter should be fixed to the skin of the child with a suture and covered by an occlusive-type dressing, which should be changed as needed with meticulous technique by the neurosurgical staff. When these drains are eventually removed, it is often necessary to place a 5-0 nylon suture at the puncture site to stop a transient CSF leak. Frequent ultrasound scans should be carried out during all phases of treatment to assess ventricular size. Although the author is aware that in some units, the pediatric specialist carries out the placement of such external drainage catheters, he firmly believes that the placement and management of such a drainage apparatus should be carried out under the

HYDROCEPHALUS AND MYELOMENINGOCELE

Once the decision to operate on a newborn with a myelomeningocele has been made, an important early surgical decision that needs to be made is how to manage the associated hydrocephalus. If the baby has been born with a large head and full fontanelle, and if computed tomography (CT) scanning or ultrasound has confirmed the presence of significant ventriculomegaly, uncomplicated healing of the myelomeningocele dural closure will be facilitated by immediate CSF diversion. The author had previously used closed ventricular drainage in this situation, maintaining this system until back healing had progressed to the point at which it was believed to be safe to proceed with ventriculoperitoneal shunting. We now carry out shunting simultaneously with myelomeningocele repair because it corrects the hydrocephalus, eliminates additional administration of anesthesia, and shortens the patient's hospital stay. Also, it has not resulted in an increased rate of morbidity or infection. If significant hydrocephalus is present at birth, we place a shunt after repair of the myelomeningocele if the repair has proceeded uneventfully, dural closure is secure, and the subarachnoid space is uncontaminated. Because the infant remains prone for several days after repair in this situation, the shunt is usually placed through an occipital burr hole.

NEONATAL TRAUMA

Most neonatal head trauma is related to either birth trauma or child abuse, and very little operative intervention has been necessary since CT and ultrasound scanning of neonates have come into regular use. Acute epidural and subdural hematomas are rare and are dealt with by craniotomy or craniectomy, as in older children. Epidural hematomas are often focal, being sharply delimited by the dural attachments at the cranial sutures. The posterior fossa is a common site of neonatal intracranial hematoma, characteristically involving the subdural space both above and below the tentorium. In neonates, the tentorium and dura of the posterior fossa are laced with large venous sinuses; lateral shear stress across the tentorium during delivery may rupture some of these sinuses or tear bridging veins from the cerebellum, leading to hematomas within the tentorium that can rupture through it and bleed into adjacent structures, causing subdural or cerebellar hematomas. It is difficult to be certain of the best neurosurgical treatment for these lesions, because when they are recognized, the child may be in extremis and die regardless of therapy. With more frequent use of CT and ultrasound scanning of neonates, these lesions are being seen in neurologically stable children with greater frequency. If the mass effect from the hematoma is negligible and the child is neurologically stable or improving, the clot is best left alone. Bleeding from the tentorium is difficult to control, and venous sinuses may be very large. Also, if there is no appreciable mass effect, careful observation with follow-up scanning is probably the safest method of treatment. If surgery is necessary, the child should be operated on in the prone position with the head flexed to provide good visualization of the tentorium. Thorough preparation should be made for clip ligation of the venous sinuses, and blood should be made available for immediate replacement as surgery is carried out.

VEIN OF GALEN MALFORMATIONS

Vein of Galen malformations are detected when an intracranial bruit is heard in a newborn with intractable heart failure. Very rarely, subarachnoid hemorrhage or hydrocephalus secondary to mass effect and aqueduct occlusion is the initial symptom.[1] Surgical management of children in heart failure is extremely difficult and is directed toward correcting the cardiac failure by decreasing the blood flow through the lesion. In neonates, the arterial feeders to the vein of Galen are usually numerous and originate at least partly from the medial and posterior choroidal arteries and the anterior and posterior cerebral arteries. Careful, complete selective preoperative cerebral angiography is essential and must be performed at a facility with specific expertise in pediatric neuroradiology, as well as the capability to use interventional techniques to eliminate as many feeding vessels as possible.

The surgical positioning and approach used depend on the number and location of the arterial feeders. A bilateral exposure is commonly required in neonates, and this approach is best carried out with the child in a supine, semi-sitting position, using a transcallosal approach to the area of the fistulae. Deliberate hypotension should be avoided because any hypoperfusion of coronary circulation that is already compromised may lead to irreversible myocardial ischemia. Those centers in which intraoperative cardiac arrest with hypothermia is used as a surgical adjunct in neonates with these lesions have almost always reported dismal results, and, at present, the use of interventional techniques to ameliorate the signs and symptoms of cardiac failure seems to be the most promising therapy for vein of Galen malformation in the neonate. Although the mortality rate approaches 80 percent in this group of unfortunate children, the occasional spectacular result indicates that these techniques merit further refinement and utilization.

OCCIPITAL ENCEPHALOCELE

The variable size and complexity of occipital encephaloceles make generalizations regarding their surgical repair difficult. The initial question inevitably posed to the neurosurgeon is whether or not this often grotesque lesion should be repaired at all. This decision depends on the extent of other congenital anomalies, the relative size of the encephalocele versus that of the remaining normal cranium, and the configuration of the so-called normal cranium. Over the past decades, studies such as air ventriculography and arteriography have been used to elucidate how much of the normal brain has been involved in the encephalocele; certainly, the most graphic test currently in use is magnetic resonance imaging (MRI), which enables the cerebral deformity to be assessed and other associated brain anomalies to be clearly identified. Vascular anatomy of the lesion can often be determined from the MRI or MR angiographic protocols, making formal arteriography unnecessary. Virtually all children with large encephaloceles are retarded to varying degrees, and a large percentage develop hydrocephalus that requires treatment during the first several months of life—facts that must also be taken into consideration before initiating treatment.

Our policy is to repair the majority of these lesions unless the associated brain and somatic anomalies are severe or the lesion is so large that its repair would involve sacrifice of a major portion of cerebral tissue. An issue that may lend urgency to making the decision to operate is related to the quality of epithelialization of the sac and whether or not there is a CSF leak. If the skin over the distal sac is thin or eroded or if a CSF leak is present, repair must be carried out within the first 24 hours of life in order to avoid meningitis. Because ventricular shunting is so often required subsequently, avoiding meningitis at this stage of the child's treatment is of utmost importance.

Repair is almost always carried out with the child in the prone position, using the precautions in positioning outlined previously (Fig. 100–3). Occasionally, a small lesion can be operated on with the child in the lateral position and the surgeon seated behind the patient. Because this position is often preferred by the anesthesiologist because it allows easy access to the airway, we make every effort to use it if the size of the lesion permits. As with an adult patient in the lateral position, a baby's brachial plexus must not be stretched by excessive downward traction on the uppermost shoulder, and the axillary nerve should be protected by placing a large roll in the axilla to prevent excessive pressure from being placed on the lateral aspect of the humerus. The child's head can be elevated 10 to 15 degrees, but not so high that an air embolus might occur. In these midline lesions, the potential for rapid bleeding from large venous sinuses always exists, and the patient's blood must be cross-matched and replacement blood be made available before surgery begins. It is frequently observed, however, that the anticipated bleeding from the midline venous sinuses rarely occurs, perhaps due to their distortion by the encephalocele or their frequent passage beneath the tentorium and confluens of sinuses instead of above or through them.

A vertical elliptic incision around the base of the lesion is outlined high enough on the sac to provide enough residual scalp for easy closure without tension. It is carried cephalad and caudal to the lesion to provide room for additional supratentorial or infratentorial exposure, should it be necessary, and to identify normal tissue planes. The bony and pericranial defect at the uppermost portion of the encephalocele is identified initially, the plane between the dural sac and the underlying skull and pericranium bluntly dissected, and the skin and dura sharply incised high on the sac around its circumference. If the lesion is small, it may be possible to preserve the arachnoid membrane surrounding the herniated brain and to reduce the entire contents of the sac into the cranial cavity. CSF cultures should be taken during the repair, particularly if there has been CSF leak prior to surgery. If the brain hernia cannot be reduced or if it is too large for this maneuver to be considered, the arachnoid is opened and the extracalvarial tissue amputated using suction and bipolar cautery. If venous and arterial channels are encountered in this gliotic tissue, every attempt should be made to preserve them, although it is often difficult to do so. When hemostasis has been obtained, the dura is trimmed and closed in a watertight fashion with a running suture of 4-0 braided monofilament nylon, silk, or Vicryl. A Valsalva maneuver is performed to check for leaks in the dural closure, and pericranium flaps can be fashioned and closed over the dura if desired. The scalp is sutured in two layers, if possible, with Vicryl in the galea and nylon in the skin. No attempt is made to repair the bony defect at this time, because it often becomes less significant in size as the child grows. A head-wrap dressing is applied and changed daily to check for the presence of subcutaneous accumulation of CSF or CSF leaks through the incision, the presence of either of which may indicate developing hydrocephalus. The child's head circumference should be monitored daily and a follow-up ultrasound, CT, or MRI scan obtained before the child's discharge from the hospital to serve as a baseline for further observation.

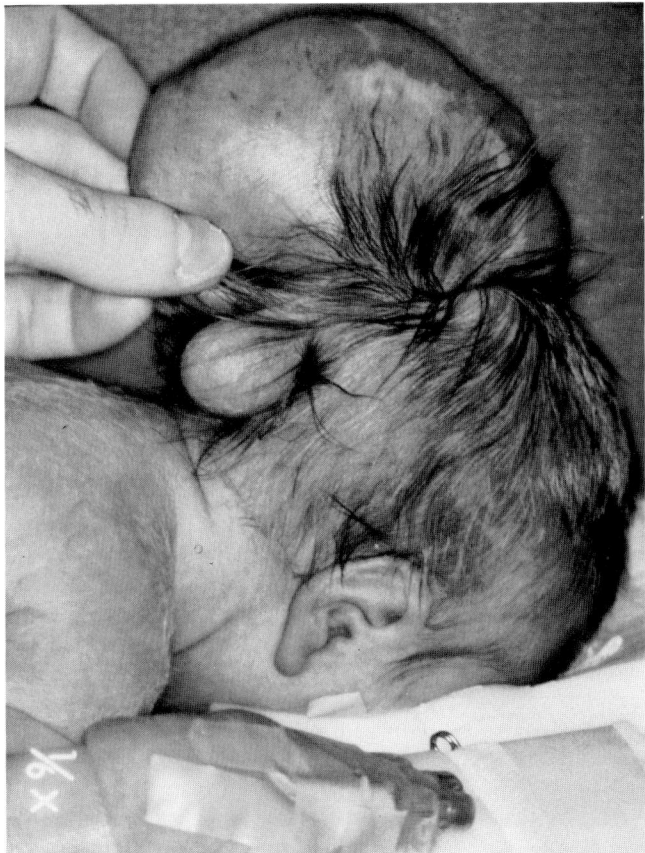

FIGURE 100–3. A baby with an occipital encephalocele in the prone position for surgery. Note padding of the face with adhesive foam. It is difficult to shave the area around the encephalocele without injuring the delicate skin on its base and sides, and this hair need only be trimmed with a clipper or scissors before the preparation begins. An assistant may need to support a pedunculated lesion during the skin preparation with sponges or with a suture or towel clip placed through redundant tissue.

FRONTONASAL ENCEPHALOCELE

Frontonasal encephaloceles should be treated as early as possible considering the child's general medical condition. Children with basal frontal encephaloceles in the pharynx or nares are at risk of developing meningitis because of direct inoculation of the meninges with nasal flora. The mass of the encephalocele can be large enough to obstruct the airway, and attempts to pass airways or endotracheal tubes through the nares or pharynx may rupture the encephaloceles, resulting in potentially dire consequences. Prophylactic tracheostomy should be considered in such situations. In certain patients, it may be extremely difficult to be certain whether the pharyngeal or nasal masses are encephaloceles, because tomograms and CT scans of this area of children are often difficult to interpret. The most helpful preoperative test is probably an MRI study in the coronal and sagittal planes, although a CT scan with and without enhancement by intrathecal metrizamide clarifies more effectively the bony anatomy and its relationship to the encephalocele.

Sincipital encephaloceles at the root of the nose or projecting into the orbit are less of an emergency in a neonate, and surgical correction can be postponed for several weeks until the anesthetic risks are somewhat reduced. The earlier these lesions are repaired, however, the less influence the lesion will have on subsequent orbital and nasal disfigurement, and repair should not be unduly delayed. A craniofacial team approach, including plastic, otolaryngologic, and ophthalmologic surgeons, represents optimal management of this problem in the majority of these patients, but the fragility of the cranial and nasal bones in the neonate limits the amount of reconstruction possible at this stage.

The surgical approach to both the basal and sincipital lesions is similar. A bicoronal skin incision is used, and the scalp is reflected forward; bilateral frontal craniotomies are performed, and the dura is opened across the supraorbital margin bilaterally. The anterior sagittal sinus is ligated with 2-0 suture material, and intradural exploration is carried out. Care must be taken to identify and preserve an intact olfactory tract and bulb, if they can be visualized, when the frontal lobes are elevated. Brain herniation through the bony defects is usually readily identified, and the brain hernia is amputated, hemostasis is secured, and a dural flap or pericranial graft is sutured in place over the bone defect. A cranial bone graft can be placed over the bone defect as well, and the repair site is buttressed with fibrin glue to help hold it in place and minimize the risk of CSF leak. It is advisable to use care in attempting aspirate or remove the tissue that has herniated into the nasal cavity to avoid inadvertent rupture of the encephalocele and the contamination of the intracranial contents with nasal flora.

DANDY-WALKER MALFORMATION

The Dandy-Walker malformation is one of the more common causes of hydrocephalus that is apparent in the first several weeks of life. In neonates, the resultant hydrocephalus is clinically similar to hydrocephalus resulting from other causes; the major surgical consideration in these patients is in the choice of the appropriate method for treating the hydrocephalus.

The CT and MRI diagnosis is based on a finding of lateral ventricular dilatation and a large posterior fossa containing a small anterior and superiorly displaced cerebellum with an open fourth ventricle extending into a large retrocerebellar CSF collection. The vermis should be absent on sagittal MRI. Supratentorial anomalies, such as agenesis of the corpus callosum, may also be seen. Differentiation between a retrocerebellar arachnoid cyst and the Dandy-Walker malformation occasionally can be difficult, but the visualization of a covered fourth ventricle that is normal in size and position relative to the cerebellar hemispheres rules out Dandy-Walker malformation.

Regardless of the precise anatomic configuration, the surgical approach to be used in these children is best determined by the anatomic configuration revealed by MRI. Direct surgical removal of the cyst has been advocated in the past, but the majority of these patients will eventually require shunting despite cyst surgery, because wide fenestration of the cyst or removal of its walls fails to alleviate the malabsorption of CSF over the cerebral hemispheres that is part of this syndrome.[2]

The most important finding on MRI study is aqueduct patency. If the aqueduct is occluded and the posterior fossa cyst appears to be isolated from the lateral ventricular system, shunting of both the cyst and the lateral ventricles is required. The author believes that both compartments need to be drained via a single valve so that the pressure is maintained similarly both above and below the tentorium; this goal is accomplished by placing a catheter in both the lateral ventricle and the cyst, and connecting them with a T connector above a single valve and distal peritoneal catheter. If the aqueduct is patent, however, a shunt placed directly into the cyst in the posterior fossa via a lateral suboccipital burr hole has been the treatment of choice for the author; the capacious area of the cyst, which is relatively free of choroid plexus, seems to lead to longer shunt patency. Children with Dandy-Walker malformation tend to tolerate shunt malfunction poorly, and questionable shunt function, therefore, should be evaluated promptly and the MRI study repeated if there is a question regarding communication between the cyst and the lateral ventricles. Occasionally, ventriculographic study through the shunt using water-soluble contrast agents may be necessary to help sort out these issues if the MRI is not diagnostic.

CHIARI II MALFORMATION

The treatment of symptomatic Chiari II malformation in a neonate with a myelomeningocele remains highly controversial. There is general agreement regarding symptomatology.[3] These babies, having undergone repair of their myelomeningocele and often with a shunt in place, develop laryngeal stridor, difficulty in feeding, and occasionally opisthotonos or limb spasticity. Laryngoscopy reveals vocal cord weakness or paralysis. Brainstem auditory-evoked potential recordings are often abnormal or show sequential deterioration. MRI vividly depicts the typical cramped posterior fossa, with small, vertically-oriented tentorium, caudal displacement of the fourth ventricle and brainstem, downward prolongation of cerebellar vermian tissue, and medullary kinking. Ultrasound study of the foramen magnum can demonstrate impaction of cerebellar tissue and possibly cystic enlargement of the fourth ventricle or hydromyelia.

In a child with symptomatic Chiari malformation, ventricular shunt function must be assessed by any appropriate method because the symptoms of the Chiari II malformation

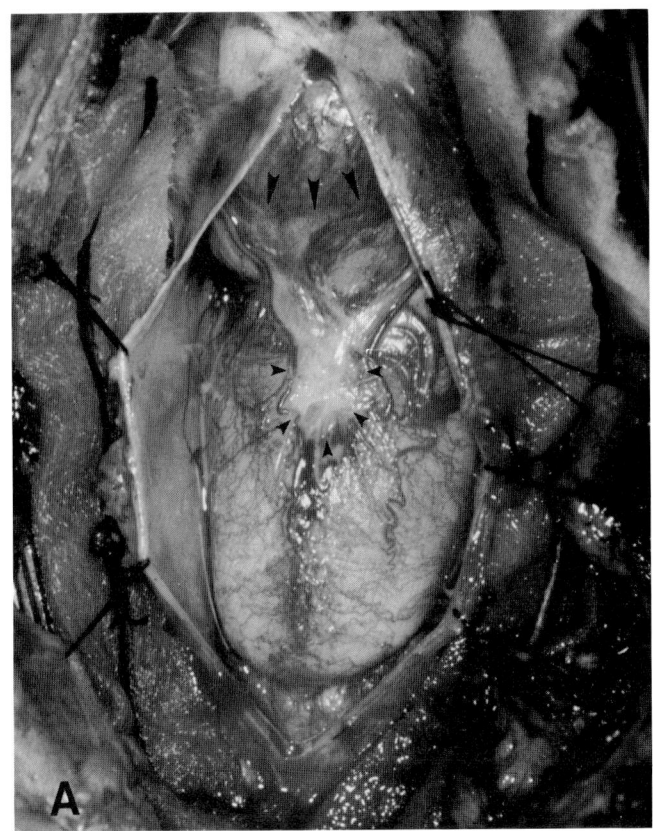
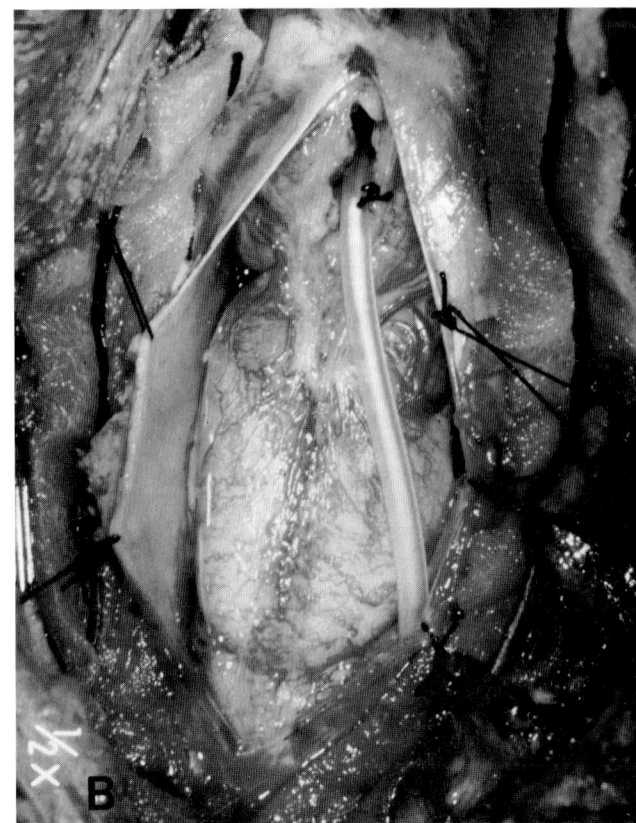
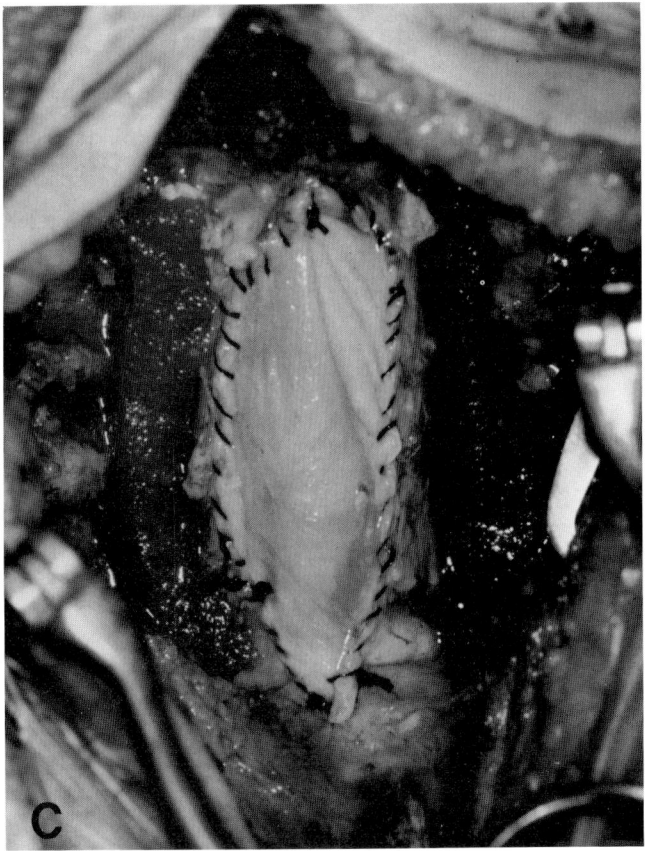

FIGURE 100–4. (A) Appearance of a Chiari II malformation after cervical laminectomy and opening of the dura. The midline cerebellar peg is relatively short in this patient, extending to C1 only. The downwardly displaced medulla is swollen and cystic from syringobulbia. The edge of the medullary kink is noted at the inferior portion of the exposure. The impression made on the herniated cerebellar tissue by the fibrous ligaments and thickened dura at the cervicomedullary junction is easily visible (large arrowheads), as is the scarred and occluded foramen of Magendie (small arrowheads). (B) A midline opening has been made in the pia of the vermis peg, and under magnification, dissection is carried through dysgenetic cerebellum into the fourth ventricle. Care must be taken that this opening is made through the cerebellum above the foramen of Magendie and not through the caudal medulla or spinal cord. If scarring is not too dense, the actual occluded foramen can be visualized by noting a tuft of externalized choroid plexus, which frequently marks its location. A Silastic catheter is placed into the fourth ventricle, threaded cephalad toward the aqueduct, led out into the cervical subarachnoid space inferiorly, and secured with a 6-0 suture through its wall into the coagulated pia of the cerebellum. The obex was not visualized in this patient. (C) A graft of lyophilized dura has been sewn into the opening in the dura.

can be exacerbated or mimicked by hydrocephalus that is not adequately treated. The MRI must be carefully reviewed to determine whether or not compression at the foramen magnum can indeed be implicated in the development of the Chiari symptoms, because in certain children with myelomeningocele, the deranged anatomy and severe caudal displacement of the brainstem itself may be the major cause of the child's presentation; no amount of decompression of the foramen magnum and cervical canal will ameliorate this anatomic change, and surgery will be futile. If shunt malfunction has been ruled out and compression has been demonstrated on the MRI study, surgery for the Chiari malformation itself is performed with the baby in the prone position. It is usually not necessary to remove any substantial amount of the suboccipital bone at the time of surgery, and in fact, the very short distance between the foramen magnum and the low torcular makes this bony removal occasionally hazardous. Cervical laminectomy is carried out to a level required to decompress the swollen herniated cerebellar tissue and brainstem based on the preoperative radiographic studies. The dura must be opened to decompress the brainstem and spinal cord because compression of the brainstem is also caused by a thickened dura and ligaments at the junction of the posterior fossa and cervical dura (Fig. 100–4A).

This portion of the surgery can also be hazardous because venous channels within the dura will bleed copiously and rapidly if opened. Prior to opening the dura, the surgeon should ascertain that the scrub nurse has clips of appropriate size in readiness, and the anesthesiologist should be informed of the possibility that large venous sinuses might be encountered. If they are inadvertently opened, these venous channels can be clipped or oversewn with nonabsorbable suture. In addition to the bony and dural decompression, it is important to attempt to re-establish normal CSF circulation in this area by opening the occluded foramen of Magendie. This structure can usually be identified at the base of the dysmorphic midline cerebellar peg (Fig. 100–4A), where tufts of choroid plexus and areas of increased vascularity can also be frequently seen. If the region of the foramen cannot be identified with certainty, a midline opening is made in the lower portion of the herniated cerebellar tissue directed slightly cephalad under the microscope. The elongated, low-lying fourth ventricle can then be entered; preoperative MRI studies or intraoperative ultrasound are helpful guides during this maneuver. Because hydromyelia can be a prominent part of the clinical syndrome, the obex should be identified, if possible, and the opening of the central canal occluded with a plug of muscle tissue. To keep the foramen of Magendie open and to permit circulation of CSF outside the ventricular system rather than down into the central canal, we place a Silastic catheter into the fourth ventricle, threading it cephalad into the ventricle, and placing the distal end in the dorsal cervical subarachnoid space. The catheter is anchored by placing a 6-0 suture through its walls into cauterized pia on the cerebellar peg adjacent to the opened foramen. A dural graft of lyophilized dura is then placed to maintain wide decompression of the area (Fig. 100–4B and C).

Postoperatively, these babies need continued monitoring in the intensive care unit. Their respiratory and feeding status remains fragile, and tracheostomy may still be necessary despite successful surgery. The long-term results of this surgical procedure in neonates remain controversial, with some reports indicating excellent results and others noting dismal outcome. It is the author's opinion that the operation is rarely required, and that when it is contemplated, it must be rigorously supported by evidence of compression on MRI.

REFERENCES

1. Hoffman HJ, Chuang S, Hendrick EB, et al: Aneurysms of the vein of Galen. Concepts in Pediatric Neurosurgery 3:52, 1983
2. Sawaya R, McLaurin RL: Dandy-Walker syndrome. Clinical analysis of 23 cases. J Neurosurg 55:89, 1981
3. Venes JL, Black KL, Latack JT: Preoperative evaluation and surgical management of the Arnold-Chiari II malformation. J Neurosurg 64:363, 1986

SECTION XV

Epilepsy

CHAPTER 101

Diagnostic Operative Techniques in the Treatment of Epilepsy: Grids and Strip Electrodes

Allen R. Wyler

Strip and grid electrodes are implantable intracranial devices used for recording bioelectrical central nervous system activity as well as for electrically stimulating underlying cortex to determine cortical function. Grid and strip electrodes differ only in shape: a strip is a single linear array of 2 to 16 electrode contacts (Fig. 101–1), whereas a grid has parallel rows of electrode contacts (Fig. 101–2). Both grid and strip electrodes can be constructed by a suitably trained laboratory technician[1] or are commercially available either as standard arrays or custom arrays designed for specific needs. They are made from biologically inert materials and can be compatible with computed tomography (CT) and magnetic resonance imaging (MRI).

The indications and implantation techniques for strip electrodes and grids are quite different, and therefore each one is discussed separately in this chapter.

STRIP ELECTRODES

INDICATIONS

The indication for placement of subdural strip electrodes is the same as those for depth electrodes: to explore and confirm the site of seizure onset by recording seizure activity directly from the brain's surface. Exploration is performed when a patient is assumed to have focal epilepsy and the location of the seizure focus is unknown. A common example is a patient who, on long-term electroencephalographic (EEG) or video monitoring, is found to have complex partial seizures, but in whom localization of the site of seizure onset cannot be determined. Because patients with complex partial seizures are assumed to have focal epilepsy, and because in most nonlesional cases the seizures originate from either the temporal or frontal lobes, strip electrodes are implanted in a standard exploratory montage to allow sampling of electrical data from both lobes bilaterally.

Confirmatory recordings are indicated in cases in which confounding discrepancies exist among localizing data accumulated during the presurgical evaluation. Typically, a patient has a potentially epileptogenic structural lesion in one region of cortex, but the extracranial EEG monitoring suggests seizures arising elsewhere. In such an individual, strip electrodes are implanted so that ictal monitoring can confirm whether or not the epileptogenic focus is truly associated with the lesion. In my experience, in a patient in whom the epileptogenic focus is strongly suspected to be within one cerebral hemisphere, the anatomic or clinical data frequently do not localize it to either the frontal or the temporal lobe.

OPERATIVE TECHNIQUE

Although strip electrodes can be inserted epidurally,[2] I do not endorse this practice for most patients because the epidural space in the temporal fossa does not allow the electrode to be advanced far enough medially to record from the parahippocampal gyrus. Also, frontal electrodes cannot be placed along the interhemispheric cortex of the frontal lobe. These locations often should be sampled in the course of an exploratory investigation. Epidural placement of strips may be indicated if one needs to record from a patient who has had prior intracranial surgery and the subdural space is too

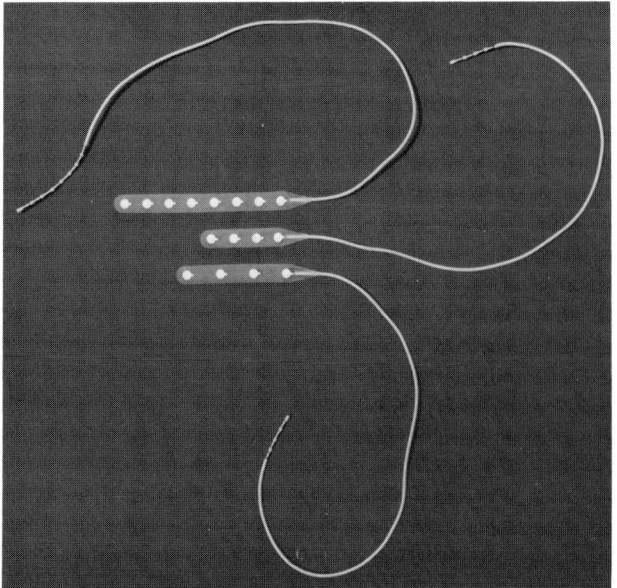

FIGURE 101–1. Examples of three strip electrodes of varying length: one 8-contact 9.5-cm, one 4-contact 6-cm, and one 4-contact 5-cm strip. (Courtesy of Ad-Tech, Inc.)

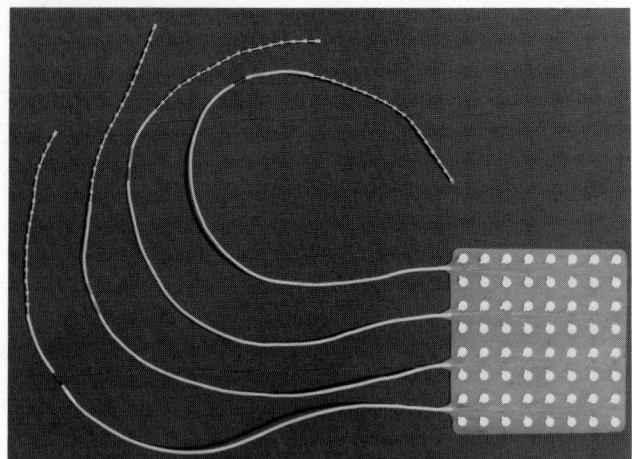

FIGURE 101–2. Example of a 64-contact (8 × 8) grid electrode array with 1-cm interelectrode separation.

scarred to allow passage of the electrodes without risk of damage to the cortex.

Strip electrodes are surgically implanted with the patient under general anesthesia. A small skin incision (no larger than is necessary for making a cranial burr hole) is made at the desired location, and a standard-sized burr hole is drilled through the skull. Dural bleeding is controlled with a bipolar coagulator, and the dura is then opened with a cruciate incision. Foreign bodies, such as bone wax or absorbable gelatin sponge (Gelfoam) are not used, because they theoretically increase the chances of infection. Although some surgeons[3] use mannitol, hyperventilation, or both, to shrink the brain, I have found these practices unnecessary.

During the surgical procedure, the electrodes are kept covered until each is needed for insertion. The electrode is then rinsed in irrigation solution before insertion. A No. 3 Penfield dissector is used to depress the cortex and guide the electrode into the subdural space and its proper trajectory. The dura is not closed. The electrode wires are tunneled with a large-bore needle to exit the skin several centimeters from the burr hole incision. Initially, electrodes were fabricated in our own laboratory and had an individual wire for each electrode contact. Since then, electrodes produced by Ad-Tech Corporation (Racine, WI) have all wires incorporated into a monostrand cable (Fig. 101–1). This design simplifies the passing of the wires transcutaneously and decreases cerebrospinal fluid (CSF) leakage postoperatively. We do not place a cable-retaining suture in the scalp as others have suggested,[3] because in our experience, this practice increases the risk of breaking the electrode cable if it is pulled inadvertently during a seizure. Rather than rely on such retaining sutures, we have had excellent results from the use of the monostrand electrodes shown in Figure 101–1; these cable unions break apart easily if tugged. Because we are interested in the site of seizure onset rather than late generalized activity, we prefer that the cable becomes detached instead of broken or that the electrode becomes dislodged or displaced. The wounds are closed in layers with Vicryl sutures in the deep fascia and subcutaneous layer, and with staples for the skin. The wound is dressed with Telfa and is covered by Selofix.

Early in our experience, we routinely recorded data from each electrode strip in the operating room before the wound was closed. This was especially important when we fabricated our own electrodes. Because we have had no recording problems from commercially available electrodes, we have long ago abandoned this procedure.

The patient is taken to the recovery room where anteroposterior and lateral skull x-ray studies or a CT scan is obtained to confirm the electrode positions. However, with the CT scan, the basal temporal electrodes are often difficult to visualize unless special thin cuts (2 mm) are taken through the middle fossa region. Although MRI-compatible strip electrodes are available, they are not easily visualized on MRI.

An ABD dressing is placed over the wounds, and the head is wrapped with a Kerlix dressing. During the first 3 days after implantation, CSF commonly leaks around the electrode wires. Because of this, the Kerlix-ABD dressing is changed as often as needed by use of sterile techniques. The original Selofix covering is not changed until either the subdural strip electrodes are extracted or the staples are removed 1 week postoperatively.

ELECTRODE POSITIONING

For most routine exploratory implants we prefer using a standard montage with four burr holes[1,4] that are opened bilaterally over the temporal and frontal lobes. The temporal burr holes are located just anterior to the ear and superior to the zygoma. Through these holes a four-contact 6-cm strip is directed medially so that the most distal electrode contact records from the parahippocampal gyrus. A second four-contact 6-cm strip is inserted through the same burr holes and directed posteriorly and laterally to overlay to the middle temporal gyrus. If an occipital focus is suspected, an eight-contact 9-cm (or even 16-cm) strip electrode can be introduced posteriorly through the temporal burr hole to sample the lateral occipital cortex in place of the 6-cm lateral temporal strip. The reason for the placement of the medial and lateral temporal strips is to determine whether seizure onset is from medial or lateral temporal cortex or from both areas simultaneously (thus termed a *regional temporal* onset). This information is important for the planning of appropriate surgery as well as for the prediction of seizure outcome from surgery. For example, patients with mesial temporal seizure onsets are more likely to be seizure free after surgery than are those with lateral temporal onsets. For some surgeons, the site of temporal onset influences the type of surgery subsequently performed.

Bifrontal burr holes are made at 4 to 6 cm anterior to the coronal suture and just lateral to midline. A four-contact 5-cm strip is placed medially, down the interhemispheric fissure, to record from the medial frontal lobe and cingulate gyrus. This medial frontal strip can be directed anteriorly or posteriorly, depending on where one wishes to record. "Inverted T" or "L-shaped" electrodes are also available for recording from this region of cortex. An eight-contact 9-cm strip is directed from the frontal burr hole toward the ipsilateral eye, so that the most distal electrodes record from the orbital frontal cortex while the remainder of contacts sample a wide expanse of frontal lobe. More than two strips can be inserted through each burr hole, but in practice, we seldom insert more than three strip electrodes through one burr hole.

The array of bilateral temporal and frontal electrodes samples cortical activity from regions that include most epileptogenic foci. More recently, if a temporal lobe focus is very strongly suspected, we have omitted the frontal burr holes and placed an eight-contact strip (in addition to the two temporal lobe strips) over the lateral frontal lobe from the temporal burr hole.[4] Although some surgeons place only bilateral temporal strip electrodes in some patients strongly believed to have temporal lobe foci, this practice is discouraged. The frontal lobe always should be recorded because simultaneous frontal and temporal lobe onset carries a poor seizure outcome prognosis, possibly indicating that the epileptogenic focus is outside the temporal lobe. Also, complex partial seizures of frontal lobe onset misleadingly acquire the clinical characteristics of temporal lobe seizures as they spread temporally. In these circumstances, strip electrodes placed only over the temporal lobes, based on the clinical characteristics of the seizures, would miss their frontal lobe origination. In basal frontal lobe epilepsy, interictal discharges can be anterior or basal temporal in distribution, as in temporal lobe epilepsy, thereby confounding the problem even more.

Bilateral strip electrodes are routinely inserted. The need for bilateral strip electrodes is self-evident from the exploratory recordings of patients who have nonlateralized seizure onsets on extracranial EEG studies. In other cases, however, the reasons for using bilateral electrodes may not be as obvious. In all patients, bilateral strip electrodes subserve comparative EEG observations that are often crucial for identification of the side on which seizures are arising. Importantly, bilateral electrode placement appropriately precludes any chance that electrodes might have been inadvertently placed only on the side to which seizures had spread rather than on the side of onset. Regardless of what might be anticipated, some patients' seizures arise unilaterally on an unsuspected side. Even when existing clues strongly suggest a unilateral epileptic focus, bilateral strip electrodes occasionally identify bilaterally independent seizure onset, or in other cases, complex partial seizures that begin bitemporally. Of significant prognostic value is the finding that patients with bilaterally simultaneous temporal lobe seizure onsets in strip electrode recordings do not have adequate seizure relief after temporal lobectomy.[4] Lastly, in temporal lobe epilepsy, bilateral strip electrode placements furnish important data, such as the interhemispheric propagation time. Lieb and colleagues[5] reported that poor postsurgical seizure relief was associated with seizure propagation to the contralateral side in less than 5 seconds, whereas good outcomes were associated with propagation times of greater than 50 seconds. Although the data of Lieb and colleagues were derived from studies with depth electrodes and are most applicable for patients suspected of having mesial temporal lobe foci, we have found that the same conclusions are valid for seizures of temporal lobe origin recorded by subdural strip electrodes.[4] Therefore, because bilateral electrodes can provide crucial prognostic information in addition to focus localization, all cases require them. Our bias is that when a frontal lobe epileptogenic focus is suspected, mesial temporal strip electrodes should also be included.

ELECTROENCEPHALOGRAPHIC MONITORING

At most comprehensive epilepsy centers, the EEG and video monitoring rooms are used only for long-term EEG monitoring and are not used by general medical or surgical patients. Patients are taken directly from the recovery room to one of these monitoring rooms, and recordings are begun on the day of electrode implantation. In some centers, patients with large grid electrodes stay in the intensive care unit for 24 to 48 hours of observation because the grid electrode can act as a significant mass, and cerebral edema can occur from removal of cortical draining veins during grid placement. This has not been a problem with subdural strip electrodes.

A reference electrode is affixed to the scalp (parietal vertex, P_z) with collodion. Because of the voltage difference of the EEG at the scalp and the brain, the scalp reference is rarely active, which allows the routine use of referential scalp electrodes. The subdural strip electrodes are connected to their cables.

The EEG data from all contacts should be recorded, if possible. Initially, we used only 16 channels but found that if all electrodes were recorded from, we more frequently obtained a clearer demonstration of focal onset. Therefore, we now routinely use 32 channels on all strip electrode patients. Most centers now have at least 32-channel recording capability per patient, and 64 channels are preferable. For example, if only two of four electrode contacts of each temporal lobe strip are used, a seizure might appear to have a regional onset within one temporal lobe. However, if all four electrode contacts of the same strip are sampled, the same seizure might be quite focal in its onset. Also, as noted earlier, electrode sampling should not be obtained from temporal or frontal strips only; unless there is a compelling reason to the contrary, EEG data should be recorded from homologous contacts of bilateral strips.

Most subdural strip electrodes can be removed percutaneously in the patient's room after administration of a sedating intravenous dose of lorazepam. Because of concerns about transmission of acquired immunodeficiency syndrome and Creutzfeldt-Jakob disease, the strips are discarded after one use.

Controversy exists over the relative accuracy of ictal and interictal strip electrode recordings. Little has been published on this issue; however, recent data show that interictal spikes are most often bilateral and diffuse and seldom lateralize focally to the region of the surgical focus.[4] In a small number of cases, extremely focal interictal spiking (i.e., to one temporal lobe) can accurately localize an epileptogenic focus but still may falsely lateralize 2 to 5 per cent of the time. These data strongly support the concept that for invasively recorded data, a well-defined focal ictal onset more closely corresponds to the location of the epileptogenic focus than does interictal spiking. However, severe alterations of normal background rhythms also can be localizing and should be brought into consideration when records are evaluated.

COMPLICATIONS

The morbidity in patients in whom strip electrodes are implanted is low. The primary concern in these patients is infection. However, few complications have been reported. Wyler and associates[1] reported one minor brain abscess and one cortical contusion in 28 patients early in the development of the technique. Rosenbaum and coworkers[3] had no morbidity for 50 patients whose electrodes were implanted for an average of 7 days. Wyler and coworkers[6] reported initial results from an ongoing prospective study to evaluate the morbidity of subdural strip electrodes in general and the use of prophylactic antibiotics in particular. They divided 350 consecutive patients into two groups, one receiving antibiotics throughout the entire time electrodes were in place, and the other receiving antibiotics in one bolus the morning of electrode insertion. They found an overall infection rate of 0.85 percent, with no difference between the two groups. The third arm of the study showed a 3 percent infection rate when no antibiotics were given. Our policy is to give one dose of antibiotics immediately before strip implantation.

Other reported complications have been accidental extraction of electrodes, cortical contusion, subdural empyema, and superficial wound infection.[7-10] Many of these complications are minor and cause no long-term problem.

ADVANTAGES AND DISADVANTAGES

Subdural strip electrodes have advantages and disadvantages compared with depth electrodes. The advantages are that (1) they are easier to implant than depth electrodes because they do not require the equipment or expertise needed for stereotaxic surgery; (2) they require less time to implant; thus, the total operating room and anesthesia costs are less than for depth electrodes; (3) they can cover larger expanses of cortex than can depth electrodes; and (4) they appear to have a lower risk of mortality and morbidity than do depth electrodes.[11]

The disadvantage of subdural strip electrodes is their inability to record from the hippocampus and amygdala. Therefore, some researchers have claimed that they are inferior for evaluating patients for temporal lobe surgery.[8, 11] Reports from other centers[3, 7, 9, 12, 13] have shown that subdural strip electrodes can provide sufficient data from which accurate surgical decisions can be made. In two studies, EEG data were recorded simultaneously from both depth and subdural strip electrodes;[14, 15] both the subdural electrodes and the depth electrodes localized the seizure onsets.

GRID ARRAYS

INDICATIONS

Grid electrodes are implanted when the lateralization of an epileptogenic focus is known unequivocally (because grids require a craniotomy for implantation and are not easily placed bilaterally) and when the purpose of the investigation is to localize precisely the extent of an epileptogenic focus. The grid electrode array is also often used to map cortical function so that the surgeon may maximize removal of an epileptogenic focus while preserving cortical function. Frequently, a person with a benign tumor or other obvious structural lesion near the motor or speech cortex requires grid electrode implantation. In this circumstance, the surgeon may implant the grid array, monitor the seizure onset, and map the boundaries of the motor cortex[16, 17] and its relationship to the focus.[12, 16, 18, 19]

OPERATIVE TECHNIQUE

A craniotomy is required for implantation of a grid array. Because most grids have from 40 to 64 contacts (five to eight rows of eight electrodes), they may be sizable. The location of the craniotomy is obviously dependent on the site of the presumed epileptogenic focus. The craniotomy opening should be large because a wide expanse of cortex must usually be sampled. The use of mannitol, hyperventilation, or both, is discouraged because it may give a false sense of space within the cranium. The dura is opened, and the grid is inserted to cover as much of the suspected cortex as possible (Fig. 101–3). Sometimes, placing the entire grid into the required position without causing some buckling of the array is impossible. If adjusting the grid slightly does not smooth it out, a few contacts from a corner may need to be cut off with heavy suture scissors to produce a smooth fit. Once the grid is in place, care is taken to bring the leads out through the dural incision without causing depression of the grid. Often use of one to several strip electrodes is necessary to sample additional cortex from areas inaccessible to the grid, such as within the interhemispheric fissure or basal temporal lobe.[12] As many strips as needed should be used for appropriate sampling of suspected cortex.

Each multicontact lead is tunneled through the skin for several centimeters and should not be brought directly through the craniotomy wound. After all leads have been tunneled, the dura is loosely closed with several interrupted silk sutures, the bone flap is sutured into place, and the scalp is closed in layers, with Vicryl for the galeal closure and staples for the skin. A standard head dressing is then applied.

RECORDINGS

Some centers move the patient to the neurosurgical intensive care unit for the first night after surgery. My own prac-

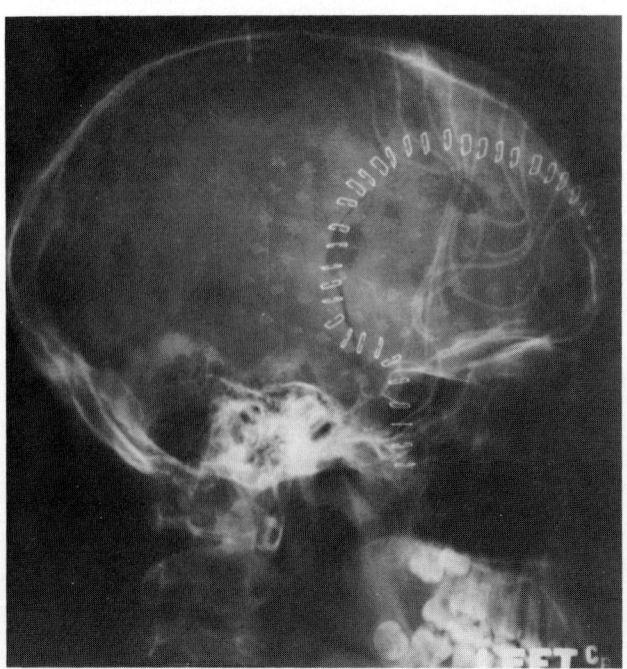

FIGURE 101–3. Lateral skull x-ray study of an 8 × 8 contact grid electrode implanted to cover the lateral cortex and the pole of the right frontal lobe. Individual electrode contacts are difficult to see without looking closely because of the thinness of AD-Tech grids.

tice is to move the patient directly from the recovery room to the monitoring room and have the electrodes connected to the EEG monitor. Often, several more electrode contacts than EEG channels are available to record, especially if additional strips have been placed. We sample as wide an area of cortex as possible. After the first seizure, the most active regions and those most likely to be involved with the seizure onset may be more apparent. Once this information is determined, the inactive contacts may be dropped, and those EEG channels can be used to sample a higher density of contacts within the region of interest. No set number of seizures needs to be recorded; this number depends on the clinical judgment of those involved in the surgical decision-making process. At our center, we rely more on ictal data, especially the recordings taken just before, during, and immediately after the seizure onset rather than late seizure recordings and interictal recordings. Seizure onsets that occur within seconds to minutes after cessation of a previous seizure are disregarded because they may be misleading.

CORTICAL MAPPING

Often, in addition to discovering the location of the epileptogenic cortex, one must also determine its relationship with functional, or "eloquent," cortex. This discrimination requires mapping of the cortex underlying the grid.[12, 17–19] The technique is similar to that performed in the operating room, as described in Chapter 106. This technique requires the use of a testing protocol appropriate to the cortical region to be investigated, which often requires the collaboration of a neuropsychologist trained in cortical function. The grid is transformed to a numeric matrix that depends on the number of contacts placed.

We use a Grass stimulus generator. Other stimulation units are available commercially; however, stimuli must be given by a constant-current generator, which controls the current density if studies of stimulation threshold are to be made. We stimulate between two adjacent electrodes rather than to a common ground because this method controls the current flow more precisely. Bipolar pulses at approximately 50 Hz may be used. As we stimulate the cortex, we monitor surrounding EEG activity to observe for cortical after-discharge to ensure that disruption of function is directly correlative to the stimulation and not to focal after-discharge. The amount of current needed to produce an effect varies between patients and between cortical regions. Enough current should be used to produce a reliable effect without causing current to spread to dura, which might result in discomfort. Occasionally, we have noted pain when current spreads to a nearby cortical vessel. In such cases, a particular contact may not be able to be mapped.

Implanted grid arrays are excellent tools for identification of the position of sensorimotor cortex with somatosensory evoked potentials. The rationale and technique have been reviewed by Allison and colleagues,[20] and clinical experience in using grids for this purpose has been discussed by others.[16, 21, 22]

GRID REMOVAL

Once sufficient data are obtained to plan an appropriate resection, the grid must be removed. If resective surgery is then planned, the grid's relationship to the underlying cortex must be kept exact during the reopening of the craniotomy, which is one of the reasons for securing the edges of the grid to the dura during the initial closure. The patient is placed in the operating position, and the head (including the grid's electrode leads) is prepared with povidone-iodine (Betadine) for 5 minutes. The electrode leads are stretched slightly and cut with heavy scissors as close to the skin edge as possible, and the cut end is allowed to retract back below the skin surface. This practice allows little contaminated lead to be pulled through the skin tunnel once the scalp and bone flap have been opened.

The head is then reprepared with povidone-iodine. The head is draped, and the craniotomy wound is opened. The bone flap is removed and placed in a bowl of irrigation solution with antistaphylococcal antibiotics. The approximating sutures around the dural opening are cut, and the dura is opened, while the grid is left still sutured to the dural edges. The exact relationship between the grid contacts and the underlying cortical topography is then drawn out on a sterile note pad, on which distinguishing vessels or abnormalities are mapped. Once the surgeon has a definite extrapolation of the matrix findings to the underlying cortex, the grid is removed and discarded. The surgeon must then change gloves and copiously irrigate the craniotomy site before proceeding with the resection. Again, before the wound is closed, it should be generously irrigated. The efficacy of prophylactic antibiotics is neither proved nor disproved in these cases. We give one dose of gentamycin before the grid is inserted, but not thereafter unless an infection complicates the implantation. The use of foreign bodies, such as gelatin sponge or bone wax, during the implantation or resective surgery is discouraged.

COMPLICATIONS

The commonest complication of grid implantation is infection. The second commonest problem is the grid itself acting as a mass lesion. If this happens, the grid should be removed immediately. This complication occurs most commonly in children, in whom the subdural space is minimal. The next commonest complication is subdural hematoma from damage to a bridging vein during implantation. However, with extreme care, these complications can be minimized.

REFERENCES

1. Wyler AR, Ojemann GA, Lettich E, Ward AA Jr: Subdural strip electrodes for localizing epileptogenic foci. J Neurosurg 60:1195–1200, 1984
2. Kuzniecky R, Faught E, Morawetz R: Electroencephalographic correlations of extracranial and epidural electrodes in temporal lobe epilepsy. Epilepsia 32:335–340, 1991
3. Rosenbaum TJ, Laxer KD, Vessely M, Smith BW: Subdural electrodes for seizure focus localization. Neurosurgery 19:73–81, 1986
4. Weinand ME, Wyler AR, Richey ET, et al: Long-term ictal monitoring with subdural strip electrodes: Prognostic factors for selecting temporal lobectomy candidates. J Neurosurg 77:20–28, 1992
5. Lieb JP, Engel J Jr, Babb TL: Interhemispheric propagation time of human hippocampal seizures: I. Relationship to surgical outcome. Epilepsia 27:286–293, 1986
6. Wyler AR, Walker G, Somes G: The morbidity of long-term seizure

monitoring using subdural strip electrodes. J Neurosurg 74:734–737, 1991
7. Smith JR, Flanigin HF, King DW, et al: Analysis of a four-year experience with depth electrodes and a two-year experience with subdural electrodes in the evaluation of ablative seizure surgery candidates. Appl Neurophysiol 50:380–385, 1987
8. van Veelen CWM, Debets RM, van Huffelen AC, et al: Combined use of subdural and intracerebral electrodes in preoperative evaluation of epilepsy. Neurosurgery 26:93–101, 1990
9. Blom S, Flink R, Hetta J, et al: Interictal and ictal activity recorded with subdural electrodes during preoperative evaluation for surgical treatment of epilepsy. J Epilepsy 2:9–20, 1989
10. Devinsky O, Sato S, Kufta CV, et al: Electroencephalographic studies of simple partial seizures with subdural electrode recordings. Neurology 39:527–533, 1989
11. Spencer SS: Depth versus subdural electrode studies for unlocalized epilepsy. J Epilepsy 2:123–127, 1989
12. Luders H, Hahn JF, Lesser RP, et al: Basal temporal subdural electrodes in the evaluation of patients with intractable epilepsy. Epilepsia 30:131–142, 1989
13. Wyler AR, Richey ET, Hermann BP: Comparison of scalp to subdural recordings for localizing epileptogenic foci. J Epilepsy 2:91–96, 1989
14. Spencer SS, Spencer DD, Williamson PD, Mattson RH: Combined depth and subdural electrode investigation in uncontrolled epilepsy. Neurology 40:74–79, 1990
15. Spencer SS, Williamson PD, Spencer DD, Mattson RH: Human hippocampal seizure spread studied by depth and subdural recording: The hippocampal commissure. Epilepsia 28:479–489, 1987
16. Uematsu S, Fisher RS, Gordon B, et al: Motor and sensory cortex in humans: Topography studied with chronic subdural stimulation. Neurosurgery 31:59–72, 1992
17. Lee BI, Luders H, Lesser RP, et al: Cortical potentials related to voluntary and passive finger movements recorded from subdural electrodes in humans. Ann Neurol 20:32–37, 1986
18. Goldring S, Gregorie EM: Surgical management of epilepsy using epidural electrodes to localize the seizure focus. Review of 100 cases. J Neurosurg 60:457–466, 1984
19. Lesser RP, Luders H, Klem G, et al: Extraoperative cortical functional localization in patients with epilepsy. J Clin Neurophysiol 4:27–53, 1987
20. Allison T, McCarthy G, Wood CC, et al: Human cortical potentials evoked by stimulation of the median nerve: I. Cytoarchitectonic areas generating short-latency activity. J Neurophysiol 62:694–710, 1989
21. Wood CC, Spencer DD, Allison T, et al: Localization of human sensorimotor cortex during surgery by cortical surface recording of somatosensory evoked potentials. J Neurosurg 68:99–111, 1988
22. Uematsu S, Lesser RP, Gordon B: Localization of sensorimotor cortex: The influence of Sherrington and Cushing on the modern concept. Neurosurgery 30:904–913, 1992

CHAPTER 102

Diagnostic Operative Techniques in the Treatment of Epilepsy: Depth Electrodes

Andre Olivier

This chapter describes the principles and technique of depth electrode, implantation and recording in patients undergoing investigation for intractable epilepsy. The term *depth electrode* is a misnomer because this type of recording is never confined to the deep structures of the brain and always involves intermediate and superficial cortical structures. The term *stereoelectroencephalography*, coined by Bancaud and coworkers,[1] probably corresponds better to the technique we describe.

The purpose of the stereotactic recording technique is to provide a three-dimensional survey of the electrical activity of brain areas to confirm or exclude the presence of a suspected epileptic focus. Originally based on the method of Talairach and Bancaud and colleagues,[1-5] our procedure of stereoencephalography has evolved to incorporate the newer techniques of cerebral recording and imaging as they became available.[6-12] The combination of electrodes implanted long term with a seizure-detection computer program is a powerful tool to determine the side and site of seizure onset when such a focus is suspected but not proven.[13-21]

The development of the technique described is based on the author's experience with 178 consecutive patients who underwent such intracranial recording. Over the years, the technique has been in constant evolution as a result of newer imaging technology.[6, 10, 11, 22, 23] However, the principles and indications have remained practically unchanged.

HISTORICAL OVERVIEW OF DIRECT BRAIN RECORDING

The first efforts to demonstrate the electrical activity of the brain were based on direct intracranial recording. By 1875, Caton had clearly demonstrated the existence of cerebral electricity by implanting electrodes in the gray matter of monkeys through openings in the skull and by studying the fluctuation of the electrical currents with a galvanometer.[24, 25]

Kaufman was the first to formulate the hypothesis that epileptic attacks would be accompanied by abnormal electrical discharges. To test this postulate, he studied the brain potentials in experimentally produced epilepsy in dogs.[24, 26]

Much later, Berger made his first observations in humans.[24, 27] Berger's initial studies were carried out in a subject harboring a cranial bone defect. Berger was later able to detect electrical potentials at the surface of the intact skull and in 1929 proposed the term *electroencephalogram* (EEG) to describe brain waves and their fluctuations.[27]

Mussen's main interest in devising the first human stereotactic apparatus was to detect the abnormal electrical activity of the brain caused by the presence of a tumor.[28] It took a long time for Mussen's idea to be realized. Meanwhile, direct recording of epileptic activity during craniotomy for epilepsy became possible. Electrocorticography was probably carried out first by Foerster and Altenburger, who published their results in 1935.[29] In subsequent years, developments in electrocorticography were mainly due to the efforts of Penfield and Jasper,[30] and Ajmone Marsan and Baldwin.[31] In the 1950s, several studies using direct surface cortical recording and simultaneous depth recording in patients with temporal lobe epilepsy were performed during craniotomies for epilepsy surgery.[30]

In 1947, Hayne and associates[32] reported on their preliminary experience in stereotactic recording from the scalp and the subcortical nuclei in patients with epilepsy. They later demonstrated that independent seizure activity can occur both in the cortex and subcortical structures, thereby showing the inherent value of depth recording in the study of human epilepsy.[32]

In 1949, Wycis and coworkers[33] also reported on the simultaneous recording of thalamic and cortical potentials in schizophrenic and epileptic patients. In addition, a large number of patients with schizophrenia and epilepsy were studied with depth electrodes by Heat and colleagues[34] in the early 1950s. However, these studies did not address specifically the localizational aspect of the EEG.

The state of the art of depth electrode recording in humans was summarized in a symposium held at the Mayo Clinic in 1953. Goals and limitations were similar to those of today.[35, 36]

Talairach, Bancaud, and collaborators[1-5] made extensive use of intracranial recording with stereotactic electrodes, or "stereoelectroencephalography." Most of their studies were based on "acute recording," with electrodes introduced orthogonally in a double-grid system while the patient was under general anesthesia. Their approach was based on anatomic data provided by the imaging modalities then available, namely ventriculography and angiography. They attempted to establish a close correlation between electrical discharges, clinical manifestations, and anatomic localization, and they explored all surgical candidates with this approach.

Although the Paris school insisted that all surgical candidates should be investigated by the stereoencephalographic technique, the approach used at the Montreal Neurological Institute was different. Intracranial recording was used only in instances in which localized seizure onset was suspected in patients with ambiguous data. The procedure has been used in 19 percent of the author's personal surgical cases, that is, in 178 of 942 patients who later underwent a craniotomy for epilepsy.

In 1963, Crandall and coworkers[37] were probably the first to systematically use depth electrodes to determine which of the two temporal lobes was responsible for seizure onset in patients with temporal lobe epilepsy. This was to become possibly the clearest indication for depth electrode investigation if the side of seizure onset remains unclear after standard investigation.[19, 38, 39]

Other modalities of intracranial recording, such as epidural and subdural strips and grids, became popular in the mid 1980s and are presented elsewhere in this volume. Our purpose is not to discuss the relative value of these methods. Epidural and subdural recording combined with depth electrodes is an integral part of stereoelectroencephalography. In this technique, the number of recording sites on the brain surface is reduced (to avoid burr holes and craniotomies) and increased within cerebral structures to obtain a better three-dimensional display of the epileptic activity.

INDICATIONS FOR INTRACRANIAL RECORDING (Tables 102–1 to 102–3)

Before intracranial recording is considered, a well-defined hypothesis of localization must be established. This hypothesis is based on the results of conventional investigative procedures, namely brain imaging and all modalities of standard EEG recording, including sphenoidal leads. The localization hypothesis must be clear and reasonable because the intracranial recording cannot be used to "go fishing" for a focus. Depth electrodes are unnecessary when all the modalities of investigation indicate a single predominant epileptogenic area. Depth electrodes can be used to further delineate the area of onset and early propagation of a seizure as suggested by clinical, imaging, and EEG data but not clearly confirmed by extracranial EEG.

The suspected zone of onset must be covered by placing electrodes in strategic structures, and additional electrodes must be placed when the clinical, imaging, and EEG data suggest that other regions could also be responsible for the seizures. The recording may confirm that seizures arise in several cortical areas and from both sides of the brain, thus precluding surgery.

MAIN INDICATIONS FOR DEPTH ELECTRODE IMPLANTATION (see Table 102–1)

There are two broad categories of indications for intracranial recording.[19, 39–42] The first is ambiguity of lateralization, in which the hemisphere or the lobe of the brain from which the seizures arise must be determined. The second is clear lateralization of the seizure process but a persistent intrahemispheric ambiguity of focus. In some cases, both the lateralization and the intrahemispheric localization may be unclear.

Ambiguity of Hemispheric Lateralization

In our experience, the commonest indication for depth electrode use has been in patients with bitemporal epilepsy who have the bitemporal syndrome.[19, 39, 40] This syndrome is characterized by the presence of one or several of the following: bilateral interictal discharges arising in both temporal areas simultaneously or in alternance over a period of time, ictal discharges contralateral to the maximal interictal anomalies, and seizures being recorded with an unclarified side of onset. The presence of a structural or atrophic lesion contralateral to the maximal epileptic activity can also be an indication[43] (see Table 102–4).

In patients presenting this syndrome, cerebral electrodes

Table 102–1. INTRACEREBRAL ELECTRODES

Advantages
Clarifies a problem of hemispheric lateralization (e.g., so-called bitemporal cases)
Clarifies a problem of localization within one hemisphere (e.g., frontal vs temporal)
Can be combined easily with computer recording techniques:
　Tracing devoid of recording artifacts
　Large number of attacks recorded
Study of epileptic threshold by stimulation
　Basic neurophysiologic data obtained by stimulation and recordings
Disadvantages
Risks and complications of a neurosurgical procedure
Costs in time, personnel, and material
Prolonged and intensive care for one patient, possibly to the detriment of other patients

Table 102–2. MAIN INDICATIONS FOR DEPTH ELECTRODES

Ambiguity of hemispheric localization
　Bitemporal epilepsy
　Bifrontal epilepsy
　Biooccipital epilepsy (rare)
Ambiguity of intrahemispheric localization
　Parietocentrofrontal
　Frontotemporal
　Occipitotemporal

Table 102–3. DEPTH ELECTRODE CONTRAINDICATIONS

Lack of a working hypothesis about localization from clinical and electroencephalographic (EEG) data
Incomplete investigation
　Serial EEGs
　Decrease in medication
　Sphenoidal electrodes and sleep activation
　Seizure monitoring
　Neuropsychological studies
　Imaging studies
Lack of technical facilities
　Stereotactic data acquisition systems
Patient's unsatisfactory motivation

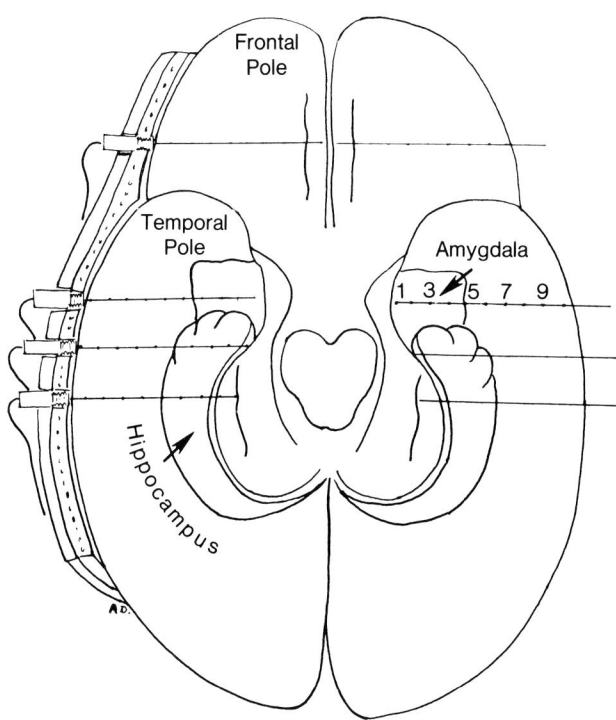

FIGURE 102-1. Example of electrode placement in both temporal and frontal lobes (numbers indicate sites of recording along the electrode array).

(Fig. 102-1) have repeatedly shown that in most cases, one temporal lobe is clearly predominant in the onset and early propagation of the seizures.[15, 19, 22, 39, 44] Following an anterior temporal cortical resection, including the amygdala and various extents of the hippocampus, some of these patients previously rejected for surgery have shown a decrease in their seizure activity comparable to that of the so-called unilateral cases.

Ambiguity of Intrahemispheric Localization

Another common indication for intracranial recording is ambiguity of localization of a focus within one hemisphere when clear hemispheric lateralization exists. Such ambiguity may reside between the frontal lobe and the temporal lobe or the temporal lobe and the occipital lobe. The ambiguity may involve not only the frontal lobe itself and its various subdivisions but also the central and parietal areas. Finally, patients suspected of having secondary generalized epilepsy in which a primary focus is strongly suspected but unproved can also be considered for such an investigation.

In extratemporal epilepsy, the main indications for intracranial (stereoencephalographic) recording are the following: (1) difficulty with lateralization (usually frontal), (2) determination of a lead area for seizure onset in secondary generalized seizures, (3) determination of seizure onset across the central area in the presence of parietocentrofrontal discharges, and (4) determination of seizure onset in cases of frontotemporal or occipitotemporal ambiguity.

TECHNIQUE OF INTRACRANIAL ELECTRODE PLACEMENT

The overall procedure for intracranial electrode placement is carried out in two stages. Stage I is called "stereotactic localization" and consists of stereotactic brain imaging. Its purpose is to obtain and integrate brain images for the selection of targets and to determine the eventual position of recording sites in relation to specific brain structures. This stage takes into account all clinical, metabolic, imaging, and EEG data already available. Stage II is the implantation of the electrodes after repositioning of the stereotactic frame. These two procedures are usually carried out a few days apart.

STEREOTACTIC SYSTEM AND APPARATUS

Any stereotactic apparatus that allows for a lateral orthogonal approach can be used to insert electrodes. The stereotactic apparatus used at the Montreal Neurological Institute was designed for depth electrode implantation and brain tumor biopsies (OBT frame and apparatus: Tipal Instruments, Montreal, Canada)[66, 68, 72, 73, 74] (Figs. 102-2 to 102-5).[6] With this apparatus, either a lateral orthogonal or an arc-radius approach may be used. The lateral orthogonal approach is more useful for the placement of most intracerebral electrodes and is performed with the help of orthogonal carriers (Figs. 102-4 and 102-5). There are two types of these carriers, depending on the type of electrodes used: a single-headed carrier is used for home-made electrodes with no built-in pin connector and introduced on target through a brain cannula (see Fig. 102-4). For commercial electrodes with built-in pin connectors, a double-headed carrier is used (see Fig. 102-5).[45]

The frame is made of an aluminum base, to which a removable front plastic bridge is incorporated. The base ring supports four vertical plastic pillars. Metric scales are incorporated in the horizontal, vertical, and transverse bars. The entire frame is nonmagnetic, nonconductive, and compatible with computed tomography (CT) and magnetic resonance imaging (MRI).[6-9] The side, front, and back bridges support the fiducial marker plates for digital angiography, CT, and MRI (see Figs. 102-2 and 102-6). These fiducial markers for CT consist of two Z-shaped metallic rods incorporated

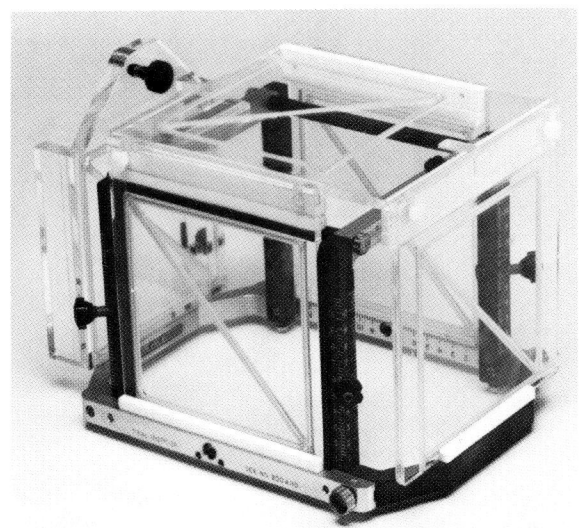

FIGURE 102-2. Stereotactic OBT frame with fiducial MRI plates in place.

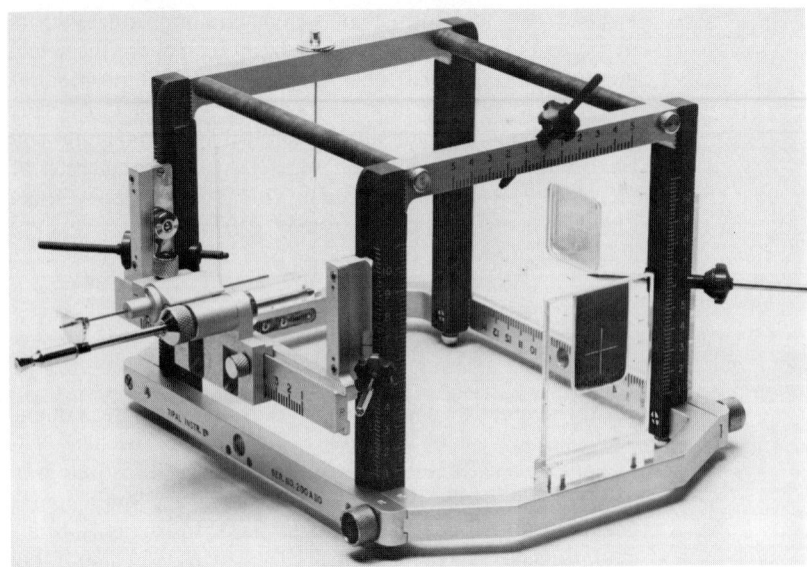

FIGURE 102-3. Stereotactic OBT apparatus with plates and electrode carriers in place.

into Plexiglas plates, whereas those for MRI consist of Z-shaped tubes filled with a solution of copper sulfate (see Fig. 102-2).[6,7,9] The marker plates for digital angiography contain four metallic dots, readily identifiable on both lateral and anteroposterior projections (see Fig. 102-3). These fiducial markers are located at predetermined positions in relation to the frame coordinates. Computer software can readily provide the coordinates of any point within the volume of the frame.

The light weight and compactness of the frame make it convenient to move the patient to the different imaging units within the hospital. Sets of measurement pins with length indicators are used to reposition the frame exactly at the time of the implantation procedure. The overall procedure is always carried out in two stages so that the electrode target sites can be selected with the greatest accuracy possible and the morphologic and functional data can be integrated. This

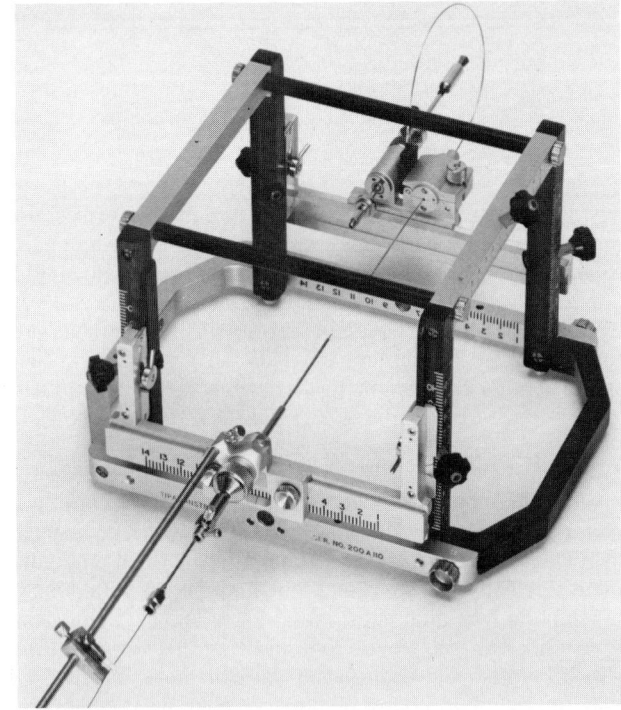

FIGURE 102-5. On one side, the single-headed carrier showing the homemade electrode inserted through the cannula, which is immobilized on target by an alligator clamp. On the other side is the double-headed carrier with a commercial electrode guided by a stylet.

approach also takes care of the unavoidable delays in carrying smoothly the various imaging modalities and also minimizes the risks of infection if the entire procedure has to be performed the same day.

STAGE I: STEREOTACTIC LOCALIZATION

Placement of Stereotactic Frame

For stage I, the hair is clipped but not shaved. At each fixation site, a small button of scalp is removed with a sharp

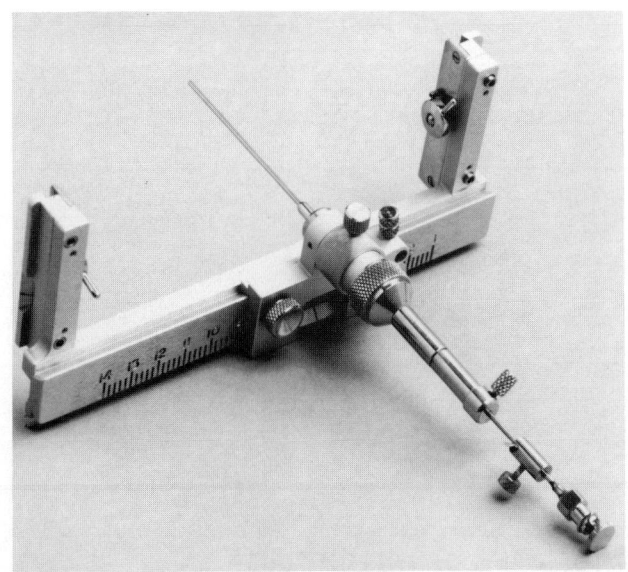

FIGURE 102-4. Sliding sidebar and carrier with brain cannula in place.

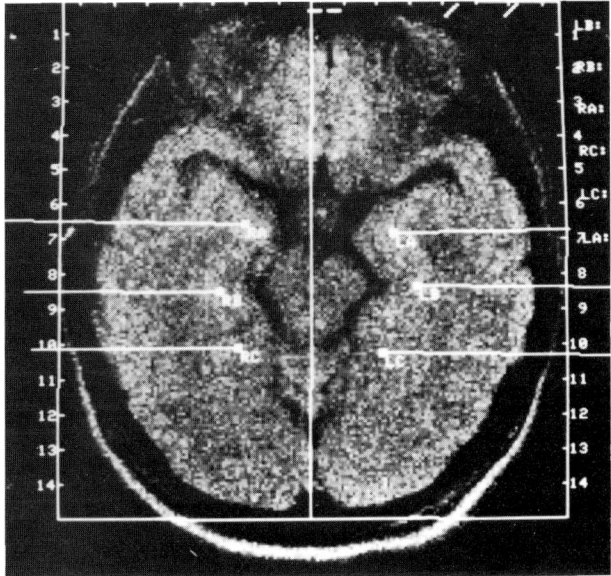

FIGURE 102–6. MRI section in the temporal plane.

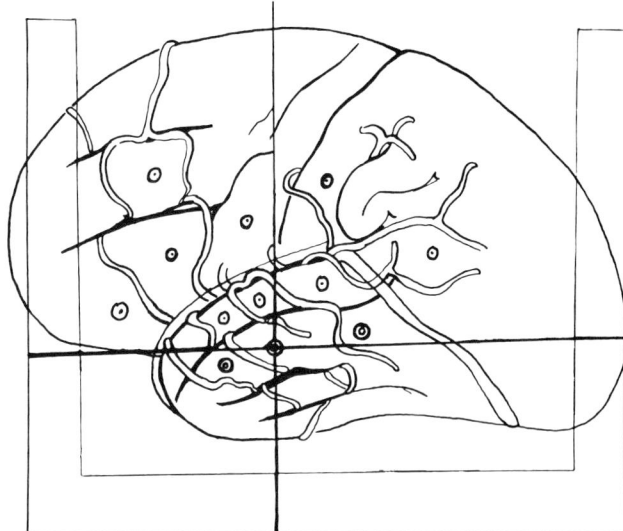

FIGURE 102–7. Angiography diagram showing the purpose of arteriovenous angiography, i.e., identification of structures and avoidance of major blood vessels.

metal punch, and a battery-powered drill is used to make a small hole (2 mm) in the outer table of the skull. The frame is eventually fixed to the head with three carbon pins inserted in the holes. These pins will be reintroduced in the same holes during stage II (implantation).

Control X-Rays

Because the procedure is performed in two stages, lateral x-ray films must be obtained before leaving the operating room. These films are used as control for the reapplication of the frame before electrodes are placed. Traditionally, these x-rays have been performed in a "teleradiologic" setting, that is, at a focal distance of 4.5 m with the help of a frame mirror and laser beam centering device. This method was used to perform direct measurement on nonmagnified head structures. Today, any distance can be used, as long as all parameters of magnification and angulation remain identical between the first and the second control films.

Stereotactic Digital Angiography

Once the stereotactic frame has been affixed to the head, the patient is brought to the radiology suite. The angiography reference plates are affixed to the frame, and a transfemoral carotid angiography is performed. During the procedure, the head and frame are kept immobilized on the frame support.

The purpose of stereotactic angiography is twofold: first, to indicate the position of major veins and arteries, and second, to provide indirect visualization of cerebral sulci and circonvolutions (Figs. 102–7 and 102–8). The position of each individual marker in relation to cerebrovascular structures can be registered easily by a computer program, with rapid display of any target coordinates by movement of a pointer on the chosen target. The computer software can also display the frame scales, the target labels, and the trajectory of any electrodes. It can also transfer data from the lateral to the anteroposterior projection and vice versa. We have used stereotactic digital subtraction angiography (DSA) in all our depth electrode procedures since January 1984. Its advantages over conventional angiography are numerous. The frame itself and the skull can be subtracted, while a grid corresponding to the frame scales can be superimposed over the anatomic structures. Optimal arterial and venous phases can be easily selected and precisely superimposed, a long and tedious procedure before the advent of DSA. Distal target sites, points of entrance over the cortex, and electrode trajectory are achieved with electrode reconstruction showing each one of the recording sites along the electrode shaft.

One of the striking advantages of DSA is the elimination of the need for teleradiology, a procedure that necessitated a complex physical installation. Since about 1955, all angiographic studies at Montreal Neurological Institute are carried out in stereoscopic condition. In every patient, we have systematically used the superimposed arterial and venous phases of the stereoscopic angiogram. Stereoscopic angiography is carried out with an image intensifier by shifting the tube seven degrees between two serial exposures. Stereoscopic

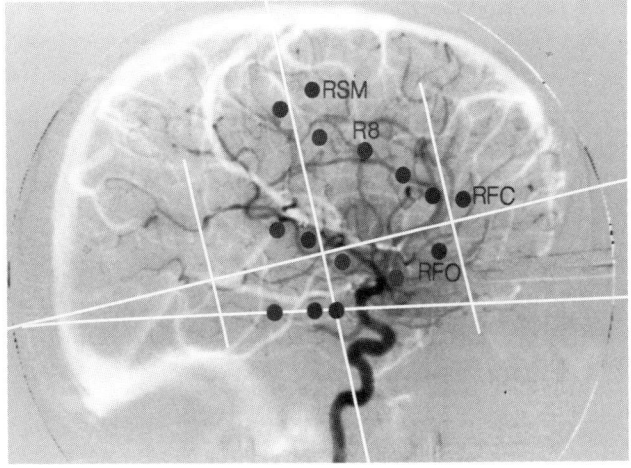

FIGURE 102–8. Arteriovenous angiogram corresponding to Figure 102–9 also showing the callosal grid and the electrode positions.

display of the angiogram is now an integral part of the software for depth electrode planning.[46]

After angiography, the patient is brought to the MRI suite for further imaging studies with the frame in place. The capacity of MRI to demonstrate both the arteries and the veins will probably render obsolete the use of DSA in the placement of electrodes. MR angiography currently provides high resolution for the arterial phase but unsatisfactory resolution of venous structures for the placement of electrodes.[47, 48]

Identification of Structures by Angiography

Stereoscopic arteriovenous angiography is used to accurately localize almost any cortical structure by revealing their gyral and sulcal patterns. The recognition of distal targets, such as the mesial surface of the first frontal gyrus and the cingulate gyrus, is relatively easy by this approach, but the identification of the mesial temporal structures is more difficult.[12] We use this approach extensively to localize the position of all the sulci over the central cortex (Figs. 102–7 and 102–8). For instance, the position of the central sulcus, a crucial landmark in the selection of surface target sites, is routinely established by arteriovenous angiography. It is absolutely essential to work with stereoscopic films in order to appreciate the use and value of this approach. Thus, for each target site, an optimal avascular corridor can be defined for the entrance, trajectory, and termination of each electrode.

Stereotactic Magnetic Resonance Imaging

The advent of MRI has brought a revolution in the field of stereotaxy.[6, 9] MRI became particularly useful in the implantation of depth electrodes (Fig. 102–9).[7] For the first time, structures used as frequent targets, such as the amygdala and the hippocampus, became directly visible. The possibility of displaying structures in the three planes of space was also fully exploited. Until the advent of MRI, most structures were localized indirectly, that is, with the help of angiography or by reference to other structures or landmarks. CT scanning, although useful, has never provided the necessary

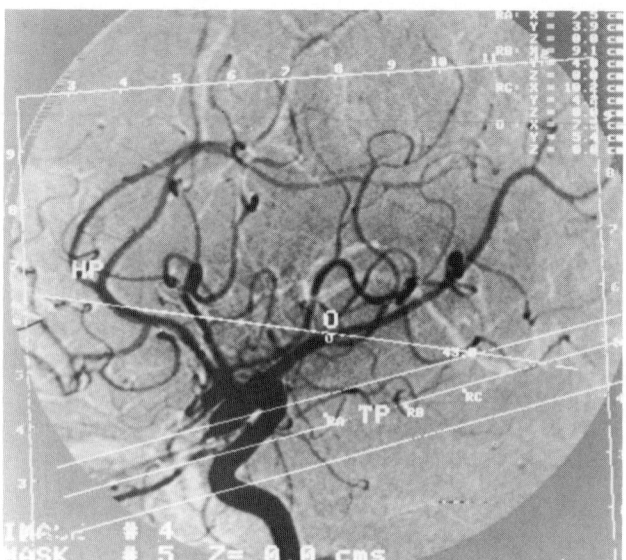

FIGURE 102–10. Stereotactic arteriovenous angiography showing the temporal plane (TP). HP = horizontal, RA = right amygdala, RB = right hippocampus, RC = right parahippocampus.

resolution for accurate localization of structures (Fig. 102–10).

Computer Work Station and Software

The design of the computer work station and stereotactic software have made brain mapping and the selection of targets a pleasant task. The work station is equipped with two computer screens, which permit the simultaneous study of the MRI and the stereoscopic angiography. The computer program allows the display of the frame grids and scale, the immediate calculation and display of target coordinates, and the visualization of electrodes and of each recording site in relation to specific cerebral structures (see Fig. 102–1).

Brain Mapping: Cross Correlation Between MRI and DSA

With the advent of MRI, striking cerebrovascular correlations become possible between MRI and DSA.[7, 49, 50] Brain mapping consists of displaying and studying the topographic cerebrovascular anatomy by combining the MRI and DSA data (see Figs. 102–7 and 102–9). Structures of crucial importance, such as the central sulcus, are usually identified first on angiography and then correlated with MRI. Once the central sulcus is localized, it is used for the subsequent identification of such structures as the precentral and postcentral gyri and the sulci of the frontal lobe.[23, 51, 52] In the temporal lobe, targets such as the amygdala, the anterior hippocampus and parahippocampus are now directly and easily identified with MRI (see Fig. 102–1).

Proportional Callosal Grid

The usefulness of a proportional grid system for stereotaxy was illustrated by the considerable interest generated for the system developed by Talairach and his collaborators,[3] which was based on the anterior and posterior commissures, which

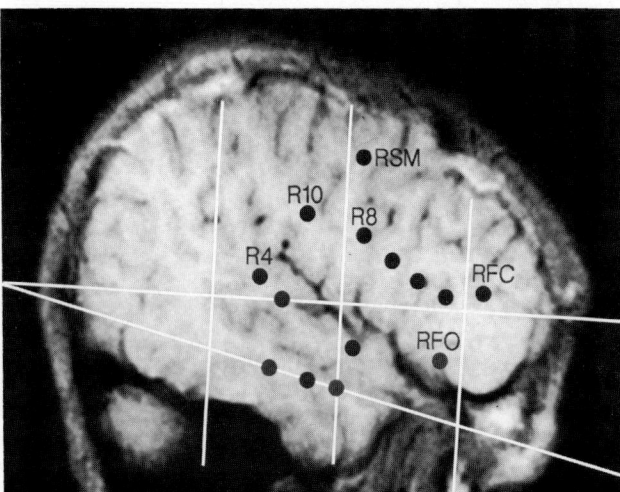

FIGURE 102–9. A display of the callosal grid over the convexity of the hemisphere and the position of various cortical and subcortical electrodes, as seen on MRI.

could be visualized on ventriculography. Over the past several years, we have developed and used extensively a proportional grid system based on the corpus callosum, a structure with a close and steady relationship with the hemisphere that is easily seen on MRI.[75]

The role of the callosal grid is to facilitate the identification of the cortical and subcortical structures, to localize small epileptogenic lesions, and to define optimal planes of section for MRI. It is also used in the planning of stereoencephalography, that is, in the comprehensive placement of depth electrodes and in the localization of the zone of maximal epileptic activity.

Construction (Fig. 102–11)

The corpus callosum can be indirectly but clearly identified in reference to the pericallosal artery and the internal cerebral vein on the combined arterial and venous phases of DSA. It can also be directly and easily visualized on an MRI midsagittal section. Hence, the corpus callosum can be used as a common anatomic landmark for both modalities; it permits the exact superimposition of two different images of the same structure in the midsagittal plane and makes integration of these two modalities a rather simple task. A series of anatomic landmarks and planes, the horizontal plane, the anterior callosal plane, the posterior callosal plane, and the midcallosal plane, can be established in relation to the corpus callosum (Fig. 102–11). The point of crossing of the midsagittal, horizontal, and midcallosal planes represents the central point of the brain. Any target or plane determined with this reference system on MRI can be transferred to DSA.

Integration of PET with MRI and DSA

Positron-emission tomography (PET) with fluorine-18-2-deoxyglucose can provide useful metabolic data in the investigation of the candidate for epilepsy surgery. With PET, interictal hypometabolism or reduced blood flow in the region of the epileptic focus is found in 70 to 80 percent of patients with complex partial seizures.[53–55] However, in contrast to DSA and MRI, PET has a relatively poor anatomic resolution. The combination or integration of these techniques is thus highly desirable. Such an approach could, for instance, demonstrate an area of high signal on T2-weighted MRI images, hypometabolism on PET, and an active epileptiform focus in the depth electrode, all related to recognizable structures. Using the stereotactic approach, we were able to integrate DSA, MRI, and PET images in stereotactic conditions[7, 49, 50] for intracranial recording as early as 1985. Structures that are difficult to delineate with certainty on PET, such as the brainstem, amygdala, and hippocampus, were clearly visualized by the superimposition and integration of these two modalities. Today, the integration of MRI and PET images is a much simpler task.[56]

Selection of Targets

Because the number of electrodes to be inserted is necessarily limited, selection of target sites must be rational and meticulous. The electrodes must be placed in areas known for their low threshold for seizures[61–64] and in areas that may be particularly involved in specific cases (see Figs. 102–6 and 102–12). The trajectory of the electrodes through specific structures, that is, their three-dimensional relationship, must be considered for the maximal EEG information to be obtained (Fig. 102–13). Each lobe and region of the brain requires a specific anatomic coverage. Finally, the selection of targets must take into consideration the vascular arterial and other anatomy along the path of penetration (see Fig. 102–8).

Stereotactic Coverage of the Temporal Lobe with Intracranial Electrodes

Several methods of depth electrode implantation have been used for the temporal lobe. In the lateral orthogonal approach, three depth electrodes are usually inserted through the second temporal gyrus and directed horizontally to the amygdala, the anterior hippocampus, and the parahippocampus gyrus (see Figs. 102–12 to 102–14). Each electrode array has a recording site at each 5-mm interval. Thus, a single electrode must survey activity from distal target sites, such as the amygdala, hippocampus, and parahippocampus, as well as from the intermediate buried sulcal cortex and from the surface of the second temporal gyrus. In addition, a series of four to five epidural (cortical) electrodes is placed along the superior temporal gyrus (see Fig. 102–8). It is sometimes also important to place electrodes at the junctional zone, that is, at the transition between the temporal and occipital lobes both on the lateral and median borders.

Because each depth electrode is in fact a strain of several electrodes (one recording site every 5 mm) (Figs. 102–13 and 102–14), such an arrangement provides a three-dimensional set-up for recording that is likely to capture any seizure arising in the temporal lobe.

Occipitotemporal Approach

The occipitotemporal approach has been used extensively by Ribstein,[57, 65] mostly with a free-hand approach, and more recently by Spencer, who used the stereotactic technique.[41] The goal of this approach is to follow the overall angulation

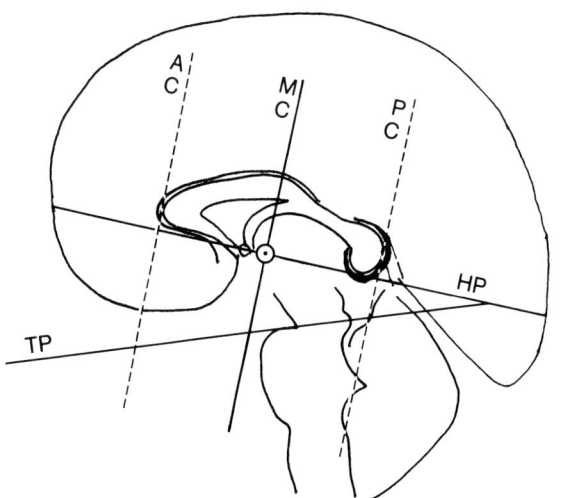

FIGURE 102–11. The callosal grid with principal planes. HP = horizontal, MC = midcallosal, TP = temporal, AC = anterior callosal, PC = posterior callosal planes.

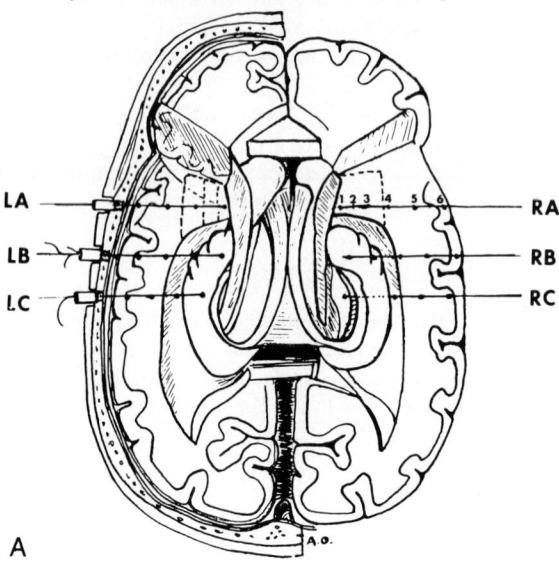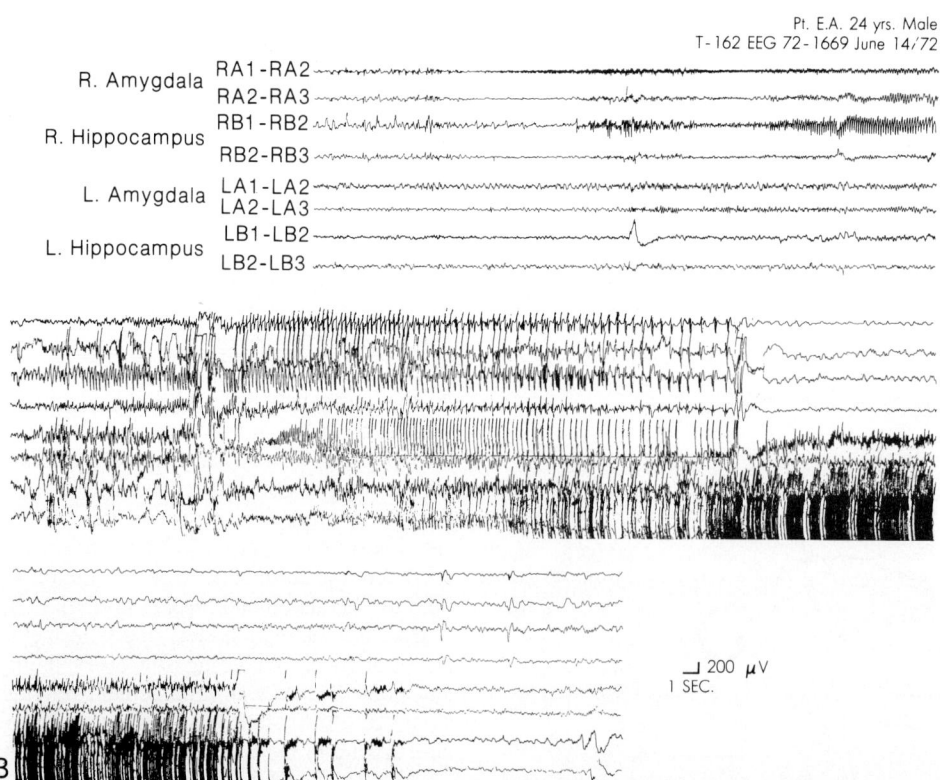

FIGURE 102–12. (A) Typical symmetric placement of electrodes in both temporal lobes. RA = Right amygdala, RB = right hippocampus, RC = right parahippocampal gyrus; LA = left amygdala, LB = left hippocampus, LC = left parahippocampal gyrus. (B) Example of spontaneous clinical seizure.

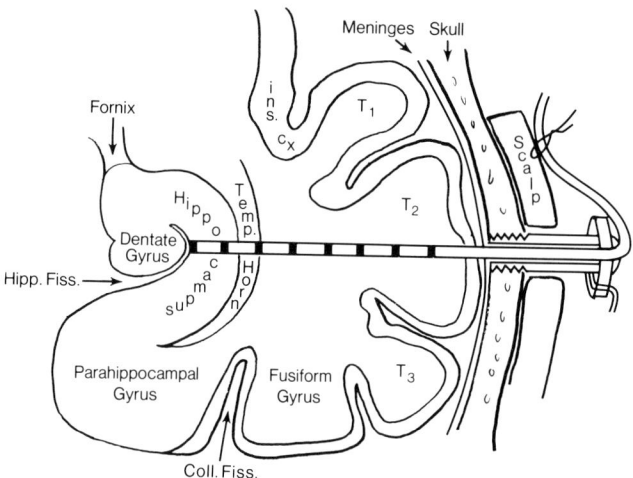

FIGURE 102–13. Showing electrode inserted in temporal lobe. See mode of fixation of the electrode with hollow peg and acrylic.

and configuration of the hippocampus and amygdala. It also provides information from the posterior temporal and occipital areas, but not from the surface of the temporal lobe. It is also unlikely that one single electrode will provide optimal specific information from several structures, such as the hippocampus, parahippocampus, and amygdala. This approach can be used when a stereotactic system does not allow for an easy lateral orthogonal approach.

Frontotemporal Approach

The frontotemporal approach is mainly vertical, with a path that comes through the frontal lobe and a distal target in the amygdala and hippocampus. With this approach, the electrode comes in close vicinity or in contact with insular blood vessels and presents greater risks. This trajectory should be avoided.

Coverage of the Frontal Lobe with Intracranial Electrodes (see Figs. 102–8 and 102–15)

Because of the very large size of the frontal lobe, seizure onset within it can remain poorly localized. Adequate coverage of the frontal lobe is more difficult than for the temporal lobe. We usually use three arrays of horizontal electrodes, implanted orthogonally. One orbital electrode goes through the third frontal gyrus in front of the insular vessels and reaches the mesial surface of F1 (first frontal gyrus). An anterior cingulate electrode passing through the second frontal gyrus is usually inserted into the anterior or superior cingulate gyrus. A third frontal electrode is passed through the second frontal gyrus and directed to the intermediate portion of the mesial surface of F1 and the anterior extent of the supplementary motor area. The supplementary motor area is best reached with a parasagittal electrode inserted along the superior frontal gyrus and recording from its mesial surface (Fig. 102–15) The anterior mesial and orbital area can be monitored with a more vertical parasagittal anterior electrode. Various montages of epidural epicerebral electrodes can be used to cover specific cortical structures over the frontal lobe.

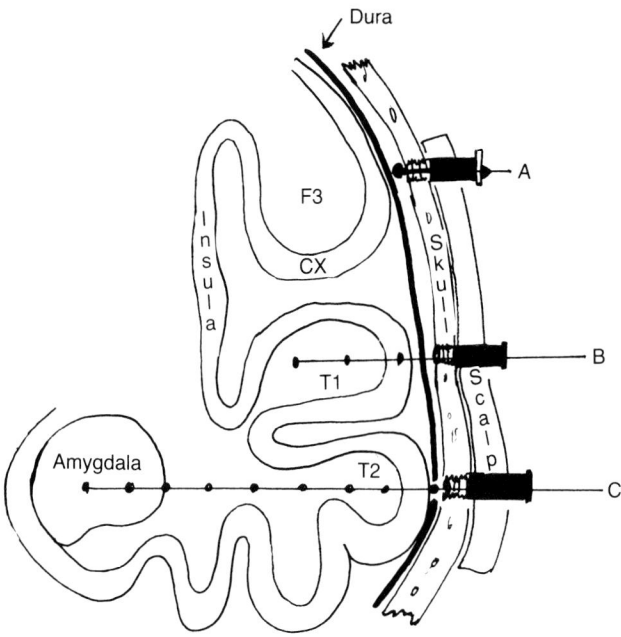

FIGURE 102–14. The principle of SEEG. (A) Surface cortical electrodes are left over the epidural space. (B) Intermediate and (C) depth electrodes are also inserted and fixed through a hollow peg.

Coverage of the Central Area

No depth electrodes are used in the central area. Cortical electrodes (surface epidural electrodes) are placed over both the precentral and the postcentral gyri and the precentral and postcentral area. When cortical electrodes are used, a mini-

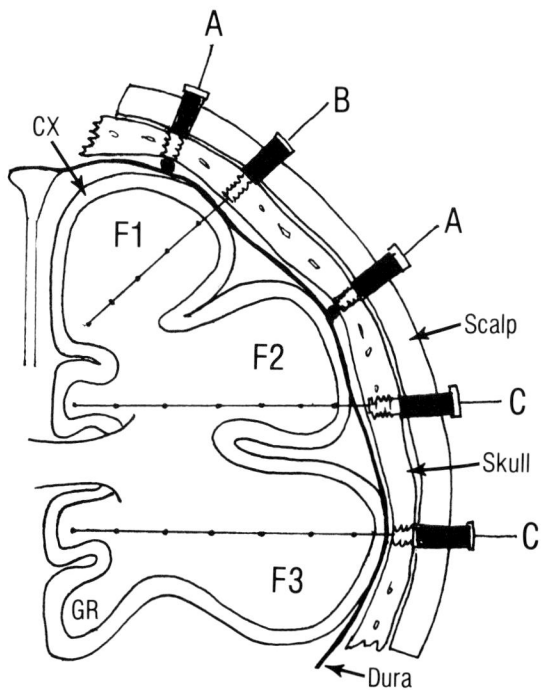

FIGURE 102–15. The type of coverage of the frontal lobe. A = Epidural cortical electrode, B = intermediate electrode, C = depth electrodes, F1 = first frontal gyrus, F2 = second frontal gyrus, F3 = third frontal gyrus, GR = gyrus rectus.

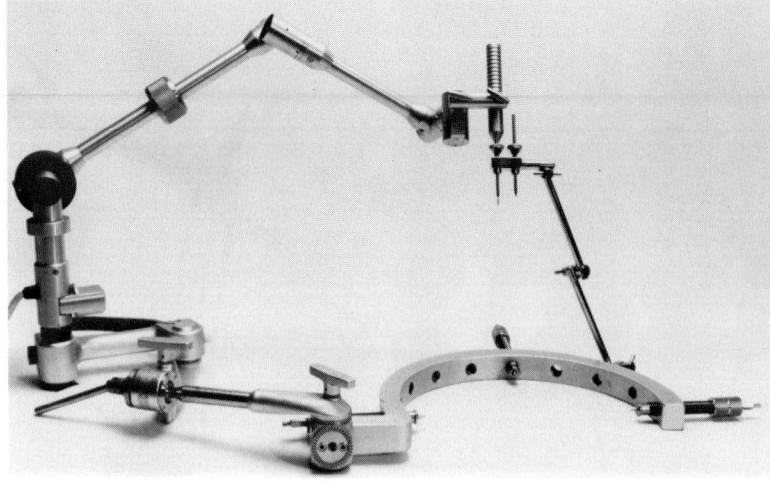

FIGURE 102–16. The system of frameless stereotaxy that can be used to insert the surface cortical electrodes and to verify the trajectory of electrode inserted within the electrode carrier.

mum of four to five electrodes must be used in chain montages to provide adequate recording. For an investigation over the central area, we use three rows of four electrodes, covering precisely the precentral, central, and postcentral areas. The placement of a large number of surface electrodes disposed in a grid fashion is now made much simpler by use of the technique of frameless stereotaxy with a wand system (see Figs. 102–8, 102–15, and 102–16).[52, 58]

Coverage of the Occipitoparietal Area

Depth electrodes can be inserted from the lateral approach into the occipital lobe with distal targets in both the supracalcarine (cuneus) and infracalcarine (lingual gyrus).[21] As already mentioned, other workers have used an occipital approach to direct electrodes toward the mesial structures of the temporal lobe. Such an approach does not permit recording in the primary occipital cortex, which is possible with the lateral orthogonal approach.

Parietal electrodes directed at the precuneus of the mesial parietal cortex can also be inserted by the lateral orthogonal approach or by a parasagittal vertical approach.

STAGE II: IMPLANTATION OF ELECTRODES

When all the various targets and trajectories have been selected and the coordinates calculated, the patient is brought back to the operating room, and the frame is replaced in the very same position in which the various initial imaging studies were conducted. The frame is affixed with the help of the premeasured pins, which are kept under separate cover between the two procedures (see Fig. 102–3). The head itself is fixed to the stereotactic chair by a specially devised head clamp, which goes around the frame itself (Fig. 102–17). The frame is not used as a head-fixating device.[59] The head clamp is also used to mount a stereotactic guide for frameless placement of electrodes.[23]

The procedure of implantation is identical for each target site. In our experience, the orthogonal approach is preferred because of its simplicity and the fact that it uses the angiographic information. However, any angle can be selected when the arc-radius approach is used. The depth of penetration to the target is established with a phantom ruler, which indicates the distance of the target from the midline of the frame. We now use a technique of frameless stereotaxy for all nonorthogonal and surface cortical electrodes (see Fig. 102–16).[23, 52]

Stereotactic Carriers and Electrodes

Two types of electrodes can be used. Commercially available electrodes with built-in pin connectors and stylets are inserted with the help of a double-headed stereotactic carrier (see Fig. 102–3). These electrodes, directed on target with an inner stylet, are usually faster to insert than the electrodes

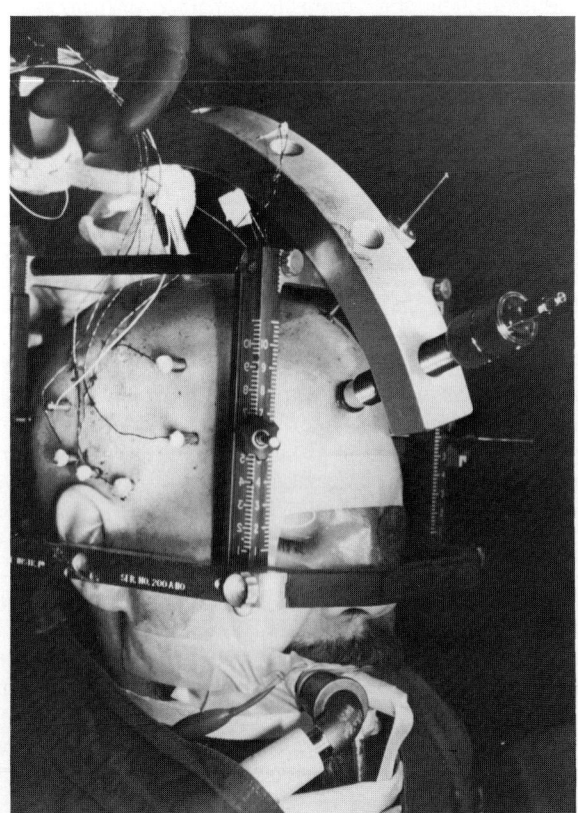

FIGURE 102–17. The head clamp, stereotactic frame, and electrode fixation at termination procedure.

that are devoid of connectors and inserted with the help of a metal cannula. Some of these commercial electrodes are MRI compatible, which makes verifying the accuracy of the placement easier. The electrodes most frequently used at the Montreal Neurological Institute are custom-made flexible strands of stainless steel wires with nine recording sites located 5 mm apart. They are introduced through a metal brain cannula mounted on a single-headed orthogonal carrier (see Figs. 102–4 and 102–5).

Step-by-Step Procedure for Insertion of Electrodes

At each target site, the stereotactic carrier is brought on target along its vertical and horizontal axis (see Figs. 102–3 to 102–5). A series of maneuvers are then repeated at each one of these target sites, through the collar chuck of the carrier.

Step 1. Scalp Punch

A sharp-edged metal cannula is used as a punch to remove a small, 3-mm scalp button. Once the core of soft tissues has been removed down to the bone, it is left undisturbed.

Step 2. Skull Trephination

Skull trephination is performed with a 3-mm twist drill. Battery-powered drills using a range of zero to 300 rpm are preferred. The lower the revolution, the better the characteristic "catch" of the inner table will be felt. The drill bit must be equipped with a strong "stopper" to prevent plunging through the dura. To perforate the skull safely and accurately, the bone thickness should be assessed for each target site so that smooth dural landing can be performed.

Step 3. Peg Insertion

Hollow bony pegs are used for electrode fixation (see Fig. 102–17). The electrodes are anchored to these pegs with acrylic or with a clamp device. Their role is essential to immobilize the electrode in place; otherwise, the electrode would move and cause damage to cerebral tissue along its path. These pegs are gently hammered in the outer table of the skull. These anchoring pegs may vary in length, according to the site of electrode placement, but they are generally 15 mm long. Pegs 25 mm in length are used to go through the temporalis muscle for the amygdala target. The pegs can also be screwed in, but this process is more time consuming than hammering.

Step 4. Dural Perforation

Perforation of the dura is carried out through the peg with a sharp probe that is insulated except for its tip. Gentle steady pressure is exerted while the coagulating current is applied against the dura. Cerebrospinal fluid leak is often seen at this stage and does not need particular attention.

Step 5. Insertion of Electrodes

The depth of penetration to reach the target is established with a phantom ruler, which indicates the distance of the target from the midline of the frame. A metal brain cannula is first introduced on target. If resistance is encountered at the dura, the cannula is gently rotated until the characteristic yielding is obtained. The cannula is then pushed on target by turning it 15 degrees side to side. The stylet is then removed and replaced by the recording electrode that is immobilized on target with an alligator clamp. The cannula is then withdrawn while the electrode remains on target (see Fig. 102–5).

Step 6. Fixation of Electrode

Fixation of the electrode to the peg is performed with acrylic (Fig. 102–17). The acrylic should be confined to the tip of the peg and not pushed too far inside so that the electrode can be easily removed. Whenever feasible, an acrylic bridge is made between adjacent pegs to provide maximal stability for each peg and electrode.

Placement of Commercial Electrodes

The placement of these electrodes follows a series of steps similar to that already described. The electrode equipped with a pin connector is pushed on target with a stylet that is usually inserted within the tubular electrode. For these electrodes, we have devised a double-headed carrier. One of the heads is used to make the twist drill hole, and the second is used for the actual placement of the electrodes, after lateral displacement of the first carrier along the horizontal plane and replacement by the second carrier. This carrier is then opened to free the electrodes and the pin connectors (see Fig. 102–5).

Placement of Cortical Electrodes (Epidural)

Because depth electrodes record from a rather limited volume of tissue along the electrode strands, covering wider areas of the cerebral hemisphere with additional surface electrodes is often necessary. Cortical electrodes are used in chain montages to record cortical activity from the epidural space. The stereotactic localization method using MRI and angiography described earlier is used to place the recording tip of these epidural electrodes precisely over any predetermined cortical location or structure (see Figs. 102–7, 102–9, and 102–15). For this reason, we prefer to use the term *cortical* electrodes. Surface cortical electrodes are particularly useful to record over crucial surfaces, such as the motor or speech centers, that preclude the use of intracerebral electrodes. At the Montreal Neurological Institute, this type of electrode is preferred over subdural strips because of its greater anatomic accuracy and ease of insertion. These electrodes can be used to form loose or compact grids over the convexity of the hemisphere.[69, 72]

Epidural cortical electrodes are inserted in the same way as the intracerebral electrodes, according to stereotactic coordinates. By use of DSA and MRI, the exact position of the gyri and sulci of the convexity can be recognized, and thus, the epidural peg can be placed exactly where desired in relation to the specific gyri (see Figs. 102–7 and 102–9). Over the past 2 years, our technique has evolved so that all the cortical electrodes and all nonorthogonal electrodes are inserted with the help of frameless stereotactic techniques (see Fig. 102–16).[50, 52, 58]

To insert the epidural cortical electrodes, a scalp button is removed with the scalp punch, and the initial steps are identical to the technique of depth electrode placement. The bone is perforated, and care is taken not to perforate the dura. A hollow peg is inserted, and a specially insulated electrode with a recording ball tip is placed in contact with the dura by moving a cap along the wire, which itself is adapted to the peg (Fig. 102–18A and B). Final immobilization to the screw is also achieved with acrylic (see Fig. 102–17). An acrylic bridge joining each peg is fashioned to provide greater stability.

Electrode Placement with Frameless Stereotaxy

During the placement of depth and surface cortical electrodes using the OBT (Olivier, Bertrand, and Tipal) stereotactic frame, we have been able to use a viewing wand (ISG Allegro Viewing Wand System: ISG Technologies, Mississauga, Ontario) within the carrier of the frame itself to display the pathway and destination of the electrodes. We have also used the wand to actually insert the electrode toward its target, along any angle in its pathway. In such a case, we used a clamp device designed for use in conjunction with the frameless system (see Fig. 102–16). This device is composed of an articulated arm with twin chucks. Its purpose is to store the memory of angulation provided by the wand and to provide the necessary support for the transcutaneo-osseous trephination. One chuck maintains angulation, and the other provides the necessary support for safe and precise trephination.

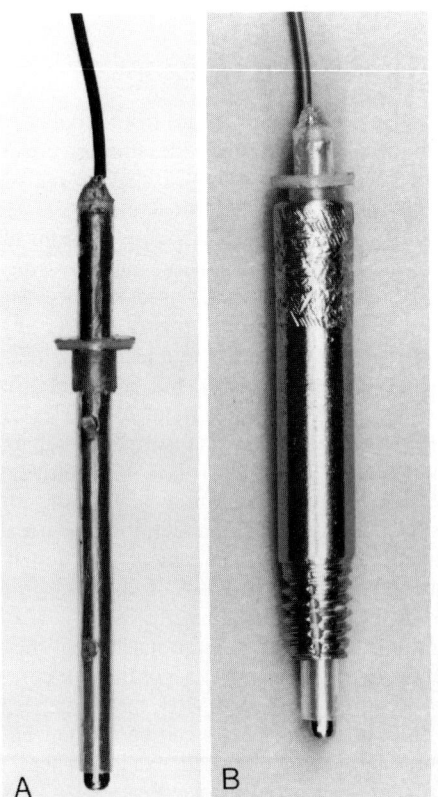

FIGURE 102–18. (A) Epidural cortical electrode. (B) The cortical electrode is inserted inside the cranial peg.

In this way, we have been able to take full advantage of the three-dimensional reconstruction of the Allegro software for volume rendering and color coding of target structures.[23, 52]

Electrode Montage and Recording

Each electrode is identified with a tag affixed to its extremity. It is then connected to the recording apparatus with a coaxial cable. Since 1972, we have used a computer-based system of automatic seizure detection devised by Ives and coworkers.[13, 14, 16] Recognized through a specific window of frequency and voltage, the seizure itself is automatically recorded as well as the electrical events preceding the seizures, during a 2-minute period. With this system, a large number of seizures can be recorded and studied in a relatively short period of time, as long as the patient is actually producing spontaneous seizures. Further development of the recording system has rendered possible spike detection and counting phase studies to determine leads from various electrodes.[60]

PATIENT MONITORING

Once the intracranial electrodes have been inserted, the patient undergoes continuous night-and-day EEG and video monitoring, the purpose of which is to record as many as possible of the typical seizures.

While being monitored with depth and cortical electrodes, the patient undergoes a period of intense physical and emotional stress. The entire team must be aware of this fact. The patient must be given regular breaks, during which the patient should undergo physiotherapy and breathing exercises.

Psychological and psychiatric monitoring is crucial because many of these patients are likely to develop psychotic postictal episodes as well as depressive features, especially if the recording period is prolonged and concrete positive results are still lacking. It is very important to take care of the patient's psychological well-being. Because these recording periods typically last from 10 to 20 days, a psychiatrist and a physiotherapist must be involved in the care of the patient. The patient must also be kept aware of the progress of his or her study. Patients with frequent seizures, especially with bitemporal epilepsy, are at risk for developing amnesia, confusion, and psychosis. Patients producing no seizures while being recorded are at risk of developing depression and agitation. Close monitoring of the antiepileptic medication in relation to the seizure frequency is also of crucial importance. Such medication is usually slowly tapered. Extreme care should be taken in lowering the medication in patients with past history of status epilepticus.

STIMULATION OF DEPTH ELECTRODES

A single session of stimulation is carried out with the goal of identifying areas of lowest threshold and of reproducing the patient's subjective aura. To avoid any kindling effect, only one session of stimulation is carried out. Stimulation through stereotactic depth electrodes can provide fundamental information on the role of specific deep structures of the human brain.[40, 71] Thus, our observations[61] have provided

Table 102–4. PRESENTATION OF BITEMPORAL EPILEPSY

Bilateral interictal discharges
Seizures recorded contralateral to the interictal activity
Seizures recorded with unclarified side of onset
Lesion contralateral to the side of epileptic activity

evidence that unless the limbic structures (amygdala and hippocampus) are activated, either in the course of a spontaneous seizure or through artificial electrical stimulation, psychic experimental phenomena do not occur. This was true not only for emotional responses but also for complex visual and auditory hallucinations, activation of memory recall, and illusions of familiarity.[61] We have not used stimulation studies for the determination of seizure onset but more as confirmatory evidence of the anatomic substratum of a seizure. Recording of spontaneous seizures remains the best indication of true seizure onset location.

HEAD DRESSING AND DRESSING CARE

A large head dressing is used to protect the skull pegs and the electrodes in the event of a major convulsive seizure. These dressings are changed regularly, and the sites of electrodes are kept cleaned.

REMOVAL OF ELECTRODES

Removal of electrodes is carried out with the patient under neuroleptanalgesia. Each recording wire is cut 1 cm from the peg. The acrylic is then broken and the wire pulled out with a clamp. Each individual wound is irrigated with an antibiotic solution and closed with a suture that is long and single to facilitate its retrieval and removal. The stitches are removed on the tenth postoperative day to permit good closure of each wound. The hair is not shaved. Whenever possible, a control MRI is performed to evaluate any potential damage caused by the electrode and to further determine the accuracy of the electrode placement.

COMPLICATIONS AND SIDE EFFECTS

In the author's series of 178 patients who received depth electrodes, the following complications have occurred.[67] Three cases of intracranial infection have been encountered.

Table 102–5. RESULTS OF SURGERY IN 86 PATIENTS WITH BITEMPORAL DISCHARGES INVESTIGATED WITH DEPTH ELECTRODES*

Class	Success (%)	Comment
I	55	⎫
II	08	⎬ 76% success from classes I through III
III	13	⎭
IV A	15	Relative success
IV B	09	Failure

*> 1.5 years of follow-up.

Two cases of brain abscesses have necessitated evacuation, without subsequent complications. Two cases of superficial scalp and subdural infections were treated with antibiotics without complications. None of the 178 patients was given prophylactic antibiotic therapy for the surgery or for the recording period.

Vascular complications have been limited to a single case of subdural hematoma, which occurred from a contusion of a frontal vein in a young patient with significant bilateral frontal lobe atrophy. The hematoma was evacuated through a small craniectomy without sequelae. No mortality and no neurologic deficit has been encountered in the entire series.

RESULTS

Positive results of depth electrode studies depend on the clarity and soundness of the working localization hypothesis at the onset. To illustrate the benefits that can be derived with depth electrodes, we have considered the results in a series of 86 patients whose conditions were considered inoperable without depth electrodes because they presented bitemporal anomalies or bitemporal syndrome (Table 102–4). In these patients, the hypothesis was that the seizures arose in one temporal lobe and not in the other. Secondarily, the procedure was performed to confirm that the seizures arose from the limbic structures.

Table 102–5 shows the results obtained for these patients without consideration of the modality of temporal resection.

These patients represent 16 percent of a series of 523 patients who had a minimum follow-up of 1.5 years. When the "success" group, or the 76 percent who were seizure free or had a decrease of more than 90 percent, is added to the relative success group, the 15 percent whose seizures decreased 50 to 90 percent, about 90 percent of the patients had a significant decrease in their seizure tendency. When the results are analyzed according to the various modalities of temporal resections, we can conclude that the study with depth electrodes in patients with bitemporal anomalies who were considered unsuitable for surgery has provided results not significantly different than those in patients with unilateral anomalies who were operated on without depth electrodes.

REFERENCES

1. Bancaud J, Dell MB: Techniques et méthode de l'exploration fonctionnelle stéréotaxique des structures encephaliques chez l'homme (cortex, sous-cortex, noyau gris centraux). Rev Neurol 101:213–227, 1959
2. Talairach J, Bancaud J: Stereotaxic exploration and therapy in epilepsy, in Vinken PJ, Bruyn GW (eds): The Epilepsies. Handbook of Clinical Neurology, vol 15. Amsterdam, North Holland, 1974, pp 758–782
3. Talairach J, Bancaud J, Szikla G, et al: Approche nouvelle de la neurochirurgie de l'épilepsie: Méthodologie stéréotaxique et résultats thérapeutiques. Neurochirurgie 20 (suppl):1–240, 1974
4. Talairach J, David M, Tournoux P: L'Exploration Chirurgicale Stéréotaxique de Lobe Temporal Dans L'Épilepsie Temporale. Paris, Masson, 1958
5. Munari C: Stereoencephalography: A rational basis of neurosurgical therapy of partial epilepsies, in Broggi G (ed): Rationale Basis of the Surgical Treatment of Epilepsies. J Libbey & Cy, 1988, pp 121–138
6. Olivier A, Peters TM, Bertrand G: Stereotaxic systems and apparatus for use with MRI, CT and SDA. Appl Neurophysiol 48:94–97, 1985
7. Olivier A, Peters TM, Clark JA, et al: Intégration de l'angiographie

numérique, de la résonance magnétique, de la tomodensitométrie et de la tomographie par émission de positrons en stéréotaxie. Rev EEG Neurophysiol Clin 17:24–43, 1987

8. Peters TM, Clark JA, Pike B, et al: Stereotactic surgical planning with magnetic resonance imaging, digital subtraction angiography and computed tomography. Appl Neurophysiol 50:33–38, 1987
9. Peters TM, Clark JA, Olivier A, et al: Integrated stereotaxic imaging with CT MR imaging and digital subtraction angiography. Radiology 161:821–826, 1986
10. Henri CJ, Collins L, Peters TM: Multi-modality image interpretation for stereotaxic surgical planning. Med Phys 18:167–177, 1991
11. Peters TM, Olivier A: CT-aided stereotaxy for depth electrode implantation and biopsy. Can J Neurol Sci 10:166–169, 1983
12. Olivier A, Peters TM, Clark JA, et al: The role of digital angiography in stereotaxy. Comptes Rendus de la Réunion de l'Association des Neurochirurgiens de Langue Française. Paris, December 1984
13. Ives J, Thompson CJ, Gloor P, et al: The on-line computer detection and recording of spontaneous temporal lobe epileptic seizures from patients with implanted depth electrodes via a radio telemetry link. Electroencephalogr Clin Neurophysiol 37:205, 1974
14. Gotman J: Automatic recognition of interictal epileptic activity in prolonged EEG recordings. Electroencephalogr Clin Neurophysiol 46:510–520, 1979
15. Gloor P, Olivier A, Ives J: Prolonged seizure monitoring with stereotaxically implanted depth electrodes in patients with bilateral interictal temporal epileptic foci. How bilateral is bilateral epilepsy? in Wada JA, Penry JK (eds): Advances in Epileptology. The Tenth Epilepsy International Symposium. Raven Press, 1980, pp 83–88
16. Olivier A, Gloor P, Ives J: Investigation et traitement chirurgical de l'épilepsie bitemporale. Union Med Can 109(2):247–250, 1980
17. So N, Olivier A, Andermann F, et al: Results of surgical treatment in patients with bitemporal epileptiform abnormalities. Ann Neurol 25:432–439, 1989
18. Olivier A, Gloor P, Ives J, et al: Stereoencephalographic Evaluation of Patients with Intractable Bitemporal Lobe Epilepsy, in Proceedings of the American Association of Neurological Surgeons, Miami, April 1974
19. Olivier A, Gloor P, Andermann F, Quesney LF: The place of stereotactic depth electrode recording in epilepsy. Appl Neurophysiol 48:395–400, 1985
20. Palmini A, Andermann F, Dubeau F, et al: Occipito-temporal epilepsies: Evaluation of selected patients requiring depth electrode studies and rationale for surgical approaches. Epilepsia 34:84–96, 1993
21. Olivier A, Gloor P, Andermann F, Ives J: Occipito-temporal epilepsy studied with stereotactically implanted depth electrodes and successfully treated by temporal resection. Ann Neurol 11:428–432, 1982
22. Olivier A, Gloor P, Ives J: Stereotaxic Seizure Monitoring in Patients with "Bitemporal Epilepsy." Indications, Techniques and Results, in Proceedings of the American Association of Neurological Surgeons (#14), Toronto, April 1977
23. Olivier A, Germano I, et al: Frameless stereotaxy for surgery of the epilepsies: Preliminary experience. J Neurosurg 1994, in press
24. Brazier MA: A History of the Electrical Activity of the Brain. London, Pitman, 1961
25. Caton R: The electric currents of the brain. BMJ 2:278, 1875
26. Kaufman PY: Electrical phenomena in the cerebral cortex (in Russian). Obroz Psikhiat Nevrol Eksper Psikhol (St Petersburg) 7–8:403–404, 513–535, 1912
27. Berger H: (1873–1941) Uber das Elektrenkephalogramm des Menschen. Arch Psychiatr Nervenkr 87:527–570, 1929
28. Olivier A, Bertrand G, Picard C: Discovery of the first human stereotactic instrument. App Neurophysiol 46:84–91, 1983
29. Foerster O, Altenburger O: Electrobiologische vorgange an der menschlischen hirnrinde. Dtsch Zeitsch Nervenheilk 135:277–288, 1935
30. Penfield W, Jasper H: Epilepsy and Functional Anatomy of the Human Brain. Boston, Little Brown, 1954
31. Ajmone Marsan C, Baldwin M: Surgical series in temporal lobe epilepsies. Electrocorticography, in Baldwin M, Bailey P (eds): Temporal Lobe Epilepsy. Springfield, IL, Thomas, 1958, pp 368–395
32. Hayne RA, Belinson L, Gibbs FA: Electrical activity of subcortical areas in epilepsy. Electroencephalogr Clin Neurophysiol 1:437–445, 1949
33. Wycis HT, Lee AJ, Spiegel EA: Simultaneous records of thalamic and cortical potentials in schizophrenics and epileptics. Confin Neurol 9:264–272, 1949
34. Heat RG, Mickle WA, Monroe RR: Characteristics of recordings from various specific nuclear masses in the brain of psychotic and non-psychotic patients. Trans Am Neurol Assoc 80:17–21, 1955
35. Dodge HW, Bailey AA, Bicford GR, et al: Neurosurgical and neurologic applications of depth electrography. Mayo Clin Proc 28:188–191, 1953
36. Bickford RG: The application of depth electrography in some varieties of epilepsies. Electroencephalogr Clin Neurophysiol 8:526–527, 1956
37. Crandall PH, Walter RC, Rand RW: Clinical applications of studies on stereotactically implanted electrodes in temporal lobe epilepsy. J Neurosurg 20:827–840, 1963
38. Olivier A, Gloor P, Ives J, et al: Chronic multiple depth electrodes in "bitemporal epilepsies." A clinical appraisal of 10 patients (abstract). Can J Neurol Sci 2:339
39. Olivier A, Gloor P, Quesney LF, Andermann F: The indications for and the role of depth electrode recording in epilepsy. Appl Neurophysiol 46:33–36, 1983
40. Ives J, Thompson CJ, Gloor P: Seizure monitoring: A new tool in electroencephalography. Electroencephalogr Clin Neurophysiol 41:422–427, 1981
41. Spencer SS: Depth electroencephalography in selection of refractory epilepsy for surgery. Ann Neurol 9:207–214, 1987
42. Spencer SS: Depth electrodes. Surgical treatment of epilepsy. Epilepsy Res Suppl 5:135–145, 1992
43. Sammaritano M, de Lotbiniere A, Andermann F, et al: False lateralization by surface EEG of seizure onset in patients with temporal lobe epilepsy and gross focal cerebral lesions. Ann Neurol 21:361–369, 1987
44. So N, Gloor P, Quesney LF, et al: Depth electrode investigations in patients with bitemporal epileptiform abnormalities. Ann Neurol 25:423–431, 1989
45. Olivier A: Stereotaxic double headed carrier for insertion of depth electrodes. J Neurosurg 65:258–259, 1986
46. Henri CJ, Collins L, Peters TM, et al: Three-dimensional interactive display of medical images for stereotactic neurosurgical planning. Pro SPIE: Medical Imaging III 1092:67–74, 1989
47. Takahashi AM, Peters TM, Henri CJ, et al: Three-Dimensional Acquisition and Display of Magnetic Resonance Angiograms. RSNA Annual Meeting, Chicago, December 1992, Scientific Exhibit 11-020 Radiology, 185(P):299, 1992
48. Pike BG, Hu BS, Glover GH, Enzmann DR: Magnetization transfer time-of-flight magnetic resonance angiography. Magn Reson Med 25:372–379, 1992
49. Olivier A, Marchand E, Peters TM, et al: Anatomical Cross-Correlation Between PET, MRI and DSA Images, in Proceedings of the Second International Meeting of Magnetic Resonance Imaging in Medicine Montreal, pp 805–806, 1986
50. Olivier A, Marchand E, Peters TM, Tyler J: Depth electrodes implantation at the Montreal Neurological Institute and Hospital, in Engel J Jr (ed): Surgical Treatment of the Epilepsies. New York, Raven Press, 1987, pp 595–602
51. Lehman R, Olivier A, Moreau J-J, Tampieri D: Use of the callosal grid system for preoperative identification of the central sulcus, in Lunsford LD, Gildenberg PL, Franklin PO (eds): Proceedings of the American Society for Stereotaxic and Functional Neurosurgery 58:1,179–188, 1992
52. Olivier A, Lacerte D, Germano I, et al: The ISG System: Clinical experience with frameless stereotactic surgery. Experience with 100 consecutive cases, in Gildenberg PL, Tasker R (eds): Stereotactic and Functional Neurosurgery. New York, McGraw Hill, in press
53. Engels J JR, Kuhl DE, Phelps ME, et al: Interictal cerebral glucose metabolism in partial epilepsy and its relation to EEG changes. Ann Neurol 12:510–517, 1982
54. Theodore WH, Newmark ME, Sato S, et al: ^{18}F-Fluorodeoxyglucose positron emission tomography in refractory complex partial seizures. Ann Neurol 14:429–437, 1983
55. Och RF, Yamamoto Y, Gloor P, et al: Correlation between the positron emission tomography measurement of glucose metabolism and oxygen utilization with focal epilepsy. Neurology 34:(suppl 1):125, 1987
56. Evans AC, Marrett S, Collins L, Peters TM: MRI-PET correlation in three dimensions using a volume-of-interest (VOI) atlas. J Cereb Blood Flow Metab 11:A69–A72, 1991
57. Ribstein M: Exploration du cerveau humain par électrodes profondes. Electroencephalogr Clin Neurophysiol 16:1–130, 1960
58. Olivier A: ISG: Allegro Wand Frameless Stereotaxy. Chicago, December 1992
59. Olivier A, Bertrand G: A new head clamp for stereotactic and intracranial procedures. Appl Neurophysiol 46:272–275, 1985

60. Gotman J: Recognition and analysis, in Gotman J, Ives J, Gloor P (eds): Long-Term Monitoring in Epilepsy (EEG Suppl 37). New York, Elsevier Scientific Publications 1985, pp 133–145
61. Gloor P, Olivier A, Quesney LF, et al: The role of limbic system in experiential phenomena of temporal lobe epilepsy. Ann Neurol 12:129–144, 1982
62. Gastaut H, Vigouroux R, Naquet R: Lésions épileptogènes amygdalo-hippocampiques provoquées chez le chat par injection de "crème d'alumine." Rev Neurol 87:607–609, 1952
63. Feindel W, Penfield W: Localization of discharge in temporal lobe automatism. Arch Neurol Psychiatry 72:605–630, 1954
64. Jasper H: Round-table discussion on depth recording. Electroencephalogr Clin Neurophysiol 8:533, 1956
65. Walker AE, Ribstein M: Chronic depth recording in focal and generalized epilepsy: An evaluation of the technique. Arch Neurol Psychiatry 78:44–45, 1957
66. Olivier A, de Lotbiniere A: Stereotactic techniques in epilepsy. Neurosurgery. State of the Art Reviews 2,1:257–285, 1987
67. Espinoza A, Olivier A: Morbidity of chronic recording with intracranial depth electrodes in 170 patients. Proceedings of the Eleventh Meeting of the World Society for Stereotactic and Functional Neurosurgery, vol 62/63, 1994, in press
68. Peters TM, Clark JA, Pike BG: A personal computer based workstation for the planning of stereotactic neurosurgical procedures, in Kelly P (ed): Computers in Stereotactic Neurosurgery. Boston, Blackwell Scientific Publications, 1990, pp 195–208
69. Olivier A, Palmini A, Gloor P, Quesney FL: Chronic Stereotactic Electrocorticography. Ste-Adèle, Eastern EEG Association, 1990
70. Halgren E, Walter RD, Cherlow DG, Crandall PH: Mental phenomena evoked by electrical stimulation of the human hippocampal formation and amygdala. Brain 101:83–117, 1978
71. Jasper HH, Rasmussen T: Studies of clinical and electrical responses to deep temporal stimulation in man with some considerations of functional anatomy, in The Brain and Human Behaviour, 1958, 316–334
72. Olivier A, Bertrand G: Stereotaxic Implantation of Depth Electrodes for Seizure Monitoring. A Manual for the Neurosurgical and Anaesthesia Residents, the Operating Room and the X-Ray Technicians. Montreal, MNI Publications, 1982
73. Olivier A, Bertrand G: Stereotaxic device for percutaneous twist-drill insertion of depth electrodes and for brain biopsy. J Neurosurg 56:307–308, 1982
74. Peters TM, Olivier A, Bertrand G: The role of computed tomographic and digital radiographic techniques in stereotaxic procedures for electrode implantation and mapping and lesion localization. Proceedings of the American Society of Stereotaxic and Functional Neurosurgery. Durham, NC, 1983, Appl Neurophysiol 46:200–205, 1983
75. Olivier A, Marchand E, Ethier R, et al: A proposed anatomical methodology for MR scanning based on the corpus callosum. Proceedings of the Second International Meeting of Magnetic Resonance Imaging in Medicine, Montreal, 1986, pp 807–810

CHAPTER 103

Temporal Lobe Operations for Drug-Resistant Epilepsy

Robert G. Grossman
Winifred J. Hamilton

Complex partial seizures (CPS) are the most common form of seizure disorder, accounting for approximately 50 percent of newly diagnosed cases of epilepsy.[1] Approximately one-third of patients with CPS have unsatisfactory control of their seizures with antiepileptic drug therapy,[2] and many patients exhibit signs of drug toxicity at the doses that they must take to reduce the frequency of seizures. Frequent seizures and the side effects of medications may lead to secondary problems for patients with CPS, including intellectual impairment and social and psychological disturbances.[3] For many patients with CPS, anterior temporal lobectomy offers the possibility of a seizure-free, or nearly seizure-free, life and a reduced dependency on antiepileptic drugs.

The purpose of this chapter is to describe in detail and illustrate an operative technique for anterior temporal lobectomy, as well as to briefly discuss the issues involved in the selection of patients for surgery.

PATIENT SELECTION FOR TEMPORAL LOBECTOMY

It is beyond the scope of this chapter to fully discuss the variety of protocols that are used at different centers to select patients for anterior temporal lobectomy.[4, 5] Briefly, there are two general criteria for patient selection: (1) the demonstration of intractability of the seizures to medical management and (2) the concordance of electrophysiologic, neurologic, neuropsychological, and imaging data that indicate the right or the left anterior temporal lobe as the site of origin of the patient's characteristic seizures. The necessary conditions in this concordance are the demonstration of the site of seizure origin during three or more of the patient's typical seizures and the localization of that site to structures that can be removed without producing unacceptable deficits. This demonstration requires correlation of the behavioral pattern of the seizure with electrical recordings from the temporal lobes, as well as recordings from the frontal, occipital, and parietal lobes.

The correlation of video recording of behavior and cerebral electrical activity is carried out initially with recording of temporal lobe activity, generally with sphenoidal electrodes, using standard scalp electrode locations. The findings of such recordings fall into one of four categories: (1) localization of the seizures to either the right or the left temporal lobe; (2) bilateral localization of the origin of the seizures; (3) posterior temporal or extratemporal, usually frontal, localization of the origin of the seizures; and (4) the inability to localize the site of onset of the seizures. In our experience, approximately 60 percent of patients who have undergone sphenoidal recording have had recordings that fall into categories 1 to 3. Patients with recordings in category 1 are candidates for further investigation for surgery. Patients with recordings in category 4 are candidates for direct recording from the temporal lobe. To accomplish this, we use depth electrodes that are stereotactically inserted into the anterior hippocampus via a lateral temporal approach. We use a single electrode on each side; other groups use multiple electrodes.[6] An alternative method of depth recording is to penetrate the hippocampus along its anteroposterior axis via an occipital approach.[7] Subdural strip electrodes are probably the most widely used method of direct recording from the temporal lobe.[8] Each of these methods has its own benefits and risks.

The next step in patient selection is to determine the concordance of the site of seizure origin with other evidence of temporal lobe pathology, obtained from magnetic resonance imaging (MRI), positron-emission tomography (PET), and single photon–emission computed tomography (SPECT) studies, as well as from neuropsychological testing. The final step is to determine the risk of the surgery producing speech or memory deficits, on the basis of the data from neuropsychological testing and from the testing of memory during the suppression of temporal lobe function produced by intracarotid amobarbital (Amytal) injection (Wada's test).

RESECTION OF THE TEMPORAL LOBE FOR CONTROL OF COMPLEX PARTIAL SEIZURES

EXTENT OF TISSUE RESECTION

A discussion of the technique of anterior temporal lobectomy for the treatment of CPS should consider (1) the anatomic structures within the temporal lobe that should be excised, (2) the preoperative planning for the surgery, and (3) the intraoperative techniques for performing the resection.

With respect to the first point (i.e., the structures to be excised), epileptic discharges can be recorded in patients with CPS from the lateral temporal neocortex (the superior, middle, inferior, and fusiform temporal gyri), the parahippocampal gyrus, the hippocampal formation (Ammon's horn), the insula, the amygdala, and the uncus. All of these structures are possible sites for resection for seizure control. Four questions about the resection of these structures to obtain control of CPS should be considered: (1) Which of these anatomic structures must be excised to obtain seizure control? (2) Which specific areas and volumes of these structures must be removed? (3) What are the neurologic and neuropsychological deficits that can result from these resections? (4) What are the risks and benefits of alternative techniques for performing the resections?

Definitive answers cannot be given to these questions at the present time. The number of temporal lobectomies that have been performed worldwide and reported in detail is still small, and the lack of uniform criteria for patient selection, the grading of outcome, postoperative verification with MRI scanning of the structures removed, and the description of the pathology of the resected tissue has made it difficult to compare surgical series. The organization of a common data base for temporal lobe surgery should provide a basis for answering these questions.[9]

With this perspective in mind, in this chapter a surgical technique is described for the removal of a limited portion of the anterior lateral temporal neocortex, the anterior 3 cm of the parahippocampal gyrus, the anterior 3 cm of the hippocampal formation, and the amygdala. This operation, which is based on the use of microsurgical methods, represents an evolution in technique from the classic temporal lobectomy, in which a much larger area of the lateral temporal lobe was resected. The operation can be considered to hold an intermediate position between a classic lobectomy, and an amygdalo-hippocampectomy[10] as discussed in Chapter 104 of this volume. In radical hippocampectomy, discussed in Chapter 105 of this volume, the hippocampus is removed more posteriorly than the operation described here, while approximately the same amount of lateral temporal neocortex is removed.

The technique described in this chapter has been used in 125 consecutive anterior temporal lobectomies, of which 121 have been followed for periods of time from 6 months to 13 years (Table 103–1). Resection of these structures in the manner described here has provided excellent control of seizures (defined as a reduction in the frequency of seizures of 95 percent or more) in 97 percent of patients with classic Ammon's horn sclerosis (AHS) and in 80 percent of patients with a ganglioglioma, with no mortality and minimal morbidity. The relationship of outcome to the pathology of the resected tissue strongly suggests that the extent of temporal lobe resection necessary for the control of CPS varies with the underlying neuropathology that causes the seizures. Ammon's horn sclerosis is the pathologic change that is found most frequently in temporal lobectomy specimens. AHS is found in 50 to 60 percent of specimens in most series, followed in frequency by gangliogliomas in 20 to 30 percent of cases, then followed by neuronal loss and gliosis in a pattern not characteristic of AHS in about 10 percent of patients.[11–13] Cavernous angiomas, gliomas, and other structural lesions of the temporal lobe comprise the remainder of the pathologic substrates of CPS. It is possible that a more extensive resection of temporal tissue than described here may be needed to achieve control of seizures in some patients with gangliogliomas and with diffuse pathologic changes in the temporal lobe. It is also possible that a more limited resection than described here, such as stereotactic ablation of the anterior portion of Ammon's horn, might give equally good results in the control of CPS in patients with AHS.

Table 103–1. OUTCOME BY PATHOLOGY FOLLOWING ANTERIOR TEMPORAL LOBECTOMY FOR COMPLEX PARTIAL SEIZURES
(Follow-up Range: 6 months–13 years, N = 121)

Pathology	Outcome Category			
	1 (%)	2	3	4
Classical AHS (N = 58)	56 (97)	1	0	1
Possible AHS* (N = 11)	4 (36)	4	1	2
Atypical AHS (N = 2)	2 (100)	0	0	0
AHS and ganglioglioma (N = 3)	3 (100)	0	0	0
Ganglioglioma (N = 30)	24 (80)	3	1	2
Nonspecific changes (N = 9)	4 (44)	2	3	0
Miscellaneous tumor (N = 4)	4 (100)	0	0	0
Vascular malformations (N = 2)	2 (100)	0	0	0
Infarct (N = 2)	1 (50)	0	1	0
Total number	100	10	6	5
Percentage	83	8	5	4

*Insufficient specimen for pathologic diagnosis. Preoperative data and histology of the portions of the specimen received suggest AHS.
Outcome categories: 1 = ≥ 95-percent reduction in seizures; 2 = 75- to 94-percent reduction in seizures; 3 = 50- to 74-percent reduction in seizures; and 4 = < 50-percent reduction in seizures.

PREOPERATIVE PREPARATION OF THE PATIENT

The patient's anticonvulsant drug regimen is continued up to the time of surgery, with the exception of valproic acid or its derivatives, which may interfere with platelet function. The patient is typed and cross-matched for 2 units of blood as a precautionary measure, but transfusion is rarely needed. Blood loss occurs almost exclusively during the opening of the craniotomy and at its closure, and the loss rarely exceeds 100 ml. Corticosteroids (dexamethasone, 10 mg) are given at the time of the induction of anesthesia and, after surgery, at a dose of 4 mg every 6 hours for 3 days. An antibiotic is given at the start of surgery and for 24 hours after surgery.

ANESTHESIA

All of the temporal lobectomies in our series have been performed with the patient under general anesthesia. The anesthetic agents used at the present time are isoflurane and nitrous oxide, supplemented with fentanyl. Muscle paralysis is obtained with vecuronium. As indicated earlier, there are benefits and risks that are specific to each of the choices that can be made with respect to particular operative techniques. The use of general anesthesia precludes testing for localization of speech during the surgery. However, the risk of producing language dysfunction is small if only a limited portion of the lateral temporal neocortex is resected and the arterial supply and the venous drainage of the cortex are respected, as discussed later. The benefits of general anesthesia include the certainty of lack of movement of the patient during microsurgery, which is performed adjacent to the brainstem, and absolute control of the patient's airway.

ELECTROCORTICOGRAPHY

A full discussion of the role of electrocorticography as a guide to surgical resection is beyond the scope of this chapter. Electrocorticography has classically been used as a guide to tailoring the extent of the resection. We have used electrocorticography primarily for correlation with outcome and only to a minor extent in tailoring the resection.

If the surgery is performed with the patient under general anesthesia, prior to the performance of electrocorticography, the nitrous oxide is discontinued and the isoflurane concentration is reduced to 0.3 percent. The concentrations of anesthetic gases are monitored with mass spectroscopy. Recordings are obtained from the lateral temporal lobe, parahippocampal gyrus, insula, and hippocampus prior to and after tissue resection. Interictal spike discharges have been recorded from one or more of these structures in the majority of patients with varying pathologies. After a standardized resection has been completed, the majority of patients have exhibited residual spike discharges in tissue adjacent to the resection. Bordering spike-generating areas have been resected if their resection required removing only a small amount of additional tissue. The presence of residual spike discharges after the final resection has not been a predictor of poor control of seizures in patients with AHS. The resection described later has produced an excellent outcome for almost all patients with AHS, including those patients exhibiting residual spike discharges. However, the presence of residual spike discharges might be an indicator for a more extensive resection in patients with other pathologic findings in whom the resection described has produced excellent seizure control in only 44 to 80 percent of patients, depending on the underlying pathology. On the other hand, the control of seizures achieved with the technique described here has a success rate that is equivalent to that achieved in most series of temporal resections, some of which have used electrocorticography as a guide for tailoring of the extent of the resection.

PATIENT POSITIONING

The position used for this resection is similar to that used for a pterional craniotomy. The patient is positioned supine, with a roll under the shoulder and the back of the table moderately elevated to bring the head above the heart. The head is slightly extended and is turned 45 degrees, to bring the frontotemporal area uppermost. The head is held in place with three-point skull fixation. The table is rotated an additional 15 to 20 degrees to make the frontotemporal area more nearly horizontal.

OPERATIVE TECHNIQUE

The procedure can be divided into four stages: (1) craniotomy; (2) resection of the anterior lateral portion of the temporal lobe; (3) microsurgical resection of the amygdala, hippocampal formation, and parahippocampal gyrus; and (4) closure. Certain considerations are of primary importance in each of these stages.

Craniotomy

The major considerations in the design of the scalp and bone flaps are providing adequate exposure of the temporal lobe and the best cosmetic result. Because the object of the operation is to return the patient to as normal a life as possible, performing a craniotomy that is virtually undetectable by the patient and by others is of psychological benefit to the patient. A modified pterional craniotomy is used, as shown in Figure 103–1, using a smaller skin flap than that described by Yasargil for the surgery of aneurysms of the circle of Willis.

The skin incision is started at the hairline at the anterior portion of the superior temporal line, carried back along the temporal line to a point above the ear, and extended down along the anterior border of the ear to the root of the zygoma. The position of the superficial temporal artery should be identified by palpation prior to making the incision. The artery is avoided by an incision along the border of the ear. The outer layer of the fascia of the temporalis muscle is incised sharply below its insertion on the superior temporal line to leave a small cuff of fascia for reattaching the temporalis muscle. The posterior limb of the fascial incision is carried down to the root of the zygoma using scissors. The temporalis muscle fibers are incised with cutting current to expose the root of the zygoma, which is the posterior basal limit of the craniotomy (Fig. 103–1B, perforation 6). The anterior limb of the temporalis fascia incision is carried along the superior temporal line to expose the frontal process of the zygomatic bone. This exposure can usually be accomplished without extending the scalp incision onto the side of the forehead by cutting the galea with fine scissors beneath the skin. The temporalis muscle is elevated from the skull. The scalp and temporalis muscle, which is not separated from the galea, form a single flap, which is retracted with fishhook retractors attached to springs (Fig. 103–2A).

A free bone flap is made. The flap is cut with a Gigli saw superiorly and with a high-speed cutting burr inferiorly close to the zygoma. When the bone is replaced, it fits securely and without producing a hollow temporal contour. Three skull openings, about 3 cm apart, are made inferior to the superior temporal line with a perforator (Fig. 103–1B, perforations 1 to 3). A Kerrison rongeur is used to slightly enlarge the openings, to bevel the inner table of the bone, and to cut a channel for the passage of a Gigli saw. The dura is stripped away from the under surface of the skull with a modified #3 Penfield elevator. A Gigli saw is passed between adjacent perforations, and beveled cuts are made. The three inferior perforations are made with a 5-mm cutting burr and a high-speed drill. Perforations 4 and 5 straddle the outer third of the sphenoid wing. Perforation 4 is made on the hollow posterior surface of the frontal process of the zygomatic bone. Perforation 5 is made on the suture at the junction of the sphenoid wing and the temporal bone. Perforation 6 is made in the temporal bone at the root of the zygoma. A 3-mm cutting burr is used to cut a channel between perforations 5 and 6, and then between perforations 4 and 5, where

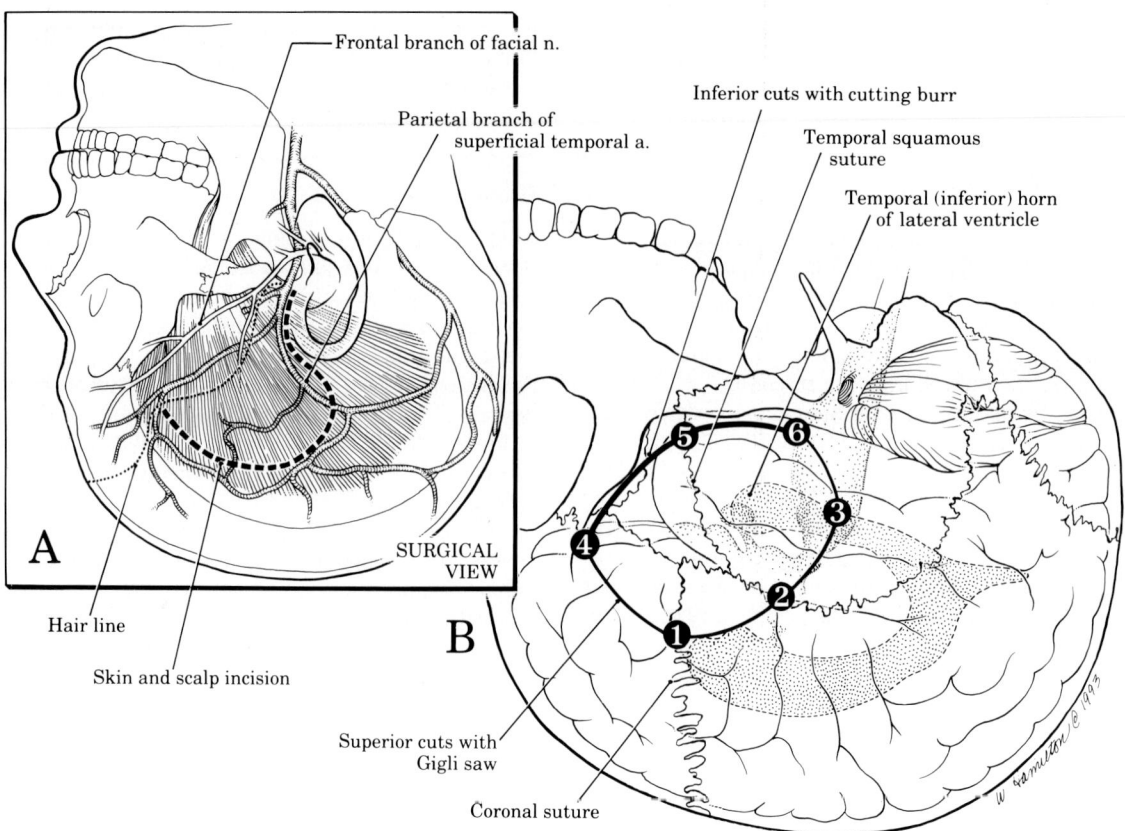

FIGURE 103–1. Right anterior temporal lobectomy. Operative orientation from the surgeon's perspective. (A) Scalp incision. (B) Position of the craniotomy in relationship to important anatomic structures, and the order in which skull perforations are made.

the middle meningeal artery may be encountered in the bone. The final cutting of the bone is performed with a 1-mm burr.

The bone flap is then elevated, and the middle meningeal artery is identified, cauterized, and cut. It is not necessary to drill down the lateral aspect of the sphenoid wing, as is done for exposure of the circle of Willis. Preserving the sphenoid wing preserves the normal temporal contour. Twist-drill holes are made in the margins of the craniotomy, and the dura is tacked up to the bone with 4-0 sutures. The dura is opened in a horseshoe-shaped flap, retracted back over the temporalis muscle, and protected with moist cottonoids to reduce shrinkage. The inferior frontal gyrus and 5 to 6 cm of the temporal lobe are exposed by the craniotomy. Electrocorticography may be carried out at this time from the lateral temporal lobe and from the frontal lobe with coronet or grid electrodes and from the undersurface of the temporal lobe with strip electrodes.

Resection of the Anterior Lateral Temporal Lobe

The major considerations in this portion of the operation are to avoid excision of too much of the lateral temporal lobe and interruption of arteries and veins supplying the more posterior portions of the temporal lobe. Language deficits developing after temporal lobectomy can result from interruption of branches of the middle cerebral artery, which leave the sylvian fissure and course over the superior and middle temporal gyri within the anterior 4 cm of the temporal lobe to ultimately supply the more posterior cortex. The superior portion of the resection should be tailored to avoid interrupting such vessels. The vein of Labbé lies at a distance of 4 to 6 cm from the temporal tip, and the vein should not be disturbed. The extent of the lateral temporal resection should be kept as small as possible compatible with exposure of the hippocampus in the floor of the temporal horn of the lateral ventricle. Planning of the resection should not be completely based on measurement of the length of resection along the long axis of the temporal lobe, particularly in children. The entire configuration of the temporal fossa should be assessed, and the resection should be kept anterior to the petrous ridge. The area of the brain to be resected is demarcated by thin sheets of rubber covered with moist cottonoids.

The initial resection is made along the superior temporal gyrus, using a fine microblade or microscissors to cut the pia-arachnoid (Fig. 103–2A and B; incision 1). Microbipolar cautery is used to coagulate vessels, and a fine suction tip is used to remove tissue. The incision is started at about 2 cm from the temporal tip and is inclined slightly laterally (toward the floor of the middle fossa) through the white matter of the superior temporal gyrus. At a depth of 1 to 2 cm, the gray matter of the cortex is encountered, and a small amount of cerebrospinal fluid (CSF) is usually recognized, indicating that the line of resection is passing along the sylvian fissure and the subarachnoid space of the insula. The incision is then carried posteriorly to a distance of 3.5 to 4 cm from the temporal tip.

The direction of the incision is then taken at a right angle to cross the long axis of the temporal lobe, and the incision

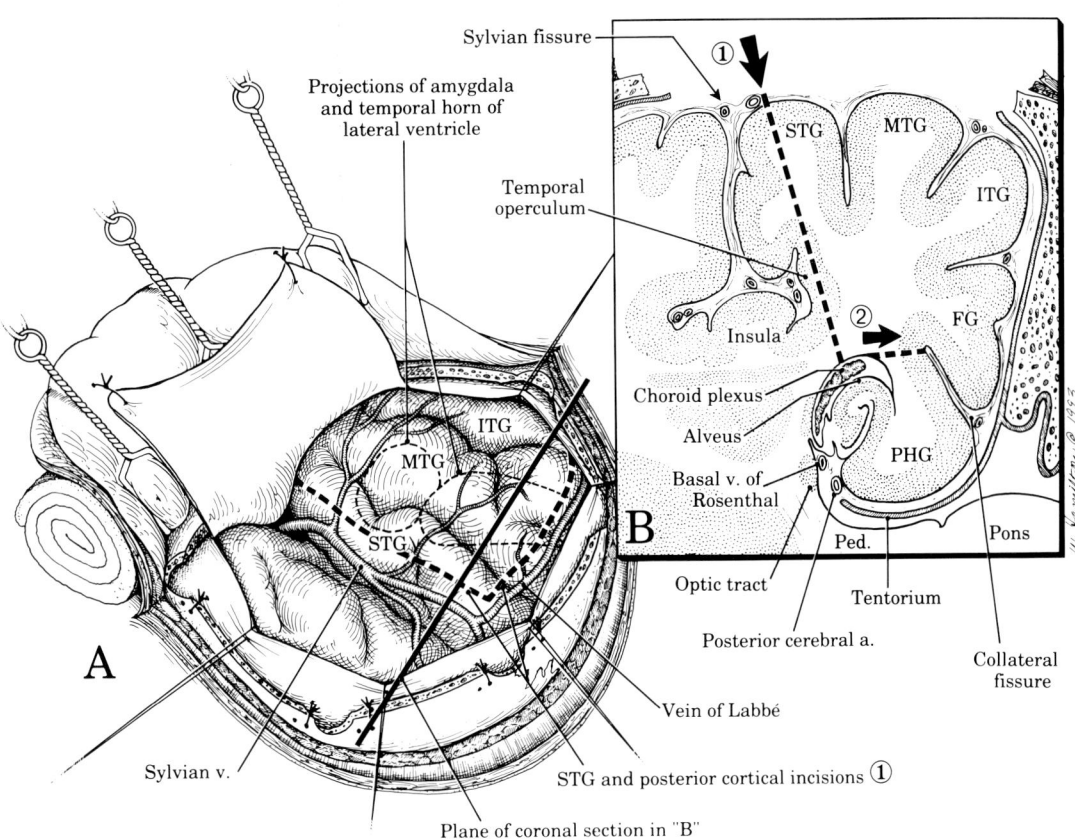

FIGURE 103–2. Lateral temporal resection. (A) Exposure of the lateral temporal lobe. The positions of the amygdala and the temporal horn of the lateral ventricle are indicated, as are the cortical incisions. (B) A coronal section through the right temporal lobe approximately 1 cm posterior to the tip of the hippocampal pes viewed from a posterior-to-anterior perspective. Cortical incision #1 through the STG is angled slightly laterally (toward the floor of the middle fossa) through the gray matter of the temporal operculum to the temporal horn of the lateral ventricle. FG = fusiform gyrus, ITG = inferior temporal gyrus, MTG = middle temporal gyrus, Ped. = peduncle, PHG = parahippocampal gyrus, STG = superior temporal gyrus.

is carried across the middle and inferior temporal gyri. The incision is carried deep into the gyri and is angled slightly posteriorly until the temporal horn of the lateral ventricle is entered. A small cottonoid is placed in the horn. Semisharp dissection through the white matter with a Freer dissector is useful in finding the temporal horn. The depth of the temporal horn from the cortical surface should be determined from the MRI scan; it almost always lies at a depth of 3.5 cm. Measurement of the depth of the incision with a ventricular cannula marked at 3.5 cm is useful as the incision is made.

The removal of tissue causes the anterior temporal lobe to retract away from the sphenoid wing, and the superior temporal gyrus incision is now extended up to the temporal tip. Veins draining from the sylvian fissure into the sphenoparietal sinus are preserved. The lateral temporal lobe is then removed by dissection in the white matter at the level of the temporal horn parallel to the cortical surface (Fig. 103–2B; incision 2). This incision will reach the collateral fissure and the fusiform gyrus on the floor of the middle fossa. Incision of the pia-arachnoid of the fusiform gyrus is started posteriorly and is carried anteriorly. The lateral temporal lobe is lifted upward, and the most anteromedial portion of the cortex is removed subpially. The pia-arachnoid of the anteromedial cortex is cut, and the specimen is removed. The insula and the hippocampus areas are exposed. Recording is carried out from these structures and from the frontal and temporal lobes adjacent to the resection.

Resection of the Amygdala, Hippocampus, and Parahippocampal Gyrus

This part of the operation is performed with the aid of the operating microscope. The major consideration is to avoid injury to the posterior cerebral artery. An understanding of the vascular anatomy of the temporal lobe is essential. There is an excellent illustration of this anatomy in the paper by Yasargil and associates on amygdalo-hippocampectomy.[10] A second consideration is that a large amount of CSF is removed by suction during this stage of the surgery, which results in the cortex falling away from the dura and the stretching of draining cortical veins. This problem can result in avulsion of the posterior inferior temporal veins that drain into the petrosal sinus, causing profuse hemorrhage. Therefore, replacement of CSF should be carried out frequently by irrigation of the basal cisterns with saline or artificial CSF.

A third precaution is to avoid compressing the medial aspect of the temporal horn with a retractor blade, which can damage the basal ganglia beneath it. The use of extremely stable self-retaining retractors with tapered blades greatly facilitates this portion of the operation. The most anterior portion of the temporal horn is held open, with the retractor blades placed on the medial and lateral walls (Fig. 103–3B). The walls are protected with rubber strips (not shown in the figure). An incision is made with bipolar cautery and suction from the tip of the choroid fissure to the anteromedial edge of the mesial temporal lobe (Fig. 103–3B, incision 3). The incision is carried through the amygdala, which is removed by aspiration, down to the pia-arachnoid of the anterior medial parahippocampal cortex. Through the pia-arachnoid, it is possible to see the tentorial edge and incisura, and the oculomotor nerve and posterior cerebral artery (Fig. 103–3C). The pia-arachnoid is cut over the tentorium.

The retractors are then moved posteriorly to the level of the choroid plexus. A third retractor is placed posteriorly against the overlying temporal lobe to facilitate exposure. The medial retractor is placed on the choroid plexus, which is retracted gently, thereby exposing the pia-arachnoid of the choroid fissure. The fimbria and alveus are then removed from the body of the hippocampus with suction (Fig. 103–3C). The aspiration of these structures reveals the edge of the hippocampal fissure. A veil of arachnoid extends from the choroidal fissure into the hippocampal fissure. The arachnoid surrounds a vein 3 to 4 mm in diameter (Fig. 103–3A and C). The vein is coagulated, and the vein and the arachnoid are cut with microscissors (Fig. 103–3A and D, incision 5). This incision exposes the superior edge of the subiculum (Fig. 103–3D). Arterial branches also enter the hippocampal fissure posterior to the vein, and if the posterior hippocampus is resected, these vessels also are coagulated and cut.

The posterior cerebral artery and its branches that supply the undersurface of the temporal lobe have a variable relationship to the subiculum. The posterior cerebral artery can be strongly attached to the subiculum and can lie laterally. Great care should be taken to ascertain the course of the posterior cerebral artery as it courses posteriorly from the anterior incisura, where it can be easily seen. The hippocampus and subiculum could be removed en bloc at this point by detaching the subicular pia-arachnoid from the vasculature covering it. However, it is safer to remove these structures with a subpial subicular incision. This incision traverses the subiculum and reaches the pia-arachnoid of the parahippocampal gyrus (Figs. 103–3A and 3E, incision 6). To perform this incision, the hippocampus and parahippocampal gyrus are retracted slightly laterally so that they lie on the tentorium (Fig. 103–3E). The subicular incision is started anteriorly at the rostral edge of the tentorium and is carried down to the tentorium (Fig. 103–3E). The incision is continued posteriorly, keeping the incision on the tentorium. As branches of the posterior cerebral artery are encountered in the pia-arachnoid of the subiculum, they are coagulated and cut. The incision is carried posteriorly for 3 cm from the anterior tip of the pes in the temporal horn. The resection extends about 1 cm posterior to the vein entering the hippocampal fissure. This incision frees the medial edge of the specimen. To completely detach the specimen, an incision is made at right angles to the long axis of the hippocampus through the parahippocampal gyrus and the hippocampus (Fig. 103–3E, incision 7, and Fig. 103–3F).

In the great majority of patients in our series, the uncus has not been removed. The uncus can be removed subpially with suction, taking care not to damage fine perforating vessels going to the brainstem from the posterior communicating, choroidal, and posterior cerebral arteries.

Electrical recording from the hippocampal stump and other structures is carried out at this point. Cut surfaces are then covered with a single layer of oxidized regenerated cellulose (Surgicel).

Closure

The subarachnoid space is filled with saline. The dura is closed in a watertight fashion with running continuous 4-0 nonabsorbable sutures. Occasionally, a small patch graft of lyophilized human dura or pericranium is required to obtain watertight closure. An epidural drain is placed. The bone flap is secured in position with 3-0 Vicryl sutures passed through the twist-drill holes in the bone flap and in the skull. The temporalis muscle is closed with 2-0 Vicryl, and the muscle fascia closed with another layer of 2-0 Vicryl. The perforator openings are small, and they are covered by the closure of the fascia. The galea is closed with 3-0 Vicryl, and the skin is closed with staples.

OUTCOME

COMPLICATIONS

Serious complications following anterior temporal lobectomy are rare.[14] Of the 125 consecutive anterior temporal lobectomies in our series, there were no deaths, infections, need for large blood transfusions, or hemiparesis after surgery. Transient paresis of cranial nerves III or IV was seen in three patients. Three patients in our series exhibited aphasias, which improved over time.

Contralateral superior quadrantanopia has been reported to occur in approximately 50 percent of patients following classic temporal lobectomy.[14] This field defect is thought to result from interruption of the optic radiation fibers in Meyer's loop in the temporal lobe. The incidence of a field defect is lower when the amount of lateral temporal lobe resected is restricted to 3.5 to 4 cm.

SEIZURE CONTROL

Accurate comparison of outcomes among various centers is difficult because different methodologies are used to select patients and to assess outcome. A 1991 survey conducted by Engel and associates included outcome statistics on 3579 patients from 100 epilepsy centers who underwent anterior temporal lobectomy for CPS between 1986 and 1990.[9] Of these patients, 2429 (67.9 percent) were seizure free following surgery and 860 (24.0 percent) were improved.

In our series of 121 patients who underwent anterior temporal lobectomy for CPS and who have been followed for periods ranging from 6 months to 13 years (Table 103–1), 100 patients (83 percent) experienced a 95-percent or better reduction in their seizures following surgery. As a group, the patients with classic AHS (hippocampal sclerosis in CA1, CA3, CA4, and the dentate gyrus) had the best outcome. Among the 58 patients with classic AHS, 56 (97 percent) experienced a 95-percent or better reduction in seizures following surgery. Of these 56 patients, 36 (64 percent) were entirely free of auras and seizures, and 16 (29 percent) had

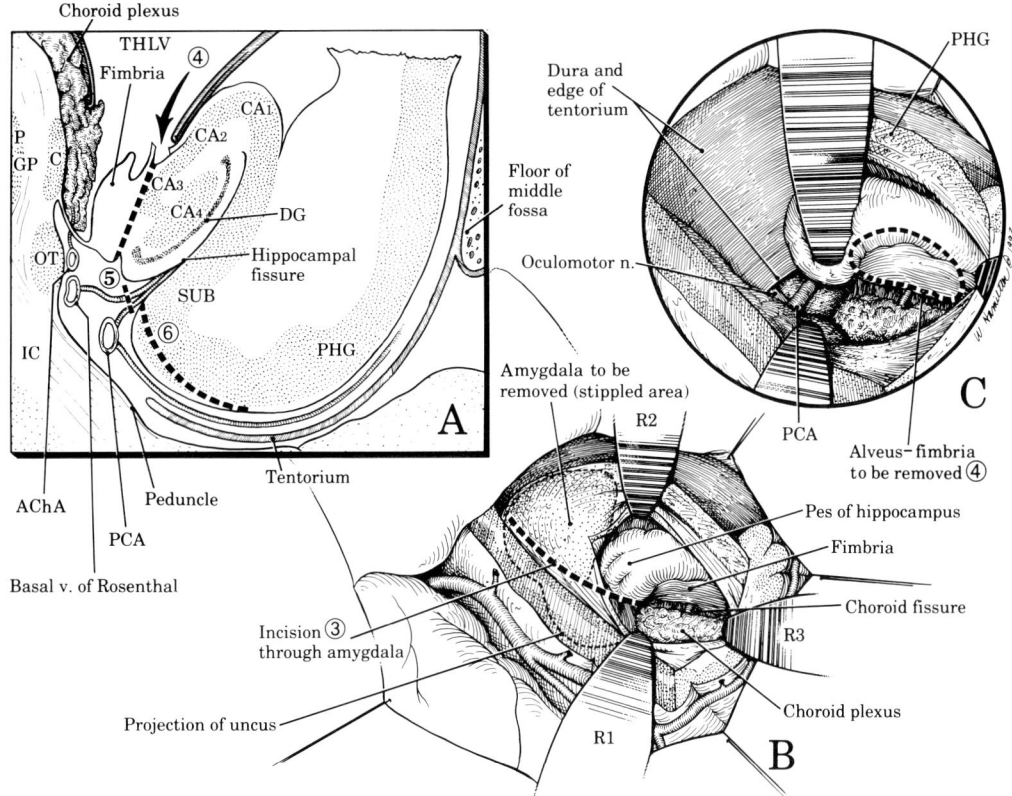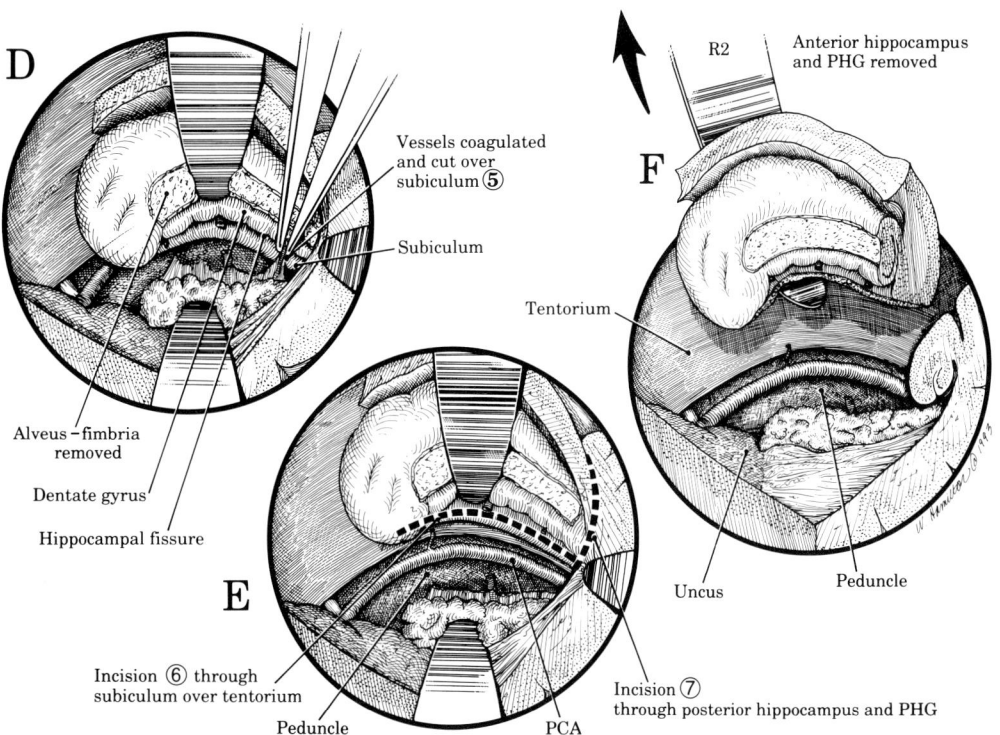

FIGURE 103–3. Microsurgical resection of the amygdala, hippocampus and parahippocampal gyrus. (A) Coronal section of the right mesial temporal lobe viewed from a posterior-to-anterior perspective showing orienting anatomy and incisions. (B) Exposure of the amygdala and the hippocampus following removal of the anterior lateral temporal lobe. The temporal horn is opened, showing the pes of the hippocampus and the choroid plexus. Incision #3, from the choroid fissure through the amygdala, is indicated; the stippled area will be removed with suction. (C) The amygdala and anterior medial parahippocampal gyrus have been removed, revealing the tentorium, PCA, and oculomotor nerve. The dotted line indicates incision #4 into the alveus. (D) The alveus-fimbria has been removed. The vein entering the hippocampal fissure is coagulated and cut, working over the subiculum. (E) The hippocampus is retracted very slightly laterally over the tentorium. The position of the PCA is kept in mind as the hippocampal specimen is detached medially (incision #6), and posteriorly (incision #7). (F) The anterior hippocampus and parahippocampal gyrus are removed. AChA = anterior choroidal artery, C = tail of the caudate, CA1 to CA4 = areas of Ammon's horn (cornu ammonis) of the hippocampus, DG = dentate gyrus, GP = globus pallidus, IC = intercommissural fibers, OT = optic tract, P = putamen, PCA = posterior cerebral artery, PHG = parahippocampal gyrus, R1 to R3 = retractors 1 to 3, SUB = subiculum, THLV = temporal horn of the lateral ventricle.

rare seizures or auras with identifiable precipitating causes only, generally as a result of stopping anticonvulsant medication. Of the 56 AHS patients with excellent results following surgery, 39 (70 percent) were taking significantly reduced levels of antiepileptic medication at the time of their most recent follow-up, including eight patients (21 percent) who had been able to stop antiepileptic medications entirely. If all patients with a pattern of hippocampal sclerosis (classic AHS; probable AHS, but insufficient specimen for pathologic diagnosis; atypical AHS; and AHS and a ganglioglioma; N = 74) are considered as a group, 65 (88 percent) experienced a 95-percent or better reduction in the frequency of their seizures.

As noted earlier, patients with pathologic findings other than AHS in general did slightly less well. Of the patients with a ganglioglioma (N = 30), who represent the second largest group of patients, 24 (80 percent) experienced a 95-percent or better reduction in the frequency of seizures. Approximately one-quarter of these patients were able to discontinue antiepileptic medications. Patients whose specimen displayed nonspecific changes (N = 9) had the poorest outcome, with 4 (44 percent) experiencing a reduction of 95 percent or better in the occurrence of seizures postoperatively.

NEUROPSYCHOLOGICAL OUTCOME

A loss of material-specific memory is noted in most patients who undergo an anterior temporal lobectomy that includes the excision of mesial temporal structures. In our series of patients, a comparison of preoperative and postoperative testing revealed that verbal memory was more affected than spatial memory and that, as expected, a decline in verbal memory was more likely to occur following a left temporal resection. Patients with a right-sided resection or with pathologic findings of AHS exhibited the least postoperative memory decline. This second finding concurs with a study by Hermann and colleagues, in which they found that patients with moderate or severe hippocampal sclerosis had significantly less change in their memory following anterior temporal lobectomy than did patients with no or mild hippocampal sclerosis.[15]

A significant increase in attention span and in perceptual organization was seen in nearly all patients with AHS and in most patients with a left-sided procedure following surgery. This is probably the reason that intelligence scores were modestly higher in most patients following surgery, although the change was not statistically significant. Other series have reported similar findings.[16] In our series, AHS patients showed greater improvement in intelligence scores following surgery than did patients with other types of pathology, although patients with AHS typically had slightly lower intelligence scores preoperatively.

Patients who were seizure free following surgery generally reported significantly decreased levels of anxiety and depression, as well as a greater sense of self-confidence and independence. For many patients, obtaining a driver's license was particularly important and allowed them to expand their educational, employment, and social choices significantly. Patients with long-standing emotional and social problems often improved less than would be expected based on the postoperative control of their seizures, a finding that has been reported in other series as well.[17]

REFERENCES

1. Hauser WA: The natural history of temporal lobe epilepsy, in Lüders HO (ed): Epilepsy Surgery. New York, Raven Press, 1992, pp 133–141
2. Juul-Jensen P. Epidemiology of intractable epilepsy, in Schmidt D, Morselli PL (eds): Intractable Epilepsy. New York, Raven Press, 1986, pp 5–11
3. Trimble MR: Psychiatric aspects of epilepsy. Psychiatr Dev 5:285–300, 1987
4. Engel J Jr, Levesque M, Crandall PH, et al: The epilepsies, in Grossman RG, Hamilton WJ (eds): Principles of Neurosurgery. New York, Raven Press, 1991, pp 319–358
5. Walsh AR, Ojemann GA: Anterior temporal lobectomy for epilepsy. Clin Neurosurg 38:535–547, 1992
6. Engel J Jr, Henry TR, Risinger MW, et al: Presurgical evaluation for partial epilepsy: Relative contributions of chronic depth-electrode recordings versus FDG-PET and scalp-sphenoidal ictal EEG. Neurology 40:1670–1677, 1990
7. Spencer SS, Spencer DD, Williamson PD, Mattson RH: The localizing value of depth electroencephalography in 32 patients with refractory epilepsy. Ann Neurol 12:248–253, 1982
8. Weinand ME, Wyler AR, Richey ET, et al: Long-term ictal monitoring with subdural strip electrodes: Prognostic factors for selecting temporal lobectomy candidates. J Neurosurg 77:20–28, 1992
9. Engel J Jr, Van Ness PC, Rasmussen TB, Ojemann LM: Outcome with respect to epileptic seizures, in Engel J Jr (ed): Surgical Treatment of the Epilepsies, 2nd ed. New York, Raven Press, 1993, pp 609–621
10. Yasargil MG, Teddy PJ, Roth P: Selective amygdalo-hippocampectomy: Operative anatomy and surgical technique, in Symon L, Brihaye J, Guidetti B, et al (eds): Advances and Technical Standards in Neurosurgery. New York, Springer-Verlag, 1985, pp 93–123
11. Armstrong DD, Bruton CJ: Postscript: What terminology is appropriate for tissue pathology? How does it predict outcome? in Engel J Jr (ed): Surgical Treatment of the Epilepsies. New York, Raven Press, 1987, pp 541–552
12. Duncan JS, Sagar HJ: Seizure characteristics, pathology, and outcome after temporal lobectomy. Neurology 37:405–409, 1987
13. Vinters HV, Armstrong DL, Babb TL, et al: The neuropathology of human symptomatic epilepsy, in Engel J Jr (ed): Surgical Treatment of the Epilepsies, 2nd ed. New York, Raven Press, 1993, pp 593–608
14. Pilcher WH, Roberts DW, Flanigin HF, et al: Complications of epilepsy surgery, in Engel J Jr (ed): Surgical Treatment of the Epilepsies, 2nd ed. New York, Raven Press, 1993, pp 565–581
15. Hermann BP, Wyler AR, Somes G, et al: Pathological status of the mesial temporal lobe predicts memory outcome from left anterior temporal lobectomy. Neurosurgery 31:652–657, 1992
16. Dodrill CB, Hermann BP, Rausch R, et al: Neuropsychological testing for assessing prognosis following surgery for epilepsy, in Engel J Jr (ed): Surgical Treatment of the Epilepsies, 2nd ed. New York, Raven Press, 1993, pp 263–271
17. Hermann BP, Wyler AR, Somes G: Preoperative psychological adjustment and surgical outcome are determinants of psychosocial status after anterior temporal lobectomy. J Neurol Neurosurg Psychiatry 55:491–496, 1992

CHAPTER 104

Amygdalo-Hippocampectomy for Drug-Resistant Temporal Lobe Epilepsy

C. E. Polkey

The object of this chapter is to discuss the place of selective amygdalo-hippocampectomy in the treatment of drug-resistant epilepsy of temporal lobe origin so that the best seizure control is obtained with minimal morbidity and mortality and with regard to the other temporal lobe resections available.

The development and diversification of unilateral temporal lobe resections for drug-resistant epilepsy has been dependent on the philosophies behind the detection of seizure origin and technical advances in neurosurgery. These resections evolved from the superficial corticectomies performed by the early pioneers based on electrical evidence,[1] to more extensive resections involving the mesial temporal structures,[2] including the realization of the importance of pathology in determining outcome.[3] There has always been an element of idiosyncrasy in the precise limits of temporal lobe resections, as has been recently shown in reviews of the extensive Montreal experience.[4,5] Recently, new developments have focused on the mesial temporal structures with the revival of selective amygdalo-hippocampectomy by Wieser and Yasargil,[6] and the new procedure of extended hippocampal removal described by Spencer and his colleagues.[7] The numerous alternatives present a bewildering array of possibilities to those unfamiliar to the field and an intriguing intellectual challenge to others. Therefore, it is important to compare the procedure of selective amygdalo-hippocampectomy with alternative temporal lobe resections, as well as to review the various techniques of performing amygdalo-hippocampectomy.

The genesis and propagation of temporal lobe seizures is a complex subject in itself. It is clear from the results of various temporal lobe resections that there is a definite but imprecise relationship between pathology and the origin of the electrical seizures. In contrast to other parts of the cortical mantle, surgery that involves only removal of the lesion is not always efficient in the temporal lobe. Cascino and associates found low rates of seizure relief after lesionectomy within the temporal lobe compared with other parts of the cortical mantle.[8] Therefore, judgments have to be made about the correct surgical procedure considering both the structural pathology and the neurophysiologic findings in any particular case.

Cognitive function, especially recent memory, forms a major part of the normal function of the temporal lobe, together with some less well-defined effects on personality. Therefore, it is necessary to consider the possible effect of any proposed resection on these functions in each patient. This is especially important because physical neurologic disability or death are relatively rare sequelae to modern temporal lobe surgery, whereas intellectual change is more common; although intellectual change is rarely devastating, it can still be disabling.

SELECTION CRITERIA

It is appropriate to deal briefly with the selection criteria for temporal lobe surgery and how these help determine which patients are suitable for amygdalo-hippocampectomy. None of the various temporal lobe resections rely on a single mechanism for the control or relief of seizures. Indeed a number of mechanisms may be invoked that include the removal of structural pathology, the disruption of neuronal connections and pathways, and a reduction in the mass of epileptogenic neurones available to participate in the seizure. These last two neuronal mechanisms are of particular importance in the temporal lobe. Recent studies have shown that the neuronal connections of the amygdala to other parts of the brain are more extensive than has been previously realized, as summarized by Olivier.[9] Some specialists also believe that there is an amplifying circuit between the deep structures in the hippocampus and the lateral neocortex whose interruption can help reduce the frequency of seizures.[10] This factor may provide the explanation for the limited success of neocortical resection, including the modern results reported by Hardiman and colleagues.[11]

PREOPERATIVE INVESTIGATION

For reasons already given, the general assessment of patients for temporal lobe surgery is covered and, subsequently, indications are given as to which findings favor amygdalo-hippocampectomy. Such investigation is essentially a multidisciplinary task. All investigations must start with a detailed clinical history, which should include a thorough scrutiny of previous clinical notes, enquiry about handedness, evidence from observers regarding the nature and frequency of the seizures, educational background, and a history of any psychiatric or behavioral disturbances. Briefly, the interictal history may suggest the causes for pathology in the temporal lobe, and the ictal history may enable one to localize the origin of the seizures within the brain. Not all partial seizures originate in the temporal lobe. Those with a prolonged initial phase are more likely to do so, whereas those with a tendency for rapid secondary generalization are more likely to be frontal in origin. However, secondary generalization, or the occurrence of generalized seizures as well as partial seizures, are not necessarily a contraindication to successful temporal lobe surgery. Except in the case of severe and obvious pathology, neurologic signs are usually absent. A more detailed discussion of these points is found in our review of surgery for epilepsy.[12]

At this point, it is important to introduce the twin concepts of concordance and redundancy in the assessment of patients for resective surgery for epilepsy. Concordance means that the clinical and neurophysiologic data, structural and functional brain imaging, and neuropsychological profile all point to a common target. Redundancy ensures that if such a target exists, it should be identified with minimal effort. This is especially important because after the basic clinical evaluation, further tests may involve an element of discomfort and risk for the patient and also may be extremely costly. It also explains why one center may use one test in preference to another because both may provide the same results through different methods.

In our own center, we use phased management, in which the patients proceed from one phase to another, the tests becoming more complex with each phase until a definite decision is made to operate or the patient is regarded as inoperable. In Table 104–1, the fates of 105 patients entering the preoperative assessment program are summarized.

PHASE 1A

This phase comprises a detailed clinical history and examination, followed by a routine and sleep electroencephalogram (EEG) with appropriate electrode placements, a neuropsychological profile,[13] and preliminary structural brain imaging according to a locally agreed-on protocol sufficient to detect a discrete lesion in the temporal lobe or mesial temporal sclerosis. Although magnetic resonance imaging (MRI) is preferred because of the high detection rate for discrete lesions and the improved detection rate for mesial temporal sclerosis, fourth-generation computed tomography (CT) scans can give useful results, especially if the slices are appropriately angled.[14]

At this point, it is probably useful to make a distinction between focal discrete lesions in the temporal lobe, such as cavernous hemangiomas, low-grade glial tumors, and dysembryoplastic neuroepithelial tumors and more subtle lesions, such as cortical dysplasia and mesial temporal sclerosis. This distinction is of importance because, in practice, a certain laxity can be accepted in the neurophysiologic criteria for surgery in the presence of a discrete focal lesion.

Without laboring the point, it is essential that all these preliminary investigations should be performed in a manner that meets high standards and in such a way as to answer the question being asked in a positive manner, where possible.

CASE REPORT 1: DISCRETE LESION

SR is a right-handed schoolboy who was 9 years of age at operation. The child has had epilepsy since age 5 years, partial complex seizures nonlateralizing, over 50 per month. A calcified mass was found on CT scan in the right temporal region (Fig. 104–1). A widespread abnormality was discovered with a scalp EEG, with interictal spikes found on the right. Verbal IQ 119, Performance IQ 109.

The child underwent a right amygdalo-hippocampectomy on July 7, 1987. The diagnosis was astrocytoma.

During the first 2 years after surgery, the child experienced an occasional aura but no seizures. No AED since January 1990. SR has made normal progress and attends a normal school. The child was last seen 5 years after surgery.

PHASE 1B

This phase is used to lateralize between left and right and also to establish localization of the seizures within the hemisphere and, where possible, distinguish between medial and lateral seizure foci in the temporal lobe. Three kinds of tests are involved—functional brain imaging, carotid amobarbital (Amytal) testing, and invasive neurophysiological testing with videotelemetry.

Functional brain imaging can be achieved in a number of ways, most of which relate to interictal examination, although single photon–emission computed tomography (SPECT) is probably only useful in ictal examination. FDG-PET has been in use for many years, initially by Engel and colleagues, who have described lateralized hypometabolism in relation to electrical foci in the temporal lobe.[15–17] Wieser and colleagues have also described the preoperative findings in patients subsequently admitted to undergo selective amygdalo-hippocampectomy and the postoperative changes in these patients. They note that the area of hypometabolism indicated by the PET scan is always larger than the proposed area of resection and that, not only does it persist for at least 1 year after surgery, but the hypometabolism and its persistence bear no relation to outcome.[18, 19] With SPECT, there is a reliable lateralization and even localization within the temporal lobe, provided that ictal SPECT is used, but this examination does involve injection of the HMPAO within a short time of the beginning of the seizure.[20–23] It is hoped that magnetic resonance spectroscopy will become useful in the future, but at present, it is only a research tool.[24, 25]

The Wada test should now be considered. In the traditional form of this test, sodium amytal is injected into one internal carotid artery, and the speech and memory functions of that

Table 104–1. FATE OF 105 PATIENTS ENTERING EPILEPSY SURGERY PROGRAM FOR ALL OPERATIONS

Management Phase	Number of Patients	Fate		
		Operate	Reject	To Next Phase
1A	105	35	5	65
1B	65	30	10	25
II	25	15	10	—

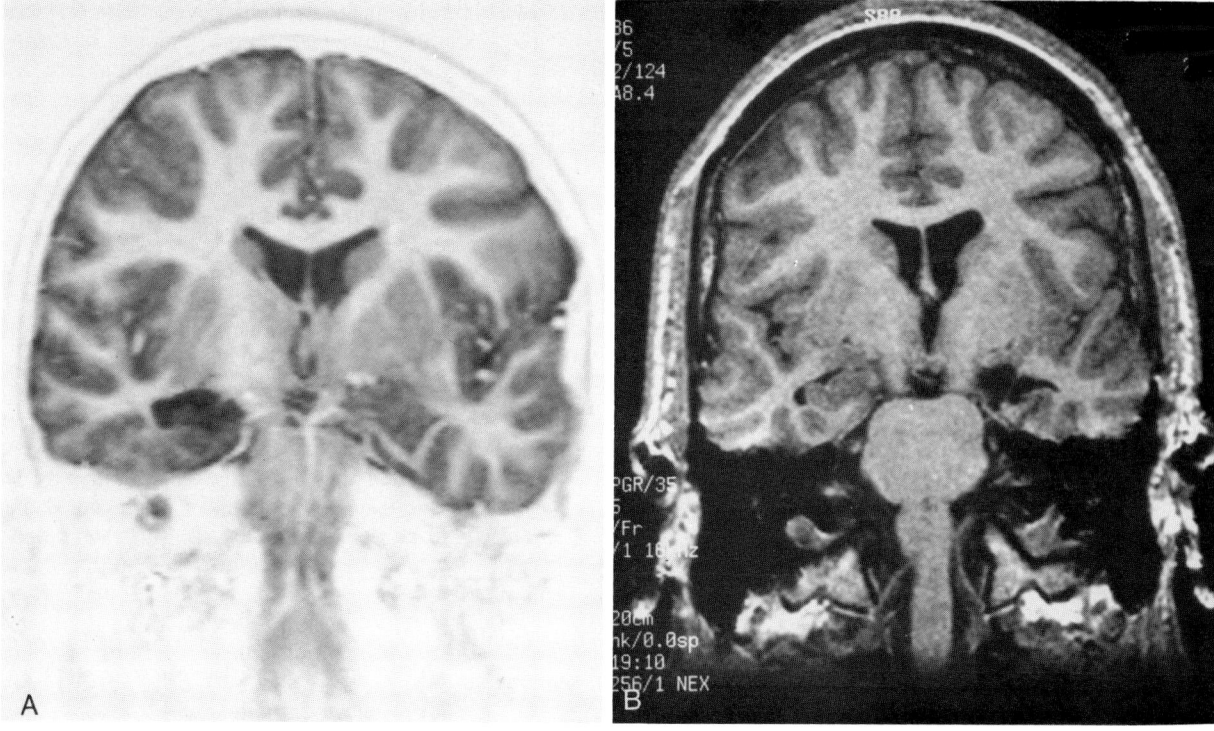

FIGURE 104–1. Postoperative coronal MRI scans showing the extent of the amygdalo-hippocampectomy. (A) Patient SR; (B) another patient who had MTS in the specimen.

hemisphere are examined during the few minutes that it is under the influence of the drug. There are numerous variations as to how this test is performed.[26] In addition, there are a number of selective carotid Amytal tests that aim to restrict the distribution of the Amytal to smaller vessels supplying only the hippocampus or parts thereof.[27, 28] It is difficult to demonstrate that these tests, which can be more difficult and dangerous than the traditional test, have any advantage when it comes to comparing the results of acting on the findings of the tests. There is evidence from animal experiments, imaging studies following stroke, and the results of surgery that both the deep temporal structures and the neocortex play a part in normal short-term memory.[29] This proposition relates to normal function and does not take any account of the influence of temporal lobe pathology on the distribution of memory between the temporal lobes. We have shown some time ago that the material-specific cognitive deficit that occurs as a result of unilateral temporal lobectomy (which was first described by Milner[30]) depends on the underlying pathology. When one temporal lobe is rendered nonfunctional from an early age, as for example with mesial temporal sclerosis following a febrile convulsion, then there is little intellectual penalty following unilateral temporal lobectomy.[13] However, in patients in whom there is normal temporal lobe function, it would seem to be an advantage to preserve the lateral neocortex during temporal lobe resection.

By means of invasive neurophysiologic methods, it is possible to establish the precise origin of seizures within the temporal lobe. A controversy is beginning to arise as to whether there is any need to carry out these sophisticated investigations if one can show that there is unilateral temporal lobe pathology through the use of MRI imaging. In the next few years, a series may be published describing the selection of patients for temporal lobe resection on structural imaging grounds alone. In that case, it may be necessary to reverse our present view that for a restricted operation, such as amygdalo-hippocampectomy, it is probably necessary to perform invasive tests in the absence of the discrete focal pathology described earlier to prove the mesial origin of the seizures with neurophysiologic evidence.[31]

The most convenient way to perform the examination is by using videotelemetry with foramen ovale electrodes, which was first described by Wieser and colleagues.[32] Multicontact electrodes are inserted on each side through a cannula passed through the foramen ovale while the patient is under general anaesthesia, so that the electrodes come to lie against the medial side of the temporal lobe. Wieser validated the findings for these electrodes by examining recordings from temporal lobe depth electrodes in the same patient. By this means, he was able to establish that there is a mesiobasal onset for the seizures, which he regarded correctly as an essential condition for amygdalo-hippocampectomy in the absence of a discrete focal abnormality on structural imaging.

CASE REPORT 2: MESIAL TEMPORAL SCLEROSIS WITH FORAMEN OVALE TELEMETRY

MM was aged 22 years at operation. It was noted that the patient suffered a 20-minute febrile convulsion at 1 year of age. PCS since aged 3 years with an epigastric aura and dysphasia. The patient has an average of 15 seizures per month. CT was not helpful, VIQ 80, PIQ 81. The patient had bilateral memory deficits. Wada's test showed that the patient was left hemisphere dominant, with memory in both hemispheres. Scalp EEG and FO videotelemetry showed that the left medial temporal region was the origin for the patient's seizures.

A left amygdalo-hippocampectomy was performed on February 9, 1988. The tissue diagnosis was mesial temporal sclerosis.

During the first 2 years following surgery, the patient experienced occasional auras, which decreased in frequency and had no seizures. AED was reduced. MM went on to become a nurse; there was no gross intellectual change. The patient was last seen 4 years after surgery.

PHASE II

If these tests fail to clarify the issue, and it is believed that surgery has not been totally ruled out, then it may be necessary to proceed to complex invasive neurophysiology employing some form of depth electrode or possibly subdural strip exploration of the temporal lobe. Again, there is a very large variety of ways in which this procedure can be achieved, and this will be fully covered in later chapters. Our own preference is to use a combination of subdural and depth electrodes, which was first described by Van Veelen and others.[33] Among the 42 patients who underwent amygdalo-hippocampectomy between 1987 and 1992, three were operated on without invasive neurophysiology, the remaining 39 patients were investigated with foramen ovale electrodes, and five of these required further investigation with subdural and depth electrodes.

CASE REPORT 3: AMYGDALO-HIPPOCAMPECTOMY SELECTION WITH DEPTH ELECTRODES

CM was aged 34 years at operation and is a left-handed typist. Prolonged FC occurred at aged 15 months. She has had chronic epilepsy since she was 23 years of age (1977). She has stomach aura and pcs. The patient suffers from 20 attacks per month. VIQ 99, PIQ 111. There is impairment of the patient's visuospatial memory. When the Wada test was performed, it was discovered that the patient was right hemisphere dominant for speech. CT was not helpful. Scalp telemetry revealed a right temporal focus. FO electrodes, left onset with rapid switch to right. Subdural and depth electrodes confirmed onset of the seizure in the left hippocampus, with a rapid switch to the right.

A left amygdalo-hippocampectomy was performed on November 10, 1988. The tissue diagnosis was mesial temporal sclerosis. The patient has been free of seizures since the operation. She is on carbamazepine to keep her driver's license. The patient was last seen 4 years after surgery.

MANAGEMENT DECISIONS

At the end of this preoperative evaluation, which in spite of the brief summary given here may be long and difficult, the multidisciplinary team may be in a position to make a recommendation regarding the site and the nature of the surgical resection.

In making this recommendation, the results of the tests described can be related to one of three areas:
1. The presence of a discrete focal structural lesion in one temporal lobe,
2. Evidence of a functional deficit in one temporal lobe,
3. Evidence of seizure onset in one temporal lobe and the location of that seizure onset within the temporal lobe.

With this evidence, the following decision tree can be used:
I. Does the evidence favor one temporal lobe as the surgical target, or does it indicate the involvement of extratemporal cortex, which requires a combined approach?
II. If the evidence favors one temporal lobe, is there a discrete focal structural lesion within that temporal lobe?
   A. If so, is that lesion within an area that can be encompassed by a selective amygdalo-hippocampectomy?
   B. If so, is there evidence of cognitive function within that temporal lobe that requires the surgeon to attempt to minimize cognitive damage?
   Note: If there is no cognitive function to be preserved, a larger resection may be preferred for other reasons, such as ease of access. It should also be noted that if there is a discrete structural lesion in the lateral neocortex, it may often be desirable to resect the mesial temporal structures as well for reasons mentioned earlier.
III. If no discrete focal lesion is found within the temporal lobe, is there evidence for unilateral seizure onset in one temporal lobe?
   A. If there is evidence for unilateral seizure onset, is that onset mesial, lateral, or diffuse?
   B. If that onset is mesial, what is the cognitive function in that temporal lobe? If there is salvageable memory, then selective amygdalo-hippocampectomy may be considered.

REGIONAL SURGICAL ANATOMY

The surgical anatomy for amygdalo-hippocampectomy is among the most difficult in the brain to deal with because of both the multiplicity of structures involved and the wide range of variations encountered. This is so before consideration is given to the distortions produced by shrinkage of the area from scarring or atrophy, or space-occupying lesions in the tissue.

Whatever approach is used, the structures that are removed, at least in part, are the amygdala (amygdaloid nucleus), hippocampus, and parahippocampal gyrus. Whereas the structures in close relation to the amygdala limit the amount of tissue that can be removed, in the case of the hippocampus and the parahippocampal gyrus, the position and size of the approach incision limit the amounts of tissue that can be removed, at least if the intention to limit damage to the surrounding tissue, notably the temporal neocortex, is to be maintained.

The amygdala lies in the roof of the anterior part of the temporal horn of the ventricular system. Its important relationships to other anatomic features are on its medial and anterior aspect, and therefore, farthest away from the operator's approach. These anatomic features are the caudate nucleus and the optic tract, and in safeguarding these structures, complete removal is impossible. The amygdala is largely anterior to the hippocampus, although on coronal slices, it is level with the pes.

The hippocampus is a complex structure whose medial

and superior aspects are covered with ependyma and form part of the temporal horn and the boundaries of the crural and ambient cisterns. The inferior and lateral boundaries of the hippocampus are related to other temporal lobe structures. Inferiorly, the hippocampus is continuous with the uncus and parahippocampal gyrus and, laterally, with the collateral sulcus and inferior temporal gyrus. In its midportion, the choroid plexus is located immediately next to the hippocampus on its medial edge. It is clear from the above-mentioned discussion that the parahippocampal gyrus is immediately bordered by the hippocampus and is itself related inferiorly to the structures within the subarachnoid cisterns, which are discussed later, and the floor of the middle fossa once the incisural edge is passed.

The remainder of the regional anatomy is best considered in relation to the subarachnoid cisterns and to the major blood vessels and blood supply because these are the areas that have to be entered and the elements that have to be safeguarded in performing the procedure. The microsurgical anatomy of this area has been described in detail by both Yasargil[34] and Renella,[35] and I am indebted to their work for this shortened description.

The cisterns involved in the formation of the sylvian fissure are important when the approach described by Yasargil is used but are irrelevant to other approaches and, therefore, do not need further detailed discussion. However the remaining cisterns, which are encountered whatever approach is used, are important. The crural cistern runs between the medial surface of the uncus and the cerebral peduncle, and opens into the ambient cistern. Although cranial nerve III (oculomotor nerve) is not within this cistern, it must be remembered that the nerve runs across the anterior end of the incisura. The crural cistern contains the anterior choroidal artery. The ambient cistern is located around the lateral aspect of the cerebral peduncle. It extends from the lateral mesencephalon medially to the parahippocampal gyrus laterally. The width of this cistern varies with the width of the incisura, and there is a tendency in some circumstances for the mesiobasal structures to bulge into this area. The ambient cistern is by far the more important because it is relevant whatever approach is used for amygdalo-hippocampectomy, or even for more extensive temporal lobe resections. It contains the proximal part of the posterior cerebral artery, the posterior choroidal vessels, and the mesencephalic part of the basal vein.

The major vessels in this area are important in this operation for two reasons— first because they are the vessels from which the arterial supply and venous drainage of the region derive, and second, because they and therefore the areas that they supply, may be in danger in the course of the dissection. The branches of the middle cerebral artery are important in planning the entry point in the transsylvian approach. Renella[35] gives a good account of the variations.

The anterior choroidal artery originates from the internal carotid artery distal to the origin of the posterior communicating artery. Renella gives a detailed description of the subsequent course of the vessel and its branches.[35] Many branches lead to structures other than the hippocampus and should not be damaged. It is known that there is a reciprocal relationship between the blood supply to the hippocampus from the anterior choroidal artery and the posterior choroidal vessels derived from the posterior cerebral artery.[35] The anterior choroidal artery travels through the carotid cistern and then through the crural cistern, and after crossing the ambient cistern, it runs into the choroid fissure and thence into the choroid plexus. Branches to the hippocampus arise from these last two segments of the artery. Yasargil emphasizes that only the lateral branches from the artery should be divided.[34]

The posterior cerebral artery was found to have an anomalous origin in 18 percent of the specimens examined by Renella.[35] Krayenbühl and Yasargil divided the course of the vessel into four segments, of which the first two, P1 and P2, are relevant to this description.[35a] The P1 segment runs from the origin from the basilar artery to its junction with the posterior communicating artery, the P2 segment, from there to the origin of the inferior temporal arteries. The vascular supply to the mesial temporal structures arises from the P1 and P2 segments; the arteries supplying the hippocampus, from the P2 segment via the posterior choroidal arteries; and the arteries to the parahippocampal gyrus, from the P3 segment.

The venous drainage of this area is complex and was finally described by Huang, who showed that eventually they all drain to the basal vein.[34, 36]

ANESTHETIC CONSIDERATIONS AND AIDS TO SURGERY

The anesthetic considerations are the same as those of any simple intracranial procedure, and the presence of a mass lesion is usually not relevant. Yasargil has recommended the use of a lumbar cerebrospinal fluid (CSF) drain, but we have not found this to be essential. Because we use intraoperative corticography, we are in the habit of using routine prophylactic antibiotics but this is a matter of choice. We have not found it necessary to use dexamethasone routinely. Anticonvulsant medication is omitted on the morning of surgery and is restored as soon as possible thereafter, and we have not experienced frequent or difficult problems with postoperative seizures. The premedication, provided it achieves adequate sedation and antisialogogue action, is a matter of preference. The usual anesthetic monitors and techniques are used with the patient paralyzed and ventilated. There is no indication for or possibility of conducting this procedure with the patient under local anesthesia. Two units of cross-matched blood are routinely obtained for this operation but are seldom used. In our practice, we use corticography routinely and occasionally use this study as a method of finally deciding which temporal lobe resection to perform. However, in general, cortigraphy is not necessary.[37]

SURGICAL TECHNIQUE

A number of approaches have been described, and in general, there is little difference among them. The two most well-known approaches are transcortical and transsylvian. There is a theoretical advantage to the transsylvian approach of Yasargil because more frontal fiber connections are divided. The original approach by Niemeyer was transcortical,[38] and many other surgeons have adopted the transcortical rather than the more difficult and restricting transsylvian approach. Therefore, the operation can be viewed in two stages—(1) the initial method of exposure and (2) the method of dealing with the mesial temporal structures after they have been exposed. The transsylvian approach obviates the need for a large neocortical incision, although there is no evidence that this is an advantage. At present, no information on surgical series comparing the two approaches has been published. Renella describes a number of approaches[39] but does not indicate subsequently which approach was used in the small number of patients who underwent the operation. Yasargil has emphasized that this operation is essentially a microsurgical procedure and requires careful microsurgical technique to minimize mortality and morbidity. Acute corticographic recording at operation is probably not required, although we have had useful experience with it.[37]

In an interesting comparison of the approaches used in studies of fixed hemispheres, Goncalves-Ferreira and his colleagues have shown that, whereas the transsylvian approach is farthest from the hippocampus, it traverses neural tissue of the least thickness (Fig. 104–2).[40]

EXPOSURE

Transcortical Approach

For the transcortical approach, the position of the head is the same as that used for a standard approach to the temporal lobe for a lobectomy. Our preference is for a five-point flap based on the floor of the middle fossa, as indicated by the root of the zygoma, and the floor of the anterior fossa, as indicated by the external angular groove. Again, the opening of the dura does not need detailed description. The positioning of the transcortical access varies from one operator to another. In 1987, Olivier described an approach through the anterior part of the superior temporal gyrus (T1) but has subsequently reverted to the original Niemeyer approach through the middle temporal gyrus (T2), using an incision 2 to 3 cm long, centered about 4 cm from the pole.[41]

When stereotactically guided volumetric removal of the hippocampus is being carried out, the approach will vary but entry is frequently through some part of the temporal neocortex.

Transsylvian Approach

Yasargil and associates state that they considered the transcortical and subtemporal approaches but rejected them, the first because of the inevitable cortical damage and the second because of the excessive retraction. Therefore, they adapted the pterional transsylvian approach used for aneurysm surgery. The position of the head in this approach is different. It is secured in a pin headrest, and it should be inclined 35 degrees toward the opposite side and adjusted so that the malar is the highest point. This is important because in order to carry out the approach, it is essential that the sylvian fissure is vertical. Yasargil describes the technical details of the approach well. The sphenoid wing has to be drilled away for best exposure. The pterional craniotomy used by Yasargil will be familiar to most readers and is described elsewhere in this book. The sylvian fissure is opened, and the area of the circular sulcus described by Yasargil is identified. Through a 20-mm incision, the amygdala and then the hippocampus are identified. The vascular landmarks and other details of this approach are to be found in the accounts by Yasargil and Renella.[34, 35] It is important to identify the site of this incision correctly, because if it is too near the temporal pole, the operation becomes much more difficult.

RESECTION

From this point on, once the exposure has been made, the resection involves the same maneuvers. Yasargil's approach precludes the use of the Cavitron ultrasonic aspirator (CUSA) because of the restricted access. For this reason, his description of the operative maneuvers is more detailed. Also, the order of removal is changed. In Yasargil's approach, the amygdala is encountered first on the way to the temporal horn and its partial removal facilitates the visualization of the temporal horn and hippocampus. He describes a piecemeal removal of this area, which may appear gray or grayish brown, reminding one that in the medial or mediobasal direction, the optic tract is eventually encountered. Olivier, on the other hand, notes that the amygdala is visualized after the main hippocampal specimen has been removed and suggests that from the transcortical approach, it can be removed dorsally up to the middle cerebral artery. Both Yasargil and Olivier agree that a vital step in the removal of the hippocampus is the identification of the hippocampal sulcus (called sulcus choroideus by Yasargil) and Ammon's horn artery or arteries, which run into the hippocampus and which may originate from both the anterior and posterior choroidal arteries. A detailed discussion of the variations has been given by Renella.[35] Yasargil commences his hippocampal removal at this point anteriorly, where the anterior choroidal artery is identified and safeguarded. Only the lateral branches from the artery are divided. Papaverine may be applied locally to the area of the anterior choroidal trunk after the dissection in this area has been completed to minimize spasm.

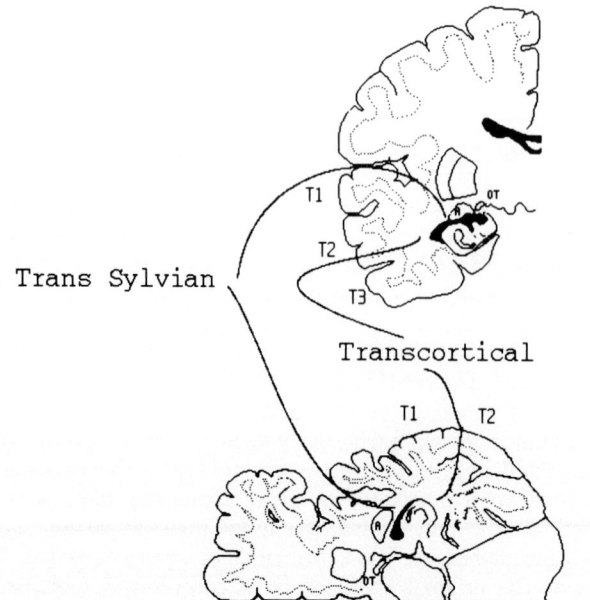

FIGURE 104–2. Transsylvian and transcortical approaches on schematic coronal and axial slices. A = amygdala, OT = optic tract.

The dissection proceeds posteriorly from this point until the hippocampus is divided posteriorly across its tail, usually at the end of the P2 portion of the posterior cerebral artery, which will have been visualized under the arachnoid of the ambiens cistern. This layer of arachnoid is a very important barrier in all temporal lobe resections and seldom is broached even by tumorous lesions. The dissection then proceeds anteriorly but laterally at the level of the collateral sulcus and including the parahippocampal gyrus until, passing around the pes hippocampus, it joins the starting point, and the specimen can then be removed. Provided care is taken to respect the appropriate anatomic boundaries and to identify and divide small arteries and veins to and from the specimen, the resection is virtually avascular. I agree with Yasargil that in the transsylvian approach, it is neither possible nor prudent to put brain retractors inside the cortical incision, although I have found it useful to use a self-retaining retractor to hold the frontal lobe and a hand-held retractor to restrain the temporal cortex above the incision. Although Yasargil and Teddy describe how up to 4 cm of hippocampus can be removed by this route, we have found that in our patients, between 1.5 and 2 cm are removed. This discrepancy may result from the difference in pathology, with a higher proportion of patients with sclerosis appearing in our series. After removing the bulk of the hippocampus, it is possible to remove more from the distal stump before concluding the operation. After the resection is complete, careful hemostasis is carried out in the cavity. I have found that a light pack of cotton wool and patience are best.

When the resection is being carried out under stereotactic guidance, then presumably the boundaries of the resection are determined by brain imaging study.

MAJOR INTRAOPERATIVE COMPLICATIONS

Vascular injury is the most important complication to be feared from this operation. In the transsylvian approach, the M1 portion of the middle cerebral artery is at risk, especially with the limited access. It has to be protected from retraction, accidental injury, and trauma associated with applying diathermy to adjacent vessels. Similarly, in dissecting the hippocampus free, care must be taken to identify the vessels in the ambient cistern positively and early, and to take care in dealing with the small vessels that pass to the hippocampus to avoid damage to more major vessels.

The next important problem, especially for the novice, is maintenance of the correct orientation, especially during the initial exposure and approach. This factor can be more difficult with the transsylvian approach, in which correct orientation of the head is important. In all approaches, early and positive identification of the temporal horn and the hippocampus is essential.

Finally, it is important to recognize when the pathology is too large or located too posteriorly to be dealt with by this route.

Avoidance of these problems depends on careful preoperative planning, correct positioning of the patient, and careful microsurgical technique.

POSTOPERATIVE MANAGEMENT

Because we routinely use acute electrocorticography, we also administer antibiotics perioperatively, usually for up to 4 days postoperatively, although this measure may not be necessary in shorter operations. The usual postcraniotomy neurologic observations are necessary. Our policy with regard to the administration of steroids has already been stated. Infection or hemorrhage within the surgical wound is managed appropriately.

Even with the most careful surgical technique, there is bound to be some swelling at the surgical site. This swelling may manifest itself as a mild weakness or dysphasia, if the operation is in the dominant hemisphere, which is usually transient and does not require treatment. It is wise to check these findings by CT scan to ensure that they are not due to a hematoma at the surgical site. There is also the possibility of focal seizures affecting the face or arm, so-called neighborhood fits. We have not seen these seizures with selective amygdalo-hippocampectomy, and they are more likely to occur with the larger temporal lobe resections.

The period of anesthesia and recovery may deprive the patient of his or her usual anticonvulsant drugs, and occasionally, this may result in seizures in the immediate postoperative period, especially because some of the more common anticonvulsant drugs are not available in parenteral form.

RESULTS

The results of an operation of this kind may be viewed from several angles. Clearly, the relief of seizures is the most obvious, together with neurologic deficit and early and late mortality. However, one must also consider the patient's quality of life, which is affected by changes in intellectual function and is reflected in personality to some extent. Although many authors have mentioned the procedure as one of the alternative types of temporal lobe resection,[41] apart from the series described by Wieser and Yasargil, whose most recent assessment was in 1991,[31] other authors have described only small numbers of patients. Our own unpublished series comprises 41 patients operated on between 1987 and 1992, and forms part of a larger series embracing all kinds of temporal lobe resections. The results from various series have to be interpreted in light of the pathology responsible for the temporal lobe disease because, as with other temporal lobe procedures, the result is related to the pathology. Finally, it is also necessary to have a common outcome scale, and the scale proposed by Engel[42] is used here. The size and position of the lesion may be of importance. Although Yasargil describes being able to remove up to 4 cm of hippocampus, this procedure is not easy, and Wieser and associates estimate that the reoperation rate in their series is around 5 percent.[31] We have certainly encountered lesions that, because of their posterior location, could not be removed by the transsylvian route. On one occasion, we have had to reoperate to remove the lesion by a standard lobectomy, and on another occasion, we have had to change to performing a lobectomy during the procedure. There has been one other patient in our series who underwent a standard lobectomy 5 years after having undergone an unsuccessful selective amygdalo-hippocampectomy; a lesion that was not made visible by brain imaging was found in the lobectomy specimen.

Table 104–2. SEIZURE OUTCOME FROM SELECTIVE AMYGDALO-HIPPOCAMPECTOMY IN VARIOUS SERIES

Series	Seizure Free (%)	90% Reduction (%)	Not Improved (%)
Ilae, TL	57.3	90.1	9.9
Ilae, AH	60.1	81.5	18.5
Renella	61	93	7
Zurich	59	78	22
Zurich, NL*	43	68	32
Maudsley	34	83	17

*Wieser's figures when nonlesional cases are excluded. Note results with casual cases among this group are still excellent (73 percent seizure free).[31]

SEIZURE RELIEF

Apart from our own series, there are only three published sources of information about the results of this operation. These sources are the summary of the Global Survey, carried out for the International League Against Epilepsy; the results of the Zurich group[31]; and those published by Renella. The results are summarized and compared with those of standard temporal lobectomy in Table 104–2. In a postoperative study of 30 patients, Wieser and coworkers have shown that the larger the volume of the resection, the better the outcome. They also found that it was important to carry out an adequate removal of the parahippocampal gyrus and subiculum.[43] Certainly, the influence of pathology on these results has to be taken into account in the Zurich series,[39] and in Renella's series, there is a preponderance of nonsclerotic discrete lesions. In 215 patients operated on in Zurich, some kind of discrete lesion was found in 144 (67 percent), gliosis including the results of encephalitis in another 37 patients (17 percent), and no structural lesion in the remaining 34 patients (16 percent).[31] By contrast, in our series, selective amygdalo-hippocampectomy is used in conjunction with other temporal lobe resections in the way described earlier. Between 1987 and 1992, a total of 153 temporal lobe resections were carried out. Sixty-six percent of these procedures were standard temporal lobectomies using the Falconer en bloc method,[44] 7 percent were extended temporal lobectomies using Spencer's technique,[7] and the remaining 27 percent, consisting of 41 patients, were selective amygdalo-hippocampectomies using the transsylvian approach. However, in contrast to the other temporal resections, the definitive pathology in these patients was mesial temporal sclerosis, both from the preoperative assessment and from the neuropathologic examination of the specimens. Although 73 percent of these patients showed this pathology, it was present in only 37 percent of patients who underwent lobectomies. In both series, there were patients with nonspecific findings—22 percent of the patients undergoing selective amygdalo-hippocampectomy and 18 percent of the patients undergoing temporal lobectomies. As expected, our results with regard to seizure relief from selective amygdalo-hippocampectomy are similar to those found with mesial temporal sclerosis in the temporal lobe series, shown in Table 103–3.

COMPLICATIONS

The Zurich series[31] has a very low complication rate, with only one patient developing hemiparesis in over 200 cases and no visual field defects. Renella reports two instances of transient hemiparesis in 62 patients.[35] In the 42 patients in our series, there is one patient with permanent hemiplegia; two patients with transient weakness, which improved; one patient with hemianopia; and unfortunately, one patient who suffered an obscure ischemic process starting 10 days after surgery and resulting in a persistent vegetative state. Almost all of the complications in our group were due to ischemic problems, which are the principal acute hazard in this operation.

With regard to adverse effects on intelligence and personality, these complications are less easy to evaluate. The Zurich series reported no adverse effects on cognitive function in those patients in whom the operation reduced the frequency of the seizures.[31] Renella's findings in a smaller group of 22 patients have shown that the operation reduced intellectual performance in left-sided procedures and improved it in right-sided procedures. When the operation was unsuccessful, an adverse effect was found.[35] Recently, an analysis of cognitive function was made in 42 patients undergoing temporal lobe surgery, 19 of whom had undergone en bloc lobectomy and 23 of whom had undergone selective amygdalo-hippocampectomy. The study was undertaken to test the hypothesis that selective amygdalo-hippocampectomy produced less impairment of cognitive function than en bloc temporal lobectomy. This was found to be true when the resection involved the temporal lobe that mediated the function tested; however, when the operation was on the temporal lobe that did not mediate the tested function, the result was the reverse.[45] We also have unpublished data that suggest that when an amygdalo-hippocampectomy is carried out on a temporal lobe that has failed a classic Wada test, this procedure has an adverse but not devastating effect on cognitive function if the operation involves the dominant temporal lobe. However, there is no effect when the operation is on the nondominant side. This raises interesting concepts that cannot be conveniently discussed here. Renella observes that the operation had little effect on the psychosocial circumstances of their patients. In our small series, there have been no adverse personality effects. Of particular interest is the anecdotal observation that there have been no cases of depression among these patients, whereas depression occurs frequently in patients subjected to nondominant temporal lobectomy.

DISCUSSION

Perhaps the best way to approach the indications and contraindications for this operation is from the original rationale

Table 104–3. SEIZURE OUTCOME IN PATIENTS WITH PROVEN MESIAL TEMPORAL SCLEROSIS TREATED BY TEMPORAL LOBECTOMY OR AMYGDALO-HIPPOCAMPECTOMY OVER THE SAME TIME PERIOD

Seizure Outcome	Temporal Lobectomy		Selective AH	
	N. Patients	Percent	N. Patients	Percent
1A seizure free	7	24	6	22
1 seizure free (Engel)	9	31	12	44
Improved	21	72	24	89
Not improved	8	28	3	11

of Wieser and Yasargil. Yasargil noted that a better result was obtained with regard to seizure control if the removal included the hippocampus and amygdala as well as the gross lesion.[35] Wieser identified and defined the concept of mesiobasal limbic epilepsy and proposed selective amygdalo-hippocampectomy as a logical solution to this condition. Wieser also proposed that the operation might be useful for palliative purposes in patients in whom the mesial temporal structures were not necessarily the sole origin but a principal participant in the epileptogenic pathway.[46]

A subsidiary consideration is the cognitive function of the temporal lobe to be operated on. When there is no evidence of function in that temporal lobe, with all the function located on the contralateral side, then there is no advantage to a restricted operation. Spencer and associates claim that there was no cognitive deficit following their extended lobectomy.[7]

As far as the technique of operation is concerned, the theoretical claims made by Yasargil and Wieser for their approach are difficult to sustain. There is no doubt that in inexperienced hands, this approach is more difficult to perform and is more likely to result in less efficient removal of tissue with greater hazard. The place of the stereotactically guided amygdalo-hippocampectomy is not yet defined but requires considerable capital investment. The removal of these structures by stereotactic use of a beam of external radiation or by using the gamma knife is still in its experimental phase.[47]

INDICATIONS FOR SELECTIVE AMYGDALO-HIPPOCAMPECTOMY

Indications for selective amygdalo-hippocampectomy are provided in the following list:

1. A lesion confined to the medial temporal structures that can be removed or destroyed through a restricted cortical approach.

2. Evidence of unilateral mesial onset of partial complex seizures from one temporal lobe, obtained by appropriate invasive neurophysiologic techniques and videotelemetry.

3. Indications that some of the patient's memory function was subserved by the operated temporal lobe.

CONTRAINDICATIONS FOR SELECTIVE AMYGDALO-HIPPOCAMPECTOMY

Contraindications for selective amygdalo-hippocampectomy are as follows:

1. A lesion that is outside of the mesial temporal structures.

2. A lesion that is confined to the medial temporal structures but is too large to be removed or destroyed through a restricted incision or too posterior for access. In these cases, consideration should be given to Spencer's extended temporal lobectomy.[7]

3. A patient in whom neurophysiologic evidence indicates that onset is in the region of the temporal lobe.*

4. A patient in whom the contralateral temporal lobe carries all or most of the recent memory function.*

5. A patient in whom the majority of the memory function is carried in the operated temporal lobe (i.e., the patient has failed the Amytal test, and there is no evidence of a structural lesion in that temporal lobe). Such patients are likely to have a poor result with regard to seizure relief and, as a result, suffer considerable deterioration in cognitive function. Such risks are greater in the dominant temporal lobe.

SUMMARY

Unilateral selective amygdalo-hippocampectomy is an operation that still has a limited place in the treatment of drug-resistant epilepsy of temporal lobe origin. The initial enthusiasm for the procedure has not been sustained, and in a center offering a comprehensive range of surgical procedures, it is probably applicable in its present form to approximately 15 to 20 percent of patients.

REFERENCES

1. Bailey P: Surgical treatment of psychomotor epilepsy. Five year follow-up. South Med J 54:299–301, 1961
2. Jensen I: Temporal lobe surgery around the world. Acta Neurol Scand 52:354–373, 1975
3. Falconer MA: Genetic and related aetiological factors in temporal lobe epilepsy. Epilepsia 12:13–31, 1971
4. Rasmussen T, Feindel W: Temporal lobectomy: Review of 100 cases with major hippocampectomy. Can J Neurol Sci 18:601–602, 1991
5. Feindel W, Rasmussen T: Temporal lobectomy with amygdalectomy and minimal hippocampal resection: Review of 100 cases. Can J Neurol Sci 18:603–605, 1991
6. Wieser HG, Yasargil MG: Die ''Selektiv Amygdala-Hippokampektomie'' als chirurgische Behandlung du medio-basal Limbischen Epilepsie. Neurochirugia 25:39–50, 1982
7. Spencer DD, Spencer SS, Mattson RH, et al: Access to the posterior medial temporal structures in the surgical treatment of temporal lobe epilepsy. Neurosurgery 15:667–671, 1984
8. Cascino GD, Kelly PJ, Sharbrough FW, et al: Long-term follow-up of stereotactic lesionectomy in partial epilepsy: Predictive factors and electroencephalographic results. Epilepsia 33:639–644, 1992
9. Olivier A: Relevance of removal of limbic structures in surgery for temporal lobe epilepsy. Can J Neurol Sci 18:628–635, 1991
10. Siegfried J: Les pacemakers neurologiques: Bilan de trois decennies. Neurochirugie 37:81–85, 1991
11. Hardiman O, Burke T, Phillips J, et al: Microdysgenesis in resected temporal neocortex: Incidence and clinical significance in focal epilepesy. Neurology 38:1041–1047, 1988
12. Polkey CE, Binnie CD: Neurosurgical Treatment of Epilepsy, in Laidlaw J, Richens A, Chadwick D (eds): A Textbook of Epilepsy, 4th ed. Edinburgh, Churchill Livingstone, 1993, pp 561–611
13. Powell GE, Polkey CE, McMillan TM: The new Maudsley series of temporal lobectomy I: Short term cognitive effects. Br J Clin Psychol 24:109–124, 1985
14. Adams CBT, Anslow P, Molyneaux A, Oxbury J: Radiological detection of surgically treatable pathology, in Engel J (ed): Surgical Treatment of the Epilepsies. New York, Raven Press, 1987, pp 213–233
15. Engel J, Henry TR, Risinger MW, et al: Presurgical evaluation for partial epilepsy: Relative contributions of chronic depth-electrode recordings vs FDG-PET and scalp-sphenoidal ictal EEG. Neurology 40:1670–1677, 1990
16. Debets RM, Van Veelen CMW, Maquet P, et al: Quantitative analysis of 18/FDG-PET in the presurgical evaluation of patients suffering from refractory partial epilepsy. Comparison with CT, MRI, and combined subdural and depth electrodes. Acta Neurochir (Wien) 50:88–94, 1990
17. Swartz BE, Tomiyasu U, Delgado Escueta AV, et al: Neuroimaging in temporal lobe epilepsy: Test sensitivity and relationships to pathology and postoperative outcome. Epilepsia 33:624–634, 1992

---

*In the instance of contraindications 3 and 4, a temporal lobectomy is preferred for various reasons, which have already been discussed.

18. Wieser HG, Hajek M, Leenders KL: PET findings before and after selective amygdalo-hippocampectomy. Second International Epilepsy Symposium 1992, p 41 (Abstract)
19. Wieser HG, Hajek M, Leenders KL: PET findings before and after selective amygdalo-hippocampectomy. Cleveland Symposium 1990, p 41
20. Rowe CC, Berkovic SF, Sia STB, et al: Localisation of epileptic foci with postictal single photon emission computed tomography. Ann Neurol 26:660–668, 1989
21. Rowe CC, Berkovic SF, Austin MC, et al: Visual and quantitative analysis of interictal SPECT with technetium-99m-HMPAO in temporal lobe epilepsy. J Nucl Med 32:1688–1694, 1991
22. Jabbari B, Van Nostrand D, Gunderson CH, et al: EEG and neuroimaging localisation in partial epilepsy. Electroencephalogr Clin Neurophysiol 79:108–113, 1991
23. Rowe CC, Berkovic SF, Austin MC, et al: Patterns of postictal cerebral blood flow in temporal lobe epilepsy: Qualitative and quantitative analysis. Neurology 41:1096–1103, 1991
24. Breiter SN, Barker PB, Mathews VP, et al: Proton spectroscopy in patients with seizure disorder. ASNR 30TH Annual Meeting 1992, p 82 (Abstract)
25. Kuzniecky R, Elgavish GA, Hetherington HP, et al: In vivo 31P nuclear magnetic resonance spectroscopy of human temporal lobe epilepsy. Neurology 42:1586–1590, 1992
26. Rausch R: Role of the neuropsychological evaluation and the intracarotid sodium amobarbital procedure in the surgical treatment of epilepsy. In Theodore WH (ed): Surgical Treatment of Epilepsy. (Epilepsy Res. Suppl. 5.), Amsterdam, Elsevier Science Publishers B.V., 1992, pp 77–86
27. Jack CR, Nichols DA, Sharbrough FW, et al: Selective posterior cerebral amytal test for evaluating memory function before surgery for temporal lobe seizure. Radiology 168:787–793, 1988
28. Wieser HG, Valvanis A, Roos A, et al: "Selective" and "superselective" temporal lobe Amytal tests: I Neuroradiological, neuroanatomical and electrical data, in Manelis J (ed): Advances in Epileptology, Vol. 17. New York, Raven Press, 1989, pp 20–27
29. Polkey CE, Channon SL: Memory and temporal lobe surgery: A review. J Roy Soc Med 83:100–103, 1990
30. Milner B: Psychological aspects of focal epilepsy and its surgical management, in Purpura DP, Penry JK, Walter RD (eds): Neurosurgical Management of the Epilepsies. New York, Raven Press, 1975, pp 299–332
31. Wieser HG: Selective amygdalo-hippocampectomy: Indications and follow-up. Can J Neurol Sci 18:617–627, 1991
32. Siegfried J, Wieser HG, Stodieck SRG: Foramen ovale electrodes: A new technique enabling presurgical evaluation of patients with mesiobasal temporal lobe seizures. Appl Neurophysiol 48:408–417, 1985
33. Van Veelen CMW, Debets C, Van Huffelen AC, et al: Combined use of subdural and intracerebral electrodes in preoperative evaluation of epilepsy. Neurosurgery 26:93–101, 1990
34. Yasargil MG, Teddy PJ, Roth P: Selective amygdalo-hippocampectomy. Operative anatomy and surgical technique, in Symon L (ed): Advances and Technical Standards in Neurosurgery, 12th ed. Wien, Springer-Verlag, 1985, pp 93–123
35. Renella RR: Morphology of the temporo-medial region, in Microsurgery of the Temporo-Medial Region. Wien, Springer-Verlag, 1989, pp 1–48
35a. Krayenbühl H, Yasargil MG: Cerebral Angiography, 2nd ed. London, Butterworth's, 1968
36. Huang YP, Wolf BS: The basal cerebral vein and its tributaries, in Newton TH, Potts DG (eds): Radiology of the Skull and Brain. St Louis, Mosby, 1974, pp 2111–2154
37. Polkey CE, Binnie CD, Janota I: Acute hippocampal recording and pathology at temporal lobe resection and amygdalo-hippocampectomy for epilepsy. J Neurol Neurosurg Psychiatry 52:1050–1057, 1989
38. Niemeyer P: The transventricular amygdala-hippocampectomy in temporal lobe epilepsy, in Baldwin M, Bailey P (eds): Temporal Lobe Epilepsy, Springfield, Charles C Thomas, 1958, pp 461–482
39. Renella RR: Surgery of the temporo-medial region, in Microsurgery of the Temporo-Medial Region. Wien, Springer-Verlag, 1989, pp 122–157
40. Goncalves-Ferreira G, Melancis JL, Andrade M, et al: 1992. (Unpub)
41. Olivier A: Temporal resections in the surgical treatment of epilepsy, in Theodore WH (ed): Surgical Treatment of Epilepsy. (Epilepsy Res. Suppl. 5.), Amsterdam, Elsevier Science Publishers BV, 1992, pp 175–188
42. Engel J: Outcome with respect to epileptic seizures, in Engel J (ed): Surgical Treatment of the Epilepsies. New York, Raven Press, 1987, pp 553–571
43. Siegel AM, Wieser HG, Wichmann W, Yasargil MG: Relationship between MR-imaged total amount of tissue removed, resection scores of specific mediobasal limbic subcompartments and clinical outcome following selective amygdalo-hippocampectomy. Epilepsy Res 6:56–65, 1990
44. Falconer MA: Anterior temporal lobectomy for epilepsy, in Logue V (ed): Operative Surgery, Vol. 14, Neurosurgery. London, Butterworths, 1971, pp 142–149
45. Goldstein LH, Polkey CE: Short-term cognitive changes after unilateral temporal lobectomy or unilateral amygdalo-hippocampectomy for the relief of temporal lobe epilepsy. J Neurol Neurosurg Psychiatry 56:135–140, 1993
46. Wieser HG: Selective amygdalo-hippocampectomy for temporal lobe epilepsy. Epilepsia 29:S100–S113, 1988
47. Bardia-Solorio JL, Barcia JA, Hernandez G, et al: Radiosurgery of epilepsy. Acta Neurochir 117:109, 1992 (Abstract)

CHAPTER 105

Temporal Lobe Operations for Epilepsy: Radical Hippocampectomy

Dennis D. Spencer
Werner K. Doyle

Temporal lobectomy is the most common surgical procedure performed for the treatment of medically refractory epilepsy. This operation has evolved in parallel to our growing knowledge of the epilepsies and our understanding of the pathophysiology and pathoanatomy of the most common form of refractory epilepsy. Our understanding and tools have advanced so that we can offer selected patients a better than 85 percent chance of safely eliminating their seizures without causing them neurologic harm. The neurosurgical approach we have adopted reflects the evolution of our understanding of this disease and undoubtedly will continue to change as we learn more about the problem and develop new ways to define it. Therefore, before describing the surgical technique, we review the historical as well as the modern neurosurgical perspectives that provide the rationale for this procedure.

HISTORY OF EPILEPSY SURGERY AND TEMPORAL LOBECTOMY

Bouchet and Cazauvielh[1] described, in 1825, gross visible and palpable abnormalities of hippocampal specimens obtained at autopsy from patients suffering from "alienation epilepsy." This was the first evidence linking the most common form of focal epilepsy to a pathologic substrate. In another autopsy study, Sommer[2] in 1880 described gliosis and pyramidal cell loss within the hippocampus of epileptics and hypothesized that this finding was responsible for their epilepsy. In 1872, Hughlings Jackson[3] suggested that hyperexcitable brain adjacent to temporal lobe lesions was responsible for epilepsy, and in 1888, he pointed out the association of the "dreamy state" and the classic auras of taste, smell, and epigastric sensations to temporal lobe lesions.[4] He did not, however, mention medial temporal sclerosis in connection with his findings.[5]

Neurosurgery helped to provide the link between medial temporal pathology and seizures, by correlating the efficacy of seizure control by directed surgical resections with the resected tissue's histopathology. Surgery for epilepsy was pioneered by Horsley, who in 1886 began excising visible cortical scars.[6] Cortical excision and partial lobectomy was continued by Foerster.[7] It was Bailey and Gibbs,[8] however, in 1951, who popularized the resection of the temporal lobe using electrographic data, limiting their resection to lateral temporal cortex. On the basis of their experience, they eventually recommended temporal lobectomy back to the level of the central sulcus, noting enough success in controlling seizures to recommend the procedure.[8] Penfield also adopted intraoperative electrocorticography and based the extent of his temporal lobectomy on electrocorticography performed during an awake craniotomy.[9] He would resect all portions of the temporal lobe that showed interictal spiking, removing the anterior hippocampus only if it was grossly or electrically abnormal.[10] Penfield and his associates[10, 11] noted more successful outcome with more complete resection of the medial structures (amygdala and anterior hippocampus).

With this new surgical experience, the significance of the mesial abnormalities were appreciated. In 1953, Earle and associates[12] described diffuse atrophic changes in the inferior medial portion of the temporal lobe in two thirds of their epilepsy patients who underwent temporal lobectomy. Margerison and Corsellis[13] added to this understanding by finding hippocampal sclerosis in 22 of 26 patients diagnosed with temporal lobe epilepsy. They also noted that hippocampal sclerosis occurred unilaterally in 80 percent of their cases.[13] Morris[14] described intraoperative abnormal electrographic discharges originating from the amygdala and anterior hippocampus, pointing out that pathologic changes were most noticeable in these structures. He proposed that the "standard temporal lobectomy" should include 6.5 cm of the lateral cortex, the uncus, the amygdala, and 2 to 4 cm of the anterior hippocampus. This proposal was echoed by Walker[15] in his description of the standard temporal lobectomy. Falconer and Cavanagh[16] then described detailed pathology in the en bloc temporal lobe resections they performed. The atrophy and gliosis Falconer and his associates[16–18] found included and extended beyond the hippocampus, leading them to call the abnormality mesial temporal sclerosis (MTS). They also noted that patients exhibited a better prognosis if either MTS or a lesion was discovered within the resection specimen.[18–20] Falconer essentially directed his resection to the hippocampal formation rather than the temporal neocortex, and this approach served as the model for most technical modifications that followed.

The classic neurosurgical approaches were also altered by the adoption of stereotactic depth recordings, introduced by Bancaud and Talairach.[21, 22] This technique provided accurate intracranial pathoelectrophysiologic localization of partial epilepsies. Crandall[23] also adopted the standardized en bloc resection, because it was especially suited for clinical research. He was able to correlate electrophysiologic studies, which included depth electrodes, to epileptogenic brain he resected.[23, 24] Studies using intracranial monitoring demonstrated that medial basal limbic seizures were the most common and responsive to therapy.[25-27] By defining onset areas for certain seizures more accurately, it permitted more selective surgical intervention and improved surgical efficacy.

Modern neuroimaging and electrographic localization improved the clinician's ability to identify focal seizure onsets generated from discrete areas of the medial basal region of the temporal lobe.[22, 28-31] Patient selection was much better defined. As a consequence, it became apparent that resections of medial basal structures were found to be more effective than those limited to the lateral cortex,[32, 33] and classic anterior temporal lobectomy came to be regarded as an unnecessarily extensive operation in treating patients who demonstrated defined seizure origin only within mesial basal limbic structures.[34] This led to the procedure of selective amygdalohippocampectomy and anteromedial temporal resection to treat the forms of epilepsy that were not related to gross structural lesions.[25, 27, 34, 35] The anterior medial temporal resection (AMTR) is described in this chapter.

EXPERIMENTAL AND CLINICAL EVIDENCE FOR MEDIAL TEMPORAL PATHOLOGY: RATIONALE FOR MEDIAL TEMPORAL RESECTION

Early surgical procedures were mainly lateral temporal neocortical resections, which yielded many unsuccessful or only partially successful results. It was observed that reoperation in these failures, which included resection of the medial structures, resulted in further benefit to these patients. This observation demonstrated that removal of the medial structures was important, but not necessarily sufficient, for seizure control.[8, 36-38] Later studies have suggested that the extent of medial basal resection is the primary determinant of the outcome of temporal lobectomy in patients with intractable seizures and a unilateral temporal epileptogenic focus, irrespective of the size of the lateral cortical resection.[39, 40]

Long-term invasive electrophysiologic monitoring revealed that the majority of ictal events observed in temporal lobe epilepsy originated in the medial temporal lobe, often entirely within the hippocampus.[27] Electrographic ictal localization, especially if invasive studies such as depth and subdural electrodes are used, is accepted as the single most accurate method to identify the region of seizure onset.[41-43] Use of interictal spikes was advocated historically and is still advocated by some contemporary neurosurgeons to define cortical resection.[44] Interictal spikes have not, however, been equated precisely with ictal foci or any specific pathology within the resected tissue they define.[43, 45] This is not unexpected, considering that interictal spikes may represent synaptically mediated events propagated from distant abnormal sites.[46] Epileptiform spiking is also nonspecific, because it has been described in non-epileptics.[47] Given that seizures in medial temporal lobe epilepsy begin almost always in the hippocampus, and an entorhinal cortex (ERC) in which pathologic changes are most common, interictal spikes emerging from histologically normal temporal neocortex cannot be used as the sole means of outlining the resection of a potential epileptogenic zone. This explains the historically higher incidence of failures when this approach was used as the only means of defining the surgical resection.

Unilateral hippocampal atrophy identified by high-resolution magnetic resonance imaging (MRI) has been correlated with neuronal loss and sclerosis of the subsequently resected structure.[48, 49] It is not unexpected, therefore, that hippocampal atrophy seen on MRI also correlates to a good prognosis after temporal lobectomy ipsilateral to the atrophy. Magnetic resonance imaging has become very important in helping to identify medial temporal pathoanatomy in nonlesional temporal epilepsy patients before surgical resection.

Neuronal loss, gliosis, and histochemical changes are identified in the hippocampal formation removed from the patients most often cured of their temporal lobe epilepsy.[50] The extent of neuronal loss, gliosis, and histochemical changes in nonlesional epilepsy is quantitatively different for medial temporal epilepsy associated with lesions and other epilepsies.[51, 52] Not only is the neuronal loss more severe, but synaptic reorganization is present in medial temporal lobe epilepsy and is not present in other forms of temporal lobe epilepsy. Some changes identified in MTS probably are more than secondary effects of seizures and likely represent changes that are themselves epileptogenic.

The hippocampus is vulnerable to becoming epileptogenic from neurotoxins, antimetabolites, head trauma, anoxia, ischemia, and intracranial infection.[53] Several endogenous and exogenous excitatory amino acids seem to have a role in epileptogenisis through damage to the medial limbic structures.[54-56] Excitotoxic injury during severe febrile convulsions occurring in early childhood may initiate the changes that eventually lead to the onset of complex partial seizures in adolescence. Not only are the amygdala ERC and hippocampus likely to be the epileptogenic region, they also have intimate neuronal connections with the remaining limbic system that are undoubtedly essential for the seizure propagation. Primate pathway studies demonstrate concentrated input to the hippocampal formation via the entorhinal cortex and reveal substantial efferents from the hippocampus through the fimbria and subicular pathways. This finding accounts for the widespread neocortical innervation of areas that could serve as the basis for the varied behavioral expressions of generated seizures.[57, 58] Although the injured hippocampus may have a low threshold for recruiting, synchronization, and amplification to create a seizure discharge, the anatomic integrity of the temporal lobe is necessary for the full expression of a temporal lobe seizure. For this reason, a lateral temporal resection may be curative or palliative in some instances, despite medial temporal pathology.[25, 44, 59-60] The amygdala also has important relay connections to the limbic system.

Neuropathologic, neuroanatomic, and neurophysiologic findings all identify abnormalities in the medial temporal structures, specifically the hippocampus.[51, 52, 62] Therefore, medial resection removes the majority of the epileptogenic substrate. Evidence has accumulated suggesting the extent to which the medial structures should be resected. Depth electrodes placed down the long axis of the hippocampus have shown that electrical abnormalities are usually found throughout the body of the hippocampus, and less often is there a distinct segment of the hippocampus that initiates the seizure. Pathologic abnormalities seen in resected hippocampi also reflect a diffuse area of disease. And in approximately 20 percent of patients with unilateral temporal lobe epilepsy studied with depth electrodes, the abnormal electrical foci were in the posterior portions of the hippocampus not routinely resected by standard lobectomies.[63–65] The need to include the posterior portions of the hippocampus in the medial resection was met by a more radical hippocampectomy that still preserved the lateral temporal cortex. There are other surgical options, reviewed later, representing variations of opinion of the extent of medial resection necessary and sufficient for success, and representing different approaches to minimize functional disruption of overlying cortex. However, they all have the common goal of medial temporal resection, specifically of the hippocampus.

SURVEY OF MEDIAL TEMPORAL RESECTIVE PROCEDURES

COMMON GOALS

The neurosurgeon's goal is to localize and define portions of the nervous system that are pathologic and, by a surgical means, improve the patient's compromised neurologic function. Most temporal lobectomies performed are resections based upon noninvasive predictors of hippocampal pathology and upon chronic EEG recordings of ictal events rather than intraoperative interictal recordings of lateral temporal cortex. Patient selection has become more uniform among the centers as the clinical pathology is better understood. Our patient selection is reviewed later in this chapter. The following survey lists different strategies for ablating the epileptic focus. Each represents a different bias in terms of the extent of resection deemed necessary and sufficient for success as well as avoidance of functional and anatomic areas in order to limit neurologic deficits.

STEREOTACTIC SURGERY

One drawback of transcortical approaches is the possible morbidity related to the excessive resection of nonepileptogenic cortex in order to gain safe access to deeper structures. Open stereotactic selective amygdalohippocampectomy[66] is described as a method to overcome this problem. Although the technique was developed for removal of neoplastic lesions, it has been utilized in selective resections of the amygdala-hippocampal complex in patients with temporal lobe epilepsy.[67] A lateral transcortical temporal approach employing a stereotactic, computer-based image-directed system is described. According to its advocates, this method offers selective resection with very limited superficial cortical resection, avoiding eloquent cortex and without exposing important vascular elements. No large series using this technique is as yet available to compare efficacy of seizure control and neurologic outcome. Also, the inherent great expense of the system and large capital investment in technical staff prohibits its wide use.

There are also isolated reports of stereotactic ablations of medial structures in the literature.[68–71] They are limited to relatively small areas of anatomy, however, and usually have poor results. No formal modern series comparable to those of open craniotomies is available.

TRANS-SYLVIAN APPROACH

Wieser and Yasargil and their colleagues,[25, 35, 72] reported a series of patients who underwent selective unilateral amygdala-hippocampectomy for drug-resistant temporal lobe epilepsy. Their operation was very selective, including only the amygdala, uncus, and hippocampus posteriorly to the level of the superior colliculus. With their trans-sylvian approach, lateral temporal cortex was not resected. Detailed neuropsychological testing was not reported for these patients, but the authors thought that in general there were fewer functional deficits than in a comparable group that they treated with larger temporal lobectomies.

The trans-sylvian approach is technically demanding.[25] In addition to limitations associated with the very restrictive exposure, there is a significant risk of morbidity related to dissection through the sylvian fissure. This involves risk of damage to the sylvian veins, branches of the middle cerebral arteries, the anterior choroidal artery, and the branches of the posterior cerebral artery.[66] The vessels themselves need not be damaged, because vasospasm alone could result in hemiparesis or hemianopia.

LATERAL NEOCORTICAL CORTESECTOMY/ TRANSCORTICAL TRANSVENTRICULAR HIPPOCAMPECTOMY

Niemeyer,[73] in 1958, presented histologic abnormalities mostly within the hippocampus of temporal lobes removed by standard temporal lobectomy and provided the rationale for the procedure he went on to describe. He developed a transventricular amygdalectomy and a 3-cm hippocampectomy performed through a 2-cm middle temporal gyrus incision. This technique suffers from limited exposure and does not allow for en bloc excisions.

SUBTEMPORAL APPROACH

The subtemporal approach is also technically complex because it entails removing zygomatic process removal to the inferior middle fossa. For rare cases of tumor in the dominant hemisphere, this may be considered, but alternative approaches, notably awake temporal lobectomy with functional mapping, are available.[35]

ANTERIOR MEDIAL TEMPORAL RESECTION

The extent of lateral temporal resection in our AMTR is limited to the temporal pole to provide access for a generous resection of the medial structures. If lateral ictal events are recorded or a lateral lesion is imaged preoperatively, then resection may not be directed to the medial structures. Details of the procedure are described here. Because it is still unclear how much of the parahippocampus, amygdala, entorhinal cortex, and hippocampus is necessary and sufficient to define the epileptogenic region for resection, we remove as much as possible without causing neurologic harm. Then, maximal efficacy is ensured with one surgical procedure.

This method's advantages are similar to those of the other approaches described. They all preclude intraoperative electrocorticography, and the limited anterior temporal pole resection makes language mapping unnecessary in the dominant hemisphere. Operations can then be performed under general anesthesia. Also, with this approach, visual field cuts can often be avoided or, if present, do not exceed an upper quadrantanopsia.

Other advantages of this procedure, which the other methods do not all share, are similar to those Crandall[23] outlined when he adopted his standardized en bloc resection. AMTR is well suited for clinical research. Standardized AMTR permits scientific assessment of intact tissue from an en bloc resection and allows assessment of surgical outcome without the confounding variations inherent in varied tailored resections. Standardized procedures permit studies of induced changes in neuropsychological and psychosocial function, validation of presurgical criteria, and correlation of the pathology in the resected tissue to new assessment criteria and modalities. Our data indicate that a radical resection of the medial temporal structures controls seizures in approximately 85 percent of patients and is accomplished without additional neurologic morbidity. Therefore, AMTR has proven efficacy as good as or better than that of other contemporary methods reported.

ANTERIOR MEDIAL TEMPORAL LOBECTOMY PERFORMED AT YALE

PATIENT SELECTION

Patient selection involves identifying patients with medically refractory epilepsy in whom a region causing all of a patient's habitual seizures can be localized. The patient becomes a candidate for surgery if this region can be removed safely. Therefore, functional identification of anatomic areas involved in the resection and a prediction of the neurologic and neuropsychologic effects of a resection are critical to the selection process. Phased evaluation at Yale involves a series of progressively more invasive studies. Details of this evaluation have been described elsewhere[61, 126] and are summarized here (Table 105-1). The phased evaluation at Yale is designed for the evaluation of all cases of medically refractory epilepsy.

Patients who satisfy generally accepted criteria for medically refractory epilepsy[74-77] undergo phase I of the evaluation, which consists of a complete medical, neurologic, and psychiatric history and examination. Neuropsychologic testing, high-resolution MRI with three-dimensional rendering and volumetric analysis of the hippocampus, and baseline EEG are routinely performed. Formal visual field evaluation, positron-emission tomography (PET), SPECT, and sometimes CT scans are included in this portion of the workup.

Table 105-1. Phased Evaluation of Patients with Medically Refractory Epilepsy

Phase I	History, medical, neurological, psychiatric examinations
	Neurophysiological assessment
	CT with and without contrast
	MRI
	Formal visual fields evaluation
	Baseline EEG
	Continuous audio/video EEG monitoring to record a minimum of three spontaneous seizures
Phase II	Cerebral angiogram
	Left and right cerebral amytal testing
Phase III	Depth and subdural electrodes—number and placement dependent on prior evaluation
	Continuous audio/video EEG monitoring to record at least three spontaneous seizures
	Stimulation and evoked potentials through subdural and depth electrodes for mapping functional cerebral areas
Phase IV	Mapping of speech and motor areas when indicated
	Evoked potentials
	Cortical resection or callosal section

Continuous audio-video EEG monitoring of at least three spontaneous habitual seizures is obtained.

In a clinical conference, neurosurgeons, neurologists, neuropsychologists, and other members of the epilepsy surgery team review the data to determine whether the patient is a viable surgical candidate. Such a conference takes place after each phase.

Phase II of the evaluation involves a cerebral angiogram and intracarotid sodium amytal test.[78] The information gathered from this study is essential to the decision-making process because of the important functional information it provides. Lateralization of speech dominance and memory function and prediction of residual memory capacity following a lobectomy cannot be obtained any other way at the present time.

Phase III is undertaken if (1) the data up until now are not concordant in defining a clear focal area of seizure origin such as the medial temporal lobe or (2) additional functional localization such as speech mapping is required. Several options are available, depending on the specific information sought. Stereotactically placed depth electrodes or subdural strip electrodes placed through burr holes can be used to lateralize and localize seizure onset. This long-term intracranial monitoring is similar to phase I audio-video EEG monitoring, with the intention of capturing ictal and interictal events from the sampled intracranial sites. Direct stimulation and evoked potential mapping using the electrodes may be performed to acquire functional and neuropsychological data. Often, when functional mapping is desired, a large grid array is placed, via a craniotomy, over the area to be studied. This is usually in a setting in which a neocortical focus is suspected. The grid is used for electrographic localization and functional mapping using stimulation techniques. We also have a series of patients in whom depth and subdural strips localize the seizure focus to a neocortical area, which requires repeat phase III evaluation using a large electrode array for better localization. In most cases, grid removal, which involves re-exploration of the craniotomy, is accompanied by resection.

The final phase (phase IV) is the definitive neurosurgical

procedure. Though it is most often AMTR under general anesthesia, phase IV may also involve, when appropriate, speech and motor mapping during an awake craniotomy. Although evoked potential motor and sensory mapping can be accomplished with the patient under general anesthesia, speech localization and other specialized neuropsychological mapping such as verbal memory assessment must be done using local anesthesia if it was not accomplished with a chronic subdural grid. Cortical resection other than AMTR, subpial transection, and callosal section are other procedures included in phase IV.

SOME SPECIFIC SELECTION CONSIDERATIONS

Our selection of patients with medial temporal epilepsy (MTE) for surgery has been greatly influenced by high-resolution MRI. Because MTE is associated with focal anatomic pathology (atrophy due to cell loss) we and others have adopted imaging as an important factor in our evaluation. Magnetic resonance imaging allows us to offer more than 50 percent of presenting patients with refractory focal epilepsy either lesion removal or AMTR without depth or subdural electrodes, a marked decrease from the 90 percent intracranial monitoring rate before MRI.[26] MRI alone, however, is not sufficient for selection; concordance of additional clinical data is still essential. Audio-video EEG must record at least three typical seizures documenting electroclinical correlation with the location of the anatomic pathology shown on MRI. Also, results of neuropsychological testing should not disagree with the other localizing data. Of course, the case must also fulfill the criteria for medical intractability. Patients who are shown on imaging not to have a mass of hippocampal atrophy and whose additional clinical data provide conflicting information undergo placement of depth and subdural electrodes for further evaluation.

SURGICAL PROCEDURE

The operation of anterior medial temporal lobectomy for temporal lobe epilepsy due to MTS evolved from 1980 to 1985[27, 45, 59] and currently takes the following form.

Patient preparation for this procedure is similar to that for most elective craniotomies. No change in the preoperative antiepileptic drug regimen is made. Use of perioperative antibiotics and steroids is at the discretion of the surgeon. We have gone through several changes in our steroid regimens and have found that moderate perioperative doses (Solu-Medrol, 125 mg IV q6h) with a rapid 5-day postoperative taper has been of benefit to minimize symptoms such as headache that prevents early patient mobilization. Although there may be a theoretical advantage to using perioperative steroids to minimize traumatic injury, we have not noticed any significant differences in outcome compared with our early experience of performing this procedure without steroids.

The operation is usually performed using general anesthesia. The patient is supine, in a slightly flexed position, and a blanket roll is placed under the appropriate shoulder. The head, in three-pin fixation, is turned laterally so that the line of the zygoma is at an angle of about 10 degrees to the floor. This slight angle allows for an unobstructed microscopic line of sight along the length of the temporal horn and the hippocampus during the latter stages of the operation.

A standard temporal craniotomy is performed, exposing about 9 cm of the temporal lobe. The skin incision is begun on the superior aspect of the zygoma about 1.5 cm anterior to the tragus and carried superiorly over the ear to the mastoid vertex line, where it curves gently just superior to the temporal squamosa and inferior to the temporal muscle insertion. The incision may stop at the hairline or may extend medially along the hairline to the midline if more frontal exposure is required. Effort is always made to preserve the superficial temporal artery to maximize preservation of the scalp flap's blood supply. The temporalis muscle can be turned in one piece with the skin, and flapped anteriorly, or it can be incised radially beginning at the area of the posterior zygoma, extending to the temporalis insertion, and continuing along the insertion, to leave a rim of temporalis fascia that is used to re-approximate the muscle during closure. A free frontotemporal bone flap is then elevated. Its anteroposterior extent should be at least 6 cm along the temporal bone. The superior boundary of the bone flap should be designed to expose the sylvian fissure and orbital frontal region. The temporal bone is rongeured as close to floor of the middle fossa as possible without violating the mastoid air cells. If the air cells are opened, they are immediately packed and isolated from the wound. The dura is tented peripherally and opened in a rectangular manner with the superior portion as a base, and an additional dural incision is made toward the temporal tip for exposure of the pole.

The surface of the temporal lobe is inspected, with attention directed to the draining veins. These are not interrupted except for those veins at the anterior temporal tip and inferior aspect of the inferior temporal gyrus and occipitotemporal gyrus. The vein of Labbé is routinely saved. The remainder of the operation consists of taking two or three separate resection specimens, depending on the shallowness of the middle fossa and the extent of the temporal lobe atrophy.

The first stage of the resection consists of incising the cortex in a line that extends 3 to 3.5 cm from the tip of the temporal lobe, along the superior margin of the middle temporal gyrus. This incision line should then curve across the middle and inferior temporal gyri, stopping typically at the occipitotemporal gyrus or including a portion of this gyrus. The superior margin of this resection is the inferior arachnoid of the superior temporal gyrus, which is not violated. The temporal pole is resected en bloc. The depth of the resection is approximately 3 cm, designed to approach the temporal horn but not enter it, thus creating a block of tissue measuring approximately 3 cm^3. This cube of tissue is then submitted for histologic examination, and the second stage of the procedure begins.

All exposed surfaces of the brain are covered with a collagen sponge, and two self-retaining retractors are positioned, one to retract the superior temporal gyrus and the other placed on the cut surface of the middle and inferior temporal gyri of the posterior portion of the resection bed. The ultrasonic aspirator is then placed on a relatively low setting, the white matter overlying the temporal horn is dissected, and the horn is entered. This maneuver provides an important landmark and allows orientation of the dissection away from the optic tract. The incision is carried anteriorly and medially across the anterior fibers of the temporal stem and the junction of the middle and superior third of the amygdala toward the lesser wing of the sphenoid. Dissection is further carried medially and inferiorly to the incisura of the tentorium, where the uncus of the parahippocampus is identified and an ultrasonic aspirator is used to gently dissect and remove the uncus from the arachnoid overlying the carotid artery and the optic and third nerves. The incision along the uncus of the parahippocampus is carried posteriorly over the arachnoid to the anterior midbrain. At this point, the dissection ends medially and anteriorly, and the superior self-retaining retractor is inserted deeper to gently retract the remaining fibers of the temporal stem, superior temporal gyrus, and the superior aspect of the cut amygdala.

Attention is now turned to the posteroinferior aspect of the incision, where the occipital temporal fasciculus is identified and incised posteriorly, joining the temporal horn to the floor of the middle fossa. This incision is extended with bipolar coagulation and ultrasonic aspiration, following the curve of the hippocampus but not violating it. The posterior dissection is curtailed when the hippocampus begins to curve medially and the arachnoid of the medial occipital temporal gyrus can be identified. As this dissection continues, the neocortical self-retaining retractor is curved and inserted along the line of dissection until the lateral temporal neocortex can be gently elevated, exposing the length of the hippocampus, the parahippocampus, and the medial aspect of the occipitotemporal gyrus. With the two retractors now in proper position, the operating microscope is brought into the operative field, and the remaining dissection is carried out under magnified vision.

Through the microscope, attention is directed again to the incision along the uncus. One can easily identify the thick white bands anterior to the arachnoid of the midbrain, which represent the uncinate fasciculus and the anterior commisure. These fibers are divided with the ultrasonic aspirator, care again being taken not to violate the arachnoid overlying the midbrain. This incision is carried posteriorly to join the choroidal fissure and the choroid plexus. At this point, depending on the bulk of the medial structures present in the middle fossa, one may resect the anterior occipitotemporal gyrus and the amygdala using bipolar coagulation and ultrasonic aspiration in a second en bloc excision; this is submitted for histologic examination. Only the hippocampus and the parahippocampus now remain. Depending on the overall anatomy of the temporal lobe and the extent of exposure, this second en bloc resection could have been included in the previously removed anterior temporal pole specimen.

The small vessels irrigating the medial parahippocampus and hippocampus emanating from the posterior cerebral artery and the anterior choroidal artery are identified. These vessels from the posterior cerebral artery lie in the arachnoid of the hippocampal fissure and are coagulated in the fissure singly and divided with microscissors. Irrigating vessels from the anterior choroidal artery that supply the hippocampus are coagulated as they enter the structure and then are cut sharply. As the dissection continues in a posterior direction, the arachnoid posterior to the brain stem and overlying the posteromedial parahippocampus becomes visible and is preserved. The arachnoid just lateral to the incisura is coagulated and incised. The hippocampus can now be gently elevated away from the brain stem (flipped at its attachments of remaining arachnoid and perforating vessels supplying it). The fimbria, easily identified as it streams from the alveus, is freed from the arachnoid overlying the thalamus with a microdissector.

The dissection continues under microscopic vision with further division of smaller perforating vessels from the posterior cerebral artery. This large artery can now be easily seen under the arachnoid. The hippocampus is followed as it approximates the superior colliculus of the midbrain. At this point, the incision from the middle fossa floor is joined to the incision of the posterior body of the hippocampus, and the medial structures, including the parahippocampus and hippocampus, are removed en bloc. At the end of the dissection, one should be able to identify, from superior to inferior, the choroid plexus, the arachnoid overlying the inferior aspect of the thalamus and optic tract and the lateral aspect of the midbrain, the coagulated arachnoid and vessels of the hippocampal fissure, the arachnoid overlying the posterior cerebral artery, and the medial edge of the tentorium. The fourth nerve may sometimes be seen running just lateral to the incisural edge, the third nerve is identified anteriorly and medially, again beneath the arachnoid, with the carotid artery in the most anterior position of the resection bed. Meticulous hemostasis is obtained, the retractors are removed to allow the lateral temporal cortex to settle into position, the dura is closed completely with interrupted sutures, the bone is wired into position, and the muscle and scalp are closed in layers. A subgaleal drain is rarely necessary.

We routinely perform electrocorticography for research purposes but do not use the data to tailor the resection. For intraoperative electrocorticography, anesthetic considerations become more important. Isofluorane is kept at a stable end-tidal concentration of 0.25 percent. Anesthesia is supplemented only with a muscle paralyzer and fentanyl. Nitrous oxide is not used until after all electrocorticography has been accomplished.

The patient is mobilized as rapidly as possible, usually sitting in a chair on the first postoperative day. There are otherwise no special postoperative management issues, except re-initiating the preoperative antiepileptic drug regimen as soon as possible, making up for the oral doses missed during the anesthesia, and maintaining appropriate blood levels of the antiepileptics. Antiepileptic drug dosages may require adjustment, but typically, we continue the same regimen for at least 6 months, usually waiting 1 year before we consider weaning the patient from one drug in the setting of a polydrug regimen. It is not until a patient has 2 years of seizure-free history that cessation of antiepileptic medical management is considered.

FINDINGS

Neuronal counts have been determined in over 100 patients undergoing selective anteromedial temporal lobectomy (AMTL). In these cases, we have compared nonlesional temporal lobectomies in patients with temporal lobe epilepsy (TLE), with hippocampi resected during surgery directed at medial temporal gliomas. Cells in the CA1–4 fields and the granule cells in the dentate were counted with a modification of the technique described by Dam[79, 80] and the results were compared with cell counts of age-matched autopsy specimens.[81] In specimens without tumors, there was more than a 50 percent loss of neurons and a concomitant gliosis in all CA fields as well as in the dentate. Although cell loss was present in the hippocampi near tumors, this finding was not statistically different from the cell counts in autopsy controls.[51] DeLanerolle and colleagues[52] used immunohistochemistry techniques to study this tissue and noted a loss of specific cell types. They described profound loss of the hilar interneuron population staining for somatostatin (SS) and neuropeptide-Y (NPY) in over 80 percent of the nontumor medial temporal lobe specimens (we call this group cryptogenic temporal lobe epilepsy, CTLE). Also, profuse sprouting of NPY and dynorphin (DYN) fibers into the dentate molecular layer accompanied this cell loss. This reorganization of fibers around the dentate gyrus was not observed in the autopsy controls or in hippocampi removed from epileptic patients harboring a temporal lobe tumor.

The profound cell loss associated with CTLE can be observed in vivo using volumetric analysis of the hippocampus and temporal neocortex with MRI. Early results show a strong direct correlation between cell counts and hippocampal volumes.[48, 49, 82] Hippocampal volumes have also been directly related to surgical outcome. More atrophic cases correlate with a better outcome.[83]

OUTCOME AND PREDICTORS OF SUCCESS

SUCCESS

The two important predictors of surgical success are the ability to select the surgical candidate with unilateral temporal lobe epilepsy and the ability to locate the temporal lobe epileptogenic region and thus to determine which portion of the temporal lobe to remove so seizure control is optimized and neurologic and cognitive deficits are minimized.[45] This information is usually obtained during the phased evaluation already described.

We are still analyzing our outcome data at the time of this writing. It has become clear, however, that a particular descriptive pattern has the highest likelihood of seizure-free outcome. This patient's profile is characteristic of the usual medial temporal lobe epilepsy patient (CTLE). He or she (there is no sexual predominance):

- Is typically between 20 and 30 years old
- Has developed intractable complex partial seizures in adolescence (average age 11 years)
- Frequently has a history of a childhood febrile seizures (60 percent)
- Has MRI volumetric studies revealing hippocampal or temporal lobe atrophy
- Demonstrates unilateral electrographic seizure onset in the hippocampal-entorhinal cortex, either inferred from surface EEG or documented from depth and subdural intracranial studies
- Has 50 percent or more neuronal loss and concomitant gliosis in all CA fields and in the dentate granule cell layer without changes in the subiculum and entorhinal cortex
- Has immunohistochemical studies showing somatostatin and neuropeptide-Y interneuron loss in the dentate hilum as well as selective fiber sprouting in the dentate
- Has hippocampal slice electrophysiology showing abnormal bursting in dentate granule cells

Anterior medial temporal lobe resection of 68 patients with these characteristics yielded an 87 percent success in seizure control after at least 1 year of follow-up.

Comparing success rates among different surgical techniques or among different epilepsy centers is difficult because uniform criteria for success or general outcome have not been established. Typically, outcome of surgery for temporal lobe epilepsy is reported with respect to seizure frequency, usually independent of whether patients remain on anticonvulsant medication.[84] Efforts have been recently made to include other social and personal factors in outcome classification schemes, because social, familial, psychiatric, and employment issues are recognized as also very important in describing the overall outcome and success. Good outcome could be considered quite individualized. For example, a rare seizure in one individual may represent a dramatic improvement in the patient's life, whereas in another patient, even one rare seizure could have a dramatic negative effect. Classification schemes and postoperative outcome for temporal lobe resective surgery from various series found in the literature, as well as perioperative factors that influence postoperative seizure control, are reviewed by Primrose and Ojemann.[84] The authors point out that outcome reports from various centers often depend on variables reflecting the center's surgical philosophy. Outcome for a particular procedure may be directly related to the patient selection process. Therefore, direct comparisons between published series must be viewed with caution.

A binary classification scheme—being either seizure-free or not seizure-free—offers valuable information for comparing outcome series, because it is the seizure-free category that has the largest potential impact on a patient's life. Neuropsychological and general well-being of the patient seems to show the most improvement only in the seizure-free setting.[85]

We have defined a good (successful) outcome as remaining seizure-free for at least 1 year, allowing for immediate postoperative seizures as well as for rare auras, with or without postoperative medical therapy. One-year outcome statistics reveal that with AMTR, 57 of 68 (84 percent) of the CTLE patients have seizure control. As a comparison, patients with TLE due to temporal lobe tumor had an 86 percent seizure-free outcome.

PROGNOSTIC SIGNIFICANCE OF EARLY POSTOPERATIVE SEIZURES

Early postoperative seizures are common. They may be a consequence of falling anticonvulsant levels occurring in the acute postoperative period[86] or of the epileptogenicity of the remaining tissue, which was exacerbated by the surgical resection or they may stem from the acute metabolic changes associated with general anesthesia and craniotomy. Whereas a seizure in the first 24 to 36 hours following surgery may not represent surgical failure, the presence of habitual seizures postoperatively does suggest remaining epileptic substrate representing the original disorder. Generally, the occurrence of acute perioperative seizures has been minimized, because it was believed that they do not have predictive value with respect to outcome.[87] A study by Luders and associates,[88] however, indicated that seizures within the first week of surgery predicted a greater likelihood of recurrence of epilepsy in 2 years. How soon after surgery and under what circumstances (low antiepileptic drug levels, fever, electrolyte changes, etc.) these postoperative seizures occurred are most likely important in long-term outcome prediction, but this issue has not been investigated. Postoperative auras have also not been adequately studied as to their prognostic significance.

SURGICAL FAILURES AND THEIR PATHOETIOLOGY

In the majority of surgical failures, seizures recur within the first year after surgery, often as early as the first weeks or months.[87-89] Seizure recurrence increases progressively with the length of follow-up, but being seizure-free 1 year after surgery is an excellent predictor of continued seizure-free outcome.[88] Engel[87] reports that 79 percent of patients who were seizure-free at 1 year remained seizure-free at 5 years, and 63 percent at 10 years. These statistics do not relate to AMTL as described herein; our own long-term outcome is being reviewed.

There are several reasons for surgical failure in any surgically treated epilepsy patient. Such patients undoubtedly have a predisposition to epileptogenicity, either genetic or acquired, and therefore they have a continued predisposition for seizure recurrence.[90] A satisfactory resection of one epileptogenic region may result in failure when another excitable site becomes active.[91, 92] This may also be the etiology for the unexplained recurrences observed in patients after many years free of seizures. An error in localizing the epileptogenic area during the preoperative evaluation directs the wrong surgical removal and could be another cause of failure. Localization error in presumed TLE cases may occur when seizure onset in the lateral temporal neocortex, in an extratemporal location, was not recognized and addressed. This represents a failure of patient selection or true bitemporal epilepsy, a surgical technical failure. The most important reason for surgical failure is insufficient excision of epileptogenic brain or, in the setting of a lesion, incomplete resection of an epileptogenic structural lesion. This accounts for the majority of cases of recurrent refractory epilepsy. In TLE patients, Olivier et al[93] recognized the role of retained mesial structures in patients with failed temporal lobectomy. Wyler and colleagues[94, 95] also reported a large series of reoperations, concluding that insufficient resection at the first operation was the reason for failure. Awad and associates[91] are also in agreement with these above explanations; the majority of their patients had persistent epileptogenicity related to inadequate resection, retained mesiotemporal structures, or retained epileptogenic structural lesions. Other patients had foci at more remote sites or diffuse epileptogenicity in the residual temporal lobe.[96]

WORKUP FOR SEIZURE RECURRENCE

We treat surgical failures aggressively. Each patient undergoes repeat evaluation with anatomic and metabolic imaging and video EEG monitoring, and the surgical pathologic profile is carefully reviewed. In patients treated for tumors, seizure recurrence usually precedes radiographic evidence of tumor recurrence by approximately 6 months.[97]

ROLE OF REOPERATION

In patients in whom amygdalo-hippocampectomy had failed, Wieser[98] reoperated using a standard anterior temporal lobectomy and reported a 50 percent success rate. Short-term and medium-term seizure control has been accomplished in most of the reported cases of reoperation.[91-95] Nearly half of reported patients in another series have remained seizure-free for periods of up to 72 months, and another third showed worthwhile improvement in seizure frequency despite severe intractable seizures before reoperation.[91, 96]

NEUROPSYCHOLOGICAL AND NEUROLOGIC SEQUELAE

With resective surgery involving the hippocampus and lateral temporal lobe, one would expect possible sequelae such as visual field defects, deterioration in memory function, and fluent dysphasias. The visual field defect in a patient who has an anterior temporal lobectomy is usually a superior quadrantanopia contralateral to the operated side.[99] The visual loss becomes more hemianoptic as the lateral incision is placed more posteriorly.[100-102] The posterior location of the optic radiation fibers is variable, but as a rule, patients acquire more than an upper quadrant visual field defect when an incision is made more than 5 cm from the temporal tip. By limiting our lateral cortical resection to only that sufficient to allow entry into the temporal ventricular horn (3 to 3.5 cm from the temporal tip), we typically observe only a partial superior quadrantanopia or often no field defect at all. Homonymous hemianopia has not occurred.

Dysnomia and other fluent speech errors elicited by stimulation are found in quite variable locations on the lateral temporal cortex of the dominant hemisphere.[103] Resecting these positive stimulation areas is thought to result in some degree of permanent fluent dysphasia. Preserving one gyrus between the cortical incision and the most anteriorly located site of the speech error avoids a permanent speech deficit. In our experience using stimulation in awake patients, we have rarely found fluent speech represented more anteriorly than 5.5 cm on the middle temporal gyrus and 4.5 cm on the superior temporal gyrus, as measured from the anterior temporal tip.[27, 103] This is well beyond our posterior resection margin, and the superior temporal gyrus is always preserved. Hermann and colleagues[104] have studied language function in patients with medial temporal epilepsy who underwent anterior temporal lobe resection modeled after our description. These authors found that AMTL of the dominant hemisphere can be accomplished without intraoperative or extraoperative language mapping with no measurable compromise of language function. They also demonstrated that patients rendered seizure-free by any surgical procedure demonstrated significant gains in several language areas, whereas patients who continued to experience even some seizures showed no improvements in language function.[105]

Historically, the hippocampal model of human memory was elaborated by Penfield and Milner,[107] who observed that bilateral hippocampal ablation produced permanent complete amnesia. They also found that the dominant hippocampus served verbal memory function and the nondominant hippocampus served nonverbal (i.e., visual-spacial) memory function and that the extent of unilateral hippocampal ablation seemed to relate to the severity of the memory deficit.[106, 107] This is contrary to our findings that patients who underwent extensive unilateral hippocampectomy did not produce either amnesia for specific material or memory impairment greater than that occurring with traditional partial hippocampectomy.[27]

Temporal lobe memory mechanisms seem not to be exclusively confined to medial temporal structures.[25, 27] Ojemann recently reviewed the occurrence of verbal memory deficits after dominant hemisphere temporal lobectomies and found that they correlate with the extent of lateral, but not medial, resection.[103] All of these findings suggest that it may be the relationship between the lateral cortex and the medial structures that must be preserved in order to avoid memory deficits.[108, 109]

It is known that seizure activity and anticonvulsants may depress cognitive functions[110–115] and that following surgical control of seizures, selected cognitive functions improve. The improvements are due to the elimination of ictal disturbances and to reduction in medications. The most common improvements are those related to general measures of cognition, such as intelligence quotient and learning, or to selective functions associated with brain regions outside the resected area.[34, 116–119] There is, then, growing evidence that a limited anterior temporal resection in either hemisphere does not produce significant long-term adverse neurologic or neuropsychologic sequelae and that the result of a seizure-free status may even improve the patient's neuropsychologic baseline status.

TRANSIENT SEQUELAE AND COMPLICATIONS OF AMTR

Complications are not common. General complications of neurosurgical procedures occur that are common to all intracranial operations, and specific neurologic complications are associated with AMTR. General complications include acute postoperative hemorrhage, retraction injury, wound infection, and the usual perioperative sequelae, such as anesthetic and medication intolerance, deep vein thrombosis, and infections of the bladder, lung, or intravascular lines.

TRANSIENT DEFICITS

Complications associated with AMTR and other temporal lobectomy procedures for TLE are considered separate from transient deficits, which are often seen. Penfield[120] described ''neuro-paralytic edema,'' which contributed to transient deficits he observed. Whether it is retraction injury or functional damage from temporary ischemic conditions, if functional cortex is manipulated, then transient neurologic dysfunction may result. Such deficits include memory impairment, decreased spontaneous speech, and anomias. Transient diplopia, ptosis, or pupillary dilatation results from manipulation of the third and fourth cranial nerves just under the arachnoid of the perimesencephalic cisterns and the tentorial edge. These transient deficits most often clear within several days.[121]

COMPLICATIONS AND PERMANENT DEFICITS

Temporal lobectomy usually produces some degree of permanent contralateral superior quadrantanopia. Anything less than a contralateral upper quadrant defect should not be considered a complication.

In 1961, Penfield et al[122] presented eight patients who developed a postoperative hemiplegia that they called ''manipulation hemiplegia.'' They believed this to be a consequence of traction on the middle cerebral artery perforators that resulted in vasospasm and infarction of their vascular territory.[122, 123] In more than 300 temporal lobe procedures, Girvin has had only one patient with postoperative hemiplegia, which was due to infarction within the internal capsule; this was attributed to injury of the anterior choroidal artery.

FUTURE TRENDS

METABOLIC IMAGING

PET and SPECT imaging have contributed to the understanding of epileptogenic brain regions. As ligands for specific receptors or neuronal subpopulations become available, more precise localization of epileptogenic regions and improved patient selection are anticipated. Intraoperative metabolic imaging using optical methods to topographically record cortical blood flow is being investigated by Ojemann. Activated and spontaneous SPECT, whereby metabolic abnormalities associated with epileptogenic areas can be enhanced, is an example of new metabolic imaging ideas currently under investigation.[60, 124, 125]

FAST ECHO PLANAR FUNCTIONAL IMAGING

It has now become possible to image differential blood flow using MRI. Coupling this imaging modality to specific stimulation protocols offers the possibility of localizing visual cortex, motor and sensory cortex, and speech and memory areas with excellent accuracy using this noninvasive tool.[133–136] Temporal lobe function, functional cortex localization, and perhaps abnormal pathophysiologic localization will be of tremendous help in patient selection and surgical planning. The amytal angiogram may be relegated to historical interest with the advent of functional imaging using MRI.

There is growing enthusiasm for performing epilepsy surgery in younger patients. Many believe that if seizure activity can be abolished early in a patient's life, the psychological and psychiatric impacts of a prolonged seizure disorder may be minimized.[127] It is reasonable to suspect that if seizures are controlled early in life, the gradual deterioration of cognitive and intellectual functions, the progressively disordered social and behavioral situation, and the irreversible personality changes, all of which lead to problems in family, school, and vocation, may be avoided.[128–132] As epileptologists and epilepsy surgeons gain a better understanding of the evolution of the disease process from a child's febrile convulsion to an adolescent's refractory epilepsy, earlier recognition and treatment of TLE seems likely.

SUMMARY

The Yale anterior medial temporal lobectomy was designed for resection of the posterior hippocampal epileptogenic region with preservation of lateral neocortex. Its multiple advantages, however, have prompted us to use it in most of our patients with unilateral temporal lobe epilepsy and variably extensive hippocampal disease. Minimizing lateral and maximizing medial temporal lobe removal eliminates electrocorticography and speech mapping, permitting all temporal lobectomies to be performed using general anesthesia. Study of the resected hippocampus reveals that there are at least two forms of medial temporal lobe epilepsy, characterized by history and by the degree of neuronal cell loss, gliosis, and reorganization within the hippocampus. There is also TLE associated with a structural lesion, usually a low-grade tumor. AMTL was designed for the treatment of medial temporal lobe epilepsy, and by offering en bloc resection of the medial structures, this operation is ideal for experimental and clinical studies in which the anatomically intact pathologic substrate is required.

Our follow-up period is longer than 1 year, and we are in the process of evaluating long-term efficacy. Thus far, the patients who have undergone AMTL have had excellent seizure control, small visual field defects, and fewer and shorter-lived speech deficits. Neuropsychological testing reveals no additional deficits resulting from our modified temporal lobectomy compared with the standard operation. Most patients have had less impairment in visual-spatial perception than was common with the more standard lobectomy. Because of these encouraging results, we have adopted anterior medial temporal lobectomy as a ''standard'' operation for medial temporal lobe epilepsy.[27]

REFERENCES

1. Bouchet, Cazauvielh: De l'épilepsie considérée dans ses rapports avec l'aliénation mentale. Recherche sur la nature et le siège de ces deux maladies; mémoire qui a remporte le prix au concours établi par M. Esquirol. Arch Gen Med 9:510–542, 1825
2. Sommer W: Erkrankung des ammonshorn als aetiologisches moment der epilepsie. Arch Psychiatr Nervenkr 10:631–675, 1880
3. Jackson JH: On a particular variety of epilepsy (''intellectual aura''), one case with symptoms of organic brain disease, in Taylor J (ed): Selected Writings of John Hughlings Jackson. London, Hodder and Stoughton, 1931, pp 385–405
4. Jackson JH: Brain 11:179, 1888
5. Falconer MA: Mesial temporal (Ammon's horn) sclerosis as a common cause of epilepsy: Aetiology, treatment, and prevention. Lancet 2:767–770, 1974
6. Falconer MA, Taylot DC: Surgical treatment of drug-resistant epilepsy due to mesial temporal sclerosis. Arch Neurol 19:353–361, 1968
7. Foerster O: Zur pathogenese und chirurischem Behandlung der Epilepsie. Zentrabl Chir 52:531–549, 1925
8. Bailey P, Gibbs FA: The surgical treatment of psychomotor epilepsy. JAMA 145:365–370, 1951
9. Foerster O, Penfield W: The surgical basis of traumatic epilepsy and results of medical operation. Brain 53:99–119, 1930
10. Penfield W, Jasper H: Epilepsy and the functional anatomy of the human brain. Boston, Little Brown, 1954, pp 739–817
11. Penfield W, Baldwin M: Temporal lobe seizures and technique of subtotal temporal lobectomy. Ann Surg 136:625–634, 1952
12. Earle KA, Baldwin MA, Penfield W: Incisural sclerosis and temporal lobe seizures produced by hippocampal herniation at birth. Arch Neurol Psychiatry 69:27–42, 1953
13. Margerison JH, Corsellis JAN: Epilepsy and the temporal lobes: A clinical, electroencephalographic and neuropathological study of the brain in epilepsy, with particular reference to the temporal lobes. Brain 89:499–530, 1966
14. Morris AA: Temporal lobectomy with removal of uncus, hippocampus, and amygdala. Arch Neurol Psychiatry 79:479–496, 1956
15. Walker AE: Surgery for epilepsy, in Magnus O, Lorentz de Haas AM (eds): Handbook of Clinical Neurology, Vol 15. Amsterdam, North Holland, 1974, pp 39–757
16. Falconer MA, Cavanagh JB: Clinicopathological considerations of temporal lobe epilepsy due to small focal lesions. Brain 82:483–504, 1956
17. Falconer MA, Hill D, Meyer A, et al: Treatment of temporal-lobe epilepsy by temporal lobectomy: A survey of findings and results. Lancet 1:827–835, 1955
18. Falconer MA, Serafetinides EA, Corsellis JAN: Etiology and pathogenesis of temporal lobe epilepsy. Arch Neurol 10:233–248, 1964
19. Engel J, Driver MV, Falconer MA: Electrophysiological correlates of pathology and surgical results in temporal lobe epilepsy. Brain 98:129–156, 1975
20. Falconer M, Hill D, Pampliglione G: Discussion on the surgery of temporal lobe epilepsy. Proc Roy Soc Med 46:965–976, 1953
21. Bancaud J, Talairach J: Macro-stereoelectroencephalography in epilepsy, in Remond A (ed): Handbook of Electroencephalography and Clinical Neurophysiology, Vol 10 B: Stereoelectroencephalography. Amsterdam, Elsevier, 1975, pp 3–33
22. Talairach J, Bancaud J, Szikla G, et al: Approche nouvelle de la neurochirurgie de l'épilépsie. Methodologie stéreotaxique et résultats thérapeutiques. Neurochirurgie [Suppl] 20:1–240, 1974
23. Crandall PH: Standard *en bloc* anterior temporal lobectomy, in Spencer D, Spencer S (eds): Surgery for Epilepsy. Boston, Blackwell Scientific, 1991, pp 118–129
24. Lieb JP, Engel J, Brown WJ, et al: Neuropathological findings following temporal lobectomy related to surface and deep EEG patterns. Epilepsia 22:539–549, 1981
25. Wieser HG, Yasargil MG: Selective amygdalohippocampectomy as a surgical treatment of mesiobasal limbic epilepsy. Surg Neurol 17:445–457, 1982
26. Spencer SS, Williamson PD, Spencer DD, Mattson RH: Human hippocampal seizure spread studied by depth and subdural recordings: The hippocampal commissure. Epilepsia 28:479–487, 1987
27. Spencer DD, Spencer SS, Mattson RH, et al: Access to the posterior medial temporal lobe structures in the surgical treatment of temporal lobe epilepsy. Neurosurgery 15:667–671, 1984
28. Levesque MF, Zhang J, Wilson C, et al: Stereotactic investigation of limbic epilepsy using a multimodal image analysis system. J Neurosurg 73:792–797, 1990
29. Peters TM, Clark JE, Olivier A, et al: Integrated stereotaxic imaging with CT, MR imaging and digital subtraction angiography. Radiology 161:821–826, 1986
30. Van Veelan CWM, Depets RMC, van Huffelen AC, et al: Combined use of subdural and intracranial electrodes in preoperative evaluation of epilepsy. Neurosurgery 26:93–101, 1990
31. Zhang J, Levesque MF, Wilson C, et al: Multimodal imaging for stereotactic surgery. Radiology 175:435–441, 1990
32. Green JR, Duisbery REH, McGrath WB: Focal epilepsy of psychomotor type. J Neurosurg 8:157–172, 1951
33. Van Bruen JM, Ajmone-Marsan C, Mutsuga C: Temporal lobe seizures with additional foci treated by resection. J Neurosurg 45:596–607, 1975
34. Wieser HG: Selective amygdalo-hippocampectomy: Indications, investigative technique and results, in Symon L, et al (eds): Advances and Technical Standards in Neurosurgery, Vol 13. New York, Springer, 1986, pp 39–133
35. Yasargil MG, Teddy PJ, Roth P: Selective amygdalohippocampectomy: Operative anatomy and surgical technique, in Symon L, et al (eds): Advances and Technical Standards in Neurosurgery, Vol 12. New York, Springer, 1985, pp 93–124

36. Penfield W, Erickson TC: Epilepsy and Cerebral Localization. Springfield, IL, Charles C Thomas, 1941
37. Penfield W, Paine K: Results of surgical therapy for focal epileptic seizures. Can Med Assoc J 73:515–531, 1955
38. Olivier A, Tanaka T, Andermann F: Reoperations in temporal lobe epilepsy. Epilepsia 29:678, 1988
39. Nayel MH, Awad IA, Luders H: Extent of mesiobasal resection determines outcome of temporal lobectomy for intractable epilepsy. Epilepsia 31:678, 1990
40. Awad IA, Katz A, Hahn JF, et al: Extent of resection in temporal lobectomy for epilepsy. I: Interobserver analysis and correlation with seizure outcome. Epilepsia 30:756–762, 1989
41. Engel J, Rausch R, Lieb JP, et al: Correlation of criteria used for localizing epileptic foci in patients considered for surgical therapy of epilepsy. Ann Neurol 9:215–224, 1981
42. Spencer SS: Intracranial recording, in Spencer D, Spencer S (eds): Surgery for Epilepsy. Boston, Blackwell Scientific, 1991, pp 54–65
43. Goldring S: Epilepsy surgery. Clinical Neurology 31:369–389, 1984
44. Ojemann GA: Temporal lobectomy tailored to electrocorticography and funcitonal mapping, in Spencer D, Spencer S (eds): Surgery for Epilepsy. Boston, Blackwell Scientific, 1991, pp 137–145
45. Spencer D: Anterior temporal lobectomy: Directing the surgical approach to the pathologic substrate, in Spencer D, Spencer S (eds): Surgery for Epilepsy. Boston, Blackwell Scientific, 1991, pp 129–137
46. Wyler AR: Comment (temporal lobectomy), in Spencer D, Spencer S (eds): Surgery for Epilepsy. Boston, Blackwell Scientific, 1991, pp 148–149
47. Chatrian GE: Paroxysmal patterns in "normal" subjects, in Rimond A (ed): Handbook of Electroencephalography and Clinical Neurophysiology, Vol 6A. Amsterdam, Elsevier, 1976, pp 114–123
48. Jack CR, Sharbrough FW, Twomey CK, et al: Temporal lobe seizures: Lateralization with MR volume measurements of the hippocampal formation. Radiology 175:423–429, 1990
49. Lencz T, McCarthy G, Bronen RA, et al: Quantitative magnetic resonance in temporal lobe epilepsy: Relationship to neuropathology and neuropsychological function. Ann Neurol 31:629–637, 1992
50. Babb TL, Brown WJ, Pretorius J, et al: Temporal lobe volumetric cell densities in temporal lobe epilepsy. Epilepsia 25:729–740, 1984
51. Kim JH, Guimaraes PO, Shen MY, et al: Hippocampal neuronal density in temporal lobe epilepsy with and without gliomas. Acta Neuropathol 80:41–45, 1990
52. DeLanerolle NC, Kim JH, Robbins RJ, et al: Hippocampal interneuron loss and plasticity in human temporal lobe epilepsy. Brain Research 495:387–395, 1989
53. Meencke HJ, Veith G: Hippocampal sclerosis in epilepsy, in Luders H: Epilepsy Surgery. New York, Raven Press, 1991
54. Griffiths T, Evans MC, Meldrum BS: Intracellular calcium accumulation in rat hippocampus during seizures induced by bicuculline or L-allylglycine. Neuroscience 10:385–395, 1983
55. Olney JW: Excitatory transmitters and epilepsy-related brain damage. Int Rev Neurobiol 27:337–362, 1985
56. Sloviter RS, Dempster DW: "Epileptic" brain damage is replicated qualitatively in the rat hippocampus by central injection of glutatmate or aspartate but not by GABA or acetylcholine. Brain Res Bull 15:39–60, 1985
57. Insauti R, Amaral DG, Cowan WM. The entorhinal cortes of the monkey: II: Cortical afferents. J Comp Neurol 264:356–395, 1987
58. Van Hoesen FW, Pandya DN, Butters N: Some connections of the entorhinal (area 28) and perirhinal (area 35) cortices of the rhesus monkey. II: Frontal lobe afferents. Brain Res 95:25–38, 1975
59. Spencer DD, Inserni J: Temporal lobectomy, in Luders H: Epilepsy Surgery. New York, Raven Press, 1991, pp 533–545
60. Hardiman O, Coughlan A, O'More B, et al: Interictal spike localization with methohexitone; preoperative activation and surgical followup. Epilepsia 28:335–339, 1987
61. Spencer DD: Epilepsy surgery protocol at Yale (Appendix E), in Luders H (ed): Epilepsy Surgery. New York, Raven Press, 1991, pp 800–802
62. Masukawa LM, Higashima M, Kim JH, et al: Epileptiform discharges evoked in hippocampal brain slices from epileptic patients. Brain Res 493:168–174, 1989
63. Ray CD: A new multicontact, multipurpose depth probe: First experimental results. Mayo Clin Proc 40:781–790, 1965
64. Spencer SS: Depth electroencephalography in selection of refractory epilepsy for surgery. Ann Neurol 9:207–214, 1981
65. Spencer SS, Spencer DD, Williamson PD, et al: Value of depth electroencephalography in 32 refractory epileptic patients. Ann Neurol 21:248–253, 1982
66. Kratimenos GP, Pell MF, Thomas GT, et al: Open stereotactic selective amygdalohippocampectomy for drug resistant epilepsy. Acta Neurochir 116:150–154, 1992
67. Kelly PJ, Sharbrough FW, Kall BA, et al: Magnetic resonance imaging–based computer assisted stereotactic resection of the hippocampus and amygdala in patients with temporal lobe epilepsy. Mayo Clin Proc 62:103–108, 1987
68. Talairach J, Stikla G: Destruction partielle amygdalo-hippocampique par l'yttrium 90 dans le traitement de certaines épilépsies à expréssion rhinencéphalique. Neurochirugie 11:233–240, 1965
69. Turner EA: A new approach to unilateral and bilateral lobectomies for psychomotor epilepsy. J Neurosurg Psychiatry 26:285–299, 1963
70. Narabayashi H, Mizutami T: Epileptic seizures and the stereotactic amygdalotomy. Confin Neurol 32:289–297, 1970
71. Spiegel ER, Wycis HT, Baird HW: Pallidectomy and pallidoamygdalotomy in certain types of convulsive disorders. Arch Neurol Psychiatry 80:714–728, 1958
72. Wieser HG, Yasargil MG: Die "selektive Amygdala Hippokampektomie" als Chirurgische Behandlungsmethode der mediobasal-limbischen Epilepsie. Neurochirurgia 25:39–50, 1982
73. Niemeyer P: The transventricular amygdala-hippocamptectomy in temporal lobe epilepsy, in Baldwin M, Bailey P (eds): Temporal Lobe Epilepsy. Springfield, IL, Charles C Thomas, 1958, pp 461–482
74. Walter RD: Principles of clinical investigation of surgical candidates. Adv Neurol 8:49–58, 1975
75. Spencer SS: Surgical options for uncontrolled epilepsy. Neurologic Clinics 4:669–695, 1986
76. Rossi GF: Considerations on the principles of surgical treatment of partial epilepsy. Brain Res 95:395–402, 1975
77. Williamson PD, Wieser HG, Delgado-Escueta AV: Clinical characteristics of partial seizures, in Engel J (ed): Surgical Treatment of the Epilepsies. New York, Raven Press, 1987, pp 101–120
78. Wada J, Rasmussen T: Intracarotid injection of sodium amytal for lateralization of cerebral speech dominance; experimental and clinical observations. J Neurosurg 17:266–282, 1960
79. Dam AM: Epilepsy and neuronal loss in the hippocampus. Epilepsia 21:617–629, 1980
80. Dam AM: Hippocampal neuron loss in epilepsy and after experimental seizures. Acta Neurol Scand 66:601–642, 1982
81. Williamson A, McCormick CA, Shepard CM, et al: Intracellular recordings from epileptic human dentate granule cells show evidence of hyperexcitability. Epilepsia 31:625, 1990
82. Lencz T, McCarthy G, Bronen R, et al: Hippocampus in temporal lobe epilepsy: Correlation of presurgical MRI volumetrics with postsurgical cell counts. Epilepsia 31:667, 1990
83. Jack CR, Sherbough FW, Cascino J, et al: Magnetic resonance image–based hippocampal volumetry: Correlation with outcome after temporal lobectomy. Ann Neurol 31:138–146, 1982
84. Primrose DC, Ojemann GA: Outcome of resective surgery for temporal lobe epilepsy, in Luders H (ed): Epilepsy Surgery. New York, Raven Press, 1991, pp 601–611
85. Herman BP, Wyler AR, Ackerman B, et al: Short-term psychological outcome of anterior temporal lobectomy. J Neurosurg 71:327–334, 1989
86. Friel P, Clarke H, Ojemann G, et al: Decreased anticonvulsant levels after epilepsy surgery. Epilepsia 28:588, 1987
87. Engel J: Outcome with respect to epileptic seizures, in Engel J (ed): Surgical Treatment of the Epilepsies. New York, Raven Press, 1987, pp 553–571
88. Luders H, Murphy D, Dinner D, et al: Prognostic value of epileptic seizures occuring in the first week after surgery for epilepsy. Epilepsia 29:679, 1988
89. Swanson TH, Hirschorn KA, Cascino GD, et al: Outcome of patients with early seizures after epilepsy surgery. Epilepsia 30:728, 1989
90. Andermann E: Multifactorial inheritance of generalized and focal epilepsy, in Anderson VE, Hauser WA, Penry JK, et al (eds): Genetic Basis of the Epilepsies. New York, Raven Press, 1982, pp 355–374
91. Awad IA, Nayel MH, Luders H: Second operation after the failure of previous resection for epilepsy. Neurosurgery 28:510–518, 1991
92. MacDonald DB, Hirschorn KA, Sharbrough FW, et al: Second surgery for intractable partial epilepsy: Mayo Clinic experience. Epilepsia 30:727, 1989
93. Olivier A, Tanaka T, Andermann F: Reoperations in temporal lobe epilepsy. Epilepsia 29:678, 1988

94. Wyler AR, Herman BP, Richey ET: Results of reoperation for failed epilepsy surgery. J Neurosurg 71:815–819, 1989
95. Wyler AR, Herman BP, Richey ET: Results of reoperation for failed epilepsy surgery. Epilepsia 30:728, 1989
96. Awad IA, Wingkum EC, Nayel MH, et al: Surgical failures and reoperation, in Luders H (ed): Epilepsy Surgery. New York, Raven Press, 1991, pp 679–685
97. Spencer DD, Spencer SS, Williamson PD, et al: Intracranial masses in patients with refractory partial epilepsy. Neurology 34:432–436, 1984
98. Wieser HG: Selective amygdalo-hippocampectomy for temporal lobe epilepsy. Epilepsia 29(suppl 2):S100–S113, 1988
99. Van Buren JM: Complications of surgical approaches in the diagnosis and treatment of epilepsy, in Engel J (ed): Surgical Treatment of the Epilepsies. New York, Raven Press, 1987, pp 465–475
100. Falconer MA, Wilson JD: Visual field changes following anterior temporal lobectomy: Their significance in relation to "Meyer's" loop of the optic radiation. Brain 81:1–14, 1958
101. Marino R, Rasmussen T: Visual field changes after temporal lobectomy in man. Neurology 18:825–835, 1968
102. Katz A, Awad IA, Kong AK, et al: Extent of resection in temporal lobectomy for epilepsy. II: Memory changes and neurologic complications. Epilepsia 30:763–771, 1989
103. Ojemann G: Individual variability in cortical localization of language. J Neurosurg 50:164–169, 1979
104. Hermann BP, Wyler AR, Somes G: Language function following anterior temporal lobectomy. J Neurosurg 74:560–566, 1991
105. Hermann B, Wyler AR: Comparative results of dominant temporal lobectomy under general or local anesthesia: Language outcome. Epilepsia 29:668, 1988
106. Milner B: Psychological aspects of focal epilepsy and its neurosurgical management. Adv Neurol 8:299–321, 1975
107. Penfield W, Milner B: Memory deficit produced by bilateral lesions in the hippocampal zone. Arch Neurol Psychiatry 79:475–497, 1958
108. Spencer DD, Spencer SS, Mattson RH, et al: Access to the posterior medial temporal lobe structures in the surgical treatment of temporal lobe epilepsy (comments). Neurosurgery 15:667–671, 1984
109. Schwarz SS, Spencer DD, Novelly RA, et al: Preservation of verbal and pictorial memory after anteromedial temporal lobectomy and radical hippocampectomy for temporal lobe epilepsy. Epilepsia 29:678, 1988
110. Dodrill CB: Diphenylhydantoin serum levels, toxicity, and neuropsychological performance in patients with epilepsy. Epilepsia 16:593–600, 1975
111. Matthews CG, Harley JP: Cognitive and motor-sensory performance in toxic and nontoxic epileptic subjects. Neurology 25:184–188, 1975
112. Rausch R, Lieb JP, Crandall PH: Neuropsychological correlates of patterns of depth spike activity in epileptic patients. Arch Neurol 35:699–706, 1978
113. Schmidt D: Toxicity of anti-epileptic drugs, in Pedly TA, Meldrum BS (eds): Recent Advances in Epilepsy, No 3. Edinburgh, Churchill-Livingstone, 1986, pp 211–233
114. Schmidt D: Adverse effects of antiepileptic drugs in children. Cleve Clin J Med 56(Suppl part 1):S132–S139, 1989
115. Wilkus RJ, Dodrill CB: Neuropsychological correlates of the electroencephalogram in epileptics. I: Topographic correlates of the average rate of epileptiform activity. Epilepsia 17:89–100, 1976
116. Hermann BP, Wyler AR, Richey ET: Wisconsin Card Sorting Test performance in patients with complex partial seizures of temporal lobe origin. J Clin Exp Neuropsychol 10:467–476, 1988
117. Novelly RA, Augustine EA, Mattson RH, et al: Selective memory improvement and impairment in temporal lobectomy for epilepsy. Ann Neurol 15:64–67, 1984
118. Rausch R, Crandall PH: Psychological status related to surgical control of temporal lobe seizures. Epilepsia 23:191–202, 1982
119. Nadig T, Wieser HG: Problems of learning and memory: Comparison of performances before and after surgical therapy, in Wieser HG, Elger CE (eds): Presurgical Evaluation of Epileptics. Heidelberg, Springer, 1987, pp 91–93
120. Penfield W: Pitfalls and success in surgical treatment of focal epilepsy. Br Med J 1:669–672, 1958
121. Walczak TS, Radtke RA, McNamara JO, et al: Anterior temporal lobectomy for complex partial seizures: Evaluation, results and long-term follow-up in 100 cases. Neurology 40:413–418, 1990
122. Penfield W, Lende RA, Rasmussen T: Manipulation hemiplegia: An untoward complication in the surgery of focal epilepsy. J Neurosurg 18:760–776, 1961
123. Helgason CM, Bergen D, Bleck D, et al: Infarction after surgery of focal epilepsy: Manipulation hemiplegia revisited. Epilepsia 28:340–345, 1987
124. Hufnagel A, Burr W, Elger CE, et al: Localization of the epileptic focus during methoxital-induced anesthesia. Epilepsia 33:271–284, 1992
125. Wyler AR, Richey ET, Atkinson RA, et al: Methoxital activation of epileptogenic foci during acute electrocorticography. Epilepsia 28:490–494, 1987
126. Spencer SS, Schwartz S, Spencer DD: The treatment of epilepsy with surgery. Merritt Putnam Q 5:3–19, 1988
127. Wyllie E: Pediatric epileptology: That children may someday live free of seizures. Cleve Clin J Med 56(suppl part I):S9, 1989
128. Falconer MA: Reversibility by temporal lobe resection of the behavioral abnormalities of temporal lobe epilepsy. N Engl J Med 289:451–455, 1973
129. Glaser GH: Limbic epilepsy in children. J Nerv Ment Dis 144:391–397, 1967
130. Glaser GH: Epilepsy: Neuropsychological aspects, in Arieti S (ed): American Handbook of Psychiatry, Vol 4. New York, Basic Books, 1975, pp 314–355
131. Penry JK, Daly DD (eds): Complex Partial Seizures and Their Treatments. Adv Neurol 11:1–1, 1975
132. Glazer GH: Treatment of intractable temporal lobe-limbic (complex partial seizures) by temporal lobectomy. Ann Neurol 8:455–459, 1980
133. Belliveu JW, Kennedy DN Jr, McKinstry RC, et al: Functional mapping of the human visual cortex by magnetic resonance imaging. Science 254:716, 1991
134. Kwong KK, Belliveu JW, Chesler DA, et al: Dynamic magnetic resonance imaging of human brain activity during primary sensory stimulation. PNAS 89:5675, 1992
135. Bandettini P, Wong E, Hinks R, et al: Time course EPI of human brain function during task activation. Magn Reson Med 25:390, 1992
136. Ogawa S, Tank DW, Menon R, et al: Intrinsic signal changes accompanying sensory stimulation: Functional brain mapping with magnetic resonance imaging. PNAS 89:5951, 1992

CHAPTER 106

Awake Operations with Mapping in Epilepsy

George A. Ojemann

This chapter describes two somewhat unusual intraoperative techniques that are useful in planning some cortical resections. The first is a technique for localizing eloquent cortex, sites essential for motor or language function in an individual patient, using electrical stimulation mapping. Although it was developed in the context of surgery for epilepsy, this technique is applicable to any resection close to eloquent areas, including resections for intrinsic tumors and vascular lesions, in which the goal is to maximize the extent of the resection with minimal risk of motor or speech deficits. The second is a technique for intraoperative identification of epileptic tissue, likely to be the site of seizure generation in patients with medically intractable epilepsy, using recording of interictal spikes (IIS) on the electrocorticogram (ECoG). This technique, too, was developed for epilepsy surgery but is also of value in increasing the probability of seizure control after lesion resections, when seizure control is a major problem. This is especially true for temporal lobe resections. Both techniques can be used with the patient under general anesthesia, with certain limitations, except that there is no intraoperative technique for individually localizing language in that setting. However, general anesthesia interferes with the accuracy of both techniques to some extent, so that ideally they are used in awake patients. Thus, this chapter begins with a discussion of the author's present technique of craniotomy in awake patients. Both stimulation and ECoG recording can also be used with chronically implanted subdural electrodes and extraoperative recording and stimulation. Although that technique is not described in detail here, the relative usefulness of intraoperative or extraoperative techniques in different patients is discussed.

TECHNIQUE OF AWAKE CRANIOTOMY

The advent of propofol intravenous anesthesia has made awake craniotomy much easier for both the patient and the surgeon.[1] About the only demand now made on the patient is that he or she should hold still for 1 to 2 hours while awake. Thus, the technique can be easily used in children of 12 or older and in most adolescents and adults. It can also be safely used in the presence of an intracranial mass, although the brain will be slightly tighter than is usually observed with modern endotracheal anesthesia, and it may be necessary to be slightly more aggressive with the use of intravenous osmotic agents in that setting compared with that of general anesthesia.

We now use only the lateral position with propofol. In that position, we have not had difficulties maintaining an airway; problems with maintaining the airway have occurred in patients in the supine position. The patient is positioned while awake with particular attention to his or her comfort. The head rests on a foam donut, and skeletal fixation is not used. Propofol anesthesia is then induced intravenously. Once the patient is asleep, a local anesthetic field block is placed, using a mixture of equal volumes of 0.5 percent lidocaine and 0.25 percent bupivacaine (Marcaine), both with 1:200,000 epinephrine. Propofol is not a particularly good analgesic, so the patient under anesthesia will often show more reaction to the placement of this block than will an awake patient. Thus, we use the same technique, making the first injections slowly through a needle, initially 30-gauge, at sites near the major scalp nerves and then completing the block around the entire area of the planned incision. Use of small amounts of intravenous fentanyl is of value in reducing responses to placement of the block. If the incision is to extend to the root of the zygoma, the insertions of the temporalis muscle are also infiltrated. The scalp incision and craniotomy then proceed in the usual manner. Once the dura is exposed, dural pain sensation is blocked by intradural injection of small quantities of the local anesthetic on each side of the middle meningeal artery, using the 30-gauge needle. A clamp is placed on the skull at the edge of the craniotomy, not only to provide a place to attach ECoG recording equipment but also to provide a handle to control the head if the patient becomes restless.

At this point, all pain-sensitive structures have been blocked with local anesthetics, and the noisy bone removal completed with the patient asleep. The lateral surface of the brain, of course, is insensitive to pain or touch. We usually awaken the patient before opening the dura, unless that opening is expected to be very tedious, for example when extensive pial-dural adhesions are anticipated. Patients are usually conversant within 7 to 12 minutes of stopping the propofol. At that time, they are reminded that they are in the operating room and should not move their head without first asking. The longest period before awakening in our experience has been 30 minutes. The patient usually awakens abruptly, a major advantage of propofol, and there is commonly no period of confusion when the propofol anesthesia has lasted no more than 1 to 1.5 hours. Recovery after longer periods of propofol anesthesia is usually slower, with a greater chance of a period of confusion. Propofol is also not a particularly good antiepileptic agent. Occasionally, we have observed clinical signs of spontaneous seizures in severe epileptics who are put to sleep with propofol. Short-acting benzodiazepines or barbiturates may be needed to control those seizures, but use of those drugs will interfere with subsequent recording and stimulation.

IDENTIFYING ELOQUENT CORTEX WITH ELECTRICAL STIMULATION MAPPING

The location of eloquent areas is mainly a concern in planning cortical resections in central portions of the hemisphere, and in the language-dominant hemisphere, posterior frontal, and posterior temporal-inferior parietal areas. Although language is usually lateralized to the left hemisphere, statistically independent of handedness,[2] when there is any question about unusual language lateralization, this factor should be established preoperatively with the intracarotid amobarbital perfusion test.[3] Whether location of language areas is important in planning anterior temporal resections in the dominant hemisphere is controversial (and has recently been reviewed).[4] There are no randomized studies to resolve this issue, but a report of consecutive series of anterior temporal lobectomies with or without identification of language areas suggested that there was a slightly greater risk of a postoperative language deficit in the series conducted without identification of language areas, although the difference was small.[5,6]

Eloquent areas can be identified either anatomically or functionally. However, the anatomic landmarks that identify rolandic cortex (i.e., vertically oriented gyri with a U shape at the sylvian fissure) are often difficult to discern through the intact pia, and they may be distorted or displaced by tumors. Common anatomic landmarks for avoiding language areas in the dominant hemisphere are the pterion for frontal resections, and for temporal resections, the line of rolandic cortex, or the vein of Labbé, or 4 to 4.5 cm from the temporal tip sparing superior gyrus. When language areas are individually identified by stimulation mapping, findings indicate that these landmarks unnecessarily restrict resections for many patients and do not avoid essential language areas in some other patients.[7]

The standard technique for individually identifying functionally important areas is electrical stimulation mapping. At present, there are no other established techniques to obtain this information, although optical imaging of the intrinsic signal[8,9] is a promising intraoperative technique, while identification of local blood flow changes during language measures in individual subjects with positron-emission tomography (PET) or dynamic magnetic resonance imaging (MRI) may eventually provide this information through the intact skull. In stimulation mapping, an electric current is applied to the cortical surface. This procedure produces a variety of effects, both exciting neurons and en passage fibers as well as blocking their function. These effects can produce excitation and inhibition locally or at a distance.[10] Thus, the effects of stimulation cannot be easily predicted physiologically but rather must be determined empirically. In the quiet patient, responses are readily evoked from primary motor and somatosensory cortex (localized movements or dysesthesias), somewhat more rarely from primary visual cortex (localized phosphenes), and infrequently from primary auditory cortex. Stimulation of other cortical areas produces no response at currents below the threshold for afterdischarges, although in patients with temporal lobe epilepsy, larger currents associated with afterdischarge occasionally evoke the interpretive and experiential response studies by Penfield and his associates.[11-13] However, if the patient engages in an ongoing measure of language, stimulation of some dominant hemisphere cortical areas outside primary cortices will disrupt language performance. Presumably, the predominant effect of stimulation at those sites is a disruption of function, probably by depolarization blockade. This is the technique of stimulation mapping of language initially developed by Penfield.[14] The choice of language measure to use with stimulation mapping is somewhat controversial. Penfield used object naming. This method also has the advantage as a screening measure for language function because all aphasic syndromes include deficits in naming. This is the language measure most often used by the author.[7] However, others have used reading measures as a screening test.[15]

For the surgeon, the important aspects of stimulation mapping are how localized the effects are and how reliably those effects predict the effect of resecting cortex. Imaging of the changes in the intrinsic signal that indicate where the stimulating current is altering neurons has shown that with bipolar cortical surface stimulation as used by the author, the changes are confined to tissue between the electrodes in both humans[9] and animals.[16] Behaviorally, both sensorimotor and language effects of stimulation are usually localized on a scale of millimeters to a few centimeters. Threshold sensorimotor effects with direct cortical stimulation are usually confined to a few millimeters on each side of the central sulcus, showing the classic homocular pattern of localization. Sites where stimulation repeatedly evokes naming errors are often confined to several separate cortical sites, each 1 to 2 cm² in extent, often with sharp boundaries (Fig. 106–1).[7] However, although they are often localized in an individual patient, these sites related to naming by stimulation are in somewhat different places in different patients (Fig. 106–2).[7] This variability in exact location of language areas indicates that only the most posterior portion of inferior frontal gyrus, immediately in front of face motor cortex, is essential in a large proportion of patients. Elsewhere, including any portion of the entire Wernicke area, essential language areas are present in not much more than one-third of patients. This substantial variability is one of the strongest arguments for using mapping function in each patient rather than depending on anatomic landmarks derived from population studies.

Evidence that sites identified as important to naming by stimulation mapping predict language effects of a resection are derived from several studies. In resections for epilepsy, Ojemann[17] found that when anterior temporal resections came within 2 cm along a continuous gyrus of a site where stimulation evoked repeated object naming errors, testing with a sensitive aphasia battery 1 month after operation showed subtle language changes that were not present when the resection had not come within 2 cm. Moreover, these changes were not related to the size of the resection, the degree of seizure control, or the patient's preoperative verbal abilities. In temporal lobe tumor resections, Haglund and associates[18] found that when the resection came within 5 mm of a site showing repeated naming errors with stimulation,

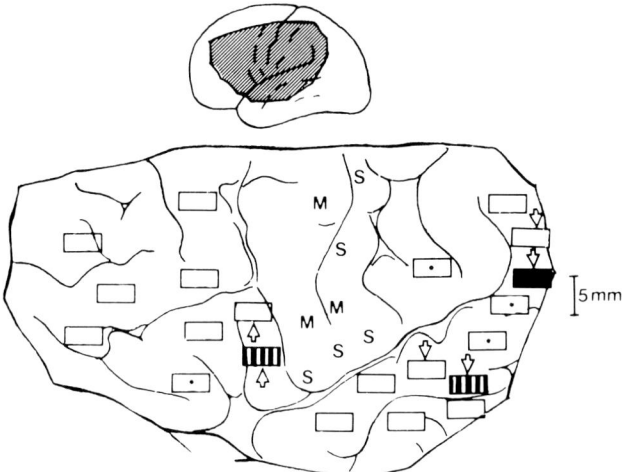

FIGURE 106–1. Localization of stimulation-evoked changes in naming in lateral cortex of left-dominant hemisphere of a 24-year-old woman. Each stimulation site is represented by rectangle. Filled or striped rectangles = repeated naming errors evoked there. Dot = single naming error evoked. Arrows identify nearby sites on contiguous gyri—one with repeated errors, the other without. Stimulation with 4-second trains of 60-Hz 2.5 msec total duration biphasic pulses at 8 mA between pulse peaks, delivered in a bipolar manner across 1-mm electrodes, separated by 5 mm. Naming error rate in absence of stimulation 0. M, S = site of evoked motor or sensory responses identifying rolandic cortex. (From Ojemann GA: Brain organization for language from the perspective of electrical stimulation mapping. Behav Brain Sci 6:189–230, 1983.)

about one-third of patients had permanent postoperative clinically evident aphasia, whereas when these sites were 15 mm or more from the margin of the resection, no patient had even temporary clinically evident aphasia. Very large resections in classic language cortex have not been followed by postoperative aphasias when stimulation mapping demonstrated all essential sites for naming elsewhere.[7] Thus, stimulation and lesions seem to identify the same cortical sites as essential to language. Interestingly, surface cortical stimulation predicts effects of resections that include both surface and buried cortex, suggesting that essential language areas are rarely, if ever, located only in buried cortex.

Stimulation mapping has been useful for investigation of the human cortical organization, particularly for language and memory.[19] Some of those findings have implications for planning resections very close to eloquent areas. Patterns of localization of perisylvian sites essential for naming differed between males and females, with a subset of females tending to have fewer temporoparietal naming sites, including a small group who seemed to have only frontal sites.[7] Patients who were verbally brighter tended to have naming sites in middle temporal gyrus, whereas those with poorer verbal skill tended to have naming sites in superior temporal gyrus. Highly localized perisylvian essential sites for naming have been identified in children as young as 4 years of age. When perisylvian stimulation effects on different language measures are examined, the general rule seems to be that slightly different cortical areas are essential for different language dimensions. Different sites seem to be essential for naming in two different languages[17, 20–22] including sign and oral languages.[23, 24] Different sites are often essential for naming or reading[17, 25] or for recent verbal memory.[26] In a few special settings, it may be useful to map localization of some of these other functions, for example in a patient heavily dependent on a second language or on reading skill. Avoiding cortical sites related by stimulation to recent verbal memory has been shown to be of value in decreasing the likelihood of a postoperative memory deficit in epilepsy patients who fail intracarotid amytal assessment of memory function.[26, 27] Stimulation mapping has also identified sites where repeated language errors are evoked in the supplementary motor area, on the medial and superior surfaces of posterior frontal lobe,[14, 28, 29] and on the basal surface of temporal lobe[15] in the dominant hemisphere. However, in contrast to perisylvian sites, resection of these areas apparently results in only a transient language deficit. In addition, stimulation mapping has been used to investigate localization of visuospatial functions in the nondominant hemisphere,[30] but these findings have not been used to plan resections.

TECHNIQUE OF INTRAOPERATIVE STIMULATION MAPPING

Several technical factors are important to successful stimulation mapping:

1. Mapping is difficult beyond the edges of the craniotomy. The exposure then should be generous and should include likely locations of functionally important areas.
2. Sites where language is located must be identified, because only then does the absence of language changes indicate cortex that can be resected with a low risk of aphasia. This also requires that the exposure include areas that are likely sites for language.
3. The stimulating current must be sufficiently large to alter function in cortex, but not so large as to evoke a seizure.
4. The patient must make few errors on the language

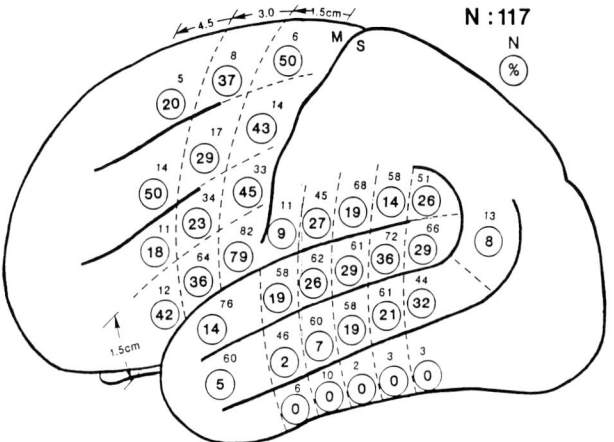

FIGURE 106–2. Variability in language localization in lateral cortex of left hemisphere derived from stimulation mapping during naming in 117 nonaphasic patients, all left dominant for language. Individual patient maps aligned to motor cortex and end of sylvian fissure. The cortex is then divided into arbitrary zones identified by dashed lines. Upper number in each zone is number of patients with sites of stimulation within that zone. Lower number in circle is percent of those patients with sites of repeated naming errors. Only one zone, the inferior frontal cortex just in front of face motor area, shows naming changes in over half the sample. (From Ojemann G, Ojemann J, Lettich E, Berger M: Cortical language localization in left-dominant hemisphere. J Neurosurg 71:316–326, 1989.)

measure in the absence of stimulation. Only a few samples of stimulation effect at any one site can be obtained. If there are many errors in the absence of stimulation, errors during stimulation may be random events and not related to stimulation effects at that site. The author regularly obtains three samples of stimulation effect at each site. For errors on all samples to have less than a 5-percent probability of being random events, the error rate in the absence of stimulation must not exceed 40 percent. Thus, stimulation mapping is of limited value in severely aphasic patients. Patients with mild aphasias may not be able to name with a low enough control error rate, but they may be able to read single words or can be continuously engaged in conversation during stimulation, although neither technique seems to be as satisfactory as naming for localizing language.

The only parameters of stimulation varied in the author's technique are the current level and train duration. All stimulations use 60-Hz trains of biphasic pulses, each phase 1 msec in duration, delivered from a constant current stimulator across 1-mm stainless steel bipolar ball electrodes placed 5 mm apart. Most other contemporary stimulation techniques use somewhat shorter pulses, often 0.3 msec for each phase, and some use 30-Hz frequency but are otherwise similar. Levels of electrical charge that produce histologic changes in tissue have been extensively studied in animals.[31] Histologic examination of stimulation sites in resected human cortex does not show any changes in the author's patients (unpublished data). Moreover, patients' performance in the absence of stimulation does not deteriorate after repeated stimulations. Both these findings indicate that stimulation at the indicated parameters does not permanently alter cortex.

After the patient is awakened and the dura opened, ECoG recording is undertaken. At the completion of this recoding, the afterdischarge threshold is established for the area of cortex to be sampled with language mapping. A small current, commonly 2 ma between pulse peaks, is applied for 4 seconds to cortex adjacent to an ECoG electrode; in the case of temporal exposures, thresholds are first determined for more posterior electrodes. This stimulation is repeated at increasing currents until afterdischarges are evoked, the patient reports a response, or an arbitrary upper limit on current is reached, usually 10 ma between pulse peaks for direct cortical stimulation. The current is then reduced 2 ma below that afterdischarge threshold, and the threshold at the next most anterior electrode is determined. After all electrodes are sampled, a process that requires 5 to 10 minutes, a current is selected for mapping that is at the lowest threshold for afterdischarge. The main reason for establishing the afterdischarge threshold is to avoid evoking a seizure. A brief train of afterdischarge after a stimulus train is usually not a problem. However, afterdischarge thresholds occasionally are less than 2 ma. Using larger currents in such patients is likely to evoke a seizure. However, using that small a current in other patients with higher thresholds may not alter cortical function, resulting in unreliable mapping.

Sensorimotor cortex is then identified. The author uses stimulus trains beginning at 2 ma, asking the patient for any evoked sensory responses, while an assistant looks for any overt movements. Current is increased at 1-ma intervals until responses are obtained. The site of each positive response is identified with a sterile numbered ticket. Other surgeons have used electromyographic responses to single pulses to identify motor areas.[31] Motor cortex can also be identified with stimulation of the patient under general anesthesia, so long as the patient is not paralyzed. However, patient responses under general anesthesia are much less focal, no sensory information is available, and tongue movements are difficult to identify. Recording of somatosensory evoked responses provides an alternative technique for identifying sensory cortex while the patient is under general anesthesia,[32] but in patients who are awake, that procedure requires more time and provides less information than stimulation mapping.

Following identification of the rolandic cortex, sterile numbered tickets are placed across the remaining cortex that is to be sampled during naming. The patient then begins the naming task. The author uses slide pictures of common objects to elicit naming, showing each slide at 4-second intervals on a back-projecting slide projector. A 4-second stimulation train is applied to one of the sites identified by a ticket at the appearance of the second or third slide. An assistant records the patient's responses and the number of the site stimulated. Another site is stimulated 2 or 3 slides later, until all sites have been sampled once. The process is then repeated in a different order two more times, so that stimulation effects on naming have been determined three times for each site. Sites with repeated naming errors are considered essential for language. With this technique, stimulation effects on naming can be determined for 20 sites in 20 minutes. Stimulation mapping with other language measures follows this same general plan, although the relation of applying the current to the behavioral measures may vary, especially when assessing memory. Our specialized and rather time-consuming protocol for assessing cortical stimulation effects on the input, storage, or retrieval phases of recent verbal memory has been published.[26]

INTRAOPERATIVE ELECTROCORTICOGRAPHY TO IDENTIFY EPILEPTIC AREAS

There are a number of different approaches to identifying the tissue that must be resected to control seizures in patients with medically intractable epilepsy.[4] In the approach used by the author, intraoperative recording of the residual interictal epileptiform activity (IIS) present in an awake patient on full antiepileptic medication is used to identify that tissue. Use of IIS for this purpose is controversial. Evidence supporting the value of IIS as a marker for epileptic tissue include the colocalization of IIS and sites of seizure onset in animal models of epilepsy, and usually, although not invariably, in human epilepsy, the evidence that a localized interictal epileptic focus is a major predictor of postoperative seizure control[33] and that persisting IIS following a resection decreases the chances of seizure control.[34] Recording of IIS can be performed with the patient under general anesthesia, but all anesthetic agents alter the ECoG and IIS patterns. If recordings are to be made with the patient under general anesthesia, the patient is paralyzed and the anesthetic lightened significantly. In the author's view, it is even better to record the ECoG in the awake patient with no anesthesia at the time of the recording. Propofol alters the ECoG when it is administered, but those effects very rapidly clear when it is discontinued.

Use of intraoperative recording of IIS in resections in

patients with intractable seizures associated with a lesion is also controversial. Unquestionably, lesion resection alone will control seizures in some patients and is usually adequate for patients whose seizures are controlled with antiepileptic medications. However, a recent meta-analysis of published results of lesion resections, with or without the additional resection of tissue with IIS on the ECoG in patients with intractable seizures and at least 2-year follow-up after operation, demonstrated that substantially more patients were free of seizures after resections including the abnormal tissue shown on the ECoG, almost regardless of the type of lesion.[35] This was particularly true for lesions in temporal lobe. At that location, tissue at a substantial distance from the lesion and uninvolved with it often has IIS, particularly the medial temporal structures, including hippocampus. If the presenting problem is intractable seizures, it is the author's view that resection of a temporal lesion should certainly use epilepsy surgery techniques, including ECoG recording, and these techniques should ideally be used in extratemporal lesion resections in such patients.

TECHNIQUE OF INTRAOPERATIVE ELECTROCORTICOGRAPHY

The goal of the ECoG recording is to delineate the full extent of IIS. To this end, subdural strip electrodes are placed over cortical areas not immediately under the craniotomy, such as basal temporal cortex, orbital frontal surface, or the medial face of a hemisphere. Recordings are obtained from lateral surface through carbon ball electrodes. The author uses referential ECoG recordings to a linked neck reference. The initial resection is designed to remove all tissue with IIS and any grossly evident lesion, unless the tissue is functionally important. The resection is usually undertaken after restarting propofol anesthesia, unless tissue very close to an area essential for language or motor functions is to be removed. Then that portion of the resection is performed while testing the patient's function, stopping the resection when the function begins to fail. If stopped at that point, any postoperative deficit is only transient.

In temporal lobe resections, the author repeats the ECoG recording after removal of the lateral cortex and opening the ventricle, placing a subdural strip on the hippocampus, and another parallel to it on parahippocampal gyrus. The location of IIS on recordings from these electrodes is used to plan the extent of the medial temporal resection. Propofol is briefly turned off for this recording, and the subsequent ECoG recording repeated after completion of the resection. The presence of IIS in some locations on this postresection ECoG, including discharges in the insula and probably the posterior parahippocampal gyrus, is not an indication for further resection. Following a resection, IIS sometimes appear at lateral cortical sites where they were previously absent. Whether or not this finding is an indication for further resection is still controversial.

COMPARISON OF INTRAOPERATIVE AND EXTRAOPERATIVE RECORDING AND STIMULATION MAPPING

In some situations, recording and stimulation require the use of chronic subdural electrodes, with these studies obtained outside the operating room. These situations include occasions when language mapping is required but the patient cannot cooperate with an awake craniotomy, as is the case with young children, or when recording of seizure onset is needed to plan the resection, as when there are widespread or multifocal IIS on scalp EEG, and particularly if these IIS overlap eloquent areas. Then it is often of value to establish the relation between the site of seizure onset and the eloquent areas. Because electrodes cannot be placed to sample the entire brain, sites of electrode placement depend on preoperative assessment of where seizures are likely to originate and where the eloquent areas of interest are likely to be located.

However, use of chronic electrode techniques exposes the patient to two operations—one to place the electrodes and one to remove them and undertake any indicated resection. The risk of both infection and the total investment of health care resources are increased when larger arrays of chronic electrodes are used, as is required for detailed mapping. If chronic electrodes are to be used in patients who could alternatively be managed with awake craniotomies, an improved outcome must be present to justify these increased risks and costs. That is not the case for adolescents and adults who require only mapping (as in lesions near eloquent areas) or who do not require intracranial ictal recording (as with patients with epilepsy and a focus clearly established by noninvasive preoperative evaluation). In the author's view, these patients are best managed with awake craniotomy.

REFERENCES

1. Silbergeld DL, Mueller WM, Ojemann GA, Lettich E: The use of propofol (Diprivan) for awake craniotomies—technical note. Surg Neurol (in press), 1993
2. Woods R, Dodrill C, Ojemann G: Brain injury, handedness, and speech lateralization in a series of amobarbital studies. Ann Neurol 23:510–518, 1988
3. Wada J, Rasmussen T: Intracarotid injections of sodium amytal for the lateralization of cerebral speech dominance. J Neurosurg 17:266–282, 1960
4. Ojemann G, Silbergeld D: Approaches to epilepsy surgery. Neurosurg Clin North Am 4:183–192, 1993
5. Herman B, Wyler A, Somes G: Language function following anterior temporal lobectomy. J Neurosurg 74:560–566, 1991
6. Barbaro N, Walker J, Laxer K: Letter: Temporal lobectomy and language function. J Neurosurg 75:830, 1991
7. Ojemann G, Ojemann J, Lettich E, Berger M: Cortical language localization in left-dominant hemisphere. J Neurosurg 71:316–326, 1989
8. Grinvald A, Frostig R, Lieke E, Hildesheim R: Optical imaging of neuronal activity. Physiol Rev 68:1285–1366, 1988
9. Haglund MM, Ojemann GA, Hochman DW: Optical imaging and epileptiform and functional activity in human cerebral cortex. Nature 358:668–671, 1992
10. Ranck J: Which elements are excited in electrical stimulation of mammalian central nervous system. A review. Brain Res 948:417–440, 1975
11. Mullan S, Penfield W: Illusions of comparative interpretation and emotion produced by epileptic discharge and by electrical stimulation in temporal cortex. Arch Neurol Psych 81:269–284, 1959
12. Penfield W, Perot P: The brain's record of auditory and visual experience—summary and discussion. Brain 86:595–696, 1963
13. Gloor PA, Olivier A, Quesney LF, et al: The role of the limbic system in experiential phenomena of temporal lobe epilepsy. Ann Neurol 12:129–144, 1982
14. Penfield W, Roberts L: Speech and brain mechanisms. Princeton, Princeton University Press, 1959
15. Luders H, Lesser R, Hahn J, et al: Basal temporal language area demonstrated by electrical stimulation. Neurology 36:505–510, 1986
16. Haglund MM, Ojemann GA, Blasdel GG: Optical imaging of bipolar cortical stimulation. J Neurosurg 78:785–793, 1993

17. Ojemann GA: Brain organization for language from the perspective of electrical stimulation mapping. Behav Brain Sci 6:189–230, 1983
18. Haglund MM, Berger MS, Lettich E, Shamseldin MS, Ojemann GA: Cortical localization of temporal lobe language sites in patients with gliomas. Neurosurgery 34:567–576, 1993
19. Ojemann G: Cortical organization of language. J Neurosci 11:2281–2287, 1991
20. Ojemann GA, Whitaker HA: The bilingual brain. Arch Neurol 35:409–412, 1978
21. Rapport RL, Tan CT, Whitaker HA: Language function and dysfunction among Chinese- and English-speaking polyglots: Cortical stimulation, Wada testing and clinical studies. Brain Lang 18:342–366, 1983
22. Black P, Ronner S: Cortical mapping for defining the limits of tumor resection. Neurosurg 20:914–919, 1987
23. Mateer CA, Polen SB, Ojemann GA, et al: Cortical localization of finger spelling and oral language. A case study. Brain Lang 17:46–57, 1982
24. Haglund MM, Ojemann GA, Lettich E, et al: Dissociation of cortical and single unit activity in spoken and signed languages. Brain Lang 44:19–27, 1993
25. Ojemann GA: Some brain mechanisms for reading, in Von Euler C, Lundberg I, Lennerstrand G (eds): Brain and Reading. New York, Macmillan, 1989, pp 47–59
26. Ojemann G, Dodrill C: Verbal memory deficits after left temporal lobectomy for epilepsy. J Neurosurg 62:101–107, 1985
27. Ojemann G, Dodrill C: Intraoperative technique for reducing language and memory deficits with left temporal lobectomy. Advances in Epileptology 16:327–330, 1987
28. Ojemann G: Localization of language in frontal cortex, in Chauvel P, Delgado-Escueta A, Halgren E, Bancaud J (eds): Frontal Lobe Seizures and Epilepsies. New York, Raven Press, 1992, pp 361–368
29. Fried I, Katz A, McCarthy G, et al: Functional organization of human supplementary motor cortex studied by electrical stimulation. J Neurosci 11:3656–3666, 1991
30. Fried I, Mateer C, Ojemann G, et al: Organization of visuospatial functions in human cortex: Evidence from electrical stimulation. Brain 105:349–371, 1982
31. Ojemann GA, Sutherling W, Lesser R, et al: Stimulation, in Engel J (ed): Surgical Treatment of the Epileptic, Vol. II. New York, Raven Press, in press, 1993
32. Woods C, Spencer D, Allison T, et al: Localization of human sensorimotor cortex during surgery by cortical surface recording of somatosensory evoked potentials. J Neurosurg 68:99–111, 1988
33. Dodrill C, Wilkus R, Ojemann G, et al: Multi-disciplinary prediction of seizure relief from cortical resection surgery. Ann Neurol 20:2–12, 1986
34. Bengzon A, Rasmussen T, Gloor P, et al: Prognostic factors in the surgical treatment of temporal lobe epilepsy. Neurology 18:717–731, 1968
35. Weber J, Silbergeld D, Winn H: Surgical resection of epileptogenic cortex associated with structural lesions. Neurosurg Clin North Am 4:327–336, 1993

CHAPTER 107

Multilobar Resections for the Control of Epilepsy

C. Munari
S. Francione
P. Kahane
D. Hoffmann
L. Tassi
G. Lo Russo
A. L. Benabid

Apparently, general agreement exists concerning the selection criteria of patients who are candidates for surgical treatment of severe, drug-resistant, partial epilepsies.[1] Several therapeutic surgical techniques are currently employed, varying from relatively limited resections,[2] such as the selective amygdalo-hippocampectomy,[3] to hemispherectomy.[4]

"Multilobar resection" is synonymous with total,[5] or functional[6] hemispherectomy.[7] In the largest published series, this kind of intervention has been performed in percentages varying from 2.5 to 11 per cent of the cases.[8] Such widely extended cortical resections are mainly performed in children with malformation-hamartomatous lesions, or encephalomalacia sequelae of anoxic-ischemic encephalopathy.[9] These resections are generally not included among the possible surgical procedures in patients with partial epilepsy that is either cryptogenic or symptomatic of a limited anatomic lesion.[10]

In fact, one of the most controversial points in epilepsy surgery is the diagnostic methodology that must be applied and, consequently, the type of cortical excision that can be performed. In patients with symptomatic partial epilepsy, the main problem consists in understanding the complex topographic and functional relationships between an anatomic (presumed to be epileptogenic) lesion and the epileptogenic area (EA), and there is no general agreement concerning the strategy to adopt. In patients suffering from cryptogenic partial epilepsies, the identification and spatial definition of the EA must be based on electrical and clinical—mostly ictal—findings.[11] Presurgical diagnostic approaches include noninvasive or invasive tools, or both. Because surgical therapeutic procedures are directly linked to the results of previously applied diagnostic protocols, one of the major diagnostic problems is the identification of the side on which ictal discharges start. For this reason, in several epilepsy surgery centers, intracerebral electrodes are bilaterally, and often symmetrically, implanted in different standardized anatomic targets,[12–15] in accordance with Gloor's[16] recent statement,

"Intracranial recordings must be designed to avoid biasing the exploration strategy in favor of one's preferred localizing hypothesis." Once the side of the intervention is decided, the extent of the removal is, in many cases, also standardized, depending on the hemispheric dominance for language. Both bilateral invasive procedures and subsequent surgical management are based on the assumption that complex partial (previously named "psychomotor") seizures are very often of temporal lobe origin, and that anterior temporal lobectomies have produced satisfactory improvements in most patients operated on by this approach.[17]

Since the 1950s, a radically different individualized approach has been elaborated by Bancaud, Talairach, and their coworkers at the Sainte Anne Hospital in Paris.[18–20] The use of stereotactically implanted multilead electrodes has been proposed as a method of verifying (either with or without evidence of an anatomic lesion) the previously elaborated hypothesis concerning the location and extent of the EA. Such hypotheses need to be supported by the electroclinical study of spontaneous seizures, and by a rigorous stereotactic and stereoscopic anatomic assessment.[21, 22] The term *stereo-electroencephalography* (stereo-EEG),[18] coined in 1962, should be distinguished from the so-called depth electrode recordings, "since the purpose of the stereo-electroencephalography is to provide a three-dimensional evaluation of the epileptogenic zone that requires placement of electrodes into deep, intermediate, and superficial planes of the brain."[7] Careful prestereo-EEG assessment of patients is probably at the origin of the two following facts:

1. Intracerebral electrodes were unilaterally implanted in more than 70 percent of patients and were implanted symmetrically bilaterally in only 7 percent in 300 investigations.[23]

2. Intracerebral electrodes were generally implanted in several lobes, with the twofold aim of recording the initial ictal discharges and correlating their early spreading with the early sequence of ictal clinical symptoms.[24, 25]

Table 107–1. CHARACTERISTICS OF 112 PARTIAL EPILEPTIC PATIENTS OPERATED ON AT THE GRENOBLE HOSPITAL BETWEEN MARCH 1990 AND JANUARY 1993

Group*				Characteristics			
	Sex, m/f	Mean Age at Intervention, years†	Mean Age at Epilepsy Onset, years†	Mean Epilepsy Duration, years†	Mean Seizure Frequency, n per month‡	Right/Left Epilepsies, n	Lesion, n (%)
A n = 112	57/55	24.5 +/− 10.8	9.5 +/− 7.9	15 +/− 8.9	31.9 +/− 50.4	78/34	75 (66.9)
B n = 23	16/7	23.9 +/− 10.4	8.4 +/− 6.6	15.5 +/− 7.7	53.3 +/− 76.2	20/3	12 (52.1)
C n = 89	41/48	24.6 +/− 11	9.7 +/− 8.2	14.9 +/− 9.2	26.4 +/− 40	58/31	63 (70.8)

*Group A = total population; group B = multilobar epilepsy; group C = unilobar epilepsy.
†Years ± standard deviation.
‡± Standard deviation.

Among several important results obtained with this methodological approach, we wish to emphasize the following:

1. The individual EA may be observed extending beyond the classic landmarks of each cerebral lobe.
2. Multilobar partial cortical resections may then be proposed and performed in patients with partial epilepsies that are either cryptogenic or associated with limited anatomic lesions, and not only in partial epileptic patients with severe, extended, hemispheric anatomic lesions (i.e., as an alternative solution to hemispherectomy).

In this chapter, we present and discuss our recently acquired experience in Grenoble (and are heavily indebted to that of the Sainte Anne Hospital), particularly with regard to the diagnostic and surgical management of multilobar—not necessarily multifocal—epilepsies.

CLINICAL FEATURES

Between March 1990 and January 1993, 112 patients underwent surgical intervention at the Grenoble Hospital for severe, drug-resistant partial epilepsy. Their general characteristics are shown in Table 107–1. Age at intervention varied from 3 to 61 years, and was under 16 years in 27 patients. Seizures began at ages varying from a few days to 49 years, with an epilepsy duration ranging from 2 to 49 years. Seizure frequency varied from 10 or more a day to several a month. Noteworthy antecedents are shown in Table 107–2.

PREOPERATIVE EVALUATION

Preoperative diagnostic procedures are summarized in Figure 107–1: the sequence of different steps clearly was decided according to the individual characteristics of each patient.

DIAGNOSTIC PROCEDURES

Noninvasive

The following data, which represent the cornerstone of our reasoning, were available in all cases: clinical interictal and ictal findings described by both the patient and the family, neurologic and neuropsychological evaluation and neuroimaging studies, including computed tomography (CT) and magnetic resonance imaging (MRI). The latter showed anatomic alterations of different types, sizes, and locations in 76 patients (lesional group), i.e., 68 percent of all cases. Single-photon emission computed tomography and positron-emission tomography was performed in one half and one third of the cases, respectively. Their results are not discussed here, because they are part of a double-blind study still in progress. Long-term video-EEG recordings were comprised of a time-synchronized audio-video-EEG system (BMSI, Campbell, USA), coupled with direct intensive surveillance, which allowed a detailed ictal clinical examination, which is mandatory for obtaining electroclinical correlates. Sixty-nine patients underwent this type of investigation.

Table 107–2. ANTECEDENTS FOUND IN THE 112 EPILEPTIC PATIENTS OPERATED ON AT GRENOBLE HOSPITAL BETWEEN MARCH 1990 AND JANUARY 1993*

Group†	Antecedents				
	FC, n (%)	PN Injury, n (%)	HT, n (%)	CNS Infection, n (%)	Others, n (%)
A	19 (17)	12 (11)	12 (11)	5 (4.5)	4 (3.6)
B	5 (22)	2 (8.7)	3 (13)	2 (8.7)	1 (4.3)
C	14 (16)	10 (11)	9 (10)	3 (3.4)	3 (3.4)

CNS = central nervous system; FC = febrile convulsions; HT = severe head trauma; PN = perinatal.
*Patients could have more than one antecedent.
†Group A = total population; group B = multilobar epilepsy; group C = unilobar epilepsy.

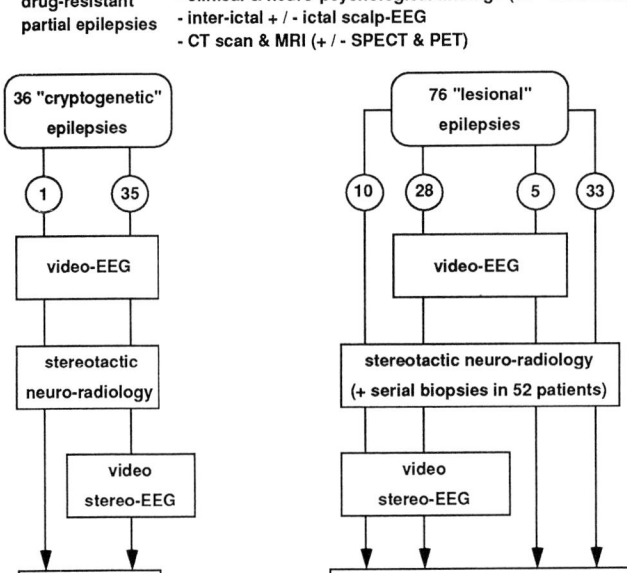

FIGURE 107-1. Presurgical and surgical strategies used in the management of 112 partial epileptic patients operated on at the Grenoble Hospital between March 1990 and January 1993. CT scan = computed tomography, MRI = magnetic resonance imaging, SPECT = 99-Tc HMPao single photon emission computed tomography, PET = 18-FDG positron emission tomography.

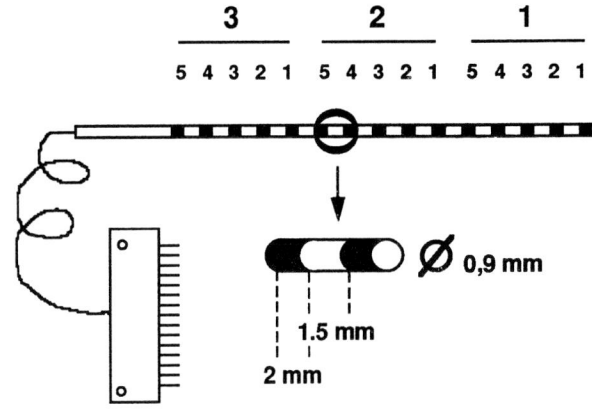

FIGURE 107-2. Technical characteristics of a 15-lead electrode and principles of numbering of each lead.

Invasive

Stereotactic and stereoscopic neuroradiologic investigations were the only invasive procedures performed in all cases.[26] In 52 of 76 patients with lesions (68 per cent), serial stereotactic biopsies were carried out[23] with the aim of obtaining a precise diagnosis of the nature of lesions too often labeled as "scars," "neonatal sequelae," or "posttraumatic injury." Intracarotid amobarbital injection (Wada test) was performed with scalp EEG monitoring in 22 patients (20 percent). Stereo-EEG investigation was judged indispensable in 73 patients (65 percent) in order to correctly define the actual extent of the EA. For each patient, the strategy of intracerebral electrode placement was defined on the basis of previously acquired clinical, electrical, and anatomic data. The cerebral structures to be investigated were selected with the twofold aim of identifying the origin of ictal discharges and detecting their early spreading. Five to 12 multilead, semirigid electrodes were percutaneously implanted stereotactically, according to the Talairach methodology,[26] and using a computer-driven robot.[28, 29] The electrodes were fixed to the bone with screws and to the skin. Each electrode comprised five, 10, or 15 leads (see characteristics on Fig. 107-2), and depth EEG recordings were obtained by bipolar recordings from contiguous leads, for which intracerebral location was particularly important to define the epileptogenic area. Although each stereo-EEG strategy is individualized, several implantation modalities may be identified.

1. In some cases, when the ictal clinical symptomatology does not correspond completely to the localization of the anatomic epileptogenic lesion (AEL), and to define the exact amount of extralesional cerebral cortex to be removed, a mostly unilobar stereo-EEG can be performed (Fig. 107-3).

2. The commonest model of stereo-EEG strategy leads to the differential diagnosis between pure temporal lobe and temporoperisylvian epilepsies in both cryptogenic (Fig. 107-4A and B) and symptomatic (Fig. 107-5A and B) cases.

3. The differential diagnosis between temporofrontal and frontotemporal seizures can be made with several modalities of electrode implantation (Fig. 107-6A and B).

4. Particular problems related to occipital seizures and the spreading of discharges may be solved by simultaneous exploration of lateral and mesial cortical areas in occipital, parietal, and temporal lobes (Fig. 107-7A and B).

5. The problem of central sensorimotor epilepsies, especially when an anatomic lesion exists, must be addressed (see Fig. 107-8). Besides the need to identify the ictal discharge onset (anteriorly, posteriorly, or in the lesion), it is necessary to study the possible modifications of somatomotor and somatosensitive pathways, also by using low-frequency (1-Hz) electrical stimulations.

This methodology can lead to the finding that in some cases, initial ictal discharges do not respect the anatomic limits of a single cerebral lobe and therefore correspond to the diagnosis of multilobar epilepsy. Among the 73 stereo-EEG procedures performed 63 (86 percent) were unilateral, of which 77 percent involved the right hemisphere only. Bilateral implantations were almost always asymmetrical in number of electrodes. The total number of implanted electrodes was 735, reflecting a mean of 10 per patient. At least one electrode was implanted in a temporal lobe in 93 percent of cases, in a frontal lobe and parietal lobe in 77 percent and in an occipital lobe in 10 percent. Three lobes were investigated, with at least one electrode per lobe, in either the right or the left hemisphere in 70 and 65 percent of cases, respectively.

CLINICAL MANAGEMENT

We first attempted to record spontaneous seizures and were successful in more than 85 percent of cases, by use of a slight and progressive reduction of antiepileptic drugs in 70 percent of these cases. Low- and high-frequency electrical stimulation was then applied, according to our clinical[30] and

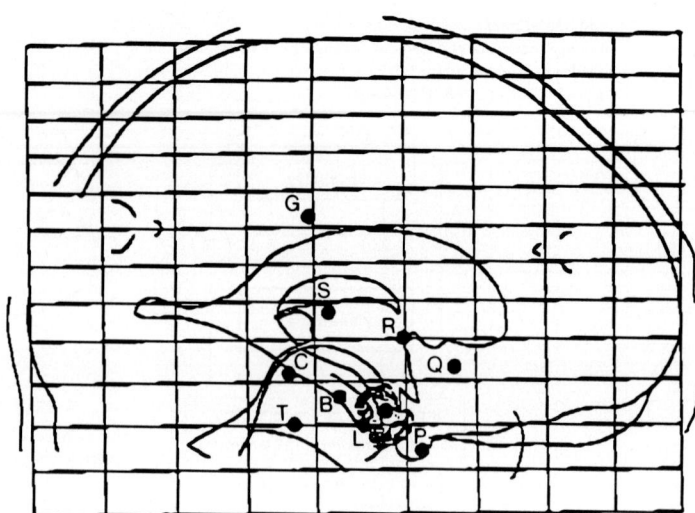
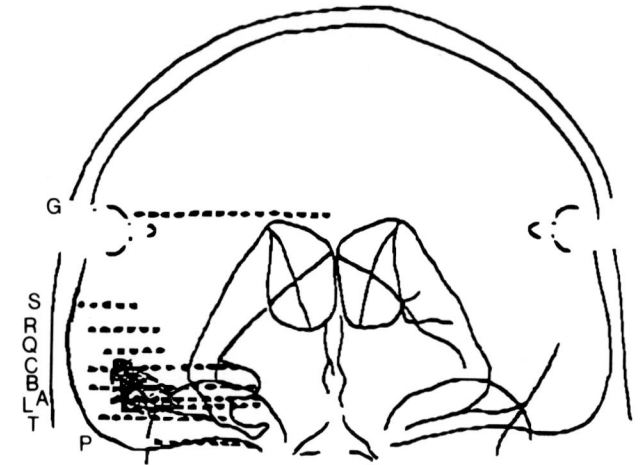

Case D.91.16
April 18, 1991

P: mesial and lateral temporopolar region

L: T5, lesion, and anterior part of T2

A: amygdala and anterior part of T2

B: midhippocampus and midpart of T2

C: posterior hippocampus and posterior part of T2

T: T4 and T3

Q: anterior part of T1

R: midpart of T1

S: posterior part of T1

P: parietal cingulate gyrus and inferior part of P2

FIGURE 107–3. Right predominantly temporal stereo-EEG study in a 28-year-old right-handed woman with a 12-year history of epilepsy associated with a right temporal astrocytoma I. Lateral and frontal view of the skull, showing the emplacement of the 11 right stereotactically implanted electrodes. The lesion is represented by dashed lines. T1, T2, T3, and T4 = first, second, third and fourth temporal convolution, P2 = second parietal convolution.

research[31] practice. The mean duration of long-term stereo-EEG recordings was 14 days (range, 4 to 18 days).

PATIENT SELECTION AND MANAGEMENT DECISIONS

WITHOUT STEREO-ELECTROENCEPHALOGRAPHY

In 39 patients (38 of the symptomatic group [50 percent] and one of the cryptogenic group), we believed that correlations between anatomic (MRI and stereotactic neuroradiology), electrical (interictal and mainly ictal scalp EEG), and clinical (interictal, ictal, and postictal) data were strong enough to propose surgical treatment, without the benefit of previous stereo-EEG. In these cases, the intervention was always confined within the limits of a single cerebral lobe (temporal: 80 percent; frontal: 10 percent; central: 7.5 percent; occipital: 2.5 percent). A pure lesionectomy was performed in 15, and it was associated to a more or less extensive corticectomy in 23 of the symptomatic patients. The limits of cortical removal were defined, in each patient, according to his or her particular anatomoelectroclinical characteristics.

WITH STEREO-ELECTROENCEPHALOGRAPHY

Stereo-EEG investigations were performed in the remaining 73 patients. An analytical study of ictal discharges showed that the anatomic origin of the ictal discharges was strictly unilobar in 44 cases (60 percent; 25 symptomatic and 19 cryptogenic). The involved lobe was temporal in 36 (82 percent), frontal in six (14 percent), central in one (2 percent), and parietal in one (2 percent). In the other 29 patients, ictal discharges originated independently in both temporal lobes in two cryptogenic cases. Because only unilateral surgical removal was possible, these cases were arbitrarily included among unilobar cases. In 5 patients, initial ictal discharges involved two lobes, but the surgical intervention was purposely limited to only one to avoid severe functional risks. Multilobar early ictal involvement was also demonstrated in the other 23 cases.

Text continued on page 1331

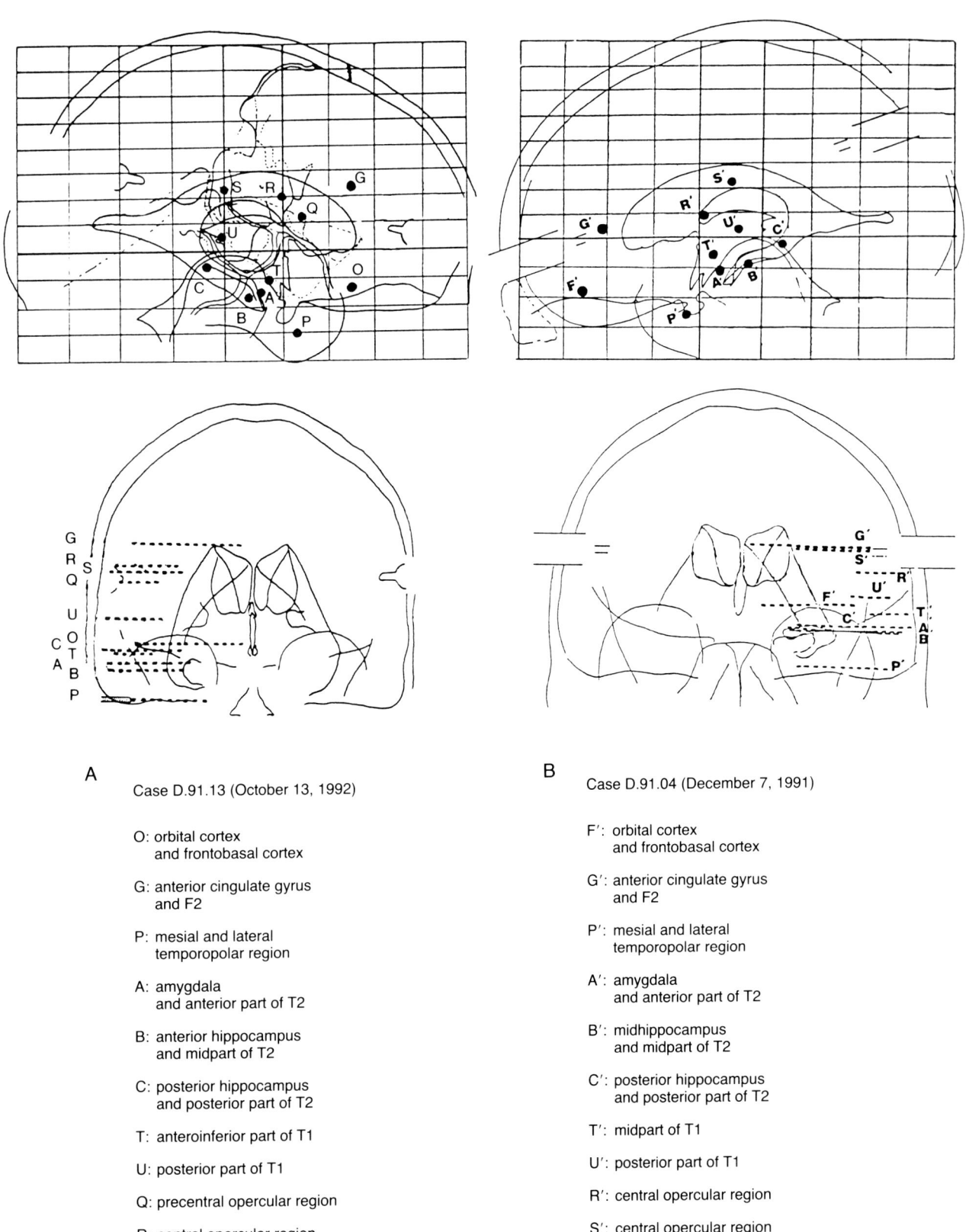

FIGURE 107-4. Temporoperisylvian stereo-EEG study in two patients suffering from a cryptogenic partial epilepsy. (A) Right exploration by means of 11 stereotactically implanted electrodes (lateral and frontal view of the skull) in a 17-year-old right-handed boy who experienced his first partial epileptic seizures at the age of 6 years. (B) Left exploration by means of 10 stereotactically implanted electrodes (lateral and frontal view of the skull) in a 21-year-old right-handed man with a partial epilepsy of 8 years' duration. T1 and T2 = first and second temporal convolution, F2 = second frontal convolution.

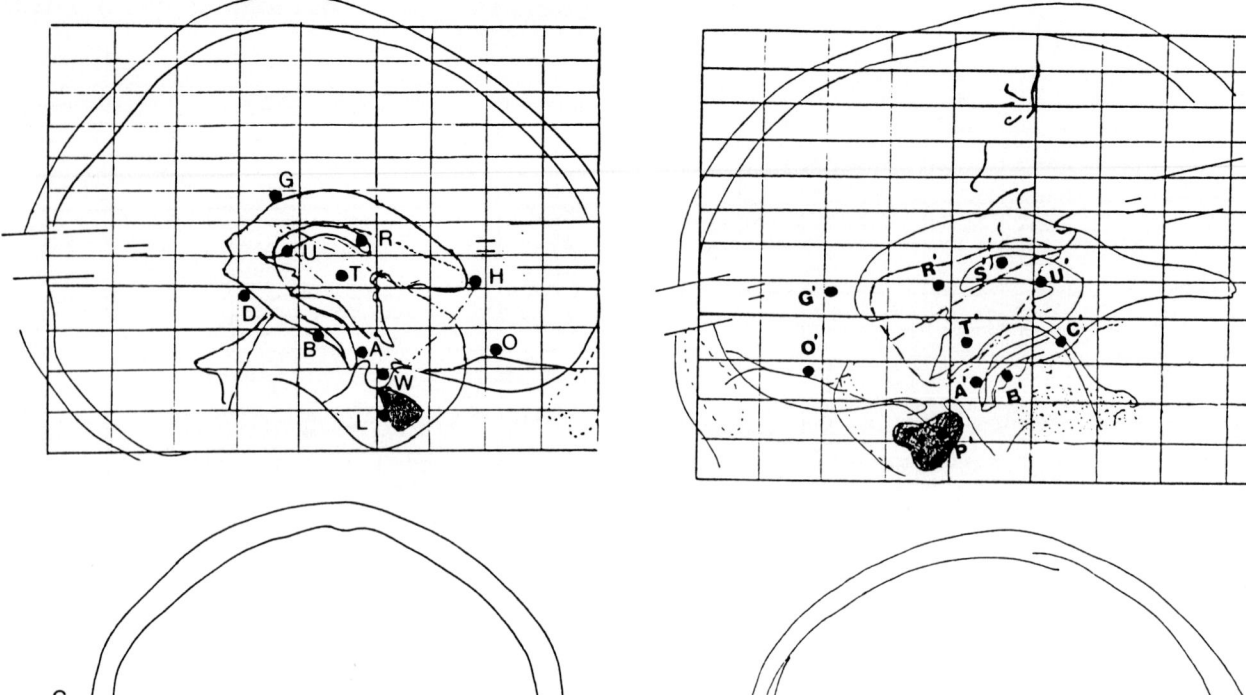

FIGURE 107–5. Temporoperisylvian stereo-EEG study in two patients suffering from a lesional partial epilepsy. (A) Right exploration by means of 11 stereotactically implanted electrodes (lateral and frontal view of the skull) in a 16-year-old right-handed girl who experienced her first partial epileptic seizures at the age of 10 years. The temporopolar lesion (dashed lines) proved to be a ganglioglioma I. (B) Left exploration by means of 10 stereotactically implanted electrodes (lateral and frontal view of the skull) in a 27-year-old right-handed man with a partial epilepsy of 11 years' duration. The temporopolar lesion (dashed lines) proved to be an astrocytoma I. T1 and T2 = first and second temporal convolution, F2 and F3 = second and third frontal convolution, P2 = second parietal convolution.

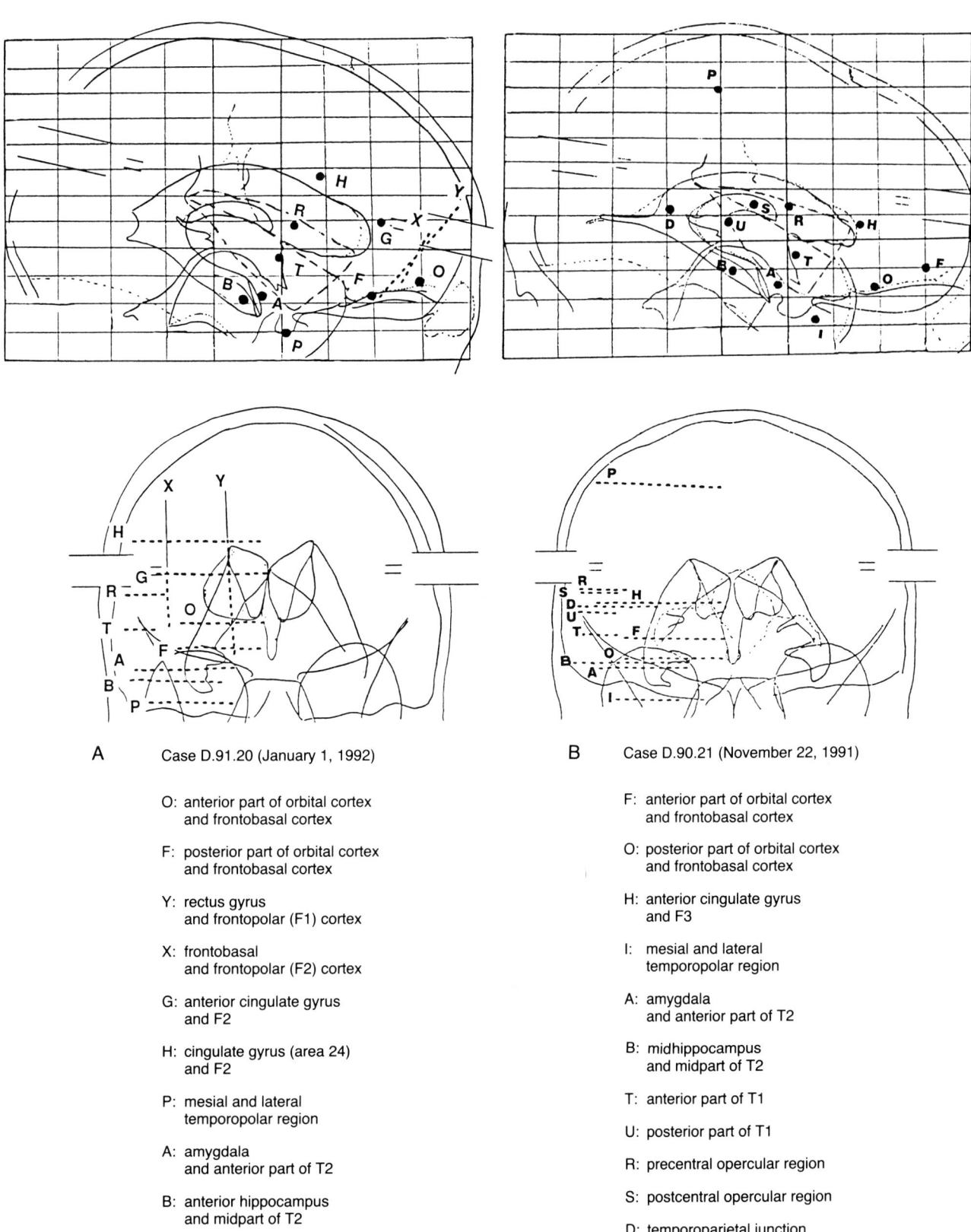

FIGURE 107–6. Frontotemporal stereo-EEG study. (A) Right exploration by means of 11 stereotactically implanted electrodes (lateral and frontal view of the skull). Real multilobar frontotemporal epilepsy (see case report of patient 16). The largely extended right frontopolar and frontobasal sequelar lesion is not represented to make the scheme more clear. (B) Right exploration by means of 12 stereotactically implanted electrodes (lateral and frontal view of the skull). Multifocal frontotemporal epilepsy (see case report of patient 10). T1 and T2 = first and second temporal convolution, F1, F2, and F3 = first, second, and third frontal convolution.

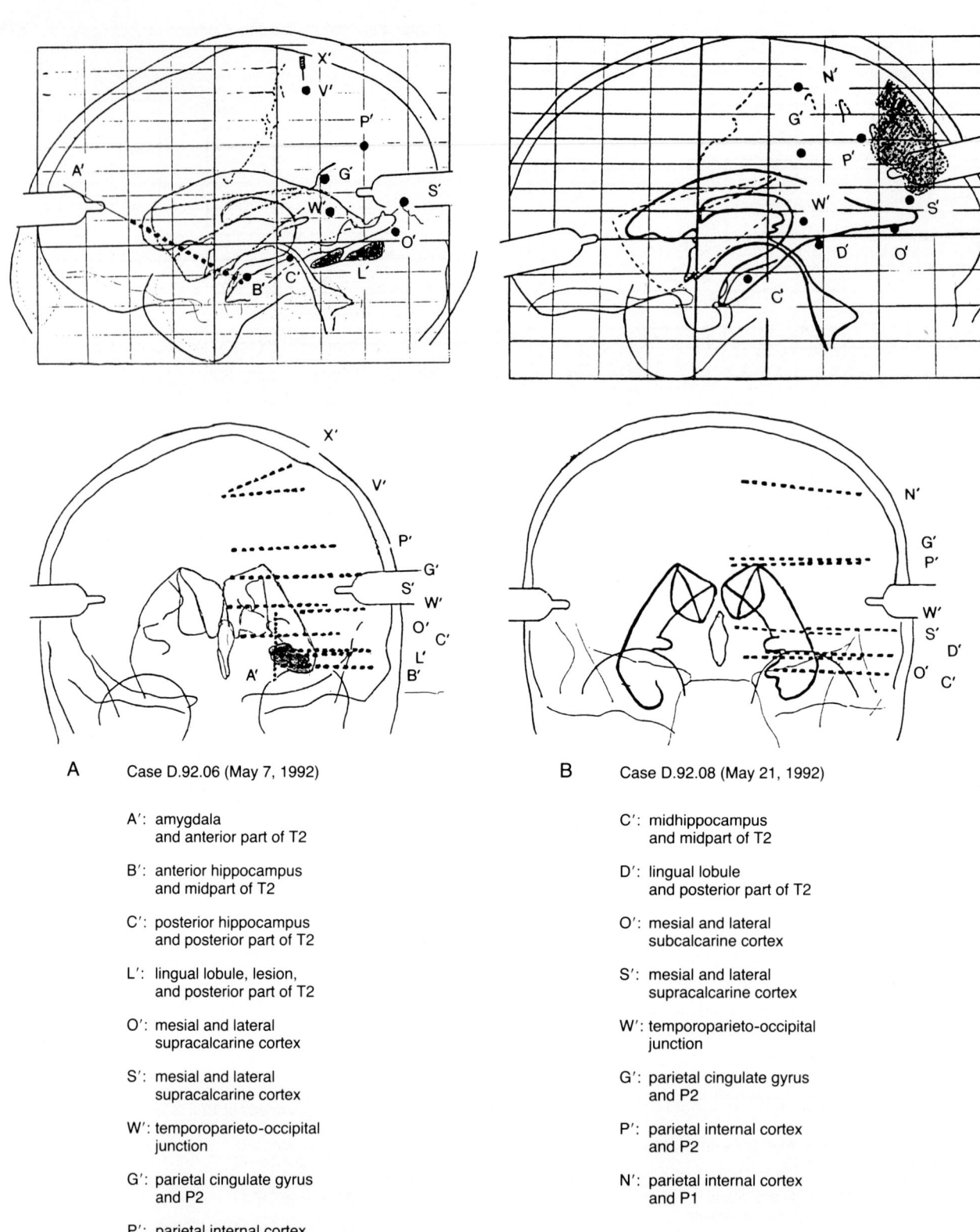

FIGURE 107-7. Occipitoparietotemporal stereo-EEG study in two patients suffering from a lesional partial epilepsy. (A) Left exploration by means of 11 stereotactically implanted electrodes (lateral and frontal view of the skull). Multifocal occipitotemporoparietal lesional (dashed lines) epilepsy (see case report of patient 21). (B) Left exploration by means of eight stereotactically implanted electrodes (lateral and frontal view of the skull) in a 44-year-old right-handed man with an epilepsy duration of 26 years. This patient was operated on 16 years earlier for a parasagittal meningioma (sequelar lesion is represented by dashed lines), but partial seizures persisted. T2 = first temporal convolution, P1 and P2 = first and second parietal convolution.

Case D.92.12

June 12, 1992

F: mesial prefrontal cortex and F1

G: anterior cingulate gyrus and F2

R: precentral opercular region

I: precentral frontal cortex

H: cingulate gyrus and precentral frontal cortex

S: central opercular region

L: lesion and ascending frontal area

M: mesial and lateral precentral frontal cortex

N: parietal cingulate gyrus and ascending parietal area

X: paracentral lobule and ascending parietal area

O: parietal internal cortex and P2

P: parietal internal cortex and P1

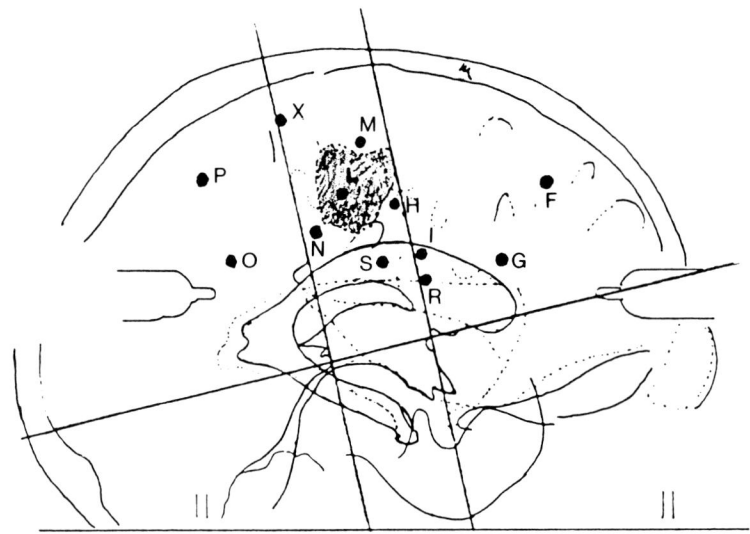

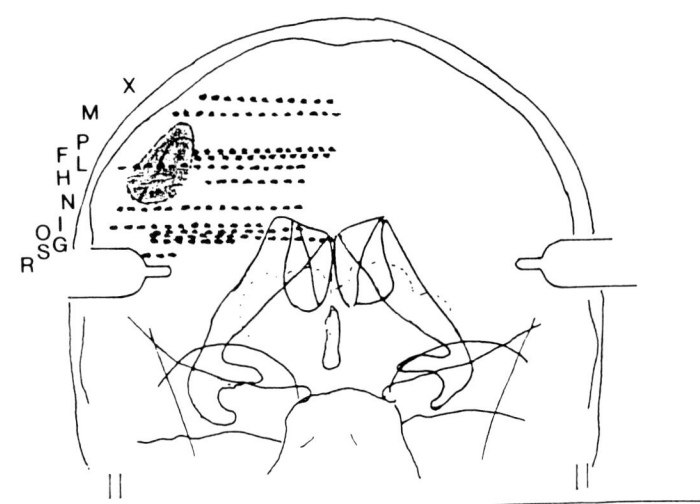

FIGURE 107-8. Right, predominantly central stereo-EEG study in a 14-year-old right-handed boy with a 13-year history of epilepsy associated with a right central gigantocellular astrocytoma (forme fruste of tuberous sclerosis). Lateral and frontal view of the skull, showing the emplacement of the 12 right stereotactically implanted electrodes. The lesion is represented by dashed lines. F1 and F2 = first and second frontal convolution, P1 and P2 = first and second parietal convolution.

Regarding the multilobar group, anatomic presurgical MRI evaluation showed no abnormalities in 11 of 23 (48 percent) multilobar patients: their conditions were considered to be cryptogenic (Table 107-3). Different kinds of anatomic lesions had been previously shown in 12 of 23 patients (52 percent) (Table 107-4). One of them (patient 23), a young boy aged 6 years, presented with anatomoclinical characteristics suggesting the diagnosis (finally histologically confirmed) of Rasmussen's syndrome. The epilepsy was considered multifocal in six patients (patients 10, 11, 20, 21, 22, and 23) because ictal discharges originated in different lobes of the same hemisphere (see Case Report 2 [Patient 21]). In 17 patients, ictal discharges almost simultaneously involved cortical areas of two or more lobes (see Case Report 1 [Patient 16]). The most important differences between this group of multilobar patients and the global population of partial epileptic patients operated on at Grenoble are (see Tables 107-1 and 107-2) the male:female (2.2) and symptomatic:cryptogenic (1.9) ratios and the seizure frequency. The predominance of the right-sided EA could be discussed as probably related to preliminary patient selection criteria.

SURGICAL MANAGEMENT

Surgical treatment of patients with severe partial epilepsy generally represents a compromise between the desire to cure each patient and the fear of creating new neurologic or neuropsychological damage. "The larger the epileptogenic cortex to be removed, the harder the compromise to be reached" can be proposed to paraphrase the quote "the larger the surgical removal, the better the result," from Rossi,[32] clearly expressed in accordance with the well-known concept of critical mass.[33]

The extent of the EA in multilobar partial epilepsies raises several particular diagnostic and therapeutic problems. With regard to diagnostic difficulties, the following are necessary:

Table 107–3. MAIN CHARACTERISTICS OF 11 CRYPTOGENIC MULTILOBAR PARTIAL EPILEPTIC PATIENTS OPERATED ON AFTER VIDEO-STEREO-EEG PROCEDURE

Patient	Sex	Age at Intervention, year	Age at Onset, year	Antecedent	Seizure Frequency, n per month	Neuro Exam	VEEG	Wada Test	SN	Location	Surgery	Follow-up, months	Outcome
1	f	18	8	FC	10	N	+	−	+	R T-Op	R T-Op	18	SF
2	m	26	11	FC	9	N	+	−	+	R T-Op	R T-Op	8	SF
3	f	34	6	CNS inf	90	N	+	−	+	R T-Op	R T-Op	2	A
4	m	17	6	PN inj–FC	12	N	+	+	+	R T-Op	R T-Op	2	SF
5	m	28	10	SNC inf	12	N	+	−	+	R T-Orb	R T-Orb	2	SF
6	m	36	28	—	5	N	+	+	+	R T-Orb	R T-Orb	1	SF
7	m	31	12	—	30	N	+	−	+	R F-T	R Orb-T	25	I
8	f	21	3	—	30	N	+	+	+	L F-T	L Orb-T	4	I
9	m	37	18	—	20	N	+	−	+	R O-T	R O-T	25	U
10	m	40	7	FC	7	N	+	−	+	R Orb-T	R Orb-T	8	SF
11	m	27	8	HT	150	N	+	−	+	R F-T	R F-T	2	I

+, yes; −, no.
A = several auras; CNS inf = central nervous sytem infection; F = frontal; FC = febrile convulsions; HT = severe head trauma; I = improved quality of life, seizure frequency, or both; L = left; N = normal; PN inj = perinatal injury; O = occipital; Op = suprasylvian opercular region; Orb = orbital cortex; R = right; SF = seizure free; SN = stereotactic neuroradiology; T = temporal; U = unchanged; VEEG = long-term video-electroencephalographic (EEG) monitoring.

1. A precise identification of the chronologic sequence of both subjective symptoms and objective clinical signs
2. A correct hypothesis regarding the spatial evolution of ictal electrical discharges to identify cortical structures that, if adequately investigated, could allow a satisfactory explanation of the clinical symptomatology
3. A millimetrical precision in defining the individual's vascular anatomy of the sulci and cortical convolutions[14, 21, 22, 34]
4. A sophisticated stereotactic methodology for safe implantation of electrodes in cortical areas with unusual vascular patterns (i.e., perisylvian, sensorimotor, and pericalcarine cortex)
5. A multichannel recording system for storing the highest possible amount of electrical information

Once such conditions are fulfilled, particular surgical problems begin:

What are the criteria for identifying the actual epileptogenic cortex?
Should only the cortical areas that are affected by the ictal discharges at the onset of the seizures be removed?
How long is the onset? One second? Five seconds? Or longer?
If the initial clinical symptomatology occurs several seconds after the onset of the electrical discharge, is removal of the symptomatogenic cortex mandatory[35] or will removing only the initially affected cortical region be sufficient?
What is the risk of removing all of the epileptogenic cortex?
What kind of neurologic and/or neuropsychological deficits can be induced? Are all of them predictable?

In this group of 23 patients, the diagnosis of multilobar epilepsy was mainly based on stereo-EEG data, corroborated

Table 107–4. MAIN CHARACTERISTICS OF 12 LESIONAL MULTILOBAR PARTIAL EPILEPTIC PATIENTS OPERATED ON AFTER VIDEO-STEREO-EEG PROCEDURE

Patient	Sex	Age at Intervention, year	Age at Onset, year	Antecedent	Seizure Frequency, n per month	Neuro Exam	VEEG	Wada Test	SN	Location	Surgery	Pathology	Follow-up, months	Outcome
12	f	26	6	FC	22	N	+	−	+	R T-P	R T-P	NMD	12	SF
13	m	10	2	—	150	N	−	−	+	R T-F	R T-Orb	astro I	24	U
14	f	19	1	—	8.5	N	−	−	++	R T-O	R T-O	astro II	25	SF
15	f	27	7	—	50	L iQ	+	−	+	R Orb-T	R T-O	astro I	30	SF
16	m	27	6	+++	6	N	+	−	+	R Orb-T	R Orb-T	gliosis	10	SF
17	m	4	0	—	45	N	+	−	++	R F-C	R F-C	TS	2	SF
18	m	14	1	—	45	L mP	−	−	+	R F-C	R F-C	FFTS	1	I
19	m	18	11	—	2	L sQ	−	−	++	R O-T-P	R O-T	DNE	18	I
20*	m	44	18	++++	10	R iQ	−	−	+	L O-P-T	L O-P	gliosis	3	SF
21*	f	14	4	HT	200	R H	−	+	+	L O-P-T	L O-P-T	Rasm	2	I
22*	m	30	16	HT	15	N	+	+	+	R T-F-C-P	R T-F-C	PPC	9	I
23*	m	7	4	—	KS	L hP	+	−	+	KS	R T-C	Rasm	4	I

+, yes; −, no; ++, with serial biopsies; +++, right frontal ependymoma operated on, then given external radiotherapy and intrathecal and general chemotherapy; ++++, right parieto-occipital meningioma.
astro = astrocytoma; C = central region; DNE = dysembryoplastic neuroepithelial tumor; F = frontal; FC = febrile convulsions; FFTS = forme fruste of tuberous sclerosis; H = hemianopia; HT = severe head trauma; hP = hemiparesis; I = improved quality of life, seizure frequency, or both; iQ = inferior quadrantanopia; KS = Kojewnikow syndrome; L = left; mP = monoparesis; N = normal; NMD = neuronal migration disorder; O = occipital; Orb = orbital cortex; P = parietal; PPC = posttraumatic porencephalic cyst; R = right; Rasm = Rasmussen's encephalitis; SF = seizure; SN = stereotactic neuroradiology; sQ = superior quadrantanopia; T = temporal; TS = tuberous sclerosis; U = unchanged; VEEG = long-term video-electroencephalographic (EEG) monitoring.
*Classified as having multifocal partial epilepsy.

by previously obtained anatomoelectroclinical information. The surgical decision tentatively took into account the risk-benefit balance and was thoroughly discussed with each patient and his or her family. The following categories were identified:

1. Total removal of the identified EA was feasible, without foreseeable risks: six patients (Patients 1, 2, 3, 4, 12, and 14).

2. A large amount, but not all, of the identified EA could be removed, thus avoiding the risks linked to a too large resection in a one-step intervention. A reintervention could be considered 18 months later, if the result was judged unsatisfactory: seven patients (Patients 5, 6, 9, 10, 15, 16, and 17).

3. The EA was correctly identified, but its complete removal could have provoked a neurologic deficit (i.e., monoparesis): the decision on the extent of removal was discussed with the patient and his or her family, who were well informed that excision could not be completed at a second intervention: three patients (Patients 18, 19, and 20).

4. The EA was, or could be, correctly defined, but its complete removal could not be proposed because of the certainty of provoking new, very severe, neurologic and/or neuropsychological or endocrine deficits. The intervention was performed in very insistent patients, with the clear aim of trying to reduce seizure frequency, and without the false hope of completely stopping them: five patients (Patients 8, 13, 21, 22, and 23).

5. The extent of the EA required a two-step intervention: two patients (Patients 7 and 11).

CHOICE OF SURGICAL APPROACH

The temporal lobe was involved in all of the 11 multilobar cryptogenic epilepsies and in nine of 12 symptomatic ones. The surgical approach was adapted to the location of the cortical areas to be removed.

BILOBAR EA (21 PATIENTS). The temporal and suprasylvian opercular areas were to be removed in four patients and temporocentral in one patient: the osteoplastic bone flap was extended from the middle fossa floor to several centimeters above the sylvian fissure. The temporal and orbital areas were to be removed in eight patients: the classic pterional approach was indicated, and care was taken to enlarge it enough to facilitate the access to the anterior and posteromesial orbital cortex. The temporal and occipital areas were to be removed in three patients: in such cases, the approach chosen depended on the areas to be predominantly removed. If only the lateral cortex needed to be resected, a classic occipitotemporal osteoplastic bone flap was performed. If the mesial structures were involved, an occipital approach provided access to the occipital ventricular horn, mainly when a visual field deficit preexisted. By a transventricular approach, mesial temporal structures could then be reached. The temporofrontal and temporoparietal areas were to be removed in one patient each: the bone flap needed to be relatively large. The frontocentral area needed to be removed in two patients: the approach varied according to whether or not removing the mesial cortex was necessary. The occipitoparietal area was to be removed in one patient.

TRILOBAR EA (TWO PATIENTS). The temporofrontocentral area was to be removed in one patient: the same method as that used for temporofrontal removal was used. The temporoparieto-occipital area was to be removed in one patient: this approach presented the same difficulties as those present in the temporo-occipital removal.

ANESTHETIC CONSIDERATIONS

In our practice, all surgical procedures are performed with the patient under general anesthesia, the electrophysiologic investigations having been previously performed, mostly during stereo-EEG. The use of barbiturates and benzodiazepines is welcome because they contribute to avoiding the risk of epileptic discharges (which increase intracranial pressure [ICP]) during surgical intervention. Because some edema may be encountered before the start of the cortical resection, mechanical hyperventilation is often employed. Prophylactic antibiotic therapy is almost always avoided.

SURGICAL TECHNIQUE

All interventions are performed with the aid of an operative microscope (magnification: $\times$ 6 to 36). There are no particular requirements for this kind of surgery, especially when the technique of en bloc removal is applied. However, we prefer to limit suction to a minimum to obtain as many unaltered specimens as possible from the resected areas. The histopathologic features can then be correlated with the previously recorded electrical activity. Several curettes of various dimensions are useful for the cutting away of mesial cortical areas (e.g., prepeduncular temporal cortex, cingulate gyrus).

Case Reports

CASE REPORT 1 [PATIENT 16]

A 25-year-old right-handed man had the following history: he was born after a normal pregnancy, and delivery was at term but was prolonged, with cyanosis. His psychomotor development was normal, and family history was unremarkable. When the patient was 6 years of age, his mother found him unconscious in the bathtub, and the patient was hospitalized for 15 days. All test results were normal, including cerebrospinal fluid assessments. One year later, the child developed an intracranial hypertension syndrome, and a right frontal tumor was discovered, partly calcified, for which an exeresis was performed. The child then underwent external radiotherapy and received intrathecal (methotrexate) and general (lomustine) chemotherapy. When the patient was 12 years of age, the seizures recurred with a frequency of one to three a day and were described as a left conjugate eye deviation, followed by secondary generalization. Treatment with carbamazepine stopped the seizures until the patient was 18, but the seizures reappeared during an attempt to reduce the medication. Since then, and in spite of numerous therapeutic medical approaches, the patient experienced ictal episodes twice a week, and their symptomatology and frequency remained unchanged.

The more frequent seizures were characterized by a sudden loss of contact, ambulation, gestural automatisms ("as if he was trying to catch things in the air"), and sometimes chewing movements; the patient could utter incomprehensible words or verbal automatisms ("go on, now I must go"), frequently rotated the trunk, most often toward the right side, and his eyes rolled toward the left. The episodes lasted 30 to 120 seconds, and the patient had no memory of the seizure. Rarely, the patient felt his seizure coming on by a sensation of cold and a piloerection on the back and thorax. Rarely, tonic-clonic generalized seizures occurred, and the patient described sometimes feeling just before them that his "brain was being crushed."

When the patient came to our center, the clinical examination was normal, and neuropsychological testing mainly showed signs of frontal dysfunction, with anamnesic troubles involving both verbal and visual material. MRI showed a large signal alteration on right frontopolar and frontobasal regions, without evidence of evolutivity. On interictal EEG, theta-delta activity and occasional spikes were recorded over the right frontotemporal region. Ictal video-EEG recording showed a right anterior seizure onset, with a spatial evolution of ictal discharge that suggested an initial frontobasal involvement with a very rapid spreading over anterior and midtemporal regions. The possibility of an orbitotemporal epilepsy was raised because electroclinical correlations clearly demonstrated that no obvious clinical signs occured once ictal discharge had begun with certainty, thus suggesting an initial involvement of the orbital cortex; and that ictal symptomatology appeared only when the discharge clearly involved the anterior and midtemporal regions and was in accordance with this electrical finding. The purpose of the stereo-EEG study was then to verify this assumption and to try to define the limits of the cortical excision (see stereotactic scheme in Fig. 107–5A): the exploration was consequently centered on the basal part of the frontal lobe and on the anterior and midpart of the temporal lobe. The most posterior electrodes in the frontal lobe (i.e., H and R) represented the posterior limits of possible exeresis because lateralized somatomotor manifestation almost certainly never occurred. The seizures recorded confirmed a frontopolar and orbitofrontal origin of ictal discharges, which became symptomatic after they spread over the inferior frontal region, the temporal pole, and the anterior and midpart of the temporal neocortical areas (Fig. 107–9A and B). Thus, the resection performed included the inferior frontal region, both internal (from the pole to the projection of electrode G) and external (from the pole to the projection of the electrodes R and H), and the temporopolar region, the uncus, and the temporal neocortex (including the first, second, and third convolution) until the projection of the electrodes T and B. The patient has been seizure free for 10 months, with a normal clinical examination and no new neuropsychological deficit.

CASE REPORT 2 [PATIENT 21]

A 15-year-old right-handed girl, who had no familial or personal antecedents, had her first seizures at the age of 4 years. The seizure was reported as a feeling of fear (resulting from terrifying visual hallucinations?), chewing and swallowing, sometimes incomprehensible talk, and frequent tonic-clonic secondary generalization. The patient could warn the people around her of the imminent seizure. Despite numerous AEDs, seizure frequency reached up to more than one per day, and other apparently different episodes occurred in the course of the illness. When the patient was referred to our center at the age of 15, ictal symptomatology could be summarized as follows:

Brief subjective episodes of "eyes trembling"

Seizures characterized by a feeling of fear, followed by unlateralized simple visual hallucinations (e.g., fog, colored circles that she tries to grab), left deviation of the right eye, subjective vertigo, late oroalimentary automatisms, and rarely, clonic jerks of the right hemibody

Sudden and isolated painful cramps located in the right calf.

A right homonymous hemianopia was the only deficit at neurologic examination. Interictal EEG showed a marked asymmetry of background activity, slower on the temporo-occipital regions of the left hemisphere, where important theta activity intermixed by sharp waves was also noted. An apparently independent slow activity could have involved the left parietal regions. T1-weighted MRI sequences showed an atrophy of the posterior part of the left hemisphere, whereas in T2-weighted sequences, a small, linear, band-shaped hyperintensity in the mesial part of left temporo-occipital junction appeared.

The clinical picture, combined with anatomic and interictal electrical features, suggested the hypothesis of a left temporo-occipitoparietal epilepsy, and a stereo-EEG investigation was planned to determine if all the different types of seizure had univocal, but probably widely extended, posterior origin. For these reasons, 11 electrodes were stereotactically implanted (see stereotactic scheme on Fig. 107–6A) to explore first the supracalcarine and subcalcarine region, the "lesion" in the lingual lobule, and the temporoparieto-occipital junction to disclose the modalities of propagation toward the parietal and temporal lobes. The existence of painful manifestations in the right lower limb led to the exploration of the ascending parietal convolution and the left paracentral lobule. Finally, the hippocampus and amygdalar region were explored to determine if the seizure could have a more anterior origin. During stereo-EEG investigation, numerous seizures were recorded. The data showed that during the seizures, characterized by fear, visual manifestations, and subjective vertigo, ictal discharges admitted a large temporoparieto-occipital origin (Fig. 107–10A). In addition, the episodes of cramps were correlated with independent parietal discharges (Fig. 107–10B). A palliative occipitotemporoparietal corticectomy was performed, including the internal and external occipital cortex, the internal occipitotemporal junction and the posterior part of the hippocampus (between the projection of the electrodes C′ and B′), and the external parietal cortex until the projection of electrode P′ and passing the projection of the electrodes G′ and W′ by 15 mm. Pathologic findings were in accordance with the diagnosis of Rasmussen's encephalitis. Since the intervention, which was performed 7 months ago, the patient continues to experience daily painful cramps, as expected, and weekly brief episodes characterized by blurred vision, more or less lateralized in the right hemifield, without loss of consciousness and rarely associated with fear. Neurologic and neuropsychological examinations are normal (excepted the pre-existent hemianopia), and the patient is very satisfied.

MAJOR INTRAOPERATIVE COMPLICATIONS AND THEIR MANAGEMENT

Candidates for surgical treatment of severe partial epilepsy are generally in very good physical condition, and their interictal ICP is not elevated.[36] Careful anesthesiologic management (mostly hyperventilation and barbiturates) can be help-

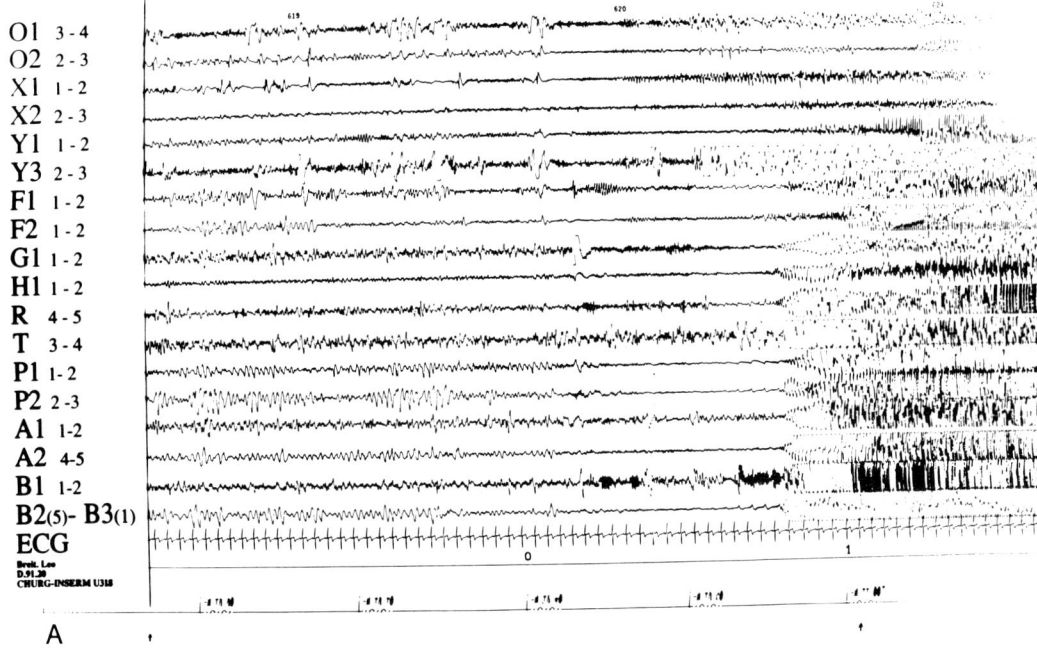

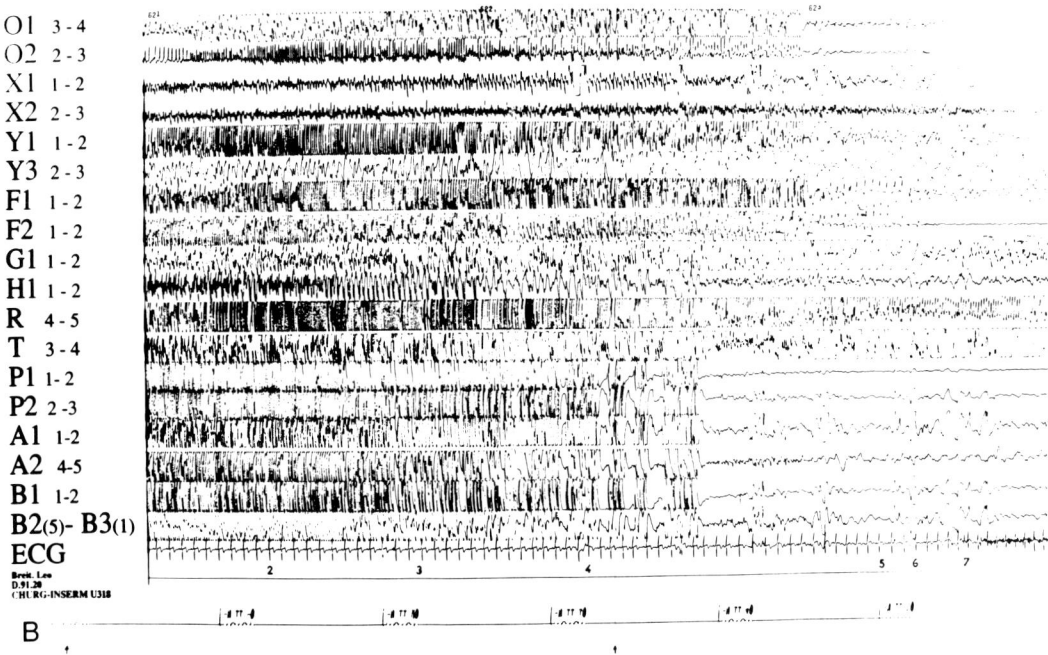

FIGURE 107–9. (A and B). Example of a multilobar epilepsy (see case report of patient 16, and stereotactic scheme on Figure 107–5A). The first electrical modification consists in the occurrence of brief sequences of low-voltage fast activity, which is particularly evident in the rectus gyrus (X1) but also in orbital cortex (F2). The involvement of the mesial frontobasal cortex occurs less than 10 seconds later. Ten seconds after, widely extended low-voltage fast activity can be appreciated, involving not only the internal and external frontobasal areas (O1, O2, X1, Y1, F1, F2) but also the frontal pole (Y3) and the temporal neocortex where the discharge is particularly tonic (P1, P2, A2, B3). The only clinical manifestation at the onset of seizure consists in deviation of the eyes, first toward the right (1), and later toward the left (2). Then, a progressive left-sided head-turning occurs (3), which stopped just before the end of ictal discharge (4). In the early postictal phase, the patient did not respond to questions (5), begins chewing (6), and presented bilateral gestural automatisms.

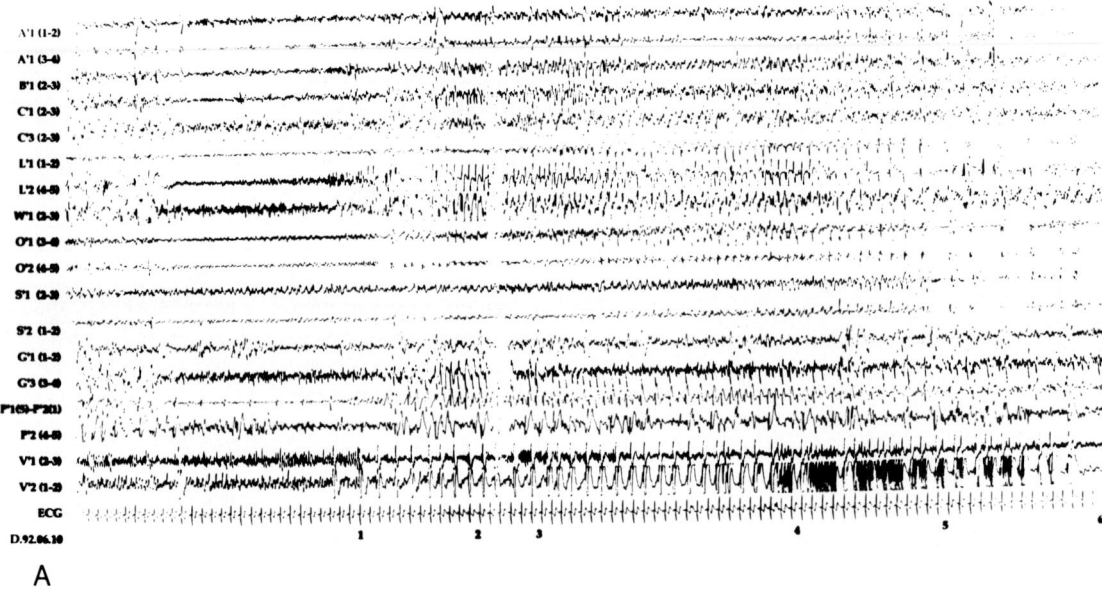

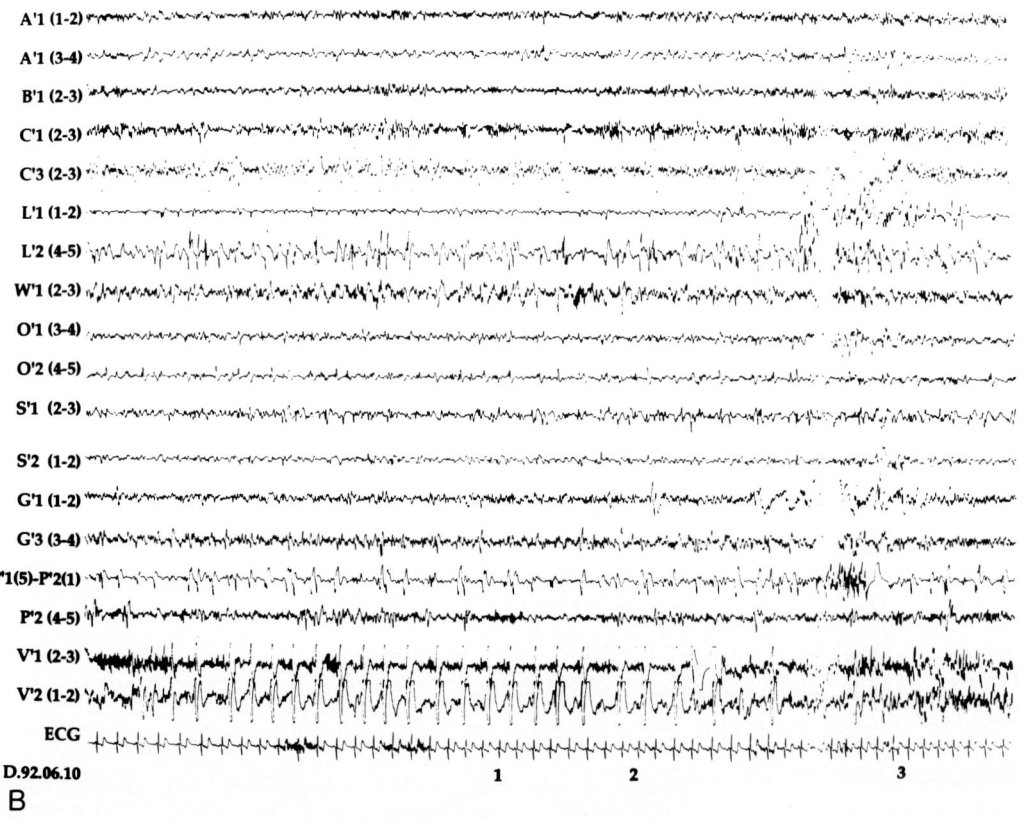

FIGURE 107–10. Example of a multifocal and multilobar epilepsy (see case report of patient 21, and stereotactic scheme in Figure 107–6A). (A) An example of a multilobar temporo-occipitoparietal seizure (onset). Low-voltage fast activity can be clearly appreciated in the lesion (L'1), but it also simultaneously involves both the perilesional areas (L'2, O'1, W'1) and the posterior parietal cortex (G'3, P'2). The involvement of the anterior and posterior part of the Ammon's horn occurs 1 second later and is less tonic, while the involvement of the post-central gyrus (V'1, V'2) occurs later, with a different electrical pattern characterized by a rhythmic spike-and-wave discharge. The patient opened her eyes when questioned (1) and stated that a seizure was about to occur (2). There also was an impression of subjective vertigo (3). Then, the patient could not respond to questions (4). (B) An example of a unilobar parietal ictal discharge in the same patient. During this other type of electroclinical seizure, the patient called the observer and explained that her cramp of the calf was about to occur (1), ascending to the thigh (2), and then disappear (3). The only electrical modification consists in a flattening of background activity associated with a rhythmic spike-and-wave discharge well localized on postcentral areas (V'1, V'2). Notably, lesional and perilesional areas are not involved.

35. Lüders HO, Engel J Jr, Munari C: General principles, in Engel J Jr (ed): Surgical Treatment of the Epilepsies, 2nd ed. New York, Raven Press, 1993, pp 137–153
36. Munari C, Andreoli A, Frattarelli M, Casaroli D: Activation par l'Amitryptiline (remarques électrocliniques à propos de 120 patients épileptiques). Rev EEG Neurophysiol 7:194–197, 1977
37. Penfield W, Jasper H: Epilepsy and the Functional Anatomy of the Human Brain. Boston, Little, Brown & Company, 1954
38. Engel J Jr: Outcome with respect to epileptic seizures, in Engel J Jr (ed): Surgical Treatment of the Epilepsies. New York, Raven Press, 1987, pp 553–571
39. Talairach J, Bancaud J: Lesions, irritative zone and epileptogenic focus. Confin Neurol 27:91–94, 1966
40. Lüders HO, Awad I: Conceptual considerations, in Lüders HO (ed): Epilepsy Surgery. New York, Raven Press, 1991, pp 51–62
41. Ojemann GA: Intraoperative tailoring of temporal lobe resections, in Engel J Jr (ed): Surgical Treatment of the Epilepsies, 2nd ed. New York, Raven Press, 1993, pp 481–488
42. Ajmone Marsan O: When are noninvasive tests enough? in Engel J Jr (ed): Surgical Treatment of the Epilepsies, 2nd ed. New York, Raven Press, 1993, pp 313–318
43. Rasmussen T, Feindel W: Temporal lobectomy: Review of 100 cases with major hippocampectomy. Can J Neurol Sci 18:601–602, 1991
44. Feindel W, Rasmussen T: Temporal lobectomy with amygdalectomy and minimal hippocampal resection: Review of 100 cases. Can J Neurol Sci 18:603–605, 1991
45. Wieser HG: Selective amygdalo-hippocampectomy for temporal lobe epilepsy. Epilepsia 29 (suppl 2):100–113, 1988
46. Primrose DC, Ojemann G: Outcome of resective surgery for temporal lobe epilepsy, in Lüders HO (ed): Epilepsy Surgery. New York, Raven Press, 1991, pp 601–611
47. Anderman F, Rasmussen T, Villemure JG: Hemispherectomy: Results for control of seizures in patients with hemiparesis, in Lüders HO (ed): Epilepsy Surgery. New York, Raven Press, 1991, pp 625–632
48. Kahane P, Francione S, Tassi L, et al: Traitement chirurgical des épilepsies partielles graves pharmaco-résistantes: Approches diagnostiques et thérapeutiques (rapport préliminaire sur trois années d'activité à Grenoble). Epilepsies 5:179–204, 1993
49. Bonis A: Long term results of cortical excisions based on stereotaxic investigations in severe drug resistant epilepsies. Acta Neurochir Suppl (Wien) 30:55–66, 1980
50. Andermann F, Salanova V, Olivier A, Rasmussen T: Occipital lobe epilepsy in children—Electroclinical manifestations, surgical indications and treatment, in Andermann F, Beaumanoir A, Mira L, et al (eds): Occipital Seizures and Epilepsies in Children. London, John Libbey, 1993, pp 213–220
51. Kuzniecky R, Cascino GD, Palmini A, et al: Structural neuroimaging, in Engel J Jr (ed): Surgical Treatment of the Epilepsies, 2nd ed. New York, Raven Press, 1993, pp 197–209
52. Munari C, Musolino A, Blond S, et al: Stereo-EEG exploration in patients with "intractable epilepsy": Topographic relationships between a lesion and the "epileptogenic areas," in Schmidt D, Morselli PL (eds): Workshop on Intractable Epilepsy. Experimental and Clinical Aspects. New York, Raven Press, 1986, pp 129–146
53. Fried I, Cascino G: Lesional surgery, in Engel J Jr (ed): Surgical Treatment of the Epilepsies, 2nd ed. New York, Raven Press, 1993, pp 501–509
54. Haddad SF, Moore SA, Menezes AH, et al: Ganglioglioma: 13 years of experience. Neurosurgery 31:171–178, 1992
55. Simard JM, Garcia-Bengochea F, Balinger WE, et al: Cavernous angioma: A review of 126 collected and 12 new clinical cases. Neurosurgery 18:162–172, 1986
56. Williamson PD: Postscript. Lessons from failures, in Engel J Jr (ed): Surgical Treatment of the Epilepsies, 2nd ed. New York, Raven Press, 1993, pp 587–591

CHAPTER 108

Cerebral Hemispherectomy for Epilepsy

Jean-Guy Villemure

Cerebral hemispherectomy, as a therapeutic procedure in humans, was first performed by Walter Dandy[1] in 1923 for the treatment of widespread glioma of the nondominant hemisphere. Close to three decades later, Krynauw[2] reported a series of "infantile hemiplegia" patients suffering from intractable seizures whom he had treated with hemispherectomy, obtaining dramatic results in seizure control and improvement in behavior. Following Krynauw's report, hemispherectomy for control of seizures in infantile hemiplegia was recognized as a valuable therapeutic procedure and practiced widely throughout the world.[3] The enthusiasm persisted until the 1960s, when following the clinical observations and the pathologic description of postoperative superficial cerebral hemosiderosis (SCH) by Oppenheimer and Griffith,[4] surgeons became reluctant to propose this operation to their patients, even though its benefit in seizure control was good.

For the next 25 years (1965–1992), modifications to anatomic hemispherectomy were proposed, all aimed at eliminating the late complication of SCH (median occurrence time of 8 years following surgery) while providing the benefit of seizure control. Multiple techniques have thus emerged, all having the same indications and, in theory, the same effect on seizure control, but aiming at reducing complications through different approaches.

Hemispherectomy refers to different technical modalities by which a cerebral hemisphere is either removed or disconnected, so that it is physiologically nonfunctional. The term is so descriptive that it is used generally, without reference to specific techniques, for the purpose of discussion.

INDICATIONS

The indications for hemispherectomy precede the choice of the surgical technique, and making the decision to operate is independent of the technique utilized. The decision to perform hemispherectomy for control of seizures results from the convergence of evidence emerging from the failure of pharmacologic control of the seizures, the patient's neurologic condition, the radiographic findings, the electroencephalographic investigation, and the suspected etiology of the seizures.[5]

SEIZURES

Patients who are considered surgical candidates for hemispherectomy have been unsuccessfully treated with anticonvulsants and either continue to have frequent seizures despite the medication or have side effects related to toxicity of the medication level necessary to control the seizures.

Different seizure patterns are observed in patient candidates for hemispherectomy; in reviewing the seizure patterns in 55 consecutive hemispherectomy patients my colleagues and I[5] observed that focal motor seizure involving the hemiplegic side predominates (over 80%); epilepsia partialis continua is usually associated with chronic encephalitis; a generalized predominantly tonic-clonic seizure pattern accounts for less than 13% of cases. It is not unusual to find more than one seizure type in candidates for hemispherectomy.

NEUROLOGIC EXAMINATION

On neurologic examination, the patient who is a candidate for hemispherectomy manifests a unilateral motor deficit that, depending on the etiologic factor and the severity of the underlying condition responsible for the seizures, ranges from a more or less severe hemiparesis to complete hemiplegia. This motor deficit is the result of a condition existing at birth or occurring early in life, or is secondary to a disease starting later in life, after normal early development, and progressing afterward. The unilateral motor deficit is characterized by the inability to perform individual finger movements and foot tapping with the affected limbs, even though the patients are able to carry out gross movements at shoulder, elbow, knee, and even hand level; such preoperative deficits are usually not worsened by hemispherectomy. In patients who have preserved ability to move the fingers individually and tap the foot, the motor deficit will be aggravated by hemispherectomy.

Over the past one to two decades, better understanding of diseases such as chronic encephalitis and Sturge-Weber syndrome has led to the consideration of hemispherectomy in patients with an incomplete motor deficit. Actually, one has to estimate the natural history of the disease responsible for the seizures to justify aggravating the neurologic condition for the benefit of better seizure control. The same rationale applies concerning visual field defect; although most candidates for hemispherectomy have hemiplegia and a homonymous hemianopsia, some patients may have intact visual fields preoperatively. In these instances, if a patient meets all the other criteria for hemispherectomy, the preoperative absence of a field defect is not an absolute contraindication to hemispherectomy.

Sensory deficits in candidates for hemispherectomy are not as striking as the motor findings. All patients have preserved, although possibly altered, cortical sensory modalities, which are rarely modified to permanent severe deficit by surgery.

Because candidates for hemispherectomy have suffered repeated seizures, usually for months to many years, owing to underlying widespread hemispheric damage, it is not surprising to find some degree of mental retardation and behavioral problems in this population. None of these features represents a contraindication to hemispherectomy, but the degree of mental retardation should be an indicator of the integrity of the so-called normal hemisphere; severe mental retardation usually reflects bilateral cerebral damage. Although Krynauw,[2] in his original series, listed abnormal behavior in infantile hemiplegia patients as an indication for hemispherectomy, we do not consider that abnormal behavior alone represents a suitable indication for hemispherectomy. It is likely that such abnormal behaviors either represent or are associated with seizures.

Speech remains a concern in the decision to proceed to hemispherectomy. In patients in whom the brain insult has occurred early in life (up to age 5 or 6 years), it is generally accepted and has been clinically demonstrated that the condition responsible for the seizures has forced speech to shift and develop in the so-called good hemisphere. There is more concern about speech in patients who are candidate for a left hemispherectomy and suffer from an acquired condition, such as chronic encephalitis, that begins after they have reached the age of 6 years. The clinician may in these instances want to perform a carotid Amytal test to obtain more precise information about speech and therefore be better able to appreciate the effect of hemispherectomy. We are aware of a few patients operated at ages 9 and 11 in whom the preoperative Amytal test demonstrated major speech localization in the hemisphere to be operated; after hemispherectomy, these patients experienced periods of mutism (lasting weeks to months) but recovered functional speech. On the basis of this experience, we do not consider possible interference with speech functions an absolute contraindication to hemispherectomy.

IMAGING

The radiologic investigation of hemispherectomy candidates usually demonstrates atrophy of the affected hemisphere. This is shown on plain skull radiograph, computed tomography (CT) scan, and magnetic resonance imaging (MRI). Positron emission tomography (PET) scan may demonstrate decreased glucose and oxygen utilization in the damaged hemisphere. Although the atrophy is usually unilateral, it may be bilateral, but it predominates in the affected hemisphere in most such cases (Fig. 108–1). In some cases of early chronic encephalitis, Sturge-Weber syndrome, hemimegalencephaly, and migrational disorder, the atrophy may not be severe. The atrophy generally manifests as an enlarged ventricle, a thin cortical mantle, atrophy of the ipsilateral cerebral peduncle, and widened subarachnoid space. Superficial calcifications should be recognized in Sturge-Weber syndrome (Fig. 108–2). An abnormal signal on MRI may be seen in migration disorder and in chronic encephalitis at an early stage.

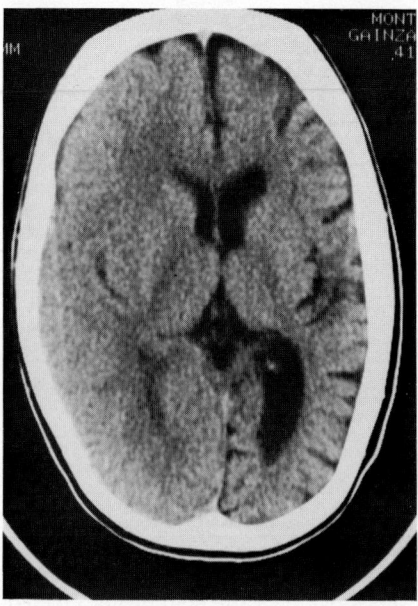

FIGURE 108–1. CT scan. Plain axial view demonstrating asymmetry of the cranial vault and cerebral hemispheres with left-sided atrophy manifested as thicker cranial vault, larger ventricle, and larger sulci.

ELECTROENCEPHALOGRAPHY

The electroencephalographic (EEG) investigation helps determine the sites of origin of seizures, the extent of the damage to the affected hemisphere, and the integrity of the good hemisphere. The EEG findings in the affected hemisphere are those of an abnormal background with widespread, low-amplitude slow wave, accompanied by multifocal, independent spikes and sharp waves. In half the patients, abnormal EEG findings are recorded from the good hemisphere; in the majority of such cases, these findings are secondary. It is important for prognosis to determine whether

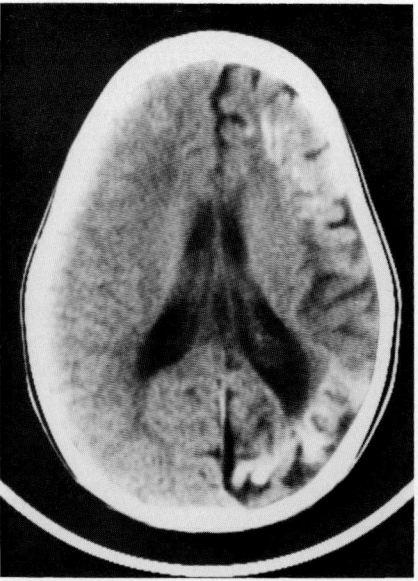

FIGURE 108–2. CT scan, plain axial view. Atrophy of the left hemisphere (enlarged sulci, large trigone) with diffuse superficial calcifications, typical of Sturge-Weber syndrome.

Table 108–1. UNDERLYING PATHOLOGY IN PATIENTS UNDERGOING HEMISPHERECTOMY FOR SEIZURES—MONTREAL NEUROLOGICAL HOSPITAL

Pathology	No. of Patients
Infantile hemiplegia	24
Encephalitis, meningitis	28
Hemimegalencephaly	5
Infarct	3
Migrational disorder	1
Head injury	6
Sturge-Weber syndrome	3
Total	70

spikes recorded from the good hemisphere are independent or secondary; when they are independent, they provide evidence of bilateral involvement and may indicate that the patient, even though helped by the operation, may not become seizure free.

ETIOLOGY

Consideration of the etiology underlying the seizure disorder is important in the decision to perform hemispherectomy, because in some instances, the operation should be done prior to the development of maximal lateralized deficit (e.g., Sturge-Weber syndrome, chronic encephalitis), whereas in other instances, the etiology might suggest bilateral cerebral damage (e.g., meningitis). Table 108–1 outlines the etiologies found in 70 consecutive hemispherectomies carried out at the Montreal Neurological Hospital. Note that about half the patients were developing normally prior to the onset of the disease responsible for the seizures that led to surgery.

HEMISPHERECTOMY TECHNIQUES

Whichever hemispherectomy technique is used, the indications remain the same, and the effect on seizure control should be identical. The various hemispherectomy techniques differ in their attempts to reduce complications, not in their rate of success in seizure control; this latter item depends primarily on patient selection and secondarily on the completeness of the hemispherectomy. Table 108–2 lists the different hemispherectomy techniques.

Table 108–2. HEMISPHERECTOMY TECHNIQUES FOR THE TREATMENT OF SEIZURES

Anatomic hemispherectomy	With basal ganglia removed
	Without basal ganglia removed
	"En bloc"
	Fragmentation
Modification to anatomic hemispherectomy	Oxford-Adams hemispherectomy
Procedures that preserve white matter	Hemidecortication
	Hemicorticectomy
Functional hemispherectomy	Classic technique
	Technical variations
Hemispherotomy	Transvertex (Delalande)
	Peri-insular (Villemure)

GENERAL FINDINGS AT SURGERY

Surgical findings depend on the etiologic condition responsible for the seizures. In expansile processes such as cystic dilatation and hemimegalencephaly, the skull might be thinner and expanded, whereas in atrophic processes, the skull is thicker and the cranial vault flat.

The cerebral hemisphere is usually hypovascular, being characterized by smaller than normal arteries and veins. In hemimegalencephaly, the tissue is vascularized normally, and there may be more volume than usual; the tissue may present an abnormally increased consistency. In patients with Sturge-Weber disease, we have not encountered difficulty with hemostasis, because the vascular anomaly is predominantly pial; the gross findings are superficial, but the tissue may be of increased consistency.

The cerebral tissue is characteristically tougher than usual in all conditions encountered. In most instances, coagulation and suction are adequate to complete the removal. Occasionally, however, the ultrasonic aspirator is useful to deal with severe gliosis. In atrophic conditions, the ipsilateral ventricle is enlarged, whereas it may be normal in early chronic encephalitis or Sturge-Weber disease and possibly smaller in hemimegalencephaly.

ANATOMIC HEMISPHERECTOMY

Anatomic hemispherectomy, described by Dandy,[1] consists in excision of the hemisphere, including the basal ganglia. It requires the occlusion of the middle and anterior cerebral arteries at the carotid bifurcation, interruption of all ipsilateral draining veins, section of the corpus callosum, and incision from the lateral ventricle to the temporal horn through the basal ganglia.

Preservation of the basal ganglia was first advocated by Gardner,[6] who modified Dandy's technique by interrupting the anterior and middle cerebral arteries distal to the lenticulostriate arteries and Heubner's artery. Whether the basal ganglia are preserved or not does not influence the motor performance postoperatively, as demonstrated by Laine and colleagues[7] and by French and associates.[8]

Anatomic hemispherectomy can be performed en bloc or in fragments, according to the surgeon's preference.[9–11]

MODIFICATIONS OF ANATOMIC HEMISPHERECTOMY

Modifications to anatomic hemispherectomy have been proposed to eliminate the complication of SCH often seen postoperatively.[4, 10–12]

Oxford-Adams Modification[13]

Following anatomic hemispherectomy, the ipsilateral foramen of Monro is occluded with a piece of muscle, to avoid mixing of bloody material from the hemispherectomy cavity with the cerebrospinal fluid and subarachnoid pathways. Furthermore, the hemispherectomy cavity is made smaller by stripping the convexity and basal dura from the bone, and tacking it to the falx and floor of the middle fossa; a large extradural space is thus created. Preventing the accumulation of blood and membrane formation by reducing the subdural hemispherectomy cavity and then preventing free communication of that cavity with the ventricular system are the principles underlying this modification.

TECHNIQUES THAT PRESERVE WHITE MATTER

Removing the cerebral cortex, which actually is the portion of the hemisphere that triggers seizures, while preserving the white matter, thus avoiding wide exposure of the ventricle, also aims at eliminating SCH. Hemidecortication[14, 15] and hemicorticectomy[16] have the same surgical principles but differ in technique.

Hemidecortication consists in excising all the cortex of one hemisphere, including subfrontal, suboccipital, and parasagittal tissue. The white matter is preserved, casting the ventricle and preventing free communication of the ventricular CSF with the surgical bed. Only the temporal horn needs to be entered to allow excision of the hippocampus.

Hemicorticectomy aims at removing all the cortex while avoiding opening the ventricle. The technique involves undermining a large portion of cortex and removing slabs of cortical tissue, leaving white matter and basal ganglia. This surgical procedure was developed to reduce the risk of hemorrhagic complication, by avoiding large exposure of the ventricle and reducing the volume of the hemispherectomy cavity.

FUNCTIONAL HEMISPHERECTOMY

Functional hemispherectomy is subtotal anatomic removal of the hemisphere by complete disconnection. The disconnection is intended to render the hemisphere physiologically unable to manifest seizures. A large volume of vascularized hemisphere is thus left in the cranial compartment but disconnected from the contralateral hemisphere and from any ipsilateral deep structure. The classic technique and its variations will be described.[15, 17–21]

Classic Technique

The procedure is performed with the patient under general anesthesia, supine on the operating table, with padding under the ipsilateral shoulder and the head parallel to the floor. Depending on the patient's age, a skull clamp may be used.

A barn-door skin flap is designed, originating at the zygoma, extending to the sagittal region at the level of the coronal suture, extending posteriorly on the midline to reach the parietal region, then aiming inferiorly toward the transverse sinus. After elevation of the skin and temporalis muscle, a bone flap is made, 1 cm lateral to the midline, to avoid dissection immediately above the superior sagittal sinus. A temporal craniectomy is carried out to allow easier access to the middle fossa. The dura is opened in a horseshoe shape and reflected to the midline.

Observation and palpation of the brain are then carried out. Independent of the condition responsible for the seizures, the brain consistency is abnormally hard, and in most

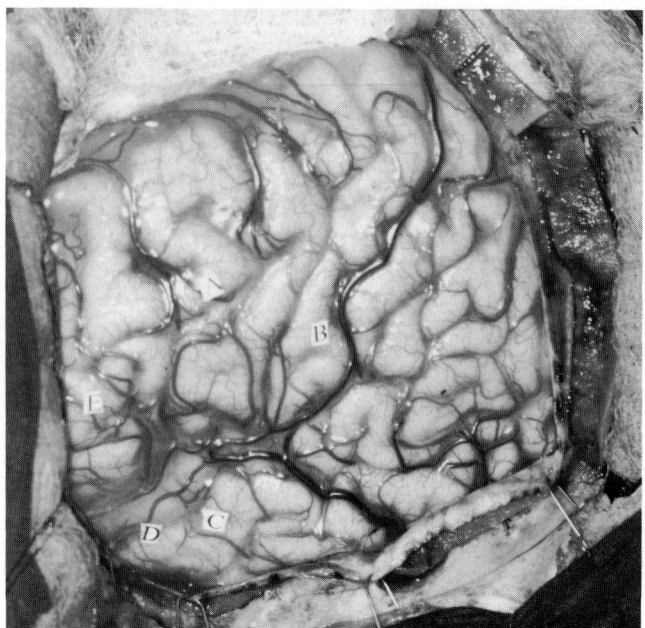

FIGURE 108–3. Operative photograph. Multiple independent epileptic foci identified by corticography (A to E), originating from the frontal, parietal, and temporal lobes.

instances, the arteries and veins are atrophic. The findings in Sturge-Weber disease are those of pial angiomatosis with the purple-red color of the surface of the brain. In hemimegalencephaly and conditions of abnormal migration, the gross appearance of the brain may be close to normal; the vascularization may be normal, and the tissue may have patchily abnormal consistency. In severe atrophy, such as the atrophy seen following a perinatal vascular accident, the ipsilateral ventricle may be extremely large; in these instances, portions of the cerebral convexity may be paper thin and translucent.

Pre-excision corticography is not essential to the operation but is useful in confirming the surface EEG findings and the presence of multifocal independent epileptic spikes (Fig. 108–3).

Functional hemispherectomy consists of four surgical steps: temporal lobectomy, excision of the central region, disconnection of the parieto-occipital lobes, and disconnection of the frontal lobe (Fig. 108–4).

Temporal Lobectomy

Temporal lobectomy may be performed first or last. It extends more posterior than the usual temporal lobectomy for partial complex seizures, so as to reach the level of the trigone. Temporal lobectomy is performed in four stages.

Stage 1: The pia over the first temporal gyrus is coagulated and incised; the gray matter and white matter of T1 are aspirated, exposing the insular cortex down to the white matter of the temporal stem.

Stage 2: Over the posterior temporal lobe, a vertical or oblique incision is made from T1 to T3. After coagulation and incision of the pia, the white matter is aspirated, and the temporal horn identified.

Stage 3: The temporal stem is sectioned with use of the bipolar coagulator with one blade in the temporal horn and one blade placed just inferior to the insular cortex. The temporal neocortex is then excised after dissection lateral to the hippocampus and coagulation and incision of the pia along the floor of the middle fossa.

Stage 4: The amygdala and hippocampus are excised via subpial aspiration and peeling of the tissue from the medial temporal pia to reach the choroidal fissure.

Excision of the Central Region

The purposes of this step are to have access to the whole corpus callosum and to isolate the frontal and parieto-occip-

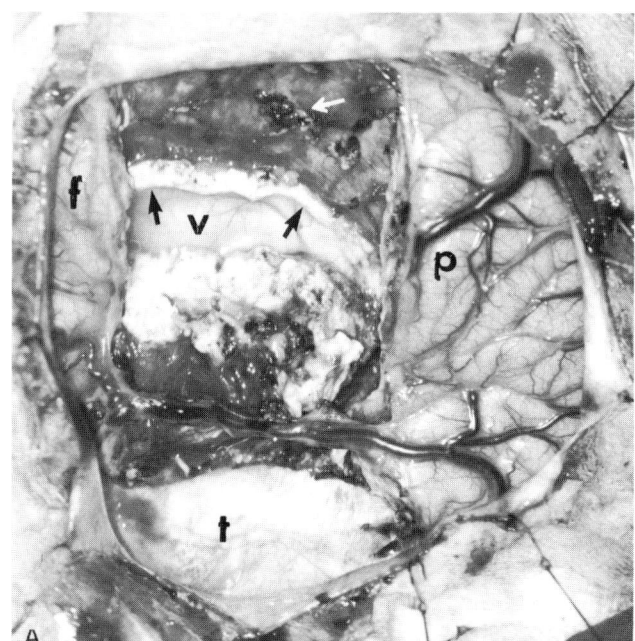

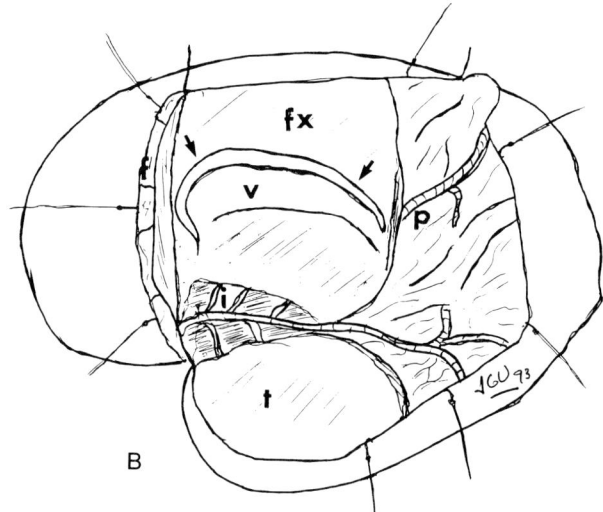

FIGURE 108–4. (A) Operative photograph demonstrating the anatomic result of the classic functional hemispherectomy (left side). Note the temporal lobectomy cavity (t), the corpus callosum widely exposed from genu to splenium (black arrows), with resection of the central region, including the parasagittal tissue (white arrow denotes falx). (B) Diagrammatic representation of classic functional hemispherectomy (left side). Excision of central region, including the parasagittal tissue (fx = falx). Exposure of the corpus callosum from the rostrum to the splenium (arrows). Frontal lobotomy and parieto-occipital lobotomies, isolating these lobes from the rest of the brain. Large temporal lobectomy (t). f = frontal lobe; i = insula; p = parietal lobe; v = ventricle.

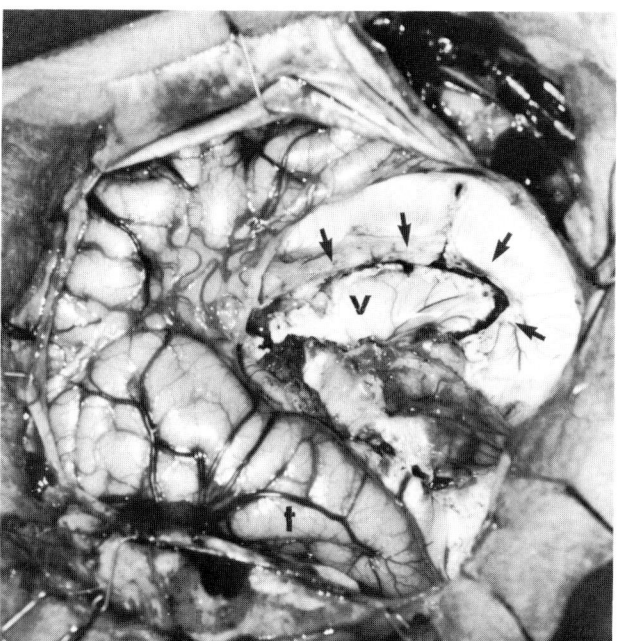

FIGURE 108–5. Operative photograph demonstrating an enlarged right lateral ventricle. Note the incision in the medial wall of the lateral ventricle (v), interrupting the fibers as they enter the corpus callosum (arrows). (Vertical incision along the falx; illustration of the callosotomy from within the ventricle, at the level of the body and genu.) t = temporal lobe.

ital lobes. The frontoparietal operculum is excised by subpial aspiration, using above the fissure of Sylvius the same technique used to excise T1. Vertical frontal and parietal incisions, theoretically projecting anterior and posterior to the corpus callosum, are then made in the cerebral convexity, reaching up to the midline. Gray matter and white matter are aspirated to the lateral ventricle inferiorly and the parasagittal pia medially. The white matter superior to the insular cortex is entered, leading to the lateral ventricle. The frontoparietal parasagittal tissue is then entered and aspirated along the falx all the way to the lateral ventricle subpially or through incision of the pia along the falx superior to the corpus callosum. A large piece of central tissue is then excised. Upon completion of this step, a portion of the callosotomy has been done (body of corpus callosum) (Fig. 108–5).

Disconnection of the Parieto-Occipital Lobes

The corpus callosum has been identified in the previous step. The thin corpus callosum and the pericallosal vessels are followed posteriorly, and with the use of suction and bipolar coagulation, from within the lateral ventricle, all fibers entering it are interrupted. This creates an incision 1 to 2 mm wide that isolates the parieto-occipital lobes from the rest of the brain. The pericallosal incision is carried posteriorly to reach the splenium of the corpus callosum. Further dissection along the medial pia is then carried out from the splenium to reach the choroidal fissure in the posterior temporal region, thus isolating the parieto-occipital lobes from any ipsilateral or contralateral connections.

Disconnection of the Frontal Lobe

The frontal lobe is disconnected in two stages. In the first stage, the white matter and gray matter of the fronto-orbital region are separated with the suction-coagulation technique, anterior to the basal ganglia, in a coronal plane. This incision reaches the pia of the orbital surface of the frontal lobe. The olfactory tract and the gyrus rectus are useful landmarks.

In the second stage, the callosotomy is completed anteriorly from within the ventricle, with interruption of all fibers from the frontal lobe entering the corpus callosum. Care is taken not to damage the pericallosal vessels, which should be identified and used as guides for the callosotomy. Once the genu and the rostrum have been identified, the incision should reach the coronal incision previously made, thereby isolating the frontal lobe in a coronal plane.

Insulectomy

When the insular cortex is to be removed, its removal is accomplished by subpial aspiration from below and from above the fissure. Identification of the underlying white matter indicates the extent of excision of the insular cortex.[22]

Technical Variations of Functional Hemispherectomy

The objective of functional hemispherectomy is to reduce the hemispherectomy cavity by preserving as much brain and subarachnoid space as possible while disconnecting the hemisphere. Variations in the original technique have been introduced and may be adapted according to the type and degree of atrophy of the hemisphere.

Reduction in Width of Central Region Removed

The removal of the central convexity and parasagittal tissue does not necessarily have to be as large as the length of the corpus callosum. Actually, through a narrower central excision, one is able to accomplish the same callosotomy from within the ventricle and isolate the frontal and parieto-occipital lobes.

Preservation of the Parasagittal Tissue

Because, once the lateral ventricle has been entered, the surgeon is able to interrupt the fibers coming into the corpus callosum from the frontal and parieto-occipital lobes as well as from the parasagittal central tissue, only the central convexity needs to be removed. The parasagittal tissue may be spared. If the corpus callosum is difficult to identify by inspection, once the lateral ventricle has been entered, we have found it useful to create an incision 2 mm wide through the parasagittal tissue, from within the ventricle, with the aim of identifying the parasagittal pia or falx. This incision, which is vertical to the plane of the corpus callosum, is then extended through the cingulate gyrus until the corpus callosum is clearly identified. The callosotomy from within the ventricle can then be accomplished.

Preservation of the Central Convexity Tissue

Not only may the width of the central region removal be reduced (anteroposterior) and the parasagittal tissue spared, but also, only a suprasylvian opening in the ventricle may be necessary to achieve the frontoparieto-occipital disconnec-

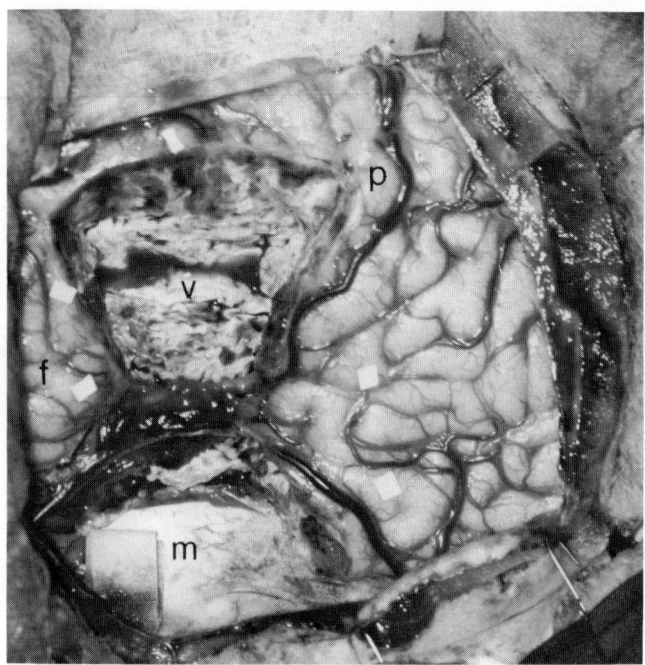

FIGURE 108–6. Operative photograph following functional hemispherectomy (variation 3). Temporal lobectomy (m), insulectomy, and suprasylvian approach to the lateral ventricle (v). See also Figure 108–8, a postoperative CT scan of same patient. p = parietal lobe; f = frontal lobe. Whte squares represent the site of the spikes recorded post-disconnection.

tion (Fig. 108–6). The larger the ventricle, the easier it is to perform this variation. Once the frontoparietal operculum has been excised, the lateral ventricle is entered via sectioning through the white matter superior to the suprasylvian insular cortex; this opening in the ventricle extends from the level of the sphenoid wing anteriorly and to the trigone posteriorly. The callosotomy as well as the frontal and parieto-occipital disconnections are accomplished through this opening.

HEMISPHEROTOMY

Hemispherotomy refers to the smallest surgical removal necessary to accomplish a hemisphere disconnection. It represents the ultimate step in the concept of functional hemispherectomy, by which the hemisphere is physiologically disconnected but anatomically preserved.

Transvertex hemispherotomy, first described by Delalande and colleagues,[23] is performed as follows. Through a high vertex craniotomy, the lateral ventricle is accessed via a frontoparietal cortical window; a callosotomy is performed from inside the lateral ventricle, the brain is transected around the thalamus, and the posterior column of the fornix is sectioned.

Peri-insular hemispherotomy (Villemure) represents a continuum of the technical variations of functional hemispherectomy.[24, 25] These variations are characterized by less suprasylvian brain removal and a rather large temporal lobectomy, allowing a physiologic disconnection of the hemisphere. With the peri-insular hemispherotomy, most of the hemisphere is anatomically preserved, including a major portion of temporal lobe. This procedure is made easier when there is a diffuse enlargement of the ipsilateral ventricle, including the temporal horn, secondary to the underlying pathologic process. The peri-insular hemispherotomy consists of two major surgical steps, creation of the suprasylvian window and of the infrasylvian window (Fig. 108–7).

The suprasylvian step corresponds to the third variation of functional hemispherectomy already described. This surgical step disconnects the whole suprasylvian portion of the hemisphere through removal of a small portion of suprasylvian brain (operculum).

The infrasylvian step aims at functionally isolating the temporal lobe; it consists of three stages that address three temporal structures: the neocortex, the amygdala, and the hippocampus. To functionally isolate the temporal lobe, the first temporal gyrus is excised in the usual manner, but as far back as the most posterior portion of the insular cortex; gray matter and white matter of T1 are aspirated subpially, exposing the insular cortex, until the white matter of the temporal stem is visualized. The white matter of the temporal stem is then transected in a plane from the level just inferior to the insular cortex to the temporal horn, and from the tip of the temporal horn to the trigone, reaching posteriorly to the suprasylvian window. The insular cortex is thus totally exposed, with the lateral ventricle seen above, the trigone posteriorly, and the temporal horn inferiorly.

The most anterior portion of T1 is then excised using the subpial aspiration technique till the uncus is reached medially. The uncus is then excised by aspiration; this step usually exposes the third cranial nerve, the proximal posterior cerebral artery, and the anterolateral pontomesencephalic junction. The amygdala is further excised superomedially until the excision appears adequate.

The anterior hippocampus is removed until the choroidal fissure is reached. The hippocampus either can be removed by aspiration and peeling or can be transected posteriorly at the level of the trigone, interrupting the fimbria-fornix. We prefer transection of the hippocampus, because it is technically easier and faster than its removal. The hemisphere disconnection is completed by joining the callosotomy incision inferior to the splenium, to the fimbria-fornix incision, by aspirating the tissue down to the medial pia and reaching the choroidal fissure posteriorly. This latter stage completes the hemispherotomy. The insular cortex is removed by aspiration when indicated.

The peri-insular hemispherotomy appears to be the surgical procedure in which the ratio of disconnection to excision of the hemisphere is the greatest technically achievable.

Case Reports

CASE REPORT 1

A 16-month-old female experienced her first seizure at age 4 months. There had been a normal pregnancy and delivery; the child exhibited left V1 and right V3 facial angiomas; her development until 4 months was described as normal. At 4 months, the patient had a febrile illness accompanied by a period of unresponsiveness without motor activity. The CT scan showed findings characteristic of Sturge-Weber syndrome. Over the following months, despite medication, the patient continued to have motor seizures involving the right side with generalization, accompanied by a progressive hemiparesis. Upon referral at age 16 months, the patient's head circumference was 44.1 cm; she exhibited a port wine nevus involving the left V1 and the right V3 distributions, a right hemianopsia on confrontation, and a flaccid right hemiparesis. She could maintain a sitting position but could not bear weight.

Three preoperative EEGs showed diffuse slow waves involving the left hemisphere. A CT scan showed diffuse atrophy of the left hemisphere, with the left lateral ventricle being larger. There were cortical calcifications predominantly in the left parieto-occipital region. An MRI scan demonstrated the same findings, with hyperintense signal of the white matter on the T2-weighted image; the corpus callosum was thinner than usual.

A left functional hemispherectomy was carried out. The superficial anatomy was normal except for the prominent nevus extending over the left side of the scalp. The whole cortical surface appeared involved by the disease process, except for a small island of normal-looking brain in the central region. The diffuse pial angiomatosis involved the parasagittal and medial temporal regions and extended from the frontal pole to the occipital pole posteriorly. In addition, there was diffuse cortical atrophy with subcortical gliosis, the white matter having a rubbery consistency. Electrocorticography performed prior to resection revealed diffuse delta wave activity with independent spiking from essentially all areas of the cortex exposed. Functional hemispherectomy disconnected the hemisphere, leaving large portions of the frontal and parieto-occipital lobes as well as the insular cortex.

There were no perioperative complications. The patho-

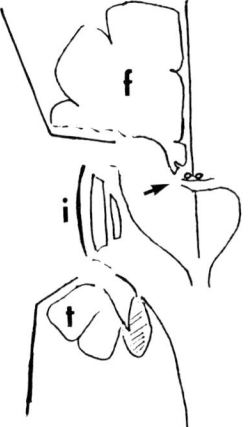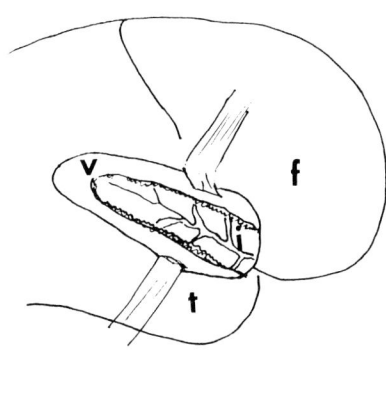

FIGURE 108–7. Diagrammatic representation of peri-insular hemispherotomy. Coronal section through the basal ganglia (drawing on the left) and lateral projection of right hemisphere (drawing on the right). Peri-insular excision allows disconnection of the whole hemisphere. Note the approach to the ventricle through the frontoparietal and temporal operculum, sectioning the corona radiata as well as the temporal stem. A callosotomy (arrow) is performed from within the ventricle (v). f = frontal lobe; i = insula; t = temporal lobe.

logic analysis confirmed the diagnosis of Sturge-Weber disease. At discharge, the patient exhibited neurologic findings identical to preoperative findings.

Five years later, the patient is off medication and has remained seizure free. She is developing very satisfactorily physically and intellectually; she engages in social activities with other children, has good learning abilities and normal speech, and is able to run despite the right hemiparesis.

CASE REPORT 2

This boy was developing normally until age 3, when he started having short episodes of pallor, sweating, coldness, and sucking movements lasting a few seconds. During the same year, he developed right focal motor seizures and generalized tonic-clonic seizures, tonic fits, drop attacks, and absence seizures. On initial investigation, CT and CSF findings were normal.

Over the next 3 years, the patient developed a right hemiparesis and started using his left hand. Despite pharmacologic treatment, the seizures continued. These were (1) focal motor seizures involving the right arm and leg, with head deviation to the right; (2) akinetic drop attacks; (3) tonic drop attacks followed by generalized convulsions, with postictal right paralysis; (4) moaning; and (5) automatisms. Seizures occurred at a frequency of four a day.

The patient was referred at age 8. The neurologic examination showed a hyperactive boy; he had a right hemianopsia, a spastic right hemiparesis, with preserved movements at major joints but inability to perform individual finger movements or foot tapping on the right. There was preservation of all the sensory modalities on the affected side, but these were altered. Reflexes were increased on the right; the gait was hemiparetic. His speech was slow but intelligible. Scalp EEGs demonstrated diffuse slow waves and multifocal independent spikes from the left hemisphere. CT scan showed diffuse left hemispheric atrophy.

The patient underwent a left functional hemispherectomy with the preoperative diagnosis of chronic encephalitis and intractable seizures. Corticography prior to removal demonstrated multiple independent epileptic spikes over the left frontal, temporal, and parietal lobes. The tissue was hard. A functional hemispherectomy was carried out through a suprasylvian window, exposing the ventricle and allowing the disconnection of the hemisphere; a temporal lobectomy was also carried out with removal of the amygdala and hippocampus (third variation of functional hemispherectomy). Because posthemispherectomy corticography demonstrated active spiking from the insular cortex, insulectomy was carried out by subpial aspiration (Fig. 108–8). The patient left the hospital with neurologic findings identical to those noted on admission and has remained seizure free and off medication for the past 3 years. His behavior as well as his learning abilities have improved.

COMPLICATIONS AND THEIR MANAGEMENT

Cerebral hemispherectomy remains a major surgical procedure even though the severe complications are now relatively rare.[26] The recognition of the late complication of superficial cerebral hemosiderosis in the mid-1960s led neurosurgeons to develop and propose surgical techniques that would reduce the rate and severity of complications associated with hemispherectomy.[13–16]

Complications occurring during surgery are rare and are

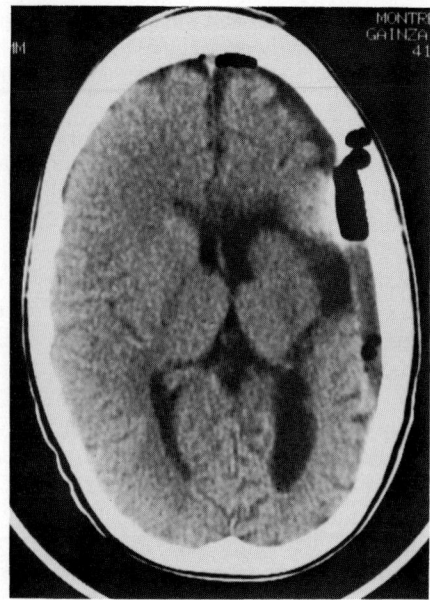

FIGURE 108–8. Postoperative CT scan, axial view, taken after the functional hemispherectomy shown in Figure 108–6. The surgical incisions can be seen in the frontal and parietal lobes, as well as the area of insulectomy.

not specific to the technique of hemispherectomy itself but rather to anatomic structures that should be preserved. We recommend, independent of the choice of technique, that the bone flap not reach the midline, so as to avoid trauma to the superior sagittal sinus and major draining veins that may be important in techniques in which a large portion of the hemisphere is anatomically spared. Occlusion of the superior sagittal sinus could manifest as major postoperative neurologic deficit and death.

Good visualization of the vascular and nervous structures are essential. Visualization is improved with fiberoptic illumination and magnification. Along the midline, in the perichiasmatic and medial temporal regions, the subpial aspiration technique is useful to decrease the risk of damage to neighboring structures.

At time of callosotomy, one has to be concerned about the contralateral pericallosal artery; the best way to avoid damaging it is to visualize the ipsilateral artery and stay outside the pericallosal cistern.

In techniques in which brain is left in situ, as many arteries and veins as possible should be preserved. This practice contributes to reducing the volume of the hemispherectomy cavity by avoiding further atrophy.

Placement of a subdural drain for 24 to 48 hours postoperatively favors the evacuation of blood debris and reduces the severity of postoperative aseptic meningitis. This is further reduced by covering the ventricular wall and filling the ventricles with cotton during surgery, as to avoid spillage of blood into the cerebrospinal fluid.

Failure to control seizures should not be regarded as a complication of the surgery, because this issue relates much more to the preoperative evaluation than to the surgical act itself. Early postoperative seizures, usually generalized in nature, that occur within 48 hours may be seen on occasions; they may be self-limited and do not preclude a good prognosis.

It is not uncommon to note *immediate postoperative fever* up to 101°F lasting for up to 10 to 12 days. It is usually accompanied by headache, lack of appetite, and malaise; this early postoperative syndrome is related to the presence of blood products mixed with cerebrospinal fluid (aseptic meningitis). It can be minimized with copious perioperative irrigation, placement of cotton pads in the ventricle during surgery, immaculate hemostasis, and postoperative subdural drainage.

Wound infection[11] and hemorrhage[7, 10, 11, 27] in the hemispherectomy cavity are among the risks of any intracranial surgical procedure, and they are rare with these procedures. They can be minimized only by strict surgical technique. Sometimes a large hematoma forms late after surgery, probably in relation to minor head injury; reducing the volume of the hemispherectomy cavity by a modified hemispherectomy technique likely decreases its incidence.

Brain shift and *brain herniation* secondary to hydrocephalus have been reported, occurring early or late after hemispherectomy.[7, 28] These complications occurred following anatomic hemispherectomy. We suspect that the incidence of such rare complications is further reduced with use of hemispherectomy techniques that leaves tissue in the cavity.

SCH was recognized and described in the mid 1960s. Oppenheimer and Griffith[4] published the postmortem findings in 3 of 17 hemispherectomy patients. The pathologic findings were those of hydrocephalus secondary to aqueductal occlusion by periaqueductal gliosis and granular ependymitis. Membranes similar to those found in chronic subdural hematomas lined the hemispherectomy cavity and the ventricles. It is postulated that repeated small subclinical hemorrhages from the membranes have been responsible for the occurrence of SCH. This late complication, occurring 4.5 to 25 years postoperatively (median 8 years), had an incidence as high as 33 percent with a mortality rate of 33 percent earlier in the Montreal Neurological Hospital series.[12] In our days, with improved radiologic evaluation, the hydrocephalus associated with this complication could be detected earlier and treated accordingly, thereby reducing the neurologic problems associated with hydrocephalus.

Hydrocephalus not secondary to SCH is also encountered as a complication of hemispherectomy. Its incidence varies according to the technique utilized and should increase with length of follow-up. The rate of hydrocephalus following hemispherectomy varies from 7 to 20 percent. It may result from the underlying cause of the seizures, such as remote head injury or infection that has altered the subarachnoid pathways, partly from the operation itself, in which blood products mix with cerebrospinal fluid, and also from the amount of subarachnoid space removed at time of surgery.[15]

It is to reduce the incidence of SCH while preserving the benefit of seizure control that modifications to anatomic hemispherectomy have emerged over the past 25 years. All the new techniques have in common reduction of the volume of the hemispherectomy cavity. In the Oxford-Adams modification, this goal is accomplished by stripping of the dura and creating a small subdural space at the expense of a larger extradural space. In the hemidecortication, hemicorticectomy, functional hemispherectomy, and hemispherotomy techniques, part of the hemisphere is left in the hemispherectomy cavity. Although the common aim is to decrease the incidence of SCH, we suspect that the incidence of large hematomas occurring early or late postoperatively should also be decreased with use of techniques that reduce the volume of dead space.

It is suspected that the long-term incidence of hydrocephalus is higher with hemispherectomy techniques in which the subarachnoid space is completely or largely removed on the operated side, and should be lower with techniques in which the subarachnoid circulatory and absorptive pathways are preserved, such as in functional hemispherectomy and hemispherotomy.

RESULTS

SEIZURE CONTROL

For the same indication, the various hemispherectomy techniques should have the same effect on seizure control. These procedures differ in surgical principles, technical steps, and complications, but they should have the same physiologic effect of reducing seizures.

In general, the effect of hemispherectomy on seizure control can be summarized as follows: 70 to 85 percent of patients remain seizure free; 15 to 20 percent have at least an 80 percent reduction in seizure frequency; and 5 to 10 percent do not show significant improvement. These results vary according to series. Indications, surgeons, techniques, underlying pathology, and length of follow-up may vary from one center to another, explaining the discrepancies. For results of specific hemispherectomy techniques, the reader should refer to the original articles.[15, 16]

In patients who continue to have seizures, the seizures usually originate from the "good" hemisphere; this outcome may or not have been predicted preoperatively.

SOCIAL EFFECTS

All patients who have preoperative behavioral problems show improvement in behavior if there is improvement in seizure control. This change may be as dramatic as having an institutionalized patient share an apartment postoperatively. Because of their improved sociability, patients integrate better to family life and to groups. The aggressiveness that preoperatively may even make a neurologic examination impossible can change to cooperation and participation by surgery.

INTELLECTUAL EFFECTS

Intellectual performance as documented by preoperative and postoperative psychological testing, improves in the majority of patients in whom seizures are better controlled. At Montreal Neurological Hospital, this has been noted to be on the order of 7 points on the full-scale IQ test. Beardsworth and Adams[29] have documented a continued improvement in intellectual abilities.

SUMMARY

Hemispherectomy for control of epilepsy is among the surgical procedures that have very good and dramatic results.

The improvement obtained through hemispherectomy in the control of pharmacologically refractory seizures is based on patient selection for this surgical procedure. The indications for surgery are developed from the critical evaluation of the patient's seizures, the neurologic examination, and imaging and EEG investigations.

Hemispherectomy techniques have been evolved to decrease the incidence of complications reported with the classic anatomic hemispherectomy, namely superficial cerebral hemosiderosis, while still providing the same benefits in seizure control. These new techniques all have a common denominator: reduction in the volume of the hemispherectomy cavity. This is accomplished at the expense of the creation of a large extradural space (Adams-Oxford modification), through decortication (hemidecortication, Hoffman; hemicorticectomy, Winston), or through a disconnection procedure (functional hemispherectomy), leading to techniques of hemispherotomy (transvertex, Delalande; peri-insular, Villemure).

Independent of the surgical technique utilized, the effect of the operation on seizure control should be identical for the same indication. Generally, 70 to 85 percent of patients undergoing hemispherectomy become seizure free postoperatively, and most of the others will show marked improvement (80 percent reduction in the frequency of seizures). Some patients (5 percent) might continue to have frequent seizures despite a thorough preoperative evaluation to rule out such results.

The choice of hemispherectomy technique should be guided by the simplicity of the operation and the lowest incidence of complications.

REFERENCES

1. Dandy WE: Removal of right cerebral hemisphere for certain tumors with hemiplegia. JAMA 90:823–825, 1928
2. Krynauw RA: Infantile hemiplegia treated by removing one cerebral hemisphere. J Neurol Neurosurg Psychiatry 13:243–267, 1950
3. White HH: Cerebral hemispherectomy in the treatment of infantile hemiplegia: Review of the literature and report of two cases. Confin Neurol 21:1–50, 1961
4. Oppenheimer DR, Griffith HB: Persistent intracranial bleeding as a complication of hemispherectomy. J Neurol Neurosurg Psychiatry 9:229–240, 1966
5. Villemure JG: Hemispherectomy, in Resor SR, Kutt K (eds): The Medical Treatment of Epilepsy. New York, Marcel Dekker, 1992, pp 243–249
6. Gardner WJ: Removal of the right cerebral hemisphere for infiltrating glioma. JAMA 12:154–164, 1933
7. Laine E, Pruvot P, Osson D: Résultats éloignés de l'hémisphérectomie dans les cas d'hématrophie cérébrale infantile génératrice d'épilepsie. Neurochirurgie 10:507–522, 1964
8. French LA, Johnson DR, Brown IA, Van Bergen FB: Cerebral hemispherectomy for control of intractable convulsive seizures. J Neurosurg 12:154–164, 1955
9. Obrador A: About the surgical technique of hemispherectomy in cases of cerebral hemiatrophy. Acta Neurochir 3:57–63, 1952
10. Griffith HB: Cerebral hemispherectomy for infantile hemiplegia in the light of late results. Ann R Coll Surg Engl 41:183–201, 1967
11. Falconer MA, Wilson PJE: Complications related to delayed hemorrhage after hemispherectomy. J Neurosurg 30:413–426, 1969
12. Rasmussen T: Post-operative superficial hemosiderosis of the brain, its diagnosis, treatment and prevention. Am Neurol Assoc 98:133–137, 1973
13. Adams CBT: Hemispherectomy: A modification. J Neurol Neurosurg Psychiatry 46:617–619, 1983
14. George RE, Hoffman HJ, Hwang PA, et al: Management of intractable seizures in unilateral megalencephaly. J Epilepsy 3(Suppl):305–313, 1990
15. Villemure JG, Adams CBT, Hoffman HJ, Peacock WJ: Hemispherectomy, in Engel J (ed): Surgical Treatment of the Epilepsies. New York, Raven Press, 1993, pp 511–518
16. Winston KR, Welch K, Adler JR, Erba G: Cerebral hemicorticectomy for epilepsy. J Neurosurg 77:889–895, 1992
17. Rasmussen T: Hemispherectomy for seizures revisited. Can J Neurol Sci 10:71–78, 1983
18. Rasmussen T, Villemure JG: Cerebral hemispherectomy for seizures with hemiplegia. Cleve Clin J Med 56(Suppl 1):62–68, 1989
19. Villemure JG: Anatomical to functional hemispherectomy from Krynauw to Rasmussen, in Theodore WH (ed): Surgical Treatment of Epilepsy. Amsterdam, Elsevier Science, 1992, pp 209–215
20. Villemure JG, Rasmussen T: Functional hemispherectomy: Methodology. J Epilepsy 3(Suppl):177–182, 1990
21. Villemure JG: Hemispherectomy techniques, in Luders HO (ed): Epilepsy Surgery. New York, Raven Press, 1992, pp 569–578
22. Villemure JG, Mascott C, Andermann F, Rasmussen T: Hemispherectomy and the insula. Epilepsia 30:5(abst), 1989
23. Delalande O, Pinard JM, Basdevant C, et al: Hemispherotomy: A new procedure for central disconnection. Epilepsia 33(Suppl 3):99–100, 1992
24. Villemure JG, Mascott C: Hemispherotomy: The peri-insular approach: Technical Aspects. Epilepsia 34(Suppl 6):48, 1993
25. Mascott C, Villemure JG: Neuroanatomical principles of peri-insular hemispherotomy: A novel variant of functional hemispherectomy for epilepsy. Epilepsia 34(Suppl 6):102–103, 1993
26. Villemure JG: Hemispherectomy: Techniques and complications, in Wyllie E (ed): The Treatment of Epilepsy: Principles and Practice. Philadelphia, Lea & Febiger, 1993, pp 1116–1119
27. Wilson PJE: Cerebral hemispherectomy for infantile hemiplegia. Brain 93:147–180, 1970
28. Cabieses F, Jeni R, Landa R: Fatal brain-stem shift following hemispherectomy. J Neurosurg 14:74–91, 1957
29. Beardsworth ED, Adams CBT: Modified hemispherectomy for epilepsy: Early results in 10 cases. Br J Neurosurg 2:73–84, 1988

CHAPTER 109

Section of the Corpus Callosum for Epilepsy

David W. Roberts

*I*n the 1930s, Van Wagenen, having made the observation that epileptic patients who subsequently sustained a stroke involving the corpus callosum often had improvement in their seizure disorders, divided the corpus callosum in a small number of patients.[1] This was followed in the early 1960s by Bogen's report of a small series of similarly operated patients with encouraging results,[2-4] and Luessenhop's comparable success in three of four children.[5,6] In 1971, Wilson chose this procedure as an alternative to hemispherectomy in a 9-year-old boy with infantile hemiplegia and demonstrated efficacy of the procedure in 20 patients warranting its wider application.[7-13]

The number of centers performing corpus callosotomy has increased dramatically over the past decade, with the majority of epilepsy centers represented at the Second Palm Desert International Conference on the Surgical Treatment of the Epilepsies (Indian Wells, CA, 1992) now offering this operation in their surgical armamentarium. Although numerous questions remain regarding optimal selection criteria and long-term prognosis, most investigators are reporting experiences confirming findings of earlier series.[14-41]

Concurrent with the clinical application of commissurotomy, an extensive body of experimental data has developed. Although the effects of callosotomy in nonprimates had been investigated earlier, Erickson's work remains a landmark for its demonstration of the major role played by the corpus callosum in the propagation of seizures in the monkey.[42] The disruption of seizure generalization by division of the commissure has been demonstrated by numerous investigators,[43-47] and these data have often been cited in support of clinical application. Data suggesting no effect or worsening of seizures following commissurotomy also exists.[36,48-51]

Since Horsley's first craniotomy for the treatment of a seizure disorder in 1886,[52] the most widely performed surgery for medically intractable epilepsy has shared the fundamental principle of removing a portion of resectable cerebral cortex presumed to represent the primary epileptogenic focus. In patients in whom such a focus can be identified, the results of operative intervention are generally rewarding; successful outcome following anterior temporal lobectomy can be achieved in 92 percent of patients selected for that procedure.[53] There is a large population of patients with poorly controlled seizures, however, in whom a resectable epileptic focus cannot be identified and who are not candidates for resection. For many of these patients, corpus callosum section may be of considerable benefit.

PATIENT SELECTION

Optimal selection criteria derive largely from preceding experience, and criteria for callosotomy continue to be defined. In patients in whom a resectable epileptogenic focus can be defined, nearly all centers would agree that a resection is the procedure of choice. The presence of such a definable focus represents perhaps the most important of exclusion criteria. The intuitive basis for proceeding with such a disconnection procedure, on the other hand, has usually rested on the presumption that propagation of the spreading seizure discharge could be disrupted and the seizure thus confined to one hemisphere. Many early patients were selected for surgery because of secondarily generalized seizures in the setting of demonstrable nondiffuse pathology, such as infantile hemiplegia. Early clinical results suggested better outcome in these patients, as well as in those with less severe but nonetheless confined disease.[7,9,11-13]

In addition to seizure disorders with secondary generalization, other generalized seizure types have been demonstrated to respond favorably to commissurotomy. Most notable among these are the atonic or akinetic seizures generally characterized by sudden drop attacks. Many series, including those of Dartmouth,[8,12] Minnesota,[19,20] and Yale,[39] have found either elimination or attenuation of this seizure type in most patients with such spells, and intractability of this seizure type in the setting of no identifiable focus for resection is the most favorable and common indication for commissurotomy. Patients incapacitated by this type of seizure should be seriously considered for callosotomy.

The distinction between truly primary generalized seizures and rapidly generalizing seizures may be exceedingly difficult clinically, and we have not excluded from surgery patients who failed to demonstrate evidence of focal onset. Also, tonic and tonic-clonic generalized seizures have been found to respond to commissurotomy and are common seizure disorders presenting for such surgery. The majority of patients in callosotomy series have presented with multiple seizure types. Surgical results in terms of seizure type have been reported[8,36,39] and are reviewed in the next section.

In an attempt to improve selection criteria, Williamson reviewed surgical outcomes from various series in terms of clinical diagnoses.[54] Classifying patients into groups of infantile hemiplegia, forme-fruste infantile hemiplegia, Rasmussen's syndrome, Lennox-Gastaut syndrome, frontal lobe epilepsy, and focal/multifocal epilepsy, he found slightly better outcomes in the first two groups but sufficient improvement to justify surgical intervention in all categories.[54]

Electroencephalographic (EEG) findings have also been correlated with surgical results. Both Geoffroy and colleagues[22] and Spencer and associates[36] have reported better results in patients with lateralized electroencephalographic abnormalities. Bilaterally synchronous epileptiform activity has been present in the majority of patients and does not represent a necessarily bad prognostic sign. The significance of bilaterally independent foci remains undetermined.

Our selection criteria include (1) medical intractability of at least 2 and usually 4 years' duration, with exhaustive anticonvulsant regimens and documented adequate serum anticonvulsant levels; (2) generalized seizures, usually but not necessarily major motor or akinetic in type; and (3) potential functional benefit if improvement in the seizure disorder is achieved. Although the likelihood of success may be lower in certain instances, we have not automatically excluded patients from surgery because of retardation, age, mixed hemisphere dominance, lack of demonstrable focal seizure onset, or bilaterally independent EEG abnormalities.

There is less consensus regarding the indications for proceeding to completion of the callosal section in those patients who have already undergone anterior section. The majority of clinical experiences with callosotomy demonstrate superior outcome with respect to seizure control in those patients who have had complete section compared with those who have had partial resection. The success rate of complete section in achieving a significant reduction in seizure frequency has been approximately twice that of partial section in several larger series.[41, 55] The question of proceeding to completion of the callosal section is a slightly different one, however, and analysis of the incremental benefit derived in patients who go on to completion is required. Review of the experiences at both Dartmouth[55] and Yale[39] demonstrates a very clear benefit in proceeding to completion in those patients with persistent generalized seizures whose response to partial section has been disappointing (discussed further in the section on results); there has been one report in which completion of the section was not associated with such benefit.[17]

SURGICAL TECHNIQUE

Review of the early commissurotomy series shows comparable success rates regardless of whether or not division of the anterior commissure or one fornix was performed at the time of corpus callosotomy.[9–13] Although there are probably individuals in whom these other structures play important roles in seizure propagation, we have restricted our procedure to division of the major commissure and underlying posterior hippocampal commissure only. Whether or not partial callosotomy is preferable to complete division as an initial procedure is less clear. At present, we are advocating partial callosotomy in most patients, with division of two-thirds to three-quarters of the corpus callosum unless there is evidence of a predominantly posterior focus. Many of these patients subsequently require completion of the callosotomy (see later), but it appears preferable to spare those not requiring complete section the effects of more extensive disconnection.

The surgery is performed with the patient under general anesthesia, and intraoperative electroencephalographic recording, when performed, has been primarily for investigative purposes. At least one surgeon has tailored his length of resection based on intraoperative EEG information,[24] but given the frequently insufficient EEG findings intraoperatively as well as the observation of subsequent seizure propagation across remaining adjacent callosal fibers, we have not adopted this practice. The patient is placed supine on the operating table, and the unturned head is secured in a Gardner head clamp. For the anterior division, the neck is left in neutral position; for the posterior division, it is flexed approximately 20 degrees. Decadron (10 mg) is administered the night before surgery and in the induction room.

We have used linear incisions and 2-inch trephinations (Figs. 109–1 and 109–2),[11, 56, 57] but the type of craniotomy is recognized as relatively unimportant. For the anterior procedure, a 9-cm transverse incision with one-third of its length across the midline is placed 2 cm in front of the coronal suture. For the posterior procedure, a similar incision and trephination is employed at the level of the parietal eminence. The placement of the craniotomy across the sagittal sinus requires increased caution but facilitates later exposure down the interhemispheric fissure. The approach is generally on the side of the nondominant right hemisphere except for those instances in which significant pathology is well lateralized to the other hemisphere.

Angiography for localization of parasagittal draining veins prior to transcallosal procedures has been advocated by some[58] but has not been a routine study in our series. Using microsurgical technique, it has always been possible to work on either or both sides of such a vein without requiring its sacrifice. Nonetheless, it is interesting and useful to note Apuzzo's observation that in 42 of 100 angiographic studies, significant veins were noted to enter the sagittal sinus within 2 cm of the coronal suture, with 70 percent of these veins posterior to that suture.[58] Angiographic information may be available in those patients who have previously undergone amytal testing, and magnetic resonance imaging (MRI) often delineates parasagittal venous structures.

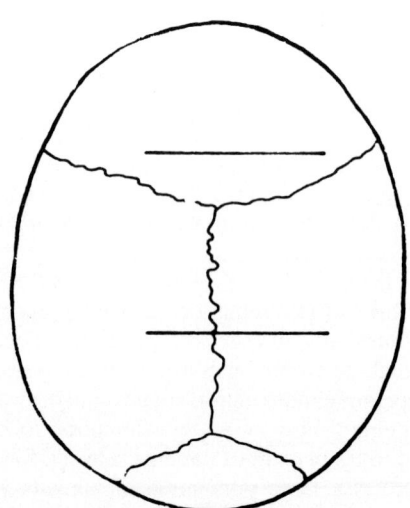

FIGURE 109–1. Anterior and posterior callosal sections are performed through respective 9-cm linear incisions and 2-inch trephinations. (From Roberts DW: Corpus callosotomy, in Reeves AG [ed]: Epilepsy and the Corpus Callosum. New York, Plenum Press, 1985, p 261.)

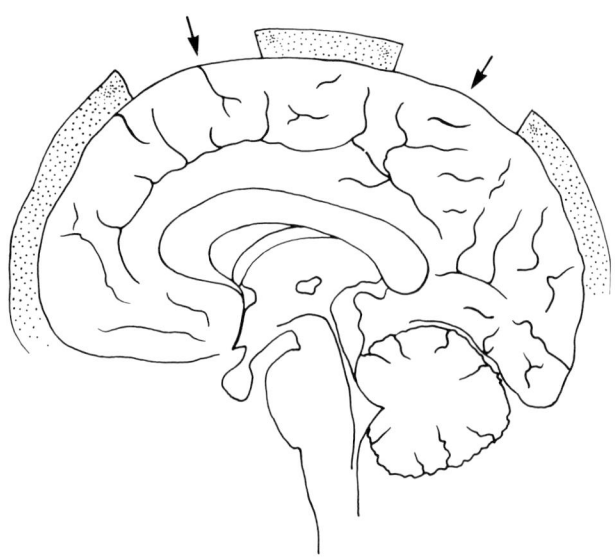

FIGURE 109–2. The anterior and posterior approaches provide direct and convenient access to the respective halves of the callosum. (From Roberts DW: Corpus callosotomy, in Reeves AG [ed]: Epilepsy and the Corpus Callosum. New York, Plenum Press, 1985, p 264.)

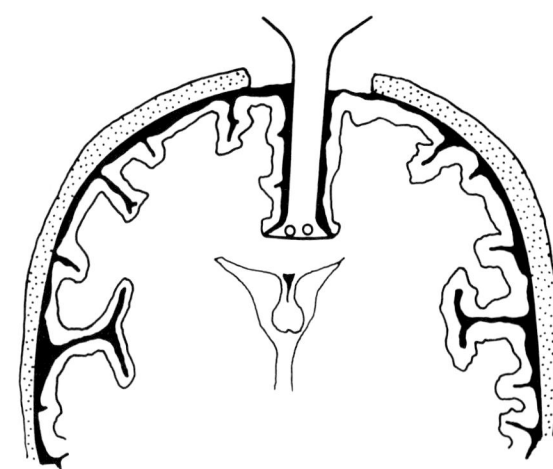

FIGURE 109–3. Minimal retraction is required on the nondominant hemisphere, if at all. Retraction of the inferior aspect of the falx and the contralateral cingulate gyrus is occasionally useful. (From Roberts DW: Corpus callosotomy, in Reeves AG [ed]: Epilepsy and the Corpus Callosum. New York, Plenum Press, 1985, p 262.)

The dura is opened in a curvilinear fashion and reflected on the sagittal sinus. Initial dissection down the interhemispheric fissure is performed under loupe magnification, and retraction is aided by the administration of mannitol (1 g/kg) during the opening. Pressed Gelfoam protects the exposed cortex, and the Greenberg self-retaining retractor is placed prior to employment of the operating microscope. A single retractor blade gently retracts the ipsilateral hemisphere, and when needed, an additional blade is used on the inferior aspect of the falx or contralateral cingulate gyrus (Fig. 109–3).

The glistening white appearance of the corpus callosum distinguishes it from the more superficial cingulate gyrus, and exposure along the length of callosum to be divided is obtained prior to entering the commissure. Adhesions between the hemispheres, especially common in the setting of previous infection or trauma, may make exposure difficult; approaching the callosum more posteriorly and using the deeper extension of the falx proves helpful in this situation. The pericallosal arteries are easily identified overlying the callosum. The actual division of callosal fibers is carried out most often between these arteries, although division lateral to these vessels, when more convenient, can be performed (Fig. 109–4).

The magnification and illumination provided by the operating microscope are invaluable during the final exposure and actual sectioning. We use the Zeiss OPMI 1H microscope on a Contraves stand. The 300-mm objective lens provides a reasonable working distance to the field; 12.5 × oculars and settings on the magnification changer of 0.4 to 1.6 are most commonly used. Small vessels supplying only the callosum itself may be coagulated using bipolar cautery. The actual division of callosal fibers is carried out using the microseptal or microsuction tip. As ultrasonic aspiration equipment becomes more refined and smaller, it may prove to be of greater utility in this step.

Early descriptions of callosal section describe the bluish appearance of the underlying ventricular ependymal surface and recommend this landmark as the limit of division.[10, 11] Over the course of our series, the advantages of identifying the midline during the division have become increasingly evident and include unequivocal assurance of completeness of fiber division, elimination of possible lateral deviation (especially in the frontal region), decreased likelihood of entering the lateral ventricle, and less operative time. A gentle sweeping from side to side of a blunt microinstrument as the callosum is nearly traversed often exposes the midline cleft between lateral ventricles (Figs. 109–5 to 109–7). Once this cleft has been identified, the remainder of the section follows easily.

The direction of actual section is not particularly important, but identification of the midline during the anterior division is easiest at the posteriormost portion of the genu or the anterior portion of the body. Subsequent division around the genu and down the rostrum is performed extraventricularly as far as possible. At this point, the rostrum is nearly

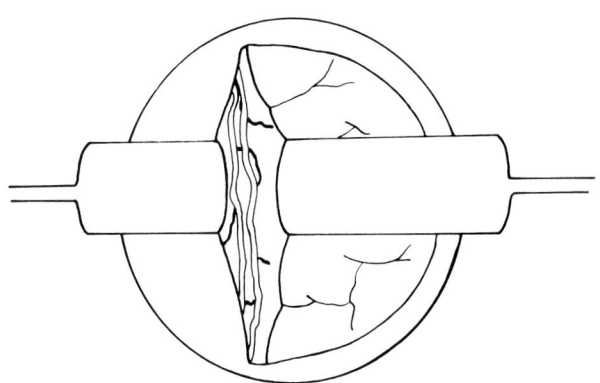

FIGURE 109–4. The pericallosal arteries are identified overlying the callosum, and the section is most often performed between them, although section lateral to these arteries may sometimes prove more convenient during part of the section. (From Roberts DW: Corpus callosotomy, in Reeves AG [ed]: Epilepsy and the Corpus Callosum. New York, Plenum Press, 1985, p 262.)

paper thin and any remaining fibers are insignificant. No attempt is made to divide the anterior commissure blindly.

Attention is now directed to the posterior extent of the division. If an attempt is being made to achieve success with a partial division, it is reasonable to carry the division through the anterior two-thirds. When the section and hemostasis is complete, a metal clip attached to a small piece of Gelfoam is placed at the posterior extent of the divided callosum. At subsequent surgery, gliosis may obscure the extent of previous resection, and such a marker has often been greatly appreciated. It has not created undesirable MRI artifacts.

Division of the posterior corpus callosum is performed in a similar fashion. As previously mentioned, the more extensive falx cerebri often aids the more posterior exposure. The fibers of the splenium are divided with similar instrumentation, and under magnification, the completeness of the section is certain. The underlying arachnoid, beneath which lie the pineal and quadrigeminal cistern, is preserved. The posterior hippocampal commissure may be indistinguishable from the adjacent callosal fibers, but this is of no practical significance because it is divided as well. If the posterior section is the initial commissurotomy procedure, a clip is left as a marker at the anteriormost extent of the section. If an anterior section has been already been performed, the previously placed clip is retrieved.

After confirmation of hemostasis, the dura is closed over Gelfilm using 4-0 Vicryl. The bone plug is secured through predrilled holes with 2-0 Ethilon, the galea aponeurosis is reapproximated using 2-0 Vicryl, and the skin is closed with either 4-0 Prolene or staples. The patient is observed in the neurosurgical observation unit overnight and is usually transferred to the neurosurgical ward the following morning. Mobilization begins immediately, and the patient is typically discharged within a week of surgery. Anticonvulsant medication generally is not altered until at least subsequent follow-up. A decision regarding completion of the callosotomy is made a minimum of 2 months after the first procedure.

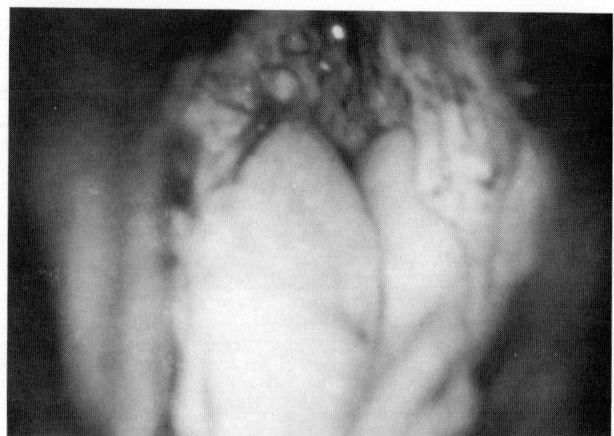

FIGURE 109–6. Intraoperative exposure of the divided genu. The ependymal surfaces of the frontal horns, the cut surfaces of the callosum, and the midline cleft are visualized (see Figure 109–5).

RESULTS

Reporting on a total of 20 patients, Wilson noted that 16 had a greater than 50-percent reduction in overall seizure frequency.[12, 13] Van Wagenen and Herren[1] reported significant improvement in nine of 10 patients, and Geoffroy[22] reported similar success in six of nine patients. Rayport[30] reported seven of nine patients significantly improved, Luessenhop[5, 6] three of four, Amacher[14] four of four, and Bouvier[16] six of six. An analysis of outcome in 183 patients from 14 centers[59] found that 5.5 percent were free of seizures, 73.5 percent improved, and 20.7 percent unimproved; the range for unimprovement was 10 to 38 percent; a follow-up survey in 1991 included 563 patients, of whom 7.6 percent were reported to be seizure free and 60.9 percent improved.[53] Although these figures are not as good as those for temporal lobectomy or extratemporal cortical resection, the patient populations are distinct, with nearly all who underwent division of the corpus callosum having failed to fulfill the selection criteria for other surgery.

The great majority of patients undergoing callosal surgery for seizure control have had multiple seizure types, and it is useful to analyze outcome in terms of seizure classification.

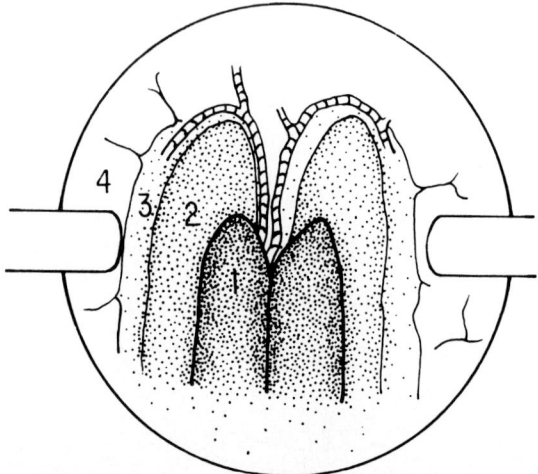

FIGURE 109–5. Division of the callosum at the level of the genu. (1) Ependymal surfaces of the frontal horns of the lateral ventricles, (2) cut surface of the genu, (3) dorsal aspect of the genu, and (4) cingulate gyrus. The anterior cerebral arteries are visualized. (From Roberts DW: Corpus callosotomy, in Reeves AG [ed]: Epilepsy and the Corpus Callosum. New York, Plenum Press, 1985, p 263.)

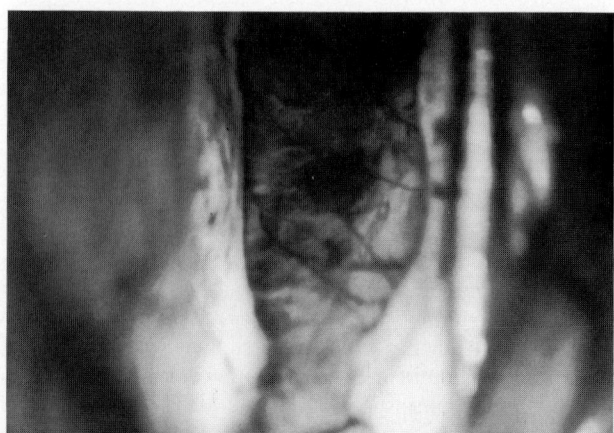

FIGURE 109–7. Intraoperative exposure of the divided splenium. The cut surfaces of the callosum and the underlying arachnoid are evident.

Table 109–1. Response of Major Seizures to Commissurotomy in the 32 of 51 Patients Who Experienced These Seizures Preoperatively

Seizure Response	Number of Patients
No seizures	14
More than 80 percent reduction in frequency	7
50 to 80 percent reduction in frequency	3
Less than 50 percent reduction in frequency	2
No reduction in frequency	6

Table 109–3. Response of Atonic Seizures to Commissurotomy in the 21 of 51 Patients Who Experienced These Seizures Preoperatively

Seizure Response	Number of Patients
No seizures	9
More than 80 percent reduction in frequency	7
50 to 80 percent reduction in frequency	2
Less than 50 percent reduction in frequency	0
No reduction in frequency	3

Tables 109–1 to 109–5 summarize outcome in the Dartmouth series of 51 patients who could be evaluated with a mean follow-up of 53.7 months and a range of 2 to 169 months.

Thirty-two of 51 patients had major motor seizures before surgery, and of these, seizures were eliminated in 14. An additional seven patients have had a reduction of greater than 80 percent in the frequency of their seizures, and three had a 50- to 80-percent reduction. Two patients have had less than 50 percent improvement; six have had no improvement in frequency, although in two patients, the seizures are less severe.

Twenty-one of 51 patients had atonic seizures, generally characterized by sudden falls to the ground. In nine patients, these seizures have been eliminated and in another seven patients, a reduction of greater than 80 percent has been achieved. Although frequency has been less successfully affected in the remaining five patients, the actual seizure has been modified in four patients from a fall to head nod or other less injurious manifestation.

Absence spells were present in 22 of 51 patients, and although the procedure was not performed for this particular seizure type, 15 patients have had elimination or greater than 80 percent reduction in frequency of these spells.

The results in focal motor epilepsy, which might be presumed to remain unaffected by a procedure thought to be effective by disruption of propagation, are indeed less successful but nevertheless interesting in this subgroup of 14 patients. Three patients demonstrated no further focal seizure activity, and an additional two patients had better than 80 percent reduction. Two patients of this group had an increase in frequency for this seizure type, and 12 patients who had not experienced focal motor seizures developed them following surgery. A worsening of this seizure type following callosotomy has been described,[38] and the possibility of the procedure resulting in a loss of an inhibitory influence has been suggested.[36, 38, 51] Our data confirm the occurrence of increased or new-onset focal seizures, but they have nearly always occurred as the attenuated remnant of previously generalizing seizure activity. In no instance, has this represented a deterioration in overall functional outcome.

Corpus callosotomy has not been advocated as a substitute for temporal lobectomy in patients eligible for that procedure, but the results with regard to complex partial seizures in 25 of 51 patients are noteworthy.[60] Eleven of 25 have had elimination of this seizure type and another three patients have had greater than 80 percent reduction in their frequency. In nine patients, the severity of the seizures has been significantly modified. The role of this procedure in patients with only complex partial seizures but in whom investigations fail to define a resectable focus remains undefined.

In a recent report of their own experience, Spencer and colleagues note comparable success rates with atonic, tonic-clonic, and myoclonic seizures.[39] In compiling reports on 330 patients from a number of institutions, they also note success rates (cure or marked improvement) for atonic seizures of 71 percent with anterior section and 74 percent with total section, for tonic-clonic seizures of 56 and 75 percent, respectively, for tonic seizures of 47 and 75 percent, and for absence seizures of 33 and 64 percent.[39]

Incremental response to completion of the callosal section in those patients whose response to anterior section has been disappointing has been noted by both the Dartmouth[55] and Yale[39] groups. Of 27 patients who had undergone anterior callosal section at our institution but continued to experience generalized seizures at a greater than desired frequency and therefore underwent completion of their section, notable improvement was found for major motor, atonic, and complex partial seizures (Table 109–6). For all seizures together, the percentage of patients obtaining an 80- to 100-percent reduction in generalized seizures improved from 29 percent following anterior section to 62 percent following completion of callosal section.[55]

Surgical complications early in this series included hydrocephalus in three, and this problem subsequently has not been encountered; the present surgical technique of remaining extraventricular may be responsible. Wound or bone flap

Table 109–2. Response of Focal Motor Seizures to Commissurotomy in the 14 of 51 Patients Who Experienced These Seizures Preoperatively

Seizure Response	Number of Patients
No seizures	3
More than 80 percent reduction in frequency	2
50 to 80 percent reduction in frequency	1
Less than 50 percent reduction in frequency	0
No reduction in frequency	6
Increased frequency	2

Table 109–4. Response of Absence Seizures to Commissurotomy in the 22 of 51 Patients Who Experienced These Seizures Preoperatively

Seizure Response	Number of Patients
No seizures	11
More than 80 percent reduction in frequency	4
50 to 80 percent reduction in frequency	3
Less than 50 percent reduction in frequency	2
No reduction in frequency	2

Table 109-5. Response of Complex Partial Seizures to Commissurotomy in the 25 of 51 Patients Who Experienced These Seizures Preoperatively

Seizure Response	Number of Patients
No seizures	10
More than 80 percent reduction in frequency	3
50 to 80 percent reduction in frequency	7
Less than 50 percent reduction in frequency	0
No reduction in frequency	5

Table 109-6. Incremental Response to Completion of Corpus Callosum Section in 27 Patients with Suboptimal Response to Anterior Callosotomy

Type of Seizure (Number of Patients with Seizure Type)	Number of Patients with at Least 80 Percent Reduction in Seizure Frequency After Anterior Section	Number of Patients with at Least 80 Percent Reduction in Seizure Frequency After Completion of Section
Major motor (21)	6	13
Atonic (16)	6	13
Focal motor (7)	1	1
Complex partial (8)	6	8

From Roberts DW, Reeves AG, Nordgren RE: The role of posterior callosotomy in patients with suboptimal response to anterior callosotomy, in Reeves AG, Roberts DW (eds): Epilepsy and Corpus Callosum, 2nd ed. New York, Plenum Press (in press).

infections occurred in three patients. Sterile meningitis was noted in three patients, and septic meningitis was documented in one patient. One patient in whom surgery and the early postoperative course had been unremarkable died from a frontal lobe infarction 12 days following surgery. A second patient died of a cardiopulmonary arrest following the development of status epilepticus, pneumonia, thrombophlebitis, and possible pulmonary embolus 3 months after surgery. The marked reduction in complication rate in the subsequent 50 patients who have undergone callosal section illustrates the learning curve and improved technique familiar to all centers.

The behavioral and neuropsychological effects of commissurotomy have been studied extensively,[61-84] the most enlightening work in this regard being that of Gazzaniga and his colleagues.[69-76, 83] The initial impression following the earliest series had been that callosotomy produced little alteration in cognitive function.[61, 62] Subsequent and more sophisticated investigations have demonstrated numerous effects of disconnection,[69, 75] but in general, it has been unusual for these effects to represent significant handicaps.

With division of the anterior corpus callosum, decreased spontaneity of speech (ranging from subtle slowing to complete mutism) and decreased use of the nondominant hand and leg (often described as either a paresis or an apraxia) are sometimes seen and usually resolve over several days. There remains discussion as to the relative contribution of surgical retraction versus acute disconnection to these changes. The great majority of patients exhibit no long-standing effects from anterior section, although exacerbation of previous lateralized deficits has been reported.[68]

Posterior callosal section, in contrast, produces a now well-recognized disconnection syndrome characterized by interhemispheric sensory dissociation. This syndrome can be demonstrated with somatosensory, auditory, and visual stimuli, with the language-dominant hemisphere not having direct access to information presented to the other hemisphere. With incomplete section, the language-dominant hemisphere may still gain access to contralateral hemisphere information, and the dissociation may not be demonstrable. With complete section, the sensory dissociation is complete and permanent.

The majority of patients in the Dartmouth series appear to have improved or remained unchanged in their level of cognitive function. This factor has usually been the result of both diminished seizure activity and decreased anticonvulsant medication. Ferrell and associates reported on formal neuropsychological testing in eight of the earliest patients and found improvement in six. The families of five patients have reported decreased cognitive ability—usually described as poorer memory or concentration—and this factor has been noted in other series as well.[66, 81] Further investigation of this finding has suggested that it may be more of an attention disorder than actual memory dysfunction,[82] although more recent investigations have documented deficits in recall as well.[83]

Speech and motor dysfunction have been frequently noted in the immediate postoperative period, but persistence of these deficits has been infrequent.[13, 36, 84] Antagonism between the right and left hemispheres, usually manifested as opposing actions of the right and left hands, has been similarly reported.[66] In only one patient of our series has this been a chronic difficulty.

SUMMARY

Although the answers to important questions regarding corpus callosotomy for intractable epilepsy continue to evolve, the experience accumulated over more than 50 years allows a number of important points to be made. Perhaps most important is the recognition that for certain patients who have failed medical management and who are not eligible for other seizure surgery commissurotomy may successfully reduce seizure frequency and severity. Atonic seizures and secondarily generalized major motor seizures are the most likely conditions to improve, but other seizure types may also respond.

Extraventricular division of the corpus callosum alone achieves the aforementioned success; complete callosotomy may not be required in all patients, and staging of the procedure remains a reasonable approach. As a microsurgical procedure, division of the corpus callosum can be safely and confidently performed.

Behavioral and neuropsychological sequelae of commissurotomy are well-recognized but uncommonly permanent disabilities. In the great majority of patients, the benefits resulting from the procedure outweigh any such adverse effects.

REFERENCES

1. Van Wagenen WP, Herren RY: Surgical division of the commissural pathways in the corpus callosum: Relation to spread of an epileptic attack. Arch Neurol Psych 44:740–759, 1940

2. Bogen JE, Fisher ED, Vogel PJ: Cerebral commissurotomy: A second case report. JAMA 194:1328–1329, 1965
3. Bogen JE, Sperry RW, Vogel PJ: Addendum: Commissural section and propagation of seizures, in Jasper HH, Ward Jr AA, Pope A (eds): Basic mechanisms of the epilepsies. Boston, Little, Brown & Company, 1969, p 439
4. Bogen JE, Vogel PJ: Cerebral commissurotomy in man: Preliminary case report. Bull Los Angeles Neurol Soc 27:169–172, 1962
5. Luessenhop AJ: Interhemispheric commissurotomy: (the split brain operation) as an alternative to hemispherectomy for control of intractable seizures. Am Surg 36:265–268, 1970
6. Luessenhop AJ, dela Cruz TC, Fenichel GM: Surgical disconnection of the cerebral hemispheres for intractable seizures. JAMA 213:1630–1636, 1970
7. Harbaugh RE, Wilson DH, Reeves AG, et al: Forebrain commissurotomy for epilepsy: Review of 20 consecutive cases. Acta Neurochir 68:263–275, 1983
8. Reeves AG, O'Leary PM: Total corpus callosotomy for control of medically intractable epilepsy, in Reeves AG (ed): Epilepsy and the Corpus Callosum. New York, Plenum Press, 1985, pp 269–280
9. Wilson DH, Culver C, Waddington M, et al: Disconnection of the cerebral hemispheres: An alternative to hemispherectomy for the control of intractable seizures. Neurology 25:1149–1153, 1975
10. Wilson DH, Reeves A, Gazzaniga M. Division of the corpus callosum for uncontrollable epilepsy. Neurology 28:649–653, 1978
11. Wilson DH, Reeves A, Gazzaniga M: Corpus callosotomy for control of intractable seizures, in Wada JA, Penry JK (eds): Advances in Epileptology: The Xth Epilepsy International Symposium. New York, Raven Press, 1980, pp 205–213
12. Wilson DH, Reeves AG, Gazzaniga MS: ''Central'' commissurotomy for intractable generalized epilepsy: Series two. Neurology 32:687–697, 1982
13. Wilson DH, Reeves AG, Gazzaniga MS, et al: Cerebral commissurotomy for control of intractable seizures. Neurology 27:708–715, 1977
14. Amacher AL: Midline commissurotomy for the treatment of some cases of intractable epilepsy. Childs Brain 2:54–58, 1970
15. Avila JO, Radvany J, Huck FR, et al: Anterior callosotomy as a substitute for hemispherectomy. Acta Neurochir 30(Suppl):137–143, 1980
16. Bouvier G, Mercier C, St Hilaire JM, et al: Anterior callosotomy and chronic depth electrode recording in the surgical management of some intractable seizures. Appl Neurophysiol 46:52–56, 1983
17. Fuiks KS, Wyler AR, Hermann BP, et al: Seizure outcome from anterior and complete corpus callosotomy. J Neurosurg 74:573–578, 1991
18. Garcia-Flores E: Corpus callosum section for patients with intractable epilepsy. Appl Neurophysiol 50:390–397, 1987
19. Gates JR, Leppik IE, Yap J, et al: Corpus callosotomy: clinical and electroencephalographic effects. Epilepsia 25:308–316, 1984
20. Gates JR, Maxwell R, Leppik IE, et al: Electroencephalographic and clinical effects of total corpus callosotomy, in Reeves AG (ed): Epilepsy and the Corpus Callosum. New York, Plenum Press, 1985, pp 315–328
21. Gates JR, Rosenfeld WE, Maxwell RE, et al: Response of multiple seizure types to corpus callosum section. Epilepsia 28:28–34, 1987
22. Geoffroy G, Lassonde M, Delisle F, et al: Corpus callosotomy for control of intractable epilepsy in children. Neurology 33:891–897, 1983
23. Huck FR, Radvany J, Avila JO, et al: Anterior callosotomy in epileptics with multiform seizures and bilateral synchronous spike and wave EEG pattern. Acta Neurochir 30(Suppl):127–135, 1980
24. Marino R Jr, Ragazzo PC: Selective criteria and results of selective partial callosotomy, in Reeves AG (ed): Epilepsy and the Corpus Callosum. New York, Plenum Press, 1985, pp 281–301
25. Murro AM, Flanigin HF, Gallagher BB, et al: Corpus callosotomy for the treatment of intractable epilepsy. Epilepsy Res 2:44–50, 1988
26. Nordgren RE, Reeves AG, Viguera AC, et al: Corpus callosotomy for intractable seizures in the pediatric age group. Arch Neurol 48:364–372, 1991
27. Oguni H, Olivier A, Andermann F, Comair J: Anterior callosotomy in the treatment of intractable epilepsies: A study of 43 patients with a mean follow-up of 39 months. Ann Neurol 30:357–364, 1991
28. Purves SJ, Wada JA, Woodhurst WB, et al: Results of anterior corpus callosum section in 24 patients with medically intractable seizures. Neurology 38:1194–1201, 1988
29. Rappaport ZH, Lerman P: Corpus callosotomy in the treatment of secondary generalizing intractable epilepsy. Acta Neurochir 94:10–14, 1988
30. Rayport M, Corrie WS, Ferguson SM: Corpus callosum section for control of clinically and electroencephalographically classified seizures, in Reeves AG (ed): Epilepsy and the Corpus Callosum. New York, Plenum Press, 1985, pp 329–337
31. Rayport M, Ferguson SM, Corrie WS: Outcomes and indications of corpus callosum section for intractable seizure control. Appl Neurophysiol 46:47–51, 1983
32. Sainte-Hilaire JM, Giard N, Bouvier G, et al: Anterior callosotomy in frontal lobe epilepsies, in Reeves AG (ed): Epilepsy and the Corpus Callosum. New York, Plenum Press, 1985, pp 303–314
33. Spencer DD, Spencer SS: Corpus callosotomy in the treatment of medically intractable secondarily generalized seizures of children. Clev Clin J Med 56(Suppl 1):S69–S77, 1988
34. Spencer SS: Corpus callosum section and other disconnection procedures for medically intractable epilepsy. Epilepsia 29(Suppl 2):S85–S99, 1988
35. Spencer SS, Elquera ED, Williamson PD, et al: Evolution of seizure types after callosotomy. J Epilepsy 4:149–156, 1992
36. Spencer SS, Gates JR, Reeves AG, et al: Corpus callosum section for uncontrolled epilepsy, in Engel J (ed): Surgical Treatment of Epilepsy. New York, Raven Press, 1987, pp 425–444
37. Spencer SS, Katz A, Ebersole J, et al: Ictal EEG changes with corpus callosum section. Epilepsia 34:568–573, 1993
38. Spencer SS, Spencer DD, Glaser GH, et al: More intense focal seizure types after callosal section: The role of inhibition. Ann Neurol 16:686–693, 1984
39. Spencer SS, Spencer DD, Sass K, et al: Anterior, total, and two-stage corpus callosum section: Differential and incremental seizure responses. Epilepsia 34:561–567, 1993
40. Spencer SS, Spencer DD, Williamson PD, et al: Effect of corpus callosum section on secondary bilaterally synchronous interictal EEG discharges. Neurology 35:1689–1694, 1985
41. Spencer SS, Spencer DD, Williamson PD, et al: Corpus callosotomy for epilepsy. I. Seizure effects. Neurology 38:19–24, 1988
42. Erickson TE: Spread of the epileptic discharge: An experimental study of the afterdischarge induced by electrical stimulation of the cerebral cortex. Arch Neurol Psychiat 43:429–452, 1940
43. Marcus EM, Watson CW: Bilateral synchronous spike wave electrographic patterns in the cat. Arch Neurol 14:601–610, 1966
44. Marcus EM, Watson CW: Symmetrical epileptogenic foci in monkey cerebral cortex: Mechanisms of interaction and regional variations in capacity for synchronous discharges. Arch Neurol 19:99–116, 1968
45. Kopeloff N, Kennard MA, Pacella BL, et al: Section of the corpus callosum in experimental epilepsy in the monkey. Arch Neurol Psychiat 63:719–727, 1950
46. Crowell RM, Ajmone Marsan C: Topographical distribution and patterns of unit activity during electrically induced after-discharge. Electroenchaphalogr Clin Neurophysiol 31(Suppl):59–73, 1972
47. Mutani R, Bergamini L, Fariello R, et al: Bilateral synchrony of epileptic discharge associated with chronic asymmetrical cortical foci. Electroencephalogr Clin Neurophysiol 34:53–59, 1973
48. Stavraky GW: Supersensitivity following lesions of the nervous system. Toronto, University of Toronto Press, 1961, pp 33–38
49. Kusske JA, Rush JL: Corpus callosum and propagation of afterdischarge to contralateral cortex and thalamus. Neurology 28:905–912, 1978
50. Reeves AG, ed: Epilepsy and the corpus callosum. New York, Plenum Press, 1985
51. Blume WT: Corpus callosum section for seizure control: Rationale and review of experimental and clinical data. Cleve Clin Q 51:319–332, 1984
52. Horsley V. Brain surgery. Br Med J 2:670–675, 1886
53. Engel Jr J, Van Ness PC, Rasmussen TB, et al: Outcome with respect to epileptic seizures, in Engel Jr J (ed): Surgical Treatment of the Epilepsies, 2nd ed. New York, Raven Press, 1993, pp 609–621
54. Williamson, PD: Corpus callosum section for intractable epilepsy: Criteria for patient selection, in Reeves AG (ed): Epilepsy and the Corpus Callosum. New York, Plenum Press, 1985, pp 243–257
55. Roberts DW, Reeves AG, Nordgren RE: The role of posterior callosotomy in patients with suboptimal response to anterior callosotomy, in Reeves AG, Roberts DW (eds): Epilepsy and the Corpus Callosum, 2nd ed. New York, Plenum Press (in press)
56. Roberts DW: Corpus callosotomy: Surgical technique, in Reeves AG (ed): Epilepsy and the Corpus Callosum. New York, Plenum Press, 1985, pp 259–267
57. Roberts DW, Rayport M, Maxwell RE, et al: Corpus callosotomy, in Engel Jr J (ed): Surgical treatment of the epilepsies, 2nd ed. New York, Raven Press, 1993, pp 519–526

58. Apuzzo MLJ, Chikovani OK, Gott PS: Transcallosal, interfornicial approaches for lesions affecting the third ventricle: Surgical considerations and consequences. Neurosurgery 10:547–554, 1982
59. Engel J Jr: Outcome with respect to epileptic seizures, in Engel J Jr (ed): Surgical Treatment of the Epilepsies. New York, Raven Press, 1987, pp 553–571
60. Roberts DW, Reeves AG: Effect of commissurotomy on complex partial epilepsy in patients without a resectable seizure focus. Appl Neurophysiol 50:398–400, 1987
61. Akelaitis AJ: Studies on corpus callosum: Higher visual function in each hemisphere's field following complete section of the corpus callosum. Arch Neurol Psychiat 45:786–796, 1941
62. Akelaitis AJ: A study of gnosis, praxis and language following section of the corpus callosum and anterior commissure. J Neurosurg 1:94–102, 1944
63. Gordon HW, Bogen JE, Sperry RW: Absence of deconnection syndrome in two patients with partial section of the neocommissures. Brain 94:327–336, 1971
64. Campbell Jr AL, Bogen JE, Smith A. Disorganization and reorganization of cognitive and sensorimotor functions in cerebral commissurotomy: Compensatory roles of the forebrain commissures and cerebral hemispheres in man. Brain 104:493–511, 1981
65. Oepen G, Schulz-Weiling R, Zimmermann P, et al: Long-term effects of partial callosal lesions: Preliminary report. Acta Neurochir 77:22, 1985
66. Ferguson SM, Rayport M, Corrie WS: Neuropsychiatric observations on behavioral consequences of corpus callosum section for seizure control, in Reeves AG (ed): Epilepsy and corpus callosum. New York, Plenum Press, 1985, pp 501–514
67. Lassonde M, Sauerwein H, Geoffroy G, et al: Effects of early and late transection of the corpus callosum in children. Brain 109:953–967, 1986
68. Sass KJ, Spencer DD, Spencer SS, et al: Corpus callosotomy for epilepsy. II: Neurologic and neuropsychological outcome. Neurology 38:24–28, 1988
69. Gazzaniga MS: The Bisected Brain. New York, Appleton-Century-Crofts, 1970
70. Gazzaniga MS, Risse GL, Springer SP, et al: Psychologic and neurologic consequences of partial and complete cerebral commissurotomy. Neurology 25:10, 1975
71. Ledoux JE, Risse GL, Springer SP, et al: Cognition and commissurotomy. Brain 100:87–104, 1977
72. Sidtis JJ, Volpe BT, Holtzman JD, et al: Cognitive interaction after staged callosal section; evidence for transfer of semantic activation. Science 212:344–346, 1981
73. Volpe BT, Sidtis JJ, Holzman JD: Cortical mechanisms involved in praxis: observations following partial and complete section of the corpus callosum in man. Neurology 32:645–650, 1982
74. Gazzaniga MS, Smylie CS: Dissociation of language and cognition: A psychological profile of two disconnected right hemispheres. Brain 107:145–153, 1984
75. Gazzaniga MS: Some contributions of the split-brain studies to the study of human cognition, in Reeves AG (ed): Epilepsy and the corpus callosum. New York, Plenum Press, 1985, pp 341–348
76. Gazzaniga MS: Perceptual and attentional processes following callosal section in humans. Neuropsychologia 25:119–133, 1987
77. Clark CR, Geffen GM: Corpus callosum surgery and recent memory. Brain 112:165–75, 1989
78. Sergent J. Furtive incursions into bicameral minds. Brain 113:537–568, 1990
79. Sergent J. Processing of spatial relations within and between the disconnected cerebral hemispheres. Brain, 114:1025–1043, 1991
80. Ferrell RB, Culver CM, Tucker GJ: Psychosocial and cognitive function after commissurotomy for intractable seizures. J Neurosurg 58:374–380, 1984
81. Zaidel E, Sperry RW: Memory impairment after commissurotomy in man. Brain 97:263–272, 1974
82. Beniak TE, Gates JR, Risse GL: Comparison of selected neuropsychological test variables pre- and postoperatively on patients subjected to corpus callosotomy. Epilepsia 26:534, 1985
83. Phelps EA, Hirst W, Gazzaniga MS: Deficits in recall following partial and complete callosum section involving the hippocampal commissure, in Reeves AG, Roberts DW (eds): Epilepsy and the Corpus Callosum. New York, Plenum Press (in press)
84. Ross MK, Reeves AG, Roberts DW: Post-commissurotomy mutism. Ann Neurol 16:11 1984

SECTION XVI

CNS Transplantation

CHAPTER 110

Transplantation in the Human Nervous System

Roy A. E. Bakay
Robert E. Breeze
Curt R. Freed

PARKINSON'S DISEASE

Central nervous system (CNS) transplantation holds tremendous potential for repair and restoration of function for the brain and spinal cord. Animal studies have clearly shown the potential for endocrinologic and neurologic functional return in both genetic and lesion-induced models of numerous neurologic diseases.[1-4] One of the most remarkably successful grafting techniques has been dopaminergic replacement in models of Parkinson's disease that use rodents[5-7] or monkeys.[8-14] Many different types of tissue are available for grafting into the CNS, and the list is expanding (Fig. 110–1).

The application of grafts into the human CNS for the treatment of Parkinson's disease was initiated in Sweden by Erik-Olof Backlund and colleagues in 1982.[15] These initial clinical trials using autologous adrenal medullary tissue were unsuccessful. Subsequent modifications by other investigators were initially reportedly successful,[16, 17] but multiple investigations could not replicate the results.[18-20] The degree of improvement is small, the degree of risks relatively large, and, worst of all, the improvement does not last. The basic principles underlying CNS transplantation have become increasingly sophisticated, and we are now more than ever clearly able to determine the reasons for the failures of the past and the need for further investigation to ensure future success.

The focus of interest has shifted to the use of fetal tissue.[21-31] Although the procedure remains investigational, reports of human fetal mesencephalic tissue being implanted into the basal ganglia of idiopathic parkinsonian or 1-methyl-4-phenyl-1, 2, 3, 6-tetrahydropyridine (MPTP) drug-induced parkinsonian patients have indicated that this technique seems to be on the correct path toward the successful relief of the symptoms of advanced parkinsonism.[22, 31] However, this technology is still evolving, and no standard technique is available. Some of the basic methodologic issues that remain to be addressed include the age of the donor tissue, the method for tissue preparation and storage, the implantation technique, the location for placement of the graft, the amount of tissue needed, and the use of immunologic suppression. The objectives of this chapter are to describe in detail the techniques that have been successfully used at the University of Colorado, to discuss the rationale behind these techniques and potential alternatives, and to identify technical modifications that are likely to develop in the future.

PATIENT SELECTION

Parkinson's disease is a progressive degenerative disorder that affects approximately 1 percent of the population over the age of 50; estimates indicate that up to 1 million people may be affected in the United States. The cardinal symptoms are resting tremor, rigidity, akinesia, and gait disturbance.[32] Although the resting tremor is the most dramatic symptom, slowness of movement (bradykinesia) and difficulty initiating movement (akinesia) represent the patient's most severe debilitating symptoms and the most difficult symptoms to treat.

Neuropathologically, the predominant finding is loss of dopaminergic cells in the substantia nigra pars compacta.[33] To produce parkinsonian symptoms, the loss of dopaminergic cells in the substantia nigra pars compacta must be 80 percent or greater. Although other lesions are present within the brain of parkinsonian patients, it is felt that most of the symptoms result from the loss of substantia nigra pars compacta dopaminergic cells. MPTP is a very specific neurotoxin that was identified as a side product of illicit drug production that affects predominantly, although not exclusively, the substantia nigra pars compacta.[34-38] An acute parkinsonian syndrome has been observed after the self-administration of MPTP.

Initially, drug therapy with levodopa appears to be extremely successful in providing the missing dopamine, but after approximately 5 years, most of the patients begin to have severe dyskinesias with on-and-off symptoms that greatly limit levodopa's effectiveness.[39] When initial symptoms occur, the use of selegiline (Deprenyl) can delay the need for replacement therapy with levodopa.[40] The problem in severe parkinsonian patients is not that they cannot form dopamine, but that they cannot store and release dopamine when needed. The fluctuation in levels of levodopa produce the on-and-off syndrome.[39, 41] Alternating between complete immobility and uncontrollable dyskinetic movements leaves these patients extremely disabled and shortens their life expectancy.

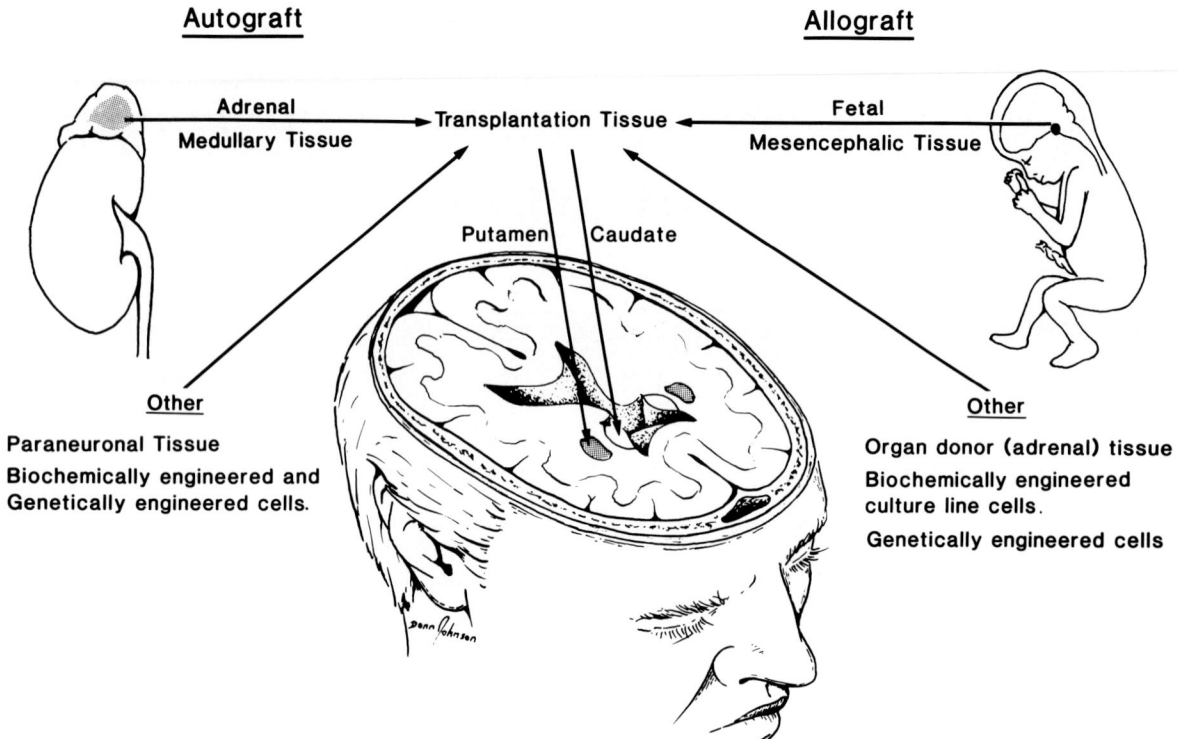

FIGURE 110–1. Both autografts and allografts have been used in the treatment of Parkinson's disease. Although the adrenal medulla has been the most commonly used tissue during the initial clinical investigations, emphasis is currently shifting to the use of fetal mesencephalic tissue. This form of therapy is evolving as more information becomes available about appropriate patient selection, targets, and transplantation techniques. (From Sladek JR Jr, Gash DM: Nerve-cell grafting in Parkinson's disease. J Neurosurg 8:337–351, 1988.)

The rationale behind fetal mesencephalic grafting is that the dopaminergic cells that are lost can be replaced by cells that are destined to produce dopamine. For this to occur, two conditions must be met. First, the appropriate-aged cells must be implanted. Immature cells may not have properly differentiated to allow satisfactory maturation to form dopaminergic cells, and cells harvested too late in development will have sent out axonal processes that when amputated during the grafting process, result in cell death. Thus, a window of time exists for proper harvesting of fetal tissue. This interval appears to be between 6 and 9 weeks for cell suspensions, based on human-to-rat CNS graft experiments.[42–45] If solid tissue pieces are implanted, the developmental window may be extended by approximately 1 week. The second condition is that the tissue must be implanted at the target site, that is, the area of denervation. Laboratory studies indicate that fetal mesencephalic cells send out their axonal processes for only several millimeters.[1–4] Whether or not reconstructive methods can be developed to allow these cells to be placed in their proper anatomic location remains to be determined.

Because of the potential risk of the procedure and the fact that patients with mild symptoms respond very well to medication, the only patients considered for this procedure have moderate-to-severe parkinsonian symptoms that are not responding well to conventional medical therapy. Evaluation of these patients is extremely difficult because of their fluctuating course and the subtlety of their symptoms. A neurologist with expertise in movement disorders is essential to the evaluation and care of these patients, both preoperatively and postoperatively. The selection criteria generally include (1) initial and persistent responsiveness to levodopa therapy, albeit a clinically unsatisfactory response; (2) good general health; (3) no neurologic disease other than parkinsonism; and (4) mental competence. Exclusion criteria include (1) computed tomographic (CT) or magnetic resonance imaging (MRI) evidence of previous stroke, (2) age greater than 75 years, (3) dementia, (4) myocardial infarction within 6 months or other significant medical conditions, (5) significant volume loss within the putamen on MRI, and (6) failure to show clinical deterioration on a drug holiday *or* absence of on-off phenomenon. The rationale for these criteria has been discussed in detail elsewhere.[46]

PATIENT ASSESSMENT

Severity of the symptoms and disability from Parkinson's disease are difficult to assess. A neurologist or a group of neurologists with specific expertise in movement disorders is essential to the the transplant team. All patients must be thoroughly examined to confirm the diagnosis of Parkinson's disease. Younger patients, shorter duration of symptoms, atypical symptoms, and a lack of response to levodopa replacement therapy all should suggest a possible error in diagnosis.

To provide a common basis for evaluation of the patient both preoperatively and postoperatively, the Core Assessment Program for Intracerebral Transplantation (CAPIT) for diagnosis and evaluation is recommended.[47] This program involves the use of the United Parkinson's Disease Rating

Scale, modified Hoehn and Yahr staging, a dyskinetic rating scale, and a self-reporting diary. Time testing and pharmacologic studies are also useful. Because of the patient's hourly and daily fluctuations, preoperative clinical evaluation should span a period of at least 3 months; during this time, medications are kept constant, and a minimum of three separate CAPIT examinations are performed in both the "on" and "off" conditions. Postoperatively, these same parameters should be evaluated in an identical setting. The CAPIT examination should be considered a minimum evaluation; most centers are adding their own measures to quantitate behavioral improvement.

Preoperative MRI should be performed to rule out any underlying pathology and to serve as a baseline for postoperative studies. Positron-emission tomography scanning with fluorodopa is becoming an increasingly important part of the preoperative evaluation. Not only does this method help to confirm the diagnosis and suggest where postoperative changes occur, it also may serve as a tool for planning graft placement.

PREPARATION OF DONOR TISSUE

Although there is general agreement that electively aborted fetuses provide the optimal donor tissue,[42–45] the ethics of this approach are complex.[48, 49] Each institution must develop its own protocols in accordance with the National Institutes of Health guidelines as well as federal, state, and local laws. The first essential requirement is that the issue of tissue donation must not be raised until the decision has been made to abort the fetus. Once permission to use the fetal tissue has been obtained, the fetal tissue must be considered an anonymous gift, negating any monetary gain, and for which the mother remains unaware as to whether or not the tissue was actually used and for whom it was actually used. This anonymity is similar to other transplant donations and it also prevents pregnancy whose goal is to donate specifically to a relative or to obtain secondary monetary gain from a third party. Because many fetuses will be unusable, this type of anonymity can be obtained. Finally, there must be no change in the indications for abortion or alteration of clinical care given on the basis of acceptance or refusal to participate in the research program.

Although spontaneously aborted fetuses have been used,[27] it is generally felt that this tissue is far less satisfactory because spontaneous first-trimester abortion fetuses frequently display chromosomal aberrations[50] and are more likely to be infected with bacteria, viruses, or protozoa.[51] Even under optimal conditions, it is not known how long the fetus has been dead; therefore, viability of this tissue would remain in doubt.

Ideally, preoperative ultrasound scanning would be performed before abortion to obtain an estimate of the crown-rump length (CRL) and Carnegie staging.[52] To obtain optimal human mesencephalic tissue, a CRL between 14 mm (Carnegie stage 17 to 18) and 28 mm (Carnegie stage 22) is sought. Although staging can be performed by examination of the products of abortion, the accuracy is decreased, and the difficulties in properly identifying tissue for staging are increased. If ultrasound is not used, the degree of development of the extremities (especially the hand) can be used to stage the fetus. The use of the last menstrual period for staging is inadequate.

The tissue is obtained through a routine suction abortion procedure, which, for ethical reasons, can be modified only if the modification does not increase the risk to the mother or adversely affect the successful completion of the abortion procedure. These simple modifications include using slightly larger bore instruments or a low-pressure aspiration technique, which are both already in clinical use. In these procedures, there is a need for greater sterility. Uterine contents are sterile, but the vaginal approach can introduce infective agents. This contamination can be reduced by swabbing the vagina and orifice to the cervix with antiseptics and using a single passage of instruments to obtain the fetal material. Because the fetus may be infected by maternal disease, maternal blood samples do need to be tested for the presence of human immunodeficiency virus, hepatitis B and C, cytomegalovirus, and syphilis. Once obtained, the fetal tissue must be rinsed multiple times with sterile saline, and cultures must be made to ensure sterility. Consultation and inclusion of an infectious disease specialist on the transplantation team are recommended.

Identification and separation of the appropriate mesencephalic tissue is a delicate and arduous task. The technique must be practiced on multiple occasions before clinical studies are performed. Absolute sterility and skilled dissection under the microscope are needed. Sterile calcium-free Hank's solution buffered at pH 7.4 with N-2-hydroxyethylpiperazine-N'-2-ethanesulfonic acid (HEPES) is used to sustain the tissue. Dissection is performed in a Petri dish against a dark background to contrast with the white embryonic tissue. Microdissection tools are essential. The forebrain is usually not found in the tissue, and the brainstem is often fractured above the spinal cord. Frequently, the fracture occurs at the mesodiencephalic juncture but can occur at the pontine or cervical flexure. The presence of tectal or cerebellar primordia constitutes landmark for orienting the brainstem in the rostral-caudal direction. Mesencephalic dopaminergic tissue lies on either side of the mesencephalic flexure. A 4- to 8-mm^3 segment of this tissue is obtained (Fig. 110–2). Once this tissue is dissected free, any meningeal attachments must be removed. In younger tissue, these attachments are extremely difficult to remove. The blood vessels outline the meninges, and with two pairs of fine Dumont forceps, this tissue can be gently removed.

Approximately 5 to 10 percent of dopamine neurons survive the transplantation process.[42] Although behavioral improvement can be obtained after transplantation of a human fetal ventral mesencephalon into a lesioned rat striatum, the human striatum is several orders of magnitude greater, and it is estimated that multiple mesencephalic donors are necessary to completely restore dopaminergic innervation to a single putamen.[25] Clinical studies in a few patients that have progressively increased the number of fetal donors have found greater behavioral improvement.

After harvesting, and under optimal conditions, the fetal tissue is implanted within 4 to 6 hours of removal. This situation is possible in Sweden, where investigators know well in advance when tissue will be harvested, and the laws allow for advanced screening.[24–26] In most other situations, however, there would be a significant delay to screen both the mother and the fetus for viruses (human immunodefi-

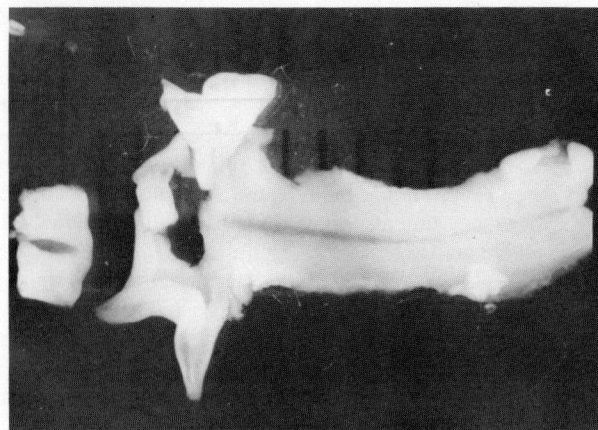

FIGURE 110-2. In this unusually well-preserved specimen, the region of the fetal mesencephalon containing the dopamine-producing cells has been dissected free of the brainstem. At fetal ages 6 and 8 weeks, a block approximately 2 × 4 × 1 mm is obtained and prepared as discussed in the text. (From Freed CR, Breeze RE, Rosenberg NL, et al: Therapeutic effects of human fetal dopamine cells transplanted in the patient with Parkinson's disease. Prog Brain Res 82:715–721, 1990.)

ciency virus, hepatitis A, B, and C, cytomegalovirus, and herpes simplex virus). In addition, most centers would evaluate the tissue for bacterial contamination not only by looking at Gram stains, but also by attempts at growing culture in media. We favor the extrusion of tissue through glass pipettes to form several "cores" (approximately 200 μm in diameter), which can be placed in F12 medium supplemented with 5-percent human placental serum (Fig. 110-3). This configuration allows the tissue to be conserved in a less traumatic method than cell suspension, while still easily transported and distributed throughout the host striatum. Maintaining the tissue in culture allows monitoring of dopamine metabolite production, performing of viral and bacterial cultures, and typing for ABO antigens (not expressed on fetal red cells but on endothelial structures). Contaminated tissue or tissue that fails to produce adequate amounts of dopamine can then be discarded. The tissue can be left in culture for 7 to 10 days without adversely affecting its viability.[53] Alternatively, the tissue may be frozen;[30] however, this technique does not appear to be as successful, and animal studies suggest that recovery of tyrosine hydroxylase–positive cells with this technique is less satisfactory.[54, 55]

The Swedish investigators prefer enzymatic and mechanical disruption of the tissue to form cell suspensions. Cell viability is frequently tested by use of small aliquots of the cell suspension and dye extrusion procedures. Staining dead cells with trypan blue is the simplest procedure; however, the use of acridine orange and ethidimide bromide to stain live and dying cells, respectively, seems to provide the best evaluation of graft viability.[56] Assessment of the portion of tyrosine hydroxylase–immunoreactive neurons on a smear also provides an estimate of success, but we believe that the evaluation from the culture media is preferable.

SURGICAL TECHNIQUE

Standard stereotactic techniques are employed, using a CT- or MRI-compatible stereotactic frame. We prefer to use the Cosman-Roberts-Wells (CRW) system, in which the standard probe carriage has been replaced by a graduated (with respect to horizontal rotation) template, to which a micromanipulator has been added to allow precise vertical movements (Fig. 110-4). The template has an array of 18 holes arranged in two columns and nine rows, with 4-mm spacing intervals, to rapidly place grafts without having to move the frame system.[58] The spacing is based on previous work that anticipates the limited axonal outgrowth of the transplanted fetal tissue.

The key target is the putamen, where dopamine depletion in idiopathic Parkinson's disease is most dramatic. The loss is bilateral, and therefore bilateral distribution over wide areas is recommended. The best results from the University of Colorado were obtained with the bilateral putamen technique.[22] However, excellent results were obtained from the Swedish group with wide, bilateral distribution of fetal tissue into both caudate and putamen.[31] It is as yet unclear whether the excellent results from Sweden were the result of the placement of tissue in the caudate as well as in the putamen (animal studies have demonstrated that different areas of the striatum produce different beneficial results), or of the use of multiple fetuses, thus increasing the number of dopaminergic cells and allowing greater distribution, or because the patients had MPTP-induced parkinsonism and not idiopathic parkinsonism, a potentially more readily treated disease entity. Hitchcock and his colleagues in England have systematically injected caudate and putamen unilaterally, and now bilaterally, and have not been able to ascertain the optimum target or targets.[23]

The University of Colorado team has developed the following surgical technique. The head ring is placed parallel to the plane that contains the major axes of both putamen. The putamen may be viewed as an ellipsoid whose major axis is

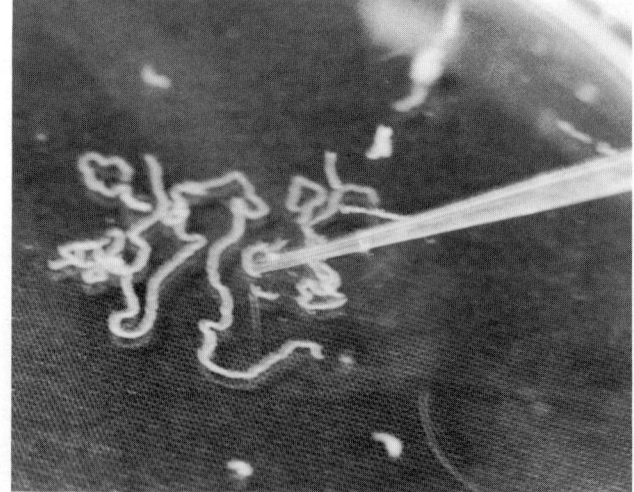

FIGURE 110-3. The fetal tissue has been extruded through a glass capillary tube (200 μ diameter) to produce cores of tissue. The cores can be cultured and the concentration of dopamine and its metabolic products measured from the culture media to ensure viable dopaminergic cells prior to the grafting. Segments of these cores are then aspirated into a needle for grafting into the brain. (From Freed CR, Breeze RE, Rosenberg NL, et al: Fetal neural implants for Parkinson's disease: Results at 15 months, in Lindvall O, Bjorklund A, Widner H [eds]: Restorative Neurology: Intracerebral Transplantation in Movement Disorders, Vol 4. Amsterdam, Elsevier Science Publishers, 1991, pp 69–77.)

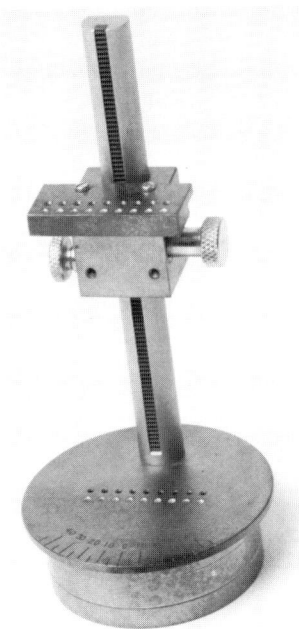

FIGURE 110-4. The rotating template and micromanipulator complex is pictured. The template has been graduated in degrees of arc with respect to horizontal rotation and is aligned in the axial plane to the long axis of the putamen as determined on CT scans. The micrometer rack adjustment allows precise tissue deposition. (From Breeze RE, Wells TH, Freed C: Implantation of fetal tissue for the management of Parkinson's disease. J Neurosurg, 1994, in press.)

oriented roughly in an anteroposterior direction when viewed in an axial section. More accurately, the major axis moves from lateral to medial as one progresses anteriorly in the axial plane. Because this hypothetical ellipsoid is "flattened," a minor axis may be defined that is normal to the major axis and is vertically oriented. This is accomplished by referring to the sagittal sections on the preoperative MRI. The subsequent error introduced by estimating this position is minimal because of the relatively short distance over which that potential angular deviation will eventually act. Once in the CT suite, 5- (thickness) × 3-mm (spacing), unenhanced, axial sections are obtained through the region of interest. The section that most closely passes through the center of the putamen is targeted. (Two different sections may be needed for targeting the right and left sides if the patient's head is not aligned favorably in the scanner.) The only coordinates obtained directly from the scanner (other than the fiducials) are the two center points, labeled C_1, and C_2 for the right and left sides, respectively. An enlarged hard copy of the targeting scans (or scans) is made. The major axes of the right and left putamen are drawn directly on the targeting scan, and the angles relative to the anteroposterior line (as defined by the fiducials and not the head or the film itself) are measured with a protractor. The lengths of the major axes are also measured to determine the number of passes that can be made in each putamen.

The patient is moved to the operating room, where the head ring is connected to the operating table in the usual fashion. The scalp is clipped, prepared, and draped in the usual fashion for stereotactic craniotomies with the CRW frame. Surgery is usually performed first on the left side of brain. The CRW frame is locked to the head ring and adjusted to correspond to the coordinates of C_2. A pointer is passed through the reference hole center (nearest to the micromanipulator) of the template (see Fig. 110-4). The arc is adjusted so that the pointer can be placed at approximately the level of the coronal suture. The lateral adjustment is placed on the value that corresponds to the arithmetically derived midpoint of the two lateral target values, and the carriage system is moved so that the pointer can be placed directly over the midline. The lateral adjustment is then returned to the value determined for C_1. This maneuver corrects for the potentially nonorthogonal alignment of the head within stereotactic space. Additional correction within the coronal plane is generally not necessary, because the approximately vertical orientation of the minor axis. This orientation can be confirmed on the preoperative MRI, and adjustments can be made, if necessary. Finally, the template is rotated to the angle measured directly from the targeting image (generally, about 12 degrees if the head is orthogonal to the fiducials).

The patient remains awake and communicative throughout the procedure. After infiltration with a local anesthetic, a gentle S-shaped incision (oriented in the anteroposterior direction) is made. With a pointer passing through the holes on the template, the exact locations of the most anterior and posterior trajectories are marked, allowing for the precise placement of the scalp incision and, subsequently, the precise placement of the craniotomy. A free bone flap measuring approximately 4 × 3 cm and elliptical in shape is fashioned with a high-speed craniotome. The dura is opened in a linear fashion and is held apart with stay sutures.

The implantation system consists of two cannulae (Fig. 110-5). The outer cannula is constructed of 17-gauge hypodermic stock that tapers to a 19-gauge needle. Both the outer cannula and its stylet are rounded and polished to minimize brain tissue injury during implantation. The larger cannula extends down to 25 mm above target. The inner cannula is fashioned from a rounded, 23-gauge needle (outer diameter, 0.64 mm) with a standard Luer lock. When passed completely into the outer cannula, the inner cannula extends 25

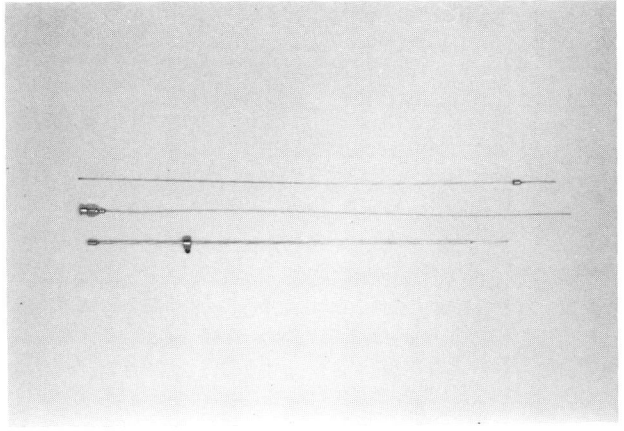

FIGURE 110-5. The outer cannula (top), inner cannula and stylet (bottom) are pictured. The outer cannula is passed through the brain with the stylet inserted. When the stylet is removed and the inner cannula inserted, the tip of the inner cannula extends about 25 mm beyond the tip of the outer cannula. (From Breeze RE, Wells TH, Freed C: Implantation of fetal tissue for the management of Parkinson's disease. J Neurosurg, 1994, in press.)

mm beyond the outer cannula. The size of the implantation tract must be less than 1 mm in diameter.[21, 24] The micromanipulator is adjusted so that the tip of the inner cannula will be located 5 mm beyond the target at maximum penetration. The target point for the micromanipulator is set at an arbitrary number, and the stop on the outer cannula is adjusted accordingly on the phantom base before surgery. The outer cannula, with the stylet in place, is passed into the brain parenchyma. The design of the cannula is such that the stiffest (17-gauge) portion of the cannula traverses the gap between the template and the brain. The thinner (19-gauge) portion traverses the cortex and deep white matter (Fig. 110–6A). The tip of the outer cannula stops several millimeters above the putamen. Only the inner cannula penetrates the putamen (Fig. 110–6B).

A core of tissue is aspirated into the inner cannula, which has been preloaded with a buffered solution. A 10-μl syringe is connected to the inner cannula. The inner cannula is passed through the outer cannula, eventually piercing the substance of the putamen. The micromanipulator is used to slowly withdraw the entire outer cannula–inner cannula assembly while the plunger of the syringe is simultaneously advanced. The volume injected into the inner cannula is approximately the same as the volume in which the core is suspended. The net result is that the tissue core is left in its original position while the needle is withdrawn from around it with minimal disruption to the putamen (Fig. 110–6C). The cannula is withdrawn 10 mm over 60 seconds and is then allowed to sit for 2 minutes. This delay allows the brain parenchyma to collapse around the tissue core. The cannula is then withdrawn another 10 mm with the micromanipulator while 3 μl of buffered solution is simultaneously injected. This technique prevents a suction effect that could dislodge the tissue core if the cannula were simply withdrawn rapidly by hand. The efficacy of this injection technique has been demonstrated with transparent gelatin models and successful animal transplants (RE Breeze and CR Freed).

The most posterior position is implanted first because of its relative close proximity to the internal capsule and because the posterior putamen is the most depleted region of the basal ganglia. In theory, some error may be introduced during stereotactic procedures by shifts in the brain as air enters the subarachnoid space. Assuming that these shifts increase over time, we make the most critical passes first, when accuracy is theoretically greatest. A total of six to eight passes are made along a single line on each side. One side is completed in about 1 hour. The scalp incision is closed before the second side is approached.

POSTOPERATIVE MANAGEMENT

The need for immunosuppressant drugs in patients receiving allogeneic fetal tissue implants in the CNS has not been established. In monkey transplant experiments, rejection of fetal tissue has been uncommon.[1, 8–14, 57] We have chosen to use immunosuppression in every other patient in our series to determine if immunosuppression improves clinical outcome.[22] All patients receive perioperative anticonvulsants (phenytoin) and perioperative antibiotics (cefazolin). Parkinson medications are kept at preoperative levels. The patients are usually discharged within 72 hours.

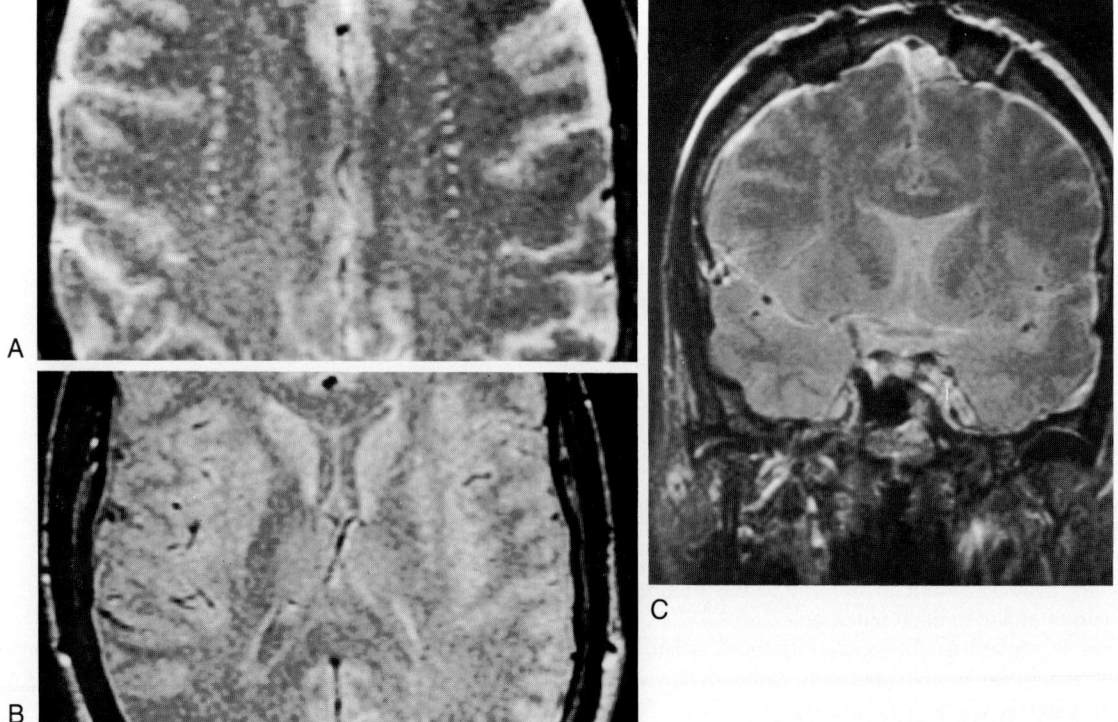

FIGURE 110–6. The tracts of the outer cannula can be seen on a T2-weighted axial MRI in the corona radiata above the putamen (A). A T1-weighted axial image obtained 3 days postoperatively through the region of the putamen illustrates the apparent absence of tissue injury despite 14 tracts through this slice (B). A coronal image demonstrates the tracts from cortex to putamen (C).

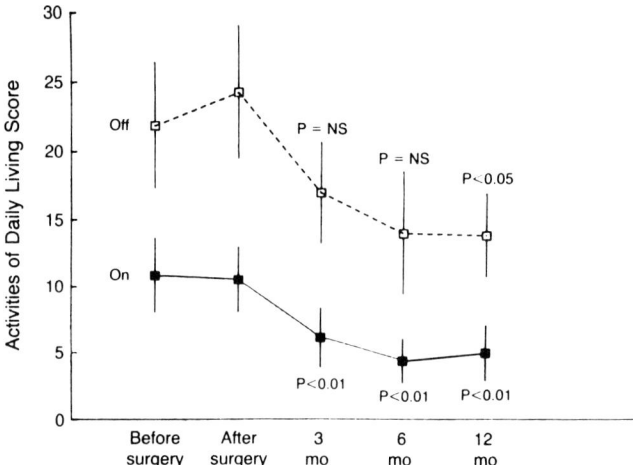

FIGURE 110–7. The activity of daily living scores of the seven patients were averaged and expressed as means + SE. Patient 2 did not distinguish on and off periods and, therefore, his scores for off periods were omitted. The phrase "after surgery" refers to an evaluation in the days after transplantation. Scores for the group improved (i.e., decreased) during both the on and the off periods, reflecting better functional capabilities under both circumstances (on this scale, 52 is the worst possible score and 0 denotes the absence of parkinsonian signs). The data were truncated at the point 12 months after surgery. The patients reported that their conditions had improved during on and off periods (p values, determined by analysis of variance with Newman-Keuls correction, refer to the difference from preoperative scores). NS denotes not significant. (From Freed CR, Breeze RE, Rosenberg NL, et al: Survival of implanted fetal dopamine cells and neurologic improvement 12 to 46 months after transplantation for Parkinson's disease. N Engl J Med 327:1549–1555, 1992.)

RESULTS

Using stereotactic CNS transplantation techniques is very safe; no deaths or major intraoperative complications have been reported. With open operative techniques, the safety of the procedure is not as good.

It is clear from all reports that improvements are delayed and gradual. Recent reports indicate that the benefits were greatest in patients with MPTP-induced parkinsonism in whom bilateral caudate putamen implantation techniques with multiple fetuses were used, and the smallest improvement occurred in patients with idiopathic Parkinson's disease who received unilateral implants into just the right caudate nucleus. However, the marked variation in technique, patient selection, and potential variability in evaluation do not lead to any firm conclusion. The University of Colorado experience reported on seven patients who demonstrated statistically significant improvements in Hoehn and Yahr scores while significantly decreasing their levodopa requirements.[22] Significant improvement in both "on" and "off" scores were also seen on the Activities of Daily Living Scale (Fig. 110–7). It is also evident from this and other reports that progressive improvement can be seen for at least 4 years.[22,31] Reports of even longer follow-up are essential for the procedure to be established. Whether or not the grafts are viable still remains to be determined because none of the parkinsonian patients has come to autopsy. Spencer and associates[30] reported on a patient who received a fetal graft for what turned out to be striatonigral degeneration and who demonstrated no evidence of tyrosine hydroxylase–positive cells at the graft site after autopsy. Position-emission tomography has demonstrated evidence of increased uptake of fluorodopa in patients whose conditions have improved.[22,31] This effect presumably results from dopamine-producing cells and processes, but other explanations are possible.

DISCUSSION

A major breakthrough in the treatment of Parkinson's disease occurred approximately 25 years ago when levodopa was demonstrated to improve the signs and symptoms of Parkinson's disease. The result was not a cure, and unfortunately, with time, the efficacy of this treatment deteriorates, and in some cases the treatment has worse effects than the disease. The use of fetal tissue transplanted into the CNS may be another breakthrough therapy that further advances our comprehensive treatment of Parkinson's disease. This therapy is in its infancy, and much more research is needed to improve the technique. Such evolution requires a team of specialists and integration with basic scientists because the major improvements are most likely to come from an understanding of the biology of the procedure rather than from an improvement in the technical aspects of the surgery. The major thrust must be to increase cell survival and integration with the host to increase the degree of functional recovery that can be achieved. Ultimately, this investigation will lead to an understanding of how the brain repairs itself and how this reparative process can be augmented to restore lost neurologic function. The goal must be establishment of a cure.

REFERENCES

1. Bjorklund A, Lindvall O, Issacson O, et al: Mechanisms of action of intracerebral neural implants: Studies on nigral and striatal grafts to the lesioned striatum. Trends Neurosci 10:509–516, 1987
2. Lindvall O: Transplantation into the human brain: Present status and future possibilities. J Neurol Neurosurg Psychiatry (Special Suppl):39–54, 1989
3. Oyesiku NM, Bakay RAE: Central nervous system transplantation, in Crockard A, Hayward R, Hoff JT (eds): Neurosurgery. Boston, Blackwell Scientific Publications, 1992, pp 448–469
4. Sladek JR Jr, Gash DM: Nerve-cell grafting in Parkinson's disease. J Neurosurg 8:337–351, 1988
5. Bjorklund A, Stenevi U: Reconstruction of the nigrostriatal dopamine pathway by intracerebral nigral transplants. Brain Res 177:555–560, 1979
6. Bjorklund A, Dunnett SB, Stenevi U, et al: Reinnervation of the denervated striatum by substantia nigra transplants: Functional consequences as revealed by pharmacological and sensorimotor testing. Brain Res 199:307–333, 1980
7. Perlow MF, Freed WF, Hoffer BJ, et al: Brain grafts reduce motor abnormalities produced by destruction of nigrostriatal dopamine system. Science 204:643–647, 1979
8. Bakay RAE, Fiandaca MS, Barrow DL, et al: Preliminary report on the use of fetal tissue transplantation to correct MPTP-induced Parkinson-like syndrome in primates. Appl Neurophysiol 48:358–361, 1985
9. Bakay RAE, Barrow DL, Fiandaca MS, et al: Biochemical and behavioral correction of MPTP Parkinson-like syndrome by fetal cell transplantation. Ann N Y Acad Sci 495:623–639, 1987
10. Bankiewicz KS, Plunkett RJ, Jacobowitz DM, et al: The effect of fetal mesencephalon implants on primate MPTP-induced parkinsonism. J Neurosurg 72:231–244, 1990
11. Dunnett SE, Annett LE: Nigral transplants in primate models of parkinsonism, in Lindvall O, Bjorklund A, Widner H (eds): Intracerebral Transplantation in Movement Disorders. New York, Elsevier Science Publishers, 1991, pp 27–50

12. Fine A, Hunt SP, Gertel WH, et al: Transplantation of embryonic marmoset dopaminergic neurons to the corpus striatum of marmosets rendered parkinsonian by 1-methyl-4-phenyl-1,2,3,6-tetrahydropyridine. Prog Brain Res 78:479–489, 1988
13. Freed CR, Richards JB, Sabol KE, et al: Fetal substantia nigra transplants lead to dopamine cell replacement and behavioral improvement in Bonnet monkeys with MPTP induced parkinsonism, in Beart PM, Woodruff G, Jackson DM (eds): Pharmacology and Functional Regulation of Dopaminergic Neurons. New York, MacMillan Press, 1988, pp 353–360
14. Redmond DE, Roth RH, Elsworth JD, et al: Fetal neuronal grafts in monkeys given methylphenyltetrahydropyridine. Lancet 17:1125–1127, 1986
15. Backlund EO, Gransberg PO, Hamberger B, et al: Transplantation of adrenal medullary tissue to striatum in parkinsonism. First clinical trials. J Neurosurg 62:169–173, 1985
16. Madrazo I, Drucker-Colin R, Diaz V, et al: Open microsurgical autograft of adrenal medulla to the right caudate nucleus in two patients with intractable Parkinson's disease. N Engl J Med 316:831–834, 1987
17. Madrazo I, Drucker-Colin R, Torres C, et al: Long-term (more than one year) evolution of patients with adrenal medullary autografts to the caudate nucleus for the treatment of Parkinson's disease, in Bunney WE Jr, Hippins H, Laakmann G, Schmauss M (eds): Neuropsychopharmacology Proceedings of the XVII CINP Congress. Berlin, Springer-Verlag, 1990, pp 118–132
18. Bakay RAE, Allen GS, Apuzzo M, et al: Preliminary report on adrenal medullary grafting from the American Association of Neurological Surgeons Graft Project, in Dunnett SB, Richards SR (eds): Neural Transplantation: From Molecular Basis to Clinical Application. Amsterdam, Elsevier Science Publishers, 1990, pp 603–617
19. Goetz CG, Olanow CW, Koller WC, et al: Multicenter study of autologous adrenal medullary transplantation to the corpus striatum in patients with advanced Parkinson's disease. N Engl J Med 320:337–341, 1989
20. Goetz CG, Stebbins GT, Klawans HL, et al: United Parkinson Foundation Neurotransplantation Registry on adrenal medullary transplants: Presurgical, and 1- and 2-year follow-up. Neurology 41(11):1719–1722, 1991
21. Freed CR, Breeze RE, Rosenberg NL, et al: Transplantation of human fetal dopamine cells for Parkinson's disease: Results at 1 year. Arch Neurol 47:505–512, 1990
22. Freed CR, Breeze RE, Rosenberg NL, et al: Survival of implanted fetal dopamine cells and neurologic improvement 12 to 46 months after transplantation for Parkinson's disease. N Engl J Med 327:1549–1555, 1992
23. Hitchcock ER, Henderson BTH, Kenny BG, et al: Stereotactic implantation of foetal mesencephalon, in Lindvall O, Bjorklund A, Widner H (eds): Intracerebral Transplantation in Movement Disorders. New York, Elsevier Science Publishers, 1991, pp 79–86
24. Lindvall O, Brundin P, Widner H, et al: Grafts of fetal dopamine neurons survive and improve motor function in Parkinson's disease. Science 247:574–577, 1990
25. Lindvall O, Rehncrona S, Brundin P, et al: Human fetal dopamine neurons grafted into the striatum in two patients with severe Parkinson's disease. Arch Neurol 46:615–631, 1989
26. Lindvall O: Prospects of transplantation in human neurodegenerative diseases. Trends Neurosci 14:376–384, 1991
27. Madrazo I, Franco-Bourland R, Ostrosky-Solis F, et al: Fetal homotransplants (ventral mesencephalon and adrenal tissue) to the striatum of parkinsonian subjects. Arch Neurol 47:1281–1285, 1990
28. Molina H, Quinones R, Alvarez L, et al: Transplantation of human fetal mesencephalic tissue in caudate nucleus as treatment for Parkinson's disease: The Cuban experience, in Lindvall O, Bjorklund A, Widner H (eds): Intracerebral Transplantation in Movement Disorders. New York, Elsevier Science Publishers, 1991, pp 99–105
29. Redmond DE, Marek KLK, Robbins RJ, et al: Human fetal substantia nigra grafts in 11 patients with Parkinson's disease: Preliminary clinical results, in Freed WJ, Rosenstein JM (eds): Restorative Neurology and Neuroscience. New York, Elsevier Science Publishers, 1992, p 231
30. Spencer DD, Robbins F, Naftolin F, et al: Unilateral transplantation of human fetal mesencephalic tissue into the caudate nucleus of patients with Parkinson's disease. N Engl J Med 327:1541–1548, 1992
31. Widner H, Tetrud J, Rehncrona S, et al: Bilateral fetal mesencephalic grafting in two patients with parkinsonism induced by 1-methyl-4-phenyl-1,2,3,6-tetrahydropyridine (MPTP). N Engl J Med 327:1556–1563, 1992
32. Miller WC, DeLong MR: Parkinsonian symptomatology: An anatomical and physiological analysis. Ann Neurol 515:287–302, 1988
33. Hassler R: Aur Pathologie de Paralysis agitans und des postenzephalitischen Parkinsonismus. J Psychol Neurol 48:387–476, 1938
34. Burns RS, LeWitt PA, Ebert MH, et al: The clinical syndrome of striatal dopamine deficiency: Parkinsonism induced by 1-methyl-4-phenyl-1,2,3,6-tetrahydropyridine (MPTP). N Engl J Med 312:1418–1421, 1985
35. Crossman AR: Primate models of dyskinesia: The experimental approach to the study of basal ganglia-related involuntary movement disorders. Neuroscience 21:1–40, 1987
36. German DC, Dubach M, Askari S, et al: 1-Methyl-4-phenyl-1,2,3,6-tetrahydropyridine-induced parkinsonian syndrome in Macaca fascicularis: Which midbrain dopaminergic neurons are lost? Neuroscience 24:161–174, 1988
37. Langston JW, Ballard PA, Tetrud JW, Irwin I: Chronic parkinsonism in humans due to a product of meperidine-analog synthesis. Science 219:979–980, 1983
38. Schneider JS, Yuwiler A, Markham CH: Selective loss of subpopulations of ventral mesencephalic dopaminergic neurons in the monkey following exposure to MPTP. Brain Res 411:144–150, 1987
39. Marsden CD, Parkes JD: Success and problems of long-term levodopa therapy in Parkinson's disease. Lancet i:345–349, 1977
40. Parkinson's Study Group: Effects of tocopherol and deprenyl on the progression of disability in early Parkinson's disease. N Engl J Med 328:176–183, 1993
41. Hoehn MM, Crowley TJ, Rutledge CO: Dopamine correlates of neurological and psychological status in untreated parkinsonism. J Neurol Neurosurg Psychiatry 39:941–951, 1976
42. Brundin P, Strecker RE, Widner H, et al: Human fetal dopamine neurons grafted in a rat model of Parkinson's disease: Immunological aspects, spontaneous and drug-induced behavior, and dopamine release. Exp Brain Res 70:192–208, 1988
43. Brundin P, Nilsson OG, Strecker RE, et al: Behavioral effects of human fetal dopamine neurons grafted in a rat model of Parkinson's disease. Exp Brain Res 65:235–240, 1986
44. Freeman TB, Spence MS, Boss BD, et al: Development of dopaminergic neurons in the human substantia nigra. Exp Neurol 113:344–353, 1991
45. Freeman RB, Kordower JR: Human cadaver embryonic substantia nigra grafts: Effects of ontogeny, pre-operative graft preparation and tissue storage, in Lindvall O, Bjorklund A, Widner H (eds): Intracerebral Transplantation in Movement Disorders. New York, Elsevier Science Publishers, 1991, pp 163–169
46. Bakay RAE: Selection criteria for CNS grafting into Parkinson's disease patients, in Lindvall O, Bjorklund A, Widner H (eds): Intracerebral Transplantation in Movement Disorders. New York, Elsevier Science Publishers, 1991, pp 137–148
47. Langston JW, Widner H, Brooks D, et al: Core assessment program for intracerebral transplantations (CAPIT). Mov Disord 7:2–13, 1992
48. Council on Scientific Affairs and Council on Ethical and Judicial Affairs: Medical applications of fetal tissue transplantation. JAMA 263:565–570, 1990
49. Advisory to the Director of the National Institutes of Health: Report of the Human Fetal Tissue Transplantation Research, Panel 2:E1. 1988, NIH, Bethesda, MD
50. Warbuton D, Stein Z, Klein J, Susser M: Chromosome abnormalities in spontaneous abortion, in Porter LH, Hook B (eds): Human Embryonic and Fetal Death. Orlando, Academic Press, 1980, pp 281–287
51. Sever JL: Infectious causes of human reproductive loss, in Porter IH, Hook B (eds): Human Embryonic and Fetal Death. Orlando, Academic Press, 1980, pp 169–175
52. O'Rahilly R, Muller F: Developmental Stages in Human Embryos. Carnegie Institution of Washington publication 637. Meriden, CN, Meriden-Stinehour Press, 1987
53. Qi J-X, Patino P, Kriek E, et al: Effects of refrigeration and tissue culture on dopamine production and transplant survival of fetal mesencephalic dopamine cells. Soc Neurosci Abstr 17:347, 1991
54. Chanaud CM, Das GD: Growth of neural transplants in rats: Effects of initial volume, growth potential, and fresh vs. frozen tissues. Neurosci Lett 80:127–133, 1987
55. Jensen S, Sorensen T, Moller AG, Zimmer J: Intraocular grafts of fresh and freeze-stored rat hippocampal tissue: A comparison of survivability and histological and connective organization. J Comp Neurol 227:558–568, 1984
56. Brundin P, Isacson O, Bjorklund A: Monitoring of cell viability in

suspensions of embryonic CNS tissue and its use as a criterion for intracerebral graft survival. Brain Res 331:251–259, 1985

57. Freed CR, Richards JB, Hutt CJ, et al: Rejection of fetal substantia nigra allografts in monkeys with MPTP-induced Parkinson's syndrome. Soc Neurosci Abstr 14(1):9, 1988.

58. Breeze RE, Wells TH, Freed, CR: Implantation of fetal tissue for the management of Parkinson's disease: A technical note. J. Neurosurgery, in press, 1994.

59. Richards, JB, Sabol KE, Kriek, EH, Freed, CR: Trained and amphetamine-induced circling behavior in lesioned, transplanted rats. J. Neural Transplantation and Plasticity 4:157–166, 1993.

CHAPTER 111

Neural Transplantation

E. R. Hitchcock

Clinical neural transplantation has been mainly applied to the treatment of Parkinson's disease, although a few reports have been published of patients with other neurodegenerative diseases receiving transplants. Neural grafting for Parkinson's disease originated in animal studies beginning in 1890, when Thompson unsuccessfully transplanted cerebral cortex from adult donor rats to the cortex of host dogs.[1] Subsequent and increasingly successful attempts demonstrated that fetal donors were more successful than adult donors, especially to younger rather than adult hosts.[2-5] Lund and Hauscha[6] demonstrated synaptic connections between embryonic grafts and neonatal host brain in 1977, and in 1978, Das and Hallas[7] successfully transplanted embryonic neural tissue into adult brain. This seminal experiment suggested that neural degenerative disease, which occurs largely in adult life, could be treated with neural transplants. Nonneural tissue can also produce reversal of deficits in animal models, probably by inducing collateral "sprouting" of processes from the host neurones[8-10] and both neural and nonneural tissue contains trophic factors.[11, 12] The response can occur within days of implantation[13, 14] and may account for the immediate response noted in some clinical studies.[15-18] Numerous animal studies support the contention that sprouting is essential for good functional recovery. Improvement in MPTP-induced parkinsonism in monkeys has been produced by caudate cavitation, nondopaminergic tissue grafting, and adrenal medullary grafts.[19, 20] (MPTP is the selective nigral toxin 1-methyl-4-phenyl-1,2,3,6 tetrahydropyridine.)

The progressive loss of dopaminergic neurons in the substantia nigra projecting to the striatum results in Parkinson's disease and its characteristic signs of resting tremor, bradykinesia, rigidity, and postural instability.

Although stereotactic thalamotomy is successful in obliterating tremor and some rigidity in Parkinson's disease, it produces little or no improvement in bradykinesia. Dopamine therapy is more successful in treating bradykinesia, although it becomes progressively less effective with increased dopamine requirements and causes increasingly severe side effects, notably dyskinesia.

The extensive dopaminergic cell loss that occurs in the substantia nigra of Parkinson's disease patients can be copied in a limited but useful rat model.[21, 22] Unilateral injections of 6-hydroxy dopamine (6-OHDA) into the ventral mesencephalon causes considerable cell loss in the substantia nigra and ventral tegmental area. The animals exhibit contralateral sensory neglect and spontaneous rotation to the side of the lesion that is increased by the administration of amphetamine; this in turn releases dopamine from the intact side. The rotation is reversed by dopamine agonists such as apomorphine, which act on supersensitized receptors in the striatum of the lesioned side. In 1979, Perlow and colleagues[23] transplanted fetal mesencephalon into the striatum of such a model, reducing the spontaneous and drug-induced rotation; Björklund and Stenevi[24] not only halted but actually reversed the rotation by this method.

ANATOMY

The nucleus caudatus and putamen comprise the striatum, which is the largest nuclear mass in the brain, the caudate and putamen appearing as a single homogenous mass that connects with other extrapyramidal centers. The putamen and the head of caudate are partly separated by the anterior limb of the internal capsule. The caudate nucleus is closely related to the lateral ventricle throughout its length, and the caudate head is continuous posteriorly with the putamen. The putamen is immediately medial to the insula and forms the outer part of the lentiform nucleus, the globus pallidus being the inner part.

The substantia nigra lies in the midbrain between the tegmentum and the cerebral peduncles. Dopaminergic neurons of the substantia nigra project into the striatum, and fibers from caudate nucleus and putamen also project in the reverse direction to the substantia nigra.

TRANSPLANTATION OF ADRENAL MEDULLARY CELLS INTO THE CENTRAL NERVOUS SYSTEM

Adrenal medullary cells synthesize catecholamine, and Freed and associates[25] showed that placing these medullary grafts into the lateral ventricle close to the denervated striatum improved drug-induced turning behavior in rats, although without any evidence of the cells extending processes. This effect may result from low levels of growth factor in the adult striatum; if nerve growth factor is added to the graft by continuous infusion or by cografting with peripheral nerve sections, the cells tend to develop a neuronal phenotype with outgrowth of processes and improvement in cell survival.[26]

Primate studies are particularly important: implantation of adrenal medulla tissue into the caudate nucleus of monkeys treated with unilateral MPTP reduces rotational asymmetry for 6 months after surgery and improves motor function in hemi-parkinsonian monkeys.[27, 28] Adrenal medullary tissue transplanted into the lateral ventricle or the striatum of rats with unilateral 6-OHDA lesions diminishes drug-induced rotation,[25, 26, 29] but grafts into rat or monkey striatum have poor survival.[27, 28, 30–33]

Chromaffin cells within the medulla produce dopamine as a noradrenaline precursor, and the dopamine levels increase when separated from the adrenal cortex. The endocrine cells are also transformed to a neuronal phenotype in the presence of trophic substances such as nerve growth factor and acidic and basic fibroblast growth factors.[34] The tissue is very dependent on nerve growth factor, but although only a small number of adrenal chromaffin cells survive striatal implantation, abundant increase in tyrosine hydroxylase (TH)-positive fibers occurs.[30] A threefold increase in the number of chromaffin cells surviving for at least 3 months and accompanying behavioral improvement has been achieved with nerve growth factor.[26] Kordower and coworkers[35] made an important observation that portions of peripheral nerve (which produce nerve growth factor), when cografted with adrenal medullary tissue into the striatum of the rhesus monkey, result in a significant increase in the survival of chromaffin cells and can produce a more than 250-percent increase in chromaffin cell survival.[36] Thus, considerable evidence exists for the presence of trophic substances that may stimulate the host dopaminergic system to sprouting of host TH-positive fibers. The consensus appears to be that although adrenal medullary tissue transplanted into the striatum can induce behavioral improvement in lesioned animals, the effect is short-term, and few cells survive. If trophic factors such as nerve growth factor are provided by infusion or by the use of cograft, then all survival is greatly improved.

ADRENAL MEDULLARY AUTOGRAFTS IN MAN

Ethical problems and practical difficulties in obtaining human neural tissue encouraged the development of the proposal by Freed and associates[25] that adrenal chromaffin cells could act as suitable donor tissue in clinical studies, permitting the use of autografts and thus avoiding the dangerous use of immunosuppression. Nonhuman primate research has a short history, but Bakay[37] pointed out that the modest improvements recorded in these studies[27, 38–40] are also seen in clinical studies[41–59] of adrenal medullary tissue grafts, whereas autopsy studies[60–63] showed minimal evidence of survival.

Backlund and coworkers[43] were the first to place adrenal medullary autografts into the caudate and putamen of patients with Parkinson's disease. These investigators used a computed tomographically (CT)-guided stereotactic procedure. They chose a target point 10 mm from the midline, 10 mm anterior to the anterior commissures, and 10 mm above the intercommissurial plane. Only one patient showed improvement, with some decrease in rigidity and akinesia over the first 6 months and a modest reduction in antiparkinsonian medication. Two years later, two additional patients were treated with adrenal medullary implants, but this time, the implants were placed into the putamen because primate studies suggested that the putamen played a more important role in motor control than the caudate and had a greater loss of dopamine content than the caudate. Two targets were chosen: one 20 mm laterally, 5 mm anterior to the anterior commissure, and 5 mm above the intercommissural plane, and the other on the same horizontal plane at the level of the anterior commissure at 25 mm from the commissure line. Some of the fragments were implanted within a steel spiral holder. Only one patient showed improvement in "on" time for about 2 months, and the second patient had serious immediate complications (peripheral vasoconstriction and hypertension), required ventilation overnight, and later developed pneumonia. No clinical rating was given for the first two patients, but they were probably stage IV Hoehn and Yahr, and the last two patients were assessed as stage IV.

Although the stereotactic method was replaced a few years later by an open procedure, most groups today use a stereotactic technique that targets the caudate or putamen using CT or magnetic resonance imaging (MRI) scanning; there is no uniformity of target placement, and coordinates for the placements are rarely given.[42]

Takeuchi and coworkers[64] performed a putaminal adrenal transplantation with the patient under general anesthesia in March 1987 in a Parkinson's disease patient, who then had improvement in akinesia and rigidity and a prolongation of the duration of the action of levodopa. A right frontotemporal skin incision was made, a bone flap turned, and the skin then closed; the left adrenal gland was removed and kept in phosphate-buffered saline at 4°C for 60 minutes. The scalp wound was reopened, the bone flap removed, and the dura opened and the sylvian fissure and insula exposed. The adrenal medulla was dissected out and macerated with phosphate-buffered saline, and the homogenate was injected into the putamen through a 2-mm-diameter brain puncture needle at a depth of 25 mm from the insula. The effect lasted for 6 months and then gradually deteriorated to the preoperative stage at 12 months.

In 1987, Madrazo and associates[65] reported the results of transplanting several small intact fragments of adrenal medulla into two patients by an open microsurgical technique into the head of the right caudate nucleus. This technique allowed the tissue to be exposed to ventricular cerebrospinal fluid (CSF). Both patients had early major improvement without complications. This report was received with great enthusiasm and awakened considerable reinterest in brain transplantation.

Several groups tried to repeat Madrazo's excellent results* but with variable success; part of the problem was the difficulty in comparing assessment techniques, selection criteria, and operative techniques. Although improvement was reported in a number of patients, many reported episodes of delusion, hallucination, and hypertension. Penn and coworkers[59] noted improvement in "on" time and reduction in dyskinesia, although antiparkinsonian medication could not be reduced; the only complications were respiratory. Lopez-Lozano and colleagues[66] reported bilateral improvement in 20 Hoehn and Yahr grade IV or V patients with parkinsonism as well a reduction in the daily dose of levodopa after

---

*See references 41, 43, 49, 53, 55, 59, 66–70.

adrenal-caudate transplantation, but they did list systemic neurologic and psychiatric complications.

Three patients had pneumonia in the first postoperative week that led to their deaths 4, 35, and 38 days after surgery. One patient required a splenectomy, another required a week's intubation and nasogastric feeding. The authors believed that the pneumonic complications probably resulted from aspiration and were associated with the subcostal approach for the adrenal exposure. One patient had a frontoparietal hematoma, which required evacuation on the second day, and another had a left parietal infarct after the onset of bilateral pneumonia. Thirteen patients had transient psychiatric disorders, including hypomania (in 1), aggressiveness (in 3), sexual dysinhibition (in 6), hallucination (in 7), delusions (in 6), and vivid dreams (in 5). These psychiatric disorders disappeared after the dosage of levodopa, carbidopa, or anticholinergic agents had been reduced. Apart from the general improvements in the features of parkinsonism, including rigidity, bradykinesia, and gait, there was an immediate decrease of 44 percent of the dosage of levodopa (carbidopa), which was necessary to reduce the toxic effects of levodopa that appeared in the postoperative period. The authors had perfused the adrenal before implantation, which permitted a more reliable separation of medulla from cortex and reduced the effects of warm ischemia. Viability of the dispersed cells of remnants of the adrenal medulla 6 to 7 hours after implantation was 85 to 87 percent.

The results of adrenal medullary grafting in human trials were generally considered disappointing, but interest revived after reports were published that some patients had moderate improvement in their parkinsonian symptoms. The United Parkinson Foundation and Registry had a large series of 61 patients, of whom 56 were followed up for 2 years: 19 percent of the group improved after 2 years, but with individual examination, the score increased to 32 percent; a significant improvement of daily "on" time occurred. However, 18 percent died during the study, and half of these deaths appeared to be related to surgery.[50]

Allen and associates[41] found that the younger and least affected parkinsonian patients had the best results, although the authors noted that of 18 patients, morbidity was mild and transient in the first 12, but four of the last six patients had serious disorders of mental state over several months. Apuzzo and colleagues[42] could not determine any preoperative characteristics that distinguished between those with good or those with poor response.

The comparatively small number of autopsy reports from adrenal transplantations all showed poor cell survival.[61–63, 71–74] Of seven reported cases,[61, 62, 71, 73] the implant could be identified in only three,[63, 72, 74] and TH-positive cells could be found in only one of these three.[74] The patient died 30 months after transplantation of adrenal medulla but had shown considerable improvement for the first 18 months: histology showed few surviving TH-immunoreactive cells but a considerable number of TH-immunoreactive fiber networks close to the implant.

INTEROPERATIVE COMPLICATIONS

Bakay[46] examined the selection criteria for grafting in Parkinson's disease patients and recorded definite age-related medical, abdominal, and intracranial complications of adrenal transplantations. He found higher complication rates in patients over 60. The American Association of Neurological Surgeons graft project[45] demonstrated considerably less morbidity from stereotactic procedures than in open: the complication rate was 13 percent with a stereotactically directed procedure and 4.8 percent with a completely stereotactic procedure. Without stereotactic guidance and with an open procedure, the intracranial complication rate was 17.8 percent.

The technique of adrenalectomy also has an important bearing on complications and mortality; retroperitoneal approaches had only 12.9-percent medical complications, compared with 25.9 percent from transabdominal exposures. Abdominal complications were greatly reduced, from 13 percent for transabdominal approaches to 4.8 percent for retroperitoneal.

Goetz and associates[49] attempted to replicate Madrazo's procedure in 19 patients and found significant improvement in some patients. Despite management by an experienced team, frequent medical complications occurred that persisted in two patients at 6 months. The investigators decided that the procedure required a "highly specialized team including a specialist in movement disorders, neurologic and general surgeons, physicians in intensive care and internal care and psychologists." This large team achieved specific functional improvement.[51] Some complications occurred: the adrenalectomy site was re-explored in one patient on the evening of surgery because of hemorrhage from the intercostal artery; another patient developed a small abscess in the cortical incision (an incidental CT finding), which was surgically removed and found to be sterile. Two patients had infections of Ommaya reservoirs inserted preoperatively, and one patient with pre-existing swallowing difficulties and dementia had a postoperative tracheostomy and subsequent gastrostomy.

TRANSPLANTATION OF HUMAN FETAL ADRENAL CELLS INTO THE CENTRAL NERVOUS SYSTEM

Madrazo and associates[57] implanted human fetal tissue from a 13-week-old fetus in the caudate of two patients with Parkinson's disease. One patient received substantia nigra, and the second patient, fetal adrenal medulla. No complications occurred, and both patients showed improvement.

Ben and colleagues[75] transplanted human adrenal medullary tissue from 24-week-old fetal tissue, which had been cultured for 1 week, into the head of each caudate nucleus in 17 patients with Parkinson's disease. All patients improved over a 3- to 18-month follow-up.

PATIENT SELECTION

Parkinson's disease should be confirmed by preferably two independent neurologists, and patients should have at least two of the following: resting tremor, cogwheel rigidity, bradykinesia, and postural reflex impairment. One of the symptoms must be bradykinesia. There should be a definite response to levodopa therapy but evidence of deterioration in the condition despite optimal treatment.

Because idiopathic parkinsonism is unusual in individuals younger than 40 years, this should probably be the lower age limit. The upper age limit is more debatable; undoubtedly with open procedures, the complication rates in patients over the age of 60 years are high, but with stereotactic procedures, the hazards are greatly reduced. Major contraindications are heart disease and arteriosclerosis, and patients with gross psychiatric disorders or dementia should not undergo the procedure because assessment and postoperative management may be extremely difficult. Previous intracranial surgery, possibly including thalamotomy, is a contraindication.

Patients who have had neoplasms should be excluded because of the admittedly remote possibility that the graft will proliferate into a tumor, making differential diagnosis difficult; in addition, the use of steroids increases the risk of neoplasia. Only one case of neoplasm has been reported, in a patient who developed a glioblastoma 8 months after surgery.[18]

The most important selection criterion is that the patient and the patient's family must be capable of understanding the aims of the study and be able to cooperate fully with the assessment.

ASSESSMENT

Ideally all or most of the Core Assessment Program for Intracerebral Transplantation (CAPIT) is used.[76] The preoperative assessment should take place over as long a period as possible consistent with the cooperation of the patient and the project's resources. Ideally, the patient should be admitted to hospital for each assessment, although this might not be possible for many reasons.

During the preoperative assessment period, drug therapy should be optimized, stabilized, and simplified, if possible; multiple prescriptions of levodopa or agonists should be gradually adjusted so that a single preparation is used. This measure is not always possible; in this case, the optimal medication should be used and adhered to throughout the preoperative assessment period.

General anesthesia is necessary to harvest the unilateral adrenal medulla, and, before this procedure, CT should be performed to ensure that bilateral adrenal tissue is present. Routine general preoperative tests, such as biochemistry assessment and chest x-ray study, should be performed. The risk of respiratory symptoms is sufficiently high, and the hazard of infected material of sufficient concern that interoperative and postoperative antibiotic treatment is a sensible precaution.

ADRENALECTOMY

The adrenalectomy should be preferably retroperitoneal rather than transabdominal because of the much lower complication rate with the former approach. After it is removed, the adrenal gland should be placed on a Petri dish, irrigated with cold saline, and then transected and divided longitudinally to reveal the whitish medullary tissue. Only a small amount of tissue is available, usually less than 1 g, and this is divided into five to six portions within 15 minutes of its removal. The portions are then handed to the neurosurgeon, who places them into the caudate cavity and fixes them with titanium clips to the ependymal wall. The general surgeons who perform the adrenalectomy and the neurosurgeons who transplant the tissue must coordinate their efforts so that operating time is reduced and as little delay as possible occurs in the dissection of the tissue.

SURGICAL PROCEDURE: OPEN

A right frontal craniotomy is made immediately anterior to the coronal suture, and a U-shaped dural opening is made based on the sagittal sinus. A catheter or brain needle is inserted into the right lateral ventricle, and the track is followed to the ventricle. Brain retractors are then inserted, and an operative microscope is used to identify the foramen of Monro, the choroid plexus, the thalamostriatal vein, and the caudate nucleus. The avascular space between the caudate veins is opened with pituitary forceps to make a 5-mm^3 cavity, into which the graft is placed and fixed with titanium clips to the ependymal wall by use of angled clip appliers. Allen and colleagues[41] held the graft in place by a gelatin sponge soaked in cryoprecipitate, and a central window was netted with fine absorbable sutures to allow the ventricular CSF to be in contact with the graft. After this step, thrombin was applied to the sponge.

SURGICAL PROCEDURE: STEREOTACTIC

There is considerably less choice in implantation site if the open procedure is used and only the head of the caudate seems to be the most feasible and least dangerous site. Using the stereotactic technique, the fragments may be introduced into the caudate, the putamen, or both.

A check x-ray study should be taken to confirm accurate cannula position before tissue transplantation, but posttransplantation radiography is probably best avoided to reduce the risk of radiation injury to the transplanted tissue.

POSTOPERATIVE MANAGEMENT

Because many of these patients are already in frail physical condition, the postoperative management must be very closely monitored because intracranial, abdominal, and medical complications may occur. A specialized team experienced in dealing with Parkinson's disease and drug therapy is essential, and intensive care and internal medicine specialists may well be needed. A sufficient number of reports of psychological disorders have been published to justify recommending a psychologist or psychiatrist as an important member of the team.

TRANSPLANTATION OF FETAL DOPAMINERGIC GRAFTS INTO THE HUMAN CENTRAL NERVOUS SYSTEM

Fetal dopaminergic grafts, however, give more consistent and sustained improvement than adrenal grafts in experimental animals,[23, 77] and findings suggest that fetal implantations are likely to be more effective in human grafting.

Lindvall[78] listed three major advantages to the use of fetal ventral mesencephalon over the use of adrenal medulla. First, although both tissues can improve rotational behavior, improvement in abnormal spontaneous behavior has been convincingly demonstrated only with nigral grafts. Second, fetal substantia nigra grafts have been demonstrated to have long-term survival, whereas the effect of adrenal medulla implantations is transient, and unless nerve growth factor is supplied effectively, the chromaffin cells atrophy. An important difference between the two grafts is the demonstration of synaptic contacts between fetal dopamine neurons and host striatum, compared with adrenal medulla cells, which release catecholamines but do not synapse.

FACTORS INFLUENCING THE TRANSPLANT

Age of Donor

The most important factors influencing the success of neural transplantation are the age of the donor and the method of tissue preparation, the site and method of the implantation, and the use of immunosuppression.

The basis for clinical transplantation has been animal work carried out mainly in rodents. This nonprimate model has obvious shortcomings but has proved useful for initial studies, which showed that a xenograft of human fetal ventral mesencephalon into immunosuppressed rats survived best if the gestational age was between 9 and 11 gestational weeks. Older tissue was less likely to survive or did so with smaller numbers of surviving cells. This finding is in accord with those of other neural transplantation studies, and the period is often termed the *transplantation window*. Most workers have chosen to follow the indications of the rodent xenograft experiments.

The species difference between nonhuman primates and human primates is clearly much less than that for rat and primate experimental findings and are of particular relevance to human studies. In 1988, the available evidence was that the primate window was wider than the rodent.[79, 80] Indeed, successful transplantation had been reported with mature primate tissue that was equivalent to third-trimester human fetuses. Experiments by the same authors reported on in 1992[81] suggested that dopaminergic cells cografted with peripheral nerve survive less well than dopamine cells from younger fetuses. United Kingdom workers therefore chose to use second-trimester human fetuses for human studies. There are several practical advantages to the use of second-trimester material; the mesencephalon is readily identified and is invariably intact in older specimens, so that large amounts of appropriate tissue can be prepared. In contrast, specimens younger than 12 weeks are often fragmented, and several fetuses must be harvested to provide sufficient material for implant. Stahl and his coworkers have had very poor return of fetal mesencephalon from over 100 specimens. Freeman and associates[82] showed that the appearance of neuritic extensions is greatly protracted in humans compared with rodents, and not all the neurons differentiate at the same time. Second-trimester mesencephalic tissue has been used by other groups.[68, 57, 83–85]

Usually, human transplantation studies using younger fetuses have needed to implant more than one fetus per patient, but workers using older fetuses have used only one.

Viability

The consensus, however, is that mesencephalic tissue of younger fetuses is less vulnerable to the process of complete cell dissociation than is that of older fetuses. However, solid fragments or large cellular aggregates are much less vulnerable, and dopaminergic cells from second-trimester human fetuses can survive with limited mechanical dissociation, as shown with in vitro experiments and cell culture.[86, 87]

Brain tissue varies in its susceptibility to tissue dispersal but has a marked sensitivity to mechanical disaggregation. Experiments with human fetal material from the second trimester showed that dispersed structures rapidly lost their viability compared with intact tissue, and the overall cell death was much greater for dispersed than for intact material. Mesencephalic tissue is more vulnerable than striatum and cortex.[86]

The effect of dissociation on older fetuses was noted earlier; Simmonds and Freed[88] saw little difference in the results of transplanting solid tissue grafts from fetuses between 11 and 17 days' gestation, apart from the fact that the younger tissue required longer periods to reproduce the maximum effect. The authors' view was "that there was a maximum donor age of approximately 15 to 16 days with dissociated cells and 17 to 18 days with solid tissue graft."

Developing central nervous system neurons are least vulnerable in the proliferative and migratory stages[89] but become more vulnerable as the cell process develops. Brundin and colleagues[90] showed that in rats, the poor survival attributed to mechanical trauma from dispersion does not occur in solid grafts, and older fetal dopamine neurons can survive well, even in xenografts. These findings suggest that injectionate is better as cell clumps because of their greater viability, and complete dispersion is harmful. In addition, if tissue is stored, it is best stored as a solid mass until immediately before transplantation.

Implantation Site

The putamen is undoubtedly more affected in Parkinson's disease than the caudate nucleus and causes many of the major clinical features. Dopamine levels in the putamen are reduced by more than 70 percent, whereas levels in the caudate nucleus may be only marginally reduced.[91, 92] The caudate, as the less severely affected nuclear mass, however, could be more responsive to a dopaminergic implant. Additionally, evidence indicates that the caudate nucleus has an initiating movement effect, whereas the putamen is more involved in fine motor tasks.

The problem of choice of site was resolved differently by different groups; some chose to use multiple site injections, often using different fetal tissue for each site. Obviously, the attribution of any response to caudate or putaminal implantation is particularly difficult in these circumstances, and the successful survival of different fetal masses induces further variability. For scientific evaluation, a single site, either caudate or putamen, is desirable, but for treatment, both sites would be logical targets. United Kingdom workers chose to conduct a series of trials designed to explore the effect of implantation sites while keeping other variables as stable as possible.

Immunology and Immunosuppression

The brain is only a relatively immunologically privileged site, and although neural allografts can survive without immunosuppression, they do not so in all circumstances.[88] This partial immunologic privilege is partly due to the low antigenicity of brain tissue and fetal neural tissue and also the blood-brain barrier, so that damage to the blood-brain barrier tends to encourage rejection. Partial survival of fetal xenografts of substantia nigra has been noted without immunosuppression,[93–95] and good graft function has been produced in MPTP-lesioned nonhuman primates without the use of immunosuppression.[80, 96]

In clinical trials, most workers have chosen to use immunosuppression. Freed and coworkers[97] used immunosuppression alternatively; three patients who did not have immunosuppression showed clinical improvement, but of the four patients treated with immunosuppression, only one showed overall improvement. The dangers of immunosuppression are well known, and careful consideration should be given to its use.

In our own studies, we have not used immunosuppression and have had no clinical or hematologic evidence of rejection, nor has there been any evidence of such rejection in the five autopsied brains available for study.

Survivability, PET, and Histology

Positron-emission tomographic (PET) studies, which may show increased dopa metabolism at the site of the transplantation, do not demonstrate the presence of surviving cells. Such information can be derived only from histologic evidence, but PET and single-photon emission computed tomography are useful indicators of graft function.

The first two patients in Lindvall and colleagues' series had mesencephalic tissue from four fetuses implanted into the caudate and two sites in the putamen. PET scans failed to detect any definite increased activity. The last two patients had three putaminal implants from four fetuses; each patient experienced some contralateral improvement in limb motor function and a definite increased uptake of ^{18}F-dopa in the putamen. Some clinical improvement was noted before the demonstration of an increased uptake.[98, 99]

Freed and associates[97, 100] performed PET studies in two patients who had mesencephalic implantations in 10 separate needle tracks of the unilateral caudate and putamen from a single fetus of 8 weeks' gestational age. Only one patient had increased activity in the putamen, although both patients showed definite clinical improvement.

Dymecki found some surviving mesencephalic cells in a patient who died 32 days after the implantation of a fetus of 10-weeks' gestational age.[95] Redmond and colleagues[101] reported finding some nigral-type neuromelanin-containing cells within the graft of one patient after death but no TH activity.

Bankiewicz and coworkers[102] demonstrated surviving neurons in four of five patients who underwent transplantation with second-trimester neurons, as well as strong "sprouting" throughout the graft area. To date, this is the only report demonstrating substantial numbers of surviving TH-positive cells in autopsy specimens.

There are some difficulties in scaling up from the rodent model. The evidence from rodent studies suggests that approximately 25,000 dopamine cells from the fetal human mesencephalon survive grafting from the striatum to immunosuppressed rats. Lindvall has calculated that because the normal human caudate and putamen nuclei are innervated by about 60,000 neurons each, the grafting of ventral mesencephalic tissue from a single fetus into one of these structures could restore 30 to 40 percent of the normal cell number.[78] Because the symptoms of parkinsonism do not appear until more than 70 percent of the dopamine neurons have degenerated,[91, 92] Lindvall postulated that tissue from one or more human fetuses implanted into a single putamen or caudate nucleus would effect some improvement in the patient's parkinsonism. However, the volume of the human putamen is 200 times that of the rat. Nevertheless, Lindvall estimates that 40 to 80 percent of the putaminal volume could be reached by the growing dopamine axons implanted along two injection tracts[78] by virtue of the greater growth capacity of the human dopamine neurons than that of the rat.

Five Parkinson's disease patients who had unilateral ventral mesencephalon implants from second-trimester fetuses survived from 18 to 24 months. Two died of cancer, two of end-stage Parkinson's disease, and one of unknown cause. Three patients had caudate implants, and two had putaminal implants with no immunosuppressants. Graft tissue was present in four of five cases, with no gross evidence of rejection in four. Sprouting of TH-positive fibers was present in two of the five patients, and neuromelanin-grafted cells were demonstrated in four of five cases. Three of the five cases had TH-positive cell survival, and two had local TH-positive sprouting.

Clinical Data

The first fetal clinical neural transplantation was performed in China by Jiang and coworkers in August 1985 but was not reported until 1987.[85] A cavity was made in the caudate nucleus, and the grafting procedure was performed 20 days later using ventral mesencephalon from a 20-week-old fetus. The procedure produced transient improvement, and there were no complications.

In September 1987, Madrazo and associates[57] used the same open craniotomy and neurosurgical procedure they used for transplantation of adrenal medullary tissue: fragments of mesencephalon were transplanted from a 13-week-old spontaneously aborted fetus into the head of the caudate nucleus of young patient with Parkinson's disease. The adrenal medulla from the same fetus was implanted into the caudate of another young patient with Parkinson's disease. There were no complications.

Madrazo and colleagues[83] reported on a total of four patients with fetal ventral mesencephalic tissue implantations whom they had followed up for 19 to 50 months. The patients' ages varied from 45 to 52 years, and their illnesses (Hoehn and Yahr stages III to IV) were of 9 to 16 years' duration. The donor tissues implanted were from single fetuses, 12 to 14 weeks' gestational age, and were implanted as intact sections of 2 × 2 × 3 mm blocks. No further division or dissociation was attempted, and the procedures were performed within 4 hours of the abortion. Immunosuppression was begun with cyclosporine, 10 mg/kg/day administered intravenously and continued postoperatively as an oral dose for 8 days. The dosage was later reduced to 5 mg/kg/day orally, which was continued indefinitely. Patients were also given prednisone, 50 mg/day for 8 days, then a reducing dosage over 6 months. Significant amelioration of rigidity, bradykinesia, postural imbalance, gait disturbances, and facial expression was reported, as was increased sensitivity to levodopa medication. One patient developed a bone flap infection and a small brain abscess, which were treated successfully with antibiotics, and another patient developed a deep thrombotic phlebitis.

In November and December 1987, Lindvall and colleagues[98] used a stereotactic technique with the patient under general anesthesia to transplant fetal ventral mesencephalon into two 48- and 55-year-old women with Parkinson's disease. Both were rated as Hoehn and Yahr stage IV in the "off" phase. Cell suspensions were obtained from four fetuses, aged 8 to 10 weeks, for each patient. Multiple injection sites were used in one caudate and two putaminal sites contralateral to the most effected extremities; both patients were treated with immunosuppression. No major clinical improvement occurred, and antiparkinsonian medication could not be reduced. The condition of one patient gradually deteriorated. PET analysis failed to show any increase in uptake of ^{18}F-dopa–derived radioactivity. Thirteen days after surgery, one patient developed symptoms of infection, which was treated successfully with antibiotics.

Two men, aged 49 and 58 years,[103] underwent grafting using a thinner cannula (1 mm). Immunosuppression was started 3 days before transplantation of tissue obtained from four fetuses aged 8 to 9 weeks. The implantation was in the anterior, middle, and posterior parts of the left putamen contralateral to the more severely affected limbs. One patient rated as Hoehn and Yahr stage III had improvement in physiologic tests and reduction of time "off," and the other patient, also rated Hoehn and Yahr stage III, showed some improvement. Both patients showed a progressive increase of tracer uptake in the grafted putamen.

Major Clinical Trials

Molina and colleagues[17] performed 30 mesencephalic implantations from single 6- to 12-week-old fetuses into the head of the caudate nucleus of Parkinson's disease patients between January 1988 and April 1990. Patients were under 55 years; had a positive response to levodopa but had severe side effects, including pronounced "on-off" phenomenon; and had insufficient clinical improvement with an antiparkinsonian drug. Clinical ratings were made during the "on" and "off" periods using the Unified Parkinson Disease Rating Scale (UPRS),[104] Northwestern Disability Scale (NUDS),[105] and the Hoehn and Yahr scale.

There was an astonishingly short time between abortion and implantation of fetal tissue, ranging from 25 to a maximum of 70 minutes and explained by the proximity of the gynecologic operating room. Patients remained in the hospital for 1 to 3 months, during which the levodopa dosage was reduced to an amount "sufficient to maintain a quality of life similar to that achieved with optimal doses before surgery."

Cyclosporine was given orally at 10 mg/kg body weight/day for the first month and then 6 mg/kg/day for up to 6 months thereafter. Immunosuppression was controlled twice weekly by estimations of plasma levels of cyclosporine, which were maintained at between 180 and 250 ng/ml.

No mortality or morbidity was reported, although a complex syndrome occurred in all patients postoperatively. This syndrome was described as "flushing of face" (including ears), neck and trunk; photophobia; repetitive yawning; gingival numbness and involuntary buccal movements; anxiety; facial and orbital pain; hypothermia; arterial hypotension; heart rate increase; polyuria; pupillary disturbances (hippus); piloerection; tremor; freezing of movements; dyskinesias; and sialorrhea. Parkinsonian symptoms began to improve after these symptoms subsided.

In April 1988, Hitchcock and coworkers[15, 106] began a pilot series of 12 patients with advanced Parkinson's disease (Hoehn and Yahr stage V). Fetal ventral mesencephalon from a single fetus (11 to 19 weeks) was implanted stereotactically into the head of the right caudate nucleus. Hitchcock[107] introduced a progressive series of clinical trials designed to determine the influence of implantation site on Parkinson's disease. A pilot series consisted of 12 patients (series I) with advanced Parkinson's disease treated by a right caudate implantation irrespective of the side with the most severe symptoms. Immediate improvement seen in some patients was attributed to dopamine release from disrupted cells.[106] Improvements in motor function during both "on" and "off" phases were sustained in three patients during a 12-month period of observation and were accompanied by significant reductions in levodopa. Time spent "on" also increased. Improvements were sustained at a lower level in three patients. No complications, morbidity, or mortality occurred, but the conditions of three patients with severe preoperative disability continued to deteriorate. Acute psychiatric reactions, which have been observed in adrenal transplantations, were not seen, although two patients, one with a preoperative history of severe depression, developed depressive symptoms 3 months postoperatively.

The following year (1989) a matched-control trial was performed: 12 patients were treated by right putaminal implantation (series II) while being compared with 12 patients (series IIIa) who were not operated on. The control group showed a steady deterioration in clinical ratings and motor function, whereas the putaminal group as a whole were stable (Fig. 111–1). Patients from series IIIb, who had earlier acted as controls (series IIIa) for the matched-control series, were then treated by right caudate implantation in 1990 and showed a marked improvement in clinical ratings and motor function; four patients were lost to follow-up.

The next year (1991), another 12 patients (series IV) were treated with bilateral caudate implantation and are still being followed up. Favorable early responses, with improvements in clinical ratings and motor function, were observed. No patients were treated with immunosuppression, and no evidence of clinical or hematologic rejection was found. Another group of patients (series V), eight of whom have been treated to date, have received bilateral caudate-putaminal implantations of fetal mesencephalon and striatum as cografts.

Freed and associates[97] reported results in seven patients who received implantations of fetal mesencephalic tissue into the caudate and putamen under local anesthesia. A CT ster-

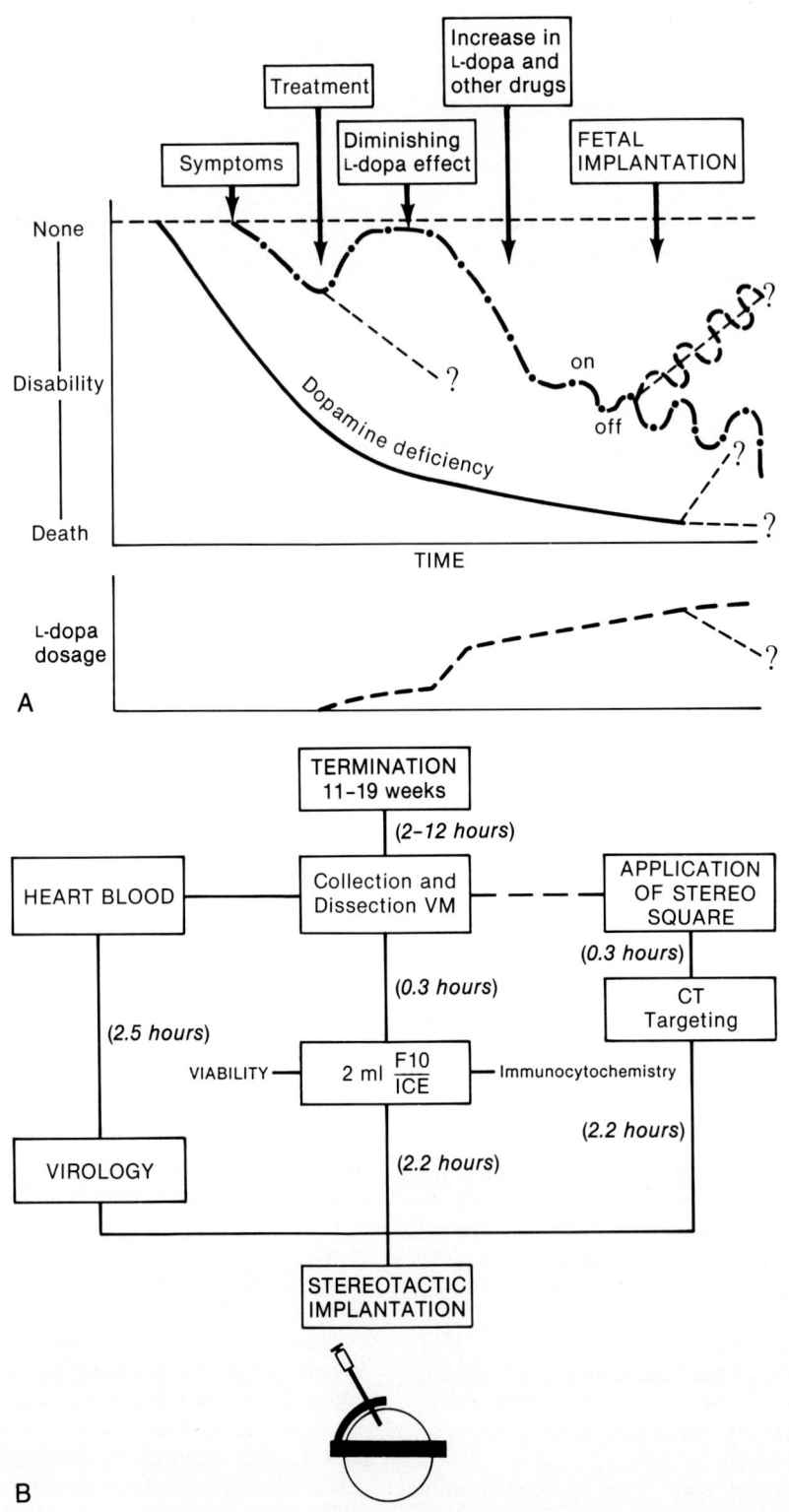

FIGURE 111-1. Outlines of transplantation strategy.

eotactic technique and multiple needle passes were used. Five patients had bilateral grafts in the putamen, and two patients, unilateral graft on the side contralateral to that of the worst symptoms. A single embryo with a gestational age of 7 to 8 weeks was used in six of the seven patients. The injection cannula consisted of a 17-gauge (1.5-mm) stainless steel outer cannula with a 19-gauge inner stylet, which was inserted to target. The stylet was then removed and replaced with a 19-gauge infusion cannula that had been preloaded with 13 μl of tissue suspension. Tissue was slowly infused at a rate of 3 μl/minute as the cannula was withdrawn. Tissue was deposited along a total distance of 15 mm in each needle tract. All patients reported improvement on the Activities of Daily Living scale, and at 6 months five of the seven patients had improvement on neurologic examination according to the UPRS and had similar improvements in the Hoehn and Yahr score and a reduction in the average drug dosage. Six patients developed drug sensitivity that necessitated a reduction in dosage. The authors concluded that immunosuppression was of uncertain value because all three of the patients who did not undergo immunosuppression had clinical improvement, whereas of the four immunosuppressed patients, only one improved.

Spencer and associates[16] reported on four patients who underwent unilateral mesencephalic implantation and compared them with a control group of similar subjects. Implanted tissue was cryopreserved in each case from one fetus of 7 to 11 weeks' gestational age. A stereotactic MRI procedure was used with two, three, or four targets 4 mm apart chosen in the head of the caudate. Procedures were performed with the patients under local anesthesia. The tissue had been stored in liquid nitrogen for up to 10 months. The tissue was kept in blocks of 0.5 to 1.0 mm^3, and after warming and rehydration, it was aspirated into a needle 1 mm in diameter and extruded along an 8-mm track to the target. Immunosuppression with cyclosporine was used for 6 months after surgery. Three of the four patients showed bilateral improvement and required a lower dose of antiparkinsonian medication, and a PET scan showed bilateral improvement of caudate dopamine. Transplant patients improved compared with their own baseline assessment, and the UPRS and symptoms improved significantly. The UPRS motor scores also improved but were not statistically significant. Patient 1 was recorded as having immediate improvement in facial mobility and mood after transplantation and thereafter progressively improving rigidity, bradykinesia, and gait. One patient failed to improve and deteriorated 4 months after surgery; histology showed striatonigral degeneration, and both grafts showed nigral-type neuromelanin but without TH activity.

These procedures have been continued and extended by these and other workers so that now more than 120 fetal transplantations for Parkinson's disease have taken place worldwide.

PROCEDURE FOR TRANSPLANTATION OF FETAL DOPAMINERGIC CELLS

Patient Selection

The selection criteria noted earlier for adrenal transplantation apply equally here. There are perhaps fewer contraindications in that the procedure is stereotactic and the added stress of adrenalectomy does not exist.

The first requirement for the procedure is that the patient has Parkinson's disease and not any other disorder, such as strionigral degeneration. This differential diagnosis requires the agreement of at least two neurologists. The criteria for acceptance in trials are

1. Parkinson's disease confirmed by two neurologists
2. Stage IV to V Hoehn and Yahr in "off" period
3. Continued deterioration despite optimal drug treatment
4. Positive response to levodopa

Ethical Protocols for Fetal Neural Transplantation

As with all experimental procedures, the patient and relatives should be kept fully informed of all aspects of the technical procedures, including the hazards and the success, if any, that can be anticipated. With increasing numbers of transplantations being performed, a rough estimate can be given of the likelihood of success and its degree. In many countries, therapeutic abortion is illegal, and only spontaneous abortion material can be obtained, but the objection to the use of this material is the frequency with which major fetal abnormalities or infection are present.

The ethical requirements of neural transplantation have been codified in Sweden and the United Kingdom. In the United Kingdom, protocols follow the recommendations of the Polkinghorne Committee.[108] One of the most important requirements is the separation between the transplanters and the clinicians performing the abortion.

Screening for Maternal and Fetal Diseases

The mothers should be screened for antibodies against human immunodeficiency virus, hepatitis B virus, cytomegalovirus, and herpes simplex virus types I and II. Some of the fetal tissue is prepared for bacteriologic culture and staining. The patient recipient should have similar screening.

First-Trimester Material

Fetal tissue (obtained 6 to 8 weeks after conception: crown-to-rump length measured by ultrasound should be 15 to 28 mm, equivalent to Carnegie stages 18 to 22) is collected from routine suction abortions. First-trimester fetuses are usually obtained by a suction abortion, and the risk of fetal contamination from the vaginal flora is reduced by a carefully aseptic technique and swabbing of the cervix with an antiseptic solution. An ultrasound scan should be performed preoperatively to determine the fetal age and intrauterine position. The cervical canal is dilated to about 15 mm, a procedure that is therefore more suitable for multipara, and the fetus is then extracted by curettage or suction. The fetal tissue is emptied into a sterile dish and immediately examined for central nervous fragments.

The material is often fragmented, and identification of brain tissue can be a major difficulty. The substantia nigra is isolated in an approximately 2 × 4 × 1 mm section, which is dissected into blocks of 0.5 to 1.00 mm^3 under sterile conditions and tested for bacterial, fungal, viral contamination.[109] Some workers use cold isotonic phosphate-bicarbonate–buffered saline with glucose (pH 7.2) and then place aliquots of 14 μl for each transplant into individual sterile tubes.[97]

Dissection Procedure for Second-Trimester Material

Immediately after expulsion, the fetus is cleansed with cold antiseptic solution and kept at 4°C. The mesencephalon is best removed by use of a posterior approach. The scalp and cartilaginous skull is removed from the occiput and posterior fossa by use of scissors and a coronal incision, and the meninges are removed. The tentorium is removed by two lateral oblique incisions to expose the posterior part of the mesencephalon, and it is convenient to remove the cerebellar hemisphere (Fig. 111–2). The mesencephalon is then removed en bloc by superior and inferior transections and transferred to a Petri dish, where the ventral mesencephalon is separated by a coronal incision. The peduncles are then excised, and the complete bloc is placed in F10 cell culture medium and kept in ice. It is then disaggregated mechanically with a 1-ml serum syringe immediately before implantation.

The viability of cells should be determined by an active dye exclusion method (Fig. 111–3) and should have a viability of between 65 and 87 percent[86]; approximately 1 to 2 percent of the cells will be dopamine neurons.[110]

Assessment

Although different groups have slightly different approaches, there appears to be general agreement that the following requirements are essential.

The assessment should be as complete as possible, and the recommended model is the CAPIT,[76] although it may be difficult to perform in its entirety, especially with large numbers of patients. Nevertheless, it is a useful guide and should be followed as much as possible (Fig. 111–4). The patient must be assessed over a preoperative period, and an important test should be performed, one in which levodopa is given at 10 PM and again the following morning. Twelve hours later, the patient undergoes an assessment of clinical and physiologic tests, after which the usual medication is given. When the medication takes effect, that is, the patient is "on," the tests are repeated. Although some variations in response occur, this is a useful basic and comparable test between different groups.

The clinical ratings used vary and include individual methods of assessment. The Hoehn and Yahr classification is used, as is the Webster Rating Scale[111] but two scales generally favored are the Northwestern Disability Scale[105] and the UPRS.[104] A 6-month period or longer of preoperative assessment is recommended and should include self-assessment diaries that record the duration of "on" and "off" periods and dyskinesia. Regular outpatient and preferably inpatient assessments of clinical state should be made using the UPRS scale, the Hoehn and Yahr scale, the Webster scale, and the Northwestern Disability Scale.

During the preoperative assessment period the drug regimen should be stabilized to optimal dosage, and, wherever possible, the treatment regimen should be simplified to include levodopa products only. If attempts at removing drugs such as bromocriptine produce deterioration, then these drugs must clearly be continued.

Videotaping has been performed by numerous workers, but it should be restricted to the videotaping of established examination techniques, such as the CAPIT. It probably contributes nothing more to analysis than a careful assessment and noting of disease rating and provides the opportunity for a number of observers to make later independent assessments. Freed and coworkers[97] devised ingenious computer-

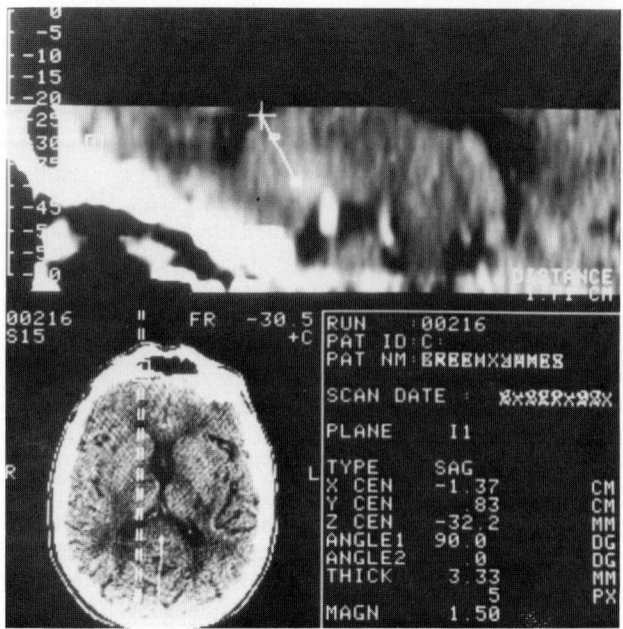

FIGURE 111–3. (Top image) CT scan through the head of the caudate nucleus. Target indicated by solid white square. (Left lower image) Horizontal CT scan through frontal horns and heads of caudate nuclei. (Right lower image) Stereotactic coordinates of target in top part of illustration were determined by using routine CT software.

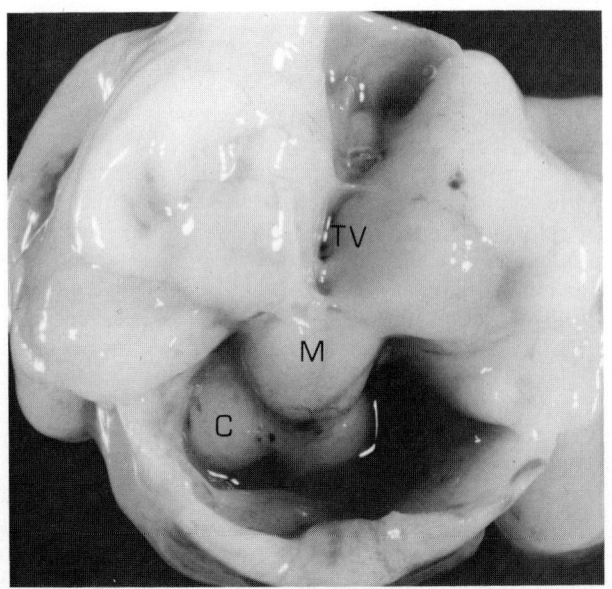

FIGURE 111–2. Human fetus. C = cerebellar, M = midbrain, TV = third ventricle. Striatum on each side of third ventricle.

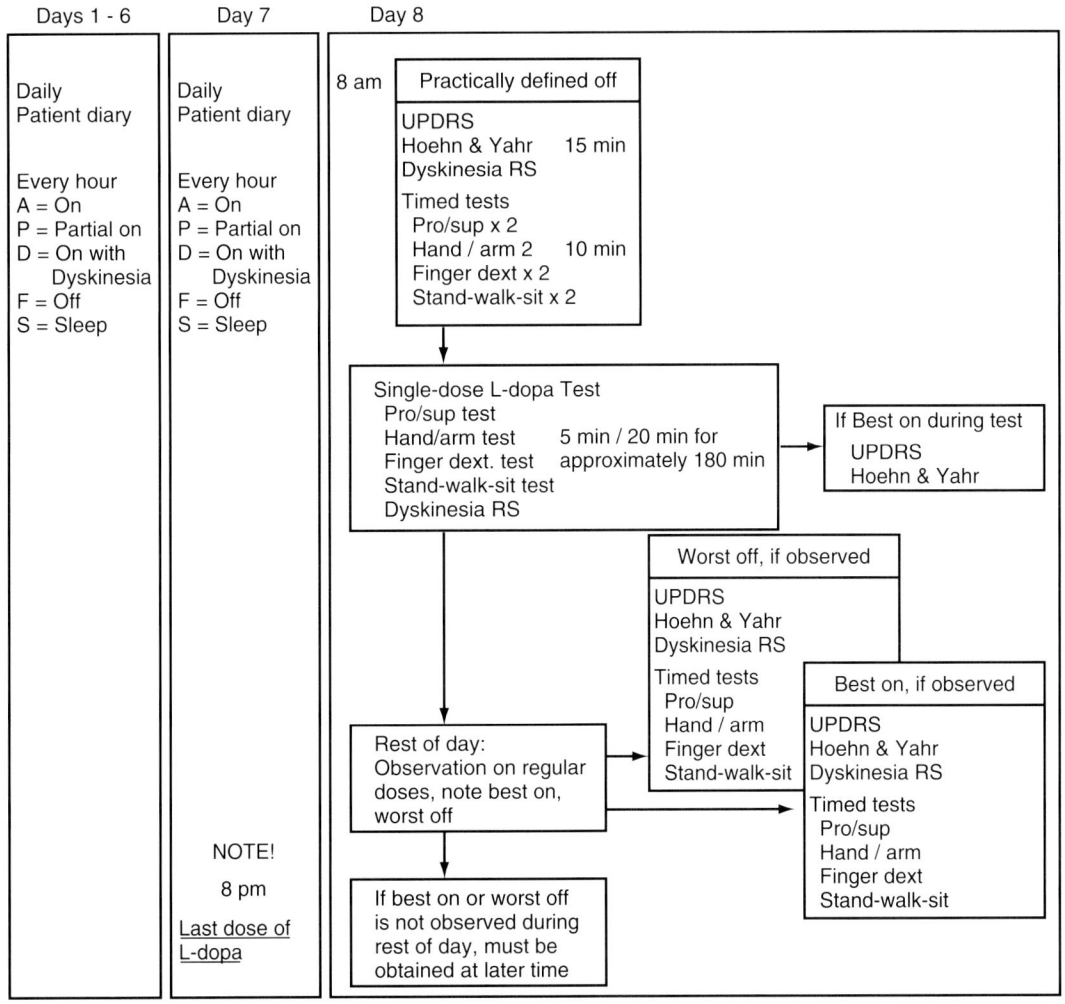

FIGURE 111–4. CAPIT: core evaluation. (From CAPIT Committee, Langston JW, Widner H, et al.: Mov Disord 7:8, 1992.)

ized and videotaped assessment methods that can be used by the patient at home.

In our own series, we have performed clinical and physiologic assessments,[106] including the UPRS and CAPIT tests (Fig. 111–4). A careful study[112] on six patients with advanced Parkinson's disease evaluated before and after implantation of fetal ventral mesencephalon to the head of the right caudate nucleus suggested that because of patient fluctuations, a combination of clinical rating scales and timing of specific limb tasks is essential. A major problem in assessment is variability between patients and within each patient, and the disease modifications produced by long-term levodopa therapy. There may be a lack of correlation between clinical rating and timed motor limb tasks, especially in those with severe disability and complex fluctuation. Specific aspects of quality of limb movement bear little relationship to the patient's symptoms, and although clinical rating scales are subjective, they remain standard methods of assessment.

Biochemical studies have been few, and the variability of catecholamine levels in CSF has discouraged many attempts to determine whether or not transplantation produces any changes.

Surgery

Implantations may be into the caudate, the putamen, or both, but the additional hazard of putaminal implantations must be recognized: there are many perforating vessels that are of greater risk in putaminal than in caudate penetration.

Few groups are now performing open procedures for fetal transplantation, although many numbers of operations were performed in this manner by Molina until recently, when she changed to a stereotactic procedure because of its greater safety and precision.

The actual operative strategy used depends on the method of fetal harvesting; if frozen or cultured cells are used,[16, 97] then operative scheduling may be arranged at a convenient time. Where fresh tissue is used, operative scheduling may be more acute but depends on local circumstances.

The stereotactic technique varies, depending on the apparatus. Few stereotactic surgeons require general anesthesia for this procedure; anesthesia imposes an additional hazard to these often vulnerable patients. After application of the stereotactic instrument, CT or MRI is performed. The surgeon may choose to use a single needle cannula track, depositing fetal material in equal portions within the caudate and putamen. Multiple cannula insertions may be made, accepting the risk of injury to perforating vessels and putaminal placements. The actual method of implantation varies between different groups, and other articles should be consulted for details; in general, however, separate aliquots of fetal material are injected at different target sites along the cannula track. When virologic tests on the fetal material are reported as normal, the patient can be transferred to the operating room and the procedure performed with the patient under local anesthesia.

The stereotactic procedure should be performed entirely with the patient under local anesthesia. The coordinates of the head of the caudate nucleus are calculated from CT or MRI with the aid of a coplanar stereotactic atlas. In practice, the head of the caudate nucleus is clearly visible on CT or MRI, and by using appropriate small sections, the putamen can also be revealed on CT and more readily on MRI (see Fig. 111–3).

The number of targets and the number of aliquots to be injected depends on the particular protocols chosen, some of which have been mentioned. Preoperative preparation of the fetal tissue is very important, as indicated under ''Factors Influencing Fetal Transplantation,'' and will depend on the surgeon's choice of whether to implant dissociated, aggregated cell suspensions or solid portions.

Bilateral implantations are likelier to be successful than unilateral, and the use of a stereotactic procedure causes no increase in morbidity or mortality. Burr holes are made, and a stainless steel cannula and obturator are advanced until they are 5 to 10 mm short of the target. The patient should be observed to determine whether or not any neurologic change has occurred after this placement. After the obturator is removed, a fine needle (Fig. 111–5) (outside diameter, 0.9 mm; inside diameter, 0.5 mm) is inserted to the target, and the position is verified by radiography.[106] The fetal material is then slowly injected at target or target sites and is then slowly withdrawn. Postimplantation radiography should be avoided because of the risk of radiation injury to fetal cells. The burrhole incision should be sutured, the stereotactic instrument removed, and the patient transferred to the ward for routine poststereotactic observations.

Improvement in severe ''off'' stages is commonly noted shortly after the implantation, but normal drug regimens should be continued unless effective transplantation results in lessened dopamine requirement. Levodopa toxicity may be manifested by delusions, hallucinations, and occasionally, hyposexuality, but this condition quickly responds to reduc-

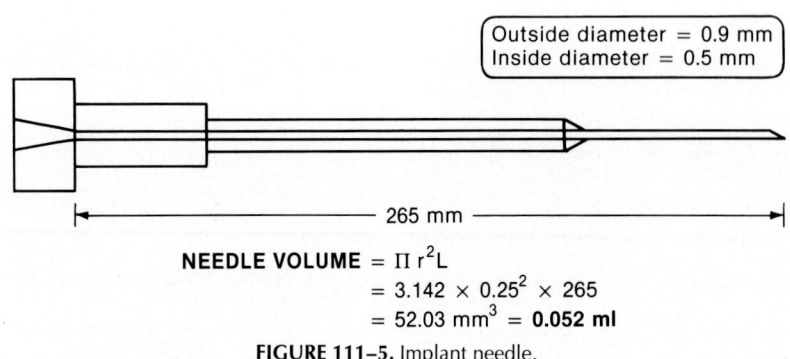

FIGURE 111–5. Implant needle.

Outside diameter = 0.9 mm
Inside diameter = 0.5 mm

265 mm

NEEDLE VOLUME = $\Pi r^2 L$
= $3.142 \times 0.25^2 \times 265$
= 52.03 mm^3 = **0.052 ml**

tions in dosage. It is unwise to adjust anticholinergic medication that has been stabilized preoperatively; it should be continued at the same dose postoperatively. Evidence indicates that immunosuppression is unnecessary and possibly harmful to graft survival[106] but those who wish to use it should consult the routine described by Spencer and associates.[16]

MRI may be performed at intervals postoperatively, and PET or single-photon emission computed tomography should be performed if available. The most important postoperative management strategy, however, is to ensure that regular assessments are performed for which the CAPIT tests are recommended.

CELL CULTURE, CRYOPRESERVATION, AND GENETICALLY ENGINEERED CELLS

The difficulties in obtaining sufficient fetal tissue to implant has encouraged an exploration of preservation of nigral cells by cell culture[97] or cryopreservation freezing[16]; with either method, a marked loss of viable neurons occurs. The possibility of producing substantial qualities of dopaminergic cells by genetic engineering is extremely attractive. Skin fibroblasts may be cultured from a host that is genetically modified to produce dopamine and theoretically could then be implanted into the host at a later date, thereby avoiding problems of rejection. Nonneuronal cells may be less effective than immortalized neurons, which would be more likely to achieve synaptic connections.

OTHER CONDITIONS

Although not strictly comparable to the ongoing process of Parkinson's disease, MPTP-induced parkinsonism in humans has provided evidence that improvements can be obtained by transplantation.[113] Human ventral mesencephalic tissue from three to four fetuses of 7 to 9 weeks' gestation was implanted at 2-week intervals into two immunosuppressed patients with severe MPTP-induced parkinsonism, and sustained improvement in motor function and greater independence were obtained. In both patients, the striatal uptake of fluorodopa increased after 1 year.

The clinical application of laboratory work to the treatment of transplantation for patients with Parkinson's disease has renewed interest in other laboratory procedures that might be applied to other neurologic diseases. An animal model of Huntington's disease produced by the injection of kainic acid into rodent[114] or primate[115] striatum shows loss of striatal neurons and motor hyperactivity that demonstrate some of the features of clinical Huntington's disease. Human fetal striatum transplanted into the striatum of such models produces improvement.[116] Similar techniques may be able to be applied in Huntington's disease itself, and a few attempts have been made with uncertain success.

Animal models of Alzheimer's disease also exist, and improvement has been obtained by transplantation of dopaminergic neurons into the striatum and transplantation of septal cholinergic neurons into the hippocampus.[117,118] The application of such simple strategies to humans is severely limited by the knowledge that Alzheimer's disease and other dementias are associated with widespread neuronal degeneration.

Successful transplantation of fetal neurons into ischemic cortex has been reported,[119,120] and isolated reports have been published on the use of fetal transplantation for the treatment of some mental disorders[121] and cortical and spinal injury in humans. The possibilities of neural grafting for spinal cord injuries or degenerations has encouraged considerable experimental work; there is evidence that embryonic transplants seem to integrate with the host's spinal cord and may encourage axonal growth.[121]

There is clearly an enormous potential for the use of neural transplantation for a large number of neurodegenerative disorders. Its use must be regarded as entirely experimental, although increasing evidence exists that improved techniques are likely to offer a reasonable chance of improvement in Parkinson's disease. The surgical procedure itself is not difficult, and its major problems are related to tissue harvesting and tissue preparation. Neurologic assessment is of prime importance, and the general constraints are such that the procedure should be performed only where there are adequate resources and experienced and expert laboratory and clinical workers.

Acknowledgments

I am grateful to Marilyn Parkes for typing the manuscript. The chapter is partly based on the experience and work of the UK Neural Transplantation Group, to whom I am grateful for support in initiating our transplantation program.

REFERENCES

1. Thompson G: Successful brain grafting. N Y Med 2:701–702, 1890
2. Das GD: Transplantation of embryonic neural tissue in the mammalian brain. Growth and differentiation of neuroblasts from various regions of the embryonic brain in the cerebellum of neonate rats. J Life Sci 93-124, 1974
3. Del Conte G: Empflanzungen von embryonalem Gewebe ins Gehurn. Beatr Path Anat Allg Pathol 42:193–203, 1907
4. Dunn E: Primary and secondary findings in a series of attempts to transplant cerebral cortex in albino rat. J Comp Neurol 271:565–582, 1917
5. Le Gros Clarke W: Neuronal differentiation in implanted foetal cortical tissue. J Neurol Neurosurg Psychiatry 3:262–272, 1940
6. Lund R, Hauscha S: Transplanted neural tissue develops connections with host rat brain. Science 193:582–584, 1976
7. Das GD, Hallas HB: Transplantation of brain tissue in the brain of adult rat. Experientia 34:1304–1306, 1978
8. Björklund A, Stenevi U: Growth of central catecholamine neurons into smooth muscle grafts in the rat mesencephalon. Brain Res 31:1–20, 1971
9. Nathaniel E, Clemente C: Growth of nerve fibres into skin and muscle grafts in rat brains. Exp Neurol 1:65–83, 1959
10. Schonfeld A, Katzman R: Autoradiographic demonstration of the central origin of regenerating fibres into iris tissue implants in the rat mesencephalon. Brain Res 197:355–363, 1980
11. Nieto-Sampedro M, Kesslak J, Gibbs R, et al: Effects of conditioning lesions on transplant survival, connectivity, and function. Ann N Y Acad Sci 495:108–119, 1987
12. Kromer L, Cornbrooks C: Identification of trophic factors and transplanted cellular environments that promote CNS axonal regeneration. Ann N Y Acad Sci 495:207–224, 1987
13. Kesslak J, Nieto-Sampedo M, Globus J, et al: Transplants of purified astrocytes promote behavioural recovery after frontal cortex ablation. Exp Neurol 92:377–390, 1986

14. Labbe R, Firl J, Mufson E, et al: Fetal brain transplants: Reduction of cognitive deficits in rats with frontal cortex lesions. Science 221:470–472, 1983
15. Hitchcock E, Clough C, Hughes R, et al: Transplantation in Parkinson's disease: Stereotactic implantation of adrenal medulla and foetal mesencephalon. Acta Neurochir Suppl(Wien) 46:48–50, 1988
16. Spencer D, Robbins R, Naftolin F, et al: Unilateral transplantation of human fetal mesencephalic tissue into the caudate nucleus of patients with Parkinson's disease. N Engl J Med 327:1541–1548, 1992
17. Molina H, Quinones R, Lazaro A, et al: Transplantation of human fetal mesencephalic tissue in caudate nucleus as treatment for Parkinson's disease: The Cuban experience, in Lindvall O, Bjorklund A, Widner H (eds): Intracerebral Transplantation in Movement Disorders. Amsterdam, Elsevier Science Publishing, 1991, pp 99–110
18. Fazzini E, Dwork AJ, Blum C, et al: Stereotaxic implantation of autologous adrenal medulla into caudate nucleus in four patients with parkinsonism. Arch Neurol 48:813–820, 1991
19. Bankiewicz K, Plunkett R, Jacobwitz D, et al: Fetal non-dopaminergic neural implants in parkinsonian primates. J Neurosurg 74:97–104, 1991
20. Plunkett R, Bankiewicz K, Cummings A, et al: Evaluation of hemiparkinsonian monkeys after adrenal autografting or caviation alone. J Neurosurg 73:918–926, 1990
21. Anden N, Dahlstrom A, Fuxe K, et al: Functional role of the nigro neostriatal dopamine neurones. Acta Pharmacol Toxicol 24:263–274, 1966
22. Ungerstedt V: Post-synaptic supersensitivity after 6-OHDA induced degeneration of the nigrostriatal dopamine system. Acta Physiol Scand 82 (suppl 367):69–93, 1971
23. Perlow M, Freed W, Hoffer B, et al: Brain grafts reduce motor abnormalities produced by destruction of nigrostriatal dopamine system. Science 204:643–647, 1979
24. Björklund A, Stenevi U: Regeneration of monoaminergic and cholinergic neurones in the mammalian central nervous system. Physiol Rev 59:62–100, 1979
25. Freed W, Morihisa J, Spoor E, et al: Transplanted adrenal chromaffin cells in rat brain reduces lesion induced rotational behaviour. Nature 292:351–352, 1981
26. Stromberg I, Herrera-Marschitz M, Ungerstedt V, et al: Chronic implants of chromaffin tissue into the dopamine-denervated striatum. Effects of NGF on graft survival, fibre growth and rotational behaviour. Exp Brain Res 60:335–349, 1985
27. Bankiewicz K, Plunkett R, Kopin I, et al: Transient behavioural recovery in hemiparkinsonian primates after adrenal medullary allografts. Prog Brain Res 78:543–550, 1993
28. Brooks-Eidelberg B, Eidelberg E, Story J, et al: Adrenal autotransplant in behaviorally trained MPTP-treated monkeys. Soc Neurosci Abstr 157:6, 1988
29. Bing G, Notter M, Hansen J, et al: Comparison of adrenal medullary, carotid body and PC12 cell grafts in 6-OHDA lesioned rats. Brain Res Bull 20:399–406, 1988
30. Date I, Felton S, Felten D: The nigrostriatal dopaminergic system in MPTP-treated mice shows more prominent recovery by syngeneic adrenal medullary graft than by allogeneic or xenogeneic graft. Brain Res 545:191–198, 1991
31. Morihisa J, Nakamura R, Freed W, et al: Adrenal medullary grafts survive and exhibit catecholamine-specific fluorescence in the primate brain. Exp Neurol 84:643–653, 1984
32. Hansen J, Bing G, Notter M, et al: Adrenal chromaffin cells as transplants in animal models of Parkinson's disease. J Electron Microsc (Tokyo) 12:308–315, 1989
33. Hansen J, Kordower J, Fiandaca M, et al: Adrenal medullary autografts into the basal ganglia of cebus monekys: Graft viability and fine structure. Exp Neurol 102:65–67, 1988
34. Gash D, Kordower J, Fiandaca M, et al: Adrenal medullary transplants in primates, in Lindvall O, Bjorklund A, Widner H (eds): Intracerebral Transplantation in Movement Disorders. Amsterdam, Elsevier Science Publishing, 1991, pp 15–25
35. Kordower J, Fiandaca M, Notter M, et al: NGF-like trophic support from peripheral nerve for grafted rhesus adrenal chromaffin cells. J Neurosurg 73:413–428, 1990
36. Date I, Felton S, Felten D: Co-grafts of adrenal medulla with peripheral nerve enhance the survivability of transplanted adrenal chromaffin cells and recovery of the host nigrostriatal dopaminergic system in MPTP-treated young mice. Brain Res 537:33–39, 1993
37. Bakay R: What have we learned from primate research? in Lindvall O, Bjorklund A, Widner H (eds): Intracerebral Transplantation in Movement Disorders. Amsterdam, Elsevier Science Publishing, 1991, pp 53–66
38. Fiandaca M, Kordower J, Hansen J, et al: Adrenal medullary autografts into the basal ganglia of cebus monkeys: Injury induced regeneration. Exp Neurol 102:76–91, 1988
39. Dubach M, Schmidt R, Martin R, et al: Transplant improved hemiparkinsonian syndrome in non-human primate: Intracerebral injection, rotometry, tyrosine hydroxylase immunocytochemistry. Prog Brain Res 78:491–496, 1988
40. Yong V, Gutman M, Kim S, et al: Transplantation of human sympathetic neurons and adrenal chromaffin cells into parkinsonian monkeys: No reversal of clinical symptoms. J Neurol Sci 94:51–67, 1989
41. Allen G, Burns R, Tulipan N, et al: Adrenal medullary transplantation to the caudate nucleus in Parkinson's disease. Initial clinical results in 18 patients. Arch Neurol 46:487–491, 1989
42. Apuzzo M, Neal J, Waters C, et al: Utilization of unilateral and bilateral stereotactically placed adreno-medullary striatal autografts in parkinsonian humans: Rationale, techniques and observations. Neurosurgery 26(5):746, 1990
43. Backlund E, Granberg P, Hamberger B, et al: Transplantation of adrenal medullary tissue to striatum in parkinsonism. J Neurosurg 62:169–173, 1985
44. Backlund E, Olson L, Seiger A, et al: Toward a transplantation therapy in Parkinson's disease. Ann N Y Acad Sci 495:658–673, 1987
45. Bakay R, Allen G, Apuzzo M, et al: Preliminary report on adrenal medullary grafting from the American Association of Neurological Surgeons graft project, in Dunnett SB, Richards SR (eds): Neural Transplantation: From Molecular Basis to Clinical Application. Amsterdam, Elsevier, 1989
46. Bakay RAE: Selection criteria for CNS grafting into Parkinson's disease patients, in Lindvall O, Bjorklund A, Widner H (eds): Intracerebral Transplantation in Movement Disorders. Amsterdam, Elsevier Science Publishing, 1991, pp 137–148
47. Bakay R, Watts R, Freeman A, et al: Preliminary report on adrenal brain transplantation for parkinsonism in man. Stereotact Funct Neurosurg 54/55:312–323, 1990
48. Bakay R, Herring A: Central nervous system grafting in the treatment of parkinsonism. Stereotact Funct Neurosurg 53:1–20, 1989
49. Goetz C, Olanow C, Koller W, et al: Multicenter study of autologous adrenal medullary transplantation to the corpus striatum in patients with advanced Parkinson's disease. N Engl J Med 320:337–341, 1989
50. Goetz C, Stebbins G, Klawans H, et al: United Parkinson Foundation Neurotransplantation Registry. Multicenter US and Canadian Database: Presurgical and 12 month follow-up, in Dunnett SB, Richards R (eds): Neural Transplantation: From Molecular Basis to Clinical Application. Amsterdam, 1993,
51. Goetz C, Tanner C, Penn R, et al: Adrenal medullary transplant to the striatum of patients with advanced Parkinson's disease: 1-year motor and psychomotor data. Neurology 40:273–276, 1990
52. Jiao S, Ding Y, Zhang W, et al: Adrenal medullary autografts in patients with Parkinson's disease. N Engl J Med 321:324–325, 1989
53. Jiao S, Zhang W, Cao J, et al: Study of adrenal medullary tissue transplantation into striatum in parkinsonism. Prog Brain Res 78:575–580, 1988
54. Kelly P, Ahlskog J, Van Heerden J, et al: Adrenal medullary autograft transplantation into the striatum of patients with Parkinson's disease. Mayo Clin Proc 64:282–290, 1989
55. Lieberman A, Ransohoff J, Berezeller P, Goldstein M: Adrenal medullary transplants as a treatment for advanced Parkinson's disease. Prog Brain Res 82:665–669, 1990
56. Lindvall O, Backlund E, Farde L, et al: Transplantation in Parkinson's disease: two cases of adrenal medullary grafts to the putamen. Ann Neurol 22:457–468, 1987
57. Madrazo I, Leon V, Torres C, et al: Transplantation of foetal substantia nigra and adrenal medulla to the caudate nucleus in two patients with Parkinson's disease (letter). N Engl J Med 318:51, 1988
58. Neal J, Apuzzo M, Waters C: Stereotactic adrenostriatal autografts for parkinsonism: Rationale, techniques and observations, in Dunnett SB, Richards SR (eds): Neural Transplantation: From Molecular Basis to Clinical Application. Amsterdam, Elsevier, 1989
59. Penn R, Goetz C, Tanner C, et al: The adrenal medullary transplant operations for Parkinson's disease: Clinical observations in five patients. Neurosurgery 22:999–1004, 1988
60. Dohan F, Robertson J, Feler C, et al: Autopsy findings in a Parkinson's

disease patient treated with adrenal medullary to caudate nucleus transplant. Soc Neurosci Abstr 14:8, 1988
61. Peterson D, Price M, Small C: Autopsy findings in a patient who had adrenal-to-brain transplant for Parkinson's disease. Neurology 39:235–238, 1989
62. Hirsch E, Duyckaerts C, Javoy-Agid F, et al: Does adrenal graft enhance recovery of dopaminergic neurons in Parkinson's disease? Ann Neurol 27:676–682, 1990
63. Hurtig H, Joyce J, Sladek J, et al: Post-mortem analysis of adrenal-medulla-to-caudate autograft in a patient with Parkinson's disease. Ann Neurol 25:607–614, 1989
64. Takeuchi J, Takebe Y, Sakakura T, et al: Adrenal medulla transplantation into the putamen in Parkinson's disease. Neurosurgery 26(3):499–503, 1990
65. Madrazo I, Drucker-Colin R, Diaz V, et al: Open microsurgical autograft of adrenal medulla to the right caudate nucleus in two patients with intractable Parkinson's disease. N Engl J Med 316:831–834, 1987
66. Lopez-Lozano JJ, Breta B, Abuscal J, et al: CPH neural transplantation group. Preparation of adrenal medullary tissue for transplantation in Parkinson's disease. A new procedure. J Neurosurg 71:452–454, 1989
67. Lopez-Lozano JJ, Brera B, Abuscal J, et al: A one-year follow-up of auto transplants of perfused adrenal medulla into Parkinson's patients. Prog Brain Res 83:653–663, 1990
68. Lopez-Lozano J, Bravo G, Brera B, et al: Can an analogy be drawn between clinical evolution of Parkinson's patients who undergo autoimplantation of adrenal medulla and those of fetal ventral mesencephalon, in Lindvall O, Bjorklund A, Widner H (eds): Intracerebral Transplantation in Movement Disorders. Amsterdam, Elsevier Science Publishing, 1991, pp 87–98
69. Olanow C, Koller W, Goetz C, et al: Autologous transplantation of adrenal medulla in Parkinson's disease: 18-month results. Arch Neurol 47:1286–1289, 1990
70. Tanner CM, Goetz CG, Gilley DW, et al: Behavioural aspects of intrastriatal adrenal medulla transplant surgery in Parkinson's disease. Neurology 38:143, 1988
71. Jankovic J, Grossman R, Goodman C, et al: Clinical, biochemical and neuropathologic findings following transplantation of adrenal medulla to the right caudate nucleus for treatment of Parkinson's disease. Neurology 39:1227–1234, 1989
72. Waters C, Itabash HH, Apuzzo MLJ, et al: Adrenal to caudate transplantation—Post-mortem study. Mov Disord 5:248–250, 1990
73. Frank F, Sturiale C, Gaist G, et al: Adrenal medullary autograft in human brains for Parkinson's disease (letter). Acta Neurochir (Wien) 94:162–163, 1988
74. Kordower JH, Cochran E, Penn R, et al: Putative chromaffin cell survival and enhanced host derived TH-fiber innervation following a functional adrenal medulla autograft for Parkinson's disease. Ann Neurol 29:405–412, 1991
75. Ben R, Ji-Chang F, Yao-Dong B, et al: Transplantation of cultured fetal adrenal medullary tissue into the brain of parkinsonian. Acta Neurochir Suppl(Wien) 52:42–44, 1991
76. CAPIT Committee, Langston JW, Widner H, et al: Mov Disord 7:2–13, 1992
77. Björklund A, Stenevi U: Intracerebral neural grafting: A historical perspective, in Björklund A, Stenevi V (eds): Neural Grafting in the Mammalian CNS. Amsterdam, Elsevier, 1985, pp 3–14
78. Lindvall O: Transplantation into the human brain: Present status and future possibilities. J Neurol Neurosurg Psychiatry (June suppl):39–54, 1989
79. Redmond E, Sladek JR, Roth R, et al: Fetal neuronal grafts in monkeys given methylphenyltetrahydropyridine. Lancet i:1125–1127, 1986
80. Sladek J, Collier T, Haber S, et al: Survival and growth of fetal catecholamine neurons transplanted into primate brain. Brain Res Bull 17:809–818, 1986
81. Collier TJ, Elsworth JD, Roth RH, et al: Peripheral nerve-dopamine neuron co-grafts in MPTP-treated African green monkeys: Preliminary observations. Restor Neurol Neurosci 4/3:163, 1992
82. Freeman TB, Spence MS, Boss BD, et al: Development of dopaminergic neurones in the human substantia nigra. Exp Neurol 113:344–353, 1993
83. Madrazo I, Franco-Bourland R, Aguilera H, et al: Open microsurgery for human brain transplantation. Experience in the treatment of Parkinson's disease, in Lindvall O, Bjorklund A, Widner H (eds): Intracerebral Transplantation in Movement Disorders. Amsterdam, Elsevier Science Publishing, 1991, pp 153–162
84. Madrazo I, Franco-Bourland R, Ostrosky-Solis F, et al: Fetal homotransplants (ventral mesencephalon and adrenal tissue) to the striatum of parkinsonian subjects. Arch Neurol 47:1281–1285, 1990
85. Jiang N, Jiang C, Tang Z, et al: Human foetal brain transplant trials in the treatment of parkinsonism. Acta Acad Med Shanghai 14:1, 1987
86. Detta A, Hitchcock E: The selective viability of human foetal brain cells. Brain Res 520:277–283, 1990
87. Dong JF, Detta A, Hitchcock ER: Direct interaction with target-derived glia enhances survival but not differentiation of human fetal mesencephalic dopaminergic neurons. 1993, in press
88. Simmonds GR, Freed WJ: Effects of intraventricular substantia nigra allografts as a function of donor age. Brain Res 530:12–90, 1990
89. Schmidt R, Björklund A, Stenevi U, et al: Intracerebral grafting of neuronal cell suspensions: III. Activity of intrastriatal nigral suspension implants as assessed by measurements of dopamine synthesis and metabolism. Acta Physiol Scand Suppl 552:19–28, 1983
90. Brundin P, Barbin G, Strecker RE, et al: Survival and function of dissociated rat dopamine neurones grafted at different developmental states or after being cultured in vitro. Dev Brain Res 39:233–293, 1988
91. Bernheimer H, Birkmayer W, Hornykiewicz O, et al: Brain dopamine and the syndromes of Parkinson and Huntington's disease. J Neurol Sci 20:415–455, 1973
92. Riederer P, Wuketich S: Time course of nigrostriatal degeneration in Parkinson's disease. J Neural Transm Gen Sect 38:277–301, 1976
93. Björklund A, Steveni U, Dunnett S, et al: Cross species neural grafting in a rat model of Parkinson's disease. Nature 298:652–654, 1982
94. Brundin P, Isacson O, Gage FH, et al: Intracerebral grafts of neuronal cell suspensions, in Bjorklund A, Stenevi U (eds): Neuronal Grafting in the Mammalian CNS. Amsterdam, Elsevier, 1985, pp 51–59
95. Dymecki J, Poltorak M, Freed WJ: The degree of genetic disparity between donor and host correlates with survival of intraventricular substantia nigra grafts. Reg Immunol 3:17–22, 1990
96. Sladek J, Redmond D, Collier T, et al: Fetal dopamine neural grafts: Extended reversal of methylphenyltetrahydropyridine-induced parkinsonism in monkeys. Prog Brain Res 78:497–506, 1988
97. Freed C, Breeze R, Rosenberg N, et al: Survival of implanted fetal dopamine cells and neurologic improvement 12 to 46 months after transplantation for Parkinson's disease. N Engl J Med 327:1549–1555, 1992
98. Lindvall O, Rehncrona S, Brundin P, et al: Human fetal dopamine neurons grafted into the striatum in two patients with severe Parkinson's disease: A detailed account of methodology and a 6-month follow-up. Arch Neurol 46:615–631, 1989
99. Sawle G, Bloomfield P, Björklund A, et al: Transplantation of fetal dopamine neurons in Parkinson's disease: PET [18F]6-1-fluorodopa studies in two patients with putaminal implants. Ann Neurol 31:166–173, 1992
100. Freed C, Breeze R, Rosenberg N, et al: Transplantation of human fetal dopamine cells for Parkinson's disease: Results at one year. Arch Neurol 47:505–512, 1990
101. Redmond DF, Leranth C, Spencer DD, et al: Fetal neural graft survival. Lancet 336:820–822, 1990
102. Bankiewicz KS, Whitwell HL, Sofroniew MV, et al: Survival of TH-positive cells and graft-induced host dopaminergic sprouting in patients with Parkinson's disease after intrastriatal grafting of fetal ventral mesencephalon. 1993, in press
103. Lindvall O: Intracerebral transplantation of fetal dopamine neurones in Sweden: Clinical experience from four patients with idiopathic Parkinson's disease, in Lindvall O, Bjorklund A, Widner H (eds): Intracerebral Transplantation in Movement Disorders. Amsterdam, Elsevier Science Publishing, 1991, pp 111–122
104. Fahn S, Elton RL, Members of the UPDRS Development Committee: United Parkinson's Disease Rating Scale, in Fahn S, Marsden CD, Calne DB, Goldstein M (eds): Recent Developments in Parkinson's Disease. Florham Park, NJ: MacMillan Healthcare Information, 1987, 2:153–163
105. Canter G, De La Torre R, Mier M: A method for evaluating disability in patients with Parkinson's disease. J Nerv Ment Dis 122:143–147, 1961
106. Hitchcock ER, Kenny BG, et al: Stereotactic implantation of foetal mesencephalon (STIM): The UK experience. Prog Brain Res 82:723–728, 1990
107. Hitchcock ER: Neural implants and recovery of function: Human work, in Rose FD, Johnson DA (eds): Recovery from Brain Damage. New York, Plenum Press, 1992, pp 67–78
108. Polkinghorne Commission: Review of the Guidance on the Research

Use of Foetuses and Foetal Material. Report of the Polkinghorne Commission HMSO CM 1989
109. Brundin P, Sauer H: Grafting human foetal tissue: A practical guide, in Lindvall O, Bjorklund A, Widner H (eds): Intracerebral Transplantation in Movement Disorders. Amsterdam, Elsevier Science Publishing, 1991, pp 171–182
110. Detta A, et al: Phenotypic plasticity of "mature" human foetal mesencephalic dopaminergic neurons and glial cells. Restor Neurol Neurosci 4:41–46, 1992
111. Webster D: Critical analysis of the disability in Parkinson's disease. Mod Treat 5:257–282, 1968
112. Henderson BTH, Kenny BG, Hitchcock ER, et al: A comparative evaluation of clinical rating scales and quantitative measurements in assessment pre and post striatal implantation of human foetal mesencephalon in Parkinson's disease. Acta Neurochir Suppl (Wien) 52:48–50, 1991
113. Widner H, Tetrud J, Rehncrona S, et al: Bilateral fetal mesencephalic grafting in two patients with parkinsonism induced by 1-methyl-4-phenyl-1,2,3 b-tetrahydropyridine (MPTP). N Engl J Med 327:1556–1563, 1992
114. Dunnett SB, Iversen SD: Learning impairments following selective kainic acid induced lesions within the neostriatum of rats. Behav Brain Res 2:189–209, 1983
115. Hantraye P, Riche D, Maziere M, et al: A primate model of Huntington's disease: Behavioural and anatomical studies of unilateral excitotoxic lesions of the caudate-putamen in the baboon. Exp Neurol 108(2):91–104, 1990
116. Wictorin K, Brundin P, Gustavi B, et al: Reformation of long axon pathways in adult rat central nervous system by human forebrain neuroblasts. Nature 347:556–558, 1990
117. Collier TJ, Gash DM, Sladek JR Jr: Transplantation of norepinephrine neurons into aged rats improves performances of a learned task. Brain Res 448(1):77–87, 1988
118. Gage F, Björklund A, Stenevi U, et al: Intrahippocampal septal grafts ameliorate learning impairments in aged rats. Science 225:532–535, 1984
119. Justice A, Deckel W, Robinson RG: Foetal neo-cortical tissue surviving transplantation into an ischaemic cortical site. Neurosci Abstr 12:1471, 1986
120. Mundrick A, Leung PPH, Bainbridge KG, et al: Neuronal transplants used in the repair of acute ischaemic injury in the central nervous system. Prog Brain Res 78:87–95, 1988
121. Clavery G, Sieradzan K, Vrbova G: Transplants of embryonic motor neurones to adult spinal cord: Survival and innervation abilities. Trends Neurosci 14:355–357, 1991

SECTION XVII

Functional Neurosurgery

CHAPTER 112

Brain Stimulation in the Management of Persistent Pain

Jan M. Gybels
Ron C. Kupers

In the early 1960s, a few neurosurgeons, inspired by the experiments of Olds and Milner[1] on the rewarding effect of electrical stimulation of the septal area in animals, attempted to treat pain in humans by stimulating these rewarding areas.[2,3] Apart from these precocious attempts, the real interest in deep brain stimulation (DBS) for the treatment of chronic pain in humans arose only at the end of the 1960s. Important incentives for this sudden interest were Reynolds' discovery of stimulation-produced analgesia (SPA) in the rat[4] and the proposal of the gate control theory by Melzack and Wall.[5]

The discovery by Reynolds that electrical stimulation of rat midbrain can produce profound analgesia without the concurrent administration of drugs opened new horizons for the treatment of chronic pain. It marked the beginning of a new era for neurosurgical pain treatment by offering an alternative to destructive and irreversible interventions. The subsequent discovery of the intimate relationship between SPA and the endogenous opioid system offered a theoretical basis for the understanding of the underlying mechanism. However, not until 1973 did the first clinical applications of periaqueductal and periventricular gray (PAG-PVG) stimulation in humans appear.[6]

The second line of interest arose from the gate control theory. According to this theory, stimulation of large-diameter fibers is capable of inhibiting nociceptive information. This idea soon found its first successful clinical applications in peripheral nerve and dorsal column stimulation. Because in certain pain syndromes, there is a lack of primary afferent fibers in the peripheral nerve or dorsal column, stimulation of the specific somatosensory relay nuclei—the ventroposterolateral and ventroposteromedial (VPL-VPM) thalamic nuclei—might offer an alternative substrate for activating the lemniscal system. The first publication on somatosensory thalamic stimulation appeared in 1973.[7] However, VPL-VPM stimulation was already being practiced by Mazars and colleagues in the early 1960s—before the proposal of the gate control theory.[8] Their theoretical framework was the theory of Head and Holmes,[9] which held that pain might be the consequence of an imbalance between protopathic and epicritic sensory functioning. Stimulation of the thalamic sensory relay nuclei would presumably increase the epicritic component and hence inhibit the protopathic inflow.

Although the initial reports on DBS were optimistic and appealing, it soon became clear that DBS was not as successful as was initially hoped. The clinical data did not fit very well with the experimental findings, and large discrepancies were noted between the results of different neurosurgical groups. Incited by the sometimes deceiving therapeutic outcome of stimulation of the classic targets, other brain structures, including the motor cortex,[10] and the Kölliker-Fuse nucleus,[11] have been recently explored for their possible role in SPA. The Kölliker-Fuse nucleus is a newcomer to the anatomy and physiology of the brain for most investigators. It lies in the upper pons ventral to the brachium conjunctivum and close to the locus coeruleus; the latter structure has been mistakenly thought to be the major source of catecholamine-containing fibers to the spinal cord. This role actually proves to be that of the Kölliker-Fuse nucleus. Hodge and coworkers[12] demonstrated that its stimulation in cats patently inhibits the response of dorsal horn cells in the cord to noxious stimuli, hence the decision of Young and colleagues to give the procedure a clinical trial. However, because only a few cases have been documented,[10,11,13] it is too early to draw any firm conclusion on the therapeutic relevance of these recently explored structures.

Brain stimulation for persistent pain is not an established method, which is why in this chapter, analysis of the clinical results is emphasized. DBS is mostly performed by neurosurgeons who have a major interest in pain and its physiopathology, and in their hands, DBS is a very safe method. Knowledge of how electrical stimulation may suppress persistent pain still remains fragmentary, and in explaining it, one is on less firm grounds than was initially thought.

CENTRAL NERVOUS SYSTEM MECHANISMS FOR PAIN MODULATION

PAG-PVG AREA

The initial report by Reynolds was soon confirmed by several other investigators (see reference 14 for a review). Subsequent laboratory investigations pointed out the close relationship between SPA and the endogenous opioid system. The development of stimulation tolerance, the existence of cross tolerance with exogenous morphine, and the reversal of SPA by naloxone were considered strong arguments for an endorphin mediation.

Electrophysiologic and anatomic studies have shown that

the analgesic effect of PAG stimulation is at least partly mediated by descending control systems (see reference 15 for a review). Because direct projections from the PAG to the dorsal horn are sparse, and lesions of the nucleus raphe magnus largely reduce the analgesia from PAG stimulation, some investigators suggested that the effect of PAG stimulation is relayed via the nucleus raphe magnus. Descending pathways from the nucleus raphe magnus to the dorsal horn have been described.[16] When activated, either by electrical stimulation or by the local administration of opioids, they exert a strong inhibitory effect on the responses of dorsal horn neurons responding to nociceptive stimulation. Recent investigations provided evidence for the existence of separate descending antinociceptive systems in the midbrain, one involving endorphinergic, and the other, monoaminergic mechanisms.[17] Several other structures have also been described to play a part in these descending inhibitory control systems. Among these structures are the habenula, the locus coeruleus, the subcoeruleus-parabrachial complex, the magnocellular part of the nucleus reticularis gigantocellularis, and the Kölliker-Fuse nucleus region.

Numerous observations made in patients, such as an increase of the endorphin content in ventricular fluid after PAG-PVG stimulation, cross tolerance between SPA- and narcotic-induced analgesia, and naloxone reversal of PAG-PVG stimulation–induced suppression of chronic pain,[18] support the animal data that pain relief by PAG-PVG stimulation is mediated by endorphin-containing neuronal systems. However, this hypothesis has been firmly challenged by Young and Chambi.[19] Using a double-blind, placebo-controlled study design, these authors failed to find evidence that PAG-PVG–induced SPA in humans is mediated by an opioid mechanism.

Stimulation of the PAG-PVG and related targets as a therapeutic tool has been largely inspired by animal experiments, which investigated nociception (acute pain), but few studies have examined the effect of stimulation in animal models of chronic pain.[20] This lack of information on chronic pain may partly explain the discrepancy between therapeutic successes in humans and analgesic efficacy in animals.

VPL-VPM AREA

As noted earlier, behavioral studies in animals prompted neurosurgeons to try to use PAG-PVG stimulation for pain alleviation in humans. In sharp contrast, little data were available for the somatosensory thalamus. The few studies that were performed failed to show SPA from the VPL-VPM nuclei.[21, 22] Experimental evidence for its presumed role in SPA was hence exclusively based on electrophysiologic data obtained from anesthetized animals. This led to the paradoxical situation that VPL-VPM stimulation was already successfully used in humans for more than two decades, before the first behavioral data in the awake animal could show VPL-induced SPA.[23]

The mechanism by which VPL-VPM stimulation abolishes chronic pain is not clear; it is not likely to result from the activation of an endogenous opioid system, because the analgesic effect of VPL-VPM stimulation is not reversed by naloxone.[18] Although investigators found that after thalamic stimulation, β-endorphin levels were more than twice the resting level, no differences in β-endorphin levels could be demonstrated between patients reporting complete pain relief and those reporting only partial relief.[24] Moreover, a much higher increase in β-endorphin levels was found after PAG stimulation.

Experimental work in the rat has shown that VPL stimulation suppresses neuronal activity evoked by noxious stimuli in the parafascicular thalamic nucleus.[25] In addition, electrical stimulation of the VPL in monkeys strongly inhibits spinothalamic tract neurons.[26, 27] Although the responses to both innocuous and noxious stimuli are inhibited, the responses to C-fiber volleys are reduced to a greater extent than are those to A-fiber volleys.[26] Therefore, some investigators have suggested that the neural substrate of VPL-VPM stimulation might lie in its capacity to inhibit spinothalamic tract cells. However, no significant descending projections from the VPL-VPM to the dorsal horn have been described. Anatomic studies have shown that spinothalamic tract neurons not only project to the thalamus but they also send axon collaterals to the PAG and nucleus raphe magnus.[28] Because stimulation of these structures may inhibit spinothalamic tract neurons, as was discussed earlier, some investigators have hypothesized that VPL-VPM stimulation antidromically activates the descending inhibitory pathways in these structures.[29] Tsubokawa and colleagues have argued that the neural basis of this VPL-VPM–induced excitation of raphe-spinal neurons involves a dopaminergic mechanism. This hypothesis has recently been supported by the clinical observation that administration of an antidopaminergic agent antagonized the analgesic effect of brain stimulation in patients with somatosensory thalamic, but not with PAG, electrodes.[30] In a recent study, stimulation of the VPL in the monkey led to a release of serotonin in the lumbar spinal cord,[31] which might favor the implication of a serotonergic mechanism.

The relevance of these experimental findings to the explanation of the analgesic effect of VPL-VPM stimulation in humans, however, remains questionable. First, VPL-VPM stimulation in humans has been shown to be an effective treatment for chronic (neuropathic) pain, whereas most animal experiments studied the effect on acute noxious stimuli in intact animals. Second, although the electrophysiologically shown inhibition of spinothalamic tract neurons lasts only milliseconds, the observed clinical pain relief after VPL-VPM stimulation can last for hours and occasionally longer.

SEPTAL AREA AND HYPOTHALAMUS

A few clinical reports have been published on the effect of stimulation in the septal area and hypothalamus. The rationale for the choice of these targets was initially the rewarding effect of septal area stimulation in animals and later, the demonstration that stimulation of these areas activates endogenous opioid mechanisms.[32] Whatever the mechanism invoked, stimulation of the medial hypothalamus in the rat can indeed suppress the hind limb withdrawal flexor reflex.[33]

PATIENT SELECTION

Just as for other neurosurgical procedures in pain control, a basic rule for considering DBS is that an organic cause should be identified for the pain syndrome, and that when several procedures are possible, preference should be given to the least invasive and least expensive one that causes the lowest morbidity and the highest comfort for the patient. Many clinical data support the hypothesis that nociceptive pain is preferentially suppressed by stimulation of the PAG-PVG, and neuropathic pain by stimulation of the VPL-VPM. Therefore, an analysis of the physiopathology of the pain syndrome is mandatory. In certain complex conditions in which neuropathic as well as nociceptive components may be involved, such as in low back pain, pharmacologic tests may be of help. For instance, because neuropathic and nociceptive pain are thought to respond differentially to opioid therapy,[34,35] testing the patient's response to a morphine infusion may be instructive. Hosobuchi[36] stated that a positive response to morphine is a prerequisite for PVG stimulation. This statement has been challenged by others.[19] However, neuropathic pain may sometimes be suppressed by barbiturate administration.[37] Hence, a test infusion with a short-acting barbiturate may be tried.

A temporary trial stimulation is the final test before a neurostimulation device is implanted. This test should have a sufficiently long duration, and the results should preferentially be evaluated by an independent third party. The aim of the test is to ensure that the pain relief is sufficient to justify implantation and that the patient is able to use the neurostimulator device properly.

PAG-PVG stimulation is mainly indicated for the treatment of nociceptive pain. Recently, the method fell somewhat in disuse for at least two reasons. First, the deceptive results of some published series of PAG-PVG stimulation made some neurosurgeons abandon this method. Second, less invasive and less expensive therapies found favor. For instance, both cancer pain and low back pain—the two commonest indications for PAG-PVG stimulation—are now often treated by spinally administered opioids. In addition, the recent plea for the use of high doses of oral opioids in cancer and even in forms of nonmalignant pain[38] is also likely to be responsible for the decline of the use of method. In the authors' opinion, DBS is rarely indicated in nociceptive cancer pain, with the possible exception of cancer of the head and neck region, which carries a sufficiently long life expectancy.

In neuropathic pain, neurostimulation procedures are the first choice. The localization of the lesion in the nervous system determines the part of the nervous system to be stimulated. Therefore, DBS is preferentially used in pain of central origin and pain in the face. However, even in cases in which the pain is of peripheral neuropathic origin, DBS may be indicated when a more peripheral location of the electrode does not succeed in providing paresthesia in the painful part of the body.

SURGICAL TECHNIQUE

Useful information regarding the surgical technique can be found in many publications, and as a reference source, a few are listed in "Selected Readings." Electrodes have been implanted in the brain for many years; this procedure is accomplished by means of a stereotactic neurosurgical procedure. Stereotactic calculations of the various targets are usually based on the results of contrast ventriculography and, more recently, computed tomographic (CT) or nuclear magnetic resonance images and atlases of stereotactic anatomy.

PAG-PVG STIMULATION SITE

Usually, multipolar electrodes are used, which allow one to choose intraoperatively the combination of contact points that produces maximal pain-suppressive effect. Because the area from which SPA can be obtained is relatively small, the crucial point in the technique is reaching the correct target.[39] Commonly used target points for PVG stimulation are those defined by Richardson and Akil:[6] $X = 10$ mm posterior to the midpoint of the AC-PC line (the line connecting the anterior commissura with the posterior commissura); $Y =$ the AC-PC line; and $Z = 2$ to 3 mm lateral to the midline. Commonly used target points for PAG stimulation are those defined by Hosobuchi and associates:[18] X and $Y =$ the iter of the aqueduct, and $Z = 2.5$ to 3.5 mm lateral to the midline of the iter of the aqueduct. Both targets seem to be equally effective for pain suppression. PVG stimulation often provides a pleasant feeling of warmth and well being at the onset, whereas PAG stimulation tends to elicit a feeling of apprehension, impending doom, and oscillopsia.[40]

Stimulation parameters differ among authors, but common values are 25 to 50 Hz, 0.1- to 1-millisecond pulse duration, and 0.5- to 2-mA intensity. To avoid stimulation tolerance, many neurosurgeons instruct their patients to stimulate only three to four times a day for a period of 15 to 25 minutes.

CASE REPORT 1:

DF suffered intractable facial pain due to a cancer of the base of the skull. This patient was operated in 1976: with the patient under local anesthesia, a 15-mm burr hole was made at the level of the left coronal suture and 5 cm from the midline. The patient was then placed in a stereotactic instrument (UTEC, Louvain), and ventriculography was performed with the patient in the sitting position, using a water-soluble nonionic iodinated contrast medium (LIPIODOL) and air (Fig. 112–1a and b). An electrode assembly, consisting of four polytetrafluoroethylene (Teflon)-coated stainless steel wires with a 1-mm bare tip separated from each other by 3 mm, was introduced. The deepest tip, to which is assigned the number 1, was then implanted at a target lying 2 mm below the commissura posterior and 2 mm to the left side of the midline (Fig. 112–1a' and 112–1b'). Stimulation between 1 and 2 (0.5 to 1 mA, frequency 30–100 Hz, 1 millisecond) first produced paresthesias in the right side of the face; then, at a higher intensity, a feeling of warmth in the right face; and at still higher intensity and low frequency (2 mA, 3 csec) a miosis of the right eye, synchronous with the frequency of the stimulating current (the left pupil could not be tested because of ophthalmoplegia). The electrode was then fixed in position by the use of polymethyl methacrylate fixed in the burr hole, and its lead was tunneled under the scalp and connected to a wire, which was led out of the skin at the right side of the head. In the first stage, lasting 10 days, the effect of stimulation of each electrode pair on clinical pain and other parameters was evaluated. In the second stage, which occurred with the patient under general anesthesia, the most effective electrode pair (2 and 3) as far as its clinical pain suppressive effect is concerned was connected to a radioreceiver implanted under the skin of the thoracic region.

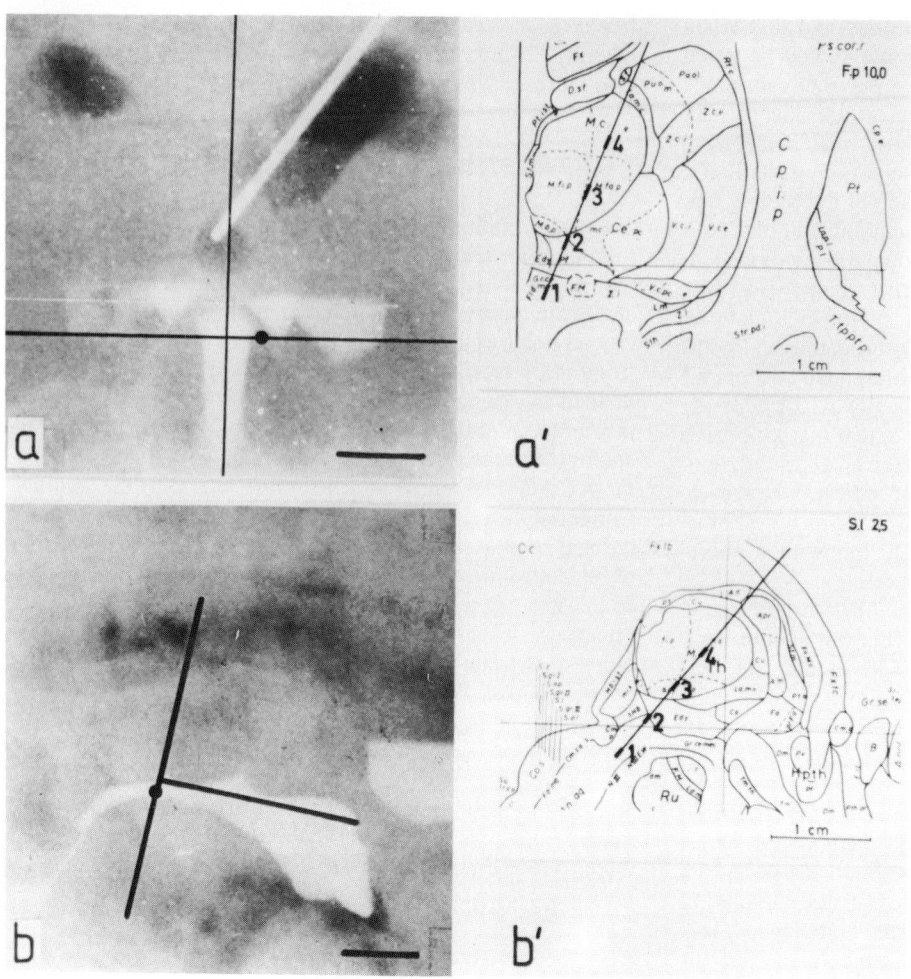

FIGURE 112–1. (a and b) AP and lateral ventriculograms with target. (a' and b') Frontal plane 10.0, and sagittal plane 2.5. (From Schaltenbrand G, Bailey P: Introduction to Stereotaxis with an Atlas of the Human Brain. Stuttgart, Thieme, 1959.)

VPL-VPM STIMULATION SITE

Monopolar electrodes are preferable for the VPL-VPM stimulation site. These electrodes are commercially available with a central stylet, which makes them less traumatizing for the brain. To obtain pain relief, the electrode should be placed in the somatotopic part of the VPL-VPM nuclei that represent the painful body site. The target is usually determined by the patient's verbal response to intraoperative stimulation. Evoked potentials, induced by peripheral nerve stimulation, alone or in combination with the patient's verbal report, may also be used for target localization. When the electrode is correctly placed, stimulation should induce paresthesiae in the painful region. However, the production of paresthesias in the painful body region is not a guarantee for success; paresthesias may cover the painful site without any effect on the pain.

Some authors, instead of aiming for the primary sensory relay nuclei, place the electrode in the afferent or efferent pathways of these nuclei, either because they believe that lemniscal stimulation is more effective[41] or that because of tissue destruction, such as that occurring in thalamic syndrome, not enough neurons are available to serve as a substratum for stimulation.[7] Just as for PAG-PVG stimulation, stimulation parameters differ among the authors, but most common values are 30 to 100 Hz, 0.2- to 1-millisecond pulse duration, and 0.1- to 0.5-mA intensity. Somatosensory thalamic stimulation is generally used at an intensity at which paresthesias are felt. Because the poststimulatory effect is generally short lasting, most patients use their stimulator most of the time.

CASE REPORT 2:

VM was operated on in 1992 for left-sided facial pain and pain in the left arm and leg after a cerebrovascular accident. A monopolar electrode (Medtronic) was implanted in the right VPL with the help of a magnetic resonance imaging (MRI)-compatible stereotactic frame (BRW, Radionics). With the patient under local anesthesia, the frame was mounted to the patient's head by use of MRI-compatible pins. The patient was then taken to an MRI scanner. The linearly polarized head coil was used. An axial topogram was taken to plan 3-mm-thick adjacent T1-weighted sagittal sections around the midline. The sagittal section on which the anterior and posterior commissures were best visualized was selected (Fig. 112–2A). Seventeen 5-mm-thick adjacent T2- and proton density–weighted axial sections were taken parallel to the line AC-PC for visualization of the thalamus and internal capsule. The MRI images were sent to a stereotactic work station in the operating room.[42] The computer calculated the three-dimensional coordinates of the anterior and posterior commissure in the midsagittal plane, as well as the length of the AC-PC line. On this line, the target was placed 2 mm anterior to CP and 14 mm right lateral. The coordinates of the entry point were measured on the skull with the help of the Brown-Roberts-

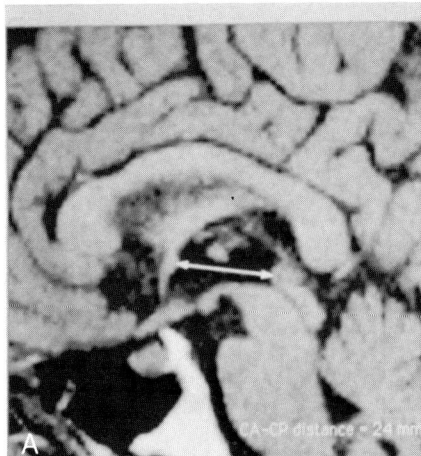 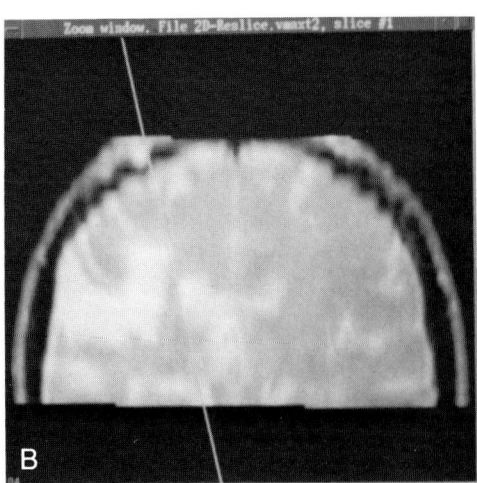

FIGURE 112–2. Case Report. (A) CA-CP as determined on MRI (T_1-weighted axial topogram). (B) Electrode trajectory through target as determined with stereotactic workstation.

Wells phantom base. The trajectory intersection was displayed on all the MRI slices, and a reslice through the trajectory was made (Fig. 112–2B). This image revealed that neither functionally important structures nor sulci were hit by the chosen trajectory. The arc system angles were calculated by the work station and installed on the frame. With the Brown-Roberts-Wells microdrive, the electrode was gradually lowered to the target in 2-mm steps, starting 10 mm above the target. After each step, the patient was stimulated, and his verbal response was reported. On target, stimulation induced paresthesias that overlapped the painful body site. The electrode was fixed in this position and connected to the stimulator in the same way as was described in Case 1.

It is well known that MRI and MR angiographic images have an inherent degree of geometric distortion. Errors of up to 8 mm are common, depending on the slice orientation and the field of view of the measurements. However, by appropriate selection of the imaging parameters, the errors can be minimized, resulting in a maximal spatial misregistration of one pixel.

RESULTS OF CLINICAL STUDIES

Because brain stimulation is not yet an established method for the treatment of persistent pain, a discerning analysis of the clinical results must be conducted. However, an objective evaluation of the clinical efficacy of brain stimulation is obscured by the lack of well-controlled studies. As already pointed out by Duncan and coworkers,[43] most of the clinical reports on DBS are case histories rather than controlled studies. The outcome measures are often too rough or uncomprehensive, which makes a rigorous statistical analysis extremely difficult. In only a few studies was an attempt undertaken to assess the effect on pain as well as on other outcome measures, such as consumption of analgesics, physical activities, and lifestyle. Moreover, practically no double-blind, placebo-controlled studies have been conducted, and only rarely has the therapeutic outcome been assessed by an uninterested third party.

GENERAL RESULTS

We reviewed the literature on DBS published up to 1993. As shown in Table 112–1, this survey comprised 37 reports, with a total of 1843 patients. In studies in which the authors reviewed their clinical data more than once, only the results of the latest of these reviews were considered. Because the way of quantifying the results differed among the authors, the following scoring system was adopted: pain relief scores of 50 percent or more and verbal ratings of excellent to good were considered successes. Patients in whom no electrode or stimulator was internalized because they did not respond favorably to trial stimulation were considered therapeutic failures. However, not all the authors reported these early treatment failures, and hence the following results overestimate the real therapeutic efficacy.

Of the 1843 patients, 51 percent (934) were considered successes. When the data obtained in neuropathic and nociceptive pain are separately analyzed, it appears that 47 percent of the 866 patients suffering neuropathic pain and 51 percent of the 469 patients suffering nociceptive pain benefited from brain stimulation. This finding seems to signify that brain stimulation is equally effective in both categories of pain. In 637 of the 1843 cases, a distinction was made between the initial results, that is, at trial stimulation, and the long-term results. In these patients, a significant decrease in therapeutic effectiveness over time was observed, namely from an initial success rate of 71 percent to a success rate at long-term follow-up of 49 percent. This difference means that in about 70 percent of the patients, the response to trial stimulation was judged as sufficient for internalization, and that of these, 70 percent showed good results at long-term follow-up. This decrease in success rate occurred both in patients with PAG-PVG stimulation (from 77 to 57 percent) and in patients with VPL-VPM stimulation (from 66 to 42 percent).

Much variability exists in the therapeutic outcome reported by the different authors. It is improbable that this variability can be accounted for by differences in pain pathology because (1) in the larger studies, the major pain syndromes are all approximately equally well represented, and (2) even

Table 112-1. RESULTS OF CLINICAL STUDIES ON BRAIN STIMULATION

Study	Patients (n)	Target	Pain Type	(%)* Success
Richardson and Akil[6]	30	PVG	N, S	70
Gybels[44]	7	PAG-PVG	S	16
Lazorthes[45]	226	PVG	N(107)	40
			S(36)	47
		VPM-IC	N(83)	28
Mazars and coworkers[46]	205	VPL-VPM	N(99)	84
			S(22)	0
		PAG-PVG	N(84)	18
Hosobuchi[47]	62	VPL-VPM	N	84
			S	0
		PAG-PVG	S	15
Mundinger and Salomao[41]	32	LM	N	53
Schvarcz[48]	6	PAG-PVG	N	100
Turnbull and coworkers[49]	18	VPL-VPM	N	57
Dieckmann and Witzman[50]	52	VPL-VPM or PVG	especially N	28
Boivie and Meyerson[51]	5	PVG	S	80
Groth and coworkers[52]	339	VPL-VPM PAG-PVG	N, S	57(74)
Plotkin[53]	60	VPL-VPM PAG	N	79
Shulman and coworkers[54]	24	VPL-VPM	N	67
Lazorthes and coworkers[55]	8	PVG	S	87
Meyerson[56]	41	VPL-VPM	N(13)	17
		PVG	N(11)	0
			S(18)	50
Siegfried[57]	61	VPL-VPM	N	78
Broggi and coworkers[58]	9	VPL-VPM	N	44 (67)
Broseta and coworkers[59]	7	VPM	N	0(86)
Hood and Siegfried[60]	8	VPL-VPM	N	50
Tsubokawa and coworkers[24]	14	VPL-IC	N, S	64
Young and coworkers[40]	29	VPL-VPM PAG-PVG	N, S	45
Kumar and Wyant[61]	18	especially PVG	N, S	78
Namba and coworkers[62]	11	VPL-VPM IC-LM	N	55
Schvarcz[63]	10	septal area	N	60
Young and coworkers[64]	48	PAG-PVG VPL-VPM	N, S	73
Baskin and coworkers[65]	9	PAG-PVG	S	89
Hosobuchi[36]	122	PAG-PVG	S	77(82)
		VPL-VPM	N	58(68)
Young and Brechner[66]	17	PAG-PVG VPL-VPM	N, S	59(94)
Levy and coworkers[67]	141	VPL-IC	N	30(61)
		PAG-PVG	S, N	32(56)
Young and Chambi[19]	52	PAG-PVG	S, N	56(87)
		VPL-VPM	N	55
Gybels and Kupers[68]	36	VPL-VPM	N	31(61)
Kumar and coworkers[69]	48	VPL-VPM	especially N	10(20)
		PAG-PVG		63(74)
Siegfried[70]	168	VPL-VPM	N	48(71)
Tsubokawa and coworkers[10]	12	motor cortex	N	75(83)
Meyerson and coworkers[13]	12	motor cortex	N	41
Tasker and coworkers[71]	13	VPL-VPM	N	31
Young and coworkers[11]	6	Kölliker-Fuse	N	50(83)

IC = internal capsule; LM = lemniscus medialis; N = neuropathic; PAG = periaqueductal gray; PVG = periventricular gray; S = somatogenic or nociceptive; VPL = ventroposterolateral; VPM = ventroposteromedial.
*Numbers in parentheses refer to initial success rates.
Adapted from Gybels JM, Sweet WH: Neurosurgical Treatment of Persistent Pain. Basel, Karger, 1989, pp 303-317.

when the results obtained in a particular diagnostic category are compared, the same variability between the authors remains. The larger and older series generally reported much more favorable results than did the smaller and more recent series. For instance, the cooperative American study (339 patients), which had a mean follow-up of 17 months, obtained a success rate of 57 percent.[52] Mazars (205 patients) and Siegfried (168 patients) reported 84- and 48-percent successes, respectively, in neuropathic pain.[46, 70] Hosobuchi (122 patients) obtained a success rate of 77 percent for PAG-PVG stimulation and 58 percent for VPL-VPM stimulation.[36] In sharp contrast, in the study by Levy and associates,[67] only 30 percent of the 84 patients suffering from neuropathic pain and 32 percent of the 57 patients suffering from nociceptive pain responded favorably to DBS. Tasker's results and our own results are in the same range: only about 30 percent of the patients were considered to be therapeutic successes.[68, 71]

Several factors have been proposed to influence therapeutic outcome and hence account for the observed variability between different authors. We briefly discuss some of them. However, most of these explanations are based on empirical observations, and they have not been confirmed in controlled studies.

Stimulation Parameters and Electrode Configuration

Mazars and coworkers[46] stated that the exact configuration of the electrode and the stimulation parameters (stimulation rate of 5 to 20 Hz instead of 30 to 100 Hz) are extremely important and may largely influence the therapeutic success. This finding, however, has not been confirmed by others. Some authors claim that the best results for VPL-VPM stimulation are obtained when the stimulation intensity is kept below the level at which paresthesias are felt[29, 46] and when only brief periods of stimulation are used.[29, 46, 72] For instance, in Siegfried and von Loveren's successful series,[72] the average daily stimulation time was less than 1 hour.

Exact Target Localization

Some investigators have argued that the large variability in therapeutic outcome may be partly attributable to differences in the exact targets *within* the somatosensory thalamus or PAG-PVG region. For sensory thalamic stimulation, the electrode must be placed in the part of the nucleus that somatotopically represents the painful zone. This estimation is usually based on the patient's verbal response to intraoperative trial stimulation. However, investigators have suggested that thalamic evoked potentials may be a better indicator for target localization. In sharp contrast with what is generally accepted, Tsubokawa[29] even reported that no correlation seems to exist between the optimal pair of electrode contact points for pain relief and that for producing paresthesias in the painful field. The problem of exact localization might also explain some of the variance observed in the results of PAG-PVG stimulation.[39, 51, 73]

Patient Selection

Because nociceptive and neuropathic pain are alleged to respond practically exclusively to PAG-PVG and VPL-VPM stimulation, respectively, a thorough knowledge of the underlying pain pathology is clearly advisable. This understanding is accomplished by a meticulous neurologic examination, CT or nuclear magnetic resonance scans, and neurophysiologic investigations. In doubtful cases, additionally, a test infusion with morphine or barbiturates can be performed. Not only the organic cause of the pain syndrome but also the psychological constitution of the patient determines the final therapeutic outcome. A minimum requirement for success is that the patient is sufficiently intelligent to understand the basic principles of DBS. However, an inappropriate psychodynamic profile of the candidate can also be a contraindication. For instance, the chance for obtaining long-term success is largely reduced in a hysterical personality or a patient with secondary sickness gain. Tasker and colleagues[71] pointed out that the clinical features of the pain may be of main importance in the therapeutic outcome. They studied the effectiveness of different surgical procedures in the treatment of intractable pain of spinal cord origin. Although neurostimulation affected steady pain in 36 percent of the cases, intermittent pain was reduced in only 16 percent of the cases, and evoked pain was not at all affected. This is an interesting finding that should be replicated in a larger series and for other pain etiologies.

RESULTS PER SPECIFIC PAIN CONDITION

With respect to the question of whether certain pain syndromes respond better to brain stimulation than others, we analyzed the data per diagnostic category. Because we were afraid that the mean success percentages might unduly reflect the (usually much better) results obtained in the larger series instead of giving a view of what is found among the authors, we also calculated median success scores. Thereto, we selected the studies in which a certain diagnostic category appeared at least four times. Then, all the results were transformed into a percent success score. In this way, the results of the smaller series got the same impact as the results of the larger studies. After this, we calculated the median value of these transformed scores. Figure 112–3 shows the results of this survey.

VPL-VPM Stimulation

AMPUTATION/STUMP OR PHANTOM LIMB PAIN. Mean success rate was 75 percent of a total of 84 reported cases. Exceptionally favorable results were reported by Mazars and coworkers.[46] In their series of 41 patients, 40 were successfully treated. Siegfried[70] reported 10 successes in 13

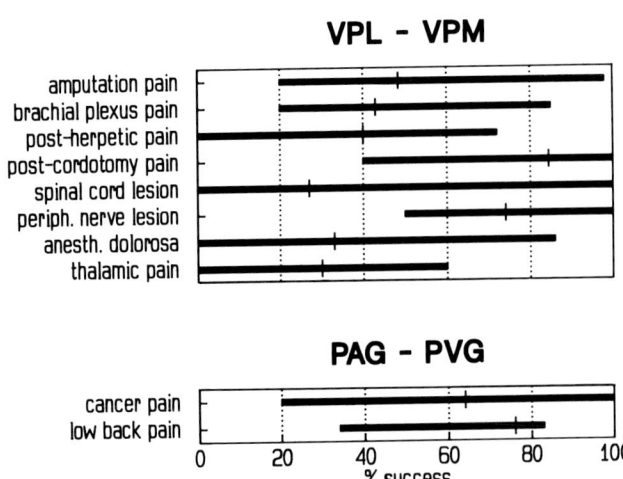

FIGURE 112–3. Results of brain stimulation per diagnostic category for VPL-VPM and PAG-PVG stimulation. The bars show the range of successes reported by the different authors. The left side of each bar represents the worst results, and the right side represents the best results. The vertical line on each bar gives the *median* success rate calculated over the different studies (see text for more details).

patients (in this section, reported success rates by Siegfried are based on the number of patients who responded favorably to trial stimulation). Much less optimistic results were reported by Lazorthes (three of 10),[45] Levy and associates (one of five)[67] and our own series (one of four).[68] Median success rate based on six studies was 48.5 percent (range, 20 to 98 percent).

BRACHIAL PLEXUS LESION PAIN. This group comprises patients with injury of the plexus as well as patients with root avulsions. Of a total of 49 patients, 27 (55 percent) were considered successes. The largest series was reported by Siegfried,[70] in which eight successes in 15 patients were obtained. Even better results were reported by Mazars and associates (11 successes of 13 patients).[46] In our own series, we obtained three successes in seven patients.[68] Median success rate based on five studies was 43 percent (range, 20 to 85 percent).

POSTHERPETIC PAIN. Of the 50 patients, 56 percent had satisfactory results. A large series of 25 patients suffering trigeminal postherpetic pain was reported by Siegfried.[70] Of these 25, 13 showed very good, and five good results (72 percent success). Mazars and colleagues[46] reported five successes in 11 patients (45 percent), and Hosobuchi, two in five.[36] According to Mazars and colleagues, patients with areas of anesthesia surrounded by wide areas of hyperpathia respond well, whereas patients with large areas of total anesthesia including most of the dermatome respond very poorly. In our own series, all five patients were considered treatment failures. Median success rate based on five studies was 40 percent (range, zero to 72 percent).

POSTCORDOTOMY PAIN. Only 26 patients have been described, of whom 19 (73 percent) responded well to DBS. Exceptionally favorable results were obtained by Hosobuchi (eight successes in nine patients)[36] and Groth and colleagues (five successes in five patients).[52] The median success rate of the four studies was 84.5 percent (range, 40 to 100 percent).

SPINAL CORD LESION PAIN. Most of the reported cases here ($n = 63$) refer to paraplegic pain. Mean success score was 35 percent. Again, favorable results were reported in the series by Mazars (four successes in four patients).[46] Less encouraging results were obtained by Lazorthes[45] and Hosobuchi[36] (two of eight patients in both studies), Tasker (three successes in 13 patients),[71] and Levy and associates (no success in seven patients).[67] The median success rate based on eight studies was 25 percent (range, zero to 100 percent).

PERIPHERAL NERVE LESION PAIN. Of the 33 patients, 73 percent responded favorably to DBS. The best results were obtained in the study by Mazars and colleagues (five successes in five patients).[46] Also, high success rates were reported by Groth and associates (77 percent)[52] and Siegfried (71 per cent).[70] The median success rate based on four studies (range, 50 to 100 percent) was 74 percent.

ANESTHESIA DOLOROSA. This comprises the largest group of patients treated with somatosensory thalamic stimulation. Of the 103 cases, 45 percent showed good results. The largest series comes from Siegfried,[70] who obtained 10 very good and six good results in a group of 24 patients suffering from facial anesthesia dolorosa (67 percent success). Failures in his series occurred in patients in whom pain complaints existed for a long time before thalamic stimulation. Excellent results were obtained by Mazars (six successes in seven patients).[46] In the study by Broseta and associates,[59] despite a very high initial success rate of six of seven patients, no long-term successes were obtained. Hosobuchi[36] reported four successes in 12 patients (33 percent), Levy and coworkers,[67] two successes in nine patients (22 percent); and in our own series we obtained two successes in six patients.[68] The median success rate over nine studies was 33 percent (range, zero to 86 percent).

THALAMIC PAIN. In the world literature, 100 cases of thalamic pain have been reported. Mean success rate was 36 percent. Mazars and colleagues[46] reported failures in all six patients with "true thalamic pain." Success rates of 18 percent (five of 28 patients) and 30 percent (six of 20 patients) have been reported by Lazorthes[45] and Levy and colleagues,[67] respectively. The most successful results were obtained by Siegfried (12 successes in 19 patients).[70] According to this author, success largely depends on the exact location of the lesion; therefore, parathalamic lesions respond better than "true" thalamic lesions. The median success rate based on seven studies was 30 percent (range, zero to 63 percent).

Despite the large variability in the reported success rates for each of the diagnostic categories, some tentative conclusions can be drawn. Pain due to peripheral nerve lesions and postcordotomy pain seem to respond to somatosensory thalamic stimulation best. The poorest results are obtained in the categories of spinal cord lesion pain, thalamic pain, and anesthesia dolorosa. It is tempting to conclude that in cases in which there is atrophy at the level of the dorsal horn and somatosensory thalamus, thalamic stimulation will result in poor outcome. It might be worthwhile to use motor cortex stimulation as an alternative in these cases.[10, 13]

PAG-PVG Stimulation

CANCER PAIN. Of 125 patients included in 11 series, 79 (63 percent) were considered successes. In the cooperative American study,[52] 22 of the 26 patients were successfully treated, whereas in the cooperative European study,[45] only 16 of 36 patients were considered successes. The median success rate was 64 percent (range, 20 to 100 percent).

LOW BACK PAIN. Pain after multiple back surgeries is by far the commonest indication for PAG-PVG stimulation. Of the 299 patients reported on in nine studies, 71 percent were considered successes. Extremely favorable results were reported in the cooperative American (79 percent successes in 82 patients) and European (83 percent successes in 24 patients) studies.[45, 52] The results by Hosobuchi[36] were similar (80 percent successes in 49 patients). In sharp contrast, Levy and associates[67] reported a success rate of only 32 percent in 47 patients. This was the only series in which the success rate was below 60 percent. The median success rate based on eight studies was 76 percent (range, 32 to 83 percent).

NEUROPATHIC PAIN. Although it is certainly not the

rule to use PAG-PVG stimulation for the treatment of neuropathic pain, some cases have been documented. In the cooperative American and European studies, respectively, 15 of 25 patients with peripheral nerve injury pain and nine of 16 patients with brachial plexus pain were successfully treated with PVG stimulation.[45, 52] In contrast, very poor results of PAG-PVG stimulation for the treatment of thalamic pain, postherpetic pain, paraplegic pain, phantom limb pain, and anesthesia dolorosa have been reported by others.[46, 70]

The following conclusions can be drawn. Low back pain seems to respond well to PAG-PVG stimulation. Unfortunately, the question of whether PAG-PVG stimulation preferentially affects the nociceptive component of low back pain has not been addressed. In view of the positive results obtained with this therapy in cancer pain, PAG-PVG stimulation could be used in patients in whom there is a moderately long life expectancy (more than 6 months) and in whom opioids provide insufficient pain relief or produce unmanageable side effects. Neuropathic pain seems not to be a good indication.

COMPLICATIONS AND SIDE EFFECTS

Provided the necessary precautions are taken, complications are rare. Occasionally, an intracranial hemorrhage or an infection may occur. In the latter case, the element of the neuroprosthesis at the site of the infection must be temporarily removed. Erosion of the hardware through the scalp, particularly in older patients, can be troublesome. After implantation of an electrode in the PAG, an oculomotor disorder can present itself, usually transiently, and the development of tolerance has been noted. In contradistinction with dorsal column stimulation, electrode migration and increase of impedance is very uncommon in DBS. In a few instances, compulsive thalamic self-stimulation has been reported.

SUMMARY

The possibility of activating more or less selectively pain inhibitory pathways without destruction of nervous tissue has tremendous appeal: indeed, unwanted side effects can be avoided, the effects of electrical stimulation are reversible, test stimulation is possible, and reliable hardware is available. There are many clinical indications that DBS can be very valuable for treating persistent pain, even in conditions in which alternative treatments have failed. Major goals to be pursued now are the search for more rigorous selection criteria and the evaluation of the results and reporting of them in a way that is accepted by the scientific community at large.

Acknowledgments

The authors are greatly indebted to Ms. Feytons-Heeren and Mr. P. De Sutter for their expert secretarial and technical assistance.

REFERENCES

1. Olds J, Milner P: Positive reinforcement produced by electrical stimulation of the septal area and other regions of the rat brain. J Comp Physiol Psychol 47:419–427, 1954
2. Heath RG, Mickle WA: Evaluation of seven years' experience with depth electrode studies in human patients, in Ramey, O'Doherty (eds): Electrical Studies on the Unanesthetized Brain. New York, Hoeber, 1960, pp 214–247
3. Gol A: Relief of pain by electrical stimulation of the septal area. J Neurol Sci 5:115–120, 1967
4. Reynolds DV: Surgery in the rat during electrical analgesia induced by focal brain stimulation. Science 164:444–445, 1969
5. Melzack R, Wall PD: Pain mechanisms: A new theory. Science 150:971–978, 1965
6. Richardson DE, Akil H: Pain reduction by electrical brain stimulation in man: II. Chronic self-administration in the periventricular gray matter. J Neurosurg 47:184–194, 1977
7. Hosobuchi Y, Adams JE, Rutkin B: Chronic thalamic stimulation for the control of facial anesthesia dolorosa. Arch Neurol 29:158–161, 1973
8. Mazars G, Mérienne L, Ciolocca C: Stimulations thalamiques intermittentes antalgiques. Note préliminaire. Rev Neurol (Paris) 128:273–279, 1973
9. Head H, Holmes G: Sensory disturbances from cerebral lesions. Brain 34:102–254, 1911
10. Tsubokawa T, Katayama Y, Yamamoto T, et al: Chronic motor cortex stimulation for the treatment of central pain. Acta Neurochir Suppl (Wien) 52:137–139, 1991
11. Young RF, Tronnier V, Rinaldi PC: Chronic stimulation of the Kölliker-Fuse nucleus region for relief of intractable pain in humans. J Neurosurg 76:979–985, 1992
12. Hodge CS, Apkarian AV, Stevens RT: Inhibition of dorsal-horn cell responses by stimulation of the Kölliker-Fuse nucleus. J Neurosurg 65:825–833, 1986
13. Meyerson BA, Lindblom U, Linderoth B, Lind G: Motor cortex stimulation as treatment of trigeminal neuropathic pain. Acta Neurochir (Wien) 117:89, 1992
14. Oliveras J-L, Besson J-M: Stimulation-produced analgesia in animals: Behavioural investigations. Prog Brain Res 77:141–157, 1988
15. Besson J-M, Chaouch A: Peripheral and spinal mechanisms of nociception. Physiol Rev 67:67–186, 1987
16. Basbaum AI, Fields HL: The origin of descending pathways in the dorsolateral funiculus of the spinal cord of the cat and rat: Further studies on the anatomy of pain modulation. J Comp Neurol 187:513–532, 1979
17. Carstens E, Culhane ES, Banisadr R: Partial involvement of monoamines and opiates in the inhibition of rat spinal nociceptive neurons evoked by stimulation in midbrain periaqueductal gray or lateral reticular formation. Brain Res 522:7–13, 1990
18. Hosobuchi Y, Adams JE, Linchitz R: Pain relief by electrical stimulation of the central gray matter in humans and its reversal by naloxone. Science 197:183–185, 1977
19. Young RF, Chambi VI: Pain relief by electrical stimulation of the periaqueductal and periventricular gray matter. Evidence for a non-opioid mechanism. J Neurosurg 66:364–371, 1987
20. Kupers R, Vos B, Gybels J: Stimulation of the nucleus paraventricularis thalami suppresses scratching and biting behaviour of arthritic rats and exerts a powerful effect on tests for acute pain. Pain 32:115–125, 1988.
21. Schmidek HH, Fohanno D, Ervin FR, Sweet WH: Pain threshold alterations by brain stimulation in the monkey. J Neurosurg 35:715–722, 1971
22. Mayer DJ, Liebeskind JC: Pain reduction by focal electrical stimulation of the brain: An anatomical and behavioral analysis. Brain Res 68:73–93, 1974
23. Kupers R, Gybels J: Electrical stimulation of the ventral posterolateral thalamic nucleus (VPL) reduces mechanical allodynia in a rat model of neuropathic pain. Neurosci Lett 150:95–98, 1993
24. Tsubokawa T, Yamamoto T, Katayama Y, et al: Thalamic relay nucleus stimulation for relief of intractable pain. Clinical results and beta-endorphin immunoreactivity in the cerebrospinal fluid. Pain 18:115–126, 1984
25. Benabid AL, Henriksen SJ, McGinty JF, Bloom FE: Thalamic nucleus ventro-postero-lateralis inhibits nucleus parafascicularis response to noxious stimuli through a non-opioid pathway. Brain Res 280:217–231, 1983
26. Gerhart KD, Yezierski RP, Fang ZR, Willis WD: Inhibition of primate spinothalamic tract neurons by stimulation in ventral posterior lateral (VPLc) thalamic nucleus: possible mechanisms. J Neurophysiol 49:406–423, 1983
27. Dickenson A: The inhibitory effects of thalamic stimulation on the

spinal transmission of nociceptive information in the rat. Pain 17:213–224, 1983
28. Giesler GJ, Yezierski RP, Gerhart KD, Willis WD: Spinothalamic tract neurons that project to medial and/or lateral thalamic nuclei: Evidence for a physiologically novel population of spinal cord neurons. J Neurophysiol 46:1285–1308, 1981
29. Tsubokawa T, Yamamoto T, Katayama Y, Moruyasy N: Clinical results and physiological basis of thalamic relay nucleus stimulation for relief of intractable pain with morphine tolerance. Appl Neurophysiol 45:143–155, 1982
30. Hosobuchi Y: Alpha-methyldopa blocks the analgesic effect of sensory thalamic stimulation in humans. Pain 5(Suppl):S274, 1990
31. Sorkin LS, McAdoo DJ, Willis WD: Stimulation in the ventral posterior lateral nucleus of the primate thalamus leads to release of serotonin in the lumbar spinal cord. Brain Res 581:307–310, 1992
32. Richardson DE: Analgesia produced by stimulation of various sites in the human beta-endorphin system. Appl Neurophysiol 45:116–122, 1982
33. Duysens J, Dom R, Gybels J: Suppression of the hindlimb flexor reflex by stimulation of the medial hypothalamus and thalamus in the rat. Brain Res 499:131–140, 1989
34. Arnér S, Meyerson BA: Lack of analgesic effect of opioids on neuropathic and idiopathic forms of pain. Pain 33:11–23, 1988
35. Kupers RC, Konings H, Adriaensen H, Gybels J: Morphine differentially affects the sensory and affective pain ratings in neurogenic and idiopathic forms of pain. Pain 47:5–12, 1991
36. Hosobuchi Y: Subcortical electrical stimulation for control of intractable pain in humans. Report of 122 cases (1970–1984). J Neurosurg 64:543–553, 1986
37. Tasker RR, Tsuda T, Hawrylyshyn P: Clinical neurophysiological investigation of deafferentation pain. Adv Pain Res Ther 5:713–738, 1983
38. Portenoy RK, Foley KM: Chronic use of opioid analgesics in nonmalignant pain: Report of 38 cases. Pain 25:171–186, 1986
39. Hosobuchi Y: Current issues regarding subcortical electrical stimulation for pain control in humans. Prog Brain Res 77:189–192, 1988
40. Young RF, Feldman RA, Kroening R, et al: Electrical stimulation of the brain in the treatment of chronic pain in man. Adv Pain Res Ther 6:289–303, 1984
41. Mundinger F, Salomao JF: Deep brain stimulation in mesencephalic lemniscus medialis for chronic pain. Acta Neurochir Suppl (Wien) 30:245–258, 1980
42. Vandermeulen D, Suetens P, Gybels J, et al: A prototype medical workstation for computer assisted stereotactic neurosurgery, in Lemke HU, Rhodes ML, Jaffe CC (eds): Computer Assisted Radiology. Berlin, Springer, 1989, pp 386–389
43. Duncan GH, Bushnell MC, Marchand S: Deep brain stimulation: A review of basic research and clinical studies. Pain 45:49–59, 1991
44. Gybels JM: Electrical stimulation of the central gray for pain relief in humans: a critical review. Adv Pain Res Ther 3:499–509, 1979
45. Lazorthes Y: European study on deep brain stimulation. Resumé, Third European Workshop on Electrical Neurostimulation, Medtronic, Paris, 1979
46. Mazars G, Mérienne L, Cioloca C: Comparative study of electrical stimulation of posterior thalamic nuclei, periaqueductal gray, and other midline mesencephalic structures in man. Adv Pain Res Ther 3:541–546, 1979
47. Hosobuchi Y: The current status of analgesic brain stimulation. Acta Neurochir Suppl (Wien) 30:219–227, 1980
48. Schvarcz JR: Chronic self-stimulation of the medial posterior inferior thalamus for the alleviation of deafferentation pain. Acta Neurochir Suppl (Wien) 30:295–301, 1980
49. Turnbull IM, Shulman R, Woodhurst WB: Thalamic stimulation for neuropathic pain. J Neurosurg 52:486–493, 1980
50. Dieckmann G, Witzmann A: Initial and long-term results of deep brain stimulation for chronic intractable pain. Appl Neurophysiol 45:167–172, 1982
51. Boivie J, Meyerson BA: A correlative anatomical and clinical study of pain suppression by deep brain stimulation. Pain 13:113–126, 1982
52. Groth K, Adams J, Richardson D, et al: Deep Brain Stimulation for Chronic Intractable Pain. Minneapolis, Medtronic, 1982
53. Plotkin R: Results in 60 cases of deep brain stimulation for chronic intractable pain. Appl Neurophysiol 45:173–178, 1982
54. Shulman R, Turnbull IM, Diewold P: Psychiatric aspects of thalamic stimulation for neuropathic pain. Pain 13:127–135, 1982
55. Lazorthes Y, Siegfried J, Gouarderes C, et al: Periventricular gray matter stimulation versus chronic intrathecal morphine in cancer pain. Adv Pain Res Ther 5:467–475, 1983
56. Meyerson BA: Electrostimulation procedures: Effects, presumed rationale, and possible mechanisms. Adv Pain Res Ther 5:495–534, 1983
57. Siegfried J: Long-term results of electrical stimulation in the treatment of pain by means of implanted electrodes (epidural spinal cord and deep brain stimulation), in Rizzi R, Visentin M (eds): Pain Therapy. Amsterdam, Elsevier, 1983, pp 463–475
58. Broggi G, Franzini A, Giorgi C, et al: Preliminary results of specific thalamic stimulation for the deafferentation pain. Acta Neurochir Suppl (Wien) 33:497–500, 1984
59. Broseta J, Roldán P, Masbout G, Barcia-Salorio JL: Chronic VPM thalamic stimulation in facial anaesthesia dolorosa following trigeminal surgery. Acta Neurochir Suppl (Wien) 33:505–506, 1984
60. Hood TW, Siegfried J: Epidural versus thalamic stimulation for the management of brachial plexus lesion pain. Acta Neurochir Suppl (Wien) 33:451–457, 1984
61. Kumar K, Wyant GM : Deep brain stimulation for alleviating chronic intractable pain. Can J Surg 28:20–22, 1985
62. Namba S, Wani T, Shimizu Y, et al: Sensory and motor responses to deep brain stimulation. Correlation with anatomical structures. J Neurosurg 63:224–234, 1985
63. Schvarcz JR: Chronic stimulation of the septal area for the relief of intractable pain. Appl Neurophysiol 48:191–194, 1985
64. Young RF, Kroening R, Fulton W, et al: Electrical stimulation of the brain in treatment of chronic pain. Experience of over 5 years. J Neurosurg 62:389–396, 1985
65. Baskin DS, Mehler WR, Hosobuchi Y, et al: Autopsy analysis of the safety, efficacy and cartography of electrical stimulation of the central gray in humans. Brain Res 371:231–236, 1986
66. Young RF, Brechner T: Electrical stimulation of the brain for relief of intractable pain due to cancer. Cancer 57:1266–1272, 1986
67. Levy RM, Lamb S, Adams JE: Treatment of chronic pain by deep brain stimulation: Long term follow-up and review of the literature. Neurosurgery 21:885–893, 1987
68. Gybels J, Kupers R: Deep brain stimulation in the treatment of chronic pain in man: Where and why? Neurophysiol Clin 20:389–398, 1990
69. Kumar K, Wyant GM, Nath R: Deep brain stimulation for control of intractable pain in humans, present and future: A ten-years' follow-up. Neurosurgery 26:774–782, 1990
70. Siegfried J. Therapeutical neurostimulation—indications reconsidered. Acta Neurochir Suppl (Wien) 52:112–117, 1991
71. Tasker RR, DeCarvalho GTC, Dolan EJ: Intractable pain of spinal cord origin: Clinical features and implications for surgery. J Neurosurg 77:373–378, 1992
72. Siegfried J, van Loveren H: Thalamic stimulation: Effects on deafferentation pain and movement disorders, in Samii M (ed): Surgery in and Around the Brain Stem and the Third Ventricle. Berlin, Springer, 1986, pp 540–546
73. Gybels J, Dom R, Cosyns P: Electrical stimulation of the central gray for pain relief in human: Autopsy data. Acta Neurochir Suppl (Wien) 30:259–268, 1980
74. Schaltenbrand G, Bailey P: Introduction to Stereotaxis with an Atlas of the Human Brain. Stuttgart, Thieme, 1959

SELECTED READINGS

Gybels JM, Sweet WH: Neurosurgical Treatment of Persistent Pain. Basel, Karger, 1989, pp 303–317
Meyerson BA: Electric stimulation of the spinal cord and brain, in Bonica JJ (ed): The Management of Pain, vol 2, 2nd ed. Philadelphia, Lea & Febiger, 1990, pp 1868–1877
Tasker RR, de Carvalho G, Dostrovsky JO: The history of central pain syndromes, with observations concerning pathophysiology and treatment, in Casey KL (ed): Pain and Central Nervous System Disease: The Central Pain Syndromes. New York, Raven Press, 1991, pp 31–58
Young RF: Brain stimulation, in Wall PD, Melzack R (eds): Textbook of Pain, 2nd ed. Edinburgh, Churchill Livingstone, 1989, pp 925–929

CHAPTER 112A

Commentary

Ronald F. Young

Drs. Gybels and Kupers have provided an excellent review of the subject of brain stimulation for the treatment of chronic pain. The authors begin with a thorough review of the basic science foundation for the application of this technique in humans. I do not agree with their statement that brain stimulation for persistent pain cannot be considered an established method. As their own review clearly indicates, brain stimulation has been in use on a regular clinical basis for well over 20 years, and initial attempts extend as far back as 30 years or more. The authors have, in fact, reviewed over 1800 patients who have undergone implantation worldwide, and considerably more patients, perhaps twice as many, have undergone implantation and have not been reported in scientific publications. I am much more in agreement with the sentiments expressed in the conclusions of this chapter, in which the authors state that "there are many clinical indications that deep brain stimulation (DBS) can be very valuable for treating persistent pain even in those conditions in which alternative treatments have failed." DBS clearly provides a potential means of treatment for patients suffering from chronic pain who are unresponsive to the usual pain therapies. When these therapies have been exhausted, DBS often offers the only therapeutic alternative. Although questions remain about the efficacy of DBS in certain chronic pain syndromes and although significant variations exist in the reported success rates from different groups using these techniques, the basic effectiveness and safety of brain stimulation for the treatment of chronic pain seems well established.

In general, I agree with the authors' comments regarding patient selection. I do not agree with the dichotomy that states that periaqueductal or periventricular gray stimulation should be applied to nociceptive pain and that sensory thalamic (VPL/VPM) stimulation should be used for neuropathic pain. Consequently, I do not agree with the authors' statements that knowing the type of pain syndrome is essential before electrode implantation. Much disagreement exists as to how a particular pain problem might be categorized as nociceptive or neuropathic. Whether categorization should be based on the type of pain described, that is, burning, for neuropathic, and other descriptors for nociceptive; whether it should be based on specific aspects of the physical examination, such as hypersensitivity to mechanical contact, allodynia, or demonstrated areas of sensory loss; or whether it should be based on radiographic studies, for instance, magnetic resonance imaging (MRI) showing tissue destruction in the thalamic syndrome, is controversial. Whether pain should be categorized as nociceptive or neuropathic based on responses to pharmacologic agents, such as opiates or barbiturates, is also controversial. Our approach has been to recommend implantation of electrodes in both periaqueductal or periventricular gray areas and VPL/VPM and to base decisions about final electrode implantation on a period of trial stimulation. With this approach, characterizing the patient's pain as nociceptive or neuropathic before electrode implantation is unnecessary.

My colleagues and I have carefully studied the usefulness of preoperative intravenous morphine infusion in the selection of patients for brain stimulation. We have found no significant difference in either our immediate or our long-term results in patients selected with or without the morphine infusion tests, and we no longer recommend this test for patient selection.

Our two most important selection criteria concern adequate prior treatment of the patient's pain syndrome and assessment of the patient's psychological status. We require that the patients have adequate treatment with pharmacologic agents, physical therapy, local anesthetic injections, acupuncture, biofeedback, and behavioral therapy, along with other treatments that may be indicated by the patient's particular pain complaint. Although we believe that all available treatments cannot be used in all patients before brain stimulation, we do believe that a reasonable trial of other treatment methods should be undertaken before DBS implantation is considered. Psychological assessment is critical, as pointed out by the authors. Patients with hysterical components to their personalities frequently show short-term benefit but rarely long-term benefit from any form of neurostimulation, including DBS. Likewise, patients with somatiform disorders, secondary gain related to their pain, and hypochondriasis rarely benefit. Preoperative testing with psychological test instruments such as the Minnesota Multiphasic Personality Inventory–II (MMPI-II) and a psychological or psychiatric interview are essential for patient selection.

I generally agree with the authors' discussion of the technical aspects of brain stimulator implantation. We now exclusively employ MRI T1-weighted sagittal and axial images. Our technique is considerably simpler than that described in the authors' illustrative case of a VPL electrode implantation. Our MRI technique involves the use of routine T1-weighted sagittal images on which the anterior and posterior commissures are identified. Axial 3-mm-thick sections are then obtained parallel to the anterior commissure–posterior commissure line. With the Leksell stereotactic system, the x, y, and z coordinates of the implantation targets can be manually calculated in a few minutes. The Leksell system is considerably easier to use than the Brown-Roberts-Wells system. The authors indicate that errors of up to 8 mm are common on MRI images, depending on slice orientation in the field of view to the measurements. We have carried out a detailed comparison of ventriculographic, computed tomographic, and MRI target localization. If accepted techniques are used to minimize MRI field distortion, we do not believe that any differences of clinical significance exist between the three techniques in determining stereotactic coordinates for brain electrode implantation. We have also carefully compared differences between the three stereotactic coordinate determination techniques and the localization of the intended target physiologically and again do not find any significant variation. We believe that the MRI technique is the easiest and safest for electrode implantation.

Our implantation technique also differs from that of the authors on many minor but nevertheless important points. First, the authors described an illustrative case of electrode implantation in the periaqueductal gray region. They suggested that a burr hole be made at the level of the coronal suture and 5 cm from the midline. We typically locate our burr hole for electrode implantation just anterior to the coronal suture and approximately 15 to 20 mm from the midline. With this technique, there is easy access to the periaqueductal and periventricular gray region, and in addition, simultaneous implantation of a second electrode through the same burr hole allows an approximately consistent parasagittal orientation between the introduced electrode and the midline, thereby providing the best access to the somatosensory thalamic nuclei.

The authors described two different types of electrodes for implantation. To my knowledge, neither one of these electrode systems is either available or approved for brain implantation in the United States. These electrodes may be acceptable in Europe, but I would not recommend their use in the United States. The electrodes available for implantation in the United States consist of platinum-iridium electrode contact surfaces of a multicontact design. To my knowledge, no stainless steel electrode or monopolar electrode is approved for implantation in the United States.

In describing the results of the various clinical studies published in the literature, the authors rightfully criticized the lack of double-blind placebo-controlled studies and those in which the therapeutic outcome has been assessed by an uninterested third party. Although these criticisms are certainly valid, they could as well be leveled at many of the surgical interventions for the treatment of pain, including other forms of neurostimulation, such as spinal stimulation, as well as drug-infusion techniques. In fact, the authors indicate that interest in DPS may be decreasing because of the use of spinal opiate infusion for treating low back pain resulting from cancerous and noncancerous conditions. In my opinion, substantially less information exists regarding the efficacy of spinal opiate infusion for treating low back pain than exists for the use of DPS in treating low back pain. The studies related to spinal opiate infusion for low back pain are also rarely double blind and are rarely placebo controlled, and rarely are the therapeutic options assessed by a disinterested third party. In addition, the length of follow-up on most of the spinal infusion studies is extremely short, whereas the follow-up studies for brain stimulation, as mentioned, extend as far as 10 to 20 years. As a consequence, I believe that the studies establishing the safety and efficacy of DPS for treating chronic pain are at least as good as those establishing the safety and efficacy of other operative interventions.

The authors correctly point out the variability in success rates reported by different groups throughout the world. I believe that this variability is related to differences in criteria for patient selection criteria and for identifying successful treatments, accuracy, and honesty of application of these criteria, length of follow-up, and use of disinterested observers. I do not believe the differences in results are related to differences in the types of pain syndromes treated nor in their distribution in the various series, nor do I believe that these differences are related to alterations in variations of techniques, implantation targets, or stimulation parameters.

My own experience includes the implantation of 394 DBS electrodes in 187 patients in the 15-year interval between 1978 and 1993. Of these 187 patients, 27 were considered to have pain purely of nociceptive origin, 74 were considered to have pain purely of neuropathic origin, and 86 were considered to have pain of mixed nociceptive and neuropathic origin. One hundred forty-two patients underwent initial electrode implantation in periaqueductal or periventricular gray regions and sensory thalamus. Thirty-five patients had electrodes implanted either unilaterally or bilaterally in the periaqueductal or periventricular gray regions alone. Four patients had electrode implantations in periventricular gray regions and the nucleus Kölliker-Fuse, three patients had electrodes implanted in the sensory thalamus alone, and three patients had electrodes placed in other combinations. Based on the results of trial stimulation, 149 patients (79.7 percent) underwent permanent electrode implantation. There were small variations in the rates of internalization of patients with nociceptive, neuropathic, and mixed pain syndromes. Long-term results were considered excellent, good, or unsuccessful. Excellent pain relief was based on the patient's description of at least 50 percent reduction in pain intensity, no use of narcotic analgesics, and physical functioning appropriate to the patient's overall general physical condition and neurologic disability. Pain relief was considered good in patients with greater than 50 percent reduction in pain intensity and some mild or intermittent use of mild narcotics, such as codeine. These patients also had appropriate levels of physical functioning. According to this assessment technique, a significantly better outcome occurred: 76 percent of patients with nociceptive pain experienced excellent or good pain relief, whereas only 49 percent of those with neuropathic pain experienced a similar level of pain relief. Patients with mixed etiologies fell between these two groups in terms of efficacy of DBS.

The long-term results are not as good when all patients who underwent DPS are considered. Using our assessment technique, 35 percent of patients with neuropathic pain obtained either excellent or good pain relief, whereas 59 percent of those with nociceptive pain syndromes achieved similar results. Patients with pain of mixed origins appeared to fare about the same as those with nociceptive pain. When all patients were considered together, 89 of the original 187 patients (48 percent) achieved excellent or good pain relief. The median follow-up of our patients is more than 7 years, and all but 15 patients have been followed up for more than 1 year since electrode implantation.

Considering the number of patients in our study, the length of time over which they have been followed up, and particularly, our results in comparison to those described by the authors and published in the world literature, the efficacy of

DPS in treating various difficult pain conditions is well established. I agree completely with the authors that refinements in selection techniques and more critical reporting of results would allow a more careful assessment of the effectiveness of DBS; nevertheless, DBS clearly offers the only available form of treatment for certain difficult painful conditions.

In my opinion, the authors have failed to sufficiently emphasize the complications associated with DPS. The complications we have experienced are described in Table 112–5. Forty-two patients (22 percent) in our series suffered some form of complication related to the electrode implantation. Complications were early, such as hemiparesis, diplopia, or sensory loss; delayed a few weeks, such as infection; or delayed many months or years, such as fractured electrodes, pain at the site of stimulator implantation, and delayed subdural hematoma. Six patients suffered permanent complications of electrode implantation, including diplopia, sensory loss, hemiparesis, and intracerebral hematoma. One death, although not directly related to electrode implantation, occurred in this series. Therefore, seven patients (3.7 percent) suffered either permanent complications or died as a result of DBS implantation. Although this is, in my opinion, an acceptably low complication rate, it emphasizes that DBS electrode implantation should be contemplated only for patients in whom a reasonable and adequate trial of other therapeutic modalities has been carried out before DBS electrode implantation.

I believe that future developments in DBS hardware are likely to improve the results and reduce complications. The authors do not discuss the use of fully implanted pulse generators for DPS. These devices have reduced the problems related to radiofrequency coupled transmitter receiver systems, which have included excessive stimulation by the patient, damage to external transmitter systems and antennas, difficulty with radiofrequency coupling for transcutaneous electrical stimulation, and the need for frequent battery replacements. The fully implanted pulse-generating systems represent an improvement over passive radiofrequency transmitter-receiver systems. Internal pulse generators with battery lives in the 3- to 5-year range are now available, and these used in conjunction with the recently available coaxial DPS electrode will provide a greater level of efficacy and reduced level of complications than the previously available DBS hardware.

In conclusion, I believe that the authors have given a fair and balanced assessment of DPS implantation for treatment of chronic pain. However, I disagree with their conclusion that DBS is not an established method for treatment of chronic pain. I believe that our own results, described in this commentary, as well as those reported in the literature, clearly support the efficacy and safety of DBS in the treatment of chronic pain. Refinements in patient selection criteria and techniques of electrode implantation and stimulation hardware should improve the safety and efficacy of DBS for the treatment of chronic pain in the future.

CHAPTER 113

Spinal Cord Stimulation for Chronic, Intractable Pain

Richard B. North

Almost 30 years ago, a new theory of pain transmission was reported, that provided a rationale for the reversible, nondestructive treatment of pain by electrical stimulation of the spinal cord. Compact solid-state electronic devices already had been developed for cardiac pacing, and this technology was adapted to stimulation of the nervous system. Technical problems were commonplace, and patient selection criteria for these procedures were not widely understood; therefore, disappointing results were common in the early application of these techniques. Implanted stimulation devices have been improved, however, and patient selection criteria have become increasingly sophisticated, leading to significantly better clinical results in contemporary practice.[1, 2]

BACKGROUND

The gate theory of pain transmission in the spinal cord, published in 1965 by Melzack and Wall, provided a theoretical rationale for the use of electrical stimulation in pain management.[3] Melzack and Wall proposed that the central transmission of neural activity signaling pain, through cells in the dorsal horn of the spinal cord, was governed by the balance of small- and large-fiber afferent input from the peripheral nervous system. An excess of small-fiber activity would open the "gate," allowing central transmission; an excess of large-fiber activity would close the gate. Because large fibers are more susceptible than small fibers to depolarization by an electrical field that is applied to a mixed population of nerve fibers, they could be recruited selectively, thereby closing the gate. Electrical stimulation of a mixed peripheral nerve could achieve this effect, but unwanted motor effects might occur at amplitudes very close to those required for a therapeutic effect. Furthermore, in clinical practice, most pain problems involve the distribution of multiple peripheral nerves. Alternatively, therefore, stimulation may be applied to the spinal cord; a population of primary afferent large fibers from multiple segments is conveniently isolated in the posterior columns. Antidromic stimulation of these primary afferents, which have collateral processes into the dorsal horn, can affect pain over a wider area.

Although the electrical stimulation techniques that follow from the gate theory have succeeded empirically, the theory itself remains controversial.[4] For example, in some pathologic circumstances, hyperalgesia is signaled by large fibers.[5]

In this situation, relief of pain by peripheral nerve or spinal cord stimulation may be explained by a frequency-related conduction block, occurring at branch points of primary afferents into dorsal column fibers and dorsal horn collateral.[6] Indeed, we have noted in clinical series that patients given a free choice of stimulator pulse repetition rate adjustments may show a disproportionate preference for a minimum rate of twenty-five pulses per second.[2] Alternative mechanisms, such as those involving dorsal horn interneurons or descending fibers, might be frequency dependent.[7–9] Other effects of spinal cord stimulation exist that are useful in the treatment of ischemic pain due to peripheral vascular disease; these effects are apparently mediated by the sympathetic nervous system.[10]

Spinal cord stimulation produces electrical fields within the spinal cord that may be modeled by finite-element computer techniques.[11, 12] The distributions of current and voltage within the spinal cord predicted by these models agree with measurements made in cadaver and primate spinal cords.[13] These models and measurements predict that an electrode's longitudinal position has the most influence in achieving the desired segmental effect. The greatest selectivity for midline, longitudinally oriented fibers occurs with bipolar stimulation, in which contacts separated by approximately 6 to 8 mm are used. Anatomic findings pertinent to spinal cord stimulation include the position of entering dorsal root fibers, which are relatively superficial within a few segments of entry.[14] Ascending fibers in the fasciculus gracilis decrease in diameter as they ascend.[15] Clinical experience corroborates these models and anatomic findings; indeed, the position and the spacing of spinal cord–stimulating electrodes are critical, and positioning of electrodes more cephalad to achieve more widespread effects commonly elicits unwanted, excessive local segmental effects.[16]

Psychophysical studies of spinal cord stimulation patients have shown subtle loss of normal sensation during stimulation, but acute pain sensibility is not affected to an extent that could lead to undesirable side effects, such as Charcot's joints.[17–19] Side effects occur increasingly as stimulation amplitude is increased and as recruitment increases; therefore, psychophysical studies should include quantitative measures of stimulation adjustment over the range of amplitudes from first perception to motor threshold.[20]

Neurochemical mechanisms underlying spinal cord stimulation have been studied in several ways. Cerebrospinal fluid analyses have shown changes in the concentration of neuro-

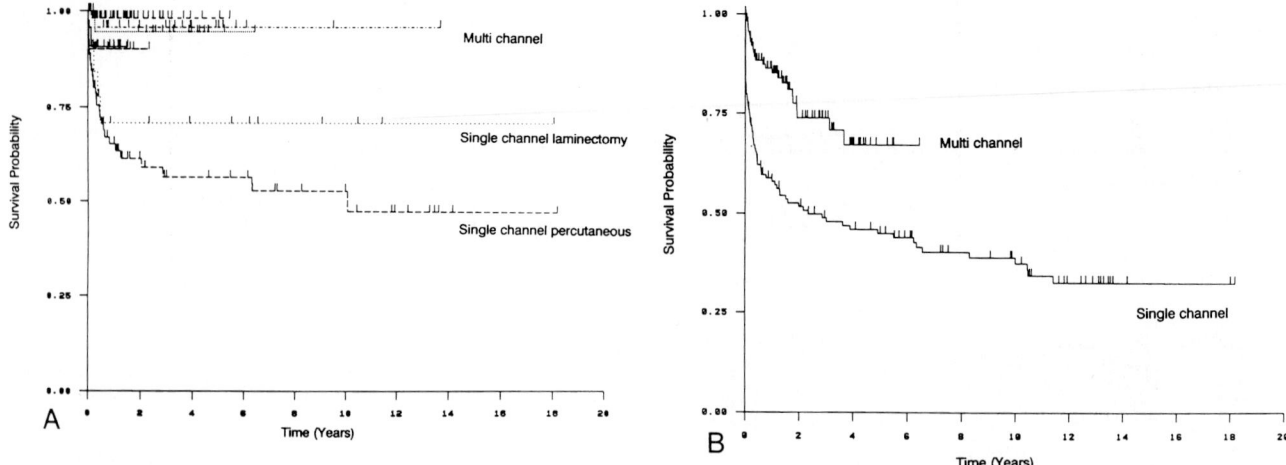

FIGURE 113–1. (A) A Kaplan-Meier survival analysis of electrode configurations used for spinal cord stimulation over the past 2 decades. The statistical end point for this analysis is a technical failure in that stimulation paresthesias no longer overlap a patient's distribution of pain, and a surgical revision of electrode position is required (whether because the electrode physically migrated or was malpositioned initially). The lowermost curve, showing the highest rate of failure, represents percutaneously inserted single contacts connected to a single-channel implant, with no provision for noninvasive adjustment of anode and cathode assignments. The middle curve represents a laminectomy electrode, likewise implanted with a single-channel, nonprogrammable device. These devices were significantly less reliable than arrays of electrodes implanted with programmable, multichannel electronics.

(B) Kaplan-Meier survival curve showing the clinical reliability of single-channel and multichannel programmable systems used for spinal cord stimulation. The statistical end point for this analysis is cessation of use of the device by the patient for any reason, including device failure without replacement and therapeutic failure (loss of pain relieving effect). The programmable, multichannel devices were significantly more successful than single-channel nonprogrammable devices. (Hazard ratio = 0.38; p <0.001). (Reproduced with permission from North RB, Kidd DH, Zahurak M, et al: Spinal cord stimulation for chronic, intractable pain: Two decades' experience. Neurosurgery 32:384–395, 1993.)

transmitters and their metabolites.[21] Pharmacologic manipulations, such as the administration of the narcotic antagonist naloxone, have shown no effect on pain relief by electrical stimulation, particularly spinal cord stimulation.[22] Animal models of neuropathic pain treated by spinal cord stimulation show apparent relief.[23]

SPINAL CORD STIMULATION DEVICES

ELECTRODE DESIGN AND PLACEMENT

The earliest applications of spinal cord stimulation for the relief of pain, first described in 1967,[24] involved high thoracic electrode placement in an attempt to treat pain in all segments caudal to the electrodes. This commonly caused excessive, uncomfortable radicular effects before the desired caudal segments were recruited. As investigators increasingly appreciated that stimulation paresthesias should overlap the distribution of pain, they adjusted electrode placements accordingly. For the treatment of low back and lower extremity pain (failed back surgery syndrome), low thoracic electrode placement most effectively isolates the painful segments.[25]

In the late 1960s and early 1970s, spinal cord stimulation electrodes were two-dimensional devices, requiring a laminectomy or laminotomy for introduction into the epidural, endodural, or subarachnoid space.[26–28] Because the ideal spinal level for electrode placement was not known a priori in an individual patient, and because longitudinal access is limited with a laminotomy performed with the patient under local anesthesia, these electrodes were problematic. Furthermore, even with technically adequate electrode placement that achieves overlap of pain by paresthesias, pain relief is not reported by patients uniformly; therefore, test stimulation with a temporary electrode is desirable.

Accordingly, in the 1970s, percutaneous techniques were developed for the placement of temporary electrodes.[29–31] These techniques were used to establish an analgesic effect before a device was permanently implanted, and also to establish the best level for electrode placement. These methods were adapted to implantation of permanent electrodes, avoiding the need for laminectomy.[19, 32] Placement of multiple individual electrodes by percutaneous technique, to achieve bipolar stimulation, was vulnerable to migration of one electrode with respect to another; this phenomenon frequently necessitates surgical revision.[19] In the early 1980s, arrays of electrodes that could be inserted through a Tuohy needle into the epidural space were developed. At the same time, methods of anchoring percutaneously placed electrodes improved, which led to improved results.[1, 33] These multicontact arrays were complemented by the development of programmable, implanted pulse generators, allowing noninvasive selection of anodes and cathodes from the array. This technology allows postoperative adjustments of electrode position (and accordingly, the pattern of stimulation paresthesias) with the patient in the erect or supine position in which the device will ordinarily be used, as opposed to the prone position, in which it is usually implanted. By comparison with early, single-channel devices, contemporary, multicontact, programmable systems rarely require surgical revision, and long-term clinical results are significantly better.[1, 2] Figure 113–1 presents these results using standard survival statistics.

Figure 113–2 shows contemporary spinal cord stimulation electrode designs for placement by percutaneous or laminectomy techniques.

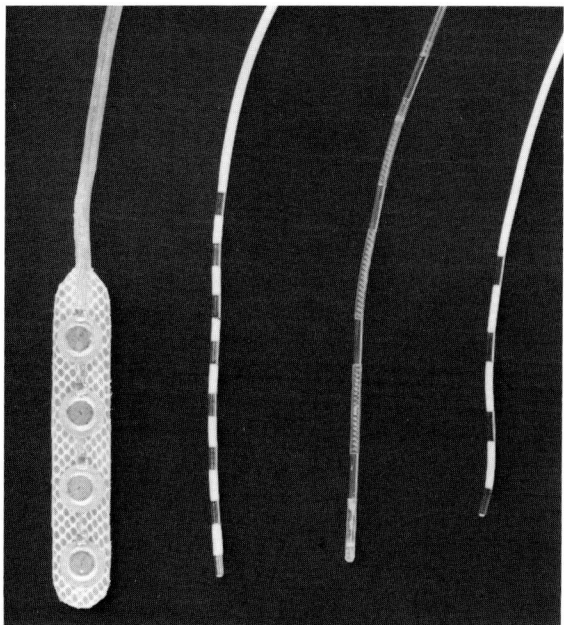

FIGURE 113-2. Contemporary spinal cord stimulation electrodes are arrays with multiple contacts. Some require laminectomy, but others may be inserted percutaneously through a modified Tuohy needle.

IMPLANTED PULSE GENERATORS

The prototype spinal cord stimulation device, used exclusively during the first decade of experience, is a passive implant powered by an externally worn radiofrequency transmitter. Totally implanted pulse generators, powered by an internal battery and capable of autonomous operation, are now available. An external device is still necessary to control these systems: the patient carries a magnet to turn the device on and off and to control the amplitude. In addition, an external programming device is used to adjust other parameters. These implants, like cardiac pacemakers, are powered by lithium primary cells. The power required for spinal cord stimulation, however, commonly exceeds that required for cardiac pacing by one or two orders of magnitude. To avoid frequent surgical replacement, careful attention must be paid to pulse amplitude, pulse width, pulse repetition rate (frequency), electrode impedance or load (determined by size and number of active contacts), and duty cycle (hours of use per day). Individual requirements may preclude the use of these devices in some cases, and in others, use of the device for its intended purpose may be compromised by concern over battery depletion. Alternatively, an externally powered, radiofrequency-coupled system contains no life-limiting components; the expense and potential morbidity of inevitable pulse-generator replacement are avoided. The obvious cosmetic advantages and convenience of a totally implanted device should be considered in this context.

Figure 113-3 shows implanted pulse generators of both externally powered, radiofrequency-coupled and totally implanted designs.

SCREENING PROTOCOLS

Neuroaugmentative techniques such as spinal cord stimulation have inherent advantages over anatomic procedures (which are intended to correct the structural abnormality causing pain) and ablative procedures (which destroy portions of the nervous system to block pain transmission). Not only are they reversible, they also may be tested preoperatively by a therapeutic trial that reproduces the long-term treatment exactly. Unfortunately, therapeutic trials of such procedures as nerve blocks and bracing provide only indirect evidence of the potential effects of alternative procedures. Percutaneous placement of a temporary epidural electrode for a therapeutic trial of spinal cord stimulation is a straightforward technique that is used to map potential electrode positions for optimal technical effect, and then to determine whether or not the response warrants permanent implantation. Indeed, most third-party payers in the United States require that "demonstration of pain relief with a temporarily implanted electrode precedes permanent implantation." This requirement may be met technically by intraoperative stimulation, proceeding to permanent implantation in a single stage.[34] An extended trial with a temporary percutaneous electrode, however, has additional advantages:

1. The patient can assess stimulation effects with a temporary system under more physiologic conditions of activity and posture outside the operating room.

2. Moving the therapeutic trial from the operating room to a fluoroscopy suite minimizes expense, while allowing the assessment of a number of anode and cathode positions and stimulation parameters.

3. If the temporary electrode is removed, rather than internalized for long-term use, the experience gained by the patient and physician with the temporary system optimizes implantation of the permanent device and expedites the procedure.

4. If a fully implanted device powered by a primary cell

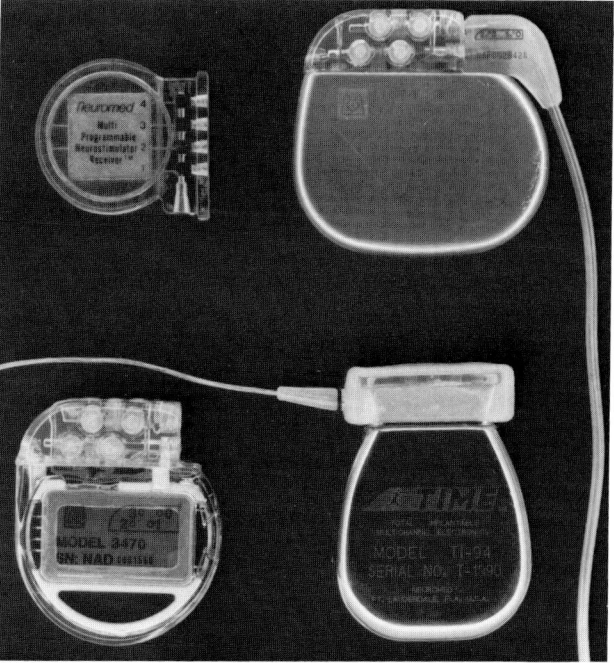

FIGURE 113-3. Contemporary implanted pulse generators used for spinal cord stimulation support multiple contacts, which may be programmed noninvasively as anodes and cathodes. Some are powered by implanted batteries (visible here); some accept or require power from an externally worn device.

is to be considered as a permanent implant, measurements with the temporary system are pertinent; if current requirements are excessive, an externally powered device may be selected instead.

A temporary electrode may be placed percutaneously and secured to the skin where it emerges from the needle tract; alternatively, an incision may be made around the needle and the lead anchored subcutaneously and connected with a percutaneous temporary cable for testing. It may be converted later to a permanent system, saving the expense of the temporary electrode. This technique has many disadvantages, however:

1. Two trips to the operating room are required—one for electrode placement and anchoring and another for removal or internalization. This requirement substantially increases the expense over that of a simple percutaneous lead.

2. The commitment on the part of the patient and physician to spinal cord stimulation and the tendency to proceed to pulse-generator implantation are greater if the electrode is anchored as for permanent implantation, in a manner that requires an incision and a second operation. This requirement partially defeats the purpose of the trial. No such commitment is involved with the use of a temporary electrode.

3. The position of an anchored temporary electrode has been established permanently; it cannot be adjusted at the bedside to assess additional positions as the patient gains experience with the system. The author routinely places a temporary percutaneous array at the most cephalad position that provides apparent overlap of pain by paresthesias without unacceptable side effects, on the basis of preliminary testing of the naive patient during placement. The array may be incrementally withdrawn at the bedside for repeated testing at more caudal positions. This time-consuming process is thereby removed from the operating room or the fluoroscopy room. Plain x-ray studies are taken, as required, to document successful repositioning.

4. Incisional pain may confuse the results of the therapeutic trial.

5. The risk of infection is greater.[16, 35]

The author routinely offers a permanent implant to patients who, after a 3-day trial with a temporary percutaneous electrode, report at least 50 percent pain relief while demonstrating stable or improved levels of activity and analgesic use. In the literature on spinal cord stimulation, the criteria for proceeding from a temporary to a permanently implanted device have varied considerably: some authors have required a percutaneous test phase lasting as long as 2 months,[36] whereas others have implanted in a single stage, with only intraoperative stimulation trials.[34] Some have required 70 to 75 percent reported pain relief;[37–39] others have required as little as 30 percent.[40] As few as 40 percent of patients undergoing temporary electrode placement have proceeded to permanent implantation.[41] Obviously, if long-term success is defined as a minimum reported percentage of pain relief (commonly 50 percent), the long-term success rate will be increased by an extended trial and a requirement for a high reported percentage of pain relief. This definition, however, arbitrarily and unduly emphasizes one of many potentially important outcome measures; other measures, such as use of other health care resources and return to productive activity or work, may not become apparent during a trial period. The potential morbidity of infection and epidural scarring (which compromises permanent device implantation) and the expense of prolonged, intensive follow-up for screening purposes must be balanced against the potential yield of a prolonged trial.

GENERAL INDICATIONS FOR SPINAL CORD STIMULATION

The criteria for the treatment for chronic, nonmalignant pain by invasive techniques, particularly implantation of a device such as a spinal cord stimulator, have been established as follows. First, a specific diagnosis has been established, providing an objective basis for the patient's complaint of pain. For example, in patients with failed back surgery syndrome, there should be objective physical findings or objective results on diagnostic imaging studies that are consistent with the reported distribution of pain; these findings should predominate over functional, nonphysiologic signs.[42] Postsurgical scarring on diagnostic imaging studies is seen even in asymptomatic patients, and neurologic findings, such as loss of deep tendon reflexes, likewise occur after successful surgery; such findings are nonspecific. In many patients with failed back surgery syndrome, the indications for the original operation are unclear from the original records and imaging studies.[43]

Second, spinal cord stimulation should be a late or last resort; alternative treatments should have been exhausted, or should be unacceptable by comparison. For example, in failed back surgery syndrome, reoperation may involve a lower yield and greater potential risks[44] and therefore may be a less desirable alternative.

Third, multidisciplinary evaluation, with specific attention to psychological issues, is important to rule out major psychiatric problems or personality disorders, significant issues of secondary gains, or major drug habituation problems.[20] Formal psychological testing has been reported to have some value in identifying subsets of patients who are poor candidates for the procedure.[45]

Last, the technical feasibility of achieving overlap of pain by paresthesias and of obtaining pain relief should be demonstrated with a temporarily implanted electrode before a permanent spinal cord stimulator is implanted. In most patients, radicular pain may be treated more easily than axial or midline pain, and neuropathic pain may be more responsive than nociceptive pain. These issues are subject to testing in individual patients by percutaneous, temporary electrode trials.

SPECIFIC INDICATIONS FOR SPINAL CORD STIMULATION

Failed back surgery syndrome has been the commonest indication for spinal cord stimulation. In patients with a chief complaint of axial low back pain, achieving pain overlap by stimulation paresthesias is difficult technically and may require complex electrode arrays and detailed psychophysical testing.[20, 46] Furthermore, axial low back pain may be mechanical or nociceptive and therefore may not respond to spinal cord stimulation as well as pain associated with nerve injury or deafferentation.[47] In the author's experience, patients in whom axial low back pain was the chief complaint have not been selected; in those with variable, secondary complaints of low back pain who have been treated, we have observed only minor associations between poor outcome and the reported percentage of low back pain.[2, 44] A complementary component of axial low back pain accordingly appears to be a minor contraindication to spinal cord stimulation; it is amenable to ongoing technical improvements and can be tested in individual patients. It has been reported that patients with complaints of unilateral lower extremity pain following low back surgery are more successfully treated,[28, 38, 48–50] but this has not been our experience.[2]

The most commonly reported application of spinal cord stimulation in Europe in recent years has been ischemic pain associated with lower extremity peripheral vascular disease.[51] Because in this disorder there are measurable changes in lower extremity perfusion and not just subjective reports of pain relief, it is unique among spinal cord stimulation applications for the treatment of pain. Spinal cord stimulation may be used in patients in whom revascularization procedures are not appropriate and in whom lower extremity pain is disabling and intractable and may lead to amputation.

Spinal cord injury patients with well-circumscribed segmental pain at the level of injury are generally good candidates for this procedure. In our experience of over 20 years, the rate of successful percutaneous trials for this condition was over 90 percent.[2] These patients, alternatively, may be candidates for dorsal root entry zone lesions, but this is an irreversible procedure that may involve sacrificing useful residual sensation and may preclude subsequent spinal cord stimulation. Patients with postcordotomy dysesthesias often respond to spinal cord stimulation, as do those with pain associated with other spinal cord lesions, such as lesions of multiple sclerosis.

Peripheral nerve injury or neuralgia, causalgia, or reflex sympathetic dystrophy respond to spinal cord stimulation in many cases.[52] In our 20-year experience, the rate of successful percutaneous trials in these patients was significantly lower than that for other conditions.[2] Nevertheless, most patients in our series proceeded to permanent implantation, so this observation is of limited clinical significance, given the availability of simple percutaneous trials.

Postamputation pain syndromes, such as phantom limb pain or stump pain usually respond to spinal cord stimulation.[53] Stump neuroma pain may be considered to be among the peripheral nerve injury syndromes discussed earlier; it often coexists with, and may be difficult to distinguish from, phantom limb pain.

Other applications for spinal cord stimulation include angina pectoris, lower extremity spasticity associated with intractable pain, and autonomic hyperreflexia.[54] These and other applications have been reported in relatively small numbers of patients and require further investigation.

CLINICAL RESULTS

The clinical results of spinal cord stimulation, as summarized in Table 113–1, have varied considerably. Patient ratings of pain and its relief are the most common outcome criteria; a minimum of 50 percent reported relief is a standard criterion for success. Often, results are expressed in terms of the number of permanent implants performed, and not the number of temporary electrodes placed for screening purposes—which may or may not be specified. In series with rates of permanent implantation as low as 40 percent,[41] adjustment for this factor is more important than in series with implantation rates exceeding 75 percent.[2] Regarding other neurosurgical procedures for the relief of pain, results are generally reported for patients who undergo the definitive procedure, and not for those who undergo screening procedures, such as myelography or diagnostic nerve blocks. However, the morbidity of these procedures is comparable to that of temporary percutaneous electrode placement. Spinal cord stimulation has the potential advantage—or disadvantage, depending on accounting methods—of a simple, low-morbidity screening test that emulates the definitive procedure.

The criteria for successful pain management include other outcome measures apart from ratings of pain and its relief: ongoing medication requirements, activities of daily living, work status, and changes in neurologic function (Fig. 113–4). The source of this information is another important consideration: interview by a disinterested third party has been reported to yield different results than physicians' office records and hospital charts.[1, 2, 55] We have always employed disinterested third-party interview methods in our reports;[1, 2, 19, 44] this methodology is reported increasingly in the literature on spinal cord stimulation.[26, 35, 48, 55–59]

COMPUTERIZED METHODS

The development of implantable electrode arrays and programmable devices has improved the technical results (overlap of pain by paresthesias) and, accordingly, the clinical results of spinal cord stimulation. The range of possible anode and cathode assignments for a multicontact array, however, becomes quite large as the number of contacts increases. Furthermore, it may be necessary to study each electrode combination over a range of pulse parameters, particularly amplitude. The range from first perception to discomfort threshold may be considered as a scale, along which the amplitude at which the painful target area is first stimulated may be quantified. Comparison between different electrode configurations and stimulus parameters should be made at identical subjective stimulus intensities along this scale.[46]

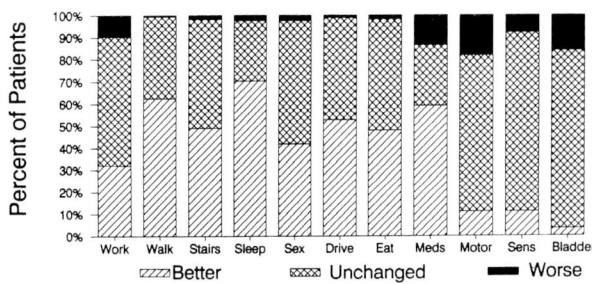

FIGURE 113–4. In our 20-year experience, the majority of patients have reported improvement in many activities of daily living. In addition, most have reported a reduction in medication requirements. Progression of neurologic symptoms has been reported infrequently (see text). (Reproduced with permission from North RB, Kidd DH, Zahurak M, et al: Spinal cord stimulation for chronic, intractable pain: Two decades' experience. Neurosurgery 32:384–395, 1993.)

Table 113–1. CLINICAL RESULTS OF SPINAL CORD STIMULATION*

Author	Number Implanted	Number Screened	Number Failed Backs	Follow-up Range	Follow-up Mean	Excellent/ Good Results (%)	Excellent/ Good FBSS Results (%)	Third-Party Follow-up
Bel and Bauer[40]	14	—	14	—	2 yr	60	60	—
Blond and coworkers[63]	58	59	59	12–72 mo	37 mo	89.5	89.5	—
Blume and coworkers[64]	20	—	20	3 yr	—	70	70	—
Broseta and coworkers[65]	11	—	—	3–20 mo	13 mo	64	—	—
Burton[26]	75	0	55	—	1 yr	59	—	y (mfr)
Burton[66]	198	—	186	—	—	43	—	—
Clark[67]	13	—	6	—	—	54	67	—
De La Porte and Siegfried[41]	36	94	36	3–96 mo	36 mo	60	—	—
De La Porte and Van de Kelft[39]	64	78	78	1–7 yr	4 yr	55	55	—
de Vera and coworkers[68]	110	124	18	—	—	75	—	—
Demirel and coworkers[69]	33	48	11	2–5 yr	—	18	—	—
Devulder and coworkers[70]	45	—	23	—	—	78	—	—
Devulder and coworkers[71]	69	—	43	≤8 yr	—	55	—	—
Erickson and Long[55]	70	10	—	≤10 yr	—	15–20	—	y (60)
Hoppenstein[30]	27	—	12	—	—	58	64	—
Hunt and coworkers[73]	13	—	5	9 mo–4 yr	—	15–31	20–60	—
Kälin and Winkelmüller[74]	—	—	77	—	—	88	88	—
Koeze and coworkers[35]	26	0	5	—	28 mo	46–62	—	y
Krainick and Thoden[75]	91	126	5	≤5 yr	—	18	—	—
Kumar and coworkers[76]	60	—	54	6–60 mo	—	62	—	—
Kumar and coworkers[48]	94	121	56	6 mo–10 yr	40 mo	66	—	y
Law[77]	81	—	—	—	—	36–80	—	—
Leclercq and Russo[78]	20	—	20	1–24 mo	—	50	50	—
LeDoux and Langford[79]	26	32	32	≤5 yr	—	76 at 1 yr	76 at 1 yr	—
LeRoy[80]	49	—	49	1–63 mo	30.7	60	—	n
Long and Erickson[56]	69	—	54	12–35 mo	—	18	—	y
Long and coworkers[81]	31	—	24	4–7 yr	—	73 at 3 yr	—	y
McCarron and Racz[82]	22	—	—	3–24 mo	—	68	—	—
Meglio and coworkers[36]	64	109	19	—	—	—	23	n
Meilman and coworkers[38]	12	20	20	≤3.5 yr	—	60	60	—
Mittal and coworkers[83]	26	31	21	—	—	46	—	—
Nielson and coworkers[57]	130	221	79	1–>35 mo	—	49	46	y
North and coworkers[1]	50	54	50	—	5.0 yr	47	47	y
North and coworkers[2]	171	205	153	2–20 yr	7.1 yr	52	—	y
Pineda[84]	76	—	56	—	—	43	43	—
Racz and coworkers[85]	26	0	18	12–42.7 mo	—	65	—	n
Ray and coworkers[49]	78	—	50	3–64 mo	19.4 mo	49	—	—
Richardson and coworkers[86]	22	36	12	1–3 yr	—	56	—	—
Richardson and Shatin[50]	136	—	136	—	45 mo	67	67	y (mfr)
Robb and Robb[87]	79	65	22	6 mo–5 yr	—	72	69	—
Sánchez-Ledesma and coworkers[47]	33	49	0	—	5.5 yr	57	—	—
Shatin and coworkers[58]	116	—	—	0.9–13.3 mo	—	74 at 6 mo	—	y (mfr)
Shealy[88]	80	0	—	7 mo–?	—	25	15–45	n
Shelden and coworkers[89]	27	—	3	—	—	—	67	—
Siegfried[90]	89	191	75	1–8 yr	~4 yr	37	—	—
Simpson[91]	56	24	7	2 wk–9 yr	29 mo	47	—	—
Spiegelmann and Friedman[59]	30	43	18	3–33 mo	13 mo	60	—	y
Sweet and Wepsic[28]	98	100	33	—	—	21–42	15–45	—
Urban and Nashold[92]	7	20	9	—	—	86	—	—
Vogel and coworkers[93]	27	50	29	>3 yr	—	18.6	—	—
Waisbrod and Gerbershagen[94]	16	—	16	6–30 mo	16 mo	75	—	—
Winkelmüller[95]	71	94	56	4 mo–7 yr	—	—	69	—
Young and Shende[96]	27	—	17	16–51 mo	—	66	—	—
Young[97]	51	14	25	12–67 mo	38 mo	65	—	—

FBSS = failed back surgery syndrome; mfr = device manufacturer; mo = month; n = no; y = yes; yr = year.
Adapted from North RB, Kidd DH, Zahurak M, et al: Spinal cord stimulation for chronic, intractable pain: Two decades' experience. Neurosurgery 32:384–395, 1993.
*The literature on spinal cord stimulation exhibits various follow-up intervals and methods, temporary electrode screening methods, and criteria for "success." Comparisons among studies or meta-analyses are difficult. An "excellent" or "good" result commonly signifies at least 50% reported relief of pain, but this is only one of many important outcome measures.

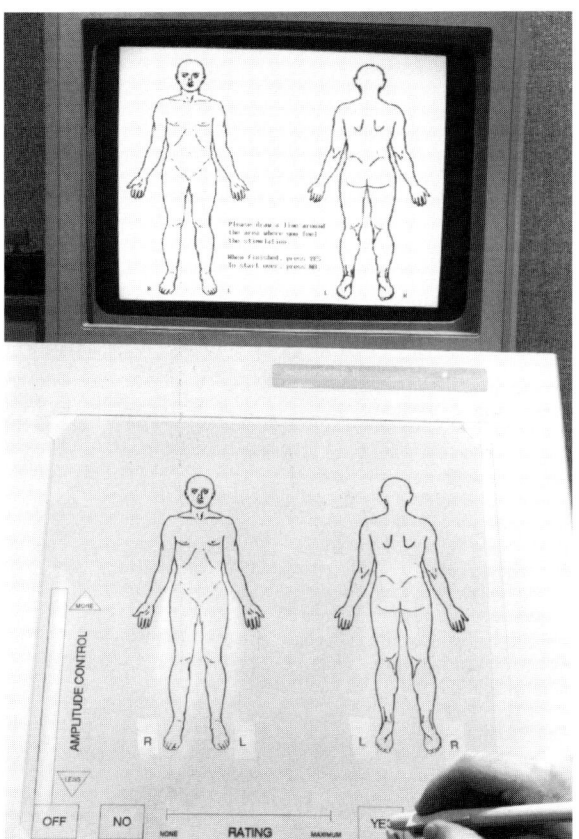

FIGURE 113–5. A personal computer graphics interface, as used by our patients to control standard, commercially available radiofrequency-coupled spinal cord stimulation implants. The controls of the device have been designed for greater use of operation than the controls of the standard radiofrequency transmitter or programming unit. The patient uses the graphics tablet to enter "pain drawings" and corresponding drawings of the distribution of stimulation paresthesias, to enter ratings using the standard 100-mm visual analogue scale, to control amplitude, and to answer yes-no questions for psychophysical studies. Overlap of pain by stimulation paresthesias is readily calculated from this graphic data, and settings are easily ranked in order for everyday clinical use by the patient.

If axial low back pain is to be targeted, precise control of the physiologic midline is important, and thresholds for bilateral stimulation should be defined.[25, 60]

Systematic, quantitative study of these effects generates a large volume of data that are best managed by computer.[25, 46, 61, 62] Data may be entered by a skilled operator who is working with the patient[25, 46] or, given suitable means of control, the patient can enter the data directly.[61, 62] Figure 113–5 illustrates a system developed for this purpose. Computerized systems that control the implanted stimulator directly allow study of novel modulation schemes and pulse sequences, which may offer advantages over the monotonic pulse sequences used for spinal cord stimulation for the past 25 years.

SUMMARY

Spinal cord stimulation has evolved into a relatively easily implemented, reversible technique with low morbidity for the management of chronic, intractable pain in selected patients. Percutaneous placement of electrode arrays supported by programmable, implanted electronics, which allow noninvasive adjustment of anode and cathode positions, has been a major technical advance. With contemporary devices, the need for surgical revision is significantly less, and clinical results have improved substantially.

REFERENCES

1. North RB, Ewend MG, Lawton MT, Piantadosi S: Spinal cord stimulation for chronic, intractable pain: Superiority of "multichannel" devices. Pain 44:119–130, 1991
2. North RB, Kidd DH, Zahurak M, et al: Spinal cord stimulation for chronic, intractable pain: Two decades' experience. Neurosurgery 32:384–395, 1993
3. Melzack P, Wall PD: Pain mechanisms: A new theory. Science 150(3699):971–978, 1965
4. Nathan PW: The gate-control theory of pain: A critical review. Brain 99:123–158, 1976
5. Campbell JN, Meyer RA: Primary afferents and hyperalgesia, in Yaksh TL (ed): Spinal Afferent Processing. New York, Plenum Publishing Corporation, 1986, pp 59–81
6. Campbell JN, Davis KD, Meyer RA, North RB: The mechanism by which dorsal column stimulation affects pain: Evidence for a new hypothesis. Pain 5:S228, 1990
7. Duggan AW, Foong FW: Bicuculline and spinal inhibition produced by dorsal column stimulation in the cat. Pain 22:249–259, 1985
8. Handwerker HO, Iggo A, Zimmerman M: Segmental and supraspinal actions on dorsal horn neurons responding to noxious and non-noxious skin stimuli. Pain 1:147–165, 1975
9. Lindblom U, Tapper N, Wiesenfeld Z: The effect of dorsal column stimulation on the nociceptive response of dorsal horn cells and its relevance for pain suppression. Pain 4:133–144, 1977
10. Linderoth B, Gunasekera L, Meyerson BA: Effects of sympathectomy on skin and muscle microcirculation during dorsal column stimulation: Animal studies. Neurosurgery 29:874–879, 1991
11. Coburn B, Sin W: A theoretical study of epidural electrical stimulation of the spinal cord: Part I. Finite element analysis of stimulus fields. IEEE Trans Biomed Eng 32:971–977, 1985
12. Holsheimer J, Strujik JJ, Rijkhoff NJM: Contact combinations in epidural spinal cord stimulation: A comparison by computer modeling. Stereotact Funct Neurosurg 56:220–233, 1991
13. Sances A, Swiontek TJ, Larson SJ, et al: Innovations in neurologic implant systems. Med Instrum 9(5):213–216, 1975
14. Dyck PJ, Lais A, Karnes J, et al: Peripheral axotomy induces neurofilament decrease, atrophy, demyelination and degeneration of root and fasciculus gracilis fibers. Brain Research 340:19–36, 1985
15. Ohnishi A, O'Brien PC, Okazaki H, Dyck PJ: Morphometry of myelinated fibers of fasciculus gracilis of man. J Neurol Sci 27:163–172, 1976
16. Law J: Spinal stimulation: Statistical superiority of monophasic stimulation of narrowly separated, longitudinal bipoles having rostral cathodes. Appl Neurophysiol 46:129–137, 1983
17. Lindblom U, Meyerson BA: Influence on touch, vibration and cutaneous pain of dorsal column stimulation in man. Pain 1:257–270, 1975
18. Marchand S, Bushnell MC, Molina-Negro P, et al: The effects of dorsal column stimulation on measures of clinical and experimental pain in man. Pain 45:249–257, 1991
19. North RB, Fischell TA, Long DM: Chronic stimulation via percutaneously inserted epidural electrodes. Neurosurgery 1:215–218, 1977
20. Law JD, Kirkpatrick AF: Pain management update: Spinal cord stimulation. Am J Pain Manage 2:34–42, 1991
21. Linderoth B, Gazelius B, Franck J, Brodin E: Dorsal column stimulation induces release of serotonin and substance P in the cat dorsal horn. Neurosurgery 31:289–297, 1992
22. Freeman TB, Campbell JN, Long DM: Naloxone does not affect pain relief induced by electrical stimulation in man. Pain 17:189–195, 1983
23. Meyerson BA, Herregodts P, Linderoth B: Enhanced flexor reflex in the mononeuropathic rat is attenuated by spinal cord stimulation. Acta Neurochir (Wien) 117:88, 1992
24. Shealy C, Mortimer J, Reswick J: Electrical inhibition of pain by stimulation of the dorsal columns: A preliminary report. Anesth Analg 46:489–491, 1967

25. Barolat G, Massaro F, He J, et al: Mapping of sensory responses to epidural stimulation of the intraspinal neural structures in man. J Neurosurg 78:233–239, 1993
26. Burton C: Dorsal column stimulation: Optimization of application. Surg Neurol 4:171–176, 1975
27. Nashold B, Somjen G, Friedman H: Paresthesias and EEG potentials evoked by stimulation of the dorsal funiculi in man. Exp Neurol 36(2):273–287, 1972
28. Sweet W, Wepsic J: Stimulation of the posterior columns of the spinal cord for pain control. Clin Neurosurg 21:278–310, 1974
29. Erickson DL: Percutaneous trial of stimulation for patient selection for implantable stimulating devices. J Neurosurg 43:440–444, 1975
30. Hoppenstein R: Electrical stimulation of the ventral and dorsal columns of the spinal cord for relief of chronic intractable pain. Surg Neurol 4:195–198, 1975
31. Hosobuchi Y, Adams JE, Weinstein PR: Preliminary percutaneous dorsal column stimulation prior to permanent implantation. J Neurosurg 37:242–245, 1972
32. Zumpano BJ, Saunders RL: Percutaneous epidural dorsal column stimulation. J Neurosurg 45:459–460, 1976
33. Leclercq TA: Electrode migration in epidural stimulation: Comparison between single electrode and four electrode programmable leads. Pain 20 (suppl 2):78, 1984
34. Feler C, Kaufman S: Spinal cord stimulation: One stage? Acta Neurochir (Wien) 117:91, 1992
35. Koeze TH, Williams AC, Reiman S: Spinal cord stimulation and the relief of chronic pain. J Neurol Neurosurg Psychiatry 50:1424–1429, 1987
36. Meglio M, Cioni B, Rossi GF: Spinal cord stimulation in management of chronic pain: A 9-year experience. J Neurosurg 70:519–524, 1989
37. Leibrock L, Meilman P, Cuka D, Green C: Spinal cord stimulation in the treatment of chronic low back and lower extremity pain syndromes. Neb Med J 69(6):180–183, 1984
38. Meilman PW, Leibrock LG, Leong FTL: Outcome of implanted spinal cord stimulation in the treatment of chronic pain: Arachnoiditis versus single nerve root injury and mononeuropathy. Clin J Pain 5:189–193, 1989
39. De la Porte C, Van de Kelft E: Spinal cord stimulation in failed back surgery syndrome. Pain 52:55–61, 1993
40. Bel S, Bauer BL: Dorsal column stimulation (DCS): Cost to benefit analysis. Acta Neurochir (Wien) 52 (suppl):121–123, 1991
41. De la Porte C, Siegfried J: Lumbosacral spinal fibrosis (spinal arachnoiditis): Its diagnosis and treatment by spinal cord stimulation. Spine 8(6):593–603, 1983
42. Waddell G, McCulloch JA, Kummel EG, Venner RM: Non-organic physical signs in low back pain. Spine 5:117–125, 1980
43. Long DM, Filtzer DL, BenDebba M, Hendler NH: Clinical features of the failed-back syndrome. J Neurosurg 69:61–71, 1988
44. North RB, Ewend MG, Lawton MT, et al: Failed back surgery syndrome: Five-year follow-up after spinal cord stimulator implantation. Neurosurgery 28:692–699, 1991
45. Daniel M, Long C, Hutcherson M, Hunter S: Psychological factors and outcome of electrode implantation for chronic pain. Neurosurgery 17(5):773–777, 1985
46. Law JD: A new method for targeting a spinal stimulator: Quantitatively paired comparisons. Appl Neurophysiol 50:436, 1987
47. Sánchez-Ledesma MJ, Garcia-March G, Diaz-Cascajo P, et al: Spinal cord stimulation in deafferentation pain. Stereotact Funct Neurosurg 53:40–55, 1989
48. Kumar K, Nath R, Wyant GM: Treatment of chronic pain by epidural spinal cord stimulation: A 10-year experience. J Neurosurg 75:402–407, 1991
49. Ray CD, Burton CV, Lifson A: Neurostimulation as used in a large clinical practice. Appl Neurophysiol 45:160–206, 1982
50. Richardson DE, Shatin D: Results of Spinal Cord Stimulation for Pain Control: Long-term Collaborative Study. Presented at American Pain Society, Poster #91240, New Orleans, LA, November 8–10, 1991
51. Broseta J, Barbera J, DeVera J, et al: Spinal cord stimulation in peripheral arterial disease. J Neurosurg 64:71–80, 1986
52. Barolat G, Schwartzman RJ, Woo R: Epidural spinal cord stimulation in the management of reflex sympathetic dystrophy. Stereotact Funct Neurosurg 53:29–39, 1989
53. Krainick JU, Thoden U, Riechert T: Pain reduction in amputees by long-term spinal cord stimulation: Long-term follow-up study over 5 years. J Neurosurg 52:346–350, 1980
54. Barolat G, Myklebust JB, Wenninger W: Effects of spinal cord stimulation on spasticity and spasms secondary to myelopathy. Appl Neurophysiol 51:29–44, 1988
55. Erickson DL, Long DM: Ten-year follow-up of dorsal column stimulation, in Bonica JJ (ed): Advances in Pain Research and Therapy, vol 5. New York, Raven Press, 1983, pp 583–589
56. Long DM, Erickson DE: Stimulation of the posterior columns of the spinal cord for relief of intractable pain. Surg Neurol 4:134–141, 1975
57. Nielson KD, Adams JE, Hosobuchi Y: Experience with dorsal column stimulation for relief of chronic intractable pain. Surg Neurol 4:148–152, 1975
58. Shatin D, Mullett K, Hults G: Totally implantable spinal cord stimulation for chronic pain: Design and efficacy. Pace 9:577–583, 1986
59. Spiegelmann R, Friedman WA: Spinal cord stimulation: A contemporary series. Neurosurgery 28:65–71, 1991
60. Law JD: Targeting a spinal stimulator to treat the "failed back surgery syndrome." Appl Neurophysiol 50:437–438, 1987
61. North RB, Fowler KR, Nigrin DA, Szymanski RE: Patient-interactive, computer-controlled neurological stimulation system: Clinical efficacy in spinal cord stimulation. J Neurosurg 76:689–695, 1992
62. North RB, Fowler KR, Nigrin DA, et al: Automated "pain drawing" analysis by computer-controlled, patient-interactive neurological stimulation system. Pain 50:51–58, 1992
63. Blond S, Armignies P, Parker F, et al: Sciatalges chroniques par désafférentation sensitive après chirurgie de la hernie discale lombaire: Aspects cliniques et thérapeutiques. Neurochirurgie 37:86–95, 1991
64. Blume H, Richardson R, Rojas C: Epidural nerve stimulation of the lower spinal cord and cauda equina for the relief of intractable pain in failed back surgery. Appl Neurophysiol 45:456–460, 1982
65. Broseta J, Roldan P, Gonzales-Darder J, et al: Chronic epidural dorsal column stimulation in the treatment of causalgic pain. Appl Neurophysiol 45:190–194, 1982
66. Burton CV: Session on spinal cord stimulation: Safety and clinical efficacy. Neurosurgery 1:164–165, 1977
67. Clark K: Electrical stimulation of the nervous system for control of pain: University of Texas Southwestern Medical School experience. Surg Neurol 4:164–166, 1975
68. de Vera JA, Rodriguez JL, Dominguez M, Robaina F: Spinal cord stimulation for chronic pain mainly in PVD, vasospastic disorders of the upper limbs and failed back surgery. Pain 5:581, 1990
69. Demirel T, Braun W, Reimers CD: Results of spinal cord stimulation in patients suffering from chronic pain after a two year observation period. Neurochirurgia (Stuttg) 27:47–50, 1984
70. Devulder J, De Colvenaer L, Rolly G, et al: Spinal cord stimulation and the relief of chronic non-malignant pain in 45 patients. Pain 5:S236, 1990
71. Devulder J, DeColvenaer L, Rolly G, et al: Spinal cord stimulation in chronic pain therapy. Clin J Pain 6:51–56, 1991
72. Hoppenstein R: Electrical stimulation of the ventral and dorsal columns of the spinal cord for relief of chronic intractable pain. Surg Neurol 4:187–194, 1975
73. Hunt WE, Goodman JH, Bingham WG: Stimulation of the dorsal spinal cord for treatment of intractable pain: A preliminary report. Surg Neurol 4:153–156, 1975
74. Kälin M-T, Winkelmüller W: Chronic pain after multiple lumbar discectomies—Significance of intermittent spinal cord stimulation. Pain 5:S241, 1990
75. Krainick JU, Thoden U: Dorsal column stimulation, in Wall PD, Melzack R (eds): Textbook of Pain. New York, Churchill Livingstone, 1989, pp 701–705
76. Kumar K, Wyant GM, Ekong CEU: Epidural spinal cord stimulation for relief of chronic pain. Pain Clin 1(2):91–99, 1986
77. Law J: Results of Treatment for Pain by Percutaneous Multicontact Stimulation of the Spinal Cord. Presented at the American Pain Society Meeting, Chicago, November 11–13, 1983
78. Leclercq T, Russo E: La stimulation epidurale dans le traitement des douleurs chroniques. Neurochirurgie 27:125–128, 1981
79. LeDoux MS, Langford KH: Spinal cord stimulation for the failed back syndrome. Spine 18:191–194, 1993
80. LeRoy PL: Stimulation of the spinal cord by biocompatible electrical current in the human. Appl Neurophysiol 44:187–193, 1981
81. Long DM, Erickson D, Campbell J, North R: Electrical stimulation of the spinal cord and peripheral nerves for pain control. Appl Neurophysiol 44:207–217, 1981
82. McCarron RF, Racz G: Percutaneous Dorsal Column Stimulator Implantation for Chronic Pain Control. Presented at North American Spine Society Meeting, Banff, Alberta, Canada, June 25–28, 1987

83. Mittal B, Thomas DGT, Walton P, Calder I: Dorsal column stimulation in chronic pain: Report of 31 cases. Ann R Coll Surg 69(3):104–109, 1987
84. Pineda A: Dorsal column stimulation and its prospects. Surg Neurol 4:157–163, 1975
85. Racz GB, McCarron RF, Talboys P: Percutaneous dorsal column stimulator for chronic pain control. Spine 14(1):1–4, 1989
86. Richardson RR, Siqueira EB, Cerullo LJ: Spinal epidural neurostimulation for treatment of acute and chronic intractable pain: Initial and long term results. Neurosurgery 5(3):344–348, 1979
87. Robb LG, Robb MP: Practical considerations in spinal cord stimulation. Pain 5:S234, 1990
88. Shealy CN: Dorsal column stimulation: Optimization of application. Surg Neurol 4:142–145, 1975
89. Shelden CH, Paul F, Jacques DB, Pudenz RH: Electrical stimulation of the nervous system. Surg Neurol 4:127–132, 1975
90. Siegfried J: Monopolar electrical stimulation of nucleus ventroposteromedialis thalami for postherpetic facial pain. Appl Neurophysiol 45:179–184, 1982
91. Simpson BA: Spinal cord stimulation in 60 cases of intractable pain. J Neurol Neurosurg Psychiatry 54:196–199, 1991
92. Urban BJ, Nashold B: Percutaneous epidural stimulation of the spinal cord for relief of pain: Long term results. J Neurosurg 48:323–328, 1978
93. Vogel HP, Heppner B, Hümbs N, et al: Long-term effects of spinal cord stimulation in chronic pain syndromes. J Neurol 233:16–18, 1986
94. Waisbrod H, Gerbershagen HU: Spinal cord stimulation in patients with a battered root syndrome. Arch Orthop Trauma Surg 104:62–64, 1985
95. Winkelmüller W: Experience with the control of low back pain by the dorsal column stimulation (DCS) system and by the peridural electrode system (Pisces), in Hosobuchi Y, Corbin T (eds): Indications for Spinal Cord Stimulation. Amsterdam, Excerpta Medica, 1981, pp 34–41
96. Young RF, Shende M: Dorsal column stimulation for relief of chronic intractable pain. Surg Forum 27:474–476, 1976
97. Young RF: Evaluation of dorsal column stimulation in the treatment of chronic pain. Neurosurgery 3:373–379, 1978

CHAPTER 114

Cerebral Lesions for Psychiatric Disorders and Pain

Jan M. Gybels
Paul R. Cosyns

Operations in the brain for psychiatric disorders are the most controversial biologic treatments in psychiatry. Physicians familiar with these treatments are convinced, from their clinical experience, that highly selective stereotactic operations on the brain can benefit some carefully selected, chronically ill psychiatric patients with a low rate of unwanted side effects. These stereotactic interventions are aimed at different brain structures. Targets that are or have been used for the treatment of obsessive-compulsive disorders (OCDs) and depression include the medial frontal subcaudate white matter, the cingulum, and the anterior part of the capsula interna; for the treatment of aggressive conduct disorders, lesions are placed in the amygdala, the intralaminar nuclei of the thalamus, the posteromedial hypothalamus, and the fundus striae terminalis. This chapter is concerned with subcaudate tractotomy, amygdalotomy, and intralaminar thalamotomy. Cingulotomy is described in Chapter 122, and anterior capsulotomy in Chapter 124.

The present discussion emphasizes the experience drawn from a multidisciplinary committee that since 1971 has supervised and coordinated functional stereotactic neurosurgery for psychiatric disorders in Belgium and the Netherlands. This experience is published in extensive detail elsewhere.[1] The attitude expressed here is taken for two reasons. Firstly, this experience reflects a practice that was adopted after 1970, the year in which the publication of *Violence and the Brain,* by Vernon Mark and Frank Ervin,[2] enhanced the already existing controversy surrounding the use of neurosurgical procedures in the management of psychiatric disorders. Secondly, because in recent years, many publications have appeared in which a greater emphasis has been placed on historical aspects and the reporting of large series than on the details of surgical technique, complications, and results, attention to matters of practical detail is appropriate in a textbook. The approach described here can serve as an example of today's attitude toward psychosurgery.

PATIENT SELECTION

Which psychiatric disorders are suitable for psychosurgery, how frequently it is used, what are the inclusion and exclusion criteria, and which decision-making procedures are recommended to fulfill ethical concerns associated with this therapy?

PSYCHIATRIC DISORDERS SUITABLE FOR PSYCHOSURGERY

During the 1940s and 1950s, psychosurgery was performed on large and disparate categories of psychiatric patients. Then, with the tremendous development of psychopharmacotherapy and new forms of psychotherapy, there was a marked reduction in the patient stream treated by psychosurgery. Despite this progress in diagnostic and therapeutic modalities, however, psychiatrists remain confronted with a residual group of highly disturbed and suffering patients for whom the psychopharmacologic and psychotherapeutic treatments have proved to be of very limited use. In countries where politics has not intruded too heavily on the decision-making process about psychosurgery, this form of treatment continues to be performed, albeit on a limited scale and on a small number of highly selected patients. In Europe, for instance, stereotactic neurosurgery for psychiatric disorders is still practiced by a small number of well-known neurosurgical teams, usually in university hospitals.

The scientific literature agrees on the following psychiatric disorders as indications, under certain circumstances, for psychosurgery: obsessive-compulsive disorders, anxiety disorders, mood disorders (unipolar as well as bipolar), and violent behavior in the mentally retarded. The caveat "under certain circumstances" is included because psychiatric diagnostic labels are necessary but not sufficient on their own for deciding to perform stereotactic surgery. In addition to the psychiatric diagnosis, the patient must fulfill several stringent criteria concerning the duration of the disorder, the personal suffering, the failure of previous, usually adequate therapies for the disorder, and the actual availability of psychiatric therapy (see discussion of patient selection). Psychosurgery, as we conceive it, is not an end in itself or a substitute for careful psychiatric treatment, but an adjunct to such treatment.

Extreme sexual aggression as an indication for stereotactic hypothalamotomy is a very controversial issue.[3] For ethical reasons, we do not accept compulsorily admitted psychiatric patients or detained delinquents as candidates for psychosurgery. Constraints from civil or judicial authorities complicate the necessary respect we owe to the essentials of the informed consent doctrine. There exist dissenting opinions on this matter, however, that argue that withholding effective treatment from a prisoner violates his or her right to treatment.[4]

Some authors undertake stereotactic operations for violent behavior in patients without a significant degree of mental retardation, or in children (from 6 to 7 years old) who are overactive, destructive, and self-mutilating even with a normal IQ.[5,6] We have no experience of psychosurgery in these situations, but stress the absolute necessity of a review board to approve the indications for surgery.

Schizophrenia is a major psychosis for which no causal treatment is currently available. Since the early period of psychosurgery, a great number of schizophrenic patients have been operated upon without showing convincing improvement. We consider schizophrenic disorder a contraindication, but authors such as Ballantine and Giriunas find it useful in "carefully selected cases . . . in whom depression, anxiety, or obsessions are very prominent accompanying symptoms."[7] Laitinen also reports positive results in schizophrenic patients in whom lesions are made in the genu of the corpus callosum (mesoloviotomy).[8]

Personality disorders are not indications for psychosurgery. The treatment of addictive behavior must be considered experimental and not an indication for stereotactic surgery in the current state of the art.

The main indications for psychosurgery are therapy-resistant and disturbing anxiety-linked behaviors, such as obsessions or compulsions, and depressive mood or aggressive behavior. Only some well-defined axis I disorders, as defined in the American Psychiatric Association's *Diagnostic and Statistical Manual of Mental Disorders*, 3rd revised edition (DSM III-R),[9] and never axis II disorders, can be taken into consideration.

INCLUSION AND EXCLUSION CRITERIA; DECISION-MAKING PROCEDURE

A review board on psychosurgery is a necessary part of the decision-making process for this form of surgery. Indeed most psychiatrists cannot, given the low basic incidence of these psychiatric cases, develop sufficient experience during their professional career to establish accurate indications for psychosurgery. Neurosurgeons, on the other hand, should not operate on psychiatric patients without adequate psychiatric expert advice and proper psychiatric follow-up care. Our committee on psychosurgery consists of an independent group of individual experts: neurosurgeons and psychiatrists from the medical schools of four different universities. It functions as a third opinion for the patient and for his or her therapist, who submits the case for review.

The following requirements are considered in each case.

- Psychosurgery is an acceptable treatment for the actual psychiatric condition of the patients (accuracy of diagnosis and intensity of patient's suffering).
- All adequate therapeutic measures have been applied and have proved to be ineffective.
- The proposed target area in the brain is appropriate.
- The proposed neurosurgeon and surgical unit are competent to perform the planned stereotactic intervention.
- Adequate preoperative and postoperative psychiatric evaluation and treatment are available.
- The patient, the nearest relative, and the therapist will consent to the treatment after being given adequate information.

The patient's informed consent is an absolute condition for psychosurgery. Some of our patients could not give it because of their psychopathology, some being too anxious to make such a decision, others too fixed in their doubts and indecision. Whenever a patient declines our advice for psychosurgery or when the patient's consent is only questionable, we always accept and respect their choices, regardless of their motivation, healthy or pathologic. Prisoners and other involuntarily committed patients cannot be considered for surgery because they are not in a position to make free choices. For incompetent patients, the legally appointed guardian and therapist in charge must give their (informed) consent, and even in these cases, the patient's consent is requested. In our practice, psychosurgical treatment requires the consent of the patient, of the nearest relative, and of the therapist as well as a positive recommendation from the committee on psychosurgery.

The clinical criteria for patients with OCDs are as follows:

- Persistent obsessions and/or compulsions of at least 4 years' duration with the symptoms constituting a source of severe personal distress and suffering for the patient and gross interference with normal daily routines.
- Failure to achieve significant and lasting positive effects with existing and usual treatment procedures over a sufficient period. Such treatments include intensive behavior therapy and psychopharmacotherapy, and the use of clomipramine at high doses for at least 3 months. A majority of patients have also received one or more courses of electroconvulsive therapy. All of our operated patients had been hospitalized during at least part of the preceding 4 years, mainly for intensive inpatient behavior therapy.
- During the course of the OCD, major depressive episodes or other mood disorders may appear; these do not constitute contraindications to psychosurgery. The diagnosis of OCD implies that the core symptomatology should be present in the absence of any significant mood change.
- Comorbidity with DSM-III schizophrenic or other psychotic disorders constitutes a contraindication for psychosurgery. Comorbidity with personality disorders of cluster B (DSM III-R), mainly the histrionic, borderline, and antisocial personality disorders, needs very close evaluation.
- The availability of intensive psychotherapeutic treatment following psychosurgery is also a prerequisite for a positive recommendation.

Physicians working in homes for mentally retarded persons may submit cases of violent behavior for review by the committee on psychosurgery. Such patients have an IQ below 50 and are irritable and hyperexcitable, with repetitive and persistent patterns of aggressive behavior against themselves and/or other persons. Their clinical records usually include several episodes of loss of control with aggressive impulses that result in serious assaults totally out of proportion to any precipitating psychosocial factor. All appropriate therapeutic and pedagogic procedures have failed to produce significant and lasting results; these include intensive psychopharmacotherapy as well as extensive behavioral and instructive measures. Seclusion and/or restraints have often been necessary for prolonged periods. The referring team, request-

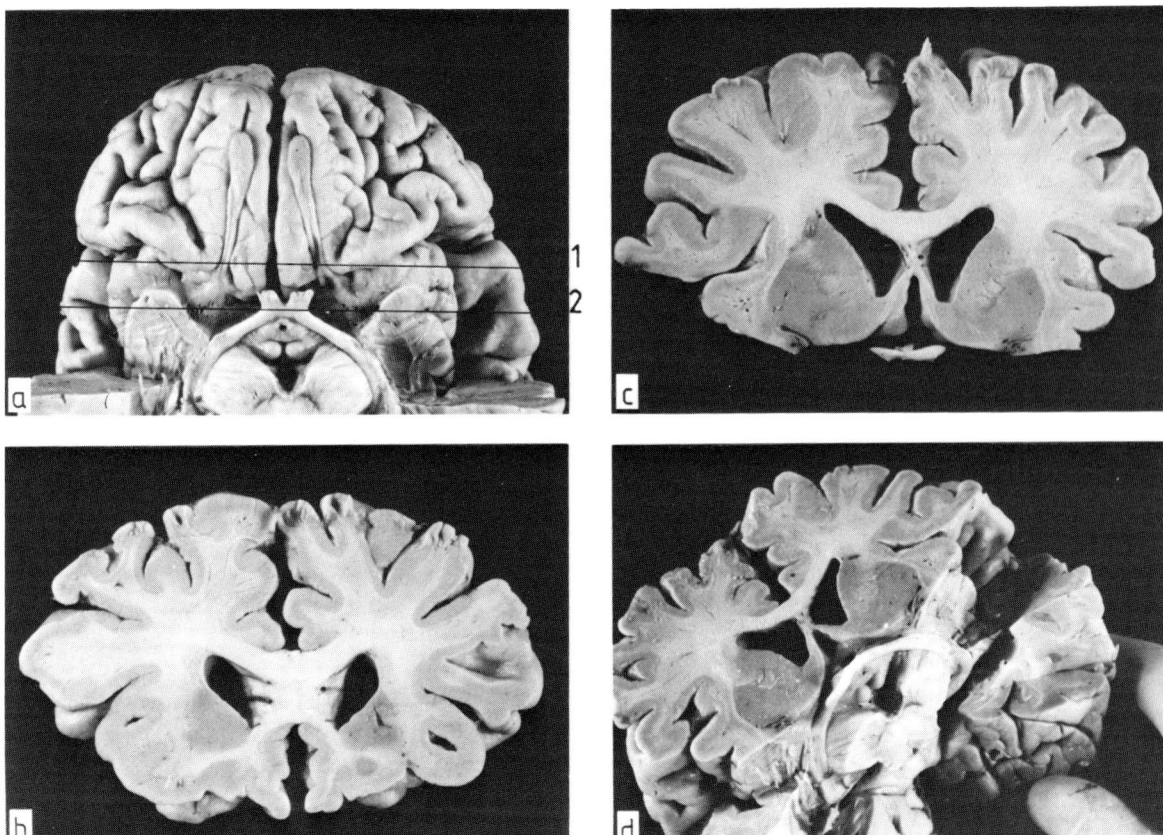

FIGURE 114–1. Dissection specimen. (a) (1) Level of target in Knight's subcaudate tractotomy and (2) level of substantia perforata anterior and substantia innominata; (b) vertical section through 1; (c) vertical section through 2; and (d) tilted view of C. (Courtesy of J. Caemaert.)

ing an opinion as to the advisability of psychosurgery, agrees to offer the patient intensive follow-up treatment and care after the surgical procedure. These patients cannot give a valid informed consent. After the approval by the committee, all necessary information is provided to the referring team and the patient's relatives, whose written consent for psychosurgery is requested.

Finally, not many statistics are available, but where they are, the actual frequency of stereotactic neurosurgery for psychiatric disorders is very low: e.g., in Belgium and The Netherlands, 0.2 per million inhabitants (1982–1991); in the United Kingdom, 0.3 per million inhabitants (1985–1989); in Australia and New Zealand, 0.2 per million inhabitants (1985–1989) (adapted from reference 10).

PSYCHOSURGERY IN OBSESSIVE-COMPULSIVE DISORDERS

For obsessive-compulsive disorders (OCDs), many targets have been used. Four procedures are accepted as being most effective: subcaudate tractotomy, cingulotomy, limbic leukotomy (subcaudate tractotomy plus cingulotomy)[11] and anterior capsulotomy.

SUBCAUDATE TRACTOTOMY

Target

In 1964, Knight[12] described the subcaudate tractotomy in which a lesion is placed in the medioposterobasal part of the frontal lobes. His rationale for this procedure was based on the favorable results, in some cases, of the orbital undercutting operation described by Scoville.[13] The area destroyed has often been called the substantia innominata, the structure situated beneath the head of the caudate nucleus in the region overlying the agranular cortex of area 13 and part of 14; neuroanatomic research has shown that the lesion is in fact anterior to the substantia innominata (Fig. 114–1).[14]

In an attempt to identify the fibers interrupted by this stereotactic intervention, Knight[12] cites the following anatomical data: "The relationship between the frontal cortex and the hypothalamus as described by Le Gros Clark and Meyer[15]; the presence of fibres from area 24 of the anterior cingulate cortex passing through the septal cortex en route to the posterior portion of area 14[16]; bilateral projections from the posterior orbital cortex of area 13 to the ventro-medial hypothalamic nuclei[17]; a projection from the amygdaloid nucleus and the lobus pyriformis sweeping up and passing into the posterior substantia before turning back and running caudally towards the hypothalamus and the dorsal medial nucleus (MD) of the thalamus from where it is relayed to the frontal cortex." Because the lesion does not penetrate the substantia innominata, it is only the amygdaloid projection to the prefrontal cortex, and mainly area 13, that is interrupted in its terminal segment after it passes through the pars magnocellularis of the thalamic dorsomedial nucleus.

Technique

For subcaudate tractotomy, target localization can be performed using either bony landmarks, air encephalography, ventriculography, and computed tomography (CT) or magnetic resonance imaging (MRI). Because most of our subcaudate tractotomies have been performed using bony landmarks, this method of target localization is described.

After fixation of the head in the stereotactic frame, bony landmarks are identified as reference structures for determining the coordinates. The target is localized 1 cm above the skull base plane (orbital roof and planum sphenoidale). It lies 5 mm anterior to the anterior border of the sella turcica (Fig. 114–2A). Initially, the target was situated at 3 mm anterior to the sella border, but since MRI showed the very near proximity of the anterior cerebral arteries, we have moved the target 2 mm more forward (Fig. 114–2B). The technique originally described by Knight[12] involves the use of radioactive yttrium 90 rods. We make the lesion by producing a series of thermocoagulations at multiple points along three trajectories, creating a lesion between 10 and 20 mm from the midline and 2 cm rostrocaudally in front of the target. The lesion is always made in one session on both sides with the patient under local or general anesthesia. If necessary, a second operation to enlarge the lesion is carried at a later time; during this second intervention, two more trajectories, 10 and 22 mm lateral to the midline and 10 mm more anterior than the first target, are used. Figure 114–2C shows a sagittal MRI scan 6 months after the stereotactic procedure, and Figure 114–2D an axial MRI scan of the same lesion 1 day after the procedure.

Knight stressed the importance of a low approach to prevent damage to the caudate nucleus. He described a case with a fatal outcome from a lesion that entered the striatum.[18] Therefore, the bilateral frontal burr holes are made as low as possible in the supraorbital region 1.5 cm from the midline. For psychological reasons, we try to achieve an almost invisible scar by placing the incision in a skin crease. The burr hole can be filled by plastic buttons or by reinsertion of the bone dust, supported in and covered by Surgicel. Sometimes, the frontal sinuses can reach so far upward that in order to avoid infection, a subcaudate tractotomy is not indicated, and an anterior capsulotomy or cingulotomy is preferable. When local anesthesia is used (the usual procedure), stimulation (pulse width 1 msec, frequency at 3 and 100 csec, and amplitude 0.1 to 2 mA) in the different target points prior to coagulation in our experience does not elicit any psychic or emotional effect. Respiratory and cardiac accelerations have been observed on stimulation in a few cases.

It should be noted that the position of the tuberculum sellae in relation to the orbitofrontal white matter is uncertain. The space between the caudate and the nucleus accumbens and the orbitofrontal gray matter is narrow, and an autopsy case has been reported in which the lesion entered the orbitofrontal gray matter in several locations.[19] Clearly, more rigorous techniques can be developed through the use of modern imaging techniques.

Surgical Complications

In a series of 30 subcaudate tractotomies, one postoperative, small intracerebral hematoma occurred beneath the frontal burr hole. This hematoma did not require operative evacuation and did not result in a lasting neurologic deficit.

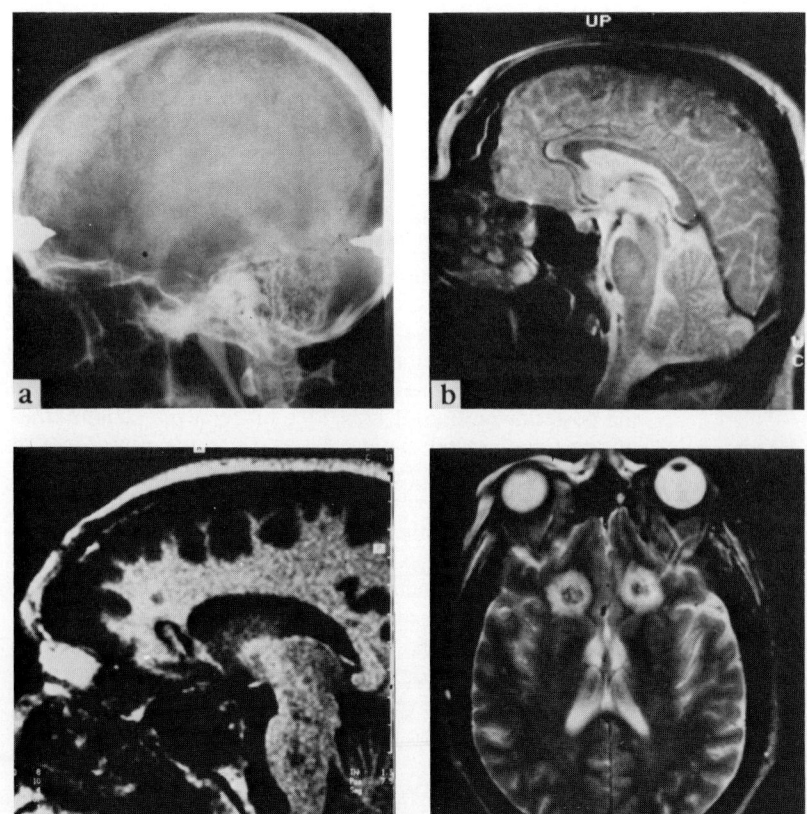

FIGURE 114–2. Case HW, 54 years old, September 1991. Subcaudate tractotomy: (a) Target as determined by bony landmarks on lateral x-ray study; (b) position of anterior cerebral arteries as seen on sagittal MRI; (c) lesion as seen on sagittal MRI, T1-weighted image, 6 months after the stereotactic procedure; (d) same lesion as seen on an axial, T2-weighted MRI, 1 day after the stereotactic procedure.

Results

We reviewed 21 successively operated cases from the first 11 years of activity of the committee on psychosurgery. Twelve patients had bifrontal stereotactic subcaudate tractotomy,[20] and 9 patients underwent progressive leukocoagulation[21] in paracingular and orbitofrontal areas. The mean age of the group, of 12 females and 9 males, was 43 years (range 27 to 65 years). Follow-up data were available for 16 of the 21 cases; at follow-up, 3 patients had died, 1 as a suicide and 2 of natural causes. Follow-up results were obtained on the average of 7 years (range 2 to 9 years) after psychosurgery.

To assess the psychiatric status of the operated OCD patients, a questionnaire was mailed during the follow-up period to the 18 operated patients and to their therapists. Specific questions in regard to target symptoms (obsessions, compulsions, anxieties, and depressive symptoms) were asked on a 6-point scoring scale, going from "the problem is over" (1 point) to "the problem is worse" (6 points). As to the target symptoms, positive developments were reported by patients and therapists. The overall obsessive-compulsive symptomatology score dropped from 5/6 to 3.5/6 at follow-up—an improvement of 26.5 percent—according to the operated patients. The evaluation of the therapists is more impressive: their scores dropped from 5.5 of 6 to 3 of 6 at follow-up—an improvement of 41 percent. The difference between patient scores before surgery and at follow-up was statistically significant for the target symptoms "obsessions" and "anxiety." In the therapist scores, the level of statistical significance was reached for the four target symptoms compulsions, obsessions, anxiety, and depression. Given the previously existing, unyielding resistance of these cases to therapeutic improvements plus the long-standing duration of disabling symptoms, the results of these psychosurgical procedures are important and noteworthy.

The same follow-up study was made of 7 OCD patients who had refused psychosurgery even though a recommendation for surgery had been approved by the committee on psychosurgery. In contrast to the findings in the operated patients, the nonoperated patients did not show any significant changes in target symptoms over a 1-year period, as reported by themselves and their therapists. A detailed statistical analysis of the scores of this patient group who refused psychosurgery revealed that any changes in the various scores failed to reach a statistical significance for all the target symptoms (compulsions, obsessions, anxiety, and depression).

Our major clinical findings and observations for the operated OCD patients can be summarized as follows:

- In a patient with positive symptomatic evolution, the improvement in anxiety and mood usually precedes that in obsessional or compulsive symptoms. The change in the latter symptoms is generally delayed, and a direct influence of stereotactic surgery on this performative aspect of behavior is generally not observed.
- Early somatic side effects are mainly a transient confusional state, probably due to local cerebral edema. This confusional state persists for a few days or weeks and, in our experience, is linked to positive long-term results. Infrequently, we also notice ataxia, oral dyskinesia, and transient urinary incontinence.
- In comparison with the patient's preoperative condition, we often note that after surgery, the patient exhibits greater sensitivity to anxiolytic and antidepressant agents; i.e., most could not tolerate postoperatively the high doses or combination of drugs they had been taking preoperatively. It may be that psychosurgery influences the sensitivity of the CNS to these drugs. Similar observations have been made in patients with bipolar affective disorder after stereotactic subcaudate tractotomy. Lovett and Shaw[22] report that in five patients (of a total of nine), drugs that were ineffective before subcaudate tractotomy appeared to become effective subsequently.
- After surgery, some patients responded favorably to previously ineffective psychotherapeutic procedures. The improvement of the anxiety level may play a key role here and we recommend restarting intensive psychological and behavior therapy after surgery.
- Transient unwanted behavioral problems or changes of personality traits were observed—a greater impulsiveness, being more "extroverted," as well as reduced reactivity and apathy. For this reason, we are very cautious about recommending psychosurgery in a patient who presents a personality disorder with a low level of acting out, such as cluster B of the personality disorders defined by the DSM III-R.[9] The organic personality disorder or postleukotomy syndrome does not occur with the actual stereotactic techniques. This "disinhibition" is difficult to appreciate from a clinical point of view. In our follow-up study, operated patients reported greater assertiveness or vitality, improved social behavior, and larger capacity to experience internal feelings and to express emotions. Lovett and Shaw[22] reported that even in bipolar affective disorders, hypomanic episodes have been more sensitive to subcaudate tractotomy than depressive episodes, and that they have either stopped or occurred in a very attenuated form.
- Delayed somatic side effects include grand mal seizures occurring several years after the operation. Among our 21 operated patients, this adverse effect occurred in 3 patients, and 2 of them had only one convulsion after alcohol abuse.
- All patients in our series underwent extensive psychological testing before surgery and at least 6 months after psychosurgery. The tests applied were Wechsler's Adult Intelligence Scale, Minnesota Multiphasic Personality Inventory, modified work learning test, and the Grassi, Hooper and Bourdon Wiersma tests. Comparison of test results obtained before and after surgery failed to reveal any significant deterioration in psychological functioning. In some patients, an improvement in IQ was noted; it was considered a result from decreased anxiety or diminished intrusion of obsessive-compulsive hindrance during the test procedure. Psychological test evidence of changes in personality as well as neuropsychological deficits could not be verified.

PSYCHOSURGERY IN AGGRESSIVE CONDUCT DISORDERS IN PATIENTS WITH PROFOUND MENTAL RETARDATION

Compared with psychosurgery for OCDs, psychosurgery for aggressive conduct disorders in patients with profound mental retardation has been performed in very few cases. The targets used in such cases have been the intralaminar

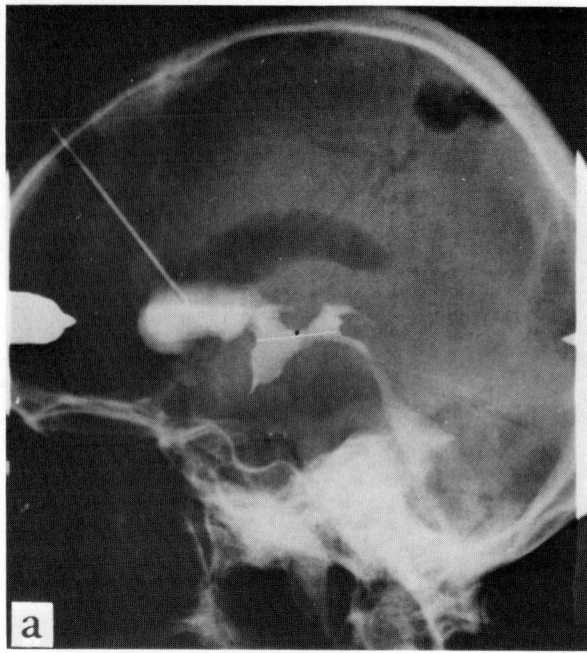 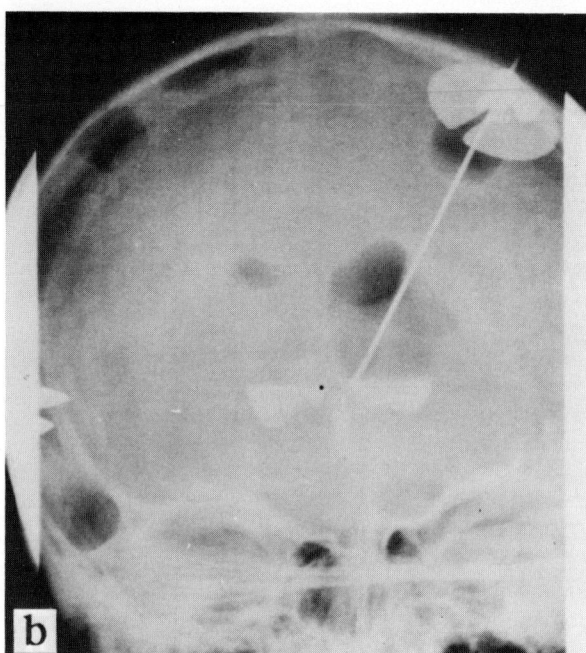

FIGURE 114–3. Case VG, 25 years old. Oligophrenia and uncontrollable aggressive disorder. Right laminotomy under general anesthesia, September 1985. (a) Lateral view and (b) AP view of air and Lipiodol ventriculography with target.

nuclei of the thalamus, the amygdala, the fundus striae terminalis and the posteromedial hypothalamus. On the basis of the recommendations of the multidisciplinary committee from The Netherlands, we have used the intralaminar and dorsomedial thalamotomy and amygdalotomy in aggressive conduct disorders.

INTRALAMINAR AND DORSOMEDIAL THALAMOTOMY

Target

Hassler and Dieckman[23] placed dorsomedial and intralaminar lesions for both hyperaggression and OCD. They hypothesized that an overactive projection truncothalamic system was producing the cogent perseverating and repetitive components of the behavior. They regarded this theory as validated by the results of their interventions.

It should be noted that the physiologic background for this theory is ill defined and speculative. The lamella medialis containing the intralaminar nuclei is situated as a thin mantle around the dorsomedial nucleus and proceeds forward along the medial border of the mammillothalamic tract of Vicq d'Azyr in the direction of the inferior thalamic peduncle. It certainly must be difficult not to damage the mammillothalamic tract. The vascular supply of the area depends on the polar thalamic artery, which runs parallel to the mammillothalamic tract, which can also be easily damaged. For these reasons, such intralaminar lesions have an inherent lack of precision and should be made only in cases of aggressive conduct disorder in patients with severe mental retardation.

Technique

Intralaminar and dorsomedial thalamotomy is most easily performed with the use of perioperative ventriculography.
We use a combination of air contrast, a positive contrast medium, and a posterior approach (Fig. 114–3). An electrode with a 5-mm bare tip is used for coagulation at 158°F during 60 seconds, creating a lesion proximately 2.5 mm thick and 5 mm long. A parieto-occipital burr hole is made so that the trajectory is angulated about 70 degrees to the AC-PC line. The target is situated 1 mm superior to the midpoint of the AC-PC line, and two trajectories are made. On a laterality of 4 mm from the midline, serial coagulations are made at target +5, target, and target −5. On a laterality of 6 mm from the midline, coagulations are made at target, target −2 and target −5. The lateral trajectory starts more dorsally in order to avoid destruction of the tractus mammillothalamicus of Vicq d'Azyr.

Because this operation is performed for hyperaggression in oligophrenic patients, it is carried out under general anesthesia. The lesions have to be made bilaterally in either one or two sessions.

Surgical Complications

In a series of 16 patients with bilateral lesions in the lamina interna and dorsomedial nucleus, the following surgical complications were seen: one temporary unilateral tremor, one gastric bleed caused by a long-existing stomach ulcer, and one supratentorial hydrocephalus 2 months postoperatively due to an aqueductal occlusion.

AMYGDALOTOMY

Target

The anatomy and physiology of the amygdala are still an object of intense study and are not the same in different animal species. Amaral and colleagues[24] have written a very extensive review of the anatomy and functional organization of the amygdaloid complex of the primate. In stereotactic surgery, use is being made of the oldest and most common subdivision that distinguishes a corticomedial nuclear group from a basolateral nuclear group. According to Narabayashi and Shima,[25] the lateral part of the corticomedial nuclear mass is the area to be destroyed for the treatment of aggressive conduct disorders. This area probably contains that part of the medial nuclear group that gives rise to a part of the stria terminalis, which itself has strong projections to the hypothalamus.

It is in this neuronal system that Burzaco's[26] target in the fundus striae terminalis and Sano and associates'[27] target in the posteromedial hypothalamus for aggressive conduct disorders are located. The medial nucleus of the amygdala receives direct inflow from the olfactory system through the lateral olfactory tract. Amygdalostriate fibers originate mainly in the basolateral nuclear group and terminate mainly in the ventral striatum and caudal part of the caudatus putamen complex.

Technique

The amygdala is quite far from the midline, and only its lateral border can be outlined on air encephalography or contrast ventriculography, through the use of temporal horn landmarks in an anteroposterior projection. The cornu Ammonis bulges from the medial side in the horn, and the lateral border of this bulge coincides approximately with the lateral border of the amygdaloid nucleus. The mediolateral dimension of the nucleus is 13 to 17 mm. The mean distance from the center of the nucleus to the midplane is 23 mm (range 21.5 to 28.5 mm), and the mean distance from the lateral border to the midplane is 30 mm (range 27 to 33 mm). The dorsoventral dimension of the nucleus is 15 to 20 mm; the ventral border is estimated to lie 2 mm above the most ventral extension of the temporal tip, along an axis drawn 2.5 mm in front of the tip of the temporal horn. Different techniques have been followed during the past 20 years. Because of the uncertainties of the landmarks, however, it is preferable to calculate the target position on MRI. Figure 114–4 depicts an amygdalotomy performed with MRI targeting using a BRW frame.

The incidence of the axial slicing is determined on a midsagittal slice, according to the line through the commissura anterior and the commissura posterior. More lateral parasagittal slices and mainly coronary slices allow for a first determination of the superoinferior z coordinate. The axial slice corresponding to the z coordinate allows one then to measure the x (lateral) and y (anteroposterior) coordinates. It has to be emphasized that MRI has an inherent degree of geometric distortion. We have analyzed this important issue by means of theoretical calculations and experiments.[28]

After the target is determined, a temporal burr hole is made that gives direct access to the T2 gyrus. A 5-mm electrode is used, and coagulation at 185°F for 60 seconds is performed, creating eight small lesions of 4 to 7 mm each. A first target, T_1, is determined, as shown in Figure 114–4, and a lesion is made at target T_1, at $T_1 - 5$ mm, at 3 mm superior to T_1, and at 5 mm lateral to the third lesion at the same height. A second target, T_2, is situated 5 mm anterior to T_1, and a lesion is made in T_2, 5 mm lateral to T_2 at the same height, 3 mm superior to the former lesion, and 5 mm lateral at the same height as the seventh lesion.

Surgical Complications

In a series of four bilateral amygdalotomies, one patient developed severe postoperative bronchopneumonia immediately after a left-sided amygdalotomy, which was performed 1 year after a right-sided amygdalotomy. She recovered from the bronchopneumonia but died 4 months later from a recurrent bilateral bronchopneumonia and a pulmonary abscess. Autopsy findings in this case demonstrated that a frontal approach to the amygdala may be dangerous. Another unexpected finding in this autopsy case is the presence of a hypothalamic hamartoma 15 mm in diameter.

Retrospectively, this lesion could have been suspected on the progressive air encephalography performed before the first procedure. Figure 114–5 shows verticofrontal slices at the level of the anterior commissure. Two small parallel lesions in the left amygdala and tiny traces of the two needle tracks through the putamen can be observed. On the right side, however, multiple small infarctions are seen in the caudate nucleus and in the putamen. Their unusual topogra-

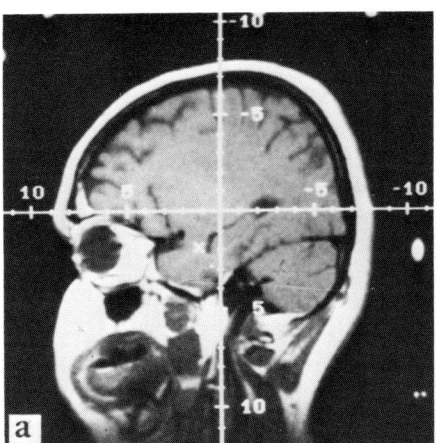 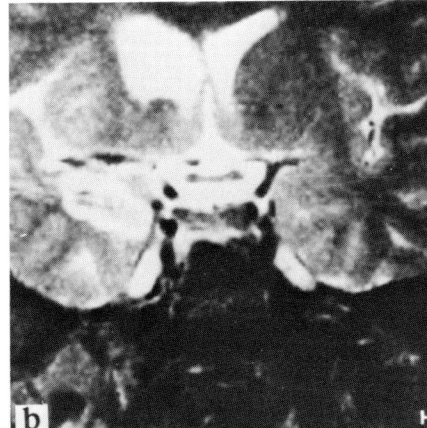 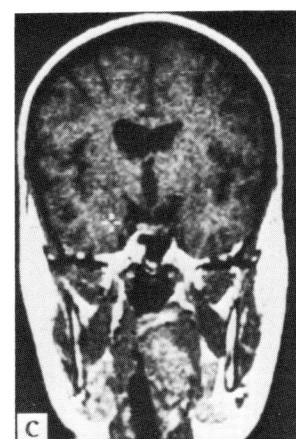

FIGURE 114–4. Case PB, 22 years old. Right amygdalotomy, under general anesthesia, January, 1988. At age 6, tuberculous meningitis. Oligophrenia and uncontrollable aggressive disorder. EEG is normal. (a and c) x and ∻ represent the localization of target T_1 as determined on MRI (T_1 acquisition); (b), MRI taken immediately after making the lesion (T_2 acquisition).

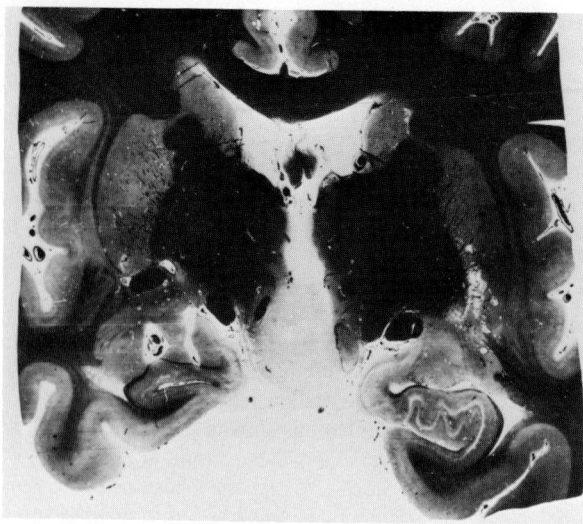

FIGURE 114–5. Case PG, 32 years old. Right amygdalotomy, May 1973; left amygdalotomy May 1974. Oligophrenia (IQ 36-51), hyperaggressivity, and generalized fits; institutionalized since age 12.

phy in the most medial and superior part of the putamen proves that they are caused by injury to the delicate tuliplike arborization of the lenticulostriate arteries bending around the putamen. This frontal approach was used because the stereotactic instrument (UTEC) available at the time (1973), designed originally for thalamotomy in Parkinson's disease, did not allow for a lateral approach. Therefore, we now prefer to reach the target from laterally perpendicular to the temporal lobe as demonstrated in Figure 114–4.

RESULTS OF PSYCHOSURGERY IN AGGRESSIVE CONDUCT DISORDERS IN PATIENTS WITH PROFOUND MENTAL RETARDATION

Because the number of patients with bilateral thalamotomy and amygdalotomy is small the results of both procedures are discussed together. This group comprises the 13 first operated patients (nine bilateral intralaminar and dorsomedial thalamotomies, four bilateral amygdalotomies) in which follow-up was sufficiently long to yield clinically relevant data.

These 13 patients with aggressive conduct disorder and mental retardation (IQ less than 50) were accepted for psychosurgical treatment. They all had protracted, severe, therapy-resistant autoaggressive or heteroaggressive behaviors. They were 9 male and 4 female institutionalized patients with a mean age of 23 years (range 10 to 37 years). In the follow-up research procedure on this group of patients, the referring (institutional) therapists were requested to indicate changes in patients' overall condition in a positive or negative sense on a 6-point rating scale (from 1, "much better," to 6, "much worse"). Additional questions dealt with changes in target symptoms, violent behavior (heteroaggression) and self-mutilation (autoaggression). The mean follow-up period was 7 years (range 4 to 11 years) after surgery.

When therapists or teams compared the actual general (overall) states of their patients now with their conditions before stereotactic surgery, they scored a mean of 2 (on a scale of 6), meaning "the patient is now better." As to the target symptoms, the following positive changes were reported: the score for heteroaggressive violent behavior dropped from 5.83 of 6 to 2.83 of 6 (an improvement of 50 percent), and the score for self-mutilation dropped from 5.33 of 6 to 2.17 of 6 (an improvement of 53 percent). Because the number of patients is small, the conclusions should be drawn with caution; given the extent of therapy resistance in this group of patients, however, the effects of psychosurgery appear very rewarding.

FRONTAL LOBE LESIONS FOR PAIN

For the second edition of their monograph *Psychosurgery,* Freeman and Watts[29] added the further title *in the Treatment of Mental Disorders and Intractable Pain.* The targets for lesions in persistent pain have been those described in this chapter in the discussion of obsessive-compulsive disorders, more particularly, cingulotomy and subcaudate tractotomy. A review can be found in Gybels and Sweet.[30] According to Ballantine and associates,[31]

The principal conclusion of practical importance from this long-term critical study is that cingulotomy for low back pain secondary to multiple operative interventions and/or arachnoiditis is a valuable addition to the armamentarium. Despite the uneasiness in the USA about malpractice actions following such surgery these operations continue at the Massachusetts General Hospital under the rigorous conditions of patient selection and care described, because they have a proven place in the treatment repertoire. The unequivocal absence of anything approaching significant deficit of basic function and the low complication rate of the stereotactic procedure are particularly attractive. We would precede any performance of cingulotomy in such cases by a full range of nondestructive operations.

For subcaudate tractotomy and inferior frontomedial leukotomy, Ballantine and associates commented, "Earlier conclusions were: that the patients leukotomized for pain seem to suffer more deficit than those leukotomized for psychosis [reference 32]. This turns out to be wrong for appropriately placed and circumscribed lesions, which may be gratifyingly beneficial."

Acknowledgments

The authors are indebted to the Members of the Committee of Psychosurgery, which since 1971 has supervised and coordinated, in Belgium and The Netherlands, functional stereotactic neurosurgery for psychiatric disorders; in particular: J. Caemaert, J. Ceha, W. Haaijman, C. van Veelen, and J. van Manen. Special thanks are due to J. Caemaert, who produced Figure 114–1 and reviewed the surgical aspects. The authors are also indebted to Ms. M. Feytons-Heeren and Mr. P. De Sutter for their expert technical assistance.

REFERENCES

1. Cosyns P, Caemaert J, Haaijman W, et al: Functional stereotactic neurosurgery for psychiatric disorders: An experience in Belgium and The Netherlands. Adv Techn Stand Neurosurg (in press)
2. Mark V, Ervin F: Violence and the Brain. New York, Harper and Row, 1970
3. Dieckman G, Schneider-Joonietz B, Schneider H: Psychiatric and neuropsychological findings after stereotactic hypothalamotomy, in cases of extreme sexual aggressivity. Acta Neurochir Suppl 44:163–166, 1988

4. Merskey H: Ethical aspects of the physical manipulation of the brain, in Bloch S, Chodoff P (eds): Psychiatric Ethics, ed 2. Oxford: Oxford Medical Publications, 1991, pp 185–214
5. Ramamurthi B: Stereotactic operation in behaviour disorders: Amygdalatomy and hypothalamotomy. Acta Neurochir Suppl 44:152–157, 1988
6. Sano K, Mayanagi Y: Posteromedial hypothalamotomy in the treatment of violent, aggressive behaviour. Acta Neurochir Suppl 44:145–151, 1988
7. Ballantine H, Giriunas I: Treatment of intractable psychiatric illness and chronic pain by stereotactic cingulotomy, in Schmidek H, Sweet WH (eds): Operative Neurosurgical Techniques, Vol II. New York, Grune & Stratton, 1988, pp 1069–1075
8. Laitinen LV: Psychosurgery today. Acta Neurochir Suppl 44:158–162, 1988
9. Diagnostic and Statistical Manual of Mental Disorders, ed 3 rev. Washington, DC, American Psychiatric Association, 1987
10. Hay P, Sachdev P: The present status of psychosurgery in Australia and New-Zealand. Med J Aust 157:17–19, 1992
11. Kelly D: Psychosurgery and the limbic system. Postgrad Med J 49:825–833, 1973
12. Knight GC: The orbital cortex as an objective in the surgical treatment of mental illness: The results of 450 cases of open operation and the development of the stereotactic approach. Br J Surg 2:114–124, 1964
13. Scoville WB: Selective cortical undercutting as a means of modifying and studying frontal lobe function in man: Preliminary report on 43 operative cases. J Neurosurg 6:65–75, 1949
14. Newcombe RL: Landmarks for lesions in the substantia innominata, in Hitchcock ER, Laitinen LV, Vaernet K (eds): Psychosurgery. Springfield, IL, Charles C Thomas, 1972, pp 289–290
15. Le Gros Clark WE, Meyer M: Anatomical relationships between the cerebral cortex and the hypothalamus. Br Med Bull 6:341–344, 1950
16. Glees P, Cole J, Whitty WM, Cairns H: The effects of lesions in the cingular gyrus and adjacent areas in monkeys. J Neurol Neurosurg Psychiatry 13:178–190, 1950
17. Le Gros Clark WE: The connexions of the frontal lobe of the brain. Lancet 1:353–356, 1948
18. Knight GC: Further observations from an experience of 660 cases of stereotactic tractotomy. Postgrad Med J 49:845–854, 1973
19. van Manen J, van Veelen CWM: Experiences in psycho-surgery in the Netherlands. Acta Neurochir Suppl 44:167–169, 1988
20. Knight GC: Bifrontal stereotaxic tractotomy in the substantia innominata: An experience of 450 cases, in Hitchcock ER, Laitinen LV, Vaernet K (eds): Psychosurgery. Springfield, IL, Charles C Thomas, 1972, pp 267–277
21. Crow HJ, Cooper R, Philips DG: Controlled multifocal frontal leucotomy for psychiatric illness. J Neurol Neurosurg Psychiatry 24:353–360, 1961
22. Lovett L, Shaw D: Outcome in bipolar affective disorder after stereotactic tractotomy. Br J Psychiatry 151:113–116, 1987
23. Hassler R, Dieckman G: Relief of obsessive-compulsive disorders, phobias and tics by stereotactic coagulation of the rostral intralaminar and medial-thalamic nuclei, in Laitinen LV, Livingston KE (eds): Surgical Approaches in Psychiatry. Lancaster, Medical and Technical Publishing Co., 1973, pp 206–212
24. Amaral DG, Price JL, Pitkänen A, Carmichael ST: Anatomical organization of the primate amygdaloid complex, in The Amygdala: Neurobiological Aspects of Emotion, Memory and Mental Dysfunction. New York, Wiley-Liss, 1992, pp 1–66
25. Narabayashi H, Shima F: Which is the better amygdala target, the medial or lateral nuclei? (for behaviour problems and paroxysm in epileptics), in Laitinen LV, Livingston KE (eds). Surgical Approaches in Psychiatry. Lancaster, Medical and Technical Publishing Co., 1973, pp 129–134
26. Burzaco JA: Fundus striae terminalis, an optional target in sedative stereotactic surgery, in Laitinen LV, Livingston KE (eds). Surgical Approaches in Psychiatry. Lancaster, Medical and Technical Publishing Co., 1973, pp 135–137
27. Sano K, Mayanagi Y, Sekino H, et al: Results of stimulation and destruction of the posterior hypothalamus in man. J Neurosurg 33:689–707, 1970
28. Michiels J, Pelgrims P, Bosmans H, et al: On the problem of geometric distortion in magnetic resonance images for stereotactic neurosurgery. Magn Reson Imag 12, 1994, in press
29. Freeman W, Watts JW: Psychosurgery in the Treatment of Mental Disorders and Intractable Pain, ed 2. Springfield, IL, Charles C Thomas, 1950
30. Gybels JM, Sweet WH: Neurosurgical Treatment of Persistent Pain. Basel, Karger, 1989, p 251
31. Ballantine HT, Bouckoms AJ, Thomas EK, Giriunas IE: Treatment of psychiatric illness by stereotactic cingulotomy. Biol Psychiatry 22:807–819, 1987
32. White JC, Sweet WH: Pain and the Neurosurgeon: A Forty-Year Experience. Springfield, IL, Charles C Thomas, 1969, p 835

SELECTED READINGS

Beck E: A cytoarchitectural investigation into the boundaries of cortical areas 13 and 14 in the human brain. J Anat 83:147–157, 1949

Bridges PK: Psychosurgery: Historical interest only or contemporary relevance (editorial). Br J Hosp Med 37:283, 1987

Brihaye J, Calliauw L, Loew F, van den Bergh R (eds): Personality and Neurosurgery. Vienna, Springer-Verlag, 1988

Cobb J, Kelly D: Psychosurgery: Is it ever justified? in Hawton K, Cowen P (eds): Dilemmas and Difficulties in the Management of Psychiatric Patients. Oxford, Oxford University Press, 1990, pp 219–230

Culliton BJ: Psychosurgery: National Commission issues surprisingly favorable report. Science 194:299–301, 1976

Hitchcock ER, Ballantine HT, Meyerson BA (eds): Modern Concepts in Psychiatric Surgery. Amsterdam, Elsevier, 1979

Hitchcock ER, Laitinen LV, Vaernet K (eds): Psychosurgery. Springfield, IL, Charles C Thomas, 1972

Insel TR: Toward a neuroanatomy of obsessive-compulsive disorder. Arch Gen Psychiatry 49:739–744, 1992

Kartsounis LD, Poynton A, Bridges PK, Bartlett JR: Neuropsychological correlates of stereotactic subcaudate tractotomy: A prospective study. Brain 114:2657–2673, 1991

Laitinen LV: Emotional responses to subcortical electrical stimulation in psychiatric patients. Clin Neurol Neurosurg 81:148–157, 1979

Laitinen LV, Livingston KE (eds): Surgical Approaches in Psychiatry. Lancaster, Medical and Technical Publishing Co., 1973

Laplane D, Levasseur M, Pillon B, et al: Obsessive-compulsive and other behavioural changes with bilateral basal ganglia lesions. Brain 112:699–725, 1989

Mindus P, Bergström K, Levander SE, et al: Magnetic resonance images related to clinical outcome after psychosurgical intervention in severe anxiety disorder. J Neurol Neurosurg Psychiatry 50:1288–1293, 1987

Modell JG, Mountz JM, Curtis GC, Greden JF. Neurophysiologic dysfunction in basal ganglia/limbic striatal and thalamocortical circuits as a pathogenetic mechanism of obsessive-compulsive disorder. J Neuropsychiatry 1:27–36, 1989

Nordahl TE, Benkelfat C, Semple WE, et al: Cerebral glucose metabolic rates in obsessive compulsive disorder. Neuropsychopharmacology 2:23–28, 1989

Poynton A, Bridges PK, Bartlett JR. Psychosurgery in Britain now. Brit J Neurosurg 1988; 2:297–306

Report and Recommendations: Psychosurgery. Washington, DC, The National Commission for the Protection of Human Subjects of Biomedical and Behavioral Research, DHEW Publication no. (OS)77-0001 and Appendix (OS)77-0002

Sweet WH, Meyerson BA: Neurosurgical aspects of primary affective disorders, in Youmans JR (ed): Neurological Surgery, ed 3. Philadelphia, WB Saunders, 1990, pp 4335–4357

CHAPTER

115

Surgical Treatment of Intractable Psychiatric Illness and Chronic Pain by Stereotactic Cingulotomy

H. Thomas Ballantine, Jr
G. Rees Cosgrove
Ida E. Giriunas

*I*ntracranial surgery for the treatment of psychiatric illness and chronic pain has been under scrutiny and criticism since 1936, when the Portuguese neurologist Egas Moniz[1] reported the results of frontal lobotomies performed by himself and his neurosurgical colleague, Almeida Lima, on 20 institutionalized, severely ill psychiatric patients. Because of this controversy, we have included in this chapter pertinent details about the history of psychiatric surgery, the rationale for its performance, and the preoperative safeguards we employ to make certain that surgical intervention is appropriate and informed consent is obtained.

In his paper, Moniz stated that 14 of 20 patients (70 percent) had shown worthwhile improvement, which led others to embrace this innovative method of treating psychiatric patients.[2] One of the most enthusiastic (destined later to become overly enthusiastic)[3] was the neuropsychiatrist Walter Freeman of Washington, DC. Three months after Moniz published his original paper, Freeman, with the neurosurgical assistance of James Watts, performed the first prefrontal lobotomy in the United States.

In 1942 Freeman and Watts[4] published a monograph entitled *Psychosurgery*, which encompassed their initial experiences with 80 prefrontal lobotomies. Subsequently, they observed that some psychiatric patients who also complained of unbearable pain were free of that complaint postoperatively. They became increasingly impressed by this finding, and the second edition of their book, published in 1950, bore the title *Psychosurgery: In the Treatment of Mental Disorders and Intractable Pain*.[5]

Early on, however, complications and undesirable side effects of this radical procedure were being reported. Tooth and Newton[6] reviewed 10,365 operations performed between 1943 and 1954. They confirmed that the rate of improvement was about 70 percent, but they also reported a 6 percent mortality rate, a 1 percent epilepsy rate, and a 1.5 percent incidence of significant personality change, often characterized by inappropriate behavior, obscene speech, and loss of social control.

These complications of the standard prefrontal lobotomy led to a search for an operation that could confer the same benefit with much less risk. More restricted frontal leucotomies were devised, such as bilateral inferior leucotomy, bimedial leucotomy, and orbital gyrus undercutting; each technique had its proponents. Then, in 1948 at the suggestion of Fulton of Yale, Cairns in England, and LeBeau in France, neurosurgeons moved away from the frontal leucotomy techniques and began to perform open anterior cingulectomies.

The introduction of stereotactic surgery revolutionized psychiatric surgery, and today, open operations are rare. In 1961, Foltz and White[7] reported the outcomes of stereotactic cingulotomies carried out for intractable pain. Encouraged by their results, we began in 1962 to employ a modification of their technique for the treatment of psychiatric illness as well as of pain.

THE CINGULATE GYRI: ANATOMIC AND PHYSIOLOGIC CONSIDERATIONS

The cingulate gyri, along with the parahippocampal gyri, are located on the medial surfaces of the cerebral hemispheres and form a "limbus" or border. This region and the structures it surrounds are often termed the "limbic lobe" of the brain. In 1937, J.W. Papez published an important paper, under the title of "A Proposed Mechanism of Emotion."[8] He postulated that the gyri cinguli, the hypothalamus, the hippocampus, and their interconnections constituted the "anatomic basis of the emotions." Over the next four decades, this theoretical region was greatly enlarged to include a myriad of anatomic entities that, taken together, form the limbic system. Figure 115–1 illustrates diagrammatically this complex arrangement.

It has been theorized that the central pathways of the emotions and the responses to them might be as follows: Sensory stimuli, both external and internal, are assembled at the brain stem and travel to the hypothalamus (HYP). From there, they may pass to the anterior thalamic nuclei (AT), and thence to the cingulum via the anterior thalamic radiations (ATR). From the cingulum, stimuli could be transmitted back to the hippocampus, mammillary bodies, and anterior thalamic nuclei via the mammilothalamic tract (MTT), and from there back to the cingulum.

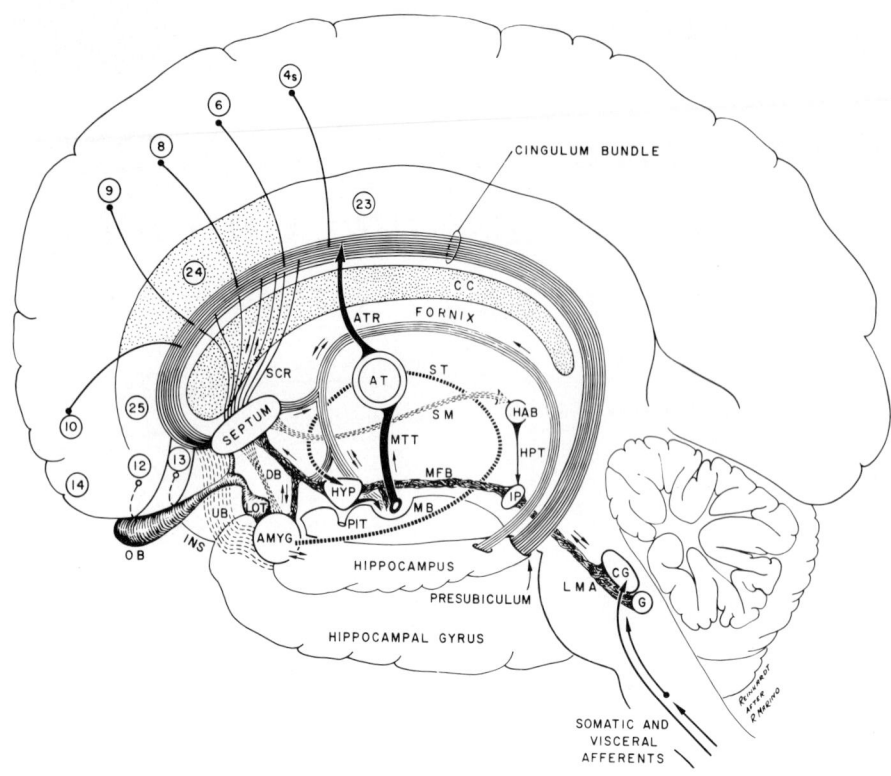

FIGURE 115–1. Schematic model of the limbic system. HYP = hypothalamus; AT = anterior thalamus; ATR = anterior thalamic radiations; MTT = mammillothalamic tract. (Reprinted from Ballantine HT Jr, Cassidy WL, Flanagan NB, et al: Stereotaxic anterior cingulotomy for neuropsychiatric illness and intractable pain. J Neurosurg 26:488–495, 1967. With permission.)

The output from this reverberating circuit is transmitted to the frontal lobes by way of several connections, the most important of which is the cingulum. In this way, the limbic system may, in the words of Papez,[8] "add emotional coloring to the psychic process."

In similar fashion, "psychic processes with emotional coloring" can be transmitted back to the limbic system, and these efferent stimuli will affect the thought processes, feelings, and behavior that are unique for each person. Although this theoretical construct may require significant modification, it is unlikely that the important role of the cingulum in the complex interplay of cognition and affect will be diminished in the future.

Neuroscientists have also delineated an interrelationship between neocortex, the limbic system, and the brain stem reticular activating system. Neurotransmitters (e.g., norepinephrine, serotonin), neuromodulators (e.g., GABA, somatostatin) and aberrant electrical neurophysiology (e.g., kindling) all mediate this complex plastic system, which appears to be responsible for the activities of thinking, mood, and behavior. Medications aimed at either enhancing neurotransmitter synthesis, inhibiting the inactivation of it, or affecting receptor sensitivity are being successfully used in treatment and in furthering our knowledge and understanding of central nervous system function.[9] Our knowledge of the central biochemical correlates of these illnesses is rudimentary, however, and there are still patients (about 20 percent of those who are disabled by affective illness) who gain little or no benefit from currently available therapeutic modalities.

Psychotropic drugs have proved to be helpful in the treatment of depression and other psychiatric illnesses and have been shown to activate receptor sensitivity and neurotransmitter concentration. For instance, the tricyclics prevent neurotransmitter re-uptake of serotonin and norepinephrine at the synapse, increasing neurotransmitter concentration at the receptor site and down-regulating beta-receptor sensitivity. These findings have encouraged many physicians to believe that alterations in neurotransmitters at the neuronal synapses play a leading, if not exclusive, role in the cause of psychiatric disorders. An observation, made by ourselves and others, that maximum improvement following limbic system surgery may not be obtained for several months has led to our hypothesis that the lesions not only affect the neuronal pathways but may also influence neurotransmitter concentrations and neuronal reorganization.

CRITERIA FOR THE SELECTION OF PSYCHIATRIC PATIENTS

It is the usual practice at our institution to accept for evaluation any person who is chronically disabled by a psychiatric illness that has not responded satisfactorily to all currently available therapies—psychotherapy, behavior modification techniques, medications, electroconvulsive therapy (ECT), etc. The duration of the illness can be of less importance than its severity. In a highly suicidal patient who has not responded to treatment, evaluation for early cingulotomy should be considered. A diagnosis of an affective disorder indicates a better prognosis than one of personality disorder or schizophrenia. However, carefully selected patients with the latter two diagnoses in whom depression, anxiety, or obsessions are very prominent accompanying symptoms and who are not severely deteriorated are likely to benefit by having those conditions modified by cingulotomy. In addition, patients with severe, disabling, and treatment-refractory obsessive-compulsive disorder are also candidates for cingulotomy.

All psychiatric patients being considered for cingulotomy must be referred by the treating psychiatrist with a written statement that all nonoperative therapies have been exhausted and, further, that if the patient is accepted for cingulotomy, the psychiatrist will be responsible for postoperative psychiatric care. Similarly, the patient must agree to return to the referring psychiatrist, with the understanding that we consider cingulotomy an adjunct to, but not a substitute for, careful psychiatric management.

In addition, both the patient and the psychiatrist must fulfill the following specific criteria before being accepted for evaluation. The referring psychiatrist must complete a form devised by the Massachusetts General Hospital (MGH) psychiatrists that provides detailed information concerning the patient's past history, present illness, family history, and all prior treatments, and copies of the patient's records must be forwarded for review. The patient must furnish assurance that someone of his or her family or acquaintance will be available to provide emotional support before, during, and after hospitalization.

Preliminary evaluation of the suitability of the patient for cingulotomy is carried out by the MGH Cingulotomy Assessment Committee, which consists of three psychiatrists (one of whom presents the case to the full Committee), two neurosurgeons, and one neurologist. The Committee must agree unanimously that the patient is a suitable candidate for operation. Alternatively, it may decide that further information is needed to clarify the diagnosis and need for operation or that additional nonoperative treatment might be helpful. Finally, the Committee may conclude that the patient is not a candidate for operation. The treating psychiatrist is informed of the Committee's decision by one of its members.

A patient who passes this first screening is then interviewed by the psychiatrist who presented the case to the full Committee, by the two neurosurgeons, and by the neurologist. This evaluation is concerned with ascertaining the diagnosis and ensuring that the patient and his or her "support person" are fully informed of the risks and possible benefits of the proposed surgery. Additionally, recent encephalogram (EEG) and magnetic resonance imaging (MRI) scans of the brain must be available. A full battery of psychological tests is also administered.

All of the "on-site" evaluators must again be unanimous in agreement that the patient meets the criteria for the cingulotomy and that the requirements of informed consent have been fulfilled. On rare occasions, these personal interviews reveal further information that cause the patient to be rejected.

Contraindications are few. Patients with pronounced hysterical or sociopathic personalities do not do well, even if presenting symptoms are appropriate. Elderly patients are at higher risk of postoperative confusion and operative complications, but cingulotomy is likely to have fewer side effects than long courses of ECT or high dosages of psychotropic drugs. Gross structural lesions demonstrated on MRI and impaired cognitive function may increase the risk of undesirable side effects and are therefore relative contraindications.

CRITERIA FOR SELECTION OF PATIENTS WITH CHRONIC PAIN SYNDROME

These are very similar to those for the psychiatric patients, in that any patient who is chronically disabled by severe pain and who has had limited or negligible response to pain-relieving procedures—such as surgery for the removal of the presumed cause of the pain, nerve blocks, pain clinic trials, and psychotropic drug trials—is accepted for evaluation. Cingulate surgery is definitely contraindicated, however, for those individuals who have pronounced hysterical or sociopathic traits.

Most patients can be managed by the operating neurosurgeon or their local referring physicians, so that, unless there is a severe depressive component to the illness, preoperative and postoperative psychiatric care is not required. Therefore, referrals from local physicians for pain management are accepted.

The patient completes a detailed pain questionnaire, which includes a pain drawing, a visual analogue scale of pain severity, a life history, a McGill-Melzack pain questionnaire, a list of 52 questions probing into the patient's personality and the influence it has on the illness, a checkoff list of 132 adjectives used to describe feelings about self, and a checkoff list (known as "SCL-90-R") of 90 problems a pain patient could be troubled by.

Patients not previously treated with psychotropic drugs are given a trial of medications, such as doxepin, 150 to 300 mg at night, with clonazepam, 1.5 to 3.0 mg in divided doses during the day.

The MGH evaluation of chronic pain patients follows the pattern delineated for the psychiatric patients. It is, however, permissible for the screening neurologist and psychiatrist to be involved in the care of pain patients before and after cingulotomy.

A close relative or friend who will provide emotional support is also required for these patients, and again, both must be fully informed of the risks and benefits of the procedure and must give consent.

Limbic system surgery should be undertaken, when indicated, in both the psychiatric and pain patients before their support systems (family unit and social environment), employment opportunities, and personality functions have been significantly and perhaps irreversibly damaged by chronic or severe dysfunction.

SURGICAL TECHNIQUES

From May 1962 to June 1991, target localization was carried out with the aid of limited air ventriculography. This method was introduced by Grantham[10] in 1951 for bimedial leucotomy. A modification was described by Foltz and White[7] in 1962, and we slightly modified their technique that same year. Since 1991, target localization using stereotactic MRI has been employed routinely, but on rare occasions, it has been necessary for technical or medical reasons to employ ventriculographic localization. Moreover, it is quite possible that surgeons wishing to carry out cingulotomy may not have access to MRI. For these reasons, both techniques are described here.

VENTRICULOGRAPHIC TARGET LOCALIZATION

Under local anesthesia or general endotracheal anesthesia, the patient is placed supine on an operating table equipped with a radiolucent head-piece and radiographic cassette holder. The head is placed in a plastic holder that allows access to the frontal region and is elevated to a 30-degree angle by flexing of the table. A 4 cm × 10 cm area of the scalp, just behind the frontal hairline is shaved. The center of this area is at the midline and 9.5 cm posterior to the nasion. After the midline is accurately identified, cross-hatches are scratched on the scalp 9.5 cm posterior to the nasion and 1.5 cm to either side of the midline. Stab wounds are made through the scalp at these points, through which the skull is also marked with twist-drill holes. The scalp is incised transversely through the points on the scalp. Bilateral burr holes are made at the twist-drill holes, and the dura and the cortex beneath the burr holes are lightly cauterized. A ventricular needle is introduced to a depth of about 2 cm, in an attempt to ascertain that no subcortical bleeding will be encountered during the introduction of the electrodes. The wound is then closed.

A plastic headband with embedded lead beads situated at 1-cm intervals is placed around the head over the orbital ridge, above the ears, and around the occiput (Fig. 115–2) to enable calculation of the amount of magnification of the fluoroscopic image.

Specially designed 17-gauge ventricular needles, electrically insulated except for the distal centimeter (Ballantine needles, Radionics, Inc., Burlington, MA), are introduced into the lateral ventricles by angling of the needles toward the external auditory meatus on the lateral view and 7 mm from the midline on the frontal view. To adequately visualize the anterior horns and the roofs of the lateral ventricles, 6 cc of air is required in each one. This can usually be accomplished by introducing 12 cc of air through one ventricular puncture.

With the use of intermittent fluoroscopic localization, and with the targets being marked on the fluoroscopic screen, the needles (now being used as thermistor-equipped electrodes) are first positioned bilaterally 1 cm above the roof of the lateral ventricles, 2.5 cm posterior to the anterior tips, and 0.7 cm on either side of the midline. After the first lesions are made, the electrodes are lowered 1 cm without changing the lateral and anteroposterior position. Lesions are made by the application of a radiofrequency current that heats the electrode tip to 85°C for 100 seconds at each position. The lesion volume is about 1 cm in diameter and 2 cm in vertical height, the inferior border being at a point about 1 mm above the lateral ventricular shadow. Figures 115–3 and 115–4 are roentgenograms showing the electrodes in place, and Figures 115–5 and 115–6 are from a postoperative MRI scan showing the areas of cingulate interruption. The air is withdrawn after the lesions are completed, and the wound is covered with a simple dressing. The length of the entire procedure is approximately 1.5 to 2.0 hours.

Repeat cingulotomies do not generally require an incision. They can usually be done under local anesthesia following preoperative medication of 5 mg of droperidol IM and 10 mg of diazepam PO; this combination provides heavy sedation from which the patient is arousable. The areas of the burr holes are shaved and sterilized. The scalp is punctured with a 15-gauge needle through which the electrodes can be inserted. If the interval since the first operation is more than a year, the inner table of the skull may have regenerated, and a twist-drill puncture is necessary. A limited ventriculogram is required, after which the electrodes are positioned as before, but 1 cm anterior to the previous lesions. If a third cingulotomy is required, the lesion can be made 1 cm posterior to the first interruption.

STEREOTACTIC MRI LOCALIZATION

Under heavy sedation, a MRI-compatible stereotactic frame is secured to the patient's head after infiltration of the

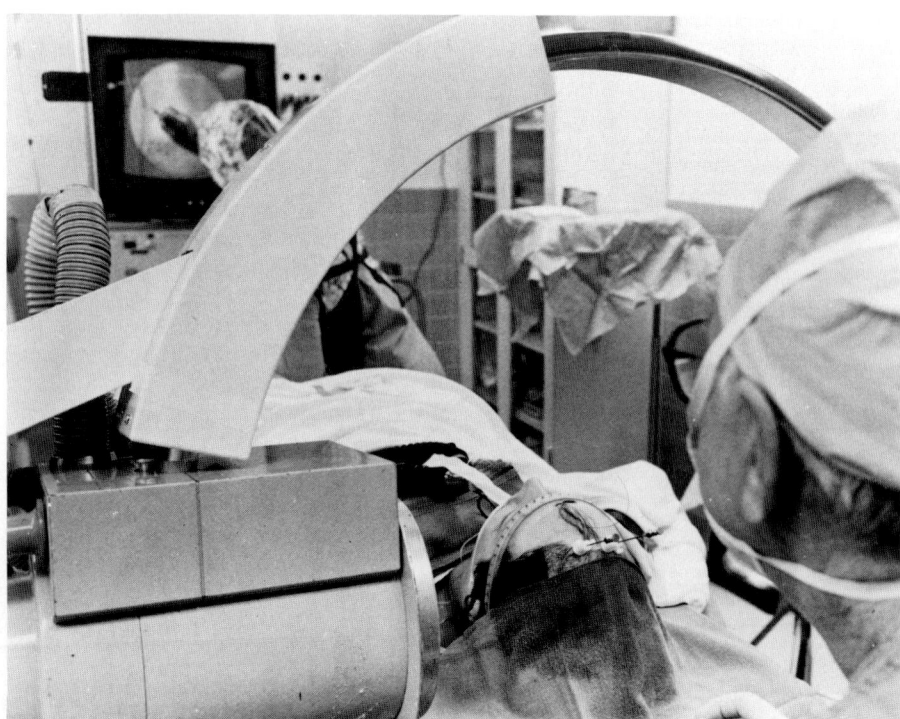

FIGURE 115–2. Stereotactic cingulotomy. Arrangement of the patient, the surgeon, the plastic headband, the C-arm fluoroscope, and screen. The needle electrodes are in position. The radiofrequency generator is at the surgeon's right.

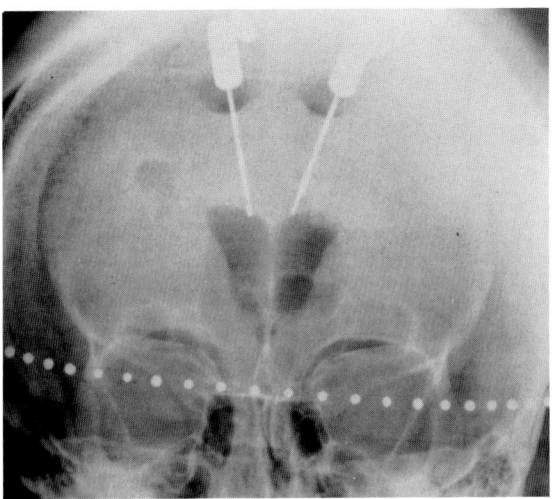

FIGURE 115-3. Anteroposterior view of the electrodes during cingulotomy. The lead beads embedded in the headband are 10 mm apart.

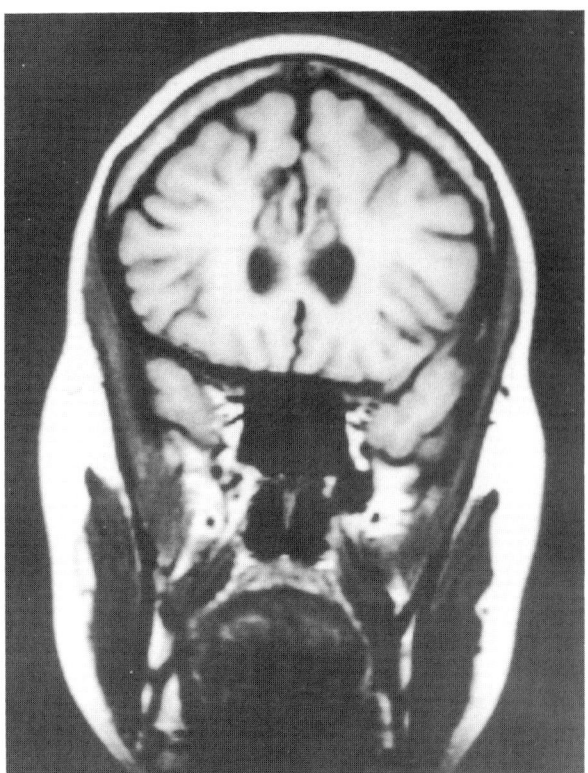

FIGURE 115-5. MRI (frontal view) showing bilateral cingulate lesions after ventriculographic localization.

pin insertion sites with local anesthesia. A T1-weighted stereotactic MRI scan is carried out (T_E 10 msec, T_R 600 msec); with the midsagittal scan used as a reference, coronal sections (4-mm thickness, 1-mm interval) are obtained in a plane parallel to the proposed trajectory of the thermocoagulation probe, spanning the entire anterior cingulum and frontal horns of the lateral ventricles. Targets are then selected from the appropriate coronal slice 2 cm posterior to the tip of the frontal horn, 7 mm from the midline, and 10 mm above the roof of the lateral ventricle.

Following calculation of the stereotactic target coordinates, the patient is returned to the operating room, where the head and stereotactic frame are prepared and draped in the usual fashion. Under local anesthesia and heavy sedation, a limited bicoronal scalp incision is made, and burr holes are placed bilaterally just anterior to the coronal suture and 2 cm from the midline. After dural opening and bipolar cauterization of the pia, a standard thermistor-equipped thermocoagulation electrode (Radionics, Inc., Burlington MA) with a 10-mm uninsulated tip is introduced to the target and heated to 85°C for 100 seconds. After adequate cooling, the electrode is advanced 10 mm, and an additional lesion is made using the same parameters to ensure complete interruption of the cingulum at the target site. The procedure is then carried out in an identical fashion on the opposite side. The scalp incision is closed, a sterile dressing applied, and the frame re-

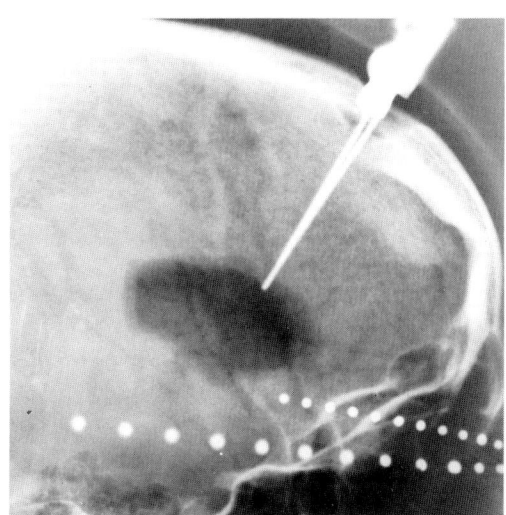

FIGURE 115-4. Lateral view of the electrodes during cingulotomy.

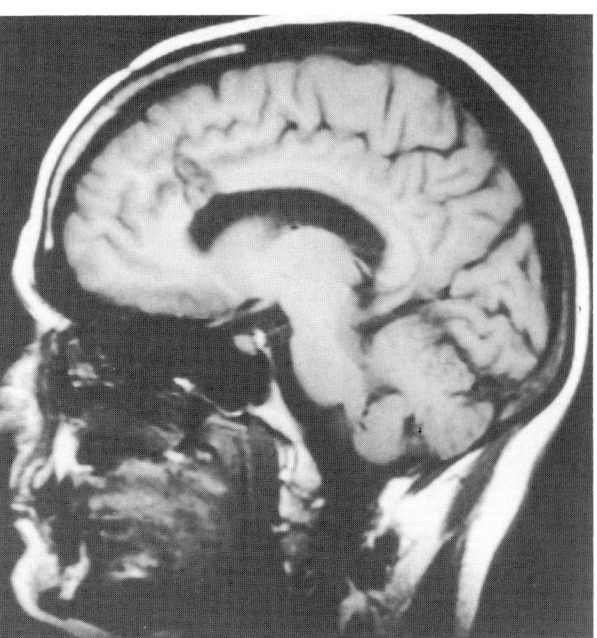

FIGURE 115-6. MRI (sagittal view) showing cingulate lesion after ventriculographic localization.

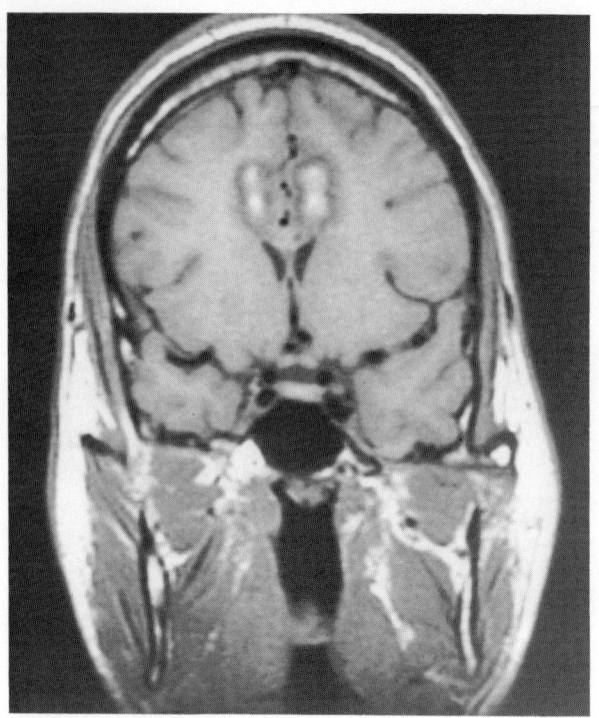

FIGURE 115–7. MRI (frontal view) showing bilateral cingulate lesions following MR localization.

moved. Figures 115–7 and 115–8 are from a postoperative MRI scan showing the lesions after MRI localization.

IMMEDIATE POSTOPERATIVE MANAGEMENT

Postoperatively, the patients are often nauseated and may develop headache, cervical pain, and fever of 100°F to 102°F, owing to air and red blood cells in the cerebral spinal fluid

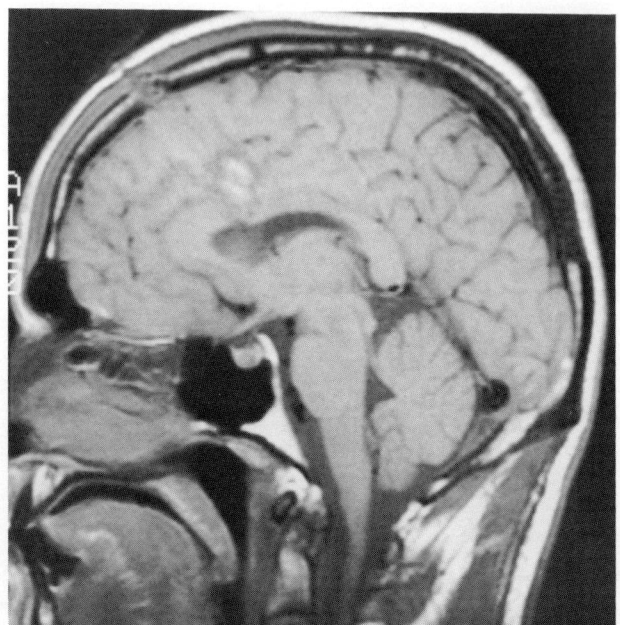

FIGURE 115–8. MRI (sagittal view) showing cingulate lesion following MR localization.

from the ventricular puncture and the resolution of the lesion's necrotic tissue. Also, bladder dysfunction (either incontinence or retention) is not uncommon. All of these side effects are treated symptomatically with appropriate medication and usually clear within 4 days. Psychiatric patients are maintained on their preoperative psychotropic medications, although usually at lower doses. Chronic pain patients are given non-narcotic analgesics along with appropriate psychotropic therapy; they do not suffer narcotic withdrawal symptoms.

LONG-TERM POSTOPERATIVE MANAGEMENT

PSYCHIATRIC PATIENTS

Most of our patients require careful, long-term psychiatric management. We ask their psychiatrists to see them weekly at first, adjusting their medications and treating them as they would any of their very sick psychiatric patients, because we consider cingulotomy not "an instant cure" but an adjunct to good psychiatric care. Medications (often at lower doses), psychotherapy, and ECT, which gave only temporary or partial relief preoperatively, are often very effective postoperatively.

The psychiatric status is usually cyclic, with gradual improvement occurring over a period of 1 month to 5 years. For the first 3 months, the low periods of these cycles are often lower than they were preoperatively. We believe this is caused by a discouragement factor, the patient feeling that the "operation failed and now there is nothing left" or "I felt normal for awhile; I cannot go through the anguish of my illness again!" The suicidal risk at this stage is high, and hospitalization is often required to protect and treat the patient.

The high periods of the cycles can occasionally result in hypomania. Lithium and often a neuroleptic are required to prevent the attack from becoming more serious. If the symptom is unrecognized and denied by the patient, however, it could become so severe that hospitalization would also be required during the acute stage.

Family members or close friends are essential in the management of postcingulotomy psychiatric patients, especially during the low and high periods of their cycles, for it is these support persons who may be required to alert the psychiatrist of the abnormal behavior.

Of the psychiatric patients we have categorized in the "well" status, 45 percent underwent more than one cingulotomy. We are, however, reluctant to perform a "double set" of lesions at the first operation, because not every patient requires it and because we believe that the absence of emotional and cognitive deficits in our series is due largely to the "staging" of the lesions. Therefore, it is our practice to perform a repeat cingulotomy after 3 months if there has been no or insufficient response to the first one. Some of our patients have had as many as three separate procedures without complications.

CHRONIC PAIN PATIENTS

Patients generally have a smooth postoperative course. Within 5 to 7 days postoperatively, they are often able to tolerate their pain without narcotic analgesics and are discharged from hospital on a psychotropic medication regimen with non-narcotic analgesics as needed. They are usually managed by the operating neurosurgeon if the depressive component of their illness is not too severe. Slow, steady improvement is concurrent with their physical and social rehabilitation, and maximum improvement seems to occur within 3 to 6 months. The assistance of family and friends in the rehabilitation process is invaluable. It is of interest that only 2 of our 23 chronic pain patients who were categorized as "well" required more than one operation.

SAFETY

As of June 1994, we had performed 820 cingulotomies on 544 patients, with no deaths and no infections. Two hemiplegias have occurred secondary to acute intracerebral hematomas caused by laceration of subcortical arteries during introduction of the ventricular needles. One patient made a complete recovery after evacuation of the clot; the other remains hemiplegic. One male patient, aged 40, developed a chronic subdural hematoma at the site of the left burr hole, which required evacuation 4 weeks after the cingulotomy. He made a complete recovery, suffered a relapse in his depression, underwent a second procedure without incident and did well, but had another relapse 4.5 years later and underwent a third cingulotomy. Six weeks after this last cingulotomy, he developed another chronic subdural hematoma, again at the site of the left burr hole. It required evacuation, and recovery was again complete without neurologic deficit.

Convulsions have occurred in seven of our patients but have been easily controlled with phenytoin. There have been no permanent neurologic behavior or intellectual deficits as a result of the cingulate lesions themselves.

EFFICACY

In 1987, we published a study of 198 of our psychiatric patients operated upon during a 20-year period and followed for 2 to 22 years (mean, 8.6 years).[11] One hundred twenty of them carried a diagnosis of affective disorder (unipolar or bipolar depression, or schizoaffective disorder), 14 suffered from disabling anxiety, 32 from obsessive-compulsive disorders, and 11 from schizophrenia, and 21 had "miscellaneous" disorders. All of the patients were disabled preoperatively; 86 (43 percent) had suicidal ideation, and 52 (26 percent) had made suicidal attempts.

In assessing the postoperative status of this group, we limited *worthwhile improvement* to apply only to those patients who were well or functioning normally on medication and/or psychotherapy or who were no longer critically ill and suicidal but still had intermittently recurring, disabling psychiatric symptoms. Using these criteria, we assigned 62 percent of our patients to the satisfactorily improved group. Another 17 percent who remained severely disabled but required less medication, spent less time in hospitals, required less psychiatric supervision, and were easier to manage were felt to have shown only *slight improvement*. The best results have been attained in patients diagnosed as having clinical depression or anxiety disorders. Eighteen (9 percent) of the entire cohort committed suicide over a mean follow-up period of 8.6 years; all had had preoperative suicidal ideation, and 13 (72 percent) had attempted suicide.[11]

We have also reviewed the postoperative status of 123 patients who underwent cingulotomy for pain. Thirty-five of them had terminal cancer, and for the first 3 postoperative months, 20 (57 percent) obtained satisfactory pain relief. Ten patients lived more than 3 months, and pain relief was sustained in only 2.

The 98 patients with noncancerous chronic pain have been followed for 1 to 21 years (mean, 7 years). There were no deaths or complications in this group, and only 3 were lost to follow-up. Severe, constant pain refractory to all the usual therapies constituted the primary indication for cingulotomy. Failed back patients are those with chronic back pain who had undergone one or more laminectomies. In the entire series, 19 percent were addicted to narcotics and 58 percent were diagnosed as suffering from one or more of the following psychiatric disorders: affective, anxiety, and personality.

The patients who were treated with cingulotomy for pain were grouped as shown in Table 115–1.

In judging whether or not the operation had conferred a worthwhile benefit we accepted any one of the following criteria:

- The patient no longer complained of pain and required no medication.
- The patient was symptom-free with minor psychotropic drugs.
- The patient was comfortable on a regimen of minor psychotropic drugs and non-narcotic analgesics.

Except for the "failed back" patients, the numbers in the other categories are too small to be of other than anecdotal value in reference to perceived benefit. Five of six patients with chronic abdominal pain were usefully improved, as were three of five patients with phantom limb pain. The operation appeared to have been of little or no help to patients suffering from tabetic, thalamic, or postherpetic pain.

On the other hand, 38 (62 percent) of 61 patients with chronic low back pain appeared to have obtained significant benefit from cingulotomy. It is again of interest that the operation was of more benefit to females than to males (77 percent versus 47 percent, respectively). Four males in this

Table 115–1. GROUPING OF PATIENTS UNDERGOING CINGULOTOMY FOR PAIN

Locus/Etiology of Pain	No. Patients
Low back	62*
Abdomen and flank	7*
Unknown	6
Miscellaneous	
Herpetic	6
Headache	3
Thalamic	3
Facial neuralgia	1
Phantom limb	5
Tabetic and "spinal"	2
Upper extremity (trauma)	3*
Total	23

*One patient in this group not followed.

group committed suicide postoperatively; three of the four carried an additional diagnosis of clinical depression.

If a satisfactory postoperative status is attained after cingulotomy for chronic pain of nonmalignant origin, it is usually permanent. This finding stands out in marked contrast to the fading of pain relief in patients operated upon for intractable cancer pain.

DISCUSSION

Although we have limited this chapter to a discussion of cingulotomy there are other approaches to the limbic system; chief among these are subcaudate tractotomy, limbic leucotomy, and anterior capsulotomy. The operative techniques and the reported results have been delineated elsewhere.[12] It should be noted, however, that anterior capsulotomy and limbic leucotomy are said to yield better postoperative outcomes than cingulotomy in cases of obsessive-compulsive neurosis.

It is because of this diversity of approaches that we prefer the term *limbic system surgery* to either *psychiatric surgery* or *psychosurgery*. Indeed, *psychosurgery* is thought by most of the general public and many physicians to refer exclusively to the outmoded and rejected prefrontal lobotomy. This semantic confusion has retarded progress and limited the acceptance and application of surgical therapy for mental illness.

In 1993, 57 years after its initial acceptance and 34 years after Moniz was awarded the Nobel Prize for its introduction, limbic system surgery remains controversial. It is imperative, therefore, that every possible precaution be taken to ensure that psychiatrically ill patients be chosen for operation only after all other generally accepted therapies have failed, that thorough preoperative evaluation is performed, that informed consent has been obtained, and that careful postoperative evaluation and management are carried out.

SUMMARY

We have presented the operative technique employed in performing 820 bilateral anterior stereotactic cingulotomies on 544 patients. There have been no deaths or infections. There is no evidence of impairment of cognition or "emotional tone" as a result of cingulate interruption. Two patients became hemiplegic, and 1 developed chronic subdural hematomas postoperatively. Seven patients reported single postoperative seizures. Subsets of 198 psychiatric and 123 chronic pain patients have been intensively evaluated over a mean follow-up period of 8.6 and 7 years, respectively. The clinical state of 79 percent of the psychiatric patients improved postoperatively, and 62 percent had achieved a satisfactory status at the time of evaluation. Of 61 chronic pain patients who met criteria for "failed back surgery," the operation was believed to have been definitely worthwhile in 38 (62 percent).

We conclude from this experience that stereotactic cingulotomy is relatively safe and effective. It should be available to the patients with severe mental illness that is refractory to all nonoperative therapies, particularly those who suffer from affective disorders. Similarly, it should be considered as a last resort for certain patients with intractable pain. Our experiences with the treatment of the "failed back syndrome" lead us to conclude that cingulotomy offers a better and safer chance for amelioration of pain than other destructive operations such as nerve root ablation and cordotomy.

REFERENCES

1. Moniz E: Tentatives Operatoires dans le Traitement de Certaines Psychoses. Paris, Masson et Cie, 1936
2. Moniz E: Prefrontal leucotomy in the treatment of mental disorders. Am J Psychiatry 93:1379–1385, 1937
3. Shutts D: Lobotomy: Resort to the Knife. New York, Van Nostrand Reinhold, 1982, pp 117–179
4. Freeman WL, Watts JW: Psychosurgery in the Treatment of Mental Disorders and Intractable Pain. Springfield, IL, Charles C Thomas, 1942
5. Freeman WL, Watts JW: Psychosurgery in the Treatment of Mental Disorders and Intractable Pain, ed 2. Springfield, IL, Charles C Thomas, 1950
6. Tooth GC, Newton MP: Leucotomy in England and Wales 1942–1954. (Reports on Public Health and Medical Subjects No. 104.) London, Her Majesty's Stationery Office, 1961
7. Foltz EL, White LE Jr: Pain "relief" by frontal cingulotomy. J Neurosurg 19:89–100, 1962
8. Papez JW: A proposed mechanism of emotion. Arch Neurol Psychiatry 38:725–743, 1937
9. Bernstein JG: Handbook of Drug Therapy in Psychiatry, ed 2. Massachusetts, John Wright—PSG Inc. Publishing, 1988, pp 1–25
10. Grantham EG: Prefrontal lobotomy for relief of pain with a report of a new operative technique. J Neurosurg 8:411–422, 1951
11. Ballantine HT Jr, Bouckoms AJ, Thomas EK, Giriunas IE: Treatment of psychiatric illness by stereotactic cingulotomy. Biol Psychiatry 22:807–819, 1987
12. Ballantine HT Jr: Neurosurgery for behavioral disorders, in Wilkins RH, Rengachary SS (eds): Neurosurgery, Vol 3. New York, Elsevier/North-Holland, 1985, pp 2527–2537

CHAPTER 116

Intraventricular Morphine in the Treatment of Pain Secondary to Cancer

Alberto Lenzi
Giuseppe Galli
Giovanni Marini

Over the past 15 years, biochemical studies, however fragmentary, have shown us that within the "human ecosystem," interdependent relationships exist between the somatic and vegetative nervous system, between neuromodulators and hormones, and also between psychic activity and the immune system.[1-3]

This ecosystem appears to have been fashioned over the course of evolution into a definite structure, the ultimate goal of which is preservation of the human species against polymorphous external aggressions. Anthropologic studies have further heightened the awareness that environmental stress can heavily influence the onset of many otherwise classically idiopathic diseases like cancer. Cancer, in fact, could very well be the end result of an imbalance between aggressive external forces and internal defense mechanisms, in which a great many factors interact in unknown proportions, producing an interference of congenital and acquired elements (either causal or voluntary), sometimes due to proneness, sometimes conditioned.

Within this complex meshwork of factors, pain is a warning signal of acute changes occurring in the physiologic homeostasis; pain is also an epiphenomenon signaling the progressive and chronic deterioration of multiple organic systems whose balanced functions ensure physical and psychological well-being.[4-6]

In the treatment of pain secondary to cancer, our prime objective is to achieve analgesia for as long as possible, using methods that provide long-lasting pain relief and, in addition, require limited surgery and create minimal injury to the nervous system's structure.[7,8]

The techniques that allow the slow infusion of microdoses of morphine into the cerebrospinal fluid (CSF) not only fulfill these requirements, they also make it easier for family members to handle a patient's pain over long periods.

MORPHINE THERAPY AND THE OPIOID SYSTEM

The analgesic effects of morphine are for the most part due to its central actions. Morphine does not significantly influence the response threshold of the nerve endings, nor the conduction of stimuli by peripheral nerves. Nevertheless, it remains rather difficult to define which centers of the nervous system are responsible for analgesia and behavioral responses.

Many of the brain's structures that are involved with pain perception and modulation are affected by morphine, yet the drug's effects on the spinal cord, the limbic system, and the periventricular and periaqueductal gray matter seem to constitute the very neurophysiologic basis of its analgesic efficacy.

The biochemical activity of opioids in providing pain relief in cancer management has been elucidated as a result of two important discoveries: the identification of specific receptors for exogenous opiates within the central nervous system, and the detection of endogenous peptide–type substances with effects similar to those of morphine. This elucidation began when Pert and Snyder of the United States and Terenius of Sweden identified the precise location of binding sites with a high affinity for opioids in the fragments of cell membrane obtained from rat brain and from the intestines of guinea pigs.[9,10]

Subsequently, many others were able to measure the density and the actual distribution of these receptors in the brain and spinal cord.[11] Classically, it has been held that two distinct pathways are involved in the perception of pain. An acute, localized pain (which is hardly diminished by opioids) is conveyed through a monosynaptic route that is phylogenetically recent, and this pain travels up the ventral spinothalamic tract and enters the ventral lateral nucleus of the thalamus, from which the neurons project out into the primary somatosensory area. Conversely, deeper pain (which is efficaciously alleviated by opioids) is conveyed through phylogenetically older, multisynaptic routes.

These multisynaptic routes are made up of groups of cells with multiple and widespread interconnections; they are interconnected by unmyelinated fibers having low conduction speed. The paleospinothalamic pathway travels up the spinal cord to reach the brain, making two important "integration stops" along the way: one at the periaqueductal gray matter level, and the second in the median area of the thalamus. The map of opioid receptor distribution corresponds to the distribution of the paleospinothalamic pathways of pain. Although a high density of receptors is also present in the amygdala, in the corpus striatum, and in the hypothalamus—regions of the brain that act together in processing the emotional components of pain—maximum receptor density is found in the substantia gelatina of the spinal cord, and also in proximity of the substantia gelatina of the spinal trigeminal nucleus.[11a, 11b]

In 1976, Martin et al[12] hypothesized the existence of three receptor subtypes, μ, κ, and σ, with initials matching those of the agonist types, i.e., morphine, ketocyclazocine, and N-allilnormetazocine.[12, 13]

Other authors report a fourth receptor, δ, specifically antagonized by D-ala-met-enkephalin. The pharmacologic picture induced by common exogenous opiates (i.e., morphine, pentazocine, and buprenorphine) appears to be the algebraic sum of the different agonist-antagonist effects carried out vis-a-vis specific receptors.[13, 14]

In 1975, Hughes and colleagues[15] were able to isolate and identify the first two analgesic peptides, met-enkephalin and leu-enkephalin, in pig brain. Soon thereafter, β-endorphin was identified, a peptide with 31 amino acids that has a structure similar to that of the met-enkephalin within it. In 1979, for the first time, Chavkin and associates[16] described dinorphin, a peptide with 13 amino acids that includes the leu-enkephalin structure.

Today, three major families of endogenous opiates are recognized.[17] Pro-opio-melano-cortin derivatives are the first major family of endogenous opiates. Their prime elements are β-endorphin, ACTH, and g-MSH. β-Endorphin is maximally concentrated in the adenohypophysis and is present in lesser amounts in the hypothalamus, amygdala, periaqueductal gray matter, and sympathetic ganglia. β-Endorphin is a very powerful agonist for μ receptors and a relatively good one for δ receptors. Polypeptides derived from pro-opio-melano-cortin play a complex yet complementary role in the body's reaction to stress. In such situations, all the polypeptides derived from this precursor are released simultaneously. Correlations among neurons containing β-endorphin, the hypothalamus, and periaqueductal gray matter all confirm the role of β-endorphin as filter-modulator of spinal pains. Projections toward the median area of the hypothalamus confirm the role of β-endorphin in regulating the hypophysis function in such a way as to maintain the body's homeostasis punctually and continuously.

Proenkephalin A derivatives are the second major family of endogenous opiates. Their prime elements are met-enkephalin and, to a certain extent, leu-enkephalin. Maximum concentration is observed in the limbic system, in the median area of the thalamus, in the amygdala, and in the substantia gelatina of the spinal cord. Enkephalin has a preferential sensitivity for δ receptors, and in part for μ receptors. Enkephalin directly acts on the cell containing these specific receptors via an inhibitory mechanism. Enkephalin released from the cell containing it triggers an increase in sodium conduction through the cell membrane, thereby partially depolarizing it. When an impulse then reaches the nerve ending, the net depolarization is lower and softer. Hence, release of the excited mediator is proportionally less. The next-receiving cell undergoes proportionally less stimulation. Thus, moment by moment, these inhibiting actions control the ascending pain pathways from the spinal cord to the brain. Substance P is considered to be the mediator of nociceptive stimuli. Enkephalins therefore act as modulators by way of presynaptic inhibitory mechanisms that manage the release of substance P in the spinal cord.[17a]

Proenkephalin B derivatives are the third major family of endogenous opiates. Their prime element is dinorphin,[18, 19] which is most concentrated around the neurohypophysis and the spinal cord. These polypeptides tend to bind with κ receptors, and at the spinal cord level, they develop an intense analgesic effect. In addition to being present in the intestinal tract and medullary tract of the adrenal gland, they are contained in different types of neurons of the central nervous system.[14, 20, 21] Although classic types of neurotransmitters (e.g., norepinephrine) hold an enzymatic synthesis at the nerve endings, are released following tonic stimuli, and undergo an enzymatic degradation or uptake, neuropeptides are produced at ribosome level in the form of long protein precursors; they are released intermittently and tend to have a long-lasting effect without uptake. Thus, the classic neurotransmission system carried out by excitation or by postsynaptic inhibition of the cell acts as an emergency signal indicating rapid changes within the organism; the neuropeptide system, in contrast, has the role of maintaining a continuous basic environment of optimal well-being and the progressive adaptation to varying input conditions, in order that the cell may rapidly return to optimal well-being. Classic peptides and neurotransmitters can coexist within the same neurons, even when confined to different compartments.[22] This coexistence, in fact, has led us to believe that peptides are of vital importance as regulators of nervous functions.

At the posterior horn of the spinal cord are located the primary sensory neurons containing substance P, somatostatin, gastrin, and cholecystokinin; spinal interneurons containing enkephalin, substance P, and neurotensin; and descending systems containing substance P, enkephalin, and serotonin. It is clear that all these play an important integrator-modulator role in afferent sensory impulses, which generally occur in this region with the fundamental presence of neuropeptides. Neuropeptides also execute a vital modulating role in hypophysis and endocrine activity via hypothalamic release or inhibitive factors of incretion.

As mentioned earlier, the human body reacts to situations of stress by releasing, from the same precursor, three functionally distinct peptides: β-endorphin, ACTH, and g-MSH. Studies conducted by Panerai[21] highlighted the fact that a state of analgesia maintained normally and continuously is the result of a balance and modulated interaction, at the receptor level, of endogenous agonist-antagonist opiates, among which are cholecystokinin and TRH.

MORPHINE INJECTIONS INTO THE CEREBROSPINAL FLUID

Since the early 1980s, microdose morphine injection into the cerebrospinal fluid (CSF) has progressively acquired a fairly well-defined place in cancer pain therapy. This trend displaces a preference for ablative techniques, which neurosurgeons had previously used to control pain of this kind, whereas general practitioners and internists often treated pain with ad libitum administration of oral or intramuscular morphine, resulting in tolerance and progressive impairment of mental faculties. Administered parenterally or orally, opiates undergo rapid metabolic inactivation by the liver.[23-25] Only a small portion of the drug reaches the specific central nervous system (CNS) receptors and, therefore, attains an analgesic effect of limited quality and duration. Conversely, morphine injected into the CSF bypasses the blood-brain barrier and reaches specific receptor sites immediately, thus making small doses of drug particularly effective.

For many years, fear of respiratory depression[26-29] hindered the general acceptance of this technique. Following proof, however, that intrathecal morphine provides intense analgesia in rats, several authors tested the effects in humans of morphine administered directly into the CSF at the extradural or subarachnoid level.[30, 31] In 1981, Leavens and colleagues[32] reported the use of intraventricular injections of morphine in four cancer patients. Our current series includes 50 patients receiving intraventricular morphine therapeutically, 119 patients receiving morphine in the spinal CSF, and 119 patients receiving morphine administered via catheter into the spinal extradural space.

The present chapter reports our experience with 50 patients suffering from neoplastic pain syndromes of the cervical and craniofacial regions. In these cases, microdoses of morphine were injected into the ventricular fluid through a catheter connected to a subcutaneous reservoir. We believe this type of drug administration offers a good way of assessing the advantages and disadvantages of the technique, even in comparison with the spinal, subarachnoid, and extradural routes.

PATIENT SELECTION

We chose patients with a presumptive life expectancy of about 6 months in whom neurosurgical procedures (e.g., thermorhizotomy, chemical rhizotomy) either had become ineffective as a result of progression of the neoplastic illness or were not indicated. All patients in this series underwent a full trial of standard analgesic treatment, both medical and surgical, and radiotherapy.

SURGICAL TECHNIQUE

A computed tomographic (CT) scan of the brain is performed in order to examine the morphology and dimensions of the cerebral ventricles and to exclude CNS involvement by the patient's disease. Subsequently, the patient is operated on in the supine position, with the neck moderately flexed. Local anesthesia is used. A right frontal arch-shaped incision is made, and a burr hole is placed 2 cm from the midline and 6 cm above the superciliary arch. The dura is opened, the right frontal horn is cannulated with a ventricular needle, and fluid is withdrawn. The ventricular needle is then replaced with a Silastic ventricular catheter (6–8 cm), connected to a 1.5-ml reservoir (Cordis Italia, Milano, Italy) (Fig. 116–1) that is placed beneath the galea. To ensure that the system is functioning perfectly, patent CSF is aspirated from the reservoir prior to skin closure.

When opiates are to be administered, the skin is disinfected repeatedly, and the reservoir is tapped transcutaneously with a 25-gauge needle connected to a 2.5-ml syringe. Half a milligram to 1 mg of morphine hydrochloride diluted in 1 ml of a 5 percent glucose solution is injected while the inner part of the system is washed with CSF to guarantee dispersion of the drug throughout the ventricle.

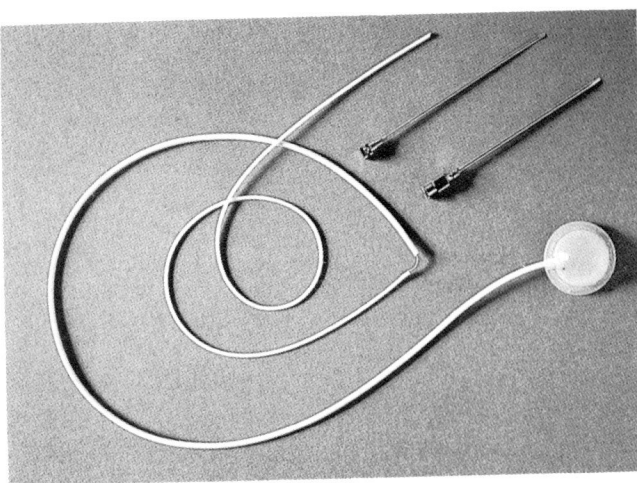

FIGURE 116–1. The ventricular needle replaced with a ventricular catheter (6 to 8 cm) and connected to a 1.5-ml reservoir (Cordis Italia, Milano Italy) is placed beneath the galea.

CASE REPORTS

Table 116–1 summarizes the type and site of the tumor in our series of 50 cases as well as the distribution, duration, and rhythm of the neoplastic pain attacks. The table also summarizes previous therapies. In 39 of 50 patients, the tumor was limited to the head and neck, tongue, larynx, parotid gland, pharynx, palatine tonsil, and oral cavity. In 4 of 12 other cases, the tumor involved the pulmonary apex (cases 4, 7, 16, and 29) or the breast (case 7), with extension into the brachial plexus. Case 34 was that of a patient suffering from bronchiogenic cancer that metastasized to the bodies of the fourth and fifth vertebrae. In 2 patients suffering from kidney tumor (cases 12 and 13), metastases reached cranial bones, causing pain in this region. Patient 18 had thyroid cancer with multiple bony metastases, and patient 33 had melanoma with multiple bony and subcutaneous metastases.

Almost all of these patients had received minor analgesic drugs (acetylsalicylic acid, ketoprofen, noramidopyrine), the efficacy of which decreased over time. Methylprednisolone was also administered occasionally. Nine patients received analgesic therapy with morphine syrup, which had poor results or unacceptable side effects. Ten patients received pentazocine as needed, often many times a day. This therapy influenced the quality of the subsequent intraventricular morphine use because of the appearance of a more or less high toxicodependence.

Of 50 patients, 44 were male and 6 were female. The mean age was 53 years. The pain classification, continuous or intermittent, was influenced, in our opinion, by the patient's personality. The pain syndrome had an average duration of 2.13 months. The use of intraventricular morphine must not begin too early, because management of these patients for long periods is difficult because of the risk of sepsis, respiratory depression, and increasing drug tolerance.

Table 116–1. ORIGIN AND CHARACTERISTICS OF PAIN AND PREVIOUS THERAPIES

Case/Patient No.	Age (yr) Sex	Etiology of Pain; Site of Tumor	Distribution; Duration of Pain	Previous Cancer-specific Treatment	Previous Analgesic Treatment
1	45, M	Tonsils; local invasion	Soft palate, pharynx, neck; 2 mo, continuous	Local resection	Minor analgesic drugs
2	50, M	Rhinopharynx; local invasion	Orofacies, neck; 3 mo, continuous	Biopsy, radiotherapy	ACTH, methylprednisolone
3	42, M	Tongue; local invasion	Oropharynx, soft palate; 3 mo, intermittent	Biopsy, radiotherapy	ACTH, methylprednisolone
4	57, M	Pulmonary apex; diffusion to brachial plexus	R arm, R cervical region, R chest wall; 1 mo, continuous	Biopsy, radiotherapy	Minor analgesic drugs
5	63, M	Tonsils; local invasion	Tongue, oropharynx, soft palate; 2 mo, continuous	Biopsy, chemotherapy	Morphine syrup
6	56, M	Pharynx; local invasion	Orofacies, neck; 5 mo, intermittent	Biopsy, radiotherapy, chemotherapy	Methylprednisolone, pentazocine
7	56, F	L breast; diffusion to brachial plexus	Upper L chest, axillary cavity, L arm, L neck; 2 mo, continuous	Mastectomy, radiotherapy	Minor analgesic drugs, alcoholic hypophysectomy
8	62, M	Tongue	Oropharynx, neck; 1 mo, continuous	Biopsy, radiotherapy	Minor analgesic drugs
9	61, M	Larynx; local invasion	Oropharynx, ear, R mastoid region; 3 mo, intermittent	Local resection, tracheostomy	Minor analgesic drugs
10	45, M	Tongue; local invasion	Oropharynx; 2 mo, continuous	Biopsy, radiotherapy	Minor analgesic drugs, pentazocine occasionally
11	64, M	Soft palate; local invasion	Orofacies, pharynx, neck; 1 mo, continuous	Biopsy, radiotherapy	ACTH, methylprednisolone
12	60, M	Kidney; multiple metastases (cranium, lungs)	Generalized; 16 mo, continuous	Nephrectomy	Morphine syrup, minor analgesic drugs
13	73, M	Kidney; multiple metastases (liver, pancreas, jaw bone)	Generalized, more severe in facial/neck region; 1 mo, intermittent	Nephrectomy	Morphine syrup
14	69, M	Tongue; local invasion	Oropharynx, R ear, neck; 2 mo, continuous	Biopsy, radiotherapy	Minor analgesic drugs, pentazocine occasionally
15	73, M	L maxillary sinus; local invasion	Orofacies, neck, L hemicranium; 4 mo, intermittent	Repeated local resections	Minor analgesic drugs
16	64, M	Pulmonary apex; multiple cranial metastases	Generalized; 1 mo, intermittent	Biopsy, chemotherapy	Minor analgesic drugs
17	46, M	Tongue; local invasion	Orofacies, R hemicranium, R neck; 3 mo, continuous	Local resection, radiotherapy	Pentazocine
18	36, M	Thyroid gland; multiple cranium/jaw metastases	Generalized (neck, cranium); 5 mo, continuous	Local resection, radiotherapy	Morphine syrup, pentazocine
19	59, M	Tongue; local invasion (jaw)	Orofacies, cranium, R neck; 9 mo, continuous	Repeated local resections, radiotherapy, chemotherapy	Morphine syrup
20	42, M	Jaw; local invasion	Orofacies, cranium, neck; 4 mo, continuous	Biopsy, radiotherapy	Morphine syrup
21	62, M	Pharynx; local invasion	Oropharynx, occipital; 2 mo, intermittent	Biopsy, radiotherapy	Minor analgesic drugs
22	77, F	Skin of the neck; local invasion	Face, L neck; 2 mo, intermittent	Biopsy, radiotherapy	Minor analgesic drugs
23	59, M	Pharynx; local invasion	Oropharynx, R neck; 5 mo, continuous	Biopsy, radiotherapy	Minor analgesic drugs
24	62, F	Tongue; local invasion (jaw)	Orofacies, neck; 5 mo, continuous	Local resection, radiotherapy	Minor analgesic drugs
25	50, F	Pharynx; local invasion	Oropharynx, neck, R hemicranium; 2 mo, intermittent	Biopsy, radiotherapy	Minor analgesic drugs, morphine syrup

Table 116–1. ORIGIN AND CHARACTERISTICS OF PAIN AND PREVIOUS THERAPIES Continued

Case/Patient No.	Age (yr) Sex	Etiology of Pain; Site of Tumor	Distribution; Duration of Pain	Previous Cancer-specific Treatment	Previous Analgesic Treatment
26	57, M	Larynx; local invasion	Neck, face, occipital area; 7 mo, continuous	Local resection, radiotherapy	Minor analgesic drugs
27	52, M	Tongue; local invasion	Orofacies, cranium; 2 mo, intermittent	Biopsy, radiotherapy	Minor analgesic drugs
28	60, M	Oral cavity	Orofacies, L neck; 3 mo, continuous	Biopsy, radiotherapy, partial resection of the jaw	Minor analgesic drugs
29	50, M	R pulmonary apex; diffusion to brachial plexus	R neck, R arm, R chest wall; 7 mo, continuous	Biopsy, radiotherapy	Minor analgesic drugs, pentazocine daily
30	62, M	Larynx; pulmonary metastases	Orofacies, neck, occipital and thoracic areas; 9 mo, continuous	Local resection, radiotherapy, chemotherapy	Morphine syrup, minor analgesic drugs
31	54, F	C2 body; oropharynx invasion	Crainofacies, L neck; 8 mo, continuous	Biopsy, radiotherapy	Minor analgesic drugs, pentazocine
32	64, M	Pharynx; local invasion	Cranium, oropharynx, L neck; 9 mo, continuous	Local resection, radiotherapy	Minor analgesic drugs
33	51, F	Skin; multiple bone/subcutaneous metastases	Generalized; 5 mo, continuous	Local resection, radiotherapy, chemotherapy	Minor analgesic drugs, epidural morphine
34	56, M	Bronchia; metastases to C4, C5 bodies	Occipital, cervical, thoracic areas; 6 mo, continuous	Biopsy, radiotherapy, laser therapy	Pentazocine daily, morphine syrup
35	59, M	L maxillary sinus; local invasion	L orofacial, cervical, occipital areas; 11 mo, continuous	Biopsy, radiotherapy	Minor analgesic drugs, L thermorhizotomy
36	70, M	Pharynx; local invasion	Oropharynx, R neck; 9 mo, continuous	Local resection, radiotherapy, chemotherapy	Minor analgesic drugs, pentazocine
37	67, M	R parotid; local invasion	R orofacies, neck; 9 mo, continuous	Biopsy, radiotherapy	Minor analgesic drugs
38	65, M	Larynx; local invasion	Oropharynx, R neck; 11 mo, intermittent	Biopsy, radiotherapy	Minor analgesic drugs
39	69, M	Pharynx; local invasion	Cranium; oropharynx, neck; 3 mo, continuous	Surgical resection, radiotherapy, chemotherapy	Minor analgesic drugs, bruprenorphine
40	66, M	Pharynx; local invasion	Orofacies, neck; 4 mo, continuous	Surgical resection, radiotherapy	Minor analgesic drugs, pentazocine
41	34, M	Thyroid; C2 body metastasis	Oropharynx, neck; 1 mo, intermittent	Biopsy, radiotherapy	Minor analgesic drugs, buprenorphine
42	56, M	Pharynx; local invasion	Orpharynx, neck; 4 mo, continuous	Biopsy, radiotherapy	Minor analgesic drugs, pentazocine
43	46, M	Rectum cancer; R lung bone metastases	R thorax, L shoulder, neck, occiput; 12 mo, continuous	Surgical resection radiotherapy	Minor analgesic drugs, buprenorphine
44	56, M	Prostate gland; multiple bone metastases	Generalized, cranium, orofacies; 7 mo, intermittent	Biopsy, chemotherapy	Minor analgesic drugs, pentazocine
45	59, M	Tongue; local invasion	Neck, orofacies, occiput; 3 mo, intermittent	Biopsy, radiotherapy, chemotherapy	Minor analgesic drugs
46	53, M	Pharynx; local invasion	Orofacies, cranium, L neck; 3 mo, continuous	Radiotherapy, biopsy, chemotherapy	Minor analgesic drugs
47	64, M	Tongue; local invasion	Occiput, R neck, orofacies; 10 mo, continuous	Surgical resection, radiotherapy	Minor analgesic drugs
48	58, M	Larynx; local invasion, diffusion to R brachial plexus	Neck, R arm polyrhizopathy; 3 mo, continuous	Surgical resection, radiotherapy, chemotherapy	Minor analgesic drugs, buprenorphine
49	57, M	Tongue; local invasion	Orofacies, neck; 3 mo, continuous	Surgical resection, radiotherapy	Minor analgesic drugs
50	61, M	Tongue; local invasion	Orofacies, R neck; 2 mo, continuous	Surgical resection, radiotherapy	Minor analgesic drugs, buprenorphine

Table 116–2. RESULTS OF INTRAVENTRICULAR MORPHINE IN NEOPLASTIC PATIENTS

Case/Patient No.	Intraventricular Morphine (mg/hr) Initial Dose	Intraventricular Morphine (mg/hr) Final Dose	Duration of Treatment (d)	Analgesia Onset (min)	Analgesia Quality	Final Evaluation	Side Effects	Notes During Treatment
1	1/24	1/24	32	10–15	Excellent	Excellent	None	No pharmacologic association
2	1/48	1/48	29	10–15	Good	Excellent	None	Minor analgesic drugs occasionally
3	1/48	1 + 1/24	274	5–10	Excellent	Excellent	Somnolence initially	Oral feeding; body weight increase; social life almost normalized; death without anguish
4	1/24	1.5/24	39	10–15	Excellent	Excellent	Constipation initially	Lucid mind, euphoria, no knowledge of imminent death
5	1/24	1/24	26	10–20	Good	Good	Emesis	Minor analgesic drugs occasionally
6	1/24	1/24	47	10–15	Excellent	Excellent	Emesis, itching	Only antiemetic drug
7	1/24	1 + 1/24	45	30	Poor	Poor	None	Treatment completely ineffective; previous alcohol neuroadenolysis
8	0.5/24	1.5/24	93	5–10	Excellent	Excellent	Emesis occasionally	Lucid mind, quiet, participation in social life; death without anguish
9	1/48	1.5/24	99	10–15	Excellent	Excellent	Emesis, itching initially	Quiet, euphoria, partial participation in social life
10	1/48	1/24	49	10–15	Excellent	Good	None	Pentazocine occasionally
11	0.5/24	1/24	67	5–10	Excellent	Excellent	Respiratory depression during the 3rd dose, reversed by naloxone	3rd dose wrongly overdosed
12	1/24	1/24	24	10–15	Good	Good	Disorientation, confusion	General condition very bad
13	0.5/24	1/24	47	5–10	Excellent	Excellent	None	Lucid mind, quiet, reasonable self-sufficiency
14	0.5/24	1/24	21	10–15	Excellent	Excellent	None	Quiet, oral feeding resumed
15	0.5/24	1/24	292	5–10	Excellent	Excellent	Urinary retention initially, dizziness	Treatment interrupted after 5 doses; weekly treatment for 2 mo; then 1 mg/24 hr
16	1/24	1/24	5	10–15	Good	Poor	None	General condition very bad
17	1/24	0.5 + 0.5/24	29	20–25	Good	Good	Emesis	Pentazocine
18	0.5/24	1/24	104	5–10	Excellent	Excellent	None	Pentazocine abstinence initially; then quiet, euphoria until death without anguish
19	0.5/24	1/24	4	15–20	Good	Good	Emesis, somnolence	Stupor, general condition very bad
20	0.5/24	1/24	195	5–10	Excellent	Excellent	Emesis for 2d	Lucid mind, quiet, social life almost normalized; death without anguish
21	0.5/24	0.5/24	238	5–10	Excellent	Excellent	None	After the 1st dose, analgesia for 2 mo; then treatment on request
22	0.5/24	1/24	249	5–10	Excellent	Excellent	Emesis initially	Lucid mind, quiet; death without anguish
23	1/24	1/24	16	15–20	Good	Good	Disorientation, stupor	General condition very bad
24	0.5/24	1/24	31	10–15	Excellent	Excellent	None	Lucid mind, quiet; death without anguish
25	1/24	1/24	25	15–20	Good	Good	None	Death without anguish
26	0.5/24	0.5/24	34	15–30	Good	Good	Disorientation, confusion	Late treatment; condition very bad
27	0.5/24	1 + 1/24	217	5–10	Excellent	Excellent	None	Lucid mind, quiet, euphoria occasionally, death without anguish

Table 116–2. RESULTS OF INTRAVENTRICULAR MORPHINE IN NEOPLASTIC PATIENTS Continued

Case/Patient No.	Intraventricular Morphine (mg/hr) Initial Dose	Intraventricular Morphine (mg/hr) Final Dose	Duration of Treatment (d)	Analgesia Onset (min)	Analgesia Quality	Final Evaluation	Side Effects	Notes During Treatment
28	1/24	1/24	85	5/10	Excellent	Excellent	None	Quiet, pain-free until last 3 d
29	0.5/24	0.5/24	23	15–20	Excellent	Good	Somnolence, confusion	Pentazocine; death from transtentorial hernia due to occipital metastases
30	0.5/24	1 + 1/24	89	5–10	Excellent	Excellent	Itching initially	Lucid mind, quiet; death without anguish
31	0.5/24	0.5/24	19	15–20	Excellent	Good	Emesis initially, somnolence, disorientation	Late treatment; condition very bad
32	0.5/24	1/24	47	10–15	Good	Good	Emesis initially	Trigeminal hyperalgic anesthesia after thermorhizotomy; tricyclic drugs
33	0.5/24	1 + 1/24	24	10–15	Excellent	Good	Constipation	Lucid mind, pain-free, but anguish
34	0.5/24	0.5/24	19	5–10	Excellent	Excellent	None	Lucid mind, quiet; sudden death while sleeping
35	0.5/24	0.5/24	137	5–10	Excellent	Excellent	None	Social life almost normalized; pain-free until death
36	0.5/24	0.5/24	56	5–10	Excellent	Excellent	Constipation	Oral feeding, quiet, lucid mind; death without anguish
37	0.5/24	0.5/24	67	5–10	Excellent	Excellent	None	Social life almost normalized; lucid mind
38	0.5/24	0.5/24	35	5–10	Excellent	Excellent	None	Quiet, lucid mind; pain-free
39	0.5/24	1/24	97	5–10	Excellent	Excellent	None	Quiet, pain-free until death
40	0.25/24	0.5/24	13	10–15	Good	Good	Somnolence	General condition very bad
41	0.5/24	0.5/24	79	5–10	Excellent	Excellent	None	Lucid mind; death without anguish
42	0.25/24	0.5/24	25	10	Good	Good	Sedation, somnolence	Pain-free until death
43	0.25/24	1/24	76	5–10	Excellent	Excellent	Nausea, vomiting	Quiet, pain-free
44	0.25/24	—	—	5	Excellent	—	Constipation	Follow-up not possible
45	0.25/24	0.5/24	27	10	Excellent	Excellent	Sedation	Quiet; death without anguish
46	0.25/24	—	—	10	Good	—	—	Follow-up not possible
47	0.25/24	0.25/24	3	10	Good	Poor	Somnolence, mental depression, anorexia	Treatment interrupted
48	0.25/24	0.5/24	43	5–10	Excellent	Excellent	None	Lucid mind, self-sufficiency until death
49	0.25/24	0.5/24	39	5–10	Excellent	Excellent	Sedation	Pain-free; death without anguish
50	0.25/24	0.25/24	27	10–15	Good	Good	None	Lucid mind, liveliness

ADDENDUM: Through 1993 we have treated a total of 134 patients with intraventricular morphine.

Conversely, therapy must not be deferred unduly when either the general clinical condition of the patient is largely compromised or the overuse of major analgesic drugs (morphine, pentazocine) has already caused a dependence that is difficult to manage.

In the first 9 patients of this series, an Ommaya reservoir was used. This was replaced by the reservoir prepared by Cordis Italia, which includes a 1.5-ml Silastic reservoir with a metal base and a ventricular catheter connected to it at a right angle; the catheter length varies from 6 to 8 cm (see Fig. 116–1).

Following introduction of this system, the patient is kept hospitalized for a 5 to 7 days, while the drug is administered and the patient is monitored with respect to response and possible side effects experienced. For home treatment, a relative or a visiting nurse can be taught how to administer the drug. All patients are monitored weekly, at the hospital if possible, or by phone from their homes.

RESULTS

Pain relief is classified as excellent (80–100 percent pain decrease), good (40–80 percent), fair (20–40 percent), and bad (less than 20 percent). Table 116–2 summarizes the initial and final doses of morphine, the time from morphine administration to onset of analgesia, analgesia quality, and side effects. The table also includes some short notes indicating the impressions and emotional evaluations of relatives, useful in underlining the efficacy of treatment, which was sometimes very good.

We administered a single dose of morphine hydrochloride, 1 mg in 1 ml of a 5 percent glucose solution, to the first patients. Analgesia, sometimes excellent (100 percent relief of pain), appeared in 5 to 30 minutes and lasted 24 to 48 hours. We later decided to decrease the initial test dose to 0.5 mg/day. This dosage represents the initial minimal dose necessary to obtain analgesia that is effective for 24 hours with very few or no side effects. In later cases, as the table shows, we started to use 0.25 mg/24 hours as the initial dose.

The best results, from the point of view of both analgesia and subjective well-being, are obtained in patients never previously treated with opioids or other major analgesic drugs. Pentazocine in particular leads rapidly to a dependence; in cases 10, 17, and 29, its previous use greatly influenced the outcome. The most encouraging result was observed in patient 18 (survival 104 days), whose pentazocine dependence was eliminated, although with difficulty. On the other hand, intraventricular morphine was completely ineffective for patient 7. In this subject, an alcohol hypophysectomy had been performed previously to relieve pain.

In 7 cases (12, 16, 19, 23, 26, 31, and 40), treatment was performed at an advanced stage, when the patients' general condition was poor, analgesia ineffective, and mentation impaired, thereby making evaluation of the therapy impossible.

Two subjects (cases 15 and 21), after the first dosages, had long periods of excellent analgesia. When their pain recurred, it was easily controlled by the infrequent administration of intraventricular morphine.

The most common side effects encountered are vomiting and itching at the beginning of the treatment; constipation appears occasionally. Loss of orientation and mental confusion are characteristically encountered among patients who undergo late operation. We believe that their mental activities were impaired by this treatment. In one patient (case 43), treatment was interrupted after 3 days because side effects (drowsiness, anorexia, moodiness) became intolerable.

One patient (case 11) experienced respiratory depression due to overdose, but this was controlled promptly with naloxone.[6, 10, 14] In three patients (cases 46, 48, and 49), follow-up was impossible.

The best results were observed in those patients whose presumptive survival time and general condition were good and who had never been treated with opioids or major analgesic drugs. Many subjects could renew their social lives and sometimes return to manual and intellectual jobs; moreover, those in whom therapy was most efficacious died without anguish.

DISCUSSION

Our experience shows that neoplastic pain of the cervical and craniofacial regions can be efficaciously controlled with microdoses of morphine injected in the ventricular fluid. In our opinion, this therapy represents a considerable improvement in the treatment of neoplastic pain of this type. Analgesia obtained by administering microdoses of morphine intraventricularly appears quickly (within 5 to 30 minutes) and is long-lasting (24 to 48 hours) when a dose of 0.5 mg is administered. The decrease of analgesic effect over the weeks or months of treatment is managed by either adjusting the interdose intervals or by increasing the daily dosage, but never exceeding a total of 2 mg/24 hours. We have not observed morphine dependence among our patients in this program. The therapeutic results are usually clearly positive or negative; when this treatment was ineffective, e.g., case 7, the administration of doses of 2.5 to 5.0 mg/24 hours did not change the ineffectiveness.

With treatment, the quality of life of many of our patients improved greatly, and often a patient described an absence of pain, not merely a dulling of the pain as generally happens when morphine is administered by other routes. In many patients, mentation was normal for a long period, sometimes until death. Other patients were often euphoric, a condition we believe to be due to the excellent quality of analgesia, removing anxiety and depression, and, perhaps, to the release of central inhibitory mechanisms.

We consider intraventricular morphine to be a therapeutic procedure specific for neoplastic pain of the cervical and craniofacial regions. Because of the technical ease of administration, the lack of major side effects, and the high quality of pain relief, this form of treatment can be extended to patients with pain from multiple bony metastases at the cervical and craniofacial regions, because morphine administered in the spinal fluid is often without efficacy, perhaps because of its excessive dilution.

Over the past few months, we have become all the more convinced that, vis-à-vis consistently valid analgesic effects, there have been some handicaps impeding the full acceptance and success of intrathecal and intraventricular morphine therapy in microdoses as a method of pain reduction.

Recently, to further improve our results, we have chosen to match therapy with life expectancy and, moreover, to strive for an improvement in the patient's quality of life. We can identify three subpopulations among our patients: those with a short, medium, and long life expectancies. The short-term group consists of patients with a probable survival of 2 to 3 weeks. In these patients, a spinal extradural catheter is used to provide daily doses of morphine (1–3 mg) at fixed intervals. In the second group, with a probable life expectancy of 1 to 2 months, and with pain localized at the soma, a subarachnoid catheter is placed at L3-L4 or L4-L5 through a Tuohy needle (14 gauge); after tunneling, the catheter is connected to a metal-base reservoir that is inserted subcutaneously on the anterior chest wall.

In the case of craniofacial and cervical pain involving cranial nerves V through IX and the first cervical roots unilaterally or bilaterally, an intraventricular catheter is inserted through a right frontal burr hole into the lateral ventricle. For these patients, a relative or nurse is carefully taught to inject the subcutaneous reservoir transcutaneously. This procedure requires meticulous asepsis and skill to avoid damaging the implanted system.

Patients in the third group have a life expectancy of more than 2 months. For this group, we suggest use of a multidose, manually operated pump to deliver the morphine, rather than daily repeat injections of a reservoir. The latter technique is difficult to manage over long periods because of the risk of sepsis, the risk of damage to the system, and the common need for a nurse to administer drugs.

The pump used for this purpose has a simple manual

Intraventricular Morphine in the Treatment of Pain Secondary to Cancer | 1439

control, allows multidoses (120 therapeutic doses in a normal regimen of 1 mg morphine per single administration), is easily reloaded, and is relatively inexpensive ($1000).

Since December 1985, in collaboration with Cordis-Europa, the Department of Neurosurgery at the University of Brescia has been using this system, which comprises a spinal catheter (76 cm) connected to a 6.5×1.5 cm pump weighing 44 g.

The pump includes (Figs. 116–2 and 116–3) a loading system composed of a Silastic dome placed between two buttons with which to periodically supply more drugs. Below it is a unidirectional valve to avoid drug reflux from the reservoir. The reservoir is a silicone-reinforced polyester membrane fixed to the sealing ring in polysulfonate. At the time of insertion, this position below the check valve is loaded with twelve 1-centigram vials of morphine hydrochloride. In the full regimen, the reservoir can hold up to 12 ml of narcotic, which equals 120 mg of morphine, equal to 120 therapeutic doses. The administration technique relies on 2 buttons, which are to be pushed in sequence; the first is lateral, the second medial. The first button transfers the desired amount of drug (e.g., 0.1 ml = 1 mg) from the reservoir to the catheter; the second, via progressive bolus, effects the actual administration of the drug into the CSF.

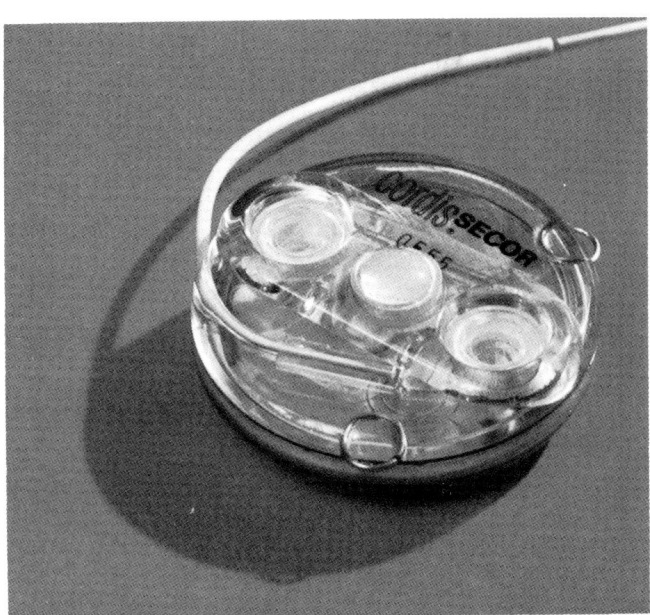

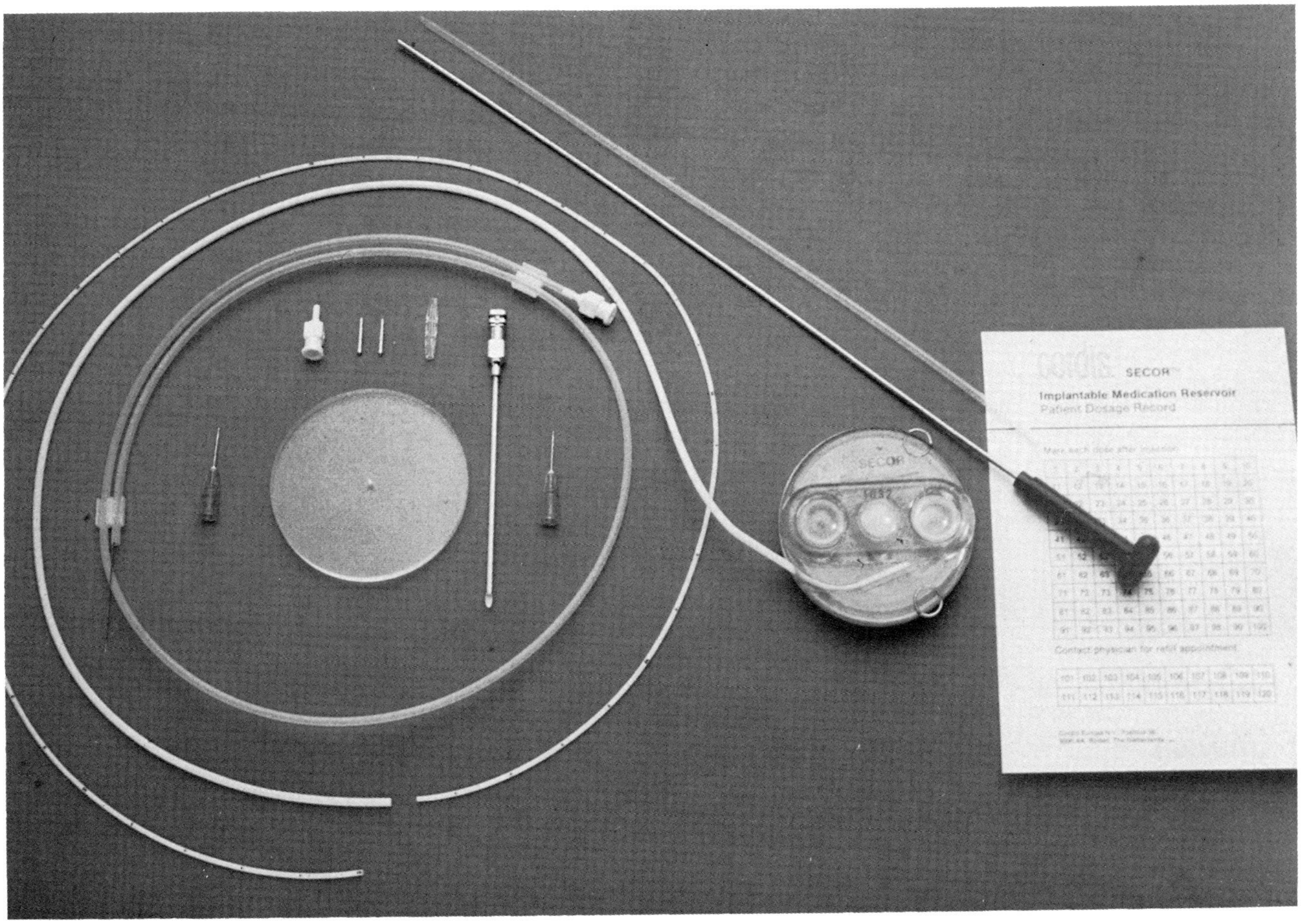

FIGURE 116–2. A spiral catheter (76 cm) is connected to a 6.5×1.5 cm pump weighing 44 g. The pump includes a loading system composed of a Siasto dome placed between two buttons.

FIGURE 116–3. Below the pump is a unidirectional valve that helps avoid drug reflux from the reservoir. The reservoir is a silicone-reinforced polyester membrane fixed to the sealing ring in polysulfonate.

An incorrect maneuver, such as inversion of the sequence, repeated depression of the same button, or the simultaneous depression of both buttons, does not permit proper administration because of the system's unidirectional flow arrangement. The spinal catheter (76 cm) is made of radiopaque Silastic. This material is inserted in the subarachnoid space at L3-L4 or L4-L5 through a Tuohy needle (14 gauge). The catheter is connected to the pump and is inserted subcutaneously on the anterior chest wall.

In the case of ventricular morphine therapy using a Secor pump, we suggest placing the pump just below the clavicle.

CLINICAL MATERIAL

To date, we have used this system in 8 cases and are impressed by the safety, simplicity of use, and reliability of this pump. We have not encountered drug overdose, incorrect administration, breakdown of parts, system failure, skin breakdown, or CSF infection.

The first patient in whom we used this system had a rectal cancer with local recurrence and involvement of the sacrum. The system was implanted December 12, 1985, and has been operating continuously for the last 9 months. The pump was reloaded 4 times. The initial dose was 1 mg morphine per day. From the third month onward, dosage was increased to 2 mg morphine per day. Analgesia, which initially was reported as being 100 percent, now remains at more than 80 percent. The patient is attentive, can walk around the house, takes walks in the garden, and cares for himself to a limited extent.

The second patient, a 75-year-old man with prostatic cancer and multiple bony metastases to the lumbar dorsal spine and the pelvis, and with metastases to both lungs and multiple costal fractures, had a system implanted February 27, 1986. Seven months later, the patient, although bedridden, was pain-free. The pump has been reloaded 3 times since its insertion.

The third patient, a 56-year-old man, has a plastocytoma involving C5, L5, the right shoulder, right tibia, pelvis, and sternum. A system that was implanted August 11, 1986, provided total pain relief during the first several weeks following its implantation but now is judged as providing relief of 80 percent of the pain.

The fourth patient, a 44-year-old man with carcinoma of the pancreas and liver metastases, had a system implanted June 28, 1986. The pump was reloaded on September 13, 1986. The patient even came personally to the hospital for supplies. He is pain-free on 2 mg morphine per day, even though severely cachectic (weight 43 kg) and intensely icteric.

SUMMARY

The manually controlled pump we have been using allows relatively easy administration of drugs into the CSF, optimal analgesic effect (because one can vary both dose and frequency of administration), reduced side effects (a result achieved by using microdoses of morphine), and a lowered risk of infection compared with systems requiring transcutaneous injection. The need to sequentially depress the two buttons (lateral and medial) for drug administration makes the presence of a professional nurse unnecessary, yet is somewhat complicated for the patient to handle alone; therefore, another person is present when the drug is given, thus avoiding the risk of overdose.

REFERENCES

1. Cannon WB: The James Lange theory of emotion. Am J Psychol 39:106, 1927
2. De Wied D: Hormonal influence on motivation learning and memory processes. Hosp Pract 11:123, 1976
3. Lazarus RS, Averill JR, Opton EM: Toward a cognitive theory of emotion, in Arnold M (ed): Feeling and Emotions. New York, Academic Press, 1970
4. Pancheri P, Biondi M: Psicologia e Psicosomatica dei Tumori. Rome, La Goliardica, 1979
5. Reich W: La Biopatia del Cancro. Milan, Sugar, 1976
6. Scarpa A: Etnomedicina. Milan, Lucisano, 1980
7. Selye H: Stress. Torino, Einaudi, 1957
8. Gianasi GC, Caruso GC: Dolore e psiche, psiche e cancro. Algos 2:46, 1985
9. Pert CB, Snyder SH: Opiate receptor: Its demonstration in nervous tissue. Science 179:1011, 1973
10. Terenius L: Endogenous peptides and analgesia. Ann Rev Pharmacol Toxicol 18:189, 1978
11. Lord JAH, Waterfield AA, Hughes J, et al: Endogenous opioid peptides: Multiple agonist and receptors. Nature 267:495, 1977
11a. Atweh SF, Kuhar MJ: Autoradiographic localization of opiate receptors in rat brain. I. Spinal cord and lower medulla. Brain Res 124:53–67, 1977
11b. Atweh SF, Kuhar MJ: Autoradiographic localization of opiate receptors in rat brain. II. The brain stem. Brain Res 129:1–12, 1977
12. Martin WR, Eades CG, Thompson JA, et al: The effect of morphine and nalorphine-like drugs in the non dependent and morphine-dependent chronic spinal dog. J Pharmacol Exp Ther 197:517, 1976
13. Wood PL: Multiple opiate receptors: Support for unique mu, delta and kappa sites. Neuropharmacology 21:487, 1982
14. Brunello M, Volterra A, Di Giulio AM, et al: Modulation of opioid system in C57 mice after repeated treatment with morphine and naloxone: Biochemical and behavioral correlates. Life Sci 34:1669, 1984
15. Hughes J, Smith TW, Kosterlitz HW, et al: Identification of two related pentapeptides from the brain with potent opiate agonist activity. Nature 258:577, 1975
16. Chavkin C, Goldstein A: Demonstration of a specific dynorphin receptor in guinea-pig ileum myenteric plexus. Nature 291:591, 1981
17. Volterra A, Brunello N, Racagni G: Recettori degli oppiacei e peptidi oppioidi endogeni. Algos 2:23, 1985
17a. Jessel TM, Iversen LL: Opiate analgesics inhibit substance P release from rat trigeminal nucleus. Nature 268:549–551, 1977
18. Chavkin C, James IF, Goldstein A: Dynorphin is a specific endogenous ligand for the kappa-opioid receptor. Science 215:413, 1982
19. Wards SJ, Portoghese PS, Takemori AE: Improved assays for the assessment of kappa- and delta properties of opiate ligands. Eur J Pharmacol 80:351, 1982
20. Imura H, Nakai Y, Nakao K, et al: Biosynthesis and distribution of opioid peptides. J Endocrinol Invest 6:139, 1983
21. Panerai AE: Sistemi peptidergici nella modulazione del dolore. Algos 3:50, 1986
22. Hokfelt T, Johansson O, Lijungdahl A, et al: Peptidergic neurones. Nature 284:515, 1980
23. Boerner U, Abbott S, Roe RL: The metabolism of morphine and heroin in man. Drug Metabol Rev 4:39, 1975
24. Wikler A: Sites and mechanism of action of morphine and related drugs in the central nervous system. Pharmacol Rev 2:435, 1950
25. Van Ree JM: Multiple brain sites involved in morphine antinociception. J Pharm Pharmacol 29:765, 1977
26. Davies GK, Tolhurst-Cleaver CL, James TL: CNS depression from intrathecal morphine (letter). Anesthesiology 52:280, 1980
27. Glynn CJ, Mther LE, Cousin MJ: Spinal narcotics and respiratory depression. Lancet 2:356, 1979

28. Boas RA: Hazards of epidural morphine. Anesthetist 2:3, 1977
29. Davies GK, Tolhurst-Cleaver CL, James TL: Respiratory depression after intrathecal narcotics. Anaesthesia 35:180, 1980
30. Lazorthes Y, Gouarderes C, Verdie GC, et al: Analgesie par injection intrathecale de morphine. Neurochirurgie 26:159, 1980
31. Pilon RN, Baker AR: Chronic pain control by means of an epidural catheter. Cancer 37:903, 1976
32. Leavens ME, Hill CS Jr, Cech DA, et al: Intrathecal and intraventricular morphine for pain in cancer patients: Initial study. J Neurosurg 56:241, 1982

CHAPTER 117

Anterior Capsulotomy for Intractable Anxiety Disorders

Per Mindus
Björn A. Meyerson

The principal therapeutic problem for psychosurgery is the optimization of the techniques to produce brain lesions of correct site, size, and configuration. Obviously, psychosurgery shares this problem with other forms of functional neurosurgery. What makes psychosurgery particularly difficult, though, is its checkered history, contemporary psychiatric controversy related to the practice of brain surgery for mental illness, the complexity of the disorders treated, and the need for very close collaboration between several specialists. In this chapter, we discuss our experience, gained over the past 20 years, with capsulotomy in otherwise intractable anxiety disorders.

INDICATIONS FOR CAPSULOTOMY IN THE TREATMENT OF ANXIETY DISORDERS

Anxiety disorders are the most prevalent, and one of the most chronic, forms of mental disorder in the general population. Despite remarkable therapeutic progress in recent years, one of five anxiety disorder patients reportedly proves unresponsive to current, up-to-date treatment, one of 10 has a chronic, deteriorating course of illness, and an undetermined small number remain so extremely disabled that they are candidates for neurosurgical intervention. Therefore, such interventions are performed, if to a very limited extent, both in the United States and in Europe,[1] although physicians and the general public have demonstrated little interest in these activities.[2, 3] An independent observer, Ellison Rodgers,[3] captured the essence of the problem, noting that "For some of the millions with intractable and disabling mental illness, surgery could be a threat but could also be a benefit that is systematically and unfairly denied them by disinterest, fear, and heavy political opposition."

Psychosurgery, a term introduced by Freeman and Watts, is an obvious misnomer because one operates on psychiatric patients, not on the psyche. More importantly, the term may be easily associated with yesterday's extensive and mutilating interventions, such as lobotomy, from which modern stereotactic interventions differ in many important ways. These types of functional neurosurgery are instead akin to those indicated in similarly incapacitating conditions, such as movement disorders, intractable epileptic seizures, or chronic pain. For these and other reasons, the authors feel that the term *psychosurgery* should be abandoned in favor of terms like *neurosurgery for mental illness.*

GENERAL GUIDELINES

The selection practices, indications, and contraindications for capsulotomy in current use at the Karolinska Hospital and elsewhere are summarized later. The general guidelines have been developed conjointly by workers in the field over several years and are consequently quite similar across sites. In brief, the guidelines include the following. The patient has been able to function adequately or almost adequately in private and professional lives at least for some years before falling ill; the illness is causing considerable suffering; because of the symptoms, the patient's psychosocial functioning is clearly reduced; the patient clearly acknowledges that he or she is ill and requests neurosurgical treatment; and the illness has been subjected to intensive and adequate psychiatric treatment for a long enough time that it is determined to be refractory to such treatment. In practice, this means a minimum of 5 years.

CURRENT INCLUSION CRITERIA FOR CAPSULOTOMY

1. The patient fulfills the current diagnostic criteria for generalized anxiety disorder, obsessive-compulsive disorder (OCD), panic disorder with agoraphobia, or social phobia, either alone or coexistent.
2. The duration of illness exceeds 5 years.
3. The disorder is causing substantial suffering.
4. The disorder is causing considerable reduction in the patient's psychosocial functioning.
5. Current treatment options tried systematically for at least 5 years have either been without appreciable effect on the symptoms or must be discontinued because of intolerable side effects.
6. The prognosis without neurosurgical intervention is considered poor.
7. The patient gives informed consent.
8. The patient agrees to participate in the preoperative evaluation program.

9. The patient agrees to participate in the postoperative rehabilitation program.

10. The referring physician is willing to acknowledge responsibility for the postoperative long-term management of the patient.

CURRENT EXCLUSION CRITERIA FOR CAPSULOTOMY

1. Age below 20 or over 65 years.
2. The patient has a complicating other, current or chronic diagnosis, for example organic brain syndrome, delusional disorder, or manifest abuse of alcohol, sedative, or illicit drugs. For a condition to qualify as "complicating," it must substantially complicate function, treatment, or the patient's ability to comply with treatment, or it must lead to serious adverse events, such as overdosage or paradoxical reactions.
3. A complicating current personality disorder (DSM) diagnosis from clusters A (e.g., paranoid personality disorder) or B (e.g., borderline, antisocial, or histrionic personality disorder) may constitute a relative contraindication. A current cluster C personality disorder (e.g., avoidant or obsessive-compulsive personality disorder) is not considered a contraindication, because it may disappear with successful treatment of the coexistent anxiety disorder.
4. The patient has a complicating, current central nervous system pathology, such as brain atrophy, dementia, or tumor.

PREOPERATIVE EVALUATION

Centers offering neurosurgical treatment for mental disorders have set up consultative teams whose task is to recommend or not recommend surgical treatment in a given case. In addition to a full account of the patient's mental and medical history, with particular emphasis on past treatment trials, the team needs the results from routine electroencephalography, cerebral computed tomography (CT) or magnetic resonance imaging (MRI), electrocardiography, routine laboratory analyses, and somatic examination, with particular emphasis on neurologic status. Neuropsychological tests, particularly those assumed to be sensitive to frontal lobe functions, should be included.

DEVELOPMENT OF CAPSULOTOMY AND ITS REGIONAL SURGICAL ANATOMY

Evidence derived from animal experimentation and lobotomy suggested that the efficacy of lobotomy resulted from interference with the connections of the orbitomedial frontal cortex and the cingulate gyri, whereas untoward intellectual and personality changes resulted from the extension of the lesions into the lateral cortex and its projections.[4] This information led Foltz and White,[5] in the United States, and later, Ballantine and coworkers[6–8] to develop the procedure of anterior bilateral cingulotomy. In Europe, different approaches were used focusing on, inter alia, the anterior limb of the internal capsule.

Meyer and Beck[9] examined autopsy brains from patients who had undergone frontal lobotomy. They found that the common denominator of those who had benefited from the procedure was the interruption of pathways contained in the anterior limb of the internal capsule and interconnecting the frontal lobes and the thalamus. In both coronal and axial sections of the brain, this part of the capsule can be easily identified as a narrow band of white matter positioned between the head of the caudate and the anterior part of the pallidum putamen. In coronal sections, the most anterior portion of the capsular white matter has a less homogeneous appearance because of the presence of thin streaks or islands of gray matter.

The French neurosurgeon Talairach and coworkers[10] were the first to report on the use of stereotactic lesions in the anterior limb of the internal capsule. They were unimpressed by the results in schizophrenia but reported satisfactory outcomes in patients with "névroses anxieuses." A few years later, the Swedish neurosurgeon Leksell used his newly developed stereotactic system to produce radiofrequency thermolesions in the internal capsules in patients with various psychiatric disorders.[11] He termed the procedure *bilateral anterior capsulotomy.*

The functional importance of the internal capsule has recently been highlighted by the notion that the pathogenesis of obsessive-compulsive symptoms may correspond to an aberrant positive feedback that is mediated partly via the extensive fiber bundles that interconnect the thalamic nuclei and the orbitofrontal cortex. These fibers pass through the anterior limb of the internal capsule.[12] In addition, the lower part of the anterior internal capsule is located very close to the substantia innominata, which is the target of another type of psychosurgical intervention used as treatment for the same disorders that often respond favorably to capsulotomy. In humans, after subcaudate tractotomy, lesions in the substantia innominata cause extensive degeneration in the ventral portion of the internal capsule.[13] The fiber degeneration could be traced back to the dorsomedial nucleus of the thalamus, which has extensive connections with various parts of the limbic system. The substantia innominata region contains neurons with wide cholinergic neocortical projections and reciprocal connections also with the orbitofrontal cortex. Some of these cells are present in islands also in the ventral part of the internal capsule.[14] Moreover, this portion of the capsule contains a large group of fibers that are efferent connections destined to the dorsomedial nucleus of thalamus, a target area used previously.[15] Finally, the internal capsules comprise fiber systems connecting the orbital cortex with the hypothalamus, the limbic system, the medial forebrain bundle, and the upper mesencephalon.[16, 17]

Gray[18] hypothesized that descending pathways from the frontal lobes to the septohippocampal system are not primarily monoaminergic, which, in his words, may account for the fact that some forms of anxiety disorders "do not respond to pharmacotherapy but can be successfully treated by lesions." Gray further proposed that the therapeutic effects of neurosurgical intervention may result from a counteraction of the direct control over emotional behavior apparently exercised by the frontal lobes, or from a change in the function of the septohippocampal comparator activities, or from both.

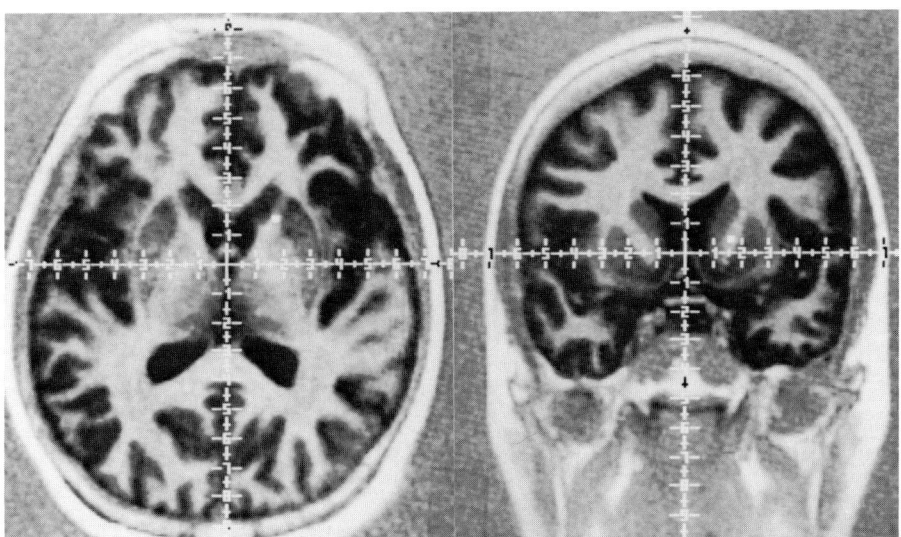

FIGURE 117-1. Stereotactic MRI. The axial image (left) was obtained from a section approximately at the level of the foramen of Monro. The target in the left anterior capsule is marked with a white dot. A coronal section (right) at the plane of the target marked on the axial image. The target corresponding to the center of the intended lesion is marked with a white dot.

SURGICAL TECHNIQUE

SURGICAL TARGET

There are no indications in the literature that any particular portion of the anteroposterior extension of the anterior limb of the internal capsule is associated with any specific function that is related to the pathogenesis of anxiety disorders, and therefore is especially suitable as a target in capsulotomy. Our target site has been placed between the anterior and middle thirds of the capsule, which is easily recognized in axial CT or MRI tomograms at the approximate level that corresponds to the foramen of Monro. This part of the capsule is generally located adjacent to the border between the putamen and globus pallidus. In a parasagittal plane, this target site approximately corresponds to half the distance between the tip of the anterior horn and the anterior commissure. In fact, these were the anatomic reference landmarks used when the localization procedure was performed with the aid of ventriculography or pneumoencephalography. In the coronal projection, the target site that corresponds to the center of the lesion should be chosen so that the basal portion of the capsule will be included in the lesion. Coronal sections of the brain further show that the anterior capsules are angled 25 to 30 degrees from the vertical plane; this angulation must be noted so that the orientation of the lesion-electrode can be adjusted to the same angles.

TARGET LOCALIZATION

Until 1976, target localization and coordinate determinations were performed with the aid of pneumoencephalography or ventriculography. However, the precision of these methods for target localization was unsatisfactory. For example, with these methods the ventricles could be dilated as a result of the presence of air, leading to a lateral dislocation of the capsules.[19] Moreover, electric stimulation generally does not provide any corroborative data as to the functional localization of the anatomic target, as is discussed later.

From 1976 to 1989, CT was regularly used for localization,[20] representing the first time that a target in stereotactic functional neurosurgery could be directly visualized. In axial CT sections, at the approximate level of the foramen of Monro, the anterior capsules are generally easy to identify. The more basal parts of the capsules are more difficult to visualize in axial sections. However, it suffices to determine the coordinates of the center of the lesion, which is generally located in an axial section where the capsules are relatively well seen. If thin and tightly packed CT slices are produced, a coronal section can be reconstructed that can provide information about the angulation of the capsules.

Since 1988, the localization procedure has been performed with MRI. In a preliminary study comprising 10 patients, CT and MRI were performed in parallel for target localization.[21] The difference between coordinates obtained with the two methods did not exceed 2 mm, and for that reason, we now feel confident to use only MRI as a routine technique for the determination of target coordinates (Fig. 117-1). A major advantage of MRI is that it provides clear images of the capsules in coronal sections in which the entire dorsoventral extension of the capsules and their angulation can be assessed (Fig. 117-2). To cover most of the capsule, the height of the lesion should be about 18 mm. For this reason, the coronal images are preferable for the determination of the Z (dorsoventral) and X (mediolateral) coordinates. In modern MRI computer programs, the coronal section corresponding to a given Y coordinate (anteroposterior, determined on an axial image) can be easily obtained. Coronal MR images obtained for the determination of X and Z coordinates are highly desirable if the operation is to be performed with a radiosurgical technique and more than one lesion in each capsule is planned. In that case, the coordinates for each of the lesions have to be determined separately if they are placed one above the other with the intention of covering most of the capsule in its dorsoventral extension.

SURGICAL PROCEDURE

In our experience, stereotactic capsulotomy is well tolerated when it is performed with the patient under local anesthesia only. Typically, these patients, although extremely anxious and tense before the procedure, afterward rarely

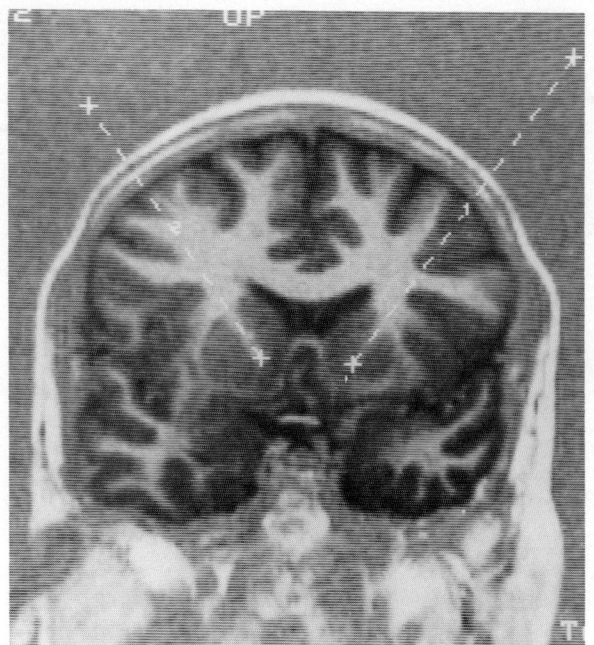

FIGURE 117–2. Stereotactic MRI, coronal section. The angulation of the anterior capsules has been determined to enable appropriate angles for the electrode trajectories.

complain about pain and discomfort experienced during the surgical intervention. However, they often find the relatively time-consuming MRI examination distressing, and effective preoperative medication is therefore advisable. We generally use 10 to 20 mg of morphine-scopolamine and 2,5 mg of droperidol administered intramuscularly, but supplementary and repeated intravenous injections with diazepam are often required. If a center-of-arch stereotactic system is used, it is wise to mark on the skin the intended site of the burr holes by using a probe attached to the electrode carrier positioned in the predetermined angle of the lesion electrode trajectory. Unless this precaution is taken, the burr holes tend to be placed too close to the midline, and the angulation of the lesion electrodes does not coincide with that of the capsules. If ordinary burr holes are made, care should be taken to replace the bone chips to minimize the cosmetic disadvantage of a permanent impression in the skull, about which some of these patients are sensitive. To produce lesions of about 15 to 18 mm in height, we use monopolar thermoelectrodes with a bare tip of 10 mm, and two partly overlapping lesions are made one above the other to produce a confluent lesion of that height (Fig. 117–3).

While the lesions are produced, in one hemisphere after the other, the alertness and orientation of the patient are checked by asking simple questions or presenting simple arithmetic problems (like counting backwards, subtracting serial threes). While the last lesion is produced, or shortly thereafter, the patient commonly becomes somewhat confused with impairment of orientation in time and space. This condition generally subsides after the first 24 hours. Agitation has never been observed.

STIMULATION AND RECORDING

In the 1970s and early 1980s, we generally performed electric stimulation in the target region before we produced the lesions. However, even when stimulation in a few patients was made simultaneously in both sides, we never observed any motor or autonomic effects, nor did the patients experience any emotional or sensory sensations, and mental symptoms, such as anxiety and obsessive thoughts, were not influenced. These negative experiences with stimulation in

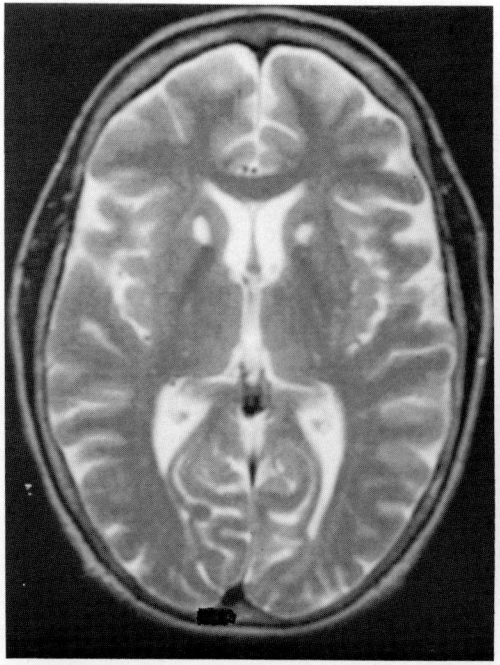
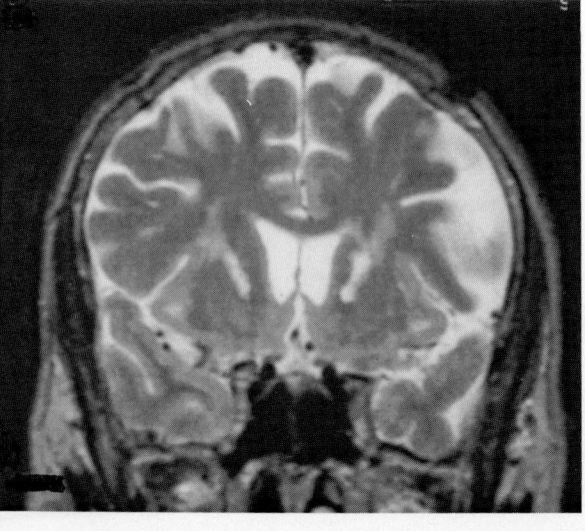

FIGURE 117–3. MRI examinations of a patient who has undergone thermocapsulotomy. The lesions in the axial section (left) appear as two white dots, and in the coronal section (right), as two white streaks.

the internal capsule are in accordance with results reported by Laitinen,[22] who found this region to be comparatively unresponsive to electric stimuli; in only seven of 21 patients was a "positive" response produced, that is, relaxation and a feeling of well-being, and these effects were usually produced from the upper part of the capsule. However, a more systematic exploration with simultaneously applied bilateral stimulation at different frequencies and high-precision monitoring of autonomic functions may provide information about an optimal site of the lesions. Perhaps electrical impedance monitoring will help to verify correct placement of the electrode tip in the internal capsule white matter. To date, no systematic study has been conducted on the usefulness of impedance monitoring, but in one study microelectrode recording has been used to identify the capsule.[23]

COMPLICATIONS

In 360 thermocapsulotomies reported in the literature, no deaths have occurred. In our own series of about 90 interventions, four patients suffered intracerebral hemorrhages. In three of these patients, the bleedings were small and accompanied by only transient symptoms of slight hemiparesis. In the fourth patient, an intraventricular hemorrhage occurred that required temporary ventricular drainage. However, this patient recovered without any neurologic sequela. Postoperative infection in the form of abscess or meningitis has not occurred. Epilepsy is a very rare complication to capsulotomy. In a series of 35 patients reported on by Bingley and Persson,[24] only one patient had seizures during the first postoperative year and required antiepileptic medication. However, that patient also presented with suspected epileptogenic abnormality in the preoperative electroencephalogram.

EARLY POSTOPERATIVE COURSE

During the first 2 to 5 postoperative days, most patients (19 of 22 patients in a series reported on by Mindus[25]) presented with occasional episodes of confusion, often occurring at night-time. In a few patients, a transitory urinary incontinence may occur. A characteristic feature of the early postoperative period is that patients are indolent and lack initiative. Often, they remain in bed without reading or listening to the radio, and many need to be encouraged to get out of bed and dressed. This period of relative lethargy is not associated with episodes of confusion, and it may last for several weeks, which is one reason why active rehabilitation has to be instituted at an early postoperative phase.

RADIOSURGICAL CAPSULOTOMY

Radiosurgery may be deployed to perform capsulotomy, a procedure referred to as gamma capsulotomy. To date, approximately 40 gamma capsulotomies have been carried out, the experience of which is considerably less than that of the thermocapsulotomy technique. In an earlier series comprising 20 gamma cases, the results were comparable to those reported after thermocapsulotomy,[26,27] which encompasses considerably larger parts of the dorsoventral extension of the capsules. In a recent series of 9 cases,[28] three small (4 × 4 mm) isocenters were used with the rationale of creating lesions of similar configuration as those of the thermolesions and further to tailor the intended irradiation field according to the individual anatomy of the patient's capsules. Moreover, for sundry reasons, the target dose was increased. Although these modifications appeared to increase the efficacy of the procedure, they also seemed to entail greater risk of side effects, because several patients manifested fatigue and apathy of long duration. For this reason, lower doses should be used in future studies.

Because of the limited experience with radiosurgery, many methodologic problems have to be further explored and solved, and of crucial importance is dose planning with regard to the radiobiologic effects. Thus, whether necrotizing doses are required or whether the same effects can be attained with lower doses is not known. Moreover, relatively little is known about the radiosensitivity of normal white or gray cerebral tissue when small volumes are irradiated with high, nonfractionated doses. If the focused irradiation is intended to cover the entire dorsoventral extension of the capsule, multiple small lesions placed one above the other are required. When multiple isocenters are planned, however, the resulting necrotizing volume is difficult to predict.[28]

RESULTS

HERNER'S STUDY

The first 116 capsulotomy patients operated on by Leksell between 1952 and 1957 were followed up prospectively by the Swedish psychiatrist Herner, who published the results in a monograph in 1961.[29] Although schizophrenia was intended to be the main indication for capsulotomy, the results in schizophrenic patients were disappointing; at follow-up after 24 to 80 months, only seven of the 64 patients were free of symptoms, and two were rated as markedly improved. Patients who are free of symptoms together with those who are much improved may be judged as having a satisfactory response to the treatment.[30] In the schizophrenic patients, this figure was 14 percent. This finding, together with the increasing clinical awareness of the antipsychotic drugs from the mid-1950s, led to the abandonment of capsulotomy in the treatment of psychotic illness. However, Herner found that the best results of capsulotomy were obtained in 18 patients suffering from what was then called *obsessional neurosis*; 50 percent of these patients were rated as having a satisfactory response to capsulotomy. Somewhat less favorable results were recorded in 15 patients with anxiety neurosis, none of whom was free of symptoms and only 20 percent were rated as markedly improved (i.e., 20 percent satisfactory result).

BINGLEY AND COWORKERS' STUDY

The favorable results in patients with refractory OCD, which is notorious for its chronicity and intractability, led Bingley and associates to select OCD patients only for capsulotomy. The operations were performed at Karolinska Hospital from 1970 to 1976. The results of the first 17 patients were reported in 1973, and the long-term results of a total of

35 patients in 1977.[30, 31] All patients were prospectively studied by two independent psychiatrists, Rylander and Bingley. Strict selection criteria were used to ensure diagnostic homogeneity. The mean age of the patients was 40 years, and more than half of them had been ill for over 17 years. Most of the patients had spent long, repeated periods in psychiatric hospitals, and all of them were reported to have undergone psychiatric treatment for several years but without appreciable effect on the patients' symptoms. Results were assessed jointly or independently by the two psychiatrists, and the patients' relatives were interviewed in all cases. After a mean follow-up of 35 months (range, 4 to 55 months), a satisfactory result was achieved in 70 percent of these severely disabled patients. Before the operation, only three patients were working full-time. At follow-up, this figure was 14, and an additional 17 were working part-time; only four patients remained incapacitated. The authors found no tendency for the patients to relapse into old symptoms with time.

LOPEZ-IBOR AND COWORKERS' STUDY

Further support for the efficacy of capsulotomy in patients with severe OCD was derived from a study by two Spanish psychiatrists, Lobez-Ibor and Lopez-Ibor Alino, who had extensive experience with an older type of frontal lobe surgery (leukotomy) in obsessive patients. They subjected their first patients to capsulotomy in 1966. After 3 years of careful observation, they were so impressed with the results of capsulotomy that they urged that it replace leukotomy. They reported the results of the first eight patients in 1972, and in 1977 (independently and simultaneously with Bingley and coworkers), the results of a total of 57 capsulotomy patients.[32] The Lopez-Ibor team wrote with regard to their patients that "this treatment means a genuine and real chance of regaining their freedom [from symptoms]."

This conclusion is of particular interest because in 1967, Lopez-Ibor and coworkers were the first to report their successful experiences with the use of clomipramine in OCD, and further, because they report having scheduled for surgery only one-tenth of the patients referred to them for evaluation. This information suggests that they were recommending only severely ill cases for capsulotomy. The Lopez-Ibor team collaborated with the neurosurgeon Burzaco,[33] who published combined data from his own study and those of Kullberg[34] and of Rylander,[26] comprising a total of 149 capsulotomy patients: satisfactory results had been reported in 72 percent of the cases.

RYLANDER'S STUDY

As mentioned earlier, two techniques for capsulotomy have been described, the conventional radiofrequency thermolesion procedure and the radiosurgical or gammacapsulotomy method described by Leksell and Backlund.[35] The experience with the gammacapsulotomy procedure is far less extensive than that with the conventional thermolesion procedure: only approximately 30 patients have been reported on in the literature,[26-28] but the results of the two procedures appear comparable.[25, 36] Whereas OCD patients only had been selected for the studies presented earlier, Rylander,[26] drawing on the early findings of Herner, extended the inclusion criteria to otherwise intractable non-OCD anxiety disorders, such as phobias. The results in the first 14 anxiety disorder patients undergoing gammacapsulotomy were reported in 1979 by Rylander, who found 71 percent of the patients to have a satisfactory response to gammacapsulotomy, a figure comparable to that reported by Bingley and coworkers[30] after thermocapsulotomy.

A CRITIQUE OF EARLIER STUDIES

FREQUENCY OF OPERATIONS

Because capsulotomy may now be regarded as a clinically established form of treatment, not all cases operated on can be expected to be reported on in the scientific literature. In some European countries, capsulotomy is known to be performed on a routine, clinical basis, albeit to a very limited extent. The numbers of capsulotomy cases published are, for this reason, probably an underestimation of the true rate (Table 117–1).

DIAGNOSTIC PRACTICES

Diagnostic practices have changed in the many years during which the capsulotomy studies were carried out. Moreover, OCD and non-OCD patients share many clinical features. Although only OCD patients are reported to have been selected in a given study, this cannot be ascertained from the reports because the diagnostic criteria used were often not reported at all or not reported in sufficient detail. Although it is true that many cases of OCD do not pose diagnostic difficulties, patients with obsessions and compulsions related to other forms of mental illness may have been operated on. This may have been the case in several studies in view of the high rate of concurrent other mental illness in OCD patients. Inspection of the clinical data of the 20 patients selected by Rylander[26] for gammacapsulotomy proves this point; according to his published data, as many as 12 patients suffered from non-OCD anxiety disorders. If the procedure has, for example, a better effect in non-OCD than in OCD patients,

Table 117–1. CAPSULOTOMY STUDIES AND NUMBER OF CASES REPORTED

Reference	n
Herner[29]	116
Martinez and coworkers[23]	12
Bingley and coworkers[30]	35
Kullberg[34]	13
Laitinen[22]	33
Vasko and Kullberg[44]	21
Rylander[26]	14
Burzaco[33]	85
Fodstad and coworkers[51]	4
Leksell and coworkers[52]	1
Mindus and coworkers[27]	7
Mindus[25]	24
Guo and coworkers[28]	11
Total	376

then the overall results may be affected by the relative proportion of the two diagnostic categories in the cohort studied. Moreover, if the results are not examined and reported separately for each group, then the differential effect, if any, of the intervention will escape observation.

Estimation of Outcome

Investigators have pointed out[2, 25] that many psychosurgical reports are problematic in that they are only retrospective, and that estimates of outcome with documented validity and reliability have not generally been available at the time of the studies. Because the interventions are performed at few centers, very few physicians are experienced in the field. Accordingly, the same clinician who was responsible for the selection and the treatment of the patients often assessed the clinical outcome also, after only a short period of observation, and with unstandardized methods of evaluation. The inherent bias problem is obvious. Most of the capsulotomy studies presented earlier are marred by at least some of these shortcomings.

Neurosurgical Techniques

The methods used, both for target localization and for lesioning, do not vary only between studies but in some instances also within studies. In one study, for example, the investigators concluded that the results did not depend on the size of the lesion, a conclusion that would appear to be invalid because the neurosurgeon was advised by the referring psychiatrists to make larger lesions in the more serious cases.[32] In addition, both monopolar and bipolar electrode configurations have been deployed producing lesions of varying sizes and forms. It is conceivable that the lack of a standardized surgical protocol has influenced the outcome.

MORE RECENT STUDIES

More recent studies at Karolinska Hospital have been designed to avoid some of the methodologic shortcomings of earlier reports by studying patients:
1. Who were uniformly selected with modern, international, operationally defined diagnostic criteria, representing both OCD and non-OCD anxiety disorders.
2. Who were operated on with standardized neurosurgical techniques.
3. In whom the clinical outcome was monitored with psychiatric evaluation methods of documented validity and reliability. These methods were used by independent assessors in prospective study designs.

These investigators argued that this design was the best solution, given the practical and ethical problems with finding, and using, nonsurgical controls or with using sham-controlled surgical studies involving craniotomy.

A PROSPECTIVE STUDY OF GAMMACAPSULOTOMY

In the first of these studies on gammacapsulotomy, a second group of seven patients with otherwise intractable anxiety disorders selected by Rylander for gammacapsulotomy were followed up prospectively for up to 7 years by two independent assessors who were not responsible for the selection and the treatment of the patients.[26, 36] The clinical morbidity was rated on modern psychiatric rating scales before surgery and again at 3 and 7 years postoperatively. Of these severely ill patients, 71 percent were rated by the two independent assessors as having a satisfactory response to gammacapsulotomy. Two additional, salient findings should be mentioned here. A statistically significant improvement occurred not only between the preoperative and the 3-year follow-up but also between the 3- and the 7-year postoperative follow-ups. This finding may be interpreted to mean that further improvement may occur even many years after surgery.

Earlier generations of CT scanners were unable to detect gammacapsulotomy lesions. For this reason, no postoperative verification could be obtained. By the time of the 7-year follow-up, however, the first MRI unit in Sweden had been installed, enabling the visualization of the gammacapsulotomy lesions with MRI. Interestingly, there was a statistically highly significant correlation between independent ratings of psychosocial functioning at the 7-year follow-up and the site and the size of the gammacapsular lesions, as determined with MRI by two independent neuroradiologists who had no access to clinical data. This was an encouraging finding for those engaged in this form of functional neurosurgery.

THE RELATIVE EFFICACY IN OCD AND NON-OCD

The team at Karolinska Hospital[20] continued to accept patients with OCD and non-OCD anxiety disorders for capsulotomy, the rationale being the considerable phenomenologic similarities and overlap between these disorders and the well-known high rates of coexistent other anxiety disorders in these diagnostic groups. The high rate of concurrent anxiety disorder in the capsulotomy cases may be assumed to be an important complicating factor contributing both to the severity and the intractability of their illnesses. In search of any differential effect of capsulotomy in OCD and non-OCD anxiety disorders, Mindus[25] compared prospectively the Comprehensive Psychopathological Rating Scale (CPRS) (a widely used psychiatric rating scale) scores of 10 OCD patients with those of 14 patients suffering from non-OCD anxiety disorders, such as generalized anxiety disorder, panic disorder with agoraphobia, and social phobia. The patients in each subgroup were rated before thermocapsulotomy and at 2, 6, and 12 months after it. The main reduction in scores was apparent already at the 2-month follow-up (t = 9.74, $p < 0.001$). From that rating session and later, there were neither significant additional reductions in scores nor significant intergroup differences. Thus, at the 12-month follow-up, the reductions in scores were of similar magnitude in both diagnostic subgroups. Both subgroups improved on the scores on the global scale included in the CPRS (the OCD subgroup: t = 2.75, $p < 0.05$; the non-OCD subgroup: t = 12.45, $p < 0.001$). Their scores on the modified Pippard[25] postoperative rating scale, which has been widely used in the field, indicated satisfactory response in 60 percent of the OCD patients and in 93 percent of the non-OCD patients.

However, four of the five poor responders were OCD patients. It appeared from this study that the results in the non-OCD group were more homogeneous with regard to outcome than in the OCD group, whose results tended to be more evenly distributed across outcome classifications. The proportion of patients rated as free of symptoms was, however, similar in both diagnostic subgroups (OCD: five of 10 or 50 percent; non-OCD: seven of 14 or 50 percent). Of the 24 patients followed up, none was rated as worse at the 12-month postoperative examination. To obtain a further estimate of the relative efficacy of capsulotomy in OCD and in non-OCD anxiety disorders, these data were combined with those of studies reporting diagnosis and outcome in sufficient detail to permit a meta-analysis.[25] The results of eight studies comprising 213 patients were accepted. Using the scores on the Pippard postoperative rating scale as the dependent measure, the two best outcome categories were contrasted to the two worst outcome categories. The results are summarized in Table 117–2.

Obviously, the data base for OCD patients is considerably larger than that for non-OCD patients, but the results appear comparable. The data suggest that both diagnostic subgroups may benefit, and, in addition, the chances should be favorable for even these severely disabled patients to obtain a clinically meaningful benefit from capsulotomy. As discussed in detail elsewhere,[25] the discrepancy between the results of Herner's study and those of later reports may well be attributed to the changes in diagnostic practices that have occurred during the many years that have passed between the studies.

LONG-TERM RESULTS OF THERMOCAPSULOTOMY IN OCD

Since the studies by Bingley and associates[30] and by Lopez-Ibor and Lopez-Ibor Alino[32] were carried out, remarkable progress has been made in the nonsurgical treatment of OCD. For this reason, it remains unclear whether their results are comparable to those of more recent studies comprising patient populations that are refractory even to current, up-to-date treatment, similar to the patients in the study reported by Mindus.[25] The methodologic weaknesses of that study, however, include the fact that the number of patients was small in each diagnostic subgroup (only 10 of 24 had OCD), and that the observation time was relatively short (1 year) after capsulotomy. For this reason, we recently conducted a study on all consecutive patients treated with thermocapsulotomy for otherwise intractable OCD at our department between 1979 and 1990. At the time of this writing, the following preliminary findings may be reported here.

During the study period, 24 patients underwent thermocapsulotomy. All candidates were preoperatively evaluated according to the same criteria described earlier and operated on by the same neurosurgeon (BAM), who used the technique for the localization of the targets and the production of the capsular lesions described earlier. Two patients were lost to follow-up. The remaining 22 patients were examined by one of us (PM) before capsulotomy, and at 3, 6, 9, 12 months, and again at an average 8 years (range, 3 to 15 years) after it. Using the obsessive-compulsive subscale of the CPRS (CPRS-OC) as the dependent measure, the investigators found a statistically highly significant symptom reduction at the 1-year follow-up compared with baseline ($t = -3.69$, $p < 0.001$, two-tailed). The findings are graphically represented in Figure 117–4. As can be seen, the main change in scores was found at the 2-month follow-up ($t = 4.03$, $p < 0.002$, two-tailed), and nonsignificant changes ($t = -1.08$, $p < 0.291$, two-tailed) were found at subsequent rating sessions up to the 8-year follow-up. Because the mean duration of the patients' illnesses exceeded 15 years, the time course of the symptom alleviation after capsulotomy is remarkable. The finding well supports our clinical impression that the effect, if any, of capsulotomy becomes clinically evident within the first 3 to 6 months. Relapse usually becomes evident within the first postoperative year.[25] No statistically significant difference was found between scores obtained at the 1- and 8-year postoperative examinations ($t = -1.08$, $p < 0.29$, two-tailed), which may be interpreted to mean that relapse into old symptoms is not expected after the 1-year follow-up and beyond. This is in agreement with the results reported previously by Bingley and colleagues.[30] In our experience, if no effect is discernible within the first postoperative 6 months, later improvement seems unlikely. If the patient has a favorable response 1 year after capsulotomy, however, improvement may continue for many years after the operation.[27, 36]

No statistically significant correlation ($r = 0.317$, $p = -2.63$) was found between preoperative and postoperative scores, a finding that may be interpreted to mean that even

Table 117–2. RESULTS OF CAPSULOTOMY CASES BY OUTCOME CATEGORIES (A+B=BEST; D+E=WORST) IN OBSESSIVE-COMPULSIVE DISORDER (OCD) AND IN NON-OCD ANXIETY DISORDER PATIENTS

| | | OCD | | | non-OCD | |
| | | A + B | D + E | | A + B | D + E |
Reference	n	n (%)	n (%)	n	n (%)	n (%)
Herner[29]	18	9 (50)	5 (28)	15	3 (20)	6 (40)
Bingley and coworkers[30]	35	25 (71)	0	—	—	—
Kullberg[34]	8	3 (34)	2 (25)	5	3 (60)	0
Rylander[26]	7	4 (57)	3 (43)	7	6 (86)	0
Burzaco[33]	85	62 (73)	4 (4)	—	—	—
Fodstad and coworkers[51]	2	2	0	—	—	—
Mindus and coworkers[27]	—	—	—	7	5 (71)	0
Mindus[25]	10	6 (60)	0	14	13 (93)	0
Total	165	111 (61)	14 (8)	48	30 (63)	6 (13)

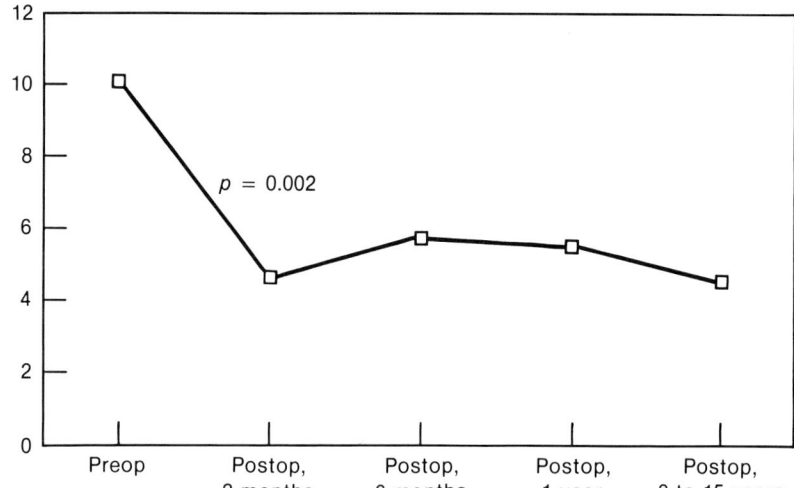

FIGURE 117–4. Ratings of clinical morbidity over time in 22 consecutive patients treated with thermocapsulotomy for intractable OCD.

the patient with the worst conceivable condition has a fair chance of obtaining a clinically meaningful response to capsulotomy. A consequence of the recent improvements in the nonsurgical treatment of OCD may be that today an even more refractory patient population is referred for neurosurgical intervention than that previously referred. Such individuals may be more difficult to treat even with neurosurgical methods. To examine this question, the patients were rank-ordered according to the preoperative and postoperative difference in their CPRS-OC scores. No statistically significant difference was found (Fisher exact probability test = 1.0, two-tailed), a finding that indicates that the efficacy of capsulotomy has remained similar over the years. The results are graphically represented in Figure 117–5. As can be seen, most of the patients improved on CPRS-OC scale, and three individuals were rated as being completely free of symptoms. We initially considered patient number five not to be a surgical candidate because of the many atypical features of her illness. Approximately 1 year later, she was again referred because she had become suicidal, and capsulotomy was carried out to save her life. Now, 11 years after the intervention, she is still symptomatic but alive and is capable of leading a life outside an institution.

In Figure 117–6, the results are shown in a more traditional way, with patients distributed according to their percentage of improvement on the CPRS-OC scale at the 8-year follow-up, compared with baseline. Five patients scored higher on this measure, that is, they were worse after, but not necessarily as a result of, capsulotomy; two patients had a minimal response; and 15 individuals were rated as having a good response to capsulotomy.

A SECOND INTERVENTION

Seven of the 22 patients underwent a second intervention. The common course for these individuals was an initial response, followed by a relapse within 3 to 6 months. The second interventions, in which the lesions were enlarged, were performed at 1 year after the first capsulotomy. Figure 117–6 shows that at least four of these seven patients benefited from the second intervention, moving from the poor response categories (which partially indicated the second intervention) to the good response categories (i.e., a more than 26-percent improvement).

Because of the nonblind nature of the study, the importance of placebo effects for the surgical results cannot be

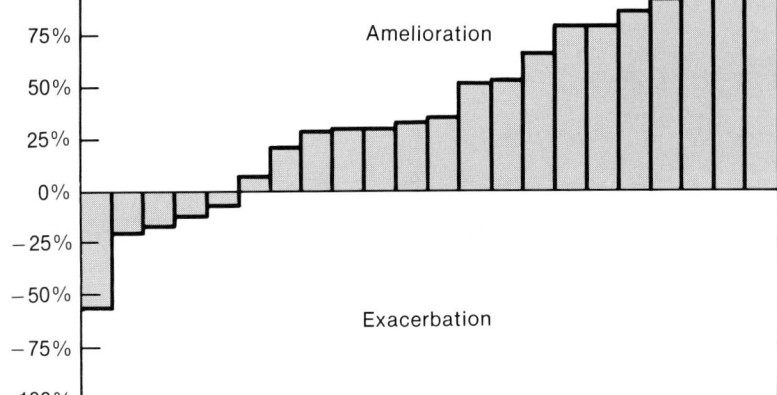

FIGURE 117–5. Percent change of obsessive-compulsive symptoms at follow-up at 8 years compared with before the operation in 22 consecutive OCD patients undergoing thermocapsulotomy.

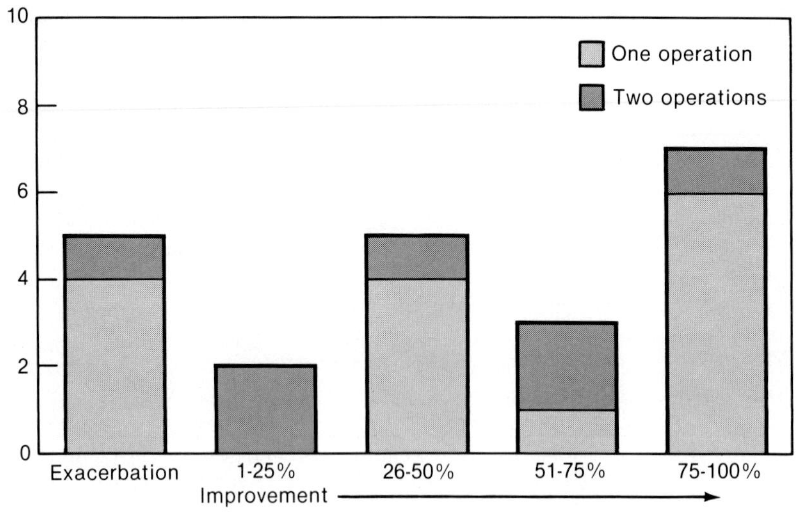

FIGURE 117-6. Distribution of clinical outcome expressed as percent improvement at follow-up compared with baseline. Same observation times and patients as in Figure 117-4.

determined. For this reason, double-blind sham-controlled trials are needed, and such a study is now under way.

THE RELATIVE EFFICACY OF PROCEDURES IN CURRENT USE

Four procedures are currently used to treat otherwise intractable anxiety disorders: cingulotomy,[37, 38] subcaudate tractotomy,[39] limbic leukotomy,[40, 41] and *capsulotomy*. In his recent review of the literature, Waziri[42] concluded that the published results were remarkably similar, but that the "data suggest that internal capsulotomy produces the best outcome, in OCD as in anxiety states." Comparisons based on published results may, at best, give only an estimate of the relative efficacy of the procedures. A direct comparison of 13 cingulotomy and 13 capsulotomy patients was published by Kullberg,[34] who found significantly ($p < 0.05$) better results in the capsulotomy group. Some evidence to the same effect was recently provided by Hay and coworkers,[43] who noted that patients with cingulotomy lesions extensive enough to involve the anterior capsule did better than those whose lesions were more restricted. Although the lesions made in capsulotomy seem to be smaller than those made in the other procedures, in the treatment of chronic, severe anxiety disorder, the outcome appears to compare favorably with that of the other procedures.

SURGICAL RISKS

COGNITIVE FUNCTIONS

The issue of negative effects of the modern interventions on cognitive functions and personality features is crucial. As is the case for any cognitive dysfunction after capsulotomy, this question has been addressed by several investigators.[26, 30, 32, 44] Using a restricted number of psychometric tests to assess approximately 200 capsulotomy patients, they found no evidence of reduced intellectual function after capsulotomy. We earlier pointed out[25] that these findings do not preclude that dysfunction in systems involving the frontal lobes may follow capsulotomy, a phenomenon that may be demonstrated with particular tests. Recent neuropsychological hypotheses concerning a biologic basis for OCD and other anxiety disorders focus on frontolimbic circuits.[12, 45] Furthermore, although the targets of capsulotomy are not placed within the frontal lobes, but instead in their connections with other parts of the brain, the operation may nonetheless be assumed to influence frontal lobe functioning. For both of these reasons, it would seem appropriate to include tests that are sensitive to frontal lobe functions. The weaknesses of the earlier studies are that the methods used were generally not specific or sensitive enough to reliably demonstrate frontal lobe pathology.

Our group recently concluded a study (Nyman & Mindus, submitted) in which an extensive neuropsychological test battery was administered to 17 patients with otherwise intractable OCD ($n = 10$) or non-OCD anxiety disorders. These patients were studied with the aim of elucidating whether there is a price, in terms of deteriorated neuropsychological performance, that the patient may have to pay for symptom alleviation.

Although extremely disabled by their illnesses at baseline, the patients performed within the normal range on most of the tests. Despite this drastic form of treatment, neuropsychological performance, as studied with current, up-to-date techniques, remained remarkably intact or even improved after capsulotomy. In five patients, however, scores reflecting perseverative behavior were commoner at follow-up, possibly indicating a dysfunction in systems involving the frontal lobes. No other neuropsychological or clinical factor distinguished this subgroup from most of the patients. From a clinical viewpoint, it may be concluded that although capsulotomy may give rise to increased perseverative behavior in occasional patients, that risk must be weighed against the risk of nonintervention in this extremely disabled, often suicidal, patient population.

From a clinical viewpoint, although this effect is not demonstrable by conventional tests, neurosurgical intervention may give rise to frontal lobe dysfunction. Therefore, the surgical candidate's cognitive functions must be evaluated; a patient with preoperative abnormal or borderline test scores may run an elevated risk for postoperative changes because any adverse effect of surgery may conceivably interact with, and add to, the effects of the persistent illness per se, and to the cumulative impact on the brain of massive earlier treatment efforts.

CAPSULOTOMY AND CREATIVITY

A quality that is difficult to evaluate by psychometric methods is creativity, such as that required in scientific and artistic work. Bingley and colleagues[30] reported on two cases that may serve as examples of the effect of capsulotomy on creativity. "An archeologist, holding a highly qualified academic position, had for 15 years suffered from an increasing obsessive-compulsive neurosis. He had been given all sorts of psychiatric treatment including several years of psychoanalysis. A few months after the operation he resumed his work at an institution. He is now very productive in his work and heads a new research project and is working on his doctor's thesis."

The other case is an artist who had been ill for 22 years and was quite disabled. "After the operation she took up her work again, and has held two exhibitions. She feels that now she can tackle the technical problems better than she could before the operation and that her creative inspiration has returned."[30]

These two patients were recently followed up. The archeologist had published his doctoral thesis in 1983. He provided documentation to show that it had been reviewed in several international scientific journals of high repute and was very well received. He continues to be productive in his work (his list of publications now contains over 160 scientific articles), he lectures frequently both nationally and internationally, and he is often seen on television and in other media discussing his recent discoveries.

The artist, now in her mid 60s, also continues to be productive. She has held several exhibitions, which could be documented with photos and other material.

The popular belief that this type of brain surgery may negatively affect creativity is not borne out by these two cases. On the contrary, both patients maintain that *their illness* prevented them from making full use of their inborn creativity.

PERSONALITY FEATURES

"Postoperative" side-effects may occur also in patients who do *not* undergo surgery. In their prospective, controlled study comparing the efficacy of intensive nonsurgical treatment with that of modified bimedial leukotomy in OCD, Tan and coworkers[46] noted brusqueness and irritability (six patients), apathy, laziness, and general blunting (two patients) among the 13 control subjects. In other words, symptoms and signs often regarded as postoperative side-effects also appeared in the nonsurgery group.

Because capsulotomy may be expected to influence, directly or indirectly, frontal lobe function and, hence, personality, it is both of theoretical and clinical interest to study personality features in patients undergoing the operation. It is well known that impulsiveness is one of the most conspicuous symptoms of frontal lobe dysfunction.[47] For this reason, a method likely to detect negative personality changes following this form of neurosurgery must cover impulsiveness and related features, such as psychopathy, hostility, and aggressiveness. One such instrument is the well-researched Karolinska Scales of Personality (KSP), developed by Schalling and coworkers,[48] which contains scales that measure traits related to frontal lobe function and scales that reflect different dimensions of anxiety proneness. Numerous studies have been performed by independent investigators who have shown the KSP to differentiate between diagnostic subgroups and to correlate significantly with biologic markers for vulnerability to certain psychopathologic conditions.

Mindus and Nyman gave the KSP to 24 consecutive patients before and 1 year after thermocapsulotomy.[49] The results of this study are shown in Figure 117–7. Before surgery, deviant scores were obtained on five of the 15 KSP scales, four of which are scales related to anxiety proneness (the SA, PA, MT, and MCA scales, see top row of graph). At 1 year after capsulotomy, statistically significant decreases were noted on eight of the scales, and normal scores were noted on all but two scales, which remained borderline. In particular, the scores on scales related to psychopathy such as impulsiveness (I), hostility (Host), and aggressiveness (Aggr, Inh A) were within the normal range. These findings after capsulotomy are in line with those of another study from the Karolinska group obtained with the Rorschach test, which were evaluated blindly and independently using modern, standardized scoring systems,[50] and permit the conclusion that negative personality changes are unlikely to occur after capsulotomy. However, these conclusions are based on observations made on groups of patients and do not preclude that negative changes may occur in individual patients.

RISK FROM NONINTERVENTION

In most studies from the field, the patients have a duration of illness that averages 15 years, a course that reveals some-

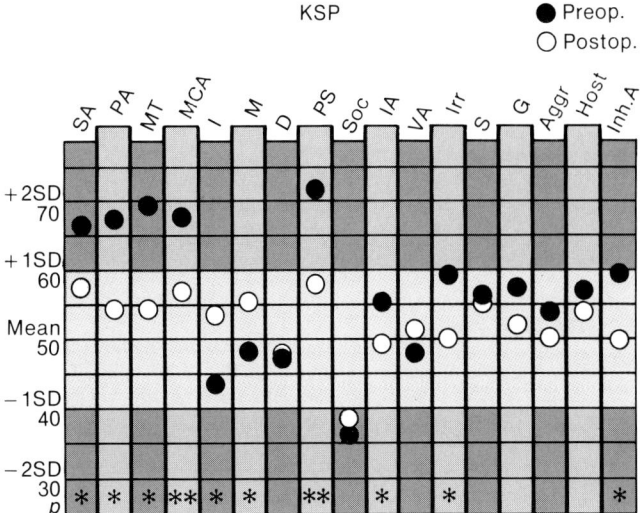

FIGURE 117–7. Scores on the Karolinska Scales of Personality (KSP) obtained before and at 1 year after thermocapsulotomy in 24 patients with incapacitating OCD and non-OCD anxiety disorders. I through Irr denotes personality scales of the inventory (see text). Scores within ± 1 SD are considered normal. *$p < 0.005$; **$p < 0.001$, two-tailed t-test between preoperative and postoperative scores, correlated data. (From Mindus P: Capsulotomy in Anxiety Disorders. A Multidisciplinary Study. [Thesis.] Stockholm, Karolinska Institute, 1991.)

thing of the prognosis. The risk for social, somatic, and mental complication, including suicide, in this group of patients cannot be overrated. A small number of cases have been described, who were eligible for intervention but never operated on, for different reasons.[25] Their conditions remained the same, and some of them later committed suicide. The physician who has a patient with chronic, disabling, and intractable anxiety disorder, in whom all therapeutic options have been exhausted, has the delicate task of weighing the risk of intervention against the risk of nonintervention. Deferring the decision to operate on a given patient may not spare the patient complications.

REFERENCES

1. Mindus P, Jenike MA: Neurosurgical treatment of malignant obsessive-compulsive disorder. Psychiatr Clin North Am 4:921–938, 1992
2. Valenstein ES: Review of the literature on postoperative evaluation, in Valenstein ES (ed): The Psychosurgery Debate. San Francisco, WH Freeman & Company 1980, p 141
3. Ellison Rodgers J: Psychosurgery—Damaging the Brain to Save the Mind. New York, Harper Collins, 1992
4. Fulton JE: Frontal Lobotomy and Affective Behavior. A Neurophysiological Analysis. New York, WW Norton, 1951
5. Foltz EL, White LE: Pain "relief" by cingulotomy. J Neurosurg 19:89–100, 1962
6. Ballantine HT Jr, Levy BS, Dagi TF, et al: Cingulotomy for psychiatric illness: Report of 13 years' experience, in Sweet W, Obrador S, Martin-Rodriguez JG (eds): Neurosurgical Treatment in Psychiatry, Pain, and Epilepsy. Baltimore, University Park Press, 1977, pp 333–353
7. Ballantine HT Jr: Neurosurgery for behavioral disorders, in Wilkins RH, Rengachary SS (eds): Neurosurgery. New York, Elsevier/North Holland Biomedical Press, 1985, pp 2527–2537
8. Ballantine HT Jr: Psychiatric surgery: its past, present and future, in Perris C, Struwe G, Jansson B (eds): Biological Psychiatry. Proceedings of the 3rd World Congress of Biological Psychiatry. Amsterdam, Elsevier/North Holland Biomedical Press, 1981, pp 1079–1086
9. Meyer A, Beck E: Prefrontal Leucotomy and Related Operations. Anatomical Aspects of Success or Failure. Henderson Trust Lecture 17. Edinburgh, London, Oliver and Boyd, 1954
10. Talairach J, Hecaen H, David M, et al: Recherches sur la coagulation thérapeutique des structures sous-corticales chez l'homme. Rev Neurol (Paris) 81:4–24, 1949
11. Leksell L: A stereotaxic apparatus for intracerebral surgery. Acta Chir Scand 99:229–233, 1949
12. Modell JG, Mountz JM, Curtis GC, Greden JF: Neurophysiologic dysfunction in basal ganglia/limbic striatal and thalamocortical circuits as a pathogenetic mechanism of obsessive-compulsive disorder. J Neuropsychiatry Clin Neurosci 1:27–36, 1989
13. Corsellis J, Jack AB: Neuropathological observations on yttrium implants and on undercutting in the orbito-frontal areas of the brain, in Laitinen LV, Livingston KE (eds): Surgical Approaches in Psychiatry. Lancaster, PA, MTP, 1973, p 90
14. Mesulam MM, Elliott JM: Neural inputs into the nucleus basalis of the substantia innominata (Ch4) in the Rhesus monkey. Brain 107:253–274, 1984
15. Leichnetz GR, Astruc J: Efferent connections of the orbitofrontal cortex in the marmoset (Saguinus oedipus). Brain Res 84:169–180, 1975
16. Nauta WJH: Circuitous connections linking cerebral cortex, limbic system, and corpus striatum, in Doane BK, Livingston KE (eds): The Limbic System. New York, Raven Press, 1986, pp 43–54
17. Nauta WJH: The problem of the frontal lobe: A reinterpretation. J Psychiatr Res 8:167–187, 1971
18. Gray JA: The Psychology of Fear and Stress. Cambridge, Cambridge University Press, 1987
19. Meyerson BA, Bergström M, Greitz T: Target localization in stereotactic capsulotomy with the aid of computed tomography, In Hitchcock ER, Ballantine HT, Meyerson BA (eds): Modern Concepts in Psychiatric Surgery. Amsterdam, Elsevier, 1979, pp 217–224
20. Meyerson BA, Mindus P: The role of anterior internal capsulotomy in psychiatric surgery, in Lunsford LD (ed): Modern Stereotactic Neurosurgery. Boston, Martinus Nijhoff Publishing, 1988, pp 353–364
21. Kihlström L, Meyerson BA, Mindus P, et al: Use of MR for target localization and dose-planning in stereotactic radiosurgical capsulotomy (abstract). Meeting of the World Society Stereotactic Functional Neurosurgery, Maebashi, Japan, 1989, p 148
22. Laitinen L: Emotional responses to subcortical electrical stimulation in psychiatric patients. Clin Neurol Neurosurg 81–83:148–157, 1979
23. Martinez SN, Bertrand C, Molina-Negro P, et al: Alteration of pain perception by stereotactic lesions of fronto-thalamic pathways. Confin Neurol 37:113–118, 1975
24. Bingley T, Persson A: EEG studies on patients with chronic obsessive-compulsive neurosis before and after psychosurgery (stereotaxic bilateral anterior capsulotomy). Electroencephalogr Clin Neurophysiol 44:691–696, 1978
25. Mindus P: Capsulotomy in Anxiety Disorders. A Multidisciplinary Study. Thesis, Karolinska Institute, Stockholm, 1991
26. Rylander G: Stereotactic radiosurgery in anxiety and obsessive-compulsive states: Psychiatric aspects, in Hitchcock ER, Ballantine HT Jr, Meyerson BA (eds): Modern Concepts in Psychiatric Surgery. Amsterdam, Elsevier/North Holland Biomedical Press, 1979, pp 235–240
27. Mindus P, Bergström K, Levander SE, et al: Magnetic resonance images related to clinical outcome after psychosurgical intervention in severe anxiety disorder. J Neurol Neurosurg Psychiatry 50:1288, 1987
28. Guo WY, Lindquist C, Kihlström L, Mindus P: Radionecrosis created in the internal capsule for psychosurgery with the gamma knife, in Guo WY: Radiological Aspects of Gamma Knife Radiosurgery. Thesis, Karolinska Institute, Stockholm, 1993
29. Herner T: Treatment of mental disorders with frontal stereotactic thermo-lesions. A follow-up of 116 cases. Acta Psychiatr Scand Suppl 66:36, 1961
30. Bingley T, Leksell L, Meyerson BA, Rylander G: Long-term results of stereotactic capsulotomy in chronic obsessive-compulsive neurosis, in Sweet WH, Obrador S, Martin-Rodriguez JG (eds): Neurosurgical Treatment in Psychiatry, Pain, and Epilepsy. Baltimore, University Park Press, 1977, pp 287–299
31. Meyerson BA: Stereotactic anterior capsulotomy in the treatment of obsessive-compulsive neurosis, in Carrea R (ed): Neurological Surgery, International Congress Series No 433. Amsterdam, Exerpta Medica, 1977, pp 307–312
32. Lopez-Ibor JJ, Lopez-Ibor Alino J: Selection criteria for patients who should undergo psychiatric surgery, in Sweet WH, Obrador S, Martin-Rodriguez JG (eds): Neurosurgical Treatment in Psychiatry, Pain, and Epilepsy. Baltimore, University Park Press, 1977, pp 151–162
33. Burzaco J: Stereotactic surgery in the treatment of obsessive-compulsive neurosis, in Perris C, Struwe G, Jansson B (eds): Proceedings of the 3rd World Congress of Biological Psychiatry. Amsterdam, Elsevier/North Holland Biomedical Press, 1981, pp 1103–1109
34. Kullberg G: Differences in effect of capsulotomy and cingulotomy, in Sweet WH, Obrador S, Martin-Rodriguez JG (eds): Neurosurgical Treatment in Psychiatry, Pain, and Epilepsy. Baltimore, University Park Press, 1977, pp 301–308
35. Leksell L, Backlund EO: Stereotactic gammacapsulotomy, in Hitchcock ER, Ballantine HR Jr, Meyerson BA (eds): Modern Concepts in Psychiatric Surgery. Amsterdam, Elsevier/North Holland Biomedical Press, 1979, pp 213–216
36. Mindus P: Capsulotomy, a psychosurgical intervention considered in cases of anxiety disorders unresponsive to conventional therapy, in Strandberg K, Beerman B, Lönnerholm G (eds): Pharmacological Treatment of Anxiety. Workshop, the Drug Information Committee of the Swedish National Board of Health and Welfare. Uppsala, Almqvist & Wiksell, Socialstyrelsen, 1988, pp 151–167
37. Ballantine HT Jr, Bouckoms AJ, Thomas EK, et al: Treatment of psychiatric illness by stereotactic cingulotomy. Biol Psychiatry 22:807–819, 1987
38. Jenike MA, Baer L, Ballantine HT Jr, et al: Cingulotomy for refractory obsessive-compulsive disorder. A long term follow-up of 33 patients. Arch Gen Psychiatry 48:548–558, 1991
39. Bartlett JR, Bridges PK: The extended subcaudate tractotomy lesion, in Sweet WH, Obrador S, Martin-Rodriguez JG (eds): Neurosurgical Treatment in Psychiatry, Pain, and Epilepsy. Baltimore, University Park Press, 1977, pp 387–398
40. Kelly D: Physiological changes during operations on the limbic system in man. Cond Reflex 7:127–138, 1972
41. Kelly D: Anxiety and Emotions. Physiological Basis and Treatment. Springfield, IL, Charles C Thomas, 1980
42. Waziri R: Psychosurgery for anxiety and obsessive-compulsive disorders, in Noyes R Jr, Roth M, Burrows GD (eds): Handbook of Anxiety.

Treatment of Anxiety, Vol. 4. Amsterdam, Elsevier Science Publishers, 1990, pp 519–535
43. Hay P, Sachev P, Cumming S, et al: Treatment of obsessive-compulsive disorder by psychosurgery. Acta Psychiatr Scand 87:197–207, 1993
44. Vasko T, Kullberg G: Results of psychological testing of cognitive functions in patients undergoing stereotactic psychiatric surgery, in Hitchcock ER, Ballantine HT Jr, Meyerson BA (eds): Modern Concepts in Psychiatric Surgery. Amsterdam, Elsevier/North Holland Biomedical Press, 1979, pp 303–310
45. Insel TR, Winslow JT: Neurobiology of obsessive-compulsive disorder. Psychiatr Clin North Am 4:813–824, 1992
46. Tan E, Marks IM, Marset P: Bi-medial leucotomy in obsessive-compulsive neurosis: A controlled serial inquiry. Br J Psychiatry 118:155, 1971
47. Stuss DT, Benson DF: Personality and emotion, in Stuss DT, Benson DF (eds): The Frontal Lobes. New York, Raven Press, 1986, p 121
48. Schalling D, Asberg M, Edman G, Oreland L: Markers of vulnerability to psychopathy: Temperament traits associated with platelet MAO activity. Acta Psychiatr Scand 16:172, 1987
49. Mindus P, Nyman H: Normalization of personality characteristics in patients with incapacitating anxiety disorders after capsulotomy. Acta Psychiatr Scand 83:283–291, 1991
50. Mindus P, Nyman H, Rosenquist A, et al: Aspects of personality in patients with anxiety disorders undergoing capsulotomy. Acta Neurochir Suppl 44: 138, 1988
51. Fodstad H, Strandman E, Karlsson B, West KA: Treatment of chronic obsessive compulsive states with anterior capsulotomy or cingulotomy. Acta Neurochir 62:1–23, 1982
52. Leksell L, Herner T, Leksell D, et al: Visualization of stereotactic radiolesions by nuclear magnetic resonance. J Neurol Neurosurg Psychiatr 48:19–20, 1985

CHAPTER 118

Neurovascular Decompression Procedures in the Surgical Management of Disorders of Cranial Nerves V, VII, IX, and X to Treat Pain

Robert H. Wilkins

VASCULAR RELATIONSHIPS OF THE CRANIAL NERVES

The cranial nerves normally have close associations with adjacent arteries and veins.[1-7] The ophthalmic artery runs along the inferior surface of the optic nerve as it enters the orbit, and the A1 segment of the anterior cerebral artery crosses the superior surface of the optic chiasm. The oculomotor nerve leaves the midbrain in close proximity to the posterior cerebral artery superiorly and the superior cerebellar artery inferiorly. The latter artery then extends around the midbrain and upper pons between, and adjacent to, the trochlear and trigeminal nerves. The anteroinferior cerebellar artery lies next to the abducens nerve as it exits from the pontomedullary junction of the brainstem and then courses posteriorly to come into close association with the facial, intermedius, and auditory nerves. The posteroinferior cerebellar artery has a variable association with the rootlets of the glossopharyngeal, vagus, and accessory nerves, and the vertebral artery may contact the hypoglossal nerve as well as some of the other lower cranial nerves.

The venous anatomy of the brainstem and cerebellopontine angle is more variable than is the arterial anatomy, but close associations often exist between the cranial nerves and these veins. The vein of the pontomesencephalic sulcus lies close to the oculomotor and trochlear nerves. The trigeminal nerve may be contacted by one or more of the tributaries of the superior petrosal vein, such as the transverse pontine vein, the pontotrigeminal vein, the vein of the cerebellopontine fissure, and the vein of the middle cerebellar peduncle. The vein of the pontomedullary sulcus courses close to the abducens, facial, intermedius, and auditory nerves, and the latter three nerves may also be contacted by the vein of the middle cerebellar peduncle and the vein of the cerebellomedullary fissure. Finally, the lateral medullary vein runs along the lateral aspect of the medulla adjacent to the entrance and exit zones of the glossopharyngeal, vagus, and accessory nerves.

Thus, both arteries and veins are normally situated in close proximity to the cranial nerves. These relationships probably vary slightly with the pulsations of the vessels, the pulsations of the cerebrospinal fluid (CSF), and the position of the head.

NEUROVASCULAR COMPRESSION AS AN ETIOLOGIC AGENT

Jannetta and others have advanced the idea that as some individuals age, their arteries elongate and their brain sags within the skull, changes that bring one or more vessels into contact with an adjacent cranial nerve.[1-14] Within each cranial nerve, a transition zone exists between central myelin (i.e., that associated with oligodendrocytes) and peripheral myelin (i.e., that associated with Schwann cells). In most of the cranial nerves, except the olfactory, optic, and acoustic nerves, this zone of transition is located within a few millimeters of the nerve's entrance into, or exit from, the brainstem.[15, 16] Jannetta and others have postulated that vascular compression of a cranial nerve leads to demyelination, especially at this zone of transition.[1-14]

Three theories have been formulated to explain how such demyelination then leads to cranial nerve dysfunction.[1-7, 9-14, 17] First, Gardner, Nielsen, and others have hypothesized that "short circuiting," or ephaptic transmission, occurs between axons in the area of demyelination, allowing "cross talk" between neighboring axons. Second, Møller has advanced evidence that focal compression and demyelination causes not only a false synapse within the nerve but also kindles an alteration within the nucleus (in this case, the facial nucleus) in patients with hemifacial spasm. Third, it has been postulated that regeneration may occur from the point of compression, with misdirection of sprouting axons such as may occur after a peripheral nerve injury in which the axons are disrupted but the epineurium remains intact.

Jannetta contends that if a cranial nerve is compressed near the brainstem by one or more adjacent blood vessels, a syndrome of hyperactive dysfunction of that nerve may develop.[1-7, 9-12] For example, compression of the trigeminal sensory root causes tic douloureux, and compression of the facial motor root causes hemifacial spasm. With continuing and worsening compression, a degree of hypoactive dysfunction may also appear, such as facial hypoesthesia and facial weakness, respectively.

Jannetta also contends that vascular compression of a cranial nerve further from the brainstem may cause a syndrome different from that caused by compression at the zone of myelin transition adjacent to the brainstem.[1-7, 9-12] For example, peripheral compression of the trigeminal nerve in the cerebellopontine angle may cause atypical trigeminal neuralgia or trigeminal neuropathy, and peripheral compression of the facial nerve in the cerebellopontine angle may cause Bell's palsy.

From these etiologic considerations has arisen the idea that a neural dysfunction syndrome caused by vascular compression should be surgically reversible. This is true for the syndromes that have the strongest evidence for vascular compression as an etiologic factor, such as hemifacial spasm.

ARGUMENTS FOR AND AGAINST THE IMPORTANCE OF NEUROVASCULAR COMPRESSION

Both the supporters and the detractors of the idea of neurovascular compression as an important etiologic factor in the development of a cranial nerve dysfunction syndrome recognize that such syndromes have other etiologies. For example, tic douloureux can be caused by a benign neoplasm in the cerebellopontine angle or by multiple sclerosis. Thus, vascular compression, if it is a significant cause of cranial nerve dysfunction, is only one of several causes.

DIFFERENTIAL SUSCEPTIBILITY OF CRANIAL NERVES TO VASCULAR COMPRESSION

For reasons that are not clear, certain cranial nerves seem to be involved by neurovascular compression more often than others. Despite their close anatomic relationships with arteries and veins adjacent to the brainstem, the oculomotor, trochlear, abducens, and hypoglossal nerves are almost never involved by compression, whereas vascular compression of the trigeminal and facial nerves is thought to be a significant cause of trigeminal neuralgia and hemifacial spasm, respectively.

Furthermore, adjacent nerves or different components of the same nerve may have different susceptibilities to vascular compression. For example, operative exposure of the trigeminal nerve at the pons in a patient with tic douloureux often demonstrates that both the main sensory root and the motor rootlets are equally compressed by the superior cerebellar artery (Fig. 118–1), yet the patient has no evidence of motor dysfunction. Trigeminal neuralgia is a condition encountered by neurologists and neurosurgeons in their daily practice; hemimasticatory spasm is a rarity. Likewise, the role of vascular compression in the etiology of hemifacial spasm seems well established, whereas vascular compression as a cause of vestibular or cochlear dysfunction is less well documented, and symptomatic vascular compression of the nervus intermedius is least proven.

ASYMPTOMATIC COMPRESSION

Because of the close anatomic associations that normally exist between cranial nerves and blood vessels and the uncommon occurrence of cranial nerve dysfunction syndromes in the general population, it is reasonable to assume that contact with, and even distortion of, nerves by adjacent blood vessels occurs without the production of symptoms or signs. Anatomic studies bear this assumption out.

The initial anatomic studies on this topic involved the inspection of fixed tissues that had been removed from the skull during the postmortem examination of subjects who had not had a known dysfunction syndrome of the appropriate cranial nerve during life. Such studies have been criticized (because of the probable alterations caused by tissue fixation and removal) as not accurately representing the actual anatomic associations present before death.

Furthermore, few pertinent observations have been reported of neurovascular relationships in asymptomatic individuals during life. Surgical exposure of the cerebellopontine angle is performed to treat a pathologic condition. If a neoplasm is present, such as a vestibular schwannoma, meningioma, or epidermoid tumor, the normal neurovascular relationships are usually distorted. If the operation is conducted for microvascular decompression of a cranial nerve, the surgeon does not ordinarily dissect other cranial nerves (unless they are immediately adjacent) sufficiently to expose their sites of entry into, or exit from, the brainstem.

GUILT BY ASSOCIATION

During the surgical treatment of a cranial nerve dysfunction syndrome, exposure of that nerve root at the brainstem does not always reveal evidence of vascular compression. An inexperienced surgeon may not expose the actual entry or exit zone of the nerve, may not recognize existing areas of vessel contact (e.g., on the side of the nerve away from the surgeon), or may alter the nerve-vessel relationships significantly during the dissection. However, even surgeons who are experienced with the technique do not always find vascular compression and are left without an etiologic explanation in those patients.[1-7, 18]

Those who doubt that neurovascular relationships have any etiologic significance think that the surgeon is simply uncovering normal nerve-vessel associations just as would be uncovered if the same operation were performed on an asymptomatic individual. The concern is that the vessels are guilty by association and not by fact. Similarly, the beneficial effects of microvascular decompression are ascribed to mild trauma to the nerve by the dissection and the insertion of material to maintain the separation of nerve and vessel or vessels.

In 1992, Hamlyn and King[19] published a study that best addressed the topic of vascular compression in asymptomatic subjects and in symptomatic patients (in this instance, patients with tic douloureux). They operated on 41 patients and documented their findings on videotape, with still color slides, and in their operative reports. They also examined 50 cadavers that were matched for age and sex with the patients in their clinical series. The same surgical techniques were used for the cadavers that were used for the patients. The first five cadavers were studied without vascular perfusion. In the next 10 cadavers, the carotid and vertebral arteries were cannulated at extracranial sites, and the transverse sinus was cannulated just distal to the torcular Herophili to establish parameters of perfusion. The final 35 cadavers were studied while the posterior circulation was perfused with a physiologic colloid solution to reproduce as closely as possible the vascular distention that would have been present during life. The authors concluded that "neurovascular compression, typified by a large vessel distorting and creating a groove in the fifth cranial nerve, was found in 37 of the 41 cases of trigeminal neuralgia.... No distortion was found in a total of 50 normal cadaveric dissections; however, on perfusion to physiological pressures, the percentage of nerves with vessels adjacent or in simple contact increased from 16 percent to 40 percent."[19]

RESPONSE TO MICROVASCULAR DECOMPRESSION

Not all patients obtain relief from an apparently adequate surgical separation of the offending vessel or vessels from the involved nerve at the brainstem. Furthermore, even among patients who obtain relief initially, the syndrome may recur, and surgical re-exploration may not reveal recurrent vascular compression.

NEUROVASCULAR DECOMPRESSION FOR DYSFUNCTION SYNDROMES OF SPECIFIC CRANIAL NERVES

Despite the concerns about etiology just discussed, in many patients with a cranial nerve dysfunction syndrome, vascular compression of that nerve at the brainstem does seem to play an important role in causation. The evidence supporting this idea is strongest with hemifacial spasm, slightly less so with tic douloureux and glossopharyngeal neuralgia, and weakest with other dysfunction syndromes. Of more practical significance, neurovascular (microvascular) decompression offers a method of treatment that usually does not produce a neurologic deficit.

FIFTH CRANIAL NERVE DYSFUNCTION

TIC DOULOUREUX (TRIGEMINAL NEURALGIA)

Diagnosis and Clinical Features

Neurovascular decompression is a useful form of treatment for tic douloureux but is considerably less effective for the treatment of other forms of facial pain. Therefore, the diagnosis must be accurate. The diagnosis of tic douloureux is based on the patient's description of the pain.

Typically, the pain has a lancinating or electrical quality that gives the patient the sensation that an exposed nerve is being manipulated, such as might be experienced when a dentist drills into the pulp of an unanesthetized tooth. The pain often originates spontaneously but may be triggered by a nonnoxious stimulus, such as a touch to some area on the same side of the face, even an area not involved by the pain. Movements of the mouth, for example, those occurring during talking or chewing, may also initiate a paroxysm of pain. The pain frequently reaches a high level of intensity (10 on a scale of 10) but usually subsides after some seconds. Although each paroxysm is relatively short in duration, such paroxysms often occur in clusters. Each paroxysm of pain is self-limited, but with repetitive clusters of tic pain, the patient may experience a less severe but more long-lasting aching discomfort in the same area of the face between paroxysms. The patient may be tortured by recurring bouts of pain for days or even months at a time, yet pain-free periods of significant duration may occur spontaneously, especially in the early course of the disorder.

Tic douloureux is more common in women than in men. It is confined to an area within the distribution of one trigeminal nerve. Although it can occur bilaterally, such occurrence is infrequent and ordinarily does not involve both trigeminal nerves simultaneously. Tic douloureux is commoner in the lower areas of the face than the upper areas and is commoner on the right side than on the left. Ordinarily, no neurologic deficits are present unless the pain results from multiple sclerosis, a tumor in the cerebellopontine angle, or some other major morphologic abnormality, such as dolichoectasia of the vertebrobasilar arterial system or an arteriovenous malformation.

Preoperative Evaluation

Because tic douloureux has several known causes, an imaging study of the brain should be obtained early in the course of management. Currently, magnetic resonance imaging (MRI) is the study that is most likely to demonstrate pertinent major morphologic abnormalities within the brain and along the course of the trigeminal nerve. In addition, with the refinement of MRI techniques, demonstrating compression of the trigeminal nerve at the pons by blood vessels of normal caliber is becoming progressively more feasible.[20]

Treatment Options

If a morphologic abnormality, such as an epidermoid tumor, meningioma, vestibular schwannoma, or arteriovenous malformation in the cerebellopontine angle, is discovered, appropriate treatment is directed toward removal of the lesion and simultaneous decompression of the trigeminal nerve, if possible. Ordinarily, this treatment results in cessation of the tic douloureux.

If the patient has a major morphologic abnormality that cannot be treated directly, or if no such abnormality is demonstrated by MRI, medical therapy is instituted to control the pain. The three medicines used most commonly for this purpose are carbamazepine (Tegretol), phenytoin (Dilantin), and baclofen (Lioresal). Carbamazepine is the most efficacious and is ordinarily tried first.

If medical therapy fails, surgical treatment is considered. The specific type of surgery recommended depends on the presumed cause of the tic douloureux, the patient's age (i.e., life expectancy) and health, and the location of the pain. Neurovascular decompression is a reasonable form of treatment if

1. The MRI shows one of the following patterns:
   a. Vascular compression of the trigeminal nerve by one or more vessels of normal caliber
   b. Vascular compression of the trigeminal nerve by vertebrobasilar dolichoectasia
   c. No abnormality identified
2. The patient is in good health, with no history to suggest multiple sclerosis, and has a reasonably long life expectancy.

The usual alternative to neurovascular decompression in these circumstances is percutaneous trigeminal rhizolysis in which a radiofrequency current or the injection of glycerol is used.[8] This procedure has low risks and ordinarily requires only one night's stay in the hospital or is performed as an outpatient procedure. However, it requires patient cooperation, it may be painful, it ordinarily causes some degree of facial hypoesthesia, and it may result in weakness of the ipsilateral muscles of mastication. If the patient's tic pain is centered about the eye, some risk exists of denervating the cornea, thereby permitting the subsequent development of keratitis.

Neurovascular decompression is a more complicated procedure that requires general anesthesia and involves greater risks of significant morbidity and even mortality. The patient ordinarily spends the night after surgery in an intensive care unit, and the total hospital stay usually ranges from 5 to 7 days. However, this procedure offers the possibility of pain relief without hypoesthesia. The patient experiences no pain during the operation, and corneal anesthesia and hemimasticatory weakness virtually never occur.

Neurovascular Decompression

PREPARATION. In the anesthesia induction area, the patient is placed in the supine position on the operating table. The patient's head is placed at the foot of the table so that the surgeon and assistant have leg room under the table during the operation and so that the circulating nurse or attendant has unimpeded access to the table's positioning controls. The initial preparations are similar to those for any craniotomy that is expected to last for 1 to 3 hours, including the placement of intravenous and intra-arterial catheters; the induction of general anesthesia and orotracheal intubation; the insertion of a urinary catheter; the administration of prophylactic antibiotics; the application of antiembolism stockings, wraps, or alternating compression devices; and the application of a Mayfield head holder. In addition, the electrodes and other paraphernalia necessary for the intraoperative monitoring of auditory and somatosensory evoked potentials are attached to the patient.

PATIENT POSITIONING. The operation can be performed with the patient in a horizontal or semisitting position.[2, 8, 11, 19, 21, 22] I prefer to use a lateral decubitus position.

After the patient has been turned to the lateral position, a lumbar puncture needle is inserted for the later drainage of CSF. A second needle is also inserted in case the first needle becomes obstructed. An axillary roll is placed at the end of the operating table, between the table and the patient's axilla. The lower shoulder extends beyond the end of the table; that arm is padded and is supported by the frame of the Mayfield head holder. The patient's head is flexed forward on the trunk, and the vertex is tilted toward the floor to maximize the surgeon's working space between the retromastoid area and the shoulder. The previously applied Mayfield head holder is fixed to its frame. To further increase the surgeon's working room, the upper shoulder is drawn toward the foot with tape, and care is taken not to stretch the brachial plexus. The entire operating table is then rotated so that the patient's head is brought upward until the operative field is parallel to the floor.

SURGICAL TECHNIQUE. The retromastoid area is clipped and shaved, and the patient and table are brought from the induction room into the operating room. As the anesthesia and evoked potential monitoring teams make their final arrangements for the operation, the operative area is prepared and draped. A linear scalp incision is made along the mastoid crease, Raney clips are applied to the skin edges, and the underlying fascial and muscular layers are divided along the same line. This step frequently necessitates coagulation and division of the occipital artery and division of the lesser occipital nerve. The soft tissues are stripped from the bone and are held apart with a self-retaining retractor. After one or two burr holes are made, bone is removed piecemeal with rongeurs, and occasionally with a drill, to create an asymmetric craniectomy measuring about 3 cm in craniocaudal length and about 2 cm at its greatest width. The superior and lateral edges of the bony opening are curved to expose the inferior margin of the transverse sinus and the medial margin of the upper sigmoid sinus. The medial edge of the craniectomy is curved somewhat in the opposite direction to permit inferomedial retraction of the lateral tentorial and upper petrosal surfaces of the cerebellum. The overall configuration of the bony opening is that of a bulging right triangle with a short side superiorly, a long side laterally, and a hypotenuse medially. Any mastoid air cells that have been opened during the performance of the craniectomy are sealed with bone wax.

As the scalp, soft tissues, and bone are opened, the patient is given mannitol (and occasionally furosemide) intravenously. Then, just before the dura mater is opened, lumbar drainage is instituted. These measures, and hyperventilation, if necessary, cause the cerebellum to fall away from the dura, which is then opened in a curved fashion parallel to the superior and lateral bony edges, about 3 to 5 mm inferior to the transverse sinus and medial to the sigmoid sinus. These superior and lateral dural edges are retracted back with temporary sutures.

The dural incision may be made before or after the operative microscope is brought into the field. However, all of the intradural manipulations should be performed under the microscope because of the accuracy and safety afforded by its illumination and magnification. Microsurgical instruments and technique should be used, and the negative pressure of the sucker should be reduced to about 80 mm Hg to prevent inadvertent injury to delicate structures, such as the trochlear nerve.

The tentorial and upper petrosal surfaces of the cerebellum are gradually and gently retracted away from the tentorium and petrous slope, respectively, as CSF is aspirated from the superior cerebellar cistern. The retractor is advanced stepwise to provide progressively deeper exposure, and an occasional bridging vein from the cerebellar surface is coagulated and divided. Ordinarily, the superior petrosal vein is encountered at or near the anteromedial end of the line of attachment of the tentorium to the petrous ridge; it drains its tributaries into the superior petrosal sinus. This vein (or veins, if there is more than one or if tributaries do not join until they are 1 or 2 mm from the sinus) must usually be coagulated and divided to permit adequate visualization of the trigeminal nerve. To prevent partially sealed venous ends from retracting and then bleeding after surgical division, each vein should be coagulated first, then cut partially to open the lumen without permitting retraction of the ends, then recoagulated on both sides of the cut, and finally, divided completely.

As the superior cerebellopontine and ambient cisterns are opened, the various components of the trigeminal nerve come into view (Fig. 118–1). The surgeon must be careful not to injure the trochlear nerve, which is parallel to the trigeminal nerve and just superior to it, or the cochleovestibular, intermedius, or facial nerves which are located in a bundle just inferior to it. To provide adequate exposure of the zone of entry into the pons of the main sensory root of the trigeminal nerve, the surgeon must place the blade retracting the cerebellum close to the cochleovestibular-intermedius-facial nerve bundle, and must take care not to injure one or more of these nerves by direct trauma, by stretch, or by interference with the circulation to the nerve or to a related structure, such as the cochlea.

The vascular relationships of the trigeminal nerve are inspected, and then the nerve and the adjacent vessels are manipulated sufficiently with blunt microdissectors to permit an inspection around as much of the circumference of the nerve root entry zone as possible. If arterial contact or compression is identified (usually by the superior cerebellar, anteroinferior cerebellar, or basilar artery), the offending artery or arteries are mobilized away from the nerve, and a pledget of material is inserted to maintain the separation (Fig. 118–2). Various materials have been used for this purpose, such as polyvinyl alcohol foam (Ivalon) or shredded polytetrafluoroethylene (Teflon) felt. I prefer polyvinyl alcohol foam, which can be cut to the dimensions required. It is soft when wet, it can be compressed to a smaller size as it is inserted, and it re-expands immediately to its cut dimensions after it is released. Its slightly rough surface ensures that it will remain in position and will be very likely to keep the vessel or vessels separated from the nerve.

Frequently, the superior cerebellar artery loops down anteromedial to the nerve, with its two or three main branches wedged in the crevice between the anteromedial surface of the nerve and the adjacent portion of the pons, and with the more distal aspects of these same branches then emerging at the superior end of the nerve-pons crevice to continue their normal arborization (see Fig. 118–1). The main trunk and the two or three main branches ordinarily can be brought up from in front of the nerve to assume a position away from the nerve superiorly; the sponge is then inserted between the nerve and the arterial tree to prevent further arterial contact (see Fig. 118–2).

If a large vein is involved, it can be mobilized as described or coagulated and divided. Small veins are handled in the latter manner. Simple coagulation without division should not be performed, if possible, because recanalization of the vein might occur with time.

If no vascular compression is identified, the main sensory root can be sectioned partially or can be compressed, rubbed, or otherwise gently traumatized to provide pain relief. If the sensory root is sectioned, the caudolateral one half to two

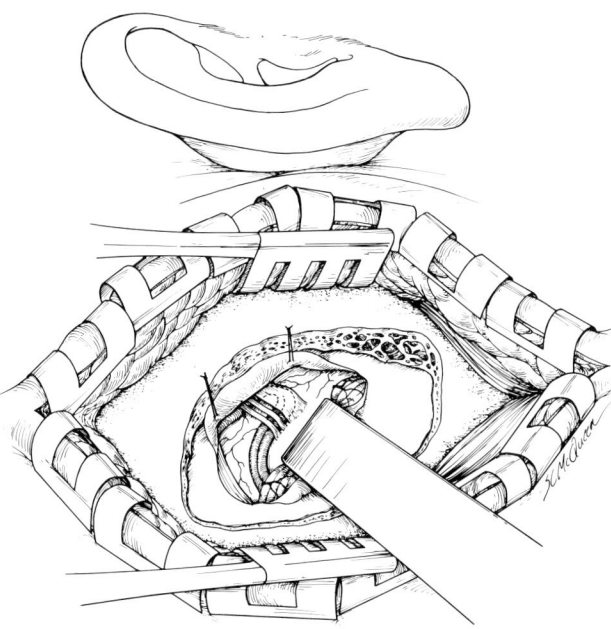

FIGURE 118–1. With the patient in a lateral decubitus position, the skin and underlying muscle have been divided in a line along the right mastoid crease. A retromastoid craniectomy has been created, and the exposed mastoid air cells have been closed with bone wax (not shown). The dura mater has been opened in a curved fashion just inferior and medial to the transverse/sigmoid sinus. With retraction of the cerebellum, the entry zone of the trigeminal nerve has been exposed. The trunk of the superior cerebellar artery and its two distal branches are seen to be wedged between the main sensory root (and two motor/sensory rootlets) of the trigeminal nerve and the adjacent pons. (Reproduced by permission from Wilkins RH: Surgical therapy of neuralgia: Vascular decompression procedures. Semin Neurol 8:280–285, 1988, Thieme Medical Publishers Inc.)

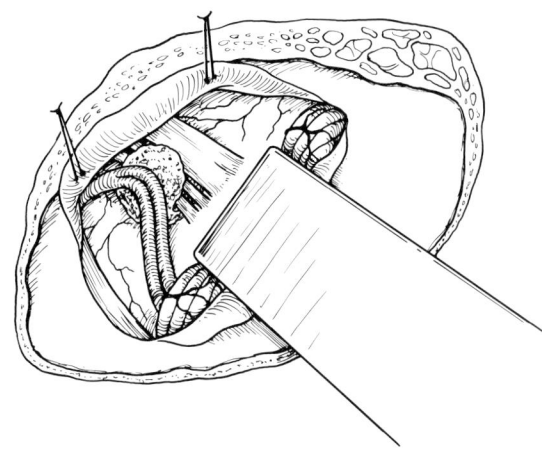

FIGURE 118–2. The trunk and distal branches of the superior cerebellar artery have been teased superiorly out of the space between the trigeminal nerve and the pons. A small pledget of Ivalon sponge has been cut to size and has been inserted to maintain the separation of the artery from the nerve and its entry zone. (Reproduced by permission from Wilkins RH: Surgical therapy of neuralgia: Vascular decompression procedures. Semin Neurol 8:280–285, 1988, Thieme Medical Publishers, Inc.)

thirds of the main sensory root is usually cut.[23] This maneuver is likely to provide pain relief, but with some sensory loss on the face—typically in the lower part of the face ipsilaterally, especially about the lips and along the side of the tongue. This loss should not result in significant corneal hypoesthesia (which might occur with sectioning of the cephalomedial portion) or trigeminal motor loss. Sectioning of a greater percentage of the main sensory root may increase the liklihood of pain relief, but it also increases the degree and extent of sensory loss, risks denervating the cornea, and increases the possibility of producing painful dysesthesia and even anesthesia dolorosa.

After the trigeminal nerve has been decompressed, cut, or traumatized, the lumbar drainage is stopped, the retractor blade is removed, the cerebellopontine angle is filled with warm irrigation solution, and the closure is begun. The dura is closed in watertight fashion, and the bone edges are rewaxed. Absorbable gelatin sponge (Gelfoam) is placed in the epidural space to fill the bony defect. The muscles, fascia, and subcutaneous tissues are closed in layers with interrupted sutures, and the skin edges are approximated with a running 4-0 nylon suture. A sterile adhesive dressing is applied, and the lumbar needles are removed. After the patient has been placed supine on the table, the head holder and evoked potential monitoring equipment are removed. The anesthetic is reversed, and the patient is taken to the recovery room.

POSTOPERATIVE CARE. The patient is monitored overnight in an intensive care unit and is usually moved to an intermediate care room the next day. Any preoperative medicines given for tic douloureux should be tapered off rather than stopped suddenly, to avoid a withdrawal syndrome. The exact schedule of this tapering depends on the amount and duration of preoperative usage. Even with continuation of the medication, however, the patient may experience tic douloureux for a while before it subsides.

The other details of postoperative care are the same as for any craniotomy. Ordinarily, recovery proceeds at a rate that permits suture removal and discharge from the hospital on the fifth postoperative day and return to full-time activities, including work, 1 month later.

RESULTS. Sweet[24] has summarized the long-term results of microvascular decompression for trigeminal neuralgia. Among 1700 patients from 17 reported series, the initial failure rate was 7 percent, and the late recurrence rate was 14 percent.

Larkins and coworkers[25] analyzed the results of such treatment for trigeminal neuralgia from one institution over a 20-year period. Although almost all of the patients had microvascular decompression, 5.5 percent had partial sectioning of the main sensory root of the trigeminal nerve instead of, or in addition to, microvascular decompression. The authors found that patient age and duration of symptoms did not affect the likelihood of pain recurrence. They divided their patients into four groups according to prior treatment and noted that the relief afforded by microvascular decompression initially and over time was the same, whether the patient had been treated previously with medication only or with a destructive procedure. The exception to these data was that evidence of trigeminal nerve damage from a prior destructive procedure was associated with a higher rate of recurrence of pain after microvascular decompression. Among 706 patients in the group who had previous treatment with medication only, 594 were followed up from 12 to 210 months (mean, 68 months) postoperatively; 76 percent had complete relief, 6.7 percent had partial relief, and 17.3 percent failed treatment. Of the 272 patients in the group with prior treatment by a destructive procedure, 241 were followed up from 12 to 214 months (mean, 77 months) postoperatively; 74.6 percent had complete relief, 4.1 percent had partial relief, and 21.1 percent failed treatment. The two groups of patients who had had a prior microvascular decompression procedure (at the same institution or elsewhere) did not fare as well. Of 116 patients in the former group, 104 were followed up for a mean of 77 months postoperatively; 50 percent had complete relief, 9.6 percent had partial relief, and 40.4 percent failed treatment. Among 23 patients in the latter group, 17 were followed up for a mean of 41 months; 47.1 percent had complete relief, 17.6 percent had partial relief; and 35 percent failed treatment.

In 1984, Piatt and Wilkins[26] reported on their results of microvascular decompression in 81 patients with tic douloureux. Of the 68 patients with definite arterial contact with the trigeminal nerve, 78 percent had excellent (72 percent) or good (6 percent) relief after a mean follow-up period of 54 months. In contrast, of the 13 patients with indefinite arterial contact or with venous contact, only 54 percent had excellent (46 percent) or good (8 percent) relief after a mean follow-up of 64 months. Furthermore, the 37 patients with anatomic distortion of the trigeminal nerve or wedging of one or more arteries between the nerve and the pons had a better outcome than the 31 with lesser forms of arterial contact. When these results for each of these four patient groups were graphed over time in Kaplan-Meier plots, it was apparent that although between 90 and 100 percent of the patients in each category obtained relief initially from microvascular decompression, a gradually enlarging number experienced recurrence of pain with time. From their own experience with 36 patients undergoing microvascular decompression for trigeminal neuralgia, Burchiel and associates[27] found that major recurrences occurred a mean of 3.5 percent annually, and minor recurrences, 1.5 percent annually.

As mentioned earlier, if arterial or significant venous compression is not identified or cannot be rectified safely during the surgical exposure of the trigeminal nerve root entry zone, the surgeon may cut part of the main sensory root. Young and Wilkins[23] found that the pain relief experienced by 83 patients treated in this fashion, after a mean follow-up of 6 years, was excellent in 48 percent, good in 22 percent, and poor in 30 percent. The failure rate for the first year was 17 percent, and it averaged 2.6 percent/year thereafter.

COMPLICATIONS. In the study by Larkins and colleagues[25] the authors tabulated the complications of their four patient groups and noted that microvascular decompression in patients who had had that procedure previously had a higher rate of temporary and permanent cranial nerve injury than in patients with prior treatment by medications or destructive procedures. The major complications in the entire group of 1117 patients included four deaths, three instances of intracranial hemorrhage, three of cerebellar edema, two of brainstem infarction, and two of hydrocephalus. Among the 139 patients with prior microvascular decompression, the repeat procedure caused permanent cranial nerve complications as follows: trigeminal nerve, 10 patients; facial nerve, two patients; and auditory nerve, two patients. The permanent cranial nerve complications in the other 978 patients included trigeminal nerve, four patients, and auditory nerve, three patients. The commonest other complications in the entire group were aseptic meningitis (in 179 patients) and CSF leakage (in 14).

Piatt and Wilkins[26] noted four major complications that resulted from their 105 posterior fossa operations for microvascular decompression or partial sensory rhizotomy of the trigeminal nerve. There was one death, from infarction in the brainstem and cerebellum, and one instance each of acute epidural hematoma, chronic subdural hematoma, and unexplained dementia. The significant unintentional cranial nerve injuries were as follows: trigeminal nerve, one patient; facial nerve, one patient; and auditory nerve, eight patients.

During the course of treating more than 250 patients with trigeminal neuralgia and more than 90 patients with hemifacial spasm via exposure of the corresponding nerve at the brainstem through a retromastoid craniectomy, we found that the occurrence of complications diminished as the surgeon gained experience with the procedure, with one exception. The incidence of profound postoperative sensorineural hearing loss after first-time microvascular decompression or partial sensory rhizotomy operations for tic douloureux or hemifacial spasm remained at 6.6 percent during the course of 152 such operations performed between 1975 and 1983; however, after the introduction of routine intraoperative monitoring of brainstem auditory evoked potentials, not a single instance of profound postoperative sensorineural hearing loss occurred after 109 similar operations performed between 1984 and 1989.[28]

In 1986, Sweet and Poletti conducted an informal survey of the complications of microvascular decompression for trigeminal neuralgia (Sweet WH, Poletti CE: Personal communication, 1986). Various complications were reported from 45 neurosurgical services. They concluded that "unless the neurosurgeon has enough experience to emphasize only his own results, he would be well advised to describe to patients a fuller range of complications than were seen in the best series."

ATYPICAL TRIGEMINAL NEURALGIA

Jannetta[10] classified two groups of patients with facial pain as having atypical trigeminal neuralgia or atypical trigeminal neuralgia with (variable) hyperautonomic dysfunction. In doing so, he has separated these conditions from tic douloureux and atypical face pain. Of practical importance, Jannetta considered atypical trigeminal neuralgia, without or with hyperautonomic dysfunction, to be caused by chronic vascular compression distal to the nerve root entry zone. In 1981, he reported that he had treated more than 75 patients with atypical trigeminal neuralgia by microvascular decompression.[10] Among 30 of these patients who were treated between 1972 and 1976 and followed up for 4 to 8 years postoperatively, 15 obtained relief of pain, and five had partial relief; one death occurred from the postoperative rupture of an undiagnosed intracerebellar arteriovenous malformation.

TIC CONVULSIF

In 1920, Harvey Cushing used the term "painful tic convulsif" to describe the association of trigeminal neuralgia with ipsilateral hemifacial spasm.[29] Cook and Jannetta[30] reported on 11 cases in 1984 and reviewed 37 more from the literature. These and other authors have noted that such patients are likely to have a structural lesion or lesions in the posterior fossa, such as a tortuous or ectatic vertebrobasilar artery complex, a cholesteatoma in the cerebellopontine angle, or simultaneous compression of the two nerves by adjacent vessels,[3] that affect the trigeminal and facial nerves. With appropriate decompression of the affected nerves, relief is expected.

SEVENTH CRANIAL NERVE DYSFUNCTION

TIC CONVULSIF

A few authors have used the term tic convulsif to mean the combination of geniculate neuralgia and hemifacial spasm. Yeh and Tew[31] described two such patients, both of whose symptoms were relieved by vascular decompression of the facial-acoustic nerve complex, including the nervus intermedius.

GENICULATE NEURALGIA

For more than 30 years, extending through 1937, J. Ramsay Hunt studied the sensory system of the facial nerve and various pain syndromes that he related to this system, forms of geniculate neuralgia.[6, 32] He classified geniculate neuralgia by suspected etiology into primary, secondary (e.g., postherpetic), and reflex forms. He also classified this condition by location of the pain into otalgic and prosopalgic forms. Subsequent physicians have found these forms of pain difficult to categorize and difficult to ascribe to dysfunction of the facial nerve and the nervus intermedius.

However, dating back to 1909, when Alfred Taylor relieved otalgia that was thought to represent "tic douloureux of the sensory filaments of the facial nerve" by surgically dividing the facial nerve, nervus intermedius, and upper fasciculus of the acoustic nerve,[33] evidence has existed that the nervus intermedius is involved in certain forms of aural pain. This evidence has accumulated from a small number of cases in which surgical sectioning of the nervus intermedius relieved the pain or stimulation of the nervus intermedius provoked the pain, or in which some other suggestive circumstance existed.

In 1969, Kempe and Smith[34] reported on a patient with geniculate neuralgia and ipsilateral hemifacial spasm that were thought to be caused by a persistent primitive acoustic artery.[34] In addition, in 1980, Ouaknine and coworkers[35] described a 48-year-old woman with a 21-year history of left geniculate neuralgia associated with left tinnitus and reduced auditory acuity, and occasional dizziness in whom a postmortem examination after her death from an unrelated cause revealed that a redundant loop of the left posteroinferior cerebellar artery was cross compressing the facial, intermediate, and cochleovestibular nerves.

However, in most cases of cranial neuralgia, the exact neurovascular relationships of the nervus intermedius are not examined. For that reason, the relative importance of vascular compression as an etiologic factor in geniculate neuralgia has not been determined.

In regard to surgical therapy, Rupa and colleagues[36] treated 18 patients with primary otalgia by a total of 31 surgical procedures. Various nerves were sectioned, singly or in combination, and microvascular decompression was performed in nine patients in whom vascular loops were discovered. However, only one patient was treated by microvascular decompression alone. The experience of Rupa and colleagues and of other surgeons has not been sufficient to permit conclusions about the possible effectiveness of microvascular decompression in the treatment of geniculate neuralgia.

CLUSTER HEADACHE (MIGRAINOUS NEURALGIA)

When episodic or chronic cluster headache becomes refractory to medical therapy, surgical treatment can be tried. Because the etiology and pathophysiology of this condition are not well understood, various approaches have been taken to surgical therapy, including sectioning of the nervus intermedius, the main sensory root of the trigeminal nerve, and the greater superficial petrosal nerve, alone or in combination.[37]

In 1986, Solomon and Apfelbaum[38] reported their experience with decompression of the facial nerve at the brainstem in five patients with chronic cluster headache. Two of the five also had decompression of the trigeminal nerve at the pons; one experienced improvement in the severity of the cluster headache, but the other did not. Of the remaining three patients, two improved. However, none of the five patients achieved complete relief.

In 1990, Morgenlander and Wilkins[37] reported the surgical treatment of 13 patients with cluster headache that was refractory to medical therapy. Interestingly, the two patients who were treated by microvascular decompression of the trigeminal nerve and sectioning of the nervus intermedius had a distinctly better outcome than the 11 patients who were treated in other ways. Although each of these two patients experienced recurrent episodes of cluster headache postoperatively, the first had been free of symptoms for 8 years and the second for 3 years when last seen postoperatively at 120 months and 135 months, respectively.

From these experiences, and from those of Jannetta, with "atypical trigeminal neuralgia with (variable) hyperautonomic dysfunction," indirect evidence exists that vascular compression of the trigeminal nerve, and perhaps the nervus intermedius, may be of etiologic significance in cluster headache. Likewise, microvascular decompression of the trigeminal nerve, alone or in combination with microvascular decompression or surgical division of the nervus intermedius, may be beneficial in the treatment of medically refractory cluster headache.

The nervus intermedius consists of interconnecting rootlets that lie between the facial nerve and the vestibular component of the acoustic nerve.[39] This complex is best approached from a superolateral direction, as provided by the surgical exposure of the trigeminal nerve described earlier in this chapter. Then, to expose the most medial aspect of the nervus intermedius, the surgeon must retract the flocculus of the cerebellum. At times, the acoustic nerve is adherent to the flocculus, necessitating division of the arachnoidal adhesions to provide adequate exposure.

NINTH AND TENTH CRANIAL NERVE DYSFUNCTION

GLOSSOPHARYNGEAL (VAGOGLOSSOPHARYNGEAL) NEURALGIA

Diagnosis and Clinical Features

Glossopharyngeal (vagoglossopharyngeal) neuralgia is a pain syndrome analogous to trigeminal neuralgia but is felt in the distribution of the glossopharyngeal nerve.[7, 40, 41] Like trigeminal neuralgia, this condition arises for no apparent reason, and the peak age of onset is between 40 and 60 years. The paroxysms of sharp, lancinating, unilateral pain occur spontaneously or can be initiated by a nonnoxious sensory stimulus or an event such as swallowing. The paroxysms frequently occur in clusters, and the clusters may recur irregularly over days, weeks, or months. Long, pain-free intervals may occur, especially at first, but the episodes of neuralgia ordinarily become more frequent with time. Usually, the pain is responsive to the same medications that are effective in the treatment of trigeminal neuralgia.

On the basis of the distribution of the glossopharyngeal nerve, glossopharyngeal neuralgia can be experienced primarily in the ear (otalgic type), primarily in the throat (pharyngeal type), or in both locations. In about 10 to 15 percent of patients, the paroxysms of pain are accompanied by bradycardia or asystole, which are thought to result from concomitant involvement of the vagus system; in turn, the bradycardia or asystole may cause syncope and even convulsions.

Like trigeminal neuralgia, glossopharyngeal neuralgia may arise because of a structural lesion affecting the glossopharyngeal nerve (secondary glossopharyngeal neuralgia) or in the absence of such a lesion (idiopathic glossopharyngeal neuralgia). However, the spectrum of structural abnormalities is somewhat different from that associated with trigeminal neuralgia. For example, the neoplasms found in patients with glossopharyngeal neuralgia are often malignant and often affect the nerve extracranially.

Glossopharyngeal neuralgia is about 70 to 100 times less common than trigeminal neuralgia. Unlike trigeminal neuralgia, glossopharyngeal neuralgia affects men as frequently as women and is more common on the left side of the head, in about a 3:2 ratio.

Glossopharyngeal neuralgia can be confused with geniculate neuralgia or with mandibular trigeminal neuralgia. Furthermore, glossopharyngeal neuralgia is accompanied by trigeminal neuralgia in about 10 percent of patients with the former disorder. The application of a topical anesthetic, such as a 10 percent cocaine solution to the region of the tonsil and pharynx, helps establish the diagnosis of glossopharyngeal neuralgia if the patient is relieved of pain for 1 to 2 hours afterward, even during swallowing and the probing of the trigger zone.

Preoperative Evaluation

After the diagnosis of glossopharyngeal neuralgia has been established by history (and anesthetic testing, if necessary), the etiology of the disorder should be identified, if possible. Physical examination may show evidence of impairment of the glossopharyngeal, vagus, and adjacent cranial nerves if the glossopharyngeal neuralgia results from a neoplasm, infection, or inflammation. Thin-slice, high-resolution computed tomography, MRI, or both, may also reveal an underlying structural lesion.

Treatment Options

When the glossopharyngeal neuralgia is found to arise from a disease process such as a neoplasm, infection, or inflammation, treatment should be directed toward the underlying disease. If this approach is not sufficient to control the pain, or if no such disease process has been uncovered, the patient should be given a trial of medication, starting with carbamazepine, in the same manner as discussed earlier in the treatment of tic douloureux.

Ordinarily, surgical treatment is reserved for patients whose pain is not controlled adequately by medication. Although various surgical approaches have been taken in the past, surgeons treat currently glossopharyngeal neuralgia in one of three ways: intracranial sectioning of the glossopharyngeal nerve and the upper vagal rootlets, percutaneous destruction of the glossopharyngeal nerve at the jugular foramen, or microvascular decompression of the glossopharyngeal nerve and vagal rootlets at the medulla oblongata.

Neurovascular Decompression

Close associations usually exist between the glossopharyngeal and vagus nerves and the posteroinferior cerebellar artery adjacent to the medulla.[42, 43] This fact may make it difficult for a surgeon to determine whether vascular compression actually exists in a patient with glossopharyngeal neuralgia whose nerves are being exposed in preparation for microvascular decompression or surgical sectioning.

Jannetta[9, 10, 12] and Laha and Jannetta[44] have fostered the idea that vascular compression of the glossopharyngeal and vagus nerves at the medulla is the cause in most cases of idiopathic glossopharyngeal neuralgia. Jannetta reported in 1980 that 15 of 17 patients who had surgical exploration of these nerves at the medulla were found to have such vascular compression (in nine cases by the posteroinferior cerebellar artery alone and in six cases by other vessels).[9] Of the two patients without documented vascular compression, one had undergone prior surgery, and the postoperative scar prevented inspection of the nerve root entry and exit zones; the other was operated on by another surgeon, and Jannetta was not present at the operation to confirm the findings.[10] In 1990, Jannetta reported on 28 patients with glossopharyngeal neuralgia, all of whom had cross compression of the glossopharyngeal and vagus nerve fascicles at the brainstem.[12]

To perform microvascular decompression, the surgeon exposes the entry and exit zones of the glossopharyngeal and vagus nerves at the medulla through a small retromastoid craniectomy. This procedure can be performed with the patient in a horizontal or a semisitting position. If the surgeon chooses to use the lateral decubitus position, the preliminary

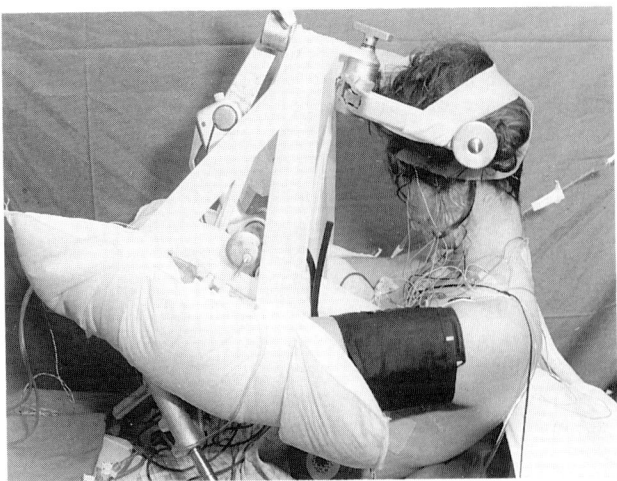

FIGURE 118–3. Semisitting (lounging) position for microvascular decompression of a cranial nerve in the posterior fossa. The patient's head is flexed forward, and the chin is rotated 10 to 15 degrees toward the side of the decompression; the head is fixed in this position with the Mayfield head holder. All pressure points are padded. The headrest of the operating table is turned down and serves as a support for the surgeon's elbows. Most of the wires shown are used for evoked potential monitoring and for the detection of muscular responses from intraoperative stimulation of the facial nerve.

steps are the same as I described earlier for tic douloureux. If the upright position is used instead (Figs. 118–3 and 118–4), the preliminary steps are the same as I have described elsewhere for hemifacial spasm.[4, 45] One of the key differences is that the patient who is placed in the semisitting

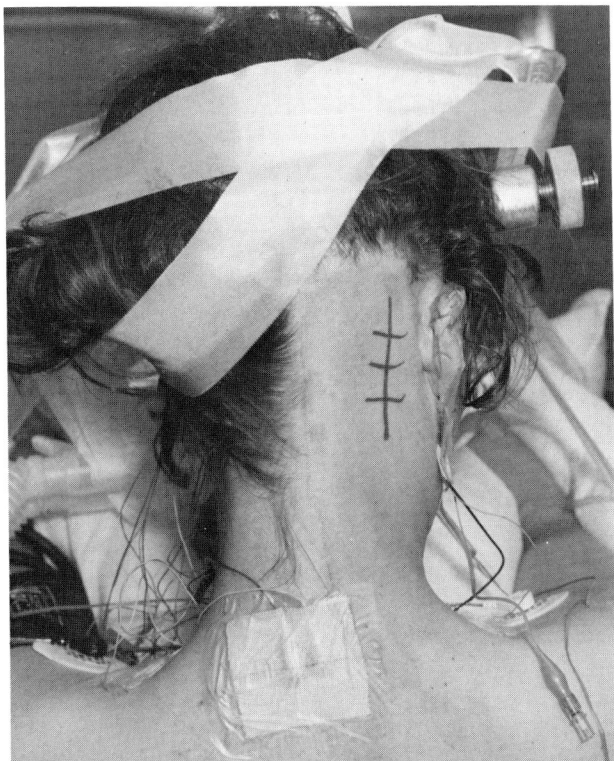

FIGURE 118–4. Semisitting (lounging) position showing the incision used for exposure of the nerve root entry and exit zones of the right facial, acoustic, glossopharyngeal, vagus, and accessory nerves.

position should have a Doppler monitor placed on the chest for detection of venous air embolism and should also have an intra-atrial catheter inserted for aspiration of air, if such embolism occurs. With either approach, the bony opening will be about the same size (2 × 3 cm) as the opening used to treat tic douloureux, but the short side of the bulging right triangle lies inferiorly rather than superiorly for this disorder. The craniectomy should be brought low enough that no residual inferior lip of bone interferes with the surgeon's line of vision. With either approach, the inferolateral aspect of the cerebellar hemisphere is retracted in a cephalomedial direction to provide the necessary degree of exposure. Intraoperative monitoring of brainstem auditory evoked potentials should be conducted to minimize the possibility of inadvertent injury to the cochlear pathways. If definite vascular compression is not identified or cannot be corrected, the surgeon can treat the glossopharyngeal neuralgia by dividing the glossopharyngeal nerve and the upper rootlets of the vagus nerve.

In 1977, Laha and Jannetta[44] described six patients with glossopharyngeal neuralgia who were treated surgically between 1971 and 1975. The ninth and tenth cranial nerves were noted to be compressed by a tortuous vertebral artery or the posteroinferior cerebellar artery at the nerve root entry and exit zones in five of the six patients. Microvascular decompression was performed in four patients, and in one of the four, the glossopharyngeal nerve and upper vagal rootlets were also cut. Among the three patients treated by microvascular decompression alone, one had relief of pain during a follow-up period of 6 months, one had incomplete relief, and one died in the immediate postoperative period from an intracerebral hemorrhage related to severe postoperative hypertension.

In 1980 and 1981, Jannetta reported an enlarged series of 11 patients with glossopharyngeal neuralgia on whom he had operated personally; nine were treated by microvascular decompression and two by nerve section.[9, 10] Of those treated by decompression, one died from a hypertensive hemorrhage, as mentioned previously. Six of the remaining eight patients had pain relief, but the follow-up lengths were not specified. Recurrences were experienced by two patients in whom small fragments of muscle were used to keep the offending vessel separated from the nerves and the medulla. Jannetta subsequently switched to using shredded polytetrafluoroethylene felt for this purpose to prevent resorption of the implanted padding. In addition to the one death, the surgical complications included one instance of temporary hypertension and four of decreased palatal function and gag reflex (two were temporary after microvascular decompression, and two were permanent after nerve section).

Individual patients or small series treated for glossopharyngeal neuralgia by microvascular decompression have been reported by a few other surgeons.[7, 41, 46] Their findings and results are generally similar to those of Jannetta.

SUMMARY

Despite questions about the exact etiologic role of neurovascular compression in tic douloureux, glossopharyngeal neuralgia, and the other disorders discussed in this chapter, and about the mechanisms by which neurovascular decompression provides benefit to patients with these conditions, such treatment does provide relief to many patients. Among the painful disorders discussed in this chapter, the cause-and-effect relationships for both etiology and therapy are most certain for tic douloureux and least certain for geniculate neuralgia and cluster headache. The twin ideas of neurovascular compression and neurovascular decompression are attractive from several standpoints, not the least of which is the possibility of ending pain without causing a neurologic deficit. However, much work is still required to clarify the many remaining points of uncertainty.

REFERENCES

1. Wilkins RH: Neurovascular compression syndromes. Neurol Clin 3:359–372, 1985
2. Wilkins RH: Surgical therapy of neuralgia: Vascular decompression procedures. Semin Neurol 8:280–285, 1988
3. Wilkins RH: Hemifacial spasm: A review. Surg Neurol 36:251–277, 1991
4. Wilkins RH: Facial nerve decompression for hemifacial spasm, in Apuzzo MLJ (ed): Brain Surgery Complication Avoidance and Management. New York, Churchill Livingstone, 1993, pp 2115–2143
5. Wilkins RH: Cranial nerve dysfunction syndromes: Evidence for microvascular compression, in Barrow DL (ed): Surgery of Cranial Nerves of the Posterior Fossa. Park Ridge, IL, The American Association of Neurological Surgeons, 1993, pp 155–163
6. Wilkins RH: Hemifacial spasm and other facial nerve dysfunction syndromes, in Barrow DL (ed): Surgery of the Cranial Nerves of the Posterior Fossa. Park Ridge, IL, The American Association of Neurological Surgeons, 1993, pp 221–232
7. Wilkins RH: Glossopharyngeal (vagoglossopharyngeal) neuralgia, in Barrow DL (ed): Surgery of the Cranial Nerves of the Posterior Fossa. Park Ridge, IL, The American Association of Neurological Surgeons, 1993, pp 245–251
8. Apfelbaum RI: Surgical management of disorders of the lower cranial nerves, in Schmidek HH, Sweet WH (eds): Operative Neurosurgical Techniques: Indications, Methods and Results, 2nd ed. Orlando, Grune & Stratton, 1988, pp 1097–1109
9. Jannetta PJ: Neurovascular compression in cranial nerve and systemic disease. Ann Surg 192:518–525, 1980
10. Jannetta PJ: Cranial nerve vascular compression syndromes (other than tic douloureux and hemifacial spasm). Clin Neurosurg 28:445–456, 1981
11. Jannetta PJ: Treatment of trigeminal neuralgia by micro-operative decompression, in Youmans JR (ed): Neurological Surgery: A Comprehensive Reference Guide to the Diagnosis and Management of Neurosurgical Problems. Philadelphia, WB Saunders, 1990, pp 3928–3942
12. Jannetta PJ: Cranial rhizopathies, in Youmans JR (ed): Neurological Surgery: A Comprehensive Reference Guide to the Diagnosis and Management of Neurosurgical Problems. Philadelphia, WB Saunders, 1990, pp 4169–4182
13. Møller AR: The cranial nerve vascular compression syndrome: I. A review of treatment. Acta Neurochir (Wien) 113:18–23, 1991
14. Møller AR: The cranial nerve vascular compression syndrome: II. A review of pathophysiology. Acta Neurochir (Wien) 113:24–30, 1991
15. Lang J, Über Bau, Länge und Gefässbeziehungen der "zentralen" und "peripheren" Strecken der intrazisternalen Hirnnerven. Zentralbl Neurochir 43:217–258, 1982
16. Skinner HA: Some histologic features of the cranial nerves. Arch Neurol Psychiatry 25:356–372, 1931
17. Gardner WJ: Cross-talk—the paradoxical transmission of a nerve impulse. Arch Neurol 14:149–156, 1966
18. Adams CBT: Microvascular compression: An alternative view and hypothesis. J Neurosurg 57:1–12, 1989
19. Hamlyn PJ, King TT: Neurovascular compression in trigeminal neuralgia: A clinical and anatomical study. J Neurosurg 76:948–954, 1992
20. Tien RD, Wilkins RH: MRA delineation of the vertebral-basilar system in patients with hemifacial spasm and trigeminal neuralgia. AJNR 14:34–36, 1993
21. Matsushima T, Fukui M, Suzuki S, et al: The microsurgical anatomy of the infratentorial lateral supracerebellar approach to the trigeminal nerve for tic douloureux. Neurosurgery 24:890–895, 1989

22. Rhoton AL Jr: Microsurgical anatomy of decompression operations on the trigeminal nerve, in Rovit RL, Murali R, Jannetta PJ (eds): Trigeminal Neuralgia. Baltimore, Williams & Wilkins, 1990, pp 165–200
23. Young JN, Wilkins RH: Partial sensory trigeminal rhizotomy at the pons for trigeminal neuralgia. J Neurosurg 79:680–687, 1993
24. Sweet WH: Trigeminal neuralgia: Problems as to cause and consequent conclusions regarding treatment, in Wilkins RH, Rengachary SS (eds): Neurosurgery, 2nd ed. New York, McGraw-Hill, 1995
25. Larkins MV, Jannetta PJ, Bissonette D: Microvascular Decompression for Recurrent Trigeminal Neuralgia. Presented at the 59th Annual Meeting of the American Association of Neurological Surgeons, New Orleans, April 23, 1991
26. Piatt JH Jr, Wilkins RH: Treatment of tic douloureux and hemifacial spasm by posterior fossa exploration: Therapeutic implications of various neurovascular relationships. Neurosurgery 14:462–471, 1984
27. Burchiel KJ, Clarke H, Haglund M, et al: Long-term efficacy of microvascular decompression in trigeminal neuralgia. J Neurosurg 69:35–38, 1988
28. Wilkins RH, Radtke RA, Erwin CW: Value of intraoperative brainstem auditory evoked potential monitoring in reducing the auditory morbidity associated with microvascular decompression of cranial nerves. Skull Base Surg 1:106–109, 1991
29. Cushing H: The major trigeminal neuralgias and their surgical treatment based on experiences with 332 gasserian operations. Am J Med Sci 160:157–184, 1920
30. Cook BR, Jannetta PJ: Tic convulsif: Results in 11 cases treated with microvascular decompression of the fifth and seventh cranial nerves. J Neurosurg 61:949–951, 1984
31. Yeh H, Tew JM Jr: Tic convulsif, the combination of geniculate neuralgia and hemifacial spasm relieved by vascular decompression. Neurology 34:682–684, 1984
32. Hunt JR: Geniculate neuralgia (neuralgia of the nervus facialis): A further contribution to the sensory system of the facial nerve and its neuralgic conditions. Arch Neurol Psychiatry 37:253–285, 1937
33. Clark LP, Taylor AS: True tic douloureux of the sensory filaments of the facial nerve. JAMA 53:2144–2146, 1909
34. Kempe LG, Smith DR: Trigeminal neuralgia, facial spasm, intermedius and glossopharyngeal neuralgia with persistent carotid basilar anastomosis. J Neurosurg 31:445–451, 1969
35. Ouaknine GE, Robert F, Molina-Negro P, et al: Geniculate neuralgia and audio-vestibular disturbances due to compression of the intermediate and eighth nerves by the postero-inferior cerebellar artery. Surg Neurol 13:147–150, 1980
36. Rupa V, Saunders RL, Weider DJ: Geniculate neuralgia: The surgical management of primary otalgia. J Neurosurg 75:505–511, 1991
37. Morgenlander JC, Wilkins RH: Surgical treatment of cluster headache. J Neurosurg 72:866–871, 1990
38. Solomon S, Apfelbaum RI: Surgical decompression of the facial nerve in the treatment of chronic cluster headache. Arch Neurol 43:479–482, 1986
39. Rhoton AL Jr, Kobayashi S, Hollinshead WH: Nervus intermedius. J Neurosurg 29:609–618, 1968
40. Rushton JG, Stevens JC, Miller RH: Glossopharyngeal (vagoglossopharyngeal) neuralgia: A study of 217 cases. Arch Neurol 38:201–205, 1981
41. Gybels JM, Sweet WH: Neurosurgical Treatment of Persistent Pain: Physiological and Pathological Mechanisms of Human Pain. Basel, S Karger, 1989, pp 91–103
42. Lister JR, Rhoton AL Jr, Matsushima T, et al: Microsurgical anatomy of the posterior inferior cerebellar artery. Neurosurgery 10:170–199, 1982
43. Rhoton AL Jr, Buza R: Microsurgical anatomy of the jugular foramen. J Neurosurg 42:541–550, 1975
44. Laha RK, Jannetta PJ: Glossopharyngeal neuralgia. J Neurosurg 47:316–320, 1977
45. Wilkins RH: Microvascular decompression of the facial nerve, in Rengachary SS, Wilkins RH (eds): Neurosurgical Operative Atlas. Baltimore, Williams & Wilkins, 1993, pp 319–328
46. Hamer J: Microneurosurgical findings of glossopharyngeal neuralgia, in Samii M (ed): Surgery in and Around the Brain Stem and the Third Ventricle. New York, Springer-Verlag, 1986, pp 285–289

SELECTED READINGS

1. Adams CBT: Microvascular compression: An alternative view and hypothesis. J Neurosurg 57:1–12, 1989
2. Barrow DL (ed): Surgery of the Cranial Nerves of the Posterior Fossa. Park Ridge, IL, The American Association of Neurological Surgeons, 1993
3. Gybels JM, Sweet WH: Neurosurgical Treatment of Persistent Pain: Physiological and Pathological Mechanisms of Human Pain. Basel, S Karger, 1989
4. Jannetta PJ: Treatment of trigeminal neuralgia by micro-operative decompression, in Youmans JR (ed): Neurological Surgery: A Comprehensive Reference Guide to the Diagnosis and Management of Neurosurgical Problems. Philadelphia, WB Saunders, 1990, pp 3928–3942
5. Morgenlander JC, Wilkins RH: Surgical treatment of cluster headache. J Neurosurg 72:866–871, 1990
6. Rovit RL, Murali R, Jannetta PJ (eds): Trigeminal Neuralgia. Baltimore, Williams & Wilkins, 1990
7. Wilkins RH: Surgical therapy of neuralgia: Vascular decompression procedures. Semin Neurol 8:280–285, 1988
8. Wilkins RH: Hemifacial spasm: A review. Surg Neurol 36:251–277, 1991

CHAPTER 119

Percutaneous Rhizotomy in the Treatment of Intractable Facial Pain (Trigeminal, Glossopharyngeal, and Vagal Nerves)

John M. Tew, Jr.
Jamal M. Taha

TRIGEMINAL NEURALGIA

The surgical treatment of trigeminal neuralgia continues to stimulate controversy, despite the fact that this condition has been recognized and treated surgically for centuries. A totally satisfactory method of treatment has never been devised. Section of a peripheral branch of the trigeminal nerve was probably the earliest form of surgical therapy. Later, intracranial section of peripheral branches[1,2] ganglion resection,[3] and retrogasserian rhizotomy were developed.[4-6] Some who questioned the need for destructive procedures[7-10] developed techniques for decompressing or compressing the posterior rootlets.

Peripheral procedures are still effective for the temporary control of chronic trigeminal pain, particularly as an early measure that provides the patient with an opportunity to test the effect of sensory deprivation.[11,12]

Based on the original observations of Dandy and Gardner,[10,13] Jannetta[14] popularized the theory that trigeminal neuralgia was caused by compression of the trigeminal root entry zone to the brainstem by vascular structures. Although the efficacy of microvascular decompression has been established, the recurrence rate associated with this operation demonstrates that it is not a curative procedure[15] in all cases.

Electrocoagulation of the trigeminal nerve was originally proposed by Kirschner in 1932.[16] Despite a report of favorable results,[17] this procedure attracted no practitioners in this country (because of complications resulting from uncontrollable spread of heat to adjacent cranial nerves and arteries) until Sweet refined the technique[18,19] with the following modifications: (1) use of a short-acting anesthetic agent, which permits the patient to awaken rapidly for sensory testing during the operation; (2) use of electrical stimulation for precise localization; (3) use of a reliable radiofrequency current for production of the lesion; and (4) use of temperature monitoring for precise control of lesion configuration. This modified procedure has become an extremely safe and popular method to partially destroy the sensory root.

PATIENT SELECTION

All patients with trigeminal neuralgia are subjected to a trial of medical therapy, beginning with carbamazepine; lioresal and phenytoin are drugs of second choice. The 75 percent of patients who fail to achieve long-term relief with medical therapy, either because of the recurrence of pain or the development of toxic side effects, are candidates for percutaneous rhizotomy. For guidelines, we refer to Garvan and Siegfried,[20] who advocated that surgery be considered for patients who have only partial relief of pain after 1 year of drug therapy and who still require medication after consumption of over 3000 tablets of a single drug.

Posterior fossa exploration and microvascular decompression are offered to patients under 65 years of age who have no medical contraindication to a major procedure. This procedure is recommended for patients with primary involvement of the ophthalmic division to avoid the complications of corneal analgesia. Computed tomography (CT) or magnetic resonance imaging exclude the rare patient in whom a tumor is a cause of trigeminal pain.[21] Angiography is not routinely used because we have found it a poor predictor of neurovascular compression.

If surgical treatment is chosen, we request that the patient and family both read and listen to an explanation of current procedures available to control trigeminal neuralgia. Frequently, the patient is advised to consult with others who have undergone major trigeminal surgery; this tactic reinforces the patient's understanding and appreciation of possible undesirable sensory loss. Differential sensory block enables the patient to experience the effect of sensory deprivation and may aid in the decision concerning surgery for atypical facial pain.

A well-informed patient can better understand possible side effects and is less likely to be disappointed postoperatively. Our policy is to let the informed patients make their own decisions regarding the mode of treatment. If a patient elects to have a destructive procedure, such as electrocoagulation, we encourage the patient to indicate the desired degree of sensory deficit. Although partial sensory loss is associated with a higher incidence of recurrence, patients usually are not reluctant to undergo repeat percutaneous rhizotomy.

TECHNIQUE: PERCUTANEOUS TRIGEMINAL RHIZOTOMY

The theoretical application of differential thermocoagulation of the trigeminal rootlets is based primarily on the work of Letcher and Goldring[22] and others.[23, 24] They demonstrated that the compound action potentials of A-delta and C fibers (nociceptive fibers) in a nerve are blocked at a lower temperature than the compound action potentials of larger A-alpha and beta fibers carrying tactile sensations. These physiologic studies showed that temperature-dependent selective destruction of A-delta and C fibers can be achieved. Despite the fact that some histologic studies showed nonselective destruction of all fibers after thermocoagulation,[25] these findings are not supported by the clinical observation of selective preservation of touch perception after radiofrequency trigeminal neurolysis in humans. This discrepancy may be explained by the nonquantitative nature of histologic studies, in which a single destroyed A-beta fiber can be more conspicuous than 10 other destroyed C fibers. Furthermore, experimental studies have demonstrated the reversibility of low current–temperature radiofrequency lesions.[23, 26]

The procedure is conducted in the radiographic suite (Fig. 119–1). The patient's oral intake is restricted 6 hours before the procedure. Atropine (0.4 mg given intramuscularly) is administered to reduce oral secretions and prevent bradycardia during the procedure. The patient lies supine with the head in the neutral position. A right-handed surgeon stands on the patient's right side, regardless of the side of the patient's pain. A 21-gauge spinal needle placed in the deltoid subcutaneous tissue acts as a reference electrode. The patient is anesthetized with an intravenous injection of 30 to 50 mg of methohexital (Brevital, Eli Lilly & Company, Indianapolis, IN). A standard 100-mm-long, 20-gauge cannula and stylet are placed in the retrogasserian portion of the trigeminal nerve. Placement is by free-hand manipulation, but a guiding device can be used. Recently, stereotatic frames and CT-guided techniques have been developed to cannulate the foramen ovale.[27, 28] These devices are not helpful in our experience. Three anatomic landmarks are chosen on the face (Fig. 119–2): (1) a point 3 cm anterior to the external auditory meatus, (2) a point beneath the medial aspect of the pupil, and (3) a point 2.5 cm lateral to the oral commissure. The first two points indicate the site of the foramen ovale, and the third is the point at which the needle penetrates the skin of the jaw. The anterior approach to the foramen ovale, as advocated by Härtel,[29] is used (Fig. 119–3). Radiographic control has been reported to be valuable, and we have effectively used the image intensifier in a lateral plane to localize the needle.[30] Using the landmarks described, we have been able to penetrate the foramen ovale either on the first attempt, in most cases, or after a simple adjustment.

An oral airway is placed between the patient's jaws to prevent the patient from involuntarily biting the finger that guides the electrode. Intravenous methohexital (Brental) is injected before needle placement. The index finger of a gloved hand is placed just inferior to the lateral pterygoid wing, and the electrode is directed into the medial portion of the foramen ovale (Fig. 119–4). This is achieved by aiming the needle toward the intersection of a coronal plane passing through a point 3 cm anterior to the tragus and a sagittal plane passing through the medial aspect of the pupil. If the needle enters the posterolateral aspect of the foramen, it may not lie within the dural investment of the trigeminal ganglion and, if advanced, probably will not reach the maxillary or ophthalmic divisions of the rootlet of the nerve. As the electrode is advanced, entrance of the needle into the foramen is signaled by a wince and a brief contraction of the masseter muscle, indicating contact with the mandibular sensory and motor fibers. Before the electrode is advanced any further, a lateral image is obtained to confirm proper placement of the electrode (Fig. 119–5A and B). Care must be taken to avoid cannulation of the superior orbital fissure anterosuperiorly or the jugular foramen posteroinferiorly, or intracranial placement of the needle through aberrant foraminae (e.g., the foramen of Vesalius, which lies anteromedial to the foramen ovale, or the innominate canal of Arnold, which lies posterior to the foramen ovale). The stylet is withdrawn to determine

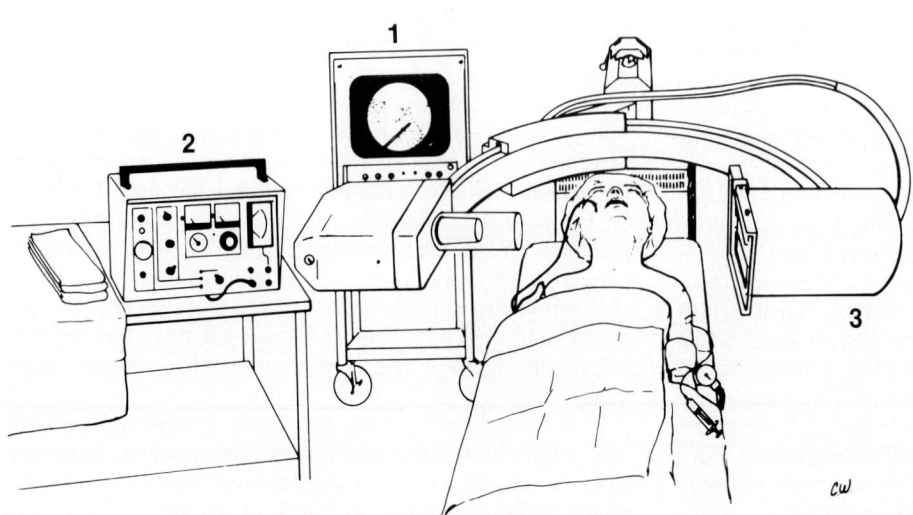

FIGURE 119–1. Operative arrangement used for stereotactic rhizotomy of the trigeminal nerve. 1 = image intensifier; 2 = radiofrequency generator; 3 = C-arm cineradiographic unit. (From Tew JM: Treatment of trigeminal neuralgia by percutaneous rhizotomy, in Youmans JR [ed]: Neurological Surgery, 2nd ed. Philadelphia, W. B. Saunders, 1982, p 3567.)

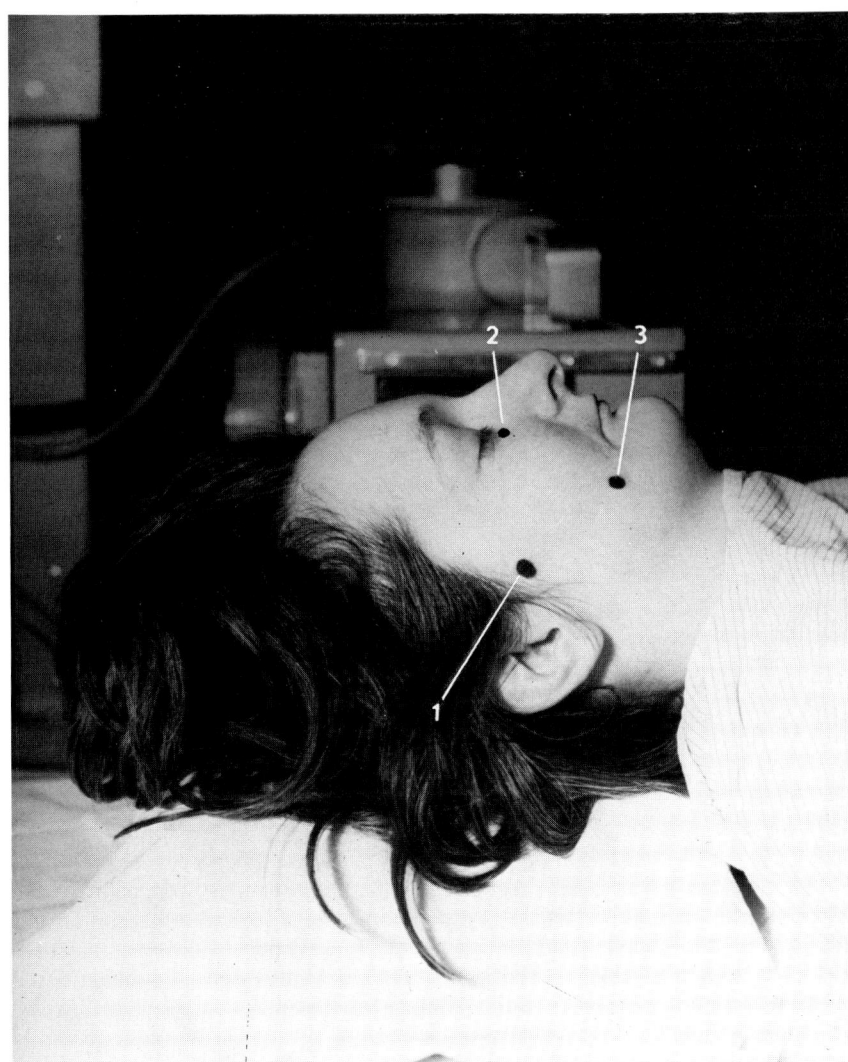

FIGURE 119–2. Anatomic landmarks for electrode placement. (From Tew JM: Treatment of trigeminal neuralgia by percutaneous rhizotomy, in Youmans JR [ed]: Neurological Surgery, 2nd ed. Philadelphia, W. B. Saunders, 1982, p 3567.)

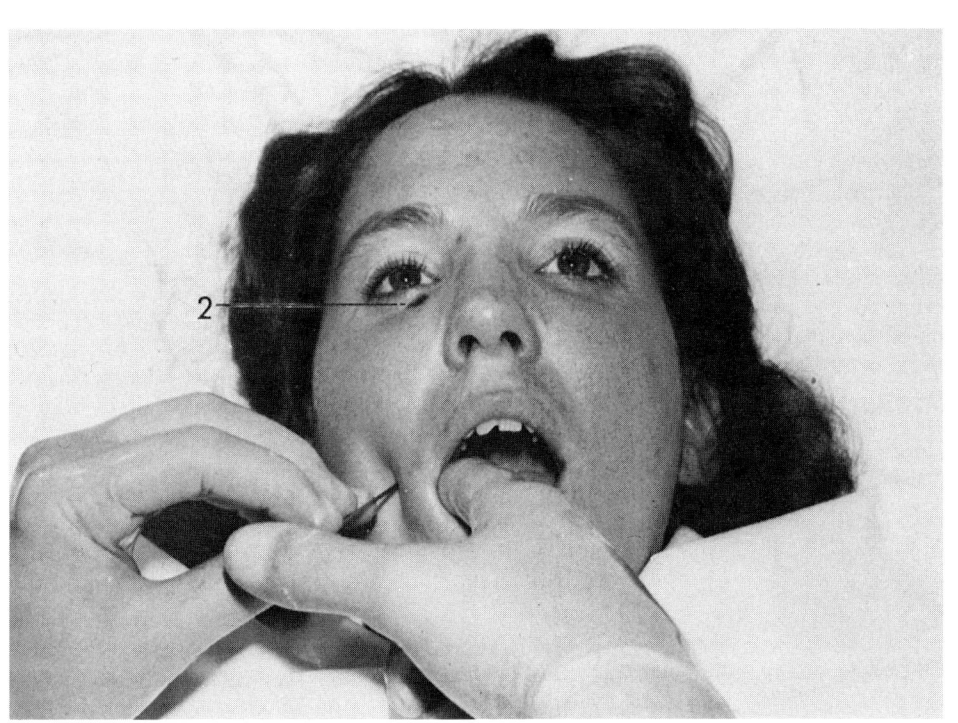

FIGURE 119–3. Needle placement according to the technique of Härtel. (From Tew JM, van Loveren: Percutaneous rhizotomy in the treatment of intractable facial pain [trigeminal, glossopharyngeal, and vagal nerves], in Schmidek HH, Sweet WH [eds]: Current Techniques in Operative Neurosurgery, 2nd ed., Philadelphia, W. B. Saunders, 1988, p 1113.)

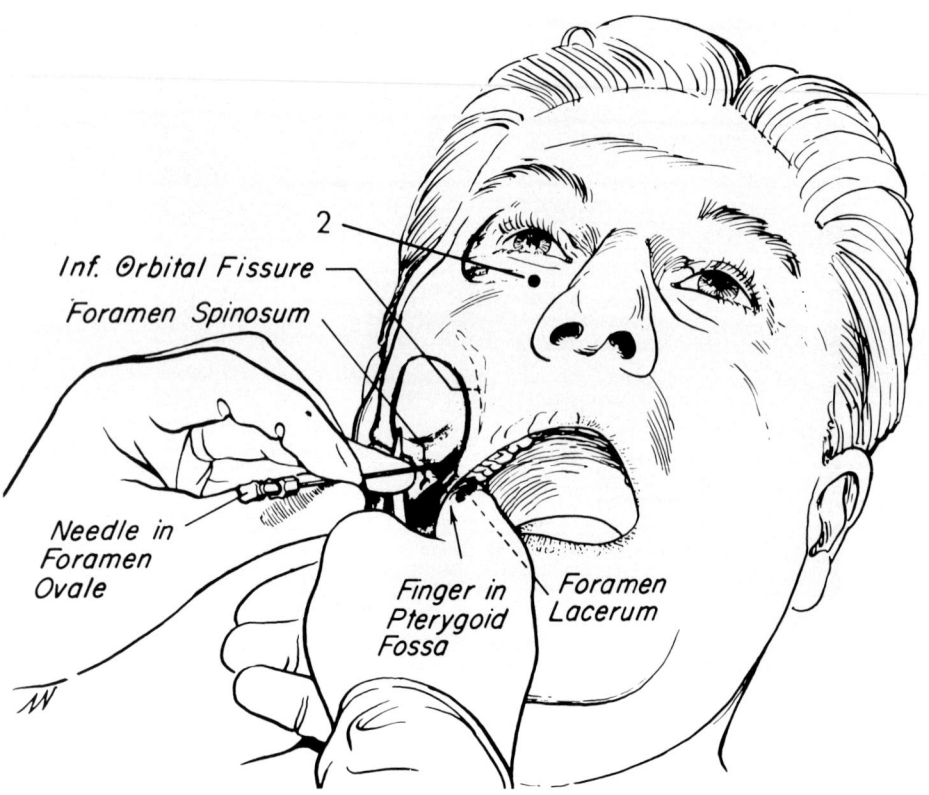

FIGURE 119–4. Free-hand placement of the electrode. The guiding finger touches the pterygoid wing. (From Tew JM: Treatment of trigeminal neuralgia by percutaneous rhizotomy, in Youmans JR [ed]: Neurological Surgery, 2nd ed. Philadelphia, W. B. Saunders, 1982, p 3567.)

whether or not the carotid artery has been penetrated, which, in our experience, has occurred on only two occasions.

Carotid artery penetration is recognized either by pulsatile blood flow through the cannula or by rhythmic fluctuation of temperature during monitoring. If the carotid artery is penetrated, the needle should be withdrawn promptly and manual pressure applied over the posterior pharyngeal space. The procedure should be discontinued and the patient allowed to recuperate for 24 to 48 hours. Ischemic complications, such as hemiparesis, and carotid-cavernous fistula have resulted from puncture of the internal carotid artery.[31] If deviated laterally, the electrode can penetrate the cartilaginous covering of the foramen lacerum and puncture the carotid artery. If the electrode is directed posterolaterally, it can pierce the carotid artery at its entrance into the petrous bone. Rish[31] noted that after the electrode passes through the foramen ovale, it can penetrate the carotid artery. This can occur if the electrode is directed anteriorly and medially into the area of the cavernous sinus (Fig. 119–6). Our anatomic studies illustrate that the carotid artery is frequently devoid of bony covering immediately ventral to Meckel's cave.

In most patients, proper positioning of the cannula within the trigeminal cistern allows free flow of cerebrospinal fluid through the needle, except in patients who have had previous surgical procedures or chemical injection. Egress of cerebrospinal fluid does not ensure that the needle lies in the proper position (retrogasserian). Cerebrospinal fluid can also be obtained from either the infratemporal subarachnoid space, if the needle is too deep, or the region distal to the gasserian ganglion, if the dural subarachnoid sleeve extends beyond the rootlets.

Electrode Localization

The cannula is calibrated to permit extrusion of the electrode in 1-mm increments. The curved electrode tip is a coil spring that carries a thermocouple, stimulator, and lesion-generating probe. When the electrode is fully inserted into the cannula, the curved tip extends 5 mm beyond the end of the cannula and projects 3 mm perpendicular to the long axis of the electrode. The cannula is insulated to the tip with polytetrafluoroethylene (Teflon) so that only the extruded portion of the electrode (zero to 5 mm) is conductive. The electrode can be rotated through a 360-degree axis for stimulation and lesion production.

Final placement of the electrode tip is determined by the patient's response to electrical stimulation. A square wave current of precisely 100 to 400 mV at 50 to 75 cycles/second and 1-millisecond's duration reproduces the paroxysmal bouts of pain that are reminiscent of trigeminal neuralgia. Stimulation can also be achieved with mild heat (<40°C). Stimulation at higher voltage (500 to 1000 mV) may be required in patients who have had previous intracranial rhizotomy or repeated alcohol injections. The response evoked serves as a reliable indicator of the probe temperature required to produce a lesion. Recently, electrodes have been developed that record trigeminal sensory evoked potentials induced by orthodromic stimulation of the three trigeminal divisions. These techniques may prove valuable in locating the tip of the electrode within the trigeminal rootlets without having to resort to a wake-up procedure.[32, 33]

After the cannula reaches the trigeminal cistern, stimulation should elicit a paroxysm of pain in the mandibular distribution. Lateral roentgenograms obtained at that time indicate whether or not the tip of the electrode lies at a point 4 to 5 mm external to the profile of the clivus. If the needle is advanced 5 mm, its tip should lie at the level of the clivus, where stimulation elicits paresthesias in the second-division rootlets. The electrode tip should not be advanced more than 8 mm deep to the profile of the clivus, because it can injure

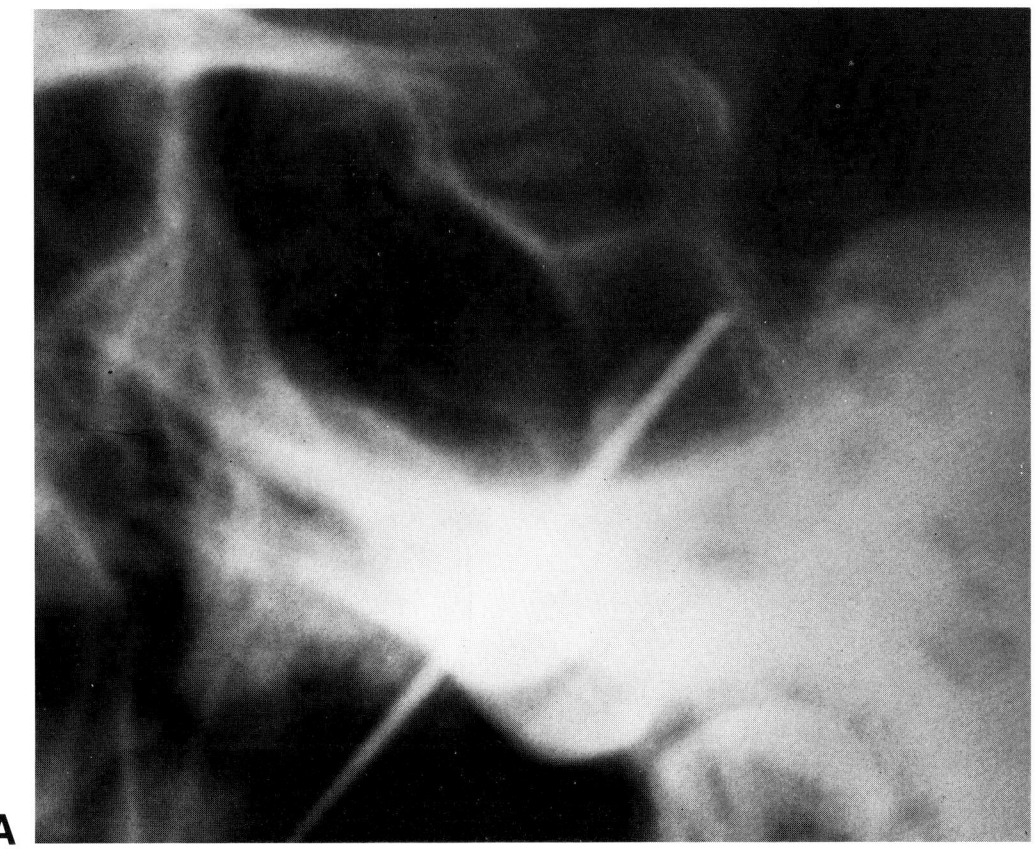

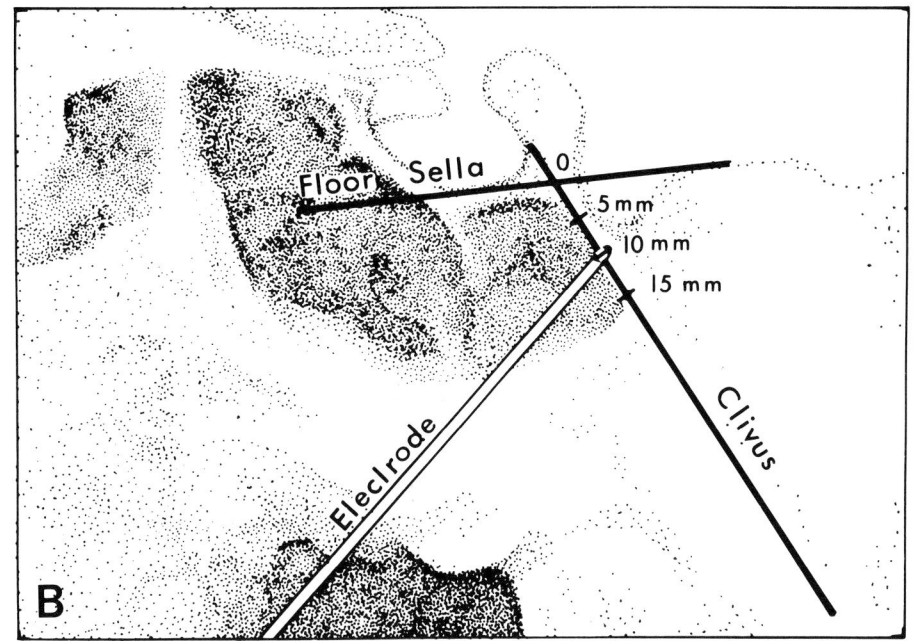

FIGURE 119–5. (A) Lateral radiograph confirming electrode placement in the foramen ovale. (B) Ideal trajectory of the electrode (5 to 10 mm below the intersection of a line drawn from the floor of the sella turcica to the clival line, or the intersection of the petrous ridge with the clivus). (From Tew JM: Treatment of trigeminal neuralgia by percutaneous rhizotomy, in Youmans JR [ed]: Neurological Surgery, 2nd ed. Philadelphia, W. B. Saunders, 1982, p 3568.)

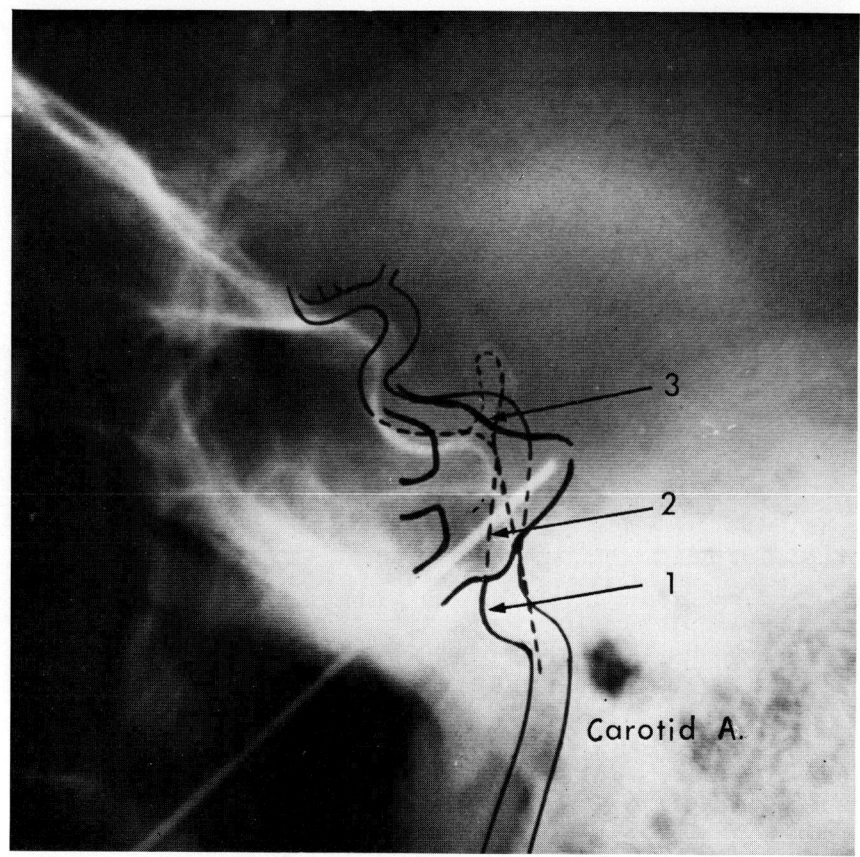

FIGURE 119–6. Composite illustration demonstrating the relationship of the carotid artery to the trigeminal ganglion and posterior rootlets. Note the location of three points of possible carotid penetration. (From Tew JM: Treatment of trigeminal neuralgia by percutaneous rhizotomy, in Youmans JR [ed]: Neurological Surgery, 2nd ed. Philadelphia, W. B. Saunders, 1982, p 3571.)

the abducens nerve in this region. Manipulation (rotation about its axis) of the curved electrode permits stimulation of different portions of the nerve (Fig. 119–7 A and B). Rotation of the electrode tip cephalad or medially provides better access to the fibers of the ophthalmic division, whereas caudal or lateral rotation contacts the mandibular fibers. This maneuverability permits precise anatomic localization in the sensory root. Sometimes, the needle must be redirected more anteromedially to bring the tip closer to the posterior clinoid for closer contact with the ophthalmic division. If the eyes move during stimulation, the cannula is too deep in the cavernous sinus or too near the brainstem. If the electrode contacts the motor root, stimulation results in masseter contraction; lateral rotation of the electrode prevents the production of a lesion that could result in motor paresis. Stimulus-evoked facial contractions indicate that the electrode is either too deep or inclined too low on the clivus or that the stimulation level is too high. Although a straight electrode was used in our first 700 cases, the advantages of the curved-tip electrode described earlier have eliminated the straight-electrode technique.

Lesion Production

The geometry of the lesions varies with the medium; reproducible lesions are 5 × 5 × 4 mm and are eccentric, with orientation toward the curve of the electrode. The electrode tip measures 0.5 mm in diameter. A thermocouple sensor is located at the tip of the electrode and provides calibration accuracy of ± 2°C over a range of 30 to 100°C.

Additional intravenous anesthetic is administered, and a preliminary lesion is produced at 60°C for 60 seconds. A facial flush (secondary to antidromic release of vasodilatory neuropeptides, such a substance P and calcitonin gene-related peptide) usually appears at this point and helps localize the region of the nerve root undergoing thermal destruction.[27, 34–36] When the patient has fully awakened, careful sensory testing of the face is conducted. Repeat lesions are produced until the desired effect is achieved. Generally, sequential lesions of 90-second duration are made by increasing the temperature 5°C with each lesion. When analgesia is approached, great care is exercised to avoid overshooting the desired result, which includes preserving the sense of touch. After a partial lesion has been produced, it is frequently possible to complete the lesion without the use of additional anesthetic agent and with the constant sensory testing that allows for fine control of denervation. The pain associated with production of the lesion is reduced because a lower temperature is required to make an effective lesion, and the curvature of the electrode avoids contact with the dura, which is the principal source of pain reception in this region. This tactic is particularly valuable when partial sensation of the cornea or other trigeminal divisions is to be preserved. The goal is usually dense hypalgesia in the primarily affected divisions.

Once the desired degree of sensory loss has been achieved, the patient is observed for an additional 15 minutes to determine if a fixed lesion has been produced. If the examination indicates a stable level of analgesia, the distribution and degree of deficit are determined by careful sensory testing. Touch perception is recorded in grams of pressure, by use of calibrated Von-Frey hairs. Masseter, pterygoid, facial, and

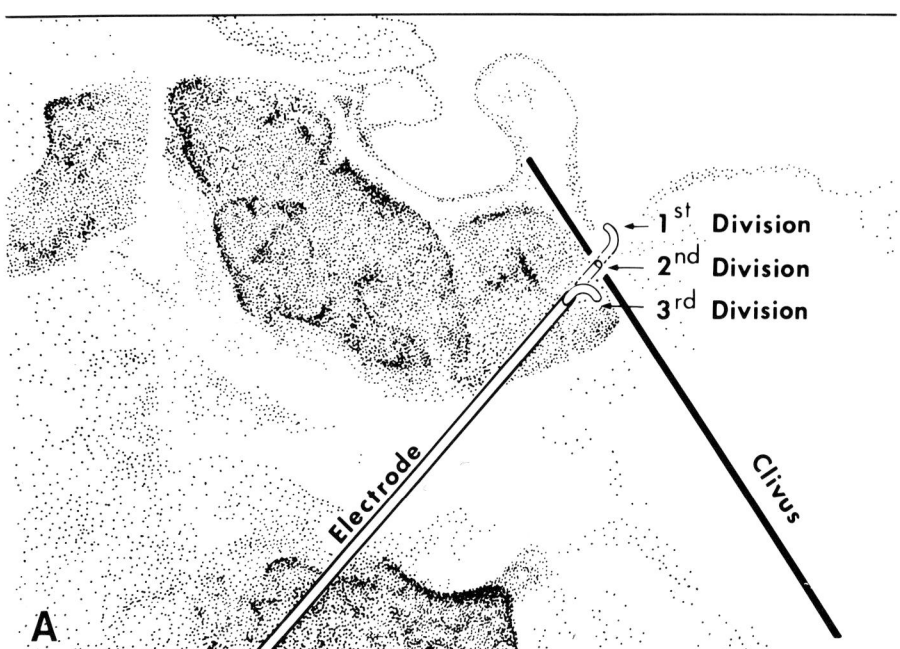

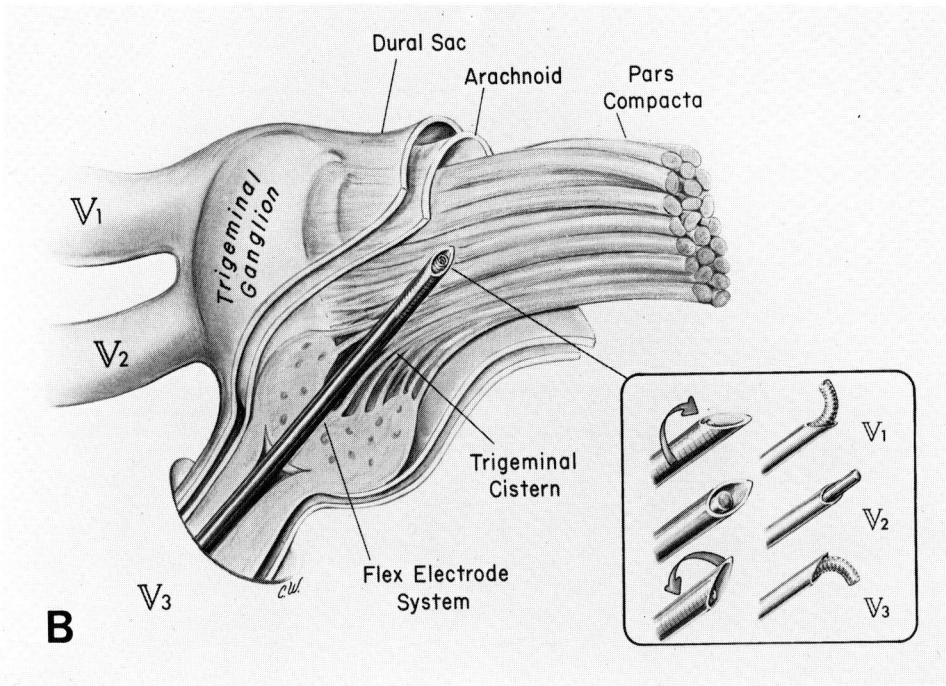

FIGURE 119–7. (A) The relationship of the electrode to the profile of the clivus. With the electrode tip at −5 mm, the third division is stimulated; at 0, the second division is stimulated, and at +5 mm deep to the clivus, the first division fibers are stimulated. The tip of the electrode should not extend more than 8 mm deep to the profile of the clivus. (B) The trigeminal rootlets and the curved electrode with thermocouple capable of producing lesions in any of the three divisions from a single position. (From Tew JM, van Loveren HR: Percutaneous rhizotomy in the treatment of intractable facial pain [trigeminal, glossopharyngeal, and vagal nerves], in Schmidek HH, Sweet WH [eds]: Current Techniques in Operative Neurosurgery, 2nd ed. Philadelphia, W. B. Saunders, 1988, p 1118.)

ocular muscle functions are recorded. The patient then is returned to his or her room and observed for 24 hours. During this period, the patient is informed of the necessity for eye care and of avoiding jaw strain, as well as the consequences of facial analgesia. Anticonvulsant medications are tapered before being discontinued.

Results

At the time of this report, more than 1500 patients have been treated surgically by percutaneous stereotactic rhizotomy. The straight electrode was used in the initial 700 cases, and the curved electrode was used in subsequent cases, with some modification of tactic and technique. The average follow-up period for all patients has been 9 years, with a range of 1 to 21 years (Table 119–1). The mean age of onset was 57 years, with a range of 10 to 95 years. The mean age at time of surgery was 65 years, with a range of 25 to 97 years.

Trigeminal neuralgia had been present for an average of 8 years and was characterized by increasingly severe episodes of paroxysmal pain and progressively shorter periods of remission. Thirty-five percent of patients had undergone a previous operation, including nerve avulsion, alcohol injection, subtotal rhizotomy, ganglionectomy, microvascular decompression, or percutaneous rhizotomy. Although approximately one third of patients had an unnecessary dental extraction or manipulation after the onset of trigeminal neuralgia, 4 percent developed the disorder immediately after dental extraction. In 4 percent of patients, multiple sclerosis was the presumed cause of their trigeminal neuralgia. The incidence of bilateral involvement was 18 percent in patients with multiple sclerosis and 5 percent in patients without multiple sclerosis. All patients had been subjected to a rigorous trial of medical therapy with either carbamazepine (Tegretol), lioresal (Baclofen), or phenytoin (Dilantin). Initial effective relief was obtained in 92 percent of the patients treated with carbamazepine and in approximately 50 percent of the patients treated with phenytoin. Lioresal has not been used as primary drug therapy. Seventy-five percent of patients eventually required a surgical procedure because of recurrence of pain or increasing side effects of medical therapy.

Follow-up results were obtained for 1200 patients (Table 119–2). At the time of evaluation, 93 percent reported excellent or good results. Pain recurred in 20 percent of patients: in 5 percent, the recurrent pain was minor and did not require medication; in another 5 percent, the pain was moderate and well controlled on medication; and in the remaining 10 percent, the pain was severe and required a surgical procedure.

Side Effects

SENSORY. All patients experience some degree of numbness in the face after a successful radiofrequency thermocoagulation procedure. Troublesome numbness and paresthesias as a result of the inherent sensory deficit proved to be the most consistent adverse side effect with both the straight and curved electrode technique, but in our early experience with the curved electrode, the incidence of this side effect was eliminated. However, with additional experience with the curved electrode in more complicated and recurrent cases, this problem is re-emerging. The overall incidence of major paresthesias (numbness that is troublesome or disturbing) was 3 percent (Table 119–3). Seventeen percent of the patients described an intermittent crawling, burning, or itching sensation that did not require treatment. Most patients

Table 119–1. CHARACTERISTICS OF 1200 PATIENTS SELECTED FOR ELECTROCOAGULATION*

Characteristic	Percent
Sex	
Female	63
Male	37
Side of coagulation	
Right	60
Bilateral	5
Division of trigeminal nerve involved	
V1	1
V2	16
V3	16
V1 and V2	15
V2 and V3	39
V1, V2, and V3	13

*Patients with multiple sclerosis were excluded. The average age of the patients was 65 years.

Table 119–2. FOLLOW-UP RESULTS OF PERCUTANEOUS STEREOTACTIC RHIZOTOMY IN 1200 PATIENTS*

Result	Description	Percent
Excellent	No tic pain, dysesthesia, or troublesome paresthesia	72
Good	No tic pain, minor dysesthesia or paresthesia	21
Fair	No tic pain, moderate dysesthesia or paresthesia	4
Poor	No tic pain, major dysesthesia or paresthesia	1
Failure	Immediate	2

*Average follow-up, 9 years. Includes patients undergoing multiple percutaneous stereotactic rhizotomies; subjective rating determined by the patient.

Table 119–3. COMPLICATIONS IN 1200 PATIENTS AFTER PERCUTANEOUS RHIZOTOMY*

Complication	Percent
Masseter weakness†	16
Pterygoid weakness	7
Dysesthesia or paresthesia (minor)	17
Dysesthesia or paresthesia (major)	3
Anesthesia dolorosa	1
Absent corneal reflex	6
With V1 pain	15
With V2 pain	5
With V3 pain	1
Keratitis	2
Diplopia	1.2
Oculomotor	0.1
Trochlear	0.5
Abducens	0.6
Meningitis	0.2
Carotid-cavernous fistula	0.1
Intracranial hemorrhage	0
Death	0

*Includes patients undergoing multiple percutaneous rhizotomies.
†Nearly all nerve palsies (motor root and extraocular) represented axonotmesis and resolved within 6 months.

readily adjusted to the sensory deficit, and the paresthesias usually diminished with time. The more active and mentally alert the patient, the fewer the disturbances of sensation reported. Older patients were more prone to this complication. Constant, severe dysesthesias in an anesthetic or analgesic zone (anesthesia dolorosa) rarely occurred with the straight electrode and occurred in only one patient (0.2 percent) with the curved electrode. Tactics to reduce dysesthesia include testing sensations continuously during lesion making, asking the patient if numbness is tolerable during the procedure, quantitating rather than qualitating numbness, and stopping lesion making if pain during thermocoagulation is no longer felt.

OCULAR. Corneal anesthesia developed in 6 percent of patients. This complication was reduced with the use of the curved electrode (Table 119–4). Neurogenic keratitis developed in 2 percent of patients. Thirty percent of this group had corneal analgesia rather than anesthesia, indicating that touch perception in the absence of pain perception does not necessarily protect against corneal ulceration. The corneal lesion was reversed in all patients by early ophthalmologic treatment. Application of a soft contact lens, meticulous eye care, and occasional tarsorrhaphy prevented permanent visual loss.

Transient diplopia occurred in 1 percent of patients. The abducens nerve located in the lateral dural wall of the cavernous sinus was the most commonly injured nerve, followed in order of frequency by the trochlear nerve and the oculomotor nerve (see Table 119–3). The duration of most persistent diplopia was 4 months. This complication was generally encountered when a lesion was created in the ophthalmic division.

MOTOR PARESIS. Paresis of muscles innervated by the motor root of the trigeminal nerve occurred in 16 percent of patients. The motor root lies medial to the ganglion and can be avoided by lateral rotation of the curved electrode if stimulation produces masseter contraction. Thus, the incidence of immediate postoperative muscle paresis was reduced from 24 to 7 percent by use of the more mobile curved electrode. In most instances, the deficit was partial and transient.

Table 119–4. COMPLICATIONS OF PERCUTANEOUS RHIZOTOMY (CURVED ELECTRODE VERSUS STRAIGHT ELECTRODE)

Complication	Patients (%)	
	Curved Electrode (500 Cases)	Straight Electrode (700 Cases)
Dysesthesia	11	27
Minor	9	22
Major	2	5
Anesthesia dolorosa	0.2	1.6
Absent corneal reflex	3	8
V1 pain	8	20
V2 pain	2	8
V3 pain	0.3	2
Keratitis	0.6	4
Diplopia	0.5	2
Masseter weakness	7	24

HERPES SIMPLEX. Lesions of herpes simplex were noted in 3 percent of patients. Because most patients were not examined after 48 hours postoperatively, this figure is undoubtedly low.

RECURRENCE OF TRIGEMINAL NEURALGIA. As the technique has become more refined, our strategy for its application has altered. The ease with which the procedure can be repeated allows production of a "light" sensory lesion as initial treatment: hypalgesia or analgesia in the primary division affected and mild hypalgesia in divisions secondarily affected or divisions harboring trigger zones. As this group of patients is followed up, their recurrence rate is expected to rise (currently 20 percent), but the rate of troublesome dysesthesias (2 percent) remains low.

DISCUSSION

The role of percutaneous stereotactic rhizotomy in the treatment of trigeminal neuralgia has been investigated and discussed by numerous authors. We present our long-term results with 1200 patients responding to follow-up after treatment by stereotactic rhizotomy using a straight electrode and subsequently the curved electrode. In our experience, the most troublesome side effects have been sensory paresthesias and trigeminal motor weakness. The rates of recurrence, reoperation, and subsequent complications are expected to increase with extended follow-up. The distinctive ability of the curved electrode tip to intimately contact the involved sensory fibers enables the production of a more effective lesion with minimal injury to adjacent noninvolved fibers. Table 119–4, which compares our results of the straight and the curved electrodes, shows a significant reduction of complications with the curved electrode, which we now use in all cases.

A review of major series with many (more than 500) patients and long follow-up periods shows the effectiveness of percutaneous radiofrequency rhizotomy in controlling pain of trigeminal neuralgia; minimal morbidity and an acceptable rate of recurrence are achieved (Table 119–5). Our earlier enthusiasm to prevent pain recurrence by creating a dense sensory lesion in the face has been replaced by a more cautious approach of creating a lighter initial lesion. Although the incidence of pain recurrence may increase, we believe that the ease of repeating the procedure justifies its use so that such complications as dysesthesia and corneal anesthesia can be minimized. The application of new tactics and technologies, such as the curved electrode, has kept morbidity statistics at a level acceptable for the continued use of this procedure, which is a standard against which other procedures are compared.

Comparison of Percutaneous Rhizotomy with Other Major Surgical Procedures

Percutaneous rhizotomy can be compared with other major surgical procedures on the basis of complications and the incidence of recurrent pain. We made no attempt to compare our results with all the series reported but selected only those that appeared to be representative. Because of variability in the number and characteristics of patients treated, follow-up

Table 119-5. RESULTS OF RETROGASSERIAN RADIOFREQUENCY THERMOCOAGULATION IN SELECTED SERIES

Series	Patients (n)	Follow-up	Patients (%)										
			Immediate Pain Relief	Recurrence	Minor Dysesthesia	Major Dysesthesia	Anesthesia Dolorosa	Absent Corneal Reflex	Keratitis	Trigeminal Motor Weakness*	Diplopia†	Perioperative Morbidity†	Mortality
Siegfried[37]	1000	5.5–8 years	100	25	NR	24	1	7	0.8	17	4	0.2	0
Fraioli and coworkers[38]	533	2 months–11 years (~6.5 years)	97	10	15	NR	1.5	3	1.9	3	0.2	0	0
Frank and Fabrizi[39]	700	> 3 years	NR	25	NR	NR	0.6	1	0	8	0.1	0	0
Broggi and coworkers[41]	1000	5–14 years	95	18	NR	5	1.5	17	0.6	10	0.5	0	0
Sweet[18, 40, 44]	702	1–33 years (~5.5 years)	99	37	16	7	2	9	3	65	0.4	0.1	0
Nugent[42, 43]	1070	1–9 years	NR	27	9	6	0.5	3.5	0.4	26	0.2	0.3	0.2
Tew and Taha	1200	1–21 years (~9 years)	98	20	17	3	1	6	2	16	1	0.3	0
Total	6205	2 months–33 years	98	23	14	8	1	7	1	17	1	0.2	0.03

NR = not reported.
*Most symptoms are transient.
†Perioperative morbidity includes meningitis (bacterial and chemical), intracranial hemorrhage, stroke, carotid-cavernous fistula, and pulmonary and cardiovascular complications.

periods, techniques, and experiences of surgeons, morbidity and recurrence data of different series may not be comparable. However, a general overview is helpful.

More patients with trigeminal neuralgia with long follow-ups have been treated with percutaneous radiofrequency thermocoagulation than with other recently practiced percutaneous techniques, such as retrogasserian glycerol injection or balloon compression. Peripheral neurectomy of any of the three peripheral branches of the trigeminal nerve must still be considered a treatment option for all surgeons who treat this condition. Glycerol rhizotomy has theoretical appeal as a mechanism to relieve pain without sensory loss; however, recent data suggest that this technique may be destructive and may require sensory denervation to avoid recurrence.[43] Table 119-6 summarizes results of several large series of patients treated with glycerol rhizotomy. Dysesthesia, which was once hoped to be eliminated with this technique, still constitutes a major complication in most series. Although this technique appears to relatively spare the motor rootlets and to a lesser extent, the corneal reflex, the recurrence rates in some series have been prohibitively high. Symptoms of chemical meningitis occasionally constitute a major perioperative morbidity.[44, 45]

Retrogasserian balloon compression, which was introduced recently, is likewise a destructive procedure that can cause dysesthesia and numbness in the face. Table 119-7 summarizes the results of several large series of patients treated with this procedure. Although preliminary results suggest a possible advantage of this technique in preserving the corneal reflex, larger studies and longer follow-up periods are needed. The relatively high incidence of carotid-cavernous fistula formation in some series[51, 52] is probably related to the large size of the needle used (14 gauge).

Among the open intracranial procedures for trigeminal neuralgia, posterior fossa exploration of the trigeminal rootlets for microvascular decompression or partial rhizotomy is most commonly practiced. Transtemporal decompression or rhizotomy procedures are now rarely performed because of their association with high rates of recurrence and complications, respectively.[9, 56] Table 119-8 summarizes the results of selected series of posterior fossa exploration for microvascular decompression or partial trigeminal rhizotomy. Microvascular decompression usually relieves trigeminal neuralgia but has a recurrence rate equal to that of percutaneous rhizotomy.[15, 62] The success of the procedure does not necessarily validate its theoretical framework; microvascular decompression may well represent a form of subtle, chronic injury of the trigeminal sensory root. Because troublesome numbness has been virtually eliminated with microvascular decompression, this procedure provides an attractive alternative to percutaneous rhizotomy, particularly in young patients. Posterior fossa exploration, however, is associated with higher

Table 119-6. RESULTS OF RETROGASSERIAN GLYCEROL RHIZOTOMY IN SELECTED SERIES

Series	Patients (n)	Follow-up	Patients (%)										
			Immediate Pain Relief	Recurrence	Minor Dysesthesia	Major Dysesthesia	Anesthesia Dolorosa	Absent Corneal Reflex	Keratitis	Trigeminal Motor Weakness	Diplopia	Perioperative Morbidity*	Mortality
Lunsford and coworkers[46]	112	4–28 months	79	17	8	6	0	0	0	0	0	2.7	0
Arias[47]	100	6–36 months	91	10	0	0	0	0	0	0	0	2	0
Dieckman and coworkers[48]	252	2–5.5 years	91	37	17	1.6	0	5	0	0	0	2	0
Saini[49]	469	1–6 years	96	92	8	5	5.5	5	5	3.4	0	0	0
Young[50]	162	6 months–5.5 years	90	19	NR	3	0	1.8	0	NR	0	0.6	0
Fujimaki and coworkers[51]	122	3–4.5 years	79	60	15	12	1.6	NR	0	NR	NR	NR	0
Total	1217	4 months–6 years	91	54	11	5	1.8	3.7	1.8	1.7	0	1	0

NR = not reported.
*Perioperative morbidity includes meningitis (bacterial and chemical), intracranial hemorrhage, stroke, carotid-cavernous fistula, and pulmonary and cardiovascular complications.

Table 119-7. RESULTS OF RETROGASSERIAN BALLOON COMPRESSION IN SELECTED SERIES

Series	Patients (n)	Follow-up	Immediate Pain Relief	Recurrence	Minor Dysesthesia	Major Dysesthesia	Anesthesia Dolorosa	Absent Corneal Reflex	Keratitis	Trigeminal Motor Weakness	Diplopia	Perioperative Morbidity*	Mortality
Meglio and coworkers[52]	74	1–3 years	93	56	NR	7	0	NR	NR	80 transient, 10 permanent	NR	1.4	0
Fraioli and coworkers[38]	159	~3.5 years	90	10	NR	7	0.6	NR	NR	7 transient, 3 permanent	0	0	0
Frank and Fabrizi[39]	212	<3 years	NR	25	NR	NR	0	0	NR	9	0.9	0.9	0
Lichtor and Mullan[53]	100	1–10 years	97	20	12	4	0	0	0	100 transient	0	2	0
Lobato and coworkers[54]	144	6 months–4.5 years	92	10	17	3	0	0	0	100 transient, 12 permanent	2.8	2	0
Peragut and coworkers[55]	70	6 months–5.5 years	98	21	11	NR	0	11	0	NR	0	0	0
Total	759	6 months–10 years	93	21	14	5	0.1	1.5	0	66 transient, 7 permanent	0.7	1	0

NR = not reported.
*Perioperative morbidity includes meningitis (bacterial and chemical), intracranial hemorrhage, stroke, carotid-cavernous fistsula, and pulmonary and cardiovascular complications.

mortality and morbidity than those resulting from percutaneous techniques. Because trigeminal neuralgia is a benign condition, posterior fossa exploration is avoided in patients who have significant risk factors for craniotomy, such as those with a physiologic age greater than 65 years or those in poor medical condition. When offering microvascular decompression procedure to a patient, one should note that a definite compression of the trigeminal nerve may be absent during posterior fossa exploration (estimated 15 percent in cumulative series); these patients usually undergo partial trigeminal rhizotomy—a procedure that carries at least the same risk of dysesthesia as a percutaneous procedure (Table 119–8).

Table 119–9 compares a series of these surgical procedures discussed. All procedures had an initial high success rate and, except for glycerol rhizotomy, had comparable recurrence rates (with the limitation of different follow-up periods). Using our curved electrode and the tactic described under technique, we were able to substantially reduce such complications as dysesthesia, anesthesia dolorosa, corneal anesthesia, and trigeminal motor weakness enough to justify the continued use of radiofrequency rhizotomy over other

Table 119-8. RESULTS OF POSTERIOR FOSSA EXPLORATION IN SELECTED SERIES

Series	Procedure	Patients (n)	Follow-up	Negative Exploration*	Immediate Pain Relief	Recurrence	Pain-Free at Last Follow-up†	Dysesthesia and Anesthesia Dolorosa	Absent Corneal Reflex	Trigeminal Motor Weakness	ICH/Infarct	Permanent Cranial Nerve Deficit‡	Perioperative Morbidity§	Mortality
Apfelbaum[57]	MVD	276		—	NR	NR	NR	NR	NR	NR	NR	NR	NR	NR
	PTR	13		—	NR	NR	NR	NR	NR	NR	NR	NR	NR	NR
	PFE	289	~4.5 years	12.5	94	12	82	0	0	0	2	2.5	16	1
Platt and Wilkins[58]	MVD	81		—	98	26	77	2.5	0	0	NR	NR	NR	NR
	PTR	22		—	95	19	86	4.5	0	0	NR	NR	NR	NR
	PFE	103	~5 years	34	97	22	73	3	0	0	3	8.8	20	1
Bederson and Wilson[59]	MVD	166		—	95	14	81	3	0	0	NR	NR	NR	0
	PTR	86		—	94	14	83	10	4.6	0	NR	NR	NR	0
	PFE	252	6 months–16 years	34	95	14	83	5.6	1.6	0	0.4	3.6	12	0
Jannetta[60]	MVD	703		—	NR	NR	NR	0	0	0	NR	NR	NR	NR
	PTR	0		—	NR	NR	NR	0	0	0	NR	NR	NR	NR
	PFE	703	≤14 years	<1	98	17	87	0	0	0	1	2.1	8	0.6
Klun[61]	MVD	178		—	96	6	93	0	0.6	NR	NR	0	NR	NR
	PTR	42		—	86	52	48	0	0	NR	NR	0	NR	NR
	PFE	220	6 months–12 years	19	97	16	85	0	0.4	0.9	0.8	0	7	1.4
Tew and Taha	MVD	70		—	99	14	90	0	0	NR	NR	0	NR	0
	PTR	30		—	94	18	87	3	6	0	NR	0	NR	0
	PFE	100	1–4 years	24	97	15	88	1	2	0	1	0	10	0
Total	MVD	1474		—	97	15	86	0.5	0.05	NR	NR	NR	NR	NR
	PTR	193		—	92	26	76	6	3	NR	NR	NR	NR	NR
	PFE	1667	6 months–14 years	15	95	17	84	1	0.4	0.1	1	3	10	0.6

ICH = intracranial hemorrhage; NR = not reported; MVD = microvascular decompression; PTR = partial trigeminal rhizotomy; PFE = posterior fossa exploration (PFE combines MVD and PTR).
*Negative exploration indicates absence of significant compression.
†Some patients have pain controlled by medications.
‡Hearing loss or facial palsy.
§Perioperative morbidity includes wound infection, meningitis, cerebrospinal fluid leakage, transient cranial nerve deficits, deep vein thrombosis, and pulmonary and cardiovascular complications.

Table 119-9. COMPARISON OF DIFFERENT PROCEDURES IN THE TREATMENT OF TRIGEMINAL NEURALGIA

Procedure*	Patients (n)	Follow-up	Immediate Pain Relief	Recurrence	Minor Dysesthesia	Major Dysesthesia	Anesthesia Dolorosa	Absent Corneal Reflex	Keratitis	Trigeminal Motor Weakness†	Permanent Cranial Nerve Deficit	ICH/Infarct	Perioperative Morbidity‡	Mortality
Radiofrequency with curved electrode (Tew)	500	1–10 years	98	20	9	2	0.2	3	0.6	7	0	0	0.5	0
Radiofrequency rhizotomy	6205	1–33 years	98	23	14	10	1.5	7	1	24	0	0	1.2	0
Glycerol rhizotomy	1217	4 months–6 years	91	54	11	5	1.8	3.7	1.8	1.7	0	0	1	0
Balloon compression	759	6 months–10 years	93	21	14	5	0.1	1.5	0	66 = transient 7 = permanent	0	0	1.7	0
Microvascular decompression	1474		97	15	0.2	0.3	0	0.05	0	NR	NR	NR	NR	NR
Partial trigeminal rhizotomy	193		92	26	5	2	1	3	0	NR	NR	NR	NR	NR
Posterior fossa exploration	1667	6 months–14 years	95	17	0.7	0.4	0.1	0.4	0	0.1	3	1	10	0.6

ICH = intracranial hemorrhage.
*Cumulative results of selected series (from Tables 119-4 to 119-8).
†In Tew and Taha's series, nearly all motor nerve palsies represented axonotmesis and resolved within 6 months.
‡Perioperative complications include wound infection, meningitis (bacterial and aseptic), cerebrospinal fluid leakage, systemic complications, transient cranial nerve deficits, and hydrocephalus.

percutaneous procedures. In our opinion, radiofrequency rhizotomy provides the most selective and graded lesion among percutaneous techniques. Compared with posterior fossa exploration, all percutaneous techniques have lower incidences of hearing loss, facial palsy, intracranial complications, perioperative morbidity, and mortality. Although not all patients undergoing posterior fossa explorations eventually have microvascular decompression, those who do may enjoy long pain relief without troublesome numbness. Because the comparison of cumulative data for different surgical procedures may not reflect the expected outcome, the surgeon should be flexible enough to offer the best procedure (percutaneous or open intracranial) for a particular patient, guided by personal experience as well as the preference of the patient.

PERCUTANEOUS COAGULATION IN OTHER PAINFUL CONDITIONS

MULTIPLE SCLEROSIS

A review of several series indicates that approximately 1 percent of patients suffering from multiple sclerosis develop trigeminal neuralgia.[63] Another perspective is that 2 to 4 percent of patients with trigeminal neuralgia have evidence of multiple sclerosis.[64] A cause-and-effect relationship is generally based on the identification of sclerotic myelin plaques on the trigeminal sensory root and descending trigeminal nucleus in several patients with this combination of disorders.[65] We have encountered 60 such patients, who constitute 4 percent of the entire group. Although trigeminal neuralgia was the initial symptom of multiple sclerosis in 5 percent of the tic–multiple sclerosis group, signs and symptoms of multiple sclerosis preceding the onset of trigeminal neuralgia had been overlooked. There is no difference in technique or results of the percutaneous method in patients with multiple sclerosis. There is always concern that pain may be caused by a central plaque not amenable to rhizotomy, but experience has not borne out these fears. Compared with patients without multiple sclerosis, patients with tic–multiple sclerosis are younger and have a much higher incidence of bilateral trigeminal neuralgia. Every effort should be made to preserve the motor root and facial sensation, thus preserving options for future contralateral treatment. Because microvascular decompression usually fails to relieve trigeminal pain in patients with multiple sclerosis,[60] this group of patients responds best to a percutaneous technique.

ATYPICAL FACIAL PAIN

Atypical facial pain is a vague diagnostic category that previously included atypical trigeminal neuralgia, dental neuralgia, neuralgia of other regional nerves (e.g., sphenopalatine, Sluder's neuralgia), postherpetic neuralgia, vascular syndromes (e.g., cluster headache, lower facial migraine), and temporomandibular joint dysfunction, but actually may be at times psychological disorders with facial somatization.[66-69] Denervation of the region of the face that harbors the pain benefits fewer than 20 percent of patients in this category, and another 20 percent are worsened by the addition of paresthesias and dysesthesias to their original complaint. We have performed percutaneous stereotactic rhizotomy on 62 such patients. Most patients are eliminated as surgical candidates by a failure to obtain relief from a test block of the trigeminal ganglion with 0.3 ml of 0.75-percent bupivacaine (Marcaine) anesthetic. However, pain caused by regional invasive tumors or carcinoma can be controlled by this technique. In patients with cluster headache (chronic migrainous neuralgia) who fail to respond to medical treat-

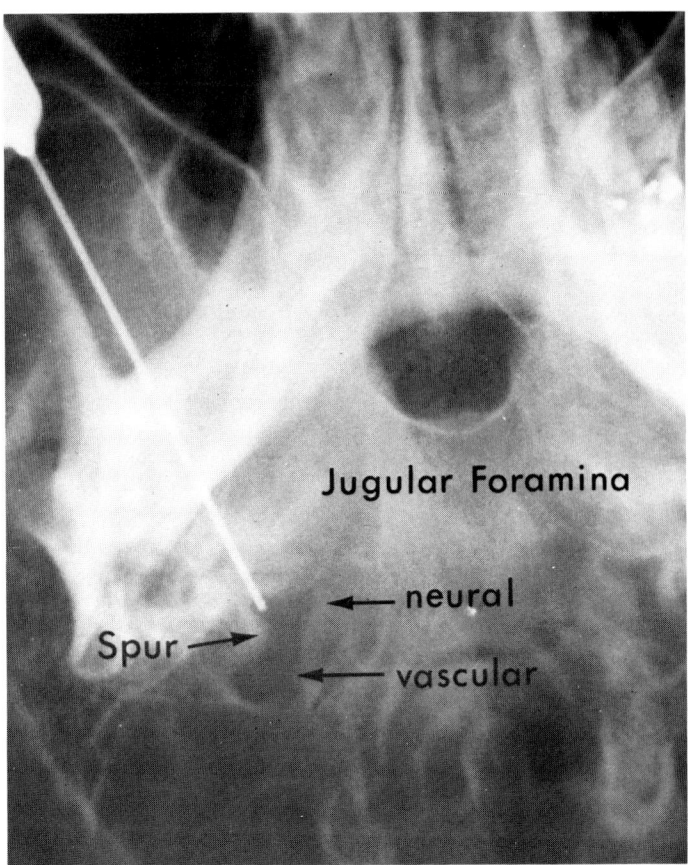

FIGURE 119-8. Needle penetrating the neural portion of the jugular foramen. Note the bony spur that divides the neural from the vascular portion. (From Tew JM: Treatment of pain of glossopharyngeal and vagus nerves by percutaneous rhizotomy, in Youmans JR [ed]: Neurological Surgery, 2nd ed. Philadelphia, W. B. Saunders, 1982, p 3610.)

ment, percutaneous radiofrequency thermocoagulation of the ophthalmic division may immediately relieve pain in 50 to 70 percent of patients and improve pain in another 10 to 30 percent.[70, 71] Better results are achieved in patients who respond to preoperative lidocaine blockade and in patients with higher levels of analgesia.[70, 71]

VAGOGLOSSOPHARYNGEAL NEURALGIA

The ratio of incidence of vagoglossopharyngeal neuralgia to that of trigeminal neuralgia is approximately 1:100 in this series. Initial therapy must be with agents documented to affect trigeminal neuralgia (e.g., carbamazepine, lioresal). Although these medications have an initial high success rate, most patients eventually experience recurring pain or side effects.[72] Surgical therapy options include intradural section of glossopharyngeal nerve and the upper vagal rootlets, microvascular decompression of the ninth and tenth cranial nerves, and percutaneous radiofrequency neurolysis of the glossopharyngeal nerve in the external nervus portion of the jugular foramen.[73–75] Safe penetration of the jugular foramen and physiologic identification of the glossopharyngeal nerve were discovered inadvertently during early experience with percutaneous rhizotomy for trigeminal neuralgia.[75] Subsequent anatomic studies elucidated appropriate facial and bony landmarks that facilitate safe, reproducible penetration of the jugular foramen. This technique has since been used by many investigators because of its technical simplicity and relative safety.

The procedure is performed in the radiography suite; small doses of methohexital are administered intravenously during painful parts of the procedure. A free-hand technique guided by lateral fluoroscopy is used similar to that described for trigeminal neuralgia. The jugular foramen is separated by an anterior fibrous or bony band into a small anteromedial pars nervosa, which contains the glossopharyngeal nerve, and a large posterolateral pars venosa, which contains the jugular bulb and the tenth and eleventh cranial nerves.[76] A basal view of the skull demonstrates that the pars nervosa of the jugular foramen is directly in line with and posterior to the foramen ovale (Fig. 119–8). The electrode entry point is 2.5 cm lateral to the oral commissure. The general target is the intersection of two planes: a sagittal plane through the pupil and a coronal plane through a point 3 cm anterior to the tragus of the ear (see Fig. 119–2). The specific target on the intersection line requires a caudal inclination of the electrode 14 degrees below the trajectory to the foramen ovale (Fig. 119–9). On true lateral fluoroscopic images, the jugular foramen is situated immediately posterior to the temporomandibular joint and anterior to the occipital condyle 27 to 33 mm below the floor of the sella (Fig. 119–10). The trajectory in the sagittal plane carries the electrode medial to the orifice of the carotid canal. Carotid artery penetration should be avoided but is not associated with significant complications unless dissection occurs or attempts at lesion generation inside the artery are made. A lateral percutaneous approach has also been described.[77] Although this approach may be useful in patients who have a tumor lying anterior to the jugular foramen, transfixing the pars nervosa from lateral to medial as such may lead to vagal nerve injury during thermocoagulation. Stereotactic frames and CT-guided percutaneous cannulation of the jugular foramen have also been used.[28, 78]

Physiologic localization is accomplished by stimulation with 100- to 300-mV current using a 1-millisecond square wave pulse at 10 to 75 Hz or with mild radiofrequency current at 40°C. This process results in pain in the ear and throat. Higher-current stimulation produces cough and contraction of the sternocleidomastoid. With the Tew tic-curved electrode (Radionics, Burlington, MA) with thermocouple tip, thermal lesions of the rootlets are started at 60°C for 90 seconds and repeated at 5°C increments until the tonsillar pharynx is analgesic and previous triggers fail to reproduce glossopharyngeal pain. Because patients can develop dangerous hypertension, hypotension, bradycardia, syncope, or even cardiac arrest if the vagal nerve or nerve of Hering are stimulated or injured,[79] hemodynamic changes should be closely monitored.

Sensory denervation of the ipsilateral gag reflex and injury to the vagal nerve may cause paralysis of the ipsilateral vocal cord, hoarseness, and dysphagia. Thus, this procedure has

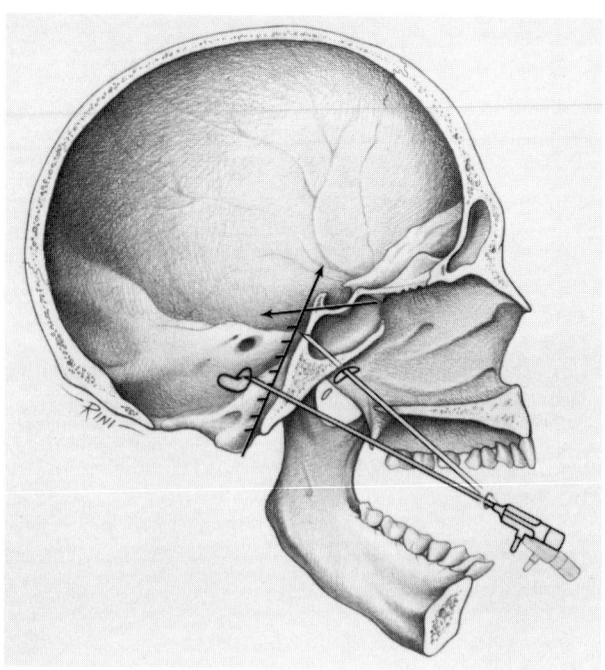

FIGURE 119–10. A lateral projection of the head. The needle is inserted 27 to 33 mm below the floor of the sella and lies posterior to the temporomandibular joint and anterior to the occipital condyle. (From Tew JM, Taha JM: Surgical management of glossopharyngeal and other uncommon facial neuralgias, in Tindall GI, Cooper PR, Barrow DL [ed]: The Practice of Neurosurgery, Baltimore, Williams & Wilkins, in press.)

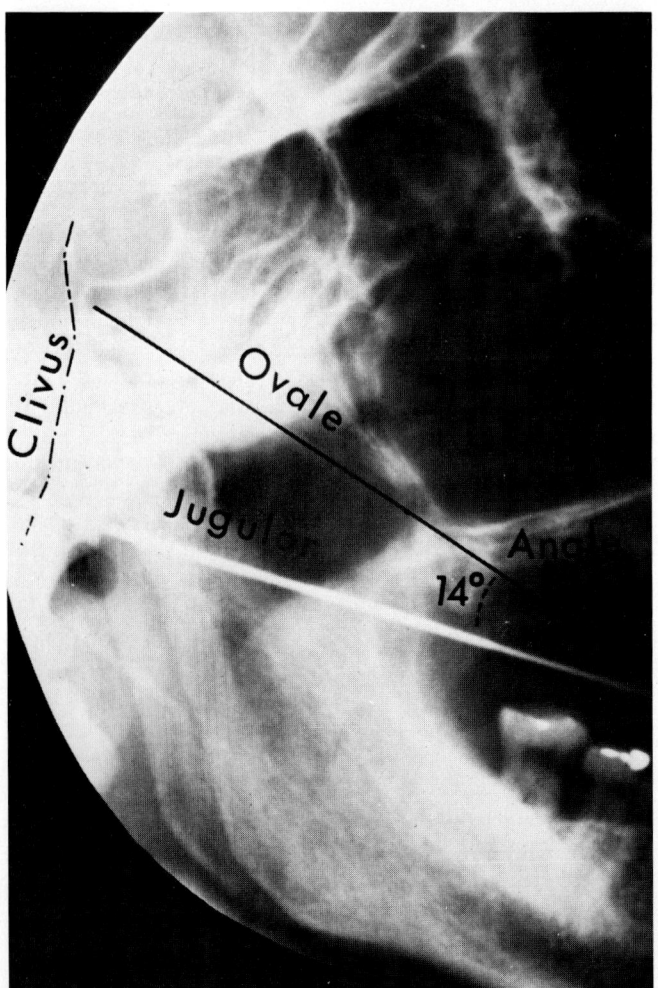

FIGURE 119–9. Composite illustration showing the trajectory of approaches to the foramen ovale and jugular foramen. The sagittal plane is identical for both procedures. (From Tew JM: Treatment of pain of glossopharyngeal and vagus nerves by percutaneous rhizotomy, in Youmans JR [ed]: Neurological Surgery, 2nd ed. Philadelphia, W. B. Saunders, 1982, p 3611.)

been largely restricted to patients with secondary neuralgia resulting from neoplasm.[75, 80, 81] Modification of physiologic monitoring during lesion generation has allowed application of this technique to patients with idiopathic glossopharyngeal neuralgia.[77, 82, 83] Accurate localization of the needle is emphasized for selective preservation of vocal cord innervation. The needle's placement should be readjusted in the following circumstances: if stimulation is achieved with more than 0.2 V or more than 48°C; if patients cough or have sternocleidomastoid contraction during stimulation; or if patients develop hypotension or bradycardia during a reversible heating test before or during lesion production. A carefully graded thermal lesion with small temperature increments and frequent neurologic examinations is essential to minimize complications.

DISCUSSION

Percutaneous radiofrequency thermocoagulation of the glossopharyngeal nerve has achieved pain relief in more than 90 percent of patients with idiopathic vagoglossopharyngeal neuralgia.[75, 82, 83] Although large series with long-term results are lacking, a low recurrence rate would be expected because the lesion is usually preganglionic and partly spreads to the vagal nerve, which can contribute to the pain. In patients with vagoglossopharyngeal neuralgia from cervicofacial tumors, 70 percent can expect pain relief or significant improvement after this procedure.[75, 80]

We have found that controlled radiofrequency thermocoagulation of the ninth and tenth cranial nerves is more difficult than that of the trigeminal nerve. Based on our experiences and those of others,[80, 81] the high incidence of hoarseness, vocal cord paralysis, and dysphagia after percutaneous radiofrequency rhizotomy limits this procedure to neuralgia of neoplastic origin and to idiopathic neuralgia in elderly patients in poor health. Other surgeons, based on their excellent results with this procedure, recommend percutaneous radiofrequency rhizotomy as the procedure of choice for idiopathic vagoglossopharyngeal neuralgia.[70, 77, 82]

SUMMARY

Percutaneous rhizotomy of the trigeminal nerve is a safe, elegant procedure when performed by experienced hands. The benign nature of disorders treated by this technique demands a procedure of similarly low morbidity and negligible mortality.

Recurrence is not a significant problem with percutaneous stereotactic rhizotomy because the procedure is easily repeated and the success rate is equal to that of the initial procedure. Higher recurrence rates are acceptable to reduce the risk of denervation paresthesias and dysesthesias. The application of percutaneous rhizotomy in other types of facial pain has also been described. Radiofrequency rhizotomy is a destructive procedure and therefore is theoretically not the ideal treatment for any condition. The widespread acceptance of this procedure underscores the deficiency in current strategies for treating facial pain and indicates that we need to continue to search for better therapeutic options.

REFERENCES

1. Hartley F: Intracranial neurectomy of the second and third divisions of the fifth nerve. N Y J Med 55:317, 1892
2. Krause F: Resection des trigeminus innerhalb der schadelhohle. Arch Klin Chir 41:821, 1892
3. Krause F: Entfernung des ganglion gasseri und des central daron gelegnen trigemenusstammes. Dtsch Med Wochenschr 19:341, 1893
4. Horsley V: Remarks on the various surgical procedures devised for the relief or cure of trigeminal neuralgia. BMJ 2:1139, 1891
5. Spiller WG, Frazier CH: The division of the sensory root of the trigeminus for the relief of tic douloureux. Univ Pa Med Bull 14:341, 1901
6. Spiller WG, Frazier CH: An experimental study of the regeneration of the posterior spinal root. Univ Pa Med Bull 16:126, 1903
7. Shelden CH, Pudenz RH, Freshwater D, et al: Compression rather than decompression for trigeminal neuralgia. J Neurosurg 12:123–126, 1955
8. Taarnhoj P: Decompression of the trigeminal root. J Neurosurg 11:299–305, 1954
9. Svien HS, Love JG: Results of decompression operation for trigeminal neuralgia four years plus after operation. J Neurosurg 16:653–655, 1959
10. Gardner WS: Concerning the mechanisms of trigeminal neuralgia and hemifacial spasm. J Neurosurg 19:947–958, 1962
11. Harris W: Alcohol injection of the gasserian ganglion for trigeminal neuralgia. Lancet 1:218, 1912
12. Harris W: An analysis of 1433 cases of paroxysmal trigeminal neuralgia (trigeminal-tic) and the end results of gasserian alcohol injection. Brain 63:209–224, 1940
13. Dandy WE: Concerning the cause of trigeminal neuralgia. Am J Surg 24:447–455, 1934
14. Jannetta P: Microsurgical approach to the trigeminal nerve for tic douloureux. Prog Neurol Surg 7:180–200, 1976
15. van Loveren H, Tew JM, Keller JT, Nurre MA: A 10-year experience in the treatment of trigeminal neuralgia: A comparison of percutaneous stereotaxic rhizotomy and posterior fossa exploration. J Neurosurg 57:757–764, 1982
16. Kirschner M: Elektrocoagulation des ganglion gasseri. Zentralbl Chir 47:2841, 1932
17. Kirschner M: Zur behandlung der trigeminus neuralgie. Dtsch Med Wochenschr 89:235, 1942
18. Sweet WH, Wepsic SG: Controlled thermocoagulation of trigeminal ganglion and results for differential destruction of pain fibers. J Neurosurg 40:143–156, 1974
19. White JC, Sweet WH: Pain and the Neurosurgeon. Springfield, IL, Charles C Thomas, 1969
20. Garvan NJ, Siegfried J: Trigeminal neuralgia—Earlier referral for surgery. Postgrad Med J 59:435–437, 1983
21. Bullett E, Tew JM, Boyd J: Intracranial tumors in patients with facial pain. J Neurosurg 64:865–871, 1986
22. Letcher FS, Goldring S: The effect of radiofrequency current and heat on peripheral nerve action potential in the cat. J Neurosurg 29:42–47, 1968
23. Brodkey JS, Miyazaki Y, Ervin FR, et al: Reversible heat lesions with radiofrequency current. J Neurosurg 21:49–53, 1964
24. Frigyesi T, Siegfried J, Groggi G: The selective vulnerability of evoked potentials in the trigeminal sensory root to graded thermocoagulation. Exp Neurol 49:11–21, 1975
25. Smith HP, McWhorter JM, Challa VR: Radiofrequency neurolysis in a clinical model. Neuropathological correlation. J Neurosurg 55:246–253, 1981
26. Brandt M: Zur chirurgischen therapie der trigeminus neuralgie. Selektive Thermokoagulation des Ganglion Gasseri. Fortschr Med 98:1699–1702, 1980
27. Arbit E, Krol G: Percutaneous radiofrequency neurolysis guided by computed tomography for the treatment of glossopharyngeal neuralgia (technical note). Neurosurgery 29:580–582, 1991
28. Laitinen L: Trigeminius stereoguide: An instrument for stereotactic approach through the foramen ovale and foramen jugulare. Surg Neurol 22:519–523, 1984
29. Härtel F: Uber die intracranielle Injektionsbehandlung der trigeminusneuralgie. Med Klin 10:582, 1914
30. Tator CH, Rowed DW: Fluoroscopy of foramen ovale as an aid to thermocoagulation of the gasserian ganglion. J Neurosurg 44:254–257, 1976
31. Rish BL: Cerebrovascular accident after percutaneous thermocoagulation of the trigeminal ganglion. J Neurosurg 44:376–377, 1976
32. McGlone F, Wells C: Preoperative monitoring during percutaneous thermocoagulation of the gasserian ganglion for the treatment of trigeminal neuralgia. Br J Neurosurg 5:39–42, 1991
33. Karol E, Sanz O, Rey R: Sensory and motor trigeminal evoked potentials to localize the position of trigeminal electrodes. Acta Neurochir (Wien) 108:110–115, 1991
34. Gonzalez G, Onofrio BM, Kerr FW: Vasodilator system of the face. J Neurosurg 42:696–703, 1975
35. Goadsby P, Edvinsson L, Ekman R: Release of vasoactive peptides in the extracerebral circulation of humans and the cat during activation of the trigeminovascular system. Ann Neurol 23:193–196, 1988
36. Tran Dinh Y, Thurel C, Cunin G, et al: Cerebral vasodilation after the thermocoagulation of the trigeminal ganglion in humans. Neurosurgery 31:658–663, 1992
37. Siegfried J: Percutaneous controlled thermocoagulation of gasserian ganglion in trigeminal neuralgia. Experience with 1000 cases, in Samii M, Jannetta P (eds): The Cranial Nerves. Berlin, Heidelberg, Springer-Verlag, 1981, pp 322–330
38. Fraioli B, Esposito V, Guidetti B, et al: Treatment of trigeminal neuralgia by thermocoagulation, glycerolization, and percutaneous compression of the gasserian ganglion and/or retrogasserian rootlets: Long-term results and therapeutic protocol. Neurosurgery 24:239–245, 1989
39. Frank F, Fabrizi A: Percutaneous treatment of trigeminal neuralgia. Acta Neurochir (Wien) 97:128–130, 1989
40. Sweet WH: Treatment of trigeminal neuralgia by percutaneous rhizotomy, in Youmans J (ed): Neurological Surgery. Philadelphia, WB Saunders, 1990, pp 3888–3921
41. Broggi G, Franzini A, Lasio G, et al: Long-term results of percutaneous retrogasserian thermorhizotomy for "essential" trigeminal neuralgia: Considerations in 1000 patients. Neurosurgery 26:783–787, 1990
42. Nugent R: Trigeminal neuralgia: Treatment by percutaneous electrocoagulation, in Wilkins RH, Rengachary SS (eds): Neurosurgery, New York, McGraw-Hill, 1985, pp 2363–2366
43. Nugent RG: Surgical treatment: Radiofrequency gangliolysis and rhizotomy, in Fromm GH, Sessle BJ (eds): Trigeminal Neuralgia: Current Concepts Regarding Pathogenesis and Treatment. Stoneham, MA, Butterworth-Heinemann, 1991, pp 159–184

44. Sweet WH: The treatment of trigeminal neuralgia (tic douloureaux). Current concepts. N Engl J Med 315:174–177, 1986
45. Lunsford D, Bennett M: Percutaneous retrogasserian glycerol rhizotomy for tic douloureux: Part 1. Technique and results in 112 patients. Neurosurgery 14:424–430, 1984
46. Lunsford D, Apfelbaum R: Choice of surgical therapeutic modalities for treatment of trigeminal neuralgia: Microvascular decompression, percutaneous retrogasserian thermal, or glycerol rhizotomy. Clin Neurosurg 32:319–333, 1985
47. Arias M: Percutaneous regrogasserian glycerol rhizotomy for trigeminal neuralgia. A prospective study of 100 cases. J Neurosurg 65:32–36, 1986
48. Dieckmann G, Bockermann V, Heyer C, Roesen M: Five-and-a-half years' experience with percutaneous retrogasserian glycerol rhizotomy in treatment of trigeminal neuralgia. Appl Neurophysiol 50:401–413, 1987
49. Saini SS: Retrogasserian anhydrous glycerol injection therapy in trigeminal neuralgia: Observations in 552 patients. J Neurol Neurosurg Psychiatry 50:1536–1538, 1987
50. Young R: Glycerol rhizolysis for the treatment of trigeminal neuralgia. J Neurosurg 69:39–45, 1988
51. Fujimaki T, Fukushima T, Miyazaki S: Percutaneous retrogasserian glycerol injection in the management of trigeminal neuralgia: Long-term follow-up results. J Neurosurg 73:212–216, 1990
52. Meglio M, Cioni B, Moles A, Visocchi M: Microvascular decompression versus percutaneous procedures for typical trigeminal neuralgia: Personal experience. Stereotact Funct Neurosurg 54:76–79, 1990
53. Lichtor T, Mullan J: A 10-year follow-up review of percutaneous microcompression of the trigeminal ganglion. J Neurosurg 72:49–54, 1990
54. Lobato R, Rivas J, Sarabina R, Lamas E: Percutaneous microcompression of the gasserian ganglion for trigeminal neuralgia. J Neurosurg 72:546–553, 1990
55. Peragut JC, Gondin-Oliveira J, Fabrizi A, Sethian M: Microcompression of the trigeminal ganglion for trigeminal neuralgia: Experience with 70 patients. Neurochirurgie 37:111–114, 1991
56. Peet MM, Schneider RD: Trigeminal neuralgia. J Neurosurg 9:367–377, 1952
57. Apfelbaum RL: Surgery for tic douloureux. Clin Neurosurg 31:358–368, 1983
58. Piatt JH, Wilkins RH: Treatment of tic douloureux and hemifacial spasm by posterior fossa exploration: Therapeutic implications of various neurovascular relationships. Neurosurgery 14:462–471, 1984
59. Bederson J, Wilson C: Evaluation of microvascular decompression and partial sensory rhizotomy in 252 cases of trigeminal neuralgia. J Neurosurg 71:359–367, 1989
60. Jannetta P: Treatment of trigeminal neuralgia by micro-operative decompression, in Youmans J (ed): Neurological Surgery. Philadelphia, WB Saunders, 1990, pp 3928–3942
61. Klun B: Microvascular decompression and partial sensory rhizotomy in the treatment of trigeminal neuralgia: Personal experience with 220 patients. Neurosurgery 30:49–52, 1992
62. Burcheil K, Clarke H, Haglund M, Loeser J: Long term efficacy of microvascular decompression in trigeminal neuralgia. J Neurosurg 69:35–38, 1988
63. Rushton JG, Olafson RA: Trigeminal neuralgia associated with multiple sclerosis. Report of 35 cases. Arch Neurol 13:383–386, 1965
64. Jensen T, Rasmussen P, Reske Nielsen E: Association of trigeminal neuralgia with multiple sclerosis: Clinical and pathological features. Acta Neurol Scand 65:182–189, 1982
65. Lazar ML, Kirkpatrick JB: Trigeminal neuralgia and multiple sclerosis: Demonstration of the plaque in an operative case. Neurosurgery 5:711–712, 1979
66. Engel GL: Primary atypical facial neuralgia: An hysterical conversion symptom. Psychosom Med 13:375–396, 1951
67. Engel GL: "Psychogenic" pain and the pain-prone patient. Am J Med 26:899–918, 1959
68. Fay T: Atypical facial neuralgia, a syndrome of vascular pain. Ann Otol Rhinol Laryngol 41:1030–1062, 1932
69. Keller JT, van Loveren H: Pathophysiology of the pain of trigeminal neuralgia and atypical facial pain: A neuroanatomical perspective. Clin Neurosurg 32:275–293, 1985
70. Gybels J, Sweet W: Neurosurgical treatment of persistent pain: Physiological and pathological mechanisms of human pain, in Gildenberg PL (ed): Pain and Headache. Basel, Switzerland, S Karger AG, 1988, pp 70–103
71. Onofrio BM, Campbell JK: Surgical treatment of chronic cluster headache. Mayo Clin Proc 61:537–544, 1986
72. King J: Glossopharyngeal neuralgia. Clin Exp Neurol 24:113–121, 1987
73. van Loveren H, Tew JM, Thomas G: Vago-glossopharyngeal and geniculate neuralgias, in Youmans J (ed): Neurological Surgery. Philadelphia, WB Saunders, 1990, pp 3943–3949
74. Jannetta P: Cranial nerve vascular compression syndromes (other than tic douloureux and hemifacial spasm). Clin Neurosurg 28:445–580, 1981
75. Tew JM Jr: Percutaneous rhizotomy in the treatment of intractable facial pain (trigeminal, glossopharyngeal, and vagal nerves), in Schmidek HH, Sweet WH (eds): Current Techniques in Operative Neurosurgery. New York, Grune & Stratton, 1977, pp 409–426
76. Rhoton A, Buza R: Microsurgical anatomy of the jugular foramen. J Neurosurg 42:541–550, 1975
77. Saker G, Ori C, Baratto V, et al: Selective percutaneous thermolesions of the ninth cranial nerve by lateral cervical approach: Report of eight cases. Surg Neurol 20:276–279, 1983
78. Arbit E, Krol G: Percutaneous radiofrequency neurolysis guided by computed tomography for the treatment of glossopharyngeal neuralgia (technical note). Neurosurgery 29:580–582, 1991
79. Ori C, Salar G, Giron G: Percutaneous glossopharyngeal thermocoagulation complicated by syncope and seizures. Neurosurgery 13:427–429, 1983
80. Lazorthes Y, Verdie J: Radiofrequency coagulation of the petrous ganglion in glossopharyngeal neuralgia. Neurosurgery 4:512, 1979
81. Sindou M, Henry JF, Blanchard P: Idiopathic neuralgia of the glossopharyngeal nerve. Study of a series of 14 cases and review of the literature. Neurochirurgie 37:18–25, 1991
82. Isamat F, Ferran E, Acebes J: Selective percutaneous thermocoagulation rhizotomy in essential glossopharyngeal neuralgia. J Neurosurg 55:575–580, 1981
83. Giorgi C, Broggi G: Surgical treatment of glossopharyngeal neuralgia and pain from cancer of the nasopharynx: A 20 year experience. J Neurosurg 61:952–955, 1984

CHAPTER

120

Surgical Management of Brainstem Vascular Malformations

John M. Tew, Jr.
Adam I. Lewis

Historically, brainstem vascular malformations were considered to be inoperable because of their deep location and intimate relationship to complex neurovascular structures.[1] Nevertheless, the natural history of this disorder suggests that over 50 percent of patients with deep-seated arteriovenous malformations (AVMs) suffer significant morbidity or death from hemorrhage.[2] With the advent of magnetic resonance imaging (MRI), more brainstem vascular malformations are being discovered. Advances in angiographic and microsurgical technique have expanded the operative domains of the neurosurgeon to include vascular malformations of the brainstem. Furthermore, intraoperative monitoring of brainstem tracts and stimulation of brainstem nuclei have helped reduce morbidity by avoiding injury to vital brainstem pathways. The authors and others have shown that surgical excision of brainstem vascular malformations is a safe and effective mode of treatment in selected patients.[3–6]

CLASSIFICATION

Intracranial vascular malformations are classified pathologically as AVMs, cavernous angiomas, venous angiomas, and capillary telangiectasias.[7] Clinically, brainstem vascular malformations may be divided into angiographically visible and occult vascular malformations.[8] AVMs and cavernous angiomas are the only vascular malformations that require operative intervention. McCormick and associates[9] reviewed 164 posterior fossa AVMs and found 38 telangiectasias. None of these lesions showed signs of hemorrhage, and all affected individuals were asymptomatic. Recently, a retrospective review of MRIs found that venous angiomas are benign lesions that should be managed conservatively.[10]

Most surgeons refer to Spetzler and Martin's[11] AVM classification for operative difficulty. In this system, there are five surgical grades based on size of the AVM, relation to eloquent neural structures, and venous drainage. Results demonstrated that with each successive grade, the percentage of patients sustaining a neurologic deficit related to surgery increased. Therefore, risk for permanent injury increases with increasingly complex vascular malformations. This grading system fails to account for the therapeutic risk associated with endovascular interventions or stereotactic radiosurgery. These two treatment modalities are playing an increasing part in AVM therapeutic considerations. A new classification and prognostic schema should be developed in consideration of embolization and radiosurgery. Moreover, vascular malformations of the brainstem defy the Spetzler and Martin classification system because venous characteristics and size have minimal relation to expected outcome.

NATURAL HISTORY

AVMs of the brainstem are rare, representing only 1 percent of all AVMs. They usually present with hemorrhage and neurologic deficit, and once symptomatic, they tend to hemorrhage repeatedly. The natural history of symptomatic AVMs demonstrates a rate of major rebleeding of 4 percent per year. Combined major morbidity and mortality is 2.7 percent per year.[2] Each hemorrhagic episode carries a 10 percent mortality rate and a 30 percent major morbidity rate. Because brainstem AVMs are located in a densely packed area of vital brain tissue and have little space for an expanding hematoma, the deficits resulting from hemorrhage here are often more devastating than those for AVMs in other locations.

CLINICAL FEATURES

The initial presentation of brainstem vascular malformations varies greatly, and the clinical course may resemble low-grade gliomas, multiple sclerosis, or inflammatory disorders. Unlike most supratentorial cryptic AVMs that present with seizures,[12] those in the brainstem present with parenchymal, subarachnoid, or intraventricular hemorrhage.

Once symptomatic, brainstem AVMs tend to hemorrhage repeatedly.[13, 14] Although cavernous angiomas also have a propensity toward recurrent hemorrhage, they rarely rupture into the subarachnoid space or the ventricular system. Further, cavernous angiomas are low-flow lesions that produce less destruction than parenchymal AVMs when they rupture[8,15]; consequently, cryptic vascular malformations tend to displace rather than destroy neural tissues.[16] In most cases, patients with cavernous angiomas recover significant neurologic function if brainstem tolerance for the mass effect of the hematoma is not exceeded. By comparison, ruptured brainstem AVMs produce larger hematomas, and patients are less likely to recover neurologic function.[15] Finally, brainstem AVMs often produce subarachnoid or intraventricular hemorrhage because they are superficial or subpial to the brainstem surface.

Clinical signs and symptoms are related to location of the malformation. In our series of 36 patients, presenting symptoms in order of frequency were diplopia, facial numbness, incoordination, gait difficulties, numbness and paresthesias, arm and/or leg weakness, and difficulty speaking and swallowing. Clinical signs included abducens and oculomotor palsy, internuclear ophthalmoplegia, nuclear facial palsy, nystagmus, facial hypoesthesia, hemisensory deficit, hyperreflexia, hemiparesis, and cerebellar ataxia. Five patients were neurologically intact on initial presentation.

PREOPERATIVE EVALUATION

Angiography is the current standard for AVM evaluation. A complete angiographic evaluation includes a four-vessel study and sequential evaluation of all phases, including arterial, capillary, and venous. This sequence gives a clear understanding of vascular dynamics of the malformation, such as rate of blood flow, differential in regional flow (arterial steal), and patterns of collateral flow. Additional information includes nidus size and configuration, as well as the position, number, and size of feeding arteries and associated aneurysms.

Because most cavernous angiomas are not visible by angiogram, MRI is the best study for preoperative evaluation. MRI of cavernous angiomas shows a consistent morphologic appearance: a central focus of mixed-signal intensity representing hemorrhage of various ages. The nidus is surrounded by a hypointense rim of hemosiderin from chronic microhemorrhages. Venous angiomas are associated with cavernous angiomas in 15 percent of cases. For both malformation types, MRI details the three-dimensional location relative to the regional brain and bony anatomy. MRI also provides information regarding the presence of hemorrhage, the relative chronology of multiple hemorrhages, and the status of regional parenchyma in terms of mass effect, edema, and injury.[17]

The high risk of damage from hemorrhage in the brainstem emphasizes the need for treatment of selected patients. Those with recurrent hemorrhage and progressive neurologic deficit are candidates for surgery. Ideally, the lesion should be superficial to the brainstem surface. When the malformation is not subpial and the patient continues to deteriorate, a corridor of noneloquent tissue can be defined by use of intraoperative monopolar stimulation of brainstem nuclei. There are no data to indicate that treatment of asymptomatic lesions is warranted. Surgical intervention, in our experience, is associated with a transient neurologic deficit in over 60 percent of cases and may not be advisable in a neurologically intact patient. We do not advocate surgery for patients with recurrent hemorrhage who have minimal or no neurologic deficits and whose malformation lies deep to the brainstem surface.

We agree with others that the best time to operate is when the condition is subacute.[18,19] Allowing time for the patient to recover from the ictus and the hematoma to organize are the principal reasons for operating within 1 to 4 weeks. The hematoma is well differentiated from the surrounding gliotic capsule, and a plane for dissection is easily defined. Operations performed emergently are avoided because the hematoma is not consolidated, the edematous neural tissue is friable, and the gliotic plane between the malformation and the brainstem is poorly defined. However, if the operation is delayed more than 1 month, the malformation may adhere to the gliotic capsule; removal of the malformation often leaves a ragged gliotic plane, which increases the potential for residual malformation. Furthermore, posthemorrhagic fibrosis occurs within the malformation after the subacute period and may require vigorous exploration and manipulation to remove.

REGIONAL SURGICAL ANATOMY

Mesencephalic AVMs are rare lesions that are usually located on the surface of the brainstem. Those that lie on the tectum produce disturbances in ocular motility and consciousness when hemorrhage occurs. More laterally placed lesions may lie at the junction of the upper fourth ventricle and the superior cerebellar peduncle in the pia-arachnoid space (above the root entry zone of the trigeminal nerve). Arterial supply arises from the superior cerebellar and anteroinferior cerebellar arteries. Contribution from the posterior cerebral artery branches is variable. Venous drainage is to the superior petrosal, mesencephalic, and superior vermian veins, and the basal vein of Rosenthal. The trochlear nerve is often entangled in the malformation.

Cerebellopontine angle AVMs are supplied primarily from anteroinferior cerebellar artery and posteroinferior cerebellar artery branches. Feeding arteries are often intertwined with cranial nerves V through XII. Usually, these AVMs maintain an extrapial or superficially subpial location and may extend into the fourth ventricle. During resection, the fourth ventricle should be inspected for residual AVM. Venous drainage is to the superior petrosal, ependymal, and pontomesencephalic veins.

Pontomedullary AVMs are often embedded in the brainstem and have a vascular supply derived from the penetrating branches of the basilar artery and branches of the anteroinferior and posteroinferior cerebellar arteries. These vessels are often indistinct from those supplying normal brain. Additionally, pontomedullary AVMs may derive their blood supply from anteroinferior cerebellar and superior cerebellar artery branches. The nidus tends to be smaller and less accessible than that of other brainstem AVMs. Venous drainage is via lateral mesencephalic and pontomesencephalic veins.

SURGICAL APPROACHES

Four surgical approaches to brainstem vascular malformations exist: superior vermian, inferior vermian, lateral cerebellar, and combined subtemporal-suboccipital transtentorial

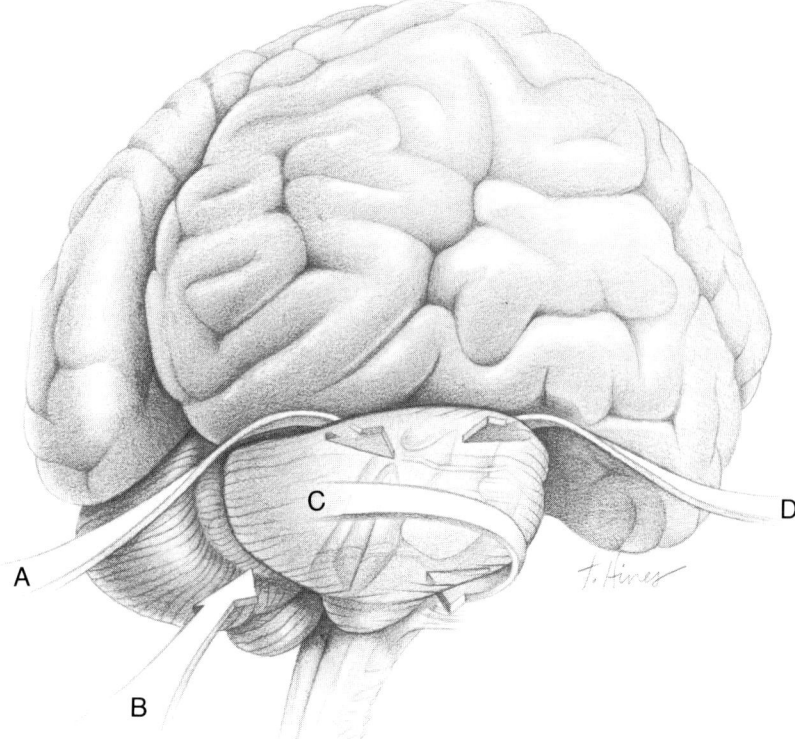

FIGURE 120–1. There are four approaches to brainstem vascular malformations illustrated in this drawing: superior vermian (A), inferior vermian (B), lateral cerebellar (C), and combined subtemporal-suboccipital transtentorial (D). The approach is dictated by the most superficial location of the malformation to the surface of the brainstem or fourth ventricle. (From Tew JM Jr, van Loveren HR: Atlas of Operative Microneurosurgery. Philadelphia, W. B. Saunders, 1994.)

(Fig. 120–1). The surgical approach is dictated by the most superficial location of the vascular malformation to the surface of the brainstem (Fig. 120–2). For midline approaches, the patient is positioned with the lesion side down to allow the widest angle of approach to the lesion and to avoid retraction of the brainstem (Fig. 120–3).

ANESTHETIC CONSIDERATIONS

Anesthesiologists serve an integral role for AVM resection. They reduce the patient's intracranial pressure, protect the brain from ischemia, and maintain hypotension during resection, which aids in hemostasis. Initially, the patient is hyperventilated to a PCO_2 of 25 to 30 mm Hg, and osmotic diuretics are administered to reduce intracranial pressure. Spinal drainage via a lumbar drain further relaxes the brain. A nitroprusside drip is titrated to mean arterial pressure of 60 mm Hg during the resection of the AVM. Induced hypotension is essential to control bleeding or intraoperative brain swelling during the resection of AVMs. Cerebral protection with etomidate or barbiturates may be given during the operation to avoid ischemia to surrounding brain tissue.

ADJUNCTS TO SURGERY

Before surgery, baseline electrophysiologic monitoring, including brainstem auditory evoked responses and somatosensory evoked potentials are obtained. Stimulation of brainstem nuclei and motor cranial nerves with a monopolar electro-

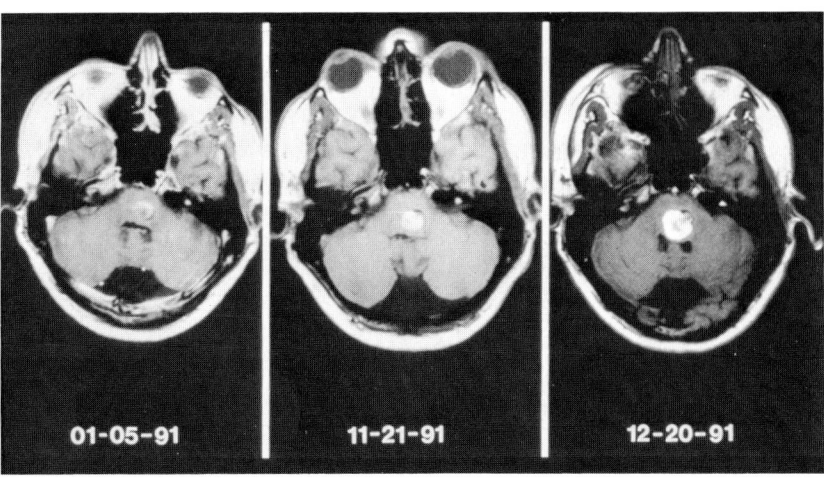

FIGURE 120–2. This series of T1-weighted MRIs demonstrates three discrete hemorrhagic episodes from a pontine cavernous angioma. After the third hemorrhage, a complete surgical resection was performed with no new neurologic deficits. Surgical therapy is indicated if there is recurrent hemorrhage or progressive neurologic deficit, or if the lesion is superficial to the brainstem surface.

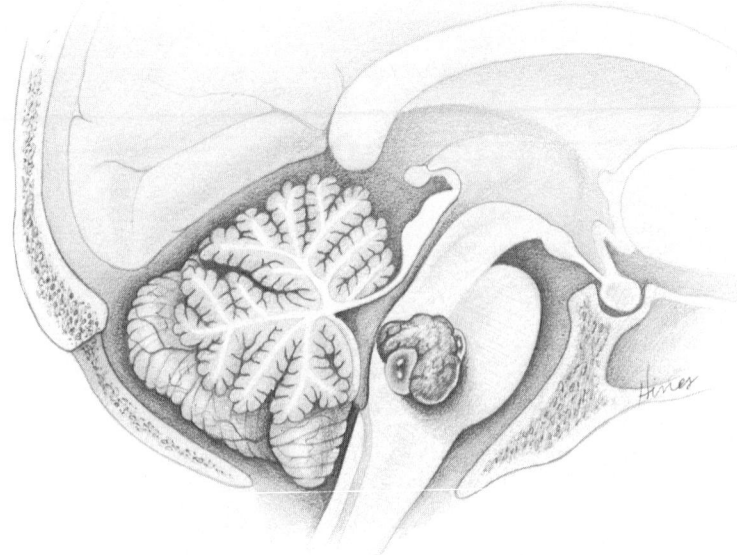

FIGURE 120-3. A sagittal view of the case presented in Figure 120-2 shows the relationship of the cavernous malformation to the fourth ventricle, pons, and cerebellum. The surgical approach to this lesion is midline with sectioning of the inferior vermis to expose the floor of the fourth ventricle. (From Tew JM Jr, van Loveren HR: Atlas of Operative Microneurosurgery. Philadelphia, W. B. Saunders, 1994.)

myogram stimulator (Xomed Nerve Integrity Monitor-2, Xomed-Treace, Jacksonville, FL) defines a corridor of noneloquent tissue and prevents injury to vital brainstem tracts. Typically, the abducens, facial, vagal, and hypoglossal nuclei are monitored and stimulated bilaterally. Real-time intraoperative ultrasound precisely locates the malformation, avoids dissection of normal tissue, and ensures a complete surgical resection. Imaging is performed with an Ultramark 9 (High Density Imaging) real-time, color-flow ultrasound system (Advanced Technology Laboratories, Bothell, WA). The ultrasonic probe with an 8-mm diameter provides a 180-degree sweep with a frequency of 7 MHz. The high-density imaging boosts the effective frequency to 14 MHz. The combined potassium-titanium-phosphate (KTP) and neodymium:yttrium-aluminum-garnet (Nd:YAG) laser (Laserscope Surgical Systems, San Jose, CA) is particularly useful in defining a plane between the malformation and normal tissue. A focusing micromanipulator with coincident helium-neon laser for coaxial aiming is attached to the microscope (Opmilas YAG, Carl Zeiss). Bypassing the handheld piece allows better visualization of deep regions in the brainstem.

Currently, preoperative embolization for brainstem AVMs is rarely possible. Catheters and guide wires are often unable to navigate the small intraluminal diameters and acute angles characteristic of feeding arteries. Also, the lack of collateral vessels poses a high risk of producing brainstem infarction from inadvertent occlusion of normal arteries. Endovascular therapy is not possible for cryptic AVMs, cavernous angiomas, or telangiectasias because they are not visualized angiographically.

Stereotactic radiosurgery is worthy of consideration for asymptomatic AVMs involving the tectum, for which surgical risk is high. No evidence exists that radiosurgery is effective for cavernous or venous angiomas and may be associated with a significant risk of radionecrosis.

SURGICAL TECHNIQUE

The goal of surgery is complete excision of the malformation to eliminate the risk of hemorrhage. The patient undergoes general endotracheal anesthesia in the supine position. An armored endotracheal tube is placed to allow the neck to be flexed, facilitating exposure to the posterior fossa. The groin is prepared, and a femoral artery sheath is placed and maintained with heparin solution under pressure for intraoperative angiography. Intraoperative angiography is not planned for patients with cavernous angiomas. The patient is placed in the lateral oblique position with the thorax elevated 15 degrees to improve venous drainage. The head is held in slight lateral extension and cervical flexion with the radiolucent Mayfield three-point fixation device for intraoperative angiography (Ohio Medical Instrument Company, Cincinnati, OH). Appropriate padding is placed, including an axillary roll for protection of the brachial plexus. A radial arterial line and urinary catheter are inserted, and pneumatic compression stockings are placed on the legs. Paired electrodes are placed in the lateral rectus, obicularis oris, vocalis muscle, and hypoglossal muscles to monitor cranial nerve nuclei. The median and auditory nerves are also selected to evaluate somatosensory and brainstem auditory evoked responses, respectively. An 18-gauge spinal needle is placed in the lumbar cistern for cerebrospinal fluid drainage, and hyperventilation to a PCO_2 of 25 to 30 mm Hg is maintained.

For tectal, pontine, and medullary vascular malformations, a midline suboccipital skin incision is made from the inion to the level of C2. A suboccipital craniotomy is performed with Midas Rex pneumatic instrumentation (Midas Rex Institute, Fort Worth, TX). The bony removal includes the foramen magnum and the posterior arch of C1. The dura is opened in a Y-shaped fashion with the incision based on the transverse sinus. The Budde halo system of flexible arm, self-retracting blades is used to expose the vermis in the midline (Ohio Medical Instrument Company, Cincinnati, OH). The cistern is opened, and the tonsils are retracted laterally with two 10-mm self-retaining retractors. For lesions of the pons or medulla, the lower one third of the vermis is split by use of the focused carbon dioxide laser energy at 10 W—which is delivered via a micromanipulator attached to the operating microscope (Fig. 120-4). For lesions of the mesencephalon, the upper vermis is sectioned. Microretractors are positioned

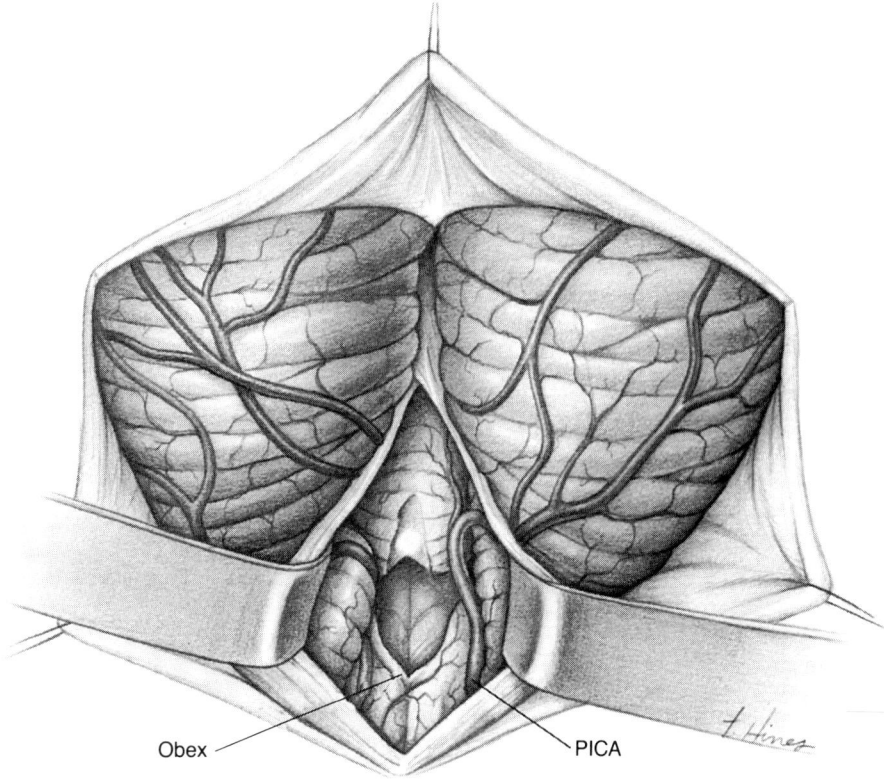

FIGURE 120–4. The dura is opened by cruciate incision. The cisterna magna is opened and the tonsils are retracted laterally with two 10-mm self-retaining retractors. After the obex is exposed, the inferior vermis between distal branches of the posteroinferior cerebellar artery (PICA) is incised with focused laser energy. (From Tew JM Jr, van Loveren HR: Atlas of Operative Microneurosurgery. Philadelphia, W. B. Saunders, 1994.)

to permit visualization from the median raphe to the lateral recesses of the fourth ventricle. In most cases, the vascular malformation is subependymal and distorts the floor of the fourth ventricle.

Monopolar stimulation of the floor of the fourth ventricle effectively maps the sixth, seventh, tenth, and twelfth cranial nerve nuclei (Fig. 120–5). In pontomedullary AVMs, the hematoma cavity is opened lateral to the seventh nerve nucleus with the carbon dioxide laser (Fig. 120–6). Suction is used to remove the liquefied portion of the cavity, and the

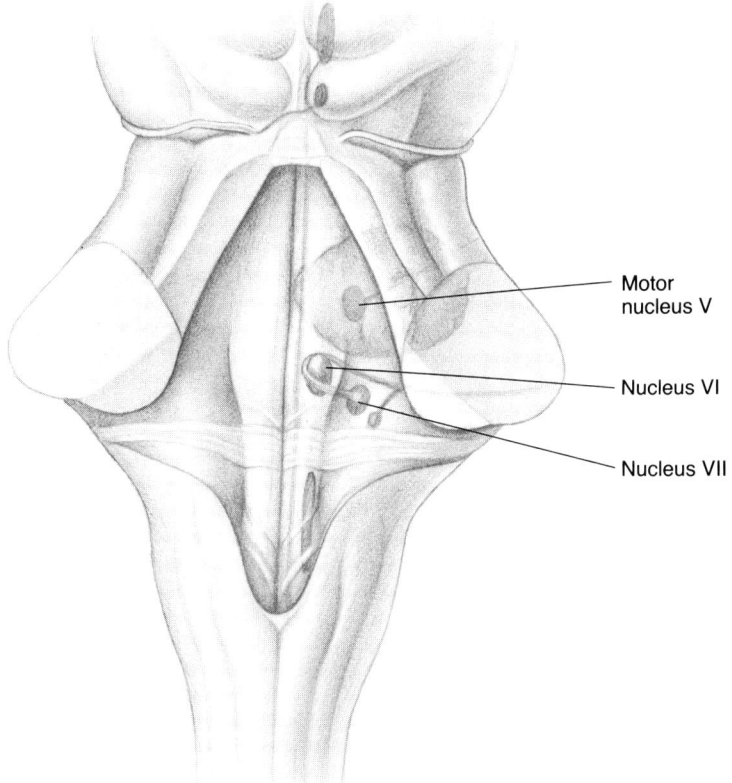

FIGURE 120–5. Anatomy of the floor of the fourth ventricle is shown in relation to the distorted appearance of the operative view. The location of the V, VI, and VII cranial nerve nuclei is mapped on the floor of the fourth ventricle by monopolar electrical stimulation in order to avoid injury during removal of the vascular malformation. In combination with somatosensory evoked potentials and brainstem auditory evoked responses, brainstem monitoring has helped reduce postoperative morbidity. (From Tew JM Jr, van Loveren HR: Atlas of Operative Microneurosurgery. Philadelphia, W. B. Saunders, 1994.)

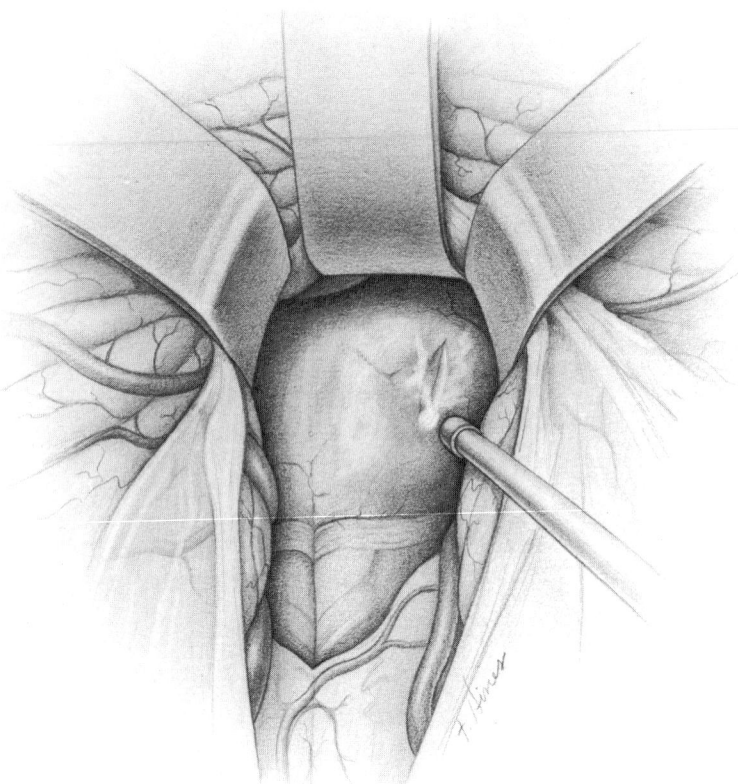

FIGURE 120–6. Retractors are positioned to permit visualization from the median raphe to the lateral recess of the right fourth ventricle. After mapping the floor of the fourth ventricle, an incision is made 1 cm superolateral to the site where stimulation elicited a facial response. (From Tew JM Jr, van Loveren HR: Atlas of Operative Microneurosurgery. Philadelphia, W. B. Saunders, 1994.)

KTP or Nd:YAG laser is used to remove the solid component. A plane of dissection is developed between the malformation and the gliotic capsule (Fig. 120–7). Feeding arteries are sacrificed while adequate venous drainage is preserved. Deep microscopic arteries that penetrate the bed of resection are obliterated with the impedance monitored bipolar forceps and laser (Fig. 120–8). Hypotension is continued throughout the dissection phase, at least until intraoperative angiography has proven that the AVM is completely excised.

Precise inspection of all bleeding points is mandatory because these vessels may have lost their autoregulation (i.e., ability to contract) and must be thoroughly obliterated by sealing of their collagen walls (Fig. 120–9). Application of a small pledget of absorbable gelatin sponge (Gelfoam) soaked with thrombin under a gently applied retractor can eliminate troublesome bleeding from capillaries and arterioles. Cavernous angiomas may be subdivided by numerous trabeculae and pockets of malformation that can become embedded and hidden from view within the gliotic capsule. Intraoperative ultrasound is a useful first step to evaluate residual AVMs and is essential to detect residual cavernous malformations. Finally, intraoperative angiography with digital subtraction in two planes is essential to document complete removal of the AVMs. Physiologic preservation of the brainstem nuclei is confirmed by stimulation with the monopolar instrument (Figs. 120–10 and 120–11).

Laterally placed vascular malformations in the cerebellopontine angle are resected through a lateral cerebellar approach. A straight incision over the mastoid notch that crosses the superior nuchal line and descends in the midline is performed. The superior and lateral myofascial cuff is retained, and the skin and muscle flaps are reflected inferiorly. A burr hole is made at the asterion, and a craniotomy is carried laterally to the edge of the sigmoid sinus and superiorly to the edge of the transverse sinus. The inferior margin extends to the foramen magnum to permit adequate decompression and removal of cerebrospinal fluid from the cisterna magna (Fig. 120–12). A cruciate incision is made in the dura after good cerebellar relaxation is achieved (Fig. 120–13). The cerebellar hemisphere is retracted medially (Figs. 120–14 to 120–16). The malformation and hematoma are dissected free from the gliotic cerebellum, and the pia-arachnoid membrane adjacent to the AVM is developed (Fig. 120–17). Numerous branches of the superior cerebellar artery and anteroinferior cerebellar artery are coagulated and incised (Figs. 120–18 to 120–22). Commonly, the AVM is entangled in the cranial nerves, but they can be preserved with precise dissection. The nidus of cerebellopontine angle AVMs usually remains superficial to the brainstem surface.

Rostral brainstem AVMs that are located laterally may be resected via the subtemporal-transtentorial approach (Figs. 120–23 and 120–24). Feeding vessels from the posterior cerebral and basilar perforating arteries are readily coagulated and excised from this approach. Initially, the temporal lobe is retracted medially and superiorly, and the tentorial margin is incised lateral to the trochlear nerve. The incision extends laterally to the superior petrosal sinus. Most of these upper prepontine AVMs are located in a pia-arachnoid plane and are readily excised. If they are embedded in the tissue of the brainstem, they may be unresectable.

An occipital burr hole for emergency ventricular aspiration is placed before closure because postoperative swelling or

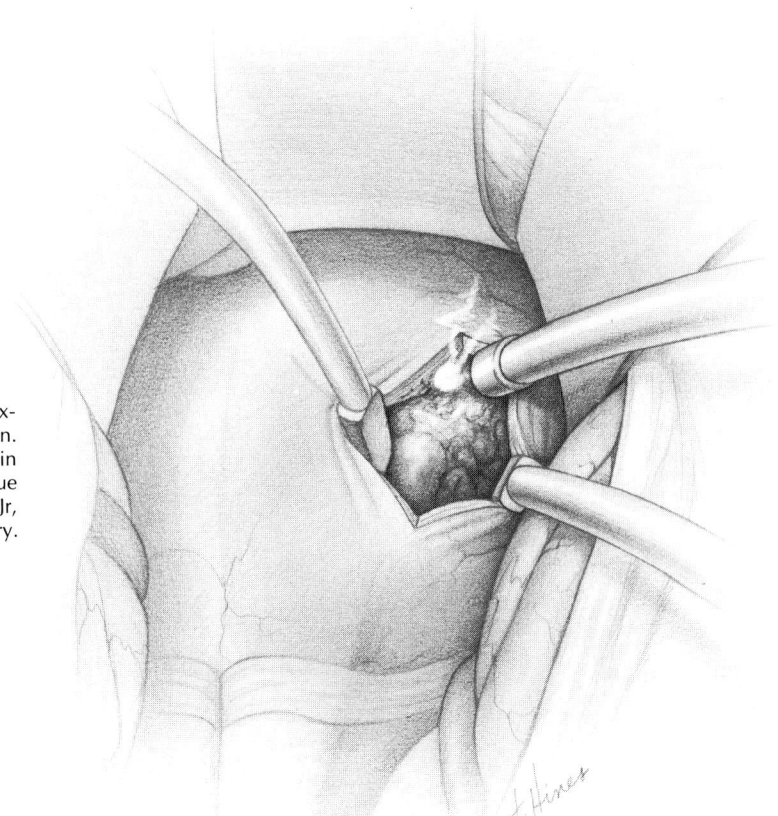

FIGURE 120–7. Opposing 2-mm retractors provide exposure of the surface of the thrombosed malformation. Later in the dissection, these retractors are very useful in allowing visualization of the entire cavity without undue manipulation of the brainstem tissues. (From Tew JM Jr, van Loveren HR: Atlas of Operative Microneurosurgery. Philadelphia, W. B. Saunders, 1994.)

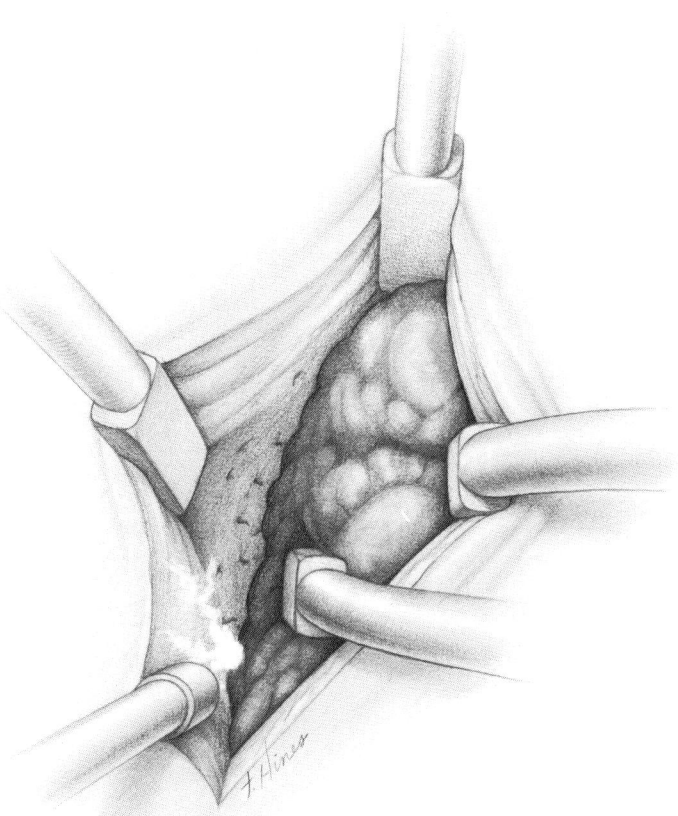

FIGURE 120–8. Initially, the liquefied portion of the hematoma is aspirated with atraumatic suction catheters. A plane is defined between the gliotic capsule and the malformation by coagulating arteriolar-like feeding arteries with bipolar forceps or laser energy. (From Tew JM Jr, van Loveren HR: Atlas of Operative Microneurosurgery. Philadelphia, W. B. Saunders, 1994.)

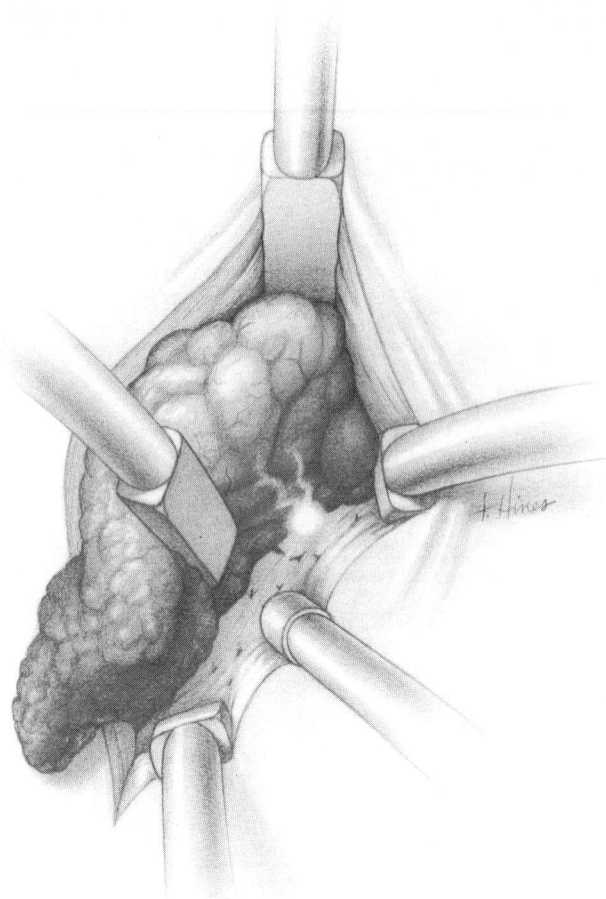

FIGURE 120-9. The lesion is reflected medially as the lateral border of the malformation is freed from the brainstem by a similar technique. The mass of the malformation is reduced by application of defocused laser energy to the surface of the malformation. (From Tew JM Jr, van Loveren HR: Atlas of Operative Microneurosurgery. Philadelphia, W. B. Saunders, 1994.)

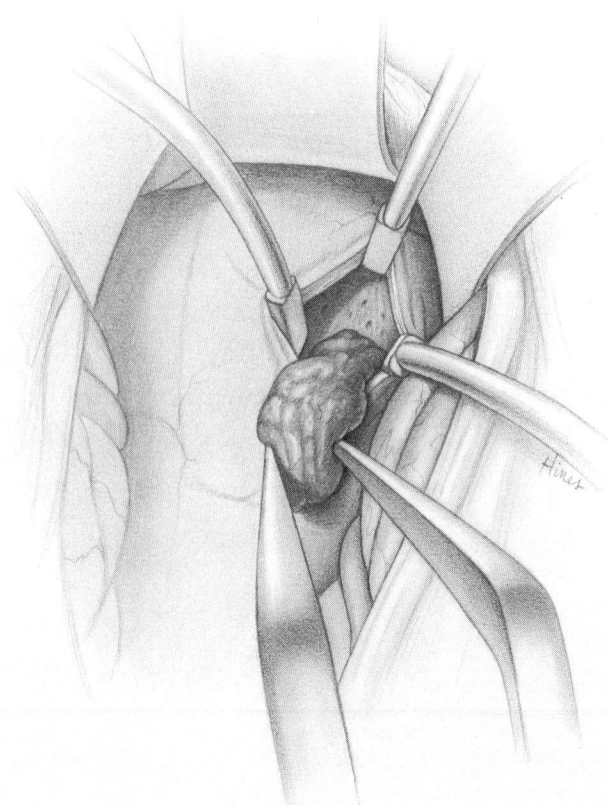

FIGURE 120-10. The shrunken malformation is removed from the cavity of the pons. The entire bed of the cavity is inspected for residual malformation. Real-time color-coded ultrasound is useful for identifying loculated areas of malformation that are embedded in the gliotic capsule. Electrophysiologic stimulation of the resection bed and floor of the fourth ventricle is repeated (after resection of the malformation) to confirm preservation of brainstem nuclei. (From Tew JM Jr, van Loveren HR: Atlas of Operative Microneurosurgery. Philadelphia, W. B. Saunders, 1994.)

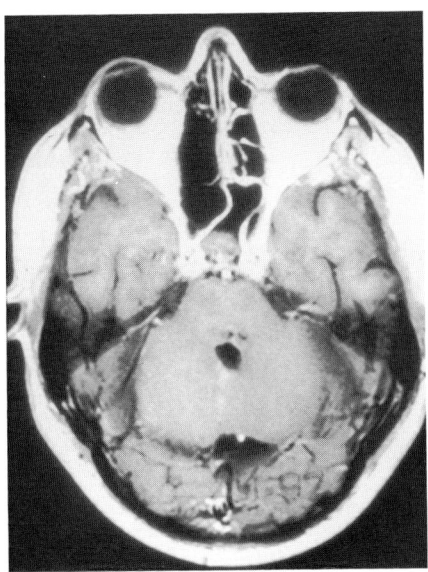

FIGURE 120–11. Postoperative T1-weighted MRI of the patient depicted in Figure 120–2 shows no residual vascular malformation.

hemorrhage can result in sudden, obstructive hydrocephalus. The dura is closed, and the bone flap is secured with stainless steel wires. Muscle, fascia, and skin are closed in layers.

ALTERNATIVE TREATMENTS

Aspiration of brainstem vascular malformations has been recommended by several authors.[20, 21] Although aspiration of the hematoma relieves mass effect and may improve recovery, it has several disadvantages: first, the risk that the probe may injure vital brainstem structures and incite new hemorrhage with puncture of the malformation[22, 23]; second, aspira-

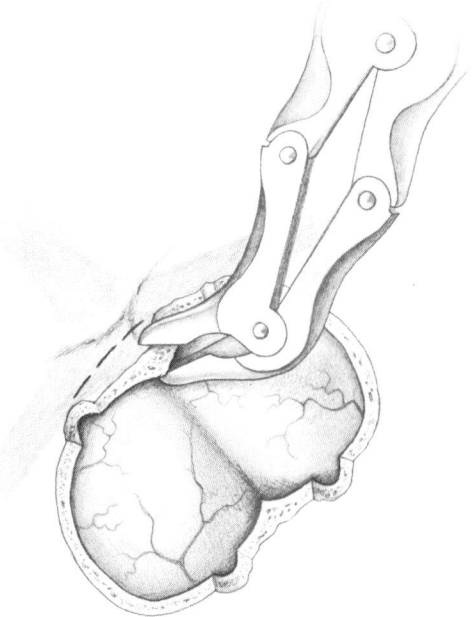

FIGURE 120–12. The bilateral suboccipital craniotomy exposes the inferior edge of the transverse sinus and 3 cm of the cerebellum on either side. The inferior margin extends to the foramen magnum to permit adequate decompression and removal of cerebrospinal fluid from the cisterna magna. (From Tew JM Jr, van Loveren HR: Atlas of Operative Microneurosurgery. Philadelphia, W. B. Saunders, 1994.)

tion of the contents may be nondiagnostic, and recurrent hemorrhage may occur[24]; and third, aspiration removes only the liquefied portion of the hematoma and not the solid portion of the malformation.[25]

Although stereotactic-guided approaches have greatly improved our ability to resect deep-seated vascular malformations, their role in surgery brainstem vascular malformations is limited.[22, 26] Stereotactic procedures do not account for pial

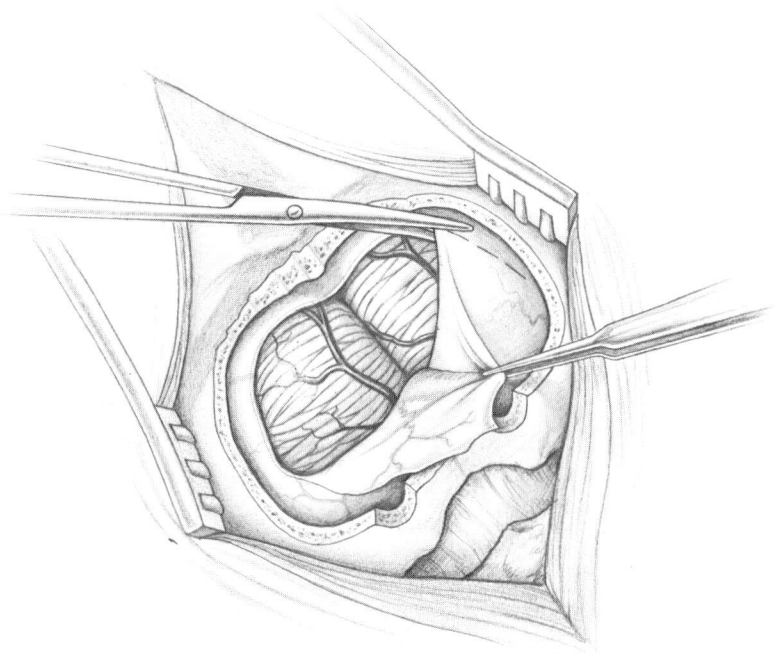

FIGURE 120–13. The dural flap is reflected on its inferior base. The skin incision has been made from 3 cm above the superior nuchal line to the midcervical spine. (From Tew JM Jr, van Loveren HR: Atlas of Operative Microneurosurgery. Philadelphia, W. B. Saunders, 1994.)

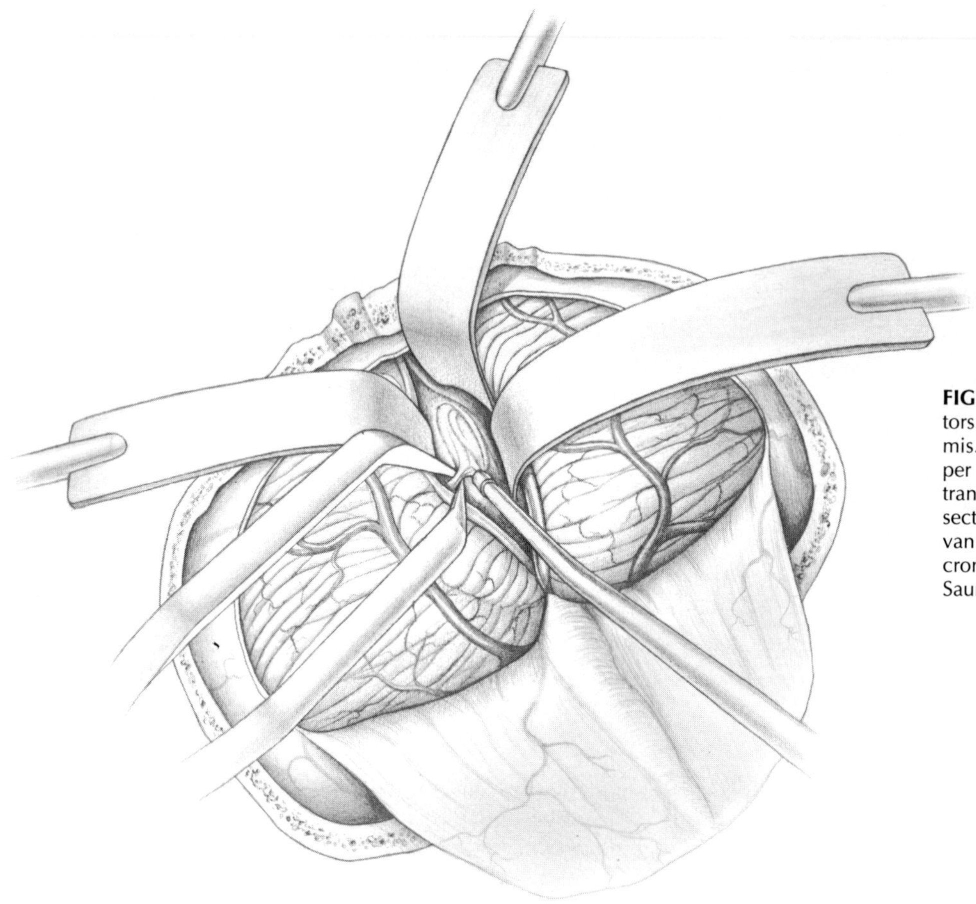

FIGURE 120–14. The self-retaining retractors are placed to expose the superior vermis. The vermis is split to expose the upper fourth ventricle. Postoperatively, a transient truncal ataxia may be seen after sectioning the vermis. (From Tew JM Jr, van Loveren HR: Atlas of Operative Microneurosurgery. Philadelphia, W. B. Saunders, 1994.)

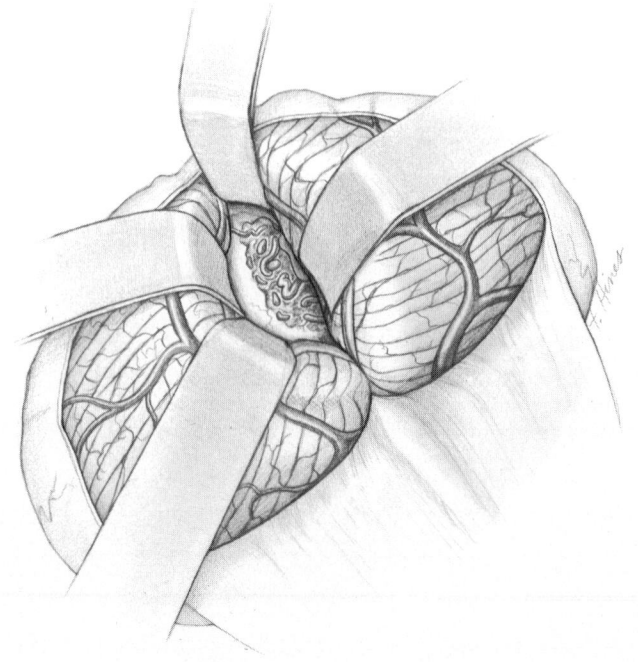

FIGURE 120–15. The retractors are positioned to expose the malformation. (From Tew JM Jr, van Loveren HR: Atlas of Operative Microneurosurgery. Philadelphia, W. B. Saunders, 1994.)

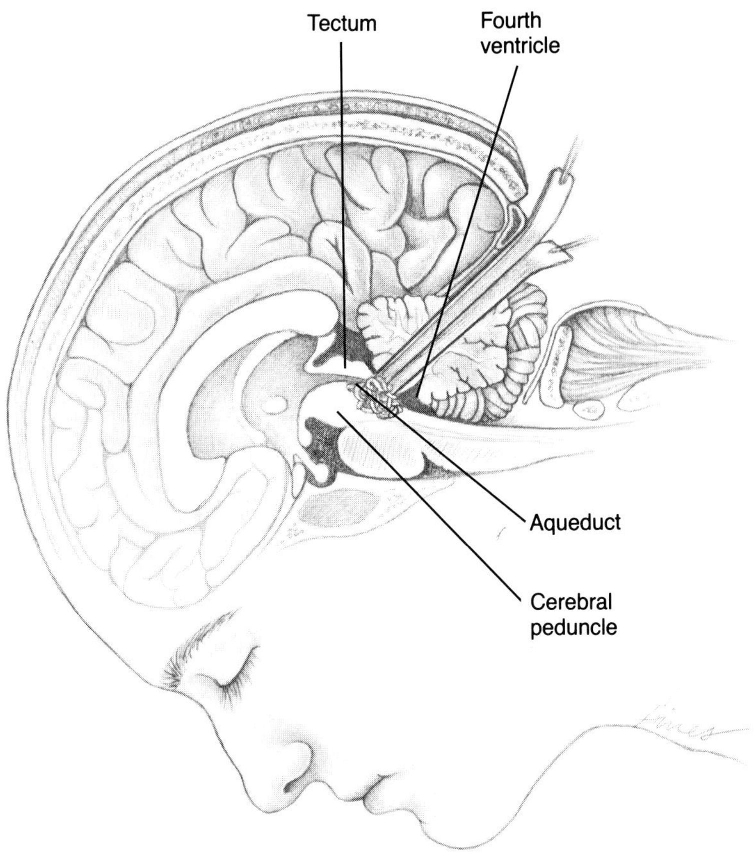

FIGURE 120–16. A sagittal view shows the relationship of the AVM to the anatomic structures: superior cerebellar peduncle, fourth ventricle, aqueduct, and tectum of the mesencephalon. (From Tew JM Jr, van Loveren HR: Atlas of Operative Microneurosurgery. Philadelphia, W. B. Saunders, 1994.)

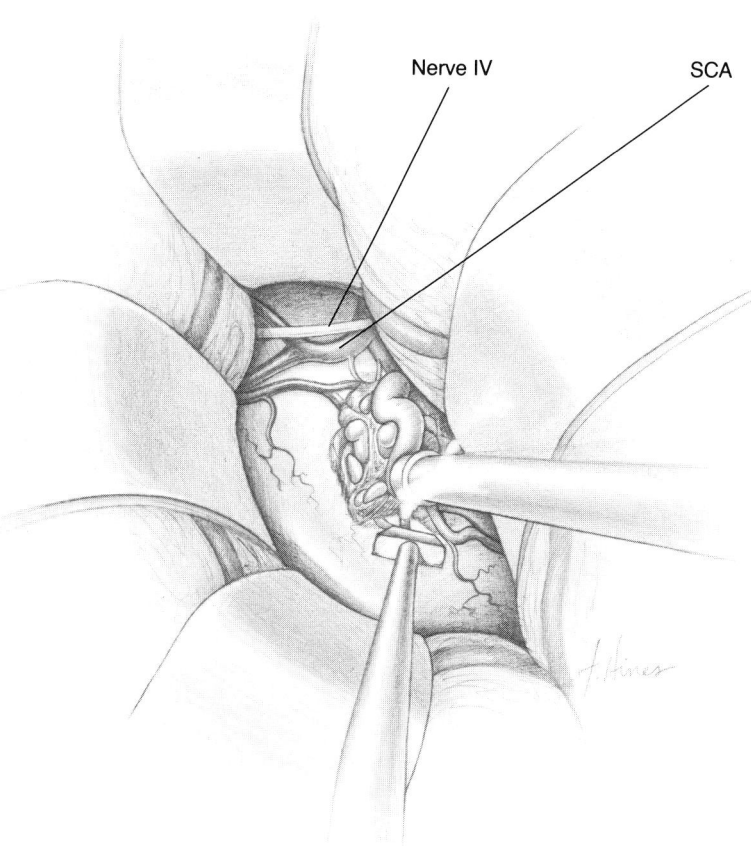

FIGURE 120–17. The same principles for supratentorial AVMs apply to those of the brainstem. Dissection begins medially and proceeds around the margin of the malformation. The fine, feeding arteries are sealed with a color-absorptive laser and bipolar forceps. Dissection is then directed upward toward the tectum, where the superior cerebellar artery (SCA) and the fourth nerve are identified. (From Tew JM Jr, van Loveren HR: Atlas of Operative Microneurosurgery. Philadelphia, W. B. Saunders, 1994.)

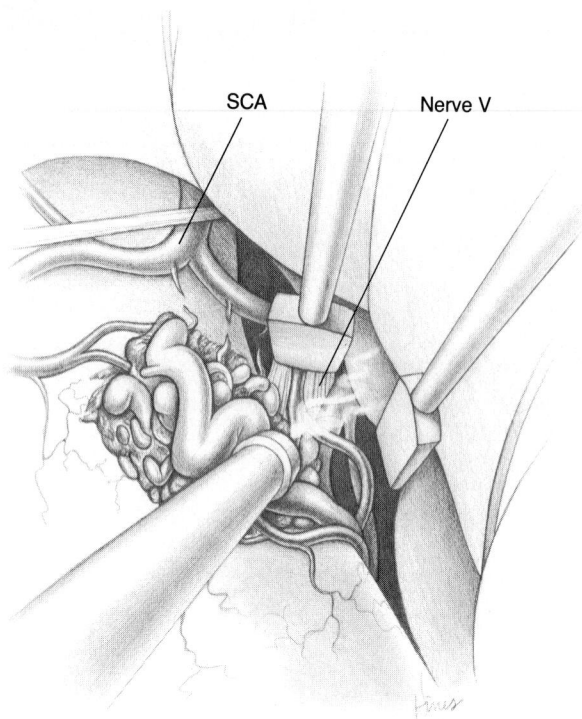

FIGURE 120–18. The cerebellum is retracted to expose the lateral aspect of the mesencephalon and pons. Feeding branches from the superior cerebellar artery (SCA) are occluded and incised. (From Tew JM Jr, van Loveren HR: Atlas of Operative Microneurosurgery. Philadelphia, W. B. Saunders, 1994.)

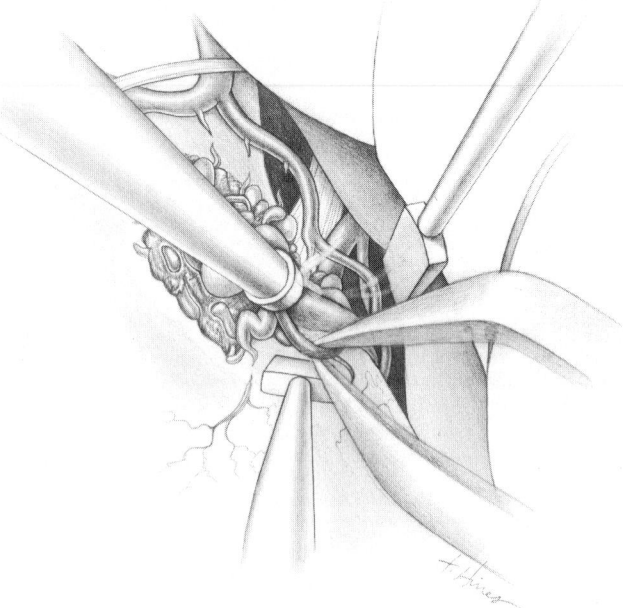

FIGURE 120–19. The trigeminal nerve and draining vein to the superior petrosal vein are identified at the lateral aspect of the pons. The primary draining vein is preserved until all feeding branches from anteroinferior cerebellar artery (AICA) are coagulated. (From Tew JM Jr, van Loveren HR: Atlas of Operative Microneurosurgery. Philadelphia, W. B. Saunders, 1994.)

planes in the posterior fossa. Coordinates plotted preoperatively may shift significantly with spinal fluid drainage, mannitol, and retraction; thereafter, these coordinates are no longer on target.

COMPLICATIONS

Intraoperative complications include hemorrhage, cerebral ischemia, and swelling of surrounding brain tissue. Despite attempts to avoid manipulation of the brainstem, gentle tamponade and exploration of the gliotic capsule may be required to stop friable deep-feeding vessels that retract during rupture. Returning to the appropriate dissection plane and compressing the malformation medially maintains a drier resection bed.

When the cerebellum suddenly becomes tense and bulging, most commonly either cerebellar venous drainage has been disturbed or the patient is not being ventilated properly. The position and patency of the endotracheal tube should be assessed, and the patient's neck position should be examined. Alternatively, obstructive hydrocephalus or occult bleeding may cause brain swelling. Tissues surrounding AVMs may be asymptomatically ischemic from the hemodynamic effects of high-volume, low-pressure shunts, which steal blood flow from them. If the arterial feeders are occluded too rapidly, loss of normal autoregulation in the surrounding ischemic areas may lead to an oversupply of blood that results in swelling and hemorrhage. Staged resection of AVMs may permit autoregulation to return to these ischemic areas and prevent this catastrophe. Spetzler and colleagues[27] have described this phenomenon under the rubric "normal perfusion breakthrough theory." In our experience breakthrough bleeding resulting from loss of cerebral autoregulation during re-

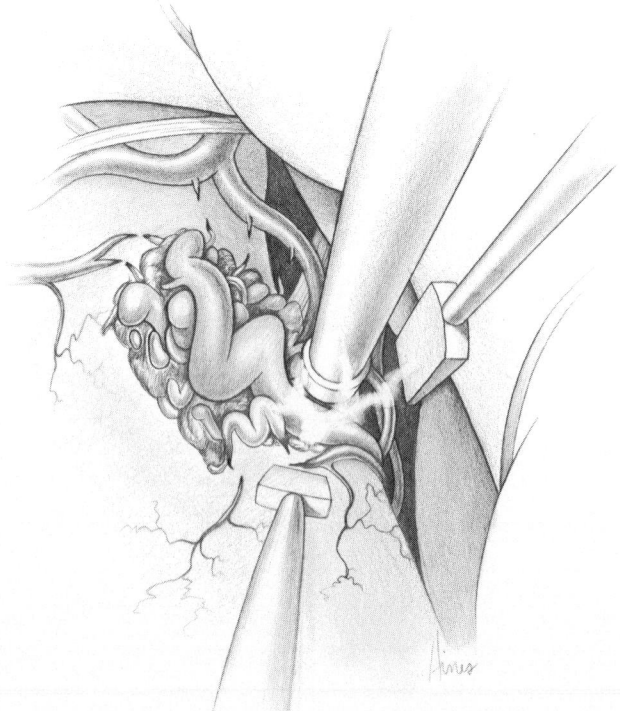

FIGURE 120–20. The primary draining vein is occluded with laser and sectioned. (From Tew JM Jr, van Loveren HR: Atlas of Operative Microneurosurgery. Philadelphia, W. B. Saunders, 1994.)

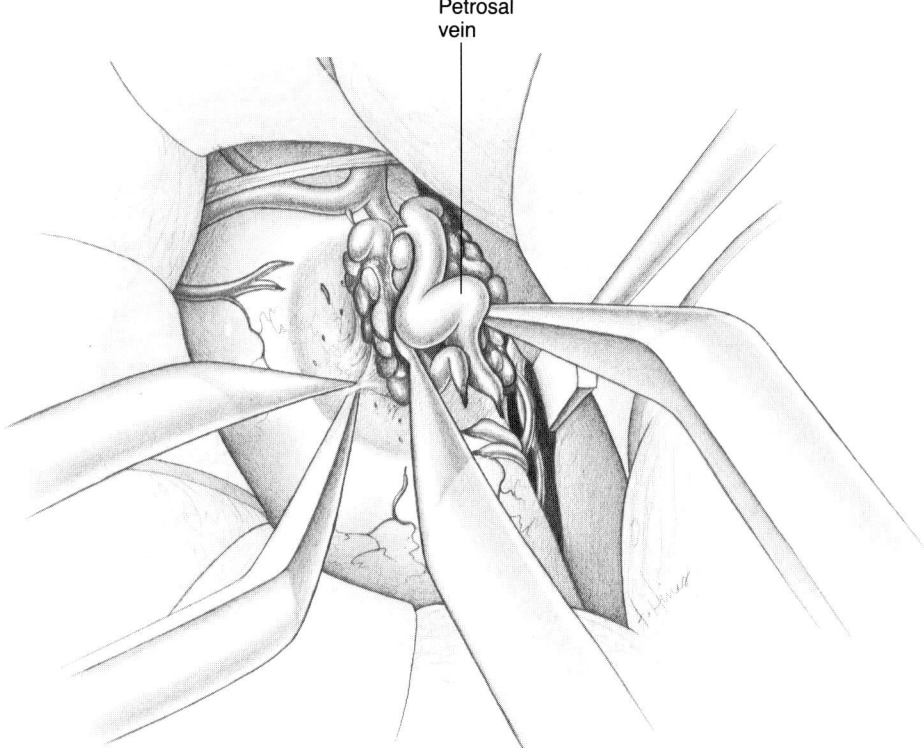

FIGURE 120-21. The bed of the malformation is inspected for bleeding sites. After the AVM is resected, the operative bed is inspected for bleeding sites. Meticulous hemostasis is essential to avoid a catastrophic postoperative hemorrhage. Intraoperative angiography is performed to ensure a complete resection of the AVM. (From Tew JM Jr, van Loveren HR: Atlas of Operative Microneurosurgery. Philadelphia, W. B. Saunders, 1994.)

moval of brainstem or deep-seated AVMs has not occurred and should be a diagnosis of exclusion. Most symptomatic ischemia results from inadvertent occlusion of normal arterial or venous vessels. Vasospasm with significant vessel stenosis is a rare cause of ischemia after surgical resection of AVMs.

Hemorrhage from poorly secured hemostasis, uncontrolled blood pressure, or residual tufts of malformation is the most devastating consequence of surgery on brainstem AVMs. A hematoma in the resection bed or cerebellum requires an urgent return to the operating room for its evacuation. Reperfusion phenomena from altered hemodynamics may cause ischemia and swelling to surrounding brain tissue. The tight confines of the brainstem tolerate very little edema formation, and transient obstructive hydrocephalus may develop. Obstructive hydrocephalus from brain swelling usually resolves and may be managed with a ventriculostomy.

POSTOPERATIVE MANAGEMENT

All patients are treated in the neuroscience intensive care unit. Complications in the postoperative period can often be anticipated and are preventable. The primary cause of postoperative hemorrhage, residual malformation, has been

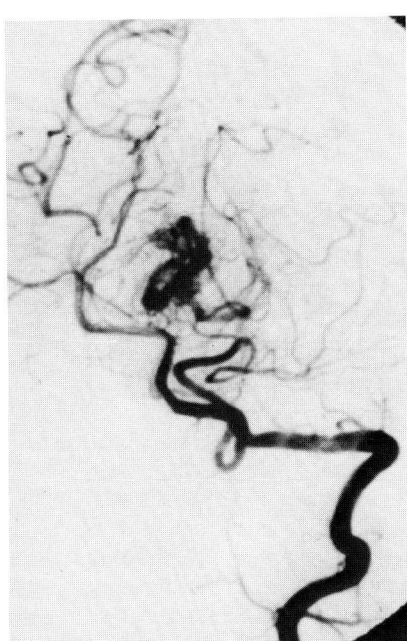

FIGURE 120-23. Vertebral angiogram in a 29-year-old woman shows a ruptured mesencephalic AVM fed by branches of the anteroinferior cerebellar artery and the superior cerebellar artery. Unlike cavernous angiomas that are intraparenchymal, brainstem AVMs are superficial or subpial in location.

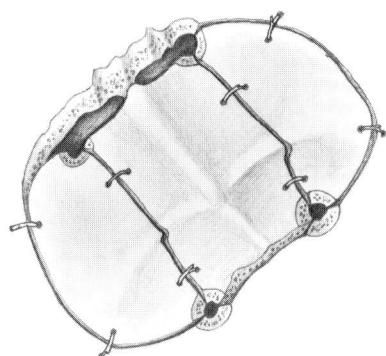

FIGURE 120-22. Closure is completed as for a bilateral suboccipital craniotomy using wires or alternatively a microplating system. (From Tew JM Jr, van Loveren HR: Atlas of Operative Microneurosurgery. Philadelphia, W. B. Saunders, 1994.)

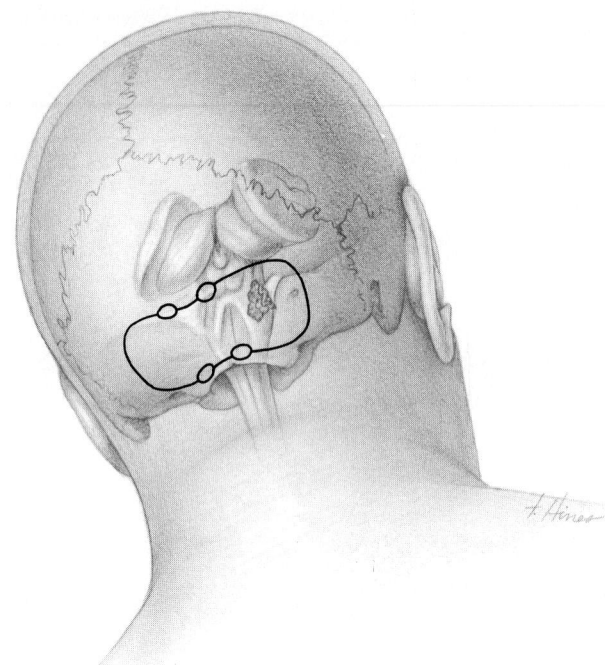

FIGURE 120-24. A lateral mesencephalic AVM located at the junction of the upper fourth ventricle and superior cerebellar peduncle is shown in relation to surrounding brainstem structures. The approach is superior vermian. (From Tew JM Jr, van Loveren HR: Atlas of Operative Microneurosurgery. Philadelphia, W. B. Saunders, 1994.)

mostly eliminated by use of intraoperative angiography and single-stage AVM removal. In the immediate postoperative period, regional cerebrovascular autoregulation may not protect the parenchyma surrounding large AVMs from reperfusion injury. We therefore maintain systemic hypotension for at least 72 hours postoperatively (mean arterial pressure, 60 to 70 mm Hg). Patients are prone to obstruction of the cerebral aqueduct from parenchymal swelling and may require steroids and a ventriculostomy. Recording of cranial nerves with injury action potentials during intraoperative monitoring alerts the surgeon to the possible need for a temporary tarsorrhaphy, tracheostomy, or gastrostomy postoperatively.

RESULTS

We have reviewed our experience (1984 to 1992) to evaluate the treatment and outcome of 36 patients with brainstem vascular malformations, 21 of whom were surgically treated and 15 of whom were conservatively treated. Among 28 cavernous angiomas, eight arteriovenous malformations, and six associated venous angiomas, most were located in the dorsal pons. Surgery was performed when the malformation was superficial to the brainstem surface or in cases of deteriorating neurologic status or repeat hemorrhage. The transvermian and lateral suboccipital approaches were used in all cases. Resection of venous angiomas was avoided. Among 21 surgical patients, 13 (62 percent) had transient worsening of their neurologic status, 5 (24 percent) suffered permanent neurologic deficits, and no mortality occurred. Permanent deficits included truncal ataxia (four patients), internuclear ophthalmoplegia (three patients), abducens palsy (two patients), paralysis of upward gaze (three patients), and nuclear facial weakness (two patients). Two patients suffered a recurrent hemorrhage from residual malformation. Overall, 19 of 21 (90 percent) surgical patients improved from their neurologic deficits and returned to independent living with good or excellent function. Of the 15 patients treated conservatively, 10 (67 percent) remained asymptomatic, three (20 percent) had minimal symptoms, and one (7 percent) suffered a major hemorrhage.

SUMMARY

Symptomatic brainstem vascular malformations have a propensity toward repeated hemorrhage. Although patients often improve substantially, nevertheless with each successive hemorrhage they are less likely to recover function. The goal of therapy is to eliminate the risk of hemorrhage without causing significant neurologic injury. Surgical excision is currently the best treatment for brainstem vascular malformations that are subpial and present with progressive neurologic deficit from recurrent hemorrhage. With appreciation for transient deficit, these lesions can be excised with acceptable permanent morbidity and no mortality.

Acknowledgment

The authors thank David Rini and Tonya Hines for illustrations and Marlene Ostrow and Mary Kemper for editorial assistance.

REFERENCES

1. Logue V, Monckton G: Posterior fossa angiomas. A clinical presentation of 9 cases. Brain 77:252–273, 1954
2. Ondra SL, Troupp H, George ED, et al: The natural history of symptomatic arteriovenous malformations of the brain: A 24-year follow-up assessment. J Neurosurg 73:387–391, 1990
3. Drake CG, Friedman AH, Peerless SJ: Posterior fossa arteriovenous malformations. J Neurosurg 64:1–10, 1986
4. Solomon RA, Stein BM: Management of arteriovenous malformations of the brainstem. J Neurosurg 64:857–864, 1986
5. Weil SM, Tew JM Jr: Surgical management of brain stem vascular malformations. Acta Neurochir (Wien) 105:14–23, 1990
6. Zimmerman RS, Spetzler RF, Lee KS, et al: Cavernous malformations of the brain stem. J Neurosurg 75:32–39, 1991
7. Russell DS, Rubenstein LJ: Pathology of Tumors of the Nervous System, 5th ed. Baltimore, Williams & Wilkins, 1989, pp 727–765
8. Abe M, Kjellberg RN, Adams RD: Clinical presentations of vascular malformations of the brain stem: Comparison of angiographically positive and negative types. J Neurol Neurosurg Psychiatry 52:167–175, 1989
9. McCormick WF, Hardman JM, Boulter TR: Vascular malformations (angiomas) of the brain, with special reference to those occurring in the posterior fossa. J Neurosurg 28:241–251, 1968
10. Garner TB, Curling OD Jr, Kelly DL, et al: The natural history of intracranial venous angiomas. J Neurosurg 75:715–722, 1991
11. Spetzler RF, Martin NA: A proposed grading system for arteriovenous malformations. J Neurosurg 65:476–483, 1986
12. Robinson JR, Awad IA, Little JR: Natural history of cavernous angioma. J Neurosurg 75:709–714, 1991
13. Humphries RP, Hendrick EB, Hoffman HJ: Arteriovenous malformations of the brainstem in childhood. Child's Brain 11:1–11, 1984

14. Scott MR, Barnes P, Kupsky W, Adelman LS: Cavernous angiomas of the central nervous system in children. J Neurosurg 76:38–44, 1992
15. Lobato RD, Rivas JJ, Gomez PA, et al: Comparison of the clinical presentation of symptomatic arteriovenous malformations (angiographically visualized) and occult vascular malformations. Neurosurgery 31:391–397, 1992
16. La Torre E, Delitala A, Sorano V: Hematoma of the quadrigeminal plate. J Neurosurg 49:610–613, 1978
17. Kashiwagi S, van Loveren HR, Tew JM Jr, et al: Diagnosis and treatment of vascular brain-stem malformations. J Neurosurg 72:27–34, 1990
18. Bertalanffy H, Gilsbach JM, Eggert HR, Seeger W: Microsurgery of deep seated cavernous angiomas: Report of 26 cases. Acta Neurochir (Wien) 13:204–207, 1991
19. Fahlbusch R, Strauss C, Huk W, et al: Surgical removal of pontomesencephalic cavernous hemangiomas. Neurosurgery 26:449–457, 1990
20. Beatty RM, Zervas NT: Stereotactic aspiration of a brainstem hematoma. Neurosurgery 13:204–207, 1983
21. Bosch DA, Beute GN: Successful stereotaxic evacuation of an acute pontomedullary hematoma. Case report. J Neurosurg 62:153–156, 1985
22. Davis DH, Kelly PJ: Stereotactic resection of occult vascular malformations. J Neurosurg 72:698–702, 1990
23. Ogilvy CS, Heros RC, Ojemann RG, et al: Angiographically occult arteriovenous malformations. J Neurosurg 69:350–355, 1988
24. Batjer H, Samson D: Arteriovenous malformations of the posterior fossa. J Neurosurg 64:849–856, 1986
25. Konovalov A, Spallone A, Makhmudov UB: Surgical management of hematomas of the brain stem. J Neurosurg 73:181–186, 1990
26. Sisti MB, Solomon RA, Stein BM: Stereotactic craniotomy in the resection of small arteriovenous malformations. J Neurosurg 75:40–44, 1991
27. Spetzler RF, Wilson CB, Weinstein P, et al: Normal perfusion pressure breakthrough theory. Clin Neurosurg 25:651–672, 1978

CHAPTER 121

Surgical Management of Thalamic–Basal Ganglia Vascular Malformations

Kenneth W. Reichert II
Adam I. Lewis
John M. Tew, Jr.

The management of vascular malformations in the thalamic–basal ganglia region continues to challenge neurologists and neurosurgeons. Because of their location near vital neural structures, these lesions have been classified as inoperable by some neurologic surgeons.[1] Treatment options include observation, embolization, radiosurgery, and surgical extirpation; however, because rupture of a vascular malformation in this critical location can lead to catastrophic intracranial hemorrhage, complete surgical removal is the preferred treatment. Drake first documented that removal of vascular malformations in the anterior and posterosuperior thalamus could be accomplished without producing devastating neurologic deficits.[2] The later reports of Solomon and Stein,[3] Shi and Chen,[4] Malik and coworkers,[5] and Matsushima and coworkers[6] confirm the successful surgical treatment of thalamic–basal ganglia vascular malformations.

In this chapter, we describe 59 patients treated for 60 vascular malformations, including 12 cavernous angiomas of the thalamic–basal ganglia region. The evaluation, management considerations, surgical techniques, and results of our experience are reviewed.

PRESENTATION

The clinical presentation of vascular malformations in the nonepileptogenic region of the deep brain is usually profound neurologic deficit secondary to hemorrhage. The clinical presentations of 60 thalamic–basal ganglia vascular malformations are illustrated in Table 121–1, and presenting deficits are summarized in Table 121–2.

EVALUATION

Patients undergo a preoperative evaluation that includes a complete neurologic and physical examination. Visual field testing is essential to evaluate the medial optic radiations often involved in lesions of this region. Neuropsychological testing, especially in dominant hemisphere malformations, is used to evaluate cognitive and memory deficits.

Computed tomography (CT) assists in the initial evaluation of acute hemorrhage to ascertain its intraparenchymal and intraventricular extension. Initial and subsequent evaluation of associated hydrocephalus is easily assessed with CT scanning. The role of magnetic resonance imaging (MRI) in the evaluation of thalamic–basal ganglia vascular malformations is essential to define the relationship of the malformation and its hemorrhage to the associated anatomic structure and ventricular system. Cerebral angiography further defines the vascular anatomy of arteriovenous malformations (AVMs), including nidus size and the differentiation of a diffuse versus a well-defined nidus. Associated vascular anomalies, especially arterial and venous aneurysms, and venous angiomas are also identified with angiography. Venous anatomy, with deep drainage and veins in the access path for the transcallosal approach, is also identified.

VASCULAR ANATOMY

Most AVMs in the thalamic–basal ganglia region are supplied by two or more major arterial systems. Table 121–3

Table 121–1. CLINICAL PRESENTATION OF THALAMIC–BASAL GANGLIA ARTERIOVENOUS MALFORMATIONS (n = 48) AND CAVERNOUS ANGIOMAS (n = 12)

Presentation	Arteriovenous Malformations		Cavernous Angiomas	
	n	%	n	%
Hemorrhage	42*	88	10†	84
Intracerebral	22	—	8	—
Intraventricular and intracerebral	13	—	2	—
Intraventricular	7	—	0	—
Headaches	3	6	1	8
Transient ischemia	1	2	0	0
Asymptomatic	2	4	1	8
Total	48	100	12	100

* Fifteen (31%) patients had multiple hemorrhages.
† Three (30%) patients had multiple hemorrhages.

Table 121–2. PRESENTING DEFICITS IN 60 THALAMIC–BASAL GANGLIA VASCULAR MALFORMATIONS

Deficit	n	%
Paralysis	33	55
Dysphasia	16	27
Hydrocephalus	14	23
Hemianopsia	14	23
Sensory	14	23
Cognitive or memory	10	17
Tremor	6	10
Ataxia	5	8
No deficit	7	12

Table 121–4. VENOUS DRAINAGE FOR 48 THALAMIC–BASAL GANGLIA ARTERIOVENOUS MALFORMATIONS

Vein	n	%
Internal cerebral vein	32	67
Vein of Galen	7	15
Thalamostriate vein	7	15
Basal vein of Rosenthal	6	13
Sylvian vein	2	4

summarizes the vascular supply of 48 AVMs. The thalamoperforate arteries, demonstrated radiographically in only 18 (38 percent) cases, were found to supply the deep aspect of all thalamic AVMs.

Venous drainage is deep and toward the midline. Solomon and Stein reported on a case of drainage to the superior sagittal sinus by way of the interhemispheric fissure,[3] but in our series, all caudothalamic malformations drained to the deep venous system. Lesions in the external capsule–striatum region are drained by the sylvian vein system. Table 121–4 summarizes the venous drainage for these 48 AVMs. Three cases of venous drainage to septal and striothalamic veins produced obstruction of the foramen of Monro, with subsequent loculated hydrocephalus.

SIZE

Nidus size ranged from 1 to 7 cm (mean, 2.8 cm). Of these, 31 (52 percent) were small (<3 cm); 25 (41 percent) were medium-sized (3 to 6 cm); and four (7 percent) were large (>6 cm).

MANAGEMENT CONSIDERATIONS

When the diagnosis of a vascular malformation is established, treatment should offer a balance between the natural history of the disease and the expected outcome of the various treatments designed specifically for each patient. Treatment options include observation, endovascular obliterative techniques, stereotactic radiosurgery, and surgery. A team approach provides the best option for the patient.

AVMs of the basal ganglia–thalamic region are rare, representing only 2 to 3 percent of all AVMs.[2] The natural history of symptomatic AVMs carries a 2- to 4-percent risk per year of recurrent hemorrhage after the first year.[7,8] A 6-percent rate of hemorrhage during the first year is reported in Wilkins' review.[8] Combined major morbidity and mortality is 2.7 percent per year.[9] Each hemorrhage episode is associated with a 10-percent risk of death and a 30-percent risk of major morbidity. Symptomatic lesions in this series tended to be associated with a higher risk of recurrent hemorrhage than were malformations in other areas of the brain. The recurrent hemorrhage rate in symptomatic thalamic–basal ganglia AVMs in our series is 5.9 percent per year. The natural history of cavernous angiomas is not completely known, but some investigators have reported that these angiomas have a less than 1-percent chance per year of hemorrhage.[10] The recurrent hemorrhage rate in symptomatic thalamic–basal ganglia cavernous angiomas in this series is 15.4 percent per year. The risk of conservative management extends over the course of the patient's lifetime and must be weighed against a presumed one-time surgical risk. The weight of evidence supports the conclusion that the natural history of ruptured and nonruptured AVMs and ruptured cavernous angiomas is not benign and warrants intervention in most circumstances. Observation as a management option for asymptomatic cavernous angiomas is supported by its more benign natural history.

The target for embolization of AVMs includes its terminal arteries, deep perforating arteries, and associated proximal aneurysms. In this study, embolization of the distal branches from the middle cerebral, anterior and posterior choroidal, P1, P2, and proximal aneurysms facilitates the safe, intraoperative removal of these lesions by preoperative control of the deep arterial supply and reduction of their vascular turgor. Elimination of the deep perforator vessels helps to decrease the risk of late operative bleeding problems and enhances the probability of complete removal.

Stereotactic radiosurgery with the gamma knife and the linear accelerator is reported to obliterate AVMs with a 79.2- to 84.1-percent success rate at 2 years.[11–14] Protection by partial obliteration of an AVM is not documented. A 3-percent permanent morbidity from radiation necrosis is reported.[15] Radiosurgery is an option for lesions that are less than 3 cm initially or those reduced to this size by embolization. The major drawbacks of radiation are the long latency between treatment and obliteration of the malformation, less than complete obliteration in 20 percent of cases, and the unknown long-term effects. Patients with thalamic–basal ganglia AVMs should be considered for stereotactic radiosurgery if their lesions are unruptured, asymptomatic, or less than 3 cm in diameter; if their lesions pose unacceptable operative risks; or if the patient prefers this treatment. Radiosurgery for cavernous angiomas cannot be recommended be-

Table 121–3. ARTERIAL SUPPLY TO 48 THALAMIC–BASAL GANGLIA ARTERIOVENOUS MALFORMATIONS

Artery	n	%
Anterior choroidal	28	58
Posterior choroidal	27	56
Lenticulostriate arteries	20	42
Thalamoperforate arteries	18	38
Pericallosal branch arteries	8	17
Posterior cerebral artery branches	4	8
Recurrent artery of Heubner	2	4

cause no evidence in the literature indicates that such treatment changes their natural history.

Surgery for thalamic–basal ganglia region vascular malformations offers the patient amelioration of disease with low morbidity. These lesions carry a 4- to 12-percent morbidity, based on Spetzler's grading system.[16] For practical purposes, lesions of the thalamic–basal ganglia region are grade III or greater because of the location in eloquent brain and deep venous drainage. All patients who have a ruptured AVM and failed radiosurgical obliteration of an AVM should be considered for surgery. Cavernous angiomas should be considered for surgical removal when they present with recurrent symptomatic hemorrhage. Vascular malformations of this region are not usually associated with epilepsy, however, the malformation or hemorrhage may extend into the cortical regions of the temporal and frontal brain. In these cases, epilepsy may be an indication for surgical treatment.

SURGICAL CONSIDERATIONS

Vascular malformations of the thalamus and caudate are located lateral and inferior to the lateral ventricle and occasionally extend into the third ventricle. Laterally placed lesions just medial to the internal capsule are most accessible. Dorsomedial and ventromedial caudothalamic lesions are more difficult to approach surgically because of the involvement of the limbic system, the hypothalamus, and the deep venous system. Central and medial lesions are the most difficult to extirpate. Thalamic–basal ganglia vascular malformations can be approached by the following approaches: transcallosal-transventricular, transcortical-transventricular, or transsylvian. Stereotactically guided craniotomy assists in locating lesions for which ventricular anatomy does not allow orientation.

TRANSCALLOSAL-TRANSVENTRICULAR APPROACH

The transcallosal-transventricular approach is preferred for vascular malformations in the lateral ventricle, choroid plexus, and dorsomedial or ventromedial caudothalamic regions. This medial approach allows access to the major arterial and venous components of the malformation before surgical removal is initiated—an advantage not offered by other exposures. A subchoroidal approach may be added to remove lesions extending into the third ventricular area. However, the transcallosal-transventricular approach offers limited lateral exposure for lesions that extend into the atrium and temporal horn region.

TRANSCORTICAL-TRANSVENTRICULAR APPROACH

The transcortical-transventricular approach offers access to laterally placed vascular malformations of the caudate and thalamus that extend to the internal capsule and proceed into the atrium and temporal horn of the lateral ventricle. This exposure avoids the medial structures previously mentioned. A frontal trajectory is undertaken for lesions in the anterior thalamus and caudate. An approach through the parietal occipital fissure to lesions located in the posterior thalamus region is preferred. The major disadvantage for this trajectory is transection of the mesial optic radiations. Many of these lesions have associated parenchymal hematoma with preoperative visual field deficits. A hematoma provides access to and aids in the dissecting of the nidus of the malformation from the surrounding brain and facilitates surgical removal. Mesial optic radiation can be spared and ample exposure gained by operating through the temporal lobe. Superior,[2] middle,[17, 18] and inferior temporal gyrus[19] approaches have been advocated. The only difficulty in using these exposures is related to the early exposure of the AVM on its lateral surface, whereas the blood supply and venous drainage are on the medial surface. Consequently, the surgeon must remove a tense malformation and may secure arterial feeders supplying the lesion only during the latter part of extirpation. Preoperative embolization and other adjunctive techniques may overcome the disadvantages of this approach.

TRANSSYLVIAN APPROACH

The transsylvian approach is preferred for lesions presenting in the area of the striatum and external capsule. Because these lesions are supplied by the middle cerebral artery, proximal control of the blood supply can be obtained with this exposure. In their experience with sylvian fissure AVMs, Sugita and colleagues[20] report difficulty in controlling the anterior and posterior choroidal arteries with this approach; a single death occurred after the removal of an AVM located in the basal ganglia. The addition of a subtemporal exposure gives access to the posterior choroidal artery. The anterior choroidal artery should be followed through the choroidal fissure to its arterial supply of the AVM. Surgical exposures of these malformations are often difficult because of their deep location, especially those located posteriorly in the dominant hemisphere.

STEREOTACTICALLY GUIDED CRANIOTOMY APPROACH

Stereotactically guided craniotomies provide an accurate approach to small vascular malformations near critical anatomic structures. The operative approach is determined by preoperative radiographic studies. The surgical corridor is ideally through a deep sulcus. Stereotactic guidance is applied through the transcortical approach for removal of the laterally placed lesions when the midline structures are not visualized. When AVMs are found in the hypothalamic or capsular regions, this technique is a valid consideration. CT or MRI are effective for localizing small malformations or their associated hematomas. Stereotactic angiography is seldom needed because CT scanning and MRI can detect even small malformations and associated hematomas; therefore, the coordinates can be generated for localization. The stereotactic device should be simple, preferably with an articulating arm or an arc that can move in and out of the operative field during surgery. The stereotactic probe defines the site of skin incision, craniotomy, cortical incision, and trajectory through the brain to the malformation surface.

ANESTHETIC CONSIDERATIONS

The assistance offered by neuroanesthesia to remove deep-seated vascular malformations is invaluable to the neurosurgeon. Preoperative preparation includes arterial, central venous, electrocardiographic, and mass spectroscopic monitoring. A lumbar-subarachnoid drain is placed to assist in cerebrospinal fluid extraction. Osmotic diuretics (mannitol, 0.5 to 1 g/kg) and loop diuretics (furosemide, 10 to 20 mg) may be given to assist in brain relaxation. Steroids (dexamethasone [decadron], 5 to 10 mg) and barbiturates (thiopental [pentothal], 3 to 5 mg/kg and etomidate, 0.2 to 0.6 mg/kg) aid in cerebral protection. Intraoperative hypotension (mean arterial pressure of 50 to 60 mm Hg) caused by nitroprusside administration is essential to decrease blood flow in the AVM, reduce hemorrhage, and allow easier surgical manipulation.

ADJUNCTS TO SURGERY

Microneurosurgery has enabled the neurosurgeon to safely resect deep-seated vascular malformations. The use of microretractors on the Budde Halo retractor system (Ohio Medical Instruments Company, Cincinnati, OH) allows the surgeon to manipulate the wall of the nidus and brain for hemostasis and visualization, keep both hands free for surgical dissection, and gain access to deep structures with minimal cerebral parenchymal retraction. The impedance-monitored bipolar (Radionics, Burlington, MA) with nonstick bayonet forceps aids in the coagulation of friable deep-feeding vessels. A separate set of bipolars is used only for AVMs to ensure maintenance of the nonstick tips. The potassium titanyl phosphate (KTP), neodymium:yttrium, aluminum, garnet (Nd:YAG), or carbon dioxide lasers are used to shrink the nidus to allow visualization around the malformation. The recently developed AVM microclips are useful for the temporary occlusion of vessels and the control of deep perforating vessels. More superficial arterial vessels may be easily coagulated.

Electrophysiologic monitoring with somatosensory and brainstem evoked responses aids the surgeon in localizing critical motor structures and assists in monitoring brain injury. Ultrasound localizes hematomas; the recent advancements of the Ultramark 9 with high-definition imaging upgrade (Advanced Technology Laboratories, Bothell, WA) enables the visualization of blood flow through cavernous angiomas. Colored Doppler ultrasonography assists in differentiating the direction of blood flow through the nidus. Intraoperative angiography is essential to documenting the complete removal of AVMs. Postoperative hemorrhage is seldom seen and repeat operation for residual malformation seldom necessary after successful intraoperative angiography.

SURGICAL TECHNIQUE

PRINCIPLES OF VASCULAR MALFORMATION RESECTION

Thalamic–basal ganglia vascular lesions are resected through techniques similar to those used for other malformations. Dissection of the AVM begins by correlation of the anatomy to diagnostic studies and proceeds to identification, isolation, and occlusion of the arterial feeders. The multiple small lenticulostriate and thalamoperforating arteries from M1, A1, P1, and P2 are reached last. Preoperative embolization of feeding arterial pedicles and intraoperative shrinkage of the nidus with color absorptive laser, bipolar coagulation, and hypotensive anesthesia greatly facilitate this dissection. Laser techniques are particularly helpful in the dissection and shrinkage of AVMs in the deep regions of the brain. The feeding vessels are obliterated by the use of bipolar coagulation and the KTP-Nd:YAG laser. Bipolar coagulation obliterates larger vessels (>0.5 mm), and the carbon dioxide laser cuts the coagulated branches. The KTP-Nd:YAG laser, which is selectively absorbed by the color red (hemoglobin), effectively closes the small, delicate perforating vessels and shrinks the overall mass of vascular tissue. Total resection of the vascular malformation in one stage is always the objective because staged procedures are associated with recurrent early hemorrhage. We recommend positioning the patient to reduce venous pressure, to decrease the need for brain retraction, and to optimize the trajectory to the lesion.

Definition of the gliotic capsule between the lesion and normal brain maintains the proper surgical plane for complete resection. Arterial supply is obliterated close to the nidus, thereby preventing destruction of normal cerebrum by chasing hemorrhaging vessels into the parenchyma. Preservation of the major venous drainage until the arterial supply is extirpated prevents rupture of the nidus from obstructive blood flow. Retraction of the malformation for exposure and nidus hemostasis allows progression to complete extirpation.

TRANSCALLOSAL-TRANSVENTRICULAR APPROACH

The transcallosal-transventricular approach is chosen for malformations located anteromedially in the caudothalamic region. After the induction of general anesthesia, a lumbar drain is placed. The thorax of the patient's nonaffected side is elevated 15 degrees with a gelatin roll, and the head of the bed is elevated 20 degrees in reverse Trendelenburg. The cranium is maintained in a radiolucent head-fixation device and rotated with the affected side down until the sagittal suture is parallel to the floor; this measure allows minimal manual retraction of the interhemispheric fissure as gravity retracts the hemisphere. The inguinal region is prepared for intraoperative angiography.

The horseshoe-shaped skin incision outlines the 4×4-cm parasagittal craniotomy, which is situated to expose the sagittal sinus for medial retraction. The position of the craniotomy is measured, with the coronal suture used for orientation, to expose the area two thirds anterior and one third posterior to the lesion. A dural incision is based on the sagittal sinus. Bridging veins to the sagittal sinus should be spared when this cranial opening is performed (Fig. 121–1). Subpial dissection can be used to mobilize veins and enhance interhemispheric exposure. Relaxation is obtained with spinal drainage and diuretics.

Under microscopic assistance, the interhemispheric dissection is performed. We prefer to use 15-mm retractors on either side of the pericallosal arteries. The corpus callosum is incised 15 to 20 mm with the aid of the KTP-Nd:YAG

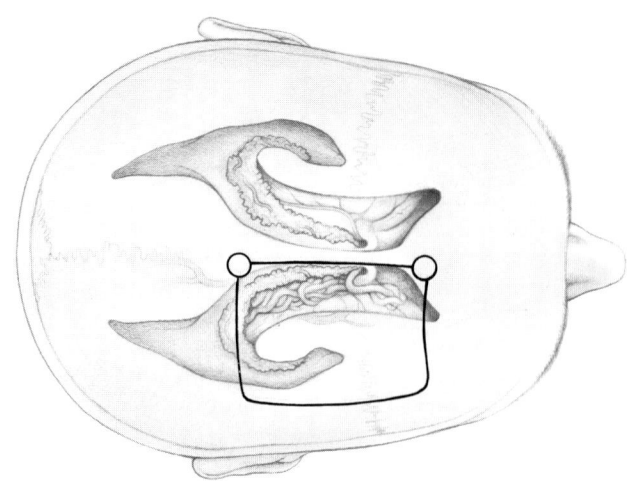

FIGURE 121-1. Craniotomy location for interhemispheric approach to medial caudothalamic vascular malformations. (From Tew JM, van Loveren HR: Atlas of Operative Microneurosurgery. Philadelphia, W. B. Saunders, 1993, p 26.)

laser (Fig. 121-2). The foramen of Monro is visualized for orientation as cerebrospinal fluid is aspirated from the ventricle. Medial caudothalamic vascular malformations are usually first visualized in the ventricle (Fig. 121-3). The patient's mean systemic blood pressure is lowered to 50 mm Hg as dissection begins.

Dissection of the nidus begins at its lateral border and proceeds along its lateral margin until the choroid plexus and malformation can be reflected medially (Fig. 121-4). Small feeding arteries and ependymal veins are coagulated and incised. The distal choroid plexus is coagulated and incised, as are posterior thalamostriate and ependymal veins. The striothalamic or caudate vein is coagulated and incised at the confluence of veins (Fig. 121-5). Intraoperative angiography is performed to document complete resection. If residual malformation is demonstrated, complete removal is accomplished in one surgical procedure.

If the malformation extends into the third ventricle, a subchoroidal approach can be used to expose the anterior third ventricle; this dissection proceeds lateral and posterior to the fornix, which should remain intact (Fig. 121-6). Dissection of the AVM proceeds by reflecting it laterally and posteriorly until the internal cerebral vein is encountered. After the entire arterial supply is removed, the internal cerebral vein is coagulated with bipolar forceps and cut. A second angiogram is performed to document complete removal.

The dura is reapproximated with interrupted sutures for a watertight closure. The craniotomy is secured in place with 28-gauge stainless steel wire. The galea is then closed with inverted interrupted suture and the skin aligned with surgical staples.

TRANSCORTICAL-TRANSVENTRICULAR APPROACH

The transcortical-transventricular approach is selected for large malformations located in the posterolateral region (thalamostriate) and extending into the atrium and posterior temporal horn. After induction of general anesthesia and lumbar drain placement, the patient is positioned supine with the thorax elevated to 15 degrees. The cranium is maintained in a radiolucent head-fixation device rotated so that the affected side is up and the sagittal suture is parallel to the floor. The

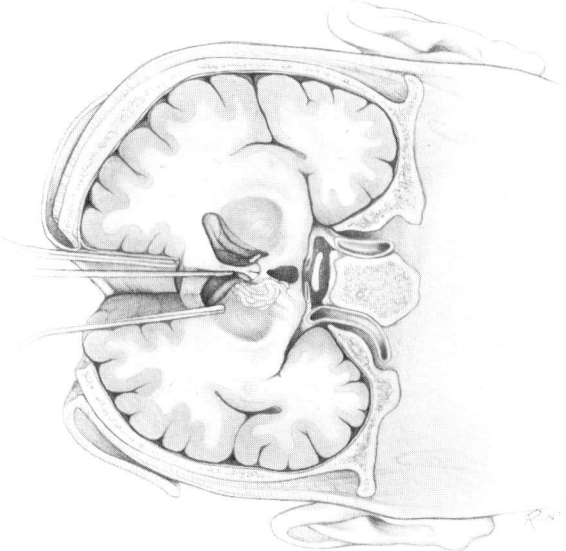

FIGURE 121-2. Coronal section demonstrates the trajectory to the malformation, hematoma, and anatomic structures. (From Tew JM, van Loveren HR: Atlas of Operative Microneurosurgery. Philadelphia, W. B. Saunders, 1993, p 262.)

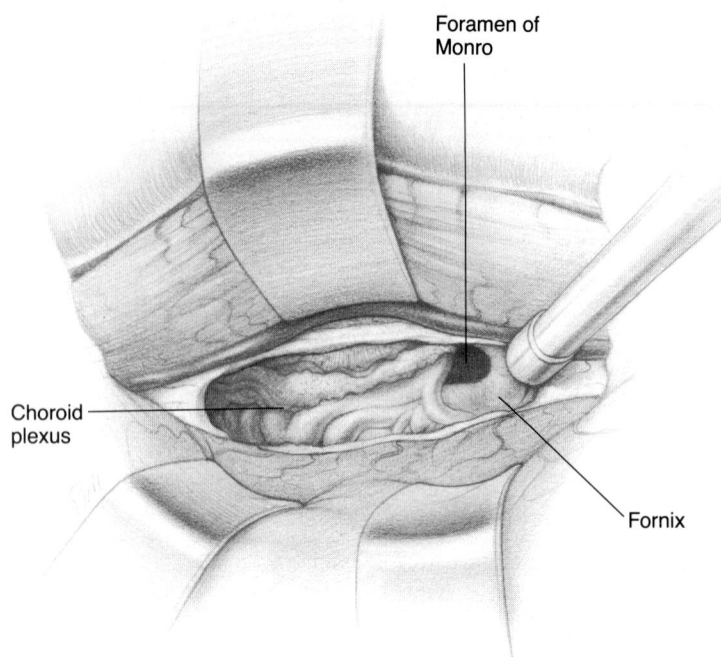

FIGURE 121–3. Interhemispheric trajectory shows intraventricular anatomy and medial aspect of AVM. (From Tew JM, van Loveren HR: Atlas of Operative Microneurosurgery. Philadelphia, W. B. Saunders, 1993, p 263.)

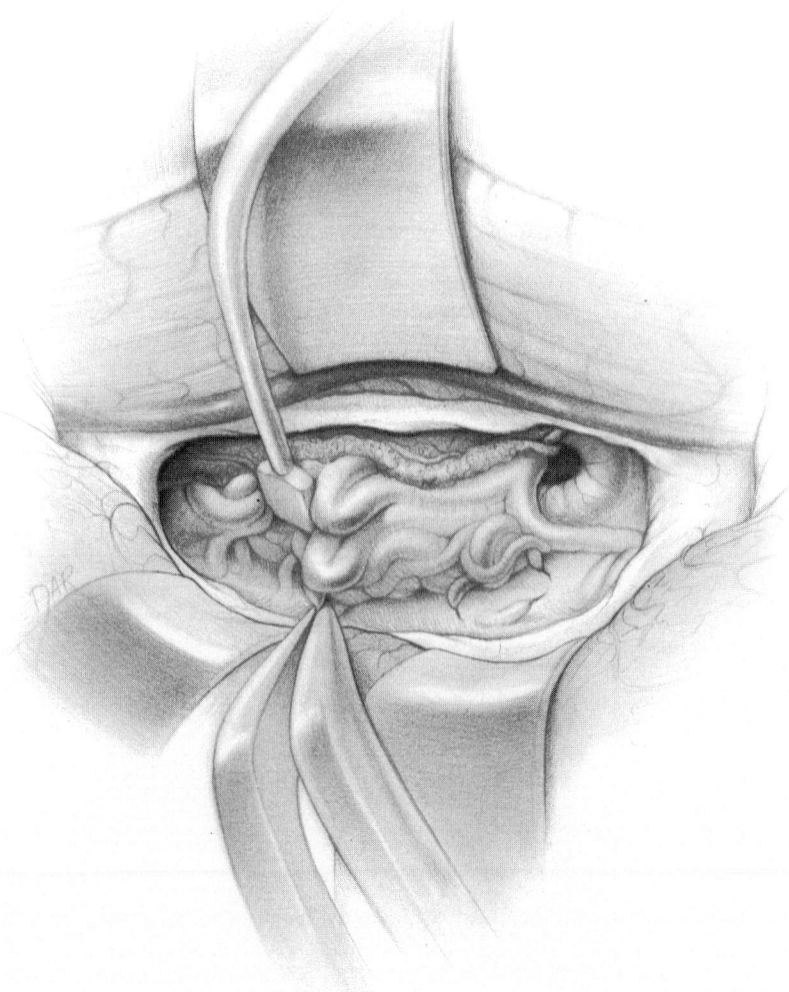

FIGURE 121–4. Lateral dissection of AVM is assisted by retracting the AVM medially with microretractors. (From Tew JM, van Loveren HR: Atlas of Operative Microneurosurgery. Philadelphia, W. B. Saunders, 1993, p 264.)

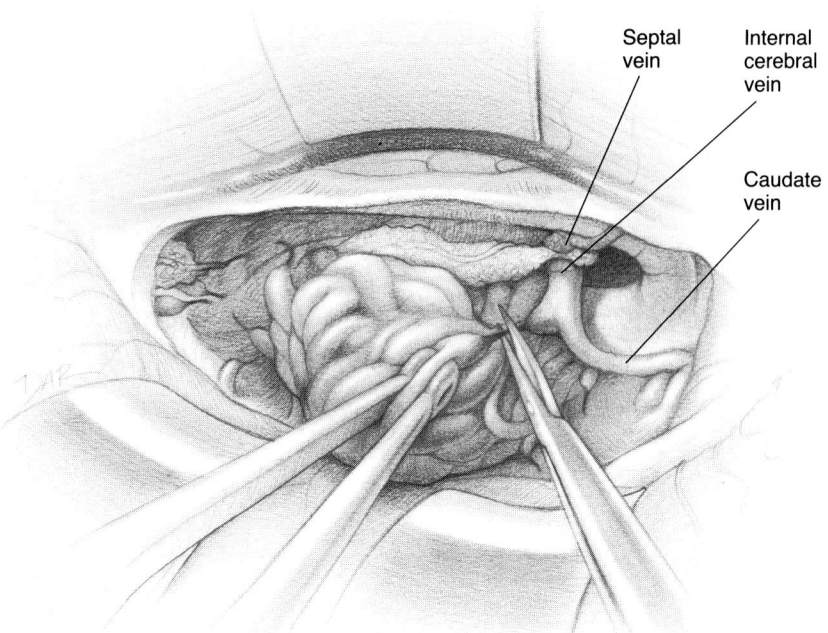

FIGURE 121–5. Medial venous anatomic structures draining AVM. (From Tew JM, van Loveren HR: Atlas of Operative Microneurosurgery. Philadelphia, W. B. Saunders, 1993, p 266.)

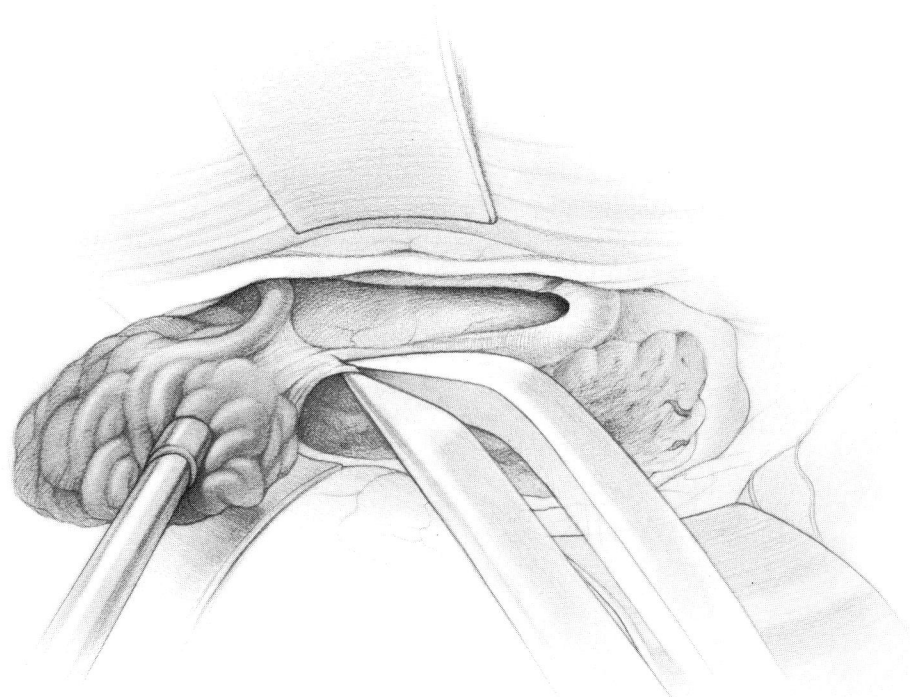

FIGURE 121–6. Subchoroidal exposure into the third ventricle allows complete excision of the AVM. (From Tew JM, van Loveren HR: Atlas of Operative Microneurosurgery. Philadelphia, W. B. Saunders, 1993, p 267.)

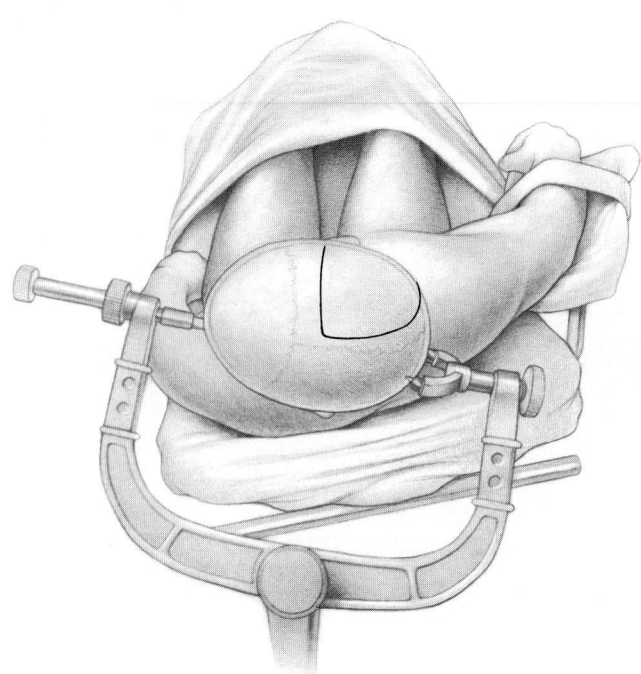

FIGURE 121–7. Surgical position for transcortical-transventricular approach to lateral caudothalamic AVM. (From Tew JM, van Loveren HR: Atlas of Operative Microneurosurgery. Philadelphia, W. B. Saunders, 1993.)

groin is prepared for intraoperative angiography (Fig. 121–7).

A parietal occipital skin flap (10 × 10 cm) is based on the inferior margin. An 8 × 8-cm bone flap ends 2 cm from the sagittal and transverse sinuses (Fig. 121–8). For frontal exposures, the lateral margin of the 10 × 10 cm skin flap is based on the sylvian fissure; the medial margin is 2 cm from the sagittal suture. The dural flap is reflected superiorly. Stereotactic guidance may also be beneficial in locating small, lateral AVMs.

To define a trajectory for exploration in parietal occipital approaches, a ventricular catheter is inserted into the sulcus of the parietal occipital fissure (Fig. 121–9) and passed through to the trigone of the ventricle. The cortical incision is made in the sulcus of the parietal occipital fissure, which is open to 30 mm and secured with four 10-mm, self-retaining retractors (Fig. 121–10). The pulvinar becomes visible in the depth of the cortical incision. Cerebrospinal fluid is aspirated from the cavity. The pulvinar, choroid plexus, and wall of the lateral ventricle are visualized by placing the retractors deeper into the cortical incision (Fig. 121–11). Mean arterial pressure is lowered to 50 mm Hg. The choroid plexus is obliterated with bipolar coagulation; the resection then proceeds inferiorly along the malformation base until the poste-

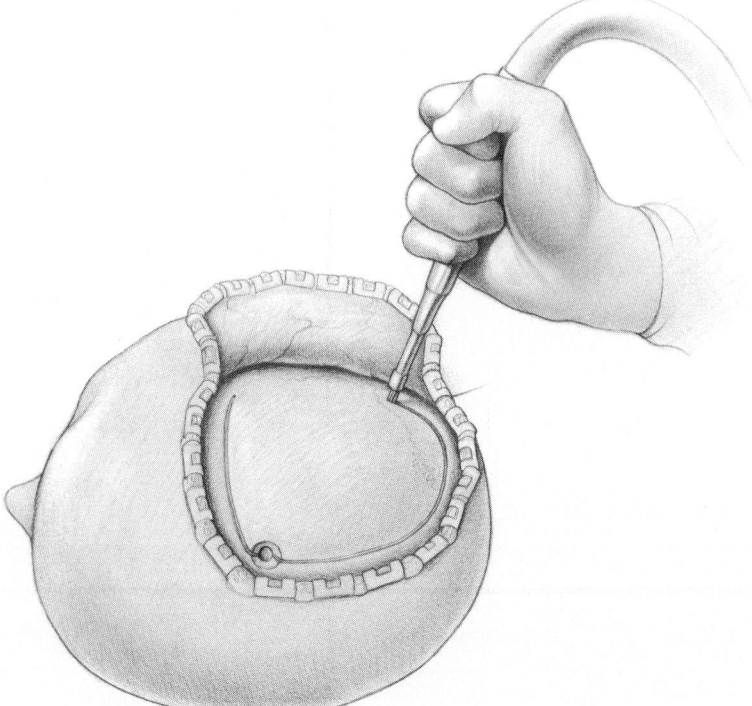

FIGURE 121–8. Skin incision and craniotomy for parietal occipital approach. (From Tew JM, van Loveren HR: Atlas of Operative Microneurosurgery. Philadelphia, W. B. Saunders, 1993, p 270.)

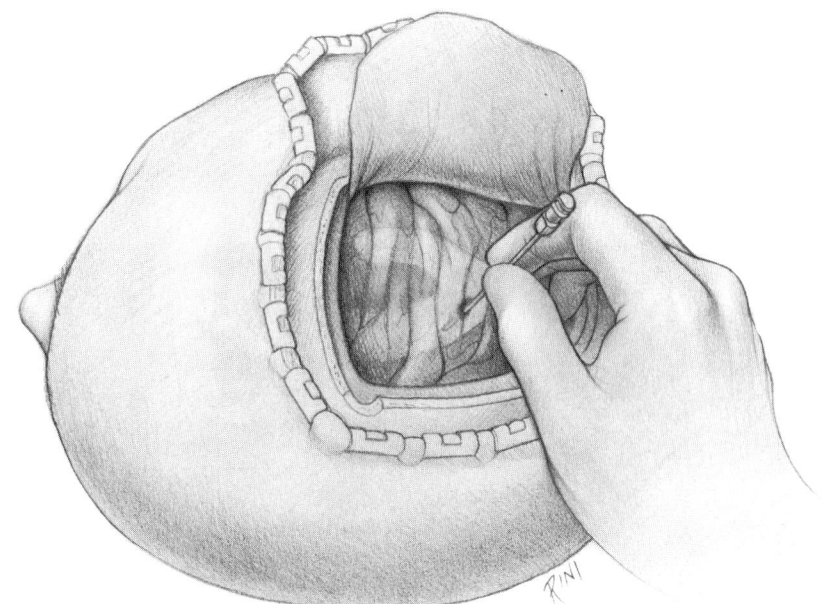

FIGURE 121–9. Dural opening and ventricular needle placement in the parieto-occipital fissure. (From Tew JM, van Loveren HR: Atlas of Operative Microneurosurgery. Philadelphia, W. B. Saunders, 1993, p 271.)

rior choroidal fissure is open (Fig. 121–12). Here, perforators from the posterior cerebral and posterior choroidal arteries are coagulated and incised. Dissection proceeds from the temporal horn across the nidus face and through the posterior hippocampus, posterior limb of the internal capsule, and thalamus, where the plane enters the lateral ventricle (Fig. 121–13). The striothalamic vein is retracted laterally as the nidus is reduced in volume (Fig. 121–14). The choroid plexus is coagulated, and the nidus mass is reflected medially to expose the foramen of Monro and the junction of the striothalamic and internal cerebral veins. The septum is then opened into the tela choroidea of the posterior third ventricle near the junction of the internal cerebral and galenic veins (Fig. 121–15). The internal cerebral vein is coagulated and excised (Fig. 121–16). After the fornix, internal cerebral vein, and wall of the third ventricle are reflected medially, the third and lateral ventricles and foramen of Monro are in view. The malformation is retracted laterally as dissection with the car-

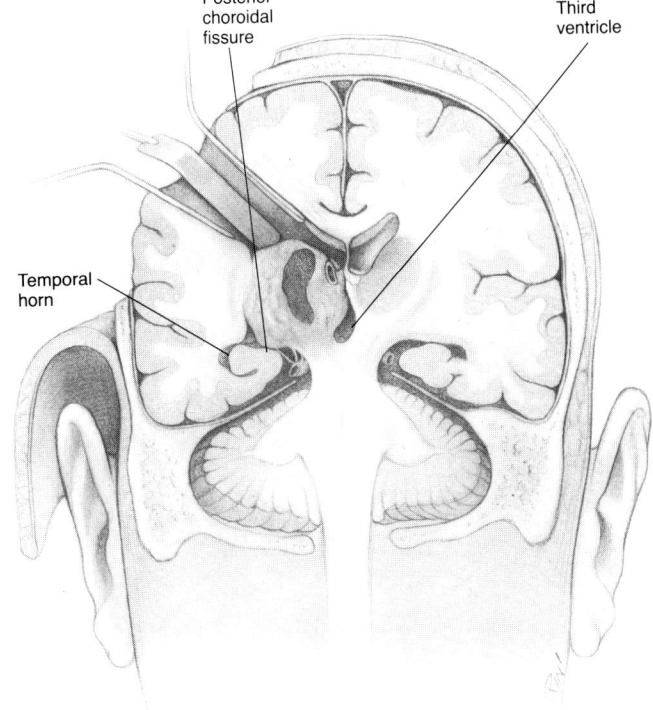

FIGURE 121–10. Coronal section illustrates the relationship of the malformation and hematoma to the ventricles, choroidal fissure, dorsal ganglia, and thalamus. (From Tew JM, van Loveren HR: Atlas of Operative Microneurosurgery. Philadelphia, W. B. Saunders, 1993, p 274.)

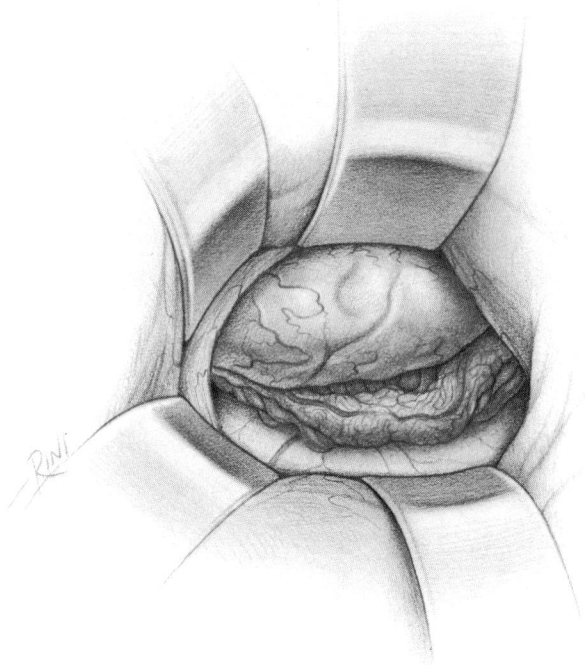

FIGURE 121–11. Transcortical view of the pulvinar, choroid plexus, and medial wall of the lateral ventricle. (From Tew JM, van Loveren HR: Atlas of Operative Microneurosurgery. Philadelphia, W. B. Saunders, 1993, p 275.)

FIGURE 121–12. The coronal section illustrates the trajectory of dissection through the temporal horn to isolate the posterior choroidal feeders and malformation base. (From Tew JM, van Loveren HR: Atlas of Operative Microneurosurgery. Philadelphia, W. B. Saunders, 1993, p 276.)

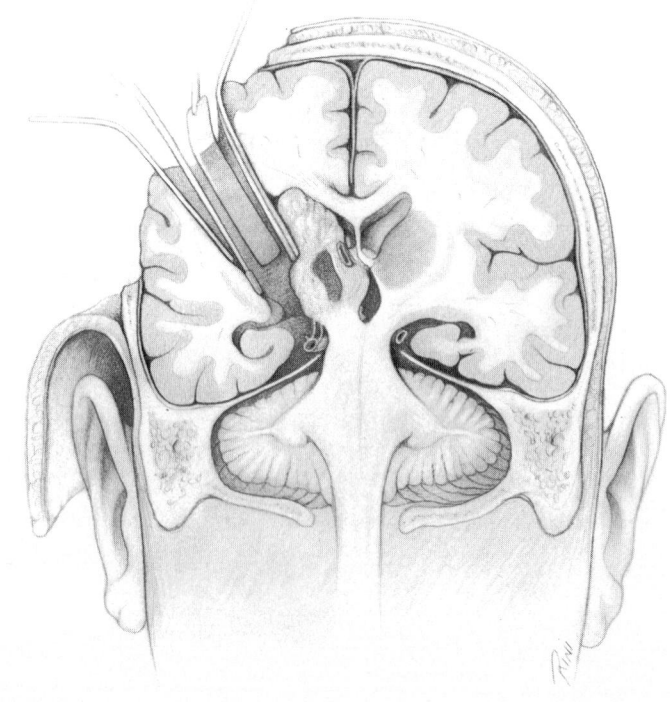

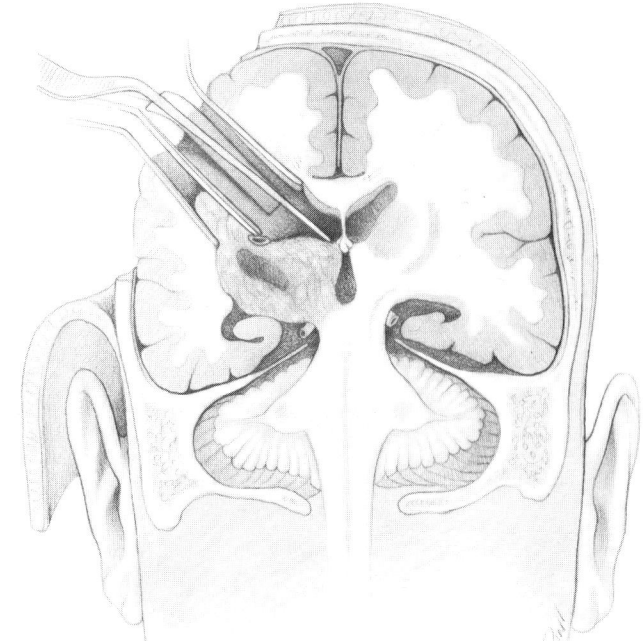

FIGURE 121–13. Coronal section shows the medial trajectory at dissection through the lateral ventricle. (From Tew JM, van Loveren HR: Atlas of Operative Microneurosurgery. Philadelphia, W. B. Saunders, 1993, p 277.)

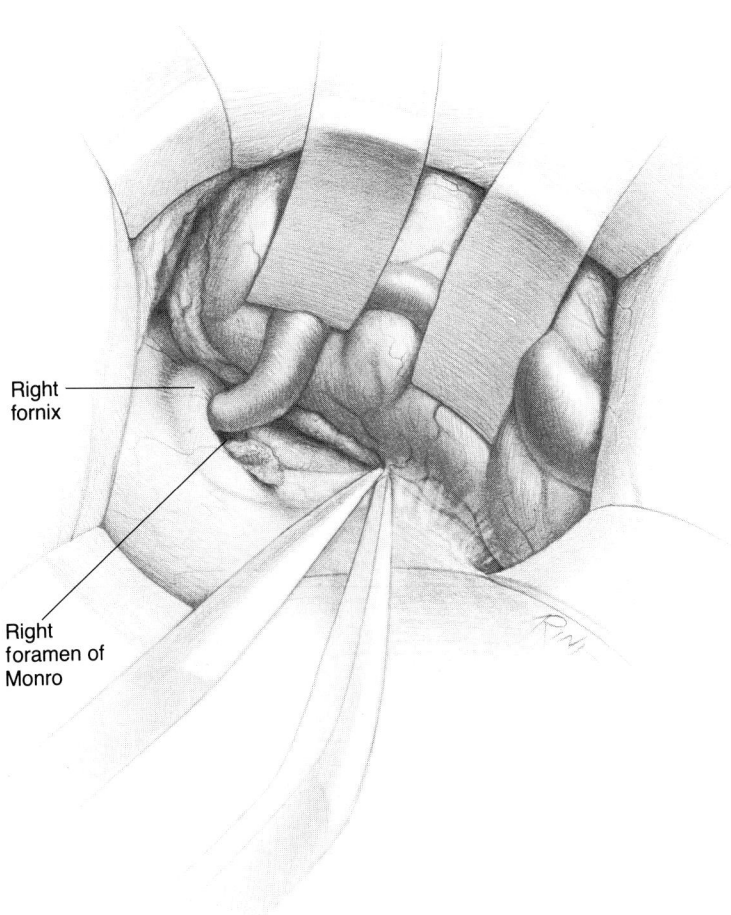

FIGURE 121–14. Lateral retraction of a dilated striothalamic vein aids in visualization of the nidus periphery. (From Tew JM, van Loveren HR: Atlas of Operative Microneurosurgery. Philadelphia, W. B. Saunders, 1993, p 278.)

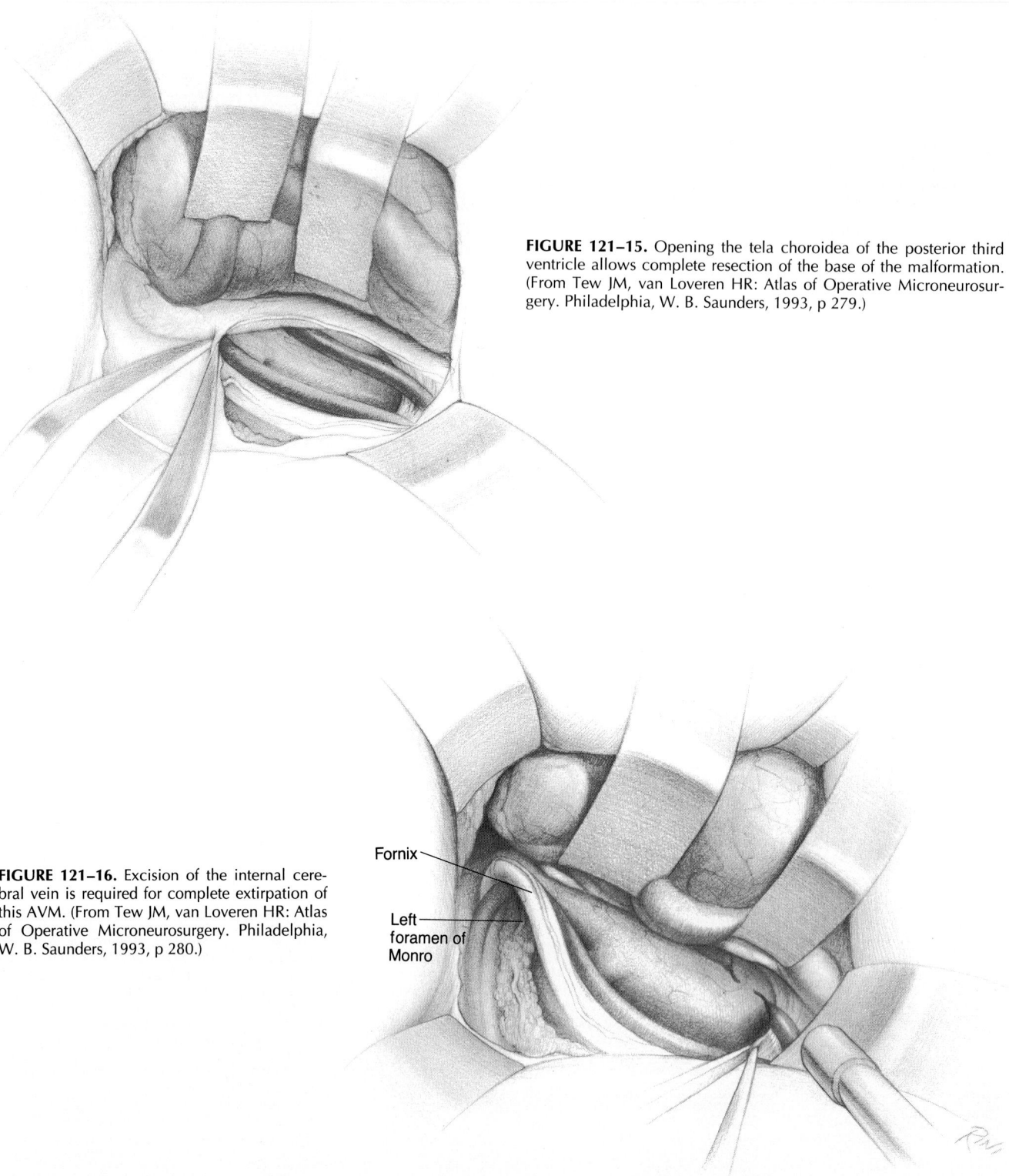

FIGURE 121–15. Opening the tela choroidea of the posterior third ventricle allows complete resection of the base of the malformation. (From Tew JM, van Loveren HR: Atlas of Operative Microneurosurgery. Philadelphia, W. B. Saunders, 1993, p 279.)

FIGURE 121–16. Excision of the internal cerebral vein is required for complete extirpation of this AVM. (From Tew JM, van Loveren HR: Atlas of Operative Microneurosurgery. Philadelphia, W. B. Saunders, 1993, p 280.)

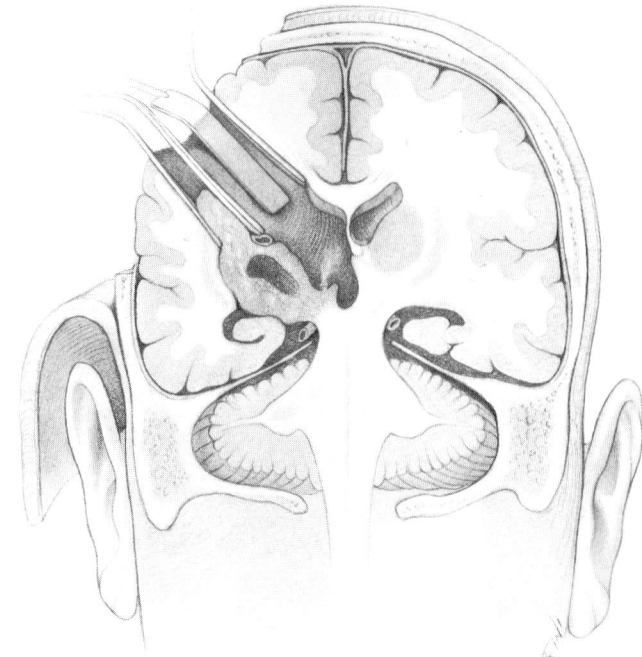

FIGURE 121–17. Coronal section shows the medial trajectory of dissection through the lateral third ventricle, floor of the lateral ventricle, and nidus base. (From Tew JM, van Loveren HR: Atlas of Operative Microneurosurgery. Philadelphia, W. B. Saunders, 1993, p 281.)

bon dioxide laser proceeds around the nidus margin (Fig. 121–17). Intraoperative angiography is performed to document complete excision.

Closure with interrupted sutures facilitates a tight dural closure. The bone flap is secured with 28-gauge wire. The galea is closed with inverted interrupted sutures, and the skin is realigned with surgical staples.

TRANSSYLVIAN APPROACH

The transsylvian approach is performed for laterally placed lesions that are fed by the branches of the anterior choroidal and middle cerebral arteries. These lesions are located in the lateral thalamus to the external capsule. With induction of general anesthesia and lumbar drain placement, the patient is positioned supine with the ipsilateral shoulder and the thorax elevated 15 degrees. The cranium is maintained in a radiolucent head-fixation device for intraoperative angiography and is rotated 45 degrees to the contralateral side. The groin is prepared for intraoperative angiography (Fig. 121–18).

A modified pterional craniotomy with a sylvian fissure extension is performed. The dura is widely excised to expose the sylvian fissure, inferior frontal lobe, and entire temporal lobe, thereby permitting wide dissection of the sylvian fissure; an infratemporal exposure is available if needed for further malformation removal. Circumferential dissection through the sylvian fissure, temporal horn, and choroidal fissure exposes the entire lesion (Fig. 121–19).

A Budde Halo self-retaining retractor system is attached to the skull-fixation device, and two 15-mm retractors are placed on opposite sides of the sylvian fissure. Cerebrospinal fluid is aspirated from the basal cisterns as the arachnoid is opened along the proximal middle cerebral artery. Mean systemic blood pressure is lowered to 50 mm Hg, and intravenous osmotic diuretics are infused to reduce intracranial volume. The sylvian veins and the M2 and M3 branches of the middle cerebral artery are identified (Fig. 121–20). An arachnoid plane is identified along the dorsal lateral aspect of the malformation. Arterial supply from the M1 branches can be isolated with bipolar coagulation. Additional retractors are placed on the medial temporal lobe as dissection continues along the lateral aspect of the malformation. The AVM is retracted medially, and draining veins are isolated from the sylvian vein as the medial aspect of the AVM is dissected. Dissection enters the medial aspect of the temporal horn, where the choroidal artery features are eliminated (Fig. 121–21). The AVM is retracted medially until the floor of the temporal horn is reached. Dissection proceeds to the posterior aspect of the AVM, permitting obliteration and incision of the posterior choroidal feeding arteries. The choroid plexus is separated from the AVM in the posterior temporal horn.

After retractors are removed from the sylvian fissure, two retractors are placed on the basal aspect of the temporal lobe (Fig. 121–22). Additional cerebrospinal fluid is withdrawn from the spinal catheter. Subpial dissection is initiated at the junction of the AVM and the inferior temporal gyrus (Fig. 121–23). The malformation is reflected inferiorly as the feeding vessels and glial connections are separated from it and as the final arterial and venous connections are divided between the basal temporal lobe and AVM. Here, the dissection joins the previous transsylvian approach. The malformation is reflected medially and retracted to expose the arterial feeding vessels that arise directly from the posterior cerebral artery. Medial branches of P2 can be coagulated and divided as they enter the malformation (Fig. 121–24). Draining veins, which course along the medial surface of the malformation, are coagulated and divided proximal to their entry into the basal vein (Fig. 121–25). The vein is incised, and the entire malformation is freed and removed. To ensure complete removal of the AVM, its cavity and exposed surfaces are inspected for bleeding sites, and intraoperative angiography is performed through the carotid and vertebral arteries.

Text continued on page 1518

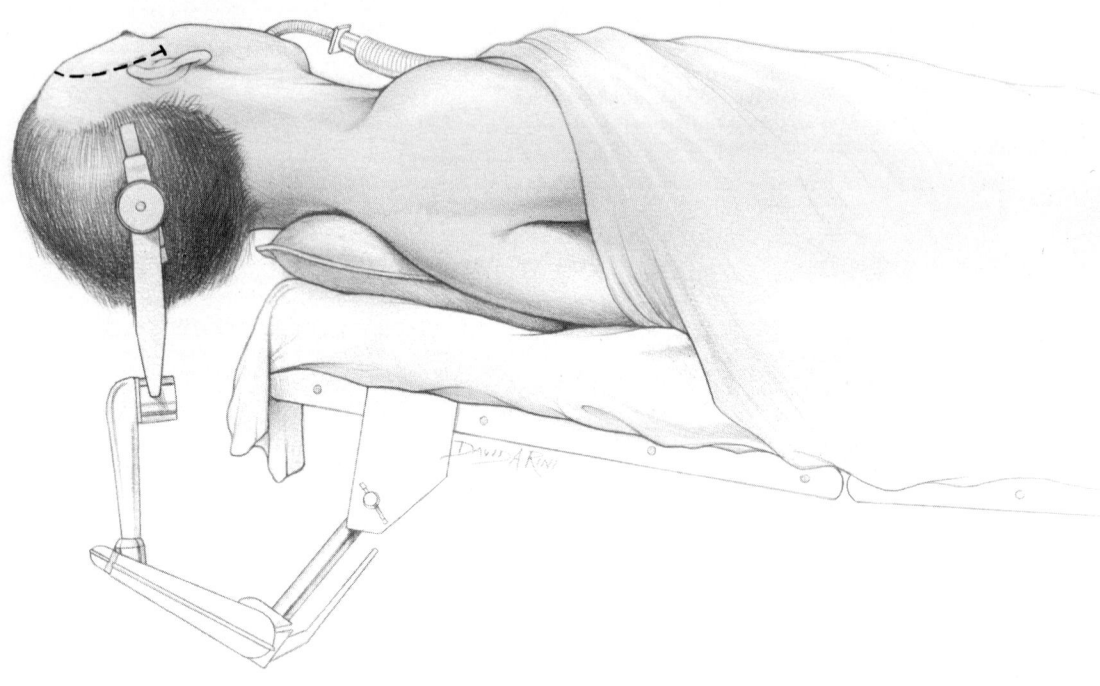

FIGURE 121–18. Patient position for transsylvian approach. (From Tew JM, van Loveren HR: Atlas of Operative Microneurosurgery. Philadelphia, W. B. Saunders, 1993, p 5.)

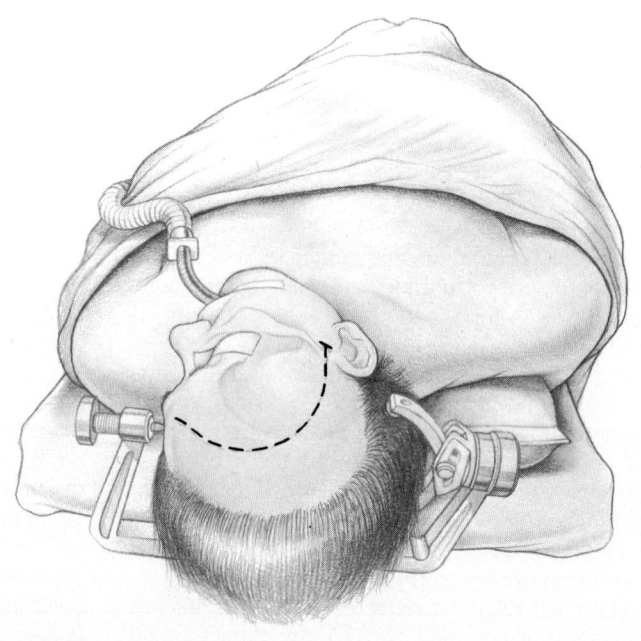

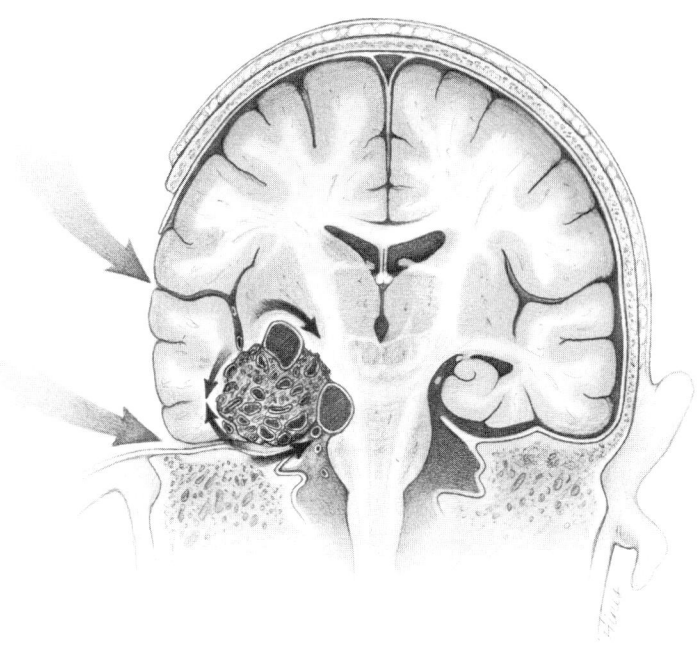

FIGURE 121–19. Coronal section shows the two trajectories needed to extirpate this medial AVM. Top arrow, transsylvian; bottom arrow, subtemporal. (From Tew JM, van Loveren HR: Atlas of Operative Microneurosurgery. Philadelphia, W. B. Saunders, 1993, p 254.)

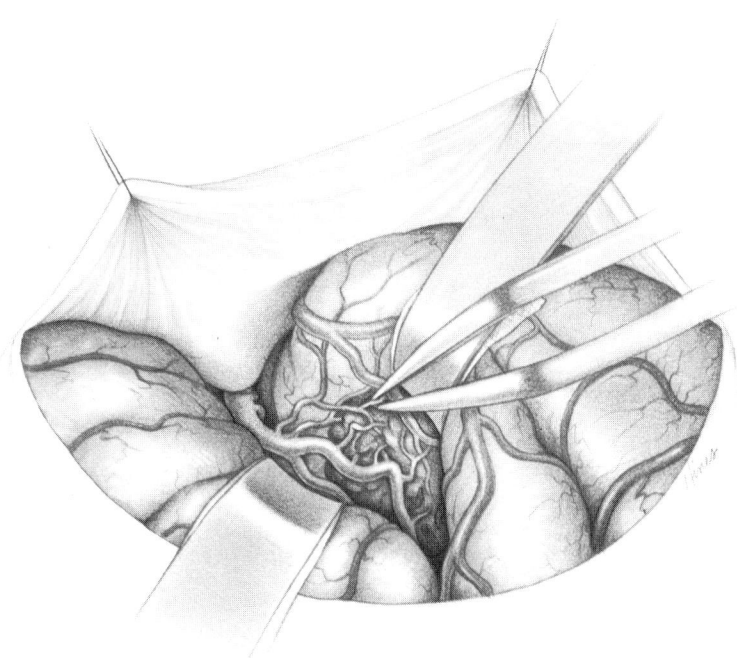

FIGURE 121–20. Transsylvian exposure allows branches from M2 and M3 to be coagulated and ligated. (From Tew JM, van Loveren HR: Atlas of Operative Microneurosurgery. Philadelphia, W. B. Saunders, 1993, p 255.)

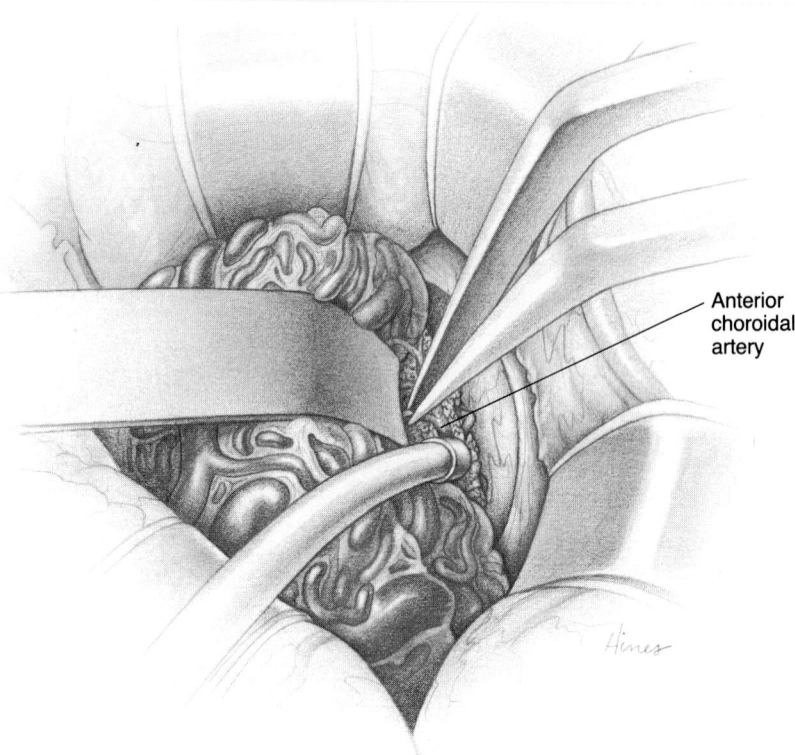

FIGURE 121–21. Medial dissection allows branches from the anterior choroidal artery to be identified and excised. (From Tew JM, van Loveren HR: Atlas of Operative Microneurosurgery. Philadelphia, W. B. Saunders, 1993, p 257.)

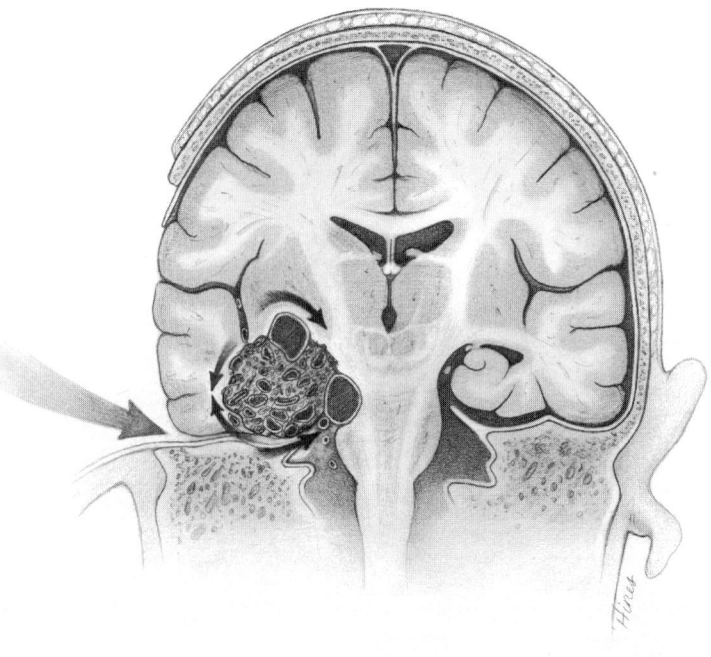

FIGURE 121–22. Coronal section demonstrates the subtemporal dissection trajectory. (From Tew JM, van Loveren HR: Atlas of Operative Microneurosurgery. Philadelphia, W. B. Saunders, 1993, p 258.)

FIGURE 121–23. Transsylvian view of the AVM with the choroid plexus at the lateral ventricle and inferior temporal gyrus exposed. (From Tew JM, van Loveren HR: Atlas of Operative Microneurosurgery. Philadelphia, W. B. Saunders, 1993, p 259.)

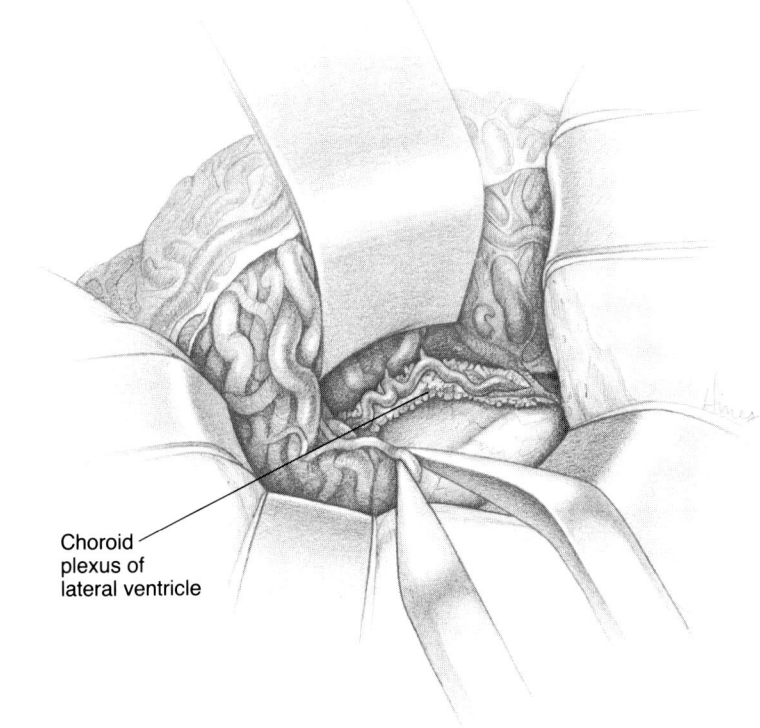

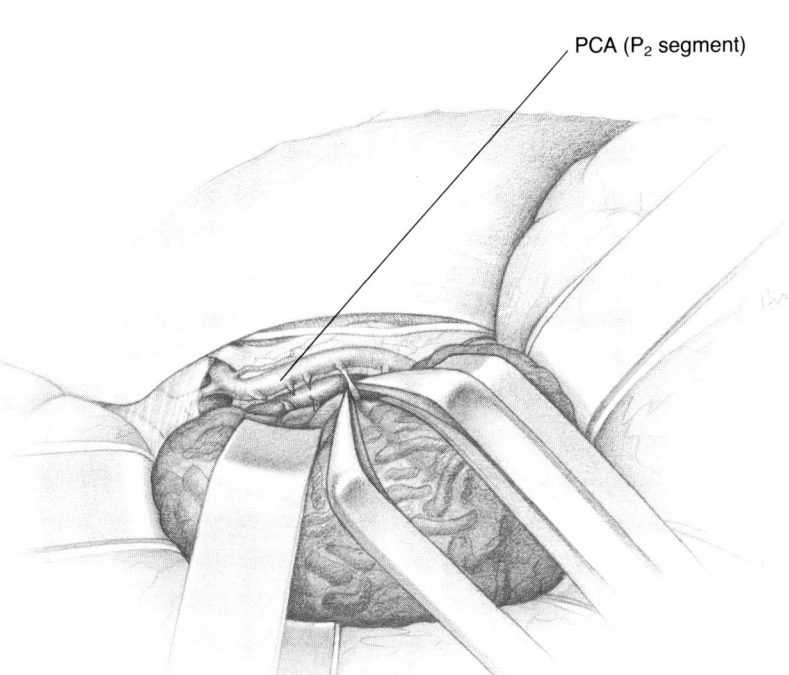

FIGURE 121–24. Subtemporal exposure allows posterior thalamoperforate arteries to be coagulated and excised. (From Tew JM, van Loveren HR: Atlas of Operative Microneurosurgery. Philadelphia, W. B. Saunders, 1993, p 259.)

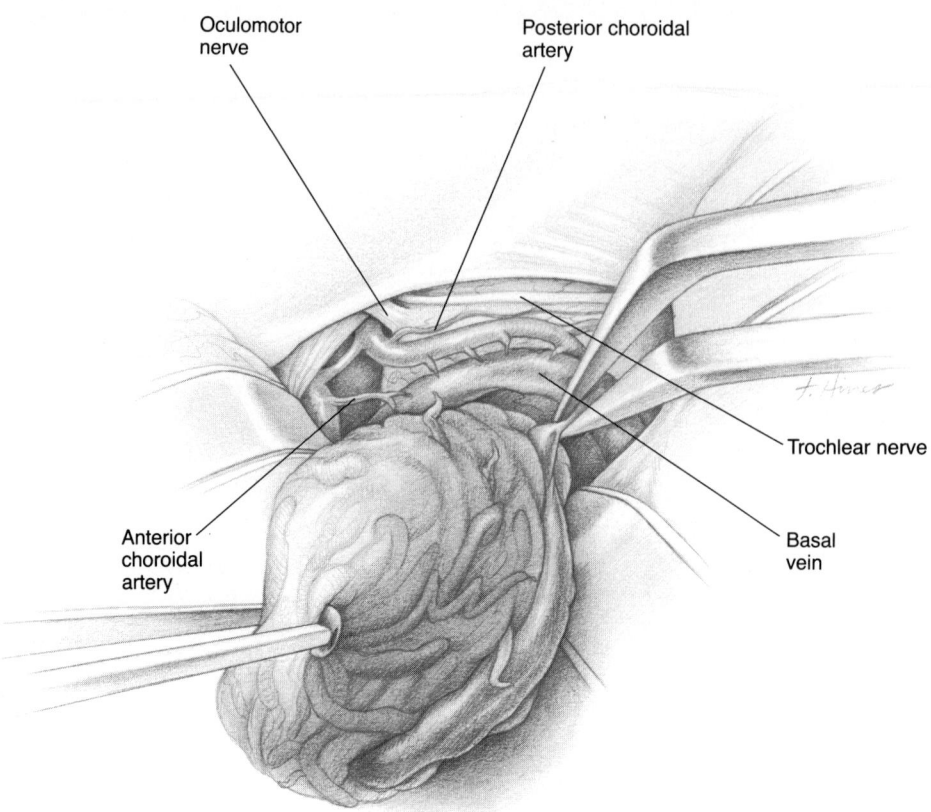

FIGURE 121–25. Removal of the AVM is complete as draining veins are taken. (From Tew JM, van Loveren HR: Atlas of Operative Microneurosurgery. Philadelphia, W. B. Saunders, 1993, p 260.)

Closure is performed as for a pterional craniotomy. The dura is closed with interrupted 4-0 Vicryl sutures, and the craniotomy flap is wired into position with two 28-gauge stainless steel wires. The temporal muscle is reattached to the superior temporal line with 2-0 Vicryl. The galea is reapproximated with 2-0 Vicryl with inverted interrupted stitches, and the skin is closed with surgical staples.

STEREOTACTICALLY GUIDED CRANIOTOMY

Stereotactically guided craniotomy is recommended for small, deep lesions distal from the midline, where localization may be difficult. Before surgery, a localizing ring is attached to the skull with the patient under local anesthesia. When the patient undergoes CT scanning or MRI, coordinates are generated for localization of the malformation. The patient is supine with the head maintained in a radiolucent head-fixation device for intraoperative angiography (Fig. 121–26). In the operating room, a craniotomy is performed with the benefit of stereotactic localization. The dura is opened, and a silicone cannula is stereotactically inserted to a predetermined point at the external border of the malformation. The cannula is cut flush with the pial surface (Fig. 121–27).

Retraction arms are attached to the arc adaptor. The pia-arachnoid plane is opened along the path of the cannula. An incision is made in the gyrus, preferably at the depth of a sulcus. The malformation is reached, and excision proceeds as previously described. A complete excision is achieved and confirmed by angiography. The dura is closed, and the bone flap is secured with stainless steel wires. Muscle, fascia, galea, and skin are closed in separate layers.

POSTOPERATIVE MANAGEMENT

Postoperative patient care includes management in the neuroscience intensive care unit. Maintenance of hypotension to a mean arterial pressure of 60 to 70 mm Hg for 72 hours assists in controlling regional cerebrovascular autoregulation, thereby protecting the surrounding parenchyma from reperfusion injury. Serial neurologic examinations are required to assess possible ischemia. The primary cause of postoperative hemorrhage has been eliminated by the use of intraoperative angiography and single-stage AVM removal. If indicated, intracranial pressure is monitored and controlled with osmotic agents, steroids, and diversion of cerebrospinal fluid. Early rehabilitation is essential because neurologic recovery may be profound. Visual field and acuity examination and neuropsychologic testing complete the postoperative evaluation.

RESULTS

The treatment of our 59 patients is summarized in Table 121–5. The ideal outcome of surgical resection of malformations in the deep brain is total removal without exacerbation of preoperative deficit or addition of a new deficit. At follow-up (range, 1 to 18 years), this status was achieved in 33 (83 percent) patients (Table 121–6).

For two patients with a malformation extending into the splenial region, splenium resection caused a visual disconnection syndrome. One patient acquired dysphasia and monoparesis of the arm as a result of injury to the internal capsule after a frontal approach. One suffered recurrent hemorrhage from a residual AVM in the perioperative period that resulted

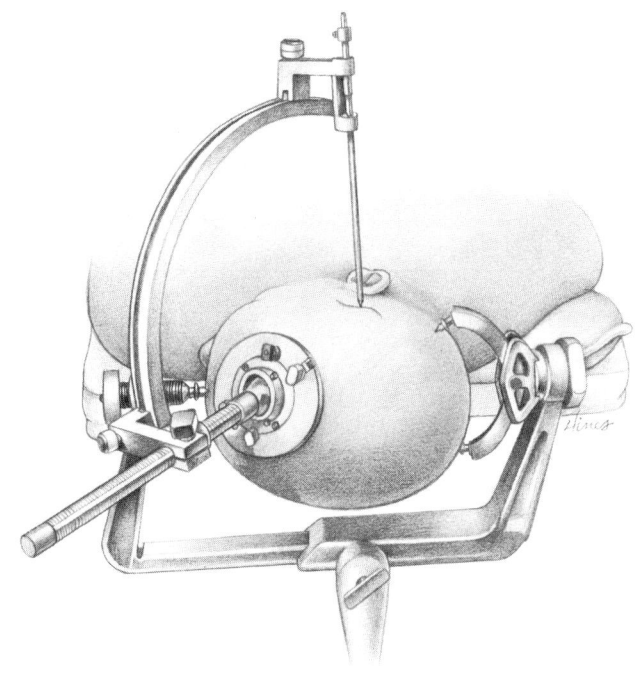

FIGURE 121–26. Intraoperative position of patient with Mayfield head holder and Pelorus stereotactic craniotomy device locating the craniotomy site and trajectory to the AVM. (From Tew JM, van Loveren HR: Atlas of Operative Microneurosurgery. Philadelphia, W. B. Saunders, 1993, p 283.)

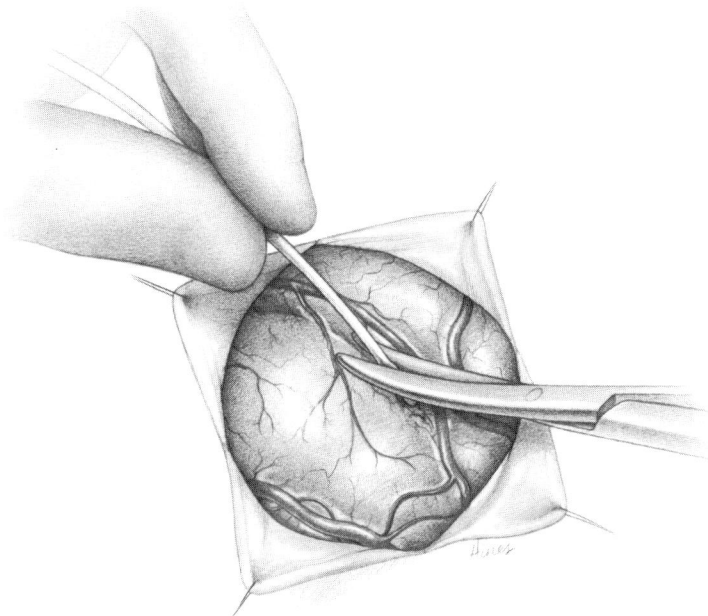

FIGURE 121–27. Silastic catheter is cut off at the cortical surface. The flexible cannula offers a safe guide to the surface of the AVM. (From Tew JM, van Loveren HR: Atlas of Operative Microneurosurgery. Philadelphia, W. B. Saunders, 1993, p 284.)

Table 121–5. TREATMENT OF 59 PATIENTS WITH ARTERIOVENOUS MALFORMATIONS

Procedure	n
Surgical*	
Transcallosal	27
Transcortical	19
Parietal	9
Frontal	10
Transsylvian	3†
Embolization	6
Stereotactic Radiation	
LINAC	4
Proton beam	3
Nonoperated	13

LINAC = linear accelerator.
*Seven patients required a second-stage operation: all of the operations were performed before the use of intraoperative angiography.
†Two patients required a combined transsylvian and transcallosal resection.

in left hemiparesis and hemianesthesia. Another patient with a pulvinar AVM who had no intraoperative complications and was neurologically intact postoperatively developed meningitis with resultant right homonymous hemianopsia and right hemiparesis. Subsequently, a ventriculoperitoneal shunting procedure was needed.

Two additional patients developed worsening of hemiparesis as a result of surgery. Despite these new deficits, four of those patients and 30 others returned to their previous occupations or educational pursuits. One patient (2 percent) who hemorrhaged from a 6-cm right caudothalamic AVM presented in a comatose state. After complete resection of his AVM, he remained vegetative and died of a respiratory complication of pneumonia.

Twenty patients have not undergone surgery in the treatment of their lesions. A summary of the complications encountered in these patients is presented in Table 121–6. Three of seven patients who underwent radiation suffered radiation injuries. Obliteration was achieved in three of the four patients who underwent LINAC and in none of the patients who underwent proton-beam treatment. The remaining untreated patients have either refused intervention or are being observed.

SUMMARY

Improved interventional neuroradiologic techniques, microsurgery, instrumentation, and neuroanesthesia have rendered deep-seated thalamic–basal ganglia vascular malformations amenable to surgical removal. Embolization has an increasing role but is still an adjuvant to surgery or stereotactic radiosurgery. The unknown long-term radiation effects and long latency period before obliteration makes radiosurgery the secondary choice of therapy for ruptured vascular malformations. The morbidity and mortality associated with malformations presenting with hemorrhage warrant surgical removal. However, because data are insufficient on unruptured malformations, the same statement may not be made for this disorder. Unruptured thalamic–basal ganglia vascular malformations should be evaluated on an individual basis and treated by observation or radiosurgical or direct surgical methods.

Acknowledgment

The authors thank Alexis Rostoker for transcription and Mary Kemper for editorial assistance.

Table 121–6. OUTCOME AND COMPLICATIONS OF SURGERY IN 40 PATIENTS AND NONSURGICAL TREATMENT IN 20 PATIENTS

Outcome	n	%
Surgical cases		
Improved	25	63
Unchanged	8	20
Worsened	6	15
Death	1	2
Complication		
Permanent deficit	6	13
Transient deficit	5	11
Recurrent hemorrhage from residual malformation*	4	9
Nonsurgical cases		
Recurrent hemorrhage(s)	10†	25
Arteriovenous malformation	7	35
Cavernous angioma	3	15
Radiation injury	3	15
Progressive neurologic deficit	3	15
Death	1	5

*No patients have had postoperative recurrent hemorrhage since the use of intraoperative angiography.
†Five patients had rebleeding.

REFERENCES

1. Luessenhop AJ, Rosa L: Cerebral arteriovenous malformations: Indications for and results of surgery, and the role of intravascular techniques. J Neurosurg 60:14–22, 1984
2. Drake CG: Cerebral arteriovenous malformations: Considerations for and experience with surgical treatment in 166 cases. Clin Neurosurg 26:145–208, 1979
3. Solomon RA, Stein BM: Interhemispheric approach for the surgical removal of thalamocaudate arteriovenous malformations. J Neurosurg 66:345–351, 1987
4. Shi Y, Chen X-C: Surgical treatment of arteriovenous malformations of the region. J Neurosurg 66:352–356, 1987
5. Malik GH, Umansky F, Patel S, et al: Microsurgical removal of arteriovenous malformations of the basal ganglia. Neurosurgery 23:209–217, 1988
6. Matsushima T, Fukui M, Kitamura K, et al: Arteriovenous malformations of the basal ganglia. Surgical indications and approaches. Neurol Med Chir (Tokyo) 28:49–56, 1988
7. Brown RD, Wiebers D, Forbes G, et al: The natural history of unruptured intracranial arteriovenous malformations. J Neurosurg 68:352–357, 1988
8. Wilkins RH: Natural history of intracranial vascular malformations: A review. Neurosurgery 16:421–430, 1985
9. Ondra SL, Troupp H, George ED, et al: The natural history of symptomatic arteriovenous malformations of the brain: A 24-year follow-up assessment. J Neurosurg 73:387–391, 1990
10. Golfinos JG, Wascher TM, Zabbiamski JM, Spetzler RF: The management of unruptured intracranial vascular malformations. BNI Q 8(3):2–11, 1992
11. Friedman WA, Bover FJ: Linear accelerator radiosurgery for arteriovenous malformations. J Neurosurg 77:832–841, 1992
12. Lunsford LD, Kondziolka D, Flickinger JC, et al: Stereotactic radiosur-

gery for arteriovenous malformations of the brain. J Neurosurg 75:512–524, 1991
13. Steiner L: Radiosurgery in cerebral arteriovenous malformations, in Fein JM, Flamm ES (eds): Cerebrovascular Surgery, vol 4. New York, Springer-Verlag, 1984, pp 1161–1215
14. Steiner L, Lindquist C: Radiosurgery in cerebral arteriovenous malformations, in Tasker RR (ed): Neurosurgery State of the Art Reviews, Stereotactic Surgery, volume 2. Philadelphia, Hanley & Belfus, 1987, pp 329–336
15. Steiner L: Treatment of arteriovenous malformations by radiosurgery, in Wilson CB, Stein BM (eds): Intracranial Arteriovenous Malformations. Baltimore, Williams & Wilkins, 1984, pp 295–311
16. Spetzler RF, Martin NA: A proposed grading system for arteriovenous malformations. J Neurosurg 65:476–483, 1986
17. U HS: Microsurgical excision of paraventricular arteriovenous malformations. Neurosurgery 16:293–303, 1985
18. Wilson CB, Martin NA: Deep supratentorial arteriovenous malformations, in Wilson CB, Stein BM (eds): Intracranial Arteriovenous Malformations. Baltimore, Williams & Wilkins, 1984, pp 184–208
19. Heros R: Arteriovenous malformations of the medial temporal lobe. Surgical approach and neuroradiological characterization. J Neurosurg 56:44–52, 1982
20. Sugita K, Takemae T, Kobayashi S: Sylvian fissure arteriovenous malformations. Neurosurgery 21:7–14, 1987

CHAPTER 122

Retrogasserian Glycerol Rhizolysis in Trigeminal Neuralgia

Bengt Linderoth
Sten Håkanson

Many patients who suffer from trigeminal neuralgia are elderly, often with concurrent diseases, and therefore there is a constant search for appropriate methods with low surgical risk, little impact on facial sensibility, and the possibility of being performed with the patient under local anesthesia. Glycerol rhizolysis, the procedure described in this chapter, is such a method. The availability of a method that can be used even in medically infirm patients may also widen the indications for surgical treatment because the usual regimen with carbamazepine, other anticonvulsants, or baclofen is known to cause severe side effects in many patients. These problems are particularly valid for patients suffering from paroxysmal facial pain associated with multiple sclerosis.

HISTORY

The discovery of the beneficial effects of glycerol in patients suffering from trigeminal neuralgia was purely accidental. During the course of the development of a procedure for producing lesions in the gasserian ganglion in patients with trigeminal neuralgia in whom the Gamma knife in Stockholm was used (Leksell stereotactic multicobalt unit), x-ray contrast medium (metrizamide) and glycerol were tried as vehicles for a radiopaque metal dust (tantalum powder). The tantalum powder was to be introduced into the retroganglionic cistern as a permanent marker to constitute a visible target for the subsequent stereotactic calculations.[1,2] The reason for choosing glycerol as the vehicle was its presumed harmless nature, being the base for the triglyceride formation in the body, and its viscosity, which makes the tantalum alluviation durable enough to allow time to deposit it in the trigeminal cistern. In fact, glycerol had earlier been used in the treatment of trigeminal neuralgia but then as a vehicle for the highly neurolytic phenol,[3] used for percutaneous treatment of trigeminal neuralgia at that time. Merely the injection of glycerol and tantalum dust in the patients abolished the paroxysmal pain before the Gamma knife procedure. On the basis of these observations, Håkanson developed the technique of treating trigeminal neuralgia by glycerol injection into the trigeminal cistern.

The first series of patients was presented in 1981.[4] The method was rapidly adopted in many neurosurgical centers. Over the years, many series of patients treated according to Håkanson's procedure, or by some variation of the original method, have been reported. The results from different series have been highly variable. In many centers, the outcome has been quite satisfactory,[5–10] and glycerol rhizolysis has continued to be the method of choice, particularly for elderly and weak patients. In other series, the results have been discouraging (Siegfried 1985: Unpublished[11]; Rhoton 1985: Unpublished;[11] Price 1985: Unpublished[12,13]) that some neurosurgeons have entirely abandoned the procedure.

In this chapter, the possible reasons for these discrepancies are examined, and a standard procedure to ensure maximum safety is described.

INDICATIONS

The main indication for rhizolysis is still classic idiopathic trigeminal neuralgia. The reason to progress to surgical treatment include deficient control of paroxysms in spite of an adequate pharmaceutical regimen, severe medication side effects, development of drug allergy or intolerance, or signs of hepatic malfunction ascribed to medication.

Paroxysmal facial pain in multiple sclerosis is another indication for glycerol rhizolysis. The initial outcome in this group of patients is as satisfactory as for those with idiopathic trigeminal neuralgia, but the long-term results are, as with other available methods, less good, as is further discussed later. Patients with signs of deafferentation should not be submitted to the procedure. However, many trigeminal neuralgia patients previously treated by other methods display signs of neural damage, such as hypesthesia, allodynia, hyperalgesia, and deafferentation pain. Such cases should be accepted for treatment only if the paroxysmal pain component dominates and after careful evaluation of the patient's sensory deficits. If such patients are accepted for glycerol rhizolysis, the procedure should be carried out with utmost care, and with only a small amount of glycerol.

The same considerations also apply to the use of the method in atypical facial pain or painful trigeminal neuropathy. In general, glycerol rhizolysis is not indicated in these cases. Only when a dominating paroxysmal component is present and the signs of deafferentation are only slight may the method be considered. Both neurosurgeon and patient should be aware of the fact that the procedure might aggravate the deafferentation picture and thereby also the constant neuropathic pain.

PREOPERATIVE EVALUATION

The preoperative examination should attempt to find the typical signs of trigeminal neuralgia and any sensory deficits, and should evaluate such elements as previous treatments, the pharmaceutical regimen, constant pain components, and ipsilateral hearing loss. Because we recommend the use of contrast medium injection in all cases, intolerance to iodine and previous adverse reactions to contrast medium should be determined. Preferentially, a MRI study, or at least computed tomography with and without contrast injection, should be performed preoperatively. The surgeon must evaluate the patient before the procedure to individualize the preoperative medication and to describe the details of the procedure to the patient to ensure good cooperation during its performance. Most patients tolerate the procedure well under local anesthesia with adequate preoperative medication, but very anxious patients may require general anesthesia. A short-acting barbiturate can also be beneficial if the surgeon has little experience with the procedure as performed with local anesthesia and may need some trials to attain proper needle placement. Performing the procedure with the patient under general anesthesia, however, is considerably more time consuming and elaborate than the local method and exposes the patient to an increased risk.

TECHNIQUE

The original technique of Håkanson has been subject to many modifications by various neurosurgeons. These variations encompass the type of anesthesia selected (general or local); the patient position and fluoroscopic projection; whether cisternography is performed or not; other modes of localization of the needle tip (electric stimulation, reactions to drip-wise injection of glycerol); the dose of glycerol used; instillation of the glycerol in one step or as minute volumes in an incremental fashion with intermittent sensory testing; trials to empty the cistern after attainment of a satisfactory effect according to the perioperative testing; and the duration of the period the patient is kept sitting with the head flexed after completion of the procedure.

Some of these modifications have resulted in less satisfactory results.[11, 13–15] We consider retrogasserian glycerol rhizolysis to be an anatomically oriented method aimed at graded lesioning of fibers in a certain locus. Thus, the localization procedure should also be anatomic, and the treatment should be meticulously performed with the use of the smallest possible volume of pure sterile glycerol considered to be effective in each case.

The procedure as it is performed at the department of neurosurgery at the Karolinska Hospital in Stockholm is described in this section.

ANESTHESIA AND SEDATION

The entire procedure is normally carried out with the patient awake and premedicated about 45 minutes before the start of the session with 5 to 10 mg of morphine hydrochloride–scopolamine administered subcutaneously and 2.5 mg of droperidol administered intramuscularly. The doses are adjusted according to the age and condition of the patient. In some cases, it is helpful to give 0.5 mg of atropine intravenously immediately before the procedure. An intravenous line with slow infusion of Ringer's solution is kept during, and for some hours after, the session.

General anesthesia using a short-acting barbiturate with endotracheal intubation is used only in particularly anxious patients. If this type is used, the anesthesia must be terminated with the patient in the sitting position with the head flexed according to the instructions of the surgeon.

The skin at the point of needle insertion and the underlying soft tissue is infiltrated with local anesthetic (e.g., lidocaine 0.5 percent).

POSITIONING

The procedure is usually performed in an x-ray suite with the patient seated in a rotatable chair, but an operating chair in an operating room and a C-arm fluoroscopic image intensifier with image-storing capacity is equally adequate.

In most cases, fluoroscopy with lateral projection is used when the cistern is punctured. Further guidance is obtained through switching to the anteroposterior projection. In rare difficult cases in which entering the proper part of the foramen ovale is a problem, the patient's head may be extended and rotated 15 to 20 degrees away from the affected side, and the fluoroscopy arm may be tilted to give an oblique projection of the skull base, including the foramen ovale. With some equipment, identifying the foramen on the fluoroscopy monitor might be difficult, but exposing the film in most cases solves the problem. If one needle already has penetrated the foramen, the identification should be easy, and a new needle can readily be inserted in the desired part of it.

ANATOMICAL LANDMARKS AND IMPORTANT STRUCTURES

The trigeminal cistern is punctured by the anterior percutaneous route via the foramen ovale, as described by Härtel.[16] After the administration of local anesthesia, a 22-gauge lumbar cannula (outside diameter, 0.7 mm; length, at least 90 mm) is inserted from a point about 3 cm lateral to the corner of the mouth. The trajectory is aimed at a point: in the lateral view, about 0.5 cm anterior to the anterior margin of the mandibular joint; in the anteroposterior view, toward the medial margin of the pupil with the eye bulb in the neutral position. Several landmarks may be used for reaching the oval foramen,[17] but in most cases, these two simple coordinates are sufficient.

Often, it is wise to direct the needle a little more medially, touching the medial wall of the foramen. The needle is then withdrawn a short distance, redirected a few millimeters more laterally, and introduced through the medial part of the foramen. Intermittent fluoroscopy is used during the entire procedure.

When the needle penetrates the foramen, the patient may experience a short spell of pain as a result of penetration of the third branch and the semilunar ganglion. The cannula should not reach beyond the clival contour as seen in the orthogonal lateral projection.

When the tip of the cannula is located inside the arachnoid of the trigeminal cistern, a spontaneous exit of cerebrospinal fluid (CSF) should occur. Because the location of the trigeminal ganglion and cistern is variable in relation to the landmarks of the base of the skull, a contrast injection has to be performed to ascertain the correct position for glycerol injection. As is discussed later, spontaneous CSF drainage, however, is not a sufficient requisite for accepting the location as intracisternal.

TRIGEMINAL CISTERNOGRAPHY

The technique we use is the same as that described by Håkanson,[18] although now, estimation of the cisternal volume is less important for the decision about what volume of glycerol to inject. The contrast medium used must be water soluable, with high radiographic attenuation, of low toxicity, and with a higher specific weight than that of CSF. The first contrast medium used was metrizamide (iodine, 300 mg/ml), but since 1986, iohexol (iodine, 300 mg/ml) has been used exclusively because it is less toxic than the former.[19] About 0.3 to 0.6 ml is injected with the patient sitting with the head slightly flexed to retain as much of the medium in the cistern as possible. If intermittent fluoroscopy is used during injection, the position of the needle tip may be estimated right away, but it should always be confirmed by x-ray films both in the lateral and anteroposterior projections. The typical appearance of the trigeminal cistern is illustrated in Figure 122–1A. Ideally, the sensory root filaments (and sometimes the motor portion) should be visualized by lateral cisternography, leaving no doubt about the intracisternal position of the tip. The typical 45-degree medial tilt of the cistern should be seen from the anteroposterior view (Fig. 122–1B). The appearance of the cistern may vary considerably from patient

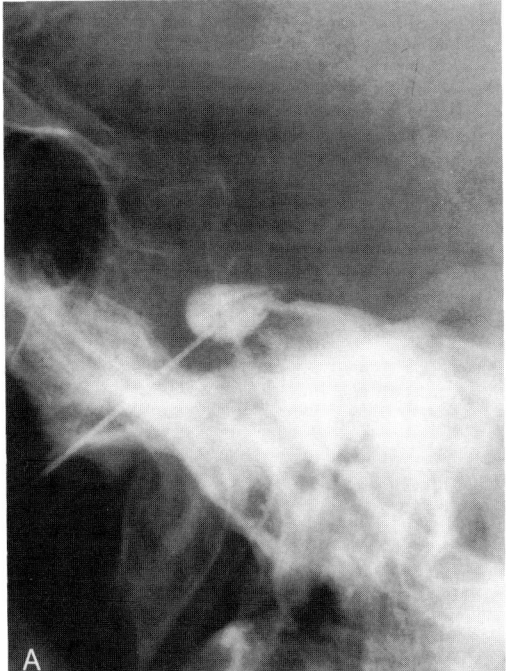
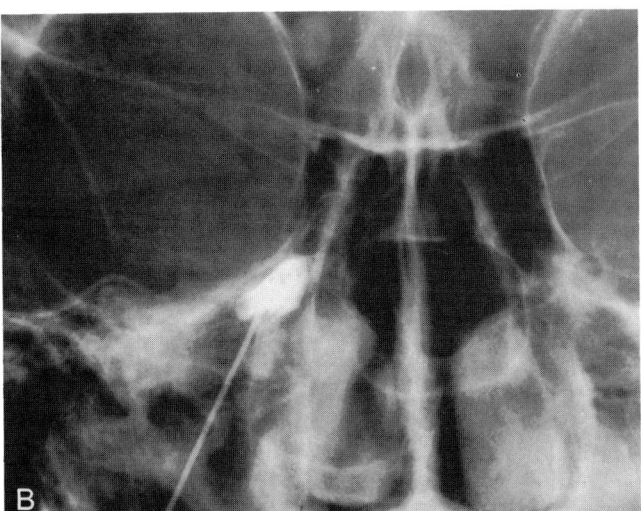
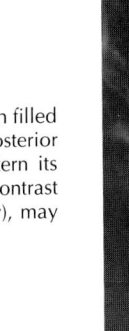

FIGURE 122–1. The typical appearance of the trigeminal cistern filled with contrast medium in the lateral (A) and in the anteroposterior projections (B). Note that the root fibers on (A) give the cistern its striped texture. In the lateral projection (C), the sparing of contrast indicates that the position of the trigeminal motor root (arrow), may be observed.

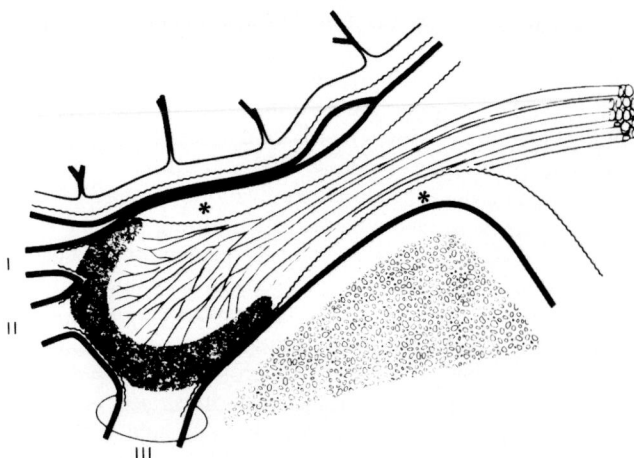

FIGURE 122–2. The different compartments in Meckel's cave. The arachnoid is drawn with a wavy line. Note the sites marked with (*), where extracisternal deposits of contrast medium and glycerol may be performed. (From Håkanson S: Trigeminal neuralgia treated by injection of glycerol into the trigeminal cistern. Neurosurgery 9:638–646, 1981.)

to patient, and it is essential that the surgeon is familiar with this anatomy. Furthermore, as is illustrated in Figure 122–2, a subdural-extracisternal compartment lies within Meckel's cave that may be injected with contrast medium. This injection takes place when contrast medium is injected without prior spontaneous CSF drainage, or if the needle is dislocated from an adequate intracisternal position during the injection, as is discussed later.

SPECIFIC DIFFICULTIES

Spontaneous CSF drainage from the needle does not guarantee an intracisternal tip location. Actually, if the cannula is placed too far laterally, the tip may be located in the subtemporal subarachnoid space and yet cause a brisk flow of CSF. The subsequent cisternography solves this problem, as is illustrated by Fig. 122–3A, which shows the proximity of the cisternal and subtemporal subarachnoid compartments in the anteroposterior projection. Figures 122–3B and C illustrate a pure subtemporal contrast injection. Our strategy in this case is to leave the first needle in place and to introduce a second needle, using the first one for guidance.

Spontaneous CSF drainage must be obtained before contrast injection. If the contrast medium is injected without this requirement being fulfilled, the deposit may well be in the extra-arachnoid subdural compartment, as is depicted in Figure 122–2.

Another problem may arise if the patient's head is not adequately tilted forward during the injection, because the contrast medium will then flow out the porus trigemini and escape to the posterior fossa, leaving the filling in the cistern

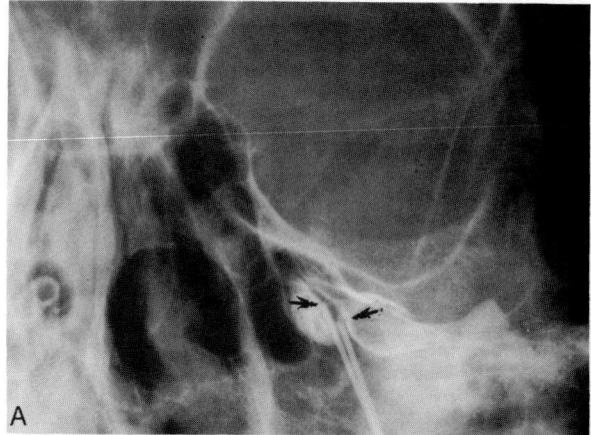

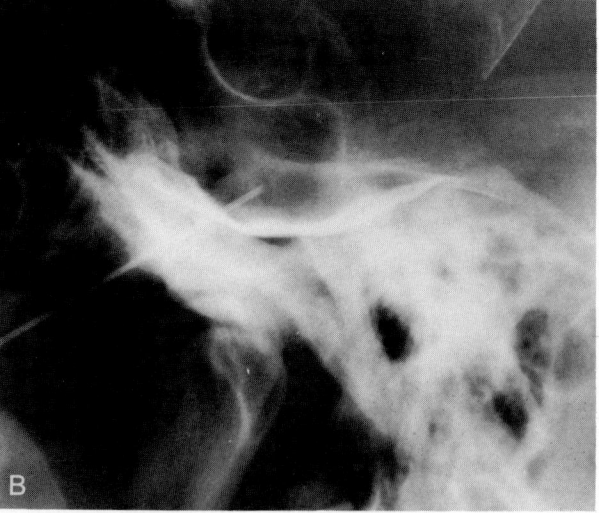

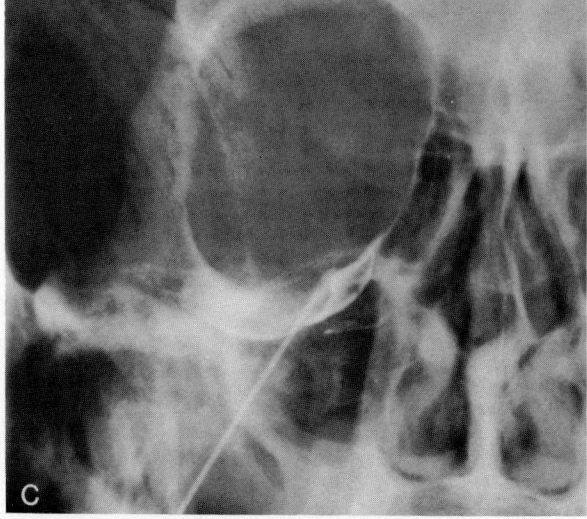

FIGURE 122–3. In the anteroposterior roentgenogram (A), in which both the trigeminal cistern and the subtemporal space have been injected with contrast medium, the proximity of these two compartments is illustrated. Medially, the contrast-filled cistern (arrow) is seen barely pierced by one of the needles in its lateral margin. Injection of contrast medium through the lateral needle yielded filling of the subtemporal space (arrow) instead. (B) The lateral roentgenogram shows a pure subtemporal contrast injection. (C) This subtemporal outflow of contrast medium in the anteroposterior projection is shown. No contrast filling of the cistern was obtained, although CSF exit was noted from the needle.

partial or too thin to confirm the correct position of the needle tip (Fig. 122–4). This situation may also result in an underestimation of the cistern volume.

CONTRAST EVACUATION. When the intracisternal position of the tip has been confirmed, the syringe is gently removed from the cannula, and the contrast medium is permitted to exit drip-wise from it. We generally evacuate the cistern by tilting the patient to the supine position. If it is difficult to evacuate all contrast medium from the bottom of the cistern to permit the glycerol to reach the lowermost root fibers, the patient can be placed in the Trendelenburg position for some minutes, a maneuver that permits the contrast medium to drain to the posterior fossa. Furthermore, the cistern may be flushed with 2 to 3 ml of sterile saline until the control x-ray film indicates that the cistern is emptied. Some of the less satisfactory results that are discussed later probably result from failure to empty the cistern in a proper way.[13, 15]

GLYCEROL INJECTION

Glycerol injection should always be performed with the patient in the sitting position to minimize spillover of the substance extracisternally. The glycerol should be anhydrous (>99.5 percent) and sterile and should be injected slowly from a 1-ml syringe. Generally, 0.18 to 0.30 ml is sufficient and we usually use around 0.20 to 0.25 ml. When the neuralgia encompasses all three branches with multiple trigger points, a somewhat larger volume is required than that used when only the third branch is involved. However, injection of volumes exceeding 0.30 ml is discouraged because of the risk of postoperative sensory deficits, (as is discussed later). Furthermore, inability to demonstrate an adequate intracisternal needle tip position precludes a subsequent glycerol injection.

BRANCH SELECTIVITY. Due to the topographic arrangements of the fibers within the cistern, some selectivity may be obtained via the following four maneuvers.

First, the volume of glycerol can be varied to fill more or less of the cistern. When the trigeminal cistern has been emptied entirely after the contrast injection, the amount of glycerol injected partly determines which branches are influenced. With the head of the patient only slightly flexed, a small volume of glycerol (0.15 to 0.20 ml) is deposited at the bottom of the cistern and mainly affect the fibers of the third and second branches. Increasing the amount of glycerol causes additional rhizolysis in the two upper portions.

Second, contrast medium may be left at the bottom of the cistern to protect the third branch. Both contrast agents used so far have specific gravities that exceed that of pure glycerol (with iodine 300 mg/ml; metrizamide, 1.329 g/l; iohexol, 1.345 g/l; as compared with glycerol, 1.242 g/l; CSF, 1.007 g/l). This, of course, implies that when deposited in the same compartment these substances replace the original CSF contents and are layered with the contrast media at the bottom and the glycerol on top of it.

With the head slightly flexed and a little contrast medium remaining at the bottom of the cistern, thus protecting the fibers of the third branch, glycerol may be gently injected to layer on top of the contrast medium. The rhizolysis then mainly engages the upper two branches.

When a patient with third-branch neuralgia is treated, no contrast medium should be allowed to remain in the cistern for the glycerol injection.

Third, the position of the tip of the needle is partly indicative of which branch will be most attained. The tip of the cannula should preferentially be positioned in the part of the cistern traversed by the root fibers to be treated. This means that for treatment of third-branch neuralgia, the optimal position is in the lower part of the cistern, whereas a first- or second-branch pain is best treated with a tip site in the upper portion.

During, or immediately after, the injection of glycerol, the patient experiences strong paresthesias (or sometimes even pain) in one or more of the divisions of the trigeminal nerve. This sensation is an indication that the substance has been deposited inside the cistern and is affecting the closest root fibers. Proper placement of the needle seems especially important in the case of reinjections, when a certain amount of adhesions inside the cistern may be present and partially prevent the drops of glycerol to sediment to the bottom.

Finally, the position of the patient's head during and after the injection also produces some selectivity of the rhizolysis. The patient should be sitting in the upright position during the injection. For first-branch neuralgia, the head should be maximally flexed (i.e., about 40 degrees) and should be kept in approximately the same position during the first hour after injection. For second-branch treatment, the flexion should be approximately 25 degrees, and for the third branch, the head should be slightly tilted laterally toward the affected side, but kept upright in the anteroposterior plane.[5]

The selectivity obtained by varying the head position has been systematically studied by Bergenheim and associates,[20, 21] who found a highly selective effect of this maneu-

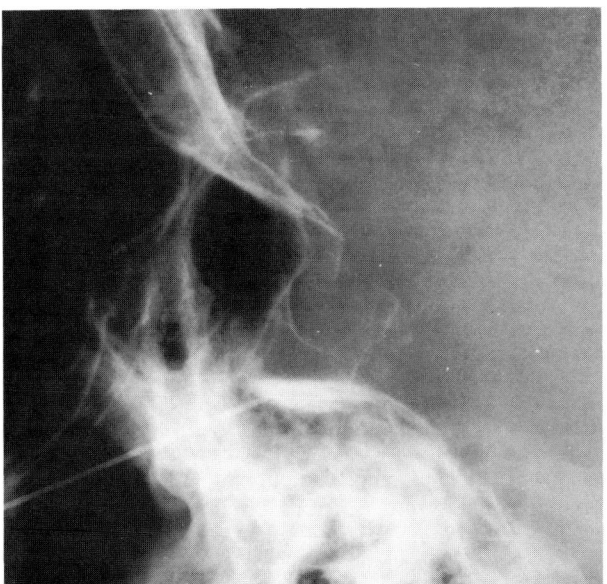

FIGURE 122–4. During contrast injection, the head of the patient should be tilted forward to prevent immediate contrast flow to the posterior fossa. In this case, the positioning of the head was not adequate, and some contrast escaped to the posterior fossa. Hence, filling of the cistern was only partial.

ver with regard to the ophthalmic branch but less selectivity for the two lower branches.

Immediately before glycerol injection, the free flow of CSF from the needle should be checked to ascertain a persisting intracisternal tip position. Dislocation is not unusual, especially if the full length of the needle must be used and the patient moves his cheek.

In certain cases, a longer needle must be used to reach the cistern. Often, thin needles (outside diameter, 0.7 mm) of adequate length are not readily available in the hospital and must be ordered separately. We discourage the use of thicker needles because larger sizes make the procedure more painful, theoretically cause more mechanical damage to the ganglion, and make the estimation of injected volume of glycerol more intricate.

A special remark must also be made about cases in which the tip of the needle is placed posteriorly in the cistern close to its clival passage. At this site an injection might be painful, and the pain may project to the eye, a reason why such a position should be avoided.

PERMANENT MARKING OF THE CISTERN

Permanent marking of the cistern is recommended and can easily be obtained by use of the original mix of glycerol and sterile radiopaque tantalum dust (Merck, Germany; grain size below 0.042 mm). About 0.5 g of tantalum is mixed with 2 ml of glycerol, and the suspension is then used for injection. The cisternal marking usually outlines the bottom (Fig. 122–5) and is of considerable help if reinjections are needed. With certain requirements fulfilled (see below), the permanent marking may replace the need for a renewed cisternography. The tantalum marking is clearly visible on x-ray many years after the injection, but there are no indications that the metal

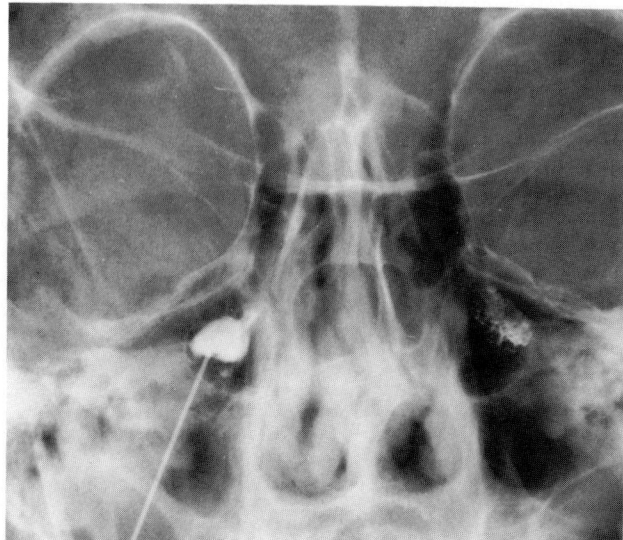

FIGURE 122–5. The trigeminal cistern on the patient's left side is permanently marked by tantalum dust lining the arachnoid of the bottom and walls of the cistern (anteroposterior view). The right cistern has been punctured and injected with contrast medium. When the cistern is marked with tantalum, the puncture and glycerol injection may be carried out without the intervening cisternography.

dust per se causes inadvertent effects, such as meningeal reactions, or otherwise influences the results of the treatment.

SPECIAL CONSIDERATIONS FOR REPEATED INJECTION

Incomplete pain relief after the initial injection seems in most cases to result from technical problems during the procedure. The high initial success rate reported in many papers (80 to 96 percent) supports this view. Reinjections should not be performed within 3 to 4 weeks after the initial trial, a criterion that excludes late responders. Before the reinjection, facial sensibility should be carefully examined. If signs of sensory impairment are found, the reinjection should be meticulously performed with the use of a minimal amount of glycerol. Alternatively, a nondestructive procedure should be considered in these patients.

When trigeminal cisternography is performed after one or more intracisternal glycerol injections, sometimes, less satisfactory outlining of the cistern is obtained. The probable cause is the formation of adhesions within the cistern that are induced by the glycerol, the contrast medium,[22] or both. The situation seems to be the same regardless of whether tantalum has been added to the substance.

If the cistern has been properly marked by tantalum dust during the initial injection and the marking is clearly visible during fluoroscopy, the reinjection may be very simple and fast. When the tip of the cannula is within the cistern, according to x-ray films in the lateral, and at least two anteroposterior projections at different angles, a spontaneous drainage of CSF through the needle confirms an intracisternal tip position. However, if no CSF exits through the cannula, a cisternography with positive contrast should be carried out.

Evacuation of the contrast medium from the cistern is facilitated by rinsing with saline.

Because of the cistern adhesions mentioned earlier, the repeated cisternography results may seem to be a little different from the initial cisternography films. This phenomenon points again to the advantage of placing the needle tip in the part of the cistern that houses the root fibers to be treated because the glycerol might be entangled by fibrotic strands that prevent it from reaching the bottom of the cistern.

In contrast to our experiences and the observations of Rappaport and Gomori,[22] Lunsford[23] noted no abnormalities of the cistern in patients undergoing repeated glycerol injections.

POSTOPERATIVE MANAGEMENT

As was mentioned earlier, after the injection, the patient should remain seated in bed upright with the head in the selected position for another hour. Some authors have tried immobilization for other periods, but no convincing evidence exists that extending the time with controlled head position increases the therapeutic effect. On the contrary, there are indications that shortening the period of fiber exposure to glycerol by actively evacuating it from the cistern may cause more extensive and less well controlled rhizolysis.[11, 20] On the other hand, Sweet has had the experience that if first-division sensory loss appears, leaving the glycerol in the

Table 122–1. RESULTS OF GLYCEROL RHIZOLYSIS

Authors	n	With Cisternography (%)	Pain Free After First Injection (%)	Total Pain Free at Follow-up (%)
Håkanson[25]	100	100	96	75
Lunsford[23]	62	100	74	66
Arias[5]	100	50	95	95
Beck and coworkers[36]	58	31	67	72
Dieckmann and coworkers[7]	252	100	91	85
Saini[28]	550	0	76*	17
Burchiel[15]	46	100	80	53
Young[8]	162	A few	90	78
Waltz and coworkers[66]	200	100	73	74
Fujimaki and coworkers[13]	122	100	80	26
North and coworkers[26]	85	0	>90	>50
Ischia and coworkers[31]	112	100	92	71
Steiger[29]	122	100	84	59

*Most failures previously treated by destructive method; otherwise, 96%.

cistern for 12 minutes or more may result in persisting corneal anesthesia. Hence, he recommends evacuating the glycerol from the cistern within 10 minutes after the onset of first-branch analgesia.[11, 24]

The latency for relief from the neuralgia varies. About half of the patients report that their paroxysms disappear immediately after the glycerol injection. In the remaining group, occasional spells may occur during the first postoperative day and sometimes for periods up to 5 days, after which the neuralgia fades away. Even longer latencies, up to 3 weeks,[23] have been reported.

An overnight hospital stay is usually required because of the heavy sedation in elderly or weak patients or because of the use of general anesthesia. In younger patients, the procedure may be performed on an outpatient basis.

Facial sensibility should be examined at least twice: during the first postoperative day and after 3 months. Patients should be encouraged to report increased body temperature during the first postoperative week, ulcers in the vicinity of the mouth, rash, eye problems, or any adverse effects that might result from the treatment. A telephone report to the surgeon about treatment effects is due at 10 days postoperatively.

The pharmaceutical regimen for the neuralgia is usually tapered off gradually during the 7 to 10 days following a successful injection. If high doses of carbamazepine are used, we usually decrease the daily intake by 100 mg every second day.

RESULTS

The treatment outcome is reviewed with respect to initial and long-term relief from the paroxysmal pain, rate of recurrence, and various complications, such as sensory disturbances, herpes eruptions, postoperative meningitis, both aseptic and bacterial. Some of the major series published so far will be examined and relevant data given in tables and text.

EVALUATION OF DIFFERENT SERIES

A major problem in the evaluation of the results of the different series is the variation in technique. Different methods have been used by different authors to ascertain an intracisternal needle position before the glycerol injection. Strategies vary from the recommended, that is, the use of cisternography,[6, 7, 23, 25] drip-wise incremental glycerol injection, and preoperative recording of sensory response,[5, 8, 26] to electric stimulation in the same way as is performed in selective thermocoagulation.[14, 27]

In some series, cisternography is not used at all[8, 26, 28]; in some, only in conjunction with treatment of first-branch neuralgia; and in others, only when no spontaneous CSF exit occurs via the cannula.[29] The extent to which cisternography is used in the series reviewed is noted in Table 122–1. In our experience, a relationship exists between the quality of the cisternography, the adequacy of needle placement, and the treatment outcome. When judging other series, of course, we have no information about the first two of these parameters.

Another important factor is the amount of glycerol used. Sometimes, the range of volumes is not explicit, and in several series, it far exceeds the original recommendations.[8, 13, 30, 31] This variation must be taken into account when the data are interpreted. The ranges of volumes of glycerol used are given in Table 122–3.

A third factor of major importance for the outcome is whether or not the patient has had some other destructive procedure before or after the glycerol rhizolysis and if information about this is given in the reports. This information is of critical importance with regard to the estimation of sensory disturbances after the procedure, and it also has an impact on the volume of glycerol to use in a specific case.

In some series, patients with diagnoses other than classic trigeminal neuralgia are included without specific notations. It is often impossible to determine this selection from the presentation of results. This information is of course most important when the outcome is judged because the results, as described later, in other facial pain conditions are often inferior to those in classic tic.

SHORT- AND LONG-TERM RESULTS

The outcome in thirteen major series with 1971 patients with long-term follow-up periods is illustrated in Table 122–1. Before the success rates are examined, it should be noted that cisternography is used as a routine for all patients in only eight of the services.[7, 13, 15, 23, 25, 29-31]

The percentage of patients enjoying immediate (within 2 weeks) relief from the paroxysmal facial pain varies between 67 and 96 percent in the different series. No clear association exists between the mere use of cisternography and success rate, either for immediate or for long-term outcome. This finding may seem remarkable against the experiences of the present authors, but it may also point to large differences in the accuracy of the cisternographic procedure.

The follow-up periods in these series vary from months to 10 years. The recurrence rates are difficult to estimate correctly because of differences in techniques of reporting and statistics. Lately, however, Kaplan-Meier analysis has been used by several authors,[15, 26, 29, 31] facilitating the interpretation of recurrences.

Recurrence in relation to length of follow-up is reviewed in Table 122–2. Roughly, within 2 years, between 2 and 50 percent of patients with a successful initial outcome experience recurrent pain. This large variation obviously casts some doubt on both the technical performance of the procedure and the follow-up methodology. However, determining how many of the patients have been reinjected and whether or not these are included in the final results is also difficult.

The original Stockholm series of 100 patients was followed up between 5 and 10 years (mean, 5 years, 4 months). At the last follow-up, 53 percent were still pain free after the first injection. Twenty-two cases had at that time been reinjected with glycerol, and 75 percent of the entire series were pain free. An additional 23 percent had only mild pains that were easy to control by pharmaceutical regimens.[32] The average volume of glycerol injected in this series was only 0.21 ml.

The average risk of recurrence in well-controlled series appears to be about 20 percent, and the rate of late reappearance of symptoms (within 5 to 10 years) may approach 50 percent. Nevertheless, because the injection can easily be repeated and carries little risk for the patient, most of the patients (>75 percent) are completely pain free after a small number of reinjections (Table 122–1). For comparison, Jannetta[33] found 80 percent of permanent pain relief in most series of microvascular decompression, 10 percent with some pain, and a 10 percent failure rate.

The most recent reports of major series of trigeminal neuralgia patients treated by glycerol rhizolysis are those of Spaziante and coworkers[34] and Lunsford and Duma,[10] which were presented at the Stockholm Meeting of the European Society of Stereotactic and Functional Neurosurgery in September 1992. Because the data are not given in full detail in the congress abstracts, they were not included in the tables presented in this chapter. The two series comprise 191 and 480 patients, respectively, and the follow-up periods were up to 10 yrs. The percentage of patients who were pain free immediately after treatment was 93 percent in the series of Spaziante and associates,[34] and the long-term follow-up revealed 77 percent[34] and 75 percent[10] pain-free individuals. No patients with anesthesia dolorosa were observed, but mild hypesthesia was found in 46 percent and 20 percent, respectively. Both authors concluded that glycerol rhizolysis is a mildly neurodestructive procedure indicated as the first therapeutic choice[34] in elderly patients, patients with multiple sclerosis, and in patients in whom other procedures, including microvascular decompression, have been unsuccessful.[10]

SIDE EFFECTS AND COMPLICATIONS

Glycerol rhizolysis, when performed by an experienced and careful neurosurgeon, should have few side effects. Only one fatal outcome has been reported.[10, 35] This patient suffered a fatal heart attack in the recovery room after the procedure. Because glycerol rhizolysis is used in patients of advanced age (the oldest in the Stockholm series is 96 years) and sometimes severely disabled patients, the number of severe complications may even seem astonishingly low.

Other serious consequences of trials to penetrate the oval foramen with a needle (e.g., intracranial hemorrhage) have been described by Sweet,[12] but these are related to the route of puncture and not to glycerol instillation per se.

The most feared consequence of neurolytic procedures, a postoperative anesthesia dolorosa, is rarely seen after glycerol rhizolysis. An exception to this is the rather heterogenous series of Saini[28] of 552 cases performed without cisternography or some other technique to confirm the localization of the needle tip before glycerol injection. In this series, the number of patients with anesthesia dolorosa was extreme: 26 (5 percent). Furthermore, 16 patients (3 percent) developed signs of disturbance of the motor function of the third branch.

Table 122–2. PAIN RECURRENCE AFTER GLYCEROL RHIZOLYSIS

Authors	n	Early Recurrence < 2 y (%)	Late Recurrence > 2 y (%)	Follow-up Range
Håkanson[25]	100	26	43	5–10 y
Lunsford[23]	62	21	*	3–28 mo
Arias[5]	100	2	10	2–3 y
Beck and coworkers[36]	58	11	*	2–40 mo
Dieckmann and coworkers[7]	252	11	37	2–5 y
Saini[28]	550	41	92	1–6 y
Burchiel[15]	46	47	75	3–44 mo
Young[8]	162	11	34	6–67 mo
Waltz and coworkers[66]	200	23	25	25–64 mo
Fujimaki and coworkers[13]	122	45	72	38–54 mo
North and coworkers[26]	85	~40	~55	6–54 mo
Ischia and coworkers[31]	112	20	26	1–5 y
Steiger[29]	122	~30	~41	1–96 mo

*Not indicated in report.

This malfunction, however, resolved within 3 to 4 months after the injection. Transient masseter weakness has also been described by others.[30, 31] Otherwise, only single cases with transitory cranial nerve dysfunction, other than the fifth, have been reported after glycerol rhizolysis. Some of these cases were reviewed by Sweet.[12]

POSTOPERATIVE FACIAL SENSORY DISTURBANCE

A disturbance of facial sensibility is not uncommon after the procedure but may last only a limited period of time: hours, a couple of days, or 1 to 2 weeks. This disturbance is not tabulated as a true side effect. More persistent alterations in the sensory function or perception within the trigeminal area are reviewed with regard to (1) postoperative slight hypesthesia, (2) severe hypesthesia, and (3) the presence of dysesthesia or allodynia. Paresthesias that are not unpleasant are not included.

HYPESTHESIA

As already stated, serious sensory disturbance, such as anesthesia dolorosa, is rare after glycerol rhizolysis except in certain series. However, transitory facial hypesthesia is a rather common phenomenon (occurring in up to 70 percent) after the procedure. Usually, the complaints vanish during the 3-month period after the operation,[5, 32] and most of the rest, within half a year.[8, 30]

The frequency of slight hypesthesia persisting for longer periods of time varies markedly between different series, as is seen from Table 122–3. In some series, only a few percent of the patients display this side effect,[5, 26] but in others, more than two thirds present with hypesthesia at follow-up.[8, 15] More severe hypesthesia and anesthesia is fortunately rare (Table 122–3) and in only one series did this effect approach 30 percent.[13] This incidence is of course not acceptable, and the authors consequently abandoned the procedure. The figures from the series of Saini,[28] Burchiel,[15] Young,[8] and Waltz and coworkers[30] must also be considered far too high (5 to 12 percent). There are at least three possible explanations for this outcome: (1) some of these patients may have had other previous or subsequent destructive procedures, (2) there may have been technical difficulties during the procedure, and (3) the volume of glycerol injected may have been too large. Sweet[12] described a case in which 1.5 ml of glycerol was injected in 0.1-ml increments, resulting in anesthesia dolorosa.

With a properly performed glycerol rhizolysis, the incidence of severe sensory disturbances should be low and should not exceed 1 percent.[7, 10, 23, 25, 32]

DYSESTHESIA

Dysesthesia, spontaneous or touch-evoked unpleasant sensations (allodynia) should occur rarely and mostly transiently after glycerol rhizolysis. In the series reviewed here, the incidence generally remains between 0 and 4 percent (Table 122–3). The series of Fujimaki and colleagues,[13] Burchiel,[15] Steiger,[29] and Saini[28] are extreme also in this respect, with frequencies between 11 and 26 percent. There is one suspected major cause of this: a previous neurodestructive procedure with a sensory disturbance not specifically recorded before the glycerol rhizolysis. Some cases may also have had procedure-induced herpetic eruptions resulting in this condition,[23] although this sequel has not been observed by us. These figures are still unacceptably high. Normally, dysthesias are present in a maximum of 2 percent of virgin cases of trigeminal neuralgia subjected to glycerol rhizolysis.[5, 7, 23, 25, 30, 36]

INFECTIOUS SIDE EFFECTS

Serious infectious complications occurring after retrogasserian glycerol rhizolysis are rare. However, reactivation of latent viral populations infesting neural tissue (notably, herpes simplex type I) seems more common than is ordinar-

Table 122–3. SENSORY COMPLICATIONS AFTER GLYCEROL RHIZOLYSIS*

Authors	n	Volume of Glycerol (ml)	Slight Hypesthesia (%)	Severe Hypesthesia (%)	Dysesthesia (%)
Håkanson[25]	100	0.2–0.3	60	0	0
Lunsford[23]	62	0.15–0.25	21†	0	3‡
Arias[5]	100	0.1–0.4	13	0	0
Beck and coworkers[36]	58	0.2–0.4	17	2	0
Dieckmann and coworkers[7]	252	0.15–0.4	20	1	2
Saini[28]	550	0.2–0.3	—	5§	11
Burchiel[15]	46	0.15–?	72	7	13
Young[8]	162	0.15–0.55	72	12	3
Waltz and coworkers[66]	200	0.2–0.6	37	7	2
Fujimaki and coworkers[13]	122	0.3–0.5	63	29	26
North and coworkers[26]	85	0.3–0.4	4	2	4‖
Ischia and coworkers[31]	112	0.4–0.5	32	0	3
Steiger[29]	122	0.2–0.35	53†	—	13

*In several series, it cannot be readily judged whether or not sensory disturbances recorded after glycerol treatment were present before the procedure. Furthermore, other destructive procedures may have been subsequently used without specific notice.
†Many with previous or additional destructive procedures.
‡After herpes reactivation.
§Only cases with previous destructive procedures.
‖Transient.

Table 122-4. INFECTIOUS COMPLICATIONS AFTER GLYCEROL RHIZOLYSIS

Authors	n	Herpes Reactivation (%)	Aseptic Meningitis (%)	Bacterial Meningitis (%)
Håkanson[25]	100	50	0	0
Lunsford[23]	62	13	3	0
Arias[5]	100	10	2	0
Beck and coworkers[36]	58	9	4	0
Dieckmann and coworkers[7]	252	77	1	1
Saini[28]	550	3	—	—
Burchiel[15]	46	5	2	2
Young[8]	162	38	0	1
Waltz and coworkers[66]	200	—	7	1
Fujimaki and coworkers[13]	122	—	—	—
North and coworkers[26]	85	—	—	—
Ischia and coworkers[31]	112	—	—	—
Steiger[29]	122	—	0	0

—, Not indicated.

ily expected. A review of the infectious complications recorded in the 13 major series earlier mentioned is given in Table 122-4.

HERPES ACTIVATION

The activation of latent herpes simplex infections is a phenomenon encountered intermittently in neurological surgery.[37] However, the viral eruption may be minor and thus easily overlooked both by the patient and the physician.

From Table 122-4, one can conclude that the incidence of herpes simplex activation after glycerol injection varies considerably between different series. The range of 3 to 77 percent of recorded postoperative viral infections probably reflects variations in accuracy of follow-up. Perioral and gingival ulcers presenting themselves during the first week after treatment are rather common, but more serious outbreaks are rare. The mouth ulcers usually require no specific therapy.

ASEPTIC MENINGITIS

Symptoms of meningitis, such as high fever, nuchal rigidity, and CSF pleocytosis, that present 24 to 36 hours after the procedure may indicate a meningeal reaction to some agent introduced into the trigeminal cistern. The CSF cultures usually are negative, and the condition is labeled aseptic meningitis. For safety reasons, patients presenting with these symptoms are often treated by high-dose intravenous antibiotics. When the negative culture results are reported, the antibiotic therapy is discontinued. These patients usually recover completely within a few days without any sequelae. If the neurosurgeon feels convinced that the reaction is of the aseptic meningismus type, he could give steroids, thereby shortening its course.[23] Aseptic meningitis is encountered with a frequency varying between zero and 7 percent (Table 122-4).

The etiology of this reaction is obscure. Both contrast agents, glycerol, tantalum dust,[23] and the extent of manipulation, that is, the number of ganglionic penetrations, have been suspected. Some authors report a diminished frequency of reactions after reduction of the amount of contrast medium.[30] In the Stockholm series, the frequency was approximately 2 percent during the metrizamide era. Since this contrast medium was exchanged for iohexol in January 1986, we have had very few cases of aseptic meningitis. That the contrast agent is the most plausible causative agent is also supported by the observations by Arias,[5] who presented a series of 100 cases in which about 50 percent were treated without previous contrast medium injection. In the group subjected to contrast injection, two cases presented with aseptic meningitis, whereas no case was found in the other group. However, aseptic meningeal reactions are observed after other manipulations of the trigeminal root as well.[33]

BACTERIAL MENINGITIS

Bacterial meningitis occurring after percutaneous puncture of the Meckel's cave is encountered with a low frequency, regardless of the intended therapeutic procedure.[32, 38] The bacterial agents responsible have most often been those occurring in the upper respiratory tract, and infections by agents of low virulence have also been described.[39] The most probable cause seems to be inadvertent (and often unrecognized) penetration of the mucosa of the oral cavity. The frequency of bacterial meningitis reported after glycerol rhizolysis varies between zero and 2 percent (Table 122-4). The frequency in the Stockholm series is steady at about 0.5 percent and seems related to the extent of manipulations during the procedure. All patients have recovered without serious sequelae after adequate treatment with antibiotics.

SPECIAL CONSIDERATIONS IN PATIENTS WITH MULTIPLE SCLEROSIS

The paroxysmal facial pains sometimes affecting patients with multiple sclerosis are usually clinically identical to those in classic trigeminal neuralgia. Therefore, all the methods used in the symptomatic treatment of trigeminal neuralgia, excluding microvascular decompression, may be used also in the treatment of facial tic in multiple sclerosis. An estimated 1 to 2 percent of patients with an established diagnosis of multiple sclerosis suffer from trigeminal neuralgia.[40–42] In different series of patients with trigeminal neuralgia, the prevalence of multiple sclerosis seems to vary considerably.

Most often, the prevalence is 2 to 4 percent, but up to 8 percent has been reported.[43, 44] Furthermore, the occurrence of bilateral facial pain is common in multiple sclerosis but is rare in idiopathic trigeminal neuralgia.

The initial success rate for percutaneous rhizolysis seems about equal for idiopathic trigeminal neuralgia and for trigeminal neuralgia in multiple sclerosis, regardless of the specific method used,[44] but the late results differ considerably between patients with the idiopathic form and patients with multiple sclerosis. The recurrence rate is much higher in the latter group, possibly because of the progressive demyelinating disease with multiple lesions within the trigeminal system. Dieckmann and coworkers[7] and Linderoth and Håkanson,[44] reported a more than 40 percent recurrence after 2 years' follow-up. This rate can be compared with that in classic trigeminal neuralgia reported earlier, about 11 percent during the same period of time in Dieckmann's series.[7] After longer follow-up periods (8 to 79 months after injection), Linderoth and Håkanson,[44] reported over 60 percent recurrent tic in the multiple sclerosis group, whereas the recurrence in the total trigeminal neuralgia group (at that time, approximately 300 patients) was 38 percent.

Elevated recurrence rates after the treatment of trigeminal neuralgia in multiple sclerosis have also been observed with selective thermocoagulation. Broggi and Franzini,[45] reported a 40 percent recurrence among multiple sclerosis patients after thermorhizotomy, as compared with 9 percent in a previous series of non–multiple sclerosis patients. However, this finding could not be corroborated by Brisman,[46] who found no significant difference in recurrences between 16 multiple sclerosis cases and 219 non–multiple sclerosis patients.

The low tolerance of patients with multiple sclerosis to pharmacologic agents (carbamazepine as well as anesthesia and sedation) merits a specific comment. Linderoth and Håkanson,[44] reported that more than 90 percent of their multiple sclerosis cases with trigeminal neuralgia complained about adverse effects of the medication. The symptoms in the multiple sclerosis group were more often an aggravation of their pre-existing symptoms than the side effects usually mentioned. Thirty-eight percent of the multiple sclerosis patients actually had to discontinue carbamazepine because of such symptoms. After the glycerol treatment, 82 percent of the patients previously on carbamazepine medication could stop taking it.

We believe that paroxysmal facial pain in multiple sclerosis should thus be more liberally treated by glycerol to save the patient from the incapacitating side effects of a heavy drug regimen. Multiple sclerosis patients are often handicapped, weak, and considered as risks during general anesthesia. The choice of a method that does not require full anesthesia is thus recommended.

PROBABLE MECHANISMS OF ACTION OF GLYCEROL

Retrogasserian glycerol rhizolysis is a purely empirical method, the beneficial effects of glycerol being discovered accidentally. There has been much debate about the putative mechanisms behind the effects of glycerol on the paroxysmal pain. It is evident from the side effects (e.g., hypesthesia) that the substance is neurolytic in the concentration used for injection. An important issue is whether or not the neurolytic effect is selective for a certain fiber spectrum. From clinical observations it is concluded that the trigger mechanism is activated by tactile stimulation and impulse propagation in large myelinated fibers.

MORPHOLOGIC EFFECTS OF GLYCEROL

Glycerol is a trivalent alcohol normally present in human tissue, where it forms the skeleton of the triglycerides.[47, 48] Glycerol readily penetrates cell membranes and actually seems to possess distinct cryoprotective properties that are beneficient to the cell. The toxicity of the substance seems to be low, and rather high doses have to be injected systemically or intrathecally to induce toxic effects.[49, 50] The neurolytic action is considered to result from its hypertonicity, a condition well known to injure nerve fibers—firstly, thin, unmyelinated, and myelinated fibers in particular.[51] The myelin sheath of the coarse fibers seems to give some transitory protection. Furthermore, length of exposure, neuron type, and the presence of demyelination may be of importance for the vulnerability of the individual fiber. For example, with longer exposures, Robertson[52] and Pal and colleagues[53] observed that myelinated fibers were particularly vulnerable and that the degree of damage correlated positively with fiber diameter.

Studies on isolated animal nerve fibers show morphologic changes after exposure of a fiber to glycerol. These changes consist of disruption of the tight junction between the Schwann cells and the axolemma, but without actual damage to the axon proper.[54] Bathing the fibers in glycerol initially caused a shrinkage of the axon with a return to the basal volume after equilibration of the substance over the cell membrane. With transfer to isosmotic conditions, the fiber swelled markedly before returning to its normal volume. Thus, marked structural changes were observed with glycerol administration, but curiously enough, the conduction properties of the treated nerve axons remained intact.[54]

After injection of glycerol intraneurally and perineurally, Håkanson and Persson[55] and Rengachary and associates[56] observed axolysis with marked myelin sheath swelling. The coarse myelinated fibers suffered the most severe damage, whereas the small-diameter myelinated and unmyelinated fibers were rather well preserved.[53] In contrast, Bremerich and Reisert,[57] found only slight histomorphologic changes after glycerol injection in the region of the oval foramen in the rat in their long-term (180 days) comparative study of axonal damage after injection of glycerol, phenolglycerin, and saline.

The damage when glycerol is injected into a cavity with isotonic body fluid is probably considerably less severe. However, Lunsford and colleagues[9] observed extensive areas of myeline degradation and axonal swelling in cats subjected to retrogasserian glycerol injections 4 to 6 weeks earlier.

The actual site of the glycerol effects has been studied by Stajcic,[58] who applied ^{3}H-labeled glycerol onto peripheral branches of the maxillary nerve and in the infraorbital canal of rats. The amount of radioactivity detected in the nerve distal to the foramen rotundum, as well as in the gasserian ganglion ipsilaterally and contralaterally, was less than 0.1 percent in all specimens. Stajcic concluded that a retrograde transport mechanism behind the effect is improbable and that the beneficial effect of the glycerol is brought about at the site of injection.

We have seen no publication of an autopsy series of trigeminal neuralgia patients treated by retrogasserian glycerol rhizolysis. There is just an anecdotal description by Sweet,[12] mentioned earlier, of a case subjected to retrogasserian glycerol injection of the extreme volume of 1.5 ml with the subsequent development of anesthesia dolorosa. At a posterior fossa craniotomy, "many months" later, the trigeminal rootlets were found to be markedly atrophic.

NEUROPHYSIOLOGIC CHANGES AFTER GLYCEROL APPLICATION

The change in osmolarity is probably the process that causes the damage to the nerve axons, and the morphologic changes seem to be minimized by a gradual alteration in the osmolarity by slow instillation and removal of glycerol from the compartment housing the axons. The functional consequences of glycerol application to normal and damaged nervous tissue is known only fragmentarily, but some observations might apply to the clinical use of the substance.

Burchiel and Russel,[59] studied the effect of glycerol applied to normal and damaged nerves in a rat neuroma model. The neuromas, produced by sectioning of the saphenous nerve, were mechano-sensitive and discharged both spontaneously and in response to light manipulation. These authors found evidence that supported the view that glycerol exerts its major action on large-diameter fibers because exposure of the injured nerve to glycerol induced a short episode of increased spontaneous firing in the nerve, a response earlier shown to originate from the myelinated fibers.

The observation by Rappaport and associates[60] that glycerol injected into neuromas was more effective than alcohol in decreasing autotomy in rats may indicate that autotomy mirrors unpleasant "tic-like" paresthesias. The mechanism, according to the authors, could be suppression of ectopic impulse barrage from the neuroma.

Sweet and coworkers[27] found that glycerol injected into the trigeminal cistern of patients abolished the late components (corresponding to the A-delta and C-fibers) in the trigeminal root potentials recorded with electric stimulation of the surface of the cheek. These recordings were made only a few minutes after the injection and thus do not permit conclusion concerning long-term effects.

Hellstrand and coworkers (Unpublished[55]) studied the effects of glycerol both on isolated frog nerve and on the trigeminal root fibers after cisternal injection in the cat. They observed a severe reduction of the evoked potentials with glycerol but a nearly total restoration after the compartment was rinsed with saline. This recoverability probably has a bearing on the clinical effects and must be taken into account when the short-term observations by Sweet and colleagues[27] are interpreted. Further, evacuation of glycerol from the cistern after a short period (5 to 20 minutes)[11, 14, 24] might, based on the knowledge that glycerol requires at least 30 minutes to equilibrate across a membrane of a living cell and according to the experimental observations mentioned earlier, induce more severe damage, especially to fine fiber systems, than a slow unloading by diffusion into the subarachnoid space.

More long-term observations of trigeminal evoked potentials have been provided by Bennett and Lunsford,[61] who investigated patients before and 6 weeks after trigeminal glycerol rhizolysis. In their study, they confirmed the earlier findings of Bennett and Jannetta[62] that the thresholds were elevated, and the evoked potentials had a markedly increased latency on the affected side in comparison with the healthy one. It was an unexpected finding when they in addition observed that these aberrations were "normalized" after the glycerol rhizolysis. Because partially demyelinated fibers are known to conduct with a slower velocity and at a lower rate,[63, 64] the authors interpreted their finding to indicate that glycerol actually selectively struck partially damaged trigeminal axons, and after their elimination, the evoked trigeminal potentials appeared "normalized."

Further long-term observations were supplied by Lunsford and colleagues,[9] who noted the clearest changes in the trigeminal evoked potentials in cats in large-diameter myelinated fibers and further that additional changes took place as late as 6 weeks after the injection.

Quantitative sensory testing using von Frey hairs, mechanical pulses, and the Marstock technique[65] also corroborates the notion that glycerol acts mainly on the large, myelinated fiber spectrum.[32]

Thus, experimental and clinical observations indicate that the effects of glycerol may result from its hyperosmolarity and that the rate of alteration of osmolarity is critical for the effect. Furthermore, the effect may be exerted via the larger myelinated fibers, notably those with previous damage to the myelin sheath, thereby possibly affecting the "trigger mechanism" for the pain paroxysms.

PLACE OF GLYCEROL RHIZOLYSIS IN THE TREATMENT OF OTHER TYPES OF FACIAL PAIN

In *painful trigeminal neuropathy* (earlier called atypical facial pain), a paroxysmal component may exist in addition to the well-known continuous neuropathic pain. The etiology varies (e.g., trauma, infection, postoperative, tumor, idiopathic) but may also include previous treatment for trigeminal neuralgia. We agree with the observations of Dieckmann and colleagues,[6] Waltz and colleagues,[66] Lunsford and Apfelbaum,[35] Rappaport,[67] and Rappaport and Gomori,[22] that glycerol rhizolysis is contraindicated in most cases, and actually may aggravate a pre-existing neuropathy. The sole exception is when the paroxysmal component is totally dominating, diminishing the quality of life for the patient and where the sensory disturbance is minimal. The diagnosis of classic trigeminal neuralgia may even have been considered earlier. In such a case, a small amount of glycerol could be injected (0.15 ml). If complete pain relief is obtained at a duration of at least 3 months, a second injection may be performed with a somewhat larger glycerol volume.

Severe, intractable *cluster headache* (migrainous neuralgia; Horton's syndrome) has also been treated by glycerol injection into the trigeminal cistern on the affected side[26, 66, 68] and Sundbärj, Personal communication, 1988). In general, the outcome has been a partial and transitory relief from the symptoms in some of the patients comparable to that achieved by other manipulations involving the trigeminal system. The conclusion is that glycerol treatment is not indicated in this condition.

INDICATIONS RECONSIDERED: RETROGASSERIAN GLYCEROL RHIZOLYSIS VERSUS OTHER OPERATIVE TREATMENTS FOR TRIGEMINAL NEURALGIA

Based on the reviews and data presented earlier, glycerol rhizolysis is considered an inexpensive method that requires little special equipment. The method seems simple, but the procedure must be meticulously performed by a surgeon with experience in the operation. The major indication remains typical idiopathic trigeminal neuralgia, particularly in patients who are elderly or weak, or who suffer from multiple sclerosis. If a young patient chooses to undergo glycerol rhizolysis in place of microvascular decompression, he may do so. However, if this patient has a rather fast recurrence, he should be urged to accept the open operation instead.

In most cases, it should be possible to affect all the trigeminal branches with some selectivity. The most problematic might be the mandibular branch. With careful technique, using the suggestions given in this chapter, it should be possible to perform rhizolysis also in that branch. In a few cases submitted to several reinjections, the adhesions inside the cistern may hamper the possibility of glycerol reaching the lowermost fibers. In such cases, selective thermocoagulation may be considered instead.

We believe that microvascular decompression in young patients without multiple sclerosis, and glycerol treatment in the elderly and weak patients are the treatments of choice for classic trigeminal neuralgia.

SUMMARY

Trigeminal glycerol rhizolysis should be offered to healthy patients in their seventies and older with classic trigeminal neuralgia, as well as to weak individuals and those suffering from multiple sclerosis. It could also be an option in younger patients who are hesitant to undergo major surgery. With meticulous technique, the method presents few problems for the patients, can be performed with the patient under local anesthesia, and carries little risk for severe side effects. The recurrence rate, although usually slightly higher than that of microvascular decompression, compares well with other percutaneous methods, particularly in view of the low risk of severe postoperative sensory disturbance.

REFERENCES

1. Leksell L: Trigeminusneuralgi. Några neurofysiologiska aspekter och en ny behandlingsmetod. Läkartidningen 68:5145–5158, 1971
2. Håkanson S, Leksell L: Stereotactic radiosurgery in trigeminal neuralgia, in Pauser G, Gerstenbrand F, Gross D (eds): Gesichtsschmerz. Schmerzstudien 2. New York, Gustav Fischer Verlag, 1979, pp 231–237
3. Jefferson A: Trigeminal root and ganglion injections using phenol in glycerine for relief of trigeminal neuralgia. J Neurol Neurosurg Psychiatry 26:345–352, 1963
4. Håkanson S: Trigeminal neuralgia treated by the injection of glycerol into the trigeminal cistern. Neurosurgery 9:638–646, 1981
5. Arias MJ: Percutaneous retrogasserian glycerol rhizotomy for trigeminal neuralgia. A prospective study of 100 cases. J Neurosurg 65:32–36, 1986
6. Dieckmann G, Veras G, Sogabe K: Retrogasserian glycerol injection or percutaneous stimulation in the treatment of typical and atypical trigeminal pain. Neurol Res 9:48–49, 1987
7. Dieckmann G, Bockermann V, Heyer C, et al: Five-and-a-half years experience with percutaneous retrogasserian glycerol rhizotomy in treatment of trigeminal neuralgia. Appl Neurophysiol 50:401–413, 1987
8. Young RF: Glycerol rhizolysis for treatment of trigeminal neuralgia. J Neurosurg 69:39–45, 1988
9. Lunsford LD, Bennett MH, Martinez AJ: Experimental trigeminal glycerol injection. Electrophysiologic and morphologic effects. Arch Neurol 42:146–149, 1985
10. Lunsford LD, Duma CH: Percutaneous retrogasserian glycerol rhizotomy: A ten-year-experience (abstract). Acta Neurochir (Wien) 117:97, 1992
11. Sweet WH: Glycerol rhizotomy, in Youmans JR (ed): Neurological Surgery, 3rd ed. Philadelphia, WB Saunders, 1990, pp 3908–3921
12. Sweet WH: Faciocephalic pain, in Apuzzo MLJ (ed): Brain Surgery: Complication Avoidance and Management. New York, Churchill Livingstone, 2053–2083, 1993
13. Fujimaki T, Fukushima T, Miyazaki S: Percutaneous retrogasserian glycerol injection in the management of trigeminal neuralgia: Long-term follow-up results. J Neurosurg 73:212–216, 1990
14. Sweet WH, Poletti CE: Problems with retrogasserian glycerol in the treatment of trigeminal neuralgia. Appl Neurophysiol 48:252–257, 1985
15. Burchiel KJ: Percutaneons retrogasserian glycerol rhizolysis in the management of trigeminal neuralgia. J Neurosurg 69:361–366, 1988
16. Härtel F: Die Leitungsanästhesie und Injectionsbehandlung des Ganglion Gasseri und der Trigeminusstämme. Arch Klin Chir 100:193–292, 1912
17. Nugent GR, Berry B: Trigeminal neuralgia treated by differential percutaneous radiofrequency coagulation of the Gasseria ganglion lesions. J Neurosurg 40:517–523, 1974
18. Håkanson S: Transoval trigeminal cisternography. Surg Neurol 10:137–144, 1978
19. Shaw DD, Bach-Gansmo T, Dahlström K: Iohexol: Summary of North American and European clinical trials in adult lumbar, thoracic and cervical myelography with a new nonionic contrast medium. Invest Radiol 20 (suppl):44–50, 1985
20. Bergenheim AT, Hariz MI, Laitinen LV: Selectivity of retrogasserian glycerol rhizotomy in the treatment of trigeminal neuralgia. Stereotact Funct Neurosurg 56:159–165, 1991
21. Bergenheim AT, Hariz MI, Laitinen LV: Retrogasserian glycerol rhizotomy and its selectivity in the treatment of trigeminal neuralgia. Acta Neurochir Suppl 58:174–177, 1993
22. Rappaport ZH, Gomori JM: Recurrent trigeminal cistern glycerol injections for tic douloureux. Acta Neurochir (Wien) 90:31–34, 1988
23. Lunsford LD: Trigeminal neuralgia: Treatment by glycerol rhizotomy, in Wilkins RH, Rengachary SS (eds): Neurosurgery. New York, McGraw-Hill, 1985, pp 2351–2356
24. Sweet WH: Retrogasserian glycerol injection as treatment for trigeminal neuralgia, in Schmidek HH, Sweet WH (eds): Operative Neurosurgical Techniques, 2nd ed. New York, Grune & Stratton, 1988, pp 1129–1137
25. Håkanson S: Retrogasserian glycerol injection as treatment of tic douloureux. Adv Pain Res Ther 5:927–933, 1983
26. North RB, Kidd DH, Piantadosi S, Carson BS: Percutaneous retrogasserian glycerol rhizotomy. J Neurosurg 72:851–856, 1990
27. Sweet WH, Poletti CE, Macon JB: Treatment of trigeminal neuralgia and other facial pains by retrogasserian injection of glycerol. Neurosurgery 9:647–653, 1981
28. Saini SS: Retrogasserian anhydrous glycerol injection therapy in trigeminal neuralgia: Observations in 552 patients. J Neurol Neurosurg Psychiatry 50:1536–1538, 1987
29. Steiger HJ: Prognostic factors in the treatment of trigeminal neuralgia: Analysis of a differential therapeutic approach. Acta Neurochir (Wien) 113:11–17, 1991
30. Waltz TA, Dalessio DJ, Ott KH, et al: Trigeminal cistern glycerol injections for facial pain. Headache 25:354–357, 1985
31. Ischia S, Luzzani A, Polati E: Retrogasserian glycerol injection: A retrospective study of 112 patients. Clin J Pain 6(4):291–296, 1990
32. Håkanson S: Surgical treatment: Retrogasserian glycerol injection, in Fromm GH, Sessle BJ (eds): Trigeminal Neuralgia. Current Concepts Regarding Pathogenesis and Treatment. Boston, Butterworth-Heinemann, 1991, pp 185–204

33. Jannetta PJ: Surgical treatment: Microvascular decompression, in Fromm GH, Sessle BJ (eds): Trigeminal Neuralgia. Current Concepts Regarding Pathogenesis and Treatment. Boston, Butterworth-Heinemann, 1991, pp 145–157
34. Spaziante R, Cappabianca P, Graziussi G, et al: Percutaneous retrogasserian glycerol rhizolysis for treatment of trigeminal neuralgia. Results in 191 patients (abstract). Acta Neurochir (Wien) 117:97, 1992
35. Lunsford LD, Apfelbaum RI: Choice of surgical therapeutical modalities for treatment of trigeminal neuralgia: Microvascular decompression, percutaneous retrogasserian thermal or glycerol rhizotomy. Clin Neurosurg 32:319–333, 1985
36. Beck DW, Olson JJ, Urig EJ: Percutaneous retrogasserian glycerol rhizotomy for treatment of trigeminal neuralgia. J Neurosurg 65:28–31, 1986
37. Nabors MW, Francis CK, Kobrine AI: Reactivation of herpesvirus in neurosurgical patients. Neurosurgery 19:599–603, 1986
38. Nugent GR: Surgical treatment: Radiofrequency gangliolysis and rhizotomy, in Fromm GH, Sessle BJ (eds): Trigeminal Neuralgia. Current Concepts Regarding Pathogenesis and Treatment. Boston, Butterworth-Heinemann, 1991, pp 159–184
39. Aspevall O, Hillebrant E, Linderoth B, Rylander M: Meningitis due to *Gemella hemolysans* after neurosurgical treatment of trigeminal neuralgia. Scand J Infect Dis 23:503–505, 1991
40. Rushton JG, Olafson RA: Trigeminal neuralgia associated with multiple sclerosis. Arch Neurol 13:383–386, 1965
41. Brett DC, Ferguson GG, Ebers GC, Paty DW: Percutaneous trigeminal rhizotomy. Treatment of trigeminal neuralgia secondary to multiple sclerosis. Arch Neurol 39:219–221, 1982
42. Jensen TS, Rasmussen P, Reske-Nielsen E: Association of trigeminal neuralgia with multiple sclerosis: Clinical and pathological features. Acta Neurol Scand 65:182–189, 1982
43. Chakravorty BG: Association of trigeminal neuralgia with multiple sclerosis. Arch Neurol 14:95–99, 1966
44. Linderoth B, Håkanson S: Paroxysmal facial pain in disseminated sclerosis treated by retrogasserian glycerol injection. Acta Neurol Scand 80:341–346, 1989
45. Broggi G, Franzini A: Radiofrequency trigeminal rhizotomy in treatment of symptomatic non-neoplastic facial pain. J Neurosurg 57:483–486, 1982
46. Brisman R: Trigeminal neuralgia and multiple sclerosis. Arch Neurol 44:379–380, 1987
47. Bunge RP: Myelin degeneration in tissue culture. Neurosci Res Progr Bull 9:496–498, 1971
48. Dulhunty AF, Gage PW: Differential effects of glycerol treatment on membrane capacity and excitation-contraction coupling in toad sartorius fibers. J Physiol (Lond) 234:373–408, 1973
49. Diechmann D: Glycerol-effects upon rabbits and rats. Indust Med 2:5–6, 1941
50. Baxter BW, Schacherl U: Experimental studies on the morphological changes produced by intrathecal phenol. Can Med Assoc J 86:1200, 1962
51. King JS, Jewett DL, Sundberg HR: Differential blockade of cat dorsal root C-fibers by various chloride solutions. J Neurosurg 36:569–583, 1972
52. Robertson JD: Structural alterations in nerve fibers produced by hypotonic and hypertonic solutions. J Biophys Biochem Cytol 4:349–364, 1958
53. Pal HK, Dinda AK, Roy S, Banerji AK: Acute effect of anhydrous glycerol on peripheral nerve: An experimental study. Br Neurosurg 3:463–470, 1989.
54. Freeman AR, Reuben JP, Brandt PW, Grundfest H: Osmometrically determined characteristics of the cell membrane of squid and lobster giant axons. J Gen Physiol 50:423–445, 1966
55. Håkanson S: Trigeminal neuralgia treated by retrogasserian injection of glycerol. Published dissertation. Karolinska Institute, Stockholm, 1982
56. Rengachary SS, Watanabe IS, Singer P, Bopp WJ: Effect of glycerol on peripheral nerve: An experimental study. Neurosurgery 13:681–688, 1983
57. Bremerich A, Reisert I: Die perineurale Leitungsblockade mit Glycerin und Phenol-Glycerin. Eine histomorphologisch-morphometrische Studie. Dtsch Zahn Z 46:825–827, 1991
58. Stajcic Z: Evidence that the site of action of glycerol in relieving tic douloureux is its actual site of application. Dtsch Zahn Z 45:44–46, 1990
59. Burchiel KJ, Russell LC: Glycerol neurolysis: Neurophysiological effects of topical glycerol application on rat saphenous nerve. J Neurosurg 63:784–788, 1985
60. Rappaport ZH, Seltzer Z, Zagzag D: The effect of glycerol on autotomy. An experimental model of neuralgia pain. Pain 26:85–91, 1986
61. Bennett MH, Lunsford LD: Percutaneous retrogasserian glycerol rhizotomy for tic douloureux: II. Results and implications of trigeminal evoked potentials studies. Neurosurgery 14:431–435, 1984
62. Bennett MH, Jannetta PJ: Evoked potentials in trigeminal neuralgia. Neurosurgery 13:242–247, 1983
63. Raminsky M, Sears TA: Internodal conduction in undissected demyelinated nerve fibers. J Physiol 227:323–350, 1972
64. Waxman SG, Brill MH: Conduction through demyelinated plaque in multiple sclerosis: Computer simulations of facilitation by short internodes. J Neurol Neurosurg Psychiatry 69:39–45, 1978
65. Fruhstorfer H, Lindblom U, Schmidt WG: Method for quantitative estimation of thermal thresholds in patients. J Neurol Neurosurg Psychiatry 39:1071–1075, 1976
66. Waltz TA, Dalessio DJ, Copeland B, Abbott G: Percutaneous injection of glycerol for the treatment of trigeminal neuralgia. Clin J Pain 5:195–198, 1989
67. Rappaport ZH: Percutaneous retrogasserian glycerol injection for trigeminal neuralgia: One year follow-up. Pain Clin 1:57–61, 1986
68. Ekbom K, Lindgren L, Nilsson BY, et al: Retrogasserian glycerol injection in the treatment of chronic cluster headache. Cephalalgia 7:21–27, 1987

CHAPTER 123

Percutaneous Trigeminal Nerve Compression

Jeffrey A. Brown
Sean Mullan

Percutaneous trigeminal ganglion compression for treatment of trigeminal neuralgia was developed in 1978, and its description was published in 1983.[1] The procedure is based on the technique of trigeminal ganglion compression performed by Shelden and colleagues[2, 3] through a temporal craniotomy. In 1952, Taarnhöj[4] reported on a series of patients treated by decompression of the posterior root, rather than by partial sectioning of it, which up until that time had been the traditional approach. Shelden and colleagues noted a similarity between those results and their own, after decompression of the second and third divisions. In both series, pain relief occurred with little or no sensory loss. Shelden and associates concluded that both procedures had in common some inadvertent disturbance or compression of the trigeminal ganglion, and they advised compression as a definitive procedure. Many confirmed the validity of the observation, and the fact that a greater sensory loss provided a higher incidence of immediate success and a lower incidence of recurrence came to be recognized. In 1959, Svien and Love[5] noted that of 91 patients treated by the Taarnhöj procedure followed up for approximately 5 years, there was an 85 percent recurrence in those who had neither subjective nor objective sensory loss, a 67 percent recurrence in those with subjective loss only, and a 36 percent recurrence in those who had both subjective and objective change. In a series of 100 patients reported on by Graf[6] in 1963, who used the Shelden operation and followed up the patients for approximately the same time, the recurrence rate was 24 percent.

Percutaneous, intracranial, radiographically controlled, compression ganglion lysis is simply the percutaneous adaptation of Shelden's concept. Several series summarizing results in more than 600 patients have now been reported.[1, 7–19] The method has several advantages over existing techniques. Like all percutaneous procedures, it eliminates the small but significant mortality and morbidity that accompany any craniotomy. Unlike other percutaneous procedures, the needle need not, and should not, pass through the foramen ovale; therefore, it eliminates a small but definite incidence of serious complications of intracranial needle penetration. It does not produce corneal anesthesia and thereby eliminates the complication of keratitis. The procedure is done with the patient under general anesthesia, thus obviating the very considerable pain, discomfort, and anxiety that are inherent in all percutaneous techniques. Any patient who has had both procedures performed readily understands this difference. Lastly, the procedure demands less skill from the operator. The needle is simply engaged in the foramen ovale under biplane radiographic control. The blunt catheter follows the third division pathway into the ganglion. No selective search occurs within the ganglion, as is true with the RF method. The same compression is used irrespective of the division or divisions involved.

TECHNIQUE

The procedure can be performed in any location in which general anesthesia can be administered. The best radiographic equipment is not always found in the operating room; it may be located in the radiology suite, or sometimes in the coronary intervention suite. Even the newest and best portable fluoroscopy units may be inadequate to define a foramen ovale in an elderly, somewhat osteoporotic, skull. Because of this, additional facilities should be available, if necessary, for conventional hard-copy radiographs. The drugs used to induce and maintain general anesthesia, which lasts about 30 to 60 minutes, are at the discretion of the anesthesiologist. Atropine or other parasympathetic blockers are not generally used.

With regard to patient position, one of the authors (SM) has consistently used the semisitting position with the neck fully extended, so that the submental vertical line is horizontal. This position enables convenient supplementation of the fluoroscopy, if necessary, by conventional radiographs taken by a wall-mounted, horizontally directed, conventional radiographic tube. Another option is to keep the patient supine. The head is placed in slight extension and in contralateral rotation (15 to 30 degrees). The vertical tube is depressed toward the feet, and the beam is angled cranially by 25 degrees. The viewing beam travels above the ramus of the mandible, medial to the coronoid process and lateral to the pterygoid plate. The foramen ovale, which appears more oval than slitlike, as in the conventional submental vertical view, is projected above the petrous apex.

A point is selected 1 cm lateral to the angle of the mouth. The skin is washed and prepared appropriately. A line is drawn with a sterile marker toward the ipsilateral pupil, and another line is directed toward a point 3 cm in front of the external auditory meatus at the level of the top of the zygoma. The foramen ovale lies directly behind the pupil, corresponding to this marker on the zygoma, and will be reached by a needle guided along the indicated planes. A liver biopsy needle (Tru-Cut Travenol) is available in most operating rooms and is thus convenient. A special thin-walled No. 14 needle or an equivalent trocar and cannula may be used. The latter is less likely to injure the middle meningeal artery or other arterial structure in the pterygoid fossa. In addition, its rounded edges make it more suitable for withdrawal of the catheter, if this is required after its first extrusion. If the catheter tip deviates from the straight direction of a needle, it is likely to get cut off by the sharp edge of the needle on withdrawal into the needle. The stylet is removed from the No. 4 Fogarty catheter, and air within the balloon is replaced by radiographic contrast (Omnipaque). The catheter is then inserted into the needle to a point marked on the shaft, to indicate when it reaches the tip of the needle. After the needle is inserted into the patient, this point of reference will be needed to determine the distance that the catheter will protrude distal to the needle tip.

The needle is first directed laterally in the soft tissues of the cheek, to ensure that it does not penetrate the mucosa into the mouth. Contaminating the procedure by inserting a finger into the mouth for confirmation of direction is not necessary. After the needle is advanced about 2 to 3 cm, the trajectory is changed to correspond with the guiding planes. From that point on, the fluoroscope is used every few millimeters to confirm directional progress. Blind or random advancement should be avoided because it will ultimately need to be corrected and because repeated needling increases the risk of subpterygoid hemorrhage. If the foramen ovale is not well visualized (with the submental beam), the spine of the sphenoid or the foramen spinosum may be identified because the foramen spinosum lies anterior and medial to the spine, and the ovale lies anterior and medial to the spinosum. A plastic skull may be kept on hand for confirmation of these relationships. If the landmarks are not clear, hard-copy radiography from a conventional machine, with the same beam plane, should be used. If the ovale is viewed clearly in the radiograph and is related to its surrounding structures, the ovale may be inferred on fluoroscopy in relation to its surroundings. The edges of the foramen may be "felt" by "stepping," advancing the needle tip in short steps into the foramen. Its position may also be inferred by touching the lateral pterygoid plate because the ovale lies immediately behind and lateral to this plate. Some resistance will be felt by the needle as though its sides were gripped, as it engages in the ovale. The force used for insertion must be gentle and should never move the freely resting head; excessive force could result in a plunge, or if the needle was wrongly directed, it could pierce the foramen lacerum and reach the carotid. Rotation of the needle to a different alignment of the bevel may facilitate introduction. Only very rarely will the needle enter a very wide foramen without the operator being clearly conscious of engagement. A needle inserted with the bevel facing down is more likely to penetrate the dura by its sharp tip than is one placed with the bevel facing up.

The fact that the needle tip has reached the emerging nerve may be evident from a sudden temporary bradycardia, which accentuates as the needle engages. This is a most useful guide, but in some patients, the needle may fully engage without bradycardia. Once engagement is felt or suspected, lateral fluoroscopy is essential to ensure that the needle does not pass through into the middle fossa. Some surgeons may commence by observing on lateral fluoroscopy the needle being directed to the point where the posterior clinoid meets the tip of the petrous pyramid. In conducting lateral fluoroscopy, the head must be positioned at right angles to the beam, or two floors of the skull or two rami of the mandible appear. The rami or skull floors must be superimposed, not overlapped. A No. 4 Fogarty balloon catheter, without its stylet, is advanced to the needle tip, as determined by an external marker. If excessive resistance to further penetration exists, the needle may not be fully engaged and might need to be advanced another 1 to 3 mm under direct radiographic control. Even when the needle is properly engaged, a slight resistance to catheter advancement may be present for the first few millimeters. Thereafter, the catheter moves easily. It is advanced 10 mm to clear the needle. At 17 mm distal to ovale, it would enter the posterior fossa. An injection of 0.3 ml of contrast quickly locates it on the fluoroscope, if necessary. This step is usually accompanied by a return or deepening of the bradycardia, which, if more than minimal, may be treated with atropine. Because the balloon is in position, the depressor response is no longer useful for location and may thus be eliminated. The balloon is further distended until it begins to protrude posteriorly through the entrance to Meckel's cave, toward the posterior fossa. In doing this, it assumes a pear shape (Fig. 123–1).

Good compression is now exerted on the posterior root (Fig. 123–2) and is usually achieved by 0.7 ml of distension, but it could require more or less, according to the size of the cave. It rarely requires more than 1 milliliter. The balloon is rated to burst at a greater distension, but the actual volume of bursting is variable. Rupture has occurred repeatedly without incident. Compression at the appropriate pear shape is maintained for 1 minute and then released. A minimum pear

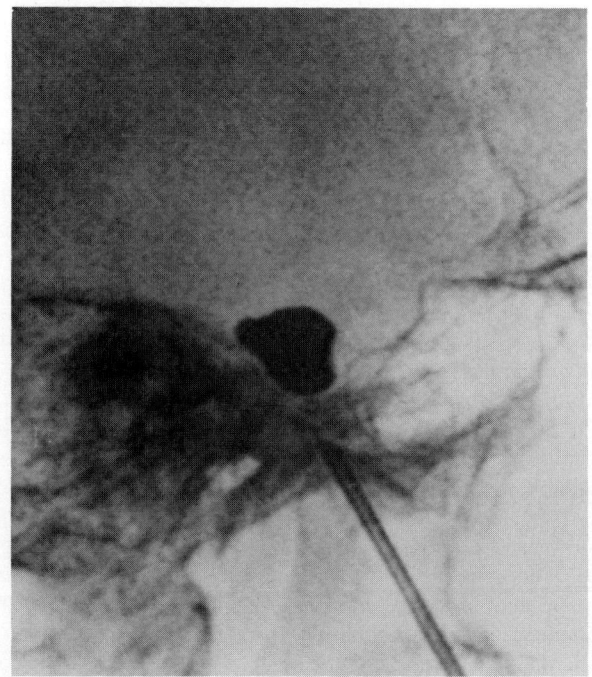

FIGURE 123–1. Typical pear shape of distended balloon. Note that bevel points up and that the needle does not enter the skull.

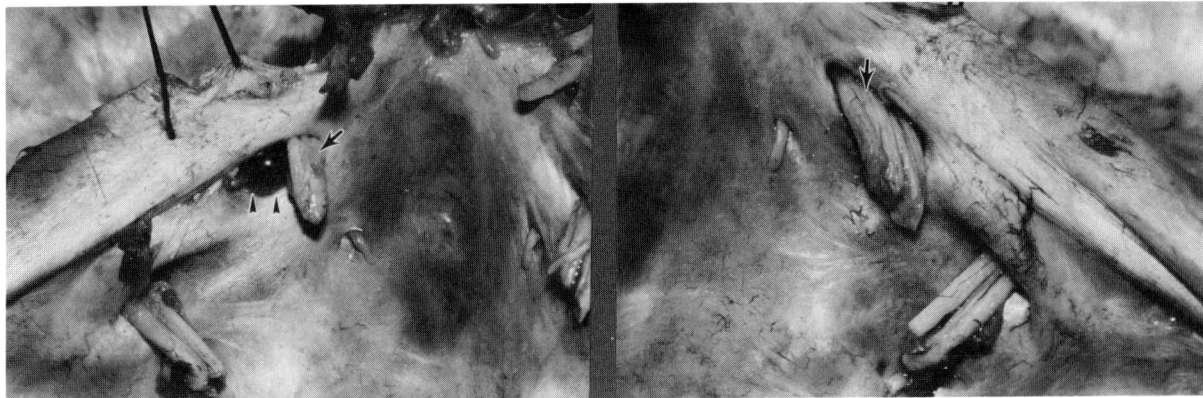

FIGURE 123-2. (Right) Arrow points to the retrogasserian trigeminal sensory and motor roots. (Left) The nerve root is compressed by the apex of the distended pear-shaped balloon.

shape and a meager bradycardia response indicates mild compression, mild hypoesthesia, and hypalgesia, and probably a shorter interval before occurrence. A good pear shape and marked bradycardia usually indicate more sensory loss and a longer lasting result. For a maximal result, the catheter tip should enter the posterior fossa and inflate in a dumbbell fashion, partly within the posterior fossa and partly within the cave. Compressions of durations longer than 1 minute probably deepen the numbness and thereby reduce the likelihood of recurrence but probably also increase the incidence of dysesthesia.

After deflation of the balloon, the needle and catheter are withdrawn, and pressure is maintained for 5 minutes at the puncture site and above the zygoma to prevent an accumulation of blood in the pterygoid space and to prevent its tracking deep to the temporal muscle. Occasionally, deep bleeding with visible swelling of the cheek appears before penetration of the foramen ovale. When this happens, it is usually best to withdraw the needle to permit a good compression of the site. The procedure can then begin again.

If the needle penetrates too far, it may pierce the dura. Although the catheter is withdrawn to the foramen ovale, it seeks this opening, and when distended, it assumes its natural rounded cylindrical shape within the dura, rather than the desired pear shape of Meckel's cave (Fig. 123–3). When this normal shape appears, we have only rarely found it possible to redirect the catheter properly during that procedure. After 3 weeks, the opening in the dura heals, and the procedure may be repeated with success. Perhaps it could be done earlier, but we lack experience with such a timeline. Rarely are caves that are scarred by alcohol now encountered, but in such cases, a balloon may not distend adequately. Pushing the catheter through into the posterior fossa, distending it to approximately 0.5 ml, then pulling it back until it engages in the neck of the cave may be possible. There, it is held in position, thereby compressing the nerve fibers.

ALTERNATIVE TECHNIQUES

TROCHAR

To avoid the possibility of subpterygoid bleeding, and to eliminate any risk of an intracranial needle problem, Gerber has used a modified No. 13 Cone trochar and cannula.[19a] The sharp trochar pierces the skin and advances with the cannula until it reaches a point 1 or 2 cm proximal to the foramen ovale. It is then replaced by a blunt trochar until it engages in the foramen.

BALLOON DISTENSION PRESSURE

The pressure within the balloon, when distended in air, is approximately 500 mm Hg. When it is distended to an identical volume and assumes the pear shape in Meckel's cave, it is approximately 1000 mm Hg. When it is distended in a fresh cadaver, a pressure of 1200 has been recorded. Thus, the effective compressing force is 500 mm Hg maintained for 1 minute.[9] This measurement can be used to determine

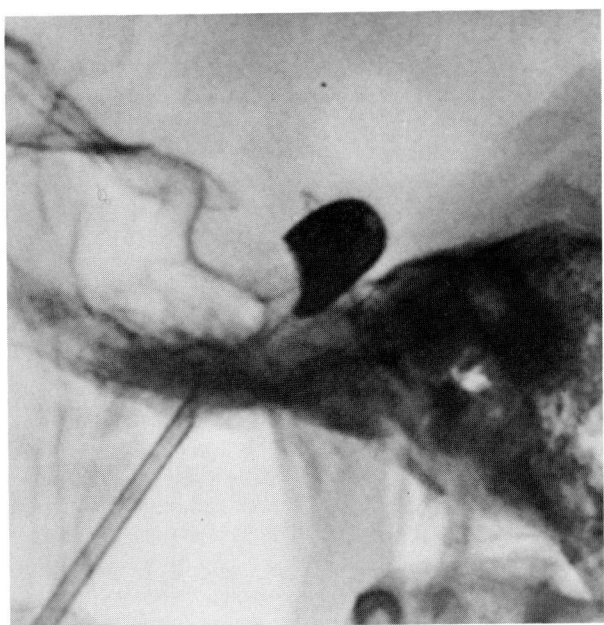

FIGURE 123-3. Cylindrical shape, indicating that the balloon is placed intradurally (or in a very large cave). The needle, which had been withdrawn slightly, had penetrated the skull in the bevel-down position, creating the dural puncture that permitted the intradural placement of the catheter.

optimal distension in some caves of large size or unusual shape in which the balloon does not assume the regular pear-shaped appearance. Such a pressure duration combination may be used to help predict the degree of sensory decrease and the duration of pain relief, but this has not been achieved. In earlier studies, compression of several minutes' duration was carried out but seemed to be associated with a greater incidence of dysesthesia and has now been abandoned.

THE PAIN REFLEX

The pain reflex has been studied in detail.[20, 21] This reflex may be completely eliminated, if thought to be undesirable, by preoperative atropine. If atropine, which produces tachycardia, is regarded as undesirable, the reflex can be eliminated by a noninvasive pacemaker, which triggers at a preset bradycardia, such as 45 beats/minute.[9] In the unprotected patient, asystole of 15 seconds or longer has been produced, necessitating in one surgeon's opinion a period of external chest compression.[7] Although such asystole has been observed on several occasions by one of the authors (SM), instant decompression and administration of atropine were the only intervention needed. In fact, the pulse will pick up in rate before there is time for the atropine to work. Nevertheless, atropine should always be available and should be given early if a patient shows a greater-than-average sensitivity of the pain reflex, as indicated by an unusual degree of bradycardia during engagement in the foramen ovale or at the beginning of compression. Atropine in these patients should not be delayed until asystole has become manifest.

TECHNICAL PROBLEMS OF NEEDLE INSERTION

In one patient with Paget's disease, and in one other without disease, entering the foramen was not possible. In earlier years, when patients who had had previous alcohol treatment were encountered, some technical difficulties of engagement were experienced.

POSTOPERATIVE SENSATION

Immediately after the procedure is completed, a good reddening of the ipsilateral conjunctiva, with or without some tearing, implies a good result. The patient awakens without pain, except for some discomfort from the site of the needle track, or a more marked localized discomfort if a hematoma is present. Because pain sensation is decreased, not absent, this local pain or discomfort can be expected. A decrease in touch and pinprick is expected on the affected side, more in the third division than in the second, and more in the second division than in the first. Little change may occur in the second division, and none may occur in the first, yet despite these findings, pain may be completely relieved in these divisions. In fact, some patients, on awakening, have a hypersensitivity to pain on the affected side, which later turns into hyposensitivity, but these patients rarely have a marked degree of sensory loss. A decrease in tickle sensation within the nostril indicates a favorable response. Corneal reflex may or may not be decreased. Compression does not selectively impair A-delta and C fibers, as does the radiofrequency lesion.[20–22] Within a few days of surgery, some patients develop a labial herpetic eruption, especially those who have had such eruptions in the past. Such a lesion can be taken as a sign of a good compression and a good outcome.

If very little or no sensory loss occurs, no relief or an early recurrence may be expected. Sometimes, despite inadequate compression, the patient may now achieve freedom from pain on a dose of carbamazepine (Tegretol) that was previously ineffective. Rarely, persistence of trigeminal pain in the first day or two may be followed by relief. This rare happening has also been noted after the Taarnhöj/Shelden procedure. Sweet records a period of relief subsequent to aborted radiofrequency (RF) procedures, although absolutely no lesion was made.[19] The patient usually finds the subjective numbness uncomfortable at first, but within 3 or 4 weeks, he or she usually adjusts to it and is no longer troubled. It is "like beginning to wear dentures or contact lenses," as one patient described it. Some patients who are obsessive-compulsive and are disturbed by anything that is not exactly perfect find it less tolerable. If such a patient is identified before the operation, the surgeon should explain that microdecompression is a valid alternative. The durations of subjective numbness and objective hypoesthesia (decreased sensitivity to touch) and hypalgesia (decreased sensitivity to pain) are quite variable but decrease considerably by 3 to 6 months. Pain does not automatically return once they disappear, nor does their persistence guarantee that there will be no recurrence. However, pain relief generally persists long after return of good sensation, apparently because good sensation does not demand a totally intact nerve. If a microvascular decompression is performed, subsequent to return of pain, the nerve at operation is seen to be considerably atrophied, despite the presence of good sensation.

MOTOR WEAKNESS

Initial motor weakness of the ipsilateral temporal and masseter muscles is almost invariable and recovers about 3 months after surgery. Most patients are unaware of it, not having used that side of their mouth for eating for many months or years. Some, especially those with a prosthesis, may be aware of malocclusion, or more rarely, of a mobile (very, very rarely painful) temporomandibular joint.

ABNORMAL SENSATIONS

Paresthesia, or abnormal feelings, may consist of pins and needles, water dripping, hands crawling, tightness, or a very mild burning sensation and has been reported in 12 percent of patients. When burning is severe, when these paresthesias become disturbing, or when hypalgesia and hypoesthesia are regarded as unpleasant, the situation is known as dysesthesia. In earlier days of the procedure, when compression was maintained for several minutes, and when patients with previous forms of treatment, such as alcohol and RF were encountered, dysesthesia was prevalent (4 percent and 5 percent, respectively), but more recently, it has virtually disappeared.

RECURRENCE

The recurrence rate for trigeminal neuralgia has been 20 percent in 5 years, with most occurring in the second year, but there has been a steady, but slow continuing recurrence up to the tenth year, when the figure will reach an estimated 30 percent. At recurrence, the patient is again given carbamazepine and usually has quite satisfactory relief at a tolerable dose. For example, one patient who had a recurrence at 8 years after surgery maintains full relief on carbamazepine 4 years later. If carbamazepine fails, the patient is given the choice of repeat procedure or, if he or she is in reasonably good health, a microvascular compression. Most have chosen another compression, having easily tolerated the subsequent mild numbness. The repeat procedure has not caused any added technical difficulties. When an older patient chooses a craniotomy and wants to have a final and definitive procedure with the least possibility of recurrence, a one-third root section (inferior third) may be added to the decompression.

MULTIPLE SCLEROSIS

Patients with multiple sclerosis are treated in the customary fashion, but knowing how much compression to give is difficult. In some patients with this disease who have had no previous treatment and who have been subjected to a posterior fossa exploration, the nerve is substantially atrophic. If a routine compression is added to such a nerve, excessive numbness could result. After one such experience, we have tended to use a lesser rather than a greater compression initially, but we have also erred on the side of inadequate compression.

BILATERAL NEURALGIA

The procedure may be carried out bilaterally, provided that the motor function of the first side is fully recovered. If substantial residual numbness is present on the first side and numbness on the other side is added, the patient may experience some subjective difficulty in handling food. We have, however, carried out a second-side procedure on a patient who had a unilateral densely numb mouth, which occurred subsequent to a classic middle fossa two-thirds root section (sparing the motor), and the patient had no distress. Usually, if significant numbness is present on the initial side, a microvascular compression might be offered on the other side. Patients with multiple sclerosis are particularly liable to have bilateral pain. In our experience, they have tolerated a bilateral staged procedure well.

LITERATURE REVIEW

A review of literature has shown that certain problems may arise when the original technique is not strictly adhered to. In one instance, death was reported after a subarachnoid hemorrhage, complicated by later hydrocephalus, multiple shunts, and shunt infection.[8] The needle had advanced beyond the foramen ovale. In another, a catheter was said to have entered the carotid artery (without complications). It is impossible to imagine doing this unless the needle had penetrated the artery.[19] In another, in which a No. 3 (smaller) Fogarty catheter was used, a high recurrence rate was reported.[14] In yet another, blindness followed a 12-minute compression.[4] The mechanism is unknown. One case of corneal anesthesia has been described.[11] Other investigators have reported performing the procedure with the patient under local anesthesia, but this method robs the procedure of one of its major benefits,[11,13] which is a pain-free intervention.

In the author's experience, complications have been minor. A sixth nerve weakness of very short duration has been observed on three occasions. Two instances of very small arteriovenous fistulae were encountered, one dural and one in the pterygoid fossa. Treatment was unnecessary because the bruit was only rarely appreciated. In a third, a persistent bruit resulted from a maxillary artery fistula. It was easily eliminated the next day by endovascular wire coil occlusion. This experience might suggest that a greater use of the trocar and cannula rather than the needle is desirable. The spontaneous resolution of such a fistula within 19 days has been reported by Revuelta and colleagues.[23]

SUMMARY

Percutaneous microcompression of the trigeminal ganglion, now in use for 14 years, has proved to be a highly effective, relatively trouble-free method of relieving trigeminal neuralgia, with a recurrence rate that approximates that of RF ganglion lysis and microvascular decompression (20 percent within 5 years). Its technique is simpler for the surgeon than the RF method, and, because it is conducted with the patient under general anesthesia, it is pain free for the patient, which is a much-appreciated benefit. The ability to keep the needle outside the skull eliminates intracranial needle complications. Reports of more than 600 cases have been published.[19]

REFERENCES

1. Mullan JF, Lichtor T: Percutaneous microcompression of the trigeminal ganglion for trigeminal neuralgia. J Neurosurg 59:1007–1012, 1983
2. Shelden CH, Pudenz RH, Freshwater DB, Crue BL: Compression rather than decompression for trigeminal neuralgia. J Neurosurg 12:123–126, 1955
3. Shelden CH, Crue BL, Coulter JA: Surgical treatment of trigeminal neuralgia and discussion of compression operation. Postgrad Med 27:595–601, 1960
4. Taarnhöj P: Decompression of the trigeminal root and the posterior part of the ganglion as treatment in trigeminal neuralgia: Preliminary communication. J Neurosurg 9:288–290, 1952
5. Svien HJ, Love JG: Results of decompression operation for trigeminal neuralgia four years plus after operation. J Neurosurg 16:653–655, 1959
6. Graf GJ: Trigeminal compression for the tic douloureux: An evaluation. J Neurosurg 20:1029–1032, 1963
7. Belber CJ, Rak RA: Balloon compression rhizolysis in the treatment of trigeminal neuralgia. Neurosurgery 20:908–913, 1987
8. Bricolo A, Dalle Ore G: Percutaneous microcompression of the gasserian ganglion for trigeminal neuralgia: Preliminary results. Acta Neurochir (Wien) 69:102, 1983
9. Brown JA, Preul MC: Percutaneous trigeminal ganglion compression for trigeminal neuralgia: Experience in 22 patients and review of the literature. J Neurosurg 70:900–904, 1989
10. Connelley TJ: Balloon compression and trigeminal neuralgia. Med J Aust 2:119, 1982

11. Esposito S, Delitala A, Bruni P, et al: Therapeutic protocol in the treatment of trigeminal neuralgia. Appl Neurophysiol 48:271–273, 1985
12. Fiume D, Scarda G, Natali G, Della Valle G: La microcompressione percutanea del ganglio di Gasser: Una nuova terapia per le nevralgie del trigemino. Riv Neurol 55(6):387–391, 1985
13. Fraioli B, Esposito V, Guidetti B, et al: Treatment of trigeminal neuralgia by thermocoagulation, glycerolization, and percutaneous compression of the gasserian ganglion and/or retrogasserian rootlets: Long-term results and therapeutic protocol. Neurosurgery 24(2):239–245, 1989
14. Fraioli B, Ferrante L, Santoro A, Di Giugno G: Recent progress in the treatment of trigeminal neuralgia: Glycerol into the trigeminal cistern and percutaneous gasserian compression by means of Fogarty's catheter. Acta Neurochir Suppl (Wien) 33:507–510, 1984
15. Lobato RD, Rivas JJ, Sarabia R, Lamas E: Percutaneous microcompression of the gasserian ganglion for trigeminal neuralgia. J Neurosurg 72:546–553, 1990
16. Meglio M, Cioni B, d'Annunziov V: Percutaneous microcompression of the gasserian ganglion: Personal experience. Acta Neurochir Suppl (Wien) 39:142–143, 1987
17. Lichtor T, Mullan JF: A 10-year follow-up review of percutaneous microcompression of the trigeminal ganglion. J Neurosurg 72:49–54, 1990
18. Spaziante R, Cappabiance P, Peca C, de Divitiis E: Subarachnoid hemorrhage and "normal pressure hydrocephalus": Fatal complication of percutaneous microcompression of the gasserian ganglion. Neurosurgery 22:148–151, 1988
19. Sweet WH: Complications of treating trigeminal neuralgia: An analysis of the literature and response to questionnaire, in Rovit R (ed): Trigeminal Neuralgia. Baltimore, Williams & Wilkins, 1990, pp 251–279
19a. Gerber AU: Needle for use during percutaneous compression of gasserian ganglia for trigeminal neuralgia; Technical note. J Neurosurg 21:45, 1989
20. Cruccu G, Inghilleri M, Fraioli B, et al: Neurophysiologic assessment of trigeminal function after surgery for trigeminal neuralgia. Neurology 37:631–638, 1987
21. Preul MC, Long PB, Brown JA, et al: Autonomic and histopathological effects of percutaneous trigeminal ganglion compression in the rabbit. J Neurosurg 72:933–940, 1990
22. Frigyesi T, Sigfried J, Brozzi G: The selective vulnerability of evoked potentials in the trigeminal sensory root to graded thermocoagulation. Exp Neurol 49:11–21, 1975
23. Revuelta R, Nathal E, Balderrama J, et al: External carotid artery fistula due to microcompression of the gasserian ganglion for relief of trigeminal neuralgia. J Neurosurg 78:499, 1993

CHAPTER 124

Complications of Percutaneous Rhizotomy and Microvascular Decompression Operations for Facial Pain

William H. Sweet
Charles E. Poletti

*I*t is our impression that in today's medicolegal climate in the United States, a sustained effort is necessary to alter the potential plaintiff/patient versus defendant/doctor adversarial relationship that is prevalent in the practice of medicine and to return it to cordial patient-doctor friendships, as in days of yore. Scrupulous honesty in describing the risks as well as the advantages of our alternative plans of action is our continuing obligation and is part of our effort to improve our public image. Hence, we have decided to republish the essential points of the chapter on complications with only minor changes.

The basic problem is that we tend to report series of patients in whom we are pleased with our results. As I survey my publications, I find that I just do not get around to publishing outcomes of my efforts if they are inferior to those already recorded. First, it is a waste of my colleagues' time to read about how I achieve inferior results. For example, I have failed to publish my techniques and results in the transfrontal removal of pituitary adenomas. It became clear that those performing transsphenoidal removals were having better results and that an article by me would not be worth reading. However, we do need to know what special vulnerabilities may be associated with our procedures and have no way of assuring that such problems are automatically reported. To remedy this deficiency with respect to the commoner invasive treatments for trigeminal neuralgia, as a pilot study, we wrote to 200 neurosurgical friends (including 50 abroad), indicating the basis for the study and requesting data from them on complications on their services or complications that they knew followed percutaneous radiofrequency lesions or microvascular decompression. To this burdensome request, 140 neurosurgeons, to whom we are most grateful, replied.

COMPLICATIONS OF PERCUTANEOUS RADIOFREQUENCY TRIGEMINAL RHIZOTOMIES

Ninety-one services provided the following data, and nearly all were not previously reported: 29 services gave their entire numbers of rhizotomies, totaling over 7000. Of lesser complications, there were 18 patients with neuroparalytic keratitis, eight with aseptic meningeal reactions (negative cultures), and five with carotid-cavernous fistulas. In three of these five cases, the Nugent type of blunt electrode protruding beyond the sharp pointed needle was used to make the heat lesion. There were 18 temporary oculomotor palsies, at least one of which was permanent; this last lesion was later shown to be caused by placement of the electrode in the inferior orbital fissure, there having been no prelesion roentgenogram. A seizure occurred during the procedure in two patients, and in one, a transient postoperative psychosis developed. In eight patients, brief asystolic periods developed during needle-electrode placement or lesion production, despite the patient's unconsciousness under intravenous anesthetic. These incidents have been properly prevented from recurring by the administration of intravenous atropine.

Hemorrhages might have been related to increased bleeding times not only because of the high doses of varied drugs for the facial pain—mostly trigeminal neuralgia—but also because these older patients were often taking anticoagulant drugs related to cardiac or cerebrovascular disease. Of 130 of our recent patients, the bleeding time was abnormal, at greater than 9½ minutes in 21 patients (16 percent ["Surgicutt" method]).

The wrong foramina which are the most difficult to avoid are inconstantly present as small openings for emissary veins only a few millimeters distant from the foramen ovale. I have entered the more frequently occurring of these two foramina nine times. The first eight times, this event occurred without incident and was followed by replacement of the electrode and making of an appropriate lesion in the same session. The radiographic appearances in the first five cases were published in 1976 and were described as resulting from penetration of an unnamed foramen. However, the ninth time, I produced a left intratemporal hemorrhage. Luckily, complete recovery from the evoked aphasia occurred within 2 weeks. The episode stimulated me to a more careful search, and I found at least three famous anatomic texts—Gray, Testut, and Paturet—that described a small "foramen or canal of

1543

Vesalius," anterior and/or medial to ovale. Only Paturet described a second small opening posterior to the lateral third of ovale, which he called the innominate foramen or canaliculus of Arnold. I have seen the canal of Vesalius on the left side in only two of six skulls I have examined, and I have found it large enough to admit an 18-gauge needle in one and a 19-gauge needle in the other. In the lateral radiographs of these skulls, the electrode lies opposite the shadow of the sella turcica, as was the case in seven of my nine in vivo cases. In the other two, the shaft projected in front of the sella turcica and might have been in the inferior orbital fissure. In all nine cases, the needle probably penetrated the temporal lobe. De Rougemont described having pierced the innominate foramen, probably with similar invasion of the temporal lobe.

Entry into the foramen lacerum has been reported and is likely to puncture the internal carotid artery, a mishap that can also occur if the inferior bony wall of the intrapetrous internal carotid canal is absent. Direct entry into the desired middle-to-medial part of the foramen ovale can be achieved by the use of fluoroscopy. It is also easily possible to enter temporal lobe or midbrain via the foramen ovale if the trajectory is too high or too far posterior. This situation can be avoided by use of the fluoroscopic unit in the lateral view as one advances the electrode by small increments.

We have seen at least nine patients in whom the electrode shaft entered the middle fossa via an opening anterior to the foramen ovale, the foramen of Vesalius, yet the much-too-anterior point might give rise on stimulation to first- or second-division paresthesias. In another case, one of the authors (WHS) obtained 16 ml of clear, colorless cerebrospinal fluid at the electrode site. Stimulation evoked a throbbing in the cheek bone at 0.30 V, 50 cycles/seconds, 1 sigma pulse duration, and heating to 48°C elicited "warmth" in the cheek bone. The x-ray films revealed the needle point to be in the pars nervosa of the jugular foramen.

OPTIC NERVE LESIONS

One patient developed pupillary dilatation, subhyaloid hemorrhage, and permanent blindness ipsilateral to the lesion in the recovery room.

One patient developed transient ipsilateral amblyopia as the lesions were being made. Four patients developed permanent complete blindness immediately after radiofrequency lesions were made. In one patient, total internal and external ophthalmoplegia occurred, and paresis occurred in nerves III, IV, and VI as well. In another patient, who had severe multiple sclerosis for 7 years, third-nerve paresis accompanied the blindness. In one of the two patients who developed only blindness without extraocular motor paresis, only two lesions were made, totaling 1 minute at 75°C.

In at least three of these four patients, after electrode placement, second-division pain occurred at electrical stimulation; this sensation was taken as adequate evidence of correct position of the electrode. Apparently, no confirmatory roentgenograms were taken in two of the four patients, because of technical failure of the radiographic equipment. Morley (Personal communication, 1986) finds it unnecessary to "resort to x-ray control for placement of the needle." However, we recommend making no lesion unless the desired responses to electrical stimulation at low threshold are accompanied by roentgenograms that in both lateral and sagittal views show the electrode shaft through the foramen ovale and the electrode tip in the expected position.

CENTRAL RETINAL ARTERY OCCLUSION

Central retinal artery occlusion occurred once in our series, in a diabetic patient.

DANGEROUS, DISABLING, OR FATAL SEQUELAE

One myocardial infarct occurred 4 days postoperatively; the 91-year-old patient died. Another myocardial infarct developed during the procedure when excessive dose of a vasodilator drug, given to prevent a rise of systolic pressure during the making of the lesion, was followed by hypotension of 24 mm Hg for 1 minute. The patient completely recovered.

Seven intracerebral (usually temporal lobe) abscesses occurred: one patient had permanent mental impairment, and three patients died. Twenty-one patients had bacterial meningitides: one patient, whose symptoms began 1 week postoperatively, died. In this patient, therapy began late in the course of the disorder. No other sequelae occurred in this patient group.

Nineteen hemorrhages (focal intracranial) occurred. In one patient, an infratemporal subdural hematoma occurred because of a needle puncture of the inferior temporal vein; when the clot was removed, the patient recovered. Three patients had hemorrhages of the ipsilateral intratemporal lobe: two died, and one was disabled (reported on earlier). Fifteen intracerebral hemorrhages occurred that were probably unrelated to the site of the electrode: eight patients died. Four patients suffered major residual sequelae (one caused by thrombocytopenia), and three patients had transitory hemiplegias. We recommend that preoperative studies be performed to assess coagulopathy, including bleeding times and monitoring of blood pressure during procedure, and that intravenous nitroprusside or other vasodilator be administered to prevent an excessive rise in blood pressure.

One arterial puncture occurred by needle-electrode; this event was followed by hemiparesis that lasted for 4 days. Five arterial subarachnoid hemorrhages occurred from the needle-electrode; two patients fully recovered, and three died—one with the needle through the infraorbital foramen into the anterior cerebral artery. In another patient, an 80-year-old woman, brisk bleeding occurred at needle placement. The bleeding was stopped and the lesion made. Six hours later, a massive subarachnoid hemorrhage occurred in the posterior and middle fossas bilaterally. We recommend stopping the procedure at once if arterial bleeding is produced—even if the bleeding is from the extracranial internal carotid artery—and resuming days later when the puncture site is healed. We have used a 20-gauge needle-electrode (cross-sectional area, 0.63 mm^2) in preference to a 19-gauge needle (cross-sectional area, 0.95 mm^2). We have never had a sequela to an arterial puncture with the 20-gauge electrode.

In at least six services (Broggi, Nugent, Siegfried, Sweet,

Table 124–1. TRIGEMINAL NEURALGIA—MICROVASCULAR DECOMPRESSION (REPORTS FROM 49 SERVICES)

Number of Cases*	Complications—Cases not previously published
Virtually no complications (9 services)	
20	3 early recurrences; pain stopped when displaced Ivalon sponge replaced; 0 complications
~150	"No major complications or deaths"
~15	0 significant complications
9	0 complications
24	0 complications
—	0 complications
"A few"	0 complications
3	0 complications
—	10 days postoperatively, sudden ipsilateral sensory loss occurred with later recovery
Moderate complications (19 services)	
—	1 temporary bilateral deafness; 1 marked intraoperative cerebellar swelling → permanent VIII with mild ataxia
26	1 CSF leak → reoperative closure; 1 temporary ipsilateral ataxia
—	1 contralateral permanent complete deafness
72	2 cerebellar hematomas, removed, patients well; temporary—1 IV; 1 VI; 1 VII; 1 ataxia
—	Some mild permanent gait disturbance; 2 temporary diplopias
~70	1 lasting total ipsilateral deafness; 1 shoulder dislocation (no previous shoulder problems)
—	1 supratentorial subdural hematoma, recovery; 2 VII, 1 VIII, all partial
24	2 permanent complete ipsilateral deafness; 1 temporary VII
—	1 permanent seventh nerve paresis
"Several hundred"	2 partial deafness; 1 cerebellar edema → reoperated temporary diplopia and ataxia; 1 CSF rhinorrhea
—	Temporary sixth nerve paresis
20	1 complete anesthesia in all 3 fifth nerve divisions, uneventful operation
20/yr	2 diplopias; some "ataxias or other cerebellar findings", some "permanent gait disturbances"
5	1 moderately painful dysesthesia
—	1 decadron-sensitive aseptic meningitis; symptoms recurred when decadron stopped—duration ~2 months
—	1 subdural hematoma at operative site, removed, recovery; 1 aseptic meningeal reaction—cleared 10 days
—	1 laceration sigmoid sinus, 2-liter blood loss, normal recovery
~50	1 lasting corneal anesthesia, 1 CSF leak requiring reoperation; 2 transient VIII; 1 laceration of transverse sinus, operation aborted
—	Several lower cranial nerve paralysis
—	Lower cranial nerve palsies
Major complications (24 services)	
—	1 lasting disabling brainstem stroke; 1 CSF leak, protracted infection, recovery; 3 lasting palsies—2 VII; 1 VII and VIII
~14	1 pontine venous thrombosis—many petrosal veins coagulated at operation; decerebrate postures all 4 limbs—almost complete recovery
~10	1 temporary IV; 1 delayed cerebellar hematoma and hypertension >3 weeks postoperatively → death
—	1 cerebellar subdural hematoma → death
—	1 "venous thrombosis and hemorrhagic infarction of cerebellum" second postoperative day
—	1 case V root in a nest of veins, all coagulated and cut → coma → death
~70	1 "moderate" brainstem stroke, minor residual; 1 disabling brainstem stroke
—	1 basilar artery rupture during operation; death
—	"Occasional case" of posterior fossa hemorrhage, cerebellar hemorrhage, cerebellar infarction, VII or VIII nerve lesion
—	Thrombosis of contralateral middle cerebral artery intraoperatively; death on second postoperative day
2	1 intraoperative contralateral basal ganglionic hemorrhage → permanent total disability. (Transverse sinus entered during operation.)
—	2 serious strokes
"Several"	1 meningitis → vasculitis → hemorrhage → death; 1 lasting complete ipsilateral deafness
111	1 cerebral infarct → death; 1 severe lasting dementia; 2 hematomas → 1 acute epidural; 1 chronic subdural both recovered; 11 significant lasting cranial nerve injuries; 11 other lesser complications with recovery
—	1 cerebellar infarct → reoperated → polymicrobial meningitis → death in healthy, 59-year-old woman
—	Awoke after event-free operation with complete loss of function in cranial nerves IV, V, VI, VII, VIII, severe ipsilateral ataxia, contralateral increased weakness and clumsiness; 2 years later, same + anesthesia dolorosa
"Very infrequently"	1 death from pontine infarction
~30	Excellent surgeons—2 deaths, males, 1 aged 31 years, 1 aged 50, uneventful operations; post mortems; necrosis of cerebellum and brainstem due to occlusion of petrosal veins
15	Multiple intraoperative intracerebral hemorrhages—confirmed at autopsy 6 days postoperatively, female, aged 55 years
"Very few"	1 totally disabling "reactive meningitis"; at reoperation "chronic hypertrophic meningitis" involving many cranial nerves; impossible to remove sponge at trigeminal nerve
30	Excellent surgeon—2 postoperative deaths in 2 healthy patients circa 50 years of age after smooth, uneventful operations
—	1 protracted wound infection, final recovery; 2 VII and 1 VII and VIII, all lasting; 1 disabling cerebellar and brainstem stroke
50	1 early postoperative death—cerebellar hematoma; 1 chronic bilateral frontal subdural hematoma with recovery
~125	2 deaths in 48 hours postoperatively; 1 superior cerebellar and postcerebral infarcts—female, late 50s, 1 quadriplegia followed by coma—female "embittered family refused autopsy." Both operations uneventful
	1 left hemiplegia after left microvascular decompression—nearly normal by 6 weeks—female
	1 left hemiparesis, left hemisensory deficit, and left homonymous hemianopia; only the hemiparesis recovered—male, aged 64 years

CSF = cerebrospinal fluid.
*A dash indicates no total number of cases stated.

Taren, Tew), each of which performed well over 1000 percutaneous retrogasserian trigeminal procedures, no lasting major extratrigeminal complication has occurred. It is easy to take a casual attitude toward the procedure because of its simplicity. The achievement of consistent success without sequelae demands scrupulous attention to detail.

Because the percutaneous method inevitably involves a risk of intratrigeminal morbidity, one does well to maximize the avoidance of significant extratrigeminal morbidity, the main advantage of this tactic.

TRIGEMINAL NEURALGIA—MICROVASCULAR DECOMPRESSION (REPORTS FROM 49 SERVICES) (Table 124–1)

Nine services reported no complications; the two largest series with these results had 24 and approximately 150 cases. In 17 services, no deaths and only moderate lasting sequelae occurred. In the nine of these that reported their numbers of operated cases, these figures varied from five to "several hundred." From 24 services came accounts of permanently disabling sequelae or deaths in 29 cases. The two largest series in this group comprised 111 and approximately 125 cases. The next largest series comprised 50 cases. The two most discouraging series involved three technically competent, distinguished neurosurgeons, who had four deaths in 60 patients, all in "healthy" individuals, three in their 50s and one aged 31, all following "smooth, uneventful operations."

SUMMARY

Although we believe that by taking appropriate precautions, one can almost eliminate the major complications and deaths from percutaneous operations, we recommend mentioning these risks to patients. How to reduce the risk of microvascular decompression is not so obvious. Perhaps the most clearcut warning is that coagulation of essential veins draining the brainstem probably led to a major infarct in four cases. Should significant blood loss occur if the transverse sinus is opened, one should consider aborting the procedure. Even if the neurosurgeon has enough experience to emphasize only his or her own results, he or she would be well advised to describe to patients the possibility of a fuller range of complications than were seen in the best series.

Acknowledgment

The authors wish to express their gratitude to the Neuro Research Foundation for its support during the preparation of the manuscript.

CHAPTER 125

Vestibular Nerve Section in the Management of Vertigo

Horace Norrell
Herbert Silverstein

During the past decade, vestibular nerve section has become an increasingly popular method of relieving inner ear vertigo. A recent survey described the results of 2820 vestibular nerve sections reported by 58 surgeons in the United States.[1] The modern trend toward interdisciplinary surgical approaches frequently combines the talents of both neurosurgeon and neurotologist during cranial nerve operations. The neurosurgeon's role in vestibular neurectomy may vary from primary surgeon to operative assistant, but in either event, the neurosurgeon must have a clear understanding of the disease process involving the vestibular system, as well as of treatment options and surgical technique. The surgical anatomy and techniques involved in vestibular nerve section are also applicable to most posterior skull base operations.

HISTORICAL PERSPECTIVE

In 1912, Frazier described one patient in whom he sectioned the eighth cranial nerve as a treatment for "aural vertigo."[2] Not until 1924, when Dandy began his surgical series, did eighth-nerve section receive more widespread attention.[3] Anatomic dissections of the eighth nerve by McKenzie in 1930 permitted him to first differentially section the vestibular nerve, preserving the cochlear nerve in 117 patients.[4]

Dandy soon adopted the selective vestibular nerve section and ultimately performed 607 eighth-nerve sections for vertiginous disorders.[5, 6] One half of the patients in Dandy's series underwent a total eighth-nerve section, resulting in a 9.2-percent incidence of permanent facial paralysis. The remaining patients who underwent neurectomy in Dandy's series experienced a 1.7-percent incidence of permanent facial paralysis, whereas McKenzie reported only a 1-percent incidence.

Even during the earliest days of vestibular nerve section for Ménière's disease, otologists were exploring alternative surgical procedures. In 1927, Portmann, a French otologist, described an operation to incise the endolymphatic sac that was based on the assumption that Ménière's disease resulted from increased endolymphatic sac pressure.[7] Endolymphatic sac surgery was further explored based on the Portmann's description of overdistention of the endolymphatic spaces (endolymphatic hydrops) in patients with Ménière's disease.

Ultimately, the endolymphatic sac was shunted into the cerebrospinal fluid of the posterior fossa.[8] Endolymphatic shunts are still popular, despite argument that the procedure is ineffective.[1, 9, 10]

In 1946, Dandy died at age 60, and at about the same time an English otologist, Cawthorne, described using the dissecting microscope to remove the membranous labyrinth as another treatment of Ménière's disease.[11] By the 1950s, labyrinthectomy and endolymphatic sac surgery had replaced vestibular neurectomy as the surgical procedure of choice for intractable peripheral vertigo. Both operations were more appealing than a craniotomy. The number of surgical cases was also reduced both by otologists' becoming more selective in choosing candidates for surgery and by the introduction of a more successful medical treatment. Patients with Ménière's disease who experienced failure after a long course of conservative therapy (usually managed by an otolaryngologist) emerged as ideal surgical candidates in the hands of the otologists. The neurosurgeon's role in the treatment of vertigo soon disappeared.

In 1961, House, a Los Angeles otologist, described a microsurgical approach to the internal auditory canal through a subtemporal, extradural route (middle fossa approach).[12] The superior and inferior vestibular nerves were exposed and could be sectioned within the depths of the internal auditory canal by drilling away the superior surface of the temporal bone, avoiding the labyrinth and facial nerves. Few neurosurgeons learned this technique, and many otologists found the exposure difficult and fraught with complications, including injury to the facial and auditory nerves and the labyrinth. The middle fossa vestibular nerve section continues to be popular among a select group of otologists.[1]

In 1972, Hitselberger and Pulec described a unique operative exposure of the posterior fossa for operations on the trigeminal nerve, the retrolabyrinthine approach.[13] An opening into the posterior fossa is created by performing a mastoidectomy and removing the bone covering the posterior fossa dura between the sigmoid sinus and the labyrinth. The procedure was further modified by Brackmann and Hitselberger in 1978 to allow many posterior cranial fossa operations.[14] While removing an intracranial glossopharyngeal neurinoma through a retrolabyrinthine exposure, Silverstein noted not only the close proximity of the dural opening to the nerves of the cerebellopontine angle but also a well-delineated cleavage plane between the cochlear and vestibular portions of the eighth nerve.[15] The opening seemed to offer a simple surgical approach with minimal cerebellar retraction, thereby permitting vestibular nerve section within the cerebellopontine angle.

During the performance of 60 retrolabyrinthine vestibular nerve sections, the occasional lack of a definite cochleovestibular cleavage plane along the eighth nerve within the cerebellopontine angle was disturbing.[16] The disadvantage of the retrolabyrinthine approach was that it did not provide the amount of exposure of the petrous bone that would permit opening of the internal auditory canal. The eighth nerve could be followed only as far laterally as the porus acusticus. This need to see and identify the nerves within the internal auditory canal led to the development of the combined retrolabyrinthine-retrosigmoid approach in 1985.[16] This exposure differs from the conventional neurosurgical posterior cranial fossa opening in that in addition to removal of the bone behind the sigmoid sinus, a limited mastoidectomy is performed to expose the entire width and length of the sigmoid sinus from its origin at the transverse sinus down to the portion just proximal to the jugular bulb. Today, this exposure is widely used for vestibular nerve section as well as for the removal of acoustic neuromas in which hearing preservation is the goal. Many skilled otologists and neurosurgeons continue to perform retrolabyrinthine or middle fossa vestibular nerve sections with results quite similar to those achieved by the combined approach.[1] As endoscopic techniques and equipment improve, the possibility of endoscopic posterior fossa vestibular nerve section remains on the horizon. In a contrast to the anecdotal results reported in earlier days of vestibular nerve sections, results today are objectively documented and established so that careful postoperative evaluation and comparisons are possible.[17]

DIFFERENTIAL DIAGNOSIS OF VESTIBULAR DISORDERS

Rarely is the neurosurgeon the initial consultant for the "dizzy patient," but it is important for the neurosurgeon to be able to establish a correct diagnosis and have an understanding of vestibular disorders. The etiology of the vertigo must be determined before any treatment is undertaken. The differentiation between peripheral and central vertigo is the first step in arriving at a diagnosis. Peripheral vertigo arises from the inner ear or vestibular nerve, whereas central vertigo's origin is the brainstem or cerebellum. History and physical examination, combined with audiovestibular testing and diagnostic imaging, results in an accurate diagnosis.

Peripheral vertigo is characterized by an intense subjective sensation of spinning, accompanied by nystagmus. The vertigo is frequently induced by positional changes, and the vertigo and nystagmus rarely persist for 30 seconds, even when position is maintained. If the provocative moves are repeated, the signs and symptoms progressively lessen with each trial (fatigability). In contrast, central positional vertigo may occur with head movements in the recumbent patient, but the patient does not have the intense vertigo experienced with peripheral disorders. The vertigo persists as long as the position is maintained and lacks latency of onset and fatigability. Peripheral vertigo can be relieved by vestibular nerve section, whereas central vertigo cannot.

Ménière's disease classically affects middle-aged adults, producing a triad of symptoms. Early symptoms include fluctuating unilateral hearing loss and tinnitus; later in the course of the disease, vertiginous attacks appear. The vertiginous attacks last from minutes to hours, disabling the victim, who prefers to lie immobilized in a dark and quiet place. Frequently, the individual vertiginous attack is preceded by a sensation of increasing pressure or fullness in the involved ear. Vertigo attacks may undergo remissions and exacerbations and finally disappear as the disease "burns out" while hearing and vestibular functions suffer progressive deterioration. Occasionally, vestibular symptoms may predominate from the start, with minimal hearing loss, a condition that leads to a diagnosis of vestibular Ménière's disease. Rarely, drop attacks (Tumarkin attacks), with or without vertigo, may occur as a manifestation of Ménière's disease.[18] Patients experiencing such attacks describe the sensation as a feeling of being pushed or shoved to the ground without loss of consciousness.

Otologic testing in patients with Ménière's disease reveals a hearing loss in the low frequencies early in the course of disease. Electronystagmography demonstrates a reduced caloric response in the affected ear, but neuroimaging studies reveal no abnormalities. Ultimately, profound hearing loss in all frequencies may occur, producing loss of serviceable hearing in the involved ear. In 15 to 40 percent of patients, the disease may ultimately involve both ears.

Most investigators agree that Ménière's disease results from endolymphatic hydrops or overdistension of the endolymphatic spaces, ultimately resulting in fibrosis of the labyrinth. The vertiginous episodes occur with the rupture of the endolymphatic membranes, allowing potassium-rich endolymph to comix with the potassium-poor perilymph. The potassium influx produces depolarization of the vestibular nerve endings, thereby producing vertigo and nystagmus. As repair proceeds, symptoms resolve, and hearing may improve to near-normal, although each attack results in progressive degenerative changes in both the cochlear and vestibular nerve endings.

The clinician must differentiate between Ménière's disease and other episodic peripheral vertigo disorders; the results of vestibular nerve section for Ménière's disease exceed the relief afforded for other conditions. Other important causes of acute vertiginous disorders include vestibular neuronitis and chronic labyrinthitis. Vestibular neuronitis occurs as a single or recurrent vertiginous episode without hearing loss. The etiology appears to be an inflammatory process, possibly viral, involving the vestibular ganglia. Chronic labyrinthitis follows middle ear inflammatory disease or trauma to the labyrinth. Chronic labyrinthitis may result in recurrent episodes of vertigo but may also be associated with chronic disequilibrium.

Benign positional vertigo must not be confused with Ménière's disease or other chronic vestibular disorders. In patients with benign positional vertigo, rapid changes in position result in brief vertiginous episodes. In the provocative test for this disorder, the patient quickly assumes the lateral supine position (Hallpike's maneuver). Symptoms occur only when the ear containing the diseased labyrinth is on the down side. Vertigo occurs, and rotatory nystagmus appears. The nystagmus is fatigable on repeated provocative testing, and the disease is frequently self-limited. Disabling or persistent symptoms may require section of the nerve to the ampulla of the posterior semicircular canal.

The role of vascular cross compression involving the vestibular nerve deserves mention. Dandy, in discussing Ménière's disease in 1937, stated, "In about 20 percent of the cases, a large artery (one of the branches of the superior-inferior cerebellar artery) lies against the nerve and, I think, is the cause of deafness and dizziness in this disease."[19] Jannetta and associates championed the cross-compression theory as the cause of vertigo that does not fit any other diagnostic profile.[20] Typical symptoms consist of a constant positional vertigo or a disequilibrium so severe that patients are disabled or constantly nauseated. Patients characteristically have motion intolerance, particularly when riding in an automobile or while pushing a shopping cart and gazing along the shelves. No demonstrable loss of auditory or vestibular function occurs. In Jannetta's opinion, vascular compression of the vestibular nerve at the brainstem is responsible for this disorder. (See commentary at the end of this chapter.) Vessels further distal along the course of the vestibular nerve are common and are not a source of the problem.

Disorders of the central nervous system, including multiple sclerosis or brainstem tumor, may produce acute central vertigo. Additional symptoms, signs, and neuroimaging study results differentiate these disorders.

Vertebral artery insufficiency rarely produces vertiginous attacks in the absence of other neurologic signs or symptoms. Acute occlusion of the labyrinthine artery may produce sudden hearing loss and vertigo, but the vertigo is self-limited once central accommodation occurs. Hearing loss is usually permanent.

Many patients complain of chronic disequilibrium without vertigo that does not fit any diagnostic description. Vestibular nerve section is not indicated in this patient group and can actually result in worsening of the patient's condition.

TREATMENT OF PERIPHERAL VESTIBULAR DISORDERS

Nonsurgical treatment forms the cornerstone of therapy for Ménière's disease and other peripheral labyrinthine disorders. Neurologists, internists, and otolaryngologists depend on vestibular depressant drugs, salt restriction, and diuretics to control symptoms. Time alone may produce a complete remission of symptoms. The unpredictability and the profound discomfort, as well as the interruption of lifestyle that accompanies the episodic vertigo attacks, compel the patient to seek surgical treatment. When the vertiginous attacks begin to interfere with everyday function, surgery becomes a consideration.

Dandy reportedly performed a vestibular neurectomy on patients with a wide variety of dizzy disorders, some within a week of the onset of the vertigo.[6] Indications for surgery today are continued intractable vertigo attacks that have not responded to multiple trials of medical treatment. Some surgeons continue to perform endolymphatic shunting as an initial surgical procedure in patients with Ménière's disease, reserving vestibular nerve section as the next step to surgical therapy.[1]

Ultimately, 20 percent of patients with Ménière's disease become surgical candidates. The selection of the initial procedure largely depends on the otologist's evaluation of the patient's hearing. With good hearing (a low speech reception threshold and high speech discrimination scores), preservation of auditory function is an additional goal of surgery; hence, selective vestibular nerve section is the procedure of choice. Because preservation of any hearing in the involved ear is important, even in patients with poor hearing, vestibular nerve section is usually the initial destructive procedure chosen. Occasionally, in a patient with very poor hearing, some surgeons choose labyrinthectomy or eighth-nerve section as the initial procedure. Poor hearing in the ear opposite to the one producing vertigo is a contraindication to vestibular neurectomy; the chance of hearing loss as a result of surgery must be considered. Bilateral Ménière's disease is another contraindication to vestibular neurectomy. Patients with ataxia or disequilibrium of central nervous system origin or a multisensory syndrome accommodate poorly after vestibular nerve section, and for these patients, the use of surgery should be discouraged.

Before surgery, all patients undergo auditory and vestibular testing (electronystagmography), including brainstem auditory evoked response testing. After surgery, auditory and vestibular studies are repeated to determine possible hearing loss and to detect any residual vestibular function. Gadolinium-enhanced magnetic resonance imaging is performed before surgery to exclude the rare tumor that mimics peripheral disease. In addition, all surgical patients undergo thin-section computed tomography of the temporal bone. For this procedure, sections 1.5-mm thick and at 1-mm intervals are taken. By use of bone windows, the temporal bone slices are reconstructed in both coronal and axial planes. These sections provide useful information on the anatomy of the labyrinth, the venous sinuses, and the internal auditory canal.

The surgical candidate must be well educated in postoperative expectations. Several preoperative sessions with a surgeon are necessary to answer all the patient's questions. The patient must understand that the major purpose of the surgery is to relieve vertiginous attacks; tinnitus will likely be unaffected, and hearing loss may continue to progress, following the natural course of Ménière's disease. The greatest fear most patients profess is facial paralysis; this consequence must be discussed frankly and openly. Unless the possibility of spinal fluid rhinorrhea and its treatment has been introduced before surgery, the uninformed patient assumes this to be a catastrophic complication if it occurs. The acute vertigo and the more subacute disequilibrium experienced after vestibular nerve section, both of which subside spontaneously, must be carefully explained. The nurses caring for the patient after surgery must also be well versed in the postoperative course. Anxiety from an inexperienced nurse can rapidly be transferred to the patient.

SURGICAL APPROACHES TO THE POSTERIOR CRANIAL FOSSA

Middle fossa vestibular nerve section is rarely in the operative repertoire of the neurosurgeon and is not described here. More recently, however, the surgical anatomy of the temporal bone has assumed greater importance to the neurosurgeon interested in skull base surgery.

Retrolabyrinthine and combined retrolabyrinthine-retrosig-

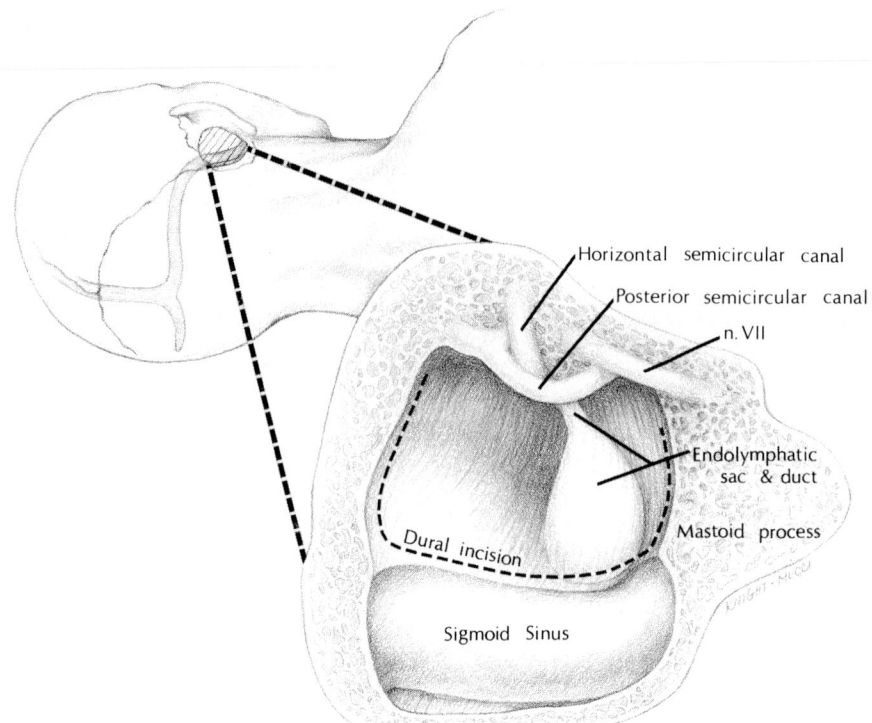

FIGURE 125–1. Removal of the right retrolabyrinthine bone exposes the sigmoid sinus and presigmoid sinus dura of the posterior fossa.

moid operations for relief of peripheral vertigo are generally performed by teams of neurosurgeons and neurotologists. The positions of the patient, the surgeon, and the anesthesiologist during the surgery are identical to those used for the retrolabyrinthine and the combined retrolabyrinthine-retrosigmoid operations. Endotracheal anesthesia is provided without neuromuscular blockade to allow facial nerve testing. Intracranial pressure is lowered by the administration of mannitol and by hypocarbia produced by controlled hyperventilation. The patient rests supine on an electrically controlled operating table, with the head turned and comfortably flexed away from the side of the surgery. Occasionally, pin-fixation head immobilization must be used, particularly in patients with very thick, short necks. The patient need not be positioned in the "park-bench" position or prone, provided that an electric operating table is available to enable rotation. The surgeon sits directly behind the patient's head, with the anesthesiologist further down on the same side of the operating table. The surgical nurse is positioned directly opposite the surgeon, and the surgical microscope base is positioned at the head of the operating table. Electronic equipment is stacked at the foot of the operating table. Intraoperative facial nerve function is monitored with electromyographic electrodes in the orbicularis oris and the orbicularis oculi muscles, along with a mechanical strain gauge sensor system, coupled with a computer.[21] Both brainstem auditory evoked potentials and direct eighth-nerve potentials are recorded during the operation. Direct eighth-nerve recordings are not considered to be an essential element in vestibular nerve section, but the use of this technique in all cases gives the surgeon a comfortable familiarity that is essential for acoustic neuroma surgery in which hearing preservation is the goal.

Retrolabyrinthine Exposure

Although the retrolabyrinthine exposure is not commonly in the neurosurgeon's armamentarium, it should be. With increasing interest in the removal of benign skull base tumors, particularly via the petrosal approach, familiarity with this surgical exposure is essential. A horseshoe-shaped retroauricular incision, with 5-cm arms and a 4-cm base located at the retroauricular crease, is made. With drilling and suction-irrigation, a complete mastoidectomy is performed to expose the entire sigmoid sinus from the superior petrosal sinus to the jugular bulb. A 1-cm edge of retrosigmoid dura is exposed to allow retraction of the sigmoid sinus. With the aid of the operating microscope, drilling is carried forward in the temporal bone beneath the descending facial nerve to expose the jugular bulb. The bone between the posterior semicircular canal and the jugular bulb must also be drilled away; this area provides a direct approach to the nerves of the cerebellopontine angle. It is unnecessary to expose the epineurium of the facial nerve or to blue-line any of the semicircular canal. The endolymphatic sac is totally exposed to its apical junction with the endolymphatic duct at the bony operculum (Fig. 125–1). Extradural landmarks enable the location of intradural structures. The eighth nerve in the cerebellopontine angle is found along an imaginary line extending from the surgeon through the crossing of the facial nerve and the posterior semicircular canal. The dura is opened superiorly to the sigmoid sinus, and the incision is extended down between the sigmoid sinus and the endolymphatic sac to the jugular bulb. The dural flap is retracted forward to cover the exposed labyrinth, and the cerebellum is gently retracted to allow opening of the cerebellopontine cistern. A special retractor permits retraction of the sigmoid

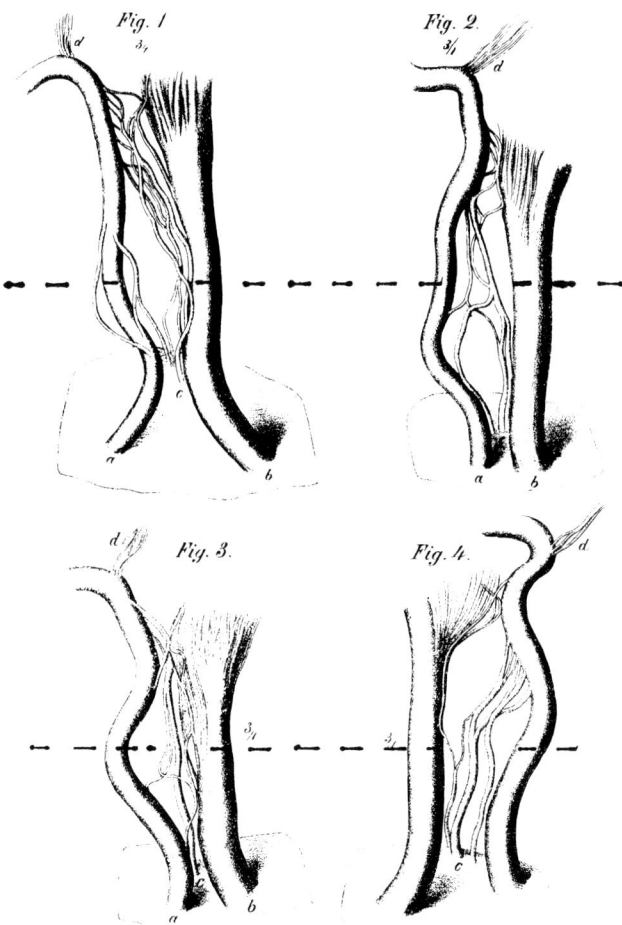

FIGURE 125–2. Dissection of nerves VII, VIII, and intermedius beginning at their emergence from the brainstem at a, b, and c, respectively, extending to their terminations within the petrous bone for nerves VIII and intermedius and to the knee of nerve VII at the point where it branches off the greater superficial petrosal nerve. Branches of the intermedius nerve unite about as often with nerve VIII as with nerve VII. Infrequently, this union occurs in the cerebellopontine cistern. The dashed line (- - -) through each drawing marks the approximate level of the opening into the internal auditory canal. (Courtesy of Bischoff EPE: Mikrospichen Analyse der Anastomosen der Kopfnerven. München J.J. Leniner 1865, Tab. XLIII, pp. 52.)

sinus along with a portion of the cerebellum to better expose the eighth nerve.[15]

Combined Retrolabyrinthine-Retrosigmoid Exposure

A linear skin incision is made 2 cm behind the mastoid tip extending from 2 cm above the lambdoid suture to well down into the neck. The occipital artery is exposed and coagulated just superficial to the bony exit of the mastoid emissary vein. A simple mastoidectomy is performed with a high-speed drill that exposes the entire length and width of the sigmoid sinus and the base of the endolymphatic sac. The superior extent of the bony opening is at the asterion, which is the usual external landmark that indicates the downward turn of the lateral sinus. A 3-cm craniectomy is then performed with rongeurs or a craniotome. The dura is incised 4 mm behind, and parallel to, the sigmoid sinus, with the ends of the dural incision curved posteriorly, thereby creating excellent exposure of the lateral cerebellar hemisphere. Forward traction on the sutures placed in the dural margin attached to the sigmoid sinus reduces the need for cerebellar retraction. In all phases of exposure, as with the retrolabyrinthine approach, the surgeon should constantly conceptualize the relationship between the bony opening landmarks and the intradural position of the cranial nerves. With the aid of the operating microscope, the cerebellum is gently retracted, and the cistern over the jugular foramen is opened, allowing the cerebellum to fall away. Retraction is rarely required after this maneuver. Rotation of the operating table away from the surgeon aids in the exposure of the eighth-nerve complex. If support of the cerebellar hemisphere is needed, it should be carried out very gently by use of a tension-operated, multijointed retractor. Sections of cut surgical glove are used between the retractor and the cerebellum to prevent instrument adhesions.

Surgical Anatomy of the Seventh and Eighth Cranial Nerves

Multiple superbly illustrated microdissections of the cranial nerves in humans were published in 1865 by Bischoff. Fig. 125–2 reproduces some of their illustrations of the seventh and eighth cranial nerves and the nervus intermedius. McKenzie's dissections led to the first practical localization of the vestibular portion of the eighth nerve in the cerebellopontine angle.[4] Using McKenzie's 1926 illustrations as an anatomic guide, a surgeon today could successfully perform a differential section of the vestibular nerve in the cerebellopontine angle. However, it is best to understand the changing anatomic relationships between the cochlear, vestibular, and facial nerves and the nervus intermedius throughout their course from the brainstem to their bony exits in the depths of the internal auditory canal. Throughout most of their course, minor individual anatomic variations occur; however, all nerves are constant in their position at the distal end of the internal auditory canal. Near the terminal end of the canal, which during surgery can be seen only by drilling away the bone that forms the posterior wall of the internal auditory canal, the superior and inferior vestibular nerves lie caudal (posterior), closest to the surgeon, obscuring the facial and cochlear nerves from view (Fig. 125–3). Terminally, the vestibular nerves are separated by the transverse (falciform) crest. Anterior to, and in front of, the superior vestibular nerve lies the facial nerve. Below the facial nerve, the cochlear nerve lies in front of the inferior vestibular nerve. As the facial nerve enters its bony canal, it is separated from the superior vestibular nerve by the vertical crest, or Bill's bar (named in honor of William House).

The inferior vestibular nerve is formed by the fusion of the saccular and posterior ampullary nerves in the depths of the internal auditory canal. The saccule (innervated by the saccular nerve) has no apparent significant physiologic function in humans, which has important implications when section of the inferior vestibular nerve is considered. After innervating the saccule, the saccular nerve enters the terminal end of the internal auditory canal through its fenestrated posteroinferior quadrant. Within 1 to 2 mm proximal to the terminal bony fenestrations, the saccular nerve is joined by the posterior ampullary nerve, which enters the posterior wall of the internal auditory canal through a small bony opening,

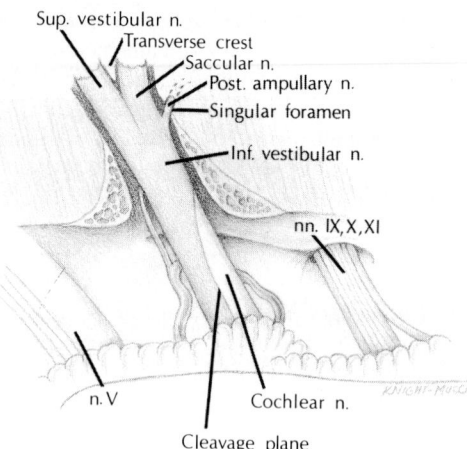

FIGURE 125–3. Within the right internal auditory canal, the superior vestibular nerve obscures the facial nerve, while the inferior vestibular nerve hides the cochlear nerve. The distance from the singular foramen to the transverse crest is 2 ± 0.7 mm; the transverse crest would not be exposed during surgery.

the singular foramen.[22] The posterior ampullary nerve (singular nerve) innervates only the ampulla of the posterior semicircular canal. Almost immediately after the inferior vestibular nerve is formed, it begins to fuse with the cochlear nerve just medial to the falciform crest. Because of this early fusion, attempts to section the entire inferior vestibular nerve, even within the depths of the internal auditory canal, carry a significant risk of injury to the cochlear nerve. By the midportion of the internal auditory canal, the inferior vestibular nerve–cochlear nerve complex and superior vestibular nerve frequently fuse into a single bundle, the eighth nerve.

As the nerves course through the internal auditory canal and the cerebellopontine cistern, rotation occurs. By the midportion of the internal auditory canal, the cochlear nerve has rotated more caudally (posteriorly) and dorsally to emerge from the porus acusticus closest to the surgeon, and the combined vestibular portions of the nerve have rotated rostrally away from the surgeon. Rotation continues so that when the nerves reach the midportion of the cerebellopontine cistern, the cochlear nerve has rotated a full 90 degrees and is within full view of the surgeon (Fig. 125–4). As the eighth nerve emerges into the cerebellopontine cistern, a fine cleavage plane usually exists between the cochlear and vestibular nerves. Subtle color difference also assists the surgeon in identifying the separate components of the eighth nerve. The vestibular portion of the nerve, rostral and closest to the trigeminal nerve, appears grayer than the inferior white cochlear component that is closest to the ninth nerve. Maintaining its rostral position, the vestibular portion of the nerve enters the brainstem rostral to the auditory portion through the middle cerebellar peduncle, and the auditory portion of the nerve enters the brainstem caudal and slightly more dorsally, where the restiform body disappears under the middle peduncle.

The facial nerve also participates in the rotation from the brainstem to its bony canal. The facial nerve emerges from the brainstem ventral and usually caudal to the eighth nerve; it is usually obscured from the surgeon's view by the eighth nerve throughout its course from the brainstem to the porus acusticus. Within the internal auditory canal, the seventh nerve rotates from caudal to rostral and from ventral to dorsal in its relationship to the cochlear portion of the eighth nerve before entering the bony facial canal. The nervus intermedius commonly originates as several twigs from the brainstem between the seventh and eighth nerves. Within the cerebellopontine cistern, the nervus intermedius fibers are intimately associated with the eighth nerve, usually attached to the ventral cleavage plane between the auditory and vestibular divisions of the nerve. In the midportion of the internal auditory canal, the nervus intermedius departs from the eighth nerve, joining the seventh nerve as it enters the facial canal.

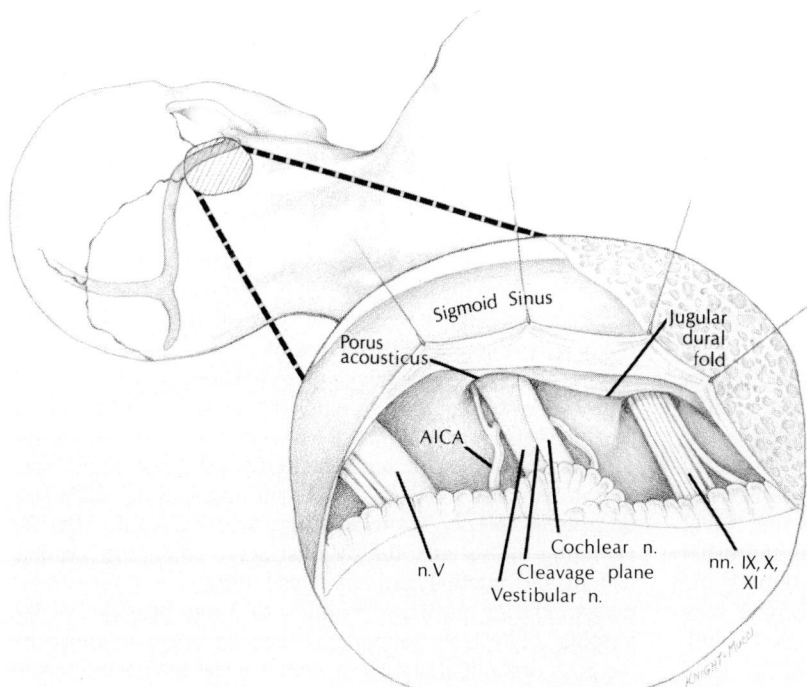

FIGURE 125–4. Nerves of the right lateral posterior cranial fossa demonstrating the cochleovestibular cleavage plane. The facial nerve is hidden beneath the eighth nerve.

A clear understanding of the rotation and changing relationship between the vestibular and cochlear portions of the eighth nerve is essential for surgeons performing surgery in the cerebellopontine angle. Before McKenzie's work, the changing position of the eighth nerve components was described but lacked practical value.[23] After the vestibular nerve section lost its popularity in the 1940s, the anatomy became less important, and more recent anatomic descriptions were misleading because they failed to note the rotation of the seventh and eighth nerves.[24] The resurrection of vestibular neurectomy and the possibility of hearing preservation during the removal of an acoustic neurinoma refocused attention on the importance of the eighth-nerve rotation.[25, 26]

Rasmussen was among the first to describe the histologic morphology of the eighth cranial nerve.[27] He demonstrated the occasional complete separation between the cochlear and vestibular portions in the eighth nerve and the total intermingling of fibers within a single trunk in other specimens. The histologic difference between the two components of the nerve accounts for the surgical color difference. The cochlear fibers are uniform in size and more compact, appearing white under surgical magnification, whereas the loose fibers of the vestibular nerve produce a grayer color. Current histologic descriptions of the cleavage plane between the cochlear and vestibular nerves vary. Silverstein and colleagues described an identifiable cleavage plane in 75 percent of specimens, realizing that in some cases vestibular fibers might still be contained within the cochlear portion of the nerve.[25] Natout and coworkers described an overlapping zone between the two divisions, in which the vestibular fibers were interspersed between the adjacent cochlear fibers.[28] Schefter and Harner studied the eighth nerve in 10 cadavers; they found no separation between the cochlear and vestibular fibers within the cerebellopontine angle in five specimens, and in the remaining cases, the eighth nerve was divided into many fascicles. No cochleovestibular cleavage plane was found in their study.[29] Surgical outcome studies tend to favor at least some separation in most patients.

Vestibular Nerve Section

The cerebellar flocculus usually covers the more medial extension of the eighth nerve and may be gently dissected away to expose a longer nerve segment. Once the nerves in the cerebellopontine angle have been identified, the cleavage plane is sought, with the surgeon being mindful that the vestibular portion of the nerve is nearest the trigeminal nerve, and the cochlear portion of the nerve is closest to the glossopharyngeal nerve. The position of the facial nerve and its relationship to the cochleovestibular cleavage plane must be immediately determined. Gentle displacement of the cochlear nerve often reveals the position of the facial nerve and allows the surgeon to determine the space separating the seventh and eighth nerves. Rarely, the seventh nerve may be adherent to the underside of the eighth nerve. Using a 2-mm mirror is also helpful in studying the ventral surface of the eighth nerve and identifying the fibers of the nervus intermedius, which may delineate the cleavage plane. An abrupt color change between the two components of the eighth nerve may be the only clue to the cleavage plane. Frequently, a tiny blood vessel courses along the cleavage planes and serves as a surgical guide. Once the cleavage plane has been identified, the divisions are bluntly separated, and care is taken not to injure the facial nerve or any of the branches of the anteroinferior cerebellar artery, particularly the labyrinthine artery. The vestibular nerve is sharply divided with microscissors. The nerve ends usually retract when the division is complete, leaving a 2-mm gap between the ends.

The dural opening for the combined retrolabyrinthine-retrosigmoid operation is 15 to 20 mm behind the dural opening for the retrolabyrinthine operation. This minor alteration in position significantly alters the surgeon's angle of approach to the nerves within the cerebellopontine cistern. From the retrolabyrinthine approach, the surgeon tends to have a more vertical view of the eighth nerve, easily permitting a perpendicular separation of the nerve. From the retrosigmoid approach, the line of sight tends to be 10 to 15 degrees off a vertical line constructed from the eighth nerve, requiring vigilance for the creation of a perpendicular nerve separation. Surgeons tend to separate the nerves along the line of sight rather than vertically, which spares vestibular nerve fibers along the ventral surface of the eighth nerve.

If a cleavage plane cannot be established, the surgeon must be prepared to drill away the posterior wall of the internal auditory canal. The surgeon must identify the endolymphatic sac along with the bony operculum covering its apex. The dura is stripped from the temporal bone between the porus of the internal auditory canal and the operculum, and care is taken not to injure the endolymphatic sac or duct. The posterior canal wall is drilled away with a diamond-coated bit. Before surgery, the position of the posterior semicircular canal and the location of the singular canal opening is determined from thin-section computed tomographic scan. Based on the radiographic measurements from the posterior margin of the porus acusticus to the opening of the singular canal, bone is removed to within 1 to 2 mm proximal to the singular canal (Fig. 125–5). Drilling beyond this depth endangers the vestibule and the posterior semicircular canal. The dural lining of the canal is sharply opened, revealing the nerves of the internal auditory canal. The opening is proximal to the transverse crest, and it is not seen. The remaining unopened posterior wall of the canal is explored with a microhook to

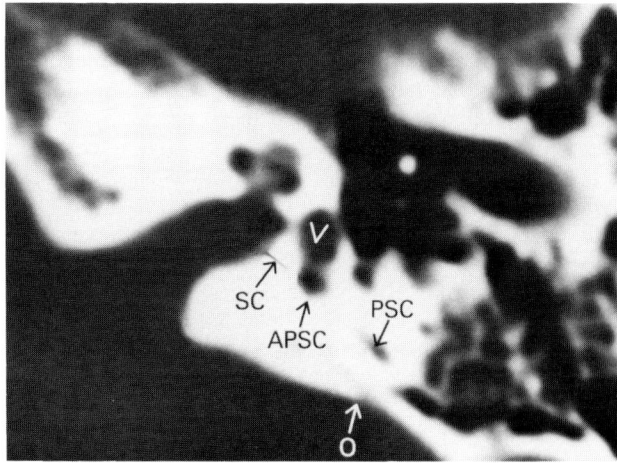

FIGURE 125–5. A computer-generated axial tomogram of the temporal bone demonstrates the singular canal (SC), the posterior semicircular posterior canal (PSC) and its ampulla (APSC), the vestibule (V), and the operculum (O) covering the endolymphatic duct.

locate the singular canal. The posterior ampullary nerve is avulsed from its canal, and the remaining inferior vestibular nerve, having no important function, is not divided, thereby avoiding injury to the cochlear nerve. The superior vestibular nerve is sectioned once the facial nerve has been identified and separated. If the vestibule or the posterior semicircular canal is opened, the fenestrations should be cautiously plugged with bone wax. Likewise, any air cells opened during the drilling must also be carefully filled with wax. The posterior fossa dura is closed, and the bony defect is filled with abdominal adipose tissue. If the retrosigmoid bone flap has been preserved, it may be replaced.

POSTOPERATIVE CARE

Immediately after surgery, patients experience acute vertigo, nausea, and vomiting quite similar to that experienced with a Ménière's attack. As central nervous system vestibular compensation occurs, vertigo rapidly resolves over 3 to 4 days, but the common complaint of disequilibrium improves more slowly. Patients with near-normal preoperative vestibular function experience the greatest immediate postoperative vertigo and nausea after labyrinthine denervation. Early ambulation appears to hasten vestibular compensation, although immediately after surgery, patients usually have a wide-based gait and a tendency to fall to the side of the vestibular nerve section. For several days after surgery, patients experience second- and third-degree nystagmus with accentuation on gaze to the side opposite the nerve section. During this time, diplopia occurs in a small number of patients. This condition is difficult to document because it rapidly clears; it appears to be either ocular dysmetria or a skew deviation. Vertigo and nausea may be suppressed by use of droperidol injections during the immediate postoperative period. As late as 1 year after surgery, some patients may experience mild transient unsteadiness after abrupt head movement.

SURGICAL COMPLICATIONS

Postoperative cerebrospinal fluid leakage occurs in fewer than 5 percent of all cases.[1] When spinal fluid is detected draining from either the wound or the nose via the eustachian tubes, spinal subarachnoid catheter drainage is immediately instituted and maintained for 3 to 5 days, and re-exploration of the surgical wound is avoided in all cases. Preoperative antibiotic administration has reduced wound infections to less than 1 percent of cases. Facial paralysis has rarely been reported.

Reduced hearing on the side of the vestibular nerve section does occur and may be complete in some patients.[1, 30] In nearly 80 percent of patients, hearing is preserved within 20 dB of their preoperative scores. Speech discrimination scores remain within 20 percent of the preoperative value in 70 percent of patients.[16, 30] Occasionally, patients develop chronic disabling headaches after opening of the internal auditory canal, and the etiology of this disturbing complication remains unexplained. Because of this complication, surgeons may be reluctant to drill away the posterior canal wall unless the cleavage plane is totally absent within the cerebellopontine cistern.

SURGICAL RESULTS

Relief of vertigo is the primary goal of vestibular nerve section. After vestibular neurectomy in patients with Ménière's disease, greater than 90 percent are either cured or significantly relieved of vertigo attacks.[16, 30] Complete cure of vertigo attacks occurs in 85 percent of cases. After vestibular nerve section in patients with vertigo attacks from labyrinthitis or vestibular neuronitis, the surgical results are slightly less impressive than in patients with Ménière's disease. Nguyen and colleagues[30] and Kemink and colleagues[31] reported only a 70-percent improvement or complete resolution of symptoms in the non-Ménière's group of patients with chronic vertigo. There is a lack of correlation between surgical outcome and the surgeon's assessment of either the completeness of the vestibular neurectomy or the clarity of the cleavage plane.

Beyond relief of vertigo, some patients report relief of chronic unsteadiness, aural pressure, and tinnitus. The possibility of relief of any one of these symptoms, no matter how troublesome, in the absence of vertigo attacks, does not justify the performance of vestibular neurectomy.

Failure of surgery to relieve vertigo attacks requires re-evaluation of vestibular function. Approximately 3 percent of patients require additional surgery. If a patient continues to have vertigo attacks arising from the side of the original surgery, a decision must be made regarding further surgery. Labyrinthectomy, transcanal eighth-nerve section, or middle fossa or posterior fossa total eighth-nerve section should be performed. All of these procedures result in hearing ablation, but the results of vertigo relief are quite good.

REFERENCES

1. Silverstein H, Wanamaker H, Flanzer J, Rosenberg S: Vestibular neurectomy in the United States—1990. Am J Otol 13:23–30, 1992
2. Frazier CH: Intracranial division of the auditory nerve for persistent aural vertigo. Surg Gynecol Obstet 15:524–529, 1912
3. Dandy WE: Ménière's disease: Its diagnosis and a method of treatment. Arch Surg 16:1127–1152, 1928
4. McKenzie KG: Ménière's syndrome: A follow-up study. Clin Neurosurg 2:44–49, 1955
5. Dandy WE: Treatment of Ménière's disease by section of only the vestibular portion of the acoustic nerve. Bull Johns Hopkins Hosp 53:52–55, 1933
6. Green RE: Surgical treatment of vertigo, with follow-up on Walter Dandy's cases. Clin Neurosurg 6:141–152, 1958
7. Portmann G: The saccus endolymphaticus and an operation for draining the same for the relief of vertigo. J Laryngol Otol 42:809–817, 1927
8. House WF: Subarachnoid shunt for drainage of endolymphatic hydrops: A preliminary report. Laryngoscope 72:713–729, 1962
9. Silverstein H, Smouha E, Jones R: Natural history versus surgery for Ménière's disease, in Fisch U, Valavanis A, Yasargil MG (eds): Neurological Surgery of the Ear and Skull Base. Berkeley, Kugler & Ghedini, 1989, pp 437–449
10. Thomsen J, Bretlau P, Tos M, Johnsen NJ: Endolymphatic sac-mastoid shunt surgery: A nonspecific treatment modality. Ann Otol Rhinol Laryngol 95:32–35, 1986
11. Cawthorne TE: The treatment of Ménière's disease. J Laryngol Otol 58:363–371, 1943
12. House WF: Surgical exposure of the internal auditory canal and its contents through the middle cranial fossa. Laryngoscope 71:1363–1385, 1961
13. Hitselberger WE, Pulec JL: Trigeminal nerve (posterior root) retrolabyrinthine selective section. Arch Otolaryngol Head Neck Surg 96:412–415, 1972

14. Brackmann DE, Hitselberger WE: Retrolabyrinthine approach: Technique and newer indications. Laryngoscope 88:286–297, 1978
15. Silverstein H, Norrell H: Retrolabyrinthine surgery: A direct approach to the cerebellopontine angle. Otolaryngol Head Neck Surg 88:462–469, 1980
16. Silverstein H, Norrell H, Rosenberg S: The resurrection of vestibular neurectomy: A 10-year experience with 115 cases. J Neurosurg 72:533–539, 1990
17. Pearson BW, Brackmann DE: Committee on hearing and equilibrium guidelines for reporting treatment results in Ménière's disease. Otolaryngol Head Neck Surg 93:579–581, 1985
18. Baloh RW, Jacobson K, Winder T: Drop attacks with Ménière's syndrome. Ann Neurol 28:384–387, 1990
19. Dandy WE: Etiological and clinical types of so-called "nerve deafness." Laryngoscope 47:594–597, 1937
20. Jannetta PJ, Moller MB, Moller AR: Disabling positional vertigo. N Engl J Med 310:1700–1705, 1984
21. Silverstein H, Rosenberg S: Surgical Techniques of the Temporal Bone and Skull Base. Malvern, PA, Lea & Febiger, 1992, pp 19–47
22. Silverstein H, Norrell H, Smouha E, Haberkamp T: The singular canal—A valuable landmark in surgery of the internal auditory canal. Otol Head Neck Surg 98:138–143, 1988
23. Courville CB: Applied anatomy of the VIIIth nerve and its environs, the cerebellopontile angle. Laryngoscope 42:415–431, 1932
24. Rhoton AL Jr: Microsurgery of the internal auditory meatus. Surg Neurol 2:311–318, 1974
25. Silverstein H, Norrell H, Haberkamp T, McDaniel AB: The unrecognized rotation of the vestibular and cochlear nerves from the labyrinth to the brain stem: Its implications to surgery of the eighth cranial nerve. Otolaryngol Head Neck Surg 95:543–549, 1986
26. Malkasian DR, Rand RW: Microsurgical neuroanatomy, in Rand RW (ed): Microneurosurgery, 2nd ed. St. Louis, CV Mosby, 1978, pp 37–70
27. Rasmussen AT: Studies of the VIIIth cranial nerve of man. Laryngoscope 50:67–83, 1949
28. Natout MAY, Terr LI, Linthicum FH Jr, House WF: Topography of the vestibulocochlear nerve fibers in the posterior cranial fossa. Laryngoscope 97:954–958, 1987
29. Schefter RP, Harner SG: Histologic study of the vestibulocochlear nerve. Ann Otolaryngol 95:146–150, 1986
30. Nguyen CD, Brackmann DE, Crane RT, et al: Retrolabyrinthine vestibular nerve section: Evaluation of technical modification in 143 cases. Am J Otol 13:328–332, 1992
31. Kemink JL, Telian SA, El-Kashlan H, Langman AW. Retrolabyrinthine vestibular nerve section: Efficacy in disorders other than Ménière's disease. Laryngoscope 101:523–528, 1991

Editorial Commentary

William H. Sweet

Norrell and Silverstein refer briefly to a 1984 publication by Jannetta and colleagues,[1] in which they describe a disorder whose symptoms consist of tinnitus, dysequilibrium, and vertigo. We may reasonably assume that the somewhat vague term *dysequilibrium* refers to any disorder or malfunction of the sensations or movements associated with any or all aspects of equilibrium. Whatever the definition of the patients' symptoms of equilibrium may be, the authors do not equivocate about their vasculoneural findings and the results of their treatment. They say, "In over 70 consecutive patients with tinnitus, dysequilibrium and vertigo, we have seen vascular compression with a precise clinicopathological correlation in every patient" (p 1170). They explain the meaning of precise clinicopathologic correlation:

1. If vertigo is present, the vascular compression is located on the vestibular portion of the eighth cranial nerve (superior or inferior nerve, or both) and at the brainstem. Vascular contacts that are more peripheral do not cause vertigo.

2. If tinnitus is present, a vessel may be compressing the cochlear portion of the eighth cranial nerve anywhere from the brainstem to the internal auditory meatus.

3. If both vertigo and tinnitus are present, the offending blood vessel is compressing both vestibular and cochlear portions of the eighth cranial nerve and therefore must be located at the brainstem (p 1704).

They say further, "In our entire series of more than 70 patients in whom the eighth nerve was decompressed to relieve tinnitus, dysequilibrium or vertigo, we have noted that tinnitus may take more than 18 months to disappear; although vertigo and dysequilibrium regress more rapidly." Jannetta's unorthodox approach to the treatment of the disorder just mentioned is matched by his equally unorthodox arithmetic calculation of his overall mortality rate for microvascular decompression of some cranial nerves. "After 160 such operations five patients died, the last dying in 1980, a 0.3-percent mortality rate." Perhaps the calculation of 3 percent might meet with more general agreement. (Olivecrona in 1961 reported a 0.4-percent operative mortality after 445 trigeminal rhizotomies in the posterior fossa).[2]

My colleague, D. Wallace, and I have been unable to find more than brief, incomplete reports purporting to show the neurovascular correlations described by Jannetta. In particular, tinnitus has been especially resistant to any sort of surgical treatment. Jannetta states that vascular contacts with the vestibular nerve away from the brainstem do not cause vertigo, whereas he finds that with the cochlear nerve, vascular compression anywhere from the brainstem to the internal auditory meatus may cause tinnitus. He was probably unaware that the anteroinferior cerebellar arterial trunk itself forms a loop in the tiny internal auditory canal, whose crowded quarters would probably lead to more pressure against the components of the eighth nerve than would the more spacious cerebellopontine cistern. Reisser and Schuknecht[3] had access to 1327 petrous portions of the human temporal bones obtained at autopsy. After special care in section of the vascular and neural structures at the porus acusticus, the temporal lobe was removed with a large bony plug cutter, fixed, decalcified, embedded in celloidin, and sectioned horizontally at 20 cm. Complete clinical histories were available with each specimen. The anteroinferior cerebellar artery was within the internal auditory canal in 160 specimens. There were nine cases of unexplained unilateral hearing loss, eight of unexplained tinnitus, 29 of vertigo unexplained by any other peripheral histopathologic correlate or central nervous system disorder, and five of endolymphatic hydrops accompanied by Ménière's disease. There was no significant correlation in any of these four groups of patients with anteroinferior cerebellar arterial loops in the internal auditory canal. Schuknecht[4] defines as a medical myth a concept of pathogenesis refuted by adequate available evidence. He places the concept of cessation of hearing loss, tinnitus, vertigo, and Ménière's syndrome by vascular compression in this category. With this point of view I am in complete agreement. Whatever phraseology one wishes to use, the conclusion that microvascular decompression has not been proved useful for any of these neuro-otologic disorders is inescapable.

REFERENCES

1. Jannetta PJ, Möller MB, Möller AR: Disabling functional vertigo. N Engl J Med 310:1700–1705, 1984
2. Olivecrona H: Trigeminal neuralgia. Triangle 5:60–69, 1961
3. Reisser C, Schuknecht HF: The anterior inferior cerebellar artery in the internal auditory canal. Laryngoscope 101:761–766, 1991
4. Schuknecht HF: Myths in neurotology. Am J Otol 13:124–126, 1992

CHAPTER 126

Open Cordotomy and Medullary Tractotomy

Charles E. Poletti

OPEN CORDOTOMY

INDICATIONS

General: Cancer Pain Below T5

We have become progressively inclined to perform cordotomy operations only on patients suffering from medically intractable cancer pain whose longevity appears limited to less than 3 years. This decision has grown from the relatively high incidence of failures 1 to 2 years after cordotomy operations and the increasing late frequency of postcordotomy painful dysesthesias. The significant instance of unavoidable complications—including motor weakness and bladder and sexual dysfunction—are further arguments against using the operation, especially bilaterally, in patients with benign disease. Accordingly, we have been reluctant to perform cordotomies in patients with peripheral nerve or spinal cord injuries, herpetic neuralgia, or chronic calcific pancreatitis, no matter how severely afflicted. With selected cancer patients, however, the operation often relieves suffering and obviates excessive use of narcotics. For these individuals, the operation should be done as a priority option. If delayed too long, the operation may not arrest or reverse extensive suffering and debilitation. For patients with markedly limited life spans, a percutaneous cordotomy is often selected.

The use of cordotomy operations is further limited by progressive decreases in the level of analgesia during the first 6 months following the operation. Often, within 3 weeks postoperatively, the level has fallen three to six segments, and at 6 months, the level may have lowered a total of six to eight segments. Thus, most surgeons agree that even with high cervical cordotomies, many patients may have no significant hypalgesia above T2-T3. Following a T2-T3 thoracic cordotomy, the level of significant permanent hypalgesia or analgesia usually is about T10. Consequently, one can usually count on a year of analgesia six to eight levels below the operation. A further consideration to make before performing the cordotomy is that often, during these postoperative 6 months in which the level of analgesia is falling, the cancer is progressing to higher levels.

More important than determining the site of the referred pain is localizing the cancerous lesion that produces the pain. For instance, one of our patients with prostatic cancer and severe, deep lateral flank pain on the right side appeared to be a good candidate for unilateral open thoracic cordotomy, until a total-body computed tomographic (CT) scan revealed a single metastasis eroding the right half of the T12 vertebra. On further direct questioning, the patient finally admitted to pain in the corresponding left lateral flank. In this case, unilateral cordotomy was no longer an option. We believe that each cordotomy operation should be individually designed primarily on the basis of the location of the cancerous lesion producing the pain.

Unilateral Somatic Cancer: Unilateral Cordotomy

Unilateral cordotomies are most effective for cancer that is not invading the viscera and for cancer that is located away from the midline and at or below the lower cervical region. Thus, excellent potential candidates are patients with cancer confined to the legs, the hips, the lateral retroperitoneal pelvic and abdominal space, the chest wall (e.g., breast cancer and Pancoast's tumor), and perhaps the lower brachial plexus. For disease below T8, we select a T2 unilateral thoracic cordotomy, which carries a lower risk than cervical cordotomy.

For cancer of the arms, as for that of the neck, nasopharynx, or face, a medullary tractotomy is worth considering instead of cordotomy, although the operative mortality and incidence of postoperative dysesthesias are slightly higher. An open C2-C3 cordotomy combined with a C2, C3, and C4 dorsal rhizotomy may relieve severe pain in the brachial plexus, upper extremity, shoulder, and neck.[1] We favor open C2-C3 cordotomy, occasionally combined with rhizotomy, over a C1-C2 percutaneous cordotomy, because of the marked anatomic variations at C1-C2 and the belief that consistently more complete, uncomplicated lesions with higher permanent levels of analgesia can be obtained using our open technique at C2-C3.

Unilateral Visceral Pain: Bilateral Cordotomy

In general, whenever a significant component of the pain is caused by disease invading the viscera, bilateral deep cordotomies are required for satisfactory relief of suffering. Often, the visceral pain from extensive cancer of the pancreas, intestine, colon, rectum, cervix, or uterus, and especially the stomach and esophagus, may be mediated by splanchnic nerves entering the spinal cord as high as T1. Many of these visceral nociceptive afferents do not cross to the other side of the spinal cord. Accordingly, in these patients, the best chance of satisfactory results rests with the highest bilateral cervical cordotomy advisable, i.e., C1-C2 percutaneous or C2-C3 open cordotomy combined with an open contralateral C5-C6 cordotomy.

Paramedian, Midline, and Bilateral Cancer: Bilateral Cordotomy

Whenever the cancer is close to the midline, unilateral cordotomy has a high probability of not securing prolonged relief. Affected patients very often become aware of severe contralateral pain shortly after surgery. Accordingly, it should be emphasized that even for paramedian cancers, it is wise to perform a bilateral cordotomy.

When bilateral cordotomies are indicated, an open cordotomy is performed at two levels, rather than a unilateral percutaneous cordotomy followed by an open operation.

ALTERNATIVES TO BILATERAL CORDOTOMY

Whenever open bilateral cordotomies are indicated, one should seriously consider various alternative operations that are available: A midline myelotomy operation may have a higher chance of relieving bilateral pain in the arms, shoulders, and neck as well as pain from bilateral visceral or extensive midline disease. In addition, midline myelotomies, compared with bilateral cordotomies, have a significantly lower incidence of later postcordotomy dysesthesias and bladder dysfunction, sleep apnea, and motor weakness.

Hitchcock[2, 3] and Schvarcz[4–6] independently have pioneered central medullary myelotomies for high bilateral disease using stereotactic techniques. These appear promising but require special expertise.

My colleagues and I[7] have developed a technically very simple nondestructive operation for intractable cancer pain in which a spinal epidural catheter is implanted for long-term administration of morphine. Using three administration systems, we demonstrated for the first time that direct spinal narcotics can be employed on a long-term basis for effective pain relief.

CONSIDERATION OF ANATOMY AND VARIATIONS

Spinal Cord

The goal of anterolateral cordotomy is to create a lesion in fibers ascending in the spinothalamic tract (STT) that carry nociceptive input from one side of the body caudal to the level of the lesion. Marked anatomic variations of the spinal cord, however, frequently impede optimal transection of the STT. Four major areas of anatomic variation that concern the surgeon are: (1) the course of the STT, (2) the course of the corticospinal tract (CST), (3) the position of the dentate insertion, and (4) the width of the spinal cord. Thus, in cordotomy as in aneurysm surgery, the individual patient's anatomy must be identified or analyzed. It often may be necessary to perform a variation of the standard operation to maximize the probability of satisfactory results.

Spinothalamic Tract

In some individuals, the STT does not appear to decussate at all. In these patients, a standard anterolateral cordotomy produces ipsilateral analgesia. Fortunately, these cases are rare. Most individuals, however, probably have a number of uncrossed nociceptive fibers; perhaps these permit the recovery of pain following cordotomy. In particular, the nociceptive fibers mediating visceral pain in many cases do not decussate fully, but instead ascend on both sides of the spinal cord. This should encourage the surgeon to perform bilateral cordotomies when visceral pain is believed to be significant.

Normally the vast majority of the nociceptive fibers do decussate, following two predictable patterns. In the first pattern, the "sacral" fibers are positioned most posterolaterally and superficially. The more rostral fibers from the lumbar, thoracic, and cervical regions ascend to assume their course more anteromedially and deeper (Fig. 126–1). The sacral fibers may lie immediately anterior to the base of the normally positioned dentate (Fig. 126–1). The cordotomy lesion therefore should first reach as far dorsally as the equator of the spinal cord, usually at the base of the dentate insertion. Beginning the lesion 1 to 2 mm anterior to this point in some individuals results in sparing of the sacral fibers.

A second relatively predictable pattern reflects the observation that pain from the superficial part of the body is relayed by fibers close to the surface of the spinal cord. Progressively deeper are the fibers mediating the sense of temperature, deep pain, and, finally, visceral pain (Fig. 126–1). Accordingly, the lesion must extend deep to the anterolateral surface of the cord, especially in patients with visceral disease. In most patients, a depth of 5 mm is required, even in the cervical region.

Perhaps most important, the lesion should include the medial and anterior portion of the anterior quadrant. It is often in this portion of the spinal cord that fibers from the anterior commissure may ascend five to six segments or more before extending far enough laterally to assume their "classic" position in the "lateral" STT. In contrast, fibers from the dorsal horn appear to cross to the anterior commissure almost immediately, i.e., at the same level or at most within one to two segments. Yet these same fibers may then ascend for five to eight segments before "crossing" fully to form the "lateral" STT. Thus, the "anterior" STT in humans consists of ascending fibers gradually coursing laterally to form the "lateral" STT. Accordingly, a lesion in the lateral anterior quadrant, albeit deep, may produce analgesia extending rostrally only eight or more segments below the lesion. In contrast, a lesion of the anterior quadrant extending to the midline may in some individuals produce analgesia to within one segment of the lesion. Thus, especially in cervical cordotomies for which a primary goal is a high permanent level of analgesia, we recommend extending the lesion at least 1 to 2 mm anterior to the most medially exiting fibers of the ventral root, i.e., within 1 to 2.5 mm of the anterior spinal artery (see Fig. 126–7). A lesion extending only as far anteriorly as the ventral root may yield a satisfactory level of analgesia in only 80 percent of patients. The technique described in the next section, in fact, usually permits a lesion of the entire anterior quadrant extending immediately to the midline anterior pial septum and anterior spinal artery. This lesion, we

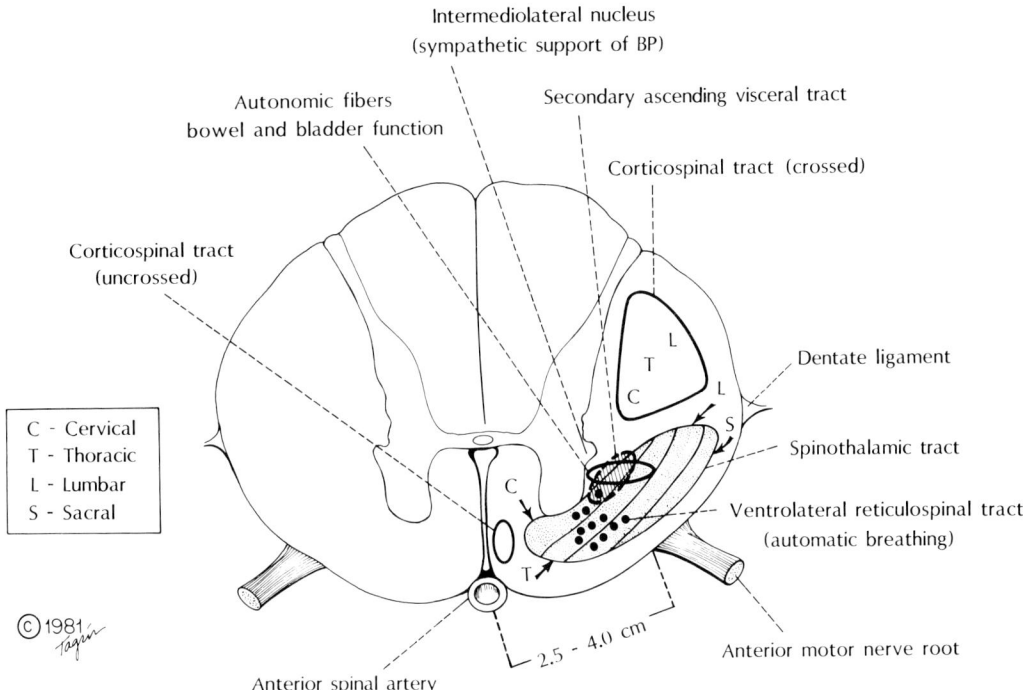

FIGURE 126–1. The spinal cord at T3 with the axon tracts relevant to making lesions of the STT. Just dorsal to the equator of the cord is the descending CST. The lesion should start about 1 mm anterior to the anterior limit of the CST. The entire STT is shown, including the anterior and lateral components. It should be emphasized that intermingled within the STT fibers are other ascending and descending tracts. Of necessity, these must be lesioned to obtain a complete lesion of the STT. These tracts intermingled at least in part with the STT include the ventrolateral reticulospinal tract, which is responsible for nonvoluntary breathing, the descending autonomic fibers for bladder and bowel sphincter control, the ascending visceral tract, and sympathetic fibers just anterolateral to their origin in the intermediolateral nucleus. In the anteromedial aspect of the cord is the uncrossed CST adjacent to the midline septum and the anterior spinal artery. Note also that the distance from the medialmost exiting motor rootlet to the anterior spinal artery and midline varies from 2.0 to 3.5 mm. (Copyright © 1981 by Edith Tagrin.)

believe, produces the highest level of analgesia feasible—usually within two and occasionally within one segment.

Corticospinal Tract

Rarely, the CST does not decussate at all. Instead, it descends uncrossed in the anterolateral quadrant of the cord. In these rare individuals, an anterolateral cordotomy would be expected to produce contralateral plegia, because these aberrant tracts are believed to finally cross near the segment of their termination on the lower motor neuron. In addition, the data of Yakovlev and Rakic[8] indicate that these abnormal patterns of the CST are probably more common than is believed. It seems reasonable to assume that there may be associated abnormalities or displacements of the normally adjacent STT.

Commonly, however, even in normal individuals, the decussating pyramidal fibers may not be fully crossed and back into the posterior aspect of the cord until the caudal half of C2. Accordingly, we are inclined to do our cervical cordotomies at C3. A C4-C5 level of analgesia, as discussed previously, may still be feasible if the lesion is extended to the midline. Clearly, when the decussation is abnormally low, careful stimulation and monitoring—even at C3—is necessary to avoid a lesion of the CST.

Dentate Insertion

The dentate ligament is formed by the joining of components of the ventral and dorsal spinal cord pia. Usually these components join to form the dentate at the equator of the cord, just anterior to the anterior extent of the CST and just posterior to the posterior extent of the sacral fibers of the SST. In a number of cases, however, as Sweet[9] has noted, the dentate origin may form anterior or posterior to this equatorial line. When it is anterior to its most common position, a lesion beginning at the dentate and extending anteriorly may not transect nociceptive fibers from the sacrum. In cases of a posterior dentate, a lesion beginning just anterior to the dentate clearly has a high probability of producing an ipsilateral motor deficit. Accordingly, the lesion should begin at the equator of the cord; irrespective of the position of the dentate. Because the equator of the rotated cord is difficult to judge, we again stress physiologic stimulation and monitoring, preferably with the patient awake.

Spinal Cord Width

The width of the spinal cord appears to vary as well, in both the thoracic and cervical regions, especially in patients with advanced cancer. In one of our patients, for instance, extensive pelvic cancer invaded the lumbosacral plexus bilaterally, producing significant sensory deficits and virtual paraplegia. In this patient, the spinal cord at T2 under the microscope measured a total width of 5.2 mm. Obviously, it would have been injudicious to try to cut the anterior quadrant to a depth of 4 to 5 mm, especially because at the time we were still using a cordotomy knife, not a blunt instrument capable of palpating the anterior midline septum adjacent to the anterior spinal artery. Accordingly, we recommend measuring the width of the spinal cord in each case and using that specific dimension to determine the approximate depth of the lesion.

PREOPERATIVE PROCEDURES

Preparations and Special Instruments

All patients are advised of the complications of cordotomy operations. When awakening the patient during the operation (wake-up anesthesia) appears appropriate, the details and alternatives are discussed with the patient, by both the surgeon and the anesthesiologist. If there is any suspicion of impaired pulmonary function contralateral to the planned lesion, a comprehensive series of pulmonary function tests are performed. When motion of the contralateral hemidiaphragm is impaired, a unilateral cervical cordotomy may trigger fatal postoperative respiratory complications by interrupting the exclusively ipsilateral descending projections of the ventrolateral reticulospinal tract (Fig. 126–1). The patient is wrapped with woven elastic bandages from the toes to the thigh to minimize the resulting operation-induced orthostatic hypotension; this is especially important when bilateral lesions are planned.

Electrophysiologic Monitoring Equipment

Because of the marked potential variability in the location within the spinal cord of both the lateral spinothalamic tract and the corticospinal tracts, we conclude that intraoperative electrophysiologic stimulation of the spinal cord combined with dorsal column–evoked responses and electromyelographic (EMG) recording are useful. In order both to stimulate in the anterior quadrant to identify the STT in the awakened patient and later to stimulate while the lesion is being made, to warn of nearby CST fibers, we use a 45-degree Jacobsen ball that is insulated except over the distal half of the ball and at the end of the handle. A standard stimulator is attached to the uninsulated end of the handle, preferably a simulator that is capable of constant current stimulation at 2 to 100 Hz. For measuring dorsal column potentials evoked by peroneal or median nerve stimulation, we use a Nicolet signal averager with bipolar epidural recording electrodes. This technique is described elsewhere.[10]

Especially in cases in which wake-up anesthesia is not used, we monitor CST function by stimulating as the lesion is being made, while looking for motor responses and elicited EMG recordings distally. A small dental mirror on a malleable shaft is used to visualize the anterior spinal artery while the lesion is being made.

OPERATIVE PROCEDURES

Anesthesia

With the improved techniques of wake-up anesthesia supplemented by local infiltration of the wound, we have discontinued the use of only local anesthetics for cordotomy operations. Wake-up anesthesia offers the opportunity to identify the SST by stimulation, to monitor bilateral motor function as the lesion is being made, and to test the extent of the induced sensory deficit before it is too late to enlarge the lesion.

A third technique, in which the patient is awake after the initial cordotomy incision, has also been described.[11] With this technique, segmental analgesia is produced (C4-T8) by blocking the dorsal roots using a single injection of epidural bupivacaine. Because normal spinal cord function is preserved and the T2 laminectomy is easily tolerated, the patient remains fully awake and cooperative for testing sensory and motor function distal to T8 after the cordotomy lesions are produced.

The operative technique described here is designed especially to maximize the probability of obtaining an optimal lesion without subjecting the patient to being awake during surgery. The goal in this technique is making as large a lesion as feasible in the anterior quadrant without transecting the CST. The lesion extends dorsally to within 1 to 2 mm of the CST, medially to the midline anterior septum, and all the way anteriorly and anterolaterally. If there is a dominant variant of the CST in the anteromedial aspect of the spinal cord, it is identified by the stimulus at the top of the Jacobsen ball. As a result, our last seven patients have been operated on under continuous general anesthesia and all have had an initial contralateral distal hemianalgesia rising to within two segments of the complete anterior quadrant cordotomy without any detectable motor weakness.

Position

For unilateral cordotomy with wake-up anesthesia, the patient can be placed in the swimmer's position, with the thorax rotated 45 degrees up from horizontal. With the spinal cord rotated 45 degrees, the operating microscope can be focused almost vertically, and the cord viewed from a transverse direction. When bilateral lesions are anticipated, or in cases in which wake-up anesthesia is not employed, the patient should be placed prone. Especially for cervical cordotomies, the head is placed in a neutral position to decrease tethering of the cord, which may occur with too much flexion. For cervical operations, the head is held in a three-pin headrest, whereas during upper thoracic operations, the head is allowed to rest on a doughnut headrest. The fully bandaged legs should be elevated on blankets, and the table set in moderate reverse Trendelenburg position. With the patient in this position, a decrease in blood pressure following bilateral lesions will indicate, as noted by Sindou (personal communication, 1981), that the depth and dorsal extent of the lesion are satisfactory.

Unilateral Cordotomy Procedure

A relatively long skin incision is made in order to provide wide lateral retraction of the skin and paraspinal muscles. This affords a view from a lateral angle of the anterior quadrant of the rotated cord.

For unilateral upper thoracic lesions the T2 and T3 laminae are exposed, whereas bilateral upper thoracic lesions call for exposure of the laminae of T2, T3, and T4. A complete laminectomy is done, extending fully laterally on the side of the planned lesion. Next, the yellow ligament above and below the laminectomy is removed, exposing the inferior edge of the rostral lamina and the superior edge of the caudal lamina. The bipolar electrodes for recording evoked potentials from bilateral peroneal nerve stimulation are inserted in the midline epidural space rostrally and caudally (Fig. 126–2).

The dura is then opened in a semicircular fashion, extending far enough laterally to allow direct visualization of the contralateral side of the spinal cord (Fig. 126–3). This permits exact measurement of the width of the spinal cord. The microscope is brought into the field. The arachnoid is opened for optimal visualization. The width of the cord is measured precisely under the microscope, and a piece of bone wax is used to mark half of the cord width from the tip of the Jacobsen ball. This measurement will be used during transection to gauge the depth of cordotomy and to allow the tip of the Jacobsen ball to reach the midline. Once the cord width has been measured, the arachnoid opening is extended laterally over the dentate ligament.

Traction of the dorsal or ventral roots during rotation of the cord may result in painful postoperative dysesthesias. The dorsal rootlets should therefore be freed from the cord to their point of exit or to the limit of the exposure. If necessary, the dorsal root should be cut to facilitate rotation, rather than risk a traction injury with postoperative hyperesthesia. As previously mentioned, in cervical cordotomies, White and Sweet[1] suggest performing bilateral rhizotomies of the three accessible dorsal roots in order to raise the level of analgesia and to decrease the postoperative incisional pain. Other workers have found that rhizotomies do not improve the results of the cordotomy.[12]

With the roots freed or cut, the cord is then rotated 45 degrees. To rotate the cord, a 4-0 silk suture is placed in two Weck clips, which are in turn placed on the dentate ligament (Fig. 126–4; see also Fig. 126–3). The silk sutures are then used to put traction on the Weck clips and the dentate for rotating the cord. If the patient is under local anesthesia and experiences pain as the cord is rotated, the dorsal root should be cut. Alternatively, cerebrospinal fluid should be aspirated, and a small cottonoid soaked in 10 percent cocaine should be applied selectively to the posterior root(s). If the root is sufficiently mobilized beforehand, however, pain during rotation is rarely elicited. With careful microsurgical dissection, the intact dentate insertion usually is strong enough to rotate the cord. If not, traction may be applied directly on the anterior root to rotate the cord. One should not be afraid to rotate the cord too far. If the anterior spinal artery along the anterior midline cannot be satisfactorily viewed, the dentate above and below the level of interest can be cut, permitting the cord to be rotated as much as 90 degrees. Electrophysiologic monitoring electrodes offer additional safety features, but we have not found their use to be mandatory if these techniques are followed as described.

Once the cord is rotated 45 degrees, a small dental mirror on a malleable handle may be used to visualize the exact course of the anterior spinal artery in the anterior midline septum and the medial limit of the exit of the ventral rootlets (Figs. 126–4 and 126–5). At the most avascular part of the exposed anterior quadrant, the tip of a No. 11 blade is inserted into the equator of the spinal cord. As noted, this is usually located immediately under the dentate insertion. The exact site of the dentate attachment can be established by observation and blunt palpation on the dentate insertion in a dorsal-to-ventral manner. Microsurgical scissors are placed in the small hole made in the pia by the No. 11 blade (Fig. 126–4). Only the pia arachnoid is then cut with the microscissors around the anterior quadrant of the cord. Cutting the pia with sharp scissors decreases the chance of avulsing the dentate attachment. Small pial vessels may be cauterized with bipolar microforceps. We incise the pia to a point 2 mm anterior to the medialmost exit of the ventral root, which should be at least 1 mm from the anterior spinal artery. An advantage of making the pial cut initially, before the lesion in the tracts, is that the natural shape of the cord is subse-

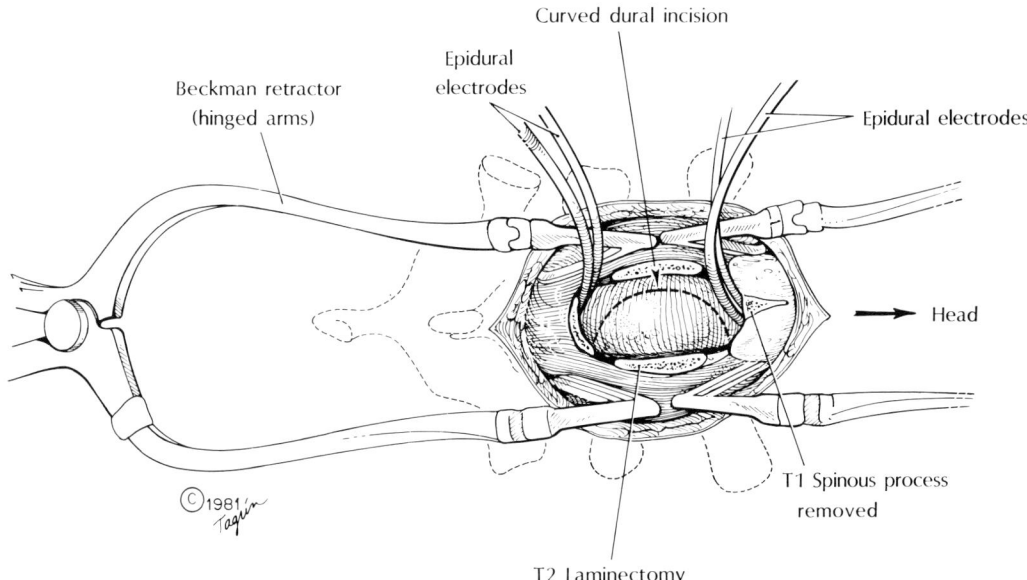

FIGURE 126–2. The spinous processes of T1, T2, and T3 are exposed. The T1 and T2 processes are removed. A complete bilateral laminectomy at T2 is shown extending far laterally on the side of the lesion. The rostral and caudal yellow ligaments are excised. The bipolar epidural electrodes are then inserted in the midline rostrally and caudally for recording sensory evoked potentials from bilateral peroneal stimulation. The projected dural incision is shown by the dotted line. (Copyright © 1981 by Edith Tagrin.)

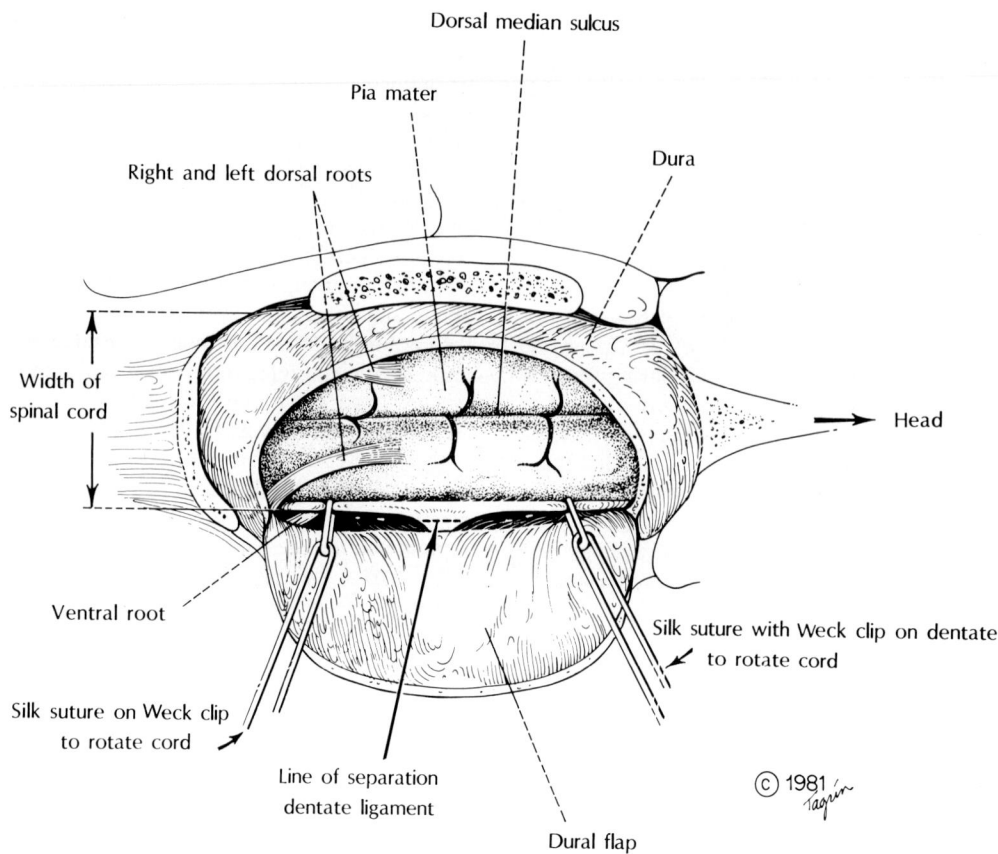

FIGURE 126–3. The dura is opened. The microscope is brought into the field. The arachnoid is dissected bilaterally. The dura contralaterally is retracted to permit direct measurement of the width of the spinal cord. Weck clips with silk sutures are applied to the dentate as shown. The arachnoid around the dorsal roots is dissected, freeing the roots to their exit point. (Copyright © 1981 by Edith Tagrin.)

quently preserved while the instrument is being inserted. Cutting the pia with a knife tends to distort the anatomy of the cord, making an accurate lesion difficult and placing indirect traction on adjacent vascular and neural structures.

With the incision in the pia, the cord is ready for cordotomy. Clearly, in making the spinal cord lesion, the two principal cautions are to avoid transecting the cortical spinal tract and to avoid damage to the anterior spinal artery and its main branches. The cortical spinal tract is particularly vulnerable to damage during cordotomy procedures, and as mentioned previously, anatomic variations limit the surgeon's ability to execute an adequate lesion without the possibility of damaging the motor system.

Our operative technique for making the lesion is unique, in that it employs the use of a blunt Jacobsen ball to simultaneously stimulate while making the lesion. The stimulator is attached to the end of the handle of the Jacobsen ball instrument. A ground electrode is inserted in the paraspinal muscles. Stimulation parameters are set for 1-msec pulses delivered at 1.5 V. Such a stimulus elicits responses in the cortical spinal tract with motion in the ipsilateral arm or leg in the asleep, unparalyzed patient when the ball tip approaches within 1 mm of the CST. The blunt-tipped instrument permits a safe traverse of the anterolateral cord all the way to the medial septum while the proximity of the instrument to the cortical spinal tract dorsally is concurrently monitored by looking for stimulation-evoked motor responses. Although the Jacobsen ball is a blunt instrument, it does not distort the very soft tissue of the cord. It has been our experience, particularly with midline myelotomies, that the Jacobsen ball is fully satisfactory for transecting spinal cord tracts.

The Jacobsen ball is inserted at the equator of the cord at the dorsalmost limit of the pial opening and is directed into the transverse axis of the cord, until the bone wax indicates that the ball is halfway across the width of the cord. Because the spinal cord has been rotated 45 degrees, the tip of the Jacobsen ball is also angled 45 degrees. Thus, during this initial motion, the shaft of the instrument is held vertically (Fig. 126–6A and B). Usually, the transverse diameter of the cord in the upper thoracic region is approximately 10 mm, so initially an incision to a depth of approximately 5 mm is indicated. In the cervical region the cord may be as wide as 16 mm, in which case an incision to 8 mm is permissible. As mentioned previously, however, the size of the cord may vary. We have seen a cord width as small as 5.2 mm in the thoracic region, presumably because of atrophy of the dorsal columns and descending cortical spinal tracts. In that particular case, it was necessary to insert the ball to only 2.5 mm in order to place the lesion at the center of the cord.

As the ball passes near the gray of the anterior horn, an ipsilateral trapezius contraction may be obtained during cervical cordotomy, and contraction of intercostal muscles during thoracic cordotomy. The presence of distal ipsilateral motor responses indicates that the stimulating Jacobsen ball is too close to the descending cortical spinal tract and must be directed more anteriorly. Redirection of the ball is most

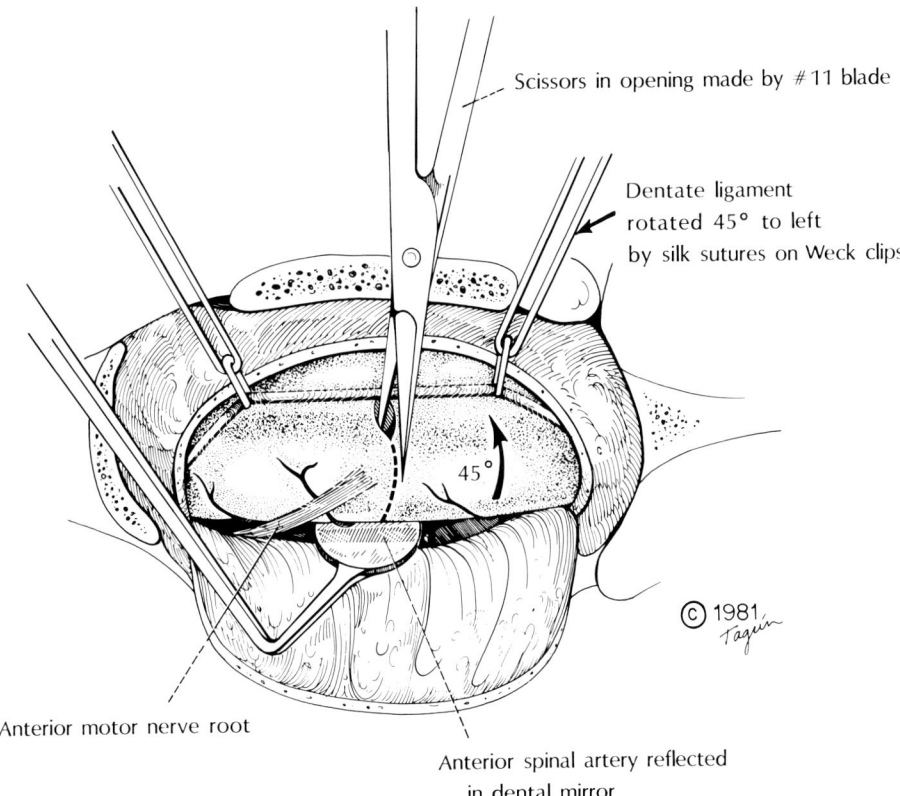

FIGURE 126–4. The dentate ligament lateral attachment has been cut. Traction is applied on the silk sutures attached by Weck clips to the dentate until the cord is rotated 45 degrees. A small dental mirror is placed ventrolaterally to permit visualization of the anterior midline septum and the course of the anterior spinal artery. The microscissors are placed into the hole made in the pia just anterior to the equator of the cord. These are used to cut the pia arachnoid around the anterior quadrant to within 1 to 2 mm of the anterior midline septum. This is usually about 2 mm anterior to the medialmost exiting ventral rootlet. (Copyright © 1981 by Edith Tagrin.)

commonly necessary when one is working in the cervical region, where the motor fibers may not be exclusively dorsal to the equator of the cord. Once the ball is in the center of the cord (Fig. 126–6B), it is drawn directly anteriorly along the palpable medial septum to the anteromedial corner of the anterior quadrant. The ball is then drawn laterally along the pia for about 1 to 2 mm until it exits from the cord at the most anteromedial extent of the pial incision (Fig. 126–7).

The ball should be drawn flush against the pia of the midline septum and the anterior quadrant. The pia is firm and can be readily palpated safely from inside the cord with the Jacobsen ball. There may be marked anatomic variation in the anteromedial portion of the anterior quadrant with a large uncrossed corticospinal tract. Should this be the case, one would expect contralateral motor responses in this region from the Jacobsen ball. We have not yet encountered such a case. Should this occur, it seems prudent to skirt this tract when making the first lesion. The ball tip of the Jacobsen instrument usually can be seen as it comes out of the pia, but if necessary, there is usually ample room to insert the mirror in order to see exactly where the ball exits. If it exits as planned, there is a very high probability that a satisfactory lesion was performed.

It is important, as shown in Figure 126–7, to make the lesion as close as possible to the midline septum. This is especially important in the cervical region, where recently crossed fibers may lie close to the septum for many levels before assuming a more lateral and dorsal position. Hardy and colleagues[13] believe that an incision extending to the midline can raise the level of resulting analgesia virtually to the level of the lesion.

Selective cervical cordotomies, i.e., partial lesions of the anterolateral quadrant, are not recommended for two reasons: first, cancer may spread to wider areas, and second, the topologic distribution of the spinal thalamic tract does not appear to be sufficiently specific for reliable results.

It should be stressed that in the cervical region, the anterior spinal artery is usually 4.5 to 5.0 mm from the center of the exit zone of the anterior nerve root. A lesion 2 mm from the midline will still be 2.5 to 3.0 mm away from the center of the exiting ventral root. Except for the danger of entry into the anterior spinal artery, there does not appear to be any disadvantage to making an incision in the medial anterior quadrant as well. We have not seen a case of contralateral motor weakness caused by transection of the uncrossed descending motor tracts.

In summary, when making the initial lesion, the surgeon should attempt to transect virtually the entire anterior quadrant of the cord from the equator anteriorly, extending to the midline.

Following the initial cordotomy lesion, the patient may be awakened in order to test the extent of the resulting analgesia as well as the integrity of motor function. Before awakening the patient, lidocaine should be injected profusely into the

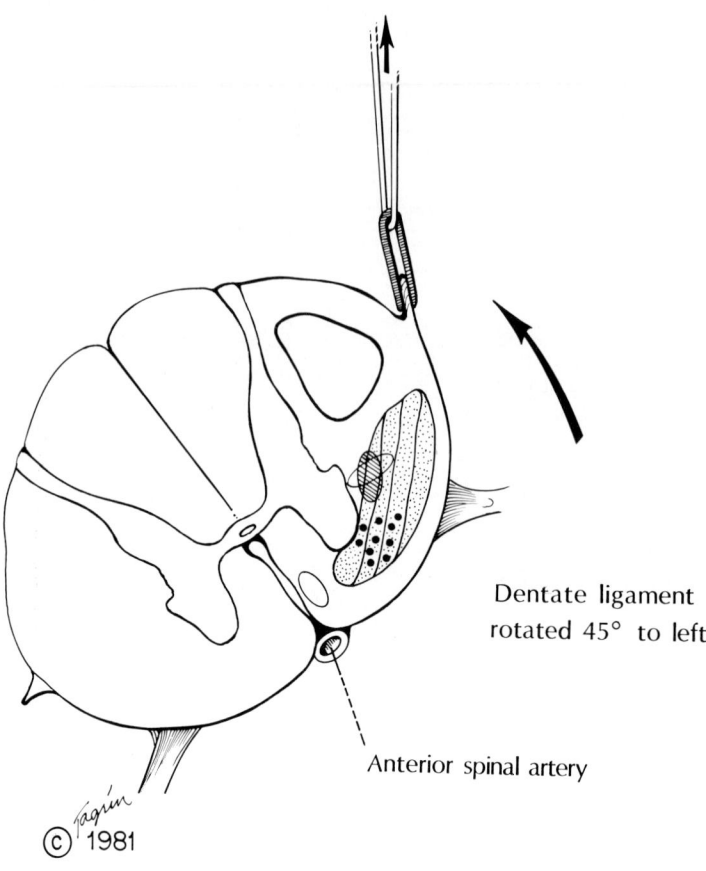

FIGURE 126–5. The orientation of the relevant tracts within the cord once it has been rotated 45 degrees. (Copyright © 1981 by Edith Tagrin.)

paraspinal muscles. When the patient awakens, pain may originate from traction on a dorsal root. This can be blocked with lidocaine or cocaine.

With the patient awake, it is advisable to test for deep visceral pain as well as for pinprick perception. This is especially important for patients in whom a significant portion of their disease lies in deep structures of the pelvis. Both legs should also be tested for motor strength, because the pyramidal tracts may not be crossed, in which case the contralateral limbs may be supplied by the spinal tract in the anterior medial quadrant with the lesion.

If the level of analgesia does not reach far enough cephalad, the lesion should be extended medially and anteriorly to include fibers adjacent to the anterior midline septum. A lesion resulting in a level of analgesia that is not sufficiently caudal, e.g., sparing the perineum and sacral distribution, should be extended closer to the equator and thus closer to the crossed cortical spinal tract. Further extensions of the initial cordotomy lesion can be made with the patient awake, because transection of the spinothalamic tract is not perceived as a painful stimulus. This arrangement permits functional monitoring of the motor system as well while the lesion is being extended.

Upon achievement of a satisfactory distribution of analgesia, the patient is re-anesthetized for closure. The Weck clips on the dentate are cut free, the cord is allowed to return to normal position, and the wound is closed.

Bilateral Cordotomy Procedure

Bilateral high cervical cordotomies are not performed because of the high risk of sleep apnea and other complications.

If bilateral analgesia is necessary, a percutaneous or open cordotomy can be done unilaterally at C2 or C3, with a contralateral cordotomy at C5-C6 performed by the posterior or anterior approach through the C5-C6 disc space. Usually, when contralateral analgesia at a high level is not mandatory, a percutaneous cordotomy is done at C2 on one side, followed by a contralateral open thoracic cordotomy at T2 or T3.

When a lower bilateral level of analgesia is satisfactory, a bilateral operation should be performed in one stage in the upper thoracic region—with one lesion at T2 and the other contralateral at T4. For this operation, the laminae at T2 and T4 are each removed as well as the spinous process of T3. The rest of the procedure is as described for unilateral cordotomy. If a previous unilateral cordotomy has been done at T3 and it becomes evident later that a contralateral lesion is indicated, the second lesion can be made at the lower margin of T1 as early as 5 to 7 days postoperatively.

POSTOPERATIVE PRECAUTIONS

Sleep Apnea

Following C2-C3 cordotomies, the patient should be placed postoperatively in the intensive care recovery room, especially because of the danger of sleep apnea. When sent back to the floor, the patient should be monitored continuously with an apnea alarm, and tidal volume should periodically be checked. The nursing staff must be alert to the possible need for prompt respiratory assistance. The potential

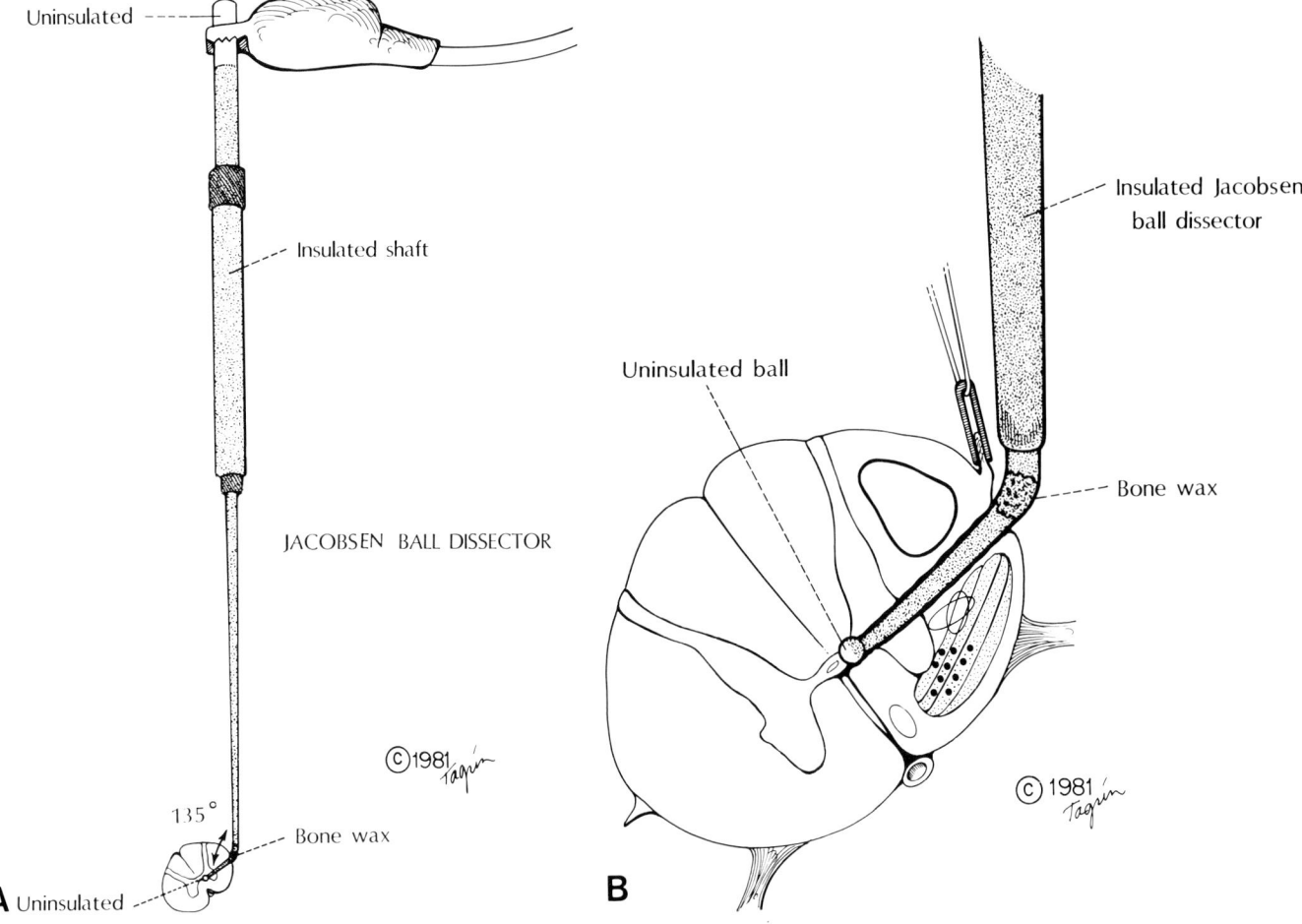

FIGURE 126–6. (A) The 45-degree Jacobsen ball tip has been inserted just anterior to the equator of the cord and, while stimulating, is slowly advanced in the transverse axis of the cord until the tip reaches the midline (i.e., until the distal part of the bone wax marker on the tip is flush against the lateral aspect of the cord). The tip should pass far enough dorsally to include the intermediolateral nucleus and all the tracts depicted in Figure 126–1 except for the crossed CST. (B) An enlarged view of the Jacobsen ball instrument after the initial insertion. Note that the distal half of the Jacobsen ball is uninsulated. Should this pass closer than 1 mm to the CST during its insertion into the cord, ipsilateral motor responses will be elicited. In this case the ball should be redirected more anteriorly. From this position, the ball is then slowly directed 90 degrees anteriorly, palpating the midline septum. (Copyright © 1981 by Edith Tagrin.)

for sleep apnea may persist for a week postoperatively, after which these precautions can be relaxed. If sleep apnea occurs after a unilateral cervical cordotomy, the patient virtually always recovers after an adequate period of assisted support.

Weakness

At the first sign of motor weakness postoperatively, we administer high-dose steroids and maintain the blood pressure, if necessary, to prevent any hypotension.

Hypotension

When bilateral lesions are made, the blood pressure must be monitored as the patient begins to mobilize—raising the head off the bed, dangling the feet, and walking. Toe-to-groin woven elastic bandage wraps may be used, along with fluid loading and antihypotensive drugs as needed. The decrease in blood pressure—even with bilateral lesions—as well as orthostatic hypotension gradually clears and is a problem only if unrecognized. A single episode of severe hypotension may compromise the blood supply significantly, particularly that to the upper thoracic cord. This ischemia may extend the lesion to the adjacent corticospinal tract.

Urinary Retention

If a Foley catheter has been placed before a bilateral procedure, a cystometrogram should be done several days postoperatively, before the catheter is removed.

OPERATIVE RESULTS

The incidence of pain relief 3 months postoperatively varies from 54 to 90 percent, with the average being 75 percent.[1, 14–18] After 18 months, the rate of relief falls to approximately 50 percent, where it remains for several years. It is generally agreed that the incidence of pain relief is greater in those patients with postoperative paresis and sphincter disturbance, suggesting a direct relation between the degree of pain relief and the extent of the lesion.

A T3 cordotomy, according to Taren and colleagues,[19] should be expected to produce a postoperative sensory level

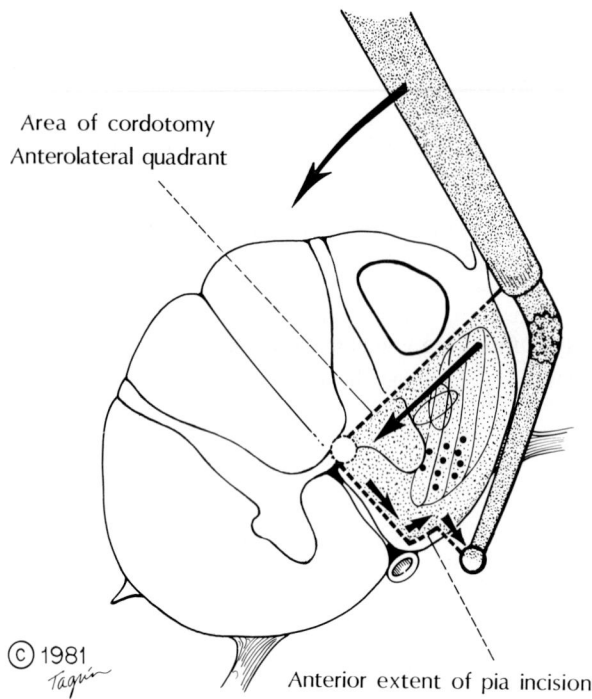

FIGURE 126-7. The tip of the Jacobsen ball has been brought 90 degrees anteriorly, palpating along the midline septum until the pia on the anterior aspect of the cord is felt. The ball is then drawn laterally along the pia until it exits from the cord at the medialmost extent of the pial incision previously made with the microscissors. (Copyright © 1981 by Edith Tagrin.)

up to T4-T5, including postoperative loss of superficial pain, temperature, deep pain, visceral pain, and itch. The permanent level, however, usually settles at T7-T10. Grant and Wood[20] report an average permanent level of analgesia or hypalgesia only up to T5 after cervical cordotomies.

In some of our cases, satisfactory and persisting relief of pain is achieved without superficial cutaneous analgesia. This dissociation between pain relief and cutaneous analgesia is seen commonly in midline myelotomies and characterizes certain thalamic lesions. Although the neurophysiologic explanation is not clear for the spinal cord, we propose that two fiber systems are involved, namely, in addition to the spinothalamic tract carrying acute pain perception, there also may be a midline multineuronal ascending system in the central gray matter of the spinal cord. This latter system may modulate a patient's ability to suppress chronic pain.

OPERATIVE FAILURES AND RECURRENCE OF PAIN

Operative Failures

The most common causes of failure to achieve satisfactory analgesia following cordotomy are as follows:

1. Failure to cut close enough to the equator of the cord, so there is sparing of the sacral representation in the spinal cord.
2. Failure to cut deep in the anterior quadrant, producing a satisfactory level of cutaneous analgesia without adequate relief of deep and visceral pain. Accordingly, in order to make sure the deep fibers carrying deep somatic visceral pain are severed, one should test these fibers intraoperatively with wake-up anesthesia. A satisfactory test for visceral pain is inflation of a Foley balloon within the bladder.
3. Insufficient extension of the lesion anteriorly and medially, resulting in a level of analgesia many segments below the level of the cordotomy.
4. Failure to cut the anterior quadrant decisively, producing an incomplete lesion with limited and patchy analgesia.
5. Performing a unilateral cordotomy when a bilateral procedure was indicated.
6. Subsequent spread of the cancer above the level of analgesia. If such spread is anticipated, a higher cordotomy should be done initially.
7. Anatomic variability of the spinal cord, resulting in an unsatisfactory lesion.

Recurrence of Pain with Fading of Analgesia

If the level of analgesia falls and islands of recovered nociception occur within a few days postoperatively, the spinothalamic fibers in the periphery of the lesion have probably been bruised but not severed. The first postoperative drop in analgesic level may be caused by recovery from direct injury by the operation, and the drop during the first week may be the result of recovery from edema and swelling. This process may explain the two-to-five-segment drop in the analgesic level during the first 2 postoperative weeks. In an excellent review on long-term follow-up of cordotomy patients, Grant and Wood[20] found that both islands and large areas of sensation returned even within a few months. It is conceivable that this recovery of pain perception is caused by collateral regeneration of new synaptic terminals[5] in short-chain internuncial neurons taking over the previous function of the long spinothalamic tract. White[21] found that 4 years after cordotomy, 54 percent of cordotomy patients had recovered pain perception; subsequent higher anterolateral cordotomies generally proved unsuccessful in re-instituting analgesia. In addition to the hypothesis of collateral sprouting, long-term fading of postcordotomy analgesia may be explained by altered synaptic and membrane excitability in pre-existing, potentially alternative nociceptive pathways. Indeed, in addition to first-order neurons ascending to medullary nuclei from the posterior columns, other neurons send efferent projections from the segmental gray matter. These may be partially responsible for conducting impulses concerned in the abnormal reference of pain. Partial support for this alternative pathway lies in the fact that stimulation of the dorsal column during midline myelotomy is often reported as painful by the awake patient.

Another hypothesis explaining the return of pain perception is that intrasegmental polysynaptic complexes form from collaterals of the crossing spinothalamic tract fibers. These may separate near the midline from the crossing spinothalamic tract fibers ascending in the spinal periaqueductal central gray matter to the reticular formation. Support for this hypothesis lies in the fact that relief of pain is experienced after midline commissural myelotomy or central myelotomy often not associated with cutaneous analgesia.

Accordingly, we believe that postcordotomy recovery of pain perception is less probably caused by spinal cord or thalamic axonal sprouting than by altered trans-synaptic excitability in pre-existing, potentially alternative nociceptive pathways.

OPERATIVE COMPLICATIONS

Mortality

The mortality in published series varies from 3 to 21 percent.[1, 14–16] It is higher for unilateral cordotomies in the cervical region involving malignant disease and still higher for bilateral cervical cordotomies. The postoperative mortality clearly is higher in cancer patients than in patients with benign disease.

Respiratory Complications

Some authors indicate that respiratory complications are the most serious concern in high cervical cordotomies. In the past, sleep apnea has been a common cause of death. Voluntary control of respiration is mediated by the cortical spinal tract, but subconscious ipsilateral respiratory movements are controlled by pathways descending deep in the centrolateral part of the spinal cord. This descending unilateral respiratory pathway is called the *ventrolateral reticulospinal tract*. Its fibers are, at least in part, intermingled with the fibers of the lateral spinothalamic tract (see Fig. 126–1). Unilateral destruction of this pathway results in little functional respiratory loss, unless contralateral respiratory function is poor. Accordingly, even for unilateral C2-C3 cordotomies, the function of the contralateral diaphragm should be evaluated preoperatively. Bilateral lesions clearly produce a high incidence of sleep apnea and death.

Postcordotomy Hypotension

Intraoperatively, there may be a sudden drop in blood pressure immediately after a cordotomy lesion has been made. Sindou (personal communication, 1981) makes the point that such a drop in pressure signifies that the lesions have been made deep enough and far enough dorsally to ensure transection of the fibers carrying visceral pain. In unilateral thoracic cordotomies, this drop is moderate and evanescent. The blood pressure usually returns to normal level by the end of wound closure. Following bilateral lesions, the drop may be marked and protracted, lasting well into the postoperative period.

Blood pressure is maintained by spinal sympathetic pathways that descend partially intermingled with the ascending STT (see Fig. 126–1). Stimulation of these fibers elevates the blood pressure and the pressure within the bladder.[22] Unlike respiratory complications, blood pressure drop is seldom a cause of death or serious morbidity unless the patient is in a sitting position when the drop occurs.

As noted, hypotension in the postoperative period may produce ischemia, especially in the thoracic region, thereby enlarging the surgical lesion and causing a new motor deficit.

Motor Weakness

Assuming that the cortical spinal tract has a relatively normal anatomy, the two principal causes of ipsilateral motor weakness following cordotomy a lesion extending too far posteriorly, which damages the crossed cortical spinal tract, and an extension too far anteromedially, which damages the anterior spinal artery with resulting ischemia. A third possible mechanism is borderline ischemia accentuated by intraoperative or postoperative hypotension. The fact that the upper thoracic cord is especially susceptible to such ischemic damage may explain why there is a higher incidence of paresis after thoracic cordotomy than after the cervical procedure.

The literature indicates that the incidence of paresis or paralysis following unilateral cordotomy varies from 0 to 11 percent,[15, 16, 23] whereas the incidence following bilateral cordotomies can run as high as 24 percent.[16] The incidence of permanent motor deficits is clearly much higher in bilateral lesions. We believe that the implementation of stimulation techniques as described decreases the incidence of paresis.

Bladder Dysfunction

Urinary bladder dysfunction after cordotomy is common. Following unilateral cordotomy, this complication is relatively uncommon (0 to 8 percent).[1, 15, 23] The disturbance usually lasts only a few days and responds well to medical management. Following bilateral cordotomies, either cervical or thoracic, the incidence of urinary dysfunction is much higher and its duration is often permanent.

When a cordotomy is done for sacral pain, sphincter disturbances are particularly likely to occur. Nathan and Smith,[24, 25] having studied the physiology of micturition and defecation, concluded that both the descending and ascending fibers responding to distension and the desire to relax sphincters are assembled in a narrow band almost crossing the equator of the cord opposite the central canal. Figure 126–1 clearly shows the high risk of bowel and bladder disturbance if a bilateral cordotomy is performed for sacral pain with the incision made close to the equator.

Sexual Dysfunction

Sweet[9] claims that the fibers involved in sexual sensation and function lie so close to those for pain (see Fig. 126–1) that sexual function is almost always impaired after unilateral cordotomy and is permanently impaired after bilateral cordotomy. Taren and colleagues[19] report that after section of the anterolateral tracts, erection and ejaculation may still occur, but sexual sensation at the moment of orgasm is lost. Sexual potency does not seem to be disturbed with unilateral cordotomy but is almost always lost following the bilateral procedure.

Dysesthesias

The abnormal sensations that may arise immediately after cordotomy, or as long as months after the operation, are sometimes divided into two groups: referred sensations and dysesthesias. Postoperatively, soreness of the skin and pain with girdle distribution may develop at or above the level of the lesion. This usually persists only for a few weeks and may be related to undue traction of the dorsal roots when the cord was rotated.

Referred sensations may be elicited by stimulation within

the analgesic area in approximately 25 percent of patients. These sensations may be felt by the patient as noxious; they are poorly localized and often referred contralaterally. After bilateral cordotomy, the sensations may be referred to an area above the level of analgesia as well as to areas of escape within the analgesic zone.

More serious are the severe constant painful dysesthesias referred to levels below the cordotomy. Their onset is usually delayed, occurring with increasing frequency as the postoperative period lengthens. Postcordotomy dysesthesias become a serious problem in approximately 6 percent of patients after 2 to 3 years. As noted, cordotomy at a higher level is not effective.

MEDULLARY TRACTOTOMY

ANATOMIC BASIS

The primary nociceptive afferents from the fifth, seventh, ninth, and tenth cranial nerves all descend in the medulla adjacent to each other, forming the descending cranial nociceptive tract (DCNT). Nature, in a degree of consideration for pain patients unparalleled in its design of the central nervous system, permits the neurosurgeon to interrupt virtually all orofacial primary nociceptive afferents by means of a single small ipsilateral lesion in the lateral dorsal medulla. Orofacial nociceptive cranial afferents, whether they enter via the fifth, seventh, ninth, or tenth cranial nerves, all descend in a compact tract, traveling caudally in the dorsolateral aspect of the medulla. At the level of the obex, this tract is bounded dorsally by the nucleus cuneatus and ventrally by the contralateral ascending spinal thalamic tract (STT). The most superficial fibers of the tract, however, do not lie on the surface of the brainstem, but are covered by the external arcuate fibers. (These fibers, important for coordination, arise from cells in the nucleus cuneatus accessorius and project to the cerebellum). The DCNT is 2 to 2.5 mm deep, its ventral margin being formed by the spinal trigeminal nucleus caudalis. In addition, the fibers within the tract have a very distinct topographic localization: Descending in the most ventral portion of the descending trigeminal tract are fibers from the first trigeminal division. Immediately ventral to these fibers are the exiting motor fibers of the eleventh cranial nerve. In turn, just ventral to these exiting motor fibers of eleventh nerve are the ascending fibers of the contralateral STT. Dorsal to the descending nociceptive fibers of the first trigeminal division are the fibers from the second trigeminal division, with the fibers from the third trigeminal division next. In turn, just dorsal to these nociceptive fibers of the trigeminal third division are the primary nociceptive fibers from the seventh nerve's nervus intermedius and, most dorsally, the descending nociceptive fibers of the ninth and tenth nerves. Finally, just dorsal to the descending tenth nociceptive fibers are the ascending ipsilateral proprioceptive fibers immediately next to the nucleus cuneatus.

Accordingly, a surgical lesion made from the dorsal limit of the ascending contralateral STT, i.e., at the line demarcated by the exiting motor rootlets of the eleventh cranial nerve, dorsally to the ventral limit of nucleus cuneatus transects first the nociceptive fibers from V1, followed by those from V2, V3, VII, IX, and X. If the lesion extends too far ventrally it will transect fibers from the contralateral STT; if too far dorsally, it will transect fibers entering the nucleus cuneatus.[1] In order to sever all the fibers from each nerve, the lesion must extend to a depth of 3 to 3.5 mm. Making such a lesion, of necessity, transects the overlying external arcuate fibers as well. Interrupting these fibers accounts for the postoperative truncal and gait ataxia.

Rowbotham, in 1938, was the first to take advantage of this configuration of the descending trigeminal nociceptive tract by performing, successfully, a trigeminal medullary tractotomy in a patient suffering from severe migrainous neuralgia involving the distribution of the first trigeminal division. It was not until 1942, however, that, on the basis of clinical observations and interpretations of Cajal's neuroanatomic drawings, Sweet recognized that the spinal descending nociceptive tract included not only nociceptive fibers descending from the trigeminal nerve but also nociceptive fibers descending from the seventh nervus intermedius and the ninth and tenth nerves. On the basis of these observations, Sweet in 1945 demonstrated that a single, slightly larger lesion in the dorsolateral medulla could interrupt virtually all primary nociceptive fibers from ipsilateral orofacial regions.

This medullary tractotomy of the DCNT, made dorsal to the exiting roots of the eleventh nerve, should be distinguished from a medullary tractotomy of the contralateral ascending STT, made just ventral to the exiting roots of the eleventh nerve. This operation, first performed by J. C. White, can be used to obtain contralateral analgesia to a dermatomal level as high as C2. Such a medullary tractotomy appears to be particularly appropriate for patients suffering from cancer invading the contralateral brachial plexus.

INDICATIONS

Even with the advent of intraventricular morphine, we believe there continues to be an occasional patient in whom a unilateral lesion of the DCNT is the best available treatment. In our experience, these patients are most likely to be suffering from a slow-growing, indolent cancer affecting only one side of the face and oropharynx. Very occasionally, a patient suffers from extremely severe periodic migrainous neuralgia that is unresponsive to conservative regimens and for which retrogasserian trigeminal rhizotomy has failed. In these patients suffering from severe periodic migrainous neuralgia, occasionally an avulsion of the greater and lesser superficial petrosal nerve has also already been made, especially in patients with marked autonomic changes: tearing, unilateral hyperhidrosis, hemicranial flush, and nasal mucosal engorgement. Another possible operation for patients suffering from periodic migrainous neuralgia has been to section the primary nociceptive afferents in the seventh nervus intermedius as well as the nociceptive fibers entering the ninth nerve and the rostral rootlets of the tenth. As shown by Bischoff's very meticulous microdissections, however, all pain fibers entering the VII-VIII root entry zone are, in fact, not confined to the discrete nervus intermedius. Not only may afferent nociceptive fibers course among the efferent motor fibers of the seventh nerve, but they may also travel within the afferents of the body of the eighth nerve. Accordingly, in patients with severe, acute disseminated periodic migrainous neuralgia, a lesion of the DCNT may be indicated. Patients with periodic migrainous neuralgia whose symptoms are confined to V1 and V2, as is typically the case, and whose neuralgia is unresponsive to caffeine-ergotamine therapy and all other medical regimens are almost certainly candidates first for a percutaneous retrogasserian trigeminal rhizotomy. Therefore, it is only patients who have a recrudescence of pain following this initial surgical procedure or spread of pain to nontrigeminal distributions who may be candidates for lesions of the DCNT.

An advantage of a DCNT tractotomy over a rhizotomy of V1 and V2 is that the tractotomy produces analgesia without anesthesia and, invariably, when made at the rostrocaudal level of the obex, preserves corneal sensation. Because the midline portion of the dura and the posterior fossa is innervated by afferent pain fibers entering the VII-VIII complex, IX, and X, it is also an advantage of the tractotomy to denervate these structures in patients with periodic migrainous neuralgia referred to the deep occipital region.

OPERATIVE PROCEDURE

Instrumentation

The only special instrument used, in addition to the standard microneurosurgical array, is the Jacobsen ball dissector described previously for use in open cordotomies. If the patient is awake, the tip of the ball can be stimulated to determine physiologically when the lesion has extended ventrally past V1 fibers into the fibers of the contralateral spinal thalamic tract, thus helping to determine the ventral limit of the V1 descending pain fibers. Similarly, the tip of the Jacobsen ball may be used to record evoked responses obtained by stimulating the dorsal column afferents from the median nerve. The sudden appearance of large evoked responses obtained by median nerve stimulation should indicate the approximation of the tip of the Jacobsen ball to the ascending dorsal fibers in nucleus cuneatus, as the lesion is extended rostrally from V3 through VII, IX, and X fibers reaching nucleus cuneatus.

Anesthesia

One can use either sustained general anesthesia or wake-up anesthesia. Satisfactory wake-up anesthesia, however, may be difficult after a prolonged exposure of the posterior fossa, especially when this is combined with a C1-C2 laminectomy in those patients in whom a dorsal rhizotomy of C1 and C2 is also desired. Accordingly, Sweet,[9] on several occasions, has done the suboccipital and upper cervical exposure in one operation and then performed a second stage in which the wound was merely reopened and the dura opened and the patient was promptly awakened after the initial lesion in the DCNT was made. With this technique, the patient may be fully satisfactorily awakened and extubated for detailed sensory testing. The patient is then put back to sleep briefly using intravenous methohexital sodium to make any required enlargement of the lesion. In our last two cases, however, both with extremely severe periodic migrainous neuralgia, I have preferred to use sustained general anesthesia and the techniques described here to obtain a fully satisfactory DCNT tractotomy.

Patient Position and Operative Technique

The patient is placed in a position halfway between lateral and prone with the head turned 45 degrees to the floor. The side of the anticipated tractotomy is placed upward, i.e., for a right-sided lesion. The patient is placed with the left shoulder on the table and nose turned down to the left toward the floor. The head of the bed is elevated 20 to 30 degrees, and the patient's head flexed forward, bringing the chin to within two fingerbreadths of the sternum. The head is held in this position with a three-point skeletal fixation headrest.

A vertical midline incision is made from the low occipital region down to the upper cervical region. The incision is extended caudally in patients in whom a concomitant dorsal rhizotomy of C1, C2 and C3 is planned. A craniectomy in the mid and low suboccipital region is made in the midline and slightly more to the side of the lesion. If only a tractotomy is planned, a laminectomy of C1 is not necessary. The dura is opened with an incision begun over the cerebellum and cerebellar tonsil on the side of the anticipated lesion. The incision is then carried down to the midline at the cervicomedullary junction and caudally at least to the level of C1—further if a rhizotomy is planned.

The microscope is then brought into the field and angled rostrally toward the inferior limit of the fourth ventricle. Retractors are placed on either side and are used to retract the cerebellar tonsils dorsolaterally until the obex is seen directly. The vermis does not have to be split. The cerebellar tonsil is then retracted further on the side of the anticipated lesion. (As noted, this is the cerebellar tonsil on the upper side, in that the patient has been positioned so that the side of the lesion is upward.)

A lesion of the DCNT may be made as far as 10 mm rostral to the obex, as advocated by Kunc, or at 2 mm below the obex, as advocated by us. The more rostral tractotomy tends to make a slightly denser lesion for people with severe cancer pain; however, it also produces more discoordination and ataxia. (The more rostral lesion interrupts more nociceptive fibers from cranial nerves VII, IX, and X but also transects more external arcuate fibers). Using microsurgical techniques, we have been satisfied with the density of our lesions made 2 mm caudal to the obex. The lesion is made in a plane transverse to the brainstem on the lateral dorsal side of the medulla, extending ventrally and dorsally. The line of demarcation between the most ventral descending fibers of V1 and the most dorsal fibers of the contralateral STT is clearly defined on the surface of the medulla by the point of exit of the roots of the eleventh cranial nerves. Accordingly, the cerebellar tip should be retracted in order to visualize at least one emerging rootlet of the eleventh nerve rostral and another rootlet caudal to the anticipated transverse level of the lesion. These may be stimulated, even in the asleep patient, to be sure they represent motor fibers of the eleventh. A line is drawn between these two exiting rootlets, and that line marks the ventral extent of the lesion. Dorsally the distinct prominences of nucleus gracilis, adjacent to the obex, and further laterally, of nucleus cuneatus can be seen. The lateral extent of the surface presentation of the eminence of nucleus cuneatus should mark the dorsomedial extent of the projected incision. Any small surface blood vessels may be teased to either side of the projected incision or cauterized very gently.

The incision is begun by using the No. 11 blade to make a very small opening in the pia-arachnoid at the lateral extent of the eminence of the nucleus cuneatus. The microsurgical scissors are then used to incise the pia-arachnoid, going laterally and anteriorly until the incision reaches the line drawn between the two exiting eleventh nerve rootlets. At this point, if the patient has been awakened, the nerves to be cut may be stimulated by mechanical pressure, as characterizes the sensitivity of these primary nociceptive afferents. Both Kunc and Sweet have used needles or sharp nerve hooks to stimulate either the fibers of the DCNT or the proprioceptive fibers ascending to the nucleus cuneatus. The patient may refer the sensations to a very focal area, permitting discrimination among V1, V2, and V3 descending fibers. When the fibers of nucleus cuneatus are stimulated mechanically, sensations are referred to the ipsilateral arm, neck, and back of the head. (Proprioceptive fibers from the lower portions of the body ascend to the nucleus gracilus.)

If the patient is awake, the lesion is extended ventrally until there is some nociceptive sensory loss in the contralateral distal lower extremity. The lesion is extended dorsomedially until there is some reference of sensation to the ipsilateral dorsal columns. The lesion should be made to a depth of only 3 mm. This is done in the current technique by putting a small piece of bone wax 3 mm up the shaft of the Jacobsen ball, and then inserting the instrument only to that depth dorsally. As in the anterior quadrant of the spinal cord, there is very little resistance even to the relatively blunt tip of the Jacobsen ball. Similarly, scarcely any bleeding occurs with this complete DCNT tractotomy. We recommend that the lesion extend ventrally at least partially into the contralateral STT and dorsally into the ascending proprioceptive fibers, to enhance the probability of a complete lasting lesion of the DCNT, because the initial lesion tends to fade in the postoperative period.

Currently, as mentioned, we are relying on these microsurgical techniques to make the tractotomy lesion with the patient under sustained general anesthesia. Additional guidance should be available in the future through advanced electrophysiologic techniques.

A medullary tractotomy of the contralateral ascending STT uses the same position and exposure, although the incision begins just ventral to the exiting rootlets of the eleventh nerve and extends more ventrally.[1,26]

COMPLICATIONS, SIDE EFFECTS, RESULTS, AND THOUGHTS FOR THE FUTURE

Clearly, this DCNT tractotomy is a major operative procedure carrying mortality and morbidity greater than those of percutaneous trigeminal rhizotomy or percutaneous glossopharyngeal rhizotomy. The worst side effect is the inevitable degree of difficulty in walking produced by this lesion. In the immediate postoperative period, patients almost invariably suffer from incoordination and lateral pulsion. As noted, this is less the case for lesions made caudal to the level of the obex. Usually by 1 month after the operation, the degree of discoordination has cleared sufficiently for patients in most occupations to have normal function. Dysesthesias as seen following spinal lesions of the STT have not been a consistent problem following lesions of the DCNT.

The degree of pain relief tends to be commensurate with the extent of the analgesia produced by the lesion. Thus, lesions producing lasting analgesia throughout the distribution of the cranial nerves have a high probability of relieving pain of either cancer or migrainous origin. Including a dorsal rhizotomy of C1, C2, and C3 improves the results in those patients whose migrainous neuralgia is not confined to orofacial regions. It is of interest that the pain of periodic migrainous neuralgia is eliminated by the DCNT tractotomy whereas the autonomic symptoms, which are characteristic of periodic migrainous neuralgia, may often persist. In several of our patients with extremely severe periodic migrainous neuralgia, who were suicidal in spite of intensive medical and psychiatric therapy and in whom radiofrequency failed, trigeminal lesions have been markedly relieved by a DCNT tractotomy. As noted, orofacial cutaneous and mucosal and corneal touch sensation is functionally preserved.

REFERENCES

1. White JC, Sweet WH: Pain and the Neurosurgeon. Springfield, IL, Charles C Thomas, 1969, pp 69, 629
2. Hitchcock ER: Stereotactic myelotomy. Proc R Soc Med 67:771, 1964
3. Hitchcock ER: Stereotactic cervical myelotomy. J Neurol Neurosurg Psychiatry 33:224, 1970
4. Schvarcz JR: Stereotactic extralemniscal myelotomy. J Neurol Neurosurg Psychiatry 39:53, 1976
5. Schvarcz JR: Functional exploration of the spinomedullary junction. Acta Neurochir (Suppl) 24:179, 1977
6. Schvarcz JR: Spinal cord stereotactic techniques re: Trigeminal nucleotomy and extralemniscal myelotomy. Appl Neurophysiol 41:99, 1978
7. Poletti CE, Cohen AM, Todd DP, et al: Clinical pain relieved by long-term epidural morphine: Two case reports with permanent indwelling systems for self-administration. J Neurosurg 55:581, 1981
8. Yakovlev PL, Rakic P: Patterns of decussation of bulbar pyramidal tracts on two sides of the spinal cord. Trans Am Neurol Assoc 91:366, 1966
9. Sweet WH: Recent observations pertinent to improving anterolateral cordotomy. Clin Neurosurg 23:80, 1976
10. Macon JB, Poletti CE: Conducted somatosensory evoked potentials during spinal surgery. Part 1: Technical aspects. J Neurosurg (in press)
11. Cowie RA, Hitchcock ER: The late results of anterolateral cordotomy for pain relief. Acta Neurochir 64:39, 1982
12. Grunert VP, Sunder-Plassmann MS: Ergebnisse der zerikalen chordotomie mit und ohne rhizotomie bei konservitiv therapie resistenten schmerzen im Schulter-Arm-Bereich. Zentralbl Neurochir 46:267, 1985
13. Hardy D, LeClereq TA, Mercky F: Microsurgical selective cordotomy by the anterior approach, in Handa H (ed): Microsurgery: International Symposium on Microsurgery. Baltimore, University Park Press, 1973
14. Brihaye J, Retif J: Comparison of the results obtained by anterolateral cordotomy at the dorsal level and at the cervical level. Neurochirurgie 7:258, 1961
15. Diemath HE, Heppner F, Walker AE: Anterolateral chordotomy for relief of pain. Postgrad Med J 29:485, 1961
16. Nathan PW: Results of antero-lateral cordotomy for pain in cancer. J Neurol Neurosurg Psychiatry 26:353, 1963
17. Dautenhahn D, Reynolds A, Darby R, et al: Thoracic epidural analgesia for open cordotomy. Anesth Analg 63:1036, 1984
18. Jack T, Lloyd J: Long-term efficacy of surgical cordotomy in intractable nonmalignant pain. Ann R Coll Surg Engl 97:102, 1983
19. Taren DA, Kahn EA, Humphrey T: The surgery of pain, in Kahn EA, Crosby EC, Schneider RC, et al (eds): Correlative Neurosurgery. Springfield, IL, Charles C Thomas, 1969

20. Grant FC, Wood FA: Experiences with cordotomy. Clin Neurosurg 5:38, 1957
21. White JC: Anterolateral cordotomy: Its effectiveness in relieving pain of non-malignant disease. Neurochirurgia 6:83, 1963.
22. Kerr FW, Alexander S: Descending autonomic pathways in the spinal cord. Arch Neurol 10:249, 1964
23. McKissock W: Second International Congress of Neurological Surgeons. International Congress Series No. 36 E27. Amsterdam, Excerpta Medica, 1961
24. Nathan PW, Smith MC: Spinal pathways subserving defecation and sensation from the lower bowel. J Neurol Neurosurg Psychiatry 16:245, 1953
25. Nathan PW, Smith MC: The centrifugal pathway for micturition within the spinal cord. J Neurol Neurosurg Psychiatry 21:177, 1958
26. Poletti CE, Ojemann RG: Stereo Atlas of Operative Microneurosurgery. Reel 19, View 3, pp 264–265, 1985

CHAPTER 127

Surgery for Hyperhidrosis and Sympathetically Mediated Pain Syndromes

Harold A. Wilkinson

In Chapter 132, Dr. Russell Hardy, Jr., and Dr. Janet Bay have reviewed the history of surgical sympathectomy and an even more detailed historical review was published by Greenwood in 1967.[2] Surgical sympathectomies were first performed in the 1890s, and techniques for both thoracic and lumbar sympathectomy were evolved over the next four decades. Early sympathectomies were performed for the treatment of epilepsy, exophthalmic goiter, spasticity, and angina pectoris. Most of these disorders proved not to be improved by sympathectomy. Several investigators documented the beneficial effects of sympathectomy for angina pectoris, vascular ischemic disorders with trophic ulcers, angina pectoris, hypertension, hyperhidrosis, and pain.[3-15] Although the advent of potent antihypertensive medications has largely eliminated the need for sympathectomy for blood pressure control, each of the other conditions continues to provide indications for sympathectomy. Angina pectoris is currently treated most commonly with medications, but the variant form Prinzmetal's angina has been shown to be refractory to most medications and to coronary vasodilation but to be quite responsive to sympathectomy.

Anatomic targets for sympathectomy are the upper thoracic sympathetic ganglia (for treatment of disorders of the upper limbs), the lower thoracic sympathetic ganglia and splanchnic nerves (for visceral abdominal pain), and lower lumbar sympathetic ganglia (for disorders of the lower extremities). The surgical options available include chemical sympathectomy, radiofrequency sympathectomy, endoscopic sympathectomy, and open surgical sympathectomy. Each of these techniques is discussed in this chapter.

Evaluating the outcome of sympathectomy is complicated by two factors: (1) determining whether the disease for which sympathectomy was done has continued to progress despite adequate sympathetic interruption and (2) the capacity for the sympathetic nervous system to reorganize or regenerate. In every large surgical series that involves long-term follow-up, the incidence of return of sympathetic functioning is as high as 10 percent, even following surgical resection of the ganglia.[12, 16-21] There are two documented cases of actual regeneration proven at surgical re-exploration, with sympatholysis being reinstituted following resection of the regenerated material.[16, 20] In 1935, Telford,[13] the pioneering sympathectomy surgeon, stated, "I do not think that any operator who has had sufficient experience of sympathectomy and has followed up his cases for some years can regard the outcome of his work as entirely satisfactory."

Nomenclature remains another impediment to analyzing the results of sympathectomy. A lengthy list of terms has been used to describe the dysautonomias or sympathetically mediated disorders.[22-24] Furthermore, published definitions are often in conflict even for the more commonly used terms, such as causalgia ("major" or "minor"), reflex sympathetic dystrophy, and Raynaud's syndrome. Some of the confusion results from the wide and often overlapping spectrum of symptoms and pathophysiology attributable to sympathetically mediated disorders and to the varying anatomic sites of those symptoms (Table 127–1). The principal manifestations are vasospasm (which is often painful), causalgia (sympathetically mediated pain without tissue destruction or ischemia), dystrophy (usually affecting joints and skin more than other tissues), coronary vasospasm (Prinzmetal's angina), and hyperhidrosis (including congenital varieties and those acquired following trauma or stroke as well as gustatory, plantar, palmar, and diffuse varieties). Sudek's atrophy (in which dystrophy predominates over pain), reflex sympathetic dystrophy, and major causalgia (both combining severe pain with dystrophic features) usually are predominantly unilateral but frequently have at least some bilateral component.[21, 22] Raynaud's syndrome (of peripheral vasospasticity) and hyperhidrosis are predominantly bilateral.

Table 127–1. SPECIFIC SYNDROMES WITH SYMPATHETICALLY MEDIATED PAIN

Syndromes with principally sympathetically mediated pain, little dystrophy or vasculopathy	Minor causalgia Shoulder/hand syndrome
Syndromes with significant circulatory problems, with variable degrees of sympathetically mediated pain	Vasospasm secondary to acute arterial occlusion Peripheral vasospastic vasculopathy; Raynaud's syndrome Peripheral structurally occlusive vasculopathies Prinzmetal's angina
Syndromes with significant dystrophic changes, with variable degrees of sympathetically mediated pain	Major causalgia Reflex sympathetic dystrophy Sudek's atrophy

INDICATIONS FOR SYMPATHECTOMY

Pathologic hyperhidrosis was the indication for one of the first reported sympathectomies, performed by Kotzareff[6] in 1920, and sympathectomy continues to be employed widely for the relief of this distressing disorder.[4, 18, 25, 33] Pathologic hyperhidrosis can interfere seriously with social relationships ("Who wants to hold hands with a wet fish?"), paperwork ("My papers are always smeared and wrinkled!"), sports ("I couldn't hold the bat!"), manual work ("I keep dropping my tools, and besides they rust too quickly!"), and housework ("I get so tired of being shocked by the toaster!"). Nonetheless, affected patients often have difficulty persuading a physician that they suffer from a significant illness. Systemic medications are rarely beneficial without major side effects, though oxybutynin (Ditropan) is at times helpful. Topical astringents and iontophoretic devices usually suffice only for patients with less severe hyperhidrosis.[18, 24, 30-34]

Thoracic surgical sympathectomy is usually highly successful for palmar hyperhidrosis, but many patients note increased sweating elsewhere, occasionally of distressing severity.[16, 18, 35, 36] Interestingly, more than one third of the patients who obtain palmar relief find that plantar sweating is also reduced, although the mechanism for this is unclear[16, 28, 35, 37] (Tables 127–2 and 127–3). For those whose plantar hyperhidrosis remains severe, supplementing thoracic sympathectomy with lumbar sympathectomy carries a risk of severe compensatory hyperhidrosis, most commonly affecting the entire trunk but at times predominantly affecting the chest, back, groin, or legs. Sympathetic denervation at T2 and T3 usually suffices for palmar hyperhidrosis, but the addition of T4 sympathectomy is said to be advisable if axillary hyperhidrosis is also distressing.[24, 30, 32, 38]

Sympathectomy for vascular disorders of the upper extremities is usually more beneficial for "essential" Raynaud's syndrome, Raynaud's syndrome secondary to use of vibrating tools, and acute vasospasm following arterial occlusions.[3, 10, 17, 19, 39-45] Results are usually less satisfactory and less long-lasting in patients with structural vasculopathies, such as collagen vasculitis, Buerger's disease, and cryoglobulinemia. It is estimated that more than 10% of patients with "primary" Raynaud's syndrome later manifest a collagen disorder.[39] Sympathectomy improves circulation only to a limited degree in patients with structural vasculopathy but can improve healing of trophic ulcers and provide relief of ischemic pain. Adequate sympatholysis of the upper extremities usually follows resection of T2 and T3 ganglia. The author's experience with stereotactic sympathectomy for vascular disease reinforces the observations well known from the experience with open surgical sympathectomy, i.e., not all vascular occlusive processes are under sympathetic control, and therefore not all symptoms can be controlled with sympathectomy.[37] Even though the acute vasospastic symptoms accompanying acute arterial occlusion respond well and maintain their response over the long term, patients with Raynaud's disease or vaso-obliterative disorders have a significant chance of suffering progression of the disease to a point no longer controllable by sympathetic interruption.

Patients with causalgic pain, or sympathetically mediated pain, can often benefit from sympathectomy, especially if there are associated dystrophic or vasospastic features.* Confirmation of a sympathetic basis for sympathetically mediated pain requires one or several diagnostic interruptions of sympathetic nerves or ganglion chains. The clinical syndromes can be quite varied but do fall into identifiable patterns (see Table 127–1). The extreme limb pain that follows acute occlusion of a major artery; angina pectoris that persists despite coronary vasodilators or angioplasty; the cold, blue, and painful hand that develops after exposure to cold; and the classic presentation of major causalgia all should be readily identifiable as most likely being associated with sympathetically mediated pain.[54] Greater diagnostic difficulty is encountered in those patients who complain of diffuse extremity pain, especially if dystrophic changes are of limited severity, who present with obstructive small-vessel disease in one or more extremities, or who present with relatively painless atrophy and dystrophy of a limb periphery. Any of these syndromes can occur in a wide array of variations, so the clinician is often challenged in making the diagnosis on a purely clinical basis. Interruption of the sympathetic supply to the affected area (lumbar or thoracic sympathetic chains or stellate ganglia) can confirm whether at least a portion of the pain is sympathetically mediated. Especially in those patients with obstructive vascular disease or significant dystrophic limb changes, much of the pain is likely to be transmitted through somatic pathways and not to be under sympathetic mediation, and postamputation pain rarely is sympathetically mediated. Furthermore, most of the painful and dystrophic syndromes occur following injury to a limb and especially following injury to a peripheral nerve, so that pain and disability secondary to the initiating injury likewise will remain after elimination of the sympathetically mediated pain component.

Much of the early experience with thoracic sympathectomy was in patients with intractable tachyarrhythmias or coronary artery pain.[5, 14, 17, 64] The advent of more effective medications sharply curtailed this application, though occasional cases prove refractory to all medications. The last decade has witnessed a rediscovery of thoracic sympathec-

Table 127–2. REMOTE CONCOMITANTS OF PALMAR HYPERHIDROSIS (RESPONSE TO 55 PATIENT QUESTIONNAIRES)

Concomitant	No. Patients Affected (%)
Plantar hyperhidrosis	19 (35)
Axillary hyperhidrosis	0
Both palmar and axillary hyperhidrosis	33 (60)
Neither	3 (5)

Table 127–3. REMOTE EFFECTS OF SYMPATHECTOMY (RESPONSE TO 55 PATIENT QUESTIONNAIRES)

Relief of Palmar Hyperhidrosis	Relief of Plantar Hyperhidrosis (No. Patients)			Relief of Axillary Hyperhidrosis (No. Patients)		
	Excellent	Partial	None	Excellent	Partial	None
Good/excellent	1	19	18	9	9	4
Partial	—	—	6	—	—	3
Poor	—	1	7	—	—	7

*See references 1, 7, 15, 22–24, 39, and 46–63.

tomy specifically for the treatment of Prinzmetal's angina, a form of angina commonly refractory to medications or coronary bypass grafting and judged likely to be due to coronary artery spasm.[37, 60, 65–72] For patients with this variant, bilateral thoracotomy or other major open sympathetic surgery under general anesthesia might be contraindicated by the cardiac disease, but they should be able to tolerate radiofrequency percutaneous surgery under supplemented local anesthesia, which carries a lower surgical risk.

Visceral pain afferents from the pancreas travel bilaterally through the splanchnic chain and through the lower thoracic sympathetic ganglia.[15, 73–75] The biliary tract is supplied by the right splanchnic nerves, and each kidney is supplied unilaterally through the splanchnic nerves. Pain from these viscera is often also transmitted through somatic nerves, often with a referred pattern of radicular pain. That component of visceral pain that can be relieved by diagnostic sympathetic blocks can often be relieved in a lasting fashion by chemical or surgical splanchnic nerve and lower thoracic sympathetic ganglion resection.* Splanchnicectomy has its greatest application in pancreatic carcinoma but is occasionally useful in chronic pancreatitis, severe biliary disease, and some types of kidney pain.

The range of nonsurgical treatments for syndromes with sympathetically mediated pain includes physical therapies, pharmacologic therapies, psychotherapy, and various anesthetic sympathetic blocks. Not all of these therapies are applicable to every syndrome. Additional forms of therapy are usually necessary for treatment of other sequelae of the initiating injury, sympathetically induced structural changes, including dystrophic and ischemic changes in arms or legs, and the psychosocial aspect of chronic disability. A series of sympathetic anesthetic blocks may produce lasting benefit, especially in cases of recent onset.[15, 49, 63] Thus, anesthetic blocks should be carried out not only to help determine whether the pain is sympathetically mediated but also in hopes of obviating surgical sympathectomy. Sympathetic fibers can be blocked along with peripheral nerves or at the level of lumbar or brachial plexus, but the resultant associated somatic sensory blockade does not permit a conclusion regarding possible sympathetic mediation of the pain. The most common anesthetic blocks of the sympathetic system itself are stellate ganglion and lumbar paravertebral blocks.

The stellate ganglion supplies sympathetic innervation to the head and neck and the sympathetic supply to the arm derives principally from T2 and T3 ganglia, not from the stellate ganglion. The reason stellate blocks are effective in producing interruption of sympathetic supply to the arm is readily apparent if the stellate injection is done with anesthetics mixed with radiographic contrast medium. Injections of greater than a few milliliters spread rapidly and widely in the paravertebral space and usually readily reach the second and third sympathetic ganglia—unless prevented from doing so by local scar (which prevents interruption of sympathetic innervation of the arm). Injecting excessive amounts of local anesthetics or allowing the local anesthetic to reach nearby cervical nerve roots can confuse the interpretation if the patient develops cutaneous sensory loss in the limb. Precise anesthetization of individual upper thoracic ganglia is important in patients whose pain persists despite partial sympathec-

tomy. To be interpretable, precise localization is necessary by radiographically guided placement of the needles and injections of very small amounts of anesthetic mixed with contrast medium.

Anesthetic injections given early in a patient's clinical course have a much greater chance of producing long-lasting or even permanent pain relief. Some instances of lasting success are encountered even in chronically persistent states of sympathetically mediated pain, so that an anesthetic sympathetic injection that produces short-term, useful relief of sympathetically mediated pain should routinely be repeated at least once—and numerous times if the resulting pain relief is of prolonged and increasing duration. The literature on surgical sympathectomy amply documents that relief of sympathetically mediated or causalgic pain is notoriously difficult to achieve adequately or permanently with sympathectomy, even though diagnostic blocks provided excellent short-term relief.

It is unclear whether sympathetically mediated pain is an efferent or an afferent phenomenon, a distinction that has therapeutic implications.[37, 55, 81, 82] Because the bulk of the sympathetic efferent supply to the arm is transmitted through the second and third ganglia, extirpation of these two ganglia usually suffices to interrupt the peripheral effects of sympathetic hyperactivity. Afferent fibers have been traced from the upper limb into the sympathetic chains from C7 to T7 ganglia, however, and consequently, complete afferent denervation conceivably could require extensive sympathectomy.[15, 49, 60, 80–84] Both electrical stimulation and mechanical stimulation of the sympathetic chain in humans have been reported to elicit pain.[66, 84] Algologists continue to debate the question of efferent versus afferent basis for sympathetically dependent pain, but two observations made during the author's sympathectomy experience argue for an efferent basis. First, during the course of nearly 1000 electrical stimulations in the vicinity of the sympathetic ganglia (admittedly, chiefly with 1-msec, 100-Hz stimuli) in conscious human patients, there have been *no* instances in which distal arm pain has been elicited or in which the patient's spontaneous causalgic pain has been reproduced, although patients commonly report acute pain or tingling in an intercostal distribution. Second, none of the patients whom the author has sympathectomized for causalgic pain and in whom pain has persisted despite effective T2 and T3 sympathectomy experienced even temporary pain relief when sympathetic interruption was extended. Three patients with persistent or recurrent pain subsequently underwent extension of sympathectomy, and eight underwent diagnostic anesthetization of the sympathetic chain at, above, or below the area of lesioning, but in none of them was pain relief achieved by more extensive sympathetic interruption.

TREATMENT OF SYMPATHETICALLY MEDIATED PAIN: SYMPATHECTOMY

Permanent or semipermanent interruption of sympathetic activity can be produced by interrupting the paravertebral sympathetic ganglion chain either through surgical dissection and resection or through chemical, thermal, or radiofrequency destruction. The human body is admirably capable of regenerating the sympathetic system, and published reports

---

*See references 1, 47, 49, 50, 52, 56–58, 60, 63, and 73–80.

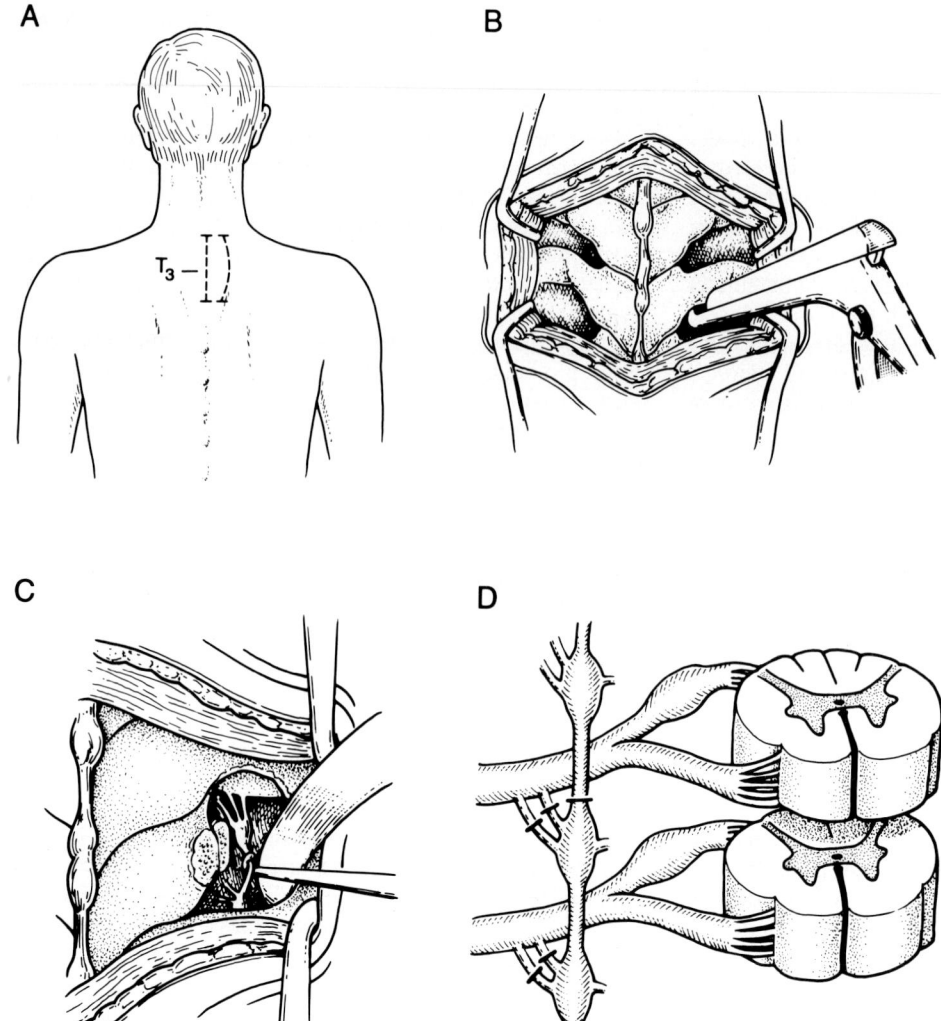

FIGURE 127–1. Interscapular approach to the thoracic sympathetic chain. (A) The skin incision is midline for bilateral exposure, but may be paramedian for a unilateral exposure. (B) The transverse process and head of the rib are resected at T2 only or for T2 and T3 ganglion resection. (C) Both the ganglion chain and its rami communicantes must be cut before removing the chain.

document regeneration even after resection of portions of the sympathetic chain.[18, 20] Most reported surgical series do not include careful long-term follow-up studies, but all document some percentage of recurrence. One well-documented follow-up study reported recurrent sympathetic activity in as many as 9.7 percent of patients followed for 3 to 8 years after open thoracic sympathectomy.[19]

The most popular surgical approaches to the thoracic sympathetic chain are interscapular, transaxillary, and supraclavicular. The lumbar chain is usually resected through a lateral retroperitoneal approach, and the splanchnic plexus through the bed of the eleventh rib. The interscapular approach involves resecting the head of one rib on each side to be sympathectomized and permits resection of T2 and T3 ganglia bilaterally through a single skin incision. The transaxillary approach involves an intercostal opening and temporary collapse of the lung. It permits only unilateral ganglion resection. Access to the T2 ganglion is at times difficult, but T3, T4, and T5 ganglia can be removed if desired. The supraclavicular approach also involves a separate incision for each side and requires dissection around the great vessels. It allows resection of stellate and T2 ganglia, but access to T3 and below may be difficult. All of these approaches to the thoracic chain carry a risk of intercostal neuralgia, and the first two may result in considerable incisional or rib pain.

The interscapular approach to the upper thoracic sympathetic chain seems to be the most popular approach used by neurosurgeons (Fig. 127–1).* A midline incision is made, centered over T2 and T3 for bilateral sympathectomy, but a paramedian straight or curved incision simplifies dissection if only a unilateral procedure is planned. Paraspinal muscles may be left in place and reflected medially. With the preoperative or intraoperative use of radiographic marking, the proximal portion of the third rib is resected on the side or sides to be sympathectomized. Completely resecting the head of the rib increases the operative complexity and postoperative pain and is not essential, although it does improve visualization of the sympathetic chain. The second and third sympathetic ganglia are found in paravertebral fat rostral and caudal, respectively, to the deep portion of the resected rib head. The chain should be cut as far as possible above and below the ganglion to ensure resection of all ganglion cells, and the rami communicantes should be sectioned to permit removal of the two ganglion segments of the chain. Placing

---

*See references 1, 3, 10, 20, 28, 49, 53, 60, 63, and 85.

metallic clips on the cut ends of the chain that are left in the patient may impede regeneration and prolong the benefit obtained. If the parietal pleura has been torn, it can usually be repaired by simple suturing, positive-pressure insufflation of the lung, and reinforcement of the suture line with gelatin foam. A chest tube is needed if the lung itself has been torn.

The transaxillary transcostal approach to the upper thoracic chain seems to be preferred by thoracic and vascular surgeons, and bilateral procedures are usually staged days to weeks apart.[16, 39, 86–89] A rib-spreading incision is made low in the axilla, usually between third and fourth ribs. The lung apex is partially compressed with a retractor to permit visualization of the thoracic chain as it lies beneath the pleura, alongside the vertebrae and near the apex of the pleural cavity. The second sympathetic ganglion not uncommonly lies above the pleural reflection away from the vertebrae, and some dissection may be necessary. In obese patients, the ganglia may not be readily apparent in the paravertebral, extrapleural fat, but palpating the space between the ventral rib heads usually gives an accurate landmark. Care must be taken not to tear the azygous veins or thoracic duct. If the lung has not been torn, as can be tested by filling the cavity with saline, it is not absolutely necessary to leave a chest tube, as long as the lung has been fully expanded under positive pressure at the time pleural closure is completed. Intercostal or mammary pain is reported to occur not infrequently following this exposure, and persistent pneumothorax, pleurisy, or empyema can be a major complication.

The third surgical alternative approach to the upper thoracic chain involves supraclavicular dissection.[89, 90] Bilateral incisions are required for bilateral sympathectomy, but both sides can be done relatively easily in a single sitting. The subclavian artery is identified; the lower stellate and upper thoracic sympathetic ganglia can be found in the fatty tissues deep and medial to this artery, usually behind the carotid and vertebral arteries, but ventral to the proximal portion of the brachial plexus. Care must be taken not to tear any of the major arteries or veins or to stretch or contuse the brachial plexus and the recurrent laryngeal and phrenic nerves. Especially in a large or obese patient, reaching the third thoracic ganglion may be difficult. Intraoperative radiography with a metallic marker may help to confirm that indeed the second and third ganglia have been exposed for resection. The apex of the parietal pleura lies near by. A chest tube is usually not needed unless a tear in the lung is documented intraoperatively or by progressive postoperative pneumothorax. Great vessel injury, hoarseness, and arm pain or weakness are among the major complications.

A transthoracic endoscopic approach to the upper thoracic sympathetic chain was described by Kux[91] in 1954 and rediscovered by four separate surgeons a quarter of a century later.[44, 92–94] This technique involves placement of a thoracoscope through the ribs, deflation of the lung, and electrolytic destruction of the sympathetic ganglion. Bilateral procedures are necessary for bilateral sympathetic interruption. The limited popularity of the original technique apparently was related to the difficulty in identifying and completely destroying the sympathetic ganglia and in reaching the T2 ganglia as well as to the high recurrence rate. Despite these problems, thoracoscopic sympathectomy is currently being re-introduced using modern endoscopic instruments and techniques, including sympathetic destruction by diathermy and laser or sympathetic chain resection using a two-port system.

In 1979, the author devised a technique for stereotactic percutaneous radiofrequency upper thoracic sympathectomy.[37, 95–98] In the ensuing 15 years, two major modifications have been made in the technique, with considerable improvement in initial and long-term results[37] (Table 127–4). In its present form, the procedure is done on a day surgery basis using local anesthesia plus neuroleptanalgesia (Fig. 127–2). Two 18-gauge radiofrequency needle electrodes are used simultaneously to reduce fluoroscopy time and to minimize periods of deep anesthesia. They are most commonly placed at the T2 and T3 paravertebral ganglia to denervate the upper limb, and bilateral procedures are commonly performed at a single session. A series of lesions are made in a rostrocaudal direction to destroy the entire fusiform ganglia, in order to reduce the frequency of late recurrences, although it is recognized that some late recurrences are inevitable even following open surgical resection.

Complications have been relatively few in a series of over 200 limbs sympathectomized. They have included a few cases of symptomatic pneumothorax and of transient intercostal neuralgia. In addition to the obvious advantage that the procedure does not require general anesthesia, the procedure can be tailored intraoperatively to the patient's needs as determined by monitoring of plethysmography and skin temperature and can easily be repeated with good results.

The lumbar sympathetic chain is approached surgically usually through a flank incision on each side to be sympathectomized (Fig. 127–3).* A muscle-splitting approach through the abdominal wall is used to reach the retroperitoneal space along the psoas muscle. The ureter is carefully elevated off the vertebral column, and the vena cava or abdominal aorta is carefully preserved at the extreme of the dissection. The sympathetic chain is identified alongside the lumbar vertebrae, and the sympathetic chain, ganglia, and rami communicantes are segmentally resected. Usually the L2 through L4 ganglia can readily be accessed, but there has been considerable debate regarding which sympathetic gan-

*See references 1, 15, 47, 49, 50, 52, 53, 56–58, 60, and 61.

Table 127–4. EXTENT OF SYMPATHECTOMY WITH EACH DEVELOPMENTAL PHASE*

Interval Sympathectomy	Sympatholysis (% limbs)					No. of Limbs
	Excellent	+	Partial	=	Combined	
Phase I						
1 Month	91	+	0	=	91	48
6 Months	81	+	11	=	93	44
2 Years	71	+	14	=	85	35
3 Years	51	+	29	=	80	35
Phase II						
1 Month	97	+	0	=	97	105
6 Months	75	+	20	=	95	101
2 Years	64	+	19	=	83	75
3 Years	58	+	17	=	75	66
Phase III						
1 Month	100	+	0	=	100	62
6 Months	94	+	6	=	100	66
2 Years	82	+	15	=	97	34
3 Years	83	+	9	=	91	23

*Extent of sympathetic denervation achieved with the three developmental phases of percutaneous thoracic sympathectomy. (Reoperated patients were counted as lost to follow-up.)

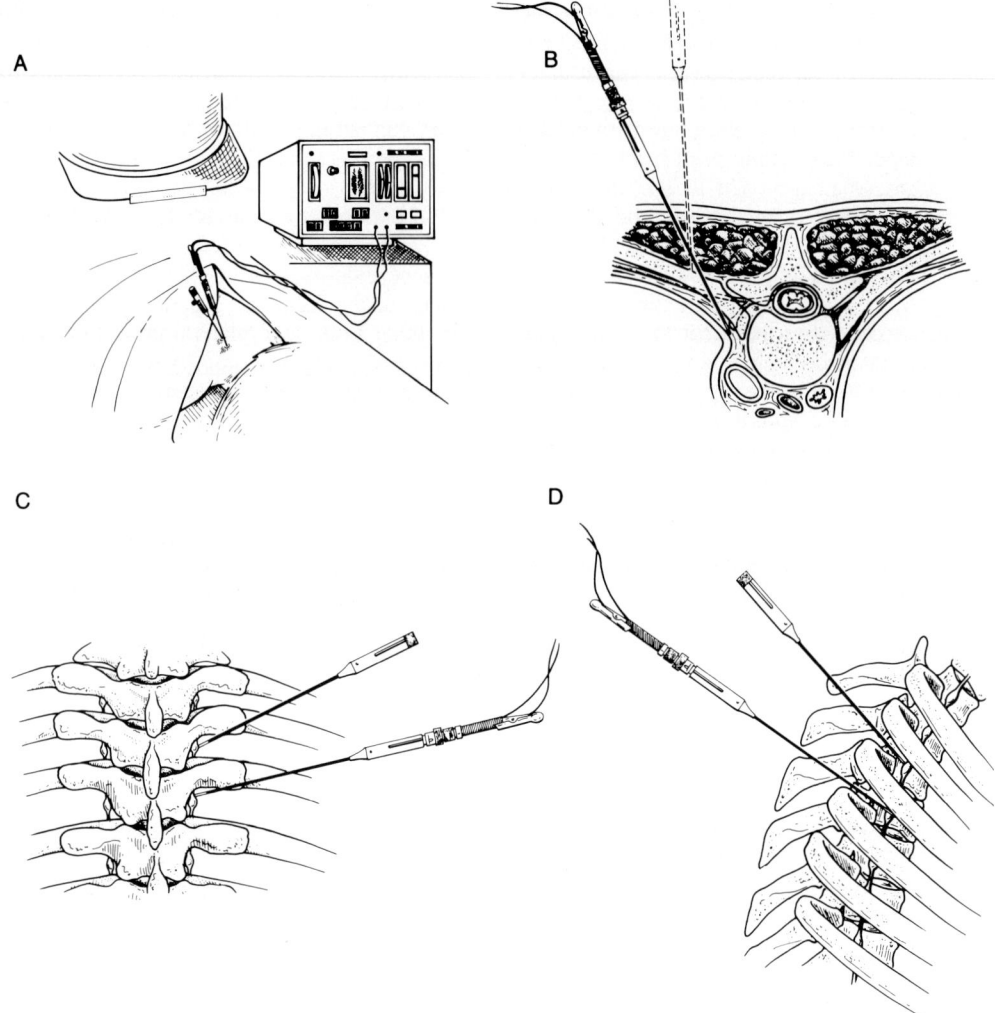

FIGURE 127–2. Percutaneous radiofrequency (RF) thoracic sympathectomy. (A) Two 18-gauge RF "tic" needle electrodes are used under C-arm fluoroscopic guidance. (B) Electrodes are placed in the extrapleural space with the bared tips in the vicinity of the sympathetic ganglia. (C and D) Electrodes are placed between the 2nd and 3rd and the 3rd and 4th ribs to lesion T2 and T3 ganglia, which lie adjacent to the mid portion of the vertebral bodies. A series of rostrocaudal lesions is necessary to ablate the entire fusiform ganglion.

glia should be included in the resection. The sympathetic preganglionic fibers arise from the lower thoracic cord and run downward to the lumbar ganglia. Many of the sympathetic efferents seem to originate in the second or third lumbar ganglia, then to pass further caudally through the chain to exit with the postganglionic rami of L4 or even L5. Although short-term sympathectomy results are good with ablation of the L2 and L3 ganglia only, it has been advocated that long-term results can be improved by including L4 or even L5. Occasional cases have been reported of recurrent sympathetic activity following L2 and L3 ganglion resection, which was then abolished by resecting L4 or even by adding L5 resection to a prior resection of L2 through L4.

Pernak and Berg[99] best described the application of radiofrequency stereotactic ablation for lumbar sympathectomy. Although others have advocated multiple lesions and extensive radiofrequency sympathectomy in the lumbar area, they have achieved considerable success with a technique in which only single lesions are made usually at the L3 sympathetic ganglia, and early outcome is monitored in terms of improved limb perfusion and increased temperature. Undoubtedly, a single lesion in the sympathetic chain is unlikely to produce permanent sympathectomy, but Pernak and Berg[99] achieve overall excellent results by integrating the sympathectomy rapidly into an aggressive restorative program for patients with low back problems.

Percutaneous alcohol or phenol sympathectomy offers the advantage of technical simplicity but carries significant potential for risk.[76–80] Thoracic alcohol sympathectomy has been uncommonly performed since Leriche[8] described inadvertent tracking of alcohol through a nerve root sheath into the subarachnoid space, causing paraplegia. Because the sympathetic ganglia are connected by rather short rami communicantes to the segmental nerves, especially in the thoracic region, and because the genitofemoral nerve courses in the retroperitoneal space near the lumbar plexus, somatic nerve injury with severe neuralgia is a potential complication. In the lumbar area, damage to adjacent arteries, ureter, or veins, and in the thoracic region, damage to the pleura, pose significant risks. Ogawa,[78] who still performs thoracic as well as lumbar alcohol sympathectomy, advocates preceding injection of sclerosing solutions with injection of radiographic

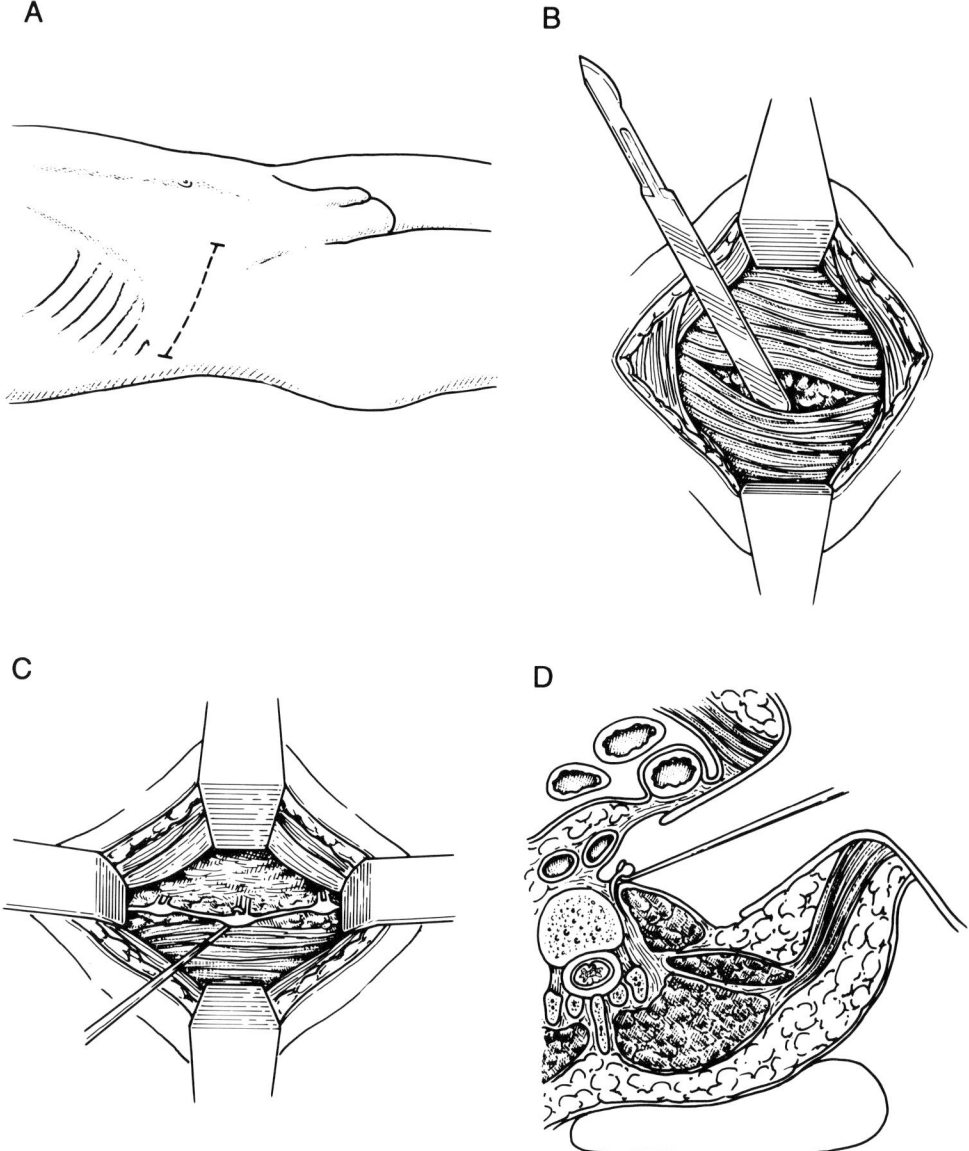

FIGURE 127–3. Lumbar surgical sympathectomy. (A) An oblique incision is made laterally over the abdomen. (B) A muscle-splitting technique is used to reach the retroperitoneal space. (C and D) The sympathetic chain is identified adjacent to the lumbar vertebrae alongside the psoas muscle, carefully avoiding the vena cava and abdominal aorta.

contrast medium to check for adequacy of contact with the planned sympathetic ganglia and to ensure that the sclerosing agent is less likely to reach and damage adjacent structures. Lumbar injections are made through paravertebral needle placement at the second or third lumbar vertebral body, and appropriate placement is gauged by injection of radiographic contrast medium (Fig. 127–4). The chemicals injected are usually 7 percent aqueous phenol, 50 percent alcohol, or absolute alcohol. The volumes injected have varied from author to author and according to the result desired, but volumes generally have varied from 3 to 8 ml.

Splanchnicectomy can be carried out by open surgical resection or chemically, using a technique quite similar to that employed for lumbar chemical sympathectomy, except that the needles are centered at L1. For open resection, the patient is positioned prone, and an oblique incision is made centered over the 11th rib, 5 or 6 cm to the right of midline (Fig. 127–5). Four to six centimeters of the rib are resected, extending from just lateral to the transverse vertebral process, and the pleura is dissected downward. Intercostal veins are ligated or clipped, and the lateral aspect of the tenth through twelfth vertebral bodies is exposed. The sympathetic ganglia are identified beneath the intercostal nerves, and ventral to them, the splanchnic nerves are identified. The splanchnic nerves may be adherent to the pleura, are usually three in number, but are quite variable in anatomy. An attempt is made to identify ninth through twelfth sympathetic ganglia. These are then isolated by clipping and cutting the sympathetic chain rostrally and caudally and dividing the rami communicantes. The splanchnic nerves are stripped as far as possible before being clipped and cut, and the whole sympathetic complex is then removed. If the pleura is torn, but not the lung, a rubber catheter can be left inside the pleura until the deep thoracic wall layers have been sutured. Suction is then applied to the catheter, which is removed while positive pressure is applied by an anesthetist. A chest tube is necessary if the lung itself has been torn. If splanchnicectomy is being carried out for pancreatic pain, a bilateral procedure must be done; it can usually be accomplished at a single sitting through right and left lateral incisions.

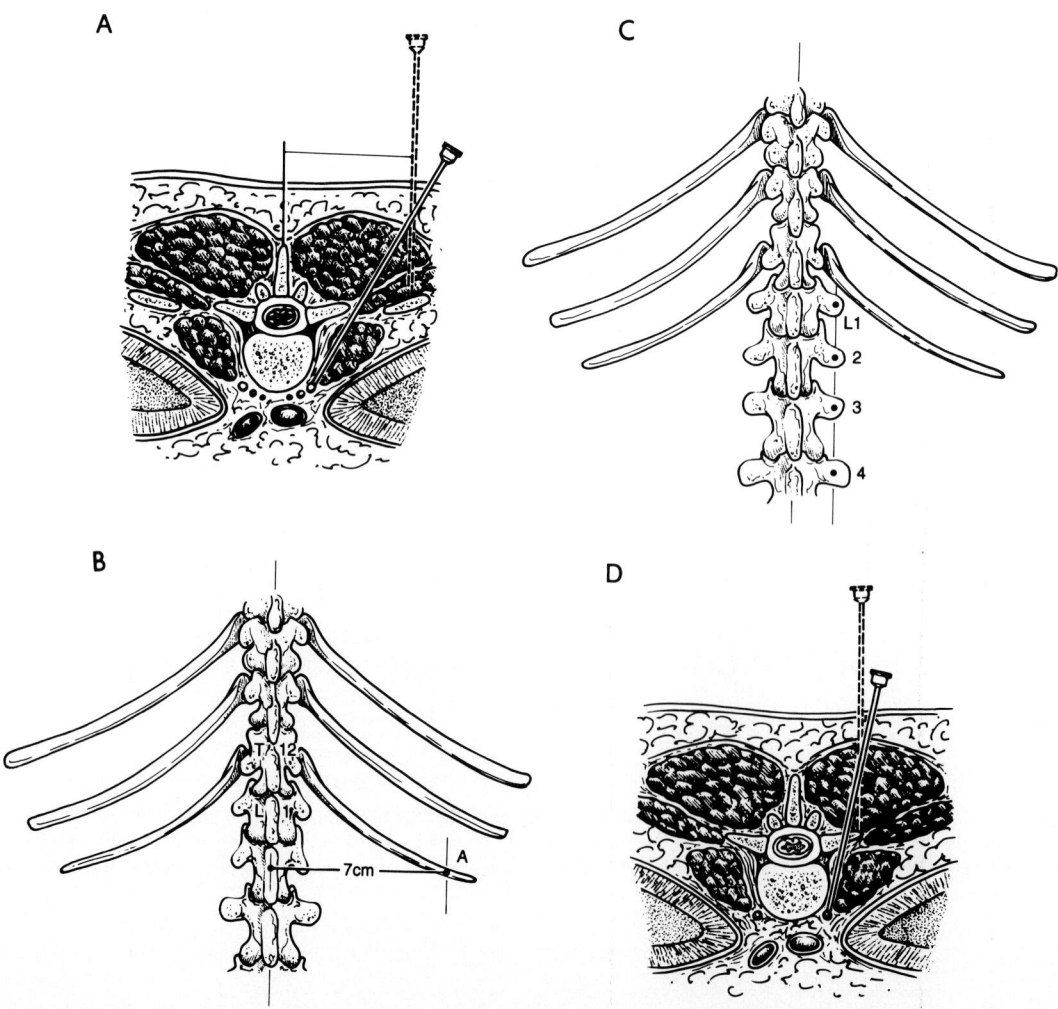

FIGURE 127–4. Lumbar or splanchnic chemical sympathectomy. (A and B) For anesthetic blocks or chemical lesioning of the splanchnic plexus, needles are placed ventrolateral to the L1 or T12 vertebra. The 12th rib is encountered by the needle about 7 cm lateral to the midline, then the needle is directed caudal and parallel to the rib at a rostromedial angle to probe the side of the vertebral body, then pass just ventral thereto. (C and D) For anesthetic blocks or chemical lesioning of the lumbar sympathetic chain, one needle may be inserted at the L3 ganglion, or individual needles at L2, L3, and L4. After contacting the transverse process, each needle is shifted caudally and placed with fluoroscopic guidance at the ventrolateral curve of the vertebral body.

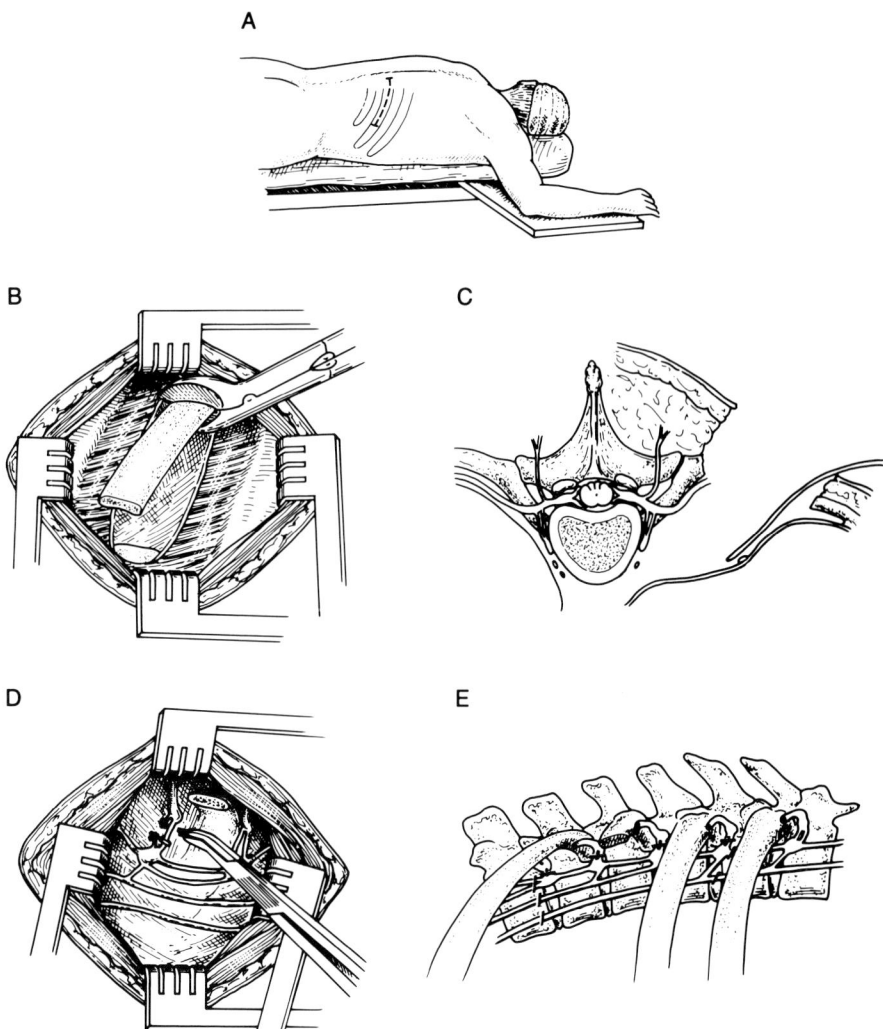

FIGURE 127-5. Surgical splanchnic sympathectomy. After making an incision over the 11th rib (A), a segment of rib lateral to the transverse process is resected; (B) the pleura is stripped from the side of the vertebrae (C), and the lower thoracic ganglia and splanchnic plexus are identified. (D and E) The lower thoracic ganglia should be resected along with sectioning of the splanchnic nerves.

OUTCOME OF SYMPATHECTOMY

Pain and disability not uncommonly persist despite successful sympathectomy, and because the sympathetic system has a tenacious propensity to regenerate, it is important in evaluating patients with persistent symptoms to determine whether or not they are or remain completely sympathectomized. A simple and fairly accurate bedside test is the starch iodine test. The part of the patient's body to be tested is painted with an iodine solution, which is allowed to dry thoroughly. Powdered cornstarch is then dusted lightly over the entire area, and the patient is placed in a hot room or beneath hot lights and is given hot liquids to drink in order to induce perspiration. Light exercising also can help to precipitate perspiration. The moisture produced allows the iodine and starch to interact, turning the white powder to black and thus delineating areas of retained sweating. Bilateral measurement of skin temperature by thermography or thermistors and measurement of limb perfusion by plethysmography can quantitate differences in sympathetically mediated functions between limbs, but is subject to considerable variables and cannot confirm whether sympathectomy is complete, especially when bilateral sympathectomy has been carried out. Variables include the extent of dystrophic and vascular changes in the limb, ambient and body temperatures, and whether or not the patient has taken vasodilating medications. Diagnostic sympathetic blocks, the most reliable way of testing for completeness of sympathectomy, should be carried out with solutions containing radiographic contrast media that can be visualized under the fluoroscope or on permanent radiographs. Testing the completeness of sympathectomy usually begins with anesthetic injections into the area of presumed sympathectomy and later adds anesthetization of adjacent sympathetic ganglia. The outcome of these diagnostic injections must be measured in terms of improvements not only in circulation and limb temperature but also in pain. Patients who continue to experience severe pain despite a sympathectomy that is already extensive rarely will obtain useful lasting pain relief from further enlargement or extension of the sympathectomy.

The results of sympathectomy for sympathetically mediated pain vary greatly according to the precise condition being treated. Sympathectomy for vascular spasm secondary to acute arterial occlusion provides nearly 100 percent long-term relief of the vasospastic component of the disorder. Sympathectomy for Raynaud's syndrome initially provides almost 100 percent relief of painful ischemic symptoms, but nearly 15 percent of patients later develop a collagen vasculopathy, and ischemic symptoms recur in nearly 25 percent of patients despite sustained sympathectomy.[39, 41, 44] Patients with ischemic obliterative vascular disorders usually obtain transient relief of pain and improved healing of necrotic and ulcerated extremities,[40, 45] but the disorder usually progresses, and ischemic symptoms eventually develop that are no longer under sympathetic mediation. Sympathectomy for Prinzmetal's angina has been carried out only in a relatively limited number of patients, although results have generally been quite good.[37, 60, 65–72]

Sympathectomies carried out for sympathetically mediated disorders characterized principally by pain with or without dystrophic features characteristically have yielded only limited success rates. Most authors report sustained pain relief in only two thirds or three fourths of patients with any of the surgical techniques.* Dystrophic features may improve steadily but usually require extensive secondary therapy. Because most of these disorders were initiated by some form of painful process, often a peripheral nerve injury, further therapy is usually necessary to restore the patients to a fully functional status, to obtain relief from persistent somatic pain, and to rehabilitate the often chronically disabled patient to a usefully functioning status.

The timing and extent of sympathectomy are also important in determining outcome. It was mentioned earlier that anesthetic sympathetic interruptions made shortly after the onset of sympathetically mediated pain states not uncommonly can provide long-term relief. Similarly, sympathectomy seems to provide a better chance of success in the patient with a syndrome characterized principally by pain when that surgery is performed earlier in the syndrome's course rather than later.[49, 60, 63] The extent of sympathectomy necessary to control sympathetically mediated pain likewise is not clear from published data. In the lumbar area, sympathectomy has ranged from single-level destruction at L2 or L3 to destruction carried from L2 through L5. In the thoracic region, destruction most commonly has been carried out at T2 and T3, but recommendations have ranged as broadly as T1 through T5.

REFERENCES

1. Hardy RW: Surgery of the sympathetic nervous system, in Schmidek HH, Sweet WH (eds): Operative Neurosurgical Techniques: Indications, Methods and Results, Vol 2. New York, Grune & Stratton, 1982, pp 1045–1061
2. Greenwood B: The origins of sympathectomy. Med Hist 11:165–169, 1967
3. Adson AW, Brown GE: The treatment of Raynaud's disease by resection of the upper thoracic and lumbar sympathetic ganglia and trunks. Surg Gynecol Obstet 48:577–603, 1929
4. Adson AW, Craig WmcK, Brown GE: Essential hyperhidrosis cured by sympathetic ganglionectomy and trunk resection. Arch Surg 31:794–806, 1935
5. Jonnesco T: Angine de poitrine guérie par la résection du sympathique cervicothoracique. Bull Acad Nat Med (Paris) 84:93, 1920
6. Kotzareff A: Résection partielle du tronc sympathique cervico droit pour hyperhidrose unilaterale (regions faciale, cervicale, thoracique et brachiale droits). Rev Med Suisse Romande 40:111–113, 1920
7. Leriche R: De la traitement de la douleur dans les cancers abdominaux et pelvieus inopérables ou récidives. Gaz Hopit Civils Milit 109:917–922, 1936

8. Leriche R, Fontaine R: Chirurgie des nerfs du coeur. J Chir (Paris) 40:508–525, 1932
9. Peet MM: Splanchnic resection for hypertension. Univ Hosp Bull (Michigan) 1:17–18, 1935
10. Smithwick RH: Modified dorsal sympathectomy for vascular spasm of the upper extremity. Am Surg 104:339, 1935
11. Smithwick RH: A technique for splanchnic resection for hypertension. Surgery 7:1–8, 1940
12. Spurling RG: Causalgia of the upper extremity: Treatment by dorsal sympathetic ganglionectomy. Ann Neurol Psychiatry 23:784–788, 1930
13. Telford ED: The technique of sympathectomy. Br J Surg 23:440–480, 1935
14. White JC, Bland EF: The surgical relief of severe angina pectoris. Medicine 27:1–42, 1948
15. White JC, Smithwick RH: The Autonomic Nervous System: Anatomy, Physiology and Surgical Application, ed 2. New York, Macmillan, 1941
16. Campbell WB, Cooper MJ, Sponsel WE, et al: Transaxillary sympathectomy: Is a one-stage bilateral procedure safe? Br J Surg 69(suppl):S29, 1982
17. Daley R: Autonomic nervous system in its relation to some forms of heart and lung disease. 1: Heart disease. Br Med J 1:173–179, 1957
18. Gjerris F, Olesen HP: Palmar hyperhidrosis: Long-term results following high thoracic sympathectomy. Acta Neurol Scand 51:167–172, 1975
19. Howng S-L, Loh J-K: Long term follow-up of upper dorsal sympathetic ganglionectomy for palmar hyperhidrosis—a scale of evaluation. Kaohsiung J Med Sci 3:704–707, 1987
20. Mattassi R, Miele F, D'Angelo F: Thoracic sympathectomy: Review of indications, results and surgical techniques. J Cardiovasc Surg 22:336–339, 1981
21. Shih CJ, Wang YC: Thoracic sympathectomy for palmar hyperhidrosis: Report of 457 cases. Surg Neurol 10:291–296, 1978
22. Kozin F, McCarthy DJ, Simms J, Genant HK: The reflex sympathetic dystrophy syndrome. I: Clinical and histologic studies: Evidence for bilaterality, response to corticosteroids and articular involvement. Am J Med 660:321–331, 1976
23. Schott GD: Mechanisms of causalgia and related clinical conditions: The role of the central and of the sympathetic nervous systems. Brain 109:717–738, 1986
24. Schutzer SF, Gossling HR: The treatment of reflex sympathetic dystrophy syndrome. J Bone Joint Surg (A) 66:625–629, 1984
25. Adar R, Kurchin A, Zwing A, Mozes M: Palmar hyperhidrosis and its surgical treatment: A report of 100 cases. Am Surg 186:34–41, 1977
26. Braeucker W: Uber die Innervation der Schweissdrusen und die Chirurgische Behandlung der Hyperhidrosis. Klin Wochenschr 7:683–686, 1982
27. Campbell WB, Cooper MJ, et al: Palmar hyperhidrosis and its surgical treatment: A report of 100 cases. Ann Surg 186:34, 1977
28. Cloward RB: Hyperhidrosis. J Neurosurg 30:545–551, 1969
29. Ellis H: Transaxillary sympathectomy in the treatment of hyperhidrosis of the upper limbs. Ann Surg 45:546, 1979
30. Greenhalgh RM, Rosengarten DS, Martin P: Role of sympathectomy for hyperhidrosis. Br Med J 1:332–334, 1971
31. Horgan K, Kderman W: Transthoracic sympathectomy in hyperhidrosis. Eur Surg Res 17(suppl 1):2, 1985
32. Price GAR: Treatment of axillary hyperhidrosis. Br Med J 2:1447, 1976
33. Sternberg A, Brickman S, et al: Transaxillary thoracic sympathectomy for primary hyperhidrosis of the upper limbs. World J Surg 6:45, 1982
34. Shelley WB: Consultations in Dermatology, vol 2. Philadelphia, WB Saunders, 1974, p 259
35. Adar R: Compensatory sweating after upper dorsal sympathectomy. J Neurosurg 51:424–425, 1979
36. Shelley WB, Florence R: Compensatory hyperhidrosis after sympathectomy. N Engl J Med 162:1056, 1960
37. Wilkinson HA: Stereotactic radiofrequency upper thoracic sympathectomy: A thirteen year experience. Surg Neurol submitted 1994
38. Sneddon IB: Treatment of axillary hyperhidrosis. Br Med J 1:1447, 1976
39. Berguer R, Smit R: Transaxillary sympathectomy (T2 to T4) for relief of vasospastic/sympathetic pain of upper extremities. Surgery 89:764–769, 1981
40. Dale WA, Lewis MD: Management of ischemia of the hand and fingers. Surgery 67:62–79, 1970

---

*See references 1, 22–24, 39, 47, 48, 50, 52, and 56–61.

41. Montorsi W, Ghringhelli C, Amoni F: Indications and results of the surgical treatment of Raynaud's phenomenon. J Cardiovasc Surg 21:203–210, 1980
42. Myers KA, Irvine WT: An objective study of lumbar sympathectomy. I: Intermittent claudication. Br Med J 1:879–883, 1966
43. Myers KA, Irvin WT: An objective study of lumbar sympathectomy. II: Skin ischaemia. Br Med J 1:943–947, 1966
44. Rosner K, Goldberg S: Der Stellewert der thorakoskopischen Sympathectomie bei der Behandlung des Raynaud-Syndrome. Z Gesamte Inn Med 34:127–128, 1979
45. Shionoya S, Barr I, Nakata Y, et al: Surgical treatment of Buerger's disease. J Cardiovasc Surg 21:777–784, 1980
46. Ascheri R, Blumel G: Zum Krankheitsbild der Sudek'schen Dystrophie. Fortschr Med 99:712–720, 1980
47. Connelly JE, Richards V: Bilateral splanchnicectomy and lumbodorsal sympathectomy for chronic relapsing pancreatitis. Ann Surg 131:58–63, 1960
48. Dawson DM, Katz M: Reflex sympathetic dystrophy. Neurology Chronicle, No 8, 1993, pp 1–6
49. Gybels JM, Sweet WH: Sympathectomy for pain, in Neurosurgical Treatment of Persistent Pain. New York, Karger, 1984, pp 257–282
50. Heisy WG, Dohn DF: Splanchnicectomy for the treatment of intractable abdominal pain. Cleve Clinic Q 34:9–25, 1967
51. Kozin F, Genant HK, Bekerman C, McCarthy DJ: The reflex sympathetic dystrophy syndrome. II: Roentgenographic and scintigraphic evidence of bilaterality and of periradicular accentuation. Am J Med 60:332–338, 1976
52. Mallet-Guy P, Beaujeu MJ: Treatment of chronic pancreatitis by unilateral splanchnicectomy. Ann Surg 60:233–241, 1950
53. Mayfield FH: Causalgia. Springfield, IL, Charles C Thomas, 1951
54. Mitchell SW: Injuries of Nerves and Their Consequences. Philadelphia, JB Lippincott, 1872
55. Ochoa J: Afferent and sympathetic roles in chronic "neuropathic" pains: Confessions on misconceptions, in Besseon JM, Guilband G (eds): Lesions of Primary Afferent Fibers as a Tool for the Study of Clinical Pain. New York, Elsevier, 1991
56. Ray BS, Console AD: The relief of pain in chronic (calcareous) pancreatitis by sympathectomy. Gynecol Obstet 89:1–8, 1949
57. Sadar ES, Cooperman MA: Bilateral thoracic sympathectomy—splanchnicectomy in the treatment of intractable pain due to pancreatic carcinoma. Cleve Clin Q 41:185–188, 1974
58. Sadar ES, Hardy RW: Thoracic splanchnicectomy and sympathectomy for the relief of pancreatic pain, in Cooperman AM (ed): Surgery of the Pancreas. St Louis, CV Mosby, 1978, pp 141–152
59. Schwartzman RJ, McLellan TL: Reflex sympathetic dystrophy: A review. Arch Neurol 44:555–561, 1987
60. Sweet WH: Sympathectomy for pain, in Youmans JR (ed): Neurological Surgery, ed 3. Philadelphia, WB Saunders, 1990, pp 4086–4107
61. de Takats G, Walter LE, Lasner J: Splanchnic nerve section for pancreatic pain. Ann Surg 131:44–57, 1950
62. Ulmer JL, Mayfield FH: Causalgia: A study of 75 cases. Surg Gynecol Obstet 83:789–795, 1946
63. White JC, Sweet WH: Pain: Its Mechanisms and Neurosurgical Control. Springfield, IL, Charles C Thomas, 1955
64. Wilkinson HA, Bryant GDN, Orgain ES: The supraventricular tachycardias: Management by interruption of cardiac sympathetics. JAMA 175:672–676, 1961
65. Baille Y, Siwalt M, Vaillant A, et al: Résultats à distance de la chirurgie de l'angor de Prinzmetal. Ann Chir 36:613–614, 1982
66. Dos SJ: Cardiac sympathectomy for angina pectoris. Ann Thorac Surg 25:178–179, 1978
67. Grodin CM, Limet R: Sympathetic denervation in association with coronary artery grafting in patients with Prinzmetal's angina. Ann Thorac Surg 23:111–117, 1977
68. Henrard L, Pierard L, Limet R: Traitement par sympathectomie thoracique de l'angor de Prinzmetal à coronaires saines. Arch Mal Coeur 75:1317–1319, 1982
69. Limet R: L'angine de Prinzmetal. Rev Med Liège 35:745–758, 1980
70. Mason DT, Spann JF, Zelis R, Amsterdam EA: Physiologic approach to the treatment of angina pectoris. N Engl J Med 281:1225–1227, 1969
71. Soots G, Warembourg H, Stankowiak C, et al: Place de la plexectomie dans le traitement de l'angor de Prinzmetal. Ann Chir 36:611–613, 1983
72. Spodick DH: Partial sympathetic denervation for variant angina pectoris. Am J Cardiol 52:1153, 1983
73. White JC: Role of sympathectomy in relief of pain, in Krayenbuhl H, Maspes PE, Sweet WH (eds): Progress in Neurological Surgery, vol 7. Basel, S Karger, 1976, pp 131–152
74. Ray BS, Neill CL: Causalgia: A centennial review. Arch Neurol 16:339–350, 1967
75. Richins CA: The innervation of the pancreas. J Comp Neurol 83:223–236, 1945
76. Cross FW, Cotton LT: Chemical lumbar sympathectomy for ischemic rest pain: A randomized, prospective controlled clinical trial. Am J Surg 150:341–345, 1985
77. Haxton HA: Chemical sympathectomy. Br Med J 1:1026–1028, 1949
78. Ogawa S: Sympathectomy with neurolytics, in Hyodo M, Oyama T, Swerdlow M (eds): The Pain Clinic IV. Utrecht, VSP Publishers, 1992, pp 138–146
79. Reid W, Watt JK, Gray TG: Phenol injection of the sympathetic chain. Br J Surg 57:45–50, 1970
80. Scott DB, Littlewood DG: Chemical lumbar sympathectomy with radiological assessment. Ann Roy Coll Surg Engl 64:135, 1982
81. Drucker WR, Hubay CA, Holden WD, et al: Pathogenesis of posttraumatic sympathetic dystrophy. Ann Surg 97:454–465, 1949
82. Homans J: Minor causalgia: A hyperesthetic neurovascular syndrome. N Engl J Med 22:870–874, 1940
83. Ray BS, Kinsey JC, Geohegan WA: Observations on the distribution of the sympathetic nerves to the pupil and extremity as determined by stimulation of the anterior roots in man. Ann Surg 118:647–655, 1943
84. Roos DB: Sympathectomy for the upper extremities: Anatomy, indications and techniques, in Rutherford RB (ed): Vascular Surgery. Philadelphia, WB Saunders, 1977, pp 623–628
85. Dohn DF, Sava GM: Sympathectomy for vascular syndromes and hyperhidrosis of the upper extremities. Clin Neurosurg 25:637–650, 1978
86. Atkins HJB: Sympathectomy by the axillary approach. Lancet 1:538–539, 1954
87. Jochimsen PR, Hartfall WG: Peraxillary upper extremity sympathectomy: Technique reviewed and clinical experience. Surgery 71:686, 1972
88. Linder F, Jenal G, Assmus H: Axillary transpleural sympathectomy: Indication, technique and results. World J Surg 7:437, 1983
89. Little JM, May J: A comparison of the supraclavicular and axillary approaches to upper thoracic sympathectomy. Aust NZ J Surg 45:143, 1975
90. Kempe L: Operative Neurosurgery, vol 2. New York, Springer-Verlag, 1970, pp 240–243
91. Kux E: Thorakoskopische Eingriffe am Nervensystem. Stuttgart, Georg Thieme, 1954
92. Kux M: Thoracic endoscopic sympathectomy by transthoracic electrocoagulation. Br J Surg 67:71, 1980
93. Malone PS, Dingnan JP, Hederman WP: Transthoracic electrocoagulation (T.T.E.C.)—a new and simple approach to upper limb sympathectomy. Irish Med J 75:20–21, 1982
94. Weale FE: Upper thoracic sympathectomy for transthoracic electrocoagulation. Br J Surg 67:71–72, 1980
95. Wilkinson HA: Hand edema after cervical fusion. JAMA 249:652, 1983
96. Wilkinson HA: Percutaneous radiofrequency upper thoracic sympathectomy: A new technique. Neurosurgery 15:811–814, 1984
97. Wilkinson HA: Radiofrequency percutaneous upper thoracic sympathectomy: Technique and review of indications. N Engl J Med 311:34–36, 1984
98. Yarzebski JL, Wilkinson HA: T2 and T3 sympathetic ganglia in the adult human: A cadaver and clinical-radiographic study and its clinical application. Neurosurgery 21:339–342, 1987
99. Pernak JM, Berg HVD: Treatment of chronic low back pain following lumbar disc operations by using thermolesion of sympathetic ganglion, in Erdmann W, Pernak J, Oyama T (eds): The Pain Clinic I. Utrecht, VNU Science Press, 1985, pp 177–186
100. Robertson DP, Simpson RK, Rose JE, Garza JS: Video-assisted endoscopic thoracic ganglionectomy. J Neurosurg 79:238–240, 1993
101. Kao MC: Video endoscopic sympathectomy using fiberoptic CO_2 laser to treat palmar hyperhidrosis. Neurosurgery 30:131–135, 1992

CHAPTER 128

Dorsal Root Ganglionectomy for Intractable Monoradicular Sciatica

Arthur Taub
Franklin Robinson
Ethan Taub

Sciatica in patients with lumbar radiculopathy caused by herniation of an intervertebral disc is often relieved by resection of herniated disc fragments. Nevertheless, chronic, intractable back pain and sciatica may persist despite surgical treatment. Approximately 3 percent of patients with surgically intractable sciatica can be shown to have sciatica of monoradicular origin.[1] In such patients, dorsal root ganglionectomy has been shown to relieve sciatica with a long-term success rate of approximately 60 percent.[1]

PATHOPHYSIOLOGY

Sciatica due to intervertebral disc herniation is a type of radicular referred pain that arises from neural impulses generated ectopically in the spinal nerve root and dorsal root ganglion as a result of mechanical irritation. Examples of this mechanism include intervertebral disc herniation, foraminal stenosis, spinal instability, and severe epidural and intradural fibrosis. Acute and chronic inflammation of neural tissue may also be partly responsible for ectopic impulse generation in these pathologic entities, and in arachnoiditis.

The objective of standard surgical therapy for sciatica is to relieve mechanical compression of the nerve root and ganglion by correction of pathologic abnormalities in adjacent nonneural structures. When such surgery fails to relieve sciatica, it may be because chronic neuropathologic changes have occurred within the spinal nerve root and dorsal root ganglion, leading to the generation of ectopic neural impulses. Whether the original causative insult to the nerve root and ganglion is brief (as in a sudden disc herniation), repetitive (as in spinal instability), or continuing (as in chronic compression by epidural scar), these neuropathologic and neurophysiologic changes may be irreversible. Thus, pain may persist even after its original cause has been removed.

The results of physiologic studies in animals[2,3] support the hypothesis that intractable sciatica is caused by pathologic abnormalities within the spinal nerve root and ganglion. A minor compressive injury of the dorsal root ganglion markedly increases the neural impulse activity produced in response to a straight-leg-raising maneuver.[2] A few dorsal root ganglion cells are normally spontaneously active; section of peripheral afferents doubles the number of spontaneously active cells.[3] In this situation, slight mechanical pressure on the dorsal root ganglion increases the frequency of impulses.[3]

The results of pathologic studies confirm the presence of chronic structural abnormalities in the spinal nerve root and dorsal root ganglion in patients with lumbar intervertebral disc herniation. In tissue obtained at autopsy[4] and by intraoperative biopsy,[1,5] abnormalities included perineurial hyperplasia and fiber degeneration in the spinal nerve root and chronic inflammation and neuronal degeneration in the dorsal root ganglion.

Such findings strongly suggest that chronic, surgically intractable sciatica arises from ectopic impulses generated in the irreversibly damaged spinal nerve root and dorsal root ganglion. Thus, when other surgical approaches have failed, a neuroablative procedure may be considered.

HISTORICAL BACKGROUND

Dorsal rhizotomy considerably antedates dorsal root ganglionectomy and has been the most commonly used neuroablative procedure in the treatment of chronic, intractable sciatica. Another technique, percutaneous radiofrequency spinal rhizotomy, was described in a previous edition of this book.[6] We briefly consider dorsal rhizotomy here to explain the origin of dorsal root ganglionectomy.

Dorsal rhizotomy for the relief of sciatica has yielded mixed results; the best results were obtained in earlier series. White and Sweet[7] reported success in nine of 12 patients (75 percent); White[8] later reported success in one additional patient as well as two late failures in the originally successful group. Of the eight patients that underwent rhizotomy at a single level, seven no longer had sciatica. Echols[9] reported that "rhizotomy stopped pain" in 34 (59 percent) of 58 patients, most of whom underwent rhizotomy at a single level. It is notable, however, that Echols's rhizotomy included section of both dorsal and ventral roots in 11 of the 58 patients; of these 11, 10 (91 percent) were relieved of pain.

Loeser[10] obtained an "initial success rate" of 75 percent and a "long-term success rate" (with follow-up of up to 10 years) of 14 percent. The series of Onofrio and Campa[11] and of Law and coworkers[12] yielded success rates of 19 and 17 percent, respectively. Hoppenstein[13] reported a short-term success rate of 73 percent in a series of 26 patients with intractable back and lower extremity pain. His patients apparently had pain of polyradicular origin; they underwent dorsal rhizotomy of "not more than two contiguous roots."

Most rhizotomies in these series were performed with exposure of dorsal rootlets within the common dural tube (so-called intradural rhizotomy). All rhizotomies were intradural in six series,[7, 8, 10-13] and "most" were intradural in one series.[9] Scoville[14] described the alternative technique of "extradural spinal sensory rhizotomy," in which the common dural tube is left intact: the dural sleeve containing the dorsal root is transected just proximal to the dorsal root ganglion. He reported a "good" result in one of two lumbar rhizotomies.

In a modification of Scoville's technique, Strait and Hunter[15] performed dorsal rhizotomy by first opening the dural sleeve and then transecting the dorsal root within it. The efficacy of surgery was assessed by a postoperative patient questionnaire consisting of three questions. In response to the question, "How are you feeling since your surgery?" 53 percent of patients reported that they felt "better." No useful conclusions can be drawn from this datum.

Segmental dysesthesia after rhizotomy was reported in some of these series. Loeser[10] stated, "Some of our patients have manifested a new type of pain in their denervated areas; others have reported the same pain as they had preoperatively." No further description or quantification was given. White[8] noted the late development of "burning or stabbing pain in a radicular distribution in the dermatomes just below the zone of anesthesia" in 5 percent of 80 patients who underwent dorsal rhizotomy for diverse indications and at diverse spinal levels. Hoppenstein[13] stated that "in almost all cases under review . . . the patients who were treated experienced severe burning or throbbing pain almost immediately after surgery or within 3 months postoperatively." Strait and Hunter[15] reported, "Causalgia or Sudeck's dystrophy were not observed. . . . The patient often complained of temporary paresthesia, which either gradually disappeared or eventually became tolerable."

Numerous investigators have sought an anatomic explanation for the frequent failure of dorsal rhizotomy to relieve sciatica and have suggested corresponding modifications in surgical technique. Schwartz[16] described fine fascicles of nerve fibers bridging spinal rootlets of adjacent cervical segments, and Pallie[17] found such bridging fascicles in the lumbosacral region as well. If left intact after dorsal rhizotomy, these fascicles might serve as a pathway for afferent signals that give rise to pain. An effort to find and divide all such fascicles was recommended.

Smith[18] theorized that the sympathetic chain might similarly serve as an accessory pathway for signals that give rise to pain. He reasoned that "simple dorsal rhizotomy may be unsuccessful in relieving pain since afferent fibers might convey pain from the spinal ganglion to the sympathetic chain and then enter the spinal cord at higher or lower levels." Accordingly, in 10 patients with intractable thoracic pain, he carried out an augmented thoracic dorsal rhizotomy, with avulsion of rami communicantes and section of the segmental (intercostal) nerve. He stated that all patients "gained relief although not from all symptoms." This procedure does not involve excision of the dorsal root ganglion, nor does it isolate the dorsal root ganglion from the central nervous system, because a segment of dorsal root distal to the ganglion is left intact, through which afferent fibers might enter the ventral root, as is discussed later. This procedure is thus not a ganglionectomy, even though it was described under that name and has been counted as such in many subsequent reviews.[19-22] An analogous procedure, involving not only section of the rami communicantes but also of the segmental nerve, is not feasible in the lumbosacral region, because an unacceptable motor deficit would result.

Coggeshall and collaborators[23, 24] offered another hypothesis and suggested another procedure. In accordance with the so-called law of Bell and Magendie, it had long been accepted that the dorsal root contained only afferent fibers, and the ventral root, only efferent fibers. This turned out to be incorrect: approximately 30 percent of all axons in the ventral root of the cat were found to be unmyelinated afferent fibers derived from the dorsal root ganglion.[23] Comparable numbers were seen in humans as later confirmed by Hosobuchi.[25] Afferent fibers in the ventral root would be left intact after dorsal rhizotomy and would provide an afferent pathway that might be responsible for persistent pain, and perhaps for postrhizotomy dysesthesia as well. Coggeshall and colleagues suggested that "dorsal root ganglionectomy, which would remove both dorsal and ventral root afferents, might be the procedure of choice for those patients where rhizotomy is contemplated."[23]

The challenge was taken up by Osgood and associates[19, 26] who described the technique of dorsal root ganglionectomy and reported encouraging preliminary results in 18 patients. Taub[1] and Pawl[27] reported good results in larger series, as did Young.[21] North and colleagues,[22] however, reported poor results in 13 patients. The results in these series and our own data are discussed further below.

SELECTION OF PATIENTS

Among patients with persistent, surgically intractable sciatica, those with monoradicular sciatica stand to benefit most from dorsal root ganglionectomy. Selection of patients with monoradicular sciatica is essential to the success of the procedure.

In some patients with polyradicular sciatica, resection of two or more dorsal root ganglia at one procedure might achieve a therapeutic benefit. In such cases, there is a higher incidence of postganglionectomy dysesthesia, which may occur at two sites simultaneously; furthermore, we have observed an unacceptable proprioceptive deficit in one such case (see "Results"). Also, a risk of an unacceptable cutaneous sensory deficit exists if adjacent ganglia are resected. For these reasons, we currently limit the procedure to resection of a single ganglion in patients with monoradicular sciatica.

Initial patient selection for dorsal root ganglionectomy is based on symptoms and signs indicative of monoradicular sciatica and the absence of potential causes of pain external to the dorsal root and the dorsal root ganglion. Among the diagnoses that are excluded are residual or recurrent intervertebral disc herniation, foraminal or lateral recess stenosis, central spinal stenosis, spinal instability, intradiscal or intraosseous infection, peripheral neuropathy, and reflex sympathetic dystrophy. To ensure that none of these is present, patients should undergo repeated neurologic examination and supplementary diagnostic studies, including some or all of the following: plain radiography or dynamic fluoroscopy of the erect lumbosacral spine in flexion and extension, with or without prior administration of a muscle relaxant; computed tomography or magnetic resonance imaging of the lumbosacral spine, with or without intravenous or subarachnoid contrast; myelography; anteroposterior and lateral hypocycloidal tomography; bone scan; and gallium scan.

Directed neurophysiologic testing is useful in some cases. Nerve conduction velocity studies may assist in excluding peripheral neuropathy. Electromyography may assist in the diagnosis and localization of radiculopathy; it may also reveal fibrillations, which are indicative of an ongoing or recurrent injury to the nerve root. Thermography may reveal patterns of temperature change that are suggestive of reflex sympathetic dystrophy.

If the clinical history, physical examination, and preliminary diagnostic studies are all indicative of monoradicular sciatica, the patient should then undergo paravertebral somatic radicular block with local anesthetic to confirm that sciatica is monoradicular and thus potentially responsive to dorsal root ganglionectomy. The technique is described later.

Patients suffering from psychosis or major affective disorders are unlikely to benefit from dorsal root ganglionectomy. We have assessed patients psychosocially primarily by repeated interview. We have also used subjective pain diagrams and self-assessment questionnaires, including the Zung Pain and Distress Index and the Minnesota Multiphasic Personality Inventory. Patients with a history of illicit or uncontrollable use of opioids or stimulants are unlikely to alter their behavior, even after relief of sciatica. Such patients may require treatment for drug addiction before they can be re-evaluated for surgery. This category does not include patients taking medication as prescribed for the relief of pain.[28] Receipt of workmen's compensation is not a contraindication to dorsal root ganglionectomy (see ''Results'').

When sciatica is reliably shown to be monoradicular by clinical examination, radiologic studies, repeated local anesthetic nerve blocks, and other studies when indicated, and when no psychiatric contraindication exists, the patient may be considered likely to benefit from dorsal root ganglionectomy.

DIAGNOSTIC RADICULAR BLOCK

As a purely diagnostic procedure, paravertebral somatic radicular block with local anesthetic should be performed at least twice, on different days, to confirm that the sciatica is monoradicular. Repeated diagnostic blocks should not be performed on a single day, because local anesthesia is of variable duration and may be unexpectedly prolonged. Under fluoroscopic guidance, a 3½-inch, 19-gauge spinal needle is placed paravertebrally so that its tip lies just lateral to the intervertebral foramen, immediately posterior to the vertebral body and just superior to the level of the intervertebral space.

In this position, the tip of the needle lies approximately 2½ inches from the skin. A 19-gauge needle should be used because a thinner needle bends and becomes difficult to place in proper position. Proper placement of the needle does not produce paresthesia, and paresthesia should not be sought as a means of verifying placement.

The clinically suspect nerve root is then blocked with a small volume of local anesthetic agent. We have generally used 7.5 ml of 1-percent lidocaine. A smaller volume is often insufficient to produce anesthesia; a greater volume may produce unintended anesthesia in adjacent segments or may block the rami communicantes or sympathetic chain, which may confound the interpretation of the results and necessitate repetition of the procedure. Neurologic examination of the affected limb is performed before, during, and after nerve root block.

The level and completeness of nerve root block are verified by observation of appropriate radicular sensory, motor, proprioceptive, and reflex deficits. The patient should report total relief of sciatica after injection of local anesthetic at a single level, beginning after an appropriate delay for the particular agent used (10 to 15 minutes for lidocaine) and lasting an appropriate time (1½ to 2 hours for lidocaine). No relief of sciatica should occur when nerve roots above and below the suspect level are blocked. Dorsal root ganglionectomy is likely to relieve sciatica only if sciatica is totally relieved by local anesthetic block of one, and only one, nerve root.

Administration of 7.5 ml of 1-percent lidocaine reliably produces both sensory and motor radicular block without blocking intraradicular sympathetic fibers. It is often desirable to assess preoperatively the severity of the proprioceptive deficit that will result from dorsal root ganglionectomy. Because this assessment cannot be made in the presence of motor block, we now also perform a differential radicular block using 7.5 ml of 0.5-percent lidocaine. This measure produces cutaneous anesthesia and proprioceptive block without motor block.

We have occasionally electrically stimulated the nerve root to be blocked by use of the same insulated hollow needle through which local anesthetic is later injected. If the tip of the needle is adjacent to the nerve root and is at the proper segmental level, electrical stimulation induces paresthesia in the same distribution as the patient's sciatica. This technique aids in positioning the needle for block. The technique is particularly helpful if extensive paravertebral scar tissue is present: in this situation, the local anesthetic agent can spread only a short distance from the site of injection, which must therefore be as close to the nerve root as possible.

Paravertebral radicular somatic block is a diagnostic procedure used in the selection of patients for surgery and is not a method of treatment. Local anesthesia is of limited duration, and symptoms always return once the anesthetic effect has subsided. It is in vain to hope that local anesthetic block, whether single or repeated, will somehow result in permanent relief of sciatica. This has never happened in our experience, which extends to more than 1500 blocks.

OPERATIVE TECHNIQUE

The patient is anesthetized, intubated, and turned to the prone or the lateral decubitus position. Blanket rolls are used

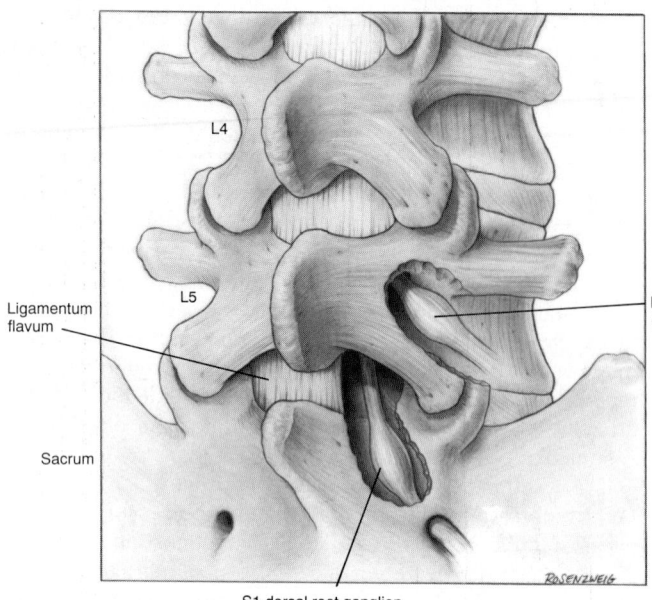

FIGURE 128–1. Bone has been resected to expose the L5 and S1 dorsal root ganglia, covered by dura mater, within the L5-S1 and S1-2 neural foramina.

for support. If the prone position is used, the surgeon stands on the same side of the patient as the ganglion that is to be removed; if the lateral decubitus position is used, the side of the ganglion is made uppermost. A prophylactic dose of cefazolin (1 g administered intravenously) is given.

A 10-cm-long incision is made in the midline at the desired spinal level, incorporating any incision from previous surgery. Cutaneous scars are excised. Dissection is carried through subcutaneous tissue to the lumbodorsal fascia, which is incised in the midline. Paraspinous muscle and ligamentous tissue are subperiosteally dissected off the spinous process and lamina and are held in check with a self-retaining hemilaminectomy retractor. We have used a variant of the Scoville retractor that is modified so that the shaft of the retractor hook has a flat surface where it abuts the spinous process. Before any bone is removed, the level of operation is confirmed by intraoperative radiography.

The dorsal root ganglion lies covered by its dural sleeve within the intervertebral foramen, usually directly inferior to the pedicle.[29] The dorsal root ganglion of a lower lumbar nerve is exposed by resection of the lateral margin of the zygapophyseal joint and several millimeters of the inferolateral margin of the overhanging pars interarticularis. The exposed segment of dural sleeve should include the entire visible swelling of the ganglion, as well as short proximal and distal segments of nerve root (Fig. 128–1). To expose the S1 dorsal root ganglion, bone resection proceeds from the L5-S1 intervertebral space. The ligamentum flavum is usually absent because of previous surgery. The S1 nerve root is identified in the interspace and is followed to the ganglion by removal of as much of the S1 hemilamina as necessary (Fig. 128–1).

Bone is resected with standard bone rongeurs. The Hall pneumatic drill with diamond burr is used when needed; carbon steel bone-cutting burrs are to be avoided when the common dural tube or nerve roots are approached. If previous surgery has included a bony fusion, the arthrodesis can usually be preserved by a keyhole exposure.

Once the nerve root and ganglion are exposed, the operating microscope is brought into the field. The field is kept free of blood by intermittent suction on cottonoid patties placed medial and lateral to the dural sleeve. Surgicel is used to control venous oozing, as necessary. The dural sleeve is incised longitudinally with a No. 11 or No. 15 scalpel blade so that the ganglion is seen along its entire extent, together with proximal and distal segments of the dorsal nerve root. The ventral nerve root is hidden from view behind the ganglion; it is separated from the dorsal root and ganglion by a thin, fibrous septum, as described by Osgood and colleagues.[26] The ganglion is mobilized with a blunt microdissector or a fine spatula, and a plane of dissection is established between it and the underlying septum (Figs. 128–2 and 128–3). Care is taken not to fillet the ganglion and create an artificial plane of dissection, because this event may result in retention of ganglionic tissue.

A standard 3- or 4-mm hemostatic clip is applied to the segment of dorsal nerve root distal to the ganglion, and the root is transected just proximal to the clip, leaving the ganglion free at its distal end. The ganglion is now held with a

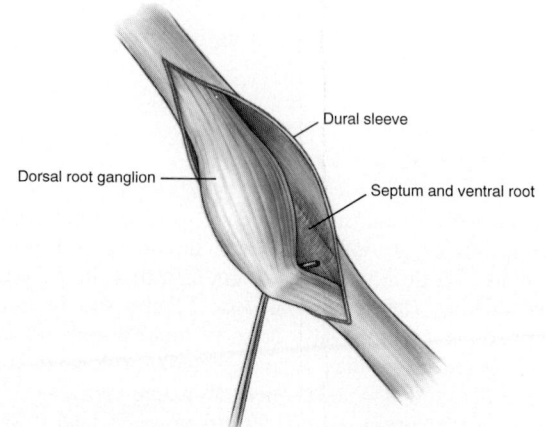

FIGURE 128–2. After the dural sleeve is opened, the dorsal root ganglion is separated from the underlying fibrous septum.

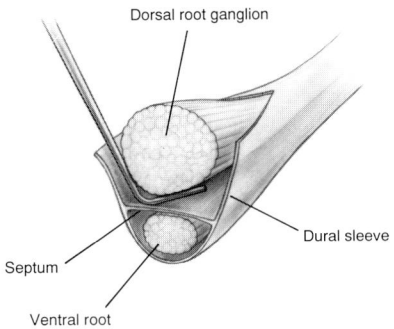

FIGURE 128–3. Cross-section of the dorsal root ganglion as it is separated from the fibrous septum.

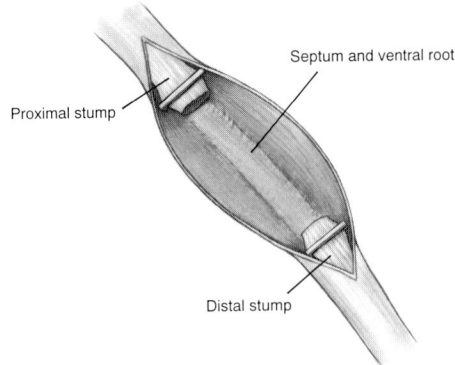

FIGURE 128–5. After removal of the ganglion, the ventral root remains intact under the septum.

fine forceps, and its undersurface is dissected off the fibrous septum under direct vision, with the dissection proceeding proximally until the proximal segment of dorsal nerve root is reached. A hemostatic clip is applied to the proximal segment (Fig. 128–4), and the ganglion is excised by transection of the proximal segment just distal to the clip. The ventral root remains intact (Fig. 128–5). The dura mater need not be closed unless a cerebrospinal fluid (CSF) leak occurs (see ''Technical Difficulties''). The field is inspected for bleeding points, hemostasis is obtained, and the wound is closed in layers in the usual fashion.

TECHNICAL DIFFICULTIES

Extensive epidural fibrosis may be present as a result of intervertebral disc disease or multiple previous operations. Fibrosis is occasionally severe enough to distort the anatomy of the nerve root and dorsal root ganglion and make the exposure difficult. In some instances, the ganglion may be more easily found, and unintentional rhizotomy avoided, by first exposing an unscarred portion of the common dural tube, and then carefully dissecting away fibrotic tissue in the medial-to-lateral direction, following the nerve root out to the ganglion.

Intraoperative leakage of CSF is seen only infrequently (<10 percent of cases), which is surprising, in view of the demonstration that the subarachnoid space is often patent as far laterally as the proximal portion of the dorsal root ganglion.[30] Perhaps meningeal inflammation resulting from the primary disease process and from prior surgery seals off the subarachnoid space nearer to the common dural tube. Leaks are readily controlled by application of a hemostatic clip to the dural edges; a small portion of the proximal dorsal root stump may be included in the clip to prevent slippage.

Electrocautery should be used sparingly within the dura mater because thermal trauma to the ventral root might result in a motor deficit. The margins of resection should include the entire visible swelling of the ganglion because retention of ganglionic tissue either proximally or distally might lead to persistence of pain after surgery.

RESULTS

Results of a series of 23 patients were reported by one of the authors (AT) in 1980.[1] This personal series now includes 61 patients who underwent dorsal root ganglionectomy in the 15-year period from 1977 to 1992. All had chronic sciatica that was unresponsive to multiple surgical procedures, including discectomy, foraminotomy, resection of epidural scar tissue, decompressive laminectomy, lumbar fusion, and sympathectomy (mean number of procedures, 3). All patients met the selection criteria outlined in ''Patient Selection,'' and were drawn from a population of approximately 3000 patients with chronic, intractable back pain and sciatica caused by lumbar disc disease. There were 33 men and 28 women, ranging from 23 to 62 years of age (mean age, 43 years; standard deviation, 9); 42 patients (69 percent) received workers' compensation.

Seventy-five dorsal root ganglia were resected, including two L3, one L4, 44 L5, two L6, and 26 S1 ganglia. Fourteen patients underwent resection of two dorsal root ganglia: seven patients at one procedure (one bilateral L5 and six bilateral S1 ganglionectomies), and seven patients at two separate procedures (one L4 and L5, and six L5 and S1 ganglionectomies). Ten patients underwent simultaneous spinal fusion for documented instability (posterolateral fusion with or without Harrington rod instrumentation). Ganglionectomy procedures were carried out by seven neurosurgeons.

Pathologic examination of 14 resected ganglia revealed nonspecific changes, including neuronal dropout and diffuse intraganglionic scarring.

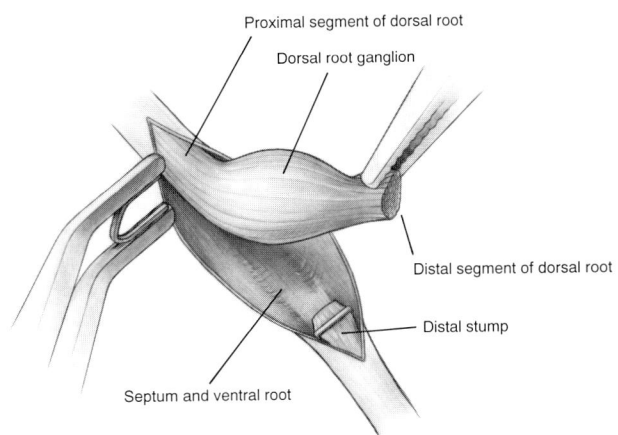

FIGURE 128–4. The distal segment of dorsal root has been clipped and transected, and a hemostatic clip is applied across the proximal segment of dorsal root.

No operative deaths occurred. The length of hospitalization when fusion was not performed ranged from 3 to 14 days (3 to 4 days in recent cases). Fusion prolonged hospitalization to as much as 1 month.

The duration of postoperative follow-up, which included serial clinical interviews and detailed neurologic examination, was less than 1 year in four patients, 1 to 4 years in 23 patients, 5 to 9 years in 14 patients, and 10 to 15 years in 20 patients.

RELIEF OF SYMPTOMS

Sciatica was markedly reduced or eliminated in 36 of 61 patients (59 percent). Of these 36 patients, 12 (33 percent) continued to have low back pain after surgery. Of the 25 patients in whom sciatica was not relieved, nine (36 percent) continued to have concomitant low back pain.

Before surgery, the 61 patients in the overall group required opioid analgesia at doses pharmacologically equivalent to a mean of 25 mg of methadone per day. The dosage required by the surgically successful group was not significantly different preoperatively (22 mg). After 1 or more years of postoperative observation, the 36 surgically successful patients required a mean methadone equivalent of 8 mg/day, and 16 of them required no opioids.

Before surgery, 39 (64 percent) of the patients were considered capable of returning to employment or to housework if ganglionectomy succeeded in relieving symptoms. Of these, 23 (59 percent, or 38 percent of the total) did return to work. The remainder were disabled primarily by persistent pain (in seven), age (in three), and unrelated illnesses (in six).

Almost invariably, if sciatica was not relieved on the first postoperative day it would not be relieved, and if it was relieved on the first postoperative day it would continue to be relieved, although an intervening period of dysesthesia might occur, as is discussed later.

Relief of sciatica was not correlated with the site of the lesion, with the duration of symptoms or the amount of opioid analgesic required preoperatively, with the presence or absence of focal or diffuse arachnoiditis as demonstrated by myelography, with the age and sex of the patient, with other illnesses, or with the operating surgeon, except in early cases. Of the 42 patients receiving workmen's compensation, 22 (52 percent) were relieved of sciatica, and 20 (48 percent) were not.

COMPLICATIONS

Technical Complications

Complications directly attributable to surgery included intradiscal infection (in one patient), pseudomeningocele (in one), resection of scar tissue only rather than the dorsal root ganglion (in one), resection of a segment of dorsal root only (in one), incomplete resection of the intended dorsal root ganglion (in six), and resection of a dorsal root ganglion adjacent to the one intended (in one, corrected at later surgery). One intraoperative dural tear was repaired without further complication.

Radicular Neurologic Deficits

Dorsal root ganglionectomy immediately produced hypesthesia and hypalgesia in a small, generally distal zone within a single dermatome. Total analgesia to pinprick was rare. The sensory deficit was always present when looked for and remained stable on serial examination, except in three patients. One patient regained sensation, as well as the original symptoms, 1 year later. Two patients regained sensation, but not symptoms, one 2 years later and one 5 years later.

Four patients developed a transient foot drop after L5 ganglionectomy and required a plastic foot brace for 1 to 2 months. Two patients developed transient painful arching of the foot after S1 ganglionectomy. No other motor abnormality was noted, except for a contralateral peroneal pressure palsy in one patient.

No proprioceptive deficits were noted after resection of a single ganglion. Resection of both the L5 and S1 ganglia produced a transient, mild, nondisabling deficit. In a single case of bilateral S1 ganglionectomy, a marked proprioceptive deficit occurred that led to repeated falls and physical injury. This deficit cleared 3 years after surgery.

One patient developed an indolent fungal infection, which eventually cleared, in the denervated S1 dermatome. No herpetic eruptions or trophic ulcerations were seen.

Postganglionectomy Dysesthesia

Incidence

Spontaneous and evoked dysesthesia in the dermatomal distribution of the resected dorsal root ganglion was seen frequently but not invariably (36 of 61 patients, or 59 percent; 46 of 75 ganglia, or 61 percent). Of 46 instances of postganglionectomy dysesthesia, 33 (72 percent) were mild or moderate and lasted 2 to 3 weeks; 11 (24 percent) were marked and lasted 3 to 6 weeks; and one (2 percent) was severe and lasted 6 weeks. In this unusual case, severe unilateral dysesthesia followed a simultaneous bilateral L5 ganglionectomy. One other instance of possible dysesthesia was difficult to assess. In three patients, mild or minimal dysesthesia persisted more than a decade after surgery but did not interfere with full activity. One of these patients intermittently required medication for suppression of dysesthesia.

Resection of two adjacent or contralateral dorsal root ganglia in a single procedure led to an additive, but not synergistic, increase in the incidence of dysesthesia. No increase in the incidence of dysesthesia occurred when the second of two ganglia was removed in a separate procedure.

Symptoms and Signs

Postganglionectomy dysesthesia occurred as a distinct clinical syndrome and was clearly different from sciatica, both subjectively and objectively. Dysesthesia could not be influenced by maneuvers used to produce sciatica. Patients in whom ganglionectomy relieved sciatica were as likely to experience dysesthesia as those whose sciatica persisted after surgery.

Dysesthesia generally began 10 to 14 days after surgery as an ache in the posterior calf (occasionally confused with thrombophlebitis; results of three venograms were negative). After this occurrence, first distal and then proximal cutaneous areas in the dermatomal distribution of the resected ganglion became hypersensitive to light touch and pinprick, which evoked intense burning pain localized to the area of the stimulus and not outlasting the stimulus. Spontaneous burning dysesthesia then arose and mounted to peak intensity over 7 to 10 days. When spontaneous dysesthesia was maximally intense, dysesthesia evoked by a tactile stimulus lasted several seconds after the stimulus was removed; a moving stimulus thus produced a lasting, invisible "trace" or "wake" on the skin. Dysesthesia ultimately resolved first proximally and then distally in the dermatome.

Grossly apparent changes in cutaneous temperature were rare; decreases in temperature were commoner than increases. The change in temperature did not correlate with the intensity or the duration of dysesthesia. We are currently studying the effects of dorsal root ganglionectomy, including postganglionectomy dysesthesia, with telethermography; this technique may disclose otherwise undetectable changes in cutaneous temperature.

Some patients in the surgically unsuccessful group postoperatively underwent diagnostic radicular block with local anesthetic and obtained temporary relief not only of sciatica but also of postganglionectomy dysesthesia. Nerve block in adjacent dermatomes had no effect. Dysesthesia could not be inhibited by pressure or noxious stimulation in the affected or adjacent dermatomes.

Diagnostic radicular block was attempted in one patient in the surgically successful group who experienced postganglionectomy dysesthesia of unusual severity. In this patient, dysesthesia was totally relieved after injection of only 3 ml of 1-percent lidocaine, but some of the local anesthetic agent had entered the systemic circulation. This observation prompted a double-blind, placebo-controlled study of the use of parenteral systemic lidocaine alone for suppression of postganglionectomy dysesthesia. Total suppression of postganglionectomy dysesthesia was obtained in all patients tested after subcutaneous (deltoid) injection of 5 to 7.5 ml of 2-percent lidocaine.[31] Dysesthesia returned when the anesthetic effect subsided. Subsequent observations indicate that lasting, uninterrupted suppression of dysesthesia may be obtained by subcutaneous injection of lidocaine every 3 to 4 hours, without adverse effects.

Treatment

Dysesthesia generally required no medication or was suppressible with the small amount of opioid given to control back pain. In more severe instances, relief was obtained with a combination of a phenothiazine (perphenazine, 2 mg given orally three times a day, or fluphenazine, 1 mg given orally three times a day) and a tricyclic agent (amitriptyline, 75 mg given orally at bedtime). One patient experienced dysesthesia of near-suicidal intensity after bilateral L5 ganglionectomy; this episode lasted 6 weeks and required at its height a combination of injectable morphine, fluphenazine, amitriptyline, and carbamazepine. In recent years, we have adopted systemic lidocaine administration as the primary treatment for postganglionectomy dysesthesia, and we have used the fluphenazine-amitriptyline combination adjunctively, when necessary.

ADDITIONAL OBSERVATIONS

In five patients who were not counted in the treatment group, dorsal root ganglionectomy was recommended, but a decision not to resect the ganglion was made intraoperatively by the surgeon. Four of these patients underwent decompressive laminectomy and discectomy, and one underwent resection of epidural scar tissue. None gained relief of sciatica.

REVIEW OF THE LITERATURE

Four other reports have been published on the use of dorsal root ganglionectomy for the relief of chronic, intractable sciatica.[19, 21, 22, 27] Their results are generally comparable to our own, with some exceptions.

Osgood and coworkers[19] carried out dorsal root ganglionectomy for diverse indications at diverse spinal levels in 18 patients. Of eight patients with intractable sciatica caused by lumbar disc disease, six (75 percent) obtained good relief of sciatica. In one of these surgically successful cases, sciatica was "much improved," but back pain persisted. Four of the eight patients underwent ganglionectomy at a single level, and four at two adjacent levels; both of the surgical failures occurred with ganglionectomy at a single level.

Pawl[27] reported on dorsal root ganglionectomy in 30 patients who had "both a unilateral sciatica and associated arachnoiditis" after "failure of lumbar disc surgery." Pawl stated that "63 percent were able to return to their premorbid activities."

Young[21] performed dorsal root ganglionectomy "for treatment of intractable pain ... in the thoracic and lumbar regions" in 33 patients. Patients underwent the procedure at multiple levels; a total of 165 ganglia were removed. Young did not state how many lumbar procedures he performed, or for what indications. He reported, "Immediate pain relief was attained in 91 percent. At the last follow-up, a mean of 30 months postoperatively, 79 percent of patients remain pain free." This series apparently consisted mainly of multilevel thoracic ganglionectomies for the treatment of pain of peripheral origin and is thus of limited significance for the present discussion of the use of dorsal root ganglionectomy in the treatment of chronic, surgically intractable sciatica.

North and coworkers[22] assessed the long-term outcome of dorsal root ganglionectomy in 13 patients with "failed back surgery syndrome." Only three patients (23 percent) reported "at least 50 percent relief of pain" at a mean of 5.5 years after surgery. In response to a questionnaire, two of the three patients said that they would not undergo the procedure again to obtain the same "overall pain relief."

What appears to be a poor outcome of dorsal root ganglionectomy in this series may be attributable to the use of inappropriate methods of follow-up and inappropriate criteria for success of treatment. Follow-up was obtained by questionnaire and by telephone interview with a nonphysician rather than by neurologic examination, which is the only way sciatica can be evaluated. Persistent pain was assessed by "standard analog pain rating methods and pain descriptors": six pain intensity scales[32] and the McGill Pain Questionnaire.[33] These instruments have no questions specifically relating to sciatica, and neither radicular pain nor sciatica is mentioned by North and colleagues in their discussion of postoperative symptoms. It cannot, therefore, be determined whether patients expressing dissatisfaction with overall pain relief in fact experienced relief of sciatica but not of other symptoms. We do not know the true success rate in this series. Success or failure of dorsal root ganglionectomy can be judged only by the extent to which it attains its single objective, the relief of sciatica.

REPORTS OF POSTGANGLIONECTOMY DYSESTHESIA

Osgood and colleagues[19] reported the occurrence of dysesthesia after dorsal root ganglionectomy in four of their 18 patients, and in two of the eight that underwent the procedure for intractable sciatica caused by lumbar disc disease. One patient had "significant, electric-like dysesthesia for 6 weeks initially"; in the other cases, dysesthesia was milder but persisted for the duration of postoperative follow-up. Increased dysesthesia was sometimes noted with micturition and defecation.

In 1980, in the first report of the series presented here,[1] Taub described postganglionectomy dysesthesia in detail.

In contrast to these reports, Young[21] noted "no complications, other than relatively prolonged wound pain," after dorsal root ganglionectomy. He stated, "Anesthesia dolorosa following either dorsal rhizotomy or dorsal root ganglionectomy is an extremely rare occurrence." No data are available on the possible occurrence of dysesthesia in the series of Pawl[27] and of North and coworkers.[22]

The mechanism of dysesthesia following dorsal root ganglionectomy for the relief of surgically intractable, monoradicular sciatica is unknown. The findings of Hosobuchi[25] are of interest. Three patients had persistent segmental dysesthesia after undergoing thoracic dorsal rhizotomy for intractable postthoracotomy pain. Thoracic dorsal root ganglionectomy was performed and resulted in disappearance of dysesthesia in two patients. In the third patient, dysesthesia disappeared immediately after ganglionectomy but later returned and persisted. These findings might suggest a role for ventral root afferent fibers in the generation of postrhizotomy dysesthesia because ganglionectomy (but not dorsal rhizotomy) disconnects these fibers from the dorsal root ganglion. If so, however, it remains unclear why dysesthesia should ever occur after ganglionectomy. It seems likelier that both postrhizotomy and postganglionectomy dysesthesia result from a pathologic response to deafferentation occurring at a more central level.

SUMMARY

Dorsal root ganglionectomy is effective in the relief of monoradicular sciatica that is caused by lumbar disc disease and persists despite repeated surgical intervention. Patients should be considered for the procedure only if sciatica is reliably demonstrated to be monoradicular by repeated diagnostic nerve root blocks with local anesthetic.

Dysesthesia in the dermatomal distribution of the resected ganglion is a characteristic consequence of dorsal root ganglionectomy; it is seen frequently but not invariably (in approximately 60 percent of cases). It is usually mild or moderate and is rarely of more than 6 weeks' duration, although mild or minimal dysesthesia may persist for years after surgery. The mechanism of postganglionectomy dysesthesia is unknown.

Dorsal root ganglionectomy was first suggested as a potential improvement on dorsal rhizotomy because of the possible existence of nociceptive input in afferent fibers of the ventral root.[23] The results of dorsal root ganglionectomy for the relief of sciatica are superior to those of dorsal rhizotomy for the relief of sciatica, as reported in most series. The only meaningful exceptions are the series of White and Sweet[7] and of Echols.[9] Conflicting data make it difficult to assess the true efficacy of dorsal rhizotomy and the true incidence of postrhizotomy dysesthesia.

The hypothesis of a role for ventral root afferents in persistent, surgically intractable sciatica is supported by the relief of sciatica obtained by Echols[9] in 10 of 11 patients by simultaneous section of dorsal and ventral roots. This procedure, however, causes a motor deficit, and dorsal root ganglionectomy does not.

We use dorsal root ganglionectomy only for the relief of persistent, surgically intractable monoradicular sciatica in selected patients. We have obtained good results in approximately 60 percent of cases. A good surgical result, although clearly beneficial, may not be the complete answer to the patient's problem. The relief of sciatica alone may sometimes restore the patient to full function, including employment, but for some patients, even when sciatica is relieved, back pain may remain a major problem and require further treatment. Moreover, dorsal root ganglionectomy has no effect on the natural history of intervertebral disc degeneration, and sciatica may recur as a result of disease at other levels. In some patients, psychosocial problems may remain to be addressed.

Acknowledgments

All patients reported here were evaluated preoperatively and followed up postoperatively by Dr. Arthur Taub. All nerve root blocks were performed by Dr. Arthur Taub.

Dorsal root ganglionectomies were performed primarily by Dr. Franklin Robinson and Dr. Isaac Goodrich, and by Drs. T. J. Arkins, L. M. Davey, S. Frankel, A. D. Greenberg, and D. Spencer. We thank Dr. I. Goodrich for demonstrating the procedure and discussing it with us, and Dr. T. J. Arkins for additional comments.

We thank David Rosenzweig of the Department of Medical Art and Photography of Cornell University Medical College for the illustrations.

REFERENCES

1. Taub A: Relief of chronic, intractable sciatica by dorsal root ganglionectomy. Trans Am Neurol Assoc 105:340–343, 1980
2. Howe JF, Loeser JD, Calvin WH: Mechanosensitivity of dorsal root ganglia and chronically injured axons: A physiological basis for the radicular pain of nerve root compression. Pain 3:25–41, 1977
3. Wall PD, Devor M: Sensory afferent impulses originate from dorsal root ganglia as well as from the periphery in normal and nerve injured rats. Pain 17:321–339, 1983
4. Lindblom K, Rexed B: Spinal nerve injury in dorso-lateral protrusions of lumbar discs. J Neurosurg 5:413–432, 1948

5. Lindahl O, Rexed B: Histologic changes in spinal nerve roots of operated cases of sciatica. Acta Orthop Scand 20:215–225, 1951
6. Uematsu S: Percutaneous electrothermocoagulation of spinal nerve trunk, ganglion, and rootlets, in Schmidek HH, Sweet WH (eds): Operative Neurosurgical Techniques: Indications, Methods and Results, 2nd ed. Orlando, Grune & Stratton, 1988, pp 1207–1221
7. White JC, Sweet WH: Pain and the Neurosurgeon: A Forty-Year Experience. Springfield, IL, Charles C Thomas, 1969, pp 459–466
8. White JC: Posterior spinal rhizotomy, in Voris HC, Whisler WW (eds): Treatment of Pain. Springfield, Charles C Thomas, 1975, pp 95–107
9. Echols DH: Sensory rhizotomy following operation for ruptured intervertebral disc: A review of 62 cases. J Neurosurg 31:335–338, 1969
10. Loeser JD: Dorsal rhizotomy for the relief of chronic pain. J Neurosurg 36:745–750, 1972
11. Onofrio BM, Campa HK: Evaluation of rhizotomy: Review of 12 years' experience. J Neurosurg 36:751–755, 1972
12. Law JD, Lehman RAW, Kirsch WM: Reoperation after lumbar intervertebral disc surgery. J Neurosurg 48:259–263, 1978
13. Hoppenstein R: A new approach to the failed, failed back syndrome. Spine 5:371–379, 1980
14. Scoville WB: Extradural spinal sensory rhizotomy. J Neurosurg 25:94–95, 1966
15. Strait TA, Hunter SE: Intraspinal extradural sensory rhizotomy in patients with failure of lumbar disc surgery. J Neurosurg 54:193–196, 1981
16. Schwartz HG: Anastomoses between cervical nerve roots. J Neurosurg 13:190–194, 1956
17. Pallie W: The intersegmental anastomoses of posterior spinal rootlets and their significance. J Neurosurg 16:188–196, 1959
18. Smith FP: Trans-spinal ganglionectomy for relief of intercostal pain. J Neurosurg 32:574–577, 1970
19. Osgood CP, Dujovny M, Faille R, Abassy M: Microsurgical lumbosacral ganglionectomy, anatomic rationale, and surgical results. Acta Neurochir (Wien) 35:197–204, 1976
20. Harris AB: Dorsal rhizotomy, in Wilkins RH, Rengachary SS (eds): Neurosurgery. New York, McGraw-Hill, 1985, pp 2430–2432
21. Young RF: Dorsal rhizotomy and dorsal root ganglionectomy, in Youmans JR (ed): Neurological Surgery, 3rd ed. Philadelphia, WB Saunders, 1990, pp 4026–4035
22. North RB, Kidd DH, Campbell JN, Long DM: Dorsal root ganglionectomy for failed back surgery syndrome: A 5-year follow-up study. J Neurosurg 74:236–242, 1991
23. Coggeshall RE, Applebaum ML, Fazen M, et al: Unmyelinated axons in human ventral roots, a possible explanation for the failure of dorsal rhizotomy to relieve pain. Brain 98:157–166, 1975
24. Coggeshall RE: Afferent fibers in the ventral root. Neurosurgery 4:443–448, 1979
25. Hosobuchi Y: The majority of unmyelinated afferent axons in human ventral roots probably conduct pain. Pain 8:167–180, 1980
26. Osgood CP, Dujovny M, Faille R, Abassy M: Microsurgical ganglionectomy for chronic pain syndromes. J Neurosurg 45:113–115, 1976
27. Pawl RP: Microsurgical Ganglionectomy for Treatment of Arachnoiditis-Related Unilateral Sciatica. Presented to the American Pain Society, Miami, 1982, as cited in Sweet WH, Gybels JM: Neurosurgical Treatment of Persistent Pain. New York, Karger, 1989, p 122
28. Taub A: Opioid analgesics in the treatment of chronic intractable pain of non-neoplastic origin, in Kitahata LM, Collins JG (eds): Narcotic Analgesics in Anesthesiology. Baltimore, Williams & Wilkins, 1982, pp 199–208
29. Cohen MS, Wall EJ, Brown RA, et al: Cauda equina anatomy: II. Extrathecal nerve roots and dorsal root ganglia. Spine 15:1248–1251, 1990
30. Lindblom K: The subarachnoid spaces of the root sheaths in the lumbar region. Acta Radiol 30:419–426, 1948
31. Taub A: Suppression of Post-Ganglionectomy Dysesthesia by Systemic Lidocaine. Presented to the American Pain Society, Washington, DC, 1986
32. Jensen MP, Karoly P, Braver S: The measurement of clinical pain intensity: A comparison of six methods. Pain 27:117–126, 1986
33. Melzack R: The McGill Pain Questionnaire: Major properties and scoring methods. Pain 1:277–299, 1975

CHAPTER 129

Percutaneous Cordotomy

R. R. Tasker

The management of chronic pain occupies an ever greater role in modern medicine, and it sometimes appears that the more one explores the problems involved, the more difficult the task becomes. One group of pain syndromes, however, has a reliable, effective, and well-studied treatment: those that depend on transmission in the spinothalamic tract in the spinal cord.

CLASSIFICATION OF CHRONIC PAIN

To put this group of pain syndromes in perspective, a pathophysiologically oriented classification of pain syndromes is proposed on the basis of existing knowledge about pain processes and observations of surgical outcome.[1-5] Entries I, II, IIIa, and IIIb in Table 129–1 constitute pain processes for which interference with transmission in pain pathways, particularly the spinothalamic tract summarized by Willis,[6] can be considered for therapy on the basis of our current understanding of pain signalling systems.

Yet, lest we feel we understand sensory physiology too well, with the notion that cordotomy is a simple, selective interruption of pain pathways, Noordenbos and Wall[7] observed the following in a patient who had suffered a penetrating wound of the spinal cord at T3 that spared a strand containing one anterolateral quadrant extending from slightly dorsal to the dentate ligament to the midline:

Paralysis below T3 with increased tendon jerks
Preservation of ability to identify temperature and pinprick only on the side contralateral to the preserved quadrant
Preservation of touch and pressure localization bilaterally
Ability to detect passive movement ipsilateral to the preserved quadrant
Preservation of pain appreciation bilaterally
Preservation of appreciation of stimuli from von Frey hairs bilaterally, sometimes at normal limits, usually at increased thresholds
Lowering of threshold for detection of von Frey hairs after repeated subthreshold stimulation

Then there is the question of the Brown-Séquard syndrome from cord hemisection, the clinical picture of which is firmly entrenched in our thinking about the cord's sensory pathways. Wall has carefully reviewed the early literature[8] and points out that Brown-Séquard, after many careful experiments, concluded that cord hemisection reduced sensitivity to contralateral sensory stimuli, as we teach today, but that it *increased sensitivity to ipsilateral stimuli*. However, when Mott repeated the experiment, he found just the opposite and confirmed his findings with Sharpey-Shafer, Jackson, and Sherrington. Brown-Séquard took due note and reviewed the issue, observing that hemisection of the cervical cord in animals induced contralateral anesthesia and ipsilateral hyperesthesia but that if a second hemisection was carried out in the thoracic cord and on the same side as the first, the contralateral anesthesia was replaced by hyperesthesia and the ipsilateral hyperesthesia, by anesthesia. Decades later, Denny-Brown noted that in monkeys, cord hemisection sometimes resulted in the one picture, sometimes the other, and showed that only partial hemisection produced contralaterally decreased sensation, whereas extending partial lesions to include half of the cord reversed the pattern of sensation, but over a period of 3 days.

In their discussion, Noordenbos and Wall[7] point out that anterolateral cordotomy restricted to the part of the cord that is anatomically occupied by spinothalamic fibers produced incomplete analgesia and that section of the entire anterolateral quadrant was necessary to achieve the greatest degree of analgesia, which was still not complete. Such optimal analgesia is associated with inability to evoke warm or cold sensations contralaterally below the cordotomy and elevated threshold to touch contralaterally. On the homolateral side, certain sensory changes have also been noted.

Table 129–1. CLASSIFICATION OF CHRONIC PAIN SYNDROMES

I Dependent on stimulation of receptors and transmission in pain pathways
    Nociceptive pain: e.g., pain from chronic arthritis, bony neoplasms
II Dependent on stimulation of receptors, transmission in sensory pathways, and perverted processing at cord level or centrally so as to signal pain perception
    Allodynia, hyperpathia, hyperesthesia in neuropathic pain
III Dependent on direct stimulation of nerve fibers and transmission in pain pathways
    a. Sciatica from disc herniation or cancerous compression of lumbosacral plexus (nociceptive pain)
    b. Spontaneous, intermittent, often lancinating, element of neuropathic pain
    c. Stimulation of a neuroma
    d. Tinel's and Lhermitte's signs
IV Not dependent on transmission in pain pathways
    a. Psychogenic pain
    b. Spontaneous, steady, usually burning, dysesthetic element of neuropathic pain
V Tic Douloureux
VI Dependent on sympathetic function
    a. Reflex sympathetic dystrophy
    b. Sympathetically maintained pain, a subgroup of the evoked element of neuropathic pain

Nathan[9] reported that after cordotomy, apart from alterations in pain and temperature perception, itch was abolished, but no deficit of mechanoreception, graphesthesia, position or vibration sense occurred and seldom no deficit of tactile sensibility occurred. He noted that total lesions of the dorsal columns do not remove appreciation of touch and pressure, and he concluded that the posterior columns are essential for discrimination in mechanoreception but that such discrimination, especially two-point discrimination, may be disturbed by lesions of the anterolateral cord.

The long tracts severed by typical cordotomy include spinothalamic, spinotectal, spinoreticular, and dorsal and ventral spinocerebellar, resulting in degeneration in such structures as the nuclei ventralis posterior lateralis, parafascicularis, centralis lateralis, nucleus cuneiformis and the periaqueductal gray in the midbrain, and reticular nuclei in the lower brainstem.[7]

A recent study by Lahuerta and colleagues[10] is interesting. In 16 patients examined after unilateral percutaneous cordotomy, pain relief did not parallel absence of pinprick appreciation, but rather, varied degrees of diminution of appreciation of skinfold pinch and cooling occurred, implicating A fibers. Less obviously, reduction of appreciation of warmth or hot pain occurred, implicating C fibers.

Interesting imaging studies are accumulating, such as the report by Di Piero and associates[11] that positron-emission tomography with radioactive C^{15} in carbon dioxide demonstrated lower regional cerebral blood flow than in normal subjects in the contralateral hemithalamus in three of four patients suffering from unilateral cancer pain. The flow was restored to normal after cordotomy, a phenomenon the authors suggested resulted from decreased thalamic synaptic activity that resulted from decreased neuronal activity projecting to, or in, the area. No cortical differences in blood flow were seen.

HISTORY OF PERCUTANEOUS CORDOTOMY

Long before pain physiology was well understood, Spiller[12] came to the conclusion, based on published experience concerning the neurologic deficit resulting from lesions of the anterolateral quadrant of the spinal cord, that relieving pain by cutting the pain pathway in the spinal cord should be possible. Spiller persuaded Martin to perform this procedure in a patient with pain caused by a tuberculoma of the cord.[13] This pioneering event spurred great interest in cordotomy performed through a laminectomy with incision of the anterolateral cord under direct vision.

The trend to minimize surgical impact and to increase precision led Mullan and his colleagues[14] to develop a technique for performing cordotomy percutaneously, by use of a needle with a radiostrontium source at its tip. The needle was inserted through the only convenient percutaneous access to spinothalamic tract, the C1-C2 (or occipital-C1) space. The difficulties of creating a radiation lesion were overcome by the introduction by Rosomoff and associates[15] of a radiofrequency lesion-making technique. This technology could easily be combined with electrophysiologic methods both for monitoring cord penetration, using electrical impedance, introduced by Gildenberg and his associates,[17] and for determining electrode position in the cord, using electrical stimulation.[18–22] To these methods, Onofrio[23] added imaging of electrode position, using myelography. Computed tomographic (CT) guidance has been described by Kanpolat and associates[24] and also by Izumi and associates.[25]

INDICATIONS FOR CORDOTOMY

Before surgical treatment for chronic pain is considered, all possible primary therapy must be exhausted and medical therapy must be evaluated. Only after drug treatment has failed, because of side effects, escalating dosages, or inefficacy, should surgical modalities be used.

CORDOTOMY VERSUS OTHER PROCEDURES

If the patient's pain warrants surgical blockade of pain transmission, what options exist other than cordotomy?

Obviously, the procedure of choice should be the one with the least impact on the patient that is most cost-effective in terms of the patient's life expectancy, the chance of success, and the likely complications.

As our understanding of modulatory mechanisms in pain physiology has increased, the use of invasive morphine infusion techniques has grown exponentially, including spinal epidural and intrathecal and intraventricular morphine infusion techniques. Infusions into the cerebrospinal fluid (CSF) usually require totally implantable refillable pumps that cannot be recycled whose high cost limits their use in cancer patients with short life expectancies. Epidural infusions can be performed with simple reservoir-cannula devices that are implanted subcutaneously, but they require repeated injections throughout the day through the same site in the skin by the patient or his attendants, thereby inviting complications, such as infection, dislodgement of hardware, and escalation of dosage beyond the capacity of the reservoir. The commonest technique employs portable external pumps for continuous intravenous infusion. Such devices have largely supplanted cordotomy in many centers, including our own, where the number of cordotomies performed have fallen from as many as 30 per year in the 1970s to three to five per year in the 1990s.

Although the use of infusion techniques represents a desirable advance in the treatment of cancer pain, it must be examined in perspective. Its use requires the patient to carry the apparatus at all times and to attend appointments continually at a health care facility. Infusion techniques also lead to complications from increasing opiate dosages that result from tolerance.

In patients who are good candidates for cordotomy, a once-only surgical procedure with a low risk and high success rate can reduce the patient's pain level such that it can be conveniently managed at home with conventional oral medication, an option frequently overlooked in current practice.

Another modulatory option is the use of long-term periventricular gray stimulation, which is thought to modulate transmission in spinothalamic pathways.[26] Unfortunately, like morphine infusions into the CSF, this technique requires the implantation of expensive equipment, although it has been used in long-term transcutaneous administration,[27] thereby avoiding the main expense of the implanted stimulator.

If a destructive procedure is considered, do alternatives to cordotomy exist? Percutaneous radiofrequency neurectomy or rhizotomy is simpler, but cancer seldom respects the domain of one or a few nerves or roots; the entire function of such structures may not be expendable; and, if the pain is caused by cancer, percutaneous access to nerves or roots may be interfered with by the cancer, as occurs in cancer at the base of the skull in patients with pain in the trigeminal territory.

Other destructive procedures are more difficult to perform or carry a greater risk than cordotomy, although occasionally, percutaneous cervical commissurotomy[28] might be considered. In properly selected patients, percutaneous cordotomy remains the treatment of choice for the treatment of pain because of its simplicity, effectiveness, and relatively low risks, whenever interruption of pain pathways is required.

The role cordotomy might play in the treatment of pain may now be examined. A review of Table 129–1 suggests that cordotomy might be considered in the treatment of the following intractable pain syndromes:

1. Pain caused by stimulation of nociceptors and transmission in spinothalamic tract by both noncancerous and cancerous disease
2. Pain caused by direct stimulation of nerve fibers that results in activation of spinothalamic tract; for example, by noncancerous compression of neural tissue, or by cancerous compression of lumbosacral and brachial plexus
3. Pain caused by ectopic impulse generation that leads to transmission in the spinothalamic tract, such as the lancinating element of neuropathic pain that is particularly common in lesions of the conus and the cauda equina
4. Allodynia, hyperpathia, and hyperesthesia

Cordotomy has seldom been used to treat disease other than malignancy because of concern about the development of postcordotomy dysesthesia or fading of the level of analgesia with time. Thus, pain caused by cancerous compression of the lumbosacral plexus is probably the commonest indication. Pain from involvement of the brachial plexus is less often an indication for two reasons: first, percutaneous cordotomy by the lateral high cervical approach cannot induce persistent analgesia consistently above the C5 dermatome, and second, most patients with cancerous involvement of the brachial plexus have pulmonary or phrenic nerve dysfunction, or both, on the side of the pain. In the latter patients, survival is dependent on pulmonary function on the side of the intended cordotomy. To produce levels of analgesia high enough to suppress the pain of brachial plexus lesions, cordotomy would likely interrupt the ipsilaterally distributed reticulospinal path, which lies adjacent to the high cervical dermatomes of the spinothalamic tract and mediates automatic respiration to the remaining lung. Such treatment would likely have disastrous consequences.[29–36]

Special reference must be made to the intermittent lancinating element of neuropathic pain. This phenomenon is most prevalent in central pain syndromes affecting the thoracolumbar region[5] and is very effectively relieved by the DREZ operation,[37] cordectomy,[38] but most conveniently, by percutaneous cordotomy.[5, 39] However, cordotomy is relatively ineffective for the steady burning, dysesthetic, or aching pain of neuropathic pain syndromes.[4]

Our own indications for percutaneous cordotomy in 398

Table 129–2. INDICATIONS FOR 398 PERCUTANEOUS CORDOTOMIES

Diagnosis	Incidence (%)
Carcinoma	
Cervix	22
Rectum	16
Colon	10
Lung	7
Breast	4
Other	22
Sarcoma	7
Cord central pain	7
Other noncancerous disorders	5

procedures are listed in Table 129–2. In recent years, the relative numbers of cases with cervical cancer appear to be diminishing.

OPEN VERSUS PERCUTANEOUS CORDOTOMY

Although proponents of open cordotomy still exist,[40] there seems to be little justification for this procedure in modern neurosurgery except in cases in which percutaneous cordotomy cannot be performed, the cord is already exposed for some other procedure, or a surgeon skilled in percutaneous cordotomy is not available.[41, 42] Many patients requiring cordotomy are too ill to travel far in pursuit of therapy.

Because the percutaneous technique subjects the patient to less impact than open cordotomy by whatever approach, mortality and morbidity are lower. A review of published experience with open cordotomy,[41] admittedly much of it in the older literature, suggested a mortality of 4 to 13.5 percent; significant paresis, 2 to 11 percent; bladder dysfunction, 3 to 23 percent; and satisfactory pain relief, 52 to 67 percent. These data can be compared with those presented below.

Although the open procedure is usually advocated in certain patients, such as children who are unable to cooperate for percutaneous cordotomy under local anesthesia, this author has performed percutaneous cordotomy with the patient under general anesthesia in 10 patients, as is discussed below, with results comparable to those of cordotomies performed with the patient under local anesthesia.

The only point of access to the cord for percutaneous cordotomy might be barred by congenital or acquired pathology, but the author has never encountered such a problem. Congenital anomalies[43–45] are well known in the cord and spinothalamic tract and can interfere with attempts to locate the spinothalamic tract; however, the author has had to resort to open cordotomy only once because of such a presumed anomaly since he learned the percutaneous technique.

The ease with which physiologic corroboration of electrode position can be achieved by the percutaneous technique with the patient under local anesthesia is a further endorsement of the percutaneous over the open technique. Finally, the ability to make a graded lesion with radiofrequency current, monitored by current flow, electrode temperature, and serial clinical testing, is impossible with the open technique.

CHOICE OF PERCUTANEOUS TECHNIQUE

Although several techniques for percutaneous cordotomy have been described, the original lateral high cervical approach of Mullan and coworkers[14] appears to have been most often employed and is the author's choice. Crue and associates[46] and Hitchcock[47] introduced a posterior high cervical approach that required the use of the Brown-Roberts-Wells and Hitchcock stereotactic frames. This author has no experience with this method, but according to Hitchcock, it can provide levels of analgesia as high as C2. Lin and coworkers[48] devised a low anterior approach specifically to avoid damage to the reticulospinal pathway that controls diaphragmatic respiration, which is the most serious complication of percutaneous cordotomy performed in the high cervical region. This technique, however, requires the cordotomy electrode to be introduced first across the disc, before the cord is impaled, so that in order to make a small alteration in the position of the electrode, the latter must be withdrawn and reinserted through the disc, a troublesome necessity. Physiologic observations and serial clinical testing may be used while the lesion is being made with the lateral high cervical approach to try to restrict a cordotomy lesion to lower body dermatomes. Because the reticulospinal tract lies adjacent to upper cervical spinothalamic dermatomes, respiratory problems are then avoided. When sparing of respiratory function is most essential, as in a patient with an apical thoracic lesion impinging on the brachial plexus and usually impairing contralateral lung and/or phrenic nerve function (the patient's respiratory function then depends on the integrity of ipsilateral lung function and control), a sufficiently high level of analgesia would not be possible with the low anterior technique to control the patient's pain.

Gybels[49] has suggested that cordotomy be considered in patients with cancer pain whose life expectancy is 2 to 5 months or longer (Table 129–3).

CONTRAINDICATIONS

Many contraindications to percutaneous cordotomy have already been mentioned. Obviously, the patient's general health must be such that he or she can be positioned supine and be subjected to intravenous sedation or intermittent general anesthesia; patients with problems such as bleeding diatheses must be excluded.

Table 129–3. GYBELS' NEUROSURGICAL INDICATIONS IN CANCER PAIN

Life Expectancy (months)	Procedure
1–2	CSF opioid infusion, percutaneous neurolytic procedures.
2–5	CSF opioid infusion, percutaneous neurolytic procedures. If these fail, cordotomy, if feasible, or other destructive surgery as the situation demands.
>5	Ablative procedures as above. PVG stimulation, CSF opioid infusion.

CSF = cerebrospinal fluid; PVG = periventricular gray.

More specifically, the patient's pain should lie below the junction of the C4-C5 dermatomes because high cervical cordotomy does not reliably produce a persistent level of analgesia higher than this. Preferably, the pain should predominate on one side, ideally in one leg, but if it is bilateral, bilateral cordotomy can be considered. We agree with Meyerson[50] that patients with midline trunk, especially perineal, pain respond in a disappointing fashion to even bilateral cordotomy.

However, the most important issue is that of respiratory contraindications. Effective respiration depends on neurologic control of breathing and the ventilatory function of the lungs. Neurologic control is directed to both the diaphragm and the intercostal muscles, the diaphragm being the most essential. Furthermore, such control is both voluntary and involuntary. Voluntary control is required when a patient is asked, for example, to take a deep breath. This act depends on innervation by the corticospinal tract and is impaired only when that structure is damaged. Survival, however, depends on unconscious breathing, not only during sleep but also during the pursuit of everyday tasks. We are not aware of, and do not voluntarily initiate, unconscious respiration; it is governed by brainstem reflexes. At the level of the cord, this function is mediated by the reticulospinal tract, which is strictly ipsilaterally distributed, meaning that if that tract is divided on one side of the cord, automatic respiration ceases in the ipsilateral lung. Loss of this automatic respiration in a single lung is not a serious event, provided that the remaining lung is functioning adequately and that its innervation for automatic respiration is intact. But if the lung contralateral to the proposed cordotomy has been totally or partially removed surgically, or if its function has been impaired by phrenic nerve paralysis or pulmonary disease, the patient may not survive loss of automatic innervation on the other side and may die from what has often been referred to as Ondine's curse. Percutaneous cordotomy by the high cervical approach should not be considered unless the patient can survive on the function of the lung on the opposite side to the cordotomy alone. As mentioned, the problem arises most often in patients with pain caused by cancerous involvement of the pulmonary apex and brachial plexus, in whom the lung is usually degraded by disease and the phrenic nerve paralyzed, as in the patient whose chest x-ray is shown in Figure 129–1. This is because the reticulospinal tract lies adjacent to the spinothalamic fibers of the upper cervical dermatomes, as shown in Figure 129–2; the necessarily high level of analgesia required to relieve the pain of the patient imaged in Figure 129–1 with Pancoast's syndrome will almost certainly damage the reticulospinal tract.

Apart from patients with apical cancer or other pulmonary disease, a second group at risk for pulmonary complications are those who have already undergone high cervical cordotomy on one side. Integrity of the reticulospinal tract on the side already operated on can be ascertained from clinical examination and is suspect if analgesia extends as high as the C4-C5-C6 dermatomes; cordotomy on the second side must not induce levels of analgesia into the cervical dermatomes lest the reticulospinal tract there also be severed. The level of analgesia may be confined to some extent to lower dermatomes, as is described under techniques, but not with certainty in every case.

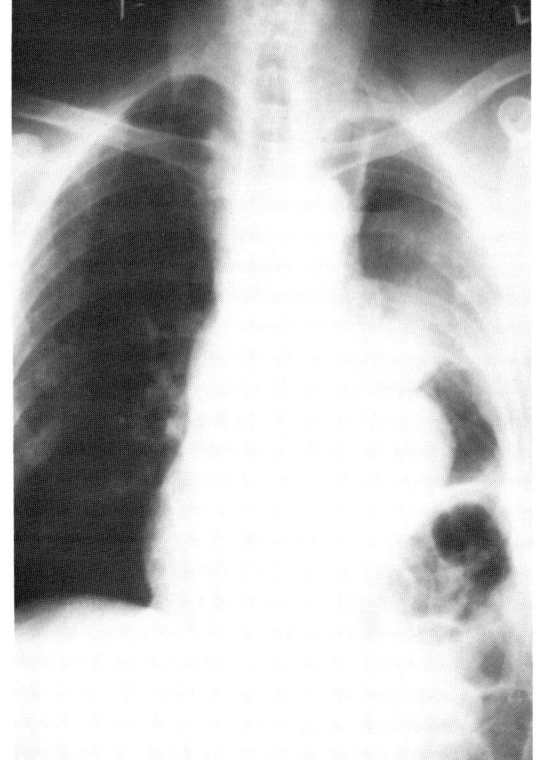

FIGURE 129–1. Anteroposterior chest x-ray study of a patient with intractable cervicobrachial pain from bronchogenic carcinoma (Pancoast's syndrome) with phrenic nerve paralysis and loss of left pulmonary tissue. A percutaneous cordotomy achieving a high enough level of analgesia to relieve the pain will interrupt the right reticulospinal path, eliminating automatic respiration in the only functioning lung.

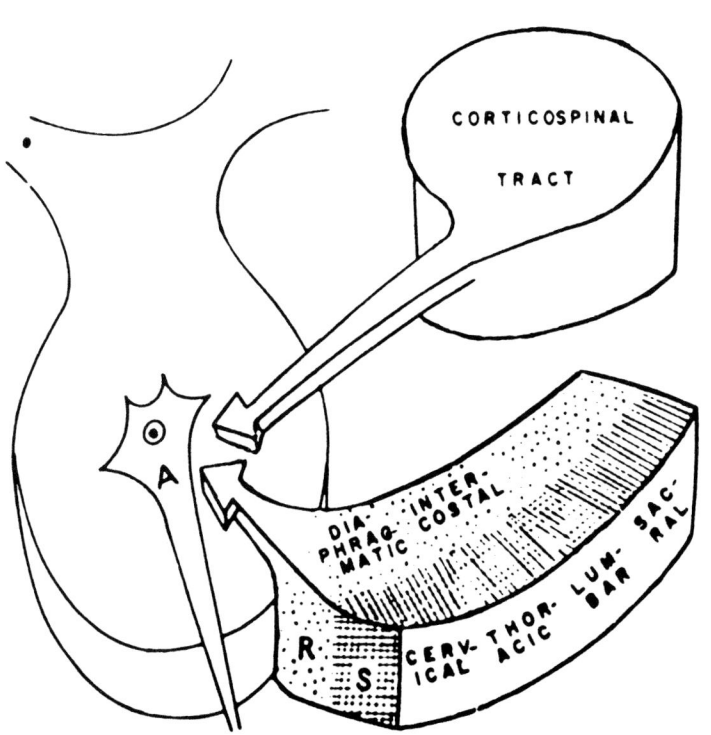

FIGURE 129–2. The relative positions of the corticospinal, reticulospinal (R), and lateral spinothalamic tracts (S) and their somatotopic organization in the human spinal cord at C1. Note that the spinothalamic fibers that originate most rostrally lie closest to the ventral horn, where they are closely associated with reticulospinal fibers that provide involuntary respiratory movement. (Reproduced with permission from Hitchcock E, Leece B: Somatotopic representation of the respiratory pathways in the cervical cord of man. J Neurosurg 27:320–329, 1967.)

ALTERNATIVES WHEN HIGH CERVICAL CORDOTOMY IS CONTRAINDICATED

For patients in whom percutaneous cordotomy is contraindicated, alternatives must be found; possibilities are listed in Table 129–4. The roles of percutaneous cordotomy by other than the lateral high cervical route and open cordotomy are indicated and have been discussed. Destructive procedures performed stereotactically or otherwise, of which mesencephalic tractotomy and medial thalamotomy are most often used, are less effective than cordotomy, expose the patient to greater mortality or morbidity, or both.[51] Frank and his associates,[52] however, advocate stereotactic mesencephalic tractotomy with at least the same enthusiasm as they do cordotomy.

The use of periventricular gray stimulation, unless performed transcutaneously with an external stimulator,[27] and implanted spinal or intraventricular morphine infusion systems, except those using a simple catheter-reservoir system, require expensive equipment that may be difficult to fund in a cancer patient with a short life expectancy.

TECHNIQUE

Successful execution of percutaneous cordotomy depends on adherence to a rigid protocol.

Table 129–4. ALTERNATIVES WHEN LATERAL HIGH CERVICAL PERCUTANEOUS CORDOTOMY IS CONTRAINDICATED

Reason for Contraindication	Alternative Procedure
Equipment or skills unavailable	Open cordotomy at T1-T2
Anomalies or disease prevent access in upper cervical region	Low anterior cervical percutaneous cordotomy
Patient uncooperative	General anesthetic
Patient has had unilateral cordotomy and has analgesia to C4-C5 level	High cervical percutaneous cordotomy with cautiously tailored lesion
	Low anterior cervical approach
	Open cordotomy at T1-T2
	Epidural spinal morphine catheter with reservoir
Patient's only functional lung and/or intact reticulospinal tract is on side of proposed cordotomy	If high level of analgesia is not required, same as in unilateral cordotomy and C4-C5 analgesia
	If high level of analgesia is required, spinal or intraventricular morphine infusion, PVG stimulation (dependent on life expectancy), stereotactic mesencephalic tractotomy, or medial thalamotomy
Analgesia above C5 required	If high level of analgesia is required, spinal or intraventricular infusion, PVG stimulation (dependent on life expectancy), stereotactic mesencephalic tractotomy, or medial thalamotomy
	High dorsal cervical percutaneous cordotomy
Patient has midline-bilateral truncal or pelvic pain	Spinal or intraventricular morphine infusion

PVG = periventricular gray.

PREOPERATIVE PREPARATION

Apart from the usual preparations for a neurosurgical procedure, the patient is brought to the operating room without presedation that would impair cooperation. Instead the patient has received the medications necessary for pain control to optimize execution of the approximately 90-minute procedure and its essential physiologic testing.

ANESTHESIA

Percutaneous cordotomy is usually performed with the patient under intravenous sedation, which should be at its maximum at two stages in the procedure: during insertion of the cordotomy electrode-needle assembly and during the making of the lesion. During the rest of the procedure, the patient should be kept comfortable but still able to report the results of physiologic testing. The patient should be lying quietly so as not to dislodge the electrode or lose the myelogram dye. Modern intravenous sedation has facilitated cordotomy, analgesia, anxiolysis, akinesis, autonomic and somatomotor areflexia, amnesia, and anesthesia and is achieved with combinations of narcotics, benzodiazepines, and intravenous anesthetic agents, such as propofol and etomidate, with adequate regional anesthesia.

POSITIONING

For optimal imaging, the patient should be positioned supine with the upper cervical spine precisely horizontal so as to entrap myelogram dye as long as possible. A strictly anteroposterior positioning is essential to eliminate parallax when the surgeon is working under image intensification; parallax results in penetration of the cord by the cordotomy electrode either anteriorly or posteriorly to the intended site. Positioning is facilitated by the use of a headholder, as shown in Figure 129–3, which, when fixed to the head of the operating table at such a height that its base constitutes a contin-

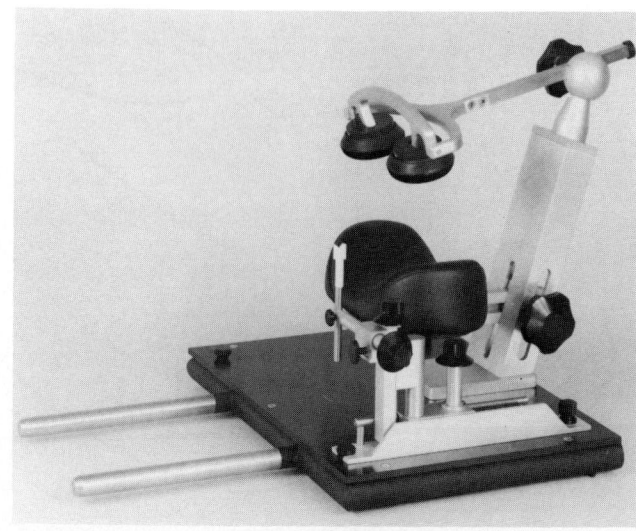

FIGURE 129–3. Head holder and mechanical stage for percutaneous cordotomy (available from Diros Technology, Toronto).

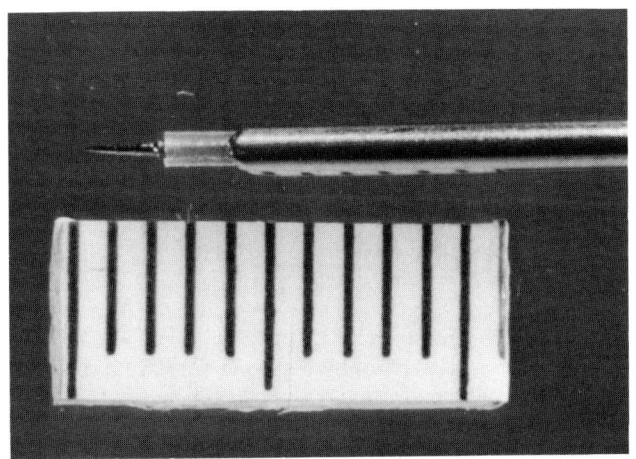

FIGURE 129–4. Percutaneous cordotomy electrode tip projecting 2 mm from introductory LP needle (scale in mm).

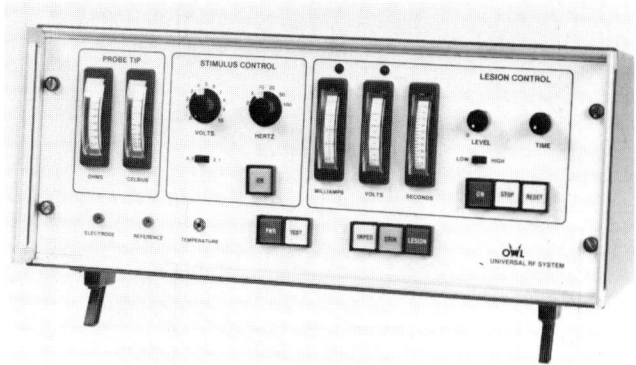

FIGURE 129–5. The OWL cordotomy system (available from Diros Technology, Toronto).

uation of the table top, holds the patient's head reasonably firmly and allows it to be raised or lowered as needed. The headholder is fitted with a three-dimensional mechanical stage to manipulate the position of the electrode and guide it to the desired location. Position is optimal when the C-arm of the image intensifier, passed under the head of the table, itself in a precisely horizontal position, yields a true lateral image of the C1-C2 interspace, into which the cordotomy electrode passes precisely horizontally. As with other procedures performed with the guidance of an image intensifier, the image should be arranged so that it moves in the same direction and plane as the operator's hands and instruments.

If surgery is performed frequently under x-ray guidance, the surgeon should wear lead-impregnated gloves to protect his or her hands.

CORDOTOMY EQUIPMENT

In addition to the headholder, a special cordotomy electrode-lumbar puncture needle assembly (Fig. 129–4) and matching electronic back-up system (Fig. 129–5) are required, such as that manufactured by Diros Technology (Diros Technology, 965 Pape Ave., Toronto, Canada M4K 3V6) or Radionics Corporation. (Radionics Corporation, P.O. Box 438, 76 Cambridge St., Burlington, MA).

The electrode provided by Diros (OWL cordotomy system) consists of a 0.4-mm, stainless steel wire insulated with shrink-fit polytetrafluoroethylene (Teflon) tubing and having an electrolytically sharpened 2-mm tip projecting beyond the tubing. This wire is matched with a thin-walled 18-gauge lumbar puncture needle so that 2 mm of polytetrafluoroethy-lene insulation projects beyond the tip of the LP needle when the electrode is locked into its hub. These dimensions are important to ensure reproducible electrical impedance readings as well as a fixed 2-mm penetration of the cord, which is arrested by the blunt end of the polytetrafluoroethylene tubing; 2 mm is the appropriate depth required to reach the spinothalamic tract. Electrodes are also available with temperature monitoring incorporated in them (Fig. 129–6). A monopolar electrode is used with a reference electrode that consists of a 23-gauge, 1.5-inch intramuscular needle inserted in the deltoid muscle on the side ipsilateral to the cordotomy. The electronic back-up system (see Fig. 129–4) is capable of measuring electrical impedance, recording temperature of the electrode tip, and delivering electrical stimulation from zero to 10 V over a range of 2 to 100 Hz, and radiofrequency current over prespecified intervals up to 90 seconds. During lesion making, current and voltage are monitored in addition to electrode tip temperature.

RADIOLOGIC LOCALIZATION AND IMPEDANCE MONITORING

After suitable preparation of the skin and, if necessary, wetting and retraction of the hair, the lumbar puncture needle is positioned precisely horizontally, as it rests on the mechanical stage of the headholder, with the image of its tip at the anteroposterior center of the C1-C2 space. It is advanced into the neck after local infiltration with 2-percent lidocaine under maximum intravenous sedation. The needle is steadily advanced, always horizontally, always aimed at the center of the C1-C2 space, as the surgeon's fingers detect penetration of neck muscles. A sense of resistance marks traversal of the ligamentum flavum and a smarter snap that of dura; penetra-

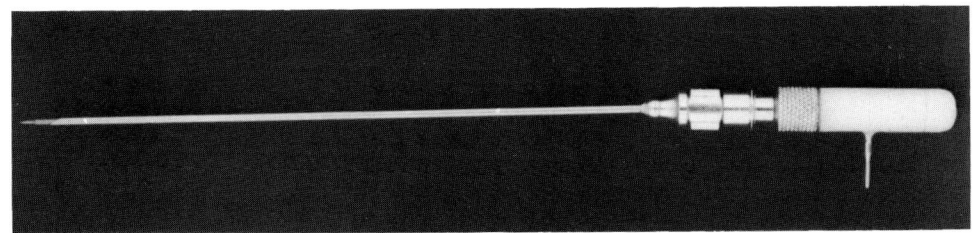

FIGURE 129–6. Percutaneous cordotomy electrode capable of temperature monitoring (available from Diros Technology, Toronto).

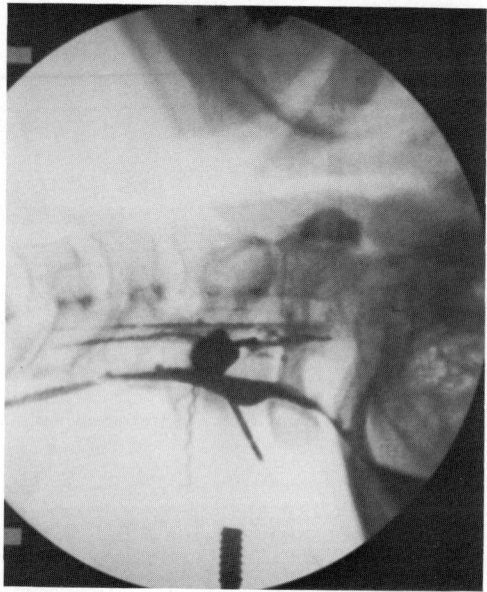

FIGURE 129–7. Lateral x-ray study showing cordotomy electrode tip just anterior to the dentate ligament (outlined with lipiodol). The ventral and dorsal root lines, anterior cord margin, and dorsal subarachnoid space are also outlined.

tion of the dura causes a brief twinge of more intense pain. The stylette of the lumbar puncture needle is periodically withdrawn to check for a flow of CSF as the needle is advanced; it is important not to go further once the subarachnoid space has been entered lest eventual control of cord penetration by the cordotomy electrode be hampered. The practice of infiltrating deeper structures with local anesthetic carries a risk of inducing a high spinal anesthetic that requires immediate intubation and ventilation for about 45 minutes, possibly with anticonvulsive therapy.

Once a flow of CSF has been obtained, an abrupt injection is made into the subarachnoid space of an emulsion consisting of equal volumes of air, CSF, and Lipiodol (ultra-fluid-ethiodinated oil with organically bound iodine, 38 percent w/w, Therapex Division E-2-EM Canada, Montreal, Canada*). A 10-cc syringe, connecting tubing, and a three-way stopcock are used for the injection. The electrode is locked into the lumbar puncture needle without loss of CSF (to avoid headache, vomiting, and loss of contrast medium), and the electrode-needle assembly is always positioned horizontally and aimed at the center of the C1-C2 space. Oil-based contrast media are essential for satisfactory cordotomy; water-soluble media provide only evanescent imaging. The contrast medium should identify the dentate ligament as a line of retained dye about the center of the C1-C2 space (Fig. 129–7), but other structures may also be visualized and cause confusion. The dorsal limit of the subarachnoid space is always seen, and sometimes, the anterior margin of the cord is seen as well. Well-defined linear images, such as the ventral and dorsal root lines, may be confused with the dentate ligament, particularly when the cord lies more ventrally or dorsally than expected. Finally, contralateral structures may sometimes also be visualized, adding to the confusion.

If the dentate ligament is not visualized, the lumbar puncture needle may be repositioned and a second injection made. In about a quarter of the procedures, visualization of the dentate ligament is not fully satisfactory, thereby increasing dependence on the physiologic corroboration of the position of the electrode.

Meyerson and von Holst[53] devised a flat-tipped cordotomy electrode that is capable of stimulating the surface of the spinal cord, enabling investigators to select the optimal site before penetration with the usual sharp electrode. The increasing difficulty of obtaining oil-based dye for myelography may be compensated for by performing cordotomy using CT guidance, as described by Kanpolat and coworkers[24] and Izumi and coworkers.[25]

Percutaneous cordotomy by the lateral high cervical approach can also be performed in the occipital C1 interspace, using the same guidelines.

Once adequate imaging has been achieved and the cordotomy electrode is locked into the hub of the lumbar puncture needle, the electrical impedance is checked. If the impedance is in excess of 400 W, suggesting that the cord has already been impaled, the position of the image of the electrode tip is checked. If it is not impinging on that of the dentate ligament, the electrode-needle assembly is carefully withdrawn until the impedance is about 400 W, signifying that the electrode tip is free in the subarachnoid space. A momentary 1- to 2-mm withdrawal of the electrode from the needle ensures disentanglement from cord structures. The lumbar needle must not be retracted too far and out of the subarachnoid space. When the electrode-needle assembly is free in the subarachnoid space, it is directed by use of the three-dimensional controls of the mechanical stage toward the image of the dentate ligament and is readvanced. As the cord is penetrated, with the electrode tip always directed toward the dentate ligament, the impedance should rise from about 400 W, a level characteristic of CSF, to 800 to 1200 W or more as the cord is impaled. During this stage, the surgeon's fingers appreciate an increased resistance, and the patient, forewarned, reports a brief twinge of pain in the neck near the needle penetration. The electrode-needle assembly is cautiously advanced to achieve a maximum impedance reading but not too far as the image of the electrode tip comes either to overlie that of the dentate ligament or to be situated very slightly anterior to it.

A common error in percutaneous cordotomy is to fail to detect cord penetration and to drive the electrode-needle assembly into the cord beyond the obstructing cuff of polytetrafluoroethylene tubing. This mishap occasionally results in neurologic complications, but the chief problem it creates is loss of control of the depth of penetration of the cord, for the resulting local contusion invalidates further impedance monitoring.

Should too deep a penetration occur, it is possible to proceed without impedance monitoring but better to direct the electrode more cephalad (even into the occipital-C1 space) or caudad in the C1-C2 interspace to attempt to find a fresh site. Localization of the percutaneous cordotomy electrode is a two-dimensional exercise at a 2-mm fixed penetration of the cord.

Sometimes, the electrode-needle assembly may pass anterior, less often posterior, to the cord, when the usual evidence of cord penetration, especially impedance rise, is not obtained.

---

*The manufacturer's instructions list drug contraindicated for intrathecal use because of the reported risk of late arachnoiditis.

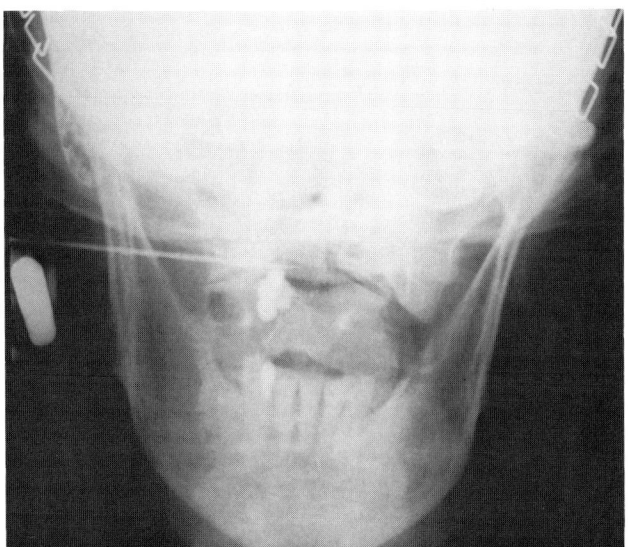

FIGURE 129–8. Anteroposterior x-ray study showing cordotomy electrode impaled in cord near midline of C1-C2 interspace.

If doubt arises about the depth of cord penetration, an anteroposterior spot x-ray to demonstrate the odontoid process through the open mouth conveniently demonstrates the position of the electrode tip. The tip, when properly positioned in spinothalamic tract, should lie at, or a few mm beyond, the midline of the dens, reflecting cord displacement by the thrust of the needle (Fig. 129–8).

PHYSIOLOGIC LOCALIZATION

Once the electrode-needle assembly is thought to be appropriately positioned, electrical stimulation is carried out. First, 2-Hz stimulation is delivered over a zero- to 10-V range, and motor responses are recorded; this recording can be performed while the patient is still too sedated to communicate readily. Table 129–5 lists possible responses and their significance. The patient may also report a "bumping" with such stimulation. It is difficult to account for the ipsilateral motor effects seen in musculature served by cervical roots when the electrode is stimulated at 2 Hz in the spinothalamic tract; they do not progress to tetanization at faster rates of stimulation. Possibly, they result from local reflexes inhibited at higher rates of stimulation.

Threshold motor responses elicited by 2-Hz stimulation in the spinothalamic tract in 136 recent cordotomies are summarized in Table 129–6. Thresholds averaged 2 to 6 V.

Once motor criteria support electrode position in the spinothalamic tract, 100-Hz stimulation is delivered over a zero- to 1-V range, with the patient alert enough to report the induced experience. Table 129–7 records the resulting responses and their significance, and Table 129–8, threshold responses obtained during 136 cordotomies with 100-Hz stimulation in the spinothalamic tract. Thresholds averaged 0.4 V.

It is always wise to increase 100-Hz stimulation to suprathreshold levels in a search for motor effects, to detect approximation of the electrode tip especially to leg corticospinal fibers, particularly if 100-Hz stimulation elicits ipsilateral paresthetic responses.

Very rarely, especially with the electrode located in the occipital-C1 space, ipsilateral paresthesias in the face occur from stimulation of the caudal trigeminal complex; ipsilateral paresthesias referred below the neck result from stimulation of the dorsal columns.

Figure 129–9 is a diagrammatic representation of the author's conception of the spinothalamic homunculus,[54] and Figure 129–10, the author's conception of the physiologic substrate of the percutaneous cordotomy technique.

Thus in the ideal cordotomy the following are observed:

1. Clear, persisting imaging of the ipsilateral dentate ligament, with the electrode tip impinging on it

Table 129–5. RESPONSES TO CORD STIMULATION AT 2 Hz

Response	Significance
No motor response 0–10 V	Defects in equipment Stimulator not turned on Patient's muscles paralyzed Gross misplacement of needle, probably not in subarachnoid space or at least outside cord
Response in contralateral side of neck, or stronger in contralateral than ipsilateral side	Electrode advanced too far
Responses in ipsilateral side of neck or accompanied by only weak response in contralateral side, often in trapezius, sternomastoid, or posterior nuchal muscles	Compatible with location either in anterior horn (especially if threshold < 1 V) or in spinothalamic tract (1–3 V) when contralateral sensory effects may be reported as well in 1 patient of 4
Responses in ipsilateral neck and upper limb	Compatible with location either in anterior horn (especially if threshold < 1 volt) or in spinothalamic tract (1–3 V) when contralateral sensory effects may be reported as well
Responses in ipsilateral upper limb or, especially, trunk or lower limb	Electrode likely in corticospinal tract

Table 129–6. THRESHOLD MOTOR RESPONSES AT 2 Hz IN SPINOTHALAMIC TRACT IN 136 RECENT CORDOTOMIES

Response (All Ipsilateral)	Incidence (%)	
Trapezius	39.8	
Trapezius and other neck, shoulder girdle muscles	1.2	
Trapezius and forearm	10.8	59.0
Trapezius and other upper limb	3.6	
Trapezius and other neck, shoulder girdle, upper limb muscles	2.4	
Trapezius, lower limb	1.2	
Posterior nuchal muscles	10.8	
Posterior nuchal and other girdle, neck muscles	2.4	
Posterior nuchal and upper limb muscles	7.2	20.4
Sternomastoid	1.2	
Lateral nuchal muscles	6.0	
Upper limb only	9.6	
No motor response	3.6	

Table 129-7. RESPONSES TO CORD STIMULATION AT 100 Hz

Response	Significance
No motor or sensory response	Defects in equipment
	Stimulator not turned on
	Patient's muscles paralyzed
	Gross misplacement of needle, probably not in subarachnoid space or at least outside cord
Tetanization of ipsilateral neck	Electrode in anterior horn
Tetanization of contralateral neck, or contralateral body below neck	Electrode has penetrated too deeply
Tetanization of ipsilateral side below neck	Electrode in corticospinal tract
No tetanization at threshold, possibly slight tetanization in ipsilateral leg at stimulation suprathreshold for contralateral sensory responses yielding a sensation of contralateral warmth, cold, rarely burning, pain or paresthesias referred usually to lower limb	Electrode is located in caudal dermatomes of spinothalamic tract where lesion tends to affect more caudal dermatomes of tract; slight risk of ipsilateral leg paresis
No tetanization, even suprathreshold, with contralateral sensory responses as above that are referred to hand	Electrode located centrally in spinothalamic tract, and lesion likely to produce extensive analgesia
No tetanization but contralateral sensory response as above in neck or upper trunk	Electrode located in most rostral dermatomes of spinothalamic tract and not likely to produce sufficient analgesia but, rather, suspended analgesia
No tetanization but ipsilateral sensory responses only	Explanation uncertain; may be subthreshold corticospinal responses; test suprathreshold stimulation
No tetanization but ipsilateral and contralateral sensory responses as above	Electrode position acceptable if suprathreshold stimulation does not induce tetanization and all other criteria are met

2. Impedance rise from about 400 to 1000 W as the cord is penetrated
3. Motor twitching at 2 Hz, 1 to 3 V in the ipsilateral neck, and sometimes also in the ipsilateral upper limb, possibly with a contralateral sensory response
4. No tetanization but a feeling of warmth or cold in the contralateral lower or upper limb at 100 Hz and 1 V or less

If less than ideal physiologic responses are obtained, the decision to make a lesion is dependent on ideal results with other features of the localization process.

If the decision is made to move the electrode, it is carefully withdrawn under impedance monitoring. Often, the impedance does not fall all the way to 400 W, a level that is characteristic of CSF, as the electrode is withdrawn a seemingly appropriate distance. Rather than risk withdrawal of the electrode-needle assembly entirely out of the subarachnoid space, it is best to unlock the electrode from the needle, keeping the needle fixed, and to withdraw the electrode back in the needle tip for a millimeter or two until the impedance falls to 400 W. The electrode is then readvanced and locked into the needle; the impedance usually remains at 400 W, indicating that it is free in the subarachnoid space. It is then ready to be manipulated (i.e., angulated) up or down through minute increments with the mechanical stage until the electrode tip impinges on the newly selected target. The whole process of localization is now repeated until acceptable physiologic responses occur. Exceptionally, more than two or three such manipulations may be necessary while the electrode-needle complex is kept within the subarachnoid space. If such repeated adjustments fail, the electrode-needle complex may be directed too anteriorly or posteriorly to allow penetration of the spinothalamic tract no matter how much angulation is employed. In that case, the whole assembly must be withdrawn from the neck, and the procedure must be begun all over again at a new penetration site.

Table 129-8. THRESHOLD SENSORY RESPONSES AT 100 Hz IN SPINOTHALAMIC TRACT IN 136 RECENT CORDOTOMIES

Response (All Contralateral)	Incidence (%)
Hot	27.4
Warm	7.7
Burning	28.2
Cold, cool	16.2
Paresthesia	1.7
Pain	6.8
Not described	12.0

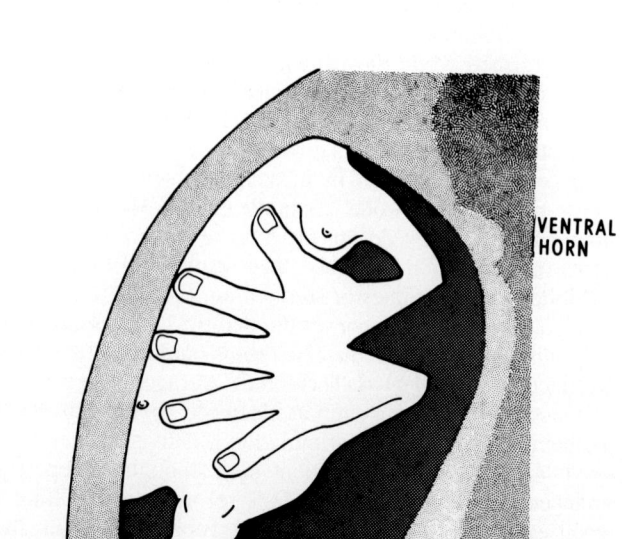

FIGURE 129-9. Somatotopographic organization of human spinothalamic tract at C1-C2.

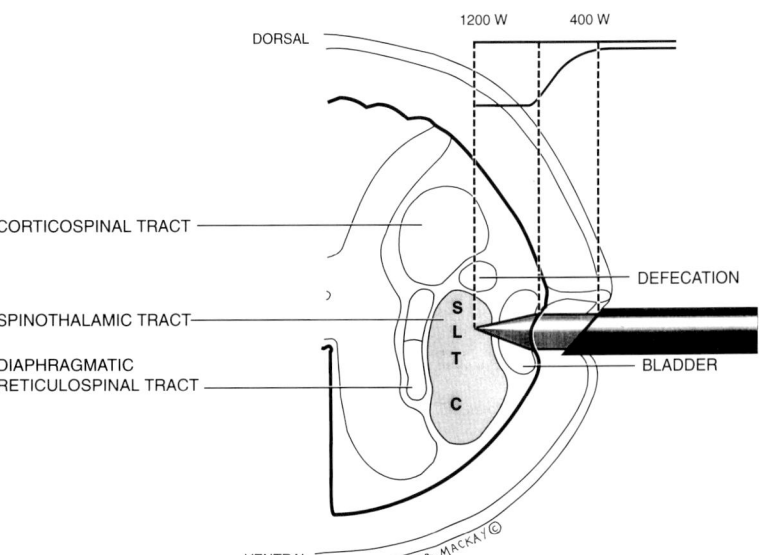

FIGURE 129–10. Percutaneous cordotomy showing impedance changes as the electrode is advanced and the anatomic relations of the spinothalamic tract. This view is oriented with the dorsal surface of the cord at the top, not as the surgeon encounters the structures with the patient in the supine position.

LESION MAKING

Once the electrode is located in the spinothalamic tract, the lesion is made. Because coagulating pia is painful, deep sedation or even brief anesthesia is again required at this stage. A minimal lesion is first made at 35 mA for 60 seconds (with the OWL equipment producing an electrode tip temperature of 60 to 75°C), following which motor and sensory function are examined as soon as the state of the patient allows. Usually, analgesia confirms proper electrode position; untoward findings, such as paresis, contraindicate lesion enlargement. Although the levels of analgesia and thermanalgesia usually match, dissociation has been reported, and minor differences in levels are common.[55, 56] If no complications occur, the lesion is enlarged in 10-mA increments to a typical maximum of 35 to 50 mA (mean, 35 mA), achieving tip temperatures of over 90°C (with the OWL equipment); serial clinical testing is repeated at each step. Because the initial lesioning coagulates the pia, enlargements can usually be made without further sedation. The maximum current and temperature are reached only over part of the 60 seconds of lesion making but probably should be maintained for at least 20 seconds to ensure an adequate lesion. Fall-off, indicating gas production around the electrode tip, which prevents further flow of current and enlargement of the lesion, occurs in about three quarters of cases in which these parameters are used. If fall-off occurs before the desired degree of analgesia is achieved, further enlargement may be made by slightly advancing the electrode-needle complex; otherwise, a new site for needle introduction is necessary, and all the above-described steps must be repeated from the beginning. In our current experience, a single lesion sufficed in 84 percent of patients, although in our first 244 cordotomies, one lesion was enough in only 61 percent of patients.

When the patient is tested at the end of the operation, there should be profound analgesia to both superficial and deep stimuli up to the desired level, and, particularly when pain affects the lower limb or pelvis, there should be no sacral sparing. If cordotomy on the opposite side is anticipated and the patient's pain is restricted to lower limbs and trunk, analgesia extending into the upper limbs is best avoided. In the operating room, examination may reveal paresis, especially in the ipsilateral lower limb, but in our experience, any patient who can still elevate the limb off the table, however weakly, will not suffer significant persistent disability. An ipsilateral Horner's syndrome (ptosis) may be noted as well as decreased excursion of the ipsilateral chest, usually transient, during involuntary respiration. Figure 129–11 illustrates a successful unilateral lesion whose dimensions fall somewhat short of those prescribed by Noordenbos and Wall.[7]

POSTOPERATIVE CARE

After the usual unilateral cordotomy, no special care is needed. The patient should remain in bed for 24 hours to minimize headache from CSF leakage, but then he or she should be assisted to walk, and some degree of unsteadiness from ipsilateral leg paresis should be anticipated. Bladder dysfunction should also be anticipated, and the patient should be catheterized as necessary until he or she is fully ambulant, when voluntary control is usually resumed. Depending on

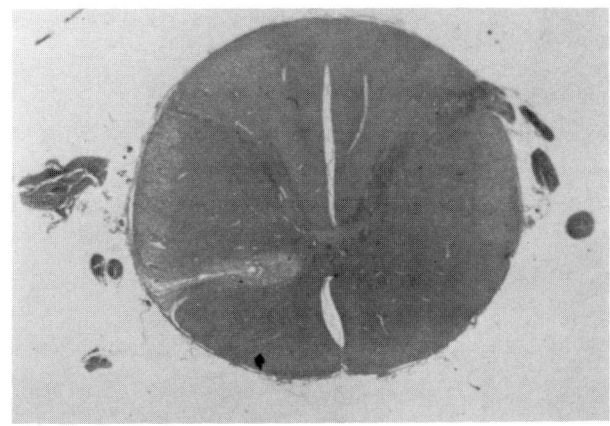

FIGURE 129–11. Transverse section of spinal cord at C1-C2 in a patient who died of his disease after unilateral percutaneous cordotomy. Hematoxylin and myelin stain.

the degree of pain relief, and with the likelihood of headache and neck pain kept in mind, analgesic medication is reduced. Opiate withdrawal, although best effected gradually, seldom results in withdrawal symptoms.

In patients who have had cordotomy on the second side or those with respiratory problems, postoperative monitoring, including that of arterial gases, in an intensive care facility is advisable for up to 3 days. Rising levels of arterial carbon dioxide particularly forewarn that ventilatory activity may be inadequate and could lead to ventilatory collapse when the medullary respiratory center ceases to respond. With ventilatory assistance, patients who develop respiratory difficulty usually recover in a few days to a week.

PERCUTANEOUS CORDOTOMY UNDER GENERAL ANESTHESIA

In children, confused patients, or others not likely to cooperate for cordotomy under local anesthesia, the procedure can be performed under general anesthesia. In fact, there are advantages to do so because positioning is facilitated and movement eliminated; muscular paralysis must be avoided so that motor effects from stimulation can be observed. The procedure is performed exactly as under local anesthesia except that perceived responses to 100-Hz stimulation are unavailable. Clinical testing for analgesia and possible paresis may be more difficult, but, with modern intravenous anesthesia techniques, the patient can usually be quickly awakened at the conclusion of the procedure.

Thus with the patient under general anesthetic, imaging, impedance monitoring, and 2-Hz stimulation are all performed as usual. If everything is in order and if no motor response is seen with 100-Hz stimulation, the lesion is made.

We have performed 10 cordotomies with the patients under general anesthesia, three on the second side. One cordotomy failed to induce analgesia, as had three previous cordotomies attempted under local anesthesia in that patient, possibly reflecting anomalous anatomy; one cordotomy produced a low level of analgesia and only partial pain relief. Seven of the nine procedures produced adequate levels of analgesia and excellent initial pain relief. The only complications were worsening of pre-existing bladder incontinence in a patient undergoing a procedure on the second side and one death from pre-existing disease (metastatic melanoma to brain and spine with paraplegia) 3 days postoperatively. Izumi and colleagues[25] reported on one case whose cordotomy was performed bilaterally in stages with the patient under general anesthesia; the patient died 1 day after surgery from gastrointestinal hemorrhage.

BILATERAL CORDOTOMY

Of the author's first 244 percutaneous cordotomies, 17.9 percent were performed bilaterally, as were 15.4 percent of the next 136. Three of the 136 were performed with the patient under general anesthetic. The technique for the second-side procedure is the same as for the first except for the following:

1. The two procedures should be performed at least 1 week apart.
2. At the time of the first procedure, analgesia in the upper cervical dermatomes should be avoided, if possible, if a second-side cordotomy is anticipated.
3. If analgesia from the first procedure extends no higher than the thoracic region, no particular precautions are necessary unless pulmonary disease is present.
4. If analgesia from the first side extends into the cervical dermatomes, cervical analgesia should be avoided on the second by restricting lesion size, by choosing a lesion site in the caudal spinothalamic dermatomes where contralateral sensations induced by 100-Hz stimulation are referred to the leg, or by performing the procedure by the low anterior cervical approach.

In a series of 136 cordotomies, 61.3 percent of patients with such lower limb sensory effects did not develop analgesia in the cervical dermatomes, whereas only 44.4 percent of those who reported stimulation-induced sensory effects in the upper limb failed to develop cervical analgesia. However, 61.2 percent of patients who developed cervical levels of analgesia had reported stimulation-induced sensory effects referred to a contralateral upper limb, 24.5 percent to a lower limb, and 14.3 percent to both, whereas 48.0 percent of patients with thoracic or lower levels of analgesia had reported upper limb, 38.0 percent lower limb, and 14.0 percent upper and lower limb sensory effects.

Two recent papers suggested that bilateral cordotomy may not be necessary as often as we might have believed. Ischia and colleagues[57] examined the results of unilateral cordotomy in 69 patients with pain caused by cancerous vertebral involvement, 47 of whom had unilateral pain. Of these, pain was totally relieved in 37 and partly in three. Seventeen patients (36 percent) were deemed as having an excellent result, and 17 (36 percent), a good result overall. Of the 22 patients with bilateral pain, 15 (68 percent) enjoyed a good result overall after unilateral cordotomy on the side opposite the worst pain.

Amano and coworkers[58] compared 161 unilateral and 60 bilateral percutaneous cordotomies and pointed out that bilateral cordotomy produced 95-percent clinically acceptable pain relief, and unilateral cordotomy produced 82-percent clinically acceptable pain relief. There was relatively little added risk in the bilateral over the unilateral group, no respiratory complications, and only a 6.7-percent incidence of urinary retention beyond the first week.

PERCUTANEOUS CORDOTOMY IN NONMALIGNANT DISEASE

Twelve percent of our cordotomies were performed for pain not caused by cancer and 7 percent for central pain of spinal cord origin.

In previous publications[59, 60] we have stressed the futility of cordotomy for the relief of pain caused by lesions in the nervous system, usually referred to as deafferentation, central, or neuropathic pain, including such pain when it is caused by cancer.[61] This issue was clearly recognized in 1969 by Rosomoff[62] and was reviewed by Tasker and Dostrovsky.[4] When the results of cordotomies in our earlier patients were reviewed, although results were similar immediately postoperatively in neuropathic and nociceptive pain (Table 129–9), we found the incidence of satisfactory longer-term pain relief to be strikingly lower in neuropathic pain.

Table 129-9. RESULTS OF PERCUTANEOUS CORDOTOMY IN PATIENTS WITH NOCICEPTIVE AND NEUROPATHIC PAIN

Type of Pain	Relief of Pain at Discharge from Hospital (%)		Relief of Pain at Latest Follow-up (%)	
	Complete	Partial	Complete	Partial
Nociceptive (n = 179)	90	6	70	12
Neuropathic (n = 15)	69	8	29	43
Mixed-neuropathic-nociceptive neuropathic element (n = 40)	72	8	53	16
Mixed-neuropathic-nociceptive nociceptive element (n = 40)	79	13	73	18

However, some patients had pain relief, and many reports in the literature described successful cordotomy in neuropathic pain syndromes.[5] Because our largest single group of such patients undergoing cordotomy had central pain caused by injuries of the spinal cord, we reviewed these patients more closely.[5] We found that they suffered from three common types of pain: steady, spontaneous pain (95 percent), intermittent, often shooting spontaneous pain (31 percent), and evoked pain (allodynia and hyperpathia) (47 percent). Intermittent pain was particularly common in patients with thoracolumbar injuries (T10-L1), whether complete or incomplete, and occurred in 57 percent of them, often shooting down one or both legs. Sixty-nine percent of the patients with cord central pain in our series who had intermittent pain had lesions in the thoracolumbar area.

When we examined the differential effects of cordotomy (in some cases by the open technique) on these three elements of cord central pain in 39 patients, steady spontaneous pain was relieved in 27 percent, intermittent spontaneous pain in 86 percent, and evoked pain in 75 percent. We concluded that destructive surgery (Nashold's DREZ procedure,[37] cordectomy,[38] and cordotomy) was statistically significantly more effective for the treatment of intermittent lancinating pain and for evoked pain than it was for steady pain; steady pain, on the other hand, responded best to chronic stimulation.

These operative results suggested that intermittent and evoked pain depended on transmission in spinothalamic pathways. In the case of intermittent pain, this transmission could arise from ectopic impulse generation, whereas in evoked pain, at least from peripheral lesions, it could result from perverted processing at the dorsal horn of normally transmitted impulses, resulting in activation of pain pathways.[63, 64]

We had, then, a rationale for selecting cordotomy to treat the intermittent shooting and evoked elements, but not the steady, usually burning or dysesthetic elements of neuropathic pain caused by cord lesions in keeping with many reports in the literature[5]; preliminary evidence suggests that the same principles apply to neuropathic pain caused by lesions other than cord lesions, an opinion also reached by Rosomoff.[62]

Finally, some patients with typically nociceptive pain not caused by cancer may be expected to respond to cordotomy in the same way as cancer patients.

RECURRENCE OF PAIN AFTER CORDOTOMY

Experience with patients undergoing cordotomy for nonmalignant disease offers the opportunity for long-term follow-up not usually possible with cancer patients. There were 39 such patients out of our series of 380 patients who underwent percutaneous cordotomy. We made a special study of 23 of these who suffered from central pain of cord origin, along with eight more who had undergone open cordotomy for this disorder. Among these 31 patients, we observed pain recurrence after intervals of 1, 1.1, 4, 5, 6, 7, 13, and 21 years, accompanied by gradual fading of the patients' analgesia. The same effect happened in one more patient with cerebral palsy after 4 years. Repetition of the cordotomy in six patients (five with cord injury, one with cerebral palsy) after 4, 4, 5, 6, 7, and 21 years restored the level of analgesia in all cases, but pain relief was recaptured only in three, an experience similar to that of Sam Lipton (Personal communication) and Nathan.[65] The explanation for these events remains a mystery because regeneration of spinothalamic tract fibers has never been demonstrated after cordotomy.

RESULTS

Success in cordotomy depends on many factors: the choice of patients (e.g., steady neuropathic pain is not relieved), the criteria used to describe success, the accuracy of the surgical technique, the length of follow-up, and the attention paid to the many reasons for pain persistence or recurrence after cordotomy. These problems are not capable of complete reconciliation between reported series.

TECHNICAL SUCCESS

First, one must examine technical success: How often was the surgeon able to locate and lesion the spinothalamic tract and how often was this adequately achieved? These data are rarely reported in the literature. In 95.5 percent of a series of 380 percutaneous cordotomies performed by the author using a standardized technique, a lesion was made in the spinothalamic tract on the first attempt—in 99 percent of patients when the results of a second attempt were included. In 2.6 percent of the 99 percent, the level of analgesia fell or faded within a few days, necessitating early repetition of the procedure. Thus, 98 percent of patients were discharged with apparently adequate analgesia that persisted until at least the first post-discharge follow-up in 93 percent. Rosomoff[62] reported that 81 percent of his *bilateral* percutaneous cordotomies were technically adequate on the first attempt, 93 percent after any repetitions.

PAIN RELIEF

However, only 88 percent of the author's procedures resulted in total pain relief, and 94.4 percent in significant relief postoperatively, whereas 72 percent resulted in total pain relief, and 84.2 percent in significant relief at latest follow-up. Thus, after 28 percent of procedures, some pain persisted in the area to which the cordotomy was directed, not to mention pain outside that area of the body, such as new pain above the level of analgesia and new or increased pain on the other side of the body.

Persistent, Recurrent, and New Postoperative Pain

In an attempt to better understand the reason for recurrent, persistent, or new pain after cordotomy, we carried out a special review of 136 procedures. After 12 percent of these, the patient continued to complain of pain on the operative side that appeared to be nociceptive in origin. In 7 percent, levels of analgesia were inadequate, but in the remaining 5 percent, the pain was unexplicable; in these patients, the pain was apparently persistent nociceptive pain below an apparently adequate level of analgesia. An additional 2 percent developed new pain above their analgesic level as a result of progression of disease. In 6.1 percent of patients, persistent pain (present preoperatively) below an apparently adequate level of analgesia had not been properly diagnosed preoperatively as constant neuropathic pain. A further 33.7 percent with some degree of persistent or new pain below an apparently adequate level of analgesia had neuropathic pain accompanying their nociceptive pain preoperatively or else developed it postoperatively from progression of cancerous damage to the lumbosacral plexus. Cordotomy selectively removed the nociceptive pain and unmasked the neuropathic pain. One percent developed postcordotomy dysesthesia.

Mirror or Ipsilateral Pain

The most interesting group was the 40.8 percent with new or worsened pain on the opposite side of the body. This phenomenon has been widely recognized and was reported in 9 percent,[66] 28 percent,[67] 36 percent,[68] 47.8 percent,[57] 56.3 percent,[69] and 63.3 percent[70] of patients. Various explanations include release by cordotomy of ipsilateral pain previously present but masked by the more severe contralateral pain[71] and various neurophysiologic phenomena.[66,67] Nathan[67] noted that of 33 patients who developed ipsilateral pain after cordotomy, nine had a potential ipsilateral cause. Nagaro and colleagues[68] reported on a patient who developed mirror pain within 6 hours of percutaneous cordotomy that worsened within a week until it reached the same level as the original pain. They observed that it was accompanied by allochiria, reference of painful pinching but not of pinprick or nonnoxious stimuli, from the analgesic to the contralateral side. The fact that the mirror pain and the allochiria were blocked by intrathecal phenol in the somatotopic area affected by the block suggested a spinal mechanism. This concept is supported by Ischia and Ischia,[72] who stated that during percutaneous cordotomy, they observed that mirror pain could be induced by pinprick until the lesion had been enlarged to an adequate size and that the same phenomenon was seen transiently for 24 to 48 hours after percutaneous cordotomy. Bowsher[66] studied three patients of 13 who had undergone successful percutaneous cordotomy but developed mirror pain, one severely. Naloxone, 0.8 mg, given intravenously to all 13 patients, increased mirror pain in one of the three who had it and induced it in another who did not suffer from it spontaneously. Bowsher concluded that such mirror pain is the result of neurophysiologic processes at the cord level. Nagaro and associates[73] studied the phenomenon of allochiria and found it in seven of 66 patients who underwent percutaneous cordotomy. Allochiria appeared immediately after induction of analgesia and disappeared when analgesia faded. It was elicited only from analgesic areas and was experienced either at the same or a more cephalad dermatomal level on the contralateral body. Each patient demonstrating allochiria also developed new contralateral, usually mirror, pain after cordotomy, and in one patient subarachnoid phenol block temporarily relieved both. Nagaro and associates proposed that both allochiria and new mirror pain depended on loss, through cordotomy, of feedback inhibition of a subsidiary pain pathway.

Postcordotomy Dysesthesia

After percutaneous cordotomy, some patients complain of usually transient burning or dysesthetic pain in the ipsilateral neck near the site of the cordotomy that is usually attributed to neuropathic pain from involvement of the C2 root. Such pain occurred in 3.1 percent of our initial 244 cases at the time of discharge from the hospital, and it persisted in 1.6 percent at later follow-up.

More serious is postcordotomy dysesthesia, usually a causalgic or dysesthetic discomfort that appears after a latent interval in all or part of the body rendered hypalgesic or analgesic. It occurred in 1 percent of our series of 136 patients who were examined for the presence of postoperative pain and in 1.5 percent of our earlier 244 patients at the time they left hospital. However, 8.6 percent complained of this problem at the time of latest follow-up, half of them to a severe degree. Typically, postcordotomy dysesthesia takes time to develop.

Postcordotomy dysesthesia is a type of central pain with all the same characteristics as other pain syndromes caused by cord lesions and may be confused with neuropathic pain caused by the patient's cancer. The latter is usually localized to an area of motor, reflex, and/or sensory change related to destruction of part of the lumbosacral plexus or of spinal roots.

Postcordotomy dysesthesia is reported in the literature in 6 percent[74] to 20 percent[76] of patients; data in many series are difficult to interpret.

Table 129–10 lists the reported incidence at the time of latest follow-up of complete and of significant but not complete relief of the pain to which the percutaneous cordotomy was directed for selected series of patients. Mirror, neuropathic, or new pain arising above a level of analgesia or postcordotomy dysesthesia, discussed earlier, are not taken into account.

COMPLICATIONS

Table 129–11 lists the author's complications and, according to the author's interpretation of the manuscripts, those reported in the literature after unilateral and bilateral percutaneous cordotomy.

Table 129-10. REPORTED PERCENTAGE OF PAIN RELIEF AFTER UNILATERAL PERCUTANEOUS CORDOTOMY

	Complete	Significant
Tasker	72	84.2
Meglio and Cioni[76]	79	—
Lahuerta and coworkers[74]	64	87
Kühner[75]	—	59
Siegfried and coworkers[77]	—	75
Lipton[78]	75	—
Ischia and coworkers[70]	—	81.1
Lorenz[79]	75	96
Amano and coworkers[58]	64	82
Ischia and coworkers[57]	—	71
Farcot and coworkers[82]	—	89

Death is nearly always the result of respiratory failure and, in the author's hands, disappeared as a complication of unilateral cordotomy once its mechanism was fully understood. Relatively high figures reported by some authors for mortality and respiratory complications reflect their aggressive use of cordotomy for pain of thoracobrachial origin in whom the risks are recognized to be high. Horner's syndrome, a cosmetic problem, is usually transient.

Cancer patients undergoing cordotomy are often terminally ill and may die of their disease within 30 days of cordotomy. Authors usually do not include such deaths in their mortality figures for cordotomy; the incidence reflects the choice of patients for surgery. In the author's series, 0.5 percent of patients died of their disease within 1 month of operation. Ischia and coworkers[80] reported such mortality in 11 percent of patients in the first week.

Thus, at present, the irreducible significant risks of unilateral cordotomy are postcordotomy dysesthesia and impairment of bladder function. The mechanism of the former is unknown; the latter results from the close approximation of the neurologic pathway for bladder control to the spinothalamic tract (see Fig. 129-10).

BILATERAL CORDOTOMY

In the author's bilateral cordotomies, 71.4 percent experienced significant bilateral relief of pain at follow-up, the square of the rate (84.2 percent) for the unilateral procedure. Ischia and colleagues[80] reported 47 percent complete relief and 59 percent significant bilateral relief in his series; Amano and colleagues, 76 percent complete relief and 95 percent significant relief; and Rosomoff,[62] 58 percent complete relief and 77 percent satisfactory relief in patients surviving 3 months.

Complications are reviewed in Table 129-11. These are largely what would be expected from patients who have undergone two cordotomies except for the respiratory risks, which account for the increased mortality, and for the greatly enhanced risk of impairing bladder function, which was seen in 12 to 58 percent.

CONCLUSION

Percutaneous cordotomy by the lateral high cervical technique is a precise, reproducible, and successful procedure if performed with a rigid protocol, affording an 84-percent rate

Table 129-11. PERCENTAGE OF REPORTED COMPLICATIONS AFTER PERCUTANEOUS CORDOTOMY

Complication	Unilateral Cordotomy								Bilateral Cordotomy					
Death from cordotomy (respiratory only)	0.3	5	4	0	0	1.4	0	0.6	1.6	10	0	27.2	0	2
Severe respiratory failure	0	—	2.6	—	—	—	—	0.6	0	20	—	29.2	0	2
Significant transient respiratory failure	0.3	—	—	3.9	—	—	—	2.4	3.2	—	—	—	0	—
Mild respiratory problems	1.2	—	—	—	—	—	—	—	1.6	—	—	4.5	—	—
Significant paresis or ataxia	1.0	4	2	2.9	8	10.1	16	—	1.6	—	1.8	13.6	0	5
Mild or transient paresis or ataxia	17.9	6.9	—	32.0	100	—	4.7	4.3	29.5	—	36.1	—	—	39
Significant worsening of bladder function	3.5	3	3	8.7	—	7.2	—	—	21.3	12	58	18.1	6.7	2
Minor, transient bladder decompensation	7.0	19	—	—	—	—	10.5	6.1	9.8	—	—	—	—	15
Transient bowel incontinence	2.1	—	—	—	—	—	—	—	9.8	—	—	—	—	—
Transient hypotension	1.8	—	—	—	—	—	—	—	8.1	40	36.1	—	—	4
Horner's syndrome	23.0*	100	—	—	—	94	42	most	23†	—	100	59	common	—
Other, significant	0.3	—	—	—	—	—	—	—	1.6	—	—	—	—	—
Other, transient, minor	0.6	—	—	—	—	—	—	—	1.6	—	—	—	—	—
Contralateral limb weakness	0	6	—	—	—	—	—	—	0	—	—	—	—	—
Reference	—	74	75	69	77	57	82	83‡	—	75	80	81	58	62

*Present in 10.9% at follow-up.
†Present in 5.0% at follow-up.
‡19 of 163 patients operated on bilaterally.

of significant relief of nociceptive pain (usually caused by cancer) per side at the time of follow-up. It is also useful (and easier to perform than the DREZ operation) for the intermittent neuralgic-like pain of thoracolumbar cord injury. Significant unavoidable complications are postcordotomy dysesthesia, which is significant in about 5 percent, and significant worsening of bladder function in 3 percent.

Success and risks in the bilateral procedure are the square of those for the unilateral, except for respiratory and bladder function.

The procedure has fallen into disuse because of the enthusiasm for morphine infusions, but it needs to be re-evaluated in appropriate cancer patients. It usually substitutes a once-only procedure for the continuous care required for morphine infusions and eliminates risks of tolerance-induced escalating drug requirements.

REFERENCES

1. Tasker RR, Organ LW, Hawrylyshyn P: Deafferentation and causalgia, in Bonica JJ (ed): Pain. New York, Raven, 1990, pp 305–329.
2. Tasker RR: Deafferentation pain, in Wall PD, Melzack R (eds): Textbook of Pain. Edinburgh, Livingstone, 1984, pp 119–132.
3. Tasker RR: Pain resulting from central nervous system pathology (central pain), in Bonica JJ (ed): Management of Pain in Clinical Practice, 2nd ed. Philadelphia, Lea & Febiger, 1989, pp 264–283
4. Tasker RR, Dostrovsky JO: Deafferentation and central pain, in Wall PD, Melzack R (eds): Textbook of Pain, 2nd ed. Edinburgh, Churchill Livingstone, 1989, pp 154–180
5. Tasker RR, DeCarvalho GTC, Dolan EJ: Intractable pain of spinal cord origin: Clinical features and implications for surgery. J Neurosurg 77:373–378, 1992
6. Willis WD: The pain system: The neural basis of nociceptive transmission in the mammalian nervous system, in Gildenberg PL (ed.): Pain and Headache, vol 8. Basel, Karger, 1985
7. Noordenbos W, Wall PD: Diverse sensory functions with an almost totally divided spinal cord. A case of spinal cord transection with preservation of one anterolateral quadrant. Pain 2:185–195, 1976
8. Wall PD: The design of experimental studies in the future development of restorative neurology of altered sensation and pain, in Dimitrijevic MR, Wall PD, Lindblom U (eds): Recent Achievements in Restorative Neurology 3: Altered Sensation and Pain. Basel, Karger, 1990, pp 197–205
9. Nathan PW: Touch and surgical division of the anterior quadrant of the spinal cord. J Neurol Neurosurg Psychiatry 53:935–939, 1990
10. Lahuerta J, Bowsher D, Campbell J, Lipton S: Clinical and instrumental evaluation of sensory function before and after percutaneous anterolateral cordotomy at cervical level in man. Pain 42:23–30, 1990
11. Di Piero V, Jones AKP, Iannotti F, et al: Chronic pain: A PET study of the central effects of percutaneous high cervical cordotomy. Pain 46:9–12, 1991
12. Spiller WG: The occasional clinical resemblance between caries of the vertebrae and lumbothoracic syringomyelia and the location within the spinal cord of the fibres for the sensations of pain and temperature. Univ Penn Med Bull 18:147–154, 1905
13. Spiller WG, Martin E: The treatment of persistent pain of organic origin in the lower part of the body by division of the anterolateral column of the spinal cord. JAMA 58:1489–1490, 1912
14. Mullan S, Harper PV, Hekmatpanah J, et al: Percutaneous interruption of the spinal pain tract by means of a strontium 90 needle. J Neurosurg 20:931–939, 1963
15. Rosomoff HL, Carroll E, Brown J, Sheptak P: Percutaneous radiofrequency cervical cordotomy: Technique. J Neurosurg 23:639–644, 1965
16. Sweet WH, Mark VH, Hamlin R: Radiofrequency lesions in the central nervous system of man and cat: Including case reports of eight bulbar pain-tract interruptions. J Neurosurg 17:213–225, 1960
17. Gildenberg PL, Zanes C, Flitter MA, et al: Impedance monitoring device for detection of penetration of the spinal cord in anterior percutaneous cervical cordotomy. Technical note. J Neurosurg 30:87–92, 1969
18. Hitchcock ER, Tsukamoto Y: Distal and proximal sensory responses during stereotactic spinal tractotomy in man. Ann Clin Res 5:68–73, 1973
19. Taren JA: Physiologic corroboration in stereotactic high cervical cordotomy. Confin Neurol 33:285–290, 1971
20. Taren JA, Davis R, Crosby EC: Target physiologic corroboration in stereotactic cervical cordotomy. J Neurosurg 30:569–584, 1969
21. Tasker RR, Organ LW: Percutaneous cordotomy. Physiological identification of target site. Confin Neurol 35:110–117, 1973
22. Tasker RR, Organ LW, Smith KC: Physiological guidelines for the localization of lesions by percutaneous cordotomy. Acta Neurochir Suppl (Wien) 21:111–117, 1974
23. Onofrio BM: Cervical spinal cord and dentate delineation in percutaneous radiofrequency cordotomy at the level of the first to second cervical vertebrae. Surg Gynecol Obstet 133:30–34, 1971
24. Kanpolat Y, Deda H, Akyar S, Bilgic S: CT-guided percutaneous cordotomy. Acta Neurochir Suppl (Wien) 46:67–68, 1989
25. Izumi J, Hirose Y, Yazaki T: Percutaneous trigeminal rhizotomy and percutaneous cordotomy under general anesthesia. Stereotact Funct Neurosurg 59:62–68, 1992
26. Richardson PE, Akil H: Pain reduction by electrical brain stimulation in man: Part II. Chronic self-administration in periventricular grey matter. J Neurosurg 47:184–194, 1977
27. Meyerson BA, Boëthius J, Carlson AM: Percutaneous central gray stimulation for cancer pain. Appl Neurophysiol 41:57–65, 1978
28. Hitchcock ER: Stereotactic cervical myelotomy. J Neurol Neurosurg Psychiatry 33:224–230, 1970
29. Hitchcock ER, Leece B: Somatotopic representation of the respiratory pathways in the cervical cord of man. J Neurosurg 27:320–329, 1967
30. Nathan PW: The descending respiratory pathway in man. J Neurol Neurosurg Psychiatry 26:487–499, 1963
31. Belmusto L, Brown E, Owens G: Clinical observations on respiratory and vasomotor disturbances as related to cervical cordotomies. J Neurosurg 20:225–232, 1963
32. Belmusto L, Woldring S, Owens G: Localization and patterns of potentials of the respiratory pathways in the cervical spinal cord in the dog. J Neurosurg 22:277–283, 1965
33. Fox JL: Localization of the respiratory pathway in the upper cervical spinal cord following percutaneous cordotomy. Neurology 19:1115–1118, 1969
34. Mullan S, Hosobuchi Y: Respiratory hazards of high cervical percutaneous cordotomy. J Neurosurg 28:291–297, 1968
35. Rosomoff HL, Krieger AJ, Kuperman AS: Effects of percutaneous cervical cordotomy on pulmonary function. J Neurosurg 31:620–627, 1969
36. Tenicela R, Rosomoff HL, Feist J, et al: Pulmonary function following percutaneous cervical cordotomy. Anesthesiology 29:7–16, 1968
37. Nashold BS Jr, Ostdahl RH: Dorsal root entry zone lesions for pain relief. J Neurosurg 51:59–69, 1979
38. Jefferson A: Cordectomy for intractable pain in paraplegia. Persistent Pain 4:115–132, 1983
39. Probst CL: Microsurgical cordotomy in 20 patients with epi-/intradural fibrosis following operation for lumbar disc herniation. Acta Neurochir (Wien) 107:30–36, 1990
40. Poletti CE: Open cordotomy medullary tractotomy, in Schmidek HH, Sweet WH (eds): Operative Neurosurgical Techniques: Indications, Methods and Results, 2nd ed. Orlando, Grune & Stratton, 1988, pp 1155–1168
41. Tasker RR: Open cordotomy, in Krayenbühl H, Maspes PE, Sweet WH (eds): Progress in Neurological Surgery. Pain, Its Neurosurgical Management, pt 11, vol 8. Basel, Karger, 1977 pp 1–14
42. Tasker RR: The merits of percutaneous cordotomy over the open operation, in Morley TP (ed): Current Controversies in Neurosurgery. Philadelphia, WB Saunders, 1976, pp 496–501
43. Morley TP: Congenital rotation of the spinal cord. J Neurosurg 10:690–692, 1953
44. Voris HC: Ipsilateral sensory loss following cordotomy. Report of a case. Arch Neurol Psychiatry 65:95–96, 1957
45. Voris HC: Variations in the spinothalamic tract in man. J Neurosurg 14:55–60, 1957
46. Crue BL, Todd EM, Carregal EJA: Posterior approach for high cervical percutaneous radiofrequency cordotomy. Confin Neurol 30:41–52, 1968
47. Hitchcock ER: An apparatus for stereotactic spinal surgery. A preliminary report. J Neurosurg 31:386–392, 1969

48. Lin RM, Gildenberg PL, Polakoff PP: An anterior approach to percutaneous lower cervical cordotomy. J Neurosurg 25:553–560, 1960
49. Gybels JM: Indications for the use of neurosurgical techniques in pain control, in Bond MR, Charlton JE, Woolf CJ (eds): Proceedings of the VI World Congress on Pain. Amsterdam, Elsevier, 1991, pp 475–482
50. Meyerson BA: Problems and controversies in PVG stimulation and sensory thalamic stimulation as treatment for pain, in Fields HL, Besson JM (eds): Progress in Brain Research 77. Amsterdam, Elsevier, 1988, pp 175–188
51. Tasker RR: Stereotactic surgery, in Wall, PD, Melzack R (eds): Textbook of Pain, 3rd ed. Edinburgh, Churchill Livingstone, 1994, pp 1137–1157
52. Frank F, Fabrizi AP, Gaist G: Stereotactic mesencephalic tractotomy in the treatment of chronic cancer pain. Acta Neurochir (Wien) 99:38–40, 1989
53. Meyerson BA, von Holst H: Extramedullary impedance monitoring and stimulation of the spinal cord surface in percutaneous cordotomy. Technical note. Acta Neurochir (Wien) 107:63–64, 1990
54. Tasker RR: Somatotopographic representation in the human thalamus, midbrain, and spinal cord. The anatomical basis for the surgical relief of pain, in Morley TP (ed): Current Controversies in Neurosurgery. Philadelphia, WB Saunders, 1976, pp 485–495
55. Sherman IC, Arieff AJ: Dissociation between pain and temperature in spinal cord lesions. J Nerv Ment Dis 108:285–292, 1948
56. Stookey B: Human chordotomy to abolish pain sense without destroying temperature sense. J Nerv Ment Dis 69:552–557, 1929
57. Ischia S, Luzzani A, Ischia A, Pacini L: Role of unilateral percutaneous cervical cordotomy in the treatment of neoplastic vertebral pain. Pain 19:123–131, 1984
58. Amano K, Kawamura H, Tanikawa T, et al: Bilateral versus unilateral percutaneous high cervical cordotomy as a surgical method of pain relief. Acta Neurochir Suppl (Wien) 52:143–145, 1991
59. Tasker RR, Organ LW, Hawrylyshyn PE: Deafferentation and causalgia, in Bonica JJ (ed): Pain Research Publications, Association for Research in Nervous and Mental Disease, vol 58. New York, Raven, 1980, pp 305–329
60. Tasker RR: Percutaneous cordotomy—the lateral high cervical technique, in Schmidek HH, Sweet WH (eds): Operative Neurosurgical Techniques. Indications, Methods and Results. New York, Grune & Stratton, 1982, pp 1137–1153
61. Tasker RR: The problem of deafferentation pain in the management of the patient with cancer. J Palliat Care 2:8–12, 1987
62. Rosomoff HL: Bilateral percutaneous radiofrequency cordotomy. J Neurosurg 31:41–46, 1969
63. Lindblom U: Assessment of abnormal evoked pain in neurological patients and its relation to spontaneous pain: A descriptive and conceptual model with some analytic results, in Fields HL, Dubner R, Cervero F (eds): Advances in Pain Research and Therapy, vol 9. New York, Raven, 1985, pp 409–423
64. Woolf CJ: Excitability changes in central neurons following peripheral damage: Role of central sensitization in the pathogenesis of pain, in Willis W (ed): Hyperalgesia and Allodynia. New York, Raven, 1992, pp 221–243
65. Nathan PW: Results of antero-lateral cordotomy for pain in cancer. J Neurol Neurosurg Psychiatry 26:353–362, 1963
66. Bowsher D: Contralateral mirror-image pain following anterolateral cordotomy. Pain 33:63–65, 1988
67. Nathan PW: Reference of sensation at the spinal level. J Neurol Neurosurg Psychiatry 19:88–100, 1956
68. Nagaro T, Kimura S, Arai T: A mechanism of new pain following cordotomy: Reference of sensation. Pain 30:89–91, 1987
69. Ischia S, Ischia A, Luzzani A, et al: Results up to death in the treatment of persistent cervico-thoracic (Pancoast) and thoracic malignant pain by unilateral percutaneous cervical cordotomy. Pain 21:339–355, 1985
70. Ischia S, Luzzani A, Ischia A, et al: Subarachnoid neurolytic block (L5-S1) and unilateral percutaneous cervical cordotomy in the treatment of pain secondary to pelvic malignant disease. Pain 20:139–149, 1984
71. Ventafridda V, DeConno F, Fochi C: Cervical percutaneous cordotomy, in Bonica JJ, Ventafridda V, Pagni CA (eds): Advances in Pain Research and Therapy, vol 4. New York, Raven, 1982, pp 185–198
72. Ischia S, Ischia A: A mechanism of new pain following cordotomy (letter). Pain 32:383–384, 1988
73. Nagaro T, Amakawa K, Kimura S, Arai T: Reference of pain following percutaneous cervical cordotomy. Pain 53:205–211, 1993
74. Lahuerta T, Lipton S, Wells JCD: Percutaneous cervical cordotomy: Results and complications in a recent series of 100 patients. Ann R Coll Surg Engl 67:41–44, 1985
75. Kühner A: La cordotome percutanée. Sa place actuelle dans la chirurgie de la douleur. Anesth Analg 38:357–359, 1981
76. Meglio M, Cioni B: The role of percutaneous cordotomy in the treatment of chronic cancer pain. Acta Neurochir (Wien) 59:111–121, 1981
77. Siegfried J, Kühner A, Sturm V: Neurosurgical treatment of cancer pain. Recent results. Cancer Res 89:148–155, 1984
78. Lipton S: Percutaneous cervical cordotomy. Acta Anaesthesiol Belg 32:81–85, 1981, with additional personal communication
79. Lorenz R: Methods of percutaneous spinothalamic tract section, in Krayenbühl H (ed): Advances and Technical Standards in Neurosurgery, vol 3. Vienna, Springer, 1976, pp 123–145
80. Ischia S, Luzzani A, Maffezzoli G: Bilateral percutaneous cervical cordotomy: Immediate and long-term results in 36 patients with neoplastic disease. J Neurol Neurosurg Psychiatry 47:141–147, 1984
81. Koulousakas A, Nittner K: Bilateral C1-C2 cordotomies. Can complications be avoided? Appl Neurophysiol 45:500–503, 1982
82. Farcot J-M, Mercky F, Tritschler J-L, Schaeffer F: Cordotomies cervicales percutanées dans les douleurs cancéreuses thoraciques primitives ou secondaires (a propos de 19 cas). Agressologie 29:87–89, 1988
83. Palma A, Holzer J, Cuadra O, Palma J: Lateral percutaneous spinothalamic tractotomy. Acta Neurochir (Wien) 93:100–103, 1988

CHAPTER 130

Microsurgical DREZotomy

Marc P. Sindou

In the 1960s, a large number of anatomic and physiologic investigations on the spinal cord[1] drew attention to the dorsal root entry zone (DREZ) as the first level of modulation for pain sensation. These works convinced the author to consider DREZ as a possible target for pain surgery and, in 1972, to undertake anatomic studies and preliminary surgical trials in humans to determine whether or not a destructive procedure at this level was feasible.[2] The first attempt at surgery in the DREZ occurred in March 1972 for the pain associated with Pancoast's syndrome. Several other patients with cancer were operated on soon after. Because the first results in the management of pain associated with certain malignancies were encouraging, we decided in the same year to attempt to perform the procedure in patients with noncancerous pain syndromes, namely, paraplegia, amputation-associated pain, and brachial plexus injury.

RATIONALE

The DREZ is defined as an anatomic entity that includes the central portion of the dorsal root, the tract of Lissauer, and the dorsal-most layers of the dorsal horn, where the afferent fibers articulate with the cells from which the ascending extralemniscal pathways originate (Fig. 130–1).[2]

THE DORSAL ROOTLETS

Each dorsal root divides into 4 to 10 rootlets of 0.25 to 1.50 mm in diameter, according to their level. Each rootlet can be considered an anatomic-functional entity, that is, a root in miniature.

Anatomic studies[3] revealed a spatial segregation of afferent fibers in the DREZ according to their sizes and destinations (Figs. 130–2 and 130–3). The lateral regrouping of the fine fibers allows them to be preferentially interrupted without destruction of the large fibers.

Whether all nociceptive fibers reach the spinal cord through the dorsal roots is unclear. Anatomic and electrophysiologic studies in animals showed that about 30 percent of the fibers in the ventral roots were afferent C axons originating from the dorsal root ganglion cells and projecting into the dorsal horn. These findings, which challenged the Bell-Magendie law, have recently been clarified. Most (but not all) of the central root afferents do not actually enter the cord through the lamina cribrosa of the ventral root but instead make a U-turn to reach the dorsal horn via the dorsal root.[4]

LISSAUER'S TRACT

The tract of Lissauer, which is situated dorsolaterally to the dorsal horn, comprises a medial part, which the small afferents enter and where they trifurcate to reach the dorsal horn, either directly or through a two-metamere ascending or descending pathway; and a lateral part, through which a large number of longitudinal endogenous propriospinal fibers interconnect different levels of the substantia gelatinosa.

The tract of Lissauer plays an important role in the intersegmental modulation of the nociceptive afferents: its medial

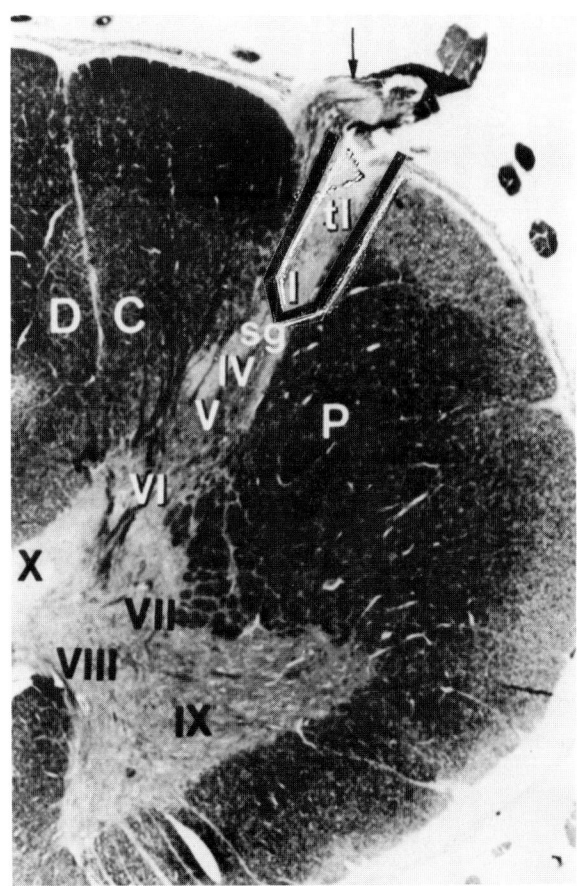

FIGURE 130–1. Rexed's lamination (I to IX). Transverse hemisection of the spinal cord at the lower cervical level with myelin stained by luxol-fuschine showing the myelinated rootlet afferents that reach the dorsal column. DC = dorsal column, P = pyramidal tract, Sg = substantia gelatinosa, tl = tract of Lissauer. The small arrow designates the pial ring of the dorsal rootlet (diameter: 1 mm). The large arrowhead shows MDT target.

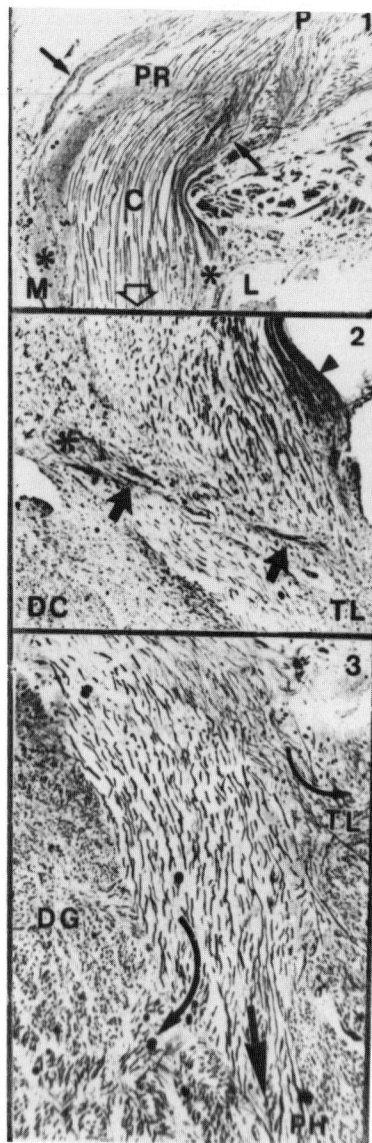

FIGURE 130–2. Course of nerve fibers at the DREZ in humans. The diameter of these cervical rootlets chosen as examples is 1 mm. Axons stained by the Bodian method. (1) Longitudinal section *before entry* into the spinal cord. At the peripheral segment (P), the large and small fibers have no particular organization. Just before the pial ring (PR), the small fibers reach the rootlet surface (arrows), mostly in the lateral region (L). In the central segment (C), the small fibers are arranged in two bundles (asterisk) located on either side of the large fibers. (2) Longitudinal section *at the entry* into the spinal cord. The large fibers constitute the center of the rootlet and run toward the dorsal column (DC). The small fibers form two bundles. One is lateral (triangle) and the other medial (asterisk). The medial portion runs obliquely across the rootlet (arrows) to reach the tract of Lissauer (TL). Thus, most of the small fibers are regrouped at the lateral region of the DREZ. (3) Longitudinal section of the rootlet with its *afferent endings* in the spinal cord. The large lemniscal fibers (thick curved arrow) are grouped medially to enter the dorsal column (DC). The large myotatic fibers (straight arrow) penetrate deeper into the posterior horn (PH) to reach the ventral horn. The small nociceptive fibers (thin curved arrow) are regrouped laterally to enter the TL. (From Sindou M: Etude de la jonction radiculomedullaire posterieure: La radicellotomie posterieure selective dans la chirurgie de la douleur. Lyon, Thesis, University Claude-Bernard, 1972; and Sindou M, Quoex C, Baleydier C: Fiber organization at the posterior spinal cord–rootlet junction in man. J Comp Neurol 153:15–26, 1974. Copyright © 1974 J Comp Neurol. Reprinted by permission of John Wiley & Sons, Inc.)

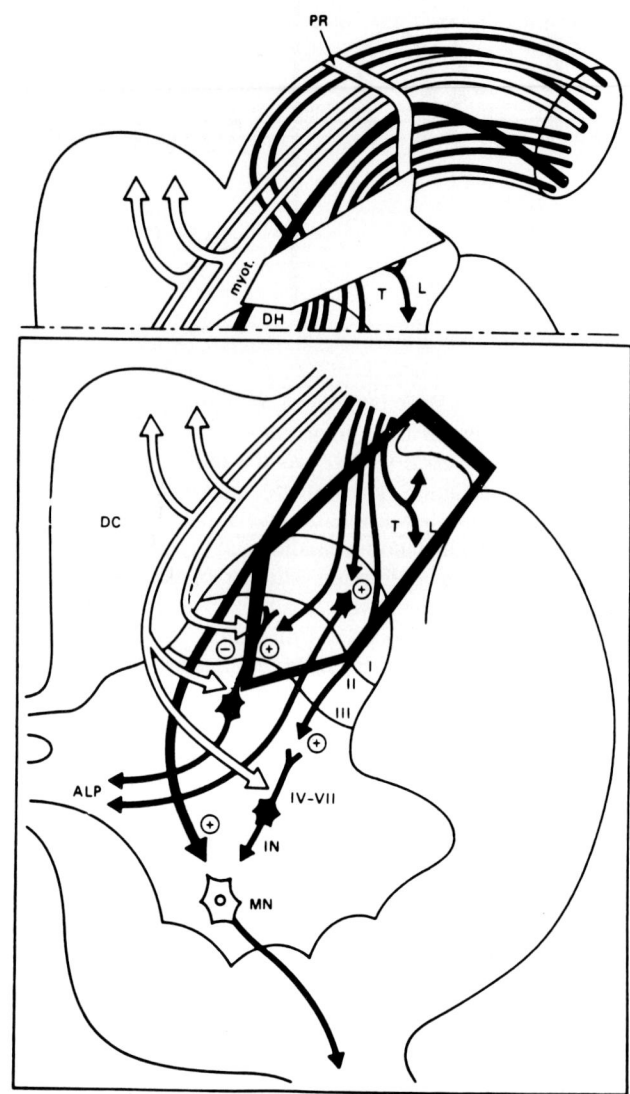

FIGURE 130–3. Schematic representation of the DREZ area and target of microsurgical DREZotomy (MDT).

(Upper Part) Each rootlet can be divided, owing to the transition of its glial support, into a peripheral and a central segment. The transition between the two segments is at the pial ring (PR), which is located approximately 1 mm outside the penetration of the rootlet into the dorsolateral sulcus. Peripherally, the fibers are mixed together. As they approach PR, the fine fibers, considered nociceptive, move toward the rootlet surfaces. In the central segment, they group in the ventrolateral portion of the DREZ to enter the dorsal horn (DH) through the tract of Lissauer (TL). The large myotatic fibers (myot) are situated in the middle of the DREZ, whereas the large lemniscal fibers are located dorsomedially.

(Lower Part) Schematic data on DH circuitry. Note the monosynaptic excitatory arc reflex, the lemniscal influence on a DH cell and an interneuron (IN), the fine fiber excitatory input onto DH cells and the IN, the origins in layer I and layers IV to VII of the anterolateral pathways (ALP), and the projection of the IN onto the motoneuron (MN). DC = dorsal column. Rexed laminae are marked from I to VI. MDT (arrowhead) cuts most of the fine and myotatic fibers, and enters the medial (excitatory) portion of LT and the apex of the dorsal horn. It should preserve most lemniscal presynaptic fibers, the lateral (inhibitory) portion of TL, and most of the DH. (From Sindou M: Etude de la jonction radiculomedullaire posterieure: La radicellotomie posterieure selective dans la chirurgie de la douleur. Lyon, Thesis, University Claude-Bernard, 1972; and Sindou M, Quoex C, Baleydier C: Fiber organization at the posterior spinal cord–rootlet junction in man. J Comp Neurol 153:15–26, 1974. Copyright © 1974 J Comp Neurol. Reprinted by permission of John Wiley & Sons, Inc.)

part transmits the excitatory effects of each dorsal root to the adjacent segments, and its lateral part conveys the inhibitory influences of the substantia gelatinosa into the neighboring metameres.[5] Thus, selective destruction of the medial part should cause a reduction in the regional excitability of the nociceptive afferents.

THE DORSAL HORN

Most of the fine nociceptive afferents enter the dorsal horn through the medial part of the tract of Lissauer and the dorsal aspect of the substantia gelatinosa. Cajal's recurrent collaterals of the large lemniscal fibers approach the dorsal horn through the ventral aspect of the substantia gelatinosa.[6] Because the dendrites of some of the spinoreticulothalamic cells make synaptic connections with the primary afferents inside the substantia gelatinosa layers, the substantia gelatinosa exerts a strong segmental modulating effect on nociceptive input. When the large lemniscal afferents within peripheral nerves or dorsal roots are altered, a reduction in the inhibitory control of the dorsal horn occurs.[1] This situation presumably results in excessive firing of the dorsal horn neurons (Fig. 130–4). This phenomenon, thought to be the origin of deafferentation pain, has been identified in patients by electrophysiologic recordings[7, 8] and has been reproduced in animal experiments.[9, 10] Destruction of these hyperactive neurons should suppress the nociceptive impulses generated in the spinoreticulothalamic pathways.

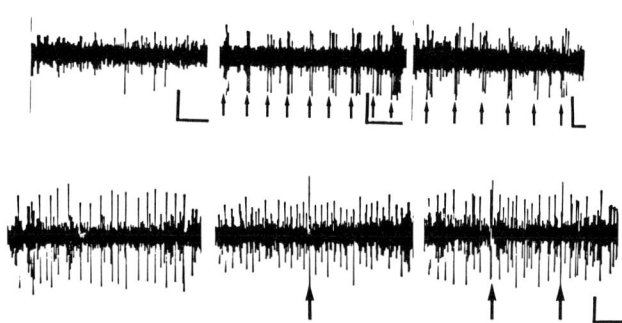

FIGURE 130–4. Dorsal horn microelectrode recordings in humans. The electrode used was a floating tungsten microelectrode that was implanted intraoperatively by free hand under the operative microscope, 5 mm in depth (i.e., in laminae IV to VI). The vertical bars are 50 μV, and the horizontal bars are 100 msec.
(Upper Trace: Normal Activity). Recordings in a non-deafferented dorsal horn (spastic patient). (Left) Almost no spontaneous activity (three spikes at random). (Middle) Spike burst discharges (arrows) evoked by regular light tactile stimulation of the corresponding dermatome and (Right) by electrical stimulation of the corresponding peripheral nerve.
(Lower Trace: Deafferentation Hyperactivity). Recordings in the L5 cord segment of a patient with pain due to a traumatic section of the hemicauda equina from root L4 to S4. (Left) Spontaneous activity of the recorded unit: continuous, regular, high-frequency discharge. (Middle) Unit during light tactile stimulation of the L4 to S1 dermatomes (arrow) and (right) during electrical stimulation of the tibial nerve (the arrows are two consecutive stimuli). Note the continuous regular discharges, which remain unaltered. (From Jeanmonod D, Sindou M, Magnin M, Baudet M: Intraoperative unit recordings in the human dorsal horn with a simplified floating microelectrode. Electroencephalogr Clin Neurophysiol 80:477–489, 1991.)

PRINCIPLES OF THE METHOD

Based on these anatomic and physiologic data, the procedure consists of a microsurgical incision and bipolar coagulations, performed ventrolaterally at the entrance of the rootlets, into the dorsolateral sulcus, and along all the spinal cord segments selected for surgery. The lesion, which penetrates the lateral part of the DREZ and the medial part of the tract of Lissauer, extends down to the apex of the dorsal horn, which is recognized by its brown-gray color. The average lesion is situated 2 mm deep and at a 45-degree angle medially and ventrally (see Fig. 130–3).

The procedure is presumed to preferentially destroy the nociceptive fibers grouped in the lateral bundle of the dorsal rootlets, as well as the excitatory medial part of the tract of Lissauer. The upper layers of the dorsal horn are also destroyed if microbipolar coagulations are performed inside the dorsal horn. The procedure is presumed to preserve at least partially the inhibitory structures of the DREZ, that is, the lemniscal fibers reaching the dorsal column, as well as their recurrent collaterals to the dorsal horn and the substantia gelatinosa propriospinal interconnecting fibers running through the lateral part of the tract of Lissauer. The method, called microsurgical DREZotomy (MDT), was conceived to prevent complete abolition of tactile and proprioceptive sensations and to avoid deafferentation phenomena.

SURGICAL ANATOMY

Working in the DREZ requires a minimal knowledge of morphologic anatomy. Details of this anatomy have been given in previous publications.[11, 12]

Poorly individualized on leaving the ganglion, the rootlets separate approximately 1 cm before they penetrate the dorsolateral sulcus. They remain joined, however, by fine leptomeningeal membranes, but these are easily separated with microdissection.

The dorsal roots, which have a mostly symmetrical distribution, show different types of division and penetration of their rootlets according to their spinal level:

1) The posterior element of C1 (1 mm in diameter) exists in 80 percent of cases.

2) The superior cervical roots (C2-C4) divide into an average of four rootlets, which are approximately 0.75 mm in diameter and are well separated from one another. Each rootlet has a cylindrical type of penetration.

3) The inferior cervical roots (C5-C8) usually divide into six rootlets, which have a diameter of 1.50 mm. They are juxtaposed against one another, and they also have a cylindrical type of penetration.

4) The thoracic roots divide into an average of five small-diameter rootlets (approximately 0.25 mm) and are very widely spaced. Penetration is filiform, or ribbon shaped.

5) The superior lumbar roots (L1-L3) divide into an average of 8 to 10 well-grouped rootlets. Often, each rootlet subdivides further into several small secondary filiform rootlets with diameters of less than 0.25 mm. They penetrate the sulcus separately. This type of penetration is called filiform penetration.

6) The lumbosacral roots (L4-S3) usually divide into seven rootlets that are approximately 1.50 mm in diameter.

At entry into the spinal cord, they are often imbricated. Penetration is usually cylindrical.

7) The sacrococcygeal roots (S4-C0), often adherent to the filum terminale, usually divide into three very slender rootlets with diameters of less than 0.25 mm. Penetration is filiform. Sometimes, coccygeal nerve bundles are included in the fibrous sheath of the filum.

Before it deeply penetrates into the spinal cord, a rootlet sometimes takes a subpial course that is superficial to but three quarters embedded in the spinal cord tissue. This course can run as long as 1 mm along the dorsolateral sulcus, and such a segment cannot be dissected, as is frequently the case in the lower part of the cord, where the rootlets are obliquely orientated.

The angulation of the DREZ lesion is determined by the axis of the dorsal horn in relation to the sagittal plane crossing the dorsolateral sulcus. According to 82 measurements (Young RF: Personal communication, 1991), the mean DREZ angle is 30 degrees at C6, 26 degrees at T4, 37 degrees at T12, and 36 degrees at L3.

The site and extent of the DREZ lesion is also determined by the shape, width, and depth of Lissauer's tract and the dorsal horn, as is shown in Figure 130–5.

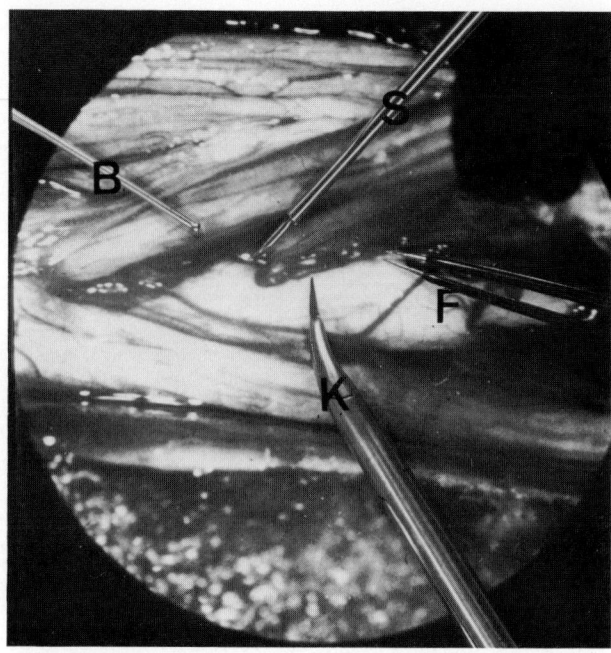

FIGURE 130–6. Technical principles of MDT and necessary instruments. Exposure of the dorsolateral aspect of the conus medullaris on the left side. The rootlets of the selected dorsal roots are retracted dorsomedially and held with a (specially designed) ball-tipped microsucker (B), used as a small hook, to gain access to the ventrolateral part of the DREZ. After division with curved sharp microscissors (S) of the fine arachnoidal filaments that stick the rootlets together with the pia mater, the main arteries running along the dorsolateral sulcus are dissected and preserved, while the smaller ones are coagulated with a pair of sharp bipolar microforceps (F). Then the incision is performed using a microknife (K), made with a small piece of razor blade inserted within the striated jaws of a curved razorblade holder (K). On average, the cut is at a 45-degree angle, descending to a depth of 2 mm. The surgical lesion is completed by performing microcoagulations under direct magnified vision at a low intensity inside the incision down to the apex of the dorsal horn. These microcoagulations are made by means of the special sharp bipolar forceps (F), which are insulated, except at the tip, over 5 mm and graduated every millimeter.

SURGICAL TECHNIQUE

Surgery is performed with the patient under general anesthesia, but with only an initial short-lasting curarization, to allow intraoperative observation of motor responses to electrical stimulation of the nerve roots. Roots are identified by electrical stimulation consisting of bipolar neurostimulation with an increasing intensity (from 0.1 to 2 mA). Stimulated ventral roots have a motor threshold at least three times lower than dorsal roots.

Standard microsurgical techniques are used with 10 to 25 × magnification. Special microinstruments for MDT have been made by Leibinger-Fischer (Freiburg, West Germany) (Fig. 130–6).

OPERATIVE PROCEDURE AT THE CERVICAL LEVEL (Fig. 130–7)

The sitting position with the patient's neck in flexion offers the surgeon a comfortable approach and lessens oozing because of the consequent lower venous pressure in the cervicocephalic region. However, the prone position, with the

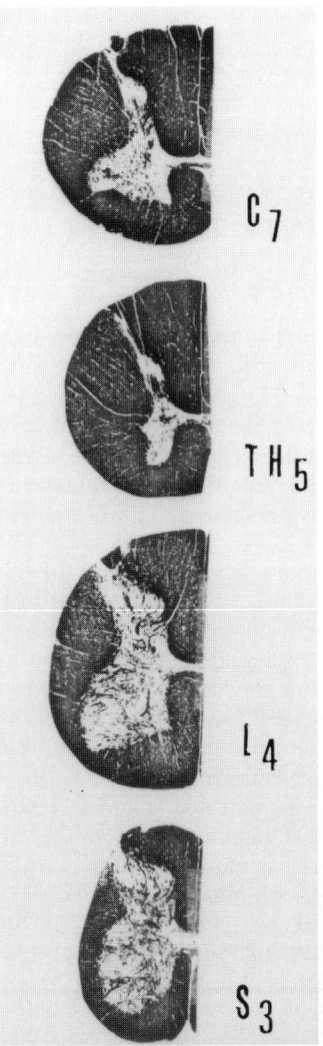

FIGURE 130–5. Variations of shape, width, and depth of the DREZ area, according to the spinal cord level.

Microsurgical DREZotomy | 1617

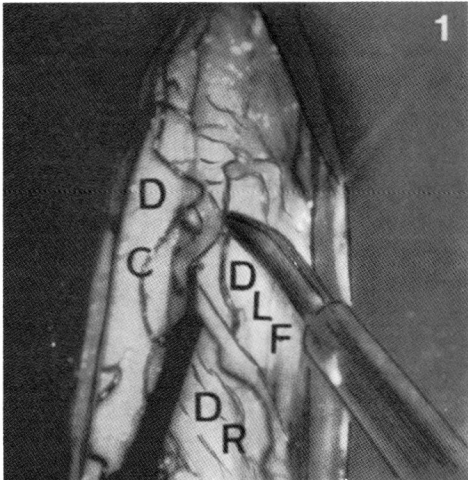

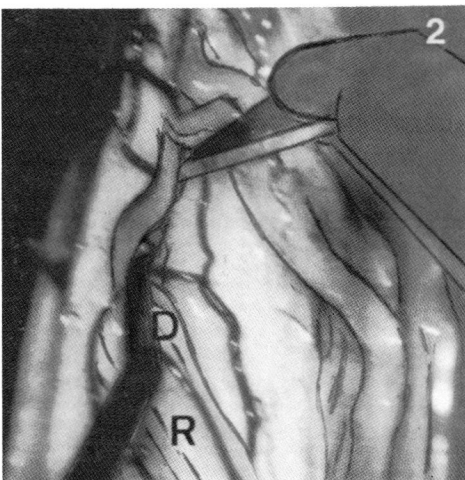

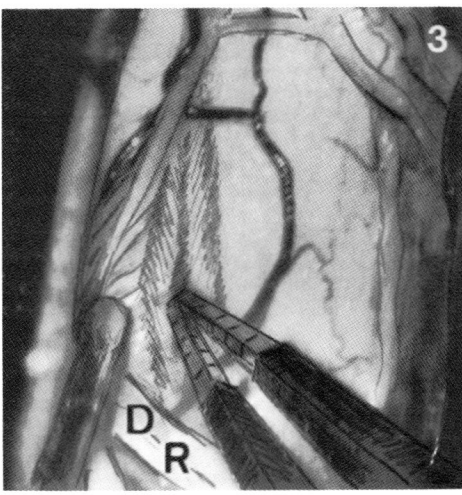

FIGURE 130-7. MDT technique at the cervical level. Exposure of the right dorsolateral aspect of the cervical cord at C6. (1) The rootlets of the selected dorsal root (DR) are displaced dorsally and medially with a hook or a microsucker to obtain access to the ventrolateral aspect of the DREZ in the dorsolateral sulcus. Using microscissors, the arachnoid adhesions are cut between cord and dorsal rootlets. DC = Dorsal cord, DLF = dorsolateral funiculus. (2) After having coagulated exclusively the tiny pial vessels, an incision of 2 mm in depth, at 45 degrees ventrally and medially, is made with a microknife in the lateral border of the dorsolateral sulcus. (3) Then microcoagulations are performed down to the apex of the dorsal horn using a sharp, graduated bipolar microforceps.

patient's head and neck flexed in the Concorde position, has the advantage of avoiding brain collapse due to cerebrospinal fluid (CSF) depletion, especially in patients with brain atrophy. Because of the lower incidence of drowsiness, mental confusion, and headaches after operation with the patient in the prone position, its use is preferred in most patients. The sitting position is still used in individuals with a short, fat neck. Whatever the position, the head is always fixed with a three-pin head holder.

The level of laminectomy is determined after identification of the prominent spinous process of C2 by palpation. A hemilaminectomy, generally from C4 to C7, with preservation of the spinous processes, allows sufficient exposure to the posterolateral aspect of the cervical spinal cord segments that correspond to the upper limb innervation, that is, the rootlets of C5 to T1 (T2).

After the dura and the arachnoid are opened longitudinally, the exposed roots and rootlets are dissected free by separation of the tiny arachnoid filaments that bind them to each other, to the arachnoid sheath, and to the spinal cord pia mater. The radicular vessels are preserved.

Each ventral and dorsal root from C4 to T1 is electrically stimulated at the level of its corresponding foramen to identify precisely its muscular innervation and its functional value. Responses are in the diaphragm for C4 (the response is palpable below the lower ribs), in the shoulder abductors for C5, in the elbow flexors for C6, in the elbow and wrist extensors for C7, and in the muscles of the hand for C8 and T1.

Microsurgical lesions are then performed at the selected levels, that is, those that correspond to the pain territory. The attachment of the rootlets to the spinal cord is sufficiently solid to allow them to be retracted posteriorly and medially to give ventrolateral access to the DREZ. The best way to retract and sustain the rootlets is to use a ball-tip microsucker. Then, the small pial vessels at this level are separated and moved, whenever possible, or coagulated by means of a sharp bipolar forceps, thus allowing the incision to be made without bleeding. The incision is made with a microknife at the entry zone of the rootlets in the dorsolateral sulcus. The incision is generally 2 mm deep into the ventrolateral part of the DREZ and Lissauer's tract and is obliquely oriented 45 degrees down to the apex of the dorsal horn, which is recognizable under the microscope by its gray-brown color. Then, the surgical lesion in the target is completed by short-duration, low-intensity microcoagulations inside the incision. Depth and extent of the lesion depend on the degree of the desired therapeutic effect and the preoperative sensory status of the patient. If the laxity of the root is sufficient, the incision is performed continuously in the dorsolateral sulcus ventrolaterally along all of the rootlets of the targeted root, thus accomplishing a sulcotomy. If not, a partial ventrolateral section is made successively on each rootlet of the root, after the surgeon has isolated each one by separation of the tiny arachnoid membranes that hold them together. Recording of surface spinal cord somatosensory evoked potentials (SEPs) by stimulation of the tibial and the median nerve can aid in checking the integrity of the dorsal column and the extent of the MDT (see Fig. 130-9), respectively.[13]

For pain due to brachial plexus avulsion, after incision of the dorsolateral sulcus, dotted microcoagulations inside the dorsal horn (at least 3 mm deep from the surface of the cord) are performed with sharp, graduated bipolar forceps at the level of the avulsed roots. Selective ventrolateral DREZ lesions are extended to the roots remaining above and below.

In brachial plexus avulsion, dissection of the spinal cord is sometimes difficult to achieve safely because of scar tissue adhering to the cord in the subarachnoid space. Atrophy, gliotic changes, or both, at the level of the avulsed roots can make the correct identification of the dorsolateral sulcus hazardous. In such cases, it is necessary to start the dissection from the remaining roots, proximal and distal to the injured area. The presence of tiny radicular vessels that enter the cord may help determine the site of the sulcus. Yellow areas corresponding to old hemorrhages on the surface of the cord or microcavities in the depth of the sulcus and the dorsal horn provide some guidance for accurately tracing the sulcomyelotomy. When the dorsolateral sulcus is difficult to find, intraoperative monitoring of the dorsal column SEPs is especially helpful.

OPERATIVE PROCEDURE AT THE LUMBOSACRAL LEVEL (Fig. 130–8)

The patient is positioned prone on thoracic and iliac supports, and the head is placed 20 cm lower than the level of the surgical wound to minimize intraoperative loss of CSF. The desired vertebral level is identified by palpation of the spinous processes or, if this is difficult, by lateral x-ray study that includes the S1 vertebra. Interspinous levels identified by a needle can then be marked with methylene blue. A laminectomy—either bilateral or unilateral, according to pain topography—from T11 to L1 or L2 is performed. The dura and arachnoid are opened longitudinally, and the filum terminale is isolated. Identification of roots is then performed by electrical stimulation.

The roots L1 and L2 are easily identified at their penetration into their respective dural sheaths. Stimulation of L2 produces a response of the iliopsoas and adductor muscles.

Identification of L3 to L5 is difficult for many reasons: (1) the exit through their respective dural sheaths is caudal to the exposure, (2) the dorsal rootlets enter the DREZ along an uninterrupted line, (3) the ventral roots are hidden in front of the dentate ligament, and (4) the motor responses in the leg to stimulation of the roots are difficult to observe intraoperatively because of the patient's prone position. Stimulation of L3 produces a preferential response in the adductors and quadriceps, of L4 in the quadriceps and L5 in the anterior tibialis.

Stimulation of the S1 dorsal root produces a motor response of the gastrocnemius-soleus group that can be confirmed later, by repeatedly checking the Achilles ankle reflex before, during, and after MDT at this level.

Stimulation of the S2-S4 dorsal roots can be assessed by recording of the motor vesical or anal response by use of

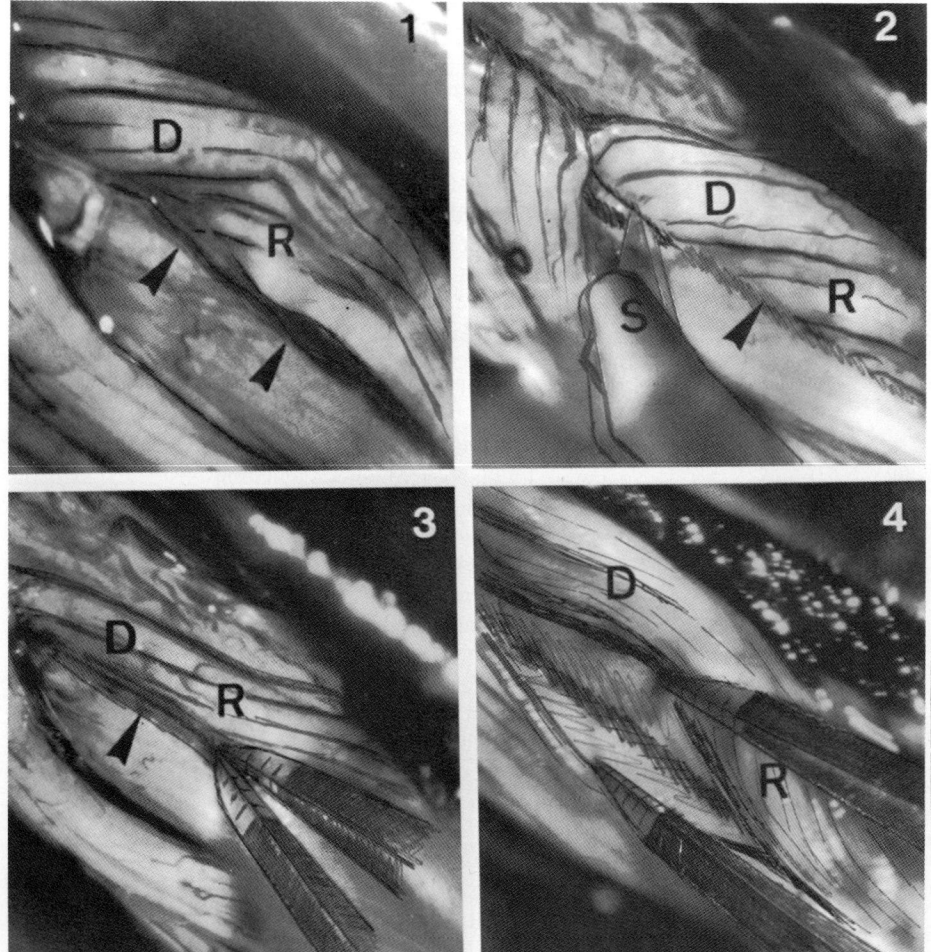

FIGURE 130–8. MDT technique at the lumbosacral level. Exposure of the left dorsolateral aspect of the conus medullaris. (1) The rootlets of the selected lumbosacral dorsal roots (DR) are displaced dorsally and medially to obtain proper access to ventrolateral aspect of the DREZ in the dorsolateral sulcus. Only the tiny pial vessels (arrows) are coagulated with a thin, pointed, bipolar microforceps. (2) A microscalpel (S) made with a small elongated fragment of a razor blade mounted on a holder is ready to start the incision, which will be at an angle of 45 degrees ventromedially and 2 mm deep (arrow: posterolateral sulcus). (3) Microcoagulations are performed inside the incision, 2 mm in depth, down to the upper layers of the dorsal horn. (4) The line of incision is opened between the two tips of the bipolar forceps and reveals its depth and the apex of the dorsal horn.

cystomanometry, recto-manometry, or electromyography of the anal sphincter. These investigations are difficult and time-consuming to perform in the operating room. We have found that measurements at the conus medullaris can be sufficient, especially for patients who already have severe preoperative impairment of their vesicoanal functions. These measurements, based on human postmortem anatomic studies, have shown that the landmark between the S1 and S2 segments is situated around 30 mm above the exit from the conus of the tiny coccygeal root.

Recordings of spinal cord surface SEPs can be useful to identify spinal cord segments and to study the effects of MDT on DREZ physiology (Fig. 130–9).[13] Stimulation of the tibial nerve gives maximal responses (dorsal horn postsynaptic potentials) in the L5-S2 segments, and stimulation of the dorsal nerve of the penis (or clitoris) in the S2-S4 segments.

All the dorsal roots of the cauda equina on one side are then displaced dorsally and medially to obtain proper access to the lateral aspect of the DREZ. A careful dissection must be carried out to cut all arachnoid adhesions, thus freeing all rootlets and related vessels. In some patients, arachnoiditis can make this dissection difficult. The posterolateral spinal artery courses along the posterolateral sulcus. Its diameter is between 0.1 and 0.5 mm and it is fed by the posterior radicular arteries and joins caudally with the descending anterior branch of the Adamkiewicz artery through the conus medullaris anastomotic loop of Lazorthes. This artery must be preserved by being freed from the sulcus. The tiny pial vessels situated on the lateral aspect of the DREZ are coagulated with a sharp microforceps and are cut with a curved microscissors. A continuous incision (i.e., a posterolateral sulcotomy) is then performed with a microscalpel. The cut must be 2 mm deep, with an angle of 45 degrees ventrally and medially, similar to that used in the cervical MDT. The borders of the incision are spread slightly apart with the forceps, so that the gray-brown color of the most dorsal part of the dorsal horn can be seen. The lesion is then completed by microcoagulations inside the cut with a graduated bipolar microforceps. A ball-tipped microsucker is used to keep the rootlets gently out of the way and to control CSF flow and bleeding.

NEUROPHYSIOLOGIC MONITORING AS AN AID TO SURGERY

Intraoperative monitoring of SEPs can be performed at the surface of the exposed spinal cord.[13, 14] Recordings of dorsal root presynaptic potentials and dorsal horn postsynaptic potentials can be useful for identification of the spinal cord segments. Potentials have a maximal intensity in C6-C7 and C8 for stimulation of the median and the cubital nerve, respectively, and in L5 to S2 and S2 to S4, for stimulation of the tibial nerve and the dorsal nerve of the penis or clitoris, respectively. Recordings of surface spinal cord SEPs can also be helpful in monitoring the surgical lesion itself. The dorsal column potentials can be monitored to determine the integrity of the ascending dorsal column fibers, especially when the dorsolateral sulcus is not clearly marked (as is common in root avulsion). In addition, the dorsal horn potentials can be monitored to follow the extent of MDT (Fig. 130–9), particularly when good sensory functions are present before surgery.

RESULTS AND INDICATIONS

CANCER PAIN

In patients with cancer pain, an effective result was obtained in 87 percent and 78 percent of the 46 and 35 patients, respectively, with DREZ lesions at the cervical (or cervicothoracic) and the lumbar (or sacral) levels. These patients

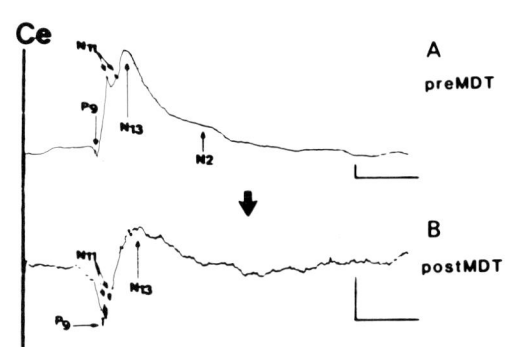
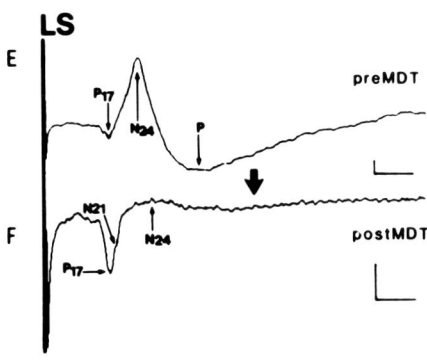

FIGURE 130–9. Effects of MDT on the evoked electrospinogram (EESG). Recordings from the surface of the dorsal column, medially to the DREZ at the C7 cervical (Ce) and the L5 lumbosacral (LS) segments, ipsilateral to the stimulation of the median and the tibial nerve, respectively, before (A) and after (B) MDT.

The initial positive event P9 (for cervical) (P17 for lumbosacral) corresponds to the farfield compound potential originating in the proximal part of the brachial (lumbosacral) plexus. The small and sharp negative peaks N11 (N21) correspond to nearfield presynaptic successive axonal events, probably generated in the proximal portion of the dorsal root, the dorsal funiculus and the large-diameter afferent collaterals to the dorsal horn. After MDT, all of these presynaptic potentials remain unchanged.

The large, slow, negative wave N13 (N24) corresponds to the postsynaptic activation of the dorsal horn by group I and II peripheral afferent fibers of the median (tibial) nerves. They are diminished after MDT (in the order of two thirds).

The later negative slow wave N2 (just visible in the cervical recording) corresponds to postsynaptic dorsal horn activity consecutive to the activation of group II and III afferent fibers. N2 is suppressed after MDT. (From Jeanmonod D, Sindou M, Mauguiere F: The human cervical and lumbosacral evoked electrospinogram. Data from intraoperative spinal cord surface recordings. Electroencephalogr Clin Neurophysiol 80:473–475, 1991.)

had topographically limited pain caused by well-localized lesions. Their survival ranged from 1 month to 4 years (mean, 13 months). Surgery was complicated by wound infection in two cases and was thought to have precipitated death in two cases.

The best indication for the use of MDT in patients with cancer is for limited pain syndromes, such as the Pancoast syndrome. For more extended cancers, high cervical spinothalamic cordotomy is preferable.

Because extensive DREZ operations at the lumbar (sacral) segments inevitably result in leg hypotonia, or sphincteric disturbances, for pain below the waist in patients able to walk, the procedure must be very restricted.

PURE NEUROGENIC PAIN

Of 139 patients with pure neurogenic pain followed up over 1 to 19 years, 87 percent benefited from surgery, and no deaths occurred. No significant neurologic complications occurred, especially as far as the dorsal column and the pyramidal tract were concerned, excepted in two cases. Detailed results have been published elsewhere.[15]

Lasting, good (more than 75 percent relief) results were achieved in patients in the following painful states:

1) In brachial plexus injuries, results were almost always good. For total pain relief, DREZ lesions must not be limited to the avulsed segments but must be extended to the adjacent remaining roots, especially if their level corresponds to the painful territory.

2) In spinal cord lesions, good effects were obtained only in patients whose pain had a "radiculometameric" distribution, that is, the pain corresponded to the level and the extent of the spinal cord lesion. Pain in the territory below the lesion, especially that located in the perineosacral area, was not favorably influenced, even if MDT was performed in the lower medullary segments. This was particularly true in patients whose pain corresponded to a permanent burning sensation and was in a totally anesthetic area. Therefore, MDT must be reserved for use in patients whose pain syndromes are related to the injured medullary segments and also the adjacent ones, if modified by consecutive pathologic processes (e.g., cavitation, gliosis, or arachnoiditis). The best indications for MDT are the same as for cordectomy: traumatic lesions of the spine below the level of T10 (as in conus medullaris), especially when pain is located in the legs rather than in the buttocks and perineum. Pain resulting from lesions of cauda equina can also be favorably influenced by MDT.

3) In peripheral nerve injuries, relief was significant only when the predominant component of pain was of the paroxysmal type (i.e., electrical shooting crises) or corresponded to allodynia (i.e., superficial provoked hyperalgesia), or both. Good results were also achieved in causalgic syndromes, even severe, as well as on the painful vasomotor components. In patients without marked preoperative deficit, DREZ lesions must not be too far extended in length and depth, because tactile and proprioceptive sensory capacities must be at least partially retained and because uncomfortable paresthesias can be avoided.

4) In postamputation painful states, phantom limb pain was stably cured only when rootlets were found avulsed. Pain in the stump was inconsistently influenced; better results were obtained when pain was of the paroxysmal or the allodynic type. In amputation patients, as well as in those with pain due to peripheral nerve lesions, that is, in patients with lesions distal to the spinal ganglion, dorsal column stimulation may be helpful. The electrodes can be inserted just above the upper level of the DREZ operation, through the same laminectomy. To be effective the lemniscal fibers central to the spinal ganglion must be functional, a state that can be tested by preoperative SEP examination.

5) In postherpetic neuralgias, only superficial pain located in the affected dermatome or dermatomes was significantly improved, especially when the pain was of the allodynic type. The permanent burning or aching deep component was not only unrelieved in most cases but was often aggravated, and patients complained of additional constrictive sensations after operation. Before deciding to perform MDT in patients with postherpetic neuralgia, even if the pain is unbearable, one must be very cautious. Although no death or postoperative neurologic complication occurred in this group, the possible vital risks in these patients, who are usually elderly, as well as eventual neurologic aggravation must be stressed, especially in patients for whom the thoracic spinal cord is the target, a common situation in postherpetic neuralgia. As a matter of fact, at this level, the tract of Lissauer is very narrow, and the dorsal horn is small and deeply situated. Identifying the exact root or roots corresponding to the herpetic lesions may be difficult. At operation, the common observation of an atrophic and gliotic aspect of the concerned roots can be helpful.

6) In our series, very few cases of pure neurogenic pain from other causes have been subjected to MDT. Therefore, we can draw no conclusions about them.

HYPERSPASTICITY WITH PAIN

Because muscular tone was diminished in the operated territories after MDT was performed for treatment of pain,[16] the procedure was applied as early as 1973 for harmful spasticity.[17] The antispastic effects can be explained by the fact that MDT, by interrupting the afferent components of the myotactic monosynaptic and the nociceptive polysynaptic reflexes, deprives the somatosensory relays of the dorsal horn of most of their excitatory inputs. MDT was performed in the lumbosacral cord (L2 down to S2 and, sometimes, S5) bilaterally in 115 paraplegic patients, 49 of whom suffered from pain from their disabling spasticity in the lower limbs, and in the cervical cord (C5 to T1) in 24 hemiplegics, 18 of whom had pain in addition to harmful spasticity in the upper limb. The excess of spasticity was significantly decreased in 85 percent of the cases. When present, pain was relieved without total loss of sensation in 88 percent in both groups, with a follow-up ranging from 2 to 19 years (mean, 7 years). Details concerning methods and results in spasticity have been published elsewhere.[18]

SUMMARY

Provided that selection of patients is rigorous, MDT can be performed with a low rate of corticospinal and dorsal column deficit. The procedure enables the sparing of some sensory functions in the operated areas, which is important in patients who retain some function in the painful territories. The distinctive feature of MDT is that it is performed at the junction between the peripheral and the central parts of the somatosensory system. This position allows the surgeon to destroy specific components in this system as a result of their spatial segregation and to act on gating mechanisms by influencing their modulatory activity toward inhibition. Electrophysiologic recordings, postoperative clinical examination, and postmortem anatomic studies (in four cases) helped confirm that the action of MDT is not simply a massive destruction of the DREZ area but is partially a "retuning" of the dorsal horn. Among a total experience of 387 personal cases operated on since 1972 for chronic pain, the best indications were

1) Topographically limited cancer pain, such as in Pancoast's syndrome.

2) Neurogenic pain resulting from
- Brachial plexus injuries, especially those with avulsion.
- Spinal cord lesions, especially for pain corresponding to segmental lesions. Pain below the lesion was not favorably influenced. Pain resulting from lesions in the conus medullaris and the cauda equina was most often significantly relieved.
- Peripheral nerve injuries, amputation, and herpes zoster, especially when the pain was predominantly paroxysmal, or it corresponded to provoked hyperalgesia, or both.

3) Hyperspasticity with pain.

REFERENCES

1. Melzach R, Wall PD: Pain mechanism. A new theory. Science 150:971–979, 1965
2. Sindou M: Etude de la jonction radiculo-médullaire postérieure: La radicellotomie postérieure sélective dans la chirurgie de la douleur. Lyon, Thesis, University Claude-Bernard, 1972
3. Sindou M, Quoex C, Baleydier C: Fiber organization at the posterior spinal cord-rootlet junction in man. J Comp Neurol 153:15–26, 1974
4. Willis WD: Pain System. Basel, Karger, 1985
5. Denny-Brown D, Kirk EJ, Yanagisawa N: The tract of Lissauer in relation to sensory transmission in the dorsal horn of spinal cord in the macaque monkey. J Comp Neurol 151:175–200, 1973
6. Szentagothai J: Neuronal and synaptic arrangement in the substantia gelatinosa. J Comp Neurol 122:219–239, 1964
7. Loeser JD, Ward AA Jr, White LE Jr: Chronic deafferentation of human spinal cord neurons. J Neurosurg 29:48–50, 1968
8. Jeanmonod D, Sindou M, Magnin M, Baudet M: Intra-operative unit recordings in the human dorsal horn with a simplified floating microelectrode. Electroencephalogr Clin Neurophysiol 72:450–454, 1989
9. Loeser JD, Ward AA Jr, White LE Jr: Some effects of deafferentation of neurons. J Neurosurg 17:629–636, 1967
10. Albe-Fessard D, Lombard MC: Use of an animal model to evaluate the origin of and protection against deafferentation pain. Pain Res Ther 5:691–700, 1983
11. Sindou M, Fischer G, Mansuy L: Posterior spinal rhizotomy and selective posterior rhizidiotomy. Prog Neurolog Surg 7:201–250, 1976
12. Sindou M, Goutelle A: Surgical posterior rhizotomies for the treatment of pain. Adv Tech Stand Neurosurg 10:147–185, 1983
13. Jeanmonod D, Sindou M: Somatosensory function following dorsal root entry zone lesions in patients with neurogenic pain or spasticity. J Neurosurg 74:916–932, 1991
14. Jeanmonod D, Sindou M, Mauguière F: The human cervical and lumbosacral evoked electrospinogram. Data from intra-operative spinal cord surface recordings. Electroencephalogr Clin Neurophysiol 80:477–489, 1991
15. Sindou M, Daher A: Spinal cord ablation procedures for pain, in Dubner A, Gebbart GF, Bond MR (eds): Proceedings of the Fifth World Congress on Pain. Amsterdam, Elsevier, 1988, pp 477–495
16. Sindou M, Fischer G, Goutelle A, Mansuy L: La radicellotomie posterieure sélective. Premiers résultats dans la chirurgie de la douleur. Neurochirurgie 20:391–408, 1974
17. Sindou M, Fischer G, Goutelle A, et al: La radicellotomie postérieure sélective dans le traitement des spasticités. Rev Neurol (Paris) 130:201–215, 1974
18. Sindou M, Jeanmonod D, Mertens P: Surgery in the dorsal root entry zone: Microsurgical Drez-tomy (MDT) for treatment of spasticity, in Sindou M, Abbott R, Keravel Y (eds): Neurosurgery for Spasticity. Wien, Springer-Verlag, 1991, pp 165–182

CHAPTER 131

Microsurgical DREZotomy in Treatment of Deafferentation Pain

James R. B. Nashold
Blaine S. Nashold, Jr.

"We must all die. But that I can save him from days of torture, that is what I feel as my great and ever new privilege. Pain is a more terrible lord of mankind than even death itself."[1]

Albert Schweitzer (1931)

Pain is the oldest symptom of disease in humans. Yet, with all the advances of medicine, it remains one of the most complex, mysterious, challenging, and rewarding to treat in patients. The history of medicine and, in particular, the history of neurosurgery, is replete with examples of the struggle between suffering and the relief of pain by the physician. The neurosurgical treatment of pain provides a unique example of the dynamic relationship between advances in our understanding of the neurophysiology of pain mechanisms and anatomy and the clinical relief of pain in patients. In no other part of neurosurgery are the rewards greater and more satisfying for the patient and the surgeon than in the diagnosis and treatment of pain. Development of dorsal root entry zone (DREZ) lesions for the treatment of brachial plexus avulsions in 1976 and the operation's expansion to treat facial pain, postherpetic pain, and other kinds of deafferentation pain is an example of the evolution of improved treatments of intractable pain based on new knowledge of the neurophysiology of pain.

The term *deafferentation pain* was first introduced in 1978 and has been defined as pain or dysesthesias caused by interruption of peripheral or central afferent input in the central nervous system. Tasker and colleagues[2] broadly defined deafferentation and stated that "while theoretically also resulting from injury to receptors, in practice it is caused by lesions of nerves, dorsal roots, spinal cord, brainstem or cerebral cortex, interruption at any anatomical level being capable of inducing pain." Neurosurgeons have been at the forefront of the treatment of deafferentation pain syndromes, starting with Bennett's first rhizotomy of dorsal roots in 1888 for the relief of pain (Fig. 131–1).[3] Since then, various surgical interventions have been used, including tractotomy, vascular decompression, percutaneous ablation, and cordotomy.

DREZ lesions were first developed in 1976 for the relief of pain in a patient with brachial plexus avulsion. Since the initial report of this procedure in 1979,[4] DREZ operations have been expanded to treat a wide range of deafferentation pain syndromes, including conus injuries, pain from paraplegia, phantom limb pain, anesthesia dolorosa, lumbosacral avulsions, peripheral nerve injuries, pain secondary to cancer or radiation, and atypical facial pain.

ANATOMY AND PHYSIOLOGY

Although the biochemical nature of deafferentation pain remains unsolved, research has begun to outline some of the basic mechanisms involved. DREZ lesions destroy Rexed's layers I to V, interrupting the secondary neurons of the spinothalamic and spinoreticular tracts. Receptors for pain fibers are concentrated in layers I, II, and V and in Lissauer's tract,

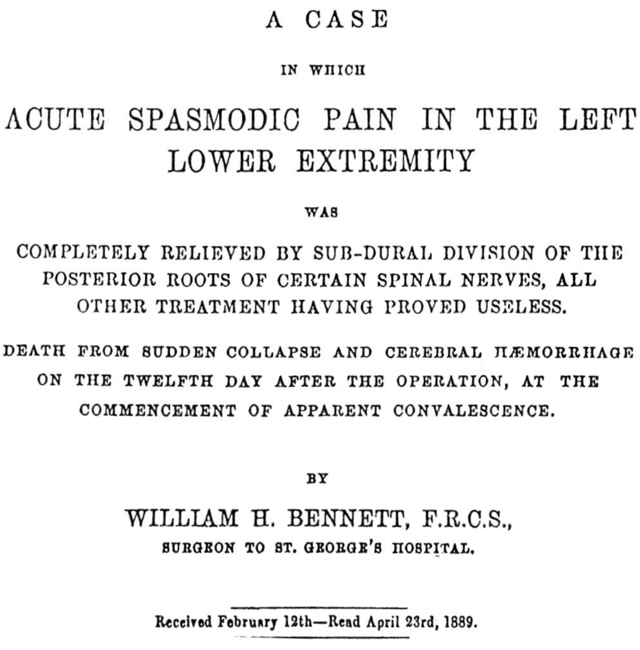

A CASE

IN WHICH

ACUTE SPASMODIC PAIN IN THE LEFT LOWER EXTREMITY

WAS

COMPLETELY RELIEVED BY SUB-DURAL DIVISION OF THE POSTERIOR ROOTS OF CERTAIN SPINAL NERVES, ALL OTHER TREATMENT HAVING PROVED USELESS.

DEATH FROM SUDDEN COLLAPSE AND CEREBRAL HÆMORRHAGE ON THE TWELFTH DAY AFTER THE OPERATION, AT THE COMMENCEMENT OF APPARENT CONVALESCENCE.

BY

WILLIAM H. BENNETT, F.R.C.S.,
SURGEON TO ST. GEORGE'S HOSPITAL.

Received February 12th—Read April 23rd, 1889.

FIGURE 131–1. Frontispiece from original article by W. H. Bennett. (From Bennett WH, cited by Abbe R: Acute spasmodic pain in the left lower extremity. Med Chir Trans 72:329–348, 1889.)

1624 | *Functional Neurosurgery*

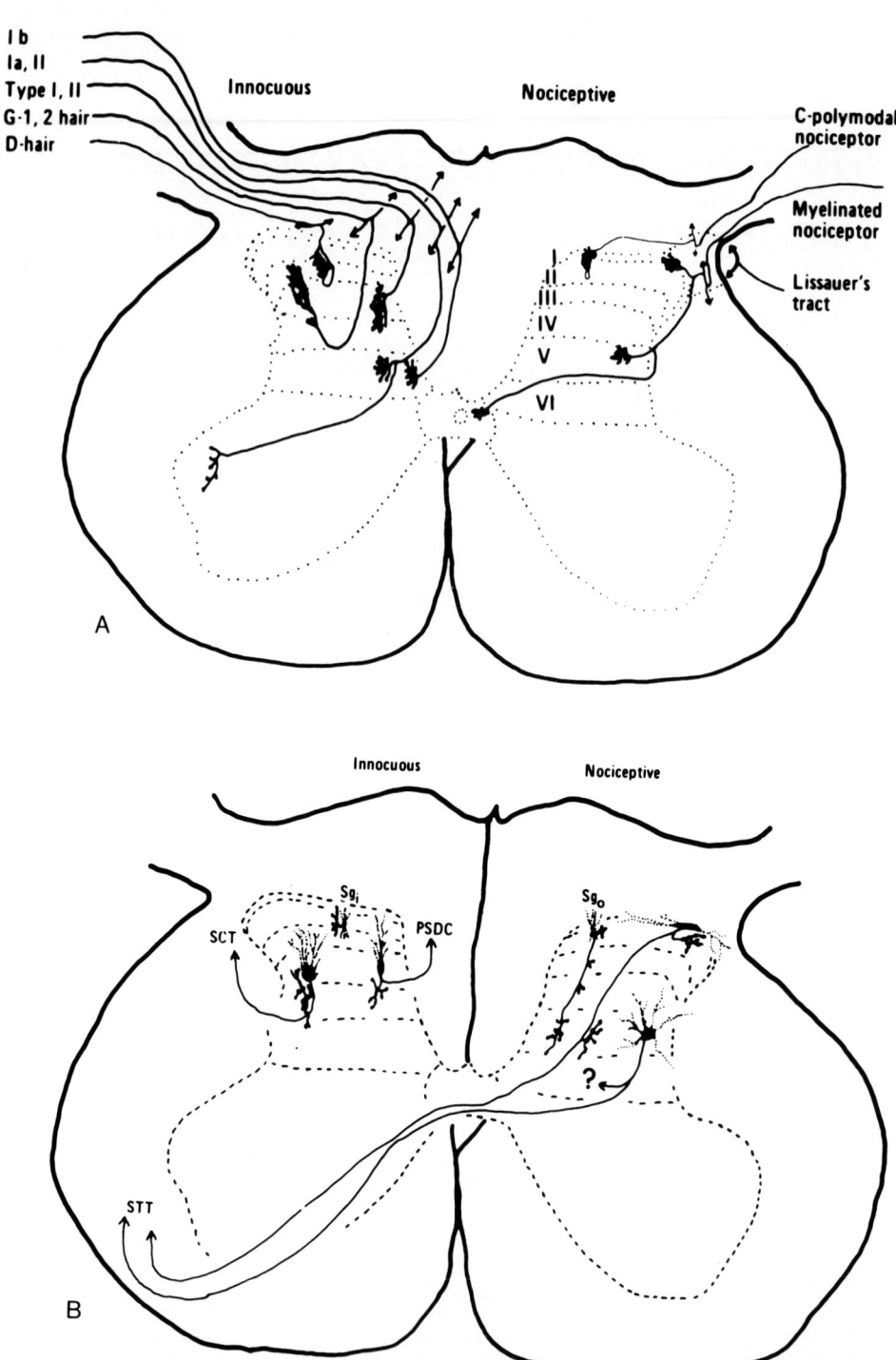

FIGURE 131–2. (A) The spinal termination regions of various primary afferent axons. The left side shows terminations of nonnociceptive afferents. Ib, Ia, and II indicate Golgi tendon organ afferents; Ia and II indicate spindle afferents. Type I and II indicate cutaneous type I and II afferent receptor types. Rexed's laminae are indicated on the right half of the cord, where nociceptor terminations are also indicated. (B) The major dendritic orientations and the major axon projections of several dorsal horn neurons. Dendrites are indicated by dotted lines, axons are indicated by solid lines, and synaptic regions are indicated by swellings in the axons. As in A, nonnociceptive neurons are shown on the left side and nociceptive neurons on the right side. SCT = Spinocervical tract, Sg_i = inner substantia gelatinosa neuron, PSDC = postsynaptic dorsal column neuron; Sg_o = outer substantia gelatinosa neuron, and STT = spinothalamic tract neuron. (From Light AR: Normal anatomy and physiology of the spinal cord dorsal horn. Appl Neurophysiol 51:78–88, 1988. By permission of S. Karger, Basel.)

a longitudinal tract of small diameter primary afferents from both dorsal horns that connects three or four spinal cord segments. The DREZ is represented in the brainstem by the trigeminal caudalis nucleus and continues caudally through the cervical, thoracic, and lumbar portions of the spinal cord to the level of the conus medullaris.[5]

The normal, uninjured DREZ maintains its neurophysiologic balance between afferent and efferent impulses under the control of excitatory and inhibitory mechanisms. With both complete and partial deafferentation, this delicate balance is destroyed. Sedivec and associates[6,7] indicated that part of the process of degeneration in the dorsal root neurons may involve the loss of dendritic spines, reorganization of dendritic structure, chromatolysis, and changes in spontaneous electrical activity. Clearly, a reorganization occurs in the DREZ neurons and receptors involved in the transmission of painful stimuli. Studies have shown that a preferential reorganization toward an increased number of nociceptive receptors occurs in the deeper layers of Rexed's laminae in the dorsal horn after deafferentation (Fig. 131–2). Numerous neurotransmitters and neuromodulators have been identified and are implicated in this process (Fig. 131–3). Excitatory

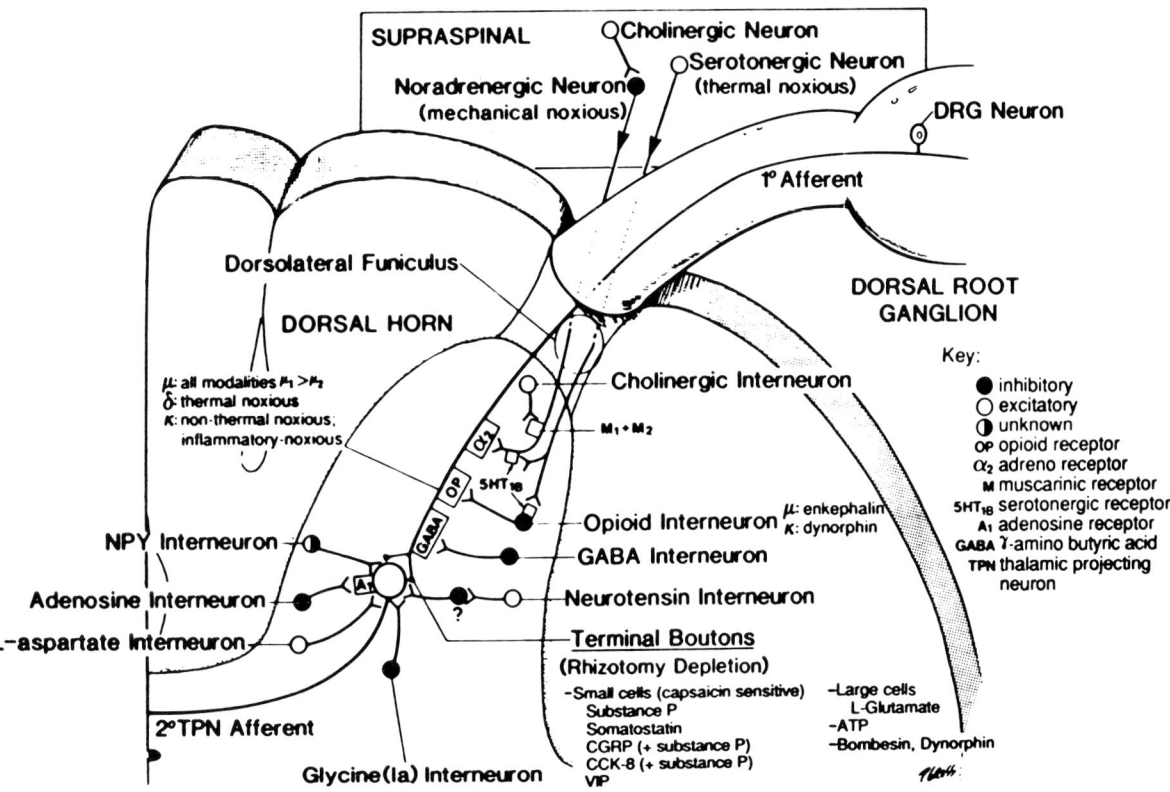

FIGURE 131–3. The neuropharmacology of the dorsal horn. (From Blumenkopf B: The general aspects of neuropharmacology of dorsal horn function, in Nashold BS, Ovelman-Levitt J [ed]: Advances in Pain Research and Therapy, vol 19. New York, Raven Press, 1991, pp 151–162.)

effects on the primary dorsal horn afferent fibers have been shown with glutamate, catecholamines, aspartate, substance P, and serotonin. Inhibitory mechanisms that down-regulate the transmission of nociception may involve glycine; gamma-aminobutyric acid; opioids like enkephalin and dynorphin; neurotensin; adenosine; somatostatin; and calcitonin gene-related peptide. Cholecystokinin and vasoactive intestinal peptide have been shown to have excitatory and inhibitory effects. In the supraspinal regions, especially in the thalamus, some neurotransmitters may have opposite effects from their actions in the DREZ on primary and secondary afferent neurons.[8–10] The sequence of exact steps of excitation and inhibition at the level of the dorsal horn and in supraspinal structures in normal states and after deafferentation remains to be elucidated. Until this has been determined, the local instillation of neurotransmitters with reliable analgesic effects remains an unrealized dream.

INDICATIONS AND PATIENT SELECTION

DEAFFERENTATION PAIN

Brachial Plexus Avulsion

Brachial plexus avulsion injuries may result from various mechanisms of action, including motorcycle and automobile accidents, gunshot wounds, or farm or other occupational accidents. Arm pain usually develops within days or weeks of the injury and is described as intense burning pain in a radicular pattern that may be exacerbated by touch or movement. Trigger spots several dermatomes away from the injured area on the neck or abdomen may cause paroxysms of pain. Depending on the chronicity and degree of the brachial plexus injured, secondary effects may include muscle wasting, dependent edema secondary to poor vascular compliance, hyporeflexia to areflexia, and poor skin care (Fig. 131–4).

Patients with brachial plexus avulsions who have not responded to pharmacologic control of their pain after at least 6 months to 1 year of treatment may be considered for DREZ lesions. A detailed history of previous treatments and surgical interventions and a thorough neurologic examination are the first steps in advising the patient about the potential for success from the DREZ operation. Accurate dermatomal, sensory maps of the involved dermatomes are important acts in the planning of operative strategies and for postoperative comparison of the levels of analgesia. Psychological evaluation and assessment of medications, with particular attention to narcotic dependence, are crucial for planning postoperative recovery.[4, 11–16]

Conus Medullaris Avulsions

Avulsions of the conus medullaris are similar to brachial plexus avulsions in their mechanism of injury and pattern of deafferented pain, and the operative planning required to treat them. Traumatic pelvic or lumbosacral injuries result from such events as motorcycle accidents, gunshot wounds, and snowmobile and automobile accidents. Spinal cord damage may range from stretch injuries to partial or complete avulsion of the lumbosacral nerve plexus. Pain is described as having a lancinating, electrical quality that begins imme-

1626 | *Functional Neurosurgery*

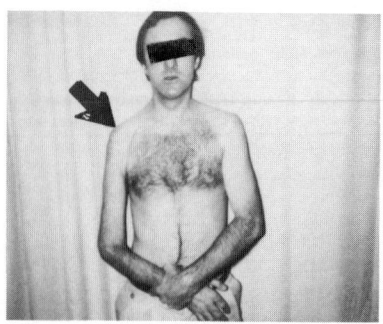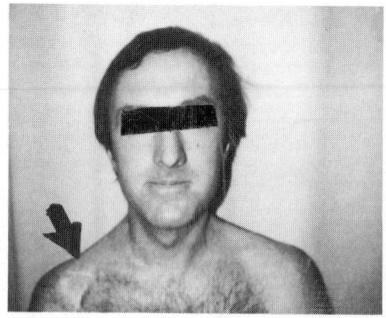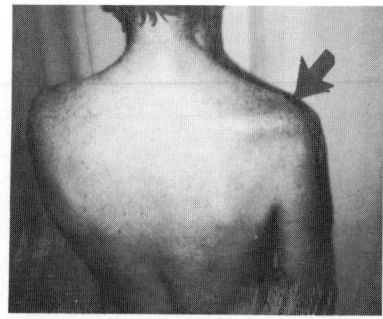

FIGURE 131–4. Patient with brachial plexus avulsion injury after a motor vehicle accident. After a DREZ operation, the patient had complete relief of his pain and has been followed up for over 7 years. The arrows indicate limb and shoulder atrophy from the accident.

diately after the accident and displays two patterns: diffuse, musculoskeletal-visceral pain or radicular, dermatomal pain. Trigger spots in adjacent dermatomes or those more distant may exist. Bladder, bowel, and sexual function may be decreased or absent and must be carefully evaluated to determine the degree of primary or secondary involvement. Dysfunction in abdominal viscera secondary to pain must be separated from primary neural compression or avulsion of nerve roots as a result of the original injury. Patients with conus avulsions tend to have more complicated postinjury problems than do those with lesions of the brachial plexus. They require intensive preoperative and postoperative management, including careful selection of surgical antibiotics.[17]

Paraplegia and Quadriplegia

Injuries resulting in paraplegia or quadriplegia are caused by a wider variety of mechanisms than those causing avulsion injuries. In addition to motorcycle or automobile accidents and gunshot wounds, injuries from diving accidents, falls, and vascular and neoplastic lesions may also cause paralysis. The development of pain may occur immediately after injury or from 6 months to more than a decade after the original injury. The pain is described as a constant burning that may or may not respect the dermatomal level of paralysis. Pain may occur at, above, or below the level of analgesia and may also be associated with intermittent paroxysms of stabbing pain and trigger areas in adjacent dermatomes or several dermatomes away.

Patients who describe a change in the level of their analgesia or pain that differs from the level of their original injury must be evaluated for the possibility of a syrinx. Our experience has shown that in as many as 15 to 20 percent of paraplegics and quadriplegics, syrinxes may contribute to their pain syndrome and complicate the picture of deafferentation. Quadriplegics may complain of lower cranial nerve dysfunction with extension of a syrinx into the lower medulla. Drainage of the cysts into the subarachnoid space of the spinal cord and DREZ lesions should be considered as surgical options. Many of these patients have undergone previous operations and may have bony vertebral fusions as well as spinal instrumentation for stabilization.[18, 19]

PERIPHERAL NERVE PAIN

Patients with central pain generally have greater relief of pain than those with peripheral pain involving the primary afferent neurons. Although two thirds of patients with brachial plexus, conus, and paraplegic injuries benefit from DREZ lesions, patients with stump pain do not respond to DREZ lesions; however, two thirds of patients with postamputation phantom limb pain receive significant relief of their pain from the DREZ operation. The original injury to the limb usually results from trauma, gangrene, or neoplasms. These patients, like paraplegics, already have undergone extensive medical treatments and at least one major surgical procedure for pain. The pain is described as aching, sharp, constant, dull, diffuse, and radicular in distribution. The onset of pain is usually immediately after injury, but its nature and intensity may have changed and be somewhat masked by secondary pain or dysesthesias from previous treatments. Patients frequently note an illusory phenomenon known as "telescoping" of extremities, like the feet and hands into the hip or shoulder, respectively. Paroxysms of pain are frequent and may be triggered by adjacent dermatome irritation, movement of the stump, or changes in the weather. In Saris and colleagues'[20] review of 22 patients, those with phantom limb pain alone were the best candidates for surgery.

Postherpetic Pain

The duration of pain from postherpetic neuralgia may range from several months to 15 years, with an average of 6 years (Fig. 131–5). All patients who received DREZ lesions had not responded to medical treatments, which included carbamazepine, amitriptyline, and transcutaneous nerve stimulation (TENS). Pain was described as burning and sharp and rarely diffuse or dull and occurred in the same distribution of the patients' herpetic scars or also involved one or two dermatomes above or below the scars, which were all located in a unilateral thoracic pattern. Hyperpathia may accompany burning pain, and hyperesthesias may be stimulated by touch and relieved by pressure.[21, 22]

Postrhizotomy or Post-thoracotomy Pain

Patients treated with multiple lumbar disc operations and dorsal rhizotomies for low back and leg pain have not significantly benefited from treatment with DREZ lesions. Pain in a radicular pattern or hypoesthesia in the L5 or S1 distribution similar to pain from a classic disc herniation may be described. Patients who had undergone rhizotomy have reported a variable pain pattern that ranges from a dermatomal pattern to burning pain after attempted surgical intervention.

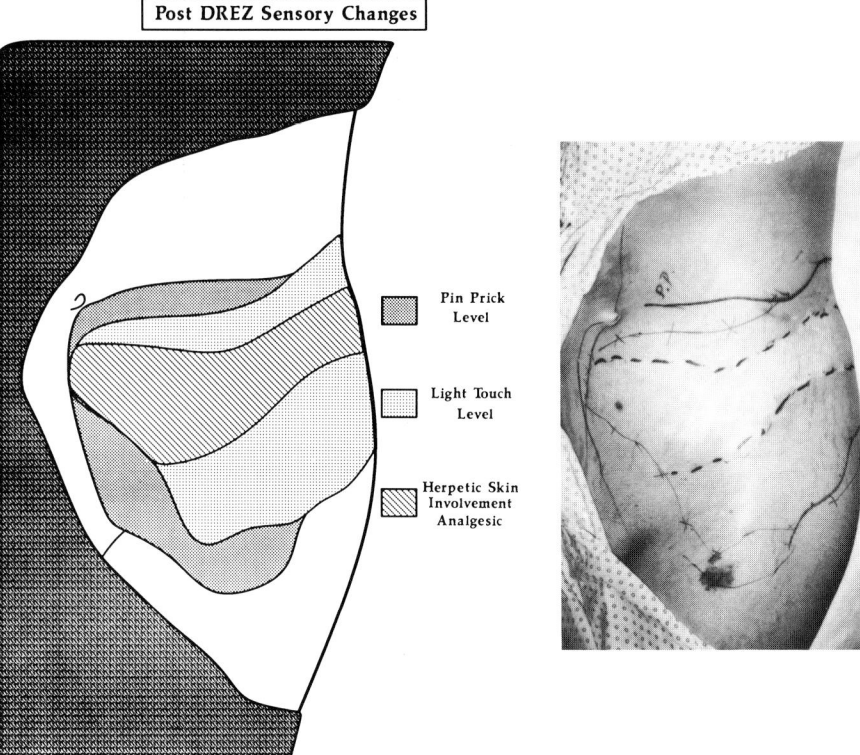

FIGURE 131–5. Patient with painful abdominal herpetic involvement. Postherpetic pain area is crosshatched. Postoperative DREZ effect showing changes in pinprick and light touch. (Right) A photograph of the patient. (Left) The same view rendered more clearly.

Hyporeflexia or areflexia and muscular wasting and atrophy may be present and may mimic an avulsion injury. Saris and associates[20] reported that less than 20 percent of 12 patients with chronic sciatica who received DREZ lesions had good results. Nashold and coworkers[23] recommend that DREZ lesions not be used for the treatment of pain from chronic sciatica. Patients with pain after thoracotomies or patients with abdominal pain do not respond well to DREZ lesions; therefore, the DREZ operation is not recommended.

Peripheral Nerves

Treatments for peripheral nerve injuries have traditionally included nonsteroidal anti-inflammatory agents, thorazine, transcutaneous nerve stimulation, and dorsal column and deep brain stimulation, with limited success.[24] Matsumura and colleagues[25] reported the successful use of DREZ lesions to treat intractable pain due to a partially injured tibial nerve. The patient had experienced a crush injury to his right foot after a traffic accident, and his second toe was amputated. Two months after the injury, burning, aching pain developed in his foot and was treated with analgesics, transcutaneous nerve stimulation, and nerve blocks without successful relief. Direct recordings of root potentials were performed in the operating room, and segmental contributions to the injured nerve were identified. Carbon dioxide laser DREZ lesions were made from L5 to S1, and the patient suffered no further foot pain and had no motor deficit. Despite the fact that only a small number of patients with peripheral nerve injuries develop intractable pain, this report indicates a potentially new application of DREZ lesions for a carefully selected group of patients with peripheral nerve injuries that contain components of deafferentation and spinal cord second-order neuron degeneration and pain.

Patients with painful reflex sympathetic dystrophy have pain relief for less than 6 months after surgery, but in 90 per cent of these patients, the pain fully returns. Local trauma is the usual cause, and pain is restricted to the arm and hand. These patients have undergone a complicated medical course with multiple pharmacologic agents, nerve blocks, and electrical stimulation. We do not recommend the DREZ operation for patients with reflex sympathetic dystrophy.

Several patients with breast cancer who have had radiation treatments to the brachial plexus were treated with DREZ lesions after suffering from burning pain in the chest and arm. These patients do not respond well to the DREZ operation, because the level of injury is in the peripheral nervous system.

Atypical Facial Pain

The treatment of atypical facial pain with DREZ lesions requires a detailed knowledge of the unique anatomy of the trigeminal nerve's nucleus caudalis (Fig. 131–6). The nucleus caudalis is the inferior third of the nucleus of the spinal trigeminal tract located in the dorsolateral portion of the medulla and extending up to the pons through the nuclei interpolaris and oralis, where it merges with the pontine main trigeminal sensory nucleus. The nucleus caudalis receives afferent fibers from all three divisions of the trigeminal nerve and is the main sensory nucleus for the ipsilateral face. Cranial nerves VII, IX, and X also send fibers to the lower component of the trigeminal nuclei. Projection fibers travel to the midbrain, thalamus, olivary nuclei, cerebellum, and the

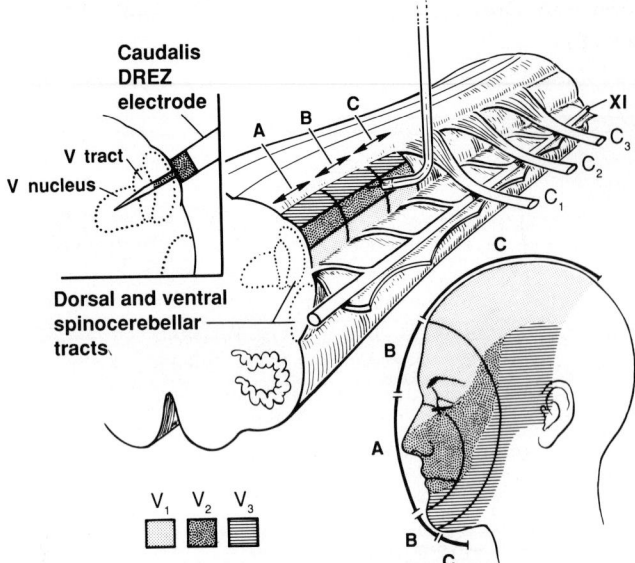

FIGURE 131–6. The relationship of the trigeminal nerve subdivisions (V_1, V_2, V_3) and the spinocerebellar tracts. The first division of the trigeminal nerve is represented nearest the spinal accessory nerve, and central regions of the face are somatotopically represented in the rostral part of the nucleus (A, B, C). The *inset* shows how the insulated caudalis DREZ electrode spares the spinocerebellar tracts. XI = 11th cranial nerve, C_1, C_2, C_3 = cervical nerve rootlets. (Adapted from Sampson JH, Nashold BS: Facial pain due to vascular lesions of the brainstem relieved by dorsal root entry zone lesions in the nucleus caudalis. J Neurosurg 77:473–475, 1992.)

more rostral trigeminal nuclei. Detailed studies of the nucleus caudalis reveal it to be round, measuring 2 mm in diameter near the obex and 0.8×1.5 mm in cross section at the C2 level. Caution is needed with the caudal-most lesions 12 mm caudal to the obex because of the close proximity of the pyramidal tract.[26, 27]

Atypical facial pain may result from a variety of pathological insults, including pontine lesions, postherpetic neuralgia, postrhizotomy, multiple sclerosis, cancer, benign neoplasms, anesthesia dolorosa, dental procedures, and vascular lesions. Most patients complain of a unilateral burning, aching, and numbness in one or all sensory divisions of the face. Trigger spots are irritated inside and outside the hyperesthetic area by touch, mouth movement, head turning, and swallowing (Fig. 131–7). Periorbital, retro-orbital and nasion pains are described as sharp and knifelike. Gag or swallowing reflexes may be decreased or absent. Patients with involvement of the pons or other wide areas of the brainstem may have associated motor, sensory, or cerebellar symptoms.[28–30]

PREOPERATIVE EVALUATION

The most important aspect of the preoperative evaluation is an accurate sensory and dermatomal map, which is the foundation for accurately placed spinal cord segment lesions and for postoperative comparison. More than one frank discussion between the patient and the surgeon may be required so that the patient is well prepared for the realities of the postoperative recovery course. Possible side effects of no pain relief, large anesthetic areas, incisional pain, and extremity ataxia resulting from the caudalis operation, as well as the management of postoperative narcotics, help the patient prepare mentally for the effects of the surgery. Such discussions are better held several days before the proposed surgery rather than the night before surgery to acclimatize the patient to the procedure.

Plain x-ray studies are obtained preoperatively on all patients to evaluate the bony anatomy of the potential operative site and to assess any spinal instrumentation or fusions that may have been performed previously. In spinal instrumentation cases, orthopedic colleagues should be consulted for advice or intraoperative assistance in removing spinal hardware and maintaining spinal stability after DREZ lesioning. Computed tomographic (CT) or magnetic resonance imaging (MRI) studies are also obtained. We prefer to use MRI because it best shows the parenchyma of the spinal cord and the presence of any syrinxes. CT myelography is helpful if a post-traumatic meningocele may be present. In the few situations in which vascular lesions are involved, cerebral angiography is necessary. Preoperative steroids are used the night before surgery, continued for 5 days postoperatively, and

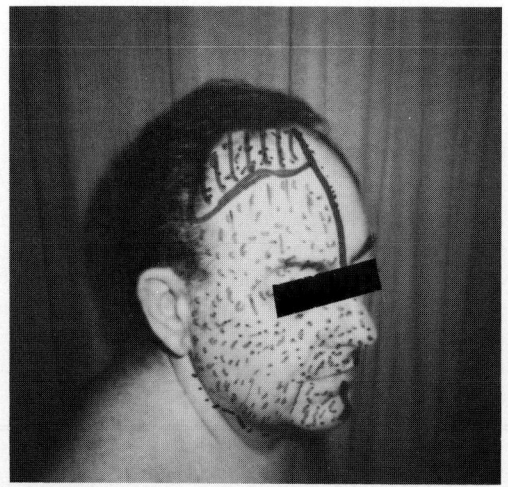 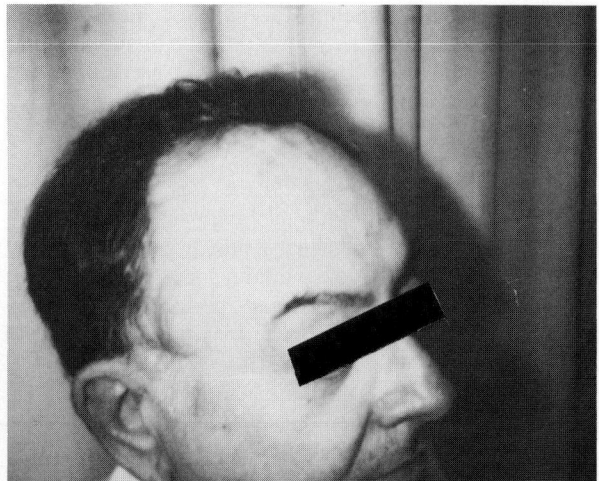

FIGURE 131–7. Photograph of a patient with postherpetic right facial pain. (Left) Before surgery. Forehead analgesia, face hyperalgesic. (Right) After surgery of caudalis DREZ, resulting in pain relief for 7 years.

gradually decreased over the last 3 days. Perioperative antibiotics are not routinely used; however, they are recommended in patients with spinal instrumentation, paraplegia, chronic urinary infections, or respiratory disease.

OPERATIVE TECHNIQUE

BRACHIAL PLEXUS AVULSION

The operative approach is to expose the level of the injured spinal cord and usually one or two segments above and below the involved area. A full laminectomy from C5 to T1 should be performed. To expose the conus medullaris, a laminectomy should be performed from T10 to L2. Whether to perform a hemilaminectomy or a full laminectomy depends on the anticipated amount of anatomic distortion because of previous operations, the original injury, and the presence of a syrinx. Generally, we prefer to perform full laminectomies when unilateral DREZ lesions are planned in the cervical region and hemilaminectomies in the thoracic level of the spine. The conus requires full laminectomy for full exposure of the cord. The approach to the nucleus caudalis is discussed later in a separate section.

All patients are placed in the prone position, and the Mayfield headholder is used for head and neck stabilization in cervical, upper thoracic (T1-T4), and trigeminal caudalis procedures. Surface electrodes for intraoperative recording are placed in the induction room, and the patients' arms are positioned at the side to permit the best access to the operative site in the cervical region.

A standard laminectomy is performed with hand-held rongeurs or the Midas Rex drill. Caution should be exercised when various drills are used to cut the bony laminae and remove the spinous processes because scar tissue from previous operations and thick, adherent dura may be torn and result in loss of the planes of anatomic dissection. If previous procedures may have distorted the layers of fascia, muscle, or bone, rongeurs provide the most control for customizing the laminectomies and avoiding unnecessary dural tears and uncontrolled epidural bleeding. If hemilaminectomies are to be performed, after the hemilamina is removed the spinous process is undercut to allow slightly more medial exposure. If rongeurs are used, the bony edges of the laminectomies may be scalloped from the bite of the instrument, and these sharp edges should be smoothed before the dura is opened. Hemostasis is critical at this stage of the opening to prevent problems once the dura is opened. Bony edges should be sealed with bone wax, all muscle bleeding should be coagulated, and the lateral gutters of the spinal canal should be carefully inspected for retracted, bleeding epidural vessels. "Cigarettes," or small rolls of Surgicel, may be placed in the gutters to aid hemostasis. Bony fragments or shavings from the laminectomy should be irrigated, and a completely dry operative field should be established.

The dura is opened in the midline, and the arachnoid should be kept intact beneath it, if at all possible. Care should be taken if the dura is opened over the site of previous operations or the site of the original injury to avoid further damage to the dorsal spinal cord. The dura may be adherent to the underlying cord from scar tissue; to arachnoid plaques, which may be very adherent; and to vascular abnormalities from postinjury revascularization. Once the dura is opened, its edges are tented up with 3–0 pop-off silk sutures placed about 1 cm apart. The caudal and rostral ends of the dural opening may be secured with ligatures of silk to prevent further extension of the dural opening beyond the operative field. The arachnoid is opened with microscissors, and its edges are tacked up to the dura with silver clips. The dura and arachnoid may be opened with the use of the operating microscope or magnified surgical lenses. Once the dura is opened, the microscope is used for all intradural work.

Rootlets injured by brachial plexus avulsion may be identified in several ways. If complete avulsion has occurred, then the dorsal roots are missing from their normal dorsolateral position on the spinal cord. If a full laminectomy has been performed, then the area of avulsion may be compared with the complementary, intact rootlets on the opposite side. The cervical roots are usually atretic, thin, gray, and avascular when compared with the normal side and usually consist of five to eight rootlets. Extensive arachnoiditis with plaques, meningoceles, and cord tissue that is spongy, soft, or gelatinous may be found once the dura has been opened.

Once the operative site has been determined by visual inspection and evoked potentials, the arachnoid is stripped off each nerve root and off the dorsum of the spinal cord to expose the lesion area. Care is taken to inspect the intended track of lesions, and blood vessels that obscure the track are dissected off and gently moved aside either medially or laterally. This action prevents interruption of the lesion-making process once it has started and provides a relatively clear avenue for access to the dorsal root entry zone (Fig. 131–8).

DREZ radiofrequency lesions are best made in the caudal to rostral direction to give the surgeon a clear view of the intended path of lesions and any abnormal anatomic areas. The Radionics DREZ electrode is used, and all radiofrequency lesions are made at 75° C for 15 seconds each. Other surgeons have reported using lasers to create the DREZ lesions, but pathology studies show that lesions with lasers are more diffuse, harder to control, and not as reproducible as radiofrequency lesions. The DREZ electrode is held at an angle of 45 degrees caudal and lateral to a line perpendicular to the axis of the spinal cord. The electrode penetrates the dorsal root entry zone to a depth of 2 mm. Pathology studies have shown that these types of lesions are oval in shape and measure 2 mm × 1 to 2 mm. Lesions should be made every 1 mm along the spinal cord, so that a four- or five-level laminectomy that exposes four spinal nerve roots should require 40 to 50 lesions. Our experience has shown that this technique of "close-packing" lesions produces the best results and that the amount of pain relief is proportional to the density of tightly placed lesions.

Blood vessels encountered along the path for lesion making should be dealt with individually. Large vessels greater than 2 to 3 mm and radicular vessels should not be sacrificed but delicately moved aside with a minimum of dissection. If this process cannot be performed safely, then one or two lesions may be skipped. Smaller surface vessels may be coagulated during lesion making, and we have not encountered any complications from the loss of these vessels. Bleeding occurring during lesion making may be stopped with small patches of Surgicel or very low current bipolar coagulation. Traumatic meningoceles are not removed (Figs. 131–9 and 131–10). The area of lesion making should be kept as dry as

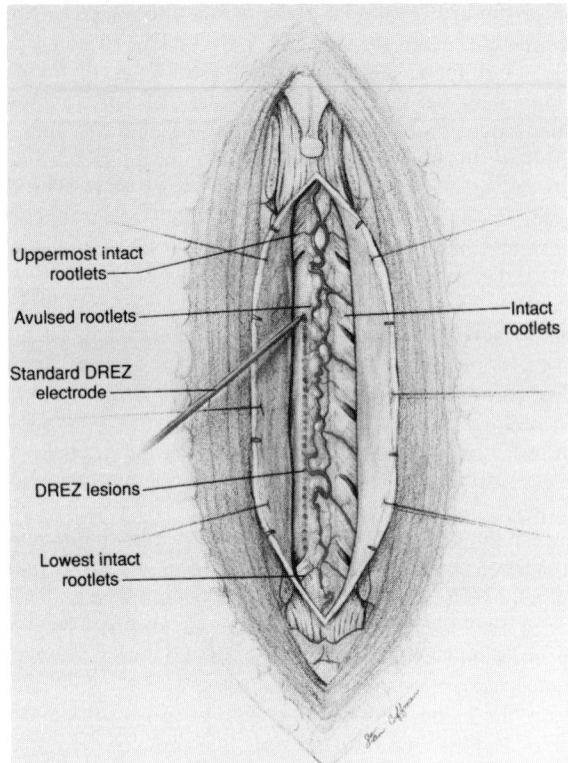

FIGURE 131–8. Operative exposure of brachial plexus avulsion. Dorsal roots are completely avulsed, and DREZ lesions are made in a caudal-to-rostral direction. (From Nashold BS, El-Naggar AO: Dorsal root entry zone (DREZ) lesioning, in Wilkins RH, Rengachary SS (eds): Neurosurgical Operative Atlas, vol 2. Baltimore, Williams & Wilkins, 1993, p 17.)

possible to create the best lesions and to minimize diffusion of heat transduction through tissue. The surgeon's assistant can suction out the ebb of cerebrospinal fluid (CSF) with a micropatty cottonoid, thereby protecting vessels and cord parenchyma from the tip of the suction. During lesion mak-

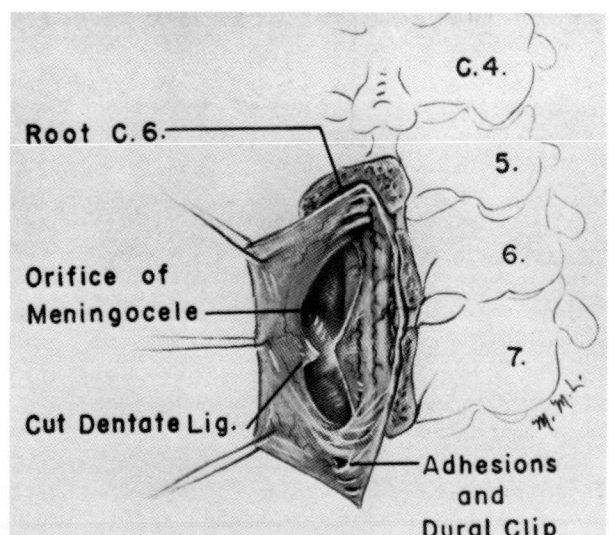

FIGURE 131–9. Meningocele showing dura and dentate ligament divided. Note absence of rootlets of spinal nerves below the sixth cervical group. (From White JC, Hanelin J: Myelographic signs of brachial plexus avulsion. J Bone Joint Surg Am 36A:113–118, 1954.)

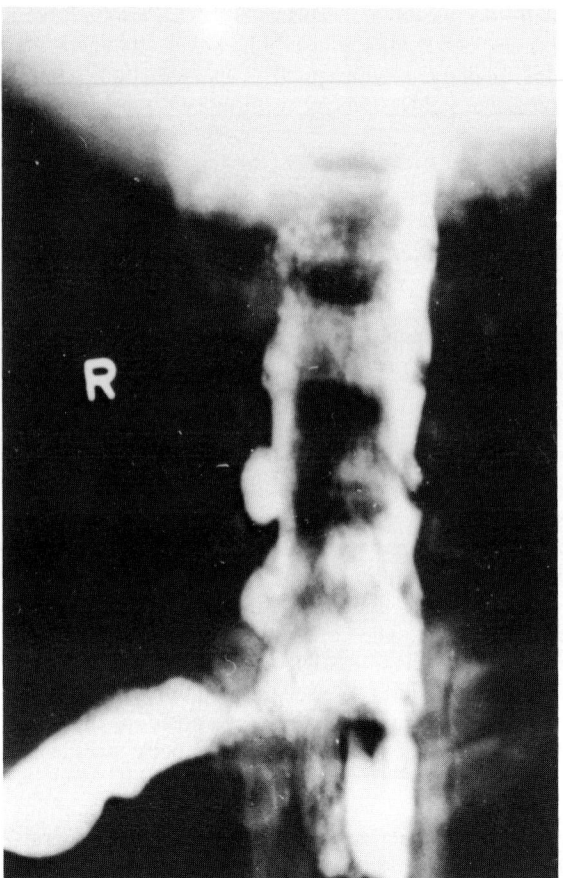

FIGURE 131–10. Cervical myelogram showing multiple postbrachial plexus avulsion meningoceles. (From Nashold BS, El-Naggar AO: Dorsal root entry zone (DREZ) lesioning, in Wilkins RH, Rengachary SS (eds): Neurosurgical Operative Atlas, vol 2. Baltimore, Williams & Wilkins, 1993, p 10.)

ing in high cervical or caudalis operations, the anesthesiologist should watch carefully for transient episodes of cardiac arrhythmias or bradycardia. Before and after each lesion, the impedance is measured and is usually less than 1200 ohms in damaged spinal cord. As the transition from injured parenchyma into more normal tissue is made, impedance readings should increase and eventually reach normal levels of 1500 ohms. We use these numbers as a guide throughout the operation and especially at the most rostral terminus of lesion making. Once consecutively normal levels of impedance are reached, and the levels correlate with the desired superior end of the treatment, lesion making is stopped.

The dura is closed in the usual fashion with 4–0 Vicryl or Prolene sutures. Dural grafts, when needed, are sutured in with Prolene. Grafts are rarely used in the cervical, thoracic, or conus operations but are more commonly employed in the caudalis closure because of the tightness of the atlanto-occipital dura. Dural tack-up sutures are a matter of surgical preference and are more helpful than other sutures in laminectomies over more than three segments. They may prevent cord compression if an epidural hematoma develops postoperatively. The remainder of the muscle, fascial, and subcutaneous layers are closed in the usual fashion. Tight closure of the fascia is extremely helpful in preventing CSF leaks from causing dehiscence of the wound and possible infection. Epidural drains are placed in the lateral gutters of the laminectomy if hemostasis is difficult or if oozing hemorrhage persists. These drains are removed on the first postoperative day.

CONUS MEDULLARIS AVULSION

Conus injuries are similar to brachial plexus avulsions except that only one or two nerve roots (L5 or S1) may be avulsed instead of three, four or five nerve roots in the cervical region. Scar tissue and previous operations, including spinal fusions and instrumentation, are more common in conus injuries than in brachial plexus injuries.

Localization of the correct thoracic vertebrae is more challenging than counting of cervical vertebrae and deserves comment because of the absence of clear local landmarks. If kyphosis exists as a result of the original injury, it helps localization of the thoracic vertebrae and the involved spinal cord level. Anteroposterior and lateral plain radiographs of the lower thoracic, lumbar, and sacral regions in one view enable the surgeon to count up from the L5 level to the proper thoracic vertebrae. Identification of the ribs as they articulate with the thoracic spine may also help.

A T11-L2 thoracolumbar laminectomy is usually performed. Large, tenacious arachnoid plaques, dural thickening, arachnoiditis, meningoceles, and bone spurs or fragments are commoner in this area than in the cervical region. Bone fragments and spurs should be removed because they may also be a source of cord compression and pain in these patients. Care should be taken to inspect each nerve root individually and its rootlets carefully to compare them with those on the normal side. The roots should be freed up of their arachnoid investments with microsurgical dissection. Lesion making should proceed in a fashion identical to the technique described earlier for brachial plexus DREZs.

PARAPLEGIA AND SYRINGOMYELIA

Traditionally, only 2 percent of paraplegics with intractable pain were thought to have syrinxes, but our experience indicates that 20 to 25 percent of paraplegics may have syringomyelia. Preoperative MRI is the best method of identifying syrinxes (Fig. 131-11). The length of the syrinx may have a single cavity or multiple cavities with or without septations. Most syrinxes are located at or above the level of the injury.

A three- or four-level laminectomy is performed to expose the damaged spinal cord at the level of injury and to expose the caudal-most part of the syrinx. Before the dura is opened, ultrasound is used to localize the syrinx. Visual inspection of the dorsal spinal cord may also indicate the level of the syrinx because of cord bulging; cord asymmetry; yellow, gray, or speckled discoloration; or effacement of the surface blood vessels. Once the dura is opened, sharp dissection should be used to free the nerve roots from their arachnoid. DREZ lesions are placed before the syrinx is opened because decompression of the syrinx may cause further distortion of the DREZ and the surrounding anatomy of the spinal cord.

The syrinx is drained through a midline dorsal myelotomy, and a soft ventricular catheter is passed along the axis of the syrinx to break down the septations and allow free communication with the subarachnoid space. For simple cysts, a syringostomy may be used for continuous drainage of the cyst. For complicated syrinxes, a T-shaped tube is placed with both arms of the T inserted into the syrinx and the vertical limb of the T cut short enough to just clear the surface of the spinal cord by several millimeters. A small, 6-0 or 7-0 nylon suture is used to anchor the protruding end of the catheter to the edge of the syringostomy (Fig. 131-12).

PHANTOM LIMB

Stump pain in patients who have had amputation is not relieved by DREZ lesions, as indicated in a series of patients reviewed by Saris and associates.[20] Sixty-seven percent of patients with phantom pain alone and one third of patients with both stump and phantom pain had good pain relief. The best results were obtained in five of six patients with post-amputation pain known to also have root avulsions. Patients with pain from traumatic amputations (35 percent) did better than those with pain secondary to cancer or gangrene. The age of patients, the length of time since their amputations, and the type of lesions made (thermal versus amperage lesions) did not affect outcome. Patients with diffuse, visceral, or truncal pain had poorer results than those with extremity or localized pain. The best candidate then for consideration of a DREZ operation to treat phantom pain after amputation is a patient with few if any previous pain procedures, phantom pain alone with no stump pain, and root avulsion from a traumatic amputation.

Patients with phantom limb pain are extremely sensitive to body position involving the amputated limb, especially when they are asleep, and care should be taken to place the patient on the operating table in a position that avoids exacerbation of their pain, even after DREZ lesions have been made. The operative technique to approach the brachial plexus or lumbosacral plexus is similar to that previously outlined for cervical and thoracolumbar laminectomies. Few if any of these patients have had previous spinal operations, fusions, or spinal instrumentation. However, because of the high incidence of traumatic amputations, meningoceles may be present. Usually, the meningoceles are at the level of the root avulsion and are found lateral to the cord and involve the nerve root sheath. Usually, the meningocele does not interfere with the dorsal approach to the cord for lesion making, and no attempt to resect or decompress the meningocele should be made. Distant trigger areas usually are not reported by patients. However, referred pain into adjacent dermatomes does occur, and DREZ lesions may be extended one or two dermatomes above the involved cord segments to make these areas analgesic.

POSTHERPETIC PAIN

Patients with postherpetic neuralgia may have excellent relief of their pain with DREZ lesions. Although these patients have usually tried extensive pharmacologic treatments, few have had prior surgery. Only half of patients with abdominal or truncal herpes benefit from the DREZ operation.

After careful sensory charts of the involved dermatomes

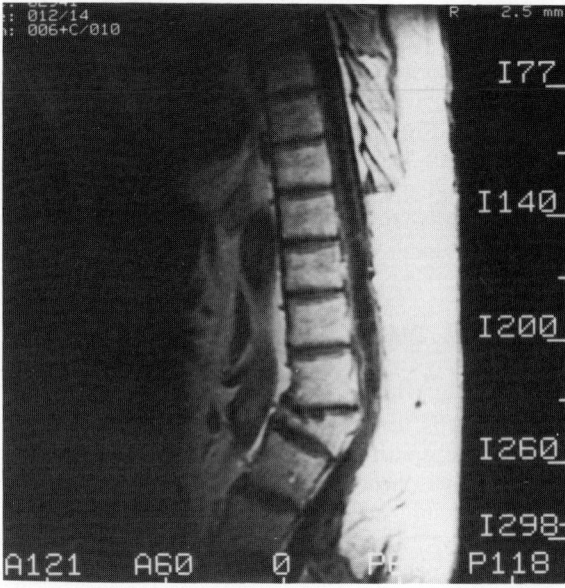 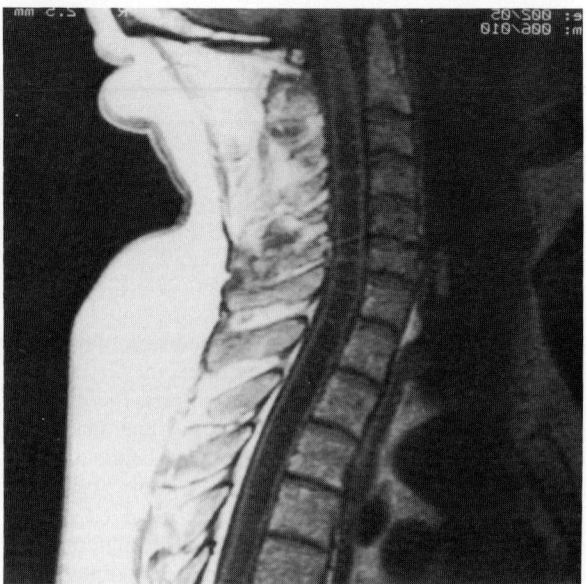

FIGURE 131–11. MRI of the spinal cord with traumatic syrinx and T12 compression in 60-year-old Vietnam veteran who suffered this injury in a helicopter crash. Cyst seen at T11-C2.

have been prepared preoperatively, a hemilaminectomy is performed to include two additional dermatomes above the involved areas. For example, if the postherpetic neuralgia involves T9 to T10, a hemilaminectomy from T7 to T10 is performed. A wider hemilaminectomy is performed, and undercutting of the spinous processes allows ample visualization of the lateral and medial dorsal spinal cord. Once the dura is opened, the affected nerve roots may appear thin, atrophic, and gray instead of off-white. However, no visual difference may exist between normal and abnormal roots.

Intraoperatively, the involved dorsal root entry segment is localized with direct spinal cord evoked potentials. By use of a percutaneous intercostal nerve root electrode, the intercostal nerve is stimulated, and recordings are made from the spinal cord at the dorsal horn. Somatosensory evoked potentials and motor evoked potentials are used intraoperatively. A more detailed discussion of this recording and localization technique follows in the section on evoked potentials and impedance in this chapter.

REFLEX SYMPATHETIC DYSTROPHY

Most patients with reflex sympathetic dystrophy do not benefit from DREZ lesions. Of 10 patients with reflex sympathetic dystrophy, only two reported good pain relief in their arms and hands from DREZ lesions. The operative technique for reflex sympathetic dystrophy is similar to that on the cervical spine for brachial plexus avulsions except that only a two- or three-level hemilaminectomy must be performed for one- or two-dermatome DREZ lesions. A hemilaminectomy may be performed instead of a full laminectomy in these cases.

POSTRHIZOTOMY AND PERIPHERAL NERVE PAIN

DREZ lesions for peripheral nerve pain are successful when they are employed on a highly selective basis. Patients undergoing this operation usually have had many previous procedures, and the lower the number of prior surgeries, the better the results. Patients with trauma-related injuries have the best results, for example, compared with patients with chronic pain from sciatica. A hemilaminectomy may be performed instead of a full laminectomy, and undercutting of the spinous process should also be performed to expose the medial cord. Bony removal should be carried out to one or two levels above the involved dermatomes. Patients with wider areas of peripheral pain that involve the entire foot instead of just an L5 or S1 distribution of pain have better pain relief if DREZ lesions are carried to two dermatomes above the affected level. Precise localization of involved cord segments is achieved via directly recorded root potentials

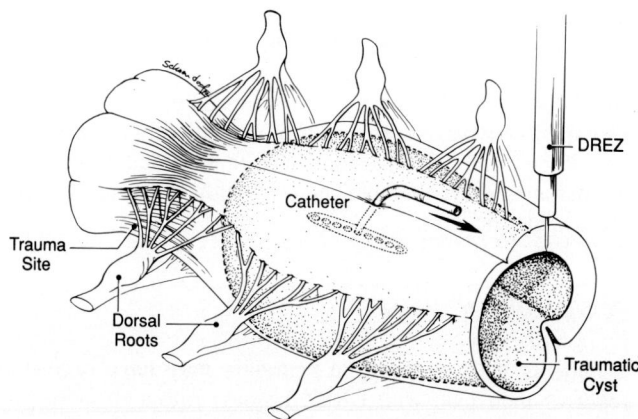

FIGURE 131–12. Traumatic cyst with syrinx-to-subarachnoid space shunt in place and DREZ electrode. (From Nashold BS, Nashold JRB: The DREZ operation, in Tindall GT, Cooper PR, Barrow D (eds): The Practice of Neurosurgery. New York, Williams & Wilkins, 1993.)

evoked by stimulation of the proximal portion of the injured nerve.

ATYPICAL FACIAL PAIN

Atypical facial pain caused by various syndromes, including refractory trigeminal neuralgia; postherpetic facial pain; orbital or dental pain; head, neck, or face pain from cancer; postradiation pain; postrhizotomy dysesthetic pain (anesthesia dolorosa); intractable migraine headaches, Wallenberg's syndrome; and vascular lesions, like basilar aneurysms and arteriovenous malformations, may be treated by DREZ lesions. Many of these patients, especially those with tic pain, have had several previous surgical procedures and present difficult clinical features that may include the classic unilateral trigeminal pain distribution or midline facial pain between the eyes, at the nasolabial folds, the lateral edges of the mouth, or at one or more teeth. Patients who have not had previous operations have better results from DREZ lesions for pain than those with previous multiple procedures. The indications for DREZ lesions need better definition in this group.

Three technical changes in the DREZ nucleus caudalis operation have recently improved this procedure. The most important innovation has been the redesign of the straight Radionics radiofrequency electrode into a right-angled electrode that permits more accurate lesion making in the nucleus caudalis without involvement of the neighboring spinocerebellar tract, thereby reducing transient postoperative ataxia. Two right-angled electrodes, one 2 mm and one 3 mm, are used because of the difference in thickness between the caudal and rostral part of the caudalis nucleus (Fig. 131–13). The 2-mm electrode is used for lesions between C2 and C1, and the 3-mm electrode is used for those from C1 to the level of the obex. The second change has been to move the anesthesia team away from the head of the table to the side of the patient, thereby permitting 180-degree access to the suboccipital exposure. The third innovation has been changing the midline suboccipital incision to a paramedian incision, dissection, and atlanto-occipital dural opening with a rostral curve that parallels the natural curve of the cervicomedullary junction.

The nucleus caudalis DREZ operation is performed through a paramedian suboccipital craniectomy and C1-C2 laminectomy (Fig. 131–14). Electrocautery is used below the skin to dissect through the subcutaneous tissue, fascia, and muscle layers, sparing the greater occipital nerve whenever possible. The soft tissue exposure is carried down to C3. Before the laminectomies are performed, the perforator drill is used to drill two burr holes lateral to the midline and 4 to 6 cm below the inion. These burr holes must be drilled first so that C1 and C2 will protect the spinal cord if the drill slips caudally off the sloping surface of the occipital bone. A Midas Rex drill or hand-held rongeurs are used to enlarge and complete the suboccipital craniectomy. Special care must be used in removal of the posterior portion of the foramen magnum, where a dense collagen-dural ring of tissue is present at the cervicomedullary junction. The laminectomies are performed in the standard fashion, and care is taken not to extend the bony C1 posterior arch removal too far laterally to involve the vertebral arteries. Large epidural venous plexuses and hemorrhage from these vessels must be avoided with careful dissection. Use of low-voltage bipolar cautery and other hemostatic techniques are employed especially in the recesses of the lateral gutters.

The dura is opened in a caudal-to-rostral direction, with a curve laterally along the natural bend of the lower medulla.

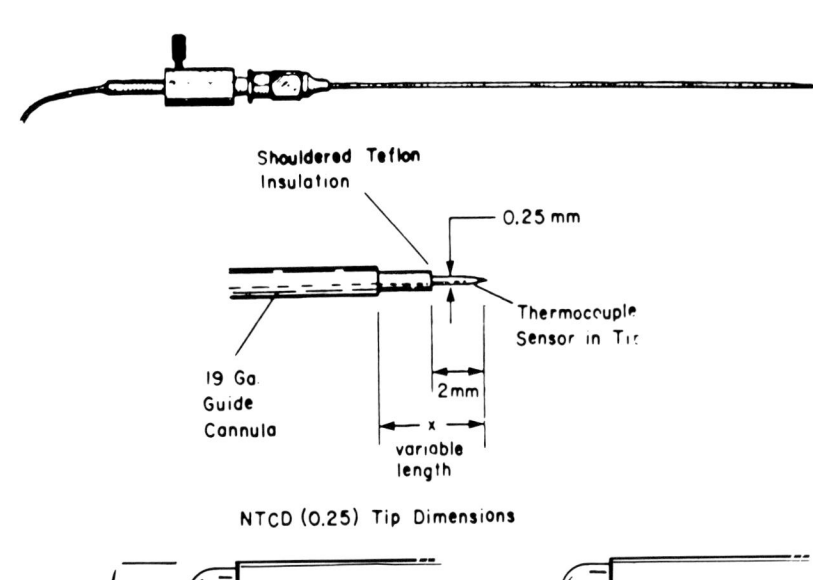

FIGURE 131–13. DREZ electrodes. (Courtesy of Radionics Corporation.) (Top) Illustration shows a 2-mm electrode for spinal DREZ. (Bottom) Lower electrodes are the new right-angled caudalis DREZ electrodes.

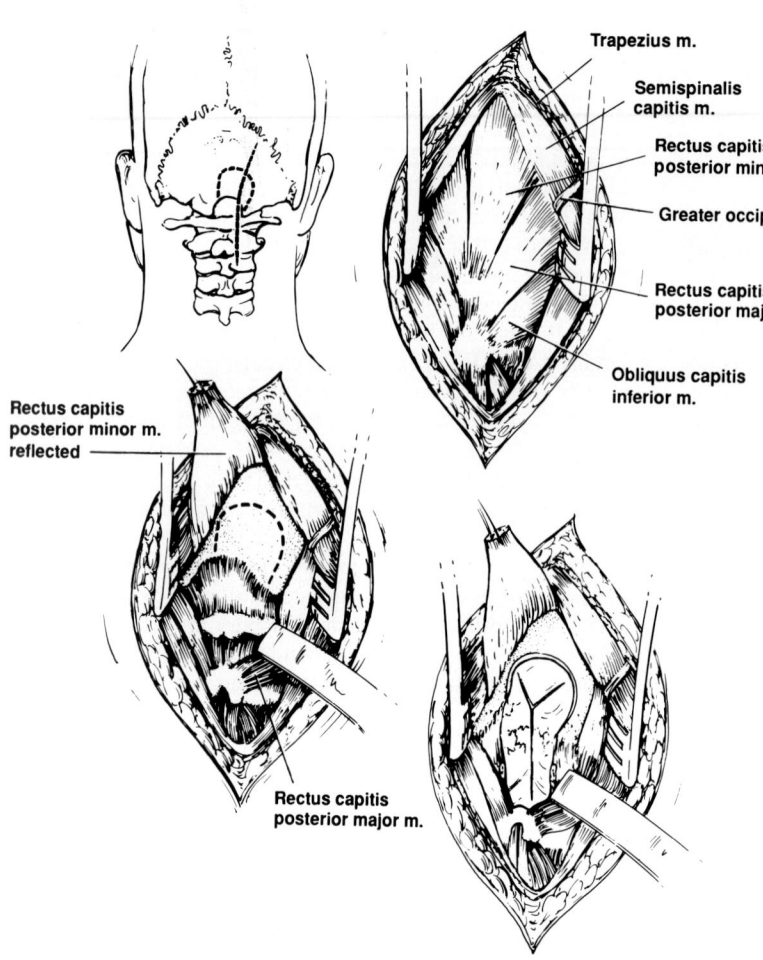

FIGURE 131–14. Unilateral exposure of the nucleus caudalis. (From Nashold BS, El-Naggar AO: Dorsal root entry zone (DREZ) lesioning, in Wilkins RH, Rengachary SS (eds): Neurosurgical Operative Atlas, vol 2. Baltimore, Williams & Wilkins, 1993, p 22.)

The dura in the suboccipital area must be slowly opened and the occipital sinus clipped off with silver clips to avoid excessive blood loss. In elderly patients, the dura in the suboccipital area may be quite thin and diaphanous and should be preserved for later closure. The size of the occipital sinus ranges widely, and the surgeon should be able to see the deeper layer of the dural-sinus wall to maintain control of the occipital sinus. During the most rostral opening of the dura, the posteroinferior cerebellar artery is found to have many different courses around the inferior cerebellum, vermis, and medulla. Occult aneurysms may be encountered and should be clipped.

Once a visual inspection of the posteroinferior cerebellar artery, the spinal accessory nerve, the dorsal roots of C1 and C2, the obex, and the vertebral arteries is completed for orientation, the DREZ lesions should be made with the El-Naggar-Nashold right-angled electrode made by Radionics (Fig. 131–15). Radiofrequency lesions are the same as for the brachial plexus and other DREZ operations; 75° C for 15 seconds. The lesions are made in a caudal-to-rostral direction, starting at the C2 dorsal rootlets in the intermediolateral sulcus with the 2-mm electrode just dorsal to where the rootlets exit the spinal cord. Lesion making is carried up to the inferior obex and the cuneate tubercle with the 3-mm electrode. Patients with midline pain syndromes of the face require extension of the lesions 1 cm above the level of the obex or require additional lesions above that level. The anesthesiologist should be warned before lesion making is begun to watch for apnea or bradycardia, which can be prevented by using atropine.

Closure of the dura is in standard fashion and may require a dural graft because the dura is usually stretched tightly over the cervicomedullary junction. Fastidious hemostasis should be achieved, and the fascia and muscle should be closed in anatomic layers.

POSTOPERATIVE MANAGEMENT

After all DREZ operations, the patients are kept in bed for 3 days with the head of the bed raised to 30 degrees on the second postoperative day. Ambulation is begun on the fourth postoperative day. Physical therapy is used for older patients to help in ambulation. Steroids are used for 5 days postoperatively, and are rapidly tapered over the last 3 days. The decision to prescribe preoperative and postoperative antibiotics is left to the surgeon's personal preference. Strict wound care and observation for CSF leaks is important. Pain medications are decreased rapidly during the first postoperative week. Careful postoperative sensory, motor, and cranial nerve examinations are performed, and the results are compared with preoperative areas of pain. CSF leaks are managed with oversewing of the skin incision, but persistent leaks lasting more than 2 days may require reinspection of the wound in the operating room.

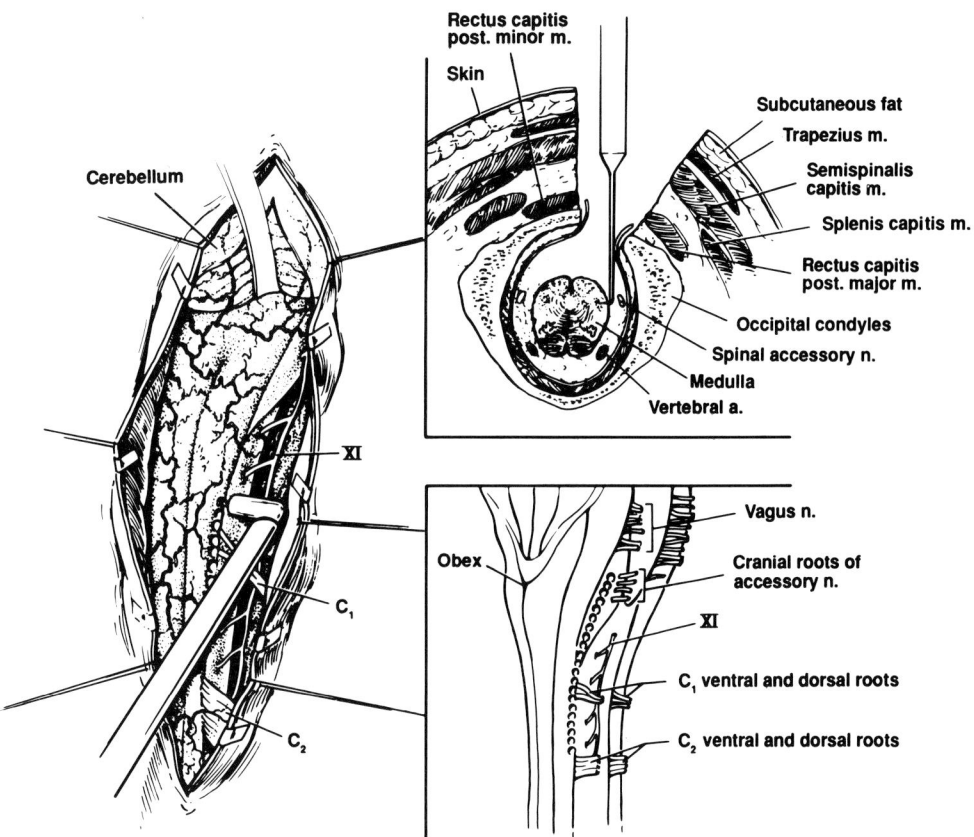

FIGURE 131–15. Precise location of lesions of the nucleus caudalis. (From Nashold BS, El-Naggar AO: Dorsal root entry zone (DREZ) lesioning, in Wilkins RH, Rengachary SS (eds): Neurosurgical Operative Atlas, vol. 2. Baltimore, Williams & Wilkins, 1993, p 23.)

INTRAOPERATIVE EVOKED POTENTIAL RECORDING AND IMPEDANCE MEASUREMENT

In brachial plexus avulsions, intraoperative recordings for spinal segment localization are not required because the area of avulsion is usually visually obvious when compared with the normal side. DREZ operations in the thoracic cord or conus medullaris require a percutaneous monopolar electrode placed preoperatively near the sciatic, posterior tibial, sural, and intercostal nerves. During surgery, an Avery Multicontact plate electrode with four platinum discs in a polyester (Dacron) web is used along the normal DREZ side. Measurement of latency and amplitude of the evoked potentials help determine the level of maximal afferent activity, which then helps to localize the involved cord segments.

Impedance levels before and after lesion making are another important intraoperative recording technique to help determine the difference between damaged spinal cord tissue and normal cord. Normal dorsal spinal cord horn impedances may range from 1200 to 1500 ohms or from 1500 to 2000 ohms. Individual numbers below these levels indicate areas of damaged spinal cord. However, absolute measurements are not as important as are trends that indicate below-average tissue impedance. Impedance should be abnormal (< 1000 ohms or < 1500 ohms in patients with high-normal levels) along most of the entire length. As damaged tissue merges into more normal tissue, the impedance progressively climbs into the normal range. Once three to four consecutive impedance levels are in the normal range and this anatomic level corresponds to the uppermost extent of the desired treatment, lesion making is terminated.

RESULTS

Our experience with over 600 patients who received DREZ procedures indicates that chronic deafferentation pain is relieved in most patients with brachial plexus avulsion injuries, postherpetic facial pain, paraplegic pain, and postamputation phantom pain of central origin. Less than 50 percent of patients with atypical facial pain who have had multiple previous procedures, chronic sciatic pain, postradiation pain, postamputation stump pain, postrhizotomy pain, and post-thoracotomy pain are helped by the DREZ operation, and they have a high recurrence of old or new forms of deafferentation pain. This finding reinforces our experience that patients with peripheral pain do less well than patients with central pain. Second DREZ procedures have shown a mixed and unpredictable relief of recurrent pain and should be avoided.

Postoperative complications include CSF leaks (in less than 1 percent), wound infections (in less than 1 percent), transient ipsilateral ataxia (40 percent), and ipsilateral upper or lower extremity weakness because of local edema secondary to lesion making (5 percent), which affects the spinocerebellar, corticospinal, or propriospinal tracts. Careful surgical techniques and attention to dural and fascial closure eliminates most CSF leaks and wound infections. The incidence of ipsilateral ataxia after nucleus caudalis DREZ lesions in the 1980s was as high as 40 to 50 percent, but it resolved over several weeks. With introduction of the right-angled electrode for nucleus caudalis DREZs, this complication has been eliminated. Two postoperative deaths of 600 patients have occurred, one in an elderly woman with facial pain who had a postoperative stroke and one in an elderly man with postherpetic thoracic pain who suffered a cerebellar hemorrhagic infarction. Care in lesion making, monitoring of evoked potentials, and fastidious hemostasis should help to control postoperative complications.

The operative technique of DREZ lesions has created a new opportunity for pain relief in patients who had little hope from traditional procedures and often faced a life of narcotic dependence. As lesion-making techniques and our understanding of the basic mechanisms of deafferentation pain syndromes continue to unfold, so, too, will the applications of this procedure.

REFERENCES

1. Schweitzer A: On the Edge of the Primeval Forest. New York, Macmillan, 1931, p 62
2. Tasker RR, Organ LW, Hawrylyshyn P: Deafferentation and causalgia, in Bonica JJ (ed): Pain. New York, Raven Press, 1980, pp 305–329
3. Bennett WH, cited by Abbe R: Acute spasmodic pain in the left lower extremity. Med Chir Trans 72:329–348, 1889
4. Nashol BS, Ostadahl RH: Dorsal root entry zone lesions for pain relief. J Neurosurg 51:59–69, 1979
5. Nashold BS: Deafferentation pain in man and animals as it relates to the DREZ operation. Can J Neurol Sci 15:5–9, 1988
6. Sedivec MJ, Caponski JJ, Mendell LM: Morphology of HRP-injected spinocervical tract neurons: Effect of dorsal rhizotomy. J Neurosci 6:661–672, 1986
7. Sedivec MJ, Capowski JJ, Ovelmen-Levitt J, Mendell LM: Changes in dendritic organization of spinocervical tract neurons following partial deafferentation. Soc Neurosci Abstr 8:755, 1982
8. Blumenkopf B: Neuropharmacology of the dorsal root entry zone. Neurosurgery 15:900–903, 1984
9. Blumenkopf B: Neurochemistry of the dorsal horn. Appl Neurophysiol 51:89–103, 1988
10. Blumenkopf B: The general aspects of neuropharmacology of dorsal horn function, in Nashold BS, Ovelmen-Levitt J (eds): Advances in Pain Research and Therapy, vol 19. New York, Raven Press, 1991, pp 151–162
11. Nashold BS, Ostdahl RH, Bullitt E, et al: Dorsal root entry zone lesions: A new neurosurgical therapy for deafferentation pain, in Bonica JJ (ed): Advances in Pain Research and Therapy, vol 5. New York, Raven Press, 1983, pp 739–750
12. Nashold BS, Higgins AC, Friedman A, et al: The DREZ operation. Modern techniques in surgery. Neurosurgery 35:1–17, 1984
13. Nashold BS, Friedman A, Bullitt E: The status of dorsal root entry zone lesions in 1987, in Clinical Neurosurgery, vol 35. Baltimore, Williams & Wilkins, 1989, pp 422–428
14. Thomas DGT, Jones SJ: Dorsal root entry zone lesions (Nashold's procedure) in brachial plexus avulsion. Neurosurgery 15:966–968, 1984
15. Rawlings CE, Rossitch E, Nashold BS: The use of limited DREZ lesions for intractable pain. Pain Manage 4:315–320, 1989
16. Nashold BS, Rossitch E, Alexander E: Dorsal root entry zone surgery for pain management. Pain Manage 6:15–23, 1991
17. Moossy JJ, Nashold BS: Dorsal root entry zone lesions for conus medullaris root avulsions. Appl Neurophysiol 51:198–205, 1988
18. Nashold BS, Bullitt E: Dorsal root entry zone lesions to control central pain in paraplegics. J Neurosurg 55:414–419, 1981
19. Nashold BS, Vierira J, El-Naggar AO: Pain and spinal cysts in paraplegia: Treatment by drainage and DREZ operation. Br J Neurosurg 4:327–336, 1990
20. Saris SC, Iacono RP, Nashold BS: Dorsal root entry zone lesions for post-amputation pain. J Neurosurg 62:72–76, 1985
21. Nashold BS, Ostdahl RH, Bullitt E: Control of pain in brachial plexus avulsion, spinal paraplegia and herpes using DREZ lesions, in Brock M (ed): Modern Neurosurgery. Heidelberg, Springer-Verlag, 1982, pp 460–463
22. Friedman AH, Nashold BS, Ovelman-Levitt J: Dorsal root entry zone lesions for the treatment of post-herpetic neuralgia. J Neurosurg 60:1258–1261, 1984
23. Nashold BS, Bullitt E, Friedman A: The place of neurosurgery in the treatment of intractable pain, in Swerdlow M, Charlton JE (eds): Relief of Intractable Pain. New York, Elsevier, 1989, pp 305–327
24. Friedman AH: Treatment of deafferentation pains following peripheral nerve injury, in Nashold BS, Ovelman-Levitt J (eds): Advances in Pain Research and Therapy, vol 19. New York, Raven Press, 1991, pp 321–330
25. Matsumura M, Shibasaki T, Negishi M, et al: Pain relief by dorsal root entry zone lesions in intractable pain due to partially injured tibial nerve. Clin J Pain 3:327–332, 1988
26. El-Naggar AO, Nashold BS: Nucleus caudalis DREZ lesions for relief of intractable facial pain, 1993, in press
27. Barr ML, Kiernan JA: The Human Nervous System. Heidelberg, Springer-Verlag, 1988, pp 131–132
28. Nashold BS, Lopes H, Chodakiewitz J, Bronec P: Trigeminal DREZ for craniofacial pain, in Samii M (ed): Surgery in and Around the Brain Stem and the Third Ventricle. Heidelberg, Springer-Verlag, 1992, pp 53–59
29. Rossitch E, Zeidman SM, Nashold BS: Nucleus caudalis DREZ for facial pain due to cancer. Br J Neurosurg 3:45–50, 1989
30. Sampson JH, Nashold BS: Facial pain due to vascular lesions of the brain stem relieved by dorsal root entry zone lesions in the nucleus caudalis. J Neurosurg 77:473–475, 1992

CHAPTER 132

Surgery of the Sympathetic Nervous System

Russell W. Hardy, Jr.
Janet W. Bay

As described in Greenwood's article, "The origins of sympathectomy,"[1] surgeons first employed sympathectomy during the last decade of the 19th century. At that time, Jonnesco performed cervical ganglionectomies for the treatment of epilepsy, exophthalmic goiter, and (somewhat later) angina pectoris. During these same years, Jaboulay and, later, LeRiche carried out sympathectomies for the relief of trophic ulcers in the lower extremity. Further interest in the operation was stimulated by the work of Royle and Hunter, who believed that sympathectomy would relieve spasticity. Although their theory was proved erroneous, observations of patients who had undergone sympathectomy led to increased use of the operation for vasospastic disease. Subsequently, this procedure was used to treat a wide variety of conditions, including angina pectoris,[2] hypertension,[3,4] and vascular disease of large and small vessels.[5-7] Currently, many of these conditions are no longer indications for sympathectomy, either because of the advent of more modern methods of treatment (as in the case of angina and hypertension) or because experience has cast doubt on the efficacy of sympathectomy (as in the treatment of claudication of vascular origin).[8]

At present, the use of sympathectomy is limited to a handful of conditions, but it remains an important surgical technique because it is uniquely effective in treating hyperhidrosis,[9] major causalgia[10-12] and some forms of minor causalgia,[13-18] shoulder-hand syndrome,[10] and certain pain of visceral origin.[19-25] Sympathectomy is also used for the treatment of ischemic ulceration, Raynaud's phenomenon, rest pain, and other sequelae of vascular insufficiency.[6,7]

This chapter discusses three separate operations. The first is upper thoracic (T2) ganglionectomy, as employed to treat hyperhidrosis and causalgia in the upper extremities. The second is splanchnicectomy combined with lower thoracic sympathectomy, which is used in the treatment of pain secondary to pancreatic cancer, or (rarely) for the pain of chronic pancreatitis, or (even more rarely) for pain of renal origin. The third is lumbar sympathectomy, as used in the treatment of major and minor causalgia in the lower extremities.

UPPER THORACIC GANGLIONECTOMY

ANATOMY

The sympathetic supply to the upper extremity is derived from preganglionic fibers leaving the cord from the second through the tenth anterior thoracic roots.[26] These fibers enter the paraspinal sympathetic ganglia via the white rami and synapse in the sympathetic chain. Postganglionic fibers leave the stellate and middle cervical ganglia to join the fifth cervical through the first thoracic roots, although the bulk of these fibers are found in the seventh and eighth cervical and first thoracic roots.[26,27]

According to the above schema, a resection of the second thoracic ganglion should be sufficient to denervate the upper extremity. It has been argued, however, that sympathetic efferents to the arm also are derived from the eighth cervical[28] and, more importantly, the first thoracic[29,30] roots. In addition, Kuntz has described communications between the third and second thoracic roots, and second and first thoracic roots, which might serve as an extraganglionic sympathetic pathway to the arm.[28-31] Finally, intermediate ganglia have been described in the spinal roots of C8, T1, and T2, which also might supply sympathetic fibers to the arm, independent of traditional pathways.[32]

If these various alternate pathways are viewed as significant, complete sympathetic denervation of the upper extremity would require resection of the middle cervical ganglion, the stellate ganglion, the second and third thoracic ganglia, and the intrathoracic nerves of Kuntz. It would also demand section of the anterior roots of T1, T2, and T3, and even then, input from anterior cervical roots might persist. In fact, such an extensive procedure has been advocated in the past,[30] and numerous authors recommend at least including the inferior portion of the stellate ganglion, in addition to T2 and T3,[10,31] to ensure a complete sympathectomy.

The sympathetic outflow to the pupil leaves the cord at T1, but contributions may also come from T2, T3, T4, and (rarely) C8.[33] These fibers then cross the stellate ganglion and synapse with postganglionic neurons in the superior cervical ganglion. Thus, procedures that require resection of the stellate ganglion will result in Horner's syndrome, although resection of the lower half of this ganglion may be performed without risking this complication.[34]

In addition, preganglionic sympathectomy (by division of the anterior spinal roots, white rami, and sympathetic chain, but with preservation of the ganglia) was at one time recommended on the grounds that this procedure would avoid "hypersensitivity" of end organs to circulating catecholamines.[35] Many now feel, however, that such hypersensitivity does not occur or is of minimal clinical significance after resection of the ganglia.[10,30]

In our experience, as well as in the experience of others, resection of the T2 ganglia has been sufficient to denervate the upper extremity and serve as adequate treatment for hyperhidrosis and causalgia.[9, 36, 37] If the lower portion of the stellate ganglion is not resected, the risk of Horner's syndrome is minimized. We have not observed hypersensitivity after T2 ganglionectomy in the treatment of hyperhidrosis, and it does not occur when postganglionic sympathectomy is performed for the treatment of causalgia (Mayfield: Personal communication; Nulsen: Personal communication).

SURGICAL APPROACHES

Many approaches to the cervical and upper thoracic chain have been employed, including posterior thoracic operations via the midline,[5, 38] paramedian,[35] or transverse[39] incisions, cervical (unilateral[40] or bilateral[41, 42]) incisions, and transthoracic[43, 44] and anterior transthoracic approaches.[45] The operation we employ is a posterior approach through a midline incision using loop magnification and headlight illumination. Lindquist and associates[46] found the operating microscope plus electrical stimulation of the chain to be useful adjuncts when the dorsal approach was used. The anterior and lateral operations have the advantage of providing excellent visualization of the sympathetic chain, but the disadvantage of the exposure being unilateral, which means that a second procedure is required if a bilateral sympathectomy is needed. The posterior paramedian approach can afford a bilateral exposure, albeit through two separate incisions. This approach may carry the disadvantage of providing less adequate visualization of the chain, and in our experience, occasional difficulties arise with the upper thoracic paramedian incision. The cervical approach can be performed through either a unilateral or a midline incision,[41] which affords bilateral exposure, but visualization of the upper thoracic ganglia may be difficult.

Recently, investigators have renewed efforts to accomplish surgical sympathectomy of the upper extremities using less invasive techniques. In 1984, Wilkinson[47, 48] reported his initial experience with radiofrequency percutaneous upper thoracic sympathectomy. Immediate postoperative results were favorable: sympathectomy was achieved in 24 of 27 limbs, and the complication rate was low and the hospital stay very brief. However, "a significant number of acute or delayed recurrences"[49] were encountered with this technique, and whether the long-term results will be competitive with those of open techniques remains to be seen.

More recently, a stereotactic technique for percutaneous, x-ray study–guided thermocoagulation of T2-T3 has been reported.[50] Excellent results were noted in the first 10 patients treated.

In addition, numerous recent reports have been published on endoscopic upper thoracic sympathectomy.[51–54] The concept is not new, having been pioneered by the Austrian surgeon, Kux.[55] His extensive experience of more than 1400 thoroscopic neurotomies performed via electrocoagulation was reported in the German literature in 1954. Favorable results have been reported with a more refined endoscopic technique by Weale,[54] Malone and colleagues,[53] and Lin.[52] (See Editorial Comment at the end of this chapter.)

Another, less invasive, technique involves the use of phenol injected percutaneously into the upper thoracic chain via computed tomographic guidance for treatment of hyperhidrosis and Raynaud's phenomenon.[56] Long-term results were not favorable: less than 50 percent of the patients achieved lasting sympathectomy.

A long-term recurrence rate of 4.1 percent has been reported for the open surgical treatment of hyperhidrosis.[57, 58] Long-term follow-up data on a larger group of patients is necessary to assess the permanence of these promising new techniques. We continue to use the dorsal operation through a midline incision because of the bilateral exposure, excellent visualization of the chain, good long-term results, and relatively low complication rate.

INDICATIONS

A T2 ganglionectomy is currently used in the treatment of essential hyperhidrosis and for major causalgia (as described originally by Weir Mitchell),[50] minor causalgia and some of its variations, and occasionally, for shoulder-hand syndrome.[59] A T2 ganglionectomy also may be employed to treat certain conditions of vascular origin.[6]

The use of sympathectomy for the treatment of essential hyperhidrosis was first described by Kotzareff.[9] Hyperhidrosis can be a source of great embarrassment and considerable disability to the patient. It may involve the entire body, including the legs and head, but symptoms are most severe and of the greatest discomfort in the upper extremities. Patients have symptoms that often date from childhood or early adolescence. Such individuals report reluctance to shake hands or touch other people, and often wear gloves to disguise their condition. The diagnosis is readily confirmed by inspection of the extremities.

Experience has confirmed the value of sympathectomy in the treatment of causalgia.[10, 12] As originally described, this condition is characterized by severe burning pain that is exacerbated by touch and appears shortly after an injury to a mixed peripheral nerve,[49] most often the median or sciatic nerve. This injury occurs most often during wartime and is relatively uncommon in civilian practice. It first may be treated by sympathetic blocks, to which a very high proportion of patients respond. In fact, response to a block is one method of establishing the diagnosis in individuals with typical symptoms. Some patients may be treated without surgery by blocks alone. If the pain recurs, however, sympathectomy may be performed, and relief of pain is obtained in a very high percentage of patients.

Sympathectomy also may be employed in the treatment of a group of ill-defined entities that are characterized by burning pain and trophic changes that may appear after peripheral nerve injury but also are associated with other conditions, including fracture, local laceration, infection,[13, 18] burns, subcutaneous injection, phlebitis, and arterial embolism. A unifying mechanism has not been postulated for these conditions, other than the suggestion that they may result from some form of sympathetic overactivity. Regardless of the etiology, some of these conditions are said to respond to sympathectomy, although the response to surgery for these conditions may well be less certain than is the response to surgery for major causalgia. Favorable response to sympathetic block selects patients who may improve after surgery,

Surgery of the Sympathetic Nervous System | 1639

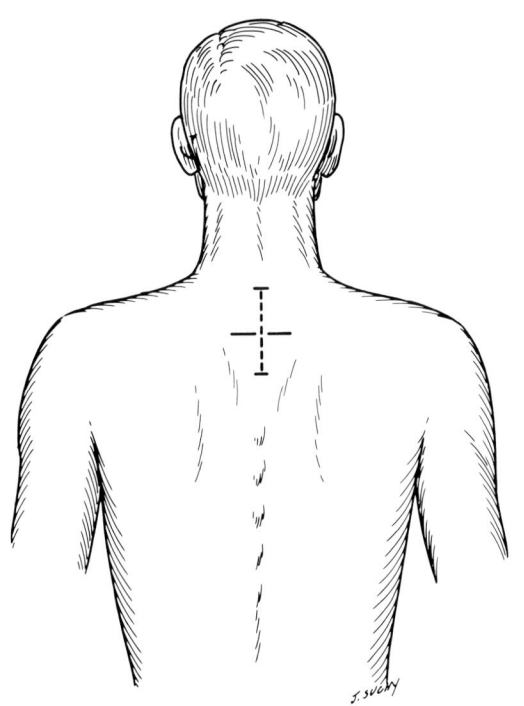

FIGURE 132–1. Location of the skin incision for a T2 ganglionectomy.

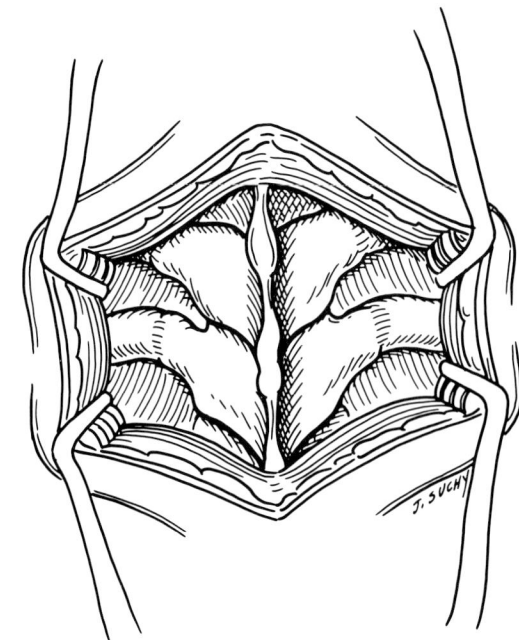

FIGURE 132–3. The completed bilateral exposure of the transverse processes of T3.

but even this is no guarantee that the operation will be successful.

OPERATIVE TECHNIQUE

The T2 ganglionectomy through a dorsal midline incision is most conveniently performed with the patient in the sitting position, although the prone position also may be used (Figs. 132–1 to 132–8). The sitting position has the advantage that an intraoperative x-ray film, confirming the level, can be obtained more conveniently than when the patient is prone. We also feel that exposure is somewhat better when the patient is erect. The principal disadvantage of the sitting position, namely air embolus, is minimal or nonexistent because the level of the costotransversectomy is at the heart.

An x-ray film is obtained before the operation, with a marker placed at the spinous process of T2. The spinous process of T2 is opposite the lamina and medial portion or the rib of T3. These structures are exposed, and confirmatory x-ray films are obtained at the T3 level. Then, the T3 transverse process and underlying rib are removed, either with a Kerrison punch or a rongeur, and care is taken to dissect free the underlying pleura. After resection of the rib and medial

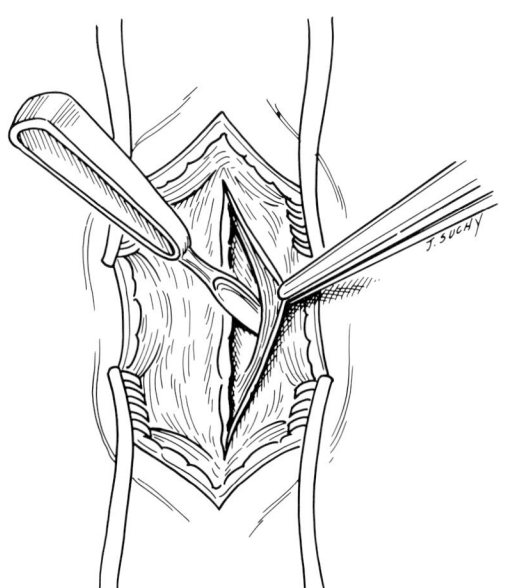

FIGURE 132–2. The beginning of the exposure of the T3 lamina and transverse process.

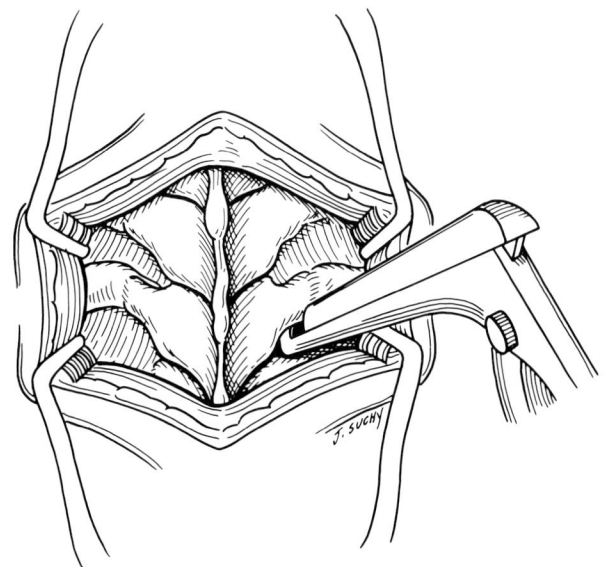

FIGURE 132–4. Resection of the T3 transverse process.

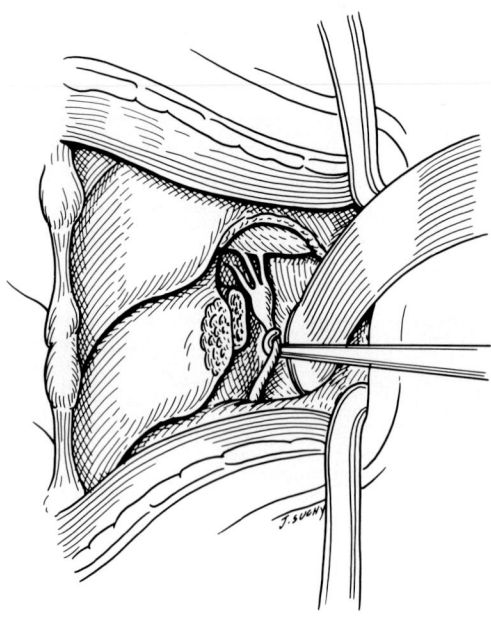

FIGURE 132-5. The T3 costotransversectomy has been completed. The nerve hook is under the sympathetic chain.

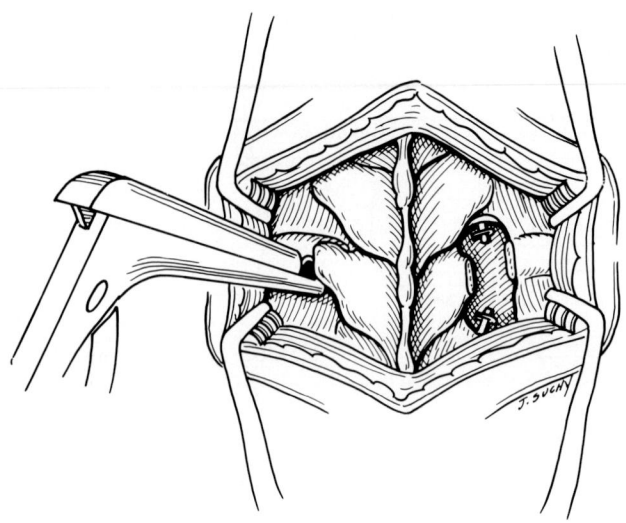

FIGURE 132-7. The contralateral T3 costotransversectomy is begun.

transverse process, the lateral border of the vertebral body is exposed by blunt dissection. The lower portion of the second rib also may need to be removed to expose the T2 ganglion. At this point, the second intercostal nerve is elevated and the sympathetic chain visualized. The communicating rami and the chain above and below the T2 ganglion are clipped and divided, and the ganglion is removed. If convenient, the T3 ganglion also may be resected. If axillary sweating is a major complaint, both the T2 and the T3 ganglia are entirely removed. A bilateral ganglionectomy is performed for hyperhidrosis ischemic disease. A unilateral procedure suffices for causalgia or reflex sympathetic dystrophy.

After resection of the ganglia and hemostasis, the incision may be closed in layers, with care being taken to obtain good closure of the deep fascia over the spinous process of T2 and T3. If a pleural tear has occurred during the course of the dissection, it may be managed by leaving a 12F red rubber catheter in place (within the leaves of the pleura) until a fascial closure is effected. The catheter then is removed with suction as the anesthetist applies positive pressure. This has been an adequate measure to avoid postoperative pneumothorax in most cases.

RESULTS

Our surgical results and complications with bilateral T2 ganglionectomy for hyperhidrosis are representative. Three hundred twenty-six patients underwent bilateral T2 ganglionectomy for hyperhidrosis at the Cleveland Clinic between 1966 and 1983. All patients had immediate relief of palmar

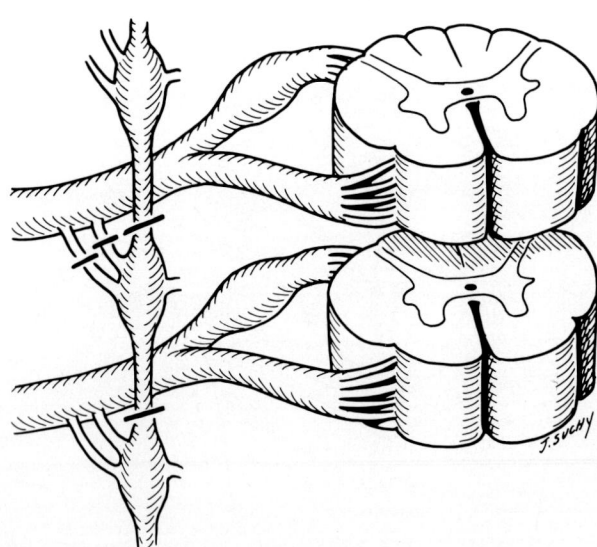

FIGURE 132-6. The extent of the sympathetic resection.

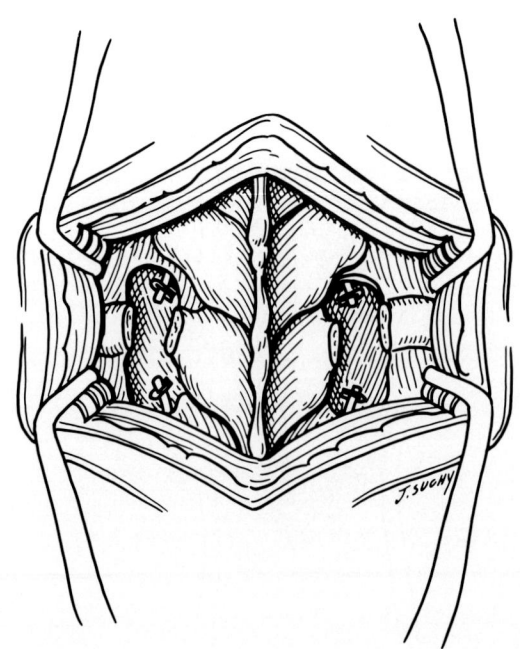

FIGURE 132-8. The complete costotransversectomy and bilateral T2 ganglionectomy.

sweating. Long-term follow-up data were obtained by questionnaire in 162 patients (49 percent). Eighty-eight percent of these patients remained satisfied with the surgical result for postoperative periods up to 15 years. Causes for dissatisfaction included compensatory sweating, intercostal neuralgia, incisional appearance, and recurrent sweating. The recurrence rate for palmar hyperhidrosis in this series was 1 percent.

COMPLICATIONS

There was no operative mortality in this group of 326 patients. Significant complications were noted in 5 percent of the patients and included wound infections (in nine), pneumonia (in two), pneumothorax (in two), cerebrospinal fluid (CSF) leak (in one), Horner's syndrome (in one), spinal cord injury (in one), and empyema (in one).

SPLANCHNICECTOMY

ANATOMY

Visceral afferents supplying the heart, pancreas, kidneys, gallbladder, and other organs have been described[37, 60, 61] and serve as a source of pain in various conditions affecting these structures.

Autonomic innervation to the pancreas is derived from the splanchnic nerves and from the vagus. Visceral afferents appear to travel exclusively through the splanchnic chain. These enter the cord via the greater splanchnic nerve after traversing the celiac ganglion. As described by Ray and Neill,[60] the pancreas receives bilateral innervation not only from the greater splanchnic nerves, which are derived from cord segments T4-T9, but also from the lesser splanchnic nerves and perhaps through the lower portion of the thoracic ganglia and the upper portion of the lumbar chains. Because the pancreas receives bilateral innervation, a bilateral operation is usually required to effect relief of pain,[22, 24] although in certain instances, a unilateral operation is said to be sufficient.[21, 25] Innervation to the biliary tracts is supplied by the right splanchnic nerves, and the nerve supply to the kidneys is also unilateral (via the lesser and least splanchnic trunks). The minor splanchnic nerves are derived from T10 and T11, and the least splanchnic nerve from T12.

Although the splanchnic nerves are divided into three separate branches, in actual practice, identification of these separate trunks may be difficult and may vary considerably from patient to patient.

Based on these anatomic considerations, the operation that we employ to denervate the pancreas is resection of the thoracic ganglia from approximately T9 through T12, together with resection of the greater, lesser, and least splanchnic nerves. Other writers have recommended a more extensive operation, including the upper lumbar ganglia, but we have not found such an extensive resection to be necessary, and removal of the upper lumbar ganglia adds technical difficulty and (in the male) the risk of sexual dysfunction.[24, 62]

INDICATIONS

Pain from pancreatic carcinoma may result from involvement of visceral afferent fibers or from pain secondary to the involvement of parietal somatic nerves. Any evidence of radicular pain suggests involvement of somatic nerves and is a contraindication to the procedure in the patient with pancreatic carcinoma. If doubt exists, the patient may be evaluated by means of a temporary splanchnic block. Frequently, we perform the operation in combination with diagnostic laparotomy. In a patient with upper abdominal and back pain and no evidence of somatic nerve involvement, a bilateral splanchnicectomy can be performed after closure of the abdominal incision and repositioning of the patient. Such a combined operation adds little to the overall morbidity of the laparotomy.

The operation also has been advocated for the pain of chronic pancreatitis,[15, 22, 25] and such pain may be relieved in certain individuals, but in our experience, the operation often fails to help the patient discontinue the use of narcotics (often because the individual develops new chronic pain at the site of operative incisions or elsewhere). Finally, a patient with benign pain of renal or biliary origin may rarely be a candidate for sympathectomy,[37] although operations for these indications are rarely performed at our institutions.

OPERATIVE TECHNIQUE

The procedure is carried out with the patient in the prone position on a laminectomy frame or with a blanket roll beneath the hips and shoulders (Figs. 132–9 through 132–16).[20] An incision is made four fingerbreadths lateral to the spinous process overlying the eleventh rib. Dissection is carried down until the rib is encountered. The periosteum overlying the rib is stripped with an elevator, and the pleura is then separated from the underlying rib with a pigtail periosteal dissector. The lateral 4 to 6 cm of rib are removed with rib cutters and

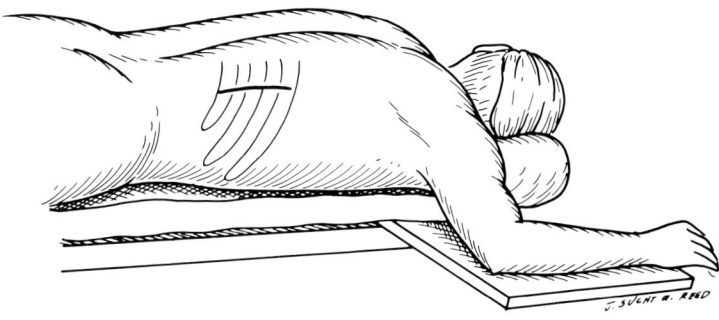

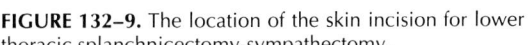

FIGURE 132–9. The location of the skin incision for lower thoracic splanchnicectomy-sympathectomy.

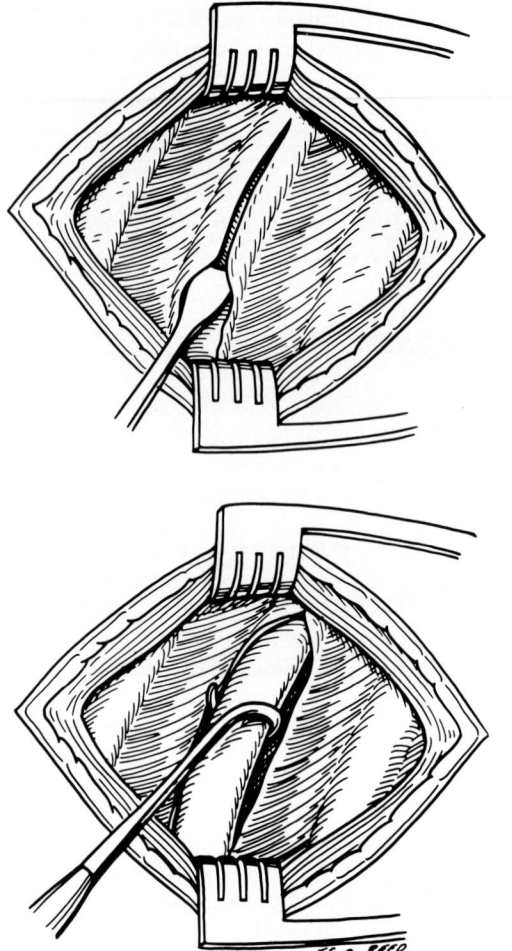

FIGURE 132–10. Subperiosteal exposure of the eleventh rib with a periosteal elevator. The underlying periosteum then is stripped with a pigtail periosteal elevator.

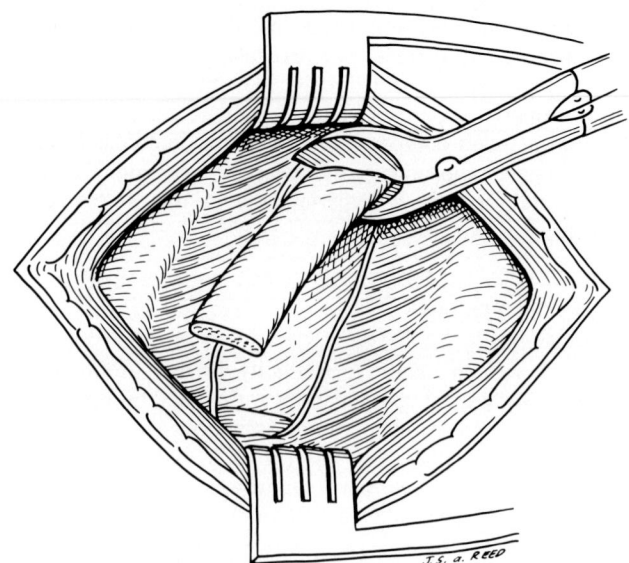

FIGURE 132–11. Resection of the eleventh rib. The underlying parietal pleura then is separated from adjacent ribs by blunt dissection.

rongeurs. The underlying pleura then is carefully dissected from the medial portion of the rib and also from the undersurface of adjacent ribs. Normally, this maneuver is not particularly difficult and can be carried out with careful finger dissection. Some large intercostal veins may be encountered as the dissection is carried out medially. These may be easily controlled with either clips or bipolar coagulation. Final dissection of the pleura from the lateral portion of the spine and the underlying surface of the rib may be carried out with Kitner dissectors. As the pleura is being retracted, it is protected beneath an abdominal sponge.

After the pleura has been swept free of the underlying surface of the rib, the remaining medial portion of the eleventh rib is removed if additional exposure is required. The exposure of the lateral portion of the adjacent vertebrae then is completed. A resection of the sympathetic ganglia and their connections, as well as the greater, lesser, and least splanchnic nerves, then is carried out. As noted earlier, the splanchnic nerves are not always constant structures, although the greater splanchnic nerve may be identified fairly reliably anterior to the sympathetic chain on the lateral margin of the vertebral bodies. As great a length of splanchnic nerve as possible is resected, together with any other branches of the lesser and least nerves that can be identified.

In addition, resection of the ganglia, T9 through T12, together with the rami communicantes, is then carried out, with the chains being divided between metal clips.

One difficulty that is sometimes encountered is that the splanchnic nerves may be difficult to find. A common cause of this is that the nerve may be swept onto the pleura and is then easily retracted along with the parietal pleura. Careful inspection of the surface of the parietal pleura usually identifies the nerve when it cannot be found adjacent to the vertebral bodies.

If the pleura is torn during the procedure, the situation may be managed by inserting a red rubber catheter through the wound and applying suction and Valsalva's maneuver during closure. If a very large tear has occurred, a chest tube may be placed at the time of closure or later, if a substantial pneumothorax is seen on postoperative films.

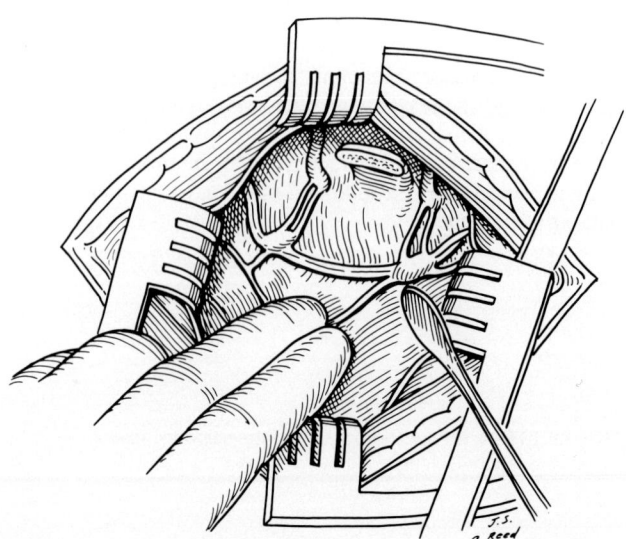

FIGURE 132–12. The exposure of the sympathetic chain and splanchnic nerves.

Surgery of the Sympathetic Nervous System | **1643**

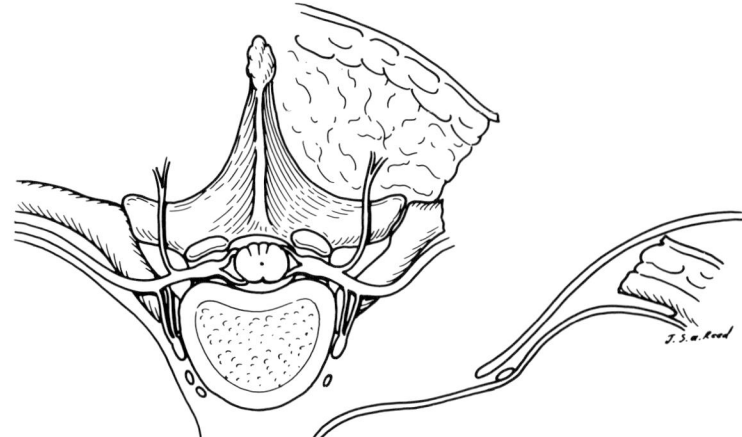

FIGURE 132–13. A cross-sectional view of the exposure. The splanchnic nerves may be inadvertently retracted with the pleura.

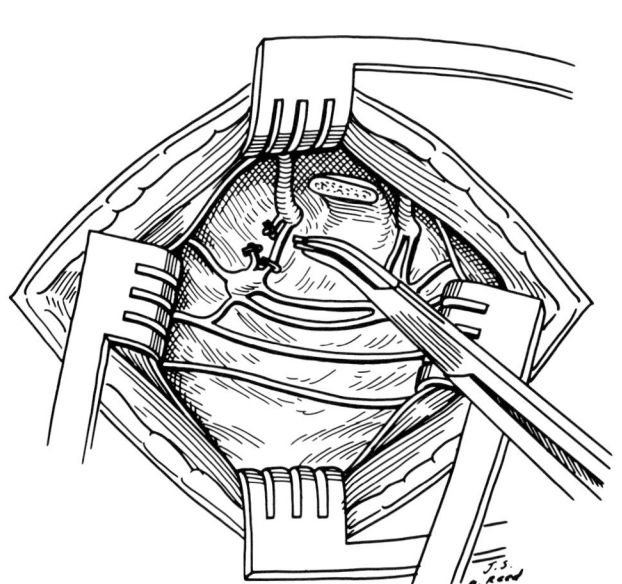

FIGURE 132–14. Resection of the sympathetic chain and splanchnic nerves.

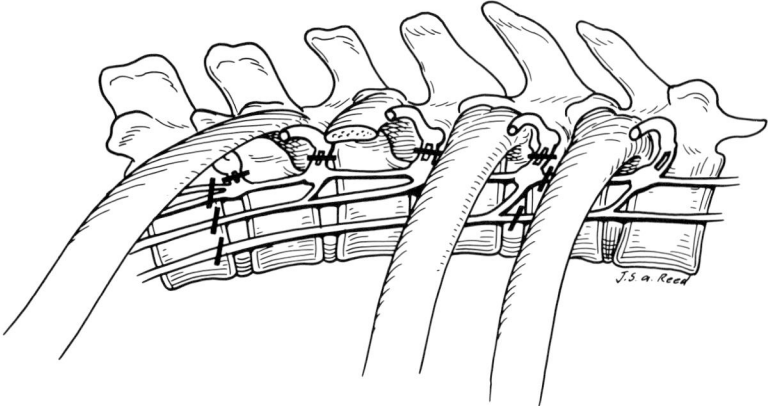

FIGURE 132–15. The ideal extent of the resection.

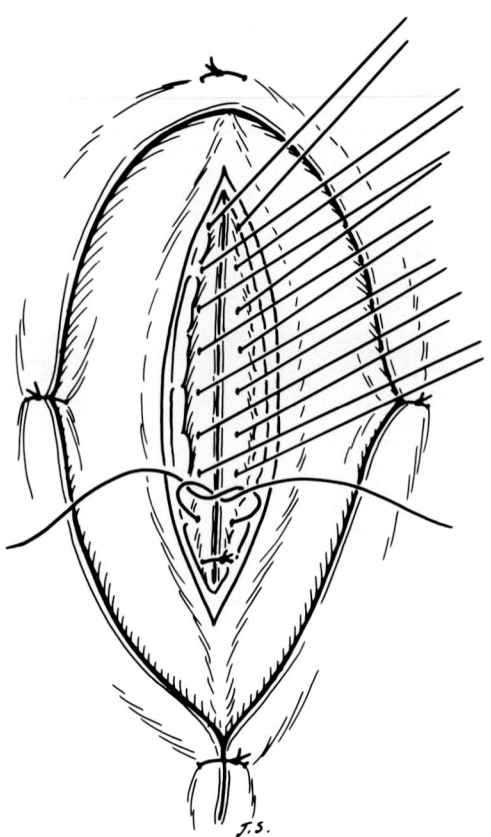

FIGURE 132-16. The layered closure of the incision.

The procedure is carried out bilaterally. As noted, it has not been our custom to divide the diaphragm and remove the L1 ganglia, as has been advocated by some.

RESULTS

In a series of 56 patients undergoing the procedure for pancreatic carcinoma, 70 percent had satisfactory relief of symptoms; 14 percent, partial relief; and 16 percent, no improvement.[23, 24] Recurrence of pain was noted in 23 percent of patients, most often in those who survived for several months; this recurrence of pain was partial and was not regarded as a severe problem. The mortality rate in patients with cancer who were undergoing combined laparotomy and splanchnicectomy was 7 percent.

COMPLICATIONS

As noted earlier, pleural tears occur occasionally and usually can be managed at the time of surgery or with a postoperative chest tube. Superficial wound infections and one case of empyema have occurred. We have not seen paraplegia as a complication of this procedure (caused by interference with the blood supply to the cord), but such catastrophes have been reported. In one patient, the use of electrocautery may have initiated a vascular thrombosis with a resulting delayed paraplegia.[63]

LUMBAR SYMPATHECTOMY

ANATOMY

The sympathetic supply to the lower extremity is derived from the five lumbar ganglia whose efferents leave the spinal canal with the L1 and L2 roots.[26, 37] Resection of the second and third lumbar ganglia should be sufficient to denervate the leg, although in a few individuals, resection of the L1, L2, and T12 ganglia has been necessary to completely abolish the pain of causalgia.[12]

INDICATIONS

The major indication for lumbar sympathectomy by the neurosurgeon is either major or minor causalgia of the lower extremity. The procedure also remains useful for the treatment of ischemic rest pain and superficial ulceration secondary to arteriosclerotic vascular disease. We have not employed this operation in the treatment of hyperhidrosis of the lower extremities.

SURGICAL TECHNIQUE

The operation may be carried out through various skin incisions. We employ the transverse incision extending

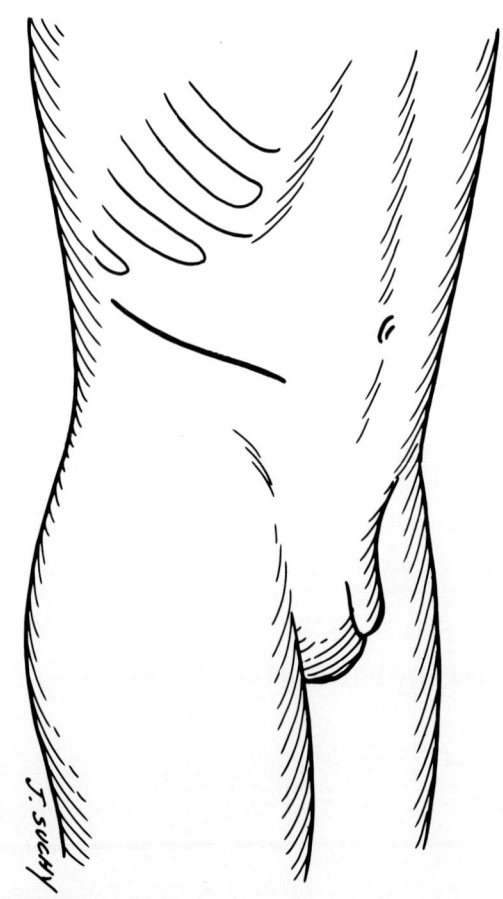

FIGURE 132-17. The incision used for lumbar sympathectomy.

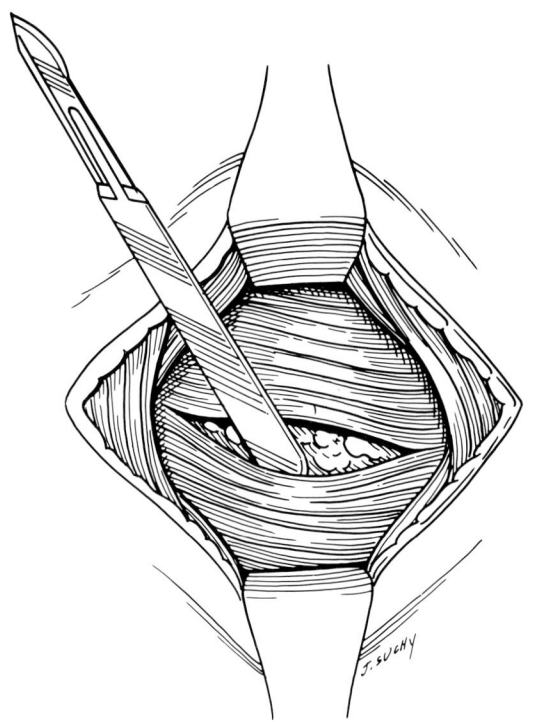

FIGURE 132-18. The abdominal muscles are divided in the direction of their fibers.

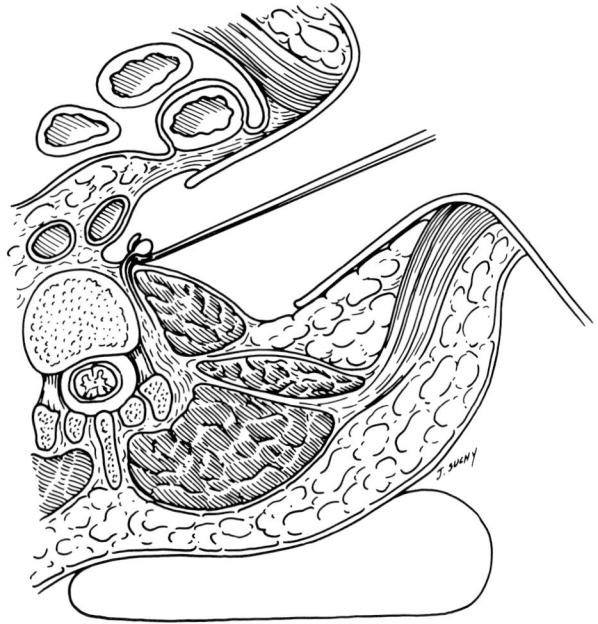

FIGURE 132-20. A cross-sectional view of the exposure following extraperitoneal retraction of the abdominal contents.

obliquely from beneath the costal margin to the right lower quadrant (Figs. 132-17 through 132-20). The external oblique, internal oblique, and transversus muscles are divided in the direction of their fibers. The peritoneum and renal fascia then are dissected free of the quadratus lumborum and iliac muscles with blunt finger dissection. Dissection then is carried medially over the anterior surface of the psoas muscle until the sympathetic chain is encountered between it and the vertebral body.

On the right side, the vena cava is encountered, and bridging veins may need to be divided and clipped or coagulated.

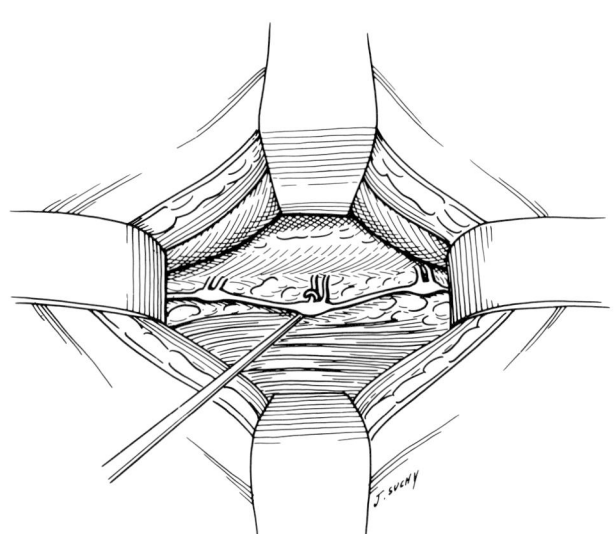

FIGURE 132-19. The sympathetic chain is identified.

On the left, the aorta may be mobilized and does not overlie the chain.

The chain is identified, and at least two ganglia are removed. The chain and rami communicantes are divided between metallic clips.

After resection of the ganglia, the muscle layers are closed separately. During this portion of the procedure, the table may be straightened to facilitate closure.

During the operation, care should be taken to identify the ureter, which is retracted medially with the kidney, and to avoid injuring somatic nerves passing through the psoas and quadratus lumborum muscles.[40, 43]

RESULTS

Peacetime experience in the treatment of causalgia in the lower extremity is limited. Excellent results, similar to those encountered in the upper arm, are generally obtained. As noted by Ulmer and Mayfield,[12] an incomplete result is obtained in some patients and may require an additional procedure to remove the L1 and T12 ganglia.

COMPLICATIONS

The major neurologic complication is the risk of sexual dysfunction if the procedure is carried out bilaterally in the male. This consideration limits its use in the treatment of hyperhidrosis and other conditions.

REFERENCES

1. Greenwood B: The origins of sympathectomy. Med Hist 11:165, 1967
2. White JC, Bland EF: The surgical relief of severe angina pectoris. Medicine 27:1, 1948

3. Peet MM: Splanchnic resection for hypertension. Univ Hosp Bull Ann Arbor Mich 1:17, 1935
4. Smithwick RH: A technique for splanchnic resection for hypertension. Surgery 7:1, 1940
5. Adson AW, Brown GE: The treatment of Raynaud's disease by resection of the upper thoracic and lumbar sympathetic ganglia and trunks. Surg Gynecol Obstet 48:577, 1929
6. Dale WA, Lewis MD: Management of ischemia of the hand and fingers. Surgery 67:62, 1970
7. Myers KA, Irvine WT: An objective study of lumbar sympathectomy: II. Skin ischaemia. BMJ 1:1943, 1966
8. Myers KA, Irvine WT: An objective study of lumbar sympathectomy: I. Intermittent claudication. BMJ 1:879, 1966
9. Dohn DF, Sava GM: Sympathectomy for vascular syndromes and hyperhidrosis of the upper extremities, in Keener EB (ed): Clinical Neurosurgery, vol 25. Baltimore, Williams & Wilkins, 1978, pp 637–650
10. Bergan JJ, Con J: Sympathectomy for pain relief. Med Clin North Am 52:147, 1968
11. Spurling RG: Causalgia of the upper extremity: Treatment by dorsal sympathetic ganglionectomy. Arch Neurol Psychiatry 23:784, 1930
12. Ulmer JL, Mayfield FH: Causalgia: A study of 75 cases. Surg Gynecol Obstet 83:789, 1946
13. Drucker WR, Hubay CA, Holden WD, et al: Pathogenesis of post traumatic sympathetic dystrophy. Am J Surg 97:454, 1959
14. Echlin F, Owens FM, Wells WL: Observations on "major" and "minor" causalgia. Arch Neurol Psychiatry 62:183, 1949
15. Hardy WG, Posch JL, Webster JE, et al: The problem of major and minor causalgias. Am J Surg 95:545, 1958
16. Homans J: Minor causalgia: A hyperesthetic neurovascular syndrome. N Engl J Med 22:870, 1940
17. McFarlane WV: Causalgic syndromes. Aust N Z J Surg 18:191, 1949
18. Wirth FP, Rutherford RB: A civilian experience with causalgia. Arch Surg 100:633, 1970
19. Connelly JE, Richards V: Bilateral splanchnicectomy and lumbodorsal sympathectomy for chronic relapsing pancreatitis. Ann Surg 131:58, 1960
20. Heisy WG, Dohn DF: Splanchnicectomy for the treatment of intractable abdominal pain. Cleve Clin J Med 34:9, 1967
21. Mallet-Guy P, Beaujeu MJ: Treatment of chronic pancreatitis by unilateral splanchnicectomy. Arch Surg 60:233, 1950
22. Ray BS, Console AD: The relief of pain in chronic (calcaneous) pancreatitis by sympathectomy. Surg Gynecol Obstet 89:1, 1949
23. Sadar ES, Cooperman AM: Bilateral thoracic sympathectomy-splanchnicectomy in the treatment of intractable pain due to pancreatic carcinoma. Cleve Clin J Med 41:185, 1974
24. Sadar ES, Hardy RW: Thoracic splanchnicectomy and sympathectomy for the relief of pancreatic pain, in Cooperman AM (ed): Surgery of the Pancreas. St. Louis, CV Mosby, 1978, pp 141–152
25. de Takats G, Walter LE, Lasner J: Splanchnic nerve section for pancreatic pain. Ann Surg 131:44, 1950
26. Pick J: The Autonomic Nervous System. Philadelphia, JB Lippincott, 1970
27. Sunderland S: The distribution of sympathetic fibres in the brachial plexus in man. Brain 71:88, 1948
28. Kirgis HD, Kuntz A: Inconstant sympathetic neural pathways. Arch Surg 44:95, 1942
29. Kuntz A, Dillon JB: Preganglionic components of the first thoracic nerve. Arch Surg 44:772, 1942
30. Ray BS: Sympathectomy of the upper extremity. J Neurosurg 10:624, 1953
31. Kuntz A: Distribution of the sympathetic rami to the brachial plexus. Arch Surg 15:871, 1927
32. Skoog T: Ganglia in the communicating rami of the cervical sympathetic trunk. Lancet 2:457, 1947
33. Ray BS, Hinsey JC, Geohegan WA: Observations on the distribution of the sympathetic nerves to the pupil and upper extremity as determined by stimulation of the anterior roots in man. Ann Surg 118:647, 1943
34. Palumbo LT: A new concept of the sympathetic pathways to the eye. Surgery 42:740, 1957
35. Smithwick RH: The rationale and technic of sympathectomy for the relief of vascular spasm of the extremities. N Engl J Med 222:699, 1940
36. Hyndman OR, Wolkin J: Sympathectomy of the upper extremity. Arch Surg 45:145, 1942
37. White JC: Role of sympathectomy in relief of pain, in Krayenbuhl H, Maspes PE, Sweet WH (eds): Progress in Neurological Surgery, vol 7. Basel, S Kargen, 1976, pp 131–152
38. Gruszkiewicz J, Doron Y, et al: Hyperhidrosis and its surgical treatment. Acta Neurochir (Wien) 81:128, 1986
39. Love JG, Jergens JL: Second thoracic sympathetic ganglionectomy for neurologic and vascular disturbance of the upper extremities. West J Surg 72:130, 1964
40. Kempe LG: Operative Neurosurgery, vol 2. Heidelberg, Springer-Verlag, 1970, pp 244–250
41. Lougheed WM: A simple technique for upper thoracic sympathectomy in patients requiring sympathectomy of the upper limb. Can J Surg 8:306, 1965
42. Moran KT, Brady MP: Surgical management of primary hyperhidrosis. Br J Surg 78:279, 1991
43. Kleinert HE, Norbert H, McDonough JJ: Surgical sympathectomy-upper and lower extremity, in Omer GE, Spinner M (eds): Peripheral Nerve Problems. Philadelphia, WB Saunders, 1980, pp 285–302
44. Ellis H: Transthoracic sympathectomy. Br J Hosp Med Jan:50, 1986
45. Palumbo LT: Anterior transthoracic approach for upper thoracic sympathectomy. Arch Surg 72:659, 1956
46. Lindquist C, Fedorcsak I, Steig PE: Electrophysiological aid in high thoracic sympathectomy for palmar hyperhidrosis. Neurosurgery 24:449, 1989
47. Wilkinson HA: Radiofrequency percutaneous upper thoracic sympathectomy. N Engl J Med 311:34, 1984
48. Wilkinson HA: Percutaneous radiofrequency upper thoracic sympathectomy: A new technique. Neurosurgery 15:811, 1984
49. Yarzebski JL, Wilkinson HA: T2 and T3 sympathetic ganglia in the adult human: A cadaver and clinical radiographic study and its clinical application. Neurosurgery 21:339, 1987
50. Chaung KS, Liou NH, Liu JC: New stereotactic technique for percutaneous thermocoagulation upper thoracic ganglionectomy in cases of palmar hyperhidrosis. Neurosurgery 22:600, 1988
51. Kao MC: Video endoscopic sympathectomy using a fiberoptic CO_2 laser to treat palmar hyperhidrosis. Neurosurgery 30:131, 1992
52. Lin CC: A new method of thoroscopic sympathectomy in hyperhidrosis palmaris. Surg Endosc 4:224, 1990
53. Malone PS, Cameron AEP, Rennie JA: The surgical treatment of upper limb hyperhidrosis. Br J Dermatol 115:81, 1986
54. Weale FE: Upper thoracic sympathectomy by transthoracic electrocoagulation. Br J Surg 67:71, 1980
55. Kux E: Thorakoskipische Eingriffe am Nerven System. Stuttgart, George Thieme Verlag, 1954
56. Dondelinger RF, Kurdziel JC: Percutaneous phenol block of the upper thoracic sympathetic chain with computed tomography guidance. Acta Radiol 28:511, 1987
57. Adar R, Kurchu A, Zweig A, Mozes M: Palmar hyperhidrosis and its surgical treatment. A report of 10 cases. Ann Surg 186:34–41, 1977
58. Hashmonai M, Kopelman D, Kein O, et al: Upper thoracic sympathectomy for primary palmar hyperhidrosis: Long-term follow-up. Br J Surg 79:268, 1992
59. Richards RL: Causalgia: A centennial review. Arch Neurol 16:339, 1967
60. Ray BS, Neill CL: Abdominal visceral sensation in man. Ann Surg 126:709, 1947
61. Richins CA: The innervation of the pancreas. J Comp Neurol 83:223, 1945
62. Whitelaw GP, Smithwick RH: Some secondary effects of sympathectomy. N Engl J Med 245:121, 1951
63. Shallat RF, Klump TE: Paraplegia following thoracolumbar sympathectomy. J Neurosurg 34:569, 1971

Editorial Comment

The Asian and Israeli populations have a much higher incidence of hyperhidrosis of the palms than do whites. Thus, Kao and colleagues reported that in a survey conducted in Taiwan, one in 300 of people between the ages 15 and 30 years had this disorder. Adar and coworkers reported an incidence of 0.15 to 0.25 percent in Israeli Jews originating in North Africa, Yemen, and the Balkans. Kao and colleagues developed a new form of treatment involving an operating thoroscope, which is a computerized compact disc camera and video system that feeds into a high-resolution television monitor. The system has a channel for applying an electrode or a fiber optic carbon dioxide laser, which makes a lesion. The system gives the surgeon a magnified view of the sympathetic trunk at the T2-T3 level. Throughout the procedure, palmar skin perfusion is monitored with a laser Doppler flowmeter, and the skin temperature is assessed on the thenar eminence with a telethermometer. Failure to induce a significant increase in these parameters after the laser lesion has been made indicates that additional laser vaporization of the sympathetic trunk is necessary.

By February 1991, *Neurosurgery* had received an account of Kao and colleagues' method and their encouraging results in 14 cases. Within 2 years, they have operated on 300 cases, each of whom had predominantly palmar but also axillary and plantar hyperhidrosis. Satisfactory relief of sweating in both hands was achieved in 287 patients (96 percent). Initially, the investigators made a T2 sympathetic ganglionic lesion; if the skin temperature and perfusion elevations were inadequate, other lesions were made at the T3 ganglia or in the trunk just below the T1 ganglion. No patient developed a persistent Horner's syndrome. A dividend benefit of substantially decreased plantar sweating occurred in 70 percent of the successful palmar group. Compensatory hyperhidrosis was described by about half the patients only when they worked in a hot, humid environment. Axillary hyperhydrosis was also present in over half of the patients and was usually helped by the same procedure, but an unacceptable degree of hyperhidrosis seen in 24 of the patients was relieved by the T2 lesion in only 19. An additional T3 lesion was required to give relief of both the sweating and the odor in the five nonresponders. In all 300 patients, recurrences 6 months later led to reoperation in four patients that revealed an almost intact trunk and ganglia; these inadequate lesions were attributed to a poor video system used in the earlier cases. Although inconsequential morbidity and no mortality occurred from the procedure, the extent to which regeneration will be a problem remains to be seen. Thus far, if good results last for 1 year, they continue for at least another year. Apparently, Kao and colleagues have developed a valuable apparatus for endoscopic surgery at many sites. It is fully described in the January 1992 issue of *Neurosurgery*.

REFERENCE

Adar R, Kurchu A, Zweig A, Mozes M: Palmar hyperhidrosis and its surgical treatment. A report of 10 cases. Ann Surg 186:34–41, 1977

CHAPTER 133

Surgical Management of Spasmodic Torticollis and Adult-Onset Dystonia

Claude M. Bertrand

Identification of a human gene responsible for torsion dystonia by Ozelius and colleagues[1] has contributed greatly to the investigation of dystonia. However, the underlying pathologic condition of the basal ganglia in adult-onset dystonia and spasmodic torticollis is still undetermined,[2–5] except in rare cases of a definite lesion within the basal structures of the brain.[6–10] Because of increasing interest in motor disorders many aspects of these diseases are now better understood, resulting in therapeutic advances. Although spasmodic torticollis is a limited manifestation of the same disease that causes adult-onset dystonia,[11, 12] differentiating between severe forms of torticollis and adult-onset dystonia is sometimes difficult.[13] Although evolution from rotational or laterocollis to dystonia with marked scoliosis of the cervicothoracic spine is unusual,[14] it was present in the history of five of 117 patients,[15] possibly because of the length of time the condition had existed and the severity of the cases referred for surgery. Likewise, spontaneous remissions did not exceed 5 percent of the cases reviewed. In both conditions, a personal or familial history of essential tremor and, occasionally, involvement of the facial musculature, is common.[16, 17] A few of our patients had siblings with torticollis.

These manifestations are not psychogenic in most cases, especially because the rhythmicity and reproducibility of the abnormal movements can be visualized by electromyography.[12, 18] Like other extrapyramidal movements, they are increased by emotion, and they disappear during sleep. Anxiety and even reactive depression may be present in a few of these patients, and an emotional shock or trauma may act as a precipitating factor. There is a natural tendency to relate the spontaneous appearance of abnormal movements to trauma, but in most cases, the relation to trauma is questionable, and a detailed inquiry may reveal that symptoms were present beforehand. In a few instances, the time interval between trauma and disorder is quite short, and onset of symptoms is rapid; however, in a review of 71 patients with idiopathic torsion dystonia and 71 control subjects, trauma as a cause was not significant.[19]

SPASMODIC TORTICOLLIS

The unqualified statement that spasmodic torticollis is a bilateral disease, which dates back to the days before electromyography, has been detrimental to the evolution of its surgical management and has led to the impression that antagonist muscles on either side are usually involved. On the contrary, in a classic case of rotational torticollis without anterocollis or retrocollis, spontaneous abnormal discharges can be found in the sternocleidomastoid on one side and the posterior cervical group, especially the splenius, on the other.[18] The contralateral antagonist muscles do not participate or may even be inhibited. Rarely, the contralateral semispinalis may contribute to rotation, but the trapezius is never involved. When the patient attempts to turn against the abnormal movements, the affected antagonist muscles may discharge instead of relax. In retrocollis, the extensors on either side, which are then synergists, evidently discharge simultaneously, whereas in laterocollis, the muscles that participate are all on the same side, for instance, the posterior cervical group with the ipsilateral sternocleidomastoid and possibly the trapezius and levator scapulae. In most instances, a combination of movements occurs, such as rotation with extension or flexion or inclination, so that the muscles that seem involved must be carefully verified because combinations vary from one patient to another. Flexion with inclination of the head to the left and rotation to the right may be caused by involvement of the left sternocleidomastoid and the ipsilateral semispinalis, whereas rotation to the right with slight inclination and extension of the occiput to the right suggests involvement of the left sternocleidomastoid combined mostly with the right splenius. In lateroretrocollis, if extension is pronounced, the contralateral semispinalis may be involved. Rarely, the sternomastoid contralateral to the movement may be discharging in an attempt to reduce the movement. Also, if muscle involvement is more diffuse, a tremor might persist after surgery. However, large movements evidently cannot occur unless the antagonists are relaxed. Unfortunately, the false impression of bilaterality has led to the use of indiscriminate bilateral symmetric denervation, such as bilateral rhizotomy, thus suppressing normal uninvolved muscles necessary for normal posture and movements.

CONSERVATIVE MANAGEMENT

Medical treatment has been greatly modified and enhanced by the general acceptance of the botulinum toxin (Botox).[20–22]

The initial treatment still involves the use of drugs, particularly trihexyphenidyl (Artane),[23] clonazepam, diazepam, as well as antidepressants, which can offer some relief, particularly in high doses.[24,25] However, the inconstant results and secondary effects of these agents have induced neurologists to resort increasingly more often to botulinum toxin injections of the muscles involved.[26] Relief of symptoms is sometimes dramatic and usually lasts from 3 to 4 months, after which the injections have to be repeated. Occasionally, transitory side effects, such as difficulty swallowing and postural instability of the head, occur. The treatment may become ineffective, sometimes because of the appearance of antibodies; otherwise, this form of treatment usually continues as long as it is satisfactory to the patient. Practically all the patients operated on in the past few years had been treated with botulinum toxin; this therapy gives the patient an impression of what can be accomplished with selective denervation. Physiotherapy and biofeedback, which probably act as a *geste antagoniste,* or counter-pressure phenomenon, may be useful, but they are infrequently successful as a long-term treatment.[27] Physiotherapy is essential after surgery, particularly to retrain the muscles that were the antagonists to the abnormal movements.

SURGICAL MANAGEMENT

Some of the techniques discussed in the previous edition of this volume have been abandoned or are at least used very infrequently for spasmodic torticollis: iontophoresis,[28] section of the frontal capsular adversive pathways,[29] thalamotomy, and pallidotomy. Although thalamotomy can sometimes produce excellent results, the target used was nucleus ventrooralis internus,[30] close to the corticobulbar fibers, with the attendant risk of dysarthria.[31] The desired hypotonia can be obtained with a more posterior lesion at the nucleus ventrointermedius (VIM) and the immediately adjoining subthalamic area, with greatly reduced risks.[32-34] Although such a lesion seems too formidable now that symptoms can be relieved with selective denervation, it should be considered with or without pallidotomy in severe forms of dystonia when all else fails.

Microvascular Lysis of the Accessory Nerve Roots

Freckmann and associates[35] suggested microvascular lysis of the accessory nerve roots, along the line of decompression of the facial nerve, even though the latter innervation is supplied by a single nerve in contrast to the multiple innervation of the posterior cervical musculature, as mentioned in a discussion by Adams.[36] In a more recent report concerning 33 patients, Freckmann and associates[37] state that "the notion that neurovascular contacts of the spinal accessory nerve roots might be of relevance as in other cranial nerve dysfunction syndromes, like hemifacial spasms, cannot be considered valid with our experience." The technique was modified and involves removing all anastomoses between the accessory nerve roots and the dorsal roots of C1 and C2. Of the 33 patients, they report excellent results in 5, good results in 10, and an improvement in 12. Three patients were unchanged, two regressed, and one died after reintervention. Paresis of lateral arm movements is mentioned in four patients. Shima and colleagues[38] in Japan reported satisfactory relief in 5 of 7 patients chosen from a group of 22. Apparently microlysis is performed quite frequently in one center in North America, but no report was obtained on the results.

Although the patients who came for selective peripheral denervation later on were evidently those in whom the symptoms were unabated following microlysis, in all six the sternocleidomastoid muscle was very active and had to be denervated peripherally; the intervention was complicated by the presence of scar tissue and the previous laminectomy. Since it has been established that any residual innervation between C1 and C5 will perpetuate abnormal movements, it is questionable that once the effect of neurapraxia is finished, there would be appreciable permanent results from such a restricted intervention, which nevertheless requires a laminectomy.

EPIDURAL CERVICAL STIMULATION

Epidural cervical stimulation has been advocated by Gildenberg[39] and more recently, by Waltz.[40] In an additional report in 1981,[41] Gildenberg suggested an initial trial period with transcutaneous stimulation. In 1987, Waltz and colleagues[42] discussed their results in 785 patients treated for various pathologies. They reported that of 66 patients with spasmodic torticollis, "marked improvement was found in 25 (37.9 percent), moderate improvement in 21 (31.8 percent) . . . ." In a double-blind study, Goetz and associates[43] found no objective evidence of improvement in 10 patients with dystonia, four of whom had spasmodic torticollis. Although the results are occasionally very good, they appear to be sporadic, but the procedure probably helps the pain that accompanies torticollis. Because epidural cervical stimulation does not require a laminectomy, it did not present a problem in the three patients who later required selective denervation.

ANTERIOR CERVICAL RHIZOTOMY

Anterior cervical rhizotomy has been modified very little since it was described by McKenzie[44] and Dandy.[45] Until a few years ago, it was the most frequently performed operation for spasmodic torticollis. Anterior cervical rhizotomy consists of sectioning of the anterior roots of C1, C2, and C3 bilaterally and part or all of the anterior root of C4 on one side, with or without section of the ascending roots of the spinal accessory nerve. Because distribution of its fibers to the trapezius and the sternocleidomastoid muscle varies, this procedure can produce an appreciable shoulder paresis; therefore, peripheral denervation is preferable.[46] In the reports published by Sorensen and Hamby (71 patients),[47] Arseni and Maretsis (52 patients),[48] Hamby and Schiffer (50 patients),[49] Tasker (47 patients),[46] and Fabinyi and Dutton (20 patients),[50] satisfactory results were reported in approximately 70 percent of the patients. Mortality was 1 to 2 percent. If an operating microscope is used, fine blood vessels can be spared and possible ischemia of the cord thereby avoided. Cervical subluxation is also rare.

In the 50 patients followed up by Hamby and Schiffer,[49]

79 percent improved, 53 percent had some residual rotation of the head, 50 percent used a cervical collar occasionally, 57 percent complained of pain in the neck and shoulders, 32 percent had dysphagia, which was usually temporary, and two patients died. These complications were probably higher in this series because of the sectioning of the ascending roots of the accessory nerves. Three recent reports should be mentioned: Hernesniemi and Keranen[51] had negative comments about their experience after rhizotomy in 12 patients. Friedman and colleagues[52] reviewed their results in 58 patients and reported that 57 percent had an excellent result, and 28 percent were significantly improved. Two deaths and three postoperative complications occurred, and one patient had an increased kyphosis. Perot[53] followed up 50 patients and concluded that "75 percent to 80 percent had been quite pleased with the result obtained." One patient had a transient myelopathy postoperatively, and two patients developed a cervical subluxation in the following year.

Reinnervation of the peripheral portion of C2 after rhizotomy, presumably from anastomoses of the cervical plexus, was found in five patients during selective denervation, two of which I had operated on a few years previously.

Anterior cervical rhizotomy with peripheral denervation of the sternocleidomastoid muscle, as indicated, was used regularly in our department until 15 years ago. Undoubtedly, it helped many patients, but it produces certain undesirable side effects, such as weakness of the neck postoperatively. Some instability of the neck as well as limitation of movements may persist. At times, this effect occurs without suppression of the abnormal movements because denervation is limited downward to C4 to protect the origin of the phrenic nerve. The posterior rami of C4 and C5 definitely contribute to the innervation of the splenius and especially of the semispinalis.

Now that electromyography, nerve blocks, and stimulation are readily available, rhizotomy, if it were still held by the surgeon as the procedure of choice, should be performed unilaterally to preserve neck stability and promote rehabilitation in patients with laterocollis and in most with rotational torticollis, when the posterior cervical group is involved only on one side. Furthermore, the roots of C1 and C2 can be sectioned extradurally, and the root of C3 can be exposed through a small hemilaminectomy by use of microscope to identify accompanying vessels.

Bilateral rhizotomy has been abandoned in our department since the advent of selective denervation because it produces too much denervation of useful antagonist muscles as well as incomplete denervation of the ones involved in the abnormal movements.

MUSCLE RESECTION

Xinkang[54] advocated selective resection of certain posterior cervical muscles together with section of the spinal accessory nerve when indicated (e.g., the splenius with section of the contralateral spinal accessory nerve for rotational torticollis). In his series, the muscles resected varied according to the type of torticollis and the results of electromyography. In 30 patients followed up for more than 1 year, the recovery was apparently permanent in 60 percent. It is contrary to our experience that resection of the splenius only abolishes movements in the synergists and that movements disappear gradually, over months, rather than immediately after surgery. Chen and coworkers[55] also reported using muscle resection successfully in the treatment of bilateral retrocollis. Muscle resection undoubtedly is accompanied by a certain amount of denervation, but denervation of the muscles involved must be complete because the least amount of residual innervation allows the abnormal movements to persist. One is tempted to agree with Maccabe[56] that "myotomy . . . is unlikely to be revived."

SELECTIVE PERIPHERAL DENERVATION

Selective peripheral denervation of the muscles involved in abnormal movements while their antagonists are spared has been the procedure used at Hôpital Notre-Dame for spasmodic torticollis for the past 14 years.[57–63] As mentioned previously, many transitional forms of spasmodic torticollis exist. The movements must be carefully analyzed, and repeated review of a videotape is desirable. In fact, obtaining a videotape together with a medical history to determine whether the patient is a suitable candidate for surgery is useful. Palpation during physical examination is helpful in determining which muscles are the main offenders. When surgery is considered, bipolar electromyograms in the presence of the neurosurgeon and a competent clinical neurophysiologist are an essential part of the investigation.[53] The needles should be placed in each muscle and proper placement ascertained from voluntary contraction of the muscle concerned. Moreover, when the record is not satisfactory and differs appreciably from the clinical picture, electromyography should be repeated with different needle placements. One must be wary of discharges originating from the platysma. Besides analyzing the tracings, both observers should compare the sound produced by the discharging muscles. Time relationships should be analyzed and permanent photographic records kept for further comparison. Simultaneous tracings should be performed in symmetric muscles, the first ones usually being the two sternocleidomastoid muscles and the two splenius muscles. Both trapezius muscles are also compared, especially to determine if and how much they are involved because they must be spared except in rare situations in which the levator scapulae can supplement and is not involved.

When the origin of the movements is in doubt, for instance, whether rotation to the right originates from the right splenius or, more rarely, from the left semispinalis, a bipolar depth electrode can be used. A bipolar electrode is also useful for studying the rectus muscles or for the obliques and the longissimus capitis. Frequently, a rhythmic tremor is present with alternate discharges of the antagonists. In this situation, the patient should be told that although selective denervation may suppress part or most of the tremor, it cannot be depended on to do so; the procedure is for the abnormal strong movements and not for the tremor. Electromyographic recordings should be obtained with the patient at rest and during active movements involving different groups of muscles. As mentioned previously, the resistance of the involved muscles to normal movements is particularly revealing.

Stimulation is used mostly to determine the point of penetration of fairly superficial motor nerves, usually the branches of the spinal accessory to the sternocleidomastoid muscle when it is to be blocked separately from the trapezius. A temporary block with 1-percent lidocaine without epinephrine can be used to determine the relative importance of the involved muscles in the abnormal movements, for instance, the right sternocleidomastoid muscle versus the left posterior cervical group in rotational torticollis or the right sternocleidomastoid muscle and the right posterior cervical group in laterocollis. We block the sternocleidomastoid muscle in most patients. Rarely is the trapezius involved in abnormal movements, except in marked laterocollis; however if it might be involved, it is also blocked to see whether or not the patient can use the levator scapulae adequately to compensate for the loss of the trapezius. The branch of the trapezius is blocked at its point of penetration into the muscle, where the horizontal and the vertical part join together at the base of the neck. About 15 ml of 1-percent lidocaine is used in this process. The sternocleidomastoid block is performed fairly deeply within the aponeurosis of the muscle and 2 inches below the mastoid to anesthetize the distal branches. The patient should be told that if the lidocaine diffuses further, in rare cases, there is a temporary block of the recurrent nerve with transitory lowering of the voice and difficulty swallowing. We now infiltrate directly into the splenius or the semispinalis in the posterior cervical region, as needed, rather than about the roots of C1 and C2 and the posterior ramus of C3. This location is used to avoid penetration of the large venous plexuses, which produced temporary nystagmus and hypotension in two patients mentioned in our initial report.[57]

Even if the blocks are sometimes incomplete, they indicate what can be expected from denervation. If blocking the sternocleidomastoid muscle produces sufficient, although partial, relief, denervation may be limited to that muscle, and the patient may be referred for physiotherapy and retraining of the antagonists, with the understanding that a more extensive procedure may be required later on. In more complex cases, many blocks are performed at different times. Rarely is more than 20 ml of 1-percent lidocaine used during one session, so the block is usually limited to one muscle group. Blocking is not used when the clinical findings and the electromyograms are definitive or if there is any history of allergy to local anesthetics. Electromyography is repeated in ambiguous cases to ensure that all the most active muscles have been detected.

SURGICAL TECHNIQUE

The surgical technique for treatment of spasmodic torticollis has evolved in the past few years and is now pretty well standardized. Because selective denervation is performed through an unusual approach and a definite plane of cleavage must be followed to obtain the necessary exposure for a complete denervation, previous experience with postmortem dissections of the neck along that plane is a prerequisite for this type of surgery. The surgeon should also visit a center where the procedure is frequently performed and should assist at preoperative examinations and electromyograms to determine the choice and extent of the denervation.

To minimize vertebral venous bleeding and to better expose the spinal accessory nerve and the posterior primary divisions in the same operating field, all patients are operated on in the sitting position with jugular catheterization, constant monitoring, and sequential pressure on the lower limbs. The sitting position has been used in more than 150 cases without complications. It certainly facilitates dissection and visualization of the fine branches of the nerves while greatly reducing the operating time. The patients are still operated on under light anesthesia, and curare is neutralized after induction to facilitate nerve stimulation. The stimulator itself is a strong, variable-current, monopolar nerve stimulator (not a disposable stimulator), to favor diffusion of the current when fine collateral branches are sought, and later on to verify that no residual innervation exists. Magnifying loupes and a head lamp are amply sufficient for visualization, and the microscope is now used only for taking pictures. The head of the patient is held erect in a standard, three-pronged head holder, is moderately flexed, and is slightly turned away from the side of the ramisectomy, so as to open the space between the occiput and C1. In cases of rotational torticollis, even those in which a meticulous verification of the denervation is included, the surgical procedure lasts between 2 and 3 1/2 hours.

Denervation of the Sternocleidomastoid Muscle

Although an incision through the crease of the neck might be preferable from a cosmetic point of view, the spinal accessory nerve is approached through an incision running from the inferior lobe of the ear and then along the trajectory of the branch of the trapezius down to the supraclavicular area. The nerve should be followed from its point of penetration in the trapezius up to the styloid process. Occasionally, recurring branches may be present below the posterior border of the sternocleidomastoid muscle coming from the trapezius branch, or at the upper limit, fine proximal branches may be present (Fig. 133–1). Besides the intrathecal connections described by Ouaknine and Nathan[64] and Gloobe and colleagues,[65] anastomotic branches may exist between the spinal accessory nerve and C1 or, more rarely, C2, but they are interrupted as the distal branches are severed.

During skin incision, care is taken to protect the great auricular nerve whenever possible to avoid temporary numbness of the ear. At the lower end of the incision, stimulation is used to identify the branch to the trapezius, which is quite superficial near the trapezius muscle. This branch must be carefully protected, but collaterals are sectioned. Dissection is then carried upward, mostly with blunt dissection, because occasional kinks occur in the course of the spinal accessory nerve. Usually, four to eight fine distal branches to the sternocleidomastoid muscle are present that may or may not join into one or two main trunks. They are sectioned and avulsed, and the proximal portion is clipped to avoid regeneration. Reinnervation was encountered in some of our earlier cases, but not enough to produce significant abnormal movements. Finally, the spinal accessory nerve must be free of all branches except for the main branch to the trapezius. The sternocleidomastoid muscle is then completely sectioned transversely to suppress residual innervation, but the aponeurosis is sutured before skin closure to maintain the contour of the neck.

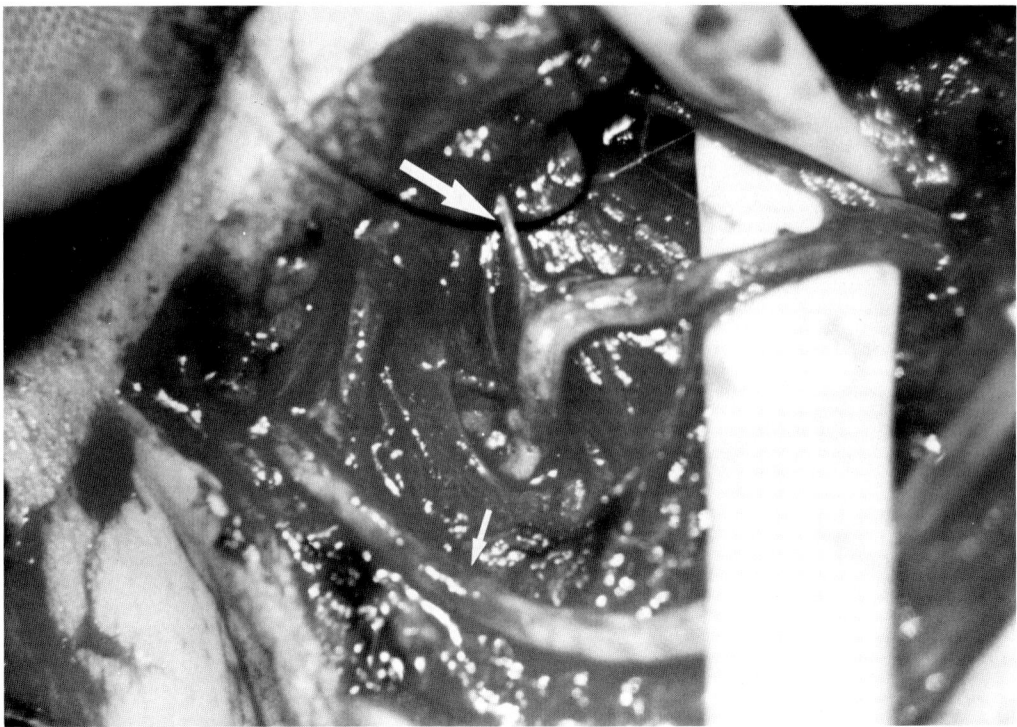

FIGURE 133-1. Photograph taken during operation showing the division of the spinal accessory nerve in two branches: one anterior (above) to the sternocleidomastoid muscle and the other (below) going to the trapezius muscle. The large arrow points to a recurrent nerve from the branch to the trapezius muscle that also innervates the sternocleidomastoid muscle. The small arrow points to a large cutaneous auricular nerve.

Peripheral Rhizotomy of C1 and C2 and Posterior Ramisectomy of C3, C4, C5, and C6

A vertical incision is made from the external occipital protuberance to the spinous process of C7. The linea alba is identified, and muscle insertions are separated along it down to the spinous process of C2. A horizontal incision is then carried out laterally from the occipital protuberance for a distance of 5 cm. This step is essential to avoid neurapraxia from excessive retraction and to visualize the proximal branches of C3 and C4. The trapezius, the semispinalis, and the splenius are sectioned near their insertion and retracted laterally, thereby exposing the occipital bone. Dissection is carried within the plane of cleavage between the undersurface of the semispinalis and the paravertebral group of muscles. The posterior primary divisions (rami) of C3, C4, and C5 course within that plane and can either be seen immediately or identified by stimulation and exposed.

The posterior arch of the atlas is denuded past the notch of the vertebral artery, under which C1 is identified. To facilitate the exposure of C1 and C2, the inferior oblique muscle is frequently sectioned and partly resected. The posterior branch of the root of C1 is followed a short distance under the vertebral artery, where it joins with the anterior branch; the root is clipped and sectioned mesial to the branches, the anterior branch is sectioned, and the posterior branch is avulsed. The posterior branch of the large root of C2 emerges between the posterior arch of the atlas and the axis. The vertebral venous plexus is coagulated to avoid possible air emboli, and the posterior branch is followed between the laminae, where it joins the anterior branch. At that point, the root is clipped, the anterior branch is sectioned, and the posterior branch is avulsed over a few centimeters. In patients with retrocollis, in whom bilateral denervation of the posterior cervical group must be carried out, the posterior branch of C1 is merely sectioned and not followed under the vertebral artery, because three patients have had temporary dysphagia after the root of C1 was totally sectioned bilaterally. Dysphagia has not occurred in bilateral denervations since only the posterior branch of the roots of C1 and C2 have been sectioned. A collateral from the vertebral artery may be present at C1 and C2, but it is rare and has been encountered only twice during surgery (Fig. 133-2).

If the plane of cleavage is satisfactory, the posterior primary divisions (rami) of C3, C4, and C5 are followed to their point of origin in the intervertebral foramen. Frequently, two or three early branches originate near the origin of the posterior ramus, at C3 and C4 (Fig. 133-3). These branches are sought with stimulation and meticulous dissection of the soft tissues lateral and anterior to the foramen. At this point, the posterior ramus is clipped near its origin and avulsed to facilitate further exposure of the area. All these little branches must be sectioned to prevent residual innervation; therefore, the muscles lateral to the articular facets must be retracted. At the level of C4, stimulation is frequently repeated to avoid damage to the anterior root and the phrenic nerve. Early collateral branches are rare at the level of C5, which is clipped as it emerges from the foramen and avulsed. The posterior ramus of C6 is very fine; on stimulation, it seems to innervate a small portion of the paravertebral muscles and probably does not contribute significantly to the abnormal movements. In patients with retrocollis, the ramisectomy is carried down to C5 bilaterally but not lower,

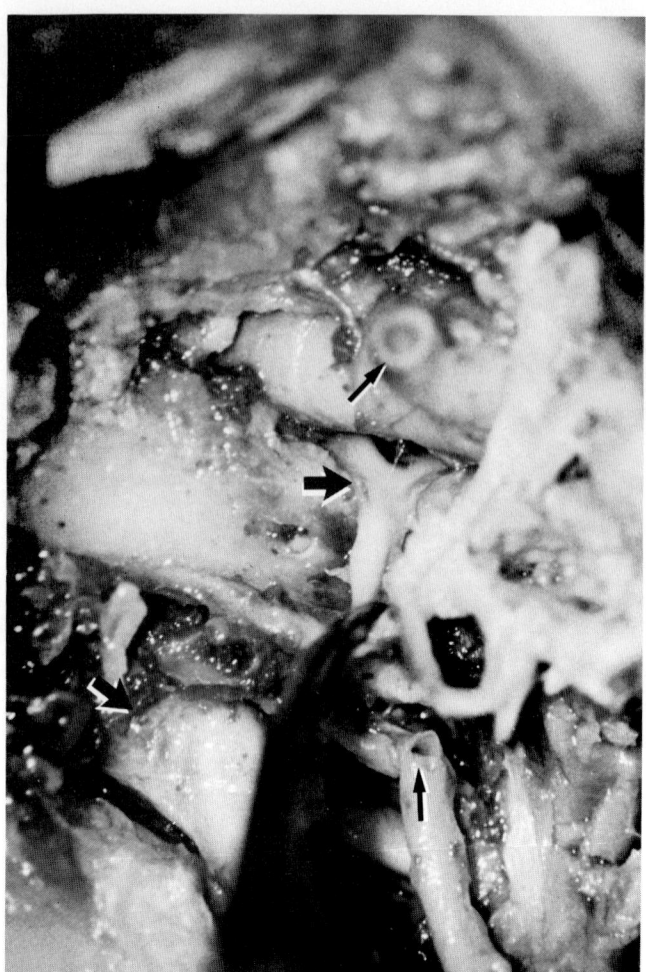

FIGURE 133–2. Microdissection on a cadaver that shows rare collateral branches of the vertebral artery (small arrows) that might be found along the roots of C1 and C2 (large arrows).

because we have found that leaving the posterior ramus of C5 on one side perpetuates some of the movements, whereas the result is excellent when the posterior ramus of C5 is removed bilaterally. In patients progressing from rotational or lateral torticollis to retrocollis, denervating the sternocleidomastoid muscle as well as both posterior cervical groups is sometimes necessary. When denervation is complete, strong stimulation at the level of the foramina must not produce any contraction of the posterior cervical group of muscles, although underlying muscles may respond.

The head is extended to facilitate closure. After hemostasis, the muscles and cervical aponeuroses are closed tightly before the skin is sutured.

The patient's head and upper body are elevated after the operation to minimize oozing. Opiate injections are given for pain for 24 to 48 hours after surgery. The patient is ambulatory the first or sometimes the second day after the operation.

PHYSIOTHERAPY

Physiotherapy is very important for restoration of normal neck movements, particularly for the antagonists to the abnormal movements and it is started 2 or 3 days after the operation. Physiotherapy is administered daily for the first week and then at least three times a week for 6 weeks, or until near-normal movements of the head occur. The therapy involves relaxation of the neck musculature, proper posture, and, mostly, retraining of the antagonists, and it strives toward full movements of the neck. In fact, after the usual ramisectomy with denervation of the sternocleidomastoid, the remaining muscles allow the patient an almost full range of movement because the anterior roots are not touched, and posterior cervical denervation is only unilateral in those cases. In patients in whom a multiple approach is required, the patient can recover a surprising range of movements with early and intensive physiotherapy and can function adequately. In our series, one such patient was a mother and a stenographer, another a school teacher, and a third, a librarian.

RESULTS

Results in 260 consecutive cases operated on for spasmodic torticollis or the cervical component of adult-onset dystonia were presented at the Second International Congress of Movement Disorders in 1992.[57] In the 117 patients reported on in the previous edition of this chapter,[15] 26 underwent a thalamotomy, pallidotomy, or both, whereas only one patient of the present group, a patient with a severe generalized dystonia, underwent a thalamotomy. Of the 260, the results of 106 (40 percent) were classified as excellent (no residual symptoms), and those of 124 (48 percent), as very good (slight residual symptoms), for a total of 238, or 88 percent (Table 133–1). More importantly, with exposure lateral to the articular facets, the percentage of total relief of symptoms has gone from 31 to 40 percent, and in the last 50 cases before this report was published, to 54 percent, although the overall rate of success was still estimated at 88 percent.

Now that total relief with preservation of near-normal movements of the neck has been amply demonstrated to be possible, one may question why 12 percent of patients continue to have an appreciable amount of movements after denervation. In a small number of these, the therapeutic possibilities are limited by severe dystonias; laterocollis with involvement of the levator scapulae or of the trapezius, if the levator scapulae cannot supplement for shoulder stability; diffuse and marked fibrosis or prolonged muscle elongation that prevents return to a normal posture; or inappropriate choice of muscles to be denervated. In two instances, rotation

Table 133–1. RESULTS IN 260 CASES AFTER SELECTIVE DENERVATION

Results, n (%)		Last 50 Cases, n (%)
Excellent	106 (40%)	27 (54%)
Very good	124 (48%)	17 (34%)
Combined	230 (88%)	44 (88%)
Fair	27 (10%)	5 (10%)
Poor	3 (1%)	1 (2%)

Excellent = no detectable abnormal movements; very good = slight deviation or slight residual movements; fair = appreciable amount of residual abnormal movements; poor = no improvement or worse.

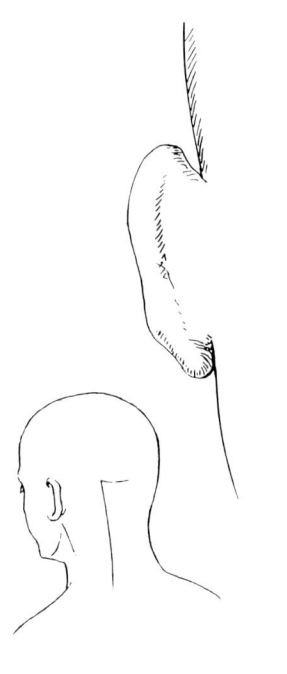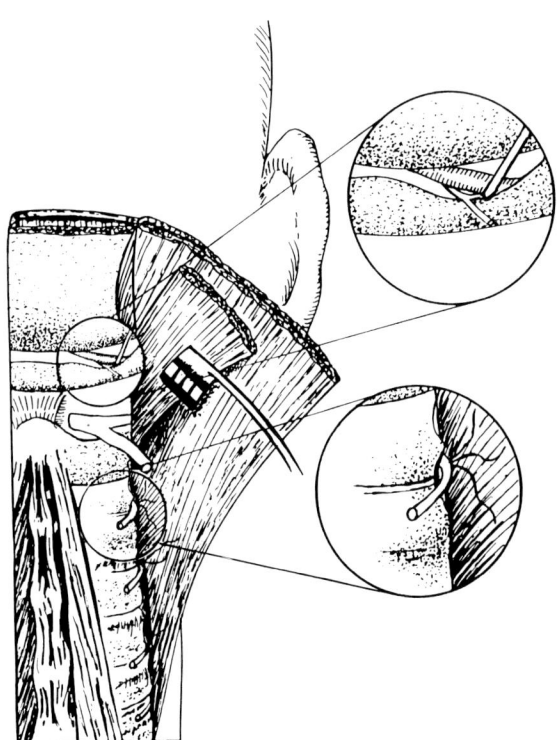

FIGURE 133–3. Surgical exposure for a right posterior cervical ramisectomy. One can see the emergence of C1 underneath the vertebral artery on the right. In the upper circle, the vertebral artery has been elevated showing the root of C1 as it divides in its anterior and posterior branches. Lower down, between the posterior arches of C1 and C2, one can see the root of C2 as it divides into its anterior and posterior branch, the latter emerging between the arches. Below, the posterior primary divisions (the rami) of C3, C4, C5, and C6 are seen as they emerge from the intervertebral foramen and come around to innervate the posterior cervical musculature. In the lower circle, the root of C3 is shown, its fine collateral branches coming out near the foramen and penetrating immediately into the muscles. If the external portion of the articular facettes are too prominent to allow visualization of the posterior portion of the foramen, they may be gouged slightly outside the articulation. The small sketch on the left shows the incision under the left ear for exposure of the left spinal accessory nerve and the posterior midline inverted L-shaped incision for the right posterior ramisectomy. (From Bertrand CM: Selective peripheral denervation for spasmodic torticollis; surgical technique, results, and observations in 260 cases. Surg Neurol 40:96–103, 1993. Copyright 1993 by Elsevier Science Publishing Co., Inc. Reprinted by permission.)

was maintained by a contralateral unopposed semispinalis. One of these has since been relieved by contralateral denervation. The contralateral semispinalis may also be the reason why a slight deviation of the head remains in some patients.

In most cases, the persisting abnormal movements probably result from residual innervation. The roots of C1 and C2 can be easily interrupted as they come off the dura. As already mentioned, the posterior primary divisions of C3 and C4, particularly the former, have fine proximal branches close to their point of emergence from the intervertebral foramen. As evident from stimulation, any residual branch can maintain innervation of the musculature, so that denervation at these levels must be very thorough. Such denervation can be achieved while the nerve supply of the deep paraspinous muscles is preserved; these muscles probably maintain ipsilateral normal movements. Because reintervention in scar tissue is not always successful, obtaining total denervation is all the more important; in fact, abnormal movements persisted in two of five of our patients after reintervention. Although the result is evident the day after operation, one must wait 6 months to confirm that it will be permanent; in a few instances, part of the relief probably resulted from neuropraxia during retraction of the muscles at operation, and part of the symptoms returned after that period of time. As reported,[15] until a few years ago, instances of a return of activity in the sternocleidomastoid muscle were reported; this activity was not sufficient to produce an appreciable amount of movement. For these reasons, the incision must allow total exposure of the spinal accessory nerve.

A third patient can be added to the two previously reported[15] as having had a poor result: this patient presented an increase in the peripheral symptoms of his dystonia after selective denervation. One patient developed a pharyngeal abscess from an infected tonsil postoperatively that required tracheostomy, tonsillectomy, and drainage of the abscess. She has had a marked relief of her abnormal movements but continues to have some limitation of lateral movements to the neck, not having benefited from early physiotherapy.

Patients with retrocollis have an excellent result from surgery now that denervation is carried to C5 bilaterally; as mentioned earlier, three patients had transitory dysphagia, but this complication can be avoided by merely sectioning the posterior branches of C1 and C2, avoiding any traction on the root, and sparing the anterior branches. Contrary to the opinion expressed in the previous edition of this chapter,[15] carrying the ramisectomy down to C5 bilaterally is necessary in these cases.

After the first 6 to 8 months after surgery, the results are well maintained over the years, which is not surprising in view of the amount of atrophy after section and avulsion of the peripheral nerves. One hundred sixty-seven patients of this group were operated on more than 5 years ago, and 64, more than 10 years ago, so the benefit may be considered to be permanent. The sequelae are rarely incommodating. Sensory loss is limited to the distribution of the greater occipital nerve and is usually not mentioned by the patient. Very few patients have complained of paresthesiae or of a sensation of tightness or fullness. Three patients reported an occasional sudden ticlike pain, which subsided a few weeks later. These patients were given carbamazepine. The greater occipital nerve could probably be spared, but one would have to ascertain that no motor innervation remains, and the manipulation may result in a higher incidence of discomfort. The marked atrophy in the back of the neck after this procedure is not apparent. Suturing the aponeurosis of the sternocleidomastoid muscle preserves a fairly normal contour of the neck, although a few patients had a cheloid at the site of the incision.

COMMENTS

Selective peripheral denervation was first used as a complement to thalamotomy[57]; however, it soon became evident that it was sufficient whenever only the neck musculature was involved. Weir Mitchell suggested a peripheral approach to C1, C2 and C3 to Keen, who reported performing one such procedure in 1891.[66] Finney and Hughson[67] wrote a very comprehensive report with excellent historical notes in 1925. They stated that McKenzie's procedure was "an unnecessary dangerous method of resection." However, without the benefit of electromyography, their procedure was no more selective than was rhizotomy. Their peripheral denervation was carried out bilaterally "to make it sufficiently comprehensive to include all the offending structures"; it was in fact a bilateral extradural rhizotomy of C1, C2, and C3. Of the 31 patients they followed up, three were unimproved, 16 were improved, and 12 were completely cured. One may presume that, in the last cases, the semi-spinalis and part of the splenius were not too involved or that the horseshoe incision denervated most of the posterior rami of C4 and C5 because they contribute actively to the innervation of these muscles. This fact is ignored by the proponents of rhizotomy.

As evidenced by the amplitude of movements that can be retained after the atlas and axis are fused, most of the movements of the head occur at the junction between the occiput and the atlas. The anterior cervical group of muscles, which is inserted at the base of the occiput close to the fulcrum, seems to contribute little to abnormal movements, except in the more severe forms of dystonia. Therefore, the muscles of special concern are the rectus muscles, the obliques, the semispinalis, the longissimus capitis, the splenius, and the sternocleidomastoid. The trapezius may be involved in inclination or extension but does not contribute to rotation.

The antagonist muscles are rarely positively involved; they are often inhibited, as confirmed by electromyography. Infrequently, the contralateral semispinalis contributes to rotation and may have to be denervated. Bilateral simultaneous discharges occur mostly in the sternomastoids. Nerve blocks can be helpful in deciding whether they are the result of resistance to the abnormal movements or are an antagonist contraction. Interestingly, the sternocleidomastoids can be denervated bilaterally, and the head will still have a fair amount of movement. In lateroretrocollis, both posterior cervical groups may contribute to extension. After bilateral ramisectomy and unilateral sternocleidomastoid denervation, the patient's head can be extended, flexed, and turned to either side. The contribution of C5 to the innervation of the posterior cervical group is quite evident; in retrocollis, leaving the posterior ramus of C5 intact on one side preserves part of the abnormal movements. In retrocollis, the anterior branch of the root of C1 is left intact to avoid dysphagia. So far, the anterior branches of C1 and C2 have been sectioned in laterocollis or rotational torticollis, but no evidence exists that they contribute significantly to the abnormal movements. The same is true of C6, which seems to have a very limited contribution to the innervation of the posterior cervical group.

Surprisingly, the area of anesthesia did not extend appreciably beyond the territory of C2 after extensive ramisectomy because the posterior primary divisions of C3, C4, C5, and C6 have mostly a motor function. This finding does not confirm the more extensive distribution suggested by Johnston[68] after his dissections, although he did find that their distribution was quite limited in the cervical area.

IMPORTANT FEATURES OF SUCCESS

The surgeon should familiarize himself or herself with the function of the various muscles of the neck singly and in combination. After examining the patient, the surgeon may mimic personally the movements of the patient while palpating his or her own muscles. For instance, during a strong rotation to the right, the left semispinalis can be felt to come into action, and it might well contribute to the preservation of normal movements of the neck after denervation of the right posterior cervical group. Hence, visiting a center in which selective denervation is performed regularly is advisable.

The following steps are important in the management of spasmodic torticollis. First, the surgeon should assess fully which muscles are involved in the abnormal movements and should confirm this with bilateral simultaneous electromyography, during which the findings can be discussed with a competent clinical electrophysiologist. For instance, as happened recently, recording may reveal that laterocollis originates from the oblique muscles rather than from the trapezius, or that the contralateral semispinalis is also involved. Second, at operation, the surgeon should expose and explore visually, and with stimulation within the muscle, insertions lateral to the intervertebral foramen for fine early branches coming from the posterior primary divisions, particularly at C3 and C4. The exposure and total section of the roots of C1 and C2 usually do not present any problem when the patient is in the sitting position. Third, the surgeon should prescribe early and active physiotherapy to restore normal or near-normal movements of the neck. Peripheral avulsion of the nervous branches seems to be an important factor in avoiding recurrences. It is comforting that after the initial period of 6 months, the result obtained is well maintained over the years. Besides avoiding an intrathecal procedure, selective denervation has the advantage over anterior cervical rhizotomy that the contour and most of the normal movements of the neck are preserved.

During the past few years, selective peripheral denervation

has been used by Arce and Russo[69] and by Davis and colleagues,[70] in the United States, and by Braun and Richter[71] in Germany, so that, including ours, well over 400 patients have been operated on. No mortality and no major complications have been reported.

ADULT-ONSET DYSTONIA

In its initial stages, adult-onset dystonia may occasionally resemble spasmodic torticollis, which is another reason not to intervene too early on patients with spasmodic torticollis or, if the symptoms are not controlled by conservative measures, to use procedures that do not leave important sequelae. The evolution of dystonia is quite different from that of spasmodic torticollis, the manifestations of which are usually stable after 2 to 3 years. In contrast with dystonia musculorum deformans of childhood, adult-onset dystonia involves primarily the axial musculature. Because the cervical component of dystonia is frequently the dominant feature, our initial approach in these cases has been selective denervation, which produced a marked relief of symptoms in eight of nine patients and a surprising amount of improvement of the compensatory scoliosis. Three had an excellent result, and five, significant relief of symptoms. In three of the nine patients, a transitory increase of their peripheral symptoms of dystonia occurred that lasted from 1 to 2 weeks. One patient with a severe, rapidly progressing dystonia had a flare-up of his symptoms following denervation. This persisted, suggesting that surgery is contraindicated when the disease is progressing actively.

Although 20 thalamotomies were performed for adult-onset dystonia between 1976 and 1981, only five were performed between 1981 and 1986, and only one in the past 3 years in our department. This decrease is probably related to the type of patients referred because of our interest in the treatment of spasmodic torticollis. However, very few reports have appeared in the literature during the past few years[72, 73] concerning the use of thalamotomy in patients with dystonia. This scarcity may be the result not only of improvement in medical treatment but also of the percentage of complications, particularly dysarthria in bilateral lesions, as reported by Andrew and associates[74] among others. Hassler and Dieckmann[75] suggested the ventro-oralis internus as the ideal target; this nucleus, which is more anterior than nucleus VIM, is closer to the corticobulbar fibers, and in our own series, the percentage of patients with dysarthria was as high as 10 percent when bilateral lesions were performed.[31] We had been impressed by the fact that bursts of discharges synchronous to peripheral muscle discharges had been obtained. However, more recently, Lenz and coworkers[73] reported single-unit activity in thalamic cells at the same frequency as the electromyographic activity in dystonia. We have obtained equally good hypotonia from lesions centered in VIM and the immediate subthalamic area, that is, in the same location that was found to be the ideal target for the arrest of tremor.[32–34] In a review of 625 patients operated on for parkinsonian or other forms of tremor, dysarthria occurred in 2 percent, and all but one resulted from bilateral lesions.[31] Such lesions situated about 3 mm posterior to the ventro-oralis internis should also be limited laterally and anteriorly, but an additional lesion can be placed in the globus pallidus internus whenever necessary. Again, the limits of the globus pallidus are ascertained by microelectrode recording. After recording before the lesion is performed, unipolar stimulation with diffusion of the current helps to identify surrounding structures, particularly the corticobulbar and the corticospinal fibers. One should consider using physiologic controls and a more posterior lesion for a thalamotomy in patients with severe involvement of the limbs not amenable to conservative therapy, as suggested by Lenz and associates.[73] The initial lesion is contralateral to the most severely involved limbs. A lesion on the other side is made a few months later if necessary.

RESULTS

Twenty-five patients were followed up: the result was extremely good in six, good in 11, fair in five, and poor in three, that is, abnormal movements were markedly relieved in two-thirds of the patients. Thirteen of these also had a ramisectomy, which helped considerably when marked inclination or extension of the head was present. In a patient with an excellent result from a unilateral lesion and a very severe persistent myoclonic type of dystonia on the other side, a contralateral lesion 1 year later was not effective. In fact, after a few weeks, the abnormal movements inexplicably reappeared on the side relieved by the previous operation. Thalamotomy with or without pallidotomy remains a useful procedure in generalized adult-onset dystonia, and it may improve functional ability, but, unfortunately, the result remains unpredictable.

SUMMARY

Selective peripheral denervation produced complete or very marked relief of symptoms in 230 (88 percent) of 260 patients with spasmodic torticollis or the cervical component of dystonia. Abnormal movements can be suppressed by peripheral denervation limited to the muscles involved with preservation of near-normal movements of the neck.

Twenty-five patients with generalized adult-onset dystonia submitted to thalamotomy, pallidotomy, or both, were reviewed. Fourteen of them also had some form of peripheral denervation. An appreciable relief of symptoms was obtained in two thirds of the patients, but the result was unpredictable. The danger of dysarthria is less than 2 percent when physiologic controls with nucleus ventrointermedius as target point are used and when thalamotomy is performed only on one side, contralateral to the greater involvement of the limbs. This method should be considered in patients with severe dystonias when conservative measures fail.

REFERENCES

1. Ozelius L, Kramer PL, Moskowitz CB, et al: Human gene for torsion dystonia located on chromosome 9q32-q34. Neuron 2:1427–1434, 1989
2. Eldrige R, Fahn S (eds): Advances in Neurology, vol 14: Dystonia. New York, Raven Press, 1976
3. Yahr MD (ed): The Basal Ganglia. Research Publications: Association for Research in Nervous and Mental Diseases, vol 55. New York, Raven Press, 1976

4. Marsden CD, Fahn S (eds): Movement Disorders. Neurology II. London, Butterworths, 1981
5. Barbeau A (ed): Disorders of Movements. Current Status of Modern Therapy, vol 8. Lancaster, PA, MTP Press, 1981
6. Isaac K, Cohen JA: Post-traumatic torticollis. Neurology 39:1642–1643, 1989
7. Hedreen JC, Sweig RN, DeLong MR, et al: Primary dystonias: A review of the pathology and suggestions for new directions of study, in Fahn S, Marsden CD, Calne D (eds): Advances in Neurology, vol 50: Dystonia 2. New York, Raven Press, 1988, pp 123–132
8. Marsden CD, Obeso JA, Zarranz JJ, Lang AE: The anatomical basis of symptomatic hemidystonia. Brain 108:463–483, 1985
9. Plant GT, Mermode AG, du Boulay EP, McDonald WI: Spasmodic torticollis due to a midbrain lesion in a case of multiple sclerosis. Mov Disord 4:359–362, 1989
10. Zweig RM, Hedreen JC, Janker WR, et al: Pathology in brainstem regions of individuals with primary dystonia. Neurology 38:702–706, 1988
11. Fahn S: Torsion dystonia: Clinical spectrum and treatment. Semin Neurol 2:316–323, 1982
12. Marsden CD: The problem of adult-onset idiopathic torsion dystonia and other isolated dyskinesias in adult life (including blepharospasm, oromandibular dystonia, dystonic writer's cramp and torticollis, or axial dystonia), in Eldridge R, Fahn S (eds): Advances in Neurology, vol 14: Dystonia. New York, Raven Press, 1976, pp 259–276
13. Fahn S: The clinical spectrum of motor tics, in Friedhoff AJ, Chase TN (eds): Advances in Neurology, vol 35: Gilles de la Tourette Syndrome. New York, Raven Press, 1982, pp 341–344
14. Taira T, Hitchock E: Torticollis as an initial symptom of adult-onset dystonia musculorum deformans. No To Shinkei 42:671–867, 1990
15. Bertrand CM: Surgical management of spasmodic torticollis and adult-onset dystonia with emphasis on selective denervation, in Schmidek H, Sweet W (eds): Operative Neurosurgical Techniques, vol 2. Orlando, Grune & Stratton, 1988, pp 1261–1269
16. Couch JR: Dystonia and tremor in spasmodic torticollis, in Eldridge R, Fahn S (eds): Advances in Neurology, vol 14: Dystonia. New York, Raven Press, 1976, pp 245–258
17. Gilbert JG: Familial spasmodic torticollis. Neurology 27:11–13, 1977
18. Podivinsky F: Torticollis, in Vinken PJ, Bruyn GW (eds): Handbook of Clinical Neurology. Amsterdam, Elsevier, 1968, pp 567–596
19. Fletcher NA, Harding AE, Marsden CD: A case control study on idiopathic torsion dystonia. Mov Disord 6:304–309, 1991
20. Tsui JK, Eisen A, Mak E, et al: A pilot study on the use of botulinum toxin in spasmodic torticollis. Can J Neurol Sci 12:314–316, 1985
21. Tsui JK, Eisen A, Stoessl AJ, et al: A double-blind study on the use of botulinum toxin in spasmodic torticollis. Lancet ii:245–247, 1986
22. Greene P, Shale H, Fahn S, et al: Treatment of torticollis with injections of botulinum toxin. Neurology 37 (suppl 1):123, 1987
23. Fahn S: High dosage anticholinergic therapy in dystonia. Neurology 33:1255–1261, 1983
24. Marsden CD, Marion N-H, Quinn N: The treatment of severe dystonia in children and adults. J Neurol Neurosurg Psychiatry 47:1166–1173, 1984
25. Lee MC: Spasmodic torticollis and other idiopathic torsion dystonias. Medical management. Postgrad Med 75:139–141, 1984
26. Jankovic J, Schawartz K: Botulinum toxin injections for cervical dystonia. Neurology 40:277–280, 1990
27. Korein J, Brudny J: Integrated EMG feedback in the management of spasmodic torticollis and focal dystonia: A prospective study of 80 patients, in Yahr MD (ed): The Basal Ganglia. Research Publications: Association for Research in Nervous and Mental Diseases, vol 55. New York, Raven Press, 1976, pp 385–424
28. Svien HJ, Cody DTR: Treatment of spasmodic torticollis by suppression of labyrinthine activity: Report of a case. Mayo Clin Proc 44:825–827, 1969
29. Mazars G, Méienne L, Chodkiewicz JP: La Chirurgie des Dyskinésies d'Orientation Céphalique. Neurochirurgie 14:745–752, 1968
30. Bertrand C: The treatment of spasmodic torticollis with particular reference to thalamotomy, in Morley T (ed): Current Controversies in Neurosurgery. Philadelphia, WB Saunders, 1976, pp 455–459
31. Bertrand C, Molina-Negro P, Martinez SN: Stereotactic targets for dystonias and dyskinesias: Their relationship to cortico-bulbar fibers and other adjoining structures, in Poirier LJ, Sourkes TK, Bédard PJ (eds): Advances in Neurology, vol 24: The Extra-pyramidal System and Its Disorders. New York, Raven Press, 1979, pp 395–399
32. Bertrand C, Hardy J, Molina-Negro P, et al: Optimum physiological target for the arrest of tremor, in Gillingham FJ, Donaldson IM (eds): Third Symposium on Parkinson's Disease. Edinburgh, Livingstone, 1969, pp 251–259
33. Velasco Francisco C, Molina-Negro Pedro, Bertrand Claude, Hardy Jules: Further definition of the subthalamic target for arrest of tremor. J Neurosurg 36:184–191, 1972
34. Bertrand C, Martinez SN, Hardy J, et al: Stereotactic surgery for parkinsonism, in Krayenbuhl H, Maspes PE, Sweet WH (eds): Progress in Neurological Surgery, vol 5. Basel, Karger S, 1973, pp 79–112
35. Freckmann N, Hagenah R, Herrmann H-D, et al: Treatment of neurogenic torticollis by microvascular lysis of the accessory nerve roots—Indication, technique and first results. Acta Neurochir (Wien) 59:167–175, 1981
36. Adams CBY: Spasmodic torticollis resulting from neurovascular compression (letter). J Neurosurg 66:635, 1987
37. Freckmann N, Hagenah R, Herrmann H-D, Müller D: Bilateral microsurgical lysis of the spinal accessory nerve roots for treatment of spasmodic torticollis—Follow-up of 33 cases. Acta Neurochir (Wien) 83:47–53, 1986
38. Shima F, Fukui M, Kitamura K, et al: Diagnosis and surgical treatment of spasmodic torticollis of 11th nerve origin. Neurosurgery 22:358–363, 1988
39. Gildenberg PL: Treatment of spasmodic torticollis with dorsal column stimulation. Acta Neurochir Suppl (Wien) 36(Suppl 24):65–66, 1977
40. Waltz JM: Surgical approach to dystonia, in Marsden CD, Fahn S (eds): Movement Disorders. Neurology II. London, Butterworths, 1981, pp 300–307
41. Gildenberg PL: Comprehensive management of spasmodic torticollis. Appl Neurophysiol 44:233–243, 1981
42. Waltz JM, Andreeson WH, Hunt DP: Spinal cord stimulation and motor disorders. Pace 10:180–204, 1987
43. Goetz CG, Penn RD, Tanner CM: Efficacy of cervical cord stimulation in dystonia. Adv Neurol 50:645–649, 1988
44. McKenzie KG: Intrameningeal division of the spinal accessory and roots of the upper cervical nerves for the treatment of spasmodic torticollis. Surg Gynecol Obstet 39:5–10, 1924
45. Dandy WE: Operation for treatment of spasmodic torticollis. Arch Surg 20:10–21, 1930
46. Tasker RR: The treatment of spasmodic torticollis by peripheral denervation: The MacKenzie operation, in Morley T (ed): Current Controversies in Neurosurgery, Philadelphia, WB Saunders, 1976, pp 448–454
47. Sorensen BF, Hamby WB: Spasmodic torticollis: Results in 71 surgically treated patients. JAMA 194:706–708, 1965
48. Arseni C, Maretsis M: The surgical treatment of spasmodic torticollis. Neurochirurgia (Stuttg) 14:177–180, 1971
49. Hamby WB, Schiffer S: Spasmodic torticollis: Results after cervical rhizotomy in 50 cases. J Neurosurg 31:323–326, 1969
50. Fabinyi G, Dutton J: The surgical treatment of spasmodic torticollis. Aust N Z J Surg 50:155–157, 1980
51. Hernesniemi J, Keranen T: Long term outcome after surgery for spasmodic torticollis. Acta Neurochir (Wien) 103:128–130, 1990
52. Friedman AH, Nashold BS Jr, Sharp R, et al: Treatment of spasmodic torticollis with intradural selective rhizotomies. J Neurosurg 78:46–53, 1993
53. Perot PL: Upper cervical ventral rhizotomy and selective section of spinal accessory rootlets for spasmodic torticollis, in Wilson CB (ed): Neurosurgical Procedures. Baltimore, Williams & Wilkins, 1992, pp 163–168
54. Xinkang C: Selective resection and denervation of cervical muscles in the treatment of spasmodic torticollis: Results in 60 cases. Neurosurgery 8:681–688, 1981
55. Chen XK, Ji SX, Zhu GH, Ma AB: Operative treatment of bilateral retrocollis. Acta Neurochir (Wien) 113:180–183, 1991
56. Maccabe JJ: Surgical treatment of spasmodic torticollis, in Marsden CD, Fahn S (eds): Movement Disorders. Neurology II. London, Butterworths, 1981, pp 308–314
57. Bertrand C, Molina-Negro P, Martinez SN: Combined stereotactic and peripheral surgical approach for spasmodic torticollis. Appl Neurophysiol 41:122–133, 1978
58. Bertrand C: Stereotactic and peripheral surgery for the control of movement disorders, in Barbeau A (ed): Disorders of Movements. Current Status of Modern Therapy, vol 8. Lancaster, MTP Press, 1981, pp 191–208
59. Bertrand C, Molina-Negro P, Martinez SN: Technical aspects of selective peripheral denervation for spasmodic torticollis. Appl Neurophysiol 45:326–330, 1982

60. Bertrand CM, Molina-Negro P: Selective peripheral denervation in 111 cases of spasmodic torticollis: Rationale and results, in Fahn S, Marsden CD, Calne DB (eds): Advances in Neurology, vol 50: Dystonia 2. New York, Raven Press, 1988, pp 638–643
61. Bertrand C, Molina-Negro P, Bouvier G, Gorczyca W: Observations and analysis of results in 131 cases of spasmodic torticollis after selective denervation. Appl Neurophysiol 50:319–323, 1987
62. Bertrand C: Cervical dystonias, particularly spasmodic torticollis, treated with selective denervation. A review after eleven years. Homenaje al Doctor Y Professor Manuel M. Velasco Suares, in Rodriguez Carbajal J, Escobar A (eds): Editorial Progreso, S.A. Mexico, 1989, pp 654–658
63. Bertrand C, Bouvier G, Molina-Negro P: Surgical treatment of spasmodic torticollis by selective denervation—A review of 260 cases. Mov Disord 7 (suppl 1):128, 1992
64. Ouaknine G, Nathan H: Anastomotic connections between the eleventh nerve and the posterior root of the first cervical nerve in humans. J Neurosurg 38:189–197, 1973
65. Gloobe H, Ouaknine G, Klausner J, Nathan H: Variations of the first cervical nerve (C1) and the spinal accessory nerve (XI) in the Cercopithecus (Cercopithecus etiopicus). J Med Primatol 3:174–184, 1974
66. Keen WW: A new operation for spasmodic wry neck. Namely, division or exsection of the nerves supplying the posterior rotator muscles of the head. Ann Surg 13:44–47, 1891
67. Finney MT, Hughson W: Spasmodic torticollis. Ann Surg 81:255–269, 1925
68. Johnston HM: The cutaneous branches of the posterior primary divisions of the spinal nerves and their distribution in the skin. J Anat Physiol 43:80–92, 1908
69. Arce C, Russo L: Selective peripheral denervation: A surgical alternative in the treatment for spasmodic torticollis. Review of fifty-five patients. Mov Disord 7 (suppl 1):128, 1992
70. Davis DH, Ahlskog JE, Litchy WJ, Root LM: Selective peripheral denervation for torticollis: Preliminary results. Mayo Clin Proc 66:365–371, 1991
71. Braun V, Richter H-P: Selective peripheral denervation in patients with spasmodic torticollis. Stereotact Funct Neurosurg 57:113–122, 1991
72. Tasker RR, Doorly T, Yamshiro K: Thalamotomy in generalized dystonia, in Fahn S, Marsden CD, Calne DB (eds): Advances in Neurology, vol 50: Dystonia 2. New York, Raven Press, 1988, pp 615–631
73. Lenz FA, Martin R, Kwan HC, et al: Thalamic single-unit activity occurring in patients with hemidystonia. Stereotact Funct Neurosurg 54/55:159–162, 1990
74. Andrew J, Fowler CJ, Harrison MJG: Stereotaxic thalamotomy in 55 cases of dystonia. Brain 106:981–1000, 1983
75. Hassler R, Dieckmann G: Stereotactic treatment of different kinds of spasmodic torticollis. Confin Neurol 32:135–143, 1970

CHAPTER 134

Neurosurgical Management of Spasticity

M. Sindou
P. Mertens

Spasticity is one of the commonest sequelae of neurologic diseases. Although spasticity can be useful in compensating for lost motor strength, it may become harmful and may lead to further functional losses. When not controllable by physical therapy and medications, spasticity can benefit from neurostimulation, intrathecal pharmacotherapy, or selective ablative procedures.

PATHOPHYSIOLOGY

As pointed out by Katz,[1] "Spasticity is something easier to recognize than characterize, and perhaps more difficult to treat successfully." In 1980, Lance[2] proposed an operational definition: "Spasticity is a motor disorder characterized by a velocity-dependant increase in tonic stretch reflexes (muscle tone) with exaggerated tendon jerks, resulting from hyperexcitability of the stretch reflex, as one component of the upper motor neuron syndrome."

According to the concept proposed by Sherrington,[3] exaggerated reflexes are caused by a release from supraspinal inhibition, resulting in an imbalance in favor of an exaggerated excitatory state at the spinal level. This notion was derived from the observation that hypertonia is an immediate consequence of decerebration.

In most human cases, spasticity develops gradually over months after a period of depressed spinal activity. Such a slow time course cannot be explained simply in terms of disinhibition of spinal circuits. Wiesendanger[4] believed that the gradual development of spasticity strongly pointed to profound reorganization of the denervated structures at the spinal level in response to the degeneration of descending fibers. These compensatory reactions are characterized by long-term changes in the synaptic transmission. Primary collaterals sprout from intact stem fibers and occupy synaptic sites vacated in the course of degeneration. Receptor supersensitivity of neurons occurs as a response to a loss of synaptic inputs. Both these mechanisms develop with a time course compatible with the development of spasticity occurring after an acute lesion.

NEUROSTIMULATION PROCEDURES

Developed in the 1970s on the basis of the gate control theory of Melzach and Wall[5] for the treatment of neurogenic pain, stimulation of the spinal cord has been partially effective in the treatment of spastic syndromes, such as those encountered in multiple sclerosis or spinal cord degenerative diseases.[6-8] For most authors, stimulation of the spinal cord is effective only when spasticity is mild and when the dorsal columns have sufficient functional fibers, as assessed by somatosensory evoked potentials. Other methods of neurostimulation, such as deep brain stimulation or cerebellar stimulation, which yield some positive results in patients with dystonic or dyskinetic syndromes, are not significantly effective for the treatment of spasticity itself.[9]

INTRATHECAL ADMINISTRATION OF BACLOFEN

To overcome the obstacle of poor transfer of baclofen through the blood-brain barrier, Penn and Kroin[10] introduced a new treatment of spasticity: direct spinal intrathecal administration of baclofen. The effectiveness of the method is linked to the presence of high concentrations of gamma aminobutyric acid–B binding sites in the dorsal horn, which allows a decrease in the necessary dosage from an average of 60 mg/day orally to an average of 100 µg/day intrathecally. To avoid daily injection by lumbar puncture, the method uses a programmable pump device, implanted subcutaneously, consisting of a reservoir containing the drug that is refilled percutaneously every 3 months and a pump that provides the desired flow. The most appropriate pump is the Synchromed pump from Medtronic Company.[11]

This method is particularly indicated for patients with severe spasticity of spinal cord origin, especially if painful spasms are present, as in advanced multiple sclerosis.[10,12]

A serious risk of intrathecal baclofen administration is overdose, which could be irreversible because of the lack of baclofen antagonists; therefore, this technique requires great care. Other complications include mechanical catheter migration or occlusion and infection, which require revision or removal of the system, respectively. The advantage of the technique is the reversibility of its effects, but high cost, necessity of periodic refilling and reprogramming, and geographic dependence are serious limitations to this conservative method.

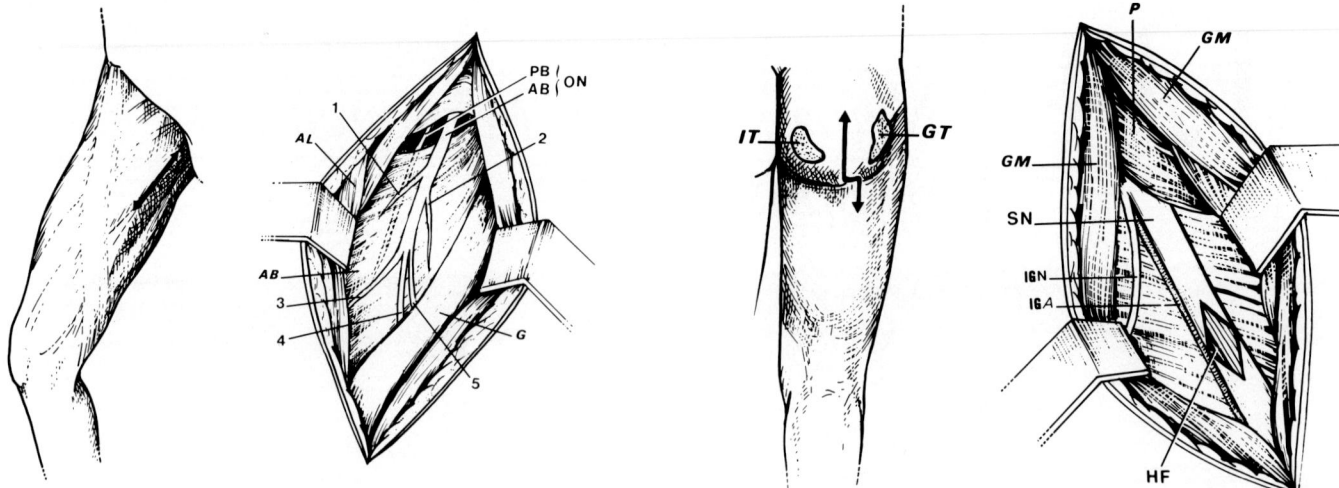

FIGURE 134–1. (Left) Obturator neurotomy. Skin incision on the relief of adductor longus muscle. Dissection of the anterior branch (AB) of the right obturator nerve (ON). The adductor longus muscle (AL) is retracted laterally and the gracilis muscle (G) medially. The nerve is anterior to the adductor brevis muscle (AB). The adductor brevis nerve (1 and 2), adductor longus nerve (3), and the gracilis nerve (4 and 5) are shown. The posterior branch (PB) of the obturator nerve lies under the adductor brevis muscle (AB).
(Right) Hamstring neurotomy. Skin incision between the ischial tuberosity (IT) and the greater trochanter (GT). Dissection of the right sciatic nerve (SN), under the piriformis muscle (P), after passing through the fibers of the gluteus maximus muscle (GM). The epineurium of the nerve is opened, and fascicles for hamstring muscles (HF) are located in the medial part of the nerve. IGN = Inferior gluteal nerve, IGA = inferior gluteal artery.

NEUROABLATIVE PROCEDURES

When spasticity cannot be controlled by conservative methods, ablative procedures must be considered. Excitability can be modified on the level of the segmental neural circuits, which are hyperactive after being deprived of their descending inhibitory influences. The surgery should be performed so that excessive hypertonia is reduced without suppression of useful muscular tone or impairment of the residual motor and sensory functions. Therefore, neuroablative techniques must be as selective as possible. Such selective lesions can be performed at the level of peripheral nerves, spinal roots, spinal cord, or the dorsal root entry zone.

PERIPHERAL NEUROTOMIES

Selective peripheral neurotomies were introduced first for the treatment of spastic deformities of the foot by Stoffel.[13] More recently, Gros and associates[14] and the authors[15] have advocated making neurotomies more selective by using microsurgical techniques and intraoperative electrical stimulation for better identification of the function of the fascicles constituting the nerve. Selectivity is required to suppress the excess of spasticity without excessive weakening of motor strength and without producing exaggerated amyotrophy. To achieve this goal, preserving at least one fourth of the motor fibers is necessary.

Neurotomies may be indicated when spasticity is localized to muscles or muscular groups supplied by a single or a few peripheral nerves that are easily accessible. To help the surgeon decide if neurotomy is appropriate, temporary local anesthetic block of the nerve with bupivacaïne can be useful. Such a test can determine if articular limitations result from spasticity, musculotendinous contractures, or articular ankyloses (only spasticity is decreased by the test). In addition, these tests give the patient a chance to appreciate what to expect from the operation.

In the management of spasticity of the lower limbs (Figs. 134–1 and 134–2), neurotomies of the tibial nerve at the popliteal region and, to a lesser extent, of the obturator nerve just below the subpubic canal, are the most commonly used, respectively, for the so-called spastic foot and for flexion–adduction deformity of the hip. Selective neurotomies of the branches to the knee flexors can also be performed at the level of the sciatic trunk through a short skin incision in the buttock.

In contrast to the lower limbs, neurotomies are seldom indicated for spasticity in the upper limbs (Fig. 134–3). However, selective fascicular neurotomies of the musculocutaneous nerve for spastic elbow flexion and of the median (and cubital) nerve for spastic hyperflexion of the wrist and fingers can be performed, provided that special care is taken with the sensory fascicles to avoid causalgic painful manifestations.

Selective neurotomies are able not only to reduce deformity but also to improve motor function by re-equilibrating the tonic balance between agonist and antagonist muscles (Fig. 134–4).

POSTERIOR RHIZOTOMIES

Posterior rhizotomy was performed for the first time for the modification of spasticity by Foerster in 1908,[16] after Sherrington demonstrated in 1898 that decerebrate rigidity in the animal model was abolished by section of the dorsal roots, that is, by interruption of the afferent input to the monosynaptic stretch and polysynaptic withdrawal reflexes. Its undesired effects on sensory and sphincter functions limited its application in the past. To diminish these disadvan-

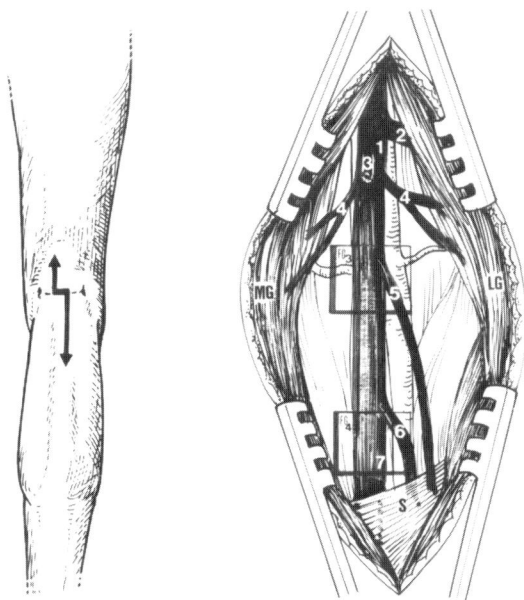 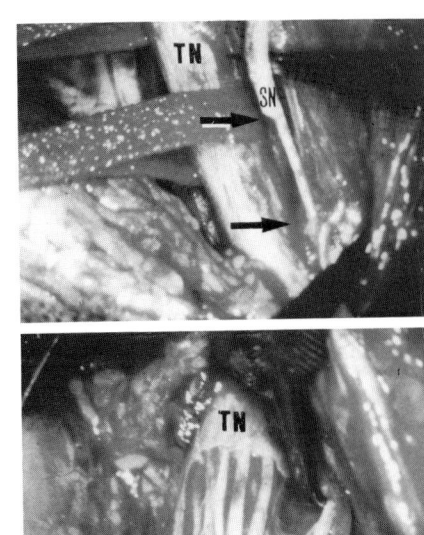

FIGURE 134–2. Selective tibial neurotomy.

(Left) Skin incision in the right popliteal fossa.

(Center) Dorsal view, showing tibial (1) and peroneal nerves (2), sural (sensory) nerve (3), and motor branches of the tibial nerve.

Equinus and ankle clonus require section of the soleus nerve (5), and if necessary, of the medial and lateral gastrocnemius nerve (4). Varus necessitates interruption of the posterior tibialis nerve (6). Tonic flexion of the toes requires section of the flexor fascicles situated inside the distal trunk of the tibial nerve (7), just above the soleus arch(es). Their precise identification apart from the sensory fascicles by electrical stimulation is of paramount importance to avoid hypoesthetic and dysesthetic disturbances, as well as trophic lesions of the plantar skin.

(Upper Right) Operative view of the resection, over 7 mm in length (between the two arrows), of two thirds of the soleus nerve (SN).

(Lower Right) Operative view of five dissected fascicles inside the distal part of the tibial nerve (TN) at the level of the soleus arch, after the epineural envelope has been opened.

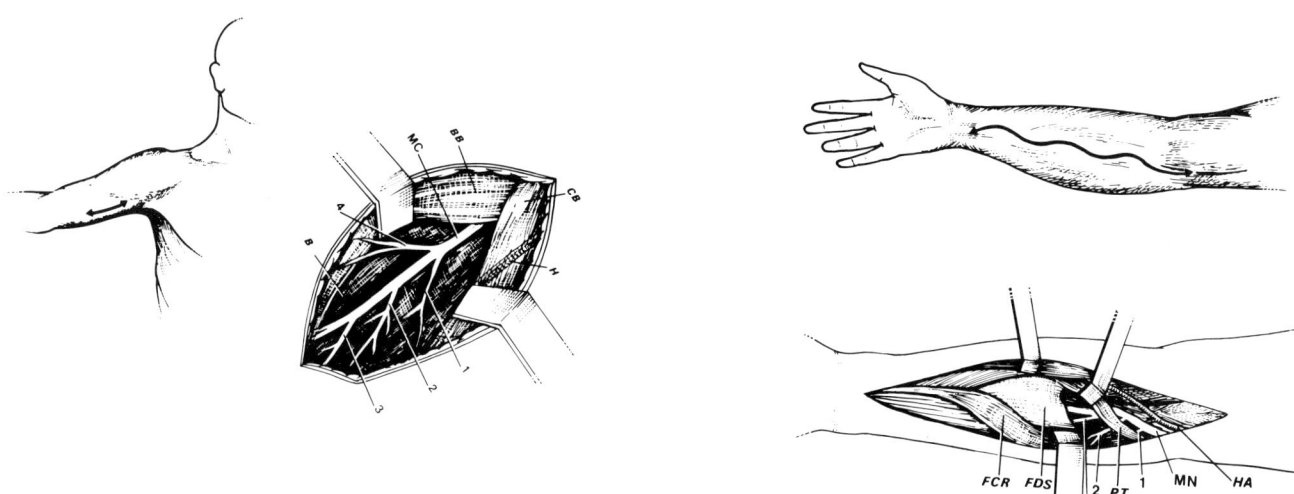

FIGURE 134–3. (Left) Musculocutaneous neurotomy. Skin incision along the medial aspect of the biceps brachii. Dissection of the right musculocutaneous nerve (MC) in the space between the biceps brachii (BB) laterally, the coracobrachialis (CB) medially, and the brachialis (B) posteriorly. Branches to brachialis (1 and 2) and to biceps brachii (3 and 4). The humeral artery (h) and the median nerve are situated medially (they are not dissected).

(Right) Median neurotomy. Skin incision on the right forearm, from the medial aspect of the biceps brachii at the level of the elbow to the midline above the wrist. During the first stage of the dissection, the pronator teres (PT) is retracted upward and laterally, and the flexor carpi radialis (FCR) is retracted medially. Branches from the median nerve (MN), before it passes under the fibrous arch of the flexor digitorum superficialis (FDS), are dissected to the pronotor teres (1), and two nerve trunks to the flexor carpi radialis, palmaris longus and flexor digitorum superficialis (2).[3] In the second stage of the dissection, the fibrous arch of the FDS is sectioned to allow the median nerve to be dissected more distally.

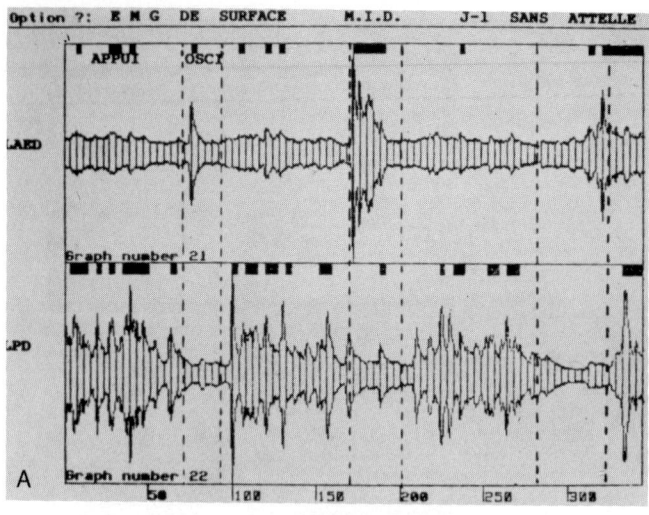
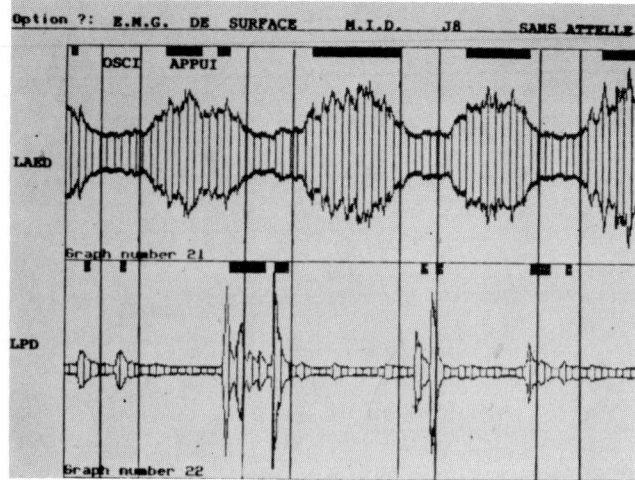
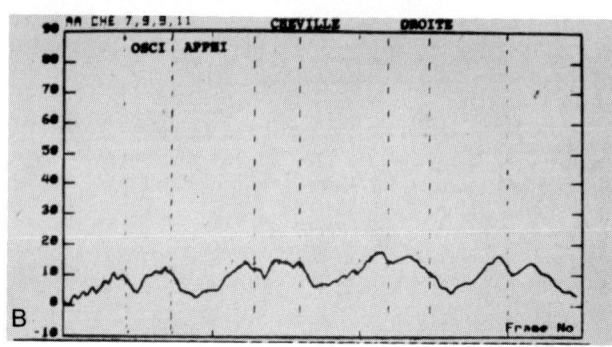
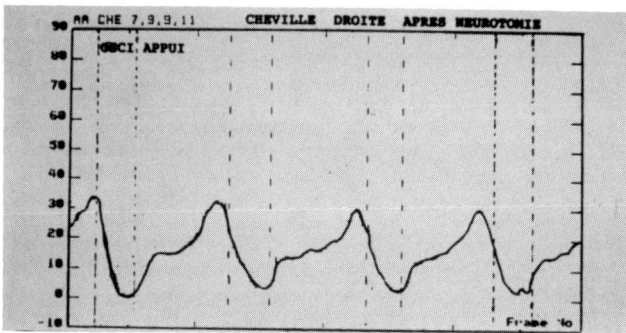

FIGURE 134-4. Movement analysis in a hemiplegic patient with a spastic foot (equinovarus) before and after selective tibial neurotomy.
(A) Surface polyelectromyography of the tibialis anterior (LAED) and the triceps surae (LPD) muscles on the spastic leg during walking. (Left) Preoperative recordings showing desynchronized activities of the triceps surae, with abnormal cocontractions of antagonist muscles: triceps surae and tibialis anterior. (Right) After selective tibial neurotomy, there is a reappearance of muscular activities in the tibialis anterior muscle, a clear decrease in triceps surae activities, and normal alternance of contractions of these muscles (i.e., triceps surae at the end of the stance phase and tibialis anterior during the swing phase).
(B) Tridimensional movement analysis of the ankle flexion-extension amplitude during the gait with VICON system.
(Left) Preoperatively, the amplitude of the spastic ankle is limited to 18 degrees of dorsal flexion.
(Right) After selective tibial neurotomy, the dorsal flexion increased to 32 degrees. Thus the tonic balance of the ankle has been reequilibrated by the selective tibial neurotomy; consequently, motor function and gait have been improved.

tages, several authors in the 1960s and 1970s attempted to develop more selective operations, especially for the treatment of children with cerebral palsy.

Posterior Selective Rhizotomy

To reduce the sensory side effects of the original Foerster method, Gros and coworkers[17] introduced a technical modification that consisted of sparing one rootlet of the five of each root, from L1 to S1. On similar principles, Ouaknine,[18] a pupil of Gros, developed a microsurgical technique that consisted of resecting one third to two thirds of each group of rootlets of all the posterior roots from L1 to S1.

Sectorial Posterior Rhizotomy

In an attempt to reduce the side effects of rhizotomy on postural tone in ambulatory patients, Gros[19] and his pupil, Privat and his colleagues[20] proposed a topographic selection of the rootlets. The surgeon prepares for the procedure by performing a preoperative assessment of useful spasticity in the abdominal, quadriceps, and gluteus medius muscles, which is related to postural tone, and harmful spasticity of hip flexors, adductors, hamstrings, and triceps surae. The first step consists of mapping of the evoked motor activity of the exposed rootlets, from L1 to S2, by direct electrostimulation of each posterior group of rootlets. Sections are planned according to the preoperative program.

Partial Posterior Rhizotomy

Fraioli and Guidetti[21] reported on a procedure of dividing the dorsal half of each rootlet of the selected posterior roots a few millimeters before their entrance into the posterolateral sulcus. Good results have been reported by the authors, without significant sensory deficit, the latter explained by the fact that partial section leaves intact a large number of fibers of all types.

Functional Posterior Rhizotomy

The neurologic search for specially organized circuits responsible for spasticity led Fasano and associates[22] to propose the so-called functional posterior rhizotomy, which is based on bipolar intraoperative stimulation of the posterior rootlets and analysis of the type of muscle responses by electromyographic recordings. Responses characterized by a permanent tonic contraction, an after-discharge pattern, or a large spatial diffusion to distant muscle groups were considered to belong to disinhibited spinal circuits responsible for spasticity. This procedure—which is especially indicated for children with cerebral palsy—has been extensively used by numerous surgical teams.[23–26] Our own adaptation of the method is illustrated in Figure 134–5.

PERCUTANEOUS THERMORHIZOTOMY AND INTRATHECAL CHEMICAL RHIZOTOMY

Percutaneous radiofrequency rhizotomy, initially performed for the treatment of pain,[27] was later applied to the treatment of neurogenic detrusor hyperreflexia[28] and of spasticity in the limb.[29–31] This method has the advantage of being less aggressive than the open procedures in very debilitated patients. It seems more appropriate for spastic disturbances limited to a few muscle groups that correspond to a small number of spinal roots, as occurs in spastic hip, which can be treated by thermorhizotomy of L2-L3. The effects are most often temporary, but the procedure can be repeated.

Intrathecal injection of alcohol was first introduced[32] for cancer pain and later was used for hypertonia in patients with severe spastic paraplegia.[33] Alcohol was then replaced by phenol (a hyperbaric solution), which is easier to control.[34–36] The best candidates for phenol intrathecal injections are paraplegic patients suffering from severe spasms who do not have useful residual movements, sphincter functions, and sensory capabilities below the level of the lesion.

LONGITUDINAL MYELOTOMY

Longitudinal myelotomy[37–39] consists of a coronal separation between the posterior and anterior horns of the lumbosacral enlargement from T11 to S2. It is performed from inside the spinal cord after a posterior commissural incision reaches the ependymal canal. Longitudinal myelotomy is indicated only for patients with spastic paraplegias with flexion spasms, when the patients have no residual useful motor control and no bladder and sexual function.

SURGERY IN THE DORSAL ROOT ENTRY ZONE

Selective posterior rhizotomy in the dorsal root entry zone (DREZ), also called microsurgical DREZotomy, was introduced in 1972[40] to treat intractable pain (see Chapter 130). Because of its inhibitory effects on muscular tone, it has been applied to patients with focalized hyperspasticity.[41–44] This method attempts to selectively interrupt the small nociceptive and the large myotactic fibers (situated laterally and centrally, respectively), while sparing the large lemniscal fibers, which are regrouped medially. It also enhances the inhibitory mechanisms of Lissauer's tract and the dorsal horn (Fig. 134–6).[5, 45]

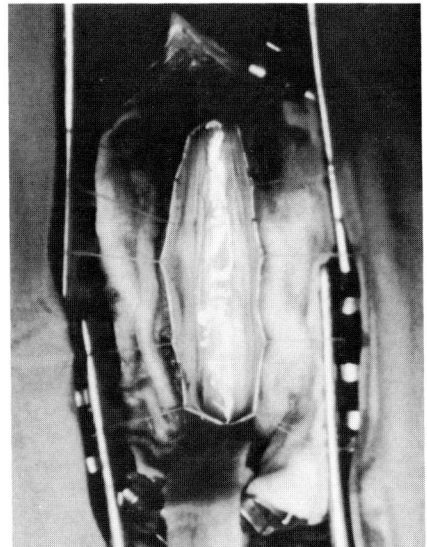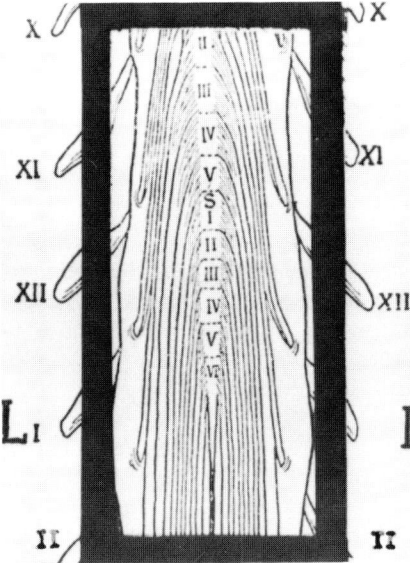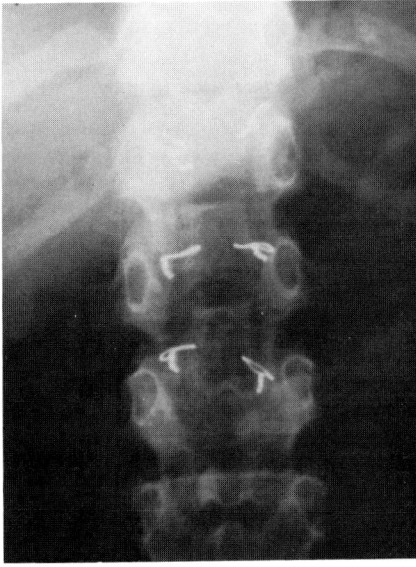

FIGURE 134–5. Lumbosacral posterior rhizotomy for cerebral palsy children. Our personal technique consists of performing a limited osteoplastic laminotomy using a power saw, in one single piece, from T11 to L1 (left). The laminae are replaced at the end of the procedure and fixed with wires (right). The dorsal (and ventral) L1, L2, and L3 roots are identified by means of the muscular responses evoked by electrical stimulation performed intradurally just before entry into their dural sheaths. The dorsal sacral rootlets are recognized at their entrance into the dorsolateral sulcus of the conus medullaris. The landmark between S1 and S2 medullary segments is located at approximately 30 mm from the exit of the coccygeal root from the conus. The dorsal rootlets of S1, L5, and L4 are identified by their evoked motor responses. The sensory roots for the bladder (S2-S3) can be identified by monitoring vesical pressure, and those for the anal sphincter (S3-S4) can be identified by rectomanometry or EMG. Surface spinal cord SEP recordings from tibial nerve (L5-S1) and pudendal nerve (S2-S3) stimulation may also be helpful.

For the surgery to be effective, a total amount of 60 percent of dorsal rootlets must be cut, of course with a different quantity cut according to the level and function of the roots involved. Also, of course, the correspondence of the roots with the muscles having harmful spasticity or useful postural tone must be considered in determining the amount of rootlets to be cut.

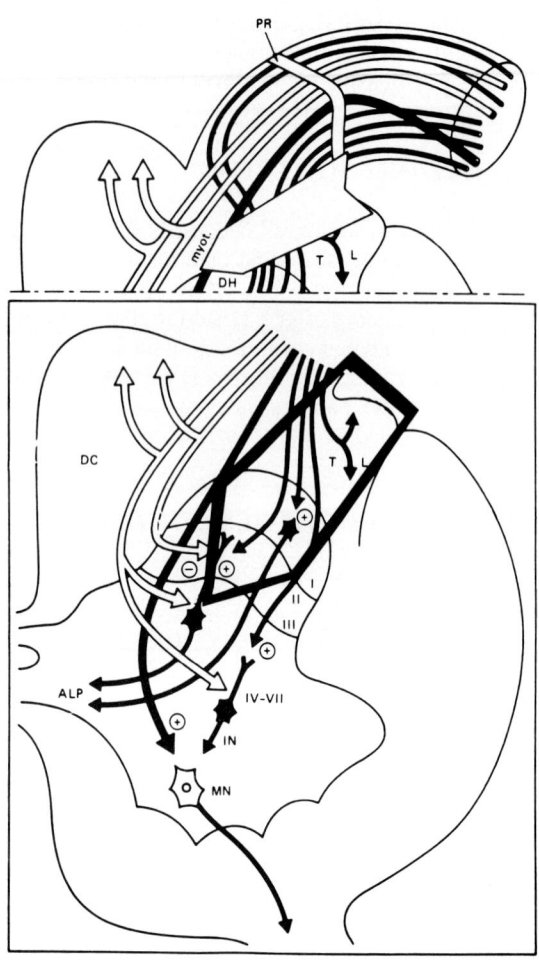
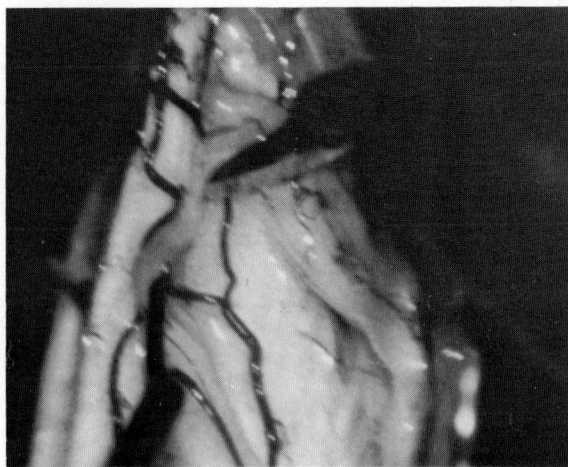
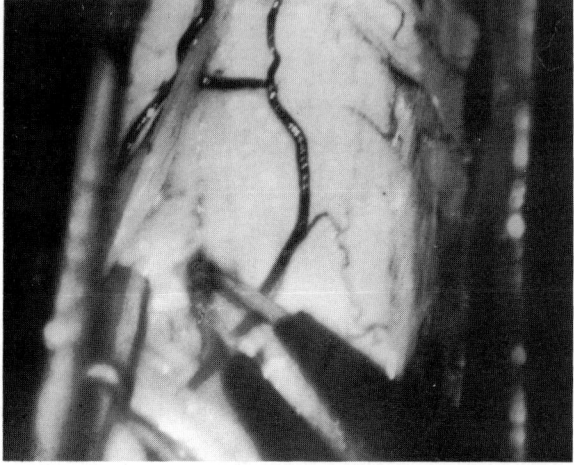

FIGURE 134–6. Micro-DREZotomy (MDT). (Left) Organization of fibers at the DREZ in humans. The large arrow shows the proposed extent of the micro-DREZOTOMY, that is, the lateral and central bundles formed by the nociceptive and myotatic fibers, as well as the excitatory medial part of the TL and the upper layers of the dorsal horn.

(Right) Technique of MDT. Example through a right cervical hemilaminectomy (the procedure for the lumbosacral roots is almost the same) (see Chapter 130). The right C6 posterior root has been retracted toward the inside to make the ventrolateral region of the DREZ accessible. The incision is performed into the dorsolateral sulcus using a small piece of razor blade (upper operative view). The incision is 2 mm deep and is made at a 45-degree angle. Then microcoagulations are created with a very sharp and graduated bipolar microforceps down to the apex of the dorsal horn (lower operative view).

Microsurgical DREZotomy, the technique of which has been detailed elsewhere,[46] consists of microsurgical incisions that are 2 mm deep and at 45-degree angles and bipolar coagulations performed ventrolaterally at the entrance of the rootlets into the dorsolateral sulcus, along all the cord segments selected for operation.

For patients with paraplegia,[47] the L2-S5 segments are approached through a T11-L2 laminectomy, whereas for the hemiplegic upper limb,[48] a C4-C7 hemilaminectomy with conservation of the spinous processes is sufficient to reach the C5-T1 segments. Identification of the metameric levels that support the harmful tonic mechanisms or correspond to the painful territories is achieved by study of the muscle responses to bipolar electrical stimulation of the anterior or posterior roots. Then, the lateral aspect of the DREZ is exposed so that the microsurgical lesions can be performed.

Microsurgical DREZotomy is indicated for spasticity in the lower limbs in disabled patients with severe hypertonic paraplegia, especially when flexion spasms, irreducible abnormal postures, or pain are present.[47] A spastic bladder can be successfully treated, provided that the detrusor is not fibrotic.[49] Microsurgical DREZotomy is also indicated in hemiplegic patients who have harmful spasticity in the upper limb.[48]

By suppressing the excess of spasticity, correcting the abnormal postures, and relieving the frequently associated pain, microsurgical DREZotomy allows physiotherapy to be resumed and, sometimes, the reappearance or improvement of useful voluntary motility.

ORTHOPEDIC SURGERY

Orthopedic procedures can reduce spasticity by means of muscle relaxation that results from tendon lengthening or from restoration of articular function when deformities have become irreducible. Current techniques for correcting excessive shortness of the muscle tendon assembly are muscular desinsertion, myotomy, tenotomy, or lengthening-tenotomy. Such techniques aim to obtain a more functional position for the limb or limbs involved. Excessive lengthening can lead to a decrease in muscular strength.

Tendon transfer has a different goal: to normalize articular orientation when it has been distorted by muscular imbalance. Transfer of spastic muscles must be avoided. If necessary, suppression of spasticity must be achieved by neurosurgical procedure before tendon transfer.

Osteotomies aim to correct bone deformation resulting from growth distortion in a child or to treat stiffened joints. Articular surgery, or arthrodesis, is indicated only when osteoarticular deformity cannot be corrected by osteotomy or tendon surgery alone. Arthrodesis must not be performed in children until they stop growing.

Orthopedic surgery can be undertaken to correct or even prevent irreducible deformities, to increase comfort in the more severely affected patients, or to improve function in those who have recovered sufficient level of voluntary motor function but only after spasticity, when present, has been reduced.

INDICATIONS FOR SURGERY

ADULTS

The following guidelines for indications for surgery in adults have been established from the literature and also from

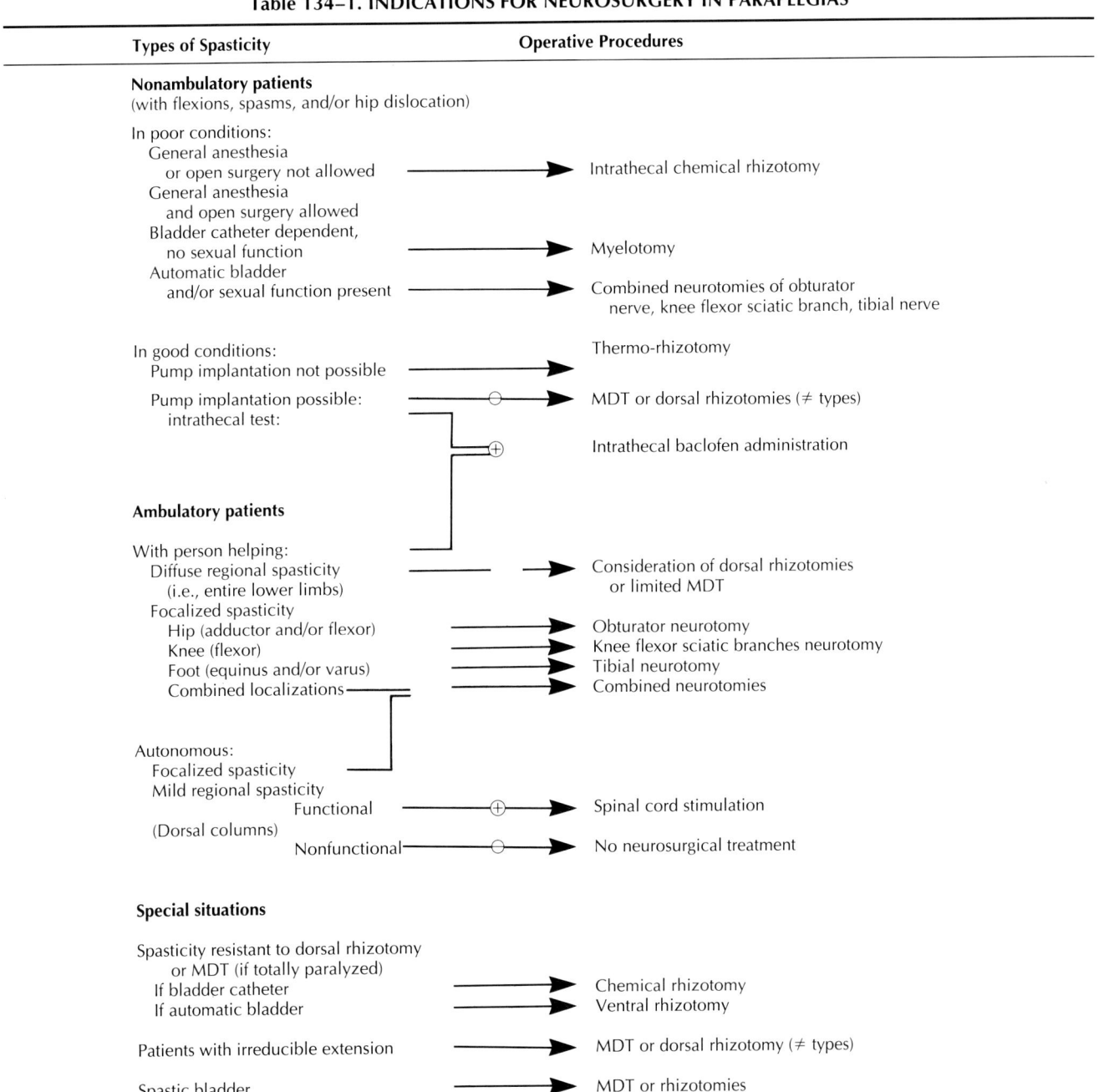

Table 134–1. INDICATIONS FOR NEUROSURGERY IN PARAPLEGIAS

MDT = microsurgical DREZotomy. ≠ = different; ⊕ = positive; ⊖ = negative.

Table 134–2. INDICATIONS FOR NEUROSURGERY IN HEMIPLEGIAS

Types of Spasticity	Operative Procedures
Lower limb	

Spastic foot
  Equinus, clonus
  Varus
  Flexion of toes
	→ Neurotomy of tibial nerve
	  Soleus (gastrocnemius) branches
	  Posterior tibialis branch
	  Flexor fascicles
	  Combined with orthopedic surgery, if needed

Tonic ambulatory foot	→ Discuss need for neurotomy of tibial nerve or no surgery at all
Upper limb	
Entire limb (or shoulder and elbow alone)	→ C_5–T_1 MDT (or C_5–C_7 MDT)
Entire limb with severe hypertonia of wrist and finger flexors	→ C_5–T_1 MDT with neurotomy of flexor fascicles of the median (and ulnar) nerve(s)
Isolated spastic hyperflexion of wrist and fingers	→ Neurotomy of median (and ulnar) flexor branches
Isolated hand in pronation	→ Neurotomy of median branches
Isolated flexion of elbow	→ Neurotomy of musculocutaneous nerve Combined with orthopedic surgery, if needed

MDT = microsurgical DREZotomy.

the authors' experience.[50, 51] This personal experience is based on the use of spinal cord stimulation (in eight cases); intrathecal baclofen infusion (in 22 cases); selective peripheral neurotomy (in 210 cases); lumbosacral dorsal rhizotomy (in 15 cases); and microsurgical DREZotomy: cervical for hyperspasticity in the upper limb (in 42 cases), lumbosacral for hyperspasticity in the lower limbs (in 93 cases), and sacral for hyperactive neurogenic bladder (in 12 cases).[46, 50, 52] Following are the guidelines for surgery in adults with spasticity:

1) Spinal cord stimulation is useful for treating spasticity of spinal cord origin, such as multiple sclerosis or degenerative diseases (e.g., Strümpell-Lorrain syndrome), provided that the spasticity is mild and the dorsal columns are still valid.

2) Intrathecal baclofen administration is indicated for paraplegic or tetraplegic patients with severe and diffuse spasticity, especially that of spinal origin. Because of its reversibility, this method can be performed before an ablative procedure is considered. However, the range between an excess of hypotonia with loss of strength and an insufficient effect is very narrow.

3) Neuroablative techniques are indicated for severe spasticity that is localized to the limbs of paraplegic, tetraplegic, or hemiplegic patients. Neurotomies are preferred when spasticity is localized to muscle groups innervated by a small number of, or a single, peripheral nerve (or nerves). When spasticity affects an entire limb, microsurgical DREZotomy is preferred. We prefer to combine several types of neuroablative procedures in the treatment of one patient, when needed. Whatever the situation and the etiology may be, orthopedic surgery must be considered only after spasticity has been reduced by physical and pharmacologic treatments first and, when necessary, by neurosurgical procedures.

Guidelines for surgical indications have been detailed elsewhere[51] and are summarized in Tables 134–1, 134–2, and 134–3. The general rule is to tailor individual treatments as much as possible to the particular problems of the patient.

CHILDREN

Surgical indications for children with cerebral palsy depend on the preoperative abilities and disabilities (see functional score in Table 134–4, modified from Abbott's classification[53]) and the functional goals of postoperative physical therapy.

Symmetrical Diplegia

When diplegia is symmetrical, selective lumbosacral posterior rhizotomies should be performed. When correctly indicated, such procedures are able to alleviate spasticity in the lower limbs, and they also have favorable "distant" effects on upper limbs (see functional score in Table 134–5), muscle tone in the trunk, speech, and swallowing. Our preference is to perform a technique that mixes the sectorial and the functional rhizotomy methods, as illustrated in Figure 134–5.

Until now, we dared not operate on patients who walked independently. However, other teams do operate on this population to improve the efficiency and cosmesis in walking. For Abbott,[53] the intervention is best delivered soon after the child has demonstrated ability to work with a therapist, that is, between the ages of 3 and 7 years.

Patients who ambulate with the help of canes or crutches, rollators or walkers, or a person can be operated on to de-

Table 134–3. INDICATIONS FOR NEUROSURGERY IN TETRAPLEGIAS

Types of Spasticity	Operative Procedures
	Try
Spinal cord, brainstem, bihemispheric lesions	→ Spinal cord stimulation, if dorsal column: functional and test ⊕
	→ Intrathecal baclofen administration with programmable implanted pump, if test ⊕
	Before deciding
	→ Neuroablative procedures in lower and/or upper limbs
	→ Complementary orthopedic surgery, if needed

Table 134-4. FUNCTIONAL SCORE: LOWER LIMBS

Score	Function
0	Normal gait
I	Independent ambulator
IA	Without any orthosis
IB	With orthosis
II	Ambulator dependent on assistive devices
IIA	Canes/crutches
IIB	Rollator/walker
IIC	Person helping
III	Quadriped crawler
IV	Belly crawler
V	Unable to locomote

crease dependence on assistance, provided that there an obvious excess of hypertonia and good strength in the antigravity muscles are present. Surgery should be delayed in children who are developing locomotion and would need only temporarily assistive devices. Quadriped crawlers, bunny hoppers, and belly crawlers can benefit from a lumbosacral posterior rhizotomy for assisted ambulation and for improved stability in the sitting position, respectively.

In totally dependent children with no locomotive abilities, surgical indications are limited to improvement of comfort and care. If mobilization of hips is painful because of joint dislocation, a microsurgical DREZotomy, from L1 to L3, can be added to the sectorial-functional posterior rhizotomy.

Asymmetrical Spasticity

For children with asymmetrical spasticity, whatever the causal mechanisms may be, a justifiable goal, although limited, can be to make the gait or the postures symmetrical. Selective peripheral neurotomies can be used to achieve this goal, especially those of the obturator and tibial types, for the spastic hip and the spastic foot, respectively.

For upper limb spasticity, the microsurgical DREZotomy procedure or selective neurotomies corresponding to the flexion muscles of the wrist and fingers, or both, may be useful.

SUMMARY

The treatment of patients with severe spasticity is both a moving and potentially dangerous field. To adequately treat these patients, a multidisciplinary approach that allows rigorous methods of assessment along with great anatomic, physiologic, pharmacologic, and surgical expertise, is necessary. Such an approach can bring enormous benefit to the disabled person.

REFERENCES

1. Katz RT: Management of spasticity. Phys Med Rehabil 67:108–116, 1988
2. Lance JW: Pathophysiology of spasticity and clinical experience with baclofen, in Feldman RG, Young RR, Koella WP (eds): Spasticity Disordered Motor Control. Chicago, Year Book, 1980, pp 185–203
3. Sherrington C: The Integrative Action of the Nervous System. London, Archibald Constable, 1906
4. Wiesendanger M: Neurobiology of spasticity, in Emre M, Benecke R (eds): Spasticity: The Current Status of Research and Treatment. Carnforth Lancaster, Parthenon Publishing Group, 1989, pp 45–61
5. Wall PD: Presynaptic control of impulses at the first central synapse in the cutaneous pathway. Prog Brain Res 12:92–118, 1974
6. Cook AW, Weinstein SP: Chronic dorsal column stimulation in multiple sclerosis. NY State Med 73:2868–2872, 1973
7. Gybels J, Van Roost D: Spinal cord stimulation for spasticity. Advances and Technical Standards in Neurosurgery, vol 15. Wien, Springer-Verlag, 1987, pp 63–96
8. Siegfried J: Treatment of spasticity by dorsal cord stimulation. Int Rehabil Med 2:31–34, 1980
9. Siegfried J, Lazorthes Y: La neurochirurgie fonctionnelle de l'infirmité motrice d'origine cérébrale. Neurochirurgie 31 (suppl 1):1–118, 1985
10. Penn RD, Kroin JS: Continuous intrathecal baclofen for severe spasticity. Lancet 2:125–127, 1985
11. Decq PH, Keravel Y: Drug pump technical description, operative procedure and post-operative management, in Sindou M, Abbott R, Keravel Y (eds): Neurosurgery for Spasticity: A Multidisciplinary Approach. Wien-New York, Springer-Verlag, 1991, pp 97–101
12. Lazorthes Y, Sallerin-Caute B, Verdie JC, et al: Chronic intrathecal baclofen administration for control of severe spasticity. J Neurosurg 72:393–402, 1990
13. Stoffel A: The treatment of spastic contractures. Am J Orthop Surg 10:611–619, 1913
14. Gros C, Frerebeau P, Benezech J, Privat JM: Neurotomie ramiculaire sélective, in Simon L (ed): Actualités en Rééducation Fonctionnelle et Réadaptation. Paris, Masson, 2, 1977, pp 230–235
15. Sindou M, Mertens P: Selective neurotomy of the tibial nerve for treatment of the spastic foot. Neurosurgery 23:738–744, 1988
16. Foerster O: On the indications and results of the excision of posterior spinal nerve roots in men. Surg Gynecol Obstet 16:463–474, 1913
17. Gros C, Ouaknine G, Vlahovitch B, Frerebeau P: La radicotomie sélective postérieure dans le traitement neurochirurgical de l'hypertonie pyramidale. Neurochirurgie 13:505–518, 1967
18. Ouaknine G: Le traitement chirurgical de la spasticité. Union Med Can 109:1–11, 1980
19. Gros C: Spasticity: Clinical classification and surgical treatment. Advances and Technical Standards in Neurosurgery, vol 6. Wien, Springer-Verlag, 1979, pp 55–97
20. Privat JM, Benezech J, Frerebeau P, Gros C: Sectorial posterior rhizotomy. A new technique of surgical treatment of spasticity. Acta Neurochir (Wien) 35:181–195, 1976
21. Fraioli B, Guidetti B: Posterior partial rootlet section in the treatment of spasticity. J Neurosurg 46:618–626, 1977
22. Fasano VA, Barolat-Romana G, Ivaldi A, Sguazzi A: La radicotomie postérieure fonctionnelle dans le traitement de la spasticité cérébrale. Neurochirurgie 22:23–34, 1976
23. Peacock WJ, Arens LJ: Selective posterior rhizotomy for the relief of spasticity in cerebral palsy. S Afr Med J 62:119–124, 1982
24. Cahan LD, Kundi MS, McPherson D, et al: Electrophysiologic studies in selective dorsal rhizotomy for spasticity in children with cerebral palsy. Appl Neurophysiol 50:459–682, 1987
25. Abbott R, Forem SL, Johann M: Selective posterior rhizotomy for the treatment of spasticity. Childs Nerv Syst 5:337–346, 1989
26. Storrs B: Selective posterior rhizotomy for treatment of progressive spasticity in patients with myelomeningocele. Pediatr Neurosci 13:135–137, 1987

Table 135-5. FUNCTIONAL SCORE: UPPER LIMBS

Score	Function
0	Normal function
I	Handling small objects possible
IA	Easily
IB	With difficulty
II	Handling big objects possible
IIA	Easily
IIB	With difficulty
III	Blocking objects possible
IIIA	Easily
IIIB	With difficulty
IV	Global movements of upper limb possible but without real useful function
V	No significant voluntary movements

27. Uematsu S, Udvarhelyi GB, Benson DW, Siebens AA: Percutaneous radiofrequency rhizotomy. Surg Neurol 2:319–325, 1974
28. Young B, Mulcachy JJ: Percutaneous sacral rhizotomy for neurogenic detrusor hyperreflexia. J Neurosurg 53:85–87, 1980
29. Kenmore D: Radiofrequency neurotomy for peripheral pain and spasticity syndromes. Contemp Neurosurg 5:1–6, 1983
30. Herz DA, Parsons KC, Pearl L: Percutaneous radiofrequency foraminal rhizotomies. Spine 8:729–732, 1983
31. Kasdon DL, Lathi ES: A prospective study of radiofrequency rhizotomy in the treatment of post-traumatic spasticity. Neurosurgery 15:526–529, 1984
32. Dogliotti A: Traitement des syndromes douloureux de la périphérie par l'alcoolisation sous-arachnoïdienne des racines postérieures à leur émergence de la moelle épinière. Presse Med 39:1249–1252, 1931
33. Guttman L: The treatment and rehabilitation of patients with injuries of the spinal cord, in History of the Second World War: Her Majesty's Stationery Office, vol Surgery. 1953, pp 422–516
34. Maher R: Relief of pain in incurable cancer. Lancet i:18–20, 1955
35. Nathan PW: Intrathecal phenol to relieve spasticity in paraplegia. Lancet ii:1099–1102, 1959
36. Kelly RE, Gauthier-Smith PC: Intrathecal phenol in the treatment of reflex spasms and spasticity. Lancet ii:1102–1105, 1959
37. Bischof W: Die longitudinale Myelotomie. Zentralbl Neurochir 2:79–88, 1951
38. Pourpre MH: Traitement neurochirurgical des contractures chez les paraplégiques post-traumatiques. Neurochirurgie 6:229–236, 1960
39. Laitinen LV, Singounas E: Longitudinal myelotomy in the treatment of spasticity of the legs. J Neurosurg 35:536–540, 1971
40. Sindou M: Etude de la Jonction Radiculo-Medullaire postérieure: La Radicellotomie Postérieure Sélective dans la Chirurgie de la Douleur. Medical Thesis, Lyon, 1972
41. Sindou M, Fischer G, Goutelle A, et al: La radicellotomie postérieure sélective dans le traitement des spasticités. Rev Neurol 130:201–215, 1974
42. Sindou M, Millet MF, Mortamais J, Eyssette M: Results of selective posterior rhizotomy in the treatment of painful and spastic paraplegia secondary to multiple sclerosis. Appl Neurophysiol 45:335–340, 1982
43. Sindou M, Pregelj R, Boisson D, et al: Surgical selective lesions of nerve fibers and myelotomies for the modification of muscle hypertonia, in Eccles J, Dimitrijevic MR (eds): Recent Achievements in Restorative Neurology: Upper Motor Neuron Functions and Dysfunctions. Basel, S Karger, 1985, pp 10–26
44. Sindou M, Abdennebi B, Sharkey P: Microsurgical selective procedures in the peripheral nerves and the posterior root-spinal cord junction for spasticity. Appl Neurophysiol 48:97–104, 1985
45. Eccles J, Eccles R, Magni F: Central inhibitory action attributable to presynaptic depolarization produced by muscle afferent volleys. J Physiol 159:147–166, 1961
46. Sindou M, Jeanmonod D, Mertens P: Surgery in the dorsal root entry zone: Microsurgical DREZotomy (MDT) for the treatment of spasticity, in Sindou M, Abbott R, Keravel Y (eds): Neurosurgery for Spasticity: A Multidisciplinary Approach. Wien-New York, Springer-Verlag, 1991, pp 165–182
47. Sindou M, Jeanmonod D: Microsurgical-DREZ-otomy for the treatment of spasticity and pain in the lower limbs. Neurosurgery 24:655–670, 1989
48. Sindou M, Mifsud JJ, Boisson D, Goutelle A: Selective posterior rhizotomy in the dorsal root entry zone for treatment of hyperspasticity and pain in the hemiplegic upper limb. Neurosurgery 18:587–595, 1986
49. Beneton C, Mertens P, Leriche A, Sindou M: The spastic bladder and its treatment, in Sindou M, Abbott R, and Keravel Y (eds): Neurosurgery for Spasticity: A Multidisciplinary Approach. Wien-New York, Springer-Verlag, 1991, pp 193–199
50. Sindou M, and Mertens P: Indication for surgery to treat adults with harmful spasticity, in Sindou M, Abbott R, Keravel Y (eds): Neurosurgery for Spasticity: A multidisciplinary approach. Wien-New York, Springer-Verlag, 1991, pp 211–213
51. Sindou M, Abbott R, Keravel Y: Neurosurgery for Spasticity: A Multidisciplinary Approach. Wien-New York, Springer-Verlag, 1991
52. Mertens P, Sindou M: Selective peripheral neurotomies for the treatment of spasticity, in Sindou M, Abbott R, Keravel Y (eds): Neurosurgery for Spasticity: A Multidisciplinary Approach. Wien-New York, Springer-Verlag, 1991, pp 119–132
53. Abbott R: Indications for surgery to treat children with spasticity due to cerebral palsy, in Sindou M, Abbott R, Keravel Y (eds): Neurosurgery for Spasticity: A Multidisciplinary Approach. Wien-New York, Springer-Verlag, 1991, pp 215–217

SECTION XVIII

Infections

CHAPTER 135

Surgical Management of Intracranial and Intraspinal Infections

R. Lewis Wright

*I*n this chapter, we consider bacterial infections of the nervous system that may require neurosurgical treatment for the control of infection or to relieve pressure on portions of the nervous system caused by the infection. These infections are mostly blood borne, but they can at times occur by direct spread from nearby infections or as a result of a surgical procedure. They are of vital importance, however, because many cases are not diagnosed until irreparable damage to the nervous system or death has occurred (Fig. 135–1). The chance of recovery is highly dependent on the degree of damage to the nervous system that has taken place before diagnosis and treatment. Patients diagnosed early in the evolution of their disease and treated promptly have the best chance of recovery. A high index of suspicion on the part of the physician treating patients with possible intracranial and intraspinal infections remains of paramount importance. Infections of the central nervous system that occur in HIV-positive patients will be discussed elsewhere in this series.

OSTEOMYELITIS OF THE SKULL

Infection of the cranial bones occasionally can spread from infections in remote areas of the body via the bloodstream. More commonly, however, the infection develops from direct spread of bacteria to devitalized areas of bone.[1] It is most often seen as an infectious complication after craniotomy or after the insertion of tongs for skeletal traction in the reduction of cervical fracture dislocations. It also can originate from infections in the adjacent paranasal sinuses or in the middle ear or can follow penetrating injuries of the cranium. *Staphylococcus aureus* is the organism most often cultured from patients with osteomyelitis of the skull. Other bacteria, either alone or in combination, can be causative organisms. Headache may vary considerably in patients with this condition, but swelling and local tenderness of the scalp usually are seen. Fever also may vary. Destruction of bone, as demonstrated on x-ray films, may not appear for up to 2 weeks after the clinical process begins. CT and MRI techniques for bone detail are useful in depicting the extent of infection.

Once osteomyelitis is diagnosed, treatment usually consists of craniectomy for removal of the infected bone and eradication of any adjacent infections in the paranasal sinuses, the middle ear, or extensions into the extradural space.

Antibiotics, whose effectiveness is determined by laboratory testing for culture and sensitivity studies, should be continued for at least 3 to 4 weeks after all evidence of active infection has subsided. External drainage for several days postoperatively is recommended. Many of these patients require subsequent cranioplasty for protection of the brain or for cosmetic purposes. This procedure should be delayed

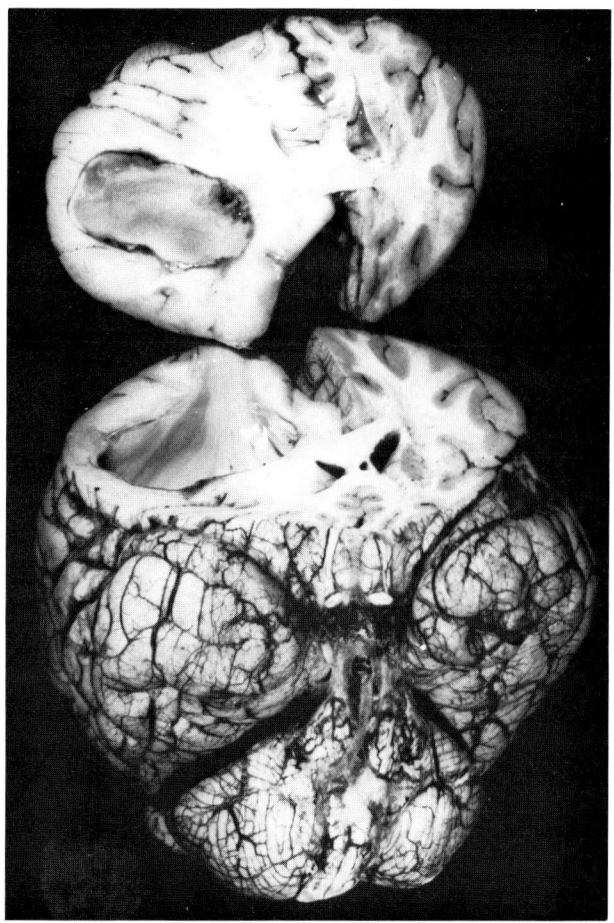

FIGURE 135–1. A postmortem photograph showing a fatal undiagnosed frontal lobe abscess. Death was caused by temporal lobe herniation.

several months to lessen the chance of recurrent infection around the implanted plastic or metal plates.

Theoretically, small areas of osteomyelitis of the skull might be treated medically with antibiotics, close clinical observation, and serial studies to document resolution and healing of the infectious process. To date, clinical experience with such cases is too scant for accurate evaluation of the effectiveness of medical treatment alone.

INTRACRANIAL EXTRADURAL ABSCESS

Intracranial extradural abscesses arise by direct spread from adjacent infections to the extradural space in patients with paranasal sinusitis, middle ear infections, and osteomyelitis of the skull.[1] These patients have fever and headache as initial complaints. As the lesion increases in size and intracranial pressure increases, lethargy occurs. In untreated patients, the infectious process can result in intradural extension with meningitis, subdural abscess, brain abscess, or thrombosis of intracranial venous sinuses.

Clinical history and x-ray films of the skull and sinuses are important in the diagnostic evaluation of these patients. CT and MRI scans show the dura and brain displaced away from the skull at the site of abscess formation. This area usually is adjacent to the site of infection in the paranasal sinuses or the middle ear.

Treatment consists of craniectomy and removal of the infectious material from the dura. External drainage for several days is warranted, and, once again, antibiotics should be continued for 3 to 4 weeks after all clinical evidence of infection has cleared.

INTRACRANIAL SUBDURAL ABSCESS

Like extradural intracranial abscesses, those in the subdural space usually arise as complications of nearby infections in the paranasal sinuses and the middle ear.[2-5] Many abscesses in patients with frontal sinusitis have spread intracranially by the venous route as thrombophlebitis. About ninety percent are supratentorial in location. Less often, they follow penetrating wounds or operative procedures. Headache, fever, and neck stiffness occur early in these patients. Seizures, principally of the focal type, are common. Many patients with subdural abscesses deteriorate rapidly over a period of hours or a few days. Profound neurologic deficit and death can occur rapidly as the process evolves. Thrombosis of underlying cortical veins can occur, but meningitis rarely complicates this infection.

This lesion usually is well demonstrated on CT or MRI scans (Fig. 135–2). Before the advent of these techniques, nuclear scans were often accurate in diagnosing the lesion, and angiograms with oblique views, if necessary, would show the subdural abscess.

The only method of treating such lesions is craniectomy or craniotomy and removal of the contents of the abscess. Heavy encapsulation does not occur, and at times portions of the thin-walled capsule must be left adhering to vital areas of the cerebral cortex. All infectious material, whether purulent or granulation tissue, should be surgically removed. Intracranial subdural abscesses are often multiloculated, and at surgery, care should be taken to make sure all pockets are drained, which can be confirmed by serial scans performed every few days. External drainage of the wound for a few days is wise. Once again, appropriate antibiotics should be continued systemically for 3 to 4 weeks.

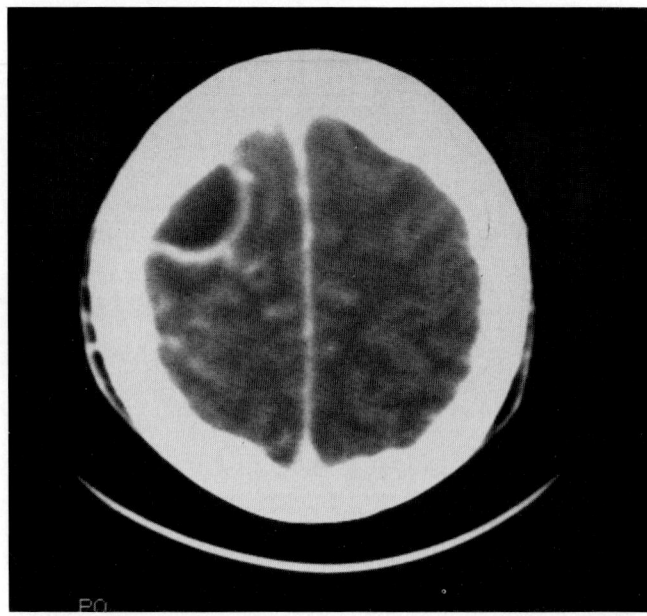

FIGURE 135–2. A CT scan demonstrating a large subdural abscess that extended from frontal sinusitis.

ABSCESS OF THE BRAIN

Brain abscesses are perhaps less common now than formerly because infections throughout the body are commonly treated with antibiotics at an early stage. There is no history of infection in one-fifth of cases.

Healthy brain tissue has long been known to be resistant to the growth of bacteria. Experimental direct inoculation of the brain with pyogenic organisms has only rarely led to abscess formation. Necrotic tissue from infarction or trauma and dead spaces left after intracranial operations have seemed to favor abscess formation.

Clinically, brain abscesses have arisen most often from septic hematogenous emboli from distant infections (particularly pulmonary infections), from adjacent foci of infection in the paranasal sinuses and the middle ear, or as complications of intracranial surgery.[6-11] Streptococci have been the organisms most often associated with brain abscess, although *S. aureus,* coliform bacilli, diphtheroids, and mixed organisms are seen.

In most patients with brain abscess, the early signs and symptoms are those of any lesion causing increased intracranial pressure: headache, somnolence, nausea, and vomiting. Seizures are common. With involvement of appropriate areas of the brain, hemiparesis, aphasia, or visual field defects may be encountered. Fever is usually absent. When the abscess arises from a septic hematogenous embolus, the abscess may develop in any one or a series of multiple sites, although these most often occur within the distribution of the middle cerebral artery and its branches. When the parent infection is

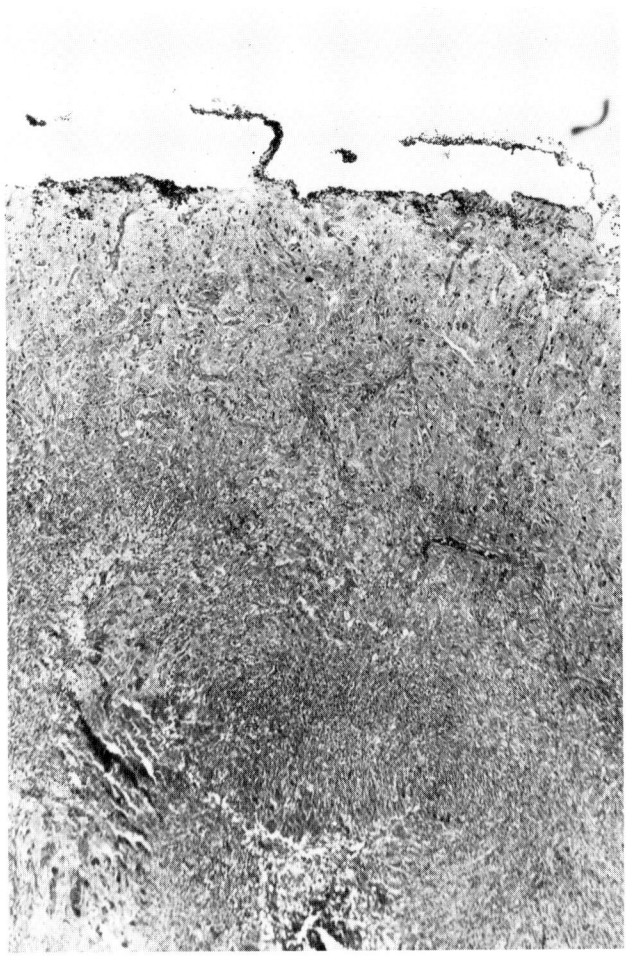

FIGURE 135-3. A photomicrograph of the wall of a brain abscess. The central area of degenerating white blood cells is surrounded by a capsule consisting of reactive astrocytes and compressed brain tissue. (Magnification: × 50.)

otogenic or in the paranasal sinuses, the brain abscess is usually nearby, having spread by direct extension intracranially or by septic thrombophlebitis. Hence, infections of the middle ear or mastoid giving rise to a brain abscess usually produce this lesion in the temporal lobe or occasionally in the cerebellum. Infections of the frontal, ethmoid, and sphenoid sinuses that produce brain abscesses usually do so in the adjacent portion of the frontal lobe.

In its early stages, a brain abscess is characterized by cerebral softening, vascular congestion, and an adjacent margin of petechial hemorrhages. Within a few days, the central portion undergoes a process of liquefaction, and a capsule begins to form. As additional time passes, the capsule wall increases in thickness. The inner layer of the abscess wall is composed of degenerating neutrophils, plasma cells, and lymphocytes enmeshed in fibrin. The outer layer is composed of compressed brain tissue and reactive astrocytes (Fig. 135-3). Edema of the surrounding brain often is marked. If untreated, most patients with brain abscesses die of increased intracranial pressure with fatal herniation of the medial temporal lobe or the cerebellar tonsils; less commonly, death is caused by rupture of the abscess and fulminating meningitis.

Alertness to the possibility of this diagnosis on the part of the attending physician has long been emphasized as an important factor in the early diagnosis of brain abscesses. Routine x-ray films of the skull can be normal or can show a significant shift of a calcified pineal gland. Sinus infections can be visualized on x-ray films. An electroencephalogram usually shows a delta focus when the abscess is superficial in location. In past years, nuclear brain scans and angiograms have shown the mass lesion in most cases, but usually these have been indistinguishable from avascular tumors or hematomas.

Modern CT and MRI scanning techniques have increased our understanding of the development of brain abscesses.[12, 13] In the early stages, a mottled area of enhancement representing the area of cerebritis is seen. With subsequent liquefaction and formation of the capsule or wall, the scan shows a ring-shaped lesion on enhancement with a central lucent area representing the area of liquefaction (Fig. 135-4). Moreover, scans provide data about the size, location, and age of the abscess and the presence of multiple abscesses.

In most cases of brain abscess surgery is required for adequate treatment. In the past, medical treatment alone of brain abscesses was condemned by many surgeons. Monitored by scans, a few successful cures by medical treatment alone have been recorded. This method should probably be limited to small, developing abscesses in which a wall has not formed and to abscesses inaccessible to surgical treatment (e.g., abscesses located in basal ganglia, and multiple small abscesses). Such patients should be followed closely with careful neurologic assessment and serial scans as appropriate drugs are administered. Antibiotics should be continued for at least 3 to 4 weeks in this group.

In a patient with a recent history of infection and findings on clinical examination and scans compatible with brain abscess, antibiotic therapy should be started promptly. Wide-

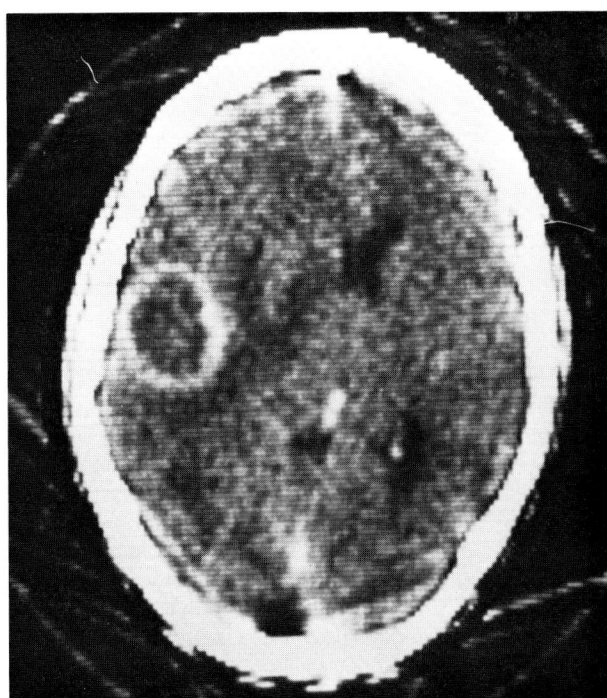

FIGURE 135-4. A CT scan of a temporoparietal abscess showing the characteristic zone of ring enhancement.

spread antibiotic coverage with agents that cross the blood-brain barrier should be used. If the organism from the parent infection is known or when cultures taken at surgery for the abscess become available, this combination may need to be modified. Edema surrounding the abscess often is marked, and the use of steroids to control cerebral edema in these patients has been of great value. When appropriate antibiotic agents are administered, the use of steroids in this situation has not led to spread of infection. Administration of corticosteroids may lead to decreased enhancement of the periphery of the abscess (the so-called ring pattern) in scans. This must not be misinterpreted as a decrease in size of the lesion.

Although the relative merits of removal versus drainage of abscesses have been debated for decades, for large encapsulated brain abscesses, surgical removal is the treatment of choice provided the lesion is in an area amenable to total removal. Brain abscesses displace the brain tissue to a marked degree, but often little brain tissue is actually destroyed. Hence, many of the neurologic defects produced by abscesses are reversible.

At craniotomy, the abscess is first aspirated as completely as possible. Large abscesses often must be opened as well to remove the contents and thereby decrease their size. The wall of the abscess then is gently dissected from adjacent white matter of the brain by use of small cottonoid patties to establish the plane between these two tissues. Gentle traction on the wall of the abscess facilitates its removal (Fig. 135–5). In large abscesses, removal of the wall is performed in a piecemeal manner, but in smaller abscesses, removal in toto may be possible. In certain situations, such as abscesses in the region of the basal ganglia and internal capsule and multiple small abscesses, simple drainage may be better treatment, and the wall of the abscess is left intact. External drainage of brain abscesses that are operated on is not necessary unless the abscess wall has been left in place. The bone flap can be replaced in these patients unless intractable cerebral edema is present. Antibiotic coverage should continue for at least 3 to 4 weeks. In patients in whom the wall or capsule of the abscess has been left intact and only simple drainage has been carried out, serial scans should be obtained. CT guided stereotactic techniques, developed in recent years, have proved useful for aspiration of small deep seated abscesses and in cases of multiple abscess formation.

SPINAL EXTRADURAL ABSCESS

Abscesses of the spinal extradural space can result from septic emboli to the extradural fat, from spread from paravertebral infections in the mediastinum or retroperitoneal space via an intervertebral foramen, or from direct extension from osteomyelitis of the spine.[14–18] Rarely, they have arisen from penetrating injuries or as complications of surgery or lumbar puncture. In recent years intravenous drug users have been identified as a group at risk for developing these infections.

Initial symptoms are local backache near the infection and the presence of fever. Involvement of adjacent nerve roots may give rise to radicular pain. Because compression of the spinal cord or cauda equina occurs, sensory and motor loss result distal to the site of compression and impairment of sphincter control develops. This process may extend over one or several vertebral segments. Rarely, the infection has extended through the entire length of the spine from the sacral to the upper cervical levels. The fact that extradural abscesses were usually dorsal to the spinal dura was first pointed out by Dandy (Fig. 135–6).[16] Perhaps as many as three-fourths are situated posteriorly in the spinal canal. Extradural fat and the extradural space are greater dorsally than either laterally or ventrally within the spinal canal.

S. aureus is the organism most often responsible for these lesions, although *Streptococcus, Pseudomonas,* and typhoid bacilli may be the causative organisms. Fungus granulomas of the extradural space also can occur; in North America, actinomycosis and blastomycosis are occasionally encountered.

In some patients, deterioration occurs quickly, within a matter of hours or a few days. In others, the disease has a prolonged course, with the clinical picture extending over a period of days or weeks. The reason for such variability is not known. Fever and leukocytosis are often absent in this latter group. Whether progression is acute or prolonged, one fact is clear; the earlier surgical decompression is carried out, the better the outlook for neurologic recovery. The cauda equina withstands pressure from abscesses as well as other mass lesions better than the spinal cord itself.

Patients suspected of having spinal extradural abscesses should undergo a careful clinical evaluation with a detailed history and general and neurologic examinations. Spinal x-ray films are indicated but are often normal, unless paravertebral abscesses or adjacent osteomyelitic areas are demonstrated. In most instances, MRI scans will identify the location and extent of the lesion. If there is some doubt, myelogram might be useful.

Surgery is necessary in almost all patients. Prompt decompressive laminectomy and removal of the abscess should be carried out. It is of vital importance that the laminectomy extend over the entire length of the abscess if good recovery is to be expected. In acute abscesses, frankly purulent material is encountered. Costotransversectomy or an anterior approach should be used in instances in which the abscess is anterior to the spinal cord. In the chronic form, only granulation tissue, which might be mistaken for a metastatic neoplasm, is found. Removal of either of these is usually possible; bacterial smears and cultures should be obtained. If acute purulence is encountered, external drainage of the wound should be performed for several days. Rarely very small abscesses in patients without significant neurological deficit have been successfully treated with antibiotics only.[19]

If an extradural abscess is suspected preoperatively, antibiotics should be begun before surgery. A choice of appropriate antibiotic is made on the basis of the antecedent infectious process. Some of the infectious chronic granulomas show no growth on culture.

SPINAL SUBDURAL ABSCESS

Abscesses of the spinal subdural space are uncommon, and most occur as extensions of infection in patients with midline congenital dermal sinuses; rarely, blood-borne cases are encountered. Local back and radicular pain may be present or absent. As the lesion increases in size, symptoms and signs of compression of the cauda equina or spinal cord ensue. With leakage into the spinal subarachnoid space, meningitis may develop.

MRI scans or a myelogram, or both, will usually outline

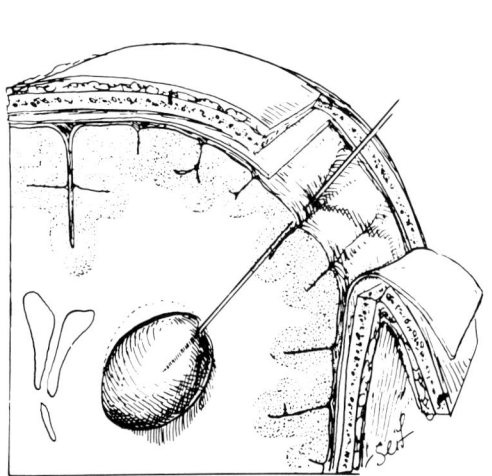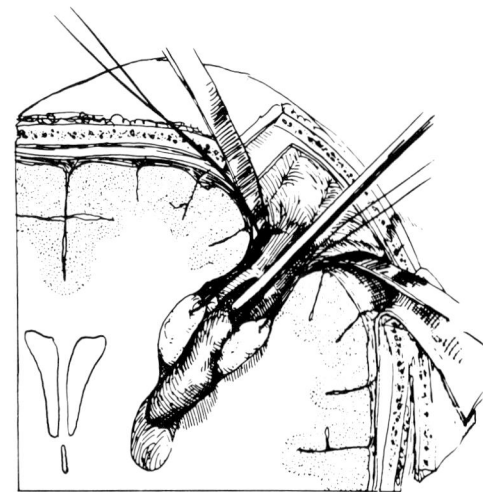

FIGURE 135–5. Technique for removing a brain abscess. Total removal can often be accomplished without resection of significant portions of the brain.

the extent. Laminectomy should extend over the length of the lesion, and external drainage should be employed for several days. The dura is probably best left open to ensure that maximal decompression is achieved. These abscesses probably never form a heavy wall or capsule. Appropriate antibiotic coverage should continue for a period of several weeks.

SPINAL INTRAMEDULLARY ABSCESS

Abscesses within the spinal cord itself are rare. These can arise via septic emboli or through penetrating injuries.[20] In the small number of cases reported, various organisms have been cultured. Progressive sensory and motor loss are the clinical picture, and pain is often absent. Systemic signs of sepsis, fever, and leukocytosis may be absent. MRI scans and myelogram will usually show a partial or complete block with evidence of widening of the spinal cord shadow. Decompression over the length of the process should be performed promptly, and aspiration with a fine needle should be performed for maximal decompression and to obtain cultures. True encapsulation of these abscesses is unlikely to occur. Once again, steroids to combat swelling and antibiotics for long periods are indicated.

OSTEOMYELITIS OF THE SPINE

Infections of the vertebral column can occur with pyogenic organisms, tuberculosis (Pott's disease), or fungi (especially actinomycosis and blastomycosis). These organisms most often reach this site via the hematogenous route. Among the pyogenic bacteria, *S. aureus* and coliform bacilli are commonest. Most cases of osteomyelitis do not concern the neurosurgeon. Compromise of the spinal cord can occur when an associated extradural abscess develops or when a bony deformity from a combined process of vertebral collapse with adjacent overgrown bone compromises the spinal canal (the so-called gibbus formation). Rarely, operative procedures on the spine can result in osteomyelitis.

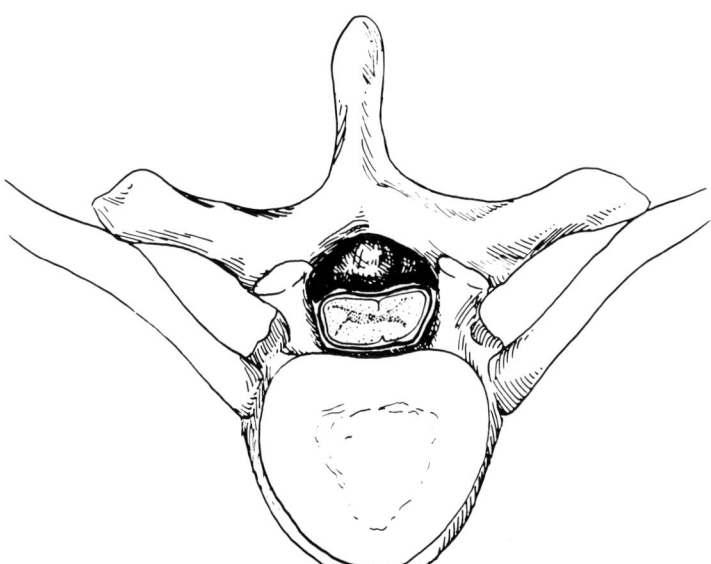

FIGURE 135–6. Most spinal extradural abscesses are characteristically located dorsal to the spinal cord.

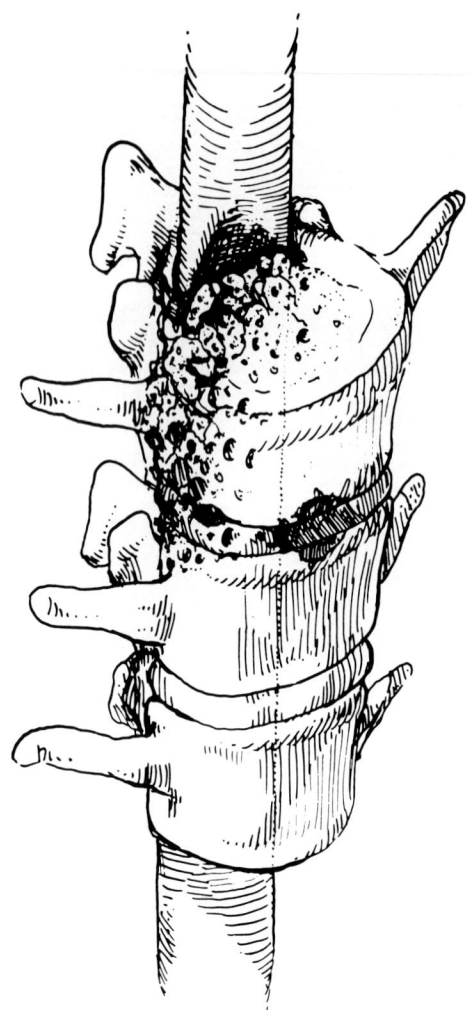

FIGURE 135-7. Osteomyelitis of the spine characteristically involves several vertebral bodies and intervening discs.

sion here, costotransversectomy (removal of bone via an oblique posterior approach, including the transverse processes, pedicles, and the involved portion of the diseased vertebral bodies) is the procedure of choice (Fig. 135-8). Anterior operations are probably best for the rare cases in which the patient has progressive paralysis from osteomyelitis of the cervical spine, and retroperitoneal bone removal can be used for the rare cases in which the patient needs lumbar decompression for gibbus formation secondary to infection in this lower area of the spine. When spinal instability is present, long-term immobilization by casts, halo devices, or braces must be provided. Antibiotics in cases of osteomyelitis should be given intravenously for a period of 4 to 6 weeks.

Many patients with mild neurologic signs of spinal cord compression associated with tuberculosis of the spine improve on a program of rest and antituberculous drugs and do not require surgery. The neurologic findings in this group must be followed up carefully.

Spinal cord symptoms can occasionally occur in infectious diseases of the spine without compression of the cord itself. These cases are caused by vascular thrombosis secondary to the inflammatory process. It is of great importance to differentiate these patients from patients with compression of the cord by the tests previously mentioned, because surgical de-

The initial complaint is back pain, usually accompanied by local tenderness and muscle spasm. Fever and leukocytosis are common.

The earliest changes are seen on lateral x-ray films of the spine; tomograms may be helpful at times. The characteristic radiographic sign is erosion of several contiguous vertebral bodies with collapse and involvement of the associated discs (Fig. 135-7). Characteristically, and for reasons unknown, metastatic tumors spare the intervertebral discs. Bone scan results are usually positive at the site of infection, and the alkaline phosphatase level is elevated in most cases.

When compression of the spinal cord occurs, a clinical history, neurologic examination, and x-ray studies are all-important in determining the cause. Narrowing of the spinal canal by vertebral collapse or gibbus formation is assessed by tomography and by scanning. In the absence of spinal stenosis in patients with osteomyelitis of the spine, an extradural abscess or granuloma is the likely cause and should be treated by the aforementioned techniques. MRI scans and at times myelogram are of utility in delineation of the process prior to surgery.

The thoracic area of the spine is most often the site of osteomyelitis. With progressive symptoms of cord compres-

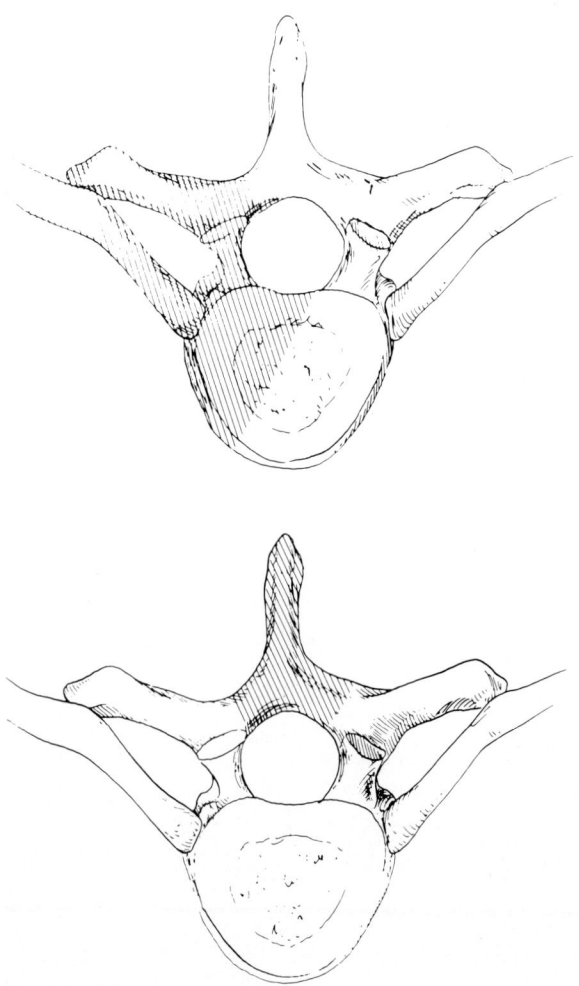

FIGURE 135-8. Areas (shaded) of bone removal in costotransversectomy (above) and laminectomy (below).

compression of the spinal cord will not benefit this group of patients.

SUMMARY

Although relatively uncommon now, infectious lesions causing dysfunction of the brain and spinal cord are neurologically devastating and sometimes fatal if they remain undetected and untreated. There is no substitute for prompt diagnosis and treatment. Modern techniques of CT and MRI scanning have made diagnosis possible at an early stage in most patients.

Proper postoperative care in all these patients may include the use of steroids when necessary to control swelling and appropriate antibiotic drugs for a prolonged period to ensure eradication of all bacteria. General supportive care, including physical therapy, is also of paramount importance.

REFERENCES

1. Woodhall B: Osteomyelitis and epi-, extra-, and subdural abscesses. Clin Neurosurg 14:239, 1966
2. Bhandari Y, Sarkari NS: Subdural empyema: A review of 37 cases. J Neurosurg 32:35, 1970
3. LeBeau J, Creissard P, Harispe L, et al: Surgical treatment of brain abscess and subdural empyema. J Neurosurg 38:198, 1973
4. Bannister G, Williams B, Smith S: Treatment of subdural empyema. J Neurosurg 55:82, 1981
5. Helfgott DC, Weingarten, K, Hartman BJ: Subdural empyema, in Scheld, Whitley, Durack (ed): Infections of the Central Nervous System. New York, Raven Press, 1991, pp 487–498
6. Ballantine HT Jr, Shealy CN: The role of radical surgery in the treatment of abscess of the brain. Surg Gynecol Obstet 109:370, 1959
7. LeBeau J: Radical surgery and penicillin in brain abscess: A method of treatment in one state with special reference to the cure of three thoracogenic cases. J Neurosurg 3:359, 1946
8. Morgan H, Wood MR, Murphey F: Experience with 88 consecutive cases of brain abscess. J Neurosurg 38:698, 1973
9. Wright RL, Ballantine HT Jr: Management of brain abscesses in children and adolescents. Am J Dis Child 114:113, 1967
10. Choudbury AR, Taylor JC, Whitaker R: Primary excision of brain abscess. Br Med J 2:1119, 1977
11. Wispelwey B, Dacey RG, Scheld WM: Brain abscess, in Scheld, Whitley, Durack (ed): Infections of the Central Nervous System. New York, Raven Press, 1991, pp 457–486
12. Britt RH, Enzmann DR: Clinical stages of human brain abscesses on serial CT scans after contrast infusion: CT, neuropathological, and clinical correlations. J Neurosurg 59:972, 1983
13. Zimmerman R: Imaging of intracranial infections, in Scheld, Whitley, Durack (ed): Infections of the Central Nervous System. New York, Raven Press, 1991, pp 887–907
14. Dandy WE: Abscesses and inflammatory tumors in the spine extradural space (so-called pachymeningitis externa). Arch Surg 13:447, 1926
15. Heusner AP: Nontuberculous spinal epidural infections. N Engl J Med 239:845, 1948
16. Gellin BG, Weingarten K, Gamache FW, Hartman BJ: Epidural abscess, in Scheld, Whitley, Durack (ed): Infections of the Central Nervous System. New York, Raven Press, 1991, pp 499–514
17. Hlavin ML, Kaminski HJ, Ross JS, Ganz E: Spinal epidural abscess: A ten-year perspective. Neurosurgery 27:177, 1990
18. Nussbaum ES, Rigamonti D, Standiford H, et al: Spinal epidural abscess: A report of 40 cases and review. Surg Neurol 38:225, 1992
19. Hanigan WC, Asner NG, Elwood PW: Magnetic resonance imaging and the nonoperative treatment of spinal epidural abscess. Surg Neurol 34:408, 1990
20. Wright RL: Intramedullary spinal cord abscess. J Neurosurg 23:208, 1965

CHAPTER 136

The Neurosurgical Management of HIV-Related Brain Lesions

E. T. Chappell
B. L. Guthrie

EPIDEMIOLOGY

The Centers for Disease Control and Prevention currently reports that approximately one million people in the United States are immunopositive for the human immunodeficiency virus (HIV). To date, 240,146 cases of acquired immunodeficiency syndrome (AIDS) have been reported, and only about 81,000 of those people are still alive.[1] Central nervous system (CNS) symptoms occur in 30 to 50 percent of AIDS cases, and as many as 90 percent have evidence of CNS disease at autopsy.[2-4] About 10 percent of AIDS patients have focal CNS lesions that might serve as a target for a stereotactic biopsy.[2,5] One-third of these patients will not have had prior manifestations of AIDS at the time they are referred for biopsy.

Intracranial disease is second only to pulmonary disease as a cause of morbidity and mortality in AIDS patients.[6] Of the approximately 10 percent of patients with focal lesions in the brain, 30 to 70 percent have *Toxoplasma gondii* abscesses, and another 15 to 30 percent have primary or metastatic CNS lymphoma.[2,5-9] The remaining 20 percent include a myriad of bacterial (e.g., *Listeria*, *Escherichia coli*), fungal (e.g., *Cryptococcus*, *Aspergillus*), and viral (e.g., HIV, herpes, cytomegalovirus) processes that can present as focal lesions on computed tomography (CT) or magnetic resonance imaging (MRI) of the brain.[2,5,9] Even the often diffuse virus-related process of progressive multifocal leukoencephalopathy frequently presents as a focal lesion.[8,9] Moreover, HIV-positive patients are also apparently susceptible to the same diseases as the HIV-negative population and therefore can have the usual primary and secondary brain tumors,[2,4,8] as well as the vascular (hemorrhage and infarction) lesions that occur in the brains of AIDS patients, and the 4 to 20 percent of biopsies from which no definite diagnosis can be made. A comprehensive list of causes of focal brain lesions in HIV-positive patients is provided in Table 136-1. Furthermore, a small percentage of AIDS patients have multiple CNS lesions of more than one etiology.[5]

PATIENT CONSIDERATIONS

Despite incubation periods of up to, and possibly greater than, 10 years as well as recent advances in treatment, AIDS remains an imminently fatal disease.[10-13] Nonetheless, potentially effective therapies exist for about 90 percent of the identifiable causes of CNS disease in AIDS patients.[2] This fact suggests the utility of brain biopsy in the diagnosis and treatment of AIDS patients with focal brain disease. Stereotactic biopsy is diagnostic in up to 96 percent of AIDS cases.[7] This and the fact that virtually all treatable AIDS-related focal brain lesions do not require resection eliminate any need for an open procedure, except in rare cases of impend-

Table 136–1. ETIOLOGIES OF FOCAL CEREBRAL LESIONS IN HIV-POSITIVE PATIENTS

Infectious
Parasites
Toxoplasma gondii
Cysticercosis
Fungi
Cryptococcus
Candida
Histoplasma
Coccidioides
Aspergillus
Mucor
Mycobacteria
Bacteria
Escherichia coli
Listeria
Nocardia
Salmonella
Spirochetes
Viruses
Cytomegalovirus
Herpes viruses
Varicella zoster
Papovavirus
Noninfectious
Neoplastic
Lymphoma (primary and secondary)
Kaposi's sarcoma
Glioma
Metastatic carcinoma
Other*
Vascular
Infarcts
Hemorrhage
Nondiagnostic

Modified from Levy and coworkers.[5]
HIV = human immunodeficiency virus.
*There is no reason to believe that HIV-positive patients are not susceptible to the same neoplastic brain diseases as the rest of the population.

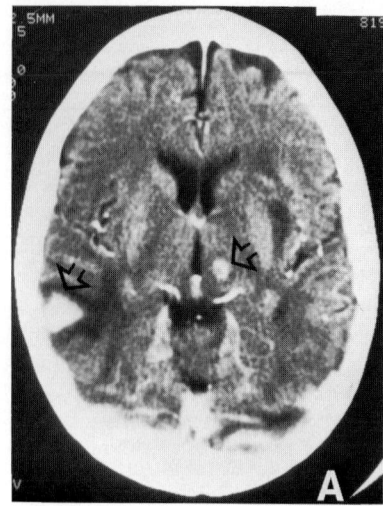 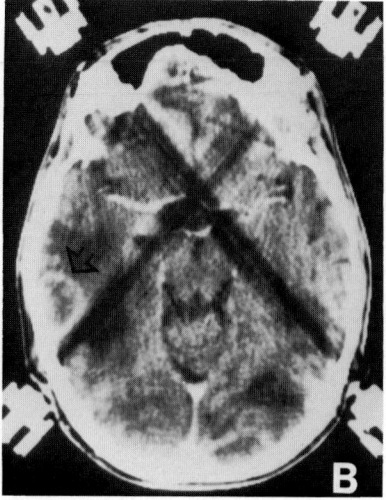

FIGURE 136–1. Contrast-enhanced CT of a 24-year-old male with AIDS. (A) These lesions (arrows) improved and then stabilized after 1 year of antitoxoplasmosis therapy. (B) After a recurrence of his symptoms 1 year later, the patient had this scan revealing a new enhancing mass on the left. Biopsies of these lesions determined that those on the right were toxoplasmosis, as expected, and the lesions on the left were determined to be lymphoma.

ing herniation due to mass effect. Furthermore, stereotactic biopsy is a low-risk procedure,[9] even in severely medically compromised patients (like many of those with AIDS), because it can usually be performed with the patient under local anesthesia.[8] In most cases, a need for definitive diagnosis and low risk to the patient are persuasive factors in the decision to undertake an invasive diagnostic procedure. On the other hand, the communicable and fatal nature of the HIV virus greatly compounds this issue and raises the questions of risk to those performing the procedure and whether or not accurate diagnosis and treatment have an effect on outcome. Questions such as these have inherent ethical overtones, but some, possibly tenuous, scientific data on these issues are available to help in the decision-making process.

RISK TO SURGEONS OPERATING ON HIV-POSITIVE PATIENTS

Solid data regarding the risk to surgeons who operate on patients who are HIV positive will never be available for several reasons. First, there is no way to be absolutely certain what other risk factors a given surgeon who contracts the virus might have and no way to be certain what operating mishaps, if any, can lead to transmission of the virus. In addition, more controversial issues, like privacy, have an effect on the reporting of such data. Notwithstanding these issues, a few relatively scientific attempts at quantifying the risk of seroconversion (becoming HIV positive) in surgeons have been reported.[14, 15] Schiff, for example, formulated a mathematical model for estimating a given surgeon's cumulative lifetime risk.[14] The model accounts for seroprevalence in the patient population; the inoculation rate, roughly based on surgical subspecialty; and the estimated probability of infection for a given procedural mishap. One survey estimated a greater than 6-percent 30-year risk in the 10 percent of surgeons considered at highest risk.[15] Even if estimates of a surgeon's risk of contracting HIV are of questionable accuracy, existing evidence raises the possibility of some risk, and any risk of contracting a fatal disease must be considered.

PREOPERATIVE EVALUATION

RADIOGRAPHIC

Accurate diagnosis and effective therapy for focal cerebral lesions in HIV-positive patients may not alter the eventual outcome; given even the slightest risk of disease transmission during an invasive procedure, the question arises as to whether the diagnosis can be made noninvasively. Although radiologists have reported an ability to make some diagnoses confidently on routine neuroimaging studies (CT and MRI), the consensus is that the definitive diagnosis must be made from pathology studies.[16–22] Dina, for example, found that if a mass in the brain of an HIV-positive patient enhanced, was unifocal, exhibited subependymal spread on CT or MRI, and was hyperdense on CT without contrast, it was never toxoplasmosis in his series of patients. However, he still recommends that these lesions undergo biopsy.[19] Despite eloquent attempts to characterize the various brain lesions seen on neuroimaging studies in HIV-positive patients, no constellation of findings is 100-percent diagnostic of any of the numerous disease entities.[21] Moreover, the possibility of multiple etiologies for multiple brain lesions cannot be ignored in these patients (Fig. 136–1).

EMPIRIC THERAPY

At best, neuroimaging is suggestive in the diagnosis of AIDS-related brain lesions. This does not mean, however, that one should proceed directly to brain biopsy. As noted earlier, most focal brain lesions in HIV-positive patients are *Toxoplasma gondii* abscesses, which generally resolve when the patient is treated with adequate doses of sulfadiazine (or clindamycin) and pyrimethamine (antitoxoplasma therapy).[24, 25] Rosenblum and associates thus proposed that stable HIV-positive patients with multiple lesions on MRI receive 2 to 3 weeks of empiric antitoxoplasma therapy.[25] If follow-up images and physical examination fail to show improvement, these authors then recommend biopsy. This regimen appears prudent, and, although 40 percent of patients cannot tolerate the therapy, leading to inadequate treatment and often to biopsy, the incidence of toxoplasmosis in biopsy series is decreasing.[8, 9] The algorithm should probably be extended to include any HIV-positive patient with one or more contrast-enhancing lesions on CT because cerebral toxoplasmosis is not always multifocal.[8] In short, a presumptive diagnosis of cerebral toxoplasma can be given confidently to an HIV-positive patient whose brain lesions resolve after administration of antitoxoplasma drugs. This regimen eliminates the need for biopsy in a population of patients who can tolerate the therapy and have no focal cerebral lesions of another etiology. However, radiographic evidence of improvement can be complicated by the concomitant administration of steroids because some lesions improve with the administration of dexamethasone or prednisone.

LABORATORY EVALUATION

Rosenblum and coworkers[25] also suggested that in the absence of mass effect, cerebrospinal fluid (CSF) should be evaluated in HIV-positive patients with focal brain lesions. However, sensitivity and specificity for most causes of HIV-related focal lesions is less than optimal.[17, 19, 24, 26–29] Only a small percentage of lymphoma patients have abnormal CSF cytology, for example.[19, 26] And although the CSF is always abnormal in toxoplasmosis patients, the findings are nonspecific.[24] In serologic tests (whether on the blood or the CSF), as expected, antibody titres are unreliable in immunocompromised patients.

SURGERY

Unable to make an accurate diagnosis by noninvasive means for an HIV-positive patient who has a focal cerebral lesion or lesions that have not responded to antitoxoplasma therapy, the primary physician must ask a surgeon to consider biopsy. Such a measure is taken if the clinician and the patient and ultimately the surgeon agree that the risk of achieving an accurate diagnosis is outweighed by the potential for improving outcome. The authors reported their experience in the management of HIV-related focal brain lesions in an attempt to define the role of brain biopsy[8] and developed an algorithm that minimizes the risk to patient and surgeon.

SURGICAL TECHNIQUE

CT-guided stereotaxis was employed for all patients in the series. Single- or double-dose administration of intravenous contrast material with and without delayed image acquisition was used. De La Paz and Enzmann suggested that double-dose delayed contrast CT provides the best results,[20] but MRI is still more sensitive and possibly more specific in the approach to HIV-related brain lesions.[16, 18, 20, 21] If a compatible stereotactic system is available, MRI guidance is a suitable alternative to CT. The efficacy of an ultrasound-guided technique prevents its exclusion as a suitable alternative as well.[30] However, this procedure involves a more involved surgical opening and thus possibly an increased risk to the surgeon and the patient.

In most cases, intravenous sedation with "monitored anesthetic care" provides adequate anesthesia. General anesthesia is used at the patient's request, if it can be tolerated. The incidence of operative complications is low, but it may be prudent to monitor patients overnight in an intensive care setting.[9]

General criteria for biopsy include the presence of an intracranial lesion that is identifiable on CT or MRI, failure of enhancing lesions to improve after at least 1 week of antitoxoplasma therapy, or a CT or MRI appearance that is highly uncharacteristic of toxoplasmosis. Finally, the patient must be able to tolerate the procedure without significant risk.

If multiple lesions are present, either the most accessible cerebral lesion in the least eloquent brain or a lesion not responding to therapy is selected. In general, specimens are taken from only one lesion, but the occasional case may warrant targeting more than one lesion (Fig. 136–1). Target sites are chosen at the center of nonenhancing or homogeneously enhancing lesions and at the hyperdense border of ring-enhancing lesions.

Specimens are given to the pathologist for intraoperative smear cytology and frozen-section histology as needed. This process is repeated until diagnostic or clearly abnormal tissue is acquired. One or more additional specimens are sent for routine histology and transmission electron microscopy. Gram stain and bacterial, viral, and fungal cultures and stains are obtained. Levy and colleagues[7] reported that the diagnostic efficacy of brain biopsy in HIV-related brain lesions can be elevated to 96 percent through the use of these and various immunohistochemical techniques performed on at least six tissue samples.

RESULTS

The records of 25 HIV-positive patients who were consecutively referred for biopsy of cerebral lesions at the George Washington University Medical Center (Washington, DC) between November 1988 and October 1990 were reviewed. The preoperative characteristics of these 25 patients are depicted in Table 136–2. Of note is that 13 of the 25 had been seropositive for HIV for a median of 34 months and were diagnosed with AIDS before presenting for brain biopsy. In the 10 other patients for which this information was available, the cerebral lesion precipitated the initial presentation for treatment and the diagnosis of AIDS. As shown in Table 136–3, this fact had great bearing on the median survival after biopsy in these patients. The patients who had previous AIDS-related disease had a considerably shorter survival time than those who were found to be HIV-positive at the time of presentation for biopsy (six versus 37 weeks). Of the 13 patients with AIDS before their biopsy, nine had lymphoma. Conversely, all patients with lymphoma had AIDS before their procedure.

A listing of the biopsy diagnoses is also provided in Table 136–3. The relatively low incidence of toxoplasmosis, the single case of a low-grade glioma (not generally considered an HIV-related lesion), and the fact that five of the biopsies provided abnormal, but nondiagnostic, tissue are facts worth noting. Also of particular interest is that more than half of the lesions that enhanced on CT were lymphoma, and progressive multifocal leukoencephalopathy was the only diagnosis made from nonenhancing lesions. In fact, whether or

Table 136–2. CHARACTERISTICS OF PATIENTS UNDERGOING STEREOTACTIC BIOPSY OF HIV-RELATED CEREBRAL LESIONS AT GWU MEDICAL CENTER (11/88–10/90, n = 25)

Characteristic	Number
Male	24
Homosexual	21
IVDA	2
Haitian	1
Female	1 (IVDA)
Age	Mean, 36 years; range, 21–53 years
*Known to have AIDS before biopsy	13 (for a median of 34 months)
*CNS lesion prompted diagnosis of AIDS	10
Karnofsky Performance Score	65 (range, 40–100)
†Median follow-up	8 weeks
Dead	17
Lost to follow-up	1

AIDS = acquired immunodeficiency syndrome; CNS = central nervous system; GWU = George Washington University; HIV = human immunodeficiency virus; IVDA = intravenous drug abuser.
*We lack this information on two patients.
†Skewed by the large number of patients who died rapidly.

not a lesion enhanced on CT correlated well with whether or not the biopsy affected the patient's therapy (Table 136–4). Sixteen of the 25 target lesions enhanced with contrast, and therapy was modified in 11 of 16 on the basis of the biopsy results. Of those 11, 10 were tumors (nine lymphomas, one low-grade astrocytoma), and the other was a herpes simplex virus infection (Fig. 136–2). These patients were either receiving antitoxoplasma therapy or awaiting a treatment plan at the time of their biopsy; thus, the results led to more appropriate therapy. The remaining five patients with contrast-enhancing lesions included two with incompletely treated toxoplasmosis and one with a cryptococcal abscess who had suffered recurrent cryptococcal meningitis. Appropriate treatment was confirmed in these three patients. Two (12.5 percent) of the 16 contrast-enhancing targets yielded abnormal, but nondiagnostic, tissue at biopsy; thus, the procedure had no impact on their treatment. In short, 87.5 percent of the patients with contrast-enhancing lesions obtained a diagnosis from their biopsy that modified or confirmed their therapy.

On the other hand, the patients with nonenhancing lesions experienced no therapeutic benefit from their biopsy. The abnormal tissue was nondiagnostic in one third of these cases, and the remainder had progressive multifocal leukoencephalopathy, for which no effective therapy exists (see Table 136–3). Only one patient suffered a complication of the procedure when a small hemorrhage with edema occurred at the operative site, leaving him somnolent for approximately 24 hours.

DISCUSSION

Several aspects of these data affect the surgeon's role in HIV-related cerebral disease. First, toxoplasmosis is the cause of CNS mass lesions in 25 to 70 percent of cases in most large series,[2, 5–7] whereas it occurred in only two of the 25 patients reported on here (8 percent, see Table 136–3). This is probably a result of the approach to CNS masses in AIDS patients outlined by Rosenblum and coworkers[25] and adopted by many practitioners who treat AIDS patients. In general, patients with contrast-enhancing lesions on CT are treated for at least 7 to 10 days with antitoxoplasma therapy as tolerated. If follow-up CT reveals an unsatisfactory response, the patient may be referred for biopsy. During this study, approximately 40 patients were treated at our institution for HIV-related focal cerebral lesions that were not referred for biopsy. About 20 of these had toxoplasmosis that responded to therapy, or the patients died during treatment. However, the remainder were treated empirically, based on presumptive (usually radiographic) diagnosis, or were not treated, based on their clinical condition or the lack of an effective therapy (13 with presumed lymphoma and seven with presumed progressive multifocal leukoencephalopathy). This result suggests a tendency on the part of the referring physicians to weigh heavily the potential for poor outcome in AIDS patients with CNS lesions against the potential benefit of having an accurate tissue diagnosis to guide appropriate therapy.

Table 136–3. RESULTS OF STEREOTACTIC BIOPSY OF HIV-RELATED CEREBRAL LESIONS AT GWU MEDICAL CENTER (11/88–10/90, n = 25)

Diagnosis	(%)	Contrast Enhancing (n)	Contrast Negative (n)	KPS (median)	Median Survival (weeks)	CNS First (unknown)*	Previous AIDS (n)
Lymphoma	36	9	—	70	6	—	9
PML	24	—	6	60	18	4 (1)	1
Toxoplasmosis	8	2	—	80	37	1 (1)	—
Low-grade glioma	4	1	—	80	74	1	—
Herpes cerebritis	4	1	—	90	8	1	—
Cryptococcoma	4	1	—	50	1	—	1
Nondiagnostic	20	2 (12.5%)	3 (33%)	55	17	3	2
Total	100	16	9	n/a	n/a	10 (2)	13
					Median Survival (weeks) 37	6	

PML = progressive multifocal leukoencephalopathy; KPS = Karnofsky Performance Score.
*It is unknown from our data whether these patients had a CNS lesion first.

Table 136–4. COMPUTED TOMOGRAPHIC APPEARANCE VERSUS IMPACT OF BIOPSY ON SUBSEQUENT TREATMENT

	Contrast Enhancing (n)	Nonenhancing (n)
Changed treatment	11	0
Confirmed treatment in progress	3	0
No help with treatment	2 (12.5%)	9 (100%)

LYMPHOMA

Outcome for AIDS-related cerebral lymphoma, for instance, justifies such a conservative tendency. Patients without AIDS who are treated aggressively for CNS lymphoma may survive a median of 13.5 months, whereas AIDS patients with CNS lymphoma invariably suffer a fulminant course and die within 3 months.[31, 32] This effect occurs regardless of whether the patients are treated and whether or not their lesions respond to therapy.[29] However, a more recent review found that HIV-positive patients with CNS lymphoma who were treated aggressively with external beam irradiation survived a median of almost 4 months, versus only 1 month if not treated.[33] The data presented earlier furthermore suggest that AIDS patients who develop lymphoma do so late in the course of their disease and usually die of systemic disease or of other AIDS-related diseases (all nine lymphoma patients had AIDS before their biopsy). In fact, despite accurate diagnosis and a full course of low-dose radiation therapy (20 to 30 Gy) in six of nine of the patients with lymphoma, the median survival was only 6 weeks (see Table 136–3) (the other three patients could not tolerate or refused radiation therapy or died before treatment could be completed). Moreover, all nine patients were treated for toxoplasmosis until their biopsy findings led to a change in therapy. These facts raise at least two questions about AIDS

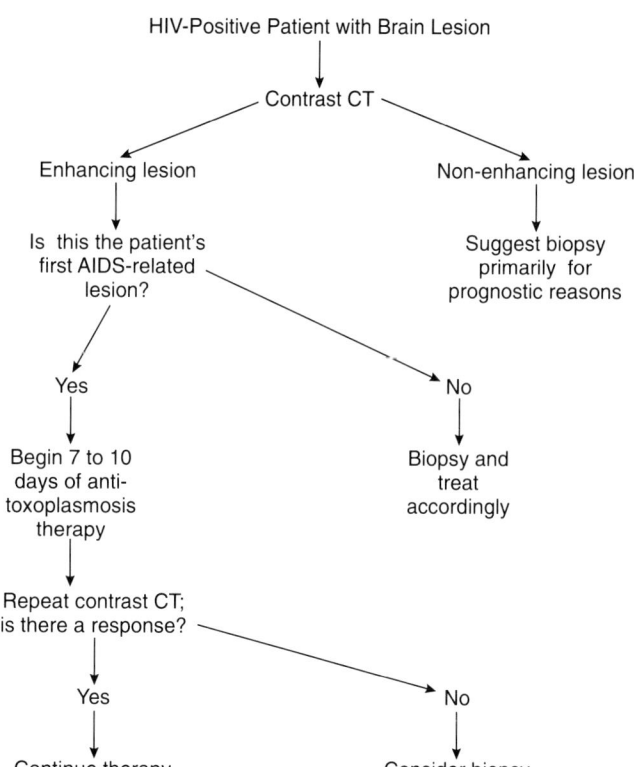

FIGURE 136–3. Proposed treatment algorithm defining the role of stereotactic biopsy in AIDS patients with cerebral lesions based on the data presented.

patients with a contrast-enhancing lesion: should the physician adopt an aggressive approach and should the physician treat empirically for toxoplasmosis or perform a biopsy immediately and treat accordingly. The answers may depend on the stage of the patient's disease and his or her wishes after being informed of the prognosis.

EFFICACY OF STEREOTACTIC BIOPSY

Stereotactic biopsy provides an accurate diagnosis in about 95 percent of cases.[34, 35] A percentage of nondiagnostic biopsies as high as that (20 percent) in the series reported on earlier can be greatly improved if the appropriate techniques are employed.[7, 36] As mentioned, these techniques have been clearly outlined by Levy and associates.[9] Immunohistochemical techniques and special stains were not routinely used in the series noted earlier, which may account for the relatively high nondiagnostic rate. However, three of the diagnoses were made by transmission electron microscopy. The small risk of not achieving a diagnosis should be considered in the decision of whether or not brain biopsy should be recommended to a patient with an AIDS-related brain lesion.

PROPOSED TREATMENT ALGORITHM
(Fig. 136–3)

Based on the data presented earlier, empiric antitoxoplasma therapy appears to be indicated for contrast-enhancing cerebral lesions in recently diagnosed HIV-positive pa-

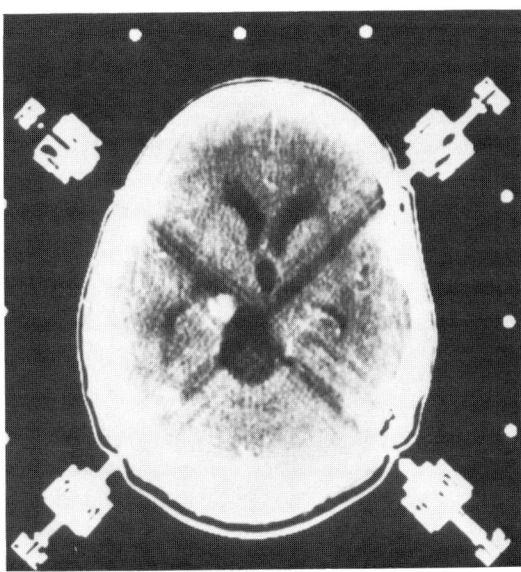

FIGURE 136–2. CT of a patient with herpes simplex viral cerebritis as an example of how even viral encephalitides can present as lesions for biopsy.

tients. However, in patients with long-standing disease and contrast-enhancing lesions for whom an aggressive approach is selected, immediate biopsy is warranted. The high incidence of lymphoma in the later stages of AIDS and the fact that many other potentially treatable etiologies are reported to cause contrast-enhancing lesions in the brains of AIDS patients both indicate such an approach. The role of biopsy in AIDS patients with nonenhancing brain lesions is less clear. Brain biopsy seldom contributes to the therapy in these patients, but it may provide prognostic information and may be required by future experimental treatment protocols. Accordingly, we have implemented the algorithm in Figure 136–3 to determine when a biopsy should be performed in AIDS patients with cerebral lesions for whom an informed decision to treat the lesion aggressively is made.

It remains to be seen whether or not such an approach effects a better outcome in patients whose therapy is altered by the results. So far, only five patients have been treated prospectively with this approach in the 2 years since the data were gathered. This low number may reflect a change in attitude regarding the approach to AIDS-related brain disease among patients and referring physicians. All but one of these patients had lymphoma and a Karnofsky Performance Score (KPS) of 90 or more. The other had a nongranulomatous chronic infectious process of uncertain etiology. The four lymphoma patients currently have a median survival of more than 4 months after having been treated with irradiation and chemotherapy as tolerated. Thus, it is still not clear whether or not an aggressive approach using the proposed algorithm will improve outcome in AIDS-related brain disease, yet it appears that the treatment algorithm has decreased the number of biopsies and increased the yield of treatable diagnoses. Both of these qualities are highly desirable in the treatment of AIDS. Real proof of improved outcome would require a randomized trial not likely to be undertaken in the current politicized atmosphere.

AGGRESSIVE VERSUS CONSERVATIVE APPROACH

Alas, the question remains as to whether or not the risk of obtaining an accurate diagnosis is outweighed by the potential for improved survival. Accurate diagnosis, and thus appropriate therapy, can be made with certainty only by obtaining tissue samples from AIDS-related brain lesions. However, patients whose lesions do not enhance on CT are apparently much less likely to have a treatable disease (our data imply they most often have progressive multifocal leukoencephalopathy). Patients with long-standing AIDS and contrast-enhancing lesions of the brain are likely to have lymphoma. Although most of these patients do poorly even with appropriate therapy, an earlier diagnosis and aggressive therapy in patients with a KPS of 90 or more may provide some survival benefit or, at least, useful information with regard to a treatment plan. The patients who are recently or simultaneously found to be HIV-positive with cerebral lesions that enhance on CT but do not respond to antitoxoplasma treatment generally survive longer and thus might benefit from targeted treatment for their cerebral disease. However, even under the best circumstances, survival is not likely to exceed a few months. Patients, referring physicians, and surgical consultants could consider this type of information when making a decision regarding diagnosis and treatment of HIV-related brain lesions.

ETHICS

A certainly fatal communicable disease like AIDS raises yet another issue in the decision-making process peculiar to such a unique circumstance, that is, whether or not the risk to the surgeon should be included in the formula. Medical ethicists have addressed the issue of physicians' obligations to treat patients with AIDS, and most feel that it is unethical for a physician to refuse to treat patients with AIDS, simply because they have the disease.[37,38] There are, however, certain "limiting factors," not the least of which is "excessive risk." As noted earlier, accurately calculating the risk of a particular surgeon performing a particular procedure on an AIDS patient is not feasible. Nonetheless, if the formula and data outlined by Schiff[14] are applied to stereotactic biopsy, an estimated range can be derived. Assuming an injury rate of one significant injury per 50 biopsies (with a seroprevalence of 100 percent), and 25 AIDS biopsies per year over 30 years of practice, the probability of contracting HIV for a surgeon performing stereotactic brain biopsies on HIV-positive patients is 0.0075. By no one's standards does this constitute excessive risk. Even this is probably an overestimate in light of the fact that inoculation during a stereotactic biopsy is extremely unlikely (no significant injuries have occurred to the authors or their assistants, associates, or local colleagues in more than 50 AIDS biopsies performed in a 4-year period at two hospitals). Performance of the procedure by one surgeon and one surgical technician exchanging virtually all blunt instruments (except needles for local anesthetic and a scalpel for scalp puncture) on a Mayo stand minimizes the chance of a significant injury. In addition, the procedure is practically bloodless, and the use of a bio-occlusive drape further reduces exposure.

The only other potentially acceptable limiting factor to a physician's obligation to treat a patient with AIDS is the issue of "questionable benefit".[33] If no reasonable chance exists that the patient will benefit from the procedure, then the physician is under no obligation to treat. In fact, the physician is obliged not to treat.

This chapter is intended to assist the physician in the complex decision of whether or not to offer brain biopsy to a given patient who presents with an HIV-related brain lesion. That each case be evaluated on an individual basis is implied, and a suggested treatment algorithm is provided should a case warrant aggressive management. To reiterate, recently diagnosed HIV-positive patients with contrast-enhancing lesions warrant a course of antitoxoplasma therapy, and biopsy might be considered if this therapy fails. Patients with long-standing disease but with a KPS of 90 or more and contrast-enhancing lesions are likely to benefit from accurate diagnosis and treatment of their cerebral disease. If the lesion is nonenhancing, the decision becomes more difficult, but in the author's experience, biopsy of these lesions is seldom helpful. The prospective efficacy of this approach remains to be quantified. Related ethical issues and, perhaps in the near future, economic issues, cannot be ignored. However, with the available information in hand, the authors hope that the patient, the referring physician, and the surgical consultant can make the best decision.

REFERENCES

1. Centers for Disease Control National AIDS Hotline: November 18, 1992
2. So YT, Beckstead JH, Davis RL: Primary central nervous system lymphoma in acquired immune deficiency syndrome: A clinical and pathological study. Ann Neurol 20:566–572, 1986
3. De Giorlami U, Smith TW, Hienin D, Hauw JJ: Neuropathology of the acquired immunodeficiency syndrome. Arch Pathol Lab Med 114(7):643–655, 1990
4. Kanzer MD: Neuropathology of AIDS. Crit Rev Neurobiol 5(4):313–362, 1990
5. Levy RM, Bresdesen DE, Rosenblum ML: Neurological manifestations of the acquired immunodeficiency syndrome (AIDS): Experience at UCSF and review of the literature. J Neurosurg 62:475–495, 1985
6. Loneragan R, Doust BD, Walker J: Neuroradiological manifestation of the acquired immunodeficiency syndrome. Australas Radiol 34:32–39, 1990
7. Levy RM, Russell E, Yungbluth M, et al: The efficacy of image-guided stereotactic brain biopsy in neurologically symptomatic acquired immunodeficiency syndrome patients. Neurosurgery 30:186–190, 1992
8. Chappell ET, Guthrie BL, Orenstein J: The role of stereotactic biopsy in the management of HIV-related focal brain lesions. Neurosurgery 30:825–829, 1992
9. Apuzzo MJ, Chnadrasoma PT, Cohen D, et al: Computed imaging stereotaxy. Experience and perspective related to 500 procedures applied to brain masses. Neurosurgery 20:930–937, 1987
10. Falloon J: Current therapy for HIV infection and its complications. Postgrad Med 91(8):115–132, 1992
11. Broder S (moderator): Antiretroviral therapy in AIDS. Ann Intern Med 113:604–618, 1990
12. Kuo JM, Taylor JM, Detels R: Estimating the AIDS incubation period from a prevalent cohort. Am J Epidemiol 133(10):1050–1057, 1991
13. Salzberg AM, Dolins SL, Salzberg C: HIV incubation times. Lancet ii(8655):166, 1989
14. Schiff SJ: A surgeon's risk of AIDS. J Neurosurgery 73:651–660, 1990
15. Lowenfels AB, Wormser GP, Jain R: Frequency of puncture injuries in surgeons and estimated risk of HIV infection. Arch Surg 124:1284, 1989
16. Rodriguez WL, Ramirez-Ronda CH: CNS involvement in AIDS patients as seen with CT and MR: A review. Bol Asoc Med P R 83(12):548–551, 1991
17. Remick SC, Diamond C, Migliozzi JA, et al: Primary central nervous system lymphoma in patients with and without the acquired immune deficiency syndrome. A retrospective analysis and review of the literature. Medicine (Baltimore) 69(6):345–360, 1990
18. Rauch RA, Bazan C III, Jinkins JR: Imaging of infections of the central nervous system. Curr Opin Radiol 4(1):43–51, 1992
19. Dina T: Primary central nervous system lymphoma versus toxoplasmosis in AIDS. Radiology 179:823, 1991
20. De La Paz R, Enzmann D: Neuroradiology of acquired immunodeficiency syndrome, in Rosenblum ML, Levy RM, Bredesen E (eds): AIDS and the Central Nervous System. New York, Raven Press, 1988, pp 121–154
21. Kupfer MC, Chi-Shing Z, Colletti PM, et al: MRI evaluation of AIDS-related encephalopathy: Toxoplasmosis vs. lymphoma. Magn Reson Imaging 8:51–56, 1990
22. Poon T, Matoso I, Tchertkoff V, et al: CT features of primary cerebral lymphoma in AIDS and non-AIDS patients. J Comput Assist Tomogr 13:6–9, 1989
23. Mariuz PR, Luft BJ: Toxoplasmic encephalitis. AIDS Clin Rev 105–130, 1992
24. Pons VG, Jacobs RA, Hollander H, et al: Nonviral infections of the central nervous system in patients with acquired immunodeficiency syndrome, in Rosenblum ML, Levy RM, Bresdesen DE (eds): AIDS and the Nervous System. New York, Raven Press, 1988, pp 263–284
25. Rosenblum ML, Levy RM, Bresdesen DE: Algorithms for the treatment of AIDS patients with neurologic disease, in Rosenblum ML, Levy RM, Bresdesen E (eds): AIDS and the Central Nervous System. New York, Raven Press, 1988, pp 389–396
26. So YT, Chaoucoir A, Davis RL, et al: Neoplasms of the central nervous system in acquired immunodeficiency syndrome, in Rosenblum ML, Levy RM, Bresdesen DE (eds): AIDS and the Central Nervous System. New York, Raven Press, 1988, pp 285–300
27. Strigle SM, Gal AA: Review of the central nervous system cytopathology in human immunodeficiency virus infection. Diagn Cytopathol 7(4):387–401, 1991
28. Weinke T, Rogler G, Sixt C, et al: Cryptococcoses in AIDS patients: Observations concerning CNS involvement. J Neurol 236–238, 1989
29. Rosenblum ML, Levy RM, Bresdesen DE (eds): AIDS and the Nervous System. New York, Raven Press, 1988
30. Di Lorenzo N, Esposito V, Lunardi P, et al: A comparison of computerized tomography–guided stereotactic and ultrasound-guided techniques for brain biopsy. J Neurosurg 75:763, 1991
31. Hochberg FH, Miller DC: Primary central nervous system lymphoma. J Neurosurg 68:835–853, 1988
32. So YT, Beckstead JH, Davis RL: Primary central nervous system lymphoma in acquired immune deficiency syndrome: A clinical and pathological study. Ann Neurol 20:566–572, 1986
33. Baumgartner JE, Rachlin JR, Beckstead JH, et al: Primary central nervous system lymphomas: Natural history and response to radiation therapy in 55 patients with acquired immunodeficiency syndrome. J Neurosurg 73:206–211, 1990
34. Friedman WA, Sceats DJ, Blake RN, Ballinger WE: The incidence of unexpected pathological findings in an image-guided biopsy series: A review of 100 consecutive cases. Neurosurgery 25:180–184, 1989
35. Kaufman HK, Catalano LW: Diagnostic brain biopsy: A series of 50 cases and a review. Neurosurgery 4:129–136, 1979
36. Zimmer C, Daeschlein G, Patt S, Weigel K: Strategy for diagnosis of *Toxoplasma gondii* in stereotactic brain biopsies. Stereotact Funct Neurosurg 56:66–75, 1991
37. Emanuel EJ: Do physicians have an obligation to treat patients with AIDS? N Engl J Med 318:1686–1690, 1988
38. Zuger A, Miles SH: Physicians, AIDS, and occupational risk. JAMA 258:1924, 1987

CHAPTER 137

Surgical Management of Tuberculous and Fungal Infections of the Nervous System

Ravi Bhatia
Rana Patir
Prakash Narain Tandon

Infection of the central nervous system (CNS) by *Mycobacterium tuberculosis* is invariably secondary to a primary focus elsewhere in the body. The avium, bovine, and atypical mycobacteria are rarely isolated from the non-immunocompromised host. The primary site is usually pulmonary, bone, and gastrointestinal tract; genitourinary sites are less common. The incidence of CNS tuberculosis is a reflection of the overall incidence of tuberculosis within a population. Tuberculosis of the nervous system, which merits the attention of a neurosurgeon, occurs in several forms, and more than one form may be present in the same individual (Table 137–1). This chapter deals only with tuberculomas and tuberculous meningitis. Pott's disease of the spine, tubercular encephalopathy, and spinal arachnoiditis are extensively described in orthopedic and neurologic texts.

The recognition of fungal meningitis, abscess, and granuloma as distinct clinical entities is fairly recent. Fungal infections of the CNS are invariably secondary to pulmonary or nasopharyngeal infection. The spread may be hematogenous or by direct contiguity, as in paranasal sinus involvement. There has also been a greater awareness and an upsurge in the incidence in both tuberculosis and fungal infections of the CNS on account of their relationship with acquired immunodeficiency syndrome (AIDS) and AIDS-related complex.

TUBERCULOSIS

Tuberculosis is a major problem worldwide, especially in developing countries. Every year, an estimated 7.1 million new cases (of all forms) and 2.6 million deaths occur in the Third World countries alone.[1] The incidence of the disease, which had declined dramatically in developed countries and to a great extent in Third World countries because of newer antituberculous drugs, has again increased with the advent of AIDS.[2] An estimated 54 percent of patients with tuberculosis in developed countries may be seropositive for the human immunodeficiency virus (HIV). The combined effect of tuberculosis and AIDS on individual patients, the health care system, and the economy will soon reach enormous dimensions. Tuberculosis has ceased to be a disease of quaint historical interest, even in countries like the United States.[3] Besides AIDS, other factors like poverty, emergence of drug-resistant strains of tuberculosis, and intravenous drug use, have contributed to the rapid spread of the disease in the past decade.[4] In Britain, the incidence of CNS tuberculosis has again increased in areas with large immigrant populations.[5] Tuberculosis in AIDS is likelier to have extrapulmonary manifestations, particularly neural tuberculosis.[4]

TUBERCULOMAS

Incidence

Although the incidence of tuberculomas or chronic granulomas has declined worldwide, tuberculosis continues to be a medical problem. For instance, in India, the number of patients treated for tuberculosis in all major centers has decreased. The King Edward Memorial Hospital in Bombay reported a figure of 30.5 percent (for the period 1957 to 1963) this figure declined to 12.1 percent (for the period 1974 to 1978). In the Madras General Hospital, the numbers declined from 20.0 percent in 1951 to 1960 to 12.2 percent in 1975 to 1979. In Christian Medical College Hospital, Vellore, there was a drop from 14.4 percent in 1949 to 1959 to 6.5 percent in 1970 to 1977. The All India Institute of

Table 137–1. TUBERCULOSIS OF THE NERVOUS SYSTEM

Anatomic Area	Manifestation
Intracranial Tuberculosis	
Parenchymal	Tuberculoma
	Abscess
	Tubercular encephalopathy
Meningeal	Chronic meningitis
Calvarial	Osteomyelitis
Spinal Tuberculosis	
Vertebral	Pott's disease of the spine
Meningeal	Arachnoiditis
Parenchymal	Tuberculoma

Medical Sciences (AIIMS) hospital, Delhi, which always had a lower percentage, showed a decline from 4.2 percent in 1965 to 1969 to 3.3 percent in 1974 to 1978.[6] A high incidence has been reported from Chile (16 percent),[7] Romania (7.3 percent),[8] and South Africa.[9] Although tuberculosis is widely prevalent in Nigeria, only 15 cases of tuberculomas were detected in a 5-year period.[10] Misdiagnosis was ruled out because a postmortem analysis of all patients dying of intracranial space-occupying lesions showed no cases of tuberculoma.

Similarly, in Taiwan, where CNS tuberculosis is common,[11] tuberculomas constituted only 1 percent of all intracranial mass lesions.[5] A combined series from several neurosurgical centers in Japan showed an incidence of only 2.6 percent.[12] In an interesting study from New York, Mayers and associates[13] reported on a series of 12 patients with tuberculomas who were all native-born Americans and long-time residents. In 1978, Armstrong and Edwards[14] reported on 49 Native American Indians or Eskimo Canadians with intracranial tuberculomas. Tuberculomas are increasingly reported in industrialized nations, such as Great Britain[15-18] and the United States,[13, 19-22] and account for 1 to 2 percent of all intracranial lesions.

Location

Tuberculomas can occur at any site in the brain (Table 137-2) but rarely occur within the spinal cord. Unusual sites of tuberculomas include dura mater, subdural space, orbital fissure, brainstem,[23, 24] pituitary gland,[25, 26] or any part of the ventricular system. Intramedullary tuberculomas are rare,[27, 28] and compared with 128 intracranial lesions, we have treated only five such cases.

Patient Age and Sex

Earlier series noted a higher incidence of tuberculosis in males than in females. However, more recently, females with tuberculomas either just outnumber males or equal them in number.[29-31] In our series, there were 66 males and 62 females. Tuberculosis is a disease of the young; 70 percent of patients are below 30 years. Tuberculomas are uncommon in children under the age of 4 years, although we have treated a 9-month-old infant with multiple tuberculomas.

Clinical Features

The signs and symptoms of tuberculomas resemble those of other intracranial space-occupying lesions. As they enlarge gradually, the clinical picture is one of a slowly progressive lesion, although in at least 50 percent of patients, the symptoms are less than 6 months in duration. Features that are of help in distinguishing tuberculomas from other brain tumors are constitutional symptoms, such as weight loss, fever or malaise, a history of active tuberculosis, a high frequency of seizures even in association with a cerebellar lesion, a positive result on the Mantoux test, and a raised sedimentation rate. Infants and young children may have an enlarging head. The clinical diagnosis is often presumptive because even in endemic areas, extracranial tuberculosis may coexist with a brain tumor. Pyrexia is variable and may not be present in more than 20 to 25 percent of patients[31] and the Mantoux test result may be negative.[9, 30] The clinical course may uncommonly show spontaneous remissions and relapses.[23] Clinical evidence of an active focus of tuberculosis, such as the lungs and lymph glands, may be present in only 33 percent of patients[30, 32] and in about 10 percent of close relatives. Rare signs include scalp swelling, cerebrospinal fluid (CSF) rhinorrhea, features of a pituitary tumor,[25, 26] unilateral proptosis, and trigeminal neuralgia.[30] The clinical picture may be confusing when multiple lesions are present. For instance, a 33-year-old woman presented with behavioral problems, homonymous hemianopsia, hemiparesis, and signs of a partial Brown-Séquard syndrome. On magnetic resonance imaging (MRI), she proved to have multiple tuberculomas in the brain and spinal cord. The diagnosis was established on a cervical lymph node biopsy and response to anti-tuberculous drugs. Intramedullary tuberculomas with no evidence of extracranial tuberculosis are clinically indistinguishable from intramedullary tumors, and the diagnosis invariably occurs at surgery or, more recently, on an MRI. Dinakar and colleagues[33] reported a spinal tuberculous granuloma in association with a congenital dermal sinus.

The nature of the immunologic compromise in AIDS increases host susceptibility to tuberculosis. Organisms belonging to the *Mycobacterium avium* complex are the commonest cause of systemic bacterial infection in AIDS patients and have been demonstrated in 50 percent of such patients coming to autopsy.[14] Because of immune suppression, abscess formation is likelier than the chronic inflammatory granuloma seen in immunocompetent patients. Seizures, headaches, and an altered mental state are common presentations, but fever is often absent. The infection is usually a reactivation of latent tuberculosis.[34]

Tuberculomas may occur in association with tuberculous meningitis or may develop during the course of treatment of tubercular meningitis with anti-tuberculous drugs, altering the clinical presentation.[4] In tubercular meningitis, symptoms of raised intracranial pressure (ICP) and development of focal neurologic signs, such as motor weakness, cerebellar signs, field defects, visual compromise, and behavioral problems in children, necessitate a search for expanding tuberculomas.

Table 137-2. LOCATION OF INTRACRANIAL TUBERCULOMAS (128 SURGICALLY VERIFIED CASES FROM 1975-1992, ALL INDIA INSTITUTE OF MEDICAL SCIENCES HOSPITAL, NEW DELHI)*

Location	Incidence (n)
Supratentorial	
Parietal	28
Frontal	26
Temporal	15
Basal ganglia or thalamus	4
Sellar or suprasellar	4
Orbital fissure	1
Total	78
Infratentorial	
Cerebellum	44
Cerebellopontine angle	3
Tentorium	1
Brainstem	2
Total	50

*Depending on the location of the major component of the lesion.

Pathologic Features

The typical tuberculoma is a solid, well-defined avascular mass with multiple nubbins extending to and compressing the surrounding brain. Typically, it is creamy white on the surface and has a pale yellow, often gritty caseating central core with a crenated margin. It has a firm collagenous capsule that at times has a pinkish appearance, which is usually referred to as the mature form of tuberculoma.[30] The immature form consists of multiple small tubercles, some with caseating or liquefied centers dispersed within an edematous brain. Severe edema, possibly caused by an allergic response,[30] may surround these tubercles. Tuberculomas vary in size from 1.5 to 8 cm, and they vary in weight. Giant tuberculomas can occupy an entire cerebral hemisphere,[32] and many adhere to the dura. The dural attachment can be very tenuous or so firm that the tumor resembles a meningioma.

Microscopically, the central zone of caseous necrosis is surrounded by tuberculous granulation tissue consisting of epithelioid cells, Langerhans giant cells, and some lymphocytes, polymorphonuclear leukocytes, and plasma cells (Fig. 137–1). Acid-fast bacilli are usually present in both these layers. The brain surrounding a tuberculoma may show degenerated nerve fibers and nerve cells, thrombosed vessels, and occasionally, swollen astrocytes and oligodendroglial cells. The changes in the small vessels can lead to microhemorrhages or microinfarcts, and these areas may coalesce.[35] Smaller satellite tuberculomas may surround the main mass.

Tuberculomas can take several unusual forms,[36, 37] representing the spectra of inflammatory reaction: (1) incipient tuberculoma, which may appear as an irregular, fleshy, gray cortical mass with associated meningeal tuberculomatosis or even grapelike clusters of tuberculoma along cerebral vessels; (2) subdural cyst overlying an intracerebral tuberculoma; (3) cystic tuberculoma; (4) tubercular abscess; (5) extensive edematous encephalopathy without a tuberculoma; (6) severe cerebral edema with a small, ''inconsequential'' tuberculoma; and (7) rarely, tuberculoma that has spread transdurally to the calvarium.

The factors that lead to a different type of tissue reaction associated with the presence of numerous live bacilli are not known. A tubercular abscess is likelier to occur in patients with AIDS (vide supra) than is a solid expanding lesion. It is also likely that previous anti-tuberculous drugs may play a role in the development of an abscess. The role of hydrolytic enzymes in liquefaction in tuberculous lesions at sites other than the brain has been extensively studied. Enzyme inhibitors from dead bacilli and necrotic tissue in caseous material have been reported to prevent liquefaction in tuberculous lesions.[38] Brain tissue that is rich in hydrolytic enzymes may release large quantities of these enzymes and produce liquefaction, allowing tubercle bacilli to proliferate.

Dastur and Dave[39] studied the ultrastructural characteristics of tuberculomas. The mononuclear cells in the reactive border zone were found to be blood monocyte–derived epithelioid cells of various forms and stages with active phagocytic capacity. In the edematous brain tissue surrounding the tuberculoma, the endothelial cells and tight junctions of the blood vessels remained intact. The single basement membrane layer of the blood vessels showed thickening but retained the usual homogeneous appearance. In contrast, the vessels in the reactive border zone of the tuberculomas showed marked proliferation of the basement membrane into several concentric layers associated with fragmentation. This proliferating fragmenting basement membrane often included infiltrating inflammatory cells. The nature of this proliferating basement membrane material was not clear, although glycoproteins appeared to be the major constituent. This proteinaceous basement membrane material may act as a newly formed antigen and thus may initiate a cellular antibody reaction, resulting in vasculitis and brain damage.

Radhakrishnan and associates[40] demonstrated immunohistochemically mycobacterial antigens in the paraffin section of 10 intracranial tuberculous granulomas. They compared the results with the conventional Ziehl-Neelsen method of staining acid-fast bacilli. In none of the 10 specimens were acid-fast bacilli demonstrable. However, mycobacterial antigens were characterized as diffusely staining, granular, brownish-pink material within the cytoplasm of giant cells and macrophages. In 14 specimens of granulomatous lesions of nontubercular etiology, immunohistochemical stains were negative for mycobacterial antigens. They believe this technique to be more sensitive than the Ziehl-Neelsen method.

Radiologic Features

Tuberculomas cannot be differentiated from other CNS tumors on plain x-ray films of the skull. Conventional radiologic investigations fail to distinguish tuberculomas from other avascular tumors of the brain. At best, a presumptive diagnosis can be made in patients with clinical features of extracranial tuberculosis as well as radiographic features in the chest. However, the absence of tuberculosis on chest radiography or a lack of clinical evidence of extrapulmonary tuberculosis does not rule out the diagnosis of a tuberculoma.[41–45] Radiologically, tubercular osteomyelitis cannot be distinguished from pyogenic osteomyelitis. The presence of calcification on conventional radiography is seldom conclusive, with the striking exceptions of the Eskimos and the North American Indians, in whom nearly 60 percent are known to have calcifications.[30] Calcification is not indicative of an inactive lesion.[28] Calcification occurs in fewer than 6 percent of tuberculomas and is rarely extensive or dense.[7, 8, 32] Cerebral angiography invariably reveals an avascular

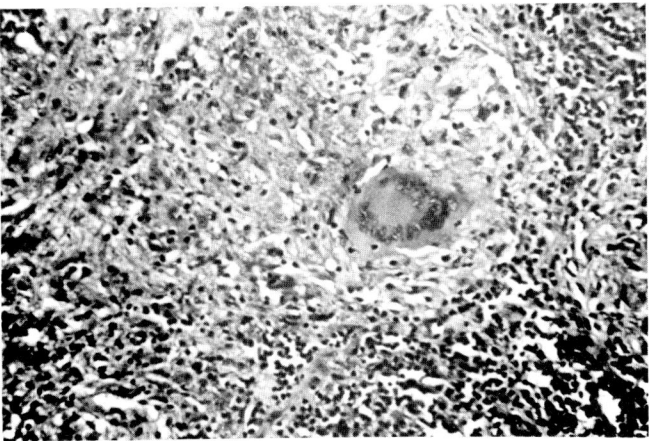

FIGURE 137–1. A photomicrograph of a typical tuberculoma with Langerhans giant cells, epithelioid cells and lymphocytes. Hematoxylin and eosin stain: magnification × 100.

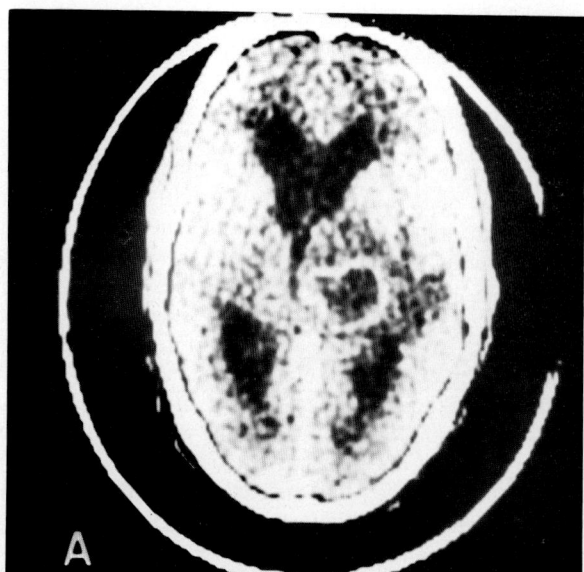

FIGURE 137–2. (A) A contrast-enhanced CT scan showing multiple rings and discs surrounded by areas of low attenuation indicating edema characteristic of tuberculosis. (B and C) Not all tuberculomas are typical. The contrast-enhanced CT scan of a 40-year-old female patient who presented with raised pressure and ataxia and who had bilateral cerebellar signs shows a high attenuating midline posterior fossa lesion, which was thought to be a glioma preoperatively and later proved to be a tuberculoma on histology.

mass, although surface tuberculomas may show some peripheral vascularity.[32, 41] An associated vascular spasm may be seen that is ascribed to tuberculous vasculitis.[42]

Computed Tomography and Magnetic Resonance Imaging

Before the advent of computed tomographic (CT) scanning, the diagnosis of an intracranial tuberculoma was established only by biopsy or after excision. With CT scanning, lesions as small as 1.5 cm in diameter can be fairly accurately identified.* These small lesions, which exist without clinical

---
*See references 9, 15, 17, 21, 23, 31, and 43–50.

evidence of elevated pressure, were excluded from earlier statistics that were based on surgical material. Reviews from South Africa,[9] India,[43, 47, 48] Hong Kong,[49] Great Britain,[15, 50] Saudi Arabia,[45] and the United States[13] have pointed out that most tuberculomas are similar in appearance (Figs. 137–2 and 137–3).

The tuberculoma CT scan image is of (1) a lesion that appears as isodense with the brain or slightly hyperdense and enhances strongly with contrast, revealing a dense, unbroken ring of enhancement; (2) in some cases, an enhancing disc or nodular mass with a regular or an irregular margin; and (3) combinations of rings and discs, which may coalesce. Uncommonly, tuberculomas may present as a nonenhancing lesion or even a strongly enhancing lesion that is indistin-

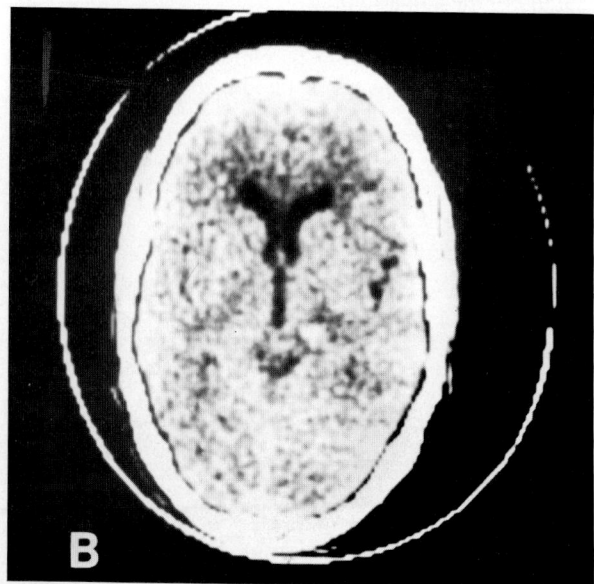

FIGURE 137–3. This patient, who had undergone a kidney transplant and was on regular immunosuppressants, developed hemiparesis over a 10-day period. (A) A contrast-enhanced scan shows a large ring-shaped lesion in the right thalamus. Stereotactic aspiration of pus revealed *Mycobacterium tuberculosis*. The patient improved rapidly on medical therapy. (B) A repeat scan shows almost complete resolution of the lesion.

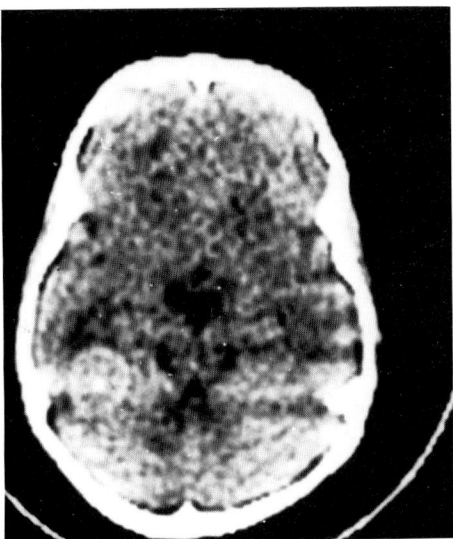

FIGURE 137-4. A contrast-enhanced scan of a 7-year-old girl with elevated intracranial pressure and cerebellar signs shows the target sign of a tuberculoma.

guishable from a meningioma. Welchman[9] noted that tuberculomas in which the CT characteristics differed from those with ring enhancement were not surrounded by brain parenchyma.

Calcification on the CT may give a characteristic picture of tuberculosis. Welchman found calcification in four of 10 tuberculomas, peripheral in one, and central in three. In the latter three cases, a peripheral ring of contrast enhancement was present, giving rise to a target sign. A central focus of enhancement in tuberculomas may occasionally be present (Fig. 137-4).

Multiplicity is common in CT scans of tuberculomas. Bhargava and Tandon[44] found that 50 to 60 percent of cases may demonstrate multiple lesions. The CT scan also picks up small lesions less than 1.5 cm in size, disc like or rings, single or multiple, having slightly increased attenuation that enhances with contrast, and surrounded by disproportionately low attenuating white-matter edema. Bhargava and Tandon[44] had labeled them "microtuberculomas." Careful review of these cases suggests that not all those lesions are tuberculous in etiology. Indian neurologists and neurosurgeons encounter these lesions frequently in children and young adults, but reports have come from other countries, too. The patients generally present with focal epilepsy and no neurologic deficit. Although some of these cases are definitely tuberculomas, as proved by biopsies, others result from a variety of causes.[51-56]

Goulatia and coworkers[51] suggested that edema and increased vascular permeability due to the seizure may be responsible for the CT appearance. Chandy and associates[54, 56] found cysticercosis as the commonest cause, and Ahuja and associates[53] noted that 12 of their 38 patients were seropositive for cysticercosis, and two were seropositive for tuberculosis. Obviously, it is not possible to arrive at a definitive etiologic diagnosis of these lesions. When first seen, they could represent tuberculomas, abscesses, cysticercus granulomas, or focal meningoencephalitis. Nearly 30 to 40 percent of these lesions may regress either spontaneously or as a result of anticonvulsant drugs alone (Fig. 137-5).

Gupta and colleagues[54] reported on the MRI results of 31 patients with intracranial tuberculomas. In all of the patients, CT scanning showed focal hypodense, hyperdense, or ring lesions. On MRI, solid tuberculomas appeared as isointense with the gray matter in the T1-weighted images and hyperintense in the T2-weighted images. On T1-weighted images, lesions with central caseous necrosis have an isointense or hypointense center with an isointense periphery, depending on the degree of central liquefaction present. On the T2-weighted image, these lesions have central hyperintensity with a hypointense periphery. The central necrosis is better visualized in the T2-weighted image, and even lesions with minimal liquefaction that appeared to be isointense in T1-weighted image are well visualized (Figs. 137-6 to 137-8). Intramedullary tuberculomas appear isointense on T1-weighted images, and on T2-weighted images, the lesion is hypointense, surrounded by a ring of hyperintensity because

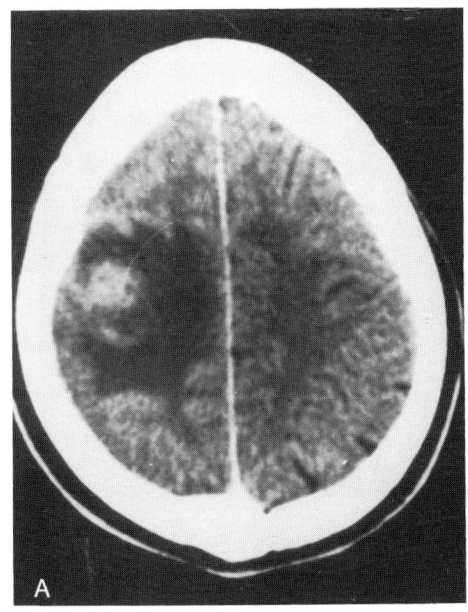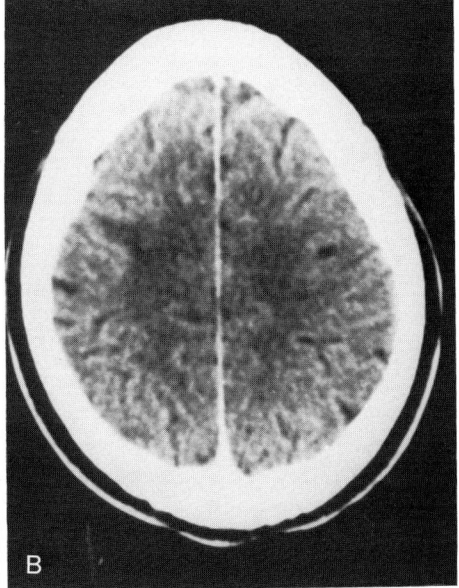

FIGURE 137-5. A contrast-enhanced CT scan of a patient who had right focal motor seizures shows (A) a disc-like lesion with disproportionate surrounding low attenuation, which has disappeared 2 months later (B) on anticonvulsants alone.

1694 | *Intracranial Infections*

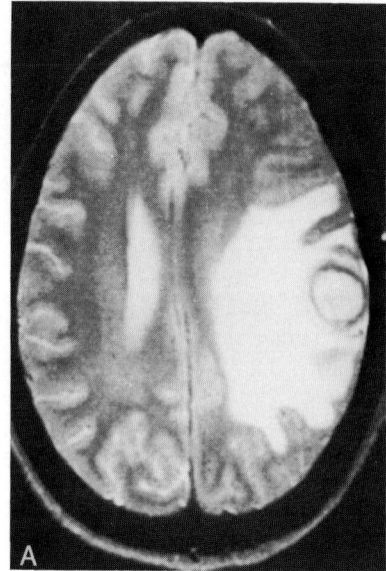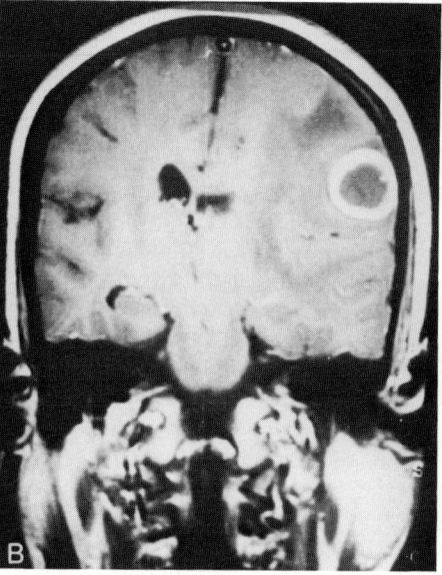

FIGURE 137–6. A 28-year-old man with intractable seizures. (A) Axial T2-weighted image (TR/TE = 2200/90) shows a left parietal lesion that has a thick low-intensity periphery (due to collagen) surrounding a central high-signal intensity (due to caseation). There is significant surrounding edema causing a mass effect. (B) Gadolinium-DTPA–enhanced coronal T1-weighted image (TR/TE = 600/15) demonstrates intense ring enhancement of the granulation tissue.

of the edema commonly accompanying these lesions (Fig. 137–9).

Medical Treatment

Antituberculous Drugs

The drugs generally prescribed nearly always come from a group of six antibiotics known to be effective in the treatment of extracranial tuberculosis (Table 137–3). The first-line agents most commonly used are isoniazide, rifampicin (rifampin), and pyrazinamide, all of which are bactericidal. Ethambutal, a bacteriostatic drug, usually cannot be given for periods longer than 3 or 4 months, but drug therapy is generally required for 16 to 18 months.[4,13,31] Ethambutal is sometimes given as a first-line agent when four drugs are given together, but it is more often used as a second-line drug. Streptomycin and ethionamide[4] are both very valuable second-line drugs. The optimal duration of treatment is not definite, because there are no reports of controlled trials in the treatment of intracranial tuberculomas or tuberculous meningitis apart from the early trials with streptomycin.[58] This is in marked contrast to the treatment of pulmonary tuberculosis, which is based on data obtained from well-controlled trials. At present, three drugs are administered for the initial 3 or 4 months, and two drugs, for an additional 14 to 16 months. Occasionally, the drug treatment may have to be prolonged. In symptomatic intracranial tuberculoma developing during treatment of tuberculous meningitis, antituberculous drugs may be prescribed in larger doses and for 18 months to 3 years.[59] Usually, the regimen involves a combination of rifampicin, isoniazid, and ethambutal for 3 to

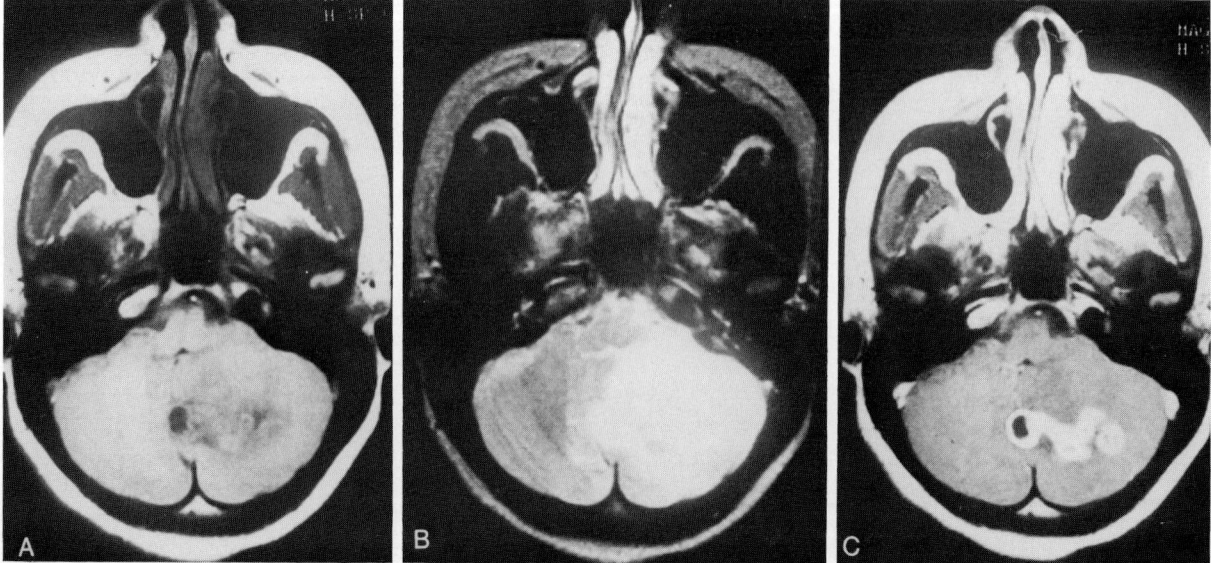

FIGURE 137–7. (A) Axial T1-weighted image (TR/TE = 600/15) shows irregular hypointensity in the vermis and adjoining cerebellar cortex with mass effect. The low-intensity focus close to the midline corresponds to the verified area of necrosis. (B) Axial T2-weighted image (TR/TE = 2200/90) shows nodular low-signal intensities with edema surrounding the lesion. (C) The gadolinium-DTPA–enhanced image (TR/TE = 600/15) demonstrates the pathology to better advantage as a cluster of ring lesions.

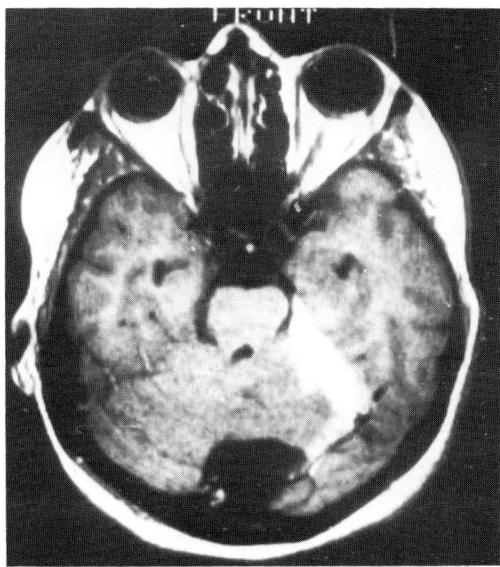

FIGURE 137–8. This MRI of a 25-year-old woman, who had headache and seizures for 5 months, has an atypical appearance. At surgery, the lesion was confirmed as a tentorial tuberculoma.

4 months, followed by isoniazid and rifampicin for an additional 14 months.

Transient disturbance in liver function is often observed in patients taking a combination of isoniazid and rifampicin. The incidence of serious liver disturbance appears to be higher in Asians.[50] Pyridoxine (10 mg/day) is invariably added to prevent peripheral neuropathy due to isoniazid.

Most intracranial tuberculomas resolve with medical therapy.[15, 21, 31, 46–50] The clinical and radiologic improvement is a result of reduction in the size of the tuberculoma and the perilesional edema. Lesions irrespective of their size usually start to regress after 4 to 6 weeks, and most tuberculomas resolve within 12 to 14 months of treatment. Some ring lesions change their character and become disc like or nodular on treatment. In general, patients with raised ICP are slower to respond than those with seizures alone.

In about one third of cases, residual evidence of the lesion is an area of calcification, sometimes just a speck of low attenuation.[31] Medical treatment may occasionally result in liquefaction of the center of the lesion without any reduction in size.[24] In some patients, the tuberculoma may either show no change or actually increase in size on antituberculous drugs.[17] Tuberculomas seem to enlarge and compress the surrounding brain without causing destruction that is usually associated with a malignant tumor; as a result, they can resolve with minimal residual deficits.

Corticosteroids

Corticosteroids are used in the presence of elevated ICP or severe cerebral edema as noted on CT scans. Treatment is seldom prolonged beyond 2 to 3 weeks, during which time the corticosteroid therapy can produce dramatic improvement in the clinical state of the patient. Occasionally, patients require steroids for a much longer period.

Anticonvulsant Medications

The high incidence of seizures with tuberculomas mandates the routine use of anticonvulsants. The drugs used are phenytoin or carbamazepine, adjusted in dosage according to serum levels of the anticonvulsant. Patients taking phenytoin and isoniazid may develop phenytoin toxicity because high levels of isoniazid in the serum can block the metabolism of the anticonvulsant.

Surgery

A tuberculoma that severely elevates ICP and threatens life or vision merits emergent surgical excision. With the exception of these lesions, most neurosurgeons familiar with tuberculomas restrict surgical intervention to (1) patients who do not respond clinically or radiologically to anti-tuberculous drugs; (2) patients whose diagnosis is in doubt, such as those with an atypical CT or MRI image of the lesion; and (3) patients with obstructive hydrocephalus.

Complete excision of tuberculomas is generally reserved for smaller lesions in noneloquent areas of the brain that have been precisely localized on both coronal and sagittal reconstruction of CT scans. Larger lesions require subtotal excision when they cause pressure-related symptoms; rarely is complete removal necessary. An insistence on total excision at the cost of an undesirable neurologic deficit is to be deprecated. In cases of multiple tuberculomas, only the largest mass need be decompressed.

An appropriate craniotomy or craniectomy is performed

Table 137–3. ANTITUBERCULOUS DRUGS

Drug	Dosage	Contraindications	Side Effects
Isoniazid	Oral/IM 300 mg/day (3–10 mg/kg)	Drug-induced liver disease	Peripheral neuritis, psychosis, optic neuritis, occasionally lupus syndrome, convulsions
Rifampicin	Oral 450–600 mg/day (10 mg/kg)	Jaundice, pregnancy	Liver toxicity, gastrointestinal symptoms, rarely shock, respiratory collapse
Ethambutol	Oral (15 mg/kg)	Optic neuritis	Optic neuritis, color blindness, peripheral neuritis
Pyrazinamide	Oral (20–30 mg/kg)	Liver damage	Hepatitis
Streptomycin	IM 1 gm/day (20–25 mg/kg)	Pregnancy	Ototoxicity, renal damage
Ethionamide	Oral (15 mg/kg)	Depression, pregnancy	Gastrointestinal disturbances

IM = intramuscular.

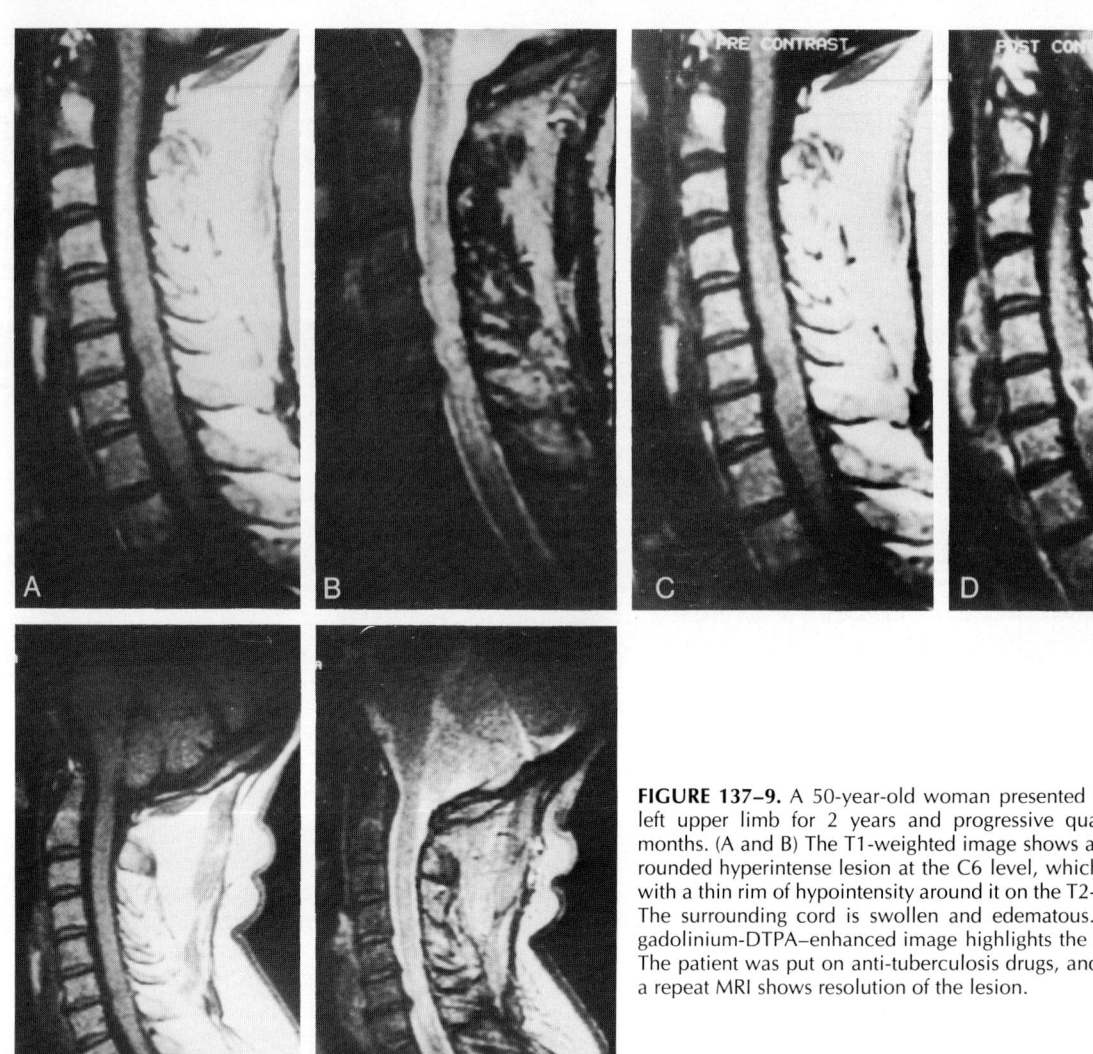

FIGURE 137–9. A 50-year-old woman presented with pain in the left upper limb for 2 years and progressive quadriparesis for 6 months. (A and B) The T1-weighted image shows an intramedullary rounded hyperintense lesion at the C6 level, which is hyperintense with a thin rim of hypointensity around it on the T2-weighted image. The surrounding cord is swollen and edematous. (C and D) The gadolinium-DTPA–enhanced image highlights the lesion. (E and F) The patient was put on anti-tuberculosis drugs, and 3 months later, a repeat MRI shows resolution of the lesion.

over the site of the lesion. A clear plane of cleavage[7, 8, 29, 30, 32, 41] exists between the firm avascular tuberculoma and the edematous brain. The edema is usually not as pronounced as that associated with metastatic deposits. Tuberculous lesions are often on the cortical surface and are adherent to the overlying dura. Although dural adhesions are usually separable with ease, the dural attachment at times can be extremely vascular, resembling meningiomas.[32] After the tumor surface is identified, it is removed piecemeal from within the confines of the granuloma. The ultrasonic aspirator is a useful aid to the decompression. En bloc removal is indicated only for small lesions. Where the center is liquefied or necrotic, aspiration of the contents is sufficient; no attempt should be made to excise the capsule. Subcortical lesions are approached through a small corticectomy with preservation of as many vessels as possible. Peroperative ultrasonography is useful to accurately localize small, deep-seated lesions. The incision is deepened until a tough gliotic layer is encountered. With the aid of magnification and illumination provided by an operating microscope, the tuberculoma is decompressed. Parts of the tuberculoma adherent to major vessels, venous sinus, or brainstem are left in situ. The practice of frontal and temporal lobectomy and ventricular punctures with instillation of streptomycin into the ventricles, if they are opened, is seldom indicated.

Steroids have been advocated when the ventricle is entered during surgery.[29] Precise localization obviates preliminary needling of the brain, and excision of edematous brain is seldom necessary to achieve decompression. After several months' administration of antituberculous drugs, the lesion may be tough in consistency and resistant to curetting. If surgical exploration is undertaken for an atypical lesion and a tuberculoma is encountered, minimal surgical manipulation is advised.

CT- or MRI-guided stereotactic biopsy and aspiration is the preferred mode of diagnosis and treatment for (1) deep-seated lesions, such as those in the thalamus or basal ganglia, and (2) tubercular abscesses or tuberculomas with a liquefied center that can be readily decompressed by this method. Atypical lesions also merit a stereotactic instead of an open biopsy. We prefer to use the Leksell frame and the Backlund biopsy kit for such procedures. Bhatia and associates[48] described 15 tuberculomas of the basal ganglia and thalamus. Two of the 15 lesions were stereotactically aspirated, yielding pus that showed acid-fast bacilli on the smear, which were confirmed as *M. tuberculosis* on culture. Although the first patient, who had earlier received a kidney transplant, improved remarkably, the second patient was left with a residual hemiparesis (see Fig. 137–3).

Chiasmal decompression may be indicated for a suprasellar tuberculoma developing during treatment for tuberculous meningitis.[60] Brainstem tuberculomas are a rarity and seldom require surgical decompression. Pandya and coworkers[24] however, reported on a case of two tuberculomas, one in the hemisphere and the other in the brainstem. The brainstem tuberculoma underwent caseation and liquefaction and required drainage.

A ventriculoperitoneal shunt may be required for a tuberculoma that causes hydrocephalus, resulting either from obstruction of CSF pathway or from associated tuberculous meningitis. Tuberculomas of the pituitary gland are very rare lesions indeed.[25, 26] We have operated on four such patients, none of whom were diagnosed preoperatively. These were all solitary lesions, and three of them were operated on through the transsphenoidal route and one via the subfrontal route. Three patients made a good recovery but required long-term thyroid supplements; the fourth patient died after a stormy postoperative period. He developed diabetes insipidus, hypothermia, and hypotension.

Results

Initial reports of mortality ranged from 10 to 27 percent for intracranial tuberculomas, but the results have improved dramatically in recent years. Harder and coworkers[45] reported no deaths in 20 cases, although two patients were lost to follow-up. In our experience of 50 consecutive cases,[31] one patient died in the hospital, and one died 2 years after treatment, probably as a result of infection with a drug-resistant organism. Both of these patients had multiple tuberculomas and markedly elevated ICP. Numerous reports have been published of patients with deep-seated inaccessible lesions and lesions in the brainstem who have enjoyed excellent recovery.

TUBERCULOUS MENINGITIS

Incidence

Tuberculous meningitis is an uncommon condition in most technologically advanced countries, but it is a major cause of morbidity and mortality in countries where pulmonary tuberculosis is still common. The incidence of tuberculosis in India is around 450 per 100,000 population; in England, 12.2 per 100,000; and in Holland and Australia, about five per 100,000.[4] Tuberculous meningitis is a disease of childhood whose highest incidence is in the first 3 years of life. It is uncommon below the age of 6 months and is rare before the age of 3 months.[61] An increasing incidence in adults has been reported in recent years, not only in technologically advanced countries[62] but also in countries like India.

The major neurosurgical interest in tuberculous meningitis is the occurrence of hydrocephalus, tuberculomas, and rarely, chiasmal arachnoiditis. Hydrocephalus is almost invariable in children who survive for more than 4 to 6 weeks and is most often caused by blockage of the basal cisterns and the sylvian fissures by tubercular exudate in the acute phase of the disease. In more chronic phases, hydrocephalus is caused by vascular adhesive arachnoiditis. In some cases, hydrocephalus may be caused by obstruction at the outlet of the fourth ventricle, less commonly, by obstruction at the level of the aqueduct either as a result of circumferential narrowing of the brainstem by exudates or as a result of an intraluminal tuberculoma. The obstruction to the CSF circulation in tuberculous meningitis often occurs at multiple sites.[61] Tuberculous meningitis may rarely be followed by the development of syringomyelia, despite appropriate chemotherapy.[63]

Problems of Diagnosis

In many patients, the diagnosis of tuberculous meningitis still poses considerable difficulties. Examination of CSF is often inconclusive, tubercle bacilli being found on direct smears in no more than 10 to 15 percent of initial samples. A notable exception was the report of Kennedy and Fallon,[62] who isolated *M. tuberculosis* in 83 percent of 52 patients. As an alternative to bacteriologic methods, several new techniques have been employed to diagnose tuberculous meningitis: (1) enzyme-linked immunosorbent assay to detect *M. tuberculosis* antigen 5 and antimycobacterial antibody in CSF of patients with tubercular meningitis,[64] (2) latex particle agglutination test,[65] and (3) polymerase chain reaction.[66] The diagnosis of tuberculous meningitis is generally made based on the presence of two or more of the following criteria: clinical evidence, evidence of CSF cellular and biochemical findings, an associated tubercular focus elsewhere in the body, and the clinical and CSF response of a suspected case to antituberculous drugs.

Imaging

Computed Tomography

Although normal scan results may be seen in the early stages of tuberculous meningitis, the following features may be demonstrable in the course of the illness: exudates in the basal cisterns, hydrocephalus, infarcts, tuberculomas, and edema in the white matter.[67–70] Contrast enhancement of the meninges is the most characteristic sign and was present in 71 percent of the 183 patients collected from four studies carried out in England, India, Hong Kong, and South Africa.[4] It was seen in the sylvian fissures and around the brainstem and tentorial cisterns. The enhancement is irregular and is unlike the sharply defined enhancement of circulating blood in normal vessels in the fissures and cisterns. This characteristic indicates inflammation and the presence of granulation tissue. Equally common was hydrocephalus involving the lateral, third, and fourth ventricles and present in the first scan in 72 percent of patients.[4] Hydrocephalus was also commoner in the medium to advanced stages of the disease.

In most cases, associated periventricular lucency indicates transependymal CSF flow caused by elevated ICP and is therefore an important sign of impending deterioration. Bullock and Van Dellen[67] pointed out that in tuberculous meningitis, periventricular lucency is likely to be a result of a spread of inflammatory process. Therefore, the degree of hydrocephalus may not reflect the degree of elevation of intraventricular pressure.

Magnetic Resonance Imaging

No consistent or characteristic signal abnormality attributed to meningeal inflammation or basal cistern exudate has been described. When hydrocephalus is present, long TR images show any associated interstitial accumulation of CSF as bilateral, rather uniform periventricular areas of increased intensity. MRI is more sensitive in demonstrating early infarcts than is CT (Fig. 137–10).[71]

Medical Treatment

The drug therapy for tuberculous meningitis and tuberculomas is similar (see Table 137–3). Short-course chemotherapy is well established for treatment of pulmonary tuberculosis but not for extrapulmonary disease. Goel and colleagues[72] reviewed 35 cases of tuberculous meningitis in which chemotherapy was given for periods less than 2 years. Short-term therapy was associated with recrudescence of tuberculous meningitis and in some cases, with the development of deep cerebral infarcts and permanent neurologic deficit. Short-term chemotherapy for tuberculous meningitis is inadequate. Controversy exists regarding the need for intrathecally administered streptomycin in the acute stage of the disease. Although the routine use of intrathecal streptomycin is advocated by some,[73] we seldom use it. It is generally accepted that steroids are a useful adjunct in treating children under 1 year of age, severely ill and toxic patients, and patients threatened with paraplegia. Intrathecal steroids have changed the course of tuberculous meningitis coexisting with associated spinal block and impending paraplegia in patients taking adequate antituberculous drugs with or without oral corticosteroids.

Surgery

Sir Hugh Cairns[74] first advocated ventricular decompression during the acute stage of tuberculous meningitis. Since then, numerous procedures have been tried, and reports have conclusively documented the efficacy of ventriculoatrial or ventriculoperitoneal shunts for this condition.[68, 75–77] The fear of spreading tubercle bacilli through the shunt is unfounded. Hydrocephalus may resolve with medical treatment alone; however, surgical diversion of CSF is indicated when hydrocephalus is associated with symptomatic elevated ICP. Surgery during the early acute stage of the disease to obviate the effects of a progressive increase of intraventricular pressure has been advocated.

Ventriculoperitoneal shunts are generally preferred to ventriculoatrial shunts because of the numerous vascular complications associated with the latter. An unusual complication of ventriculoatrial shunt that we encountered was the development of chronic pulmonary hypertension. This occurred in two adults and one child 3 to 5 years after insertion of the shunt. The probable cause is either recurrent pulmonary thromboembolism from the shunt tube in the right atrium or an autoimmune reaction to the tubercular proteins. After a shunt is inserted, a progressive reduction in size of the ventricles occurs, but the ventricles may not return to normal size. Uncommonly, although the lateral and third ventricles become smaller, the fourth ventricle remains enlarged and becomes isolated from the rest of the CSF pathways. This condition leads to pressure on the brainstem, which is treated either by deroofing the outlet of the fourth ventricle or, more often, by inserting a second shunt from the fourth ventricular cavity. Rarely, optochiasmal arachnoiditis may be responsible for the development of visual deterioration and may indicate a need for decompression of the optic nerves and chiasm.[60] Cerebral tuberculomas can develop insidiously during treatment of tuberculous meningitis,[46, 78, 79] and the patient may die as a result of elevated ICP. CT scans are helpful in

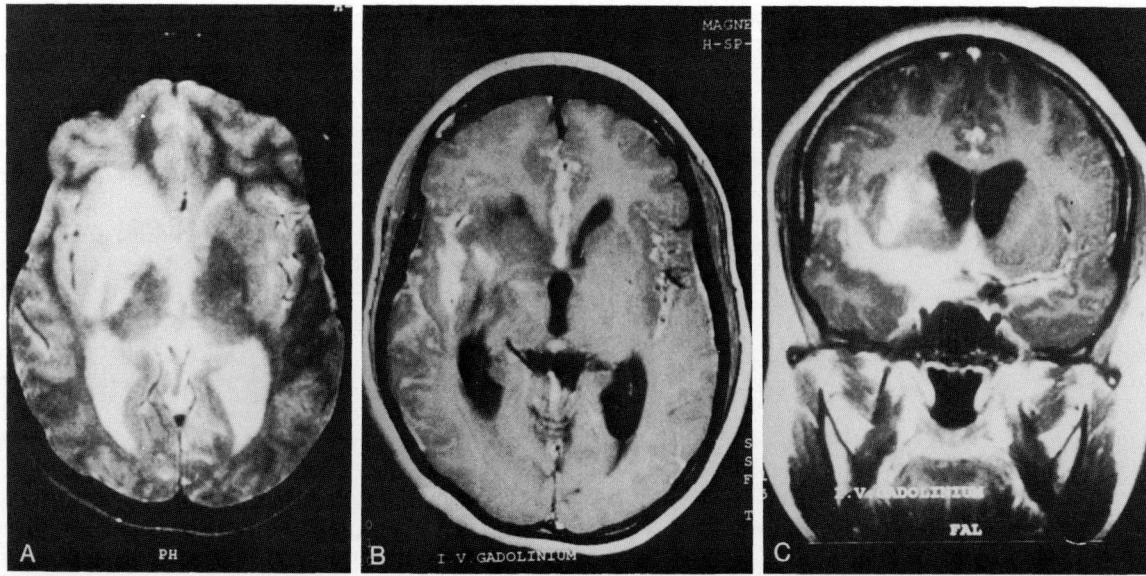

FIGURE 137–10. A 20-year-old woman with tubercular meningitis and left hemiparesis. (A) The axial T2-weighted image (TR/TE = 2200/90) shows focal areas of infarction involving the striatum, the head of the caudate, and the internal capsule. (B and C) Gadolinium-DTPA–enhanced T1-weighted axial and coronal images (TR/TE = 600/15) demonstrate enhancing exudates in the interhemispheric and sylvian fissures, which is more marked on the right side. Note also the enhancement of the leptomeninges over the brain surface.

recognizing and surgically removing these lesions. Infrequently, separate shunts are required from each lateral ventricle if a CSF block is present at the level of the third ventricle.

Results

The prognosis of tuberculous meningitis depends on the patient's level of consciousness, the presence and degree of exudates, and the presence of hydrocephalus. The presence of cerebral infarcts often precludes a good recovery. Palur and coworkers[77] reviewed 114 patients with tuberculous meningitis and hydrocephalus who underwent shunt surgery. During a long-term follow-up period ranging from 6 months to 13 years (mean, 45.6 months), the mortality rate was 20 percent for patients in grade I (headache, vomiting, fever, and neck stiffness with normal sensorium and no neurologic deficit); 34.7 percent for patients in grade II (normal sensorium, neurologic deficit present); 51.9 percent for patients in grade III (altered sensorium but easily arousable with or without dense neurologic deficit); and 100 percent for patients in grade IV (deeply comatosed, decerebrate, or decorticate posturing). Only grade at the time of admission was seen to be statistically significant in determining the final outcome ($p<0.001$). The other factors studied included age at admission, duration of altered sensorium, CSF cell count at initial examination, CSF protein level at initial examination, number of shunt revisions required, and necessity of bilateral shunts. Early shunt surgery is advocated for grade I and II patients. For patients in grade III, surgery may be performed either without a trial of external ventricular drainage or when an improvement in sensorium occurs after such a trial. All patients in grade IV should undergo external ventricular drainage, and only those who show a significant change in their neurologic status within 24 to 48 hours of drainage should undergo shunt surgery.

FUNGAL INFECTIONS

CNS infections due to fungi are much less frequent than those due to bacteria (Table 137–4). Although more than 60 species of fungi have been identified as pathogenic to humans, very few come under the purview of the neurosurgeon. They are broadly divided into two groups: pathogenic, which infect the immunocompetent host, like the dimorphic fungi; and opportunistic, which infect the immunocompromised host (Table 137–5). Susceptibility to fungal infection may result from multiple factors leading to the spread to the CNS of almost any fungus that is capable of growth at body temperature. Some of these undoubtedly can occur in otherwise normal hosts with no obvious immunocompromise. Spread of pathogenic dimorphic fungi, *Cryptococcus neoformans*, or dematiaceous fungi occur more often in elderly males.[80] In contrast, pregnant women are at greater risk for dissemination of *Coccidioides immitis* and the development of meningitis. Ethnic factors may play a role in susceptibility to coccidioidal meningitis, being higher among African-Americans, Filipinos, and Native Americans.

The presence of AIDS and immunocompromise not only increases the susceptibility to mycotic infection but also makes the effects very dramatic. Cryptococcal and candidal infections are two of the commonest fungi afflicting patients with HIV infections: 5 to 10 percent of these patients have cryptococcal meningitis or cryptococcomas.[80]

In a large percentage of cases, the diagnosis is based on the morphology of the fungus in the tissues because by the time a histologic diagnosis is made, the formalin renders the tissue unsuitable for culture. It is also impossible to distinguish between different forms of fungi with certainty, on the basis of the morphology of the lesion at surgery.

PATHOLOGIC FEATURES

C. neoformans and *C. immitis* are the commonest fungi that cause meningitis, and they may do so without any evidence of lesions elsewhere. Species of *Candida* and *Aspergillus* more commonly cause focal abscesses or cerebral infarcts. Among *Candida*, *Candida albicans* is the commonest, followed by *Candida tropicalis*. At least nine species of *Aspergillus* have been detected in the CNS and include most commonly *Aspergillus fumigatus* and *Aspergillus flavus*. *Aspergillus* and species of mucoraceous fungi may extend directly to the brain from paranasal sinuses or other contiguous sites.[80-87] They produce focal brain lesions with or without signs of meningitis. Dimorphic pathogens may cause either meningeal or focal cerebral involvement, such as granuloma or abscess. Dermatiaceous fungi are divided into two groups: those having thick-walled brown bodies (sclerotic cells) and causing characteristic skin lesions, called chromomycosis; and those that invade various sites, including the CNS, called phaeohyphomycosis. These include *Xylohypha bantiana*, a

Table 137–4. INFECTION AND INFESTATIONS OF THE BRAIN (743 SURGICALLY VERIFIED CASES FROM 1965–1992, ALL INDIA INSTITUTE OF MEDICAL SCIENCES HOSPITAL, NEW DELHI)

Type	Incidence (n)
Brain abscess	434
Tuberculomas	165
Parasitic infestations	102
Fungal infections	42
Total	743

Table 137–5. MORPHOLOGIC CLASSIFICATION OF FUNGI

Pathogenic dimorphic (hyphal/filamentous in nature and spherules or yeasts in humans)
Coccidioides immitis
Histoplasma capsulatum
Blastomyces dermatitidis
Paracoccidioides brasiliensis
Sporothrix schenckii
Encapsulated yeasts
Cryptococcus neoformans
Yeasts
Candida sp.
Dematiaceous fungi
Xylohypha (Cladosporium) bantiana
Opportunistic vasculotropic hyphae
Aspergillus sp.
Mucoraceous Zygomycetes

Adapted from Diamond RD: Fungal meningitis, in Lambert HP (ed): Infections of the Central Nervous System. Philadelphia, BC Decker, 1991, pp 229–245.

Table 137–6. FUNGI IDENTIFIED IN 45 PATIENTS IN THE NEUROLOGY AND NEUROSURGERY SERVICES OF ALL INDIA INSTITUTE OF MEDICAL SCIENCES (1965–1992)

Fungus	Patients (n)
Aspergillus	27
Cryptococcus	9
Xylohypha	4
Mucormycosis	3
Unidentified	2

rare cause of fungal brain abscess.[85, 86] The hyphal form may require the Fontana-Masson melanin-specific stain to differentiate it from *Aspergillus* sp. (see Table 137–6 for the types of fungi seen at the AIIMS hospital).

The fungi usually enter the body through the respiratory system by inhalation of aerosolized fungi, or by direct spread from the paranasal sinuses, middle ear, palate, orbit, mastoid, bone, or skin (Table 137–7). A primary focus of infection, often subclinical, is established in the lung, or the fungus may spread by contiguity. Susceptibility to infection[3] is facilitated by: (1) impaired cell-mediated immunity, as in AIDS, organ transplants, corticosteroid therapy, T-cell depletion, and lymphomas (*C. neoformans, C. immitis, Histoplasma,* and *Candida*); (2) granulocyte dysfunction, which may be qualitative, quantitative, or both, as in cytotoxic chemotherapy, hematologic malignancies, diabetes, corticosteroid therapy, malnutrition (*Aspergillus, Candida* sp., and *Mucor*); (3) blood-borne dissemination, as in drug abuse, endocarditis (especially with the use of prosthetic valves), and intravenous fluids (*Candida* sp.); and (4) contiguous infection (members of Mucorales, *Aspergillus*).

Depending on the specific infection and the host factor in the patient, fungal infections take several forms. A chronic granulomatous reaction may lead to a focal granuloma or abscess, or if in the basal meninges, obstructive hydrocephalus. Most of these patients have a long history of symptoms. In the abscence of immunocompromise, meningitis tends to be subacute or chronic. In immunocompromised patients, the course is more rapid and at times acute. The clinical features in either case may not be typical of meningitis because neck stiffness may be mild or absent. Occasionally, associated signs of spinal arachnoiditis may be present. Fever may be low grade or even absent. Rarely, basal meningitis may lead to mycotic aneurysms and subarachnoid hemorrhage. This has been reported in candidal, *Aspergillus,* coccidioidomycosis, and *Mucor* infections.[80, 88]

The second type of infection produces diffuse cerebritis, often with areas of hemorrhagic infarction of the brain, microabscess formation, and intense cerebral edema. The history in these patients is short, often less than 7 to 10 days, and the clinical suspicion of rapidly growing brain tumor or abscess is raised. The third type of infection produces signs similar to those of the second except that in addition, the patients also have an underlying serious disease.

PROBLEMS IN DIAGNOSIS

The first problem in diagnosis is that the illness is often a chronic one, lasting years, and the mildness of the initial symptoms may be misleading. Among 45 cases of fungal granuloma at the AIIMS hospital, fever was present in only nine patients, and evidence of contiguous infection in the paranasal sinuses, orbit, and skin was present in only seven (Table 137–8). Second, the CT or MRI findings in focal granulomas are not distinctive.[83, 89–91] A clue may be provided by involvement of the paranasal sinuses, the orbit, and the frontal bone. The granulomas are indistinguishable from brain tumors and even tuberculomas. Certainly, no features exist by which a fungal abscess can be distinguished from a pyogenic abscess (Figs. 137–11 to 137–13). Gupta and co-workers[91] reported an intracranial *Aspergillus* granuloma that simulated a meningioma on MRI. Third, the diagnosis of a solitary fungal granuloma is seldom made with confidence preoperatively or even intraoperatively. This granuloma has both a macroscopic and microscopic resemblance to tuberculomas. The difficulty is compounded when the fungi in the tissue are few. The presence of numerous foreign body giant cells and fibrosis and the conspicuous absence of caseation necrosis may arouse suspicion of a possible fungal etiology. Routine examination of pus from an abscess for fungi is useful, even when a pyogenic organism has been isolated.

MEDICAL TREATMENT

In the management of fungal infections of the CNS, amphotericin B and flucytosine remain the first line of drug therapy.[80, 81, 83, 87, 92–95] Amphotericin B has a wider spectrum than flucytosine and is administered intravenously, intrathecally and intraventricularly, or intracavitarily through an Ommaya or Rickham-type reservoir.[57] The starting dose is 0.25mg/kg/day; this dosage is gradually increased, if tolerated, to 1 mg/kg to reach a total dose of 2 grams over a

Table 137–7. SINUS INVOLVEMENT OF FUNGAL INFECTIONS (7 PATIENTS), ALL INDIA INSTITUTE OF MEDICAL SCIENCES (1965–1992)

Sinus	Patients (n)
Maxillary	3
Sphenoid	2
Frontal	1
Ethmoid	1

Table 137–8. CLINICAL FEATURES IN 45 PATIENTS WITH FUNGAL LESIONS (1965–1992), ALL INDIA INSTITUTE OF MEDICAL SCIENCES

Clinical Feature	Incidence (n)
Elevated intracranial pressure	29
Drowsiness	16
Seizures	10
Impaired vision	12
Fever	9
Skin lesions	2
Proptosis	3
Nasal obstruction	1
Compressive myelopathy	1

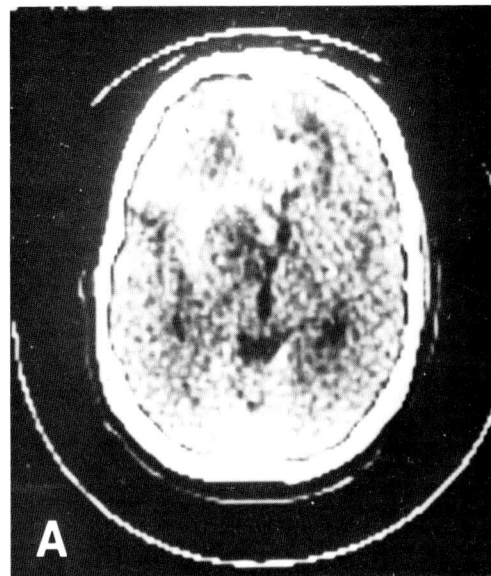
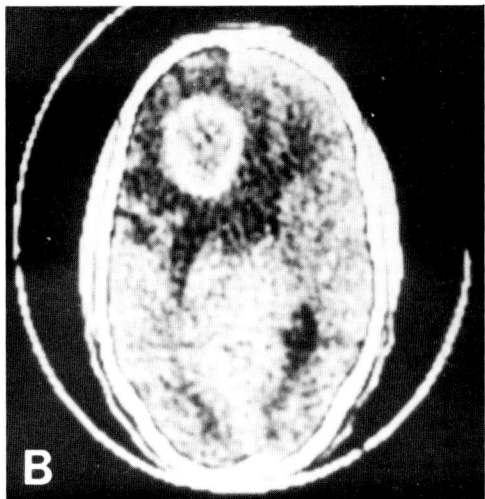

FIGURE 137–11. Aspergillosis. (A) In this patient, the aspergillosis appears as a diffuse frontal mass. (B) In this patient, the aspergillosis appears as a well-defined enhancing lesion.

period of 6 weeks. The maximum dose in severely ill patients is 1.5 mg/kg/day, given on alternate days, dissolved in 500 ml 5-percent glucose in a very slow drip. These patients usually also receive steroids. Because amphotericin B is nephrotoxic, frequent determinations of blood urea and serum creatinine levels are required. Toxicity is reduced by giving the patient an intravenous infusion of mannitol. Nausea, vomiting, fever, and hypokalemia are common side effects. Flucytosine has a narrower spectrum, is less toxic, and, unlike amphotericin B, can be absorbed orally. It is given at a dose of 150 to 200 mg/kg/day in divided doses. This drug is toxic to the liver and blood.

The imidazole group of antifungal drugs, miconazole and ketoconazole, have been used as alternatives to amphotericin B because of the toxicity of amphotericin B and because some patients are partially or completely resistant to it.[96]

Shehab and associates[97] showed good results with oral ketoconazole and intraventricular miconazole in nine children with coccidioidal meningitis. Four patients received amphotericin B earlier and had no improvement and also developed severe toxicity. Five patients were treated with only imidazoles. All the patients had ventriculitis, and ventriculoperitoneal shunts were inserted. No relapse or recrudescence occurred in a follow-up period of 82 to 90 months.

Miconazole is coupled to a castor oil carrier, which is responsible for some of the hypersensitivity reactions. The drug can be given intravenously or intrathecally.[97] Oral ketoconazole is potentially hepatotoxic and should be used with care in patients with hepatic involvement. Newer oral triazoles appear promising. Itraconazole can be given orally and seems to have fewer side effects than earlier-generation agents. It also has greater in vitro activity against *Aspergillus*.

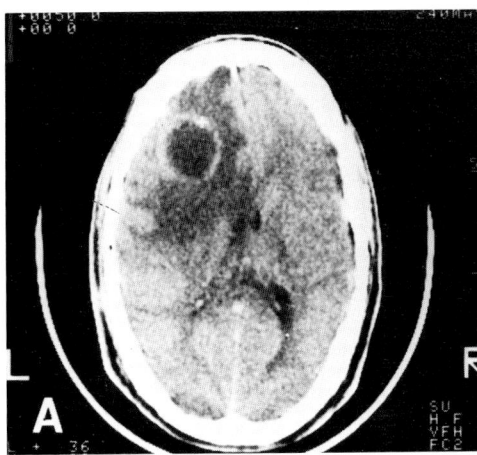
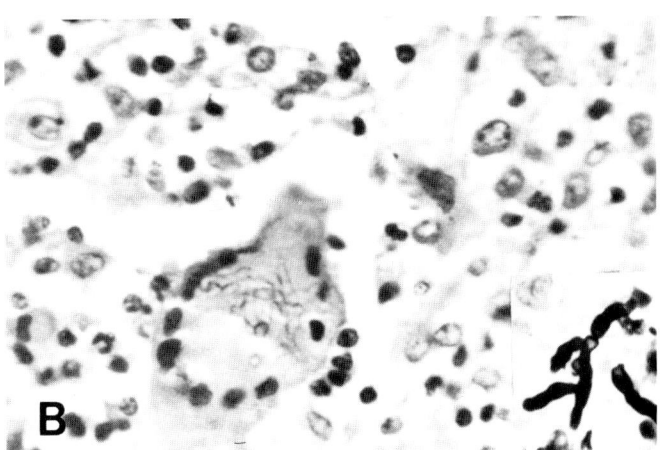

FIGURE 137–12. *Xylohypha bantiana* (Cladosporium) abscess in a 40-year-old patient. (A) A CT scan shows a typical abscess. (B) A photomicrograph of the fungal abscess. Note the giant cells containing fungal hyphae. Inset: Specimen stained with silver methiamine showing branching hyphae. Magnification: × 240.

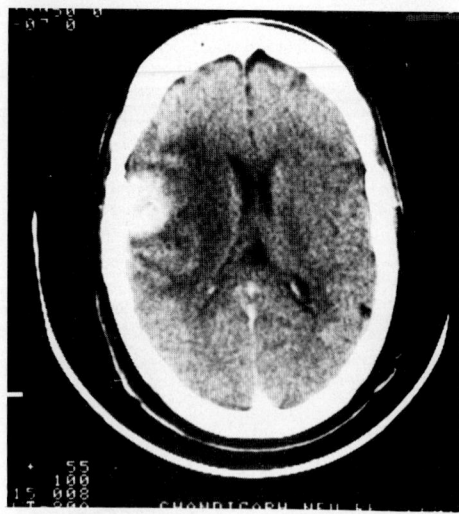

FIGURE 137-13. Cryptococcal granuloma in a 56-year-old patient. The patient had been treated for a tuberculoma, and the lack of response mandated excision.

Adjuvant therapy, like hyperbaric oxygen, has been tried with some success in patients with rhinocerebral mucormycosis.[98]

SURGERY

Surgery (Table 137-9) is indicated for focal granulomas or abscesses and for obstructive hydrocephalus. Fungal granulomas resemble tuberculomas except that they tend to have a more fibrous consistency. They often need to be cut with a knife or scissors and resist curetting. The ultrasonic aspirator is seldom of use. The clear plane of cleavage seen with tuberculomas is usually not present, and adherence to the dura is firmer, particularly to the basal dura. Unlike tuberculomas, a fungal granuloma should be completely excised whenever possible. If pus aspirated from an abscess reveals evidence of a fungal infection, the abscess needs to be excised. Deep-seated lesions in the basal ganglia and thalamus are best stereotactically biopsied or aspirated.[95, 99] Ventriculoperitoneal shunt, unilateral or bilateral, may be necessary to relieve symptoms of elevated ICP.[93, 94] Cryptococcal meningoencephalitis may appear as pseudotumor cerebri with narrowed ventricles, requiring bilateral decompression. Antifungal drugs are complementary to surgical therapy. Insertion of an Ommaya or Rickham reservoir may be required for instillation of drugs into the ventricles or into the abscess cavity.[95] Diagnosis of the intracranial lesion may be obtained when the paranasal sinuses are involved. A transsphenoidal, transethmoidal, or maxillary antrum biopsy may give a clue to the diagnosis. Occasionally, a skin lesion biopsy may be diagnostic. Fungal lesions causing compressive myelopathy are exceedingly rare. The single case occurring in our series resulted from an *Aspergillus* extradural granuloma with involvement of the vertebral body and adjacent ribs.

Results

Among 37 patients who had surgery for brain or spinal cord lesions, 12 patients died in the postoperative period, and two patients died 11 months and 2 years later, respectively. Four patients were unchanged or worse after surgery. Nineteen patients who came for regular follow-up (9 months to 10 years) after surgery have remained well. Suprisingly, four patients who did not receive antifungal drugs recovered. All of them had been operated on in the earlier years and had radical excision of the lesion.

Table 137-9. SURGICAL MANAGEMENT OF FUNGAL LESIONS IN 39 PATIENTS (1965-1992), ALL INDIA INSTITUTE OF MEDICAL SCIENCES

Excision of lesion	
Granuloma	23
Abscess*	8
Shunts†	3
Biopsy	
Transethmoidal	1
Lymph node	1
Bilateral decompression	1
Decompression of sequestrated ventricles	1
Laminectomy	1

*Two patients had preliminary aspiration.
†Two patients received shunts in addition to excision of the lesion.

Acknowledgment

We are grateful to Professor AK Banerji, who operated on many of these patients and was a constant source of new ideas on their management; to Professor RK Goulatia, for neuroradiologic assistance; and to Dr. SK Aggarwal, who has kindly provided the magnetic resonance images. The secretarial help of Ms. Poonam is gratefully acknowledged.

REFERENCES

1. Murray CJL: World tuberculosis burden. Lancet 335:1043-1044, 1990
2. Slutkin G, Leowski J, Mann J: Tuberculosis and AIDS. The effect of the AIDS epidemic on the tuberculosis problem and tuberculosis programmes. Bull Int Union Tuberc Lung Dis 63:21-24, 1988
3. Davidson PT: Tuberculosis—New views of an old issue. N Engl J Med 312:1514-1515, 1985
4. Teoh R, Humphries MJ: Tuberculous meningitis, in Lambert HP (ed): Infections of the Central Nervous System. Philadelphia, BC Decker, 1991, p 189
5. Tang LM, Swash M: Tuberculosis of the nervous system, a modern problem. J R Soc Med 78:429-432, 1985
6. Lalitha VS, Dastur DK: Tuberculosis of the central nervous system: II. Brain tuberculomas vis-a-vis intracranial space-occupying lesions, 1953-1978. Neurol India 28:202-206, 1980
7. Asenjo A, Valladeres H, Fierro J: Tuberculoma of the brain. Arch Neurol 65:146-160, 1951
8. Arseni C: Two hundred and one cases of tuberculoma treated surgically. J Neurol Neurosurg Psychiatry 21:308-311, 1958
9. Welchman JM: Computerized tomography of intracranial tuberculoma. Clin Radiol 30:567-573, 1979
10. Ohaegbulam SC, Amuta J, Saddeqi N: Tuberculoma of the central nervous system in eastern Nigeria. Tubercle 60:163-166, 1979
11. Tang LM, Chee CY, Cheng SY, et al: Neurological complications of tuberculous meningitis, in Sixth Asian and Oceanian Congress of Neurology Abstracts. Amsterdam, Excerpta Medica, 1983, pp 93-94
12. Katsura S, Suzuki J, Wada T: A statistical study of brain tumors in the neurosurgical clinics of Japan. J Neurosurg 16:570-580, 1959
13. Mayers MM, Kaufman DM, Miller MH: Recent cases of intracranial tuberculomas. Neurology 28:256-260, 1978
14. Armstrong FB, Edwards AM: Intracranial tuberculoma in native races

of Canada, with special reference to symptomatic epilepsy and neurologic features. Can Med Assoc J 89:56–65, 1963
15. Peatfield RC, Shawdon HH: Five cases of intracranial tuberculoma followed by serial computerized tomography. J Neurol Neurosurg Psychiatry 42:373–379, 1979
16. Maurice-Williams RS: Tuberculomas of the brain in Britain. Postgrad Med J 48:678–681, 1972
17. Chambers ST, Hendrickse WA, Record C, et al: Paradoxical expansion of intracranial tuberculomas during chemotherapy. Lancet i:181–184, 1984
18. Anderson JM, MacMillan JJ: Intracranial tuberculoma—An increasing problem in Britain. J Neurol Neurosurg Psychiatry 38:194–201, 1975
19. Hirsch LF, Lee SH, Silberstein SD: Intracranial tuberculoma and the CAT scan. Acta Neurochir (Wien) 45:155–161, 1978
20. Wilkinson HA, Ferris EJ, Muggia AL, et al: Central nervous system tuberculosis. A persistant disease. J Neurosurg 34:15–22, 1971
21. Leibrock L, Epstein MH, Rybock JD: Cerebral tuberculoma localized by EMI scan. Surg Neurol 5:305–306, 1976
22. Lehrer H, Venkatesh B, Girolamo R, et al: Tuberculoma of the brain (revisited). AJR 118:594–600, 1973
23. Mahanta A, Kalra L, Maheshwari MC, et al: Brain stem tuberculoma—An unusual presentation. J Neurol 227:249–253, 1982
24. Pandya SK, Desai AD, Dastur HM: Caseative liquefaction within brain stem tuberculoma under drug therapy with simultaneous regression of cerebral tuberculomas. Neurol India 30:121–128, 1982
25. Choudhary C, Mehta VS, Roy S: Tuberculoma of anterior pituitary. A case report. Neurol India 34:341–344, 1986
26. Brooks PH, Dumlao JS, Bronsky D, Waldstein SS: Hypophysial tuberculoma with hypopituitarism. Am J Med 54:777–781, 1973
27. Jena A, Banerji AK, Tripathi RP, et al: Demonstration of intramedullary tuberculomas by magnetic resonance imaging: A report of two cases. Br J Radiol 64:555–558, 1991
28. Rhoton EL, Ballinger WE Jr, Quisling R, Sypert GW: Intramedullary spinal tuberculoma. Neurosurgery 22:733–736, 1988
29. Mathai KV, Chandy J: Tuberculous infection of the nervous system. Clin Neurosurg 14:145–177, 1966
30. Dastur HM: Tuberculoma, in Vinken PJ, Bruyn GW (eds): Handbook of Clinical Neurology, vol 18. New York, Elsevier, 1975, pp 413–426
31. Tandon PN, Bhargava S: Effect of medical treatment on intracranial tuberculoma—A CT study. Tubercle 66:85–97, 1985
32. Ramamurthi B, Varadarajan MG: Diagnosis of tuberculomas of the brain. J Neurosurg 18:1–7, 1961
33. Dinakar I, Seetharam W, Leelanaidu PS, et al: Tuberculous granuloma associated with a congenital dermal sinus. Neurol India 22:207–208, 1974
34. Bishberg E, Sunderam G, Reichman LB, Kapila R: Central nervous system tuberculosis with the aquired immunodeficiency syndrome and its related complex. Ann Intern Med 105:210–213, 1986
35. Dastur DK: Neurosurgically relevant aspects of pathology and pathogenesis of intracranial and intraspinal tuberculosis. Neurosurg Rev 6:103–110, 1983
36. Sinh G, Pandya SK, Dastur DK: Pathogenesis of unusual intracranial tuberculomas and tuberculous space-occupying lesions. J Neurosurg 29:149–159, 1968
37. Sandhyamani S, Roy S, Bhatia R: Tuberculous brain abscess. Acta Neurochir (Wien) 59:247–256, 1981
38. Dannenberg AM Jr, Sugimoto M: Liquefaction of caseous foci in tuberculosis. Am Rev Respir Dis 113:257–259, 1976
39. Dastur DK, Dave UP: Further observations on the fine structure of blood vessels in neurotuberculosis: Possible significance of vasculitis with proliferated basement membrane, in Cervos-Navarro J, Betz E, Ebhardt G, Ferszt R, and Wüllenweber (eds): Advances in Neurology. Vol 20. New York, Raven Press, 1978, pp 577–589
40. Radhakrishnan VV, Mathai A, Radhakrishnan NS: Immunohistochemical demonstration of mycobacterial antigen in intracranial tuberculoma. Indian J Exp Biol 29:641–644, 1991
41. Tandon PN, Pathak SN: Tuberculosis of the central nervous system, in Spillane JD (ed): Tropical Neurology. London, Oxford University Press, 1973, pp 51–62
42. Dastur HM, Desai AD: A comparative study of brain tuberculomas and gliomas based upon 107 case records of each. Brain 88:375–396, 1965
43. Bhargava S, Tandon PN: CNS tuberculosis—lessons learnt from CT studies. Neurol India 28:207–212, 1980
44. Bhargava S, Tandon PN: Intracranial tuberculomas—A CT study. Br J Radiol 53:935–945, 1980
45. Harder E, Al-Kawl MZ, Carney P: Intracranial tuberculomas—Conservative management. Am J Med 74:570–576, 1983
46. Lees AJ, MacLeod AF, Marshall J: Cerebral tuberculomas developing during treatment of tuberculosis meningitis. Lancet i:1208–1211, 1980
47. Vengsarkar US, Pisipaty RP, Parekh B, et al: Intracranial tuberculoma and the CT scan. J Neurosurg 64:568–574, 1986
48. Bhatia R, Tandon PN, Misra NK: Inflammatory lesions of the basal ganglia and thalamus: Review of twenty-one cases. Neurosurgery 19:983–988, 1986
49. Teoh R, Humphries MJ, Hoare RD, O'Mahony G: Clinical correlation of CT changes in 64 Chinese patients with tuberculous meningitis. J Neurol 236:48–51, 1989
50. Traub M, Colchester ACF, Kingsley, Swash M: Tuberculosis of the central nervous system. Q J Med 209:81–100, 1984
51. Goulatia RK, Verma A, Mishra NK, Ahuja GK: Disappearing CT lesions in epilepsy. Epilepsia 28:523–527, 1987
52. Wadia RS, Makhale CN, Kelkar AV, Grant KB: Focal epilepsy in India with special reference to lesions showing ring or disc-like enhancement on contrast computed tomography. J Neurol Neurosurg Psychiatry 50:1298–1301, 1987
53. Ahuja GK, Behari M, Prasad K, et al: Disappearing CT lesions in epilepsy: Is tuberculosis or cysticercosis the cause? J Neurol Neurosurg Psychiatry 52:915–916, 1989
54. Chandy MJ, Rajshekhar V, Prakash S, et al: Cysticercosis causing single small CT lesions in Indian patients with epilepsy. Lancet i:390–391, 1989
55. Rajshekhar V: Etiology and management of single small CT lesion in patients with seizures: Understanding a controversy. Arch Neurol Scand 84:465–470, 1991
56. Chandy MJ, Rajshekhar VR, Ghosh S, et al: Single small enhancing CT lesions in Indian patients with epilepsy: Clinical radiological and pathological considerations. J Neurol Neurosurg Psychiatry 54:702–705, 1991
57. Gupta RK, Jena A, Singh AK, et al: Role of magnetic resonance (MR) in the diagnosis and management of intracranial tuberculoma. Clin Radiol 41:1200–127, 1990
58. Medical Research Council (Streptomycin in Tuberculosis Trials Committee): Streptomycin treatment of tuberculous meningitis. Lancet i:582, 1948
59. Teoh R, Humphries MJ, O'Mahony G: Sympatomatic intracranial tuberculoma developing during treatment of tuberculosis: A report of 10 patients and review of the literature. Q J Med 241:449–460, 1987
60. Teoh R, Poon W, Humphries MJ, O'Mahony G: Suprasellar tuberculoma developing during treatment of tuberculous meningitis requiring urgent surgical decompression. J Neurol 235:321–322, 1988
61. Tandon PN, Bhatia R, Bhargava S: Tuberculous meningitis, in Vinken PK, Bruyn GW, Klawans HL (eds): Handbook of Clinical Neurology, vol 8. Amsterdam, Elsevier Science Publisher, 1988, pp 195–226
62. Kennedy DH, Fallon RJ: Tuberculous meningitis. JAMA 241:264–268, 1984
63. Fehlings MG, Bernstein M: Syringomyelia as a complication of tuberculous meningitis. Can J Neurol Sci 19:84–87, 1992
64. Radhakrishnan VV, Mathai A: Enzyme-linked immunosorbent assay to detect *Mycobacterium tuberculosis* antigen 5 and antimycobacterial antibody in cerebrospinal fluid of patients with tubercular meningitis. J Clin Lab Anal 5:233–237, 1991
65. Shankar P, Manjunath N, Shriniwas, et al: Rapid diagnosis of tuberculous meningitis by polymerase chain reaction. Lancet 337:5–7, 1991
66. A new diagnostic test for tuberculous meningitis (editorial). Tubercle 66:157, 1985
67. Bullock MRR, Van Dellen JR: The role of cerebrospinal fluid shunting in tuberculous meningitis. Surg Neurol 18:274–276, 1982
68. Upadhyaya P, Bhargava S, Sundaram KP, et al: Hydrocephalus caused by tuberculous meningitis—Clinical picture, CT findings, and results of shunt surgery. Z Kinderchir 38:76–79, 1983
69. Bhargava S, Gupta AK, Tandon PN: Tuberculous meningitis—A CT study. Br J Radiol 55:189–196, 1982
70. Kingsley DPE, Hendrickse WA, Kendall BE, et al: Tuberculous meningitis: Role of CT in management and prognosis. J Neurol Neurosurg Psychiatry 50:30–36, 1987
71. Brown BC, Post MJD: Intracranial infections, in Atlas SW (ed): Magnetic Resonance Imaging of the Brain and Spine. New York, Raven Press, 1991, pp 520–523
72. Goel A, Pandya SK, Satoskar AR: Whither short course chemotherapy meningitis? Neurosurgery 27:418–421, 1990
73. Anonymous: Tuberculous meningitis in children. BMJ 1:1–2, 1971

74. Cairns H: Neurosurgical methods in the treatment of tuberculous meningitis with a note on some of the unusual manifestations of the disease. Arch Dis Child 26:373–386, 1951
75. Bullock MRR, Welchman JM: Diagnostic and prognostic features of tuberculous meningitis on CT scanning. J Neurol Neurosurg Psychiatry 45:1098–1101, 1982
76. Bhagwati SN: Ventriculoatrial shunts in tuberculous meningitis with hydrocephalus. J Neurosurg 35:309–313, 1971
77. Palur R, Rajshekhar V, Chandy MJ, et al: Shunt surgery for hydrocephalus in tuberculous meningitis. A long-term follow up study. J Neurosurg 74:64–69, 1991
78. Borah NC, Maheshwari MC, Mishra NK, et al: Appearance of tuberculoma during the course of TB meningitis. J Neurol 231:269–270, 1984
79. Lebas J, Malkin JE, Coquin Y, et al: Cerebral tuberculomas developing during treatment of tuberculous meningitis. Lancet ii:84, 1980
80. Diamond RD: Fungal meningitis, in Lambert HP (ed): Infections of the Central Nervous System. Philadelphia, BC Decker, 1991, pp 229–245
81. Utz JP: Fungal infection of the central nervous system. Clin Neurosurg 14:86–100, 1966
82. Mohandas S, Ahuja GK, Sood VP, et al: Aspergillosis of the central nervous system. J Neurol Sci 38:229–233, 1978
83. Mehta VS, Bhatia R, Mahapatra AK, et al: Intracranial mycotic infection in nonimmunosuppressed individuals. J Indian Med Assoc 83:185–188, 1985
84. Deshpande DH, Desai AP, Dastur HM: Aspergillosis of the central nervous system. Neurol India 23:167–175, 1975
85. Sandhyamani S, Bhatia R, Mohapatra LN, Roy S: Cerebral cladosporiosis. Surg Neurol 15:431–434, 1981
86. Banerjee U, Mohapatra AK, Sarkar C, Chaudhery R: Cladosporiosis (cerebral phoeohyphomycosis) of brain—A case report. Mycopathologia 105:163–166, 1989
87. Kelly PC: Coccidioidal meningitis, in Stevens DA (ed): Coccidioidomycosis: A Text. New York, Plenum Medical Book Company, 1980, pp 163–193
88. Ahuja GK, Jain N, Vijayaraghavan M, Roy S: Cerebral mycotic aneurysm of fungal origin. J Neurosurg 49:107–110, 1978
89. Tully RJ, Watts C: Computed tomography and intracranial aspergillosis. Neuroradiology 17:111–113, 1979
90. Harper CG: Cryptococcal granuloma presenting as a mass lesion. Surg Neurol 11:425, 1979
91. Gupta R, Singh AK, Bishnu P, Malhotra V: Intracranial aspergillus granuloma simulating meningioma on MR imaging. J Comput Assist Tomogr 14:467–469, 1990
92. Sapico FL: Dissappearance of focal cryptoccoccal brain lesion on chemotherapy alone. Lancet i:560, 1979
93. Chan KH, Mann KS, Yue CP: Neurosurgical aspects of cerebral cryptococcosis. Neurosurgery 25:44–47, 1989
94. Tang LM: Ventriculoperitoneal shunt in cryptococcal meningitis with hydrocephalus. Surg Neurol 33:314–319, 1990
95. Camarata PJ, Dunn DL, Farney AC, et al: Continuous intracavitary administration of amphotericin B as an adjunct in the treatment of aspergillus brain abscess: Case report and review of the literature. Neurosurgery 31:575–579, 1992
96. Weinstein L, Jacoby I: Successful treatment of cerebral cryptococcoma and meningitis with miconazole. Ann Intern Med 93:569–571, 1980
97. Shehab ZM, Britton H, Dunn JH: Imidazole therapy of coccidioidal meningitis in children. Pediatr Infect Dis J 7:40–44, 1988
98. Ferguson BJ, Mitchell TG, Moon R, et al: Adjunctive hyperbaric oxygen for treatment of rhinocerebral mucormycosis. Rev Infect Dis 10:551–559, 1988
99. Goodmen ML, Coffey RJ: Stereotactic drainage of *Aspergillus* brain abscess with long-term survival: Case report and review. Neurosurgery 24:96–99, 1989

SELECTED READING

Lambert HP (ed): Infections of the Central Nervous System. Philadelphia, BC Decker, 1991
Mathai KV, Chandy J: Tuberculous infection of the nervous system. Clin Neurosurg 14:145, 1966
Tandon PN, Bhatia R, Bhargava S: Tuberculous meningitis, in Vinken PJ, Bruyn GW, Klawans HL: Handbook of Clinical Neurology. Amsterdam, Elsevier Science Publishers, 1988, pp 195–226

CHAPTER 138

Neurosurgical Aspects of Neurocysticercosis

Francisco Escobedo

Most parasites that reach nervous tissue do so hematogenously. Considering the number of parasites that exist, it is surprising that so few cases of central nervous system (CNS) invasion occur. This relatively low incidence is probably the result of the protection afforded by the blood-brain barrier[1] and certain immunologic reactions that are not well understood.

The most important determinant of the incidence of parasitic diseases is the hygienic character of the environment. These diseases are seen more frequently in geographic areas in which sanitary control of the water supply, agricultural systems, and food handling is poor. A tropical climate also favors the development of some parasites, and these disorders have often been considered tropical diseases. However, parasitic disorders are being seen with increasing frequency in industrialized nations because of the migration of infected persons from endemic areas. Parasitic infections of the CNS have spread to groups and countries in which such diseases were previously rare.[2,3] Parasitic diseases affecting the CNS include amebiasis, malaria, coenurosis, echinococcosis, schistosomiasis, paragonimiasis, trichinosis, filariasis, angiostrongyliasis, *Toxocara canis* encephalitis, and gnathostomiasis. Most of these disorders are not treated surgically. The discussion in this chapter is restricted to cysticercosis, the most common of these disorders affecting the CNS, for which surgical treatment is indicated.

CYSTICERCOSIS

Human cysticercosis results when a person serves as the intermediate host of *Taenia solium*, the porcine tapeworm; the larvae develop in various body tissues. The presence of the encysted larvae in the nervous tissue, its cavities, or its coverings constitutes the disease known as neurocysticercosis. The cysts are called *Cysticercus cellulosae*.[4]

T. solium infestation is endemic in parts of Asia (India and China), Africa, Eastern Europe, Indonesia, and Latin America. Cases occur sporadically in other parts of the world. The incidence varies according to the economic and social condition, as reflected in the level of hygiene of a region, with the lower socioeconomic groups having a higher incidence of the disease.[1-5]

In Mexico, between 5 and 10 percent of all patients requiring surgery on the CNS are operated on for cysticercosis. These patients constitute approximately 25 percent of all patients operated on for increased intracranial pressure.[6] In a study we conducted at the Institute of Neurology and Neurosurgery in Mexico between 1964 and 1969, 206 cases were diagnosed: this number corresponded to 3.1 percent of all patients undergoing neurologic surgery in those years. Fifty-three percent of these patients required surgical therapy. Of the 206 cases, 153 improved, 27 remained unchanged, and 26 died.[7,8] In another study conducted between 1976 and 1986 that corresponded with the first 10 years computed tomography (CT) was used, 519 neurocysticercosis cases demanded 889 surgical operations, a figure representing 13 percent of all neurosurgical operations in that period. The increase in the number of cases is not the result of a higher incidence of the disease but of a more accessible way to diagnose the disease through CT. During the same period and at the same institution, 5.4 percent of inpatients and 10.3 percent of autopsies revealed neurocysticercosis.[9] At the National Medical Center of Mexico City, cysticerci were found in the brain of three of every 100 autopsied adults.[10] This chapter is based on our experience in the management of approximately 1000 cases of neurocysticercosis.

THE PARASITE AND ACQUISITION OF INFECTION

In the usual cycle of transmission, only the pig harbors the larval stage of *T. solium*; human beings acquire the adult tapeworm by eating undercooked pork. The larval infection is acquired through the ingestion of food contaminated with *T. solium* eggs, each of which contains an active embryo or oncosphere. The oncospheres are liberated by digestive juices. They then penetrate the wall of the small intestine and burrow into the vessels, from which they are carried to distant sites. The organisms lodge in various tissues, mainly muscle, skin, brain, and eye.[1-4]

PATHOPHYSIOLOGY

Once the embryos have arrived in the brain, they go through different biologic stages:

ENCEPHALITIC STAGE. This stage is characterized by a focal inflammatory reaction with local brain edema that could produce symptoms like headache and, in certain cases, focal seizures.

CYSTIC STAGE. If the parasites are not destroyed, they grow and develop into larvae, or cysticerci, in 60 to 70 days. This is the most common form and the best known. The typical cysticerci have an ovoid form and are about half an inch in diameter, consisting of a very fragile membrane, fluid, and a scolex with suckers and hooks. The cysts can live in tissue for long periods of time.

Cysticerci most commonly lodge in the brain and skeletal muscle. The larvae vary in size from about 5 mm to about 5 cm. Cysticerci can lodge in the parenchyma of the brain (around 60 percent), the subarachnoid space (meningobasal and cortical, in around 40 percent), the ventricular system (in around 10 percent), mixed areas (in more than 50 percent), and the spine (in nearly 1 percent).

The location, number, and size of these lesions determine the clinical manifestations.[1,6,11] The manifestations are also the result of focal and mass effect and of the inflammatory response to the cysticerci in the nervous tissue, the meninges, or the vessels; the focal effect; the mass effect; and the effect of obstruction of the foramina, ventricular system, subarachnoid space, and cisterns of the brain.

Cysts can lodge in the ventricular system and cause an obstructive hydrocephalus, either because of the cysts themselves or because of the inflammatory response they incite. Endothelial proliferation can occur in the cerebral arteries and arterioles as a result of vasculitis, and the vessel may become occluded. These processes can coexist in the same patient (Table 138–1). The combination of these factors and the distribution of the lesions makes neurocysticercosis a pleomorphic disease. Except when acute massive exposure exists, symptoms appear only after a latent period of a few years, because in most cases, viable cysts incite little inflammatory response from the host.[1,8,12]

The number of cysts, the duration of the illness, the location of cerebral cysticerci, their enlargement, and the local inflammatory response they provoke can lead to a clinical syndrome with focal neurologic manifestations, cranial nerve palsies, or a tumorlike presentation.

RACEMOSE FORM. When a group of cysts develop together and are located at the deepest portions of the fissures or at the base of the brain in the subarachnoid space, they incite chronic meningitis and arachnoiditis, after which a communicating or noncommunicating hydrocephalus frequently develops.

PARTIALLY DEGENERATED STAGE. The cyst partially degenerates, the clear fluid content becomes jellylike, and it is no longer viable.

TOTALLY DEGENERATED STAGE. Should the cysts degenerate, a lipocalcareous infiltration develops and becomes calcified, making them easier to diagnose from CT scan.[5,11]

CLINICAL SIGNS AND SYMPTOMS

The disease follows an idiosyncratic course, depending on the individual's immune response, the severity of infestation, the location of the cysts, and the size, site, and number of neurologic lesions. If the cysticerci are single or few in number and are lodged in a nonstrategic area of the brain, no signs of disease may be present, as has been seen in around 75 percent of the cases, according to necropsy series.[10] If large numbers of cysts are present or if they lodge in eloquent areas of the CNS, seizures, focal deficits, increased intracranial pressure secondary to mass effect of communicating and noncommunicating hydrocephalus, and meningitis may develop. Frequently, the predominating signs or symptoms change during the course of infection. Focal, jacksonian, or generalized seizures occur in anywhere from 30 to 92 percent of patients, depending on the reported series. Headache is practically universal in patients with hydrocephalus. Nausea, vomiting, impaired vision, confusion, dizziness, and ataxia are also common manifestations of the disease. Papilledema and changes in mental status frequently occur in patients with hydrocephalus, and focal deficits are common in those with mass lesions.[8,9,13–16]

DIAGNOSIS

The diagnosis of neurocysticercosis is established by a combination of the clinical history and physical findings, signs, and results of laboratory and serologic tests, and CT scans or magnetic resonance imaging (MRI). The neurologic signs and symptoms are nonspecific, but the finding of multiple subcutaneous cysts strongly suggests the diagnosis.

The most important clinical aspects that facilitate the diagnosis are

1. Knowledge of patient's country of origin and a history of exposure in an endemic zone
2. History of personal or family teniasis
3. Presence of chronic, persistent headache
4. Late-onset seizures[16]
5. Neurological symptoms, particularly if associated with increased intracranial pressure
6. Mental deterioration in a nonelderly patient

The cerebrospinal fluid (CSF) is usually abnormal and suggests chronic meningitis manifested as lymphocytic pleocytosis and, in some cases, CSF eosinophilia, decreased glucose level, and elevated protein level.[12]

CT is the most useful study, and the findings are diagnostic in most cases. The appearance of cerebral cysticercosis on CT scans varies and depends on the stage of the disease: a hyperdense, nodular mass is seen in the encephalitic phase; hypodense, round lesions of varying sizes sometimes surrounded by an enhanced ring are seen when the lesion is cystic (Figs. 138–1 to 138–4). In later stages of the disease,

Table 138–1. SYMPTOMS AND SIGNS OF NEUROCYSTICERCOSIS*

Focal effect
Mass effect
Inflammatory response
    On nervous tissue
    On meninges-arachnoid
    On vessels
Hydrocephalus caused by obstruction
    Of foramina
    Of aqueduct
    Of cisterns
    Of subarachnoid space

*All of these processes may coexist in the same patient.

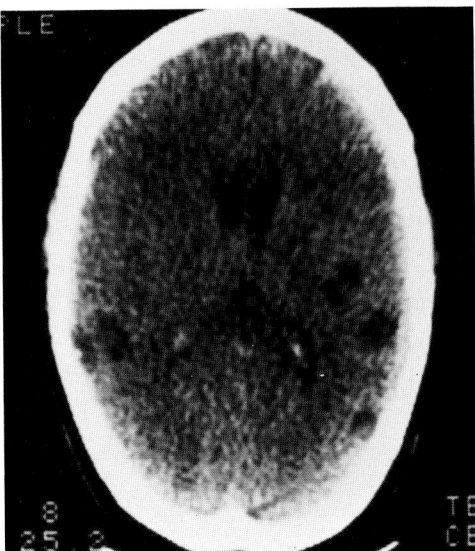

FIGURE 138–1. A noncontrast CT scan showing multiple parenchymal cysts as hypodense round lesions.

the cysts may be calcified. Some lesions can be seen on CT scans only with contrast enhancement. The diagnosis is less certain when single lesions are present or radiographic findings are nonspecific, such as in hydrocephalus. Subarachnoid or intraventricular cysts are difficult to detect with CT scans, and a positive contrast medium (metrizamide) introduced into an obstructed lateral ventricle may be required to demonstrate them.[17-22]

MRI is also very useful in making the diagnosis in most cases. The findings of cerebral cysticercosis on MRI vary according to the stage of the disease: a hyperintense, nodular mass highly surrounded by edema is seen in the encephalitic phase, hypointense round lesions of varying sizes are seen during the cystic stage (Fig. 138–5), and not so hypointense round cysts are seen during a partially degenerated phase (Fig. 138–6). The calcified cysticerci are not well demonstrated on MRI. Subarachnoid and intraventricular cysts, as well as hydrocephalus,[23] are well shown in some cases (Fig. 138–7). In cases of suspected spinal neurocysticercosis, myelography and CT scans or MRI are recommended.[17-20]

Immunologic testing of the CSF is useful in cysticercosis, in contrast with serologic testing, which is neither highly sensitive nor specific. Although numerous tests are available, there are no standardized antigens or methods. *T. solium* antigen preparations identify cross-reactive antibodies in some patients with echinococcosis, schistosomiasis, or other cestode infections. Despite these drawbacks, however, detection of antibodies in a patient with a typical clinical appearance and compatible CT or MRI findings generally establishes the diagnosis.[9, 23-25]

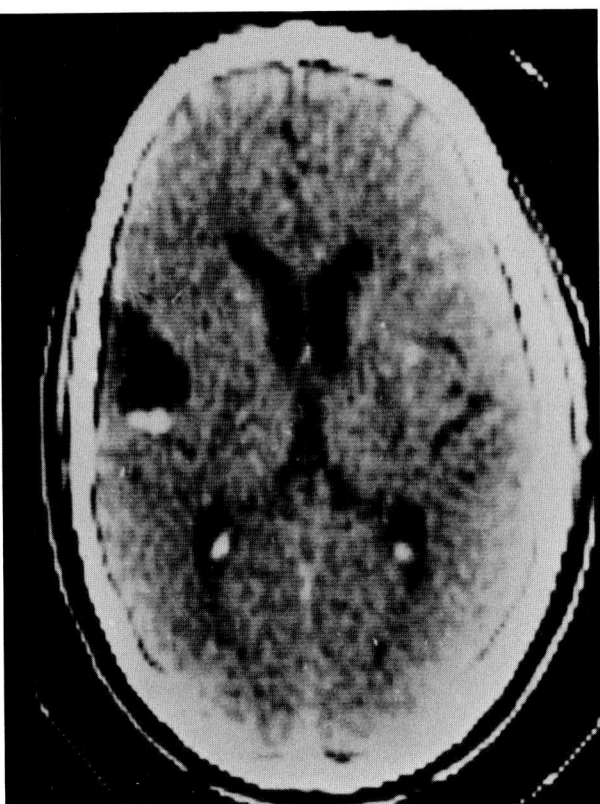

FIGURE 138–3. A CT scan of a patient with a single large cyst and calcifications.

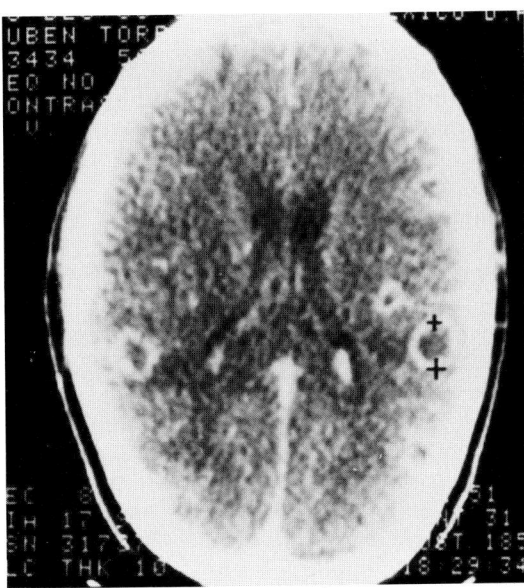

FIGURE 138–2. A contrast-enhanced CT scan of the same patient as in Figure 138–1 showing the multiple parenchymal cysts as round lesions with a ring of enhancement.

PROGNOSIS

The prognosis of cysticercosis is variable and difficult to assess, and the course and tempo of the disease may change, partly because of differences between the individuals' immunologic responses and by an increased inflammatory reaction in previously quiescent, viable cysts. Many neurocysticercosis patients are asymptomatic; their disease is discovered incidentally on radiographic studies performed for other reasons, and they have a good prognosis. Another group of patients have minimal nonspecific complaints, such as headache or dizziness, and some others have major neu-

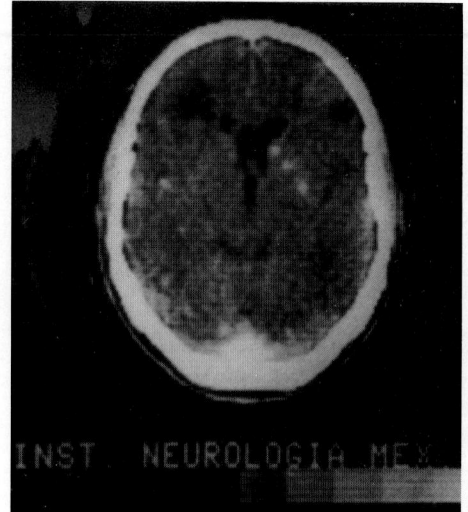
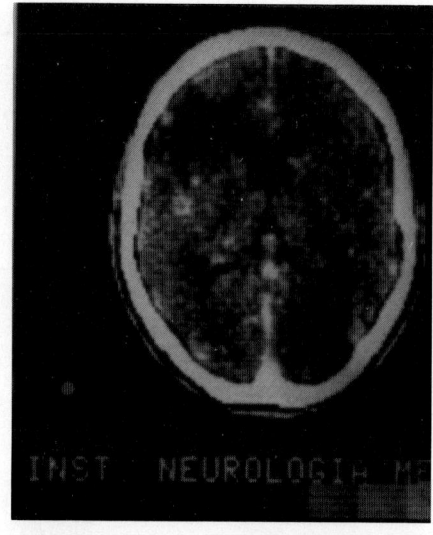
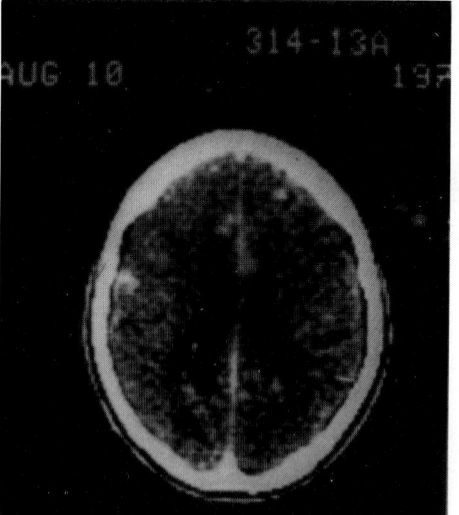
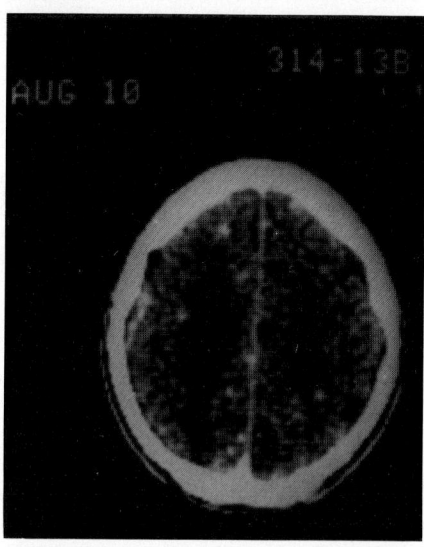

FIGURE 138–4. A CT scan of a patient with the combined form of neurocysticercotic lesions: hydrocephalus, a large cyst, multiple small cysts, partially degenerated cysts, and calcifications (dead larvae).

rologic symptoms, such as seizures, increased intracranial pressure, focal neurologic signs, mental deterioration, or involvement of the cranial nerves that requires immediate investigation because they have a serious prognosis.[22, 26]

At the National Medical Center of the Mexican Institute of Social Security, among 4250 adult autopsies carried out between 1969 and 1974, 135 cases with cerebral cysticercosis were recorded. Of these 135 cases, 81 percent displayed no neurologic symptoms, and this condition was an unexpected finding at autopsy; cerebral cysticercosis was the cause of death in the remaining 19 percent.[10]

NATURAL HISTORY AND THERAPY

Supportive therapy includes anticonvulsant medication and steroids; the latter have been reported to cause short-term and sometimes long-term symptomatic improvement.

Two antiparasitic drugs, praziquantel and albendazol, have been demonstrated to have a beneficial effect in parenchymal and cortical macroscopic viable cysts appearing on CT scans as hypodense images (Fig. 138–8), or hypointense images on MRI. These drugs interfere with the metabolism of the parasite but do not influence the calcified cysts, arachnoiditis, hydrocephalus, or subarachnoid, cisternal, or ventricular cysts associated with the disease.[27–35]

The surgical approach in the treatment of neurocysticercosis depends on the number, size, and localization of the cysticerci and the anatomopathologic characteristics of the infection. The following areas must be defined:

1. The number of cysts (single or multiple cysts).
2. The size of the cysts (more or less than 2 cm in diameter. Is there a mass effect?).
3. The location of the cysts (in the parenchyma of the brain or spinal cord; in the subarachnoid space of the base, cisterns, or convexity; in the ventricles; in the subarachnoid space of the spine; or mixed types).
4. The biologic stage of the parasite (Fig. 138–9) (encephalitic stage, viable cyst with clear fluid content, racemose type of cyst, partially degenerated cyst with jellylike content, or degenerated cyst that is calcified).
5. The secondary pathologic conditions produced in the

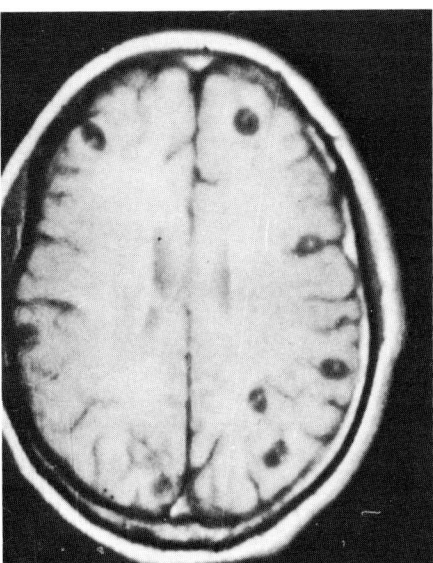

FIGURE 138–5. MRI showing multiple parenchymal cysts as round hypointense lesions. Scolex is visible as a small point in the interior of certain cysts.

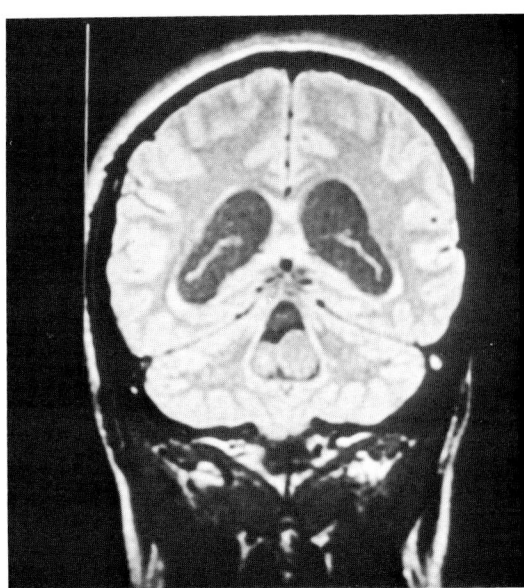

FIGURE 138–7. MRI scan in which two round lesions corresponding to cysticerci are shown in an enlarged fourth ventricle.

CNS by the presence of the cysts (Fig. 138–10) (arachnoiditis-meningitis, ependymitis, vasculitis with or without ischemic sequelae, or communicating or noncommunicating hydrocephalus).

The surgical approach varies, depending on whether larvae are situated in brain or spinal cord parenchyma or are intraventricular; whether they are single or multiple; whether they are of the cellulosae or racemose variety; and whether they are located in the cortex or in the basal subarachnoid space or both, if there is a communicating or obstructive hydrocephalus, or if an adherent arachnoiditis or ependymitis is present. Most cases involve mixed types of the disease, calcified forms with parenchymatous cysts, cisternal cysts, basilar adhesive arachnoiditis, and hydrocephalus[6, 26, 36] (Table 138–2).

To optimize the outcome of these patients, the natural history of this disease must be clearly understood, and a good CT or MRI diagnosis must be made so that the best treatment can be selected.

It is relevant to discuss the different biologic stages because they produce different damage and different clinical pictures, and they demand different therapeutic approaches.

ACUTE ENCEPHALITIC STAGE

In the acute encephalitic phase with local brain edema, if the parasites in the brain are single or few in number, the embryo could be destroyed and disappear, as could the brain edema in a few weeks.

However, if a great number of parasites arrive in the brain, the clinical picture is complicated by severe increased intracranial pressure. The diagnosis in this stage can be confirmed with CT or MRI, which would show multiple nodular masses.

The treatment should consist of steroids, antiparasitic agents, and anticonvulsants. Usually, in 6 or 8 weeks, the inflammatory process disappears, and the patient recovers. In some cases in which the number of parasites is very high, the intracranial pressure reaches critical levels without ventricular dilatation, and medical therapy has been of little value, surgical decompression by subtemporal craniotomy may be required.

CYSTIC STAGE

If the parasites are not destroyed, they grow and develop into the cystic stage, producing symptoms that vary accord-

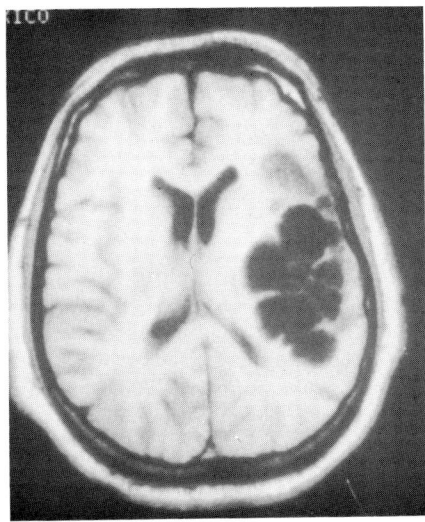

FIGURE 138–6. MRI from a patient with racemose lesions.

Table 138–2. INDICATIONS FOR SURGICAL TREATMENT OF NEUROCYSTICERCOSIS

Cysts 2 cm or larger producing focal symptoms or a mass effect
Severe increased intracranial pressure
Cysts obstructing ventricular channels
Hydrocephalus
Spinal cord compression

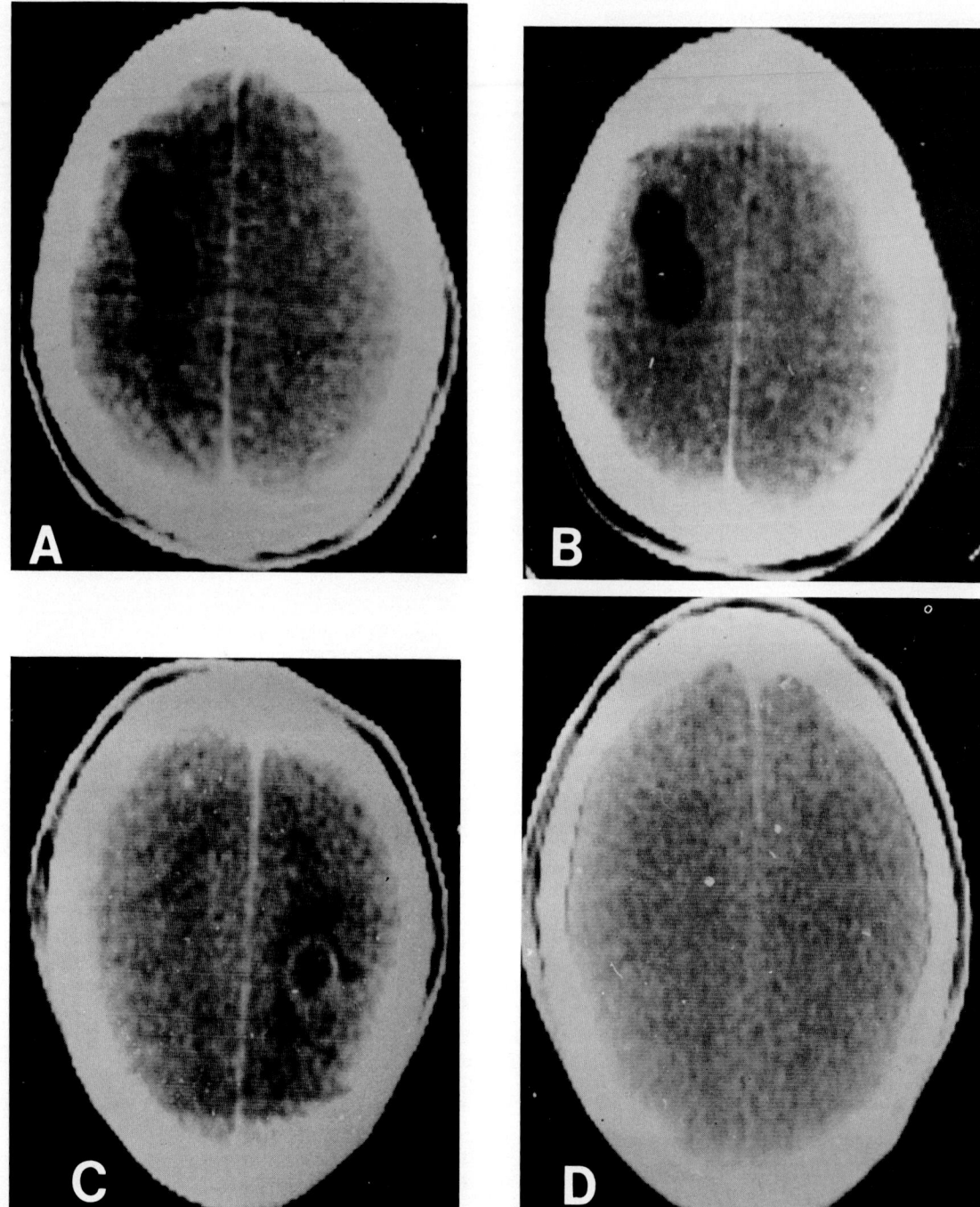

FIGURE 138–8. Contrast-enhanced CT scans before and after praziquantel therapy. (A) A large cyst 2 months before treatment, (B) the same cyst immediately before treatment, (C) the cyst 3 weeks after treatment (note the intensely enhanced ring around the lesion as a result of the inflammatory process), and (D) resolution of the lesion 3 months after treatment.

ing to the severity of the infection and the location and size of the cysts. In cases with no increased intracranial pressure, specific antiparasitic drugs (praziquantel or albendazol) should be used as the only treatment. Among this type of cyst, certain cases require surgical treatment:

Single Cysts

Cysts in the brain that produce focal symptoms, such as reluctant partial seizures, that could benefit from the extirpation of the cysticercus or cysticerci (Fig. 138–11).

Large or Racemose Cysts

Cysts 2 cm or larger or racemose lesions presenting as a tumor-like mass that are predominantly localized in the parenchyma of the cerebral hemispheres or at a major cerebral sulcus, such as the sylvian fissure. These masses could have the appearance of an enhancing ringlike abscess or tumor up to 2 to 3 inches in diameter on CT or MRI. These lesions are treated by total excision. In cases of multiple cysts, in which one large cyst appears to be primarily responsible for a focal neurologic symptom or deficit, its removal is also indicated.

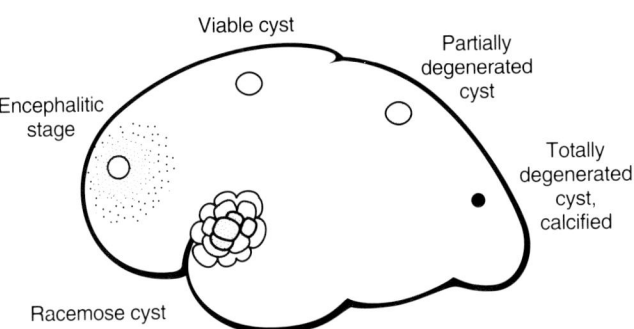

FIGURE 138–9. The biologic stage of neurocysticercosis.

The surgical approach to parenchymal or subarachnoidal cysts should be through microsurgical dissection, in which attempts are made to separate the thin-walled cyst from the surrounding nervous tissue and vessels, thereby permitting total excision. In some cases, the cyst can be extracted by aspiration or by traction with forceps. One of the reasons for failure in surgical results is the presence of inflammatory tissue that affects the wall vessels, producing vasculitis, which compromises local blood flow. Nicely extirpating the cyst is possible, but in many cases, cleaning the area of the brain from the arachnoiditis and vasculitis is not easy. We have used a carbon dioxide laser, sharply focused and at low power, to dissect and separate these structures and to extirpate as much as possible the inflammatory tissue that usually surrounds the cysts and is adjacent to vessels and adherent to nervous tissue (Fig. 138–12).

The cyst wall often is so thin and delicate that there is always the danger that the cyst will tear during dissection and its fluid contents will spill into neighboring areas of the brain. Among 114 cases of cysts that were operated on, the membranes of the extracted cyst were torn in 69 percent. Even though this complication causes concern, we have not found the spillage of cyst contents to have subsequent deleterious consequences. In most cases, steroid therapy is maintained throughout the perioperative period. If a cyst is firmly attached to surrounding structures and cannot be totally removed, the cavity is marsupialized and left as open as possible so it has a connection with the subarachnoid space.[26]

Ventricular Cysts

Cysts that migrate within the ventricular system can obstruct the foramen of Monro, the aqueduct of Sylvius, the fourth ventricle, or the cisterna magna. The larvae, when accessible, are removed to re-establish CSF flow. Because of the possibility of future inflammatory reactions to the cysts, the removal of all accessible ventricular cysts is recommended. Although most patients have multiple intraventricular cysts, a sufficient number of patients have solitary cysts, the removal of which may be curative.[18, 37]

Cysts located in the lateral or third ventricle near the foramen of Monro are reached through a frontal craniotomy and either a transcortical or a transcallosal approach. In these cases, the septum pellucidum should be fenestrated to ensure adequate bilateral ventricular drainage.

The tendency of intraventricular cysts to migrate may explain why so many tend to be found in the fourth ventricle. Imaging studies in these cases demonstrate the presence of the cysts or of a large fourth ventricle, which is sometimes disproportionately large compared with the rest of the ventricular system. This finding in a patient with cysticercosis is highly suggestive of either an isolated ventricle or an intraventricular cyst.[24]

A posterior fossa approach is performed with a suboccipital craniotomy while the patient is in the sitting position. A midline exposure permits excision of a cyst or cluster of cysts if they are at the cisterna. Many times, the cysts are blended in the middle of thick membranes, representing forms of chronic meningitis, and a creamy yellow material, representing the inflammatory response combined with dead parasites. The dissection and separation of these structures is extremely difficult (Figs. 138–13 to 138–15). Cystic masses can also be found in the cerebellopontine angle, the lateral medullary recess, and even on the cerebellar hemispheres. When cysts are located within the fourth ventricle or the cerebral aqueduct, these areas are explored after the thickened tela choroidea is opened and both cerebellar tonsils are separated (Fig. 138–16). In some cases, dividing the inferior vermis is necessary before the cyst can be extracted by gentle aspiration or traction with flat-bladed forceps on the walls of a smooth cyst. This step can be supplemented by irrigation for hydraulic dissection and a Valsalva maneuver, which assists in exposing and delivering lesions from deep recesses

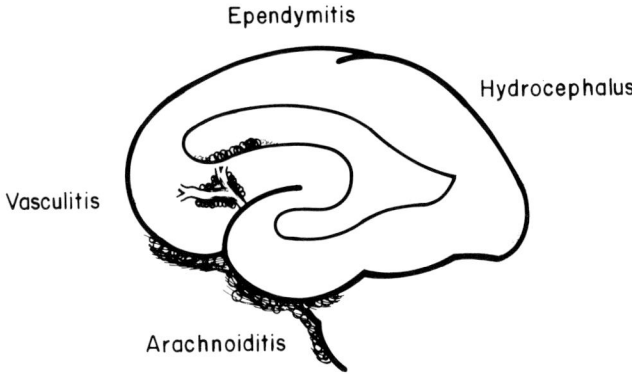

FIGURE 138–10. The secondary pathologic conditions produced by neurocysticercosis.

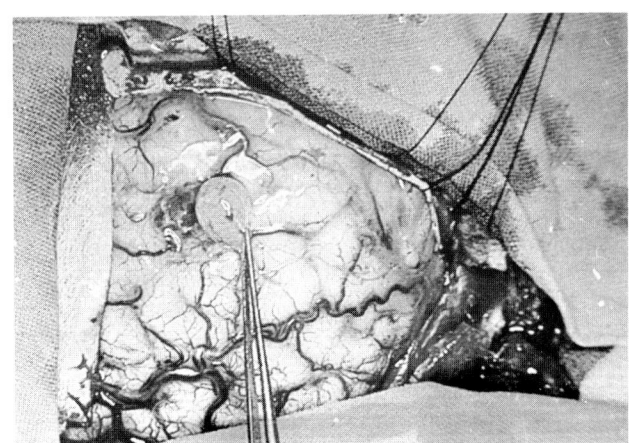

FIGURE 138–11. A cortical cyst dissected and ready for excision.

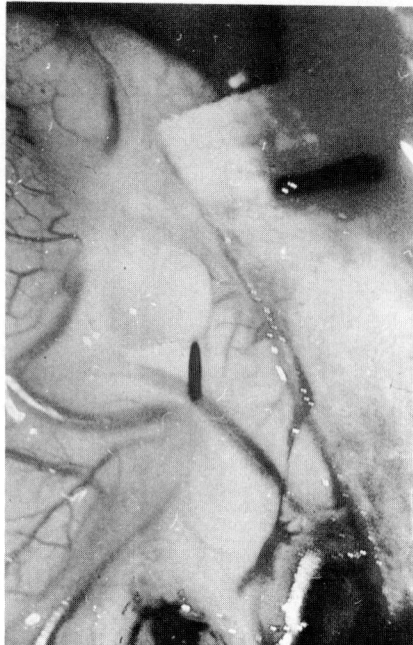

FIGURE 138–12. A cyst located in a brain fissure with an associated inflammatory reaction. This is a milky white process over the cortex and around the vessels. A thrombosed vessel also is visible in the field.

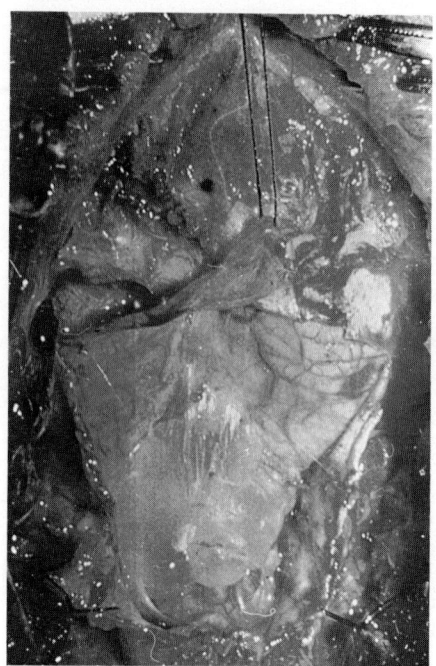

FIGURE 138–14. The suboccipital approach showing the cisterna containing several transparent cysts.

that may not have been previously suspected (Fig. 138–17). These maneuvers often re-establish CSF flow. In some cases, injecting 30 or 40 ml of saline into the lateral ventricle pushes down cysts within the ventricular system and also confirms the free flow of CSF (Fig. 138–18). If CSF flow is not re-established by these measures, a shunt should be performed immediately or within a short period of time.[26, 37, 38] In cases of deep-seated cysts in the lateral ventricles, the posterior part of the third ventricle, or the lower areas of the hemispheres, the use of a stereotactic endoscopic system to introduce forceps, suction, or cannulas for the excision or draining of the cysts should be considered.[26, 37, 39]

Hydrocephalus

In cerebral cysticercosis, the cysts are usually multiple and the inflammatory reaction widely distributed; in spite of this, many of these intraventricular cysts are removable. However, hydrocephalus or increased intracranial pressure can persist as a result of ependymitis at the foramen of Monro or at the aqueduct of Sylvius or as a result of basilar adhesive arachnoiditis, which blocks the free circulation and absorption of CSF over the base or surface of the brain. In these cases, shunting CSF into the blood stream or the peritoneal cavity is indicated. In most cases of neurocysticercosis, the CSF

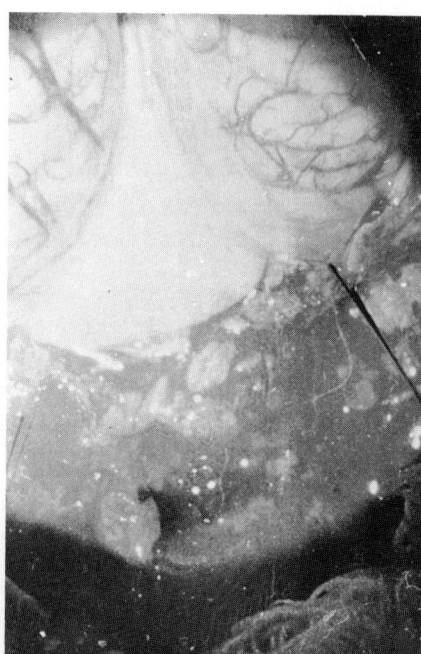

FIGURE 138–13. The suboccipital approach showing the thickened wall of the cisterna.

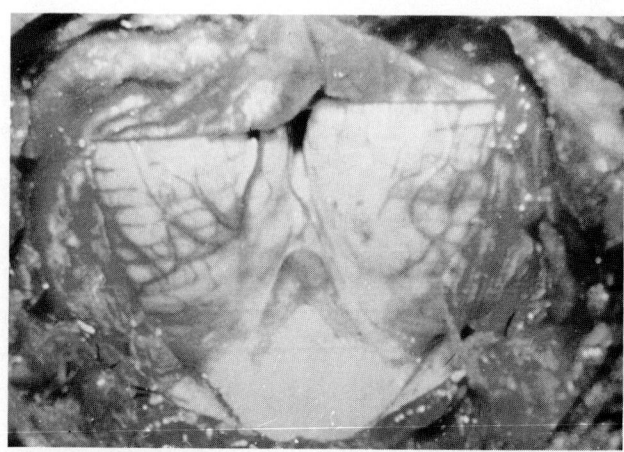

FIGURE 138–15. A cluster of cysts in the cisterna magna.

Neurosurgical Aspects of Neurocysticercosis | 1713

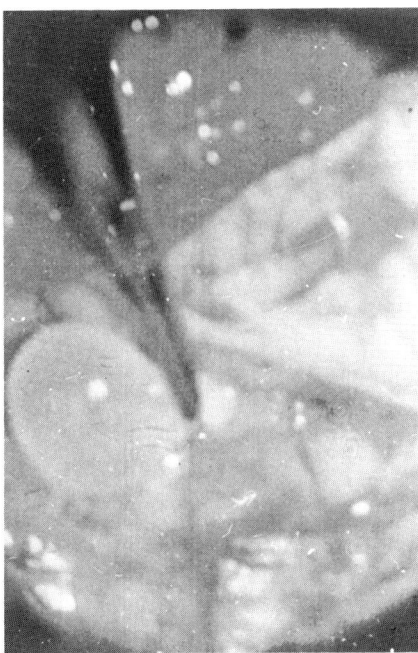

FIGURE 138–16. Extraction of a cyst from the lower part of the fourth ventricle.

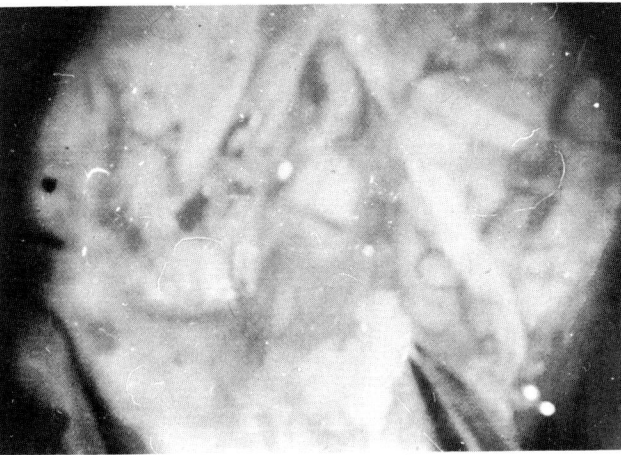

FIGURE 138–18. After the cyst has been removed from the cisterna and fourth ventricle, a creamy yellow inflammatory response (combined with dead parasites) is seen.

protein content is high, and the catheter eventually becomes occluded and requires revision. Of 448 hydrocephalic patients with neurocysticercosis in which CSF shunts were applied, systems became occluded and required revision in 42 percent; the occlusion was identified at the ventricular catheter in 65 percent, the distal catheter in 12 percent, in both catheters in 10 percent, and in an unknown place in 13 percent. Similar results were obtained with all types of shunt systems.[26]

Chiasmatic Cysts

Cysticerci located in the chiasmatic region can produce an inflammatory reaction and adhesive arachnoiditis that affects the optic nerves and chiasm. These cases are very difficult surgical problems because the chronic basilar adhesive meningitis forms a thick membrane that surrounds all the structures on the ventral surface of the brain, including the brainstem. Cysts are often blended into this mass of adhesions. These membranes are firmly attached to the optic nerves, the optic chiasm, and the internal carotid arteries. Microsurgical dissection supplemented by bipolar coagulation and, in certain cases, carbon dioxide laser can decompress these structures and remove cysts.[26]

Spinal Cysts

Cysticerci located in the spine result in symptoms that indicate injury to the spinal cord or the nerve roots. Myelography, CT, or MRI shows cysts or a block caused by arachnoiditis. In these cases, laminectomy should be performed, the dura opened, the cyst or cysts removed, and adherent membranes removed or freed up to free the neural structures.

PARTIALLY DEGENERATED STAGE

When this stage is diagnosed through CT or MRI and is not associated with increased intracranial pressure, the treatment should be through specific antiparasitic drugs (albendazol or praziquantel) that, in most cases, favor the process of destruction of the cysts already initiated. Drugs that provide symptomatic relief, such as anticonvulsants or steroids, that control the inflammatory reaction, could be required.

TOTALLY DEGENERATED STAGE

When the cysts have totally degenerated and become calcified, like an inactive foreign body, no specific treatment is indicated except anticonvulsant drugs in cases of seizures. This is the commonest form of cysticercosis found in an outpatient neurologic clinic.

Surgery is not indicated in all cases of neurocysticercosis, and when performed, it is not necessarily curative, because multiple disseminated cysts cannot be treated surgically, and the arachnoidal adhesions and cerebral vasculitis and its se-

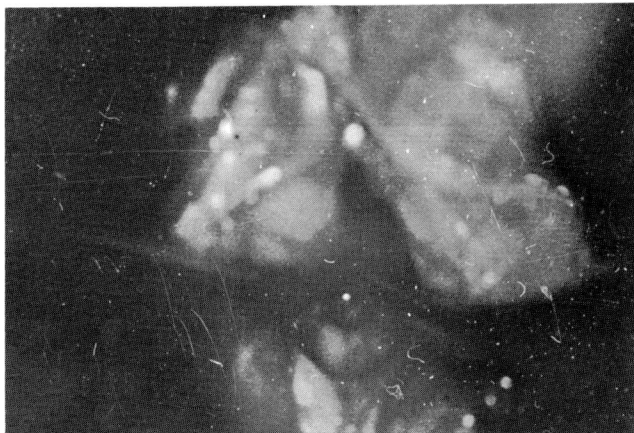

FIGURE 138–17. The suboccipital approach with separation of the cerebellar tonsils, exposure of the lower part of the fourth ventricle, and demonstration of part of a cyst.

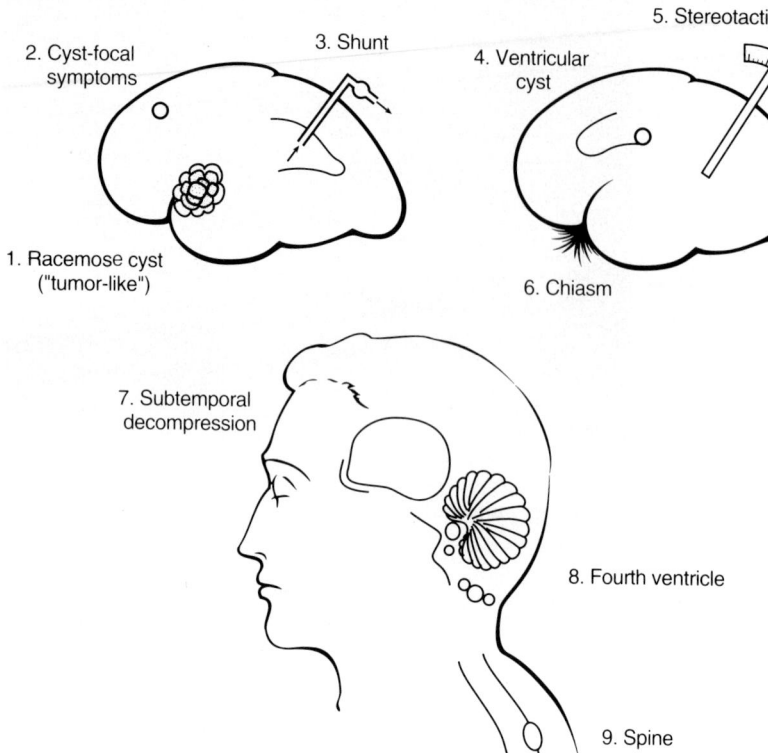

FIGURE 138–19. The different surgical approaches used to treat neurocysticercosis.

quelae may produce permanent neurologic complications. In selecting the surgical approach (Fig. 138–19), the surgeon should be aware of the possibility of an associated ependymitis and the potential for current or eventual outlet obstruction, in spite of the removal of a particular cysticercus. Direct surgical excision of one or a group of cystic lesions may be the primary therapy in most of these cases because the surgical approach treats symptomatic manifestations. Most surgical procedures are palliative. Surgery can partially and temporarily relieve increased intracranial pressure and, occasionally, the focal symptoms caused by a cortical or subcortical cysticercus, even though this is not the rule.[26, 38] Although improvement occurs, other evidence of disease precludes the idea of curing the underlying disorder surgically. Experience with ventricular shunts indicates that although they are effective for alleviating CSF blockage, the catheter eventually becomes occluded and requires revision.

Unlike the complex problems and frustrations encountered with the mixed and disseminated forms of neurocysticercosis, removal of solitary intraventricular cysts is often followed by prompt improvement and excellent recovery. Such cysts are potentially curable.

Sometimes, a patient requires several staged surgical procedures. For instance, in some cases, a shunt followed by the direct excision of cysts in the fourth ventricle or at the sylvian fissure is required; other cases require primary excision of cystic lesions and secondary shunting (Fig. 138–20).

SUMMARY

When planning the management of a patient with neurocysticercosis the physician must bear in mind the great variability of the disease. The physician must also have a clearly defined diagnosis through CT or MRI of the biologic stage of the parasite as well as of the type, number, location, and size of the lesions and the extent of the brain damage, all of which determine the therapeutic option to be used:

1. Asymptomatic calcifications: no treatment
2. Symptomatic calcifications, like seizures: anticonvulsants
3. Increased intracranial pressure: surgery (CSF shunt, cyst excision, decompression)
4. Focal neurologic symptoms associated with a cyst larger than 2 cm in diameter corresponding with the functional topography: surgery (excision)
5. Parenchymatous hypodense cysts on CT or hypointense cysts on MRI with or without scolex: antiparasitic drugs (albendazol, praziquantel)

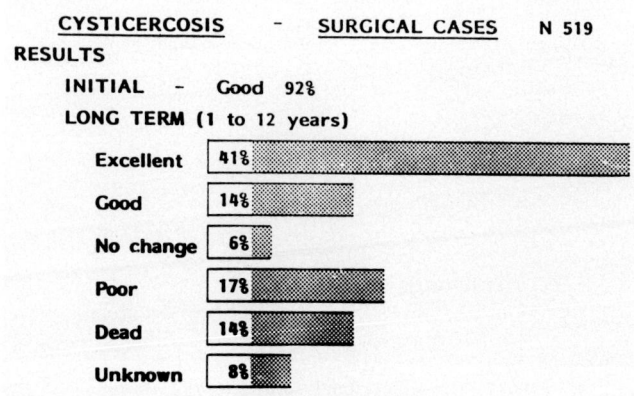

FIGURE 138–20. Initial and long-term results in 519 surgical neurocysticercosis cases.

6. Cases with severe inflammatory brain tissue reaction (on CT or MRI or in CSF) and/or vasculitis: steroids, in some cases combined with decompressive surgery and parasitic drugs (albendazol, praziquantel)

7. Spinal cysts: surgery (laminectomy, excision, decompression)

The surgical approach in the treatment of neurocysticercosis depends on the

- Number, size, and location of the cysts
- The biologic stage of the parasite
- The presence of hydrocephalus
- The inflammatory reaction of meninges, ependyma, and vessels with or without secondary ischemia

The surgical approach is different depending on whether cysts are

- Located in the parenchyma or in the ventricles
- Located in the cortex or in the subarachnoid space of the base and cisterns, or in both
- In the presence of communicating or obstructive hydrocephalus, or if adhesive arachnoiditis or ependymitis are present
- As in most cases, mixed types of the disease, like calcified forms with cysts, arachnoiditis, and hydrocephalus.

Acknowledgments

The figures relating results in surgical procedures were obtained from the study carried out by Dr. Pedro Penagos as his thesis, which was written when he was finishing his neurosurgical residency at the Instituto Nacional de Neurología y Neurocirugía in 1988.

REFERENCES

1. Escobar A, Nieto D: Cysticercosis, in Minkler J (ed): Pathology of the Nervous System, vol 3. New York, McGraw-Hill, 1972, pp 2507–2515
2. Miller BL, Goldberg MA, Heiner D, et al: Cerebral cysticercosis: An overview. Bull Clin Neurosci 48:2, 1983
3. Gardner B, Goldberg M, Douglas H, et al: The natural history of parenchymal CNS cysticercosis. Neurology 34 (suppl 1):90, 1984
4. Willms K: Cestodes, in Gorbach S, Bartlett JG, Blacklow NR (eds): Infectious Diseases. Philadelphia, WB Saunders, 1992, pp 2021–2037
5. Escobar A: The pathology of neurocysticercosis, in Palacios E, Rodríguez Carbajal J, Taveras J (eds): Cysticercosis of the Central Nervous System. Springfield, IL, Charles C Thomas, 1983, pp 27–54
6. Escobedo F, González-Mariscal G, Revuelta R, et al: Surgical treatment of cerebral cysticercosis, in Flisser A, Willms K, Lacletted P, Larralde C (eds): Cysticercosis. Present State of Knowledge and Perspectives. New York, Academic Press, 1982, pp 201–206
7. Del Brutto O, Santibañez R, Noboa C, et al: Epilepsy due to neurocysticercosis. Analysis of 203 patients. Neurology 42:389–392, 1992
8. Escobedo F, García-Ramos G, Sotelo J: Parasitic disorders and epilepsy, in Nistico G, Di Perri R, Meinardi H (eds): Epilepsy. An Update on Research and Therapy. New York, Alan R Liss, 1983, pp 227–233
9. Sotelo J, Guerrero V, Rubio F: Neurocysticercosis: A new classification based on active and inactive forms. A study of 753 cases. Arch Intern Med 145:442, 1985
10. Rabiela C, Ma T: Anatomopathological aspects of human brain cysticercosis, in Flisser A, Willms K, Laclette JP, Larralde C (eds): Cysticercosis. Present State of Knowledge and Perspectives. New York, Academic Press, 1982, pp 179–200
11. Itabashi HH: Pathology of CNS cysticercosis. Bull Clin Neurosci 48:6, 1983
12. Gajdusek C: Introduction of *Taenia solium* into West New Guinea with a note on an epidemic of burns from cysticercus epilepsy in the Ekari people of the Wissel Lakes area. P N G Med J 21:329, 1978
13. Feinberg W, Valdivia RF: Cysticercosis presenting as a subdural hematoma. Neurology 34:1112, 1984
14. Salazar A, Sotelo J, Martínez H, et al: Differential diagnosis between ventriculitis and cyst of fourth ventricle in neurocysticercosis. J Neurosurg 59:660, 1983
15. Wendy MG, Snodgrass RS: Intraparenchymal cerebral cysticercosis in children: A benign prognosis. Pediatr Neurol 1:151, 1985
16. Medina M, Rosas E, Rubio DF, Sotelo J: Neurocysticercosis as the main cause of late-onset epilepsy in Mexico. Arch Intern Med 150:325, 1990
17. Rodríguez CJ, Palacios E, Azar-Kia B, et al: Radiology of cysticercosis of the central nervous system including computed tomography. Radiology 125:127, 1977
18. Kerin D, Chi-Shing Zee, Tsai F, et al: Transventricular migration of a cysticercal cyst during pneumoencephalography. Bull Clin Neurosci 48:61, 1983
19. Kramer LD, Locke GE, Bird SE, Daryabagi J: Cerebral cysticercosis. Documentation of natural history with CT. Radiology 171:459–462, 1989
20. Mehringer CM, Hieshima G, Grinnell VS, et al: Radiologic considerations in neurocysticercosis. Bull Clin Neurosci 48:24, 1983
21. Rodríguez Carbajal J, Salgado P, Gutiérrez R, et al: The acute encephalitic phase on neurocysticercosis. Computed tomographic manifestations. AJNR Am J Neuroradiol 4:51, 1985
22. Miller B: Spontaneous radiographic disappearance of cerebral cysticercosis: Three cases. Neurology 33:1377, 1983
23. Suss R, Maravilla KR, Thompson J: Magnetic resonance imaging of intracranial cysticercosis: Comparison with CT and anatomopathologic features. AJNR Am J Neuroradiol 1986, 7:235–242
24. Ramos KM, Montoya RM, Padilla A, et al: Immunodiagnosis of neurocysticercosis. Arch Neurol 49:633–636, 1992
25. García H, Martínez M, Gilman R: Diagnosis of cysticercosis in endemic regions. Lancet 338:549, 1991
26. Escobedo F: Neurosurgical aspects of neurocysticercosis, in Schmidek H, Sweet W (eds), Operative Neurosurgical Techniques, 2nd ed. New York, Grune & Stratton, 1988, pp 93–100
27. Robles C, Chavarría M: Un caso de cisticercosis cerebral curado médicamente. Gac Med Mex 116:65, 1980
28. Botero D, Castaño S: Treatment of cysticercosis with praziquantel in Colombia. Am J Trop Med Hyg 31:811, 1982
29. Lawner PM: Medical management of neurocysticercosis with praziquantel. Bull Clin Neurosci 48:102, 1983
30. Kori SH, Olds R: PZQ therapy and NMR scans in cerebral cysticercosis. Neurology 34(suppl 1):89, 1984
31. Sotelo J, Escobedo F, Rodríguez Carbajal J, et al: Therapy of parenchymal brain cysticercosis with praziquantel. N Engl J Med 310:1001, 1984
32. Sotelo J, Torres B, Rubio Donnadieu F, et al: Praziquantel in the treatment of neurocysticercosis: Long-term follow-up. Neurology 35:752, 1985
33. Escobedo F, Penagos P, Rodríguez Carbajal J, et al: Albendazole therapy for neurocysticercosis. Arch Intern Med 147:738–741, 1987
34. Vázquez V, Sotelo J: The course of seizures after treatment for cerebral cysticercosis. N Engl J Med 327:696–701, 1992
35. Jung H, Hurtado M, Medina M, et al: Dexamethasone increases plasma levels of albendazole. J Neurol 237:279–280, 1990
36. Escobedo F: Surgical treatment of neurocysticercosis, in Palacios E, Rodríguez Carbajal J, Taveras J (eds): Cysticercosis of the Central Nervous System. Springfield, IL, Charles C Thomas, 1983, pp 114–148
37. Apuzzo MLJ, Dobkin WR, Chi-Shing Zee, et al: Surgical considerations in the treatment of intraventricular cysticercosis—an analysis of 45 cases. J Neurosurg 60:400, 1984
38. Stern EW: Neurosurgical considerations of cysticercosis of the central nervous system. J Neurosurg 55:382, 1981
39. Seigel RS, Davis LE, Kaplan RJ, et al: CT-guided aspiration of a cysticercotic thalamic cyst. Bull Clin Neurosci 48:48, 1983

SECTION XIX

Surgery of the Craniovertebral Junction and Spine

CHAPTER 139

Craniovertebral Abnormalities and Their Neurosurgical Management

John C. Van Gilder
Arnold H. Menezes

Craniovertebral junction abnormalities can be developmental, genetic, or acquired in origin.[1-3] To effectively treat these disorders when symptomatic, the clinician must have a knowledge of the embryology and the functional anatomy of the area. A myriad of abnormal neurologic findings may be present that are secondary to compression or ischemia of neural tissue. The surgical management of these disorders is dependent on precise identification of the underlying pathophysiologic condition as determined by appropriate radiologic studies. The operative treatment includes anterior and posterior approaches to the craniovertebral junction with and without bony fusion. Our experience with 716 patients treated surgically who had neurologic symptoms from craniovertebral abnormalities is the basis for management of these complex disorders. The disorders can be classified as listed in Table 139-1.

HISTORY

Subsequent to the first description of spontaneous atlantoaxial dislocation in 1830 by Bell,[4] lesions of the cervicomedullary junction have emerged from being medical curiosities to being conditions that can be effectively managed. Except for acute dislocations, the treatment of occipitoatlantoaxial joint pathologic entities was marked with failure before the era of skeletal traction. Subsequently, it was apparent that most acute and chronic dislocations could be reduced even years after the initial injury.

The early operative procedures were posterior decompression of the cervicomedullary junction with and without fusion for stabilization. Posterior decompression in patients with irreducible ventral compression of neural tissue at the craniovertebral area is often associated with a high operative risk and a low incidence of improvement: most patients are unchanged or have increased neurologic deficit.[5-8]

More recently, transpalatine-transoral[1-3, 9-19] and extrapharyngeal[20, 21] ventral operations were described for fractures, tumors, congenital abnormalities, infection, and inflammatory conditions at the cervicomedullary junction. Stabilization of the atlantoaxialoccipital joints usually has been performed by fusing of the spinal column posteriorly. The transpharyngeal route for anterior fusion has met with limited success, and further refinement of the technique may result in its future use.[20, 22-24] No single anterior or posterior surgical procedure can be used for all patients with craniovertebral abnormalities: the operation or combination of operations must be selected on an individual basis to correct the pathologic process responsible for the neurologic deficit.[1-3, 17, 25]

EMBRYOLOGY AND ANATOMY

By definition, the craniovertebral junction includes the basiocciput, the foramen magnum, the atlas, and the axis vertebra. The occipital bone is formed by fusion of four sclerotomes. The proatlas is the most caudal of the sclerotomes and loses its identity in humans. The neural arch of the primitive proatlas divides into anterior and posterior segments.[26] The former gives rise to the occipital condyles, and the latter fuses with the atlas to help form its rostral articular facets. If the posterior segment of the proatlas remains separate, the atlas has bipartite cranial articular facets, a rare anomaly that may result in horizontal instability of this joint. The proatlas also forms the dorsal portion of the C1 lateral masses and gives rise to the distal ossification center of the dens.[27]

The atlas is derived from the first cervical sclerotome as well as the proatlas. The body of the atlas as such disappears and gives origin to the dens. The anterior arch of the atlas has one center of ossification, although at times two centers may be present. The posterior arches of the atlas ossify by the age of 3 to 4 years.

The axis is developed from four primary ossification centers. The dens is formed by the C1 sclerotome, two neural arches and the body of the axis from the C2 sclerotomes, and the tip of the dens develops from the proatlas. The tip of the dens is fused with the body by the age of 12 years, and the remainder of the segments ossify and are fused by the age of 3 years.[28]

Dysgenesis of the odontoid process may encompass many congenital anomalies. Failure of the proatlas and the dens to fuse results in ossiculum terminale. Os odontoideum represents failure of the odontoid process and the axis body to

Table 139–1. CLASSIFICATION OF CRANIOVERTEBRAL JUNCTION ABNORMALITIES

Developmental anomalies of the craniovertebral junction
  Malformations of occipital bone
    Clivus segmentations
    Remnants around foramen magnum
    Basilar invagination
    Condylar hypoplasia
    Abnormal occipitoatlantal alignment
  Malformations of atlas
    Failure of atlas segmentation from occiput (assimilation)
    Atlantoaxial fusion
    Aplasia of atlas arches
  Malformations of axis
    Irregular atlantoaxial segmentation
    Dens dysplasias
      Ossiculum terminale persistens
      Os odontoideum
      Hypoplasia-aplasia
    Segmentation failure of C2-C3
  Neural dysgenesis
Genetic and acquired abnormalities of craniovertebral junction
  Abnormalities at the foramen magnum
    Basilar impression (secondary basilar invagination)
    Foraminal stenosis
    Traumatic occipitoatlantal dislocation
    Os odontoideum
    Tumors
  Atlantoaxial instability
    Errors of metabolism
    Down's syndrome
    Infections
    Inflammatory
    Traumatic atlantoaxial dislocations
    Miscellaneous

fused to the anterior margin of the foramen magnum, and the transverse process, if present, does not have a foramen for the vertebral artery. In contrast, an atlanto-occipital fusion is characterized by ankylosis between the atlas and the skull base, usually with persistence of the normal joints. The transverse process of the atlas has foramina for the vertebral arteries.

The occipitoatlantoaxial joints are complex, both anatomically and kinematically.[29, 30] Anatomically, two occipitoatlantal articulations exist. There are four atlantoaxial joints, with a common synovial lining between the dens and the anterior arch of the atlas, the dens and the transverse ligament, and between the four lateral masses. The second cervical nerve passes through the capsule of each atlantoaxial joint.

The occipitoatlantoaxial joints provide for ante-retroflexion, lateral flexion, or tilting and rotation. They therefore function as a ball-and-socket joint. Flexion-extension and lateral bending occur at the occipitoatlantal joint, and flexion-extension and axial rotation occur at the atlantoaxial joint.

The lateral atlantoaxial joints have convex articular surfaces with a horizontal orientation. Because these convex surfaces are not exactly reciprocal, a telescoping effect occurs during rotation of the head. There is relatively limited movement of the atlantoaxial joint, and head-spine motion is basically between the occipital condyles and C2. Because of the intervening C1-C2 convex joint, potential exists for decreased stability at the craniovertebral junction with extension, flexion, and rotation. Hypermobility of the occipitoatlantal joint may progressively increase in patients with congenital high cervical fusion, which may be the etiology of basilar invagination associated with Klippel-Feil abnormality.

The dens is approximated to the anterior arch of the atlas by the transverse ligament, which is anchored to the tubercle on the mesial aspect of each lateral mass of the atlas. This ligament is responsible for the stability of the atlantoaxial joint. The axis is connected to the occiput by the alar ligaments that course obliquely upward from the posterior lateral surface of the dens to the anterior and medial surface of the occipital condyles; the apical dens ligament, which continues from the medial aspect of the foramen magnum to the tip of

fuse. Hypoplasia and agenesis of the dens is the result of developmental failure of the distal ossification centers. The common pathophysiology that produces neurologic deficit with agenesis or hypoplasia of the dens is instability between the first and second cervical vertebra that results from incompetence of the cruciate ligament.

An occipital vertebra is a bony structure that is separate from the foramen magnum and incorporates the occipital condyles. The anterior arch may be partially or completely

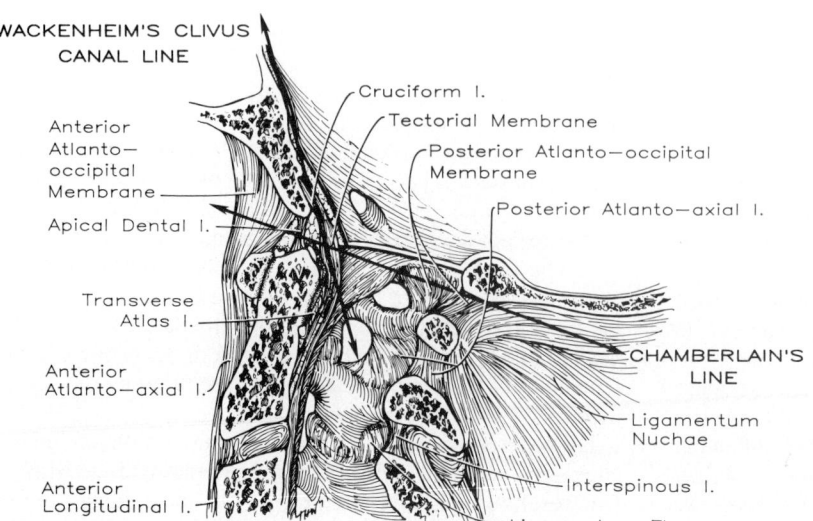

FIGURE 139–1. The anatomic relationships of the bone and soft tissue in the midsagittal plane of the craniovertebral junction.

the dens; the tentorial membrane (an extension of the deep layer to the posterior longitudinal ligament); and the cruciate ligament that consists of the transverse ligament plus triangular ascending and descending slips to the anterior rim of the foramen magnum and the axis, respectively (Fig. 139–1).

The development of the neck musculature is inadequate to supplement joint stability until the age of 8 years. Before this age, laxity of the ligamentous tissue permits excessive movement of the occipitoatlantoaxial articulations.[31, 32] Forward gliding of the skull in relation to the spine occurs if hypoplastic occipital condyles are present. This is the mechanism for the development of neurologic deficit in children who have spondyloepiphyseal dysplasia, Conradi's syndrome, or Morquio's syndrome. These syndromes are often associated with ossiculum terminale.

The lymphatic drainage to the occipitoatlantoaxial joints is through retropharyngeal glands to the deep cervical lymphatic chain. In children, because the neck musculature is not fully developed, C1-C2 subluxation may develop secondary to nasopharyngeal infections.[33, 34]

In the osseoligamentous destruction caused by rheumatoid arthritis, the synovial bursa and associated ligaments that surround the odontoid process are damaged and result in loss of stability.[35] Subluxation may occur secondary to the atlas moving anteriorly on the axis (caused by insufficiency of the cruciate ligament or fracture of the odontoid process), secondary to the atlas moving posteriorly on the axis (from erosion or fracture of the odontoid process), or by telescoping of the skull on the axis (from destruction of the axis lateral masses or apophyseal joints).[25] Chronic subluxation often results in ligamentous hypertrophy and the accumulation of granulation tissue behind the odontoid process from the hypertrophied soft tissue. Even though normal bone alignment is present on roentgenograms, there may be ventral compression of the cervicomedullary junction by soft tissue.

SIGNS AND SYMPTOMS

Cervicomedullary junction abnormalities produce a myriad of symptoms and signs, including myelopathy; brainstem, cranial nerve, and cervical root dysfunction; vascular insufficiency; or any combination of these.[1–3, 17, 36] An abnormal general appearance, usually concerning the neck, is seen with congenital abnormalities of the craniovertebral junction. The commonest congenital anomaly, atlanto-occipital fusion, has a high incidence of associated findings, consisting of low hairline, torticollis, short neck, and limitation of neck movement.[37] Similarly, the classic triad of shortening of the neck, low posterior hairline, and restriction of neck motion is described in the Klippel-Feil syndrome.[38]

Myelopathy was the commonest neurologic deficit in our series, occurring in 705 of 716 patients. The initial symptoms, such as lack of physical endurance, may be subtle, particularly in younger patients. The severity of myelopathy is variable and may present as different degrees of weakness in the upper or lower extremities. False localizing signs were common, and motor deficits included monoparesis, hemiparesis, paraparesis, tetraparesis, and quadriparesis. A myelopathy mimicking the central cord syndrome was often present in patients with basilar invagination. The pathophysiology of motor myelopathy has been attributed to repetitive trauma on the pyramidal tracts secondary to chronic compression. The false localizing signs have been attributed to stagnant hypoxia of the cervical spinal cord from venous stasis.[39]

Sensory abnormality is usually manifested by neurologic deficit relating to posterior column dysfunction and was present in 366 patients. Hypalgesia that reflected spinal thalamic tract dysfunction was unusual, occurring in only 5 percent of patients, and is usually associated with severe paralysis. Bladder incontinence was unusual, the commonest symptoms being urgency or hesitancy of urination.

Cervical root symptoms are usually manifested by suboccipital headaches in the sensory distribution of the greater occipital nerve. The dysesthesias are from irritation of the second cervical nerve as it traverses through the lateral atlantoaxial joint capsule and were present in 547 patients.

Brainstem signs included nystagmus to lateral gaze, and in 21 patients, downbeat nystagmus was present. This last finding has been well documented in cervicomedullary pathologic conditions.[40] Respiratory arrest and sleep apnea were associated with both anterior and posterior compression of the cervicomedullary junction in 13 patients, resolving in each after decompression. Dysfunction of the trigeminal, glossopharyngeal, vagus, accessory, and hypoglossal cranial nerves has been identified in our patient population, as has dysmetria, internuclear ophthalmoplegia, and facial diplegia. Tinnitus, diminished hearing, or both, were present in approximately 25 percent of the patients but was an infrequent complaint.

Symptoms attributed to vascular compromise included syncope, vertigo, episodic hemiparesis, altered level of consciousness, and transient loss of visual fields. These symptoms may be secondary to repetitive trauma of the spinal cord vessels or intermittent obstruction by angulation or stretching of the vertebral and/or anterior spinal arteries resulting from excessive mobility of an unstable atlantoaxial joint. Although several patients exhibited vascular symptoms, only 13 demonstrated angiographic evidence of vascular compromise at the craniovertebral junction.

DIAGNOSTIC INVESTIGATIONS

Several reference lines are used to evaluate plain roentgenograms in the assessment of the cervicobasilar relationships.[41] McRae's line measures the sagittal diameter of the foramen magnum from its anterior margin to its posterior margin (average, 35 mm). Towne's projection is useful for determining the transverse diameter of the foramen magnum (35 mm ± 4 mm). Chamberlain's line is a diagonal from the hard palate to the posterior margin of the foramen magnum (see Fig. 139–1). The odontoid process should not extend more than one third of its length above this line. Wackenheim's clivus-canal line is drawn along the posterior surface of the clivus (Fig. 139–1); basilar invagination is present if this line is intersected by the odontoid process. Fishgold's digastric line is measured on the frontal projection and connects the digastric grooves. The line is normally 11 mm ± 4 mm above the atlanto-occipital junction. The digastric line is the upper limit of position for the odontoid tip. Patients with abnormalities of the craniovertebral junction become symptomatic when the effective diameter of the spinal canal at the foramen magnum (from the posterior surface of the odontoid

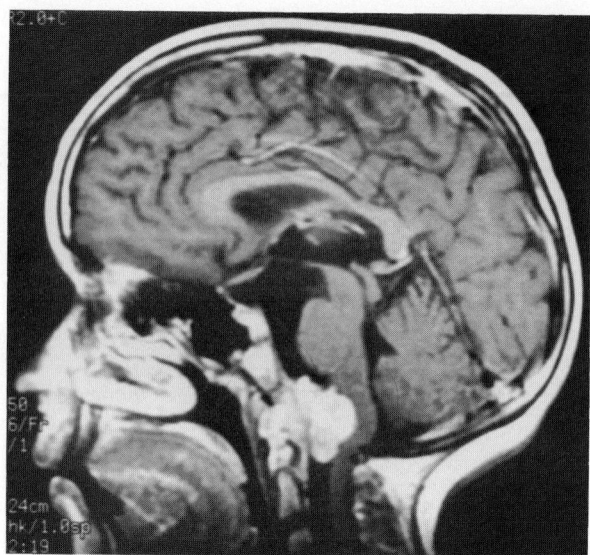

FIGURE 139–2. A midline sagittal T1-weighted magnetic resonance image with gadolinium illustrating a ventral chordoma at the cervicomedullary junction.

process to the posterior margin of the foramen magnum) is less than 19 mm.

Special radiologic procedures are necessary for the clarification of the etiology and pathophysiology of the craniovertebral abnormalities.[1–3] These examinations of the cervicomedullary junction include magnetic resonance imaging, computed tomography, and pleural directional polytomography. These studies provide complimentary information.

The most significant examination of the posterior fossa contents and spinal cord is provided by magnetic resonance imaging, which demonstrates the medulla and cervical spinal cord with great clarity. Abnormality in size and position of the cervicomedullary junction, cerebellar tonsil position, and the presence or absence of hydromyelia are demonstrated without the use of ionizing radiation (Fig. 139–2). Contrast injection of the subarachnoid space before a computed tomographic study or polytomography valuable for the correlation of a specific bone abnormality with change in the adjacent subarachnoid space. Diagnostic studies of the craniovertebral junction in the flexion-extension positions (with or without contrast material) can best be performed with plain x-ray studies or preferably tomographic examination.

OPERATIVE TECHNIQUE

No single anterior or posterior surgical procedure can be used for all patients with occipitoatlantoaxial abnormalities. The operation or combination of operations for each patient must be selected based on a complete understanding of embryology, functional anatomy, pathophysiology, and investigative radiologic abnormalities as described in the previous sections.

The treatments of craniovertebral junction abnormalities can be divided into those for deformities that can be realigned and those for deformities that cannot be realigned (Fig. 139–3). Deformities that are reducible may require immobilization by bracing or posterior fusion. Deformities that

are irreducible are divided into ventral or dorsal compression categories. In the former, the operative procedure is transoral decompression, and the latter, posterior decompression. No further surgery is necessary after decompression if the craniovertebral junction is stable. If instability is present, both ventral and posterior decompression require a posterior fusion for stability. All abnormalities can be classified into these six operative categories for treatment.[1, 5]

REDUCIBLE PATHOLOGIC CONDITION: REQUIRING IMMOBILIZATION ONLY

Forty-four patients had reducible pathologic conditions that required immobilization only as their treatment. The cause of the deformity was craniovertebral joint instability following neck infections in nine patients, posttraumatic atlantoaxial subluxations in 21 patients, and cruciate ligament tears in 14 patients.

We have purposely omitted from this discussion odontoid and atlantoaxial fractures that require fixation only because the causes and treatment of these entities are well documented in the literature.[42, 43] Although some reducible pathologic conditions can be realigned by positioning only, most require up to 15 pounds of skeletal traction with Crutchfield tongs, Gardner-Wells tongs, or a halo ring.

The halo ring with pin fixation has the advantage over other traction devices in that changing the apparatus attached to the skull is unnecessary when the patient is placed in a body brace. An acrylic vest lined with lamb's wool is preferable to the previously used plaster of Paris body cast. Lightweight metals or alloys have replaced the stainless steel rings, pins, and vertical support bars: metals such as aluminum, titanium, or graphic alloy do not distort computed tomography or magnetic resonance imaging of patients who are immobilized in such a brace. The halo brace fixation is preferred for stabilization of the craniovertebral junction because of its superiority over other methods of bracing in the rostral cervical spine.[44]

REDUCIBLE LESIONS: POSTERIOR CERVICAL FUSION

Two hundred eighty-six patients with reducible pathologic conditions had instability that required posterior cervical fu-

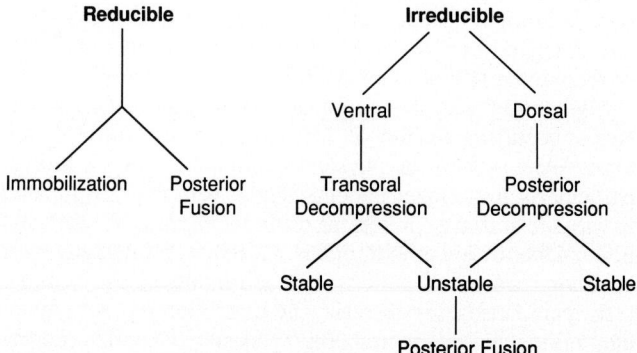

FIGURE 139–3. Algorithm for treatment of craniovertebral abnormalities.

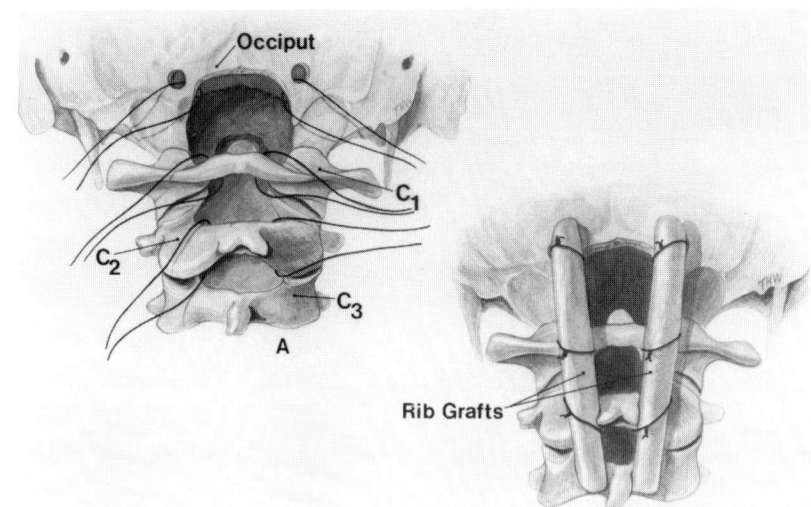

FIGURE 139-4. (A) Placement of the wires under the laminae and through the occipital bone. (B) The bone graft is secured to the occiput and laminae by twisted wire.

sion. Similar to those with reducible lesions requiring immobilization only, a few patients could be realigned with positioning only, but most required skeletal traction. In this category were 187 patients with rheumatoid arthritis and basilar invagination. One hundred seventeen had an acceptable reduction after cervical traction with use of either Gardner-Wells tongs or a halo ring apparatus. The traction is initiated at 7 pounds, followed by a graded increase up to a maximum of 15 pounds. Continuing traction for 10 to 14 days may be necessary to obtain satisfactory position for stabilization. Under certain pathologic conditions, we have not been successful in realigning the craniovertebral junction with cervical traction. These conditions include basilar invagination in which the tip of the odontoid process is 20 mm or more above the foramen magnum, fracture at the base of the dens, or complete separation of the atlas posteroanterior arches.

Operative Technique

Before administration of anesthesia, the patient is intubated while awake by use of regional block and topical anesthesia to the pharynx and larynx. After intubation, the patient is positioned on the operating table in the prone position. The head is placed in the cerebellar headrest, with the clinician ensuring that no pressure is placed about the eyes. Skeletal traction is maintained throughout the operation at between five and 10 pounds, which is sufficient to maintain satisfactory alignment of the cervicomedullary junction.

After the patient is positioned on the operating table, a lateral roentgenogram is obtained to confirm that proper occipitocervical alignment has been maintained. The neurologic examination is repeated to ensure that no significant change has occurred after positioning. The patient is then anesthetized. Pin fixation to the head is to be avoided in these patients because we have observed neurologic deterioration with pin fixation in patients with an unstable spine.

A midline incision is made from the inion to C4 down to the deep cervical fascia. The spinous processes are exposed by excision through the avascular ligamentum nuchae. With precautions taken to avoid excessive vertebral manipulation, a combination of cutting current and a two-periosteal-elevator technique (one elevator is used to retract the muscle, and the other is used for subperiosteal dissection) is used to dissect the paracervical musculature off the spinous processes and laminae in a subperiosteal plane. The suboccipital musculature is dissected from the squamous occipital bone in the subperiosteal plane by use of both cutting current and sharp-blunt dissection.

In patients with an unstable atlantoaxial articulation, fusion includes only the rostral two or three cervical vertebrae. In patients with occipitoatlantoaxial instability, the fusion includes the occiput in addition to the atlantoaxial vertebrae. A notch is placed inferiorly and superiorly on each lamina, and a hole is drilled through each side of the occipital bone lateral to the foramen magnum. Twisted 25- or 26-gauge stainless wire is placed under each lamina and through the occipital bones (Fig. 139-4). The twisted wire is prepared by bending the wire into two equal lengths, securing the bent end into a hand drill, and grasping the free ends with needle holders. The wire is twisted by turning the drill and keeping equal tension on the free wire ends. This maneuver increases the tensile strength of the wire approximately 16 times. More recently, Songar cables have been substituted for twisted wire; the advantage of these cables is that they are more pliable yet have equivalent strength when compared with the wire.

Bone donor sites are either the rib or iliac crest. The bone graft is notched adjacent to the lamina, and a notch or a hole is placed in the rostral end for the occipital wire. The graft is secured to the opposing laminar surface, or the occipital bone, or both, by twisting the ends of the wires together (Fig. 139-4). Bone chips can be placed along the fusion area for additional strength.

Patients are kept in skeletal traction for 3 to 7 days after surgery. Before ambulation they are immobilized in a halo brace and kept in the brace until the fusion is solid. The duration for immobilization is usually 3 to 4 months for atlantoaxial fusion and 6 to 12 months for occipitoatlantoaxial fusion. For the latter, less prolonged immobilization may result in nonunion, union in an abnormal position, or in patients with rheumatoid arthritis, further cranial settling with subsequent increased neurologic deficit.

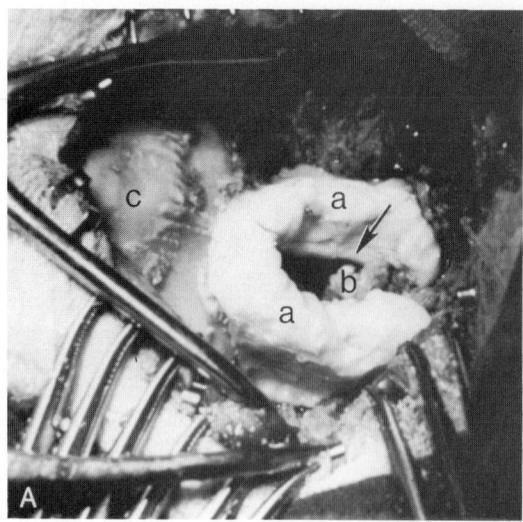
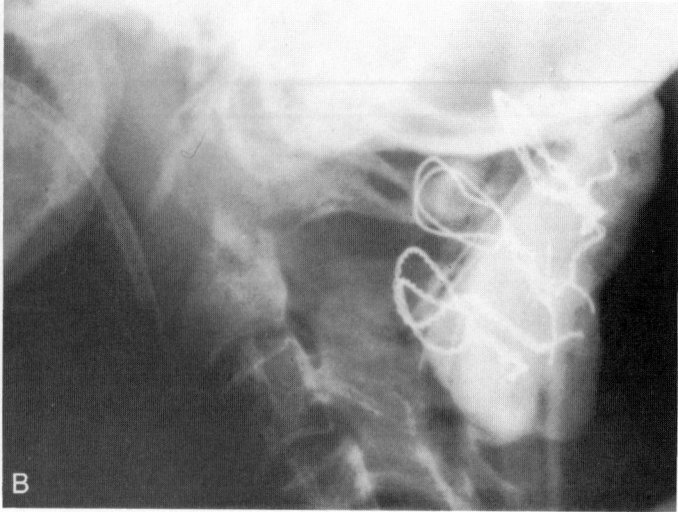

FIGURE 139–5. Intraoperative photograph illustrating acrylic overlying the bone fusion. (A) Bone graft (arrow), acrylic overlying bone graft (a), posterior arch of axis (b), and occiput (c). (B) Postoperative lateral roentgenogram 6 months following surgery.

In severely disabled patients, such as those with rheumatoid arthritis, immediate stabilization can be obtained by supplementing the bone fusion with acrylic and wire fixation.[45–47] This technique consists of placing acrylic over the bone fusion and incorporating the securing wire for the bone graft into the acrylic (Fig. 139–5). With this procedure, there is a diminished requirement for external support, allowing the use of a skull, occiput, mandibular immobilization (SOMI) brace or similar fixation apparatus for immobilization. Long-term follow-up results of this fusion technique have demonstrated satisfactory stability.

An alternative procedure for immediate fixation has been used recently that employs a Steinmann pin contoured in an inverted U shape similar to acrylic and attached to the occipital bone and vertebra with cables or wire.

POSTERIOR DECOMPRESSION WITH AND WITHOUT FUSION

The patient positioning on the operating table, the anesthesia induction technique, and the operative exposure of the spinous process and lamina are identical to the description outlined under posterior cervical fusion. A suboccipital craniectomy is performed that includes the posterior and lateral bone surrounding the foramen magnum. The lamina and spinous processes of C1-C2 and C3 are removed in a rostral-caudal direction. The laminectomy should extend laterally to the medial portion of the facets. It is important to excise all compressive soft tissue, including the constricting dural band that is frequently present in the Chiari malformation at the level of the foramen magnum.

If stabilization is necessary after laminectomy is performed, lateral interfacet fusion is used. The muscles and capsular ligaments of the C1-C2 posterior facets, or C3 posterior facets, or both, are removed with cutting current, periosteal elevators, and curets. Holes are then drilled through the inferior facet into the interfacet joint of each vertebra. If the suboccipital bone is incorporated into the fusion, a hole is drilled on each side of the occipital bone lateral to the foramen magnum. A 25- or 26-gauge stainless steel twisted wire is prepared as described in the previous section and is passed through the openings (Fig. 139–6). Passing the wire through the interfacet joint is facilitated by spreading of the joint with a Freer elevator. Either rib- or split-thickness iliac bone is placed adjacent to the facets, or occiput, or both, and is secured in place by the wires (Figs. 139–6 and 139–7). The postoperative management of the lateral fusion is identical to that described for the posterior fusion without laminectomy. The patient must remain in halo immobilization for 6 to 12 months after the procedure.

ANTERIOR TRANSORAL-TRANSPHARYNGEAL APPROACH

The goal of the transoral-transpharyngeal operation is to correct ventral irreducible compression of the cervicomedullary junction. Pharyngeal and nasal cultures are obtained 3 days before the proposed surgery to treat any pathogenic flora present with antibiotics. If normal flora is present, no antibiotics are necessary. It is prudent to have the patient's nutritional status in the best condition possible before surgery.

The patient is placed supine on the operating table with five to 10 pounds of skeletal traction to maintain alignment of the craniovertebral junction. The previously outlined techniques of intubation and administration of general anesthesia are used in these procedure. We had previously performed a tracheostomy in each patient to ensure an adequate airway postoperatively. With additional experience, we began using our current technique of inserting a malleable endotracheal tube for 24 to 48 hours postoperatively, usually rendering tracheostomy unnecessary. A gauze packing is used to occlude the pharynx to prevent blood leakage into the stomach.

The mouth is kept open with a Dingman retractor, with placement of a rubber guard over the teeth. Self-retaining retractors are attached to the frame of this instrument to depress the tongue and for lateral retraction of the oral cavity. The retraction on the tongue should be loosened intermittently during the operation to prevent lingual congestion.

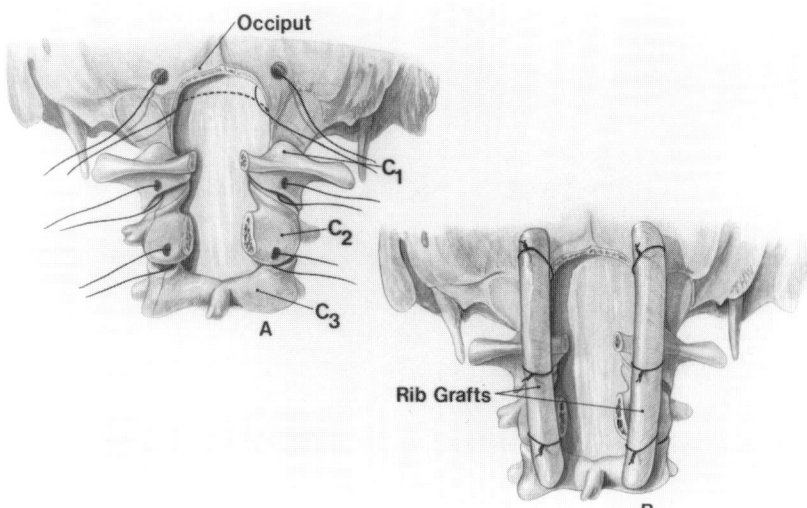

FIGURE 139–6. (A) Placement of holes and wire through the occipital bone and the C1-C2 inferior facets after laminectomy. (B) The graft is secured to the occiput and facets by wire.

The soft palate is infiltrated with 1-percent lidocaine (Xylocaine) with 1/200,000 epinephrine or normal saline, and a midline incision is made that extends from the hard palate and diverts from the midline at the base of the uvula (Fig. 139–8). This incision ensures minimal bleeding and unrestricted healing to the soft palate because the palatine artery and its accompanying palatine nerve enters the soft palate laterally and terminates in the midline. Stay sutures for retraction are placed on the soft palate flaps to allow for maximal exposure through the pharynx to the caudal portion of the clivus.

The arch of the atlas and the caudal extent of the clivus can be palpated by the surgeon through the retropharyngeal musculature. A linear midline incision is made through the posterior pharyngeal wall to the anterior longitudinal ligament and its rostral extension, the atlanto-occipital ligament.

The retropharyngeal musculature is easily separated from these ligaments, and stay sutures or a self-retaining retractor is used to maintain lateral retraction of the muscle.

After exposure of the anterior longitudinal ligament, the operating microscope is used to provide magnification and a concentrated light source. The ligament is coagulated to reduce bleeding, and the anterior body of the axis, anterior arch of the atlas, and caudal anterior clivus are exposed in the subperiosteal plane by use of a periosteal elevator (Fig. 139–9). The ventral atlantoaxial articulation is separated, and the anterior atlas is removed with a 1.5-mm footplate, 45-degree-angled punch rongeur to expose the caudal odontoid process (Fig. 139–10). The apical ligament with its attachment to the caudal clivus is removed, and if the odontoid invagination is severe, resecting a portion of the caudal clivus may be necessary. If resection of the caudal clivus is required, the tissue

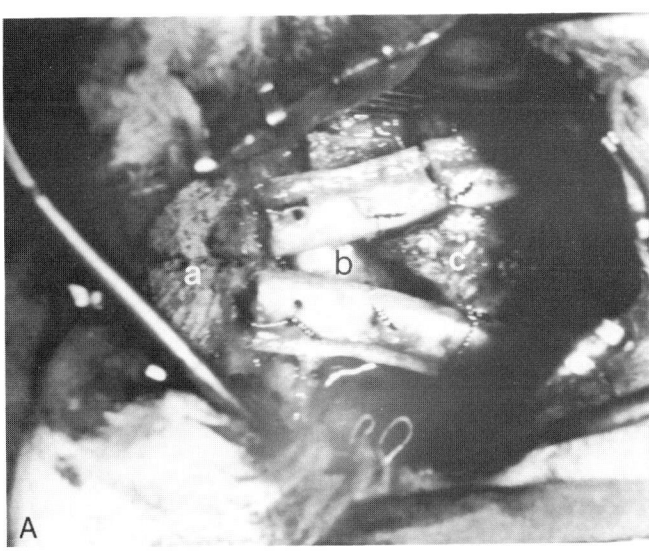
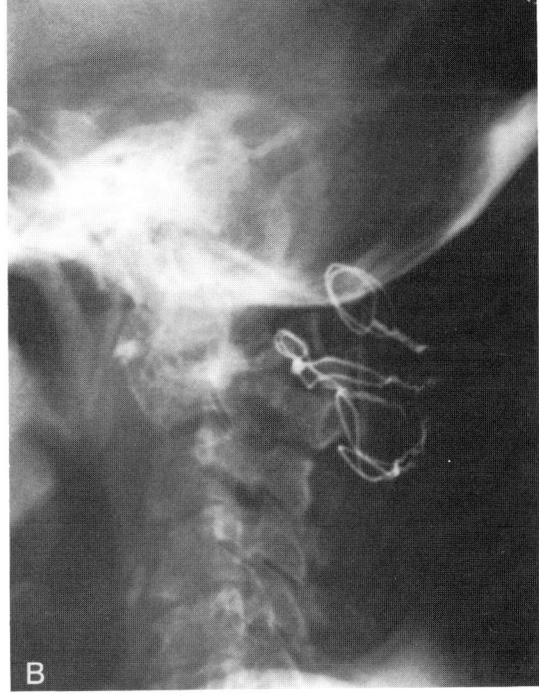

FIGURE 139–7. Operative photograph illustrating bone graft secured after C1 laminectomy and posterior-lateral enlargement of the foramen magnum. (A) Occiput (a), dura (b), and axis spinous process (c). (B) The postoperative lateral roentgenogram demonstrating alignment after surgery.

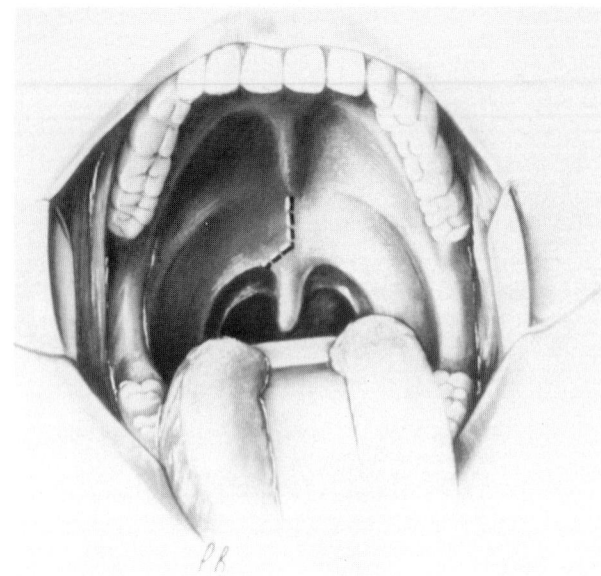

FIGURE 139–8. The midline incision in the soft palate (broken line).

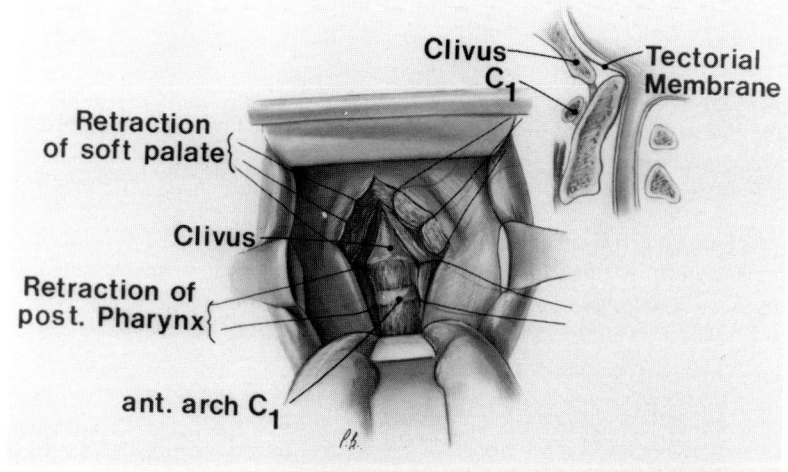

FIGURE 139–9. Exposure of the clivus, the anterior arch of the atlas, and the odontoid process. Stay sutures retract the soft palate and pharynx. The corresponding midline sagittal drawing is in the upper right inset.

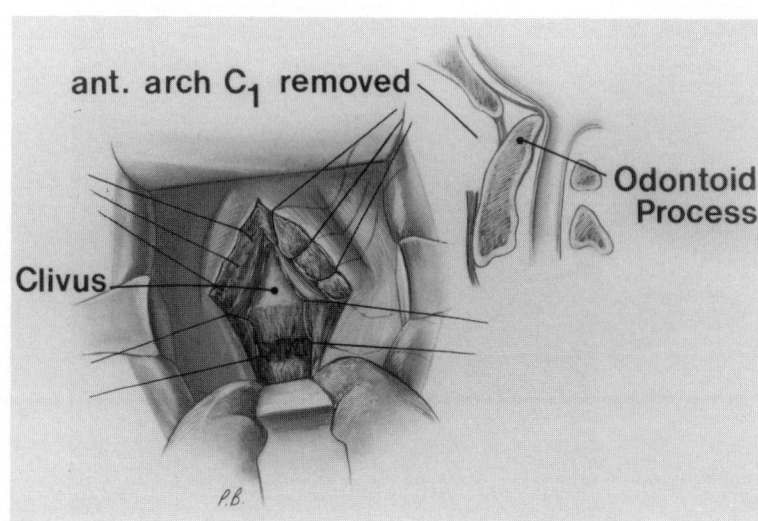

FIGURE 139–10. The operative area after excision of the anterior arch of C1 with the apical ligament intact. The corresponding midline sagittal drawing is in the inset at the upper right.

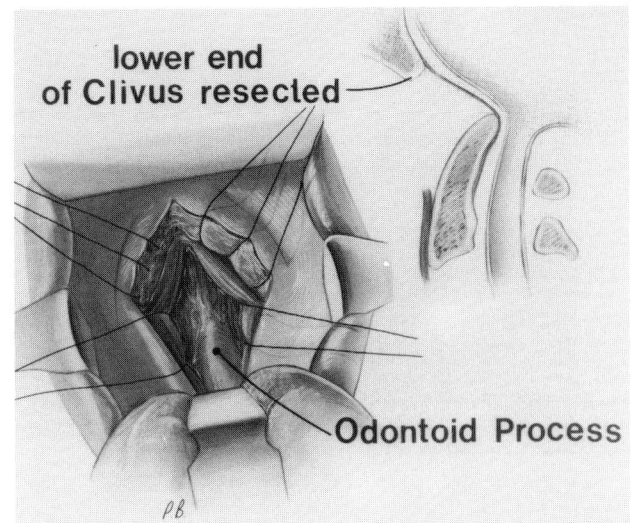

FIGURE 139-11. The operative area after excision of the apical ligament and caudal clivus to expose the odontoid tip. The corresponding midline sagittal drawing is in the inset at the upper right.

posterior to the clivus must be carefully separated from the bone because the dura can be easily penetrated, and troublesome bleeding may occur from the marginal sinus.

The surgeon should next identify the distal tip of the odontoid process by subperiosteal dissection of ligamentous tissue from its osseous ventral surface (Fig. 139-11). The bulk of the odontoid process is then removed with a steel cutting burr. A diamond burr is then substituted to remove the tip and the thin dorsal bony shell of the dens to avoid tearing the posterior soft tissue. We prefer to use a 45-degree-angled handpiece attachment to the drill to provide unrestricted visualization of the surgical field. After the posterior tissue plane at the odontoid tip is identified, the odontoid process and body of the axis are removed in a rostral-to-caudal direction for decompression of the cervicomedullary junction (Fig. 139-12).

In patients with rheumatoid arthritis and other inflammatory disorders, hypertrophy and thickening of the ligamentous tissue may be extensive. Adequate ventral decompression is not accomplished until this tissue is removed adjacent to the dura (Fig. 139-12). After identification of the dura ligamentous plane rostrally, dissection of the granulation tissue is completed in a caudal direction by sharp and blunt instrumentation. The surgeon can be assured that adequate cervicomedullary decompression has been accomplished when the pulsatile dura protrudes ventrally into the decompression site.

If the dura is torn or cerebrospinal fluid is identified, repair of the fistula can be accomplished by placing two or three layers of fascia over the rent. The fascia is harvested from the external oblique aponeurosis or fascia lata from the anterior lateral thigh. In this situation, a lumbar cerebrospinal fluid drain is inserted and maintained for 7 to 10 days after surgery. In our experience, closing the dura with sutures has not been successful and results in persistent cerebrospinal fluid leak.[48-50]

The pharyngeal musculature and aponeurosis are closed with interrupted 000 absorbable sutures in two layers. The soft tissue is approximated by closing of the nasal mucosa with interrupted sutures. Ventral mattress sutures are placed through the oral mucosa and include the muscle to ensure snug approximation. Preoperative and postoperative roent-

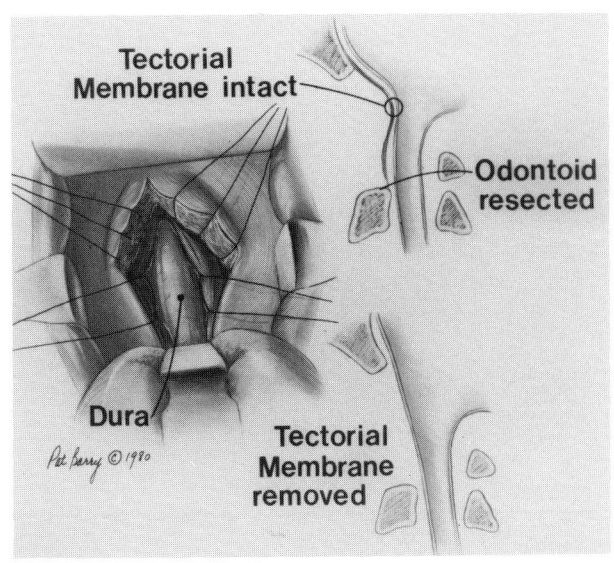

FIGURE 139-12. The operative area after removal of the dens. Following decompression, the dura should fall into the decompressed space. The sagittal drawing (upper right) illustrates failure of decompression secondary to an intact hypertrophied tectorial membrane. The sagittal drawing (lower right) demonstrates adequate decompression following removal of the ventral soft tissue. (Copyright © 1980, Pat Barry.)

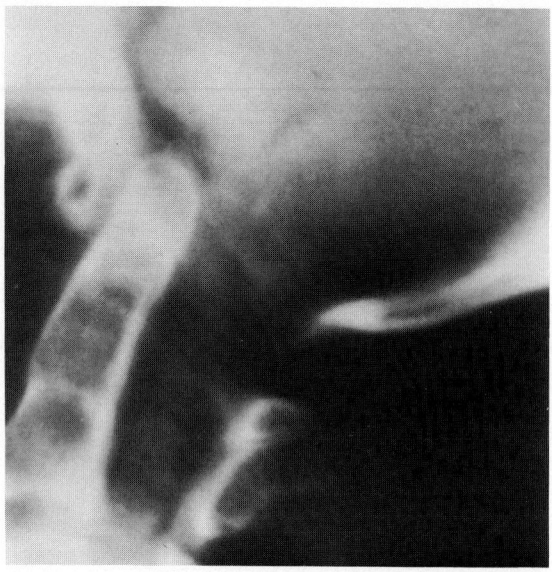
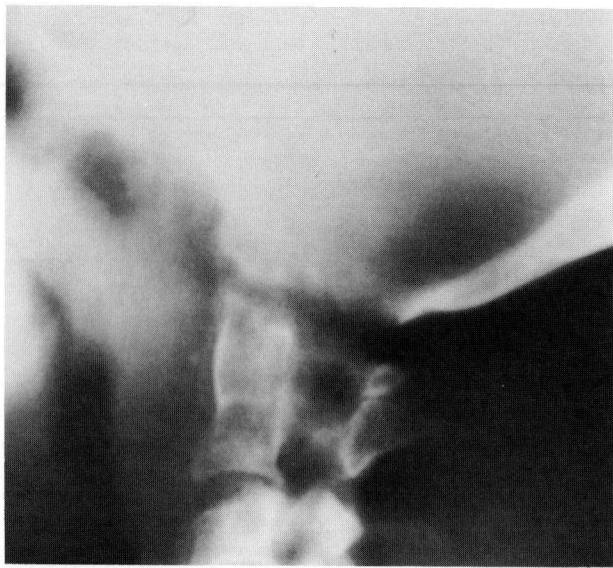

FIGURE 139–13. Preoperative lateral polytomogram illustrating basilar invagination with air contrast medium (left). Note the congenital C2-3 failure of segmentation. Postoperative polytomogram after odontoid resection (right).

genograms of basilar invagination and the odontoid resection are illustrated in Figure 139–13.

In children, the cruciate ligament and tectorial membrane must be preserved in addition to the periosteum of the dens; this measure will allow for new bone formation, and spontaneous ventral fusion has occurred in several of our cases. Similarly, spontaneous anterior bone fusion commonly occurs after posterior fusion in children.

After surgery, the patient is kept in five pounds of skeletal traction. Intravenous fluids are continued for 5 to 6 days, followed by gradually increased feedings to a regular diet by the tenth to twelfth day after surgery. Flexion-extension polytomes are obtained between 5 and 8 days postoperatively to determine craniovertebral stability. If instability is present, posterior fusion is performed as described in the previous section.

If intravenous antibiotics are used, they are discontinued 48 hours after surgery if the dura is intact. If the dura is violated and a fascial graft has been used for repair, intravenous antibiotics are continued for 14 days after surgery. If a tracheostomy is present, it is discontinued as soon as the patient's status permits.

RESULTS

Seven hundred twelve patients recovered or had improvement of their neurologic deficit after craniovertebral junction surgery. The types and incidence of these procedures are outlined in Table 139–2.

Four deaths occurred, all subsequent to transoral decompression. One patient died from sepsis secondary to uri-

Table 139–2. SUMMARY OF SURGICAL CRANIOVERTEBRAL JUNCTION TREATMENT

Stability	Compression	Operative Approach	Postoperative Stability	Posterior Fusion
Reducible 330*	—	—	—	286
Nonreducible	Ventral 256	Anterior	Stable 38	—
			Unstable 218	218
	Dorsal 130	Posterior	Stable 47	—
			Unstable 69	69

*Immobilization, n = 44

nary origin, one from brainstem abscess and meningitis, one from myocardial infarct, and one from pulmonary embolus. The ages of these patients were 66, 62, 71, and 74 years, respectively.

Complications included four cases of meningitis, each successfully treated with antibiotics and recovering without residual deficit. One patient developed cerebrospinal fluid fistula requiring reoperation and repair with a dural graft. Five patients had failure of posterior fusion, four requiring reoperation for fusion.

REFERENCES

1. VanGilder JC, Menezes AM, Dolan KD: Craniovertebral Junction Abnormalities. Mt. Kisco, NY, Futura Publishing Company, 1987
2. Menezes AH, VanGilder JC: Platybasia, basilar invagination, and cranial settling, in Apuzzo MLJ (ed): Brain Surgery Complication, Avoidance and Management. New York, Churchill Livingstone, 1993, pp 2029–2049
3. Menezes AH, VanGilder JC: Anomalies of the craniovertebral junction, in Youmans JR (ed): Neurological Surgery, 3rd ed. Philadelphia, WB Saunders, 1990, pp 1359–1420
4. Bell C: The Nervous System of the Human Body. London, Longman, Rees, Orme, Brown, & Green, 1830
5. Menezes AH, VanGilder JC, Graf CJ, et al: Craniocervical abnormalities: Comprehensive surgical approach. J Neurosurg 53:444–455, 1980
6. Dastur DK, Wadia NH, Desai AD, et al: Medullo-spinal compression due to atlanto-axial dislocation and sudden haematomyelia during decompression. Pathology, pathogenesis, and clinical correlations. Brain 88:897–924, 1965
7. Greenberg AD: Atlanto-axial dislocations. Brain 91:655–684, 1968.
8. Symonds CP, Meadows SP: Compression of the spinal cord in the neighborhood of the foramen magnum with a note on the surgical approach by Julian Taylor. Brain 60:52–84, 1937
9. Menezes AH, VanGilder JC: Transoral-transpharyngeal approach to the anterior craniovertebral junction: 10 year experience of 72 patients. J Neurosurg 69:895–903, 1988
10. Crockard HA, Calder I, Ransford AO: One stage transoral decompression and posterior fixation in rheumatoid atlanto-axial subluxation. J Bone Joint Surg Br 72:682–685, 1990
11. Apuzzo MLJ, Weiss MH, Heiden JS: Transoral exposure of the atlantoaxial region. Neurosurgery 3:201–207, 1978
12. Greenberg AD, Scoville WB, Davy LM: Transoral decompression of the atlantoaxial dislocation due to odontoid hyperplasia. Report of two cases. J Neurosurg 28:266–269, 1968
13. DiLorenzo N: Transoral approach to extradural lesions of the lower clivus and upper cervical spine: An experience of 19 cases. Neurosurgery 24:37–42, 1989
14. Hadley MN, Spetzler RF, Sonntag VK: The transoral approach to the superior cervical spine. A review of 53 cases of extradural cervicomedullary compression. J Neurosurg 71:16–23, 1989
15. Mullan S, Naunton R, Hekmatpaniah J, et al: The use of an anterior approach to ventrally placed tumors in the foramen magnum and vertebral column. J Neurosurg 24:536–543, 1966
16. Hitchcock E, Cowie R: Transoral-transclival clipping of a midline vertebral artery aneurysm. J Neurol Neurosurg Psychiatry 46:446–448, 1983
17. VanGilder JC, Menezes AH: Craniovertebral junction abnormalities, in Williams RH, Rengachery S (eds): Neurosurgery. New York, McGraw-Hill Book Company, 1993, in press
18. Moore LJ, Schwartz HC: Median labiomandibular glossotomy for access to the cervical spine. J Oral Maxillofac Surg 43:909–912, 1985
19. Hall JE, Denis F, Murray J: Exposure of the upper cervical spine for spinal decompression by a mandible and tongue splitting approach. J Bone Joint Surg Am 59:121–123, 1977
20. DeAndraek JR, MacNab I: Anterior occipito-cervical fusion using an extra-pharyngeal exposure. Am J Bone Joint Surg 51:1621–1626, 1969
21. Stevenson GC, Stoney RJ, Perkins RK, et al: A transcervical transclival approach to the ventral surface of the brain stem for removal of a clivus chordoma. J Neurosurg 24:544–551, 1966
22. Lesoin F, Pellerin P, Thomas CE III, et al: Acrylic reconstruction of an arthritic cervical spine using the transcervical-transclival approach. Surg Neurol 22:329–334, 1984
23. Estridge MN, Smith RA: Transoral fusion of an odontoid fracture. Case report. Am J Neurosurg 27:462–465, 1967
24. Fary HSY, Ong GB: Direct anterior approach to the upper cervical spine. J Bone Joint Surg 44:1588–1604, 1962
25. Menezes AH, VanGilder JC, Clark C, et al: Odontoid upward migration in rheumatoid arthritis or "cranial settling." Analysis of 45 patients. J Neurosurg 63:500–509, 1985
26. Ganguly DN, Roy KK: A study of the craniovertebral joint in the man. Anat Anz 114:433–452, 1964
27. Shapiro R, Youngberg AS, Rothman SLG: The differential diagnosis of traumatic lesions of the occipito-atlanto-axial segment. Radiol Clin North Am 11:505–526, 1973
28. Bailey DK: The normal cervical spine in infants and children. Radiology 59:712–719, 1952
29. Werne S: The craniovertebral joints. Acta Orthop Scand (suppl 23):1–50, 1957
30. White AA III, Panjabi MM: The clinical biomechanics of the occipitoatlantoaxial complex. Orthop Clin North Am 9:867–878, 1978
31. Holmes JC, Hall JE: Fusion for instability and potential instability of the cervical spine in children and adolescents. Orthop Clin North Am 9:923–943, 1978
32. Gilles RH, Bina M, Sotrel A: Infantile atlantooccipital instability. The potential danger of extreme extension. Am J Dis Child 133:30–37, 1979
33. Hess JH, Bronstein IP, Abelson SM: Atlanto-axial dislocations. Unassociated with trauma and secondary to inflammatory foci in the neck. Am J Dis Child 49:1137–1147, 1935
34. Sullivan AW: Subluxation of the atlanto-axial joint. Sequel to inflammatory process in the neck. J Pediatr 35:451–464, 1949
35. Bland JH: Rheumatoid arthritis of the cervical spine. J Rheumatol 1:319–342, 1974
36. Michie I, Clark M: Neurological syndromes associated with cervical and craniocervical anomalies. Arch Neurol 18:241–247, 1968
37. Spillane JD, Pallis C, Jones AM: Developmental abnormalities in the region of the foramen magnum. Brain 80:11–48, 1957
38. Klippel M, Feil A: Un cas d'absence des vertebres cervicales avec cage thoracique remmtant jusqu'a la base du craine. Nouv Icon Soipetriene 25:223–228, 1912
39. Taylor AR, Bymes DP: Foramen magnum and high cervical cord compression. Brain 97:473–480, 1974
40. Cogan DG, Barrows LJ: Platybasia and Arnold-Chiari malformation. Arch Ophthalmol 52:13–29, 1954
41. Dolan KD: Cervicobasilar relationships. Radiol Clin North Am 15:155–166, 1977
42. Apuzzo MLJ, Heiden JS, Weiss MH, et al: Acute fractures of the odontoid process. An analysis of 45 cases. J Neurosurg 48:85–91, 1978
43. Spine trauma in adults, in Rothman RH, Simeone FA (ed): The Spine, 3rd ed, vol II. Philadelphia, WB Saunders, 1992, pp 971–1135
44. Johnson RM, Hart DL, Simmons EF, et al: Cervical arthrosis. A study comparing their effectiveness in restricting cervical motion in normal subjects. J Bone Joint Surg Am 59:332–339, 1977
45. Duff TA: Surgical stabilization of traumatic cervical spine dislocation using methyl methacrylate. Long term results in 26 patients. J Neurosurg 64:39–44, 1986
46. Kelly DL, Alexander E Jr, Davis CH Jr, et al: Acrylic fixation of atlanto-axial dislocations. Technical note. J Neurosurg 36:366–371, 1972
47. Panjabi MM, Hopper W, White AA III, et al: Posterior spine stabilization with methyl methacrylate. Biochemical testing of a surgical specimen. Spine 2:241–247, 1977
48. Guity A, Young PH: A new technique for closure of the dura following transsphenoidal and transclival operations. J Neurosurg 72:824–828, 1990
49. Hayakawa T, Kamikawa K, Ohpishi T, et al: Prevention of postoperative complications after a transoral transclival approach to basilar aneurysm. J Neurosurg 60:276–281, 1984
50. Yamaura A, Makino H, Isobe K, et al: Repair of cerebrospinal fluid fistula following transoral transclival approach to a basilar aneurysm. Technical note. J Neurosurg 50:834–836, 1979

CHAPTER 140

Surgical Management of the Rheumatoid Cervical Spine

Robin A. Johnston
James M. Borthwick

Rheumatoid disease is a relatively common condition that has widespread systemic effects. The most important effects in the spine are in the cervical region, which demonstrates inflammatory and erosive changes in a substantial proportion of patients affected. Relatively few develop neurologic symptoms, although the effects of even a modest myelopathy superimposed on widespread arthropathy may have a devastating effect on mobility and independence. Recognition and management of this subset of the rheumatoid population has evolved over the past 25 years, improving the outlook for these patients. The days of treating such patients with bed rest and cervical immobilization are fortunately long past, and the application of better surgical techniques for access, decompression, and stabilization has been enhanced through superior imaging of the cervical spine by magnetic resonance imaging (MRI) and computed tomography (CT). Surgical decision making is always made easier by knowledge of the natural history of the condition, and this has highlighted the poor correlation between radiologic appearances and neurologic deficit. We are now beginning to address the issue of therapeutic and prophylactic surgical management. As yet, no overall agreement exists on many of the aspects of surgical treatment, including choice of surgical procedure, but management clearly can and should be tailored to meet individual patient needs. Most rheumatoid disease is managed by physicians, but there is an increasing recognition that intervention by a spinal surgeon is more likely to be effective in the early stages of cervical spine involvement. Just as in other situations in spine surgery, the less severe the neurologic deficit the more optimistic the prognosis at the time of surgery may be.

A close liaison with medical colleagues in the management of rheumatoid disease is therefore a prerequisite for good surgical decision making and for the development of effective and efficient management policies. The surgical skills required cross the old and disappearing barriers that separated neurosurgeons and orthopedic surgeons. Microsurgical access and decompression must be combined with fusion and fixation techniques to provide a comprehensive and modern management strategy. The argument for specialized practice in this type of spine surgery is compelling.

CLASSIFICATION AND PATHOLOGY

Rheumatoid disease affects between 1 and 2 percent of whites in the Western hemisphere, and women are affected considerably more frequently than men. The incidence of cervical spine involvement varies with the population studied, and estimates vary from 25 to 90 percent.[1-5] Obviously, the rate of cervical spine involvement increases with the likelihood that members of the population will be receiving surgical treatment. Most sources agree that cervical spine involvement is present in more than 80 percent of patients who have had the condition for more than 10 years, indicating a correlation between the duration and severity of rheumatoid disease and the development of cervical arthropathy.[2] The development of neurologic features is much less common and highlights the poor correlation between radiologic appearances and neurologic deficit, but other studies have shown radiologic progression both in incidence and in severity.[4,6] Pellicci and colleagues studied a population of patients in whom radiologic evidence of cervical spine involvement was initially present in 43 percent. Five years later, the incidence of radiologic involvement had increased to 70 percent. The severity of radiologic changes also increases with time, as might be expected, although this finding does not necessarily presage the development of neurologic symptoms.

In clinical practice, the association between the spine surgeon and the rheumatologist determines the level at which the screening procedure is set. The sheer number of patients with rheumatoid disease makes it impractical for spine surgeons to see all patients with radiologically determined involvement only. Clinical and radiologic screening sensitivity varies according to local practice, but accumulating evidence indicates that sensitivity should not be so low that only patients with advanced myelopathy are allowed to see the spine surgeon.

By far, the most commonly affected level is C1-C2, accounting for greater than 80 percent of all rheumatoid disease in the cervical spine. Subaxial involvement usually affects the upper to midcervical segments and may occur in combination with C1 and C2 disease. However, no level is exempt, and the synovial joints are primarily affected by the pathologic process, which also attenuates the supporting vertebral ligaments and vertebral bone density. The term *pannus* refers to an inflammatory exudate overlying the lining layer of synovial cells within the joint, but its meaning has been expanded by common usage to include the inflammatory mass of fibrous tissue formed as a result of synovial joint degeneration.

Acute inflammatory reactions and chronic erosive changes occur in the synovial tissue surrounding the odontoid process, in the joints between the occipital condyles and the lateral masses of C1, and in the similar joints between C1 and C2. Relapsing and remitting, but ultimately progressive, inflammatory erosion leads to anatomic and functional degradation of the affected joint. This degradation may be asymmetric across any one joint surface, and at any given vertebral level, considerable asymmetry may exist in the severity of involvement. Subluxation of opposing joint surfaces leads to vertebral malalignment, which usually develops over a few years. In most cases, the spinal cord can accommodate and compensate for this just as it can with other slowly developing spinal pathology. The affected joints may remain mobile or may undergo fibrous or bony ankylosis. Eventually, the joint tissues are destroyed, and the condition, at least locally, becomes inactive. In its wake, the process may leave a mass of fibrous tissue, which in the odontoid region can be responsible for spinal cord compression. Strictly speaking, this tissue is not pannus but is commonly referred to as such.

Vertebral malalignment at C1-C2 is most commonly in a forward direction, with C1 moving forward on C2. However, depending on the presence or absence of symmetry of local joint involvement, C1 may tilt laterally or even rotate on C2. If the odontoid process and ligaments become grossly attenuated, C1 may slip posteriorly on C2.[7] Destruction of the atlanto-occipital joint, or atlantoaxial joint, or both, leads to loss of height of the lateral masses of C1, with subsequent upward subluxation of the odontoid through the foramen magnum. This process is also referred to as vertical subluxation or cranial settling. In surgical planning, the direction of subluxation must be clearly ascertained and its cause understood.

The pathologic process may leave the malaligned vertebrae in a fixed position, or they may retain mobility, which could cause neurologic damage by spinal cord or nerve root compression. This instability is rarely acute, such as that associated with spine trauma, but is a more gradual process in which normal everyday movements of the cervical spine probably cause repetitive microinjuries to the cord that eventually accumulate to produce a clinical myelopathy. Ischemic cord changes are noted on a few reported autopsy cases and may result from intermittent vascular compression or rheumatoid vasculopathy.[8–10]

RADIOLOGIC INVESTIGATIONS

Initial screening of patients with rheumatoid disease is carried out by plain x-ray examination, which is less sensitive than CT or MRI (Fig. 140–1). Statistics on the radiologic incidence of cervical rheumatoid disease are compiled largely on the basis of plain x-ray examination, and one can speculate on the incidence derived from more sophisticated means. Lateral cervical views taken in flexion and extension positions are necessary to give a true reflection of the pathologic changes. Anterior subluxations may increase during flexion and reduce to almost normal alignment during extension. Normal vertebral alignment does not necessarily correlate with the absence of spinal cord compression, especially at C1-C2, where a large mass of fibrous or inflammatory tissue may replace or lie adjacent to the odontoid process

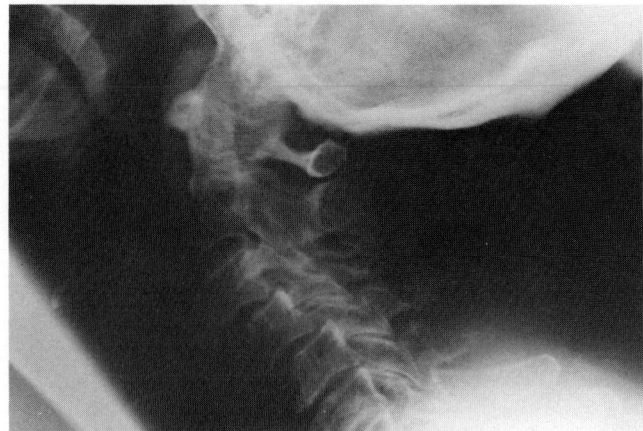

FIGURE 140–1. Subaxial rheumatoid subluxation in a stepwise fashion C3-C5.

(Fig. 140–2). The odontoid itself is best seen by an open-mouthed view, although this view may be precluded by ankylosis of the temporomandibular joints. The standard measurement of up to 3 mm between the posterior margin of the anterior arch of atlas and the odontoid process is useful but may be misleading. The size of the spinal canal is the relevant feature, and it may be compromised by soft tissue, which remains unseen on plain x-ray examination. In addition, voluntary flexion of the cervical spine may be uncon-

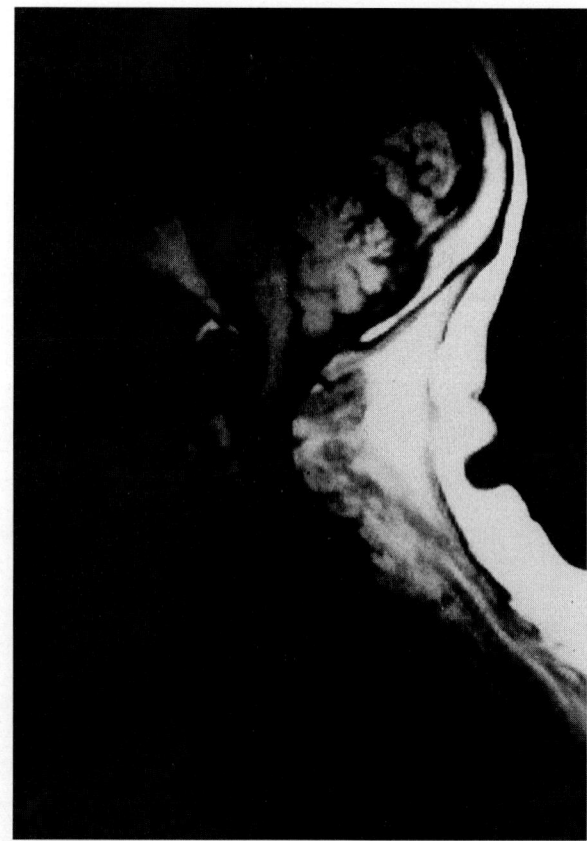

FIGURE 140–2. Magnetic resonance image; subaxial kyphosis and replacement of the odontoid process with a mass of fibrotic inflammatory tissue.

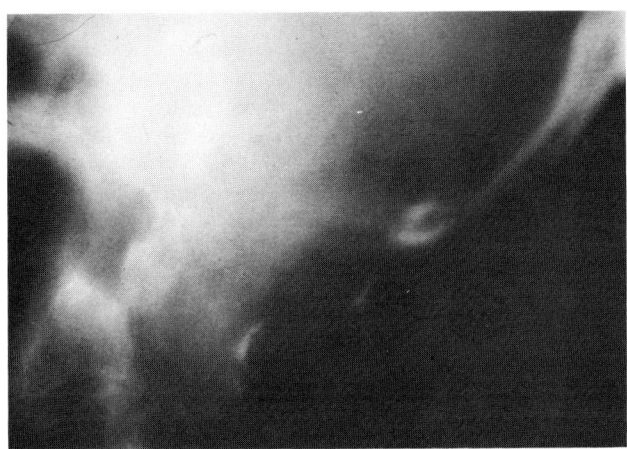

FIGURE 140-3. Plain x-ray tomogram; loss of the odontoid process and posterior subluxation of C1.

sciously limited by the patient, either because of pain or because of an awareness that excessive flexion causes neurologic symptoms, perhaps only fleeting and vague at this stage. A false sense of security may result.

Disintegration of the odontoid process warns of possible posterior subluxation at C1-C2, and asymmetric involvement of the lateral joints suggests the possibility of either rotation or lateral displacement of C1 on C2 (Fig. 140-3). Vertical subluxation may be seen on plain views, although in some patients, obtaining these views may be very difficult because of obscureness of the anatomic landmarks, such as the odontoid tip, the posterior edge of the hard palate, and the posterior rim of the foramen magnum. Many radiologic methods are available that enable determination of the degree of upward movement of the odontoid process.[11]

The commonest subaxial appearances are those produced by forward subluxation of one vertebra on the vertebra below, often associated with loss of vertebral height and erosion of the endplates. This condition may give rise to the impressive "staircase" appearance in which it must be determined whether or not the subluxation increases during flexion of the cervical spine. This process may occur at a single level or at multiple levels. Combinations of mobile and fixed subluxation can result in an increased cervical lordotic curve, a reverse or kyphotic cervical curve, or even a double-curved cervical spine. The quality of bone tissue can also be estimated by x-ray studies, which can indicate potential problems associated with surgical fixation and fusion.

Plain x-ray studies, although a valuable and relatively inexpensive means of screening the rheumatoid population, are not able to provide the detailed information required for surgical decision making and planning. Potential surgical candidates require investigation either by CT myelography or by MRI, both carried out in the flexion and extension positions.[11, 12] Both of these investigations have advantages, and the selection of which (or both) is to be used is determined by availability, quality of the imager, and personal preference. CT gives good definition of bone structure and malalignment, but it requires the use of intrathecal contrast to visualize soft tissues. Composite reformation of images in the sagittal and coronal planes is important, but these do not match the quality of MRI views in the same plane. On the contrary, only in the most modern-generation machines are horizontal magnetic resonance images as satisfactory as those produced by CT. Whichever method or methods are selected, the surgeon must know which vertebral levels are affected, what type and degree of subluxation is present, whether this subluxation is mobile or fixed, whether spinal cord compression exists, and does the cord compression reduce or increase with cervical movement (Fig. 140-4).

Software for three-dimensional image reconstruction is now widely available, but in the experience of this author, it has so far not proved to be of significant value in operative planning, perhaps because of years of cerebral reconstruction from two-dimensional images. Occasionally, vertebral angiography is required when posterior circulation insufficiency is thought to contribute to the clinical presentation, by compromise of one or other vertebral artery resulting from malalignment of C1-C2. In patients with rotation and lateral displacements at C1-C2, the surgeon must be precisely aware of the location of the vertebral arteries because these may present much closer to the midline than would otherwise be expected.

CLINICAL FEATURES AND PATIENT SELECTION

The earliest indication of cervical spine involvement is often that of midline spinal pain sometimes referred into the trapezius regions or up into the suboccipital area. The degree of radiologic involvement in patients seen at this stage may be minor, whereas other patients may be screened for cervical spine involvement, even in the absence of cervical symptoms, and show similar involvement. In this group of patients with minimal radiologic and relatively trivial symptoms, little else can be done other than be aware of the fact that the spine is involved and that deterioration may occur in the future. Attempts have been made to establish prognostic markers that identify patients who are likely to deteriorate and develop cervical myelopathy. Certain associated factors

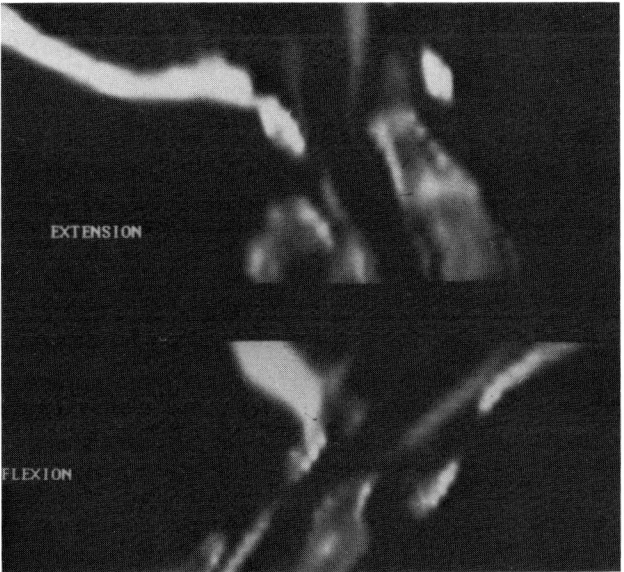

FIGURE 140-4. CT reconstruction in flexion and extension showing fixed compression of the cord by the odontoid.

have been noted, such as increased incidence of peripheral joint involvement, but these are of limited value. The use of sophisticated imaging techniques to measure cervical cord diameter may prove to be of more value. Dvorak and associates[3] observed that six of seven patients with a cord diameter of less than 6 mm in any position of the spine had signs of myelopathy. This observation begs the question as to whether other structural measurements of the cord, such as segmental volume or cross-sectional area, might be of value in identifying patients who require intervention before the development of myelopathy, to prevent the latter from developing. The same authors did not find any useful correlation between clinical myelopathy and motor evoked potentials, although changes in the latter may precede the development of clinical signs. The search for prognostic indicators will continue, but, as with cervical degenerative disease, the natural course of the illness in individual cases may not be predictable, at least in the early stages.[13]

Cervical rheumatoid myelopathy is generally present in patients who are more severely affected, and its presence affects surgical morbidity and mortality. In particular, the presence of interstitial pulmonary disease is associated with reduced postsurgical survival.[14] Evidence exists that once established, rheumatoid cervical myelopathy progresses, although the rate of progression is variable and unpredictable—a situation similar to that of cervical degenerative myelopathy.[6] Among the earliest to note this were Marks and Sharp, who found that 50 percent of their myelopathic patients died within 6 months of commencement of nonoperative treatment.[15] They noted also that not all of the deaths were directly related to neurologic causes, and that many of their patients were severely affected. This alarming observation probably contributed to the trend toward earlier and more aggressive surgical intervention.

Progressive myelopathy is one of the clearest indications for surgical intervention, but we do not know that all rheumatoid patients with myelopathy will progress and deteriorate. Evidence is accumulating that better surgical results are to be found in patients who are less severely affected neurologically and systemically at the time of surgery (Crockard: Personal communication). These findings produce increasing pressure to perform surgical procedures at an earlier time when a less complicated operation may suffice and when the general condition of the patient is more favorable. As the time of surgical intervention is made increasingly earlier, the question of preventative surgery becomes ever larger, although at present there is insufficient evidence to justify surgical intervention in patients without neurologic symptoms. Sensory symptoms comprise paresthesia, or numbness or loss of proprioception in various combinations, usually involving the upper limbs. The patient's symptoms may also suggest Lhermitte's sign, and these sensory manifestations are of prime importance in clinical diagnosis because motor weakness is considerably more difficult to determine in the presence of severe and widespread joint involvement. Grading muscle power according to the Medical Research Council, grades 0 to grade 5, is frequently difficult, inaccurate, or impossible. Symptoms such as easy fatigability or a general feeling of weakness, which is separate from the patient's appreciation of his or her normal joint symptoms, may be early indications of muscle weakness. Very careful attention to the patient's history is of paramount importance because neurologic examination can be of variable value. The presence of clearly exaggerated deep tendon reflexes confirms the diagnosis, but so often these are unobtainable because of local joint destruction. Plantar responses in particular are rarely present for this reason. An exaggerated jaw reflex may indicate medullary compression resulting from vertical subluxation of the odontoid process, but even this effect may be modified by local temporomandibular joint disease. Hyperreflexia is taken as a sign of cord damage, but Floyd and associates[16] could not correlate this event with the onset of weakness.

Recently, Rogers and coworkers[17] (personal communication) challenged the existence of cranial nerve deficits in patients with rheumatoid disease.[18] In their series of 235 patients, nystagmus was present only in patients with coexistent Chiari I malformation. Similarly, other cranial nerve symptoms, such as dysphonia or trigeminal sensory loss, may be explained on the basis of arytenoid joint involvement or upper cervical plexus radiculopathy. They note that proprioceptive deficits indicating posterior column compression play an important role in the decision of whether or not a posterior fixation should be carried out by the sublaminar wiring technique.

It is increasingly clear that preoperative clinical grading systems are useful for evaluating surgical treatment. Crockard (Personal communication) finds that the highest mortality and morbidity occurs in those patients who fall into Ranawat grade IIIB category (quadriparesis, unable to walk). More detailed classification of function and disability perhaps properly belong with the primary rheumatologic specialties, but this trend toward surgical activity analysis should be encouraged. As more and larger series are published, the risks and benefits of cervical rheumatoid surgery will become clearer.

The other major indication for surgical treatment of patients with cervical involvement is intractable suboccipital root pain. This pain results from compression or irritation of the C2 nerve root, most often caused by forward subluxation of C1 on C2. The patient complains of suboccipital pain radiating to the retromastoid region that may present suddenly, related to neck posture, or as a more continuous background pain interspersed with exacerbations. Pain is related to abnormal alignment of C1 on C2 together with active synovitis, and if medical treatment fails to relieve pain, surgical fixation has an excellent chance of achieving lasting pain resolution.

Preoperative evaluation can be difficult in patients with advanced rheumatoid disease and must take account of the systemic manifestations of the condition. These manifestations affect the degree of difficulty with which the procedure is carried out and have an effect on prognosis. The mental attitude of the patient is also important, and fortunately, despite the often prolonged history and repeated surgical intervention, these patients have, in the author's experience, a generally robust attitude. The degree of arthropathy may also have a major influence on the functional outcome, and in some advanced cases, even if the neurologic deficit can be reversed, the degree of joint involvement may preclude any useful functional recovery. For these reasons, preoperative evaluation should not be undertaken by the spine surgeon alone but should be conducted in close consultation with the relevant associated specialties.

ANESTHETIC ASSESSMENT AND MANAGEMENT

Preoperative anesthetic assessment of these patients allows the anesthetist to decide if the patient's general condition permits survival after operative intervention with minimal accompanying morbidity not specifically related to the surgery. Morbidity and mortality may be reduced by the appropriate medical management of reversible disease before surgery.

A very useful general impression is gained by obtaining an adequate medical history, which should elucidate the rapidity of deterioration in the patient's condition. A rapid decline may indicate that exercise tolerance was reasonable before the deterioration and that cardiovascular and respiratory reserve is acceptable. Alternatively, if the patient has undergone a slow and gradual decline, gauging exercise tolerance may be impossible. In some cases, exercise tolerance may be excellent, but the patient may be inactive because of other joint problems and the social circumstances in which he or she lives. Current drug therapy and the use of alcohol and tobacco should be noted, as should any relevant allergic condition.

A full medical examination of the patient should follow the history taking, and particular attention should be paid to the cardiovascular and respiratory systems. Severe anemia or cyanosis may be observed and further investigated when necessary.

Endocarditis, myocarditis, pericarditis, pericardial effusions, coronary arteritis, and conduction defects may occur in rheumatoid disease. Aortitis and valvular involvement produce aortic insufficiency, and a careful search for signs of left ventricular failure should be made. Electrocardiography and chest radiography are also carried out, and consideration is given to the use of echocardiography in appropriate patients.

Rheumatoid nodule deposition and costochondral arthritis may produce a restrictive defect in pulmonary function. Concurrent obstructive lung disease and bullous emphysematous changes may be present. Pleural effusions are common. In addition to chest radiography, measurement of forced expiratory volume and forced vital capacity, as well as arterial blood gas analysis help in the assessment of respiratory function and reserve.

Of particular interest to the anesthetist is the available access to the airway. Many patients have unstable cervical spines, and great care must be exercised during neck manipulation. Some patients have fused cervical spines, making glottic visualization difficult. Temporomandibular joint involvement makes oral access difficult or impossible, and access may be influenced by the presence or absence of dentition. Cricoarytenoid arthritis may also limit the size of the glottic opening. A grossly deviated nasal septum or the presence of nasal polyps present difficulties during nasal intubation.

Many tests can be performed in the assessment of the patient whose trachea is potentially difficult to intubate. A review by Frerk, in which a modified Mallampati test and measurement of thyromental distance were assessed, showed a high success rate in identifying patients with a difficult airway.[19]

ANESTHESIA

Patients whose cervical spines are stable and in whom there is acceptable access to the airway may be anesthetised in the conventional manner, and premedication with an oral benzodiazepine is adequate. Routine monitoring consists of electrocardiography, noninvasive arterial pressure monitoring, pulse oximetry, and capnography. After preoxygenation, anesthesia is induced by use of a short-acting intravenous agent. Once it is clear that the lungs can be inflated, a neuromuscular blocking agent is administered. The author's (JMB) choice of drugs is propofol and vecuronium. The trachea is intubated, usually orally, once full muscular paralysis is achieved. Anesthesia is maintained with inhalational agents, such as nitrous oxide and isoflurane in oxygen. Analgesia is provided by an intravenous opioid, such as morphine, and a nonsteroidal anti-inflammatory drug, such as diclofenac. At the end of the procedure, any residual neuromuscular blockade is reversed, and the patient's trachea is extubated.

Patients with unstable or fused cervical spines may be impossible to intubate by conventional means. The use of the fiberoptic intubating laryngoscope has made anesthetic management of these patients easier and safer. The author's technique is to use a drying agent, such as glycopyrronium, and an oral benzodiazepine as a premedication and then to perform fiberoptic intubation with the patient under local anesthesia, usually by the nasal route, which keeps the patient sedated but cooperative. The author's choice of agents and modes of administration are incremental morphine and midazolam for sedation, intratracheal lignocaine by cricothyroid puncture, and topical cocaine to the nasal mucosa. In most procedures, the rest of anesthesia is administered similarly to that in patients with acceptable airways.

In patients undergoing transoral odontoidectomy, some alteration in anesthetic technique is required. If the patient has cranial nerve dysfunction, brainstem compression, or both, tracheostomy may be performed at the start of the surgery to facilitate later airway protection. This procedure may be performed with the patient under local anesthesia and mask-administered general anesthesia or once the patient is intubated. Patients with poor respiratory or cardiac function who undergo surgery may benefit from a tracheostomy in the postoperative period.

Intubation is performed as discussed earlier, and the patient is then permitted to breath spontaneously from a mixture of oxygen, nitrous oxide, and a volatile anesthetic agent. Analgesia is provided by diclofenac and intravenous morphine. Additional drugs include metoclopramide for gastric motility, an H_2 antagonist to reduce gastric acidity, and a perioperative broad-spectrum antibiotic. A nasogastric tube is inserted and sutured to the nose to prevent accidental removal. Arterial pressure is monitored directly, preferably from the radial artery, but, because of the poor condition of the vasculature of these patients, a femoral line may be required. Good venous access is required. Major blood loss is uncommon, but damage to vertebral arteries and veins can occur with large blood loss over a short period of time. Urine output is measured by a catheter in the bladder. If the patient is permitted to breath spontaneously, the function of the respiratory center and the descending motor tracts can be monitored. Early warning of damage to these areas is provided in this way and allows the potential for correction before the damage becomes permanent. Neurophysiologic monitoring may be considered useful, but it is not used by the author.

Some patients do not adequately ventilate spontaneously under anesthesia for a prolonged period, but infusion techniques using propofol or ketamine may overcome this hypoventilation. When the patient cannot maintain adequate gaseous exchange, ventilating the lungs is necessary. At times of particular risk (during the removal of the odontoid and during the passage of sublaminar wires), the patient may be permitted to breath spontaneously for short periods.

After surgery, the patient is nursed in the intensive care unit and permitted to regain consciousness while receiving adequate analgesia. The tongue may rarely be swollen and potentially cause respiratory obstruction, and a degree of temporary palatal and pharyngeal dysfunction may be present, thereby increasing the risk of pulmonary aspiration. Consequently, the endotracheal tube remains in situ, and the patient breathes oxygen-enriched air via a T-piece. The trachea is usually extubated on the morning after surgery.

The patient is not permitted to eat or drink orally, and the stomach is kept empty by free drainage and hourly aspiration of the nasogastric tube. Gastric motility drugs are continued, as are the H_2 antagonists. The nasogastric tube must not be permitted to dislodge, but if it does, it should be replaced orally under direct vision to avoid trauma to the pharyngeal wound. Careful oral toilet is carried out by the nursing staff. During the first 18 to 24 hours after surgery, clear intravenous fluids are infused. After this, peripheral intravenous feeding is commenced for 2 to 3 days until oral feeding is permitted. At this stage, the patient is usually fit to return to the surgical ward.

SURGICAL ASSESSMENT

The surgeon must determine the direction of subluxation and whether it is fixed or mobile. At the C1-C2 level, it must be clear whether the subluxation is anterior, which is by far the commonest, posterior, lateral, rotational, or vertical. Anterior, vertical, and posterior subluxation may require an anterior surgical procedure in combination with the posterior approach, whereas the less common lateral and rotational subluxations usually require only posterior stabilization.

The site of cord compression may be anterior or posterior, or both, but the surgeon must determine whether or not the cord compression reduces when the vertebral alignment is returned to normal. In most cases in which the subluxation is mobile, slight extension of the cervical spine re-engages the cervical vertebrae in normal alignment, and in a substantial percentage of cases, this action reduces the compression of the spinal cord, indicating that posterior fixation-fusion in this position permits continued spinal cord decompression. In some cases, the normal vertebral alignment is still associated with soft tissue compression of the spinal cord, indicating that direct decompression by an anterior approach is necessary. In cases in which the subluxation is fixed, the site of cord compression is identified, thereby revealing the direction of the primary approach to decompress the spine (Fig. 140–4). Once the route of access is clear and the means of decompression selected, the surgeon must consider whether or not stabilization will be required at the same operation. Recent work has shown that removal of the odontoid process leads to instability in approximately 40 percent of cases, making a posterior fixation procedure almost obligatory in patients with rheumatoid disease.[20]

Where vertical odontoid subluxation is present, the tip of the odontoid process rarely passes upward beyond the lower third of the clivus, whereas in congenital anomalies of this region, extreme upward subluxation is likelier to occur. Access to the lower third of the clivus can be achieved through the transoraltranspharyngeal route. Transmaxillary access is required to reach the middle and upper thirds of the clivus, but this access is rarely required for rheumatoid disease.

If an anterior transoral approach is to be used, the patient's ability to open his or her mouth sufficiently wide is important; however, ankylosis of the temporomandibular joints may severely curtail this ability. Normal mouth opening in which the teeth are present occurs to 60 mm, or three fingerbreadths. Many rheumatoid patients are without teeth, which does facilitate access, but unless the opening is at least 40 mm (two fingerbreadths), the surgical access and room for maneuver are severely curtailed. Opening may be improved by prior surgical freeing of the temporomandibular joints. Other options include division of the mandible and retraction, or even longitudinal section of the tongue. Transmaxillary access is generally poor to the lower third of the clivus and odontoid.

The position of the vertebral arteries should be recognized at the C1 level as they emerge from the top of the vertebral artery canal and pass across the superior surface of C1. In most cases, they present no problem for either anterior or posterior surgical access to C1. However, when C1 is rotated, as can be seen on CT scan, the arteries are closer to the midline than normal.

When the subaxial spine is involved, the surgeon must obviously determine how many and which levels are affected. Degenerative and inflammatory pathology can coexist at different cervical levels. A period of cervical traction, usually little more than 72 hours, should provide radiologic evidence about the mobility and reducibility of the subaxial subluxation. In addition, repeated clinical examination indicates whether or not the patient experiences neurologic improvement when the spine is more correctly aligned. In these patients, even relatively short periods of traction and immobility may generate complications, such as joint stiffness, venous thrombosis, respiratory infection, and skin necrosis. Prolonged periods of cervical traction are not indicated for rheumatoid patients.

Both C1-C2 subluxation and subaxial subluxation can occur simultaneously, raising the difficult question of which causes more neurologic symptoms. Often with radiologic and clinical information, this is an easily soluble problem, but in some instances, it is not clear which is the more important level of compression, and major combined procedures may be indicated in these cases.

SURGICAL TECHNIQUE

The primary aims of surgical treatment of the rheumatoid cervical spine are to relieve the neurologic symptoms (including pain) and to prevent their recurrence. These goals should be achieved at minimal neurologic risk to the patient while preserving cervical spine mobility as far as possible. There are three main components to surgery of the spine: Access, decompression, and stabilization.

ANTERIOR SUBAXIAL ACCESS

The patient is positioned supine on the operating table with the shoulders, cervical spine, and occiput well supported. Care must be exercised to ensure that no involuntary and excessive movements of the cervical spine occur with the patient fully anesthetised. Positioning is initially best carried out with the patient still in a supportive external orthosis or in cervical traction. The operation may be carried out from either side, but the author almost invariably carries out anterior cervical surgery from the right side. The head is rotated approximately 15 degrees to the left, and the anesthetic tubing is positioned so that it does not interfere with perioperative x-ray studies.

For most approaches to this region for cervical degenerative disease, an oblique incision crossing the medial border of the sternocleidomastoid muscle is generally sufficient. The height of this incision depends on the level to be reached and also on the morphology of the patient's neck. For rheumatoid disease, access to several levels is usually required and for this purpose, an incision parallel to the medial border of the sternocleidomastoid muscle is preferable to the more horizontal incision. This is especially so if anterior plating is to be used to secure bone grafting across several vertebral segments. In these cases, relatively long "north-south" access is required. If access to the T1 vertebra is needed, it is facilitated by section of the sternocleidomastoid muscle approximately 1 cm above its insertion into the sternum and clavicle.

Dissection is carried through the tissue planes of the neck in a standard fashion by use of careful separation techniques with dissecting scissors, and the anterior cervical surface is soon palpated between the carotid sheath laterally and the pharynx and larynx medially. Division of the omohyoid muscle is usually required, and occasionally, dividing the superior thyroid artery between ligatures becomes necessary. Care must be taken to preserve as far as possible the internal and external laryngeal branches of the vagus nerve, the latter crossing with the superior thyroid artery in most cases. The prevertebral fascia is identified, picked up, and divided with scissors to expose the anterior longitudinal ligament, discs, and vertebral bodies, which are bordered by the medial edges of the longus colli muscles.

At this stage, identifying the correct vertebral level is necessary and is usually achieved by use of one or more lumbar puncture needles inserted a few millimeters into a vertebral disc, for the purpose of x-ray or image-intensifier identification. A small, but important, step at this point is to excise part of an identified disc by use of a knife, such that the needle can now be removed from the operative field and still leave the disc clearly identified. Retractors are carefully hooked below the medial edge of the longus colli muscle on each side. Frequently, this process involves a degree of electrocoagulation of venous vessels in this region. The upper and lower extremities of the affected vertebral segments are now clearly identified before the decompression phase of the procedure begins.

TRANSORAL ACCESS

The transoral-transpharyngeal route provides very direct and relatively uncomplicated access to the odontoid and periodontoid tissues, a procedure further facilitated if the patient has no teeth. Clearly, this field is contaminated, and achieving sterilization is unnecessary. The author uses a water-soluble iodine solution to gently swab the oral and pharyngeal tissues for a few minutes before making the initial incisions. A throat pack is inserted to prevent blood and iodine reaching the stomach and possibly causing retching or vomiting in the postoperative period.

The cervical spine should be slightly extended before this operation, and the patient may be placed in the lateral position, as described by Crockard, or in the fully supine position.[21] The former permits combined anterior and posterior surgery to occur consecutively, without requiring the surgeon to break from the procedure, turn the patient, and reprepare the area. The author prefers the fully supine position and to stand at the patient's head and be able to rotate the patient's neck slightly from side to side, as required during the operation. The supine position permits the surgeon to work either from the front, facing the patient, from the head in the upside-down position, or from the right or left sides.

A Boyle-Davis or, preferably, a Crockard ring retractor enormously facilitates access by retracting the tongue and holding open the mouth. Prolonged and excessive tongue retraction can occasionally lead to postoperative macroglossia because of edema, and this effect may be lessened by easing the retractor for a few minutes every half hour. Further specialized instrumentation includes soft palate and pharyngeal retractors.

The posterior wall of the pharynx can be easily palpated with the finger to identify the anterior tubercle of C1, which usually lies behind the soft palate. The latter may be retracted up and away toward the nasopharynx by use of specially designed retractors that fit onto the ring base. Alternatively, the soft palate may be divided for most of its length, but just before its insertion into the hard palate. The soft palate heals well if resutured carefully, but the junction of hard and soft palate is the area most at risk for wound breakdown. Division of the soft palate, if necessary, is performed with fine-point cutting electrocautery, just to one side of the midline. The sides of the soft palate can now be retracted with the pharyngeal retractors, and the posterior wall of the pharynx is exposed. This area is divided either in the midline for 2 cm above and below the anterior tubercle of C1, or alternatively, a U-shaped flap may be created. The extra crowding of the operative field when the flap is used is not outweighed by any specific advantage of this method.

Pharyngeal retractors are inserted, the deep fibers of the constrictor muscle are attached to the anterior arch of C1, and the anterior surface of the C2 body are gradually dissected laterally, thereby allowing wider exposure. Once the clean bone is exposed, the pharyngeal retractors are finally inserted, and care is taken to secure safely the armored endotracheal tube and the nasogastric tube lateral to the retractor feet, one on either side. The decompression phase of the procedure can now commence.

POSTERIOR ACCESS

For this procedure, usually, exposure of the occipital (C1-C3) region, the patient is either in the fully prone position or is held laterally, as described earlier. The cervical spine should be in the neutral or preferably, a slightly extended position. Cervical traction may or may not be in position, according to the circumstances. It is helpful and reassuring to have an x-ray study of the spine in the immediate preoperative position. The slight degree of extension produces skin folds that are a nuisance when the surgical incision is made and closed. The surgical incision runs from just below the inion as far down the cervical spine as necessary, and the musculature is dissected bilaterally through the relatively avascular midline. Vessels of the subaxial plexus are encountered around the spinous process of C2, and the dissection is carried laterally to the facet joints on each side below C2-C3.

The suboccipital bone is gradually exposed bilaterally and the foramen magnum is approached with care. Fine-needle-point electrocautery is a good method of muscle dissection. Exposure of the C1-foramen magnum level is last and is commenced in the midline, with care taken initially to identify the posterior arch of C1. In some patients with rheumatoid disease, the posterior arch of C1 is narrow and thin, whereas in others, it may be located substantially more anteriorly than normal, even in the slightly extended position of the cervical spine. In the latter case, the soft tissues of the atlanto-occipital space and the space between C1 and C2 appear to bulge posteriorly, indicating the degree of compression caused by the malalignment of C1. Care must be exercised not to disrupt the dura using electrocautery or sharp dissection, if this is preferred. The posterior arch of C1 is exposed bilaterally up to, but short of, the groove for the vertebral artery, whose location is presaged by a collection of veins. Bleeding from these is usually easily controllable with a small amount of hemostatic sponge and gentle pressure.

ANTERIOR SUBAXIAL DECOMPRESSION

The myelopathy caused by subaxial rheumatoid disease often results from stepwise malalignment of the subaxial cervical spine. Reduction of the malalignment rather than removal of a compressing bony or fibrous structure is the main mode of decompression in this situation. Realignment is produced by use of cervical traction, and in situations in which the malalignment is mobile and reducible, the patient may be placed on the operating table already in a reduced and acceptably aligned condition. In this situation, the decompression has been achieved and can be further confirmed by perioperative x-ray study.

When the malalignment is fixed or cannot be reduced to a satisfactory degree, removing one or more of the vertebral bodies to obtain satisfactory cord decompression is necessary. If a fixed irreducible kyphos is present, the kyphos needs to be excised to provide the decompression. This process may require removal of three or more vertebral bodies.

The decompression is commenced by removal of the intervertebral discs with a combination of a small-bladed knife, disc rongeurs, and small, curved or angled curettes. Having established how many vertebrae and discs need to be excised, the surgeon can now efficiently remove the vertebral bodies using a very high speed drill with various burrs that provide both end and side cutting when appropriate. This procedure is best performed with the aid of the operating microscope, especially as the posterior cortical plates are approached. These may be extensively thinned down with a cutting burr and finally flipped up with a blunt hook. Alternatively, they can be removed with a diamond-tipped burr. No osteophytes form at levels affected by rheumatoid disease. The corpectomy is carried laterally to the medial extremity of the uncovertebral joints, leaving a thin layer of lateral corticocancellous bone.

In patients with rheumatoid disease, the surgeon should probably remove what remains of the posterior longitudinal ligament, whereas this procedure is of debatable value in patients with degenerative disease. The ventral dura is exposed, and the edges of the bone resection are trimmed by use of either a small, diamond-tipped burr or a thin-based micropunch. The cranial and caudal extremities are prepared to receive bone graft by removal of the cartilaginous endplates and exposure of cancellous bone to interface with the graft.

TRANSORAL DECOMPRESSION

The anterior tubercle and arch of C1 are most easily removed with a high-speed drill with a cutting burr. Immediately posterior to this is synovial joint, which may be replaced by the fibrous product of chronic inflammation of the synovial membrane. This fibrous tissue is pale and tough, and it must be removed to expose the anterior surface of the odontoid process. Removal of the fibrous tissue can be difficult, but the author's experience using the neodymium:yttrium-aluminum-garnet contact laser indicates that this laser is particularly useful for this purpose.

The odontoid process, or what remains of it, is defined at its base, sides, and apex. The cortical bone may be of such poor quality that a blunt hook or similar instrument can easily be pushed through into the interior, which is frequently soft, poor-quality cancellous bone. The inflammatory tissue may replace part or all of the odontoid process or can separate it from the base of the C2 vertebra. Odontoid resection is achieved with the high-speed drill with both cutting and diamond-tipped burrs. Care must be exercised not to displace the odontoid posteriorly toward the cord because it may be mobile, especially if it is disconnected from the body of C2. In this situation, a specially designed odontoid-holding instrument (Codman) is helpful. The posterior cortex of the odontoid can be removed by use of a thin-based micropunch or a diamond-tipped burr. The surgeon must ensure that the odontoid apex, which often remains attached to the apical and alar ligaments, is removed. If it is inadvertently left behind, the apex will continue to cause cord compression. The ligaments are divided either with a knife or with the laser. The resection is carried inferiorly to the body of C2, and in most cases, this method is sufficient to relieve bony compression.

When the odontoid has moved vertically because of collapse of the lateral masses of C1, it usually comes to lie posterior to the lower third of the clivus. In these cases, the lower edge of the clivus must be identified by dividing and dissecting laterally the overlying mucous membrane and the insertion of the anterior longitudinal ligament. Once exposed, the lower edge of the clivus can then be gradually removed by use of either a drill or a thin-based micropunch. Approximately the lower third of the clivus can be reached and removed to gain access to the odontoid lying posteriorly.

Odontoid removal exposes the transverse component of the cruciate ligament and the remnants of the apical and alar ligaments. These areas may be markedly attenuated by the inflammatory process, or they may even be absent. Ligaments do not specifically need to be divided or removed, although this may happen during the course of the removal of posterior odontoid inflammatory tissue. This, when present in bulk, may be the prime cause of cord compression, and its removal is crucial to the completion of a satisfactory decompression. The continuation of the posterior longitudinal ligament, the membrana tectoria, lies posteriorly. This membrane can be identified but does not need to be opened or resected, although occasionally this may happen during the course of removing difficult and tough fibrous inflammatory tissue. By this stage, it should become apparent that cerebrospinal fluid (CSF) pulsations are being transmitted into the newly decompressed operative field. Inadvertent opening of the dura is uncommon in rheumatoid disease, but if it happens, a seal can be obtained with layers of fascia, muscle, and fibrin or thrombin tissue glue. A lumbar CSF drain is inserted immediately after the operation is finished, and strong consideration is given to the decision to insert a lumbar peritoneal CSF shunt 4 or 5 days later.

Closure of the pharyngeal wound is carried out in two layers, and the author prefers to use a small, strong, round-bodied needle with an absorbable suture. Closely spaced individual sutures are placed through the constrictor muscles and finally through the mucous membrane and muscle. The soft palate, when divided, should be closed in three layers, commencing posteriorly. Absorbable suture material is again preferred, and the deepest suture picks up both muscle and posterior mucous membrane. The middle layer approximates the muscle of the soft palate, and the ventral layer, both mucous membrane and muscle.

POSTERIOR DECOMPRESSION

In the author's experience, a posterior decompression rarely requires more than the removal of the posterior arch of C1, although others report the use of cervical laminectomy and fusion for subaxial rheumatoid disease.[22] The requirement for removal of the posterior arch of C1 is usually determined from preoperative imaging and is confirmed at surgical exposure by the bulging of tissues above and below a fixed anterior subluxation of C1. Passing an instrument below the posterior arch of C1 may prove difficult and dangerous in this situation. The neural arch may be severely eroded by the disease process, but even so, its removal should be carried out from the posterior surface rather than by passing punches below the arch. High-speed drills and small, fine-pointed bone nibblers are the safest instruments to use for this purpose. The resection is carried laterally until venous bleeding is encountered or the lateral surface of the dura is seen.

ANTERIOR SUBAXIAL STABILIZATION

The rheumatoid spine cannot be stabilized by an isolated Cloward operation or Smith-Robinson type of fusion procedure. Anterior cervical fusion must be combined with additional anterior instrumentation of the spine, posterior fixation-fusion, or external orthotic support. The author's (RAJ) preference is for the Smith-Robinson technique to fuse the reducible malaligned cervical spine because the cervical vertebrae frequently have lost height, making a multiple level Cloward-type procedure difficult and more prone to local collapse and further angulation. The Smith-Robinson type of graft permits the retention of much of the vertebral height and is considered to be a slightly more stable graft than the cylindrical type.

Bone strength and quality vary from satisfactory to very poor in rheumatoid disease and affects the bone fusion rate. The author's (RAJ) preference is to obtain bone grafts from the anterior iliac crest rather than to use bank bone or xenografts. However, in more severely affected patients, the harvesting of bone from the iliac crest or anywhere else adds to the morbidity of the procedure, and other options may be considered. The graft sites are carefully measured for depth, height, and width, and the bone grafts are tailored to size. They are inserted with the use of cervical traction, which is then removed, thereby producing a degree of compression that enhances bone fusion.

In recent years, the use of anterior cervical plates has increased. These plates may be used in cervical rheumatoid disease if bone quality permits (Fig. 140–5). The two main choices are the Caspar system, which employs the use of cortical screws that must penetrate both anterior and posterior

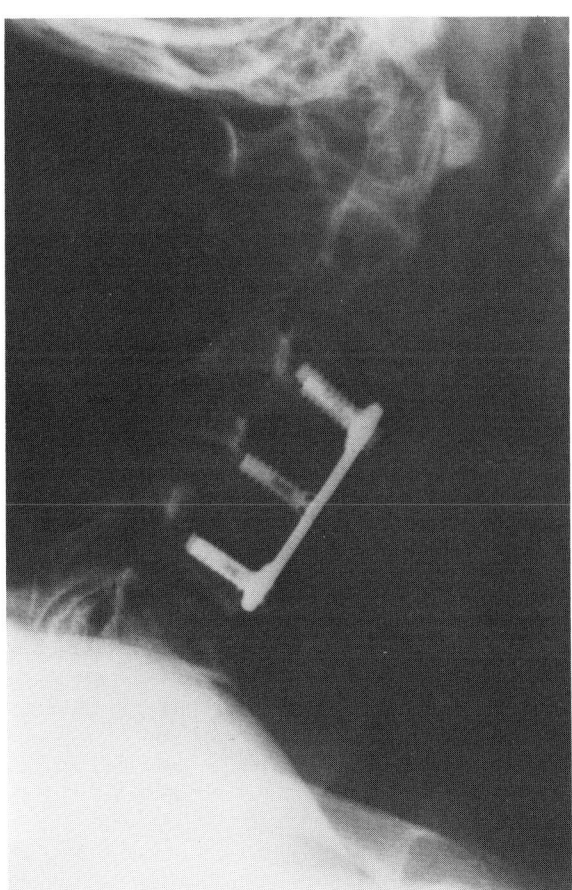

FIGURE 140–5. Subaxial subluxation fixed in alignment using a titanium plate and cancellous bone screws.

cortical plates for adequate grip, or the titanium cervical locking plate system, which uses cancellous screws of a fixed length that do not penetrate the posterior cortical plate. These plates secure the bone graft or grafts in position and add a degree of internal stability that should enhance bone fusion. As yet, there is insufficient published literature on the use of these plates in cervical rheumatoid disease, but some general observations can be made. Clearly, if bone quality is poor, the screws will be easily dislodged, and the plate will provide little, if any, stability. In patients in whom bone quality is satisfactory, the use of these plates in combination with an external orthosis may be sufficient to obviate additional posterior fixation.

In cases in which malalignment is irreducible and several vertebral bodies have been removed, replacement by a single graft of corticocancellous bone is necessary. This material is best obtained from the iliac crest and is tailored to precise length, depth, and width. It is inserted under cervical traction, which is then released to generate compression force on the graft. The graft may be keyed in, or the graft donor surfaces must be prepared flat for tight fit. In this situation, anterior plate instrumentation may be employed to secure the graft in position, according to the individual circumstances and especially, the bone quality.

POSTERIOR STABILIZATION

Most posterior stabilization procedures involve the occipital, C1, and C2 levels. After an odontoid resection, the C1-C2 level is made less stable, and particularly in patients with rheumatoid disease, posterior fixation or fusion is probably always indicated.[20] In many cases, a C1-C2 fixation is satisfactory, but in certain situations, including the suboccipital region is necessary. These situations include when the posterior arch of C1 is too attenuated by the disease to accept fixation, when a laminectomy of C1 has been carried out, and rarely when there is an occipitalized C1 vertebra. When loss of lateral mass height and vertical subluxation occurs, carrying out an occipitocervical fixation-fusion procedure is necessary. In some cases, incorporation of the C1 lamina into the fixation may prove technically difficult or excessively risky, and the surgeon may opt for the safer alternative of an occipito-C2 fusion.

The simple onlay of bone graft supported by an external orthosis is much less often used now, and in most cases, some form of internal fixation is used to enhance bone fusion. Many devices are available and for occipitocervical fusions include the Ransford loop, which is a modification of the Luque system contoured to allow wiring of the suboccipital bone. This material provides a very rigid fixation and may be extended as far down the cervical spine as necessary, even to the lowest levels. This system provides a much more rigid fixation than simple wiring with bone graft and external orthosis, which is reported to carry a pseudarthrosis rate of zero to 50 percent.[23-27] The technique described by Brattström and Granholm, in which a combination of wire, bone graft, and polymethyl methacrylate is used, is an excellent, simple, and effective method of occipitofusion, although others have abandoned this method in favor of more complex internal fixation arrangements, including shaped plates and transarticular screw fixation.[28, 29]

C1-C2 fusion procedures consist of wire fixation supplemented by bone grafting with external orthotic support. There are a wide variety of methods by which the wire can be configured, including the Gallie technique, the Brooks technique, or the method described by Roy-Camille. These techniques involve the passage of sublaminar wires at C1 or C2 or both, which requires experience, great care, and appropriate instrumentation to prevent the wire from impacting on the posterior surface of the spinal cord. The amount of space available deep to the lamina is judged from the preoperative imaging, and the presence of posterior column loss is a contraindication for this method.[17] The two main types of wire used are monofilament or multistranded cable wire, which is considerably more flexible while still incorporating high tensile strength. Passage of the multistranded wire is greatly facilitated by their flexibility. The passage of sublaminar wires at C2 and below is accomplished by the initial removal of part of the spinous processes and exposure of the midline raphe between the yellow ligaments at the interspaces. The sublaminar space is very carefully explored with a blunt-ended angled probe, the distance is assessed, and the wire is selected. The stiffer wire must be shaped to fit the contours of the cervical vertebrae, and passage of this wire is facilitated by specially designed instruments for this purpose (Codman). At all times, great care must be taken to prevent impaction on the spinal cord during passage and especially after the wires have been passed but are not yet secured into position. Removal of strands of soft tissue and ligament at the site of insertion and site of extraction of the wire makes the task easier. With the multistranded cable wire, a length of suture material may be passed initially and the flexible wire gently pulled through. When the wires are in position and looped into the selected conformation, they are tightened around the bone graft. Monofilament wire is twisted carefully up to the point at which secondary twists just begin to occur. The ends are trimmed and tucked safely down. Flexible wire needs to be tightened with the appropriate instrument and then crimped into position. Bone graft may be obtained from the posterior iliac crest and fashioned to shape, or in some cases, using bone from the spinous processes may be sufficient.

Other options for posterior fixation include titanium Halifax clamps or plates incorporating lateral mass screws. The latter are also, as with anterior plates, highly dependent on bone quality and may not be suitable in most rheumatoid patients. In the subaxial cervical spine, adjacent levels may simply be wired together by use of a sublaminar technique, although this technique is not recommended over more than two levels because the wire curves within the spinal canal if more than two levels are fixed. Interspinous wiring is another possibility but is a less secure means of internal fixation and relies heavily on external support.

Bone graft is applied to surfaces that have been decorticated by use of a high-speed drill. The rate of bone fusion is dependent on many factors, including the rigidity of the internal-external fixation, the fact that the more rigid methods of fixation are associated with higher bone fusion rates is no surprise. However, the need for any form of bone grafting has recently been called into question. It is argued that bone grafting is unnecessary, and in frail patients especially, the duration and morbidity of the operation is reduced when no bone graft is harvested (Crockard: Personal communication).

This is a stimulating challenge to accepted practice and one whose verification or refutation should be made clear in the future.

Various forms of external orthosis exist, ranging from simple cervical collars of the clerical type to Philadelphia-style collars to the skull, occiput, mandibular immunization brace and halo fixators. Each impart different degrees of fixation to the cervical spine, and the appropriate device should be selected according to the individual's needs. In some situations, no external orthotic support may be required.

OUTCOME: MORBIDITY AND COMPLICATIONS

Despite the effects of many years of systemic rheumatoid disease involving all tissues, the morbidity associated with surgery of the rheumatoid cervical spine is generally low.[21-23, 25, 30, 31] Wound dehiscence and infection are perhaps the commonest problems, but even so, they are surprisingly infrequent. Leakage of CSF after transoral surgery is a major potential problem that may require re-exploration if it does not resolve with a lumbar CSF drain. The use of fibrin-thrombin tissue glue with a lumbar CSF drain immediately after the leak is recognized at the operation effectively seals the leak and reduces the risk of fatal meningitis, which brought the earliest transoral operations into disrepute.[32, 33] Rheumatoid patients, as are other surgical patients, are prone to the complications of prolonged recumbency, including infections and venous thrombosis, but they also develop generalized joint stiffening that prolongs the recovery period. Early graduated mobilization, preferably within a unit experienced in surgery of patients with rheumatoid disease, is recommended.

Bone fusion rates in these patients tend to be lower than in those with other conditions, but a solid bone fusion may not necessarily be required in every case. Perhaps a strong fibrous union is sufficient. Santavirta and associates[2] found no correlation between clinical outcome and radiologic result.

Early postoperative mortality rates generally range from zero to 12 percent, although the cause of death is often not directly related to the surgical procedure.[22, 25, 31] Postoperative respiratory, cardiac or other major system complications reflect the generally frail nature of these patients. Increased mortality rates are associated with more severe neurologic grades (Ranawat IIIa or IIIb), as was noted by Zoma and coworkers,[23] and is strongly reinforced by Crockard (Personal communication). Santavirta and associates[2] observed that mortality risk after surgery is increased by coincident cardiac disease and by vertical subluxation of the odontoid process of greater than 3 mms. They also noted the tendency of patients classified in the worse neurologic grades to have a poor outcome and limited survival. Saway and colleagues[14] noted that the survival of postoperative patients was correlated with disease severity and, in particular, with presence of interstitial lung disease. This correlation was so strong that the role of cervical surgery at this stage needs to be carefully considered.

The neurologic gains can be considered either therapeutic or prophylactic, depending on the clinical presentation. Providing an overall estimate of neurologic improvement in this type of surgery is difficult because many of the reported series offer a variety of patients, they are often small in number, and they use different surgical procedures. Case selection, as always, probably has an influence on outcome and morbidity. Neurologic improvement usually ranges from 60 to 70 percent of patients, although in some of the earlier series, the neurologic improvement rate was higher.[34] Only when larger series are reported with outcomes correlated with preoperative neurologic grades will we have more accurate data on the efficacy of this type of surgery. The risk of neurologic deterioration is reported to be about 4 percent.

The posterior fusion procedure at C1-C2 for C2 root pain is associated with an excellent chance of successful pain relief, probably to a large extent irrespective of which method is selected for fixation-fusion.

The burgeoning interest and wealth of publications over the past 10 to 15 years concerning the surgical management of rheumatoid disease of the cervical spine reflect the role surgery plays in the treatment of these patients. This role is reasonably well defined against the background of the natural history of the condition and the likelihood of progressive myelopathy. The morbidity and mortality risks associated with surgery are becoming clear, and the greatest neurologic benefit is increasingly recognized to be associated with the lesser grades of myelopathy. It is hoped that the next few years will deliver more accurate information on the outcome of surgical management through the reporting of series containing large numbers of well-identified patients who undergo standardized surgical treatment.

The wide variety of surgical techniques available must not distract from the overriding purpose of this surgery, which is to recover or prevent neurologic deficit and to restore spinal integrity. More than one surgical technique will likely be deemed safe and successful for a given type of cervical spine involvement. It is now possible to thoroughly investigate the vertebral abnormality and to select a surgical management protocol most appropriate for the problem. Tailoring the procedure to the individual's requirement rather than applying a universal operation seems more likely to produce superior results.

As surgical management of the condition evolves, factors that are associated with a poor outcome are being more clearly identified. Treating end-stage or advanced disease certainly provides a surgical and anesthetic challenge, but simpler, safer, and more efficacious procedures might be employed at earlier stages. One of the aims of any audit of this group of patients should be to allow early identification of patients who are likely to deteriorate, although whether or not this will be possible remains to be seen. Because of this continuing uncertainty, the role of prophylactic cervical surgery remains unclear.

Acknowledgment

The contribution of Miss Helen Wilson to the preparation and completion of this chapter will never be fully recognized.

REFERENCES

1. Stevens JC, Cartlidge NEF, Saunders M, et al: Atlanto-axial subluxation and cervical myelopathy in rheumatoid arthritis. Q J Med 159:391–408, 1971

2. Santavirta S, Konttinen YT, Laasonen E, et al: Ten-year results of operation for rheumatoid cervical spine disorders. J Bone Joint Surg Br 73(B):116–120, 1991
3. Dvorak J, Grob D, Baumgartner H, et al: Functional evaluation of the spinal cord by magnetic resonance imaging in patients with rheumatoid arthritis and instability of upper cervical spine. Spine 14:1057–1064, 1989
4. Mathews JA: Atlanto-axial subluxation in rheumatoid arthritis. Ann Rheum Dis 33:526–531, 1974
5. Bland JH: Rheumatoid arthritis of the cervical spine. J Rheumatol 3:319–341, 1974
6. Pellicci PM, Ranawat CS, Tsairis P, Bryan WJ: A prospective study of the progression of rheumatoid arthritis of the cervical spine. J Bone Joint Surg Am 63(A):342–350, 1981
7. Santavirta S, Kankaanpaa U, Sandelin J, et al: Evaluation of patients with rheumatoid cervical spine. Scand J Rheumatol 16:9–16, 1987
8. Manz HJ, Luessenhop AJ, Robertson DM: Cervical myelopathy due to atlantoaxial and subaxial subluxation in rheumatoid arthritis. Arch Pathol Lab Med 107:94–98, 1983
9. Nakano KK, Schoene WC, Baker RA, Dawson DM: The cervical myelopathy associated with rheumatoid arthritis: Analysis of 32 patients with 2 postmortem cases. Ann Neurol 3:144–151, 1978
10. Hughes JT: Spinal cord involvement by C4-C5 vertebral subluxation in rheumatoid arthritis: A description of 2 cases examined by necropsy. Ann Neurol 1:575–582, 1977
11. Bell GR, Stearns KL: Flexion-extension MRI of the upper rheumatoid cervical spine. Orthopedics 14:969–974, 1991
12. Krodel A, Refior HJ, Westermann S: The importance of functional magnetic resonance imaging in the planning of stabilizing operations on the cervical spine in rheumatoid patients. Arch Orthop Trauma Surg 109:30–33, 1989
13. Dillin WH, Watkins RG: Clinical syndromes in cervical myelopathy, in Rothman RH, Simeone FA (eds): The Spine, 3rd ed. Philadelphia, WB Saunders, 1992, pp 560–564
14. Saway PA, Blackburn WD, Halla JT, Alarcon GS: Clinical characteristics affecting survival in patients with rheumatoid arthritis undergoing cervical spine surgery: A controlled study. J Rheumatol 16:890–896, 1989
15. Marks JS, Sharp J: Rheumatoid cervical myelopathy. Q J Med 199:307–319, 1981
16. Floyd AS, Learmonth ID, Mody G, Meyers OL: Atlanto-axial instability and neurologic indicators in rheumatoid arthritis. Clin Orthop Rel Res 241:177–182, 1989
17. Rogers MA, Crockard HA, Moskovich R, et al: Nystagmus and joint position sensation: Their importance in posterior occipitocervical fusion in rheumatoid arthritis. Presented at the 19th Annual Meeting, Cervical Spine Research Society, Philadelphia, December 1991
18. Toolanen G: Cutaneous sensory impairment in rheumatoid atlanto-axial subluxation assessed quantitatively by electrical stimulation. Scand J Rheumatol 16:27–32, 1987
19. Frerk CM: Predicting difficulties in intubation. Anaesthesia 46:1005–1008, 1991
20. Dickman CA, Locantro J, Fessler RG: The influence of transoral odontoid resection on stability of the craniovertebral junction. J Neurosurg 77:525–530, 1992
21. Crockard HA, Calder I, Ransford AO: One stage transoral decompression and posterior fixation in rheumatoid atlanto-axial subluxation. J Bone Joint Surg Br 72(B):682–685, 1990
22. Santavirta S, Konttinen YT, Laasonen E, et al: Ten year results of operations for rheumatoid cervical spine disorders. J Bone Joint Surg Br 73(B):116–120, 1991
23. Zoma A, Sturrock RD, Fisher WD, et al: Surgical stabilization of the rheumatoid cervical spine. J Bone Joint Surg Br 69(B):8–12, 1987
24. Wertheim SB, Bohlman HH: Occipitocervical fusion. J Bone Joint Surg Am 69(A6):883–836, 1987
25. Ranawat CS, O'Leary P, Pellicci P, et al: Cervical spine fusion in rheumatoid arthritis. J Bone Joint Surg Am 61(A):1003–1010, 1979
26. Chan CP, Ngian KS, Cohen L: Posterior upper cervical fusion in rheumatoid arthritis. Spine 17:268–272, 1992
27. Ferlic DC, Clayton ML, Leidholt JD, Gamble WE: Surgical treatment of the symptomatic unstable cervical spine in rheumatoid arthritis. J Bone Joint Surg Am 57(A):349–354, 1975
28. Brattström H, Granholm L: Atlanto-axial fusion in rheumatoid arthritis. Acta Orthop Scand 47:619–628, 1976
29. Grob D, Dvorak J, Gschwend N, Froehlich M: Posterior occipito-cervical fusion in rheumatoid arthritis. Arch Orthop Trauma Surg 110:38–44, 1990
30. Slatis P, Santavirta S, Sandelin J, Konttinen YT: Cranial subluxation of the odontoid process in rheumatoid arthritis. J Bone Joint Surg Am 71(A):189–195, 1989
31. Clark CR, Goetz DD, Menezes AH: Arthrodesis of the cervical spine in rheumatoid arthritis. J Bone Joint Surg Am 71(A):381–392, 1989
32. Hadley MN, Spetzler RF, Sonntag VKH: The transoral approach to the superior cervical spine. J Neurosurg 71:16–23, 1989
33. Crockard HA: The transoral approach to the base of the brain and upper cervical cord. Ann R Coll Surg Engl 67:321–325, 1985
34. Crockard HA, Essigman WK, Stevens JM, et al: Surgical treatment of cervical cord compression in rheumatoid arthritis. Ann Rheum Dis 44:809–816, 1985

Editorial Commentary

We thought of suggesting to the authors Johnston and Borthwick that they commit themselves to firmer recommendations as to specific courses of action in more of the situations they describe. However, we decided that the fact that they are so cautious about making firm recommendations about how to handle specific problems sends a strong message to the prospective surgeon in this field that he or she should conduct an intensive study of the literature before embarking on these operations and that he or she should then document the history, findings, operative procedure, and long-term results so that future surgeons will be treading on more assured ground.

CHAPTER 141

Microsurgery of Syringomyelia and Syringomyelic Cord Syndrome

Albert L. Rhoton, Jr.

The term *syringomyelia* has been used to refer to a chronic, relentlessly progressive syndrome that is caused by the destruction of gray and white matter beginning adjacent to the central canal of the spinal cord and is associated with an enlarging accumulation of fluid within the spinal cord. Its clinical hallmarks are atrophy and dissociated anesthesia beginning in the upper extremities. The first manifestation is often a loss of sensation to pain and temperature in the involved dermatomes (although tactile sensation remains intact) that is caused by destruction of the pain fibers crossing anterior to the central canal of the spinal cord. The area of destruction forms a cavity that then extends into the anterior horn and destroys the motor neurons and causes atrophy and weakness in the involved segments. As the disease progresses, evidence of involvement of the long motor and sensory pathways in the spinal cord often occurs as well. Scoliosis is frequently present, and neurogenic arthropathies develop in the later stages of the disorder. The location of the lesion has led to the constellation of typical neurologic findings being referred to as a central cord syndrome, and the association of these deficits with syringomyelia has led to the name *syringomyelic cord syndrome.*

The typical spinal syndrome is frequently accompanied by a dysfunction of the lower brain, in which case the syringomyelia is said to be accompanied by syringobulbia. The common manifestations of this bulbar dysfunction include upper and lower motor neuron signs in the bulbar musculature, gait difficulties caused by involvement of cerebellar and corticospinal pathways, and variable nystagmus. Operative experience in 56 patients with syringomyelic syndrome has led the author to conclude that hydromyelia, a condition in which the central canal of the spinal cord communicates with the fourth ventricle and is distended by cerebrospinal fluid (CSF), is the commonest cause of the syringomyelic syndrome, and that the Chiari malformation that invariably accompanies hydromyelia is the cause of the syringobulbic syndrome.

The syringomyelic cord syndrome is a relatively uncommon disorder. In a survey of neurologic disease in an English city, Brewis and his colleagues found a prevalence rate of 8.4 cases for each 100,000 persons.[1]

The pathologic basis of the syringomyelic cord syndrome is frequently misunderstood. Since the initial description of the clinical syndrome in the last century,[2] syringomyelia incorrectly has become synonymous with an untreatable degenerative condition, rather than correctly descriptive of a pressure distension of the spinal cord caused by a developmental anomaly. Authorities as prominent as those writing in Merritt's *Textbook of Neurology* classify syringomyelia as a degenerative process for which "there is no satisfactory treatment."[3] This misconception derives from the traditional impression that the syringomyelic type of neurologic deficit is caused by a degenerative cavitation and gliosis beginning adjacent to, but not communicating with, the central canal of the spinal cord; syringobulbia has been assumed to be caused by a rostral extension of the degenerative process into the brainstem.

The inaccuracy of this traditional concept is illustrated by the fact that not one of the more than 50 patients whom we have treated for a spontaneously appearing syringomyelic cord syndrome was found to have degenerative cavitation and gliosis within the spinal cord; approximately three fourths were caused by hydromyelia associated with a Chiari malformation (Fig. 141–1), and the remainder were caused by an intramedullary tumor.[4,5] These findings correspond with those of other reports on large series[6–11] in showing that the commonest cause of the spontaneously appearing, slowly progressive central cord deficit that we call the syringomyelic cord syndrome is distension of the spinal cord by a collection of CSF that communicates freely with the central canal of the spinal cord and, at its rostral end, communicates in turn with the fourth ventricle. This syndrome is invariably associated with a Chiari malformation or some other developmental anomaly that occludes the foramen of Magendie.

In response to these findings, Gardner put forward the hydrodynamic theory of the development of the syringomyelia by proposing that cystic dilatation of the cord, which originates in embryonic life and results from overdistension of the neural tube because of a partial or complete obstruction at the foramen of Magendie, results in slowly progressive dilatation of the central canal or a ramifying diverticulum originating in the central canal and in continuity with the spinal fluid pathways through the fourth ventricle.[7]

Earlier authors studying cavitation of the spinal cord suggested that the term *syringomyelia* be reserved for cavities unconnected with the central canal, and that pathologic dilatation of the central canal as a developmental anomaly be referred to as hydromyelia.[2,12] A review of large series of

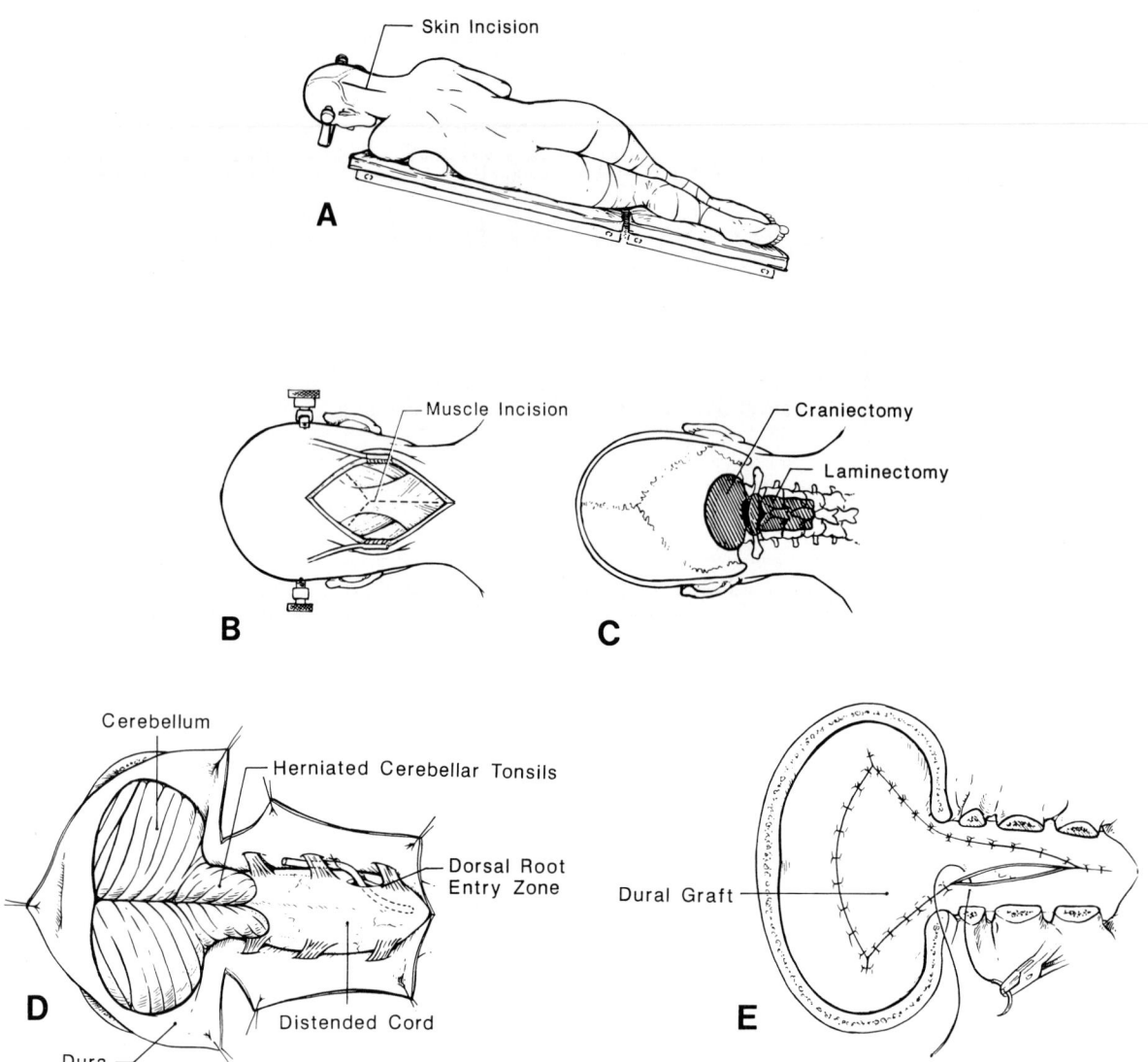

FIGURE 141-1. Surgical exposure of a Chiari malformation and hydromyelia. (A) The three-quarter prone position is used. The head is positioned higher than the feet. The face is turned 45 degrees toward the floor, and a midline skin incision is used. The side of the dorsal root entry zone to be drained is placed uppermost. (B) Site of muscle incision. A Y-shaped incision is made to provide a muscle flap attached to the superior nuchal line and inion, which facilitates closure. (C) Site of craniectomy and laminectomy. The laminectomy is extended to include C4 if a hydromyelic cavity is to be drained through the exposure. (D) Exposure of the Chiari malformation and hydromyelia. The cerebellar tonsils extend down to the level of C2. The hydromyelia has been drained through a myelotomy in the dorsal root entry zone. A silicone wick is anchored to the dura and threaded downward into the hydromyelic cavity and upward into the ventral subarachnoid space. (E) A dural graft is used to complete the closure in order to avoid constricting the cervicomedullary junction and the Chiari malformation. (Reprinted from Rhoton AL Jr, Fessler RG: Surgical treatment of Chiari malformation and hydromyelia in adults, in Wilson CB [ed]: Neurosurgical Procedures. Baltimore, Williams & Wilkins, 1992, pp 169–187. With permission.)

patients reported in the literature reveals, however, that cavities unconnected with the central canal occur rarely, except in association with intramedullary tumors.[6–11] Barnett and his colleagues[6] agree that a hydromyelic cavity is the likeliest cause of a spontaneously appearing central cord syndrome, but they refer to the condition not as hydromyelia but as communicating syringomyelia. I prefer to refer to the dynamic cord pathology associated with a Chiari malformation as hydromyelia because of the traditional association of the term syringomyelia with an untreatable degenerative disease.

In 1888, Chiari reported that most syringomyelic cavities were, in fact, hydromyelic cavities connected with the central canal of the spinal cord and were associated with the cerebellar deformity that bears his name.[12] The Chiari malformation is characterized by displacement of the cerebellar tonsils, the brainstem, and the fourth ventricle into the upper spinal canal. Because this malformation accompanies hydrocephalus and myelomeningocele in the infant, clinicians who encounter an adult with a spontaneously appearing, slowly progressive central cord syndrome—but with no history of hydrocephalus or myelomeningocele—often consider diagnoses other than a Chiari malformation and hydromyelia, when in fact that is most frequently the correct diagnosis.

In my series of patients, the second commonest cystic spinal lesion producing a syringomyelic-type cord syndrome was an intramedullary tumor associated with a cyst. The cysts did not communicate with the central canal, were not associated with a hindbrain malformation, and contained yellow or brown fluid with an elevated protein content.

Cysts can develop within the spinal cord after traumatic paraplegia, Pott's disease, and arachnoiditis.[6] Posttraumatic cysts produce a slowly ascending progressive deficit that develops long after the event and causes the acute traumatic paraplegia. Barnett and his colleagues[6] differentiated cystic lesions in the spinal cord into a noncommunicating form and a communicating form, based on whether they communicate with the central canal or with the spinal cord. The noncommunicating form was associated with an intramedullary tumor and posttraumatic paraplegia, and the communicating form resulted from persistent dilatation of the central canal under pressure associated with a developmental anomaly obstructing the foramen of Magendie. The latter is by far the commonest cause of a syringomyelic cord syndrome.

The improved understanding of the pathogenesis of syringomyelic cord syndrome that has accrued in recent years has led to a more rational approach to surgical treatment than was previously the case. This chapter focuses on patients who have the syndrome of hydromyelia associated with a Chiari malformation because it is the commonest cause of a syringomyelic cord syndrome, and because it presents the most difficult problems with respect to diagnosis and treatment.

CLINICAL FACTORS

Most central cervical cord syndromes are caused by hydromyelia associated with a Chiari malformation, which is a surgically treatable condition. For this reason, an active investigational attitude should be adopted so that the disorder is recognized and treated early because patients who have progressed beyond a certain stage of disability have little likelihood of achieving a useful recovery.

All of our patients with a Chiari malformation and hydromyelia were between the ages of 16 and 72 years. No patient had a prior history of hydrocephalus or myelomeningocele. All patients with hydromyelia had signs and symptoms referable to it, but only one-third had signs referable to the Chiari malformation. Many patients in this series, who were initially diagnosed as having untreatable degenerative disease because the size of the spinal cord (as defined on positive-contrast myelography) was normal, progressed to develop crippling deficits before a Chiari malformation with hydromyelia was discovered. In approximately one-fourth of our patients with a syringomyelic cord syndrome, the cause was a cystic intramedullary tumor. The group of patients with hydromyelia differed from the group with intramedullary tumors in that patients with hydromyelia commonly had bulbar signs, whereas those with tumors did not.

Sensory loss usually preceded lower motor neuron signs. The deficits produced by the hydromyelia ranged in severity from a minimal motor deficit or subjective sensory loss, or both, to a widespread sensory loss and quadriparesis with marked atrophy of the upper extremities and atrophy or spasticity in the lower extremities. In the early stages, the sensory deficit frequently began and was greater on one side, rather than being bilaterally symmetrical. The weakness and atrophy most commonly began and were greatest in the hands, but in three cases, shoulder-girdle involvement was so great that the arms could not be abducted at the shoulders, whereas strength in the hands was relatively preserved. In later stages, compression of the corticospinal tracts and long sensory pathways resulted in a spastic gait and sensory loss in the lower extremities. Five patients, who were followed up without surgery after the initial diagnosis because their neurologic deficits were minimal, worsened and were operated on within 1 year after the initial diagnosis.

The patients with brainstem symptoms caused by the Chiari malformation had a combination of upper and lower motor neuron signs in the bulbar musculature, gait difficulties caused by cerebellar and long tract involvement, and nystagmus. Some patients with a Chiari malformation have experienced sudden, severe respiratory stridor caused by bilateral vocal cord paralysis and a rapid onset or progression of other symptoms. Bertrand has described the mechanism for a sudden onset or change of symptoms in cases of the Chiari malformation.[13]

Although defective ventricular drainage is thought to be important in the development of hydromyelia, no patient in this series had either hydrocephalus or evidence of increased intracranial pressure.

DIAGNOSIS

RADIOLOGY

Plain films of the skull and cervical spine in patients with a Chiari malformation and hydromyelia frequently show no abnormality. In the past, it was assumed that a normal skull and cervical spine excluded the diagnosis of a Chiari malformation and hydromyelia; however, our patients infrequently had anomalies of the skull, cervical spine, or craniovertebral junction, such as a basilar impression, Klippel-Feil deformity, atlanto-occipital fusion, or widening of the anteroposterior diameter of the cervical spinal canal. In patients with an intramedullary tumor, plain x-ray films may reveal focal enlargement of the spinal cord, thinning of the pedicles and laminae, and scalloping of the vertebral bodies. In those with hydromyelia, the anteroposterior diameter of the spine may be enlarged, but none of the features of focal expansion that are seen with intramedullary tumors are present.

Magnetic resonance imaging (MRI) is the single best method for evaluating patients suspected of having a Chiari malformation and hydromyelia (Fig. 141–2). It provides information about the extent of the descent of the cerebellar tonsils and fourth ventricle into the foramen magnum and upper spinal canal, the transverse diameter and rostrocaudal extent of the hydromyelic cavity, and the size of the lateral ventricles. MRI usually provides all the information needed to plan a surgical approach to these conditions. In addition, it demonstrates the disappearance of the hydromyelic cavity with successful therapy (Fig. 141–2).

If MRI cannot be performed or does not provide the information needed for diagnosis and treatment, myelography with water-soluble contrast medium can be used in conjunction with computed tomography (CT) (Fig. 141–3). A CT scan alone shows the caudal displacement of the fourth ven-

Text continued on page 1753

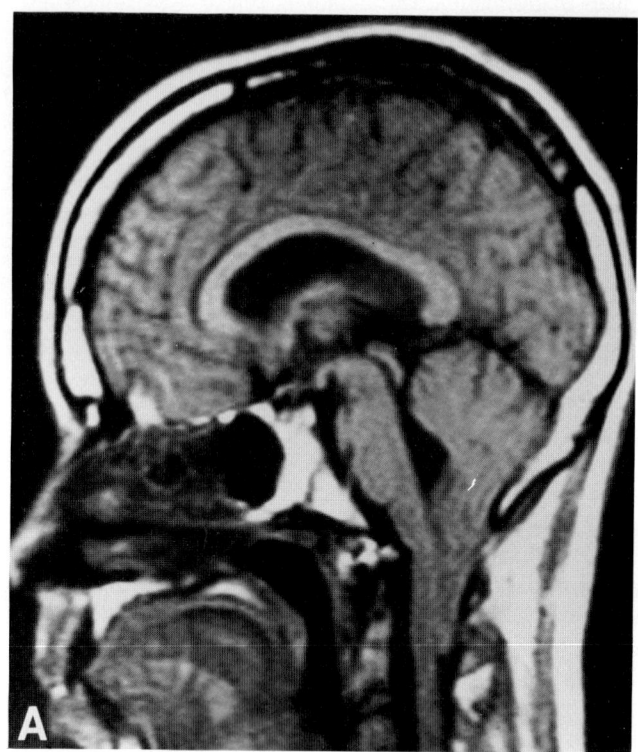
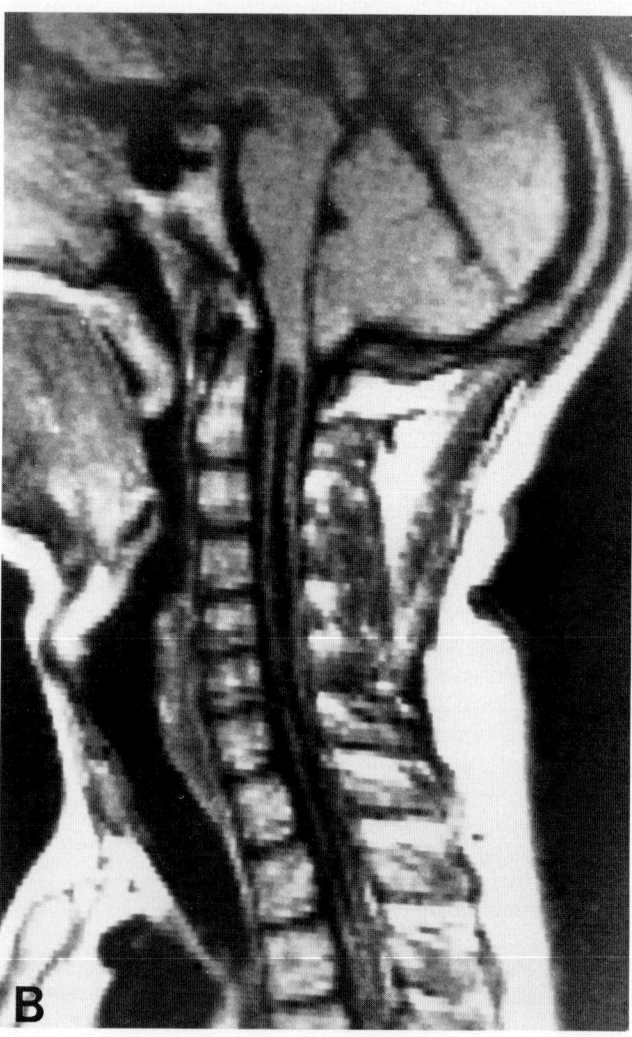

FIGURE 141–2. Magnetic resonance images of a Chiari malformation and hydromyelia from selected patients. (A) Left lateral view. Chiari malformation without hydromyelia. The cerebellar tonsils are herniated downward to the level of C-2. (B) Left lateral view. This patient with a Chiari malformation also has a hydromyelic cavity. The cavity in the spinal cord extends from the level of the foramen magnum, through the cervical region into the upper thoracic area.

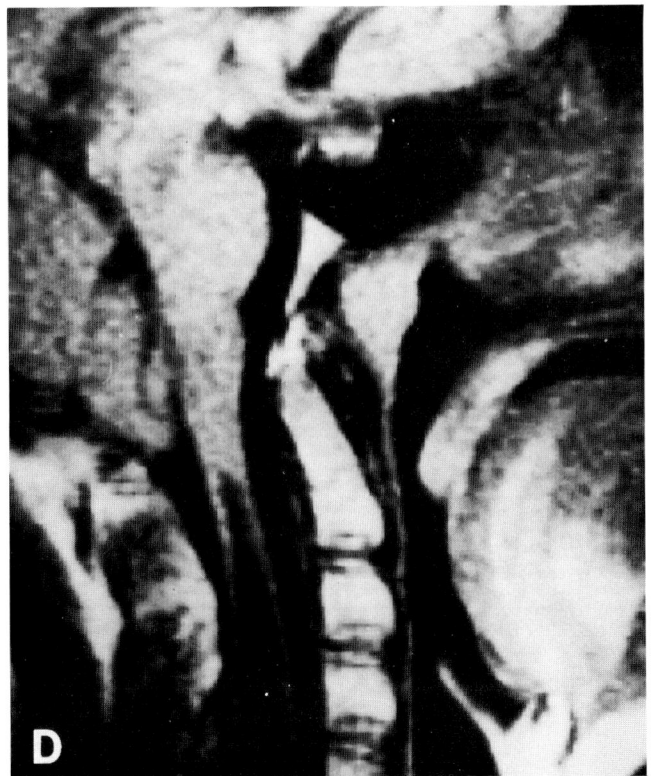
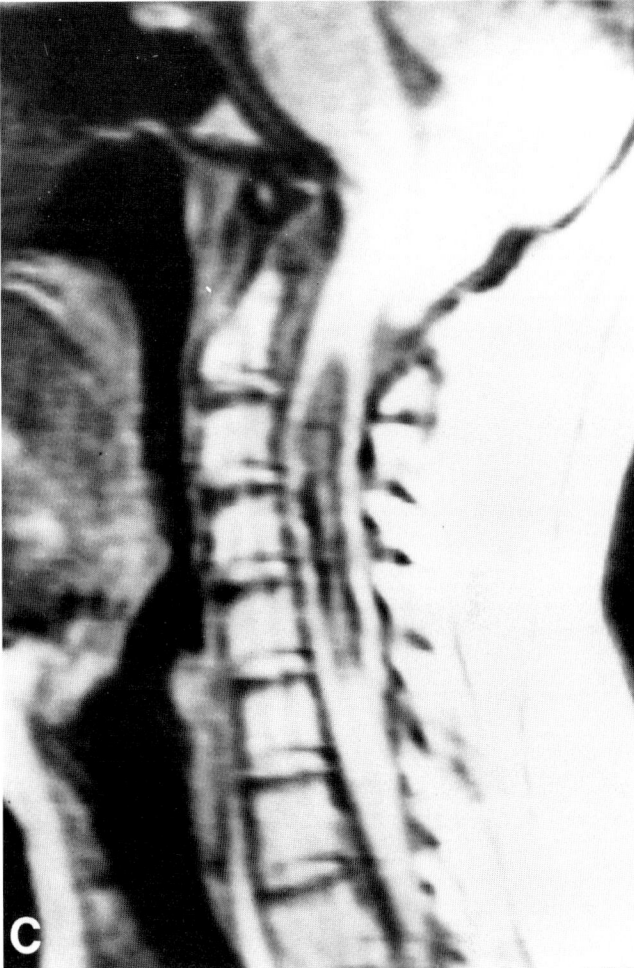
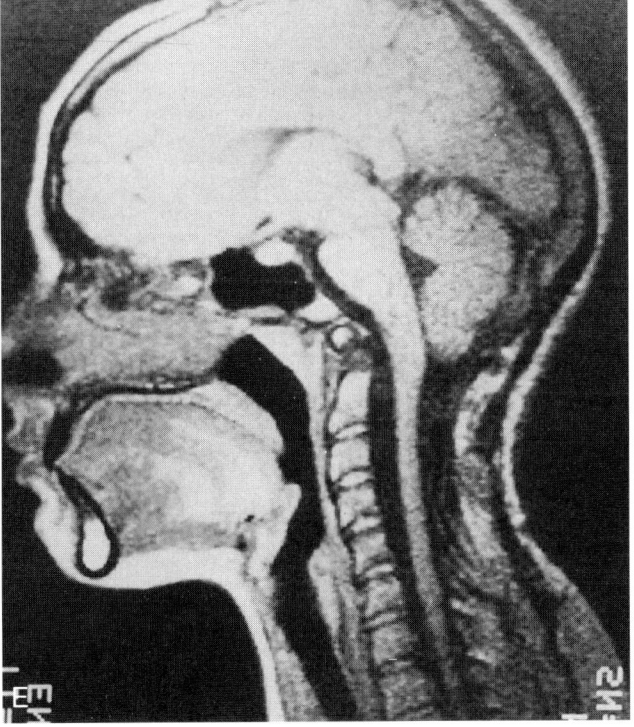

FIGURE 141–2 *Continued* (C) Left lateral view. This patient has a hydromyelic cavity with a septum in the central part of the hydromyelic cavity. (D and E) Scan from a patient before (D) and after (E) surgical treatment. (D) MRI before surgical treatment showing the Chiari malformation and the hydromyelic cavity. (E) MRI scan obtained 1 year following suboccipital craniectomy and upper cervical laminectomy and drainage of the cavity through the dorsal root entry zone. Spinal cord size has returned to normal, and the cavity within the spinal cord has disappeared.

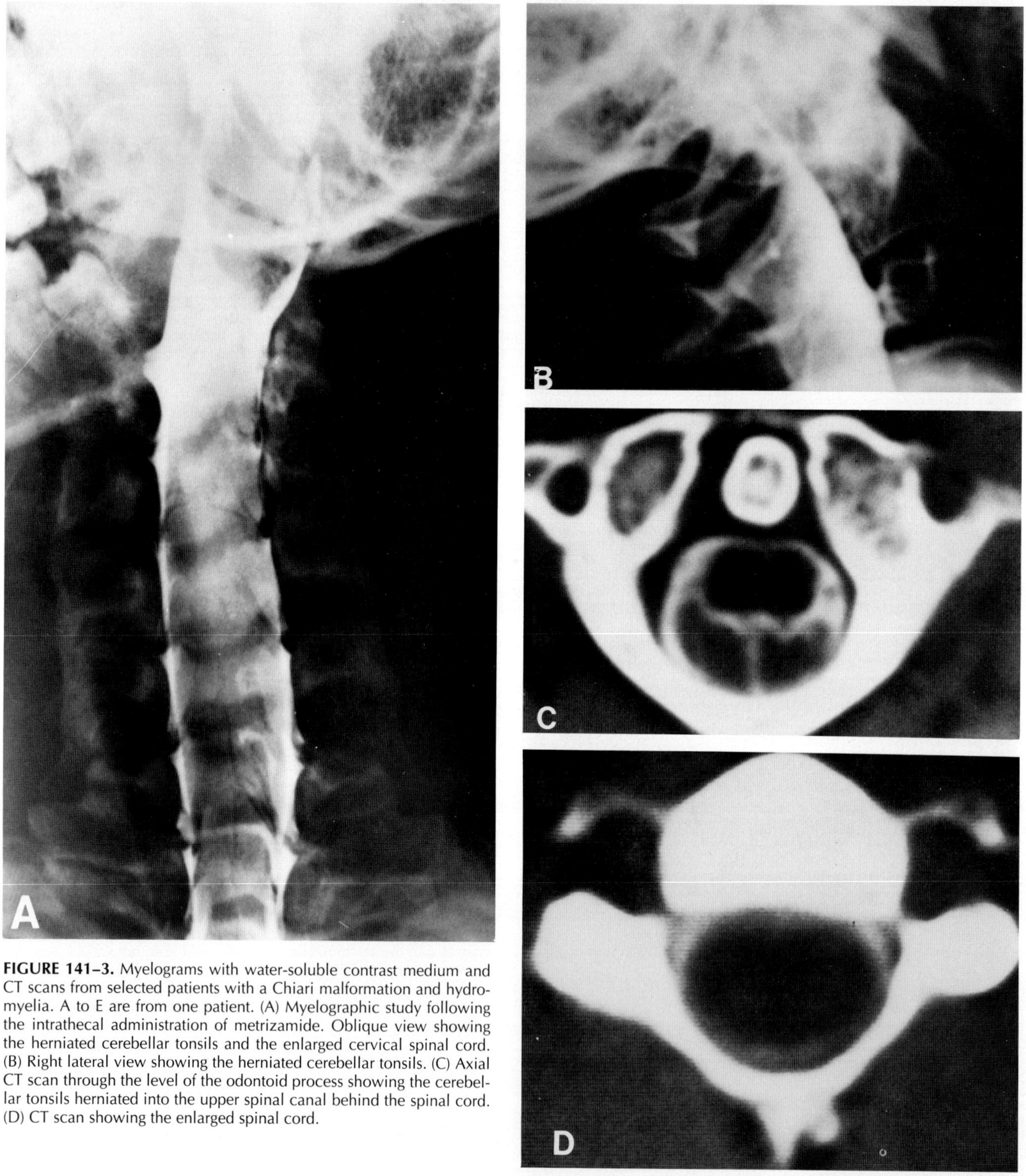

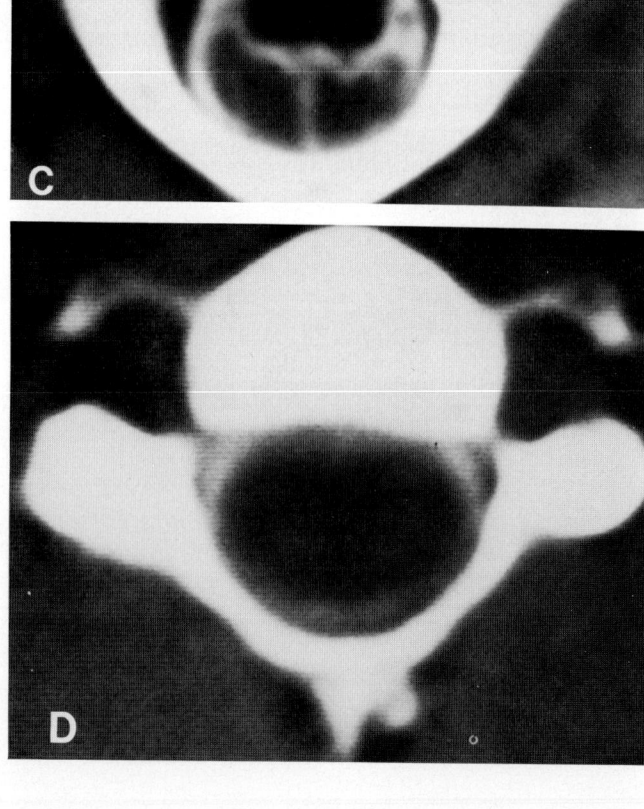

FIGURE 141–3. Myelograms with water-soluble contrast medium and CT scans from selected patients with a Chiari malformation and hydromyelia. A to E are from one patient. (A) Myelographic study following the intrathecal administration of metrizamide. Oblique view showing the herniated cerebellar tonsils and the enlarged cervical spinal cord. (B) Right lateral view showing the herniated cerebellar tonsils. (C) Axial CT scan through the level of the odontoid process showing the cerebellar tonsils herniated into the upper spinal canal behind the spinal cord. (D) CT scan showing the enlarged spinal cord.

Microsurgery of Syringomyelia and Syringomyelic Cord Syndrome | 1751

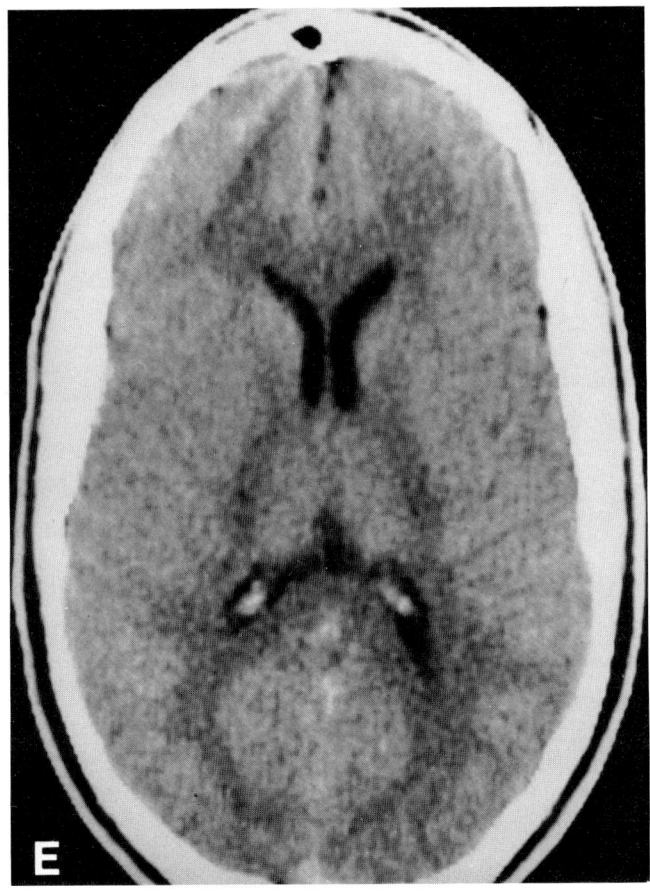

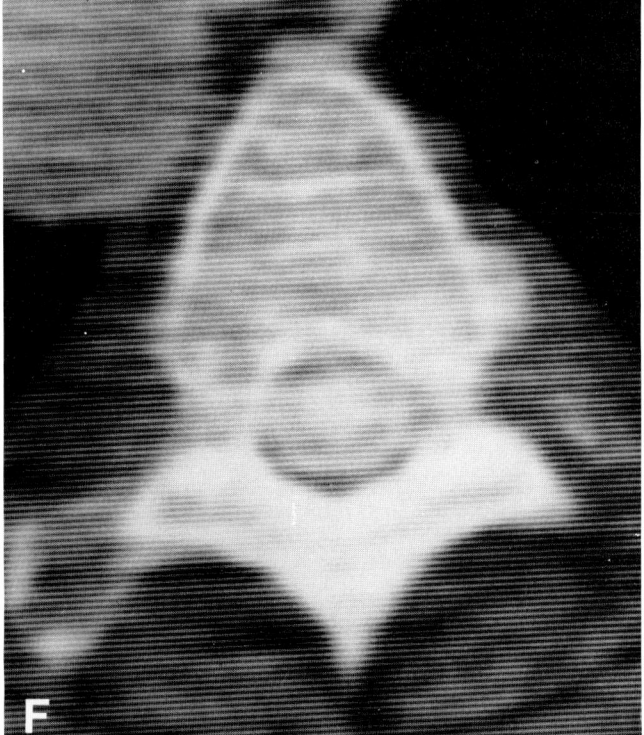

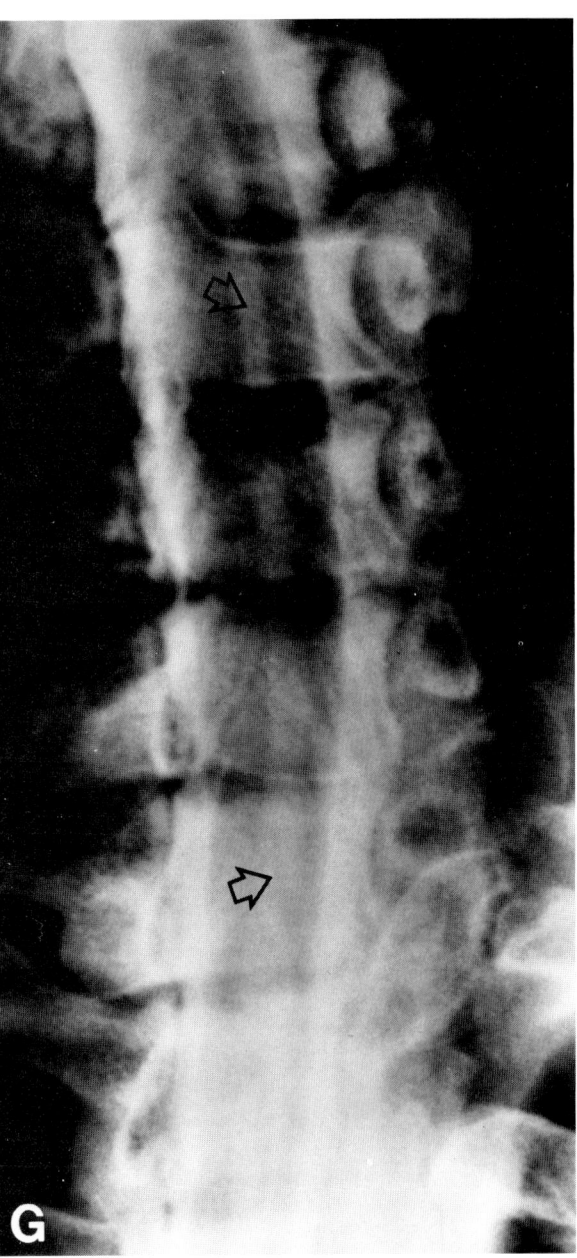

FIGURE 141–3 *Continued* (E) CT scan of head showing the lateral ventricles to be of normal size. (F) CT scan from another patient, 12 hours after intrathecal installation of metrizamide, showing the accumulation of contrast medium within the spinal cord. G to I are from another patient with a Chiari malformation. (G) During the myelogram, the metrizamide entered the hydromyelic cavity (arrows).

Illustration continued on following page

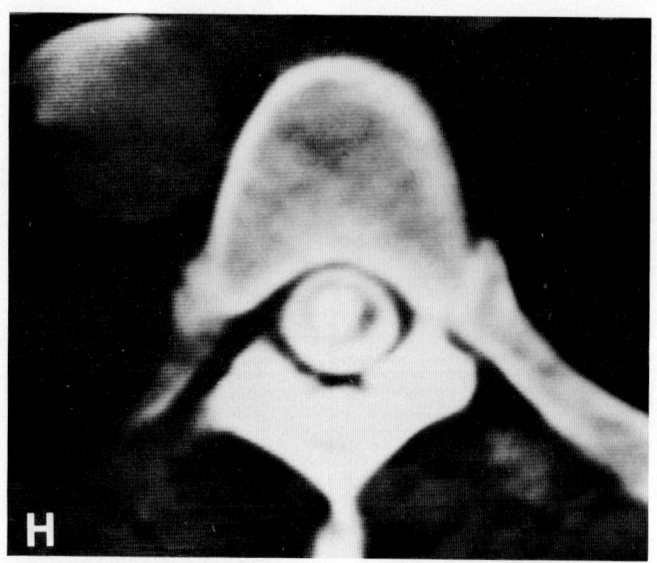
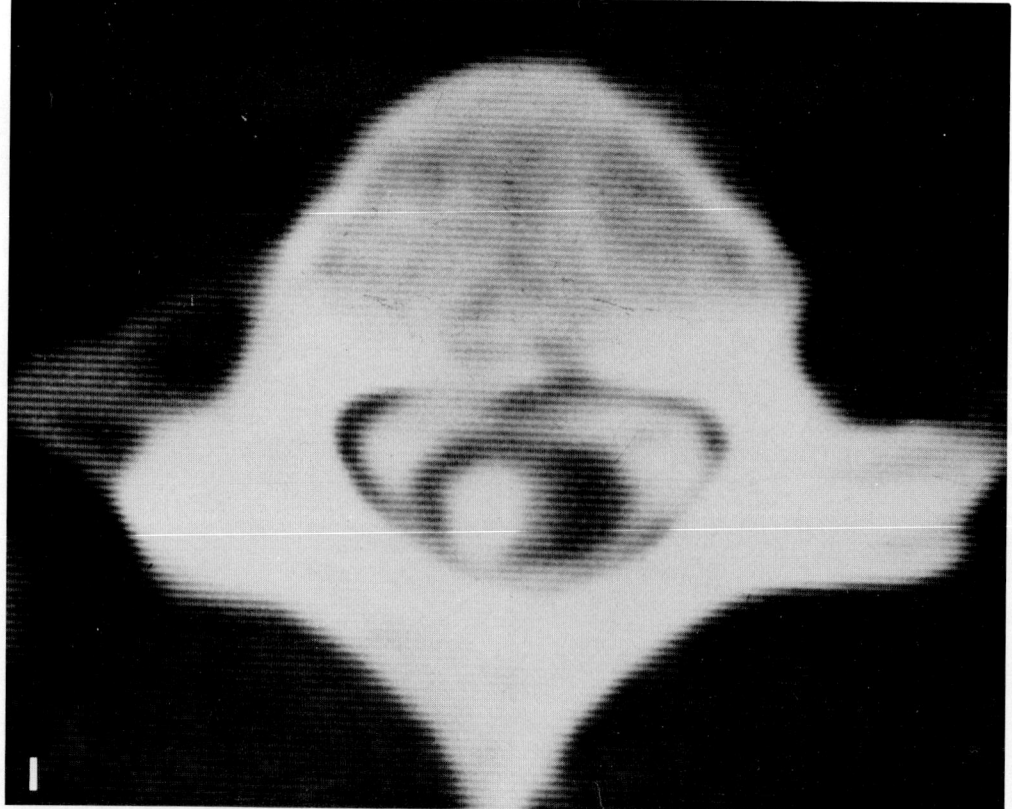

FIGURE 141–3 *Continued* (H) Axial CT scan showing the metrizamide in the hydromyelic cavity that fills the central part of the spinal cord. (I) Axial CT scan at another level, showing the cavity situated in one-half of the cord.

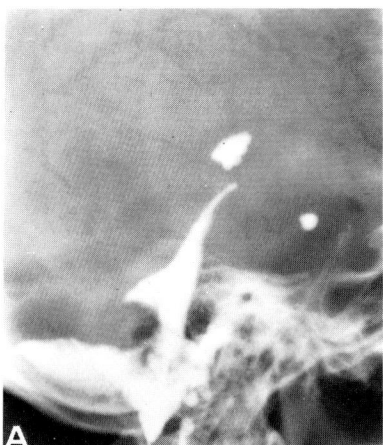
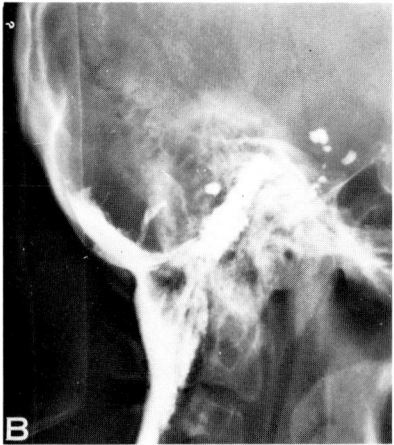
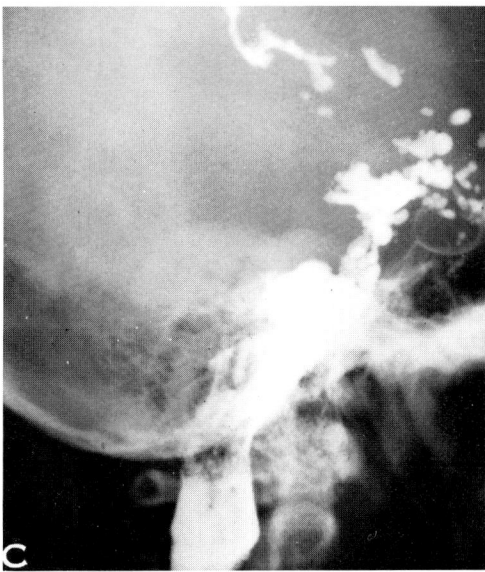

FIGURE 141–4. Myelograms, with Pantopaque, of the Chiari malformation from selected patients. (A) Normal lateral view of a Pantopaque study with the patient in the supine position. Pantopaque fills the cisterna magna and the fourth ventricle to the level of the aqueduct. (B) A Pantopaque myelogram performed with the patient in the supine position outlines the cerebellar tonsils indicative of the Chiari malformation. (C) A Pantopaque study of the foramen magnum with the patient in the supine position showing the Chiari malformation. No Pantopaque passes into the cisterna magna above the level of the foramen magnum. At surgery, dense adhesions were found in the area of the cisterna magna that bound the medulla and cerebellum to the dura. (Reprinted from Rhoton AL: Microsurgery of Arnold-Chiari malformation in adults with and without hydromyelia. J Neurosurg 45:473–483, 1976. With permission.)

tricle and cerebellar tonsils but only infrequently shows the enlarged spinal cord and the hydromyelic cavity. A CT scan performed after the intrathecal injection of metrizamide shows the tonsillar herniation and the enlargement of the spinal cord (Fig. 141–3). A CT scan delayed 8 to 24 hours after infection may show that the contrast medium has entered the cavity in the spinal cord. The hydromyelic cavity may be situated centrally or asymmetrically within the cord, and it may vary from level to level in its position (Fig. 141–3H and I). Plain x-ray films rarely show the contrast medium within the hydromyelic cavity (Fig. 141–3G).

In the past, the procedure most helpful in defining the cause of syringomyelic cord syndrome was positive-contrast myelography using iophendylate (Pantopaque) and obtained with the patient in both the prone and supine positions (Figs. 141–4 and 141–5). In patients with hydromyelia, iophendylate myelography with the patient supine outlines the Chiari malformation; frequently, the prone study reveals no abnormalities and shows normal cord size even when the patient has a large cavity that produces a marked neurologic deficit (Fig. 141–5). Many of our patients with hydromyelia were initially diagnosed as having untreatable degenerative disease, because iophendylate myelography of the cervical and thoracic regions showed that cord size was normal. In these patients, the disease had progressed, and they developed marked deficits before the correct diagnosis was established. Barnett and his colleagues[6] also noted that myelographic studies of the spinal cord alone may give normal results, even if the patient in fact has hydromyelia.

Spinal cord deficits are assumed to be caused by hydromyelia—even if the cord is of normal size or only minimally enlarged—if the neurologic deficit is typical of syringomyelia and if the myelogram with iophendylate or metrizamide or the CT scan shows the Chiari malformation. We have seen

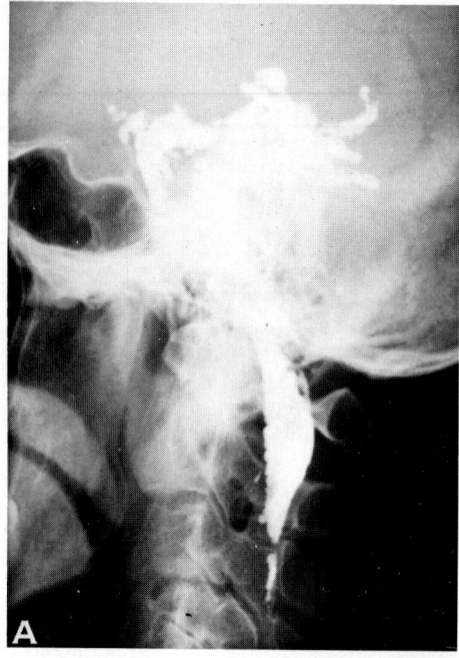
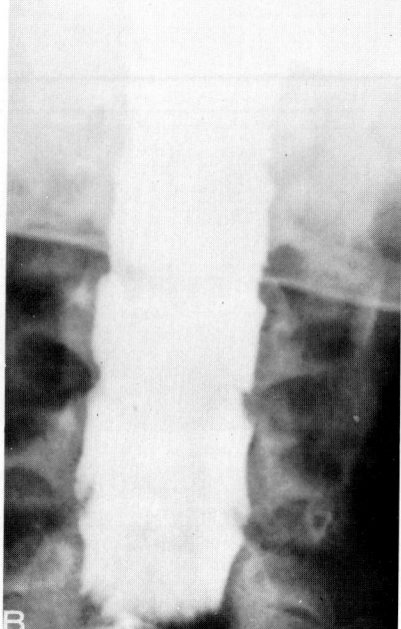
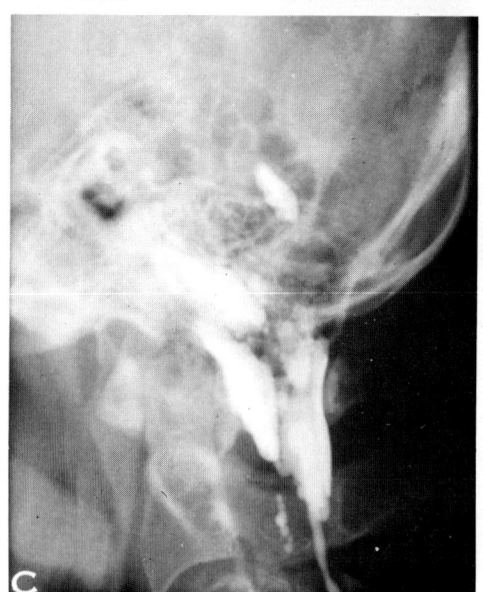
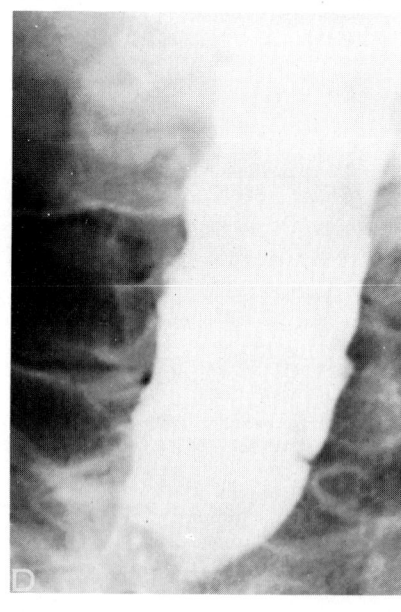

FIGURE 141–5. Myelograms with Pantopaque. A and B are from one patient; C and D are from another patient. Both patients had previous myelograms that were reported to be normal. Myelograms B and D show no striking abnormalities in the cervical regions. A diagnosis of degenerative disease had been made because the cord size appeared normal on previous myelograms. Pantopaque studies (lateral view) of the foramen magnum with both patients in the supine position (A and C) show the Chiari malformation causing obstruction to filling of the cisterna magna. The findings from supine Pantopaque myelography led to a diagnosis of Arnold-Chiari malformation with hydromyelia. (Reprinted from Rhoton AL: Microsurgery of Arnold-Chiari malformation in adults with and without hydromyelia. J Neurosurg 45:473–483, 1976. With permission.)

patients in whom deficits caused by a hydromyelic cavity were far advanced, but in whom cord diameter was normal on myelography, and we would conclude that the pia mater covering the spinal cord apparently restricts the ability of the cord to enlarge with a hydromyelic cavity.

In comparison with hydromyelia, an intramedullary tumor commonly produces a more striking picture of cord enlargement on the myelogram (Fig. 141–6). Even when an intramedullary tumor is diagnosed early, it has often caused striking enlargement of the cord and is frequently associated with an almost complete block. When present, the enlargement produced by hydromyelia is diffuse over many segments, whereas typically the enlargement caused by a tumor is more localized. Exceptions to this rule occur but are uncommon.

The author has limited experience with the use of gas myelography in the investigation of hydromyelia. The hydromyelic cord may appear thin or atrophic on air studies performed with the patient upright because the intramedullary fluid settles to the bottom of the cavity when air surrounds it. The gas delineates the cerebellar tonsils below the foramen magnum and an elongated flaccid cyst of the spinal cord. Ellertsson,[14] by tilting the patient during gas myelography, demonstrated that the hydromyelic cavity may appear flaccid or distended and may fluctuate in size, depending on the position of the patient during the study. He also showed that the enlargement of the spinal cord caused by a tumor is nonfluctuating. Pneumomyelography in patients with hydromyelia demonstrates a full cord if the study is performed with the patient's head dependent and demonstrates a thin cord when performed with the patient upright.

Angiography shows the displacement of the cerebellar tonsils associated with the Chiari malformation as defined by the descent of the posteroinferior cerebellar artery, but otherwise angiography is not helpful except to show the size of

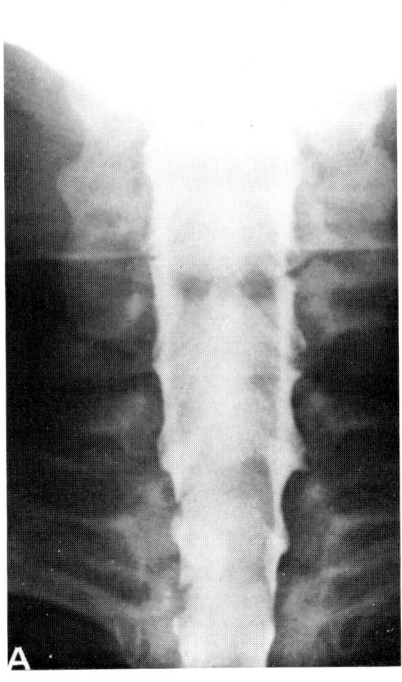
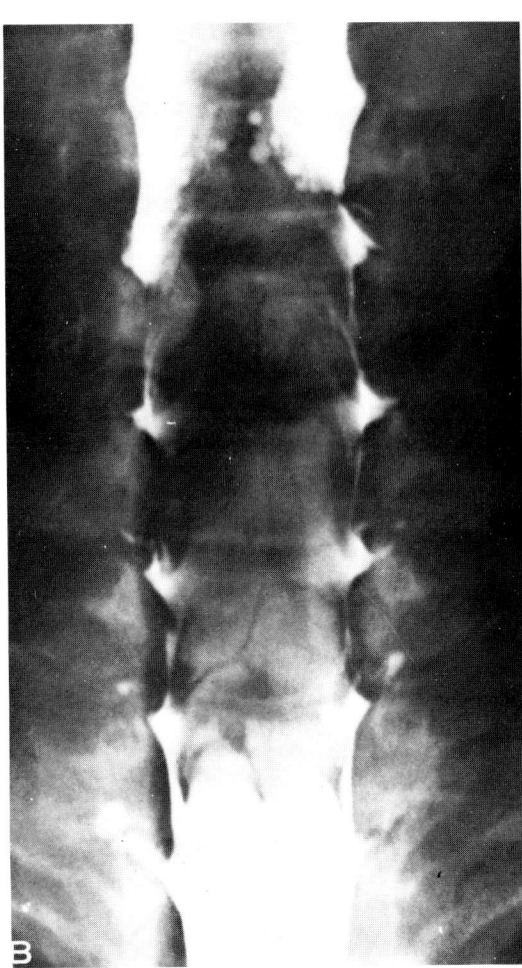

FIGURE 141–6. Myelographic studies made using Pantopaque. (A) Pantopaque study of the cervical region, showing dilatation of the cord associated with a hydromyelic deficit that is far advanced. Even in the advanced stages of hydromyelia, the myelographic picture is not as striking as one in which the obstruction is caused by an intramedullary tumor. (B) Pantopaque study showing an intramedullary tumor. The hydromyelia presents a more diffuse enlargement; tumor enlargement is more localized. (Reprinted from Rhoton AL: Microsurgery of Arnold-Chiari malformation in adults with and without hydromyelia. J Neurosurg 45:473–483, 1976. With permission.)

the lateral ventricles and to diagnostically exclude a tumor in the posterior fossa as the cause of the caudally displaced cerebellar tonsils.

SURGICAL TREATMENT AND RESULTS

CHIARI MALFORMATION WITH HYDROMYELIA

The most effective treatment for Chiari malformation and hydromyelia, in our experience, is a suboccipital craniectomy, upper cervical laminectomy, and duroplasty to decompress the Chiari malformation, followed by drainage of the hydromyelic cavity through the dorsal root entry zone into the subarachnoid space (see Fig. 141–1). If the fourth ventricle is blocked, an outlet should be established with microsurgical techniques, and the hydromyelia cavity should be drained. Decompressing the Chiari malformation alone has been advocated but, in our experience, has not been as effective as the decompression of the Chiari malformation and drainage of the syrinx. However, decompression alone has proved more effective in reducing the size of a hydromyelic cavity than drainage of the cavity alone.

In the past, the operation was performed with the patient in the semisitting position, with the neck in a neutral position. Recently, we have been using the three-quarter prone position with the table tilted to place the head slightly above the trunk. Marked flexion of the neck during surgery for Chiari malformation has been reported to increase the neurologic deficit or cause respiratory problems.[15] A suboccipital craniectomy and upper cervical laminectomy to decompress the Chiari malformation are performed through a midline skin incision (see Fig. 141–1). If only a Chiari malformation is present, the laminectomy would include C1 to C3; if hydromyelia is also present, the laminectomy would include C4 to prepare for drainage of the cavity at the C3-C4 level.

The elongated cerebellar tonsils vary in appearance from those of normal color and consistency to those that are white and firm because of scarring and gliosis (Figs. 141–7A and 141–8). The caudal loop of the posteroinferior cerebellar artery often descends to the level of C2, marking the lower margin of the cerebellar tonsils (Figs. 141–7A and 141–8A).

It is essential that the dura be opened and then closed with a dural graft that is tailored to relieve the constriction of the medulla and cerebellar tonsils (see Fig. 141–1). The degree to which the dura and arachnoid adhere to the spinal cord and medulla can be predicted from neuroradiologic studies (Fig. 141–7). If CSF can be demonstrated between the dura and the cerebellar tonsils, the meninges can be separated easily from the tonsils. If the tonsils are pressed against the dura lining the cisterna magna and no CSF can be seen between the tonsils and dura, the cerebellar tonsils may be adherent to the arachnoid and the dura. If a plaque of arach-

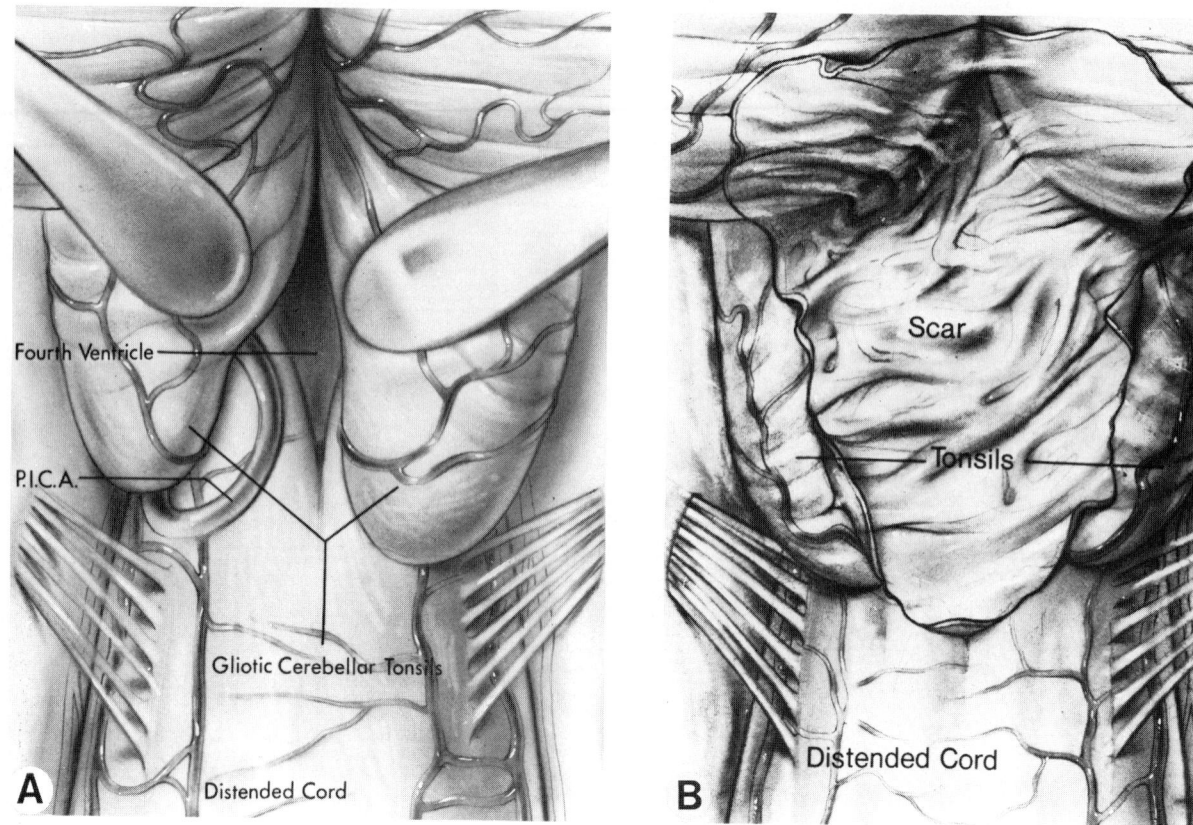

FIGURE 141–7. Abnormalities at the outlet of the fourth ventricle with the Chiari malformation. The patients are in the sitting position (see Figure 141–1). (A) Less complicated form of the Chiari malformation. The herniated gliotic cerebellar tonsils, the ascending course of the cervical nerve roots, the abnormal caudal descent of the posterior inferior cerebellar artery, the loss of normal folial patterns over the tips of the herniated cerebellar tonsils, and the elongated fourth ventricle with the distended spinal cord below are shown. (B) A more complex deformity, with occlusion of the foramen of Magendie by a plaque of scar in which the pia, dura, and arachnoid are adherent to the dorsal medulla and cerebellum, occluding the outlet of the fourth ventricle. Disconnecting this mat of scar from the neural tissue could cause injury to the medulla, the cervical spinal cord, and the structures in the floor of the fourth ventricle; for that reason, the scar is not detached. The dura is opened by incising around the net of scar, which is left attached to the pia over these vital structures. (Reprinted from Rhoton AL: Syringomyelia, in Wilson CB, Hoff JT [eds]: Current Surgical Management of Neurologic Disease. New York, Churchill Livingstone, 1980, pp 29–45. With permission.)

noid and dura is adherent to the dorsal surface of the medulla and the spinal cord, it should be left attached because an attempt to disconnect it might injure the neural tissue (Fig. 141–7B). If the foramen of Magendie is blocked, as occurs in a few cases, an outlet should be established by microsurgical techniques. Care should be taken to ensure that the dissection is far enough superior to enter the fluid cavity of the fourth ventricle rather than the cord or medulla. After the fourth ventricle is opened, a silicone wick is attached to the dura and passed upward into the new opening in the midline (Figs. 141–9 to 141–11). The silicone wick serves to maintain the patency of the outlet rather than to provide a conduit for drainage.

After the Chiari malformation has been decompressed, the syrinx is drained into the subarachnoid space through a longitudinal incision in the dorsal root entry zone at the C3–C4 level. The dorsal root entry zone between the lateral and posterior columns is selected for the myelotomy because it is consistently the thinnest area in patients with hydromyelia (Figs. 141–9 to 141–11). The natural dissection of the cavity along the dorsal root entry zone also leads to a proprioceptive deficit in the upper extremities; hence, incision here minimizes the possibility of increasing the patient's deficit because the arm fibers course in the lateral part of the posterior columns adjacent to the dorsal root entry zone.

An important consideration is whether to drain the hydromyelia through the left or the right dorsal root entry zone. Naturally, the root entry zone that has been the most severely damaged and into which the hydromyelia has dissected the closest to the cord surface is selected for the incision. The side of greater involvement can usually be predicted from the neurologic findings. The side showing the greater deficit related to the cervical sensory nerves is usually selected. High-quality MRI scans in the axial plane commonly show that the cavity has dissected further into either the left or right dorsal horn. The side with greatest damage and the one to be drained is usually placed uppermost if the patient is operated on in the three-quarter prone position.

The dorsal root entry zone myelotomy used to treat hydromyelia is different from the midline myelotomy between the gracile fasciculi (which carry the lower-extremity fibers) that is made to expose and remove an intermedullary tumor (Figs. 141–11 to 141–15). The cord usually is the thinnest on the side of the greater neurologic deficit. Before the cord is incised, a needle should be introduced into the cavity at the thinnest area to collect fluid for cell count and protein deter-

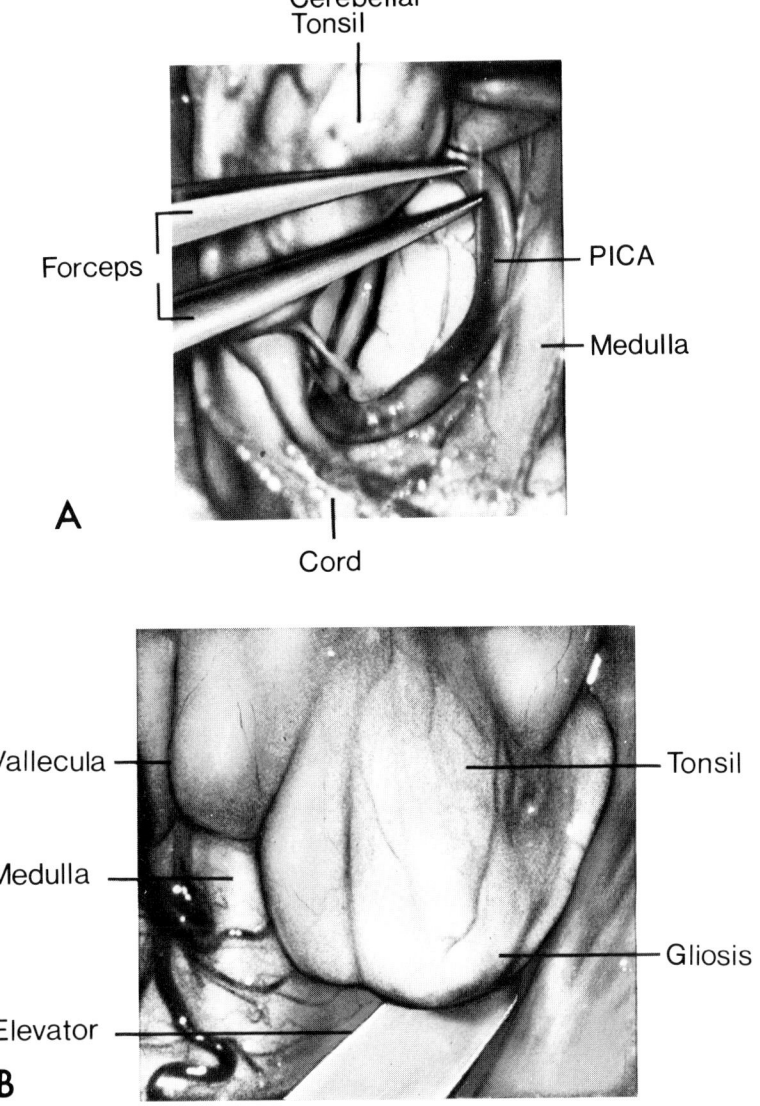

FIGURE 141-8. Posterior views of Chiari malformations through suboccipital craniectomies. The photographs were taken through the surgical microscope at 6× magnification and were retouched and labeled to increase clarity. (A) A caudal loop of the posterior inferior cerebellar artery (PICA) is displaced around the caudal margin of a herniated cerebellar tonsil. The lower margin of the tonsil was at C2. (B) The lower margin of the herniated cerebellar tonsil. Same patient as shown in Figure 141-2B. The pale color at the tip of the left cerebellar tonsil is caused by gliosis in herniated tonsillar tips. (Reprinted from Rhoton AL: Microsurgery of Arnold-Chiari malformation in adults with and without hydromyelia. J Neurosurg 45:473-483, 1976. With permission.)

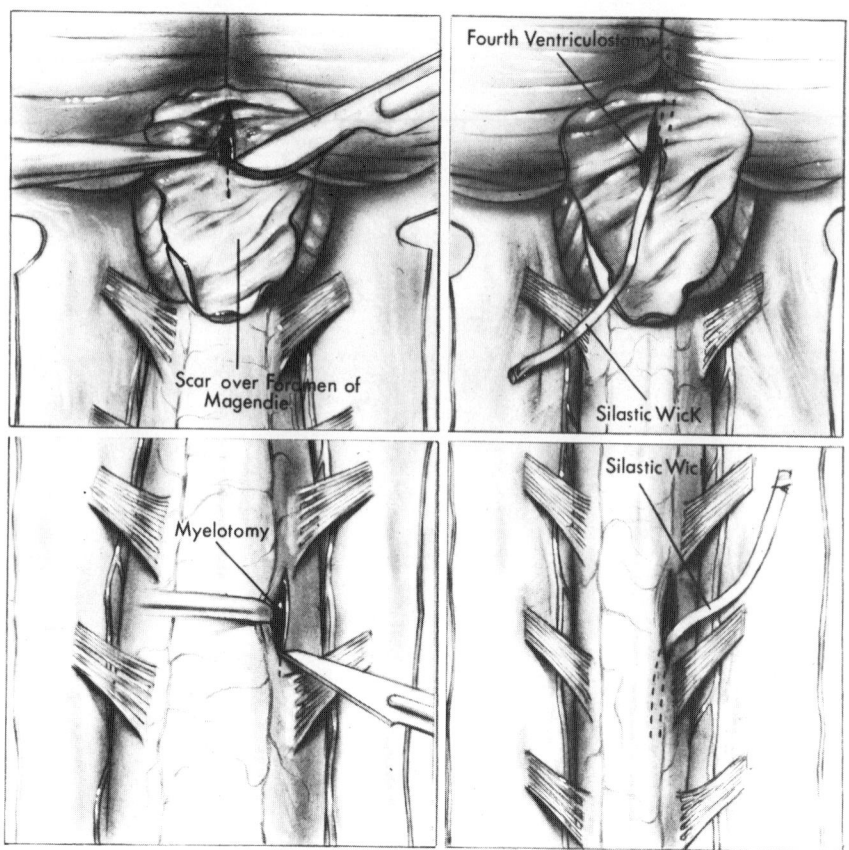

FIGURE 141–9. The surgical approach used by the author for treating a Chiari malformation with hydromyelia. A suboccipital craniectomy and upper cervical laminectomy have been performed to expose and decompress the Chiari malformation (upper right and left) and to expose the hydromyelic spinal cord (lower right and left). The foramen of Magendie is re-established by opening through the upper part of the scar into the fourth ventricle (upper left). A Silastic wick is then anchored to the dura and led through the opening into the fourth ventricle (upper right). The hydromyelic cord is decompressed by opening through the thinnest area, which is consistently through the dorsal root entry zone, using a longitudinal incision placed along the course of the entry of the dorsal roots (lower left). A Silastic wick is then anchored to the dura and led downward into the hydromyelic cavity (lower right). After the incision, the distended cord becomes smaller. (Reprinted from Rhoton AL: Syringomyelia, in Wilson CB, Hoff JT [eds]: Current Surgical Management of Neurologic Disease. New York, Churchill Livingstone, 1980, pp 29–45. With permission.)

minations. Clear CSF with a normal protein level indicates hydromyelia, whereas colored fluid or an elevated protein level indicates an intramedullary tumor. A vertical incision at least 8 mm long is made into the thinnest area along the doral root entry zone, and a silicone wick is anchored to the dura above and threaded downward into the myelotomy (see Figs. 141–9 to 141–12). The dura is closed with a triangular dural graft to ensure that the area around the Chiari malformation is not constricted.

No deaths have occurred in the author's operative series, and the neurologic deficit was increased in only two patients as a result of surgery. One patient developed a mild proprioceptive sensory loss in the right thumb that did not impair the patient in performing work that required moderate dexterity. Another patient, who was quadriparetic and bedridden before surgery, experienced a further mild loss of strength in her only functional extremity as a result of surgery. No patient has shown further progression of deficits during follow-up periods ranging from 1 to 14 years.

A careful explanation, preoperatively, about the reasonable potential benefits of the operation is helpful in obtaining an optimal result from surgical therapy. Most patients report that their functional abilities are improved by the operation, although postoperative neurologic examination usually reveals approximately the same deficit as before operation. Because of this, patients are counseled before the operation regarding the fact that the operation should stop the progression of the deficit, but that it will not restore the patient to normal. The operation commonly arrests the progression of muscle atrophy, prevents the size of areas of numbness from increasing, and may result in some improvement in strength. Most patients with preoperative pain, called anesthesia dolorosa, which is localized to areas of numbness, continue to experience exacerbations of this pain related to emotional stress, hunger, cold weather, and fatigue, after operation. Spasticity also fluctuates after surgery, under the aforementioned conditions, although, on motor testing, no further loss of strength occurs. We have also seen deformities at joints associated with muscle atrophy increase during the years after surgery, even though no further atrophy or loss of strength has occurred. MRI has provided an excellent way of following these patients. However, even when postoperative MRI shows the hydromyelia to be absent, patients may continue to experience fluctuations in pain and spasticity, even though the size of analgesic areas, extent of muscle atrophy, and loss of strength do not progress.

We have seen five patients who were treated previously with a decompressive suboccipital craniectomy and upper cervical laminectomy, plus muscle plugging of the upper end of the central canal at the obex, but who did not have drainage of the hydromyelic cavity. Their neurologic deficits continued to progress. In these cases, we performed a hemilaminectomy in the thoracic region over the lower extent of the hydromyelic cavity, drained the fluid collection through the dorsal root entry zone, and threaded a silicone wick, anchored to the dura, through the myelotomy (see Fig. 141–9).

The question arises as to whether every cord should be drained if there is a hydromyelic cavity in association with the Chiari malformation. We have a few patients in whom the decision has been made not to drain the syrinx because

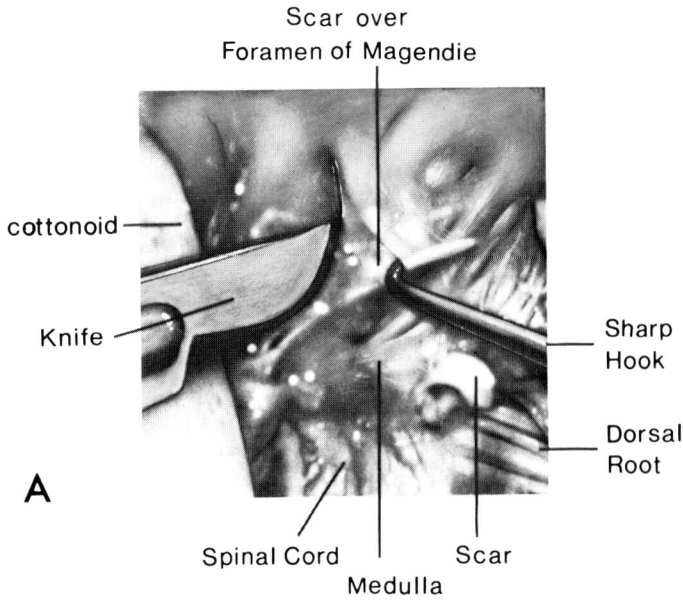

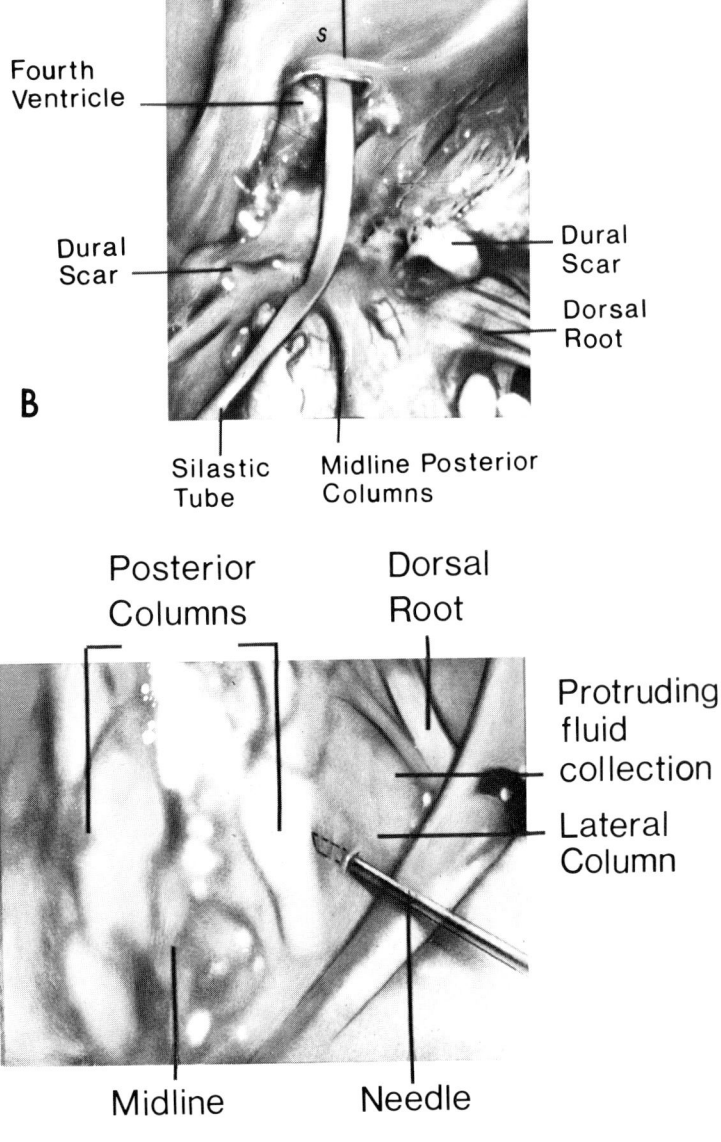

FIGURE 141–10. Posterior views of a Chiari malformation and hydromyelia through a suboccipital craniectomy and a C1-C3 laminectomy. The photographs were taken at 6× magnification through the surgical microscope and were retouched for clarity. All photographs are of the same patient. (A) The incision of the dense mat of scar over the foramen of Magendie. (B) The opening into the fourth ventricle is completed, and a Silastic tube, anchored to the dura below, is threaded rostrally. (C) A needle is introduced into the right half of the spinal cord lateral to the posterior column near the C3 dorsal root entry zone. Clear fluid was obtained. The cord was so thin in this area that the needle tip could be seen through the bulging surface.

Illustration continued on following page

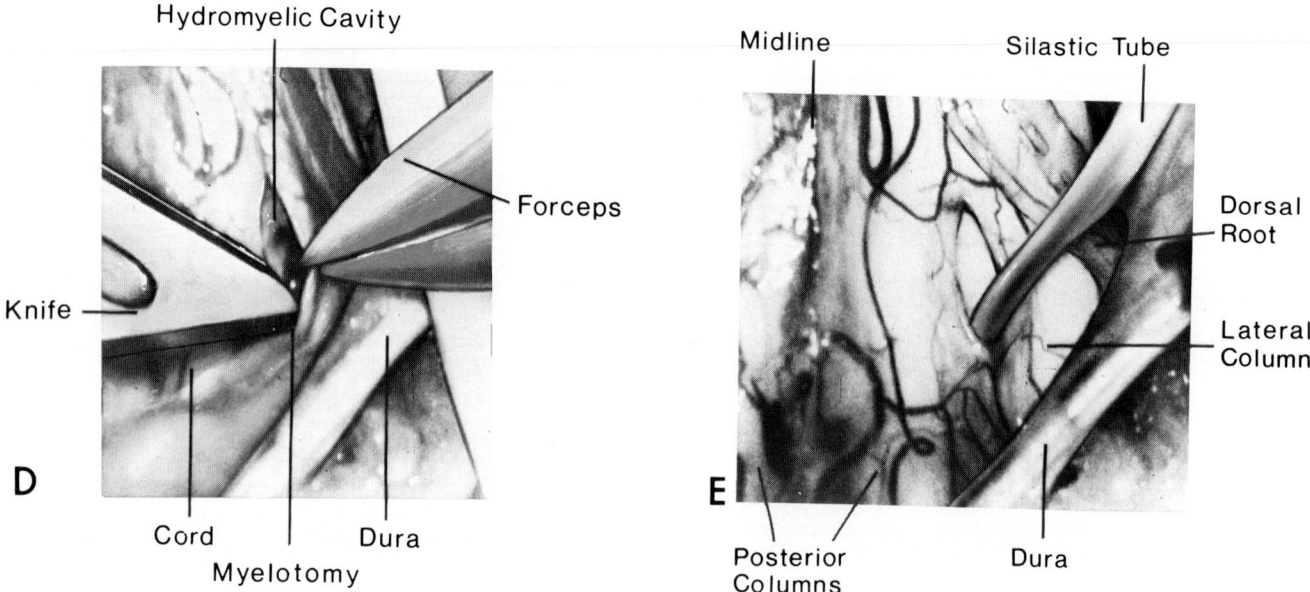

FIGURE 141–10 *Continued* (D) An incision 1 cm in length is made in the dorsal root entry zone using a No. 11 knife blade. The cord is thinner than the dura. (E) A Silastic wick is attached to the dura above and led downward into the hydromyelic cavity. (Reprinted from Rhoton AL: Microsurgery of Arnold-Chiari malformation in adults with and without hydromyelia. J Neurosurg 45:473–483, 1976. With permission.)

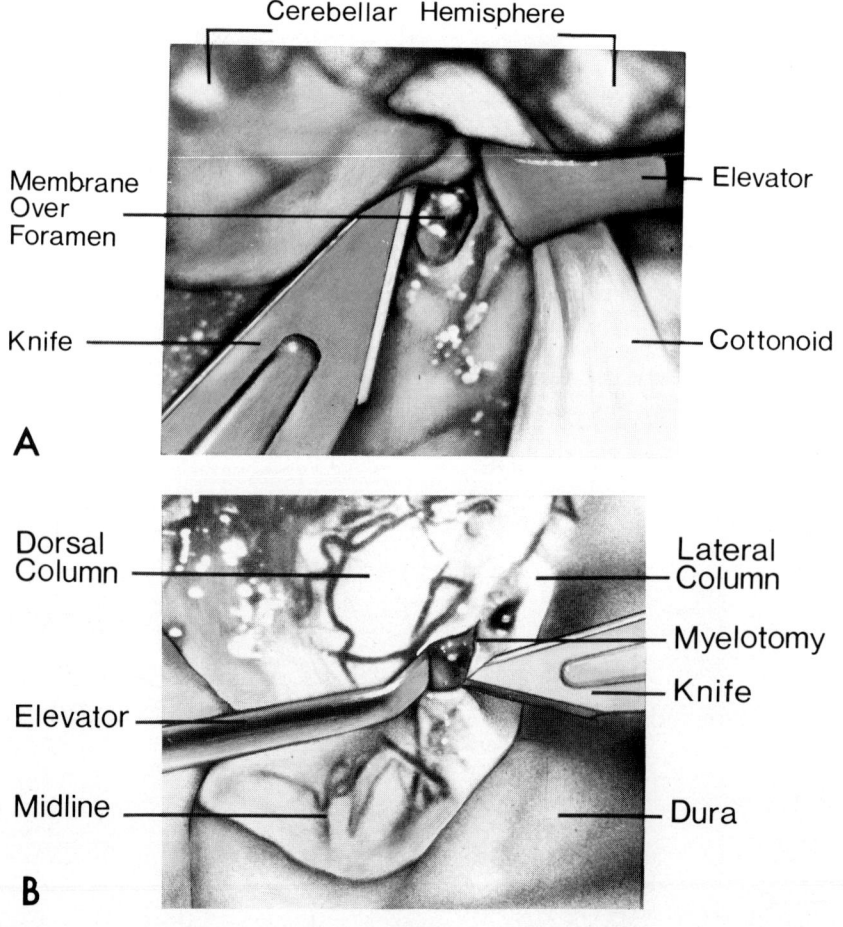

FIGURE 141–11. (A) A view through a suboccipital craniectomy of the membrane occluding the foramen of Magendie. A hydromyelia also was present, and is shown in B. The occluding membrane was incised with a No. 11 blade. (B) The cord was incised at the C3 dorsal root entry zone. The covering over the hydromyelic cavity was only as thick as a layer of dura. A Silastic wick was left in both the fourth ventricle and the cord. (Reprinted from Rhoton AL: Microsurgery of Arnold-Chiari malformation in adults with and without hydromyelia. J Neurosurg 45:473–483, 1976. With permission.)

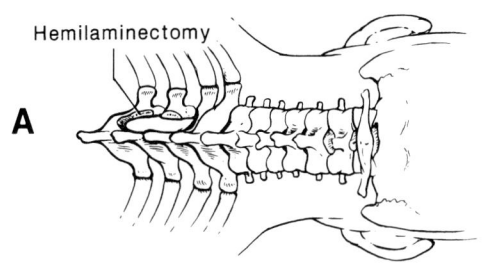
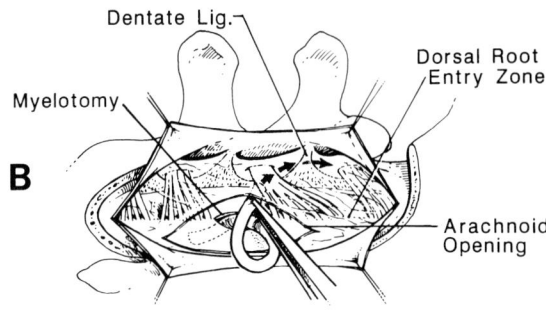
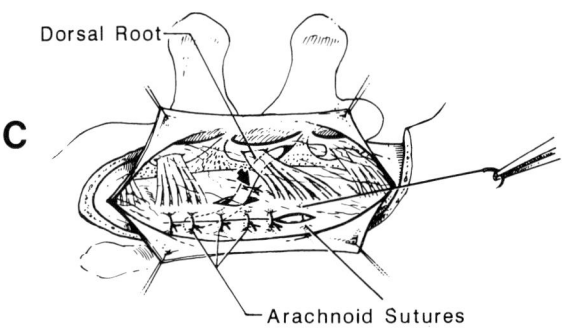

FIGURE 141–12. Dorsal root entry zone myelotomy in the upper thoracic region. This approach is used if the patient has only hydromyelia and no Chiari malformation, or if a suboccipital craniectomy and decompression of the Chiari malformation has failed to arrest the progression of a spinal cord deficit. (A) The operation is done with the patient in the prone or three-quarter prone position. The side of the dorsal root entry zone to be drained is placed uppermost if the three-quarter prone position is used. The hemilaminectomy is positioned below the cervical enlargement of the spinal cord in the upper thoracic area. (B) The myelotomy is located in the dorsal root entry zone. (C) A silicone wick is threaded downward into the hydromyelic cavity and upward into the subarachnoid space anterior to the dentate ligament. The wick is anchored to the arachnoid membrane with a fine suture, and the arachnoid membrane and dura are closed as separate layers.

the cavity was small and there was significant thickness of the cord overlying the cavity, both of which increase the risk of myelotomy. On the other hand, a dorsal root entry zone myelotomy is performed if the cord is paper thin in the area of the dorsal root entry zone, and even with moderate-sized cavities, we believe that it does add to the decompression.

INTRAMEDULLARY TUMOR

The surgical treatment of an intramedullary tumor consists of a laminectomy that is as extensive as that required to expose the abnormal cord for decompression. This step is followed by a midline myelotomy, biopsy of the tumor, and total removal of the tumor if a cleavage plane can be developed between the tumor and the neural tissue (see Fig. 141–13). Biopsy only, or incomplete removal, is followed by radiation therapy.

ALTERNATIVE TREATMENTS

Percutaneous needling of the hydromyelic cavity has been advocated as a possible mode of therapy (see Fig. 141–13)[16]; however, aspiration of fluid at surgery is followed by rapid refilling of the hydromyelic cavity from the ventricular system, and it seems unlikely that a needle track would remain patent. In treating hydromyelia, the longitudinal opening into the cord should be long enough to ensure that there is no tendency for spontaneous closure.

Gardner initially recommended surgical treatment consisting of a suboccipital craniectomy and cervical laminectomy to decompress the malformation, and plugging of the upper end of the patent central canal (at the area of the obex) with a small piece of muscle.[7,8] Subsequently, he has reported that most of the patients treated with occlusion of the upper end of the central canal later developed progressive neurologic deficits.[9] I favor making an incision between the posterior and lateral columns of the spinal cord to drain the hydromyelic cavity and have avoided risking damage to the hypoglossal and vagal nuclei, which are located at the obex near the upper end of the central canal.

Gardner and his colleagues[11] have advocated a procedure called terminal ventriculostomy (see Fig. 141–13). The terminal ventricle is the dilated portion of the central canal that extends below the tip of the conus medullaris into the filum terminale. A laminectomy is performed over the caudal limit of the fluid sac, and the filum is opened. This procedure

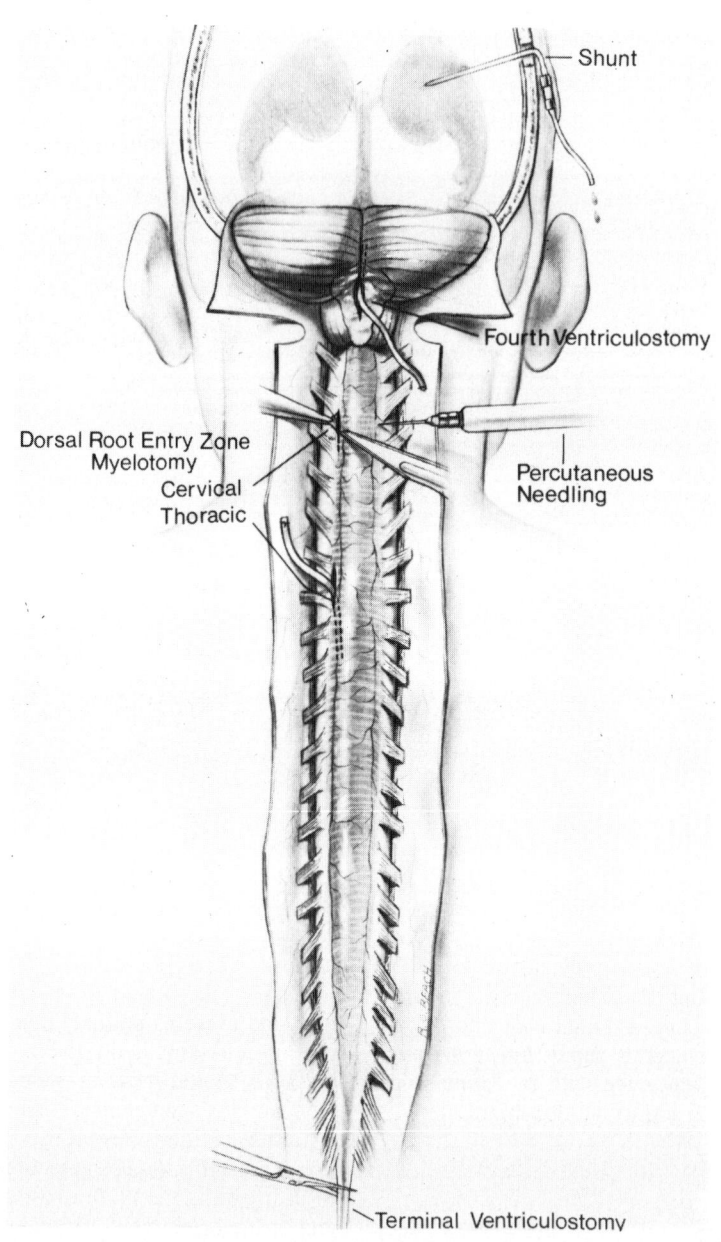

FIGURE 141–13. A summary of the different surgical techniques used to treat a Chiari malformation with hydromyelia. A cerebrospinal fluid shunt may be considered if there is significant hydrocephalus. Most adults with a Chiari malformation and hydromyelia, however, do not experience hydrocephalus. Decompression of the Chiari malformation may also be achieved by suboccipital craniectomy and upper cervical laminectomy, with insertion of a Silastic wick through a fourth ventriculostomy. Percutaneous needling of the cyst also has been advocated. We combine decompression of the Chiari malformation with a myelotomy in the dorsal root entry zone in the cervical region to drain the hydromyelic cord. If the Chiari malformation has been decompressed previously, a myelotomy of the dorsal root entry zone may be performed below the cervical enlargement in the thoracic region. If the cavity extends into the filum terminale, terminal ventriculostomy may be performed by dividing the filum terminale. (Reprinted from Rhoton AL: Syringomyelia, in Wilson CB, Hoff JT [eds]: Current Surgical Management of Neurologic Disease. New York, Churchill Livingstone, 1980, pp 29–45. With permission.)

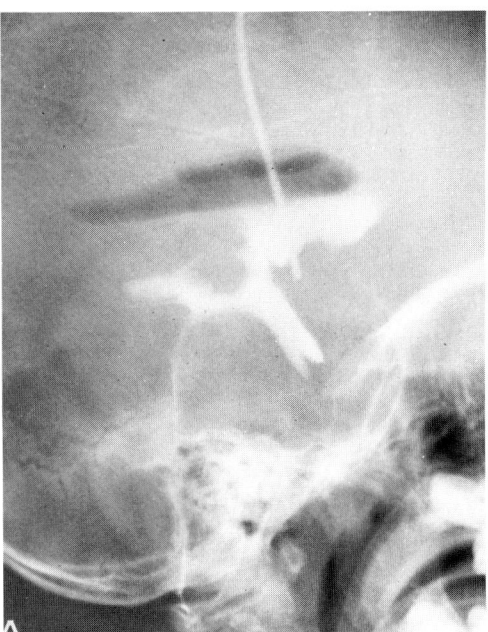
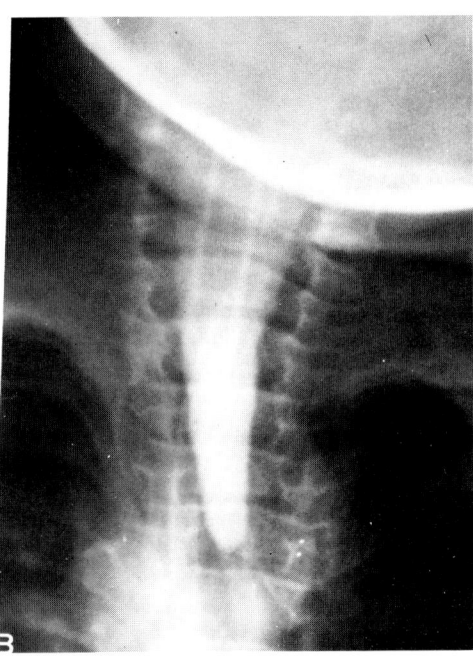

FIGURE 141–14. This infant was previously treated with a shunt for hydrocephalus. After the shunt was removed because of infection, the child developed a progressive lower motor neuron deficit in the arms. (A) Positive-contrast ventriculogram showing normal-sized ventricles (lateral view). (B) The contrast medium enters a large cavity in the cervical cord that communicates with the ventricles. (Reprinted from Rhoton AL: Microsurgery of Arnold-Chiari malformation in adults with and without hydromyelia. J Neurosurg 45:473–483, 1976. With permission.)

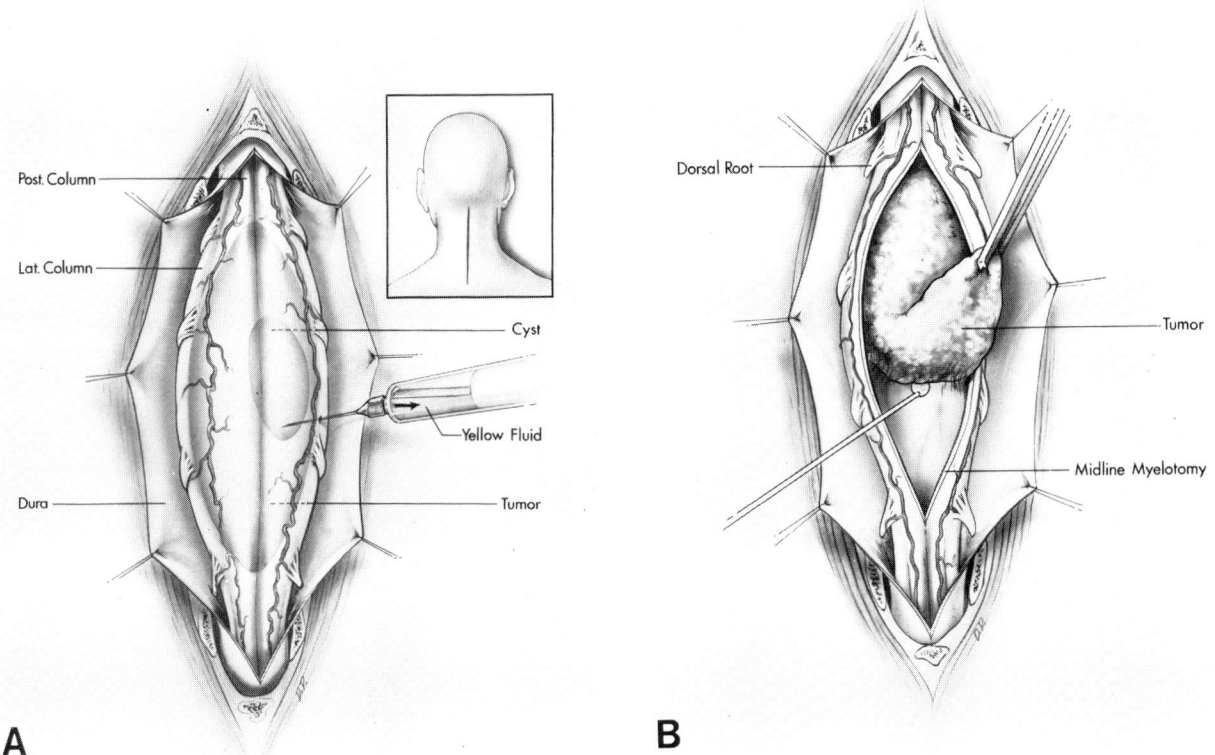

FIGURE 141–15. Exposure and removal of a cystic intramedullary tumor in the cervical region. (A) The insert (upper right) shows the position of the patient for the operation, and the incision (solid line). The illustration shows the tumor in an intramedullary location. The cyst within the tumor is being aspirated with a needle and yields yellow fluid. (B) A midline myelotomy has been performed between the posterior columns, the cleavage plane between the tumor and the spinal cord has been identified, and a small dissector is being used to remove the intramedullary tumor. The myelotomy for removal of the tumor is in the midline, while the incision for drainage of a hydromyelia is usually in the dorsal root entry zone.

does not decompress the malformation at the foramen magnum but may prove to be satisfactory if the patient has only hydromyelic symptoms. The procedure does not apply in all cases; I have seen numerous cases in which the hydromyelic cavity did not extend into the lumbar portion of the spinal cord or the filum terminalae (see Figs. 141–9 through 141–12).

Shunting of CSF from the lateral ventricle to the atrium or peritoneum has been considered as a mode of treatment (see Fig. 141–13).[17] The patients in our series, however, even those with marked hydromyelic deficits, had not significant ventricular dilatation. Furthermore, the small ventricles would make shunting difficult. In addition, our patients all had normal CSF pressure. Even if shunting were performed, a hydrostatic fluid column from the ventricles would remain and act on the cord when the patient was upright. Shunting would be indicated if the ventricles were large or if there was increased intracranial pressure.

The finding of ventricles of normal size in the present series led to the conclusion that intracavity pressure that is too low to dilate the ventricles may cause progressive cord destruction by distension. The following case of an infant supports this concept (see Fig. 141–14). After birth, this child was found to have hydrocephalus that required shunting; the shunt became infected, was removed, and was not replaced because the head and ventricular size remained normal. The child then developed a progressive, severe, lower motor neuron deficit in the arms. A second series of contrast studies showed ventricles of normal size, but positive-contrast ventriculography showed a hydromyelic cavity in the cervical cord that was hugely dilated. Thus, intracavity pressure that was too low to distend the ventricles was apparently distending the hydromyelic cord and causing a neurologic deficit in the arms. The cavity did not extend below the cervicothoracic junction.

REFERENCES

1. Brewis M, Poskanzer DC, Rolland C, et al: Neurological disease in an English city. Acta Neurol Scand 42(suppl 24):9, 1966
2. Gowers WR: A Manual of Diseases of the Nervous System, vol 1. London, Churchill, 1886
3. Merritt HH: A Textbook of Neurology, 5th ed. Philadelphia, Lea & Febiger, 1973
4. Rhoton AL Jr: Microsurgery of Arnold-Chiari malformation in adults with and without hydromyelia. J Neurosurg 45:473, 1976
5. Rhoton AL Jr, Fessler RG: Surgical treatment of Chiari malformation and hydromyelia in adults, in Wilson CB (ed): Neurosurgical Procedures. Baltimore, Williams & Wilkins, 1992, pp 169–187
6. Barnett HJM, Foster JB, Hudgson P: Syringomyelia. Philadelphia, WB Saunders, 1973, pp 6, 58, 104, 121, 312
7. Gardner WJ: Hydrodynamic mechanism of syringomyelia: Its relationship to myelocele. J Neurol Neurosurg Psychiatry 28:247, 1965
8. Gardner WJ: Myelocele: Rupture of the neural tube? Clin Neurosurg 15:57, 1968
9. Gardner WJ: Personal communication, 1978
10. Gardner WJ, Angel J: The mechanism of syringomyelia and its surgical correction. Clin Neurosurg 6:131, 1959
11. Gardner WJ, Steinberg M, Bell H, et al: Terminal Ventriculostomy in the Treatment of Syringomyelia. Presented at the Annual Meeting of the American Association of Neurological Surgeons, Miami, Florida, April 1975
12. Chiari H: über die Pathogenese der sogenannten Syringomyelie. Heilkunde 9:307, 1888
13. Bertrand G: Dynamic factors in the evolution of syringomyelia and syringobulbia. Clin Neurosurg 20:322, 1973
14. Ellertsson AB: Syringomyelia and other cystic spinal cord lesions. Acta Neurol Scand 45:403, 1969
15. Mullan S, Raimondi AJ: Respiratory hazards of the surgical treatment of the Arnold-Chiari malformation. J Neurosurg 19:675, 1962
16. Schlesinger ER, Tenner MS, Michelsen WH: Percutaneous Spinal Cord Puncture in the Analysis and Treatment of Hydromyelia. Presented at the Annual Meeting of the American Association of Neurological Surgeons, Houston, Texas, April 1971
17. Conway LW: Hydrodynamic studies in syringomyelia. J Neurosurg 27:501, 1967

CHAPTER 142

Cervicothoracic Ankylosing Spondylitis

William H. Sweet

HISTORY

Ankylosing spondylitis was first fully described by W. von Bechterew of St. Petersburg, Russia. His original accounts in 1892 in Russian, followed by papers in German in 1893 and 1897,[1–3] emphasize an increasing immobility of the entire spine as a result of ossification or calcification of all of its joints and ligaments. The title of his first detailed publication was "Re Rigidity of the Vertebral Column and its Deformity as a Special Form of Illness." The permanence of the skeletal insignias of the disease has permitted the discovery of such a skeleton in the third Egyptian dynasty around 2980 to 2900 BC

In AD 169, Connor[4] describes a segment of skeleton consisting of ileum, sacrum, five lumbar and 10 thoracic vertebrae, and three right and two left ribs bound together by bone and replacing the ligaments. The articulations were so effaced that they made one uniform continuous bone with, for example, no marks to suggest the former site of the apophyses. Boland[5] gave a fuller historical account, with references to seven probable descriptions of the disorder in the latter half of the nineteenth century.

GENERAL FEATURES

General features of ankylosing spondylitis have been given various designations: "fusion or rigidity of the vertebral column,"[3] "chronic ankylosing inflammation of the vertebral column and hip joints,"[6] "spondylosis rhizomélique,"[7] "chronic ankylosing rigidity of the vertebral column,"[8] and "chronic arthritis ankylopoetica of the vertebral column."[9] The British have been using the term *ankylosing spondylitis* for over half a century, but in 1941, the American Rheumatic Association adopted the term *rheumatoid spondylitis*.[5] Its members gradually agreed that this disorder is distinct from rheumatoid arthritis, and in December 1963, they officially capitulated and also adopted the term *ankylosing spondylitis*.

Comprehensive accounts of the clinical features of the disorder have been provided by Boland[5] and by Wilkinson and Bywaters.[10] The latter work is based on 222 hospital patients seen during 16 years, 212 of whom were followed up. The male to female ratio was 4.4:1 in this series; other investigators note a male to female predominance of as high as 10:1.[11] The first symptoms appeared before the age of 30 years in 64 percent of the cases and before the age of 40 in 89 percent. Close relatives of six percent definitely had the disorder. In 64 percent, the onset was in the sacroiliac joints or lumbar spine, giving rise to aching in the buttocks, nearly always radiating into one or both upper thighs. In three others, the radiation of pain extended into the calf or heel, in contrast to that of a protruded disc, which usually extends into the full length of the sciatic distribution. At this stage, radiographs showed ankylosis mainly of the sacroiliac and lumbar articular joints. Joints in the limbs or higher in the spine were the sites of initial involvement in the remaining third of the cases, and corresponding differences existed in the reference of pain. Those with spinal onset often noted anomalous worsening of the pain after resting and relief after activity. Some were not only awakened by pain but had to arise during the night to "limber up" before going back to sleep. Heavy exertion, however, also brought on or worsened pain in some patients. The longer the duration of the disease, the greater the extent of spinal involvement. The areas affected included the cervical spine, the area of greatest vulnerability to trauma, in 50 percent of the cases, and hips, or shoulders, or both, in 39 percent. Impaired chest expansion, often an early sign, was reduced to 5 cm or less in 96 percent and to less than half that in 62 percent of those with the disease for 20 or more years (normal = 7 cm or more). Despite ossification of the ligaments, varying degrees of osteoporosis are usually present in the bones. The spinal rigidity did not prevent 63 percent of patients from working after more than 20 years of illness.

Some of the American publications failed to discriminate this disorder from various spondylitides of inflammatory rheumatoid arthritis, and recent analyses of human leukocyte antigens (HLAs) and the biology of the major histocompatibility complex revealed a bewildering congeries of new arthritic entities. The absence of both subcutaneous rheumatic nodules and "rheumatoid factor" in the blood stream provides at least a preliminary basis for the diagnosis of ankylosing spondylitis used in this analysis. In their 92 cases, Kinsella and colleagues[12] also noted normal blood levels of antinuclear factor and antithyroglobulin.

SPECIAL FEATURES THAT INCREASE THE RISK OF SURGERY

Because spine fractures occur so much more often in young, otherwise healthy adults, surgeons may not bother to appraise intensively the general physical status of much older patients. Reduced chest expansion is an early and valuable sign of the disorder.[13] It typically involves so many systems[14] that a follow-up study of 836 such patients for an average of 13 years revealed a twofold increase in mortality for men over that of the general population.[15]

The disease may begin with bouts of intermittent fever, anorexia, weight loss, easy fatigability, and anemia. Based partly on biopsies obtained in the early stages of the disease from radiographically identified arthritis in the manubriosternal joint, Cruickshank[16] found an initial osteitis that started with villus hyperplasia of the synovium, edema and lymphocytes, plasma cells, histiocytes, and, at times, hemorrhage. Vascular fibrous granulation tissue may appear at the joint margins. Later, fibrous destruction, reactive sclerosis, and ankylosis predominate. A continuing vulnerability to an inflammatory process is suggested by bouts of acute anterior uveitis or iritis, usually unilateral, which occurs in 25 percent; such an attack may be the first symptom.[15]

An abnormal fibrotic process may appear at many sites. Thus, the aortic valvular cusps develop a fibrous thickening and focal medial necrosis leading to aortic regurgitation in three percent. Fibrous tissue may invade the atrioventricular bundle, causing conduction defects. Late in the disease, the fibrosis may involve both upper pulmonary lobes, causing cough, dyspnea, and even death from massive hemoptysis. This feature plus the immobility of the ribs may make full pulmonary function studies essential because about half of the deaths occurring after fractures of the cervical spine in these cases are from pulmonary causes. In a few patients, a major proliferation of fibrous tissue occurs in the spinal canal—at times in the thoracic region, but more often in the cauda equina.

Another long-term consequence of this malady is systemic vascular degeneration. This degeneration may cause the increased mortality relative to the general population, which is fourfold for all gastrointestinal disease, especially ulcerative colitis and other inflammatory disease of the gastrointestinal tract. The increased risk is twofold for cerebrovascular disease and is 40 percent greater for other circulatory diseases.[15] Deposition of immunoglobulin, complement, and fibrinogen in the walls of small renal vessels has been shown to be an early pathologic change in the walls of such renal vessels in biopsies of young patients with ankylosing spondylitis.[17] These changes probably account for the amyloidosis that causes uremic death in 6 percent.

The fact that the bone marrow is at special risk is evidenced by the curious complications of radiotherapy formerly given to control pain. These problems were moderately to completely relieved in 88 percent of 20 patients at 6 months by doses not exceeding 2000cGy to any one of four or five spinal fields irradiated in each patient.[10] However, a broad survey by the British Medical Research Council[18] revealed that of 100 deaths in such patients, 41 resulted from acute myelogenous leukemia and seven from aplastic anemia after radiotherapy. No deaths from leukemia or lymphoma were encountered in the 836 patients who were given no x-ray therapy and followed up an average of 13 years by Radford and coworkers.[15] The fragile character of the patients is further emphasized by the postoperative deaths of 13 of the 100 treated by spinal ostectomy or cup arthroplasty of the hip, procedures that were performed in an attempt to increase the patient's mobility.

There is a striking correlation between the B27 form of HLA and this disease; that is, it is present in only five to eight percent of the white population as a whole but is found in 90 percent of this group with this form of spondylitis. This disease is 90 times more likely to occur in an HLA-B27–positive man than an HLA-B27–negative person. Similarly, a high incidence of HLA-B27 antigen exists in those with uveitis.[19]

The genetic material encoding structures responsible for the immune response related to histocompatibility is concentrated in a small region in the short arm of chromosome 6. This region, designated the major histocompatibility complex, codes for three classes of gene products, of which class I molecules are expressed on almost all cell surfaces. They consist of one heavy (molecular weight 4500) chain and one light ($<$ 12,000) polypeptide chain. These include three reduplicated gene loci for the three groups of HLAs—these loci are designated A, B, and C.[19] The B27 marker is considered to be associated with disturbances in immune mechanisms that lead to susceptibility to rheumatic disease.[20]

Clearly, investigations to determine the presence of the often occult manifestations just described should, if feasible, precede surgery.

RADIOLOGIC FEATURES

Early radiographic changes are most likely to be seen in the pelvis and lumbar spine. Calcification at the ischial tuberosity at the origin of the hamstring muscles is illustrated in Figure 142–1, and "squaring" of the anterosuperior and anteroinferior corners of the lumbar vertebrae as seen in the lateral view is shown in Figure 142–2. The late radiographic characteristics of the various spondyloarthritides were summarized by Martel and Braunstein.[21] In the sagittal projections of the spine, a continuous vertical line of calcification joining the two rows of apophyseal joints gives rise to the typical "railway line" appearance (Fig. 142–3). In the same projection, an arc of calcification often forms a lateral boundary to the disc on each side and joins the two vertebral bodies. This is the "bamboo" type of ankylosis (Fig. 142–4). The complete calcified fusion of the intervertebral discs

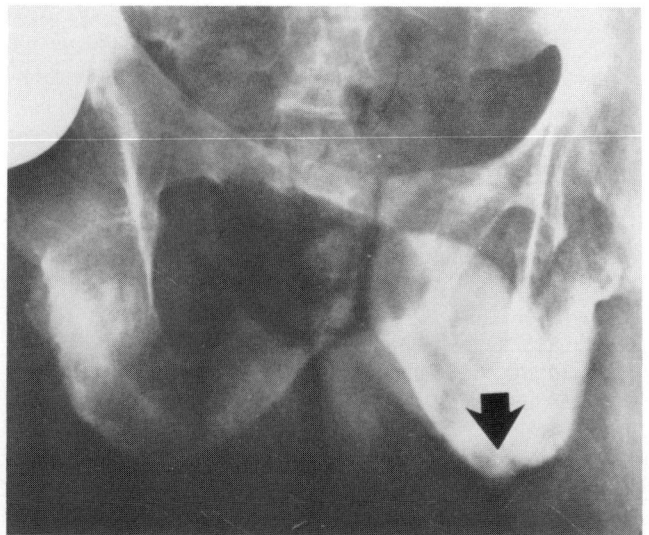

FIGURE 142–1. Early stage of lesion with erosion and sclerosis at enthesis of hamstring muscles at ischial tuberosities indicated by arrow. (From Martel W, Braunstein EM: Spondyloarthritides, in Tavares J, Ferrucci JT [eds]: Radiology. Diagnosis—Imaging—Intervention, Volume 5. Philadelphia, J. B. Lippincott, 1988, pp 2–5.)

Cervicothoracic Ankylosing Spondylitis | 1767

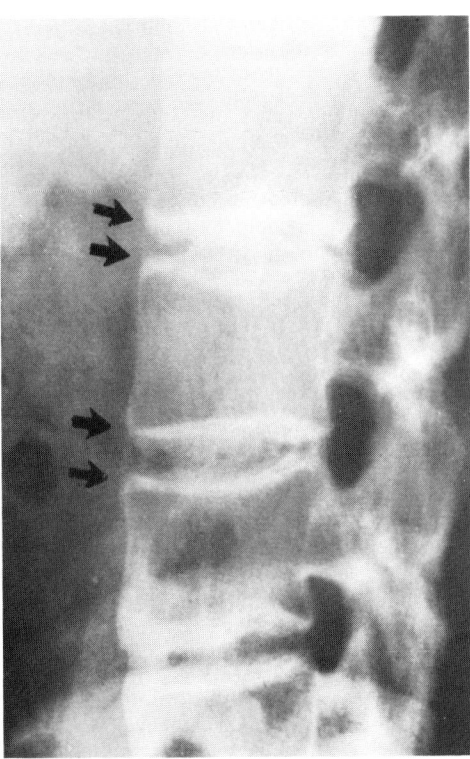

FIGURE 142-2. Early stage of lesion with *erosion* of anterior superior and of anterior longitudinal ligament, leading to "squaring of these corners." (Arrows indicate minimal lesions.) (From Martel W, Braunstein EM: Spondyloarthritides, in Tavares J, Ferrucci JT [eds] Radiology. Diagnosis—Imaging—Intervention, Volume 5. Philadelphia, J. B. Lippincott, 1988, pp 2–5.)

one fractured vertebra ensuing after a single accident. Thus, in the 23 patients of Fox and associates,[23] 28 fractures were present. Several major disasters have ensued when the second fracture, usually lower and less symptomatic, is not recognized. For example, one of the Mayo Clinic patients became paraplegic when transferred from his bed to a gurney. An L-1 fracture became displaced, and no recovery occurred after decompressive surgery and stabilization.[23] Sensory changes that might point to a second spinal lesion should be sought. As soon as feasible after the primary site of fracture has been stabilized, and until normality of the rest of the spine has been demonstrated, the patient should be treated with the same scrupulous precautions as initially.

At times, all of the calcification is so protective (and beclouds the x-ray studies) that neither the patient nor the doctor even suspects fracture. Such events have been diagnosed only when a later, more serious, fracture occurs, at times within hours after the patient has been discharged from the emergency department with a clean bill of health. In others, the transverse fracture is sufficiently incomplete so that the wearing of a sturdy, supportive collar permits adequate stabilization until bony healing, usually rapid, occurs. Unfortunately, the fracture is more often of a peculiarly dangerous type in that the break is similar to that of a long bone, that is, it is roughly horizontal through the whole spinal column. This commonly produces major dangerous mobility of the upper or the lower segment in any direction. Apparently, the tough elastic ligaments after fracture-dislocation of an otherwise normal cervical spine tend to prevent distraction and gross horizontal displacements so that simple application of skull tongs and traction in a neutral direction in the long

and the apophyseal joints usually involves the posterior longitudinal ligament but can also occur posterior to the spinal canal in the ligamenta flava and those between the spinous processes, thus uniting them. According to Cruickshank's personal studies of biopsies from 25 patients and autopsies from 12, the anterior longitudinal ligaments do not share in this calcification.[18]

However, in many cases, this ligament must have shared in the transverse disruption. This growth tends to convert the spinal column to a continuous calcified cylinder—as first described by Simmonds[22] in two postmortem specimens of the entire spine, which he macerated and then sawed in long, sagittal slices for analysis by photography and radiography. He also noted that the ribs were rigidly attached to the vertebrae and to each other by calcification at the joints and at the ligamenta costotransversaria, intratransversaria, and those between the costal tubercles, thereby accounting for the final gross reduction in inspiratory chest expansion. This extraordinary calcification is accompanied by osteoporosis of the bony vertebrae themselves. Such a spine proves prone to fracture with relatively minor trauma, especially in the cervical region. Numerous reports have been published on the ataxia of drunkenness leading to a fracture of the ankylosed cervical spine. These features also make the fractures hard to discern, and the kyphosis may interfere with magnetic resonance imaging (MRI) and computed tomography (CT) scanning. This vulnerability extends throughout the involved spine, and many investigators have reported on more than

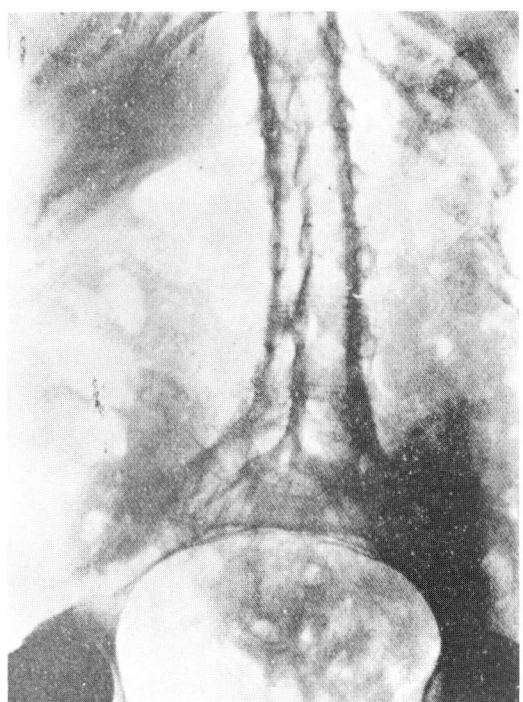

FIGURE 142-3. Late stage "railway spine" produced by continuous lines of calcification including and connecting apophyseal joints with osteoporotic vertebral bodies. (From Guttman L: Injuries of the Spine and Spinal Cord. Oxford, Blackwell Scientific Publications, 1976, p 176.)

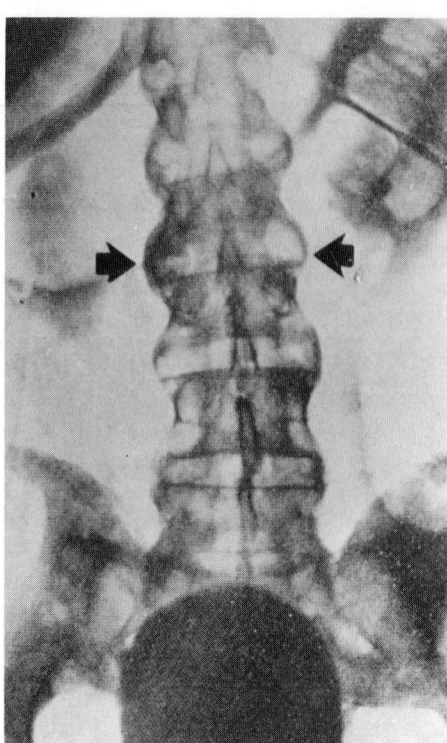

FIGURE 142–4. Late stage bamboo spine created by calcified area covering outer aspects of lumbar intervertebral discs, indicated by arrows. (From Guttman L: Injuries of the Spine and Spinal Cord. Oxford, Blackwell Scientific Publications, 1976, p 176.)

of all concerned, the procedure also caused a total transverse fracture of the lumbar spine through the disc at L2-L3, with a total permanent loss of all motor function below that level. At autopsy 7½ months later, a 2-cm diastasis bridged by callus was found between the second and third lumbar vertebral bodies. Possibly because of uncertainty as to the vigor of the operative manipulation, the lesson from this well-studied and superbly described case largely escaped notice.

Perhaps because of the relative rarity of the disorder and the lack of disabling symptoms, despite decades of its known presence in most patients, many physicians are unaware of the extraordinary propensity of the disorder for disablement. Not until trauma abruptly strikes does the physician realize what a serious set of problems a patient can present. The known presence of ankylosing spondylitis should lead at once to the suspicion of fracture. One of my patients fell while drunk just before he got into bed. Over the next several days, an increasing weakness of his right upper limb was treated as radial nerve weakness of "a Saturday night palsy." The patient had thought it best not to mention that he had been so drunk that he fell, and he added, "Besides, I didn't hurt myself when I fell." He progressed to quadriplegia and

axis of the cervical spine nearly always provides the necessary stabilization in the presence of normal cervical ligaments. Moreover, such patients are likely to be able to safely rotate their head to a useful degree because that motion occurs at the C1-C2 levels.

However, in cervical ankylosing spondylitis, the usually transverse fracture also involves the calcified ligaments extending horizontally through all elements, front to back. Most of the fractures are actually through the calcified disc. Also, the upper segment may become distracted, or separated rostrocaudally to a startling degree, moving up and away from the lower segment and causing further trauma to the cord. This distraction is likely to be worsened by modest weights of the skeletal tong traction. The injury may become still worse when the mobile upper segment slides in any direction in the horizontal plane and causes intolerable pressure on the cord. Figure 142–5 illustrates the frightful sequence that may ensue.

MANAGEMENT LEADING TO DISASTER

Some of the special problems of these patients were graphically illustrated by one of the first reported cases, that of Abdi.[9] His 47-year-old patient had both hip joint and spinal ankylosis progressing for over 20 years to minimal motion at any level from C2 to the sacrum. In an effort to give him a little motion at the hip joints, an orthopedic surgeon manipulated them under general anesthesia. The right hip remained fixed, but the left hip became mobile. To the consternation

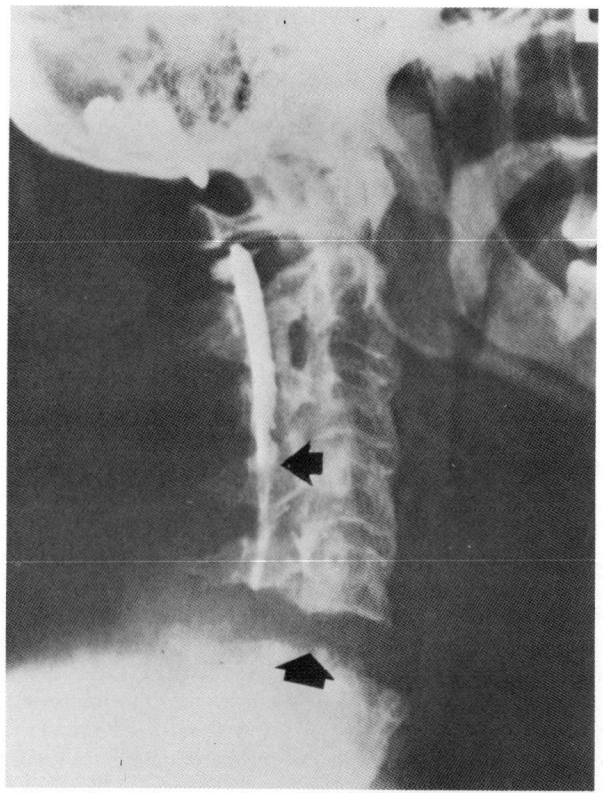

FIGURE 142–5. While drunk, a 49-year-old male fell to the floor, striking his head. He became quadriplegic at once owing to a total transverse lesion of cord at C6 from total transverse fracture through C5-C6 disc with posterior displacement of the superior aspect of the cervical spine. Traction that was increased to 100 pounds by Gardner-Wells tongs did not reduce the fracture. Myelogram of complete block at upper C4 (small arrowhead) with extreme distraction at C5-C6 disc (large arrowhead). At laminectomy, the cord was liquefied and necrotic opposite C5. Postoperatively lesions ascended one segment permanently. (From Murray GC, Persellin RH: Cervical fracture complicating ankylosing spondylitis. A report of eight cases and review of the literature. Am J Med 70:1033–1041, 1981.)

death. Some patients, such as the only one I saw as a medical student, had maintained enough bone and ligamentous continuity so that a Thomas collar worn for several weeks maintained stability of the spine until rapid healing had occurred. Pain in an upper limb but no neurologic deficit led him and me to think that the whole episode was trivial.

Such experiences do not prepare the unwary for the following vicissitudes. Bohlman[24] reported that failure to diagnose significant spine injury in his hospital's emergency room occurred in four of eight such patients; three returned later with quadriplegia. The fourth, given a tranquilizer before discharge in the emergency room, fell, became quadriplegic, and remained so. Figure 142-6 illustrates why placement of the head and upper neck in the same long axis as the body can kill the patient with a rigid cervical kyphosis. Ackerman[25] illustrated an apparatus he developed to place the traction at a proper angle to maintain reduction of a fracture in a kyphotic cervical spine, and then to keep that essential angle while the patient was being rotated from a supine to a prone attitude and back again (Fig. 142-7).

Detwiler and colleagues[26] reported on a patient with a C7-T1 subluxation and a C6 compression fracture who had a normal neurologic examination when he was first placed flat in a bed with a Philadelphia collar. The next day, he abruptly developed an incomplete neurologic lesion at the T2 level; axial traction helped at first, but later, dyspnea proceeded to respiratory arrest and fatal anoxia.

The second patient in Detwiler's study experienced only neck pain after a fall. He was transported on the usual backboard, during which his head was kept in a "neutral" position, neither flexed nor extended, a tactic continued in the hospital during examination and radiography. During this time, he became aware that flexion of his head helped, and extension toward the "neutral" position made his neck pain steadily worse. His medical attendants all assured him that they were well trained and knew they were doing the right thing; x-ray films showed a C5-C6 dislocation, and examination now revealed a total transverse lesion at C5-C6; the final result was death.[26]

Surin[27] described a special vacuum cushion into which the patient settles; it maintains the head in the proper degree of flexion during transport and examinations, and it appears to be of special value during CT and MRI, as well as when the patient is in bed.

Osgood and associates[28] reported on a 47-year-old man whose spine was fused in marked flexion for 25 years. The patient had a through-and-through horizontal fracture at the C7 body, but posterior bony elements and ligaments remained fused. The patient was neurologically intact except for pain and numbness in the left arm. The patient refused skeletal traction and was placed in a Thomas collar. One day later, the patient was neurologically normal. Then, the patient had tingling in the legs; 3 hours later, C6-C7 quadriplegia developed. Bilateral fractures of C6-C7 facets were present at the time of posterior decompression and fixation, and later, anterior fusion and stabilization were achieved and led to improvement in severe quadriparesis. The lesson learned was that the Thomas collar was inadequate, even though the fracture was initially incomplete.

Raine[29] reported on a 60-year-old women who, 2 weeks after a fall, experienced neck pain. A fracture was found at about C6 or C7, with 30-degree forward angulation. Despite

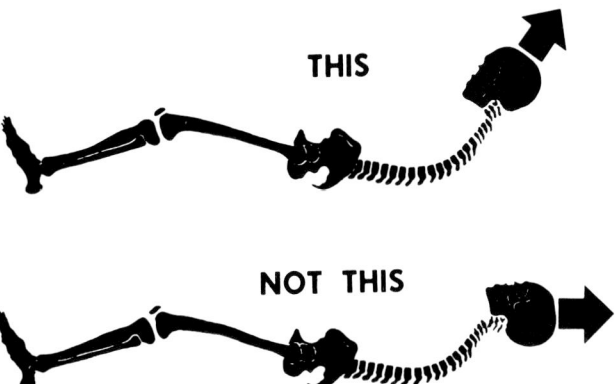

FIGURE 142-6. Proper line of traction in patients with major cervical kyphosis and fracture. Diagram illustrating why horizontal position of fracture at cervical kyphosis courts disaster. (From Young JS, Cheshire DJE, Pierce JA, et al: Cervical ankylosis with acute spinal cord injury. Paraplegia 15:133-146, 1978.)

the support of a collar, the patient developed lasting paraplegia.

A 75-year-old man, the second patient in Raine's study, fell out of wheelchair and suffered a C6 transverse fracture. The collar was not tolerated by the patient, although without it, attacks of tingling in all limbs, cyanosis, and loss of consciousness arose. Posterior fusion occurred, and death from respiratory failure occurred the next month.

Lemmen and Lang[30] reported on a drunk patient who had urinary retention and mental confusion who was admitted to the hospital and gradually developed motor but not sensory loss below C5.[30] Radiographs showed a C5 body anterior to C6, for which tongs were applied. Radiographs taken the next day showed worse distraction of C5 on C6. Sudden respiratory arrest and death occurred after the patient was turned from the face-down to the face-up position. At autopsy, all ligaments connecting C5 to C6 were torn through completely.

Bohlman[24] reported that seven of eight patients with ankylosing spondylitis cervical spine injuries had neural loss. C6-C7 injury caused subluxation and quadriplegia; tong traction was performed at once. The next day, death followed respiratory arrest while the patient was being turned during application of a Minerva jacket.[24]

The second patient in Bohlman's study had a C6-C7 injury that caused subluxation and anterior cord syndrome. Tong traction was followed by greater leg weakness. The final result was that the patient was barely able to walk.[24]

The third patient in Bohlman's study had C7-T1 subluxation and anterior cord syndrome. After laminectomy, the patient was left in tongs. Further dislocation occurred, and weakness worsened. Eventually, however, the patient made a full recovery.[24]

Osgood and colleagues[28] reported on a patient who had an injury accompanied by a loud snap in the neck; quadriparesis occurred for 24 hours, then cleared. Nine days later, C5-C6 fracture was seen through both anterior and posterior elements. Tongs at 15 pounds were applied straight horizontally. More forward slipping of C5 on C6 occurred. The patient became rapidly and permanently quadriplegic.

Osgood and associates[31] reported on a 65-year-old man whose radiographs showed through-and-through fracture-dis-

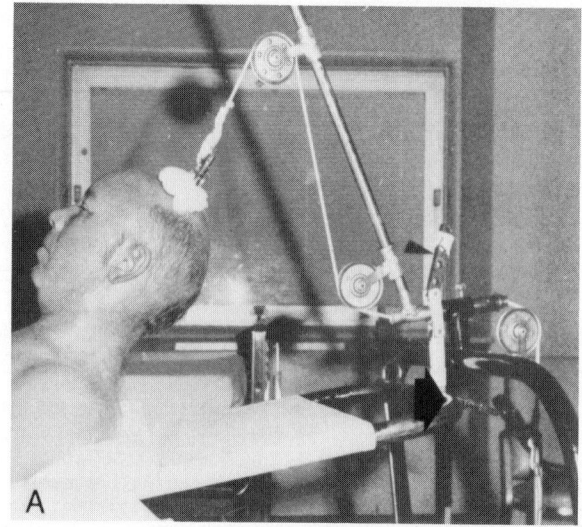
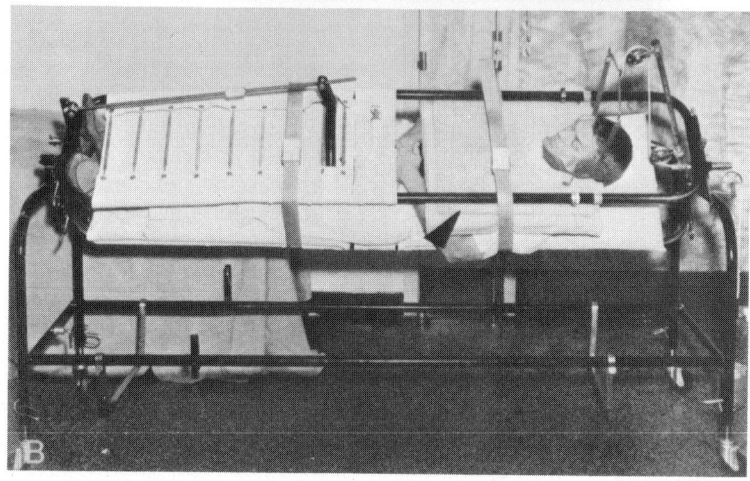

FIGURE 142–7. Proper line of traction in patients with major cervical kyphosis and fracture. (A) Fracture through body of C6 reduced by applying traction with the neck flexed 55 degrees from horizontal patient supine. Device depicted permits turning of patient through 360 degrees while maintaining this constant angle. A metal outrigger to support the pulleys is attached to the front of the bed. (B) Patient being turned to show the board supporting the chest and shoulders. Flange (arrow) prevents sliding. (From Ackerman EA. Cervical fraction in flexion. A method of maintaining constant angle prone or supine. J Bone Joint Surg 1972; 54A: 1115.)

locations at both C7-T1 and T9-10. Flaccid quadriplegia from C5 was present with maldirected traction in tongs. The patient had multiple left rib fractures, left flail chest, and left pneumothorax. Autopsy revealed spinal cord C5-T2 fragmentation and marked instability at T9-10 fracture. "Log-rolling" patient at autopsy from side to side by force applied to either shoulder caused 1- to 2-cm rotational and side-to-side dislocation of fracture margins. Epidural hemorrhage occurred at both sites.

Murray and Persellin[32] reported on a motor vehicle accident victim whose neurologic examination and x-ray studies showed the neck to be normal, but the zone below C6 was poorly seen. Repeat studies of the entire spine revealed the same result. "Electric shocks" occurred in the torso and all limbs when the patient's head was moved. Increased neck pain occurred on transfer to the bed, and motor and sensory deficits were present in both legs. CT showed a 90 percent anterior shift of C7 on T1. Tongs were applied, then laminectomy was performed, after which tongs were continued. Proper alignment was not kept. Episodes of decreased heart and respiratory rate occurred when the patient was turned on postoperative days six, nine, and 10. Pneumonia ensued, then death.

Detwiler and colleagues[26] reduced a C6-C7 subluxation by cervical flexion, but pain in this position led the patient to insist on change. Realignment in minimal extension led to total transverse cord lesion at T3; death soon followed.

In another patient in Detwiler's study, aspiration occurred while this patient was in traction, despite a functioning nasogastric tube. Respiratory arrest occurred. Emergency intubation with the patient's neck extended led to total transverse lesion at C5. Distraction and hyperextension appeared on radiograph. Death occurred soon after.[26] Clearly, tong traction has been failing because the lower and upper segments of the broken spinal column, once properly replaced, must not be allowed to move on each other. Traction tongs cannot ensure this.

The extreme variability of these patients is further illustrated by case 3 of Woodruff and Dewing.[33] This 33-year-old man, who had been completely bedridden for a year, was being turned in a Stryker frame. His head was allowed to go unsupported for "a moment"; it promptly fell into extension, causing a painful snapping sensation in the neck. Although no new neurologic abnormalities were noted at once and his fracture through the C5-C6 interspace was undisplaced, he developed increasing dysphagia and died three days later.

INDICATIONS AND RESULTS OF OPEN OPERATION

In a review of all of the published cases of this infrequent disorder that I could find in a language I could read, I encountered seven articles[26, 32, 34–38] in which clear-cut indications for early open operation in a fractured ankylosed spondylitic cervical spine were enunciated. In each, a delayed or worsening neural loss occurred after the fracture, or the spine was unstable or irreducible by traction. This stance was taken even by Hunter and Dubo,[35] whose summary of 64 such patients revealed that of those treated nonoperatively, 30 percent died, whereas 40 percent of those treated by open operation died.

I reviewed the reports on 108 patients whose fracture dislocation was between C3 and T1. Sixty-six of the patients were initially or became quadriplegic before operation. Of the 48 who did not undergo operation, eight became better, and two others were normal. Of the 18 treated by operation, not one was better or normal. There were 38 patients whose cord lesions fell short of producing complete paralysis in the legs and in some of both upper limbs. Of the 24 such patients who did not have operation, 72 percent became better or normal, whereas only 50 percent of 14 who did have an operation became better or normal. Although immobilized fracture sites tend to heal rapidly in these patients, internal fixation poses great risk in these multiply diseased patients, and the autologous grafts or metal screws, bands, straps, or wires tend to loosen in their porotic bones.

TRACTION VIA TONGS VERSUS HALO VEST

Practical directions of details of application of the halo vest are given by Young and colleagues.[39–41] Examples of the problems follow.

A 68-year-old man fell, and his forehead struck a table, causing nuchal and bilateral shoulder pain. After 4 days of bed rest, he had a mild bilateral sensorimotor loss while cranial tongs were maintaining the best possible alignment. However, a gradual increase in sensorimotor loss in all four limbs seemed beyond control. By 3 weeks after the injury, he had pneumonia, mental confusion, atrial fibrillation, dysphagia, and loss of bladder function. A halo vest was then applied, with gratifying improvement. In another month, he was at home and walking. By 13 weeks, the spine had fused at the fracture sites, and the halo was removed. At 18 months, the only anesthetic area was the right lateral thumb. Improved cervical alignment had been achieved during the healing process.

Surin reported on a quadriplegic patient in whom tongs reduced fracture, but it redislocated at once when the patient was placed in the halo vest. The fracture was kept reduced only by continuous traction near vertical on the halo ring until the fracture was healed. Unfortunately, the quadriplegia persisted.[27]

In the second patient in Surin's study, the reduced fracture was "immobilized" in a halo vest; neurologic examination results remained normal. One week later, the patient became quadriplegic in sleep. Traction on halo ring was begun at once. Only slight anterior dislocation was present at the fracture. Full motor recovery occurred in 24 hours. Traction was needed for 8 weeks.

Surin points out that the vest component of the therapy does not fit the deformed thorax, and Hunter and Dubo,[35] Weinstein and coworkers,[36] and Surin[27] all described failures of the apparatus. Two of the patients for whom treatment failed developed tetraplegia. However, these three groups of investigators and at least five others agree that the halo vest is the best approach currently available.[32, 36, 42–44]

HALO VEST

Although the halo vest accomplishes the desired objective of immobilization if the fit to the chest is tight enough, this chest compression is a major drawback because immobile ribs, pulmonary fibrosis, and pulmonary failure have been established as the commonest cause of death in the disease.

The recent comprehensive report of Rowed[42] on 21 patients recommends against axial traction prior to placement of the halo vest. Of 11 patients treated conservatively, seven are able to walk, work, or both, and two died, whereas only two of the 10 surgically treated patients have become employable. However, the two groups are not really clinically comparable. We recommend use of head and pelvic halos firmly fastened to each other as a relatively low-risk tactic to achieve stabilization after constantly monitored reduction of the fracture dislocation.

STRESS FRACTURES OR PSEUDOARTHROSES

In one of the earlier descriptions of new or worsening pain and progressive bent-over posture, a chronic rheumatoid lesion was diagnosed. However, as more cases have been studied, it is apparent that much more frequently, so-called stress fractures or pseudarthroses may develop a few months to 20 years after ankylosing spondylitis occurs in anywhere from the atlantoaxial region[45] to the lower lumbar region.[46]

At the Mayo Clinic from 1984 to 1989,[23] a period during which high-quality CT scans were in use, 23 patients with ankylosing spondylitis were seen. Investigators at this institution saw 16 stress fractures or pseudarthroses in 12 patients and 12 traumatic fractures in 11 patients, all between 33 and 71 years of age. In addition, six patients had neither fracture nor pseudarthroses, and their progressive kyphosis prevented them from seeing above a specific horizontal view line. Fox and colleagues[23] report that in the presence of fractures or pseudarthroses associated with severe spinal instability but no neurologic deficit, they do both an anterior and posterior fusion. In patients with persisting pain related to the stress fracture, Marsh[46] concluded that the rigidity occurring at all other levels concentrates all movements at the fracture site. He seeks confirmation of the diagnosis of significant pathology at this site by CT and radionuclide imaging, to which

MRI could be added. Marsh goes on to say that internal fixation without bone grafting produces immediate pain relief by rapid fracture union. These stress fractures are commoner in the lower spine and are discussed more completely in Chapter 143.

EPIDURAL AND SUBDURAL HEMATOMAS

Although I found that only one subdural and 20 epidural hematomas in patients with ankylosing spondylitis were reported in the literature, many more may have been missed because of the difficulty in performing myelograms on patients with deformed torsos and the immediate serious lesion of the cord produced by the direct trauma to it. A third reason for a higher incidence of epidural hemorrhage in the ankylosing spondylitis patient was discovered by Schneider and his colleagues,[47] who made the diagnosis on the basis of rapid deterioration in spinal cord function within a few hours of the injury in all three of their cases. The displaced fractured bone had direct access to the epidural space and poured blood into it in each case. The bleeding was so profuse that it was difficult to stop, even at operative exposure. Injury to the generous plexus of epidural veins was not the source of the bleeding. The hematoma at operation in one of their cases extended only to the C5, C6, and C7 levels and was only in the posterior half of the cord and only 4 mm thick, whereas at autopsy 14 days later, it extended from C2 to T5. The operative removal of the clot took place about 24 hours after the injury. The hematoma was removed from the other two patients about 12 hours after the trauma. Unfortunately, the clot in the third patient was 3 to 4 cm thick, surrounded the dura, and extended from C3 to C7; pneumonia killed the patient on the fourteenth postoperative day. At autopsy, no significant epidural clot was found. Only one patient, a 58-year-old with a 1.5-cm clot from C5 to T1, slowly made a full recovery.

Rowed[42] reported the high incidence of two epidural hematomas in 21 patients, one discovered at autopsy and the other in the course of removal of a herniated intervertebral disc. He also removed herniated discs from two other ankylosing spondylitis patients; in all three cases, the discs were removed because they were causing spinal cord compression.

In six other patients, a full recovery was achieved. In three of the six, recovery followed removals that were performed within about 12 hours of injury.[48–50] In another patient, the progression of neural deficit took 36 hours to reach a not quite total transverse lesion, then remained constant another 48 hours, during which a lumbar puncture showed normal dynamics, cerebrospinal fluid protein, and cell count. Nevertheless, Lowrey[51] operated, and the patient recovered about 1 year later. Hissa and associates'[52] patient had such a delayed onset and gradual worsening of his symptoms that a myelogram was not performed until the sixth day after the injury. The myelography revealed a complete block at T2, leading to removal of an epidural hematoma from T2 to T7, followed by a slow but total recovery at 2 years. One of Bohlman's[24] four cases also eventually recovered completely after a laminectomy and removal of an unexpected large epidural hematoma and a period of worsened motor power. Each of the patients of Agnetti and colleagues,[53] Osgood and colleagues,[31] and Rowed[42] and three of the patients of Bohlman[24] died respectively at 1 month, 7 days, 1 day, 1 day, and finally 18 days. The diagnosis in each was made only at postmortem. In three patients[26, 34, 54] laminectomy revealed the hematoma, delay in the removal of which partially explains the major persisting neural sequelae.

A subdural hematoma was found in one patient[55] in whom the neural deficit progressed so slowly to paraplegia that a myelogram was not performed until 1 month after the injury. The partial block was diagnosed as an intradural extramedullary defect at T12-L1. The time to major recovery from the hematoma removal was not stated.

The hope of finding a hematoma, a ruptured disc, or a bony fragment compressing the cord should lead the physician to try to obtain some form of radiographic image. Pan and coworkers[56] reported the first demonstration by MRI of a posttraumatic cervical spinal epidural hematoma, and Garza-Mercado[48] has followed with the more difficult task of securing such a study in a patient with cervical ankylosing spondylitis. The vacuum cushion of Surin[27] may help to maintain the proper position of head and neck during these studies.

The most urgent poorly solved problem is the maintenance of proper neck position for healing and in the optimal region for pulmonary prophylaxis. We are concentrating on a halo-pelvic apparatus.

Two carefully conceived recent papers present the two major divergent views on the place of laminectomy and internal stabilization—that of Fox and associates[23] is more aggressive than that of Rowed.[42]

OSTEOTOMY FOR CORRECTION OF DEFORMITY

Severe, fixed, hip flexion; lumbar spine flexion; thoracic kyphos; and cervical spine flexion or any combination of these can gradually distort the patient into a shape approaching a full circle. Although many patients continue to work despite grotesquely severe deformity, when the top of the patient's head is maintained perpendicular to the floor, chin on chest as the patient stands, then the patient cannot see ahead at all, and correction becomes a necessity. The cervical vertebrae are the most logical and the most hazardous of sites for the procedure. The orthopedic surgeon Simmons[57] has the largest experience in this country in this field.

ATLANTOAXIAL SUBLUXATION

Atlantoaxial subluxation is an uncommon feature of ankylosing spondylitis. In the series of Wilkinson and Bywaters,[10] only one of 212 patients developed atlantoaxial subluxation. Sharp and Purser[58] diagnosed this disorder in only 17 of the approximately 1000 patients with spondylitis seen in their clinic. They described these cases, plus five others, in a remarkably detailed account of each patient, which the neurosurgeon would do well to study if he or she is to treat such a rare condition. The dislocation consists of forward movement of the anterior arch of the atlas away from the odontoid process of the axis. The movement occurs as a consequence of a tear or excessive stretching of the transverse ligament, which lies against the posterior surface of the dens and attaches to bony knobs on the medial aspect of the two lateral masses of the atlas. Failure of this ligament is much commoner in rheumatoid arthritis than in AS and is related to inflammation of the associated synovial joints in this disorder. The diagnosis is made from a pair of lateral radiographs in maximal flexion and maximal extension. The principal symptom is pain in the upper cervical, suboccipital, and retrobulbar areas that is usually worsened by sudden movements or by a succession of these, as occurs during a ride on a bumpy road. Correction and stabilization of the displacement usually results in complete relief of symptoms.

Although the prescription of intensive cervical muscle exercises tends to worsen the symptoms, I have found no horror stories such as abound in the injuries to the rest of the cervical spine in ankylosing spondylitis. Radiographs show that the amount of the increased interval between the atlas and dens does not fully describe the problem in these patients. Of 19 of Sharp and Purser's[58] cases, six had intervals that were essentially normal at 2 to 4 mm, and five had intervals that were moderately increased, measuring 5 to 7 mm. The remaining eight had intervals averaging 12 mm and ranging from 8 to 17 mm.

A marked degree of fixed forward tilt of the head can also be very painful. Thus, in one patient, the atlas-dens interval in maximal flexion was normal at 3 mm, and she also had 17 degrees of forward tilt and was essentially fixed at this angle, which was still in 15-degree flexion on maximal extension. She also maintained 10 degrees of rotation of her head to the left. Her intolerable pain was almost completely relieved by skull traction and was completely eliminated by occipitocervical fusion. In another patient, the head was fixed in a complete rotary dislocation of the atlas to the right. Most of the patients have some rotation and tilting of the head in addition to a fixed forward tilt. Only two of the 22 patients had a major neurologic deficit at the time active treatment began; six had lesser deficits, and the rest were neurologically normal.

In many of the patients, the rarity of this feature of their ankylosing spondylitis led to a protracted delay in making the diagnosis. Sharp and Purser[58] found that the physician could at times make the diagnosis clinically. By pressing with the palm of one hand on the patient's forehead and the thumb of the other hand on the patient's C2 spinous process, the examiner could feel a backward sliding motion of the hand, which was best elicited by having the patient relax the neck in a semiflexed position.

RESULTS

One patient had no specific treatment because the diagnosis was not made until autopsy, although this final procedure did not occur until after a long illness that led to tetraplegia that the authors thought could have been postponed or arrested had the atlantoaxial dislocation been treated. In three others, this aspect of the disease required no treatment. Three others did reasonably well with merely a plastic or cardboard collar, but a fourth steadily worsened until his dislocation was reduced by skull traction and maintained by occipitocervical fusion. Skeletal traction followed by an autologous iliac bone graft for an occipitocervical fusion was carried out in nine of their patients. Skull traction was continued preoperatively until no further reduction occurred and was continued during the fusion operation. In some cases, the traction was continued until the graft was united. Pain from the displacement was present in all nine cases and was completely relieved in all. Cord damage in five of the nine was mild-to-moderate in four patients, who recovered from it completely, and severe in one, in whom moderate improvement occurred. Two cases with a rotary subluxation of atlas on axis were also helped substantially by specific modifications of the skeletal traction. In this disorder, symptoms are clearly amenable to major alleviation.

Acknowledgment

The author wishes to express his appreciation to the Neuro-Research Foundation for its assistance during the preparation of this manuscript.

REFERENCES

1. Bechterew W: Steifigkeit der Wirbelsäule und ihre Verkrümmung als besondere Erkrankungsform. Neurol Centralbl 12:426–434, 1893
2. Bechterew W: Akinesia Algera. Neurol Centralbl 12:531–534, 1893
3. Bechterew W: Von der Verwachsung oder Steifigkeit der Wirbelsäule. Dtsch Z Nervenheilk 11:327–337, 1897
4. Connor B, cited by Blumberg BS: Arch Rheum 1:553, 1958
5. Hollander JE (ed): Boland EW: Ankylosing spondylitis, in Arthritis and Allied Conditions. Philadelphia, Lea & Febiger, 1966, pp 633–655
6. Strumpell A: Bemerkung über die chronische ankylosierende Entzündung der Wirbelsäule und der Huftgelenke. Dtsch Z Nervenheilk 11:338–342, 1897
7. Marie P: Sur la spondylose rhizomelique. Rev Med 8:285–315, 1898
8. Fraenkel E: Über chronische ankylosierende Wirbelsäulenversteifung. Fortsch Geb Rontgenstr Nuklearmed Ergänzungsbd 7:62–90, 1903
9. Abdi O: Über ein Fall von chronischer Arthritis Ankylopoetica der Wirbelsäule. Fraktur der Wirbelsäule und Quetschung der Cauda equina. Milt Hamburgischen Staatskrank Anst 4:57–74, 1904
10. Wilkinson M, Bywaters EGL: Clinical features and course of ankylosing spondylitis. Am Rheum Dis 17:209–228, 1958
11. Calin A, Fries JF: Striking prevalence of ankylosing spondylitis in "healthy" W27 positive males and females. N Engl J Med 293:835–839, 1975
12. Kinsella TD, MacDonald FR, Johnson LG: Ankylosing spondylitis: A late re-evaluation of 92 cases. Can Med Assoc J 95:1–9, 1966
13. Hart FD, Bogdanovitch A, Nichol WD: The thorax in ankylosing spondylitis. Ann Rheum Dis 9:116, 1950
14. Calabro JJ: An appraisal of the medical and surgical management of ankylosing spondylitis. Clin Orthop 60:125–148, 1968
15. Radford EP, Doll R, Smith PG: Mortality among patients with ankylosing spondylitis not given x-ray therapy. N Engl J Med 297:572–576, 1977
16. Cruickshank B: Pathology of ankylosing spondylitis. Clin Orthop 74:43–58, 1971
17. Linder E, Pasternack A: Immunofluorescence studies on kidney biopsies in ankylosing spondylitis. Acta Pathol Microbiol 78:517–525, 1970
18. Cruickshank B: Pathology of ankylosing spondylitis. Bull Rheum Dis 10:211–214, 1960
19. Solomon G, Winchester R: Immunogenetic aspects of inflammatory arthritis, in Taveras JM, Ferrucci JT (eds): Radiology. Diagnosis—Imaging—Intervention, vol 5. Philadelphia, JB Lippincott, 1988, pp 1–4
20. Brewerton DA: HLA-B27 and the inheritance of susceptibility to rheumatic disease. Arthritis Rheum 19:656–668, 1976
21. Martel W, Braunstein EM: Spondyloarthritides, in Taveras J, Ferrucci JT (eds): Radiology. Diagnosis—Imaging—Invervention, vol 5. Philadelphia, JB Lippincott, 1988, pp 1–5
22. Simmonds M: Über Spondylitis deformans und ankylosierende Spondylitis. Fortschr Gebd Rontgenstr Nuklearmed Ergänzungsbd 7:51–62, 1903

23. Fox MW, Onofrio BM, Kilgore JE: Neurological complications of ankylosing spondylitis. J Neurosurg 78:871–878, 1993
24. Bohlman HH: Acute fractures and dislocations of the cervical spine. J Bone Joint Surg Am 61A:1119–1142, 1979
25. Ackerman EA: Cervical traction in flexion. A method of maintaining constant angle prone or supine. J Bone Joint Surg Am 54A:1114–1116, 1972
26. Detwiler KN, Loftus CM, Menezes AH, et al. Management of cervical spine injuries in patients with ankylosing spondylitis. J Neurosurg 72:210–215, 1990
27. Surin VV: Fractures of the cervical spine in patients with ankylosing spondylitis. Acta Orthop Scand 51:79–84, 1980
28. Osgood C, Martin LG, Ackerman E: Fracture-dislocation of the cervical spine with ankylosing spondylitis. J Neurosurg 39:764–769, 1973
29. Raine GET: Fractures of the cervical spine. Proc R Soc Med 63:657–658, 1970
30. Lemmen LJ, Laing PG: Fracture of the cervical spine in patients with rheumatoid arthritis. J Neurosurg 542–550, 1959
31. Osgood CP, Abbasy M, Mathews T: Multiple spine fractures in ankylosing spondylitis. J Trauma 15:163–166, 1975
32. Murray GC, Persellin RH: Cervical fracture complicating ankylosing spondylitis. A report of eight cases and review of the literature. Am J Med 70:1033–1041, 1981
33. Woodruff FP, Dewing SB: Fracture of the cervical spine patients with ankylosing spondylitis. Radiology 80:17–21, 1963
34. Grisolia A, Bell RL, Peltier LF, et al: Fractures and dislocations of the spine complicating ankylosing spondylitis. J Bone Joint Surg Am 49A:339–344, 1967
35. Hunter T, Dubo H: Spinal fractures complicating ankylosing spondylitis. Ann Intern Med 88:546–549, 1978
36. Weinstein PR, Karpman RR, Gall E, et al: Spinal cord injury, spinal fracture and spinal stenosis in ankylosing spondylitis. J Neurosurg 57:609–616, 1982
37. Malik GM, Sanders JL: Surgical treatment of rheumatoid arthritis, ankylosing spondylitis, and Paget's disease with neurologic deficit, in Schmidek HH, Sweet WH (eds): Operative Neurosurgical Techniques: Indications, Methods and Results. Philadelphia, WB Saunders, 1988, pp 1295–1306
38. Janda WE, Kelly PJ, Rhoton AL, et al: Fracture dislocation of the cervical part of the spinal column in patients with ankylosing spondylitis. Mayo Clin Proc 43:714–721, 1968
39. Young R, Thomassen EH: Step by step procedure for applying the halo ring. Orthop Rev 3(6):62–64, 1974
40. Young JS, Cheshire DJE, Pierce JA, et al: Cervical ankylosis with acute spinal cord injury. Paraplegia 15:133–146, 1977–1978
41. Young R, Murphy DJ: Step by step procedure for applying the halo vest. Orthop Rev 4:33–36, 1975
42. Rowed DW: Management of cervical spinal cord injury in ankylosing spondylitis: The intervertebral disc as a cause of cord compression. J Neurosurg 77:241–246, 1992
43. Freeman LW: Ascending spinal paralysis. Case presentation. J Neurosurg 16:120–122, 1959
44. Kiwerski J, Wieclawek H, Garwacka I: Fractures of the cervical spine in ankylosing spondylitis. Int Orthop 8:243–246, 1985
45. Martel W, Page JW: Cervical vertebral erosions and subluxations in rheumatoid arthritis and ankylosing spondylitis. Arthritis Rheum 3:546–556, 1960
46. Marsh CH: Internal fixation for stress fractures of the ankylosed spine. J R Soc Med 78:377–379, 1985
47. Schneider RC, Cherry G, Pantek H: The syndrome of acute central cervical spinal cord injury. J Neurosurg 11:546–577, 1954
48. Garza-Mercado R: Traumatic extradural hematoma of the cervical spine. Neurosurgery 24:410–414, 1989
49. Pecker J, Javalet A, Le Menn G: Spondylarthrite ankylosante et paraplégie par hématorachis extra-dural traumatique. Presse Med 68:183–184, 1960
50. Ver Brugghen A: Extradural spinal hemorrhage. Ann Surg 123:154–159, 1946
51. Lowrey JJ: Spinal epidural hematomas. Experiences with three patients. J Neurosurg 16:508–513, 1959
52. Hissa E, Boumphrey F, Bay J: Spinal epidural hematoma and ankylosing spondylitis. Clin Orthop 208:225–227, 1986
53. Agnetti V, Monaco F, Mutani R: Post-convulsive spinal epidural haematoma in ankylosing spondylitis. Eur Neurol 18:230–233, 1979
54. Fast A, Parikh S, Marin EL: Spine fractures in ankylosing spondylitis. Arch Phys Med Rehabil 67:595–597, 1986
55. Sokoloff J, Coel MN, Ignelzi RJ: Spinal subdural hematoma. Radiology 120:116, 1976
56. Pan G, Kulkarni M, MacDougall DJ, et al: Traumatic epidural hematoma of the cervical spine: Diagnosis with magnetic resonance imaging. J Neurosurg 68:798–801, 1988
57. Simmons EH: The surgical correction of flexion deformity of the cervical spine in ankylosing spondylitis, in Sherk HH, Dunn EJ, Eismont FJ, et al (eds): The Cervical Spine, 2nd ed. Philadelphia, JB Lippincott, 1989, pp 573–598
58. Sharp J, Purser DW: Spontaneous atlanto-axial dislocation in ankylosing spondylitis and rheumatoid arthritis. Ann Rheum Dis 20:47–77, 1961

CHAPTER 143

Neurosurgical Considerations in the Management of Ankylosing Spondylitis

Michael E. Miner

The skeletal remains of a person with ankylosing spondylitis have been found that date back about 5000 years. However, it was not until the latter half of the twentieth century that the clinical manifestations of ankylosing spondylitis were fully described. Ankylosing spondylitis must be considered as a systemic inflammatory disease with a genetic component in which spinal involvement is commonly present. The systemic manifestations are especially important in this disease because they may account for the major complications that may mar an otherwise successful surgical treatment. Typically, these patients seek medical attention because of indolent fevers, anorexia, and easy fatigability, or they seek ophthalmologic treatment because of anterior uveitis or iritis. The inflammatory component and consequent fibrosis may affect the aorta and the heart,[1] weakening the media of the aorta and causing aneurysms and rupture of the aorta.[2] This complication has been reported to occur during surgical procedures on the spine and after spinal fractures.[3,4] Fibrosis of the myocardium may cause conduction defects in the bundle of His and cardiac arrhythmias.[5] Pulmonary fibrosis may cause right ventricular failure with pulmonary edema,[5] apnea, and hemoptysis. A progressive decrease in chest expansion is characteristic of this disease and may result in a frozen chest wall, causing the patient to have a very restricted vital capacity.[6,7] Complications within the cardiovascular and the pulmonary systems account for the preponderance of early deaths in these patients. All patients with ankylosing spondylitis who have surgical evaluation should be carefully examined for restrictive lung disease, pulmonary fibrosis, right ventricular failure, aortic aneurysms, and conduction defects in the heart.

Patients with ankylosing spondylitis have a general proliferation of fibrous tissue that affects joints but may also affect the spinal canal and cause myelopathy or radiculopathy. Although this process may occur in the lumbar spine, it is more common in the thoracic spine, where it affects spinal cord function. This proliferation of fibrous tissue is difficult to evaluate by computed tomography (CT) but on magnetic resonance imaging (MRI) appears as a thickening of the dura and ligaments, especially affecting the ligamentum flavum, the posterior longitudinal ligament, and the ligaments of the facet joints. Although myelography is an excellent imaging study to detect neural compression, it is rarely used in these patients because patients with ankylosing spondylitis frequently have a fixed kyphotic deformity that makes lumbar puncture difficult and painful. In addition, the kyphosis makes positioning on the myelogram table difficult, and neurologic deficits following lumbar puncture have been reported.[8] The proliferation of fibrous tissue in the spinal canal is a part of the spectrum of the spinal disease that is characteristic of ankylosing spondylitis and may precede the more characteristic bony changes.

Inflammatory gastrointestinal disease, most notably ulcerative colitis, is frequently a severe problem for patients with ankylosing spondylitis. They may also develop hypertension and renal failure because this inflammatory disease also affects the renal arteries.

Ankylosing spondylitis is a progressive disease that generally comes to medical attention when people are in their 20s. Nearly two thirds of these patients are diagnosed by the age of 30, and almost 90 percent by the age of 40. Although ankylosing spondylitis is an unusual problem, it is not rare and has a prevalence of 197/100,000 in men but less than half that in women.[9] Conversely, sacroiliitis, which is one of the first symptoms that is indicative of ankylosing spondylitis, has the same prevalence in men and women.[10-12] Thus, not all people with sacroiliitis seem to progress to ankylosing spondylitis. The kyphotic spinal deformities of the thoracic and lumbar spine are overwhelmingly more frequent in men, and the surgeon tends to see older men with long-standing disease.

Most patients with ankylosing spondylitis develop a dull aching pain in the buttocks. Although the pain may radiate into the thighs, it usually does not radiate along the full course of the sciatic nerve. With thoracic and lumbar spine involvement, the patient may develop a significant flexion deformity. The initial manifestations of this disease are subtle ankyloses of the sacroiliac or facet joints in the lumbar spine, with bony erosion in the same area.[13] These two characteristics, bony erosion and sclerosis, are the early hallmarks of the spinal component of ankylosing spondylitis. The pain may be improved by mild exercise and worsened by inactivity. Patients characteristically awaken to pain, often in the middle of the night, but may improve with a moderate exercise or stretching regimen. Strenuous exercise generally worsens the pain. Ankylosing spondylitis is a progressive disease, and characteristically, the pain, stiffness, and deformity increase slowly and insidiously. Typically, the patient does not seek medical treatment for thoracic or lumbar spine deformity for 20 years or more after the initial diagnosis of ankylosing spondylitis.

This inflammatory disease is protean in its distribution in the body tissues. In evaluating patients with kyphotic deformity, Simmons and colleagues[14] found that all had an underlying muscle disease with atrophy of type I and type II muscle fibers. The components of this disease that are amenable to surgical treatment are a fixed painful deformity of the thoracic or lumbar spine, spinal fracture, spinal stenosis, or cauda equina syndrome.

The surgeons must see these patients as having complex, multifaceted medical problems requiring long-term medical management, with surgery being reserved for when these regimens fail.

FIXED SPINAL DEFORMITIES

Over time, all of these patients develop some degree of fusion of most, if not all, of their thoracic and lumbar spine. The prevention of deformity depends on long-term vigilance throughout the patient's life. Multiple x-ray studies taken on a consistent long-term basis and careful counseling with regard to positioning during sleep, awake posture, and other activities that result in the spine not remaining in a fixed position are the cornerstones of conservative spinal management. The judicious use of medications, an exercise regimen, and occasionally external orthotics are needed. Monitoring by physiatrists and rheumatologists is invaluable for these patients.

The basic disease mechanism involved in the spine with ankylosing spondylitis is an erosive inflammatory process in which the subchondral bone deteriorates; as a result, the disc space widens. The surrounding bone responds over time by becoming sclerotic around the area of inflammation. Either the erosive or the sclerotic component may become more prominent in any given patient. This spondylodiscitis was first observed by Anderson in 1937 but has only recently been noted to be an inflammatory, rather than an infective, process.[7] This disease may progress by several routes. If the sclerotic process continues, osteophytes develop between the vertebral bodies, causing bony bridging between adjacent vertebra. Although the more dramatic x-ray changes occur in the area of the vertebral body, this process occurs in the facet joints and even between the spinous processes, ultimately resulting in a fusion, which may occur over multiple segments and ultimately over the entire spine. The long-term result is that the spine becomes functionally and pathologically like a single long bone but without the strength normally associated with long bones. Fractures usually occur through the weakest point, the intervertebral disc space. The destructive process that is part of this disease may predominate but usually does not occur uniformly throughout the spine. Part of the subchondral bone of a vertebral body may be destroyed, resulting in deformity; this deformity may become incorporated in the ensuing sclerotic process, resulting in a fixed deformity.

Another mechanism responsible for the fixed deformity is chronic malpositioning of the spine. The chest wall may become restricted as a result of the ribs fusing together. One of the hallmarks of this disease is that frequently the chest wall can expand only a few centimeters during full inspiration, and during normal inspirations, only a fraction of that. This condition may result in these patients' sleeping with multiple pillows under the head and the shoulders, which may enhance the development of fixed deformities. As these patients become less able to move, they tend to exercise less and to become even more fixed in a flexed position; as a result, their center of gravity changes, causing them to bend more forward and to exaggerate the kyphosis. Ultimately, patients may become so flexed that they cannot look forward to see in front of them. This fixed position may cause patients to lose several inches in height and may cause them to be more susceptible to falls because of their limited vision.

The primary goal in the surgical correction is to get the patient into an upright posture (thus helping the patient to see forward), with the weight-bearing axis over the site of the correction, and to direct the correction at the major area of kyphosis. The main area of deformity may be anywhere in the thoracic or lumbar spine but is characteristically in the upper lumbar spine. However, the role of the patient's hip joints must be fully evaluated: the head of the femur may ankylose to the point that the patient appears to have a spinal deformity when the major problem is in the hip joints. In cases in which both the spine and the hips are contributing to the patient's deformity, the hips are generally treated first to determine whether or not their correction will offer satisfactory relief.

Patients should have full-length x-ray studies taken of their spine in the most extended upright position that they can tolerate. The chin-brow line is measured from the vertical angle, and that angle is used to determine the spinal correction. If possible, the thoracic spine should be avoided because of the risk of injuring the spinal cord and because multiple level osteotomies are frequently required. Usually, the patient has a low thoracic or lumbar center of the deformity, with loss of the lumbar lordosis. Whenever possible, the correction is carried out in the midlumbar region, at a single level below the level of the spinal cord, at the L2-L3 or L3-L4 level.

In 1945, Smith-Peterson and coworkers[15] described the first major corrective procedure that attained popularity. In that approach, the patient was laid prone on the flexed operating table, and special care was taken to have the table flexed to match the patient's deformity. Later adjustments in the procedure included having the patient lie on his or her side to avoid trying to match the position of the operating table to that of the patient. The osteotomies are performed at the facet joint and pedicles, and a wedge-shaped segment is removed on each side to allow the posterior column freedom to bend backward. The ligamentum flavum is removed at that level, and the lamina is undermined. The spine is extended by extending the operating table. This process requires disruption of the anterior longitudinal ligament and, usually, disruption of the anterior portion of the cartilaginous disc endplate. Bone grafts, taken from the spinous processes and lamina, are then placed along the denuded lamina. After 4 to 6 weeks in a plaster shell, patients wear a plaster jacket or back brace for a year or more. Unfortunately, there has been an attendant mortality rate of approximately 10 percent with this procedure and a paraplegia rate of approximately 3 percent.[16,17] The force needed to disrupt the anterior longitudinal ligament may be the cause for the untoward neurologic results. The general fragility of these patients and the difficulties with anesthetic management are the primary cause for the high mortality rate. Pulmonary complications dominate in these patients after surgery; however, this technique has been the basis for subsequent surgical procedures and has benefited many patients.

Jeffray and colleagues[17] described the closing wedge osteotomy and used transpedicular fixation in these patients. In this procedure, the posterior spine is exposed, the facet joints are identified and removed, and guidewires are passed through the pedicles. A posterior wedge of pedicle is removed with a rongeur and an osteotome. The midline posterior ligaments are removed, and the laminae are undermined with Kerrison rongeurs. The lateral masses and transverse processes are morcellated and removed. The nerve root is visualized as it passes beneath the corresponding pedicle. Angled curettes are used to compact or remove the cancellous bone of the vertebral body. The posterior wall of the body is fractured after the cancellous bone has been removed. The osteotomy is then closed while the nerves are directly visible. The anterior longitudinal ligament and cartilaginous endplate are preserved in this procedure. Pedicular screws are placed in two adjacent vertebrae and connected with contoured rods.

This procedure results in a clearer definition of the angle to be corrected and a less traumatic closure of the angle. Ample bone is available from the spinous processes, transverse processes, laminae, and body morcellation to lay along the side of the rods for fusion. The patient is placed in a plaster jacket or molded back brace with one thigh included. The external orthosis is removed at about 6 weeks. Simmons performs a similar surgical procedure but uses a Luque rectangle instead of pedicular screw fixation. Although using a Luque rectangle may be a simpler procedure, in patients with fragile bone it may be a less stable construct. The center of gravity must be changed in these procedures so that it is over the wedge osteotomy rather than in front of the posterior column, as is the case preoperatively. As the center of gravity becomes more posterior, the rate of fusion increases.

The importance of the preoperative, intraoperative, and postoperative management of these patients cannot be overemphasized. They must be intubated with extreme care, and whenever possible, an awake intubation must be considered because it allows the patient to indicate the degree of neck flexion that he or she can tolerate and diminishes the opportunity for cervical spinal cord injury. These patients are fragile and must be carefully positioned for surgery. The patients can even position themselves in the most comfortable position on the operating table, thus aiding in the determination of how to initially flex the table. The angle to be corrected should be placed directly over the break in the operating table. At this point, the patient is anesthetized. Somatosensory evoked potentials are performed continuously from the time the patient is intubated until he or she is removed from the operating table. The nerve roots at the level of the osteotomy should be included in the nerve that is stimulated. Because the bone in these patients is not strong after the osteotomy is completed, the extension of the spine must be performed with great care. Similarly, caution must be exerted to not overextend the hip joints.

Among the many potential postoperative pitfalls is the problem of postoperative ileus. Gastric tubes should be left in place until the patient is passing flatus. The pulmonary complications are the most treacherous because these patients have markedly restricted chest wall expansion, pulmonary fibrosis, and, possibly, abnormal cardiac function. We carefully evaluate pulmonary function preoperatively and expect a slow, careful, postoperative weaning from the ventilator that may take several days. Extubation is likewise more cautiously performed than in other patients because of the hazards of emergency reintubation, which is to be avoided if possible.

With extreme care in the perioperative and intraoperative management of these patients, elective surgery can be performed, and over 95 percent of patients can be expected to have a solid fusion with partial or total correction of their deformity. Even so, these are high-risk procedures, and a careful preoperative evaluation should be performed to assess pulmonary and cardiovascular function, cervical spine mobility, and general nutrition.

THORACOLUMBAR FRACTURES

The spine of patients with ankylosing spondylitis may fuse into one long bone, but the bone itself becomes osteoporotic and prone to fracture. The symptoms related to spine fractures in patients with ankylosing spondylitis may be minimal, consisting only of mild back pain. The fractures may also be very difficult to identify, even with good radiographs. X-ray studies obtained under emergency conditions are often inadequate, and patients with ankylosing spondylitis who have a history of even trivial injury should be treated as though they have a fracture until they are completely evaluated. In these patients, spine fractures may be multiple[18] and may present immediately or years after the injury. The underlying trauma may be so trivial as to go unnoticed by the patient. The largest percentage of thoracic and lumbar spine fractures in patients with ankylosing spondylitis are either through the disc space or through the adjacent remnant of the cartilaginous endplate,[19] and they appear to be extension injuries. Chance fractures through the body, pedicles, and lamina also occur, but compression fractures are uncommon in the thoracic and lumbar spine.

Fractures through the disc space are often referred to as stress fractures and are particularly likely to occur with trivial injuries. Stress fractures are more commonly seen in the thoracic and lumbar spine than in the cervical spine.[16] Chance fractures are more common in the cervical spine. Most of the fractures appear as though the spine was pulled backward and separated at either the vertebral body or the disc space. Although fractures in the cervical spine account for approximately 75 to 80 percent of the fractures seen in these patients,[7, 16] fractures in the thoracic or lumbar spine may be very treacherous and may occur after such trivial activities as transfer from a gurney in the hospital,[16] cardiopulmonary resuscitation,[20] or falls from what should be inconsequential heights. The patients who have such fractures are generally elderly. The risk of permanent neurologic damage is highest with fractures of the lower cervical spine[8, 21-24] but may also be high for patients with thoracic spinal injuries; however, these injuries occur relatively rarely and are difficult to diagnose unless the spine is dislocated. Lumbar spine fractures are associated with fewer neurologic deficits, except at the

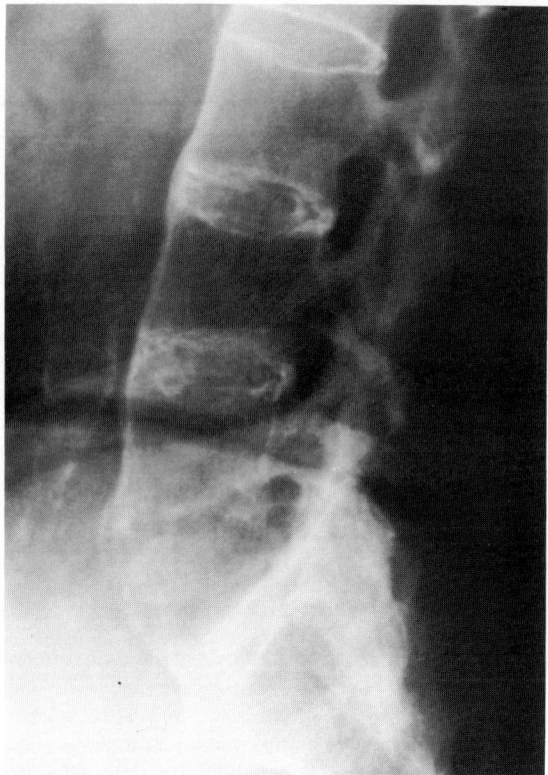

FIGURE 143–1. Anteroposterior lumbosacral spine x-ray film of the patient in Case Report 1 showing the fracture through the L5-S1 disc space. This nondisplaced stress fracture is not detectable on this film. The calcification of the posterior longitudinal ligament reveals the railroad track sign on the anteroposterior view.

that described for patients undergoing elective surgery for kyphotic deformities. Both pulmonary function testing and a thorough cardiovascular evaluation should be performed. However, many patients have had injuries to the aorta associated with thoracic and lumbar fractures, and careful attention to these injuries should precede surgical treatment. Patients with spine fractures should have the same medical evaluation as patients with fixed deformities. In almost all instances, the spine fracture can be managed nonoperatively until other problems are corrected, but great care must be taken to avoid further injury to the patients during this preoperative period.

Case Reports

CASE REPORT 1

A 56-year-old man fell from a ladder while cleaning leaves from the gutter on the first story of his house. He struck his low back and initially complained of back and shoulder pain but was reportedly neurologically intact. In the emergency room, he was found to have a clavicular and scapular fracture. He was known to have ankylosing spondylitis, and this and his complaints prompted an x-ray study of his lumbar spine (Figs. 143–1 and 143–2). He was discharged, but when he arrived home, he was unable to get out of his automobile. Friends helped him from the car and

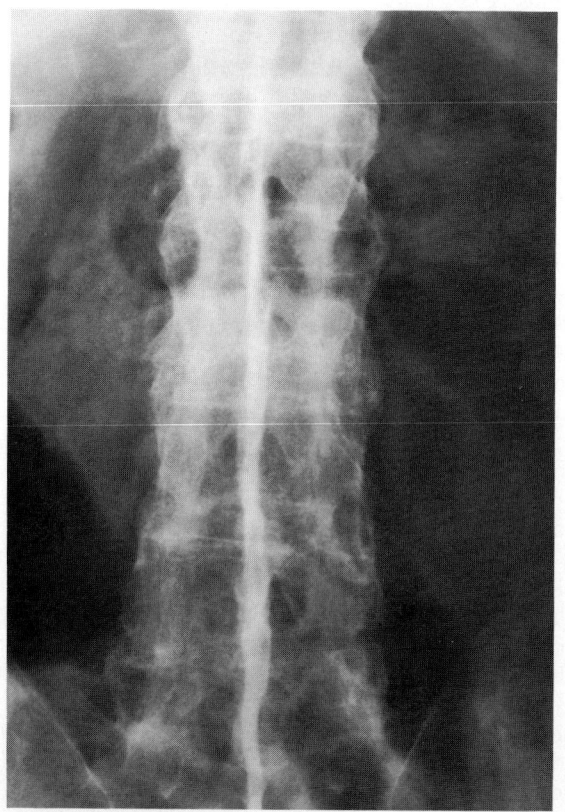

FIGURE 143–2. Companion lateral lumbosacral spine x-ray film of Fig. 143–1. This demonstrates a fracture through the L5-S1 disc space. It is nondisplaced on this lateral view as it was on the anteroposterior view. The characteristic bamboo appearance of the spine is well seen on the lateral view.

T12-L1 segment, because of the resiliency of the cauda equina compared with the spinal cord. Thorngren and associates[25] found that neurologic deficits accompanied 80 percent of cervical spine fractures but only 23 percent of thoracolumbar spine fractures. Epidural hematomas have been associated with fractures in these patients and must be considered in the diagnosis.[4] However, whether or not epidural hematomas occur more frequently in patients with ankylosing spondylitis is not clear.[7, 8, 16, 17, 25]

Fractures of the thoracic and lumbar spine may be the presenting problem in patients who are unaware that they have ankylosing spondylitis. The patients often have a history of relatively minor trauma, such as falling from a height of a few feet. The fracture may go unidentified in the emergency room, and the surgeon may be asked to see the patient only because of persistent back pain. In a patient with ankylosing spondylitis who has persistent spine pain but normal radiographic results, a radionuclide bone scan is the next appropriate test. Such scans can localize an area of interest, allowing further study with CT, MRI, or tomography. Multiple fractures are an important concern, and if obtaining radiographs of the entire spine is difficult or the radiographs are compromised, bone scanning is an alternative means of localizing an area of interest. However, bone scanning in these patients should always be viewed only as a screening test for fractures.

If possible, patients should be fully evaluated before surgical therapy is considered. Such screening should include

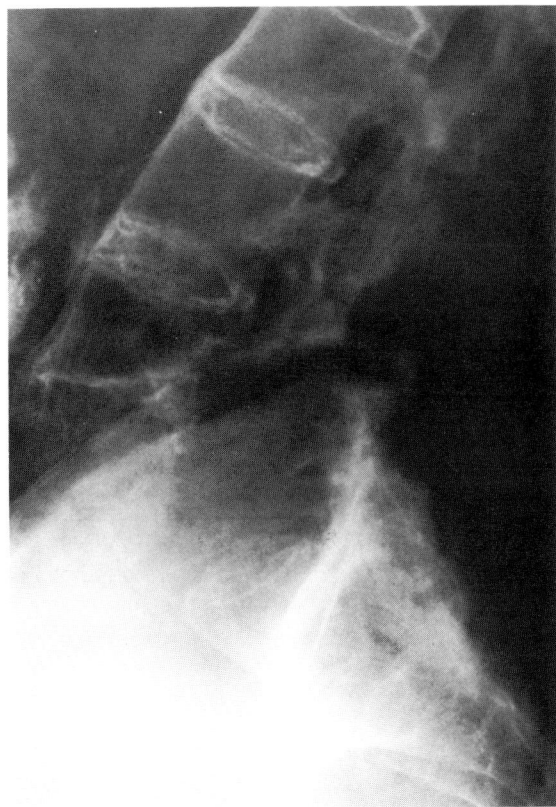

FIGURE 143-3. Lateral lumbar spine x-ray film of the patient in Case Report 1 taken 5 days after the films in Fig. 143-1 and 143-2 demonstrating marked distraction and anterior subluxation of the body of L5 on S1.

got him into a chair at home. He was unable to get out of the chair because of back pain and remained there for 2 days. He also became incontinent of stool and urine. He returned to the emergency room and was found to have a diffuse ileus but was reportedly able to move his lower extremities. He was treated in the hospital without the realization that he had a spine fracture. However, because of back pain during physical therapy, x-ray studies of the spine were performed (Fig. 143-3). He had a 3- to 4-cm dislocation of L5 on S1. However, he still had some movement in the S1 innervated muscles but had flaccid anal sphincter tone and a neurogenic bladder. Posterior fixation was performed with pedicle and sacral screws and bone grafts. This procedure was complicated by cardiac arrest, hemorrhage, pneumonia, wound infection, and cerebrospinal fluid leak. Ultimately, he was treated in a rehabilitation center but remained paraplegic.

This patient exemplifies many of the problems of patients with ankylosing spondylitis who develop lumbar spine fracture. The initial x-ray studies demonstrate a fracture, but it is subtle (see Figs. 107-1 and 107-2). The patient's ileus suggested to his physicians that he had an intra-abdominal problem, and his weakness was ascribed to his back pain. Ultimately, his persistent pain prompted evaluation. When he became subluxed during this process is unclear. The spine became so distracted that performing any type of spinal fixation was difficult. The complications that he developed were numerous and were much more severe than would have been suspected had he not had ankylosing spondylitis.

CASE REPORT 2

A 70-year-old man fell from a short step ladder at home and came to the hospital with severe back pain. He had no neurologic deficit and was unaware of having ankylosing spondylitis. He had a Chance fracture of L1 (Fig. 143-4). His pulmonary function was markedly compromised, and he was treated with bed rest for 12 weeks. He was immobilized in a back brace and was neurologically intact, able to walk without assistance, and had normal bowel and bladder function.

These two cases illustrate the point that even major fractures in the lower spine can be associated with modest or no neurologic deficit initially but that further injury can lead to major neurologic deficit. Early recognition and the difficulties that may be encountered when the diagnosis is not made early after injury are especially important features of Case 1. Case 2 illustrates that nonoperative management of these fractures can be quite successful.

TREATMENT

The treatment of spinal fractures in patients with ankylosing spondylitis is fraught with hazard. Weinstein and coworkers[8] reported a 29 percent mortality and 46 percent permanent neurologic morbidity rate in their patients. These data are consistent with the severity of the medical problems and exemplify the fragility of these patients. They also con-

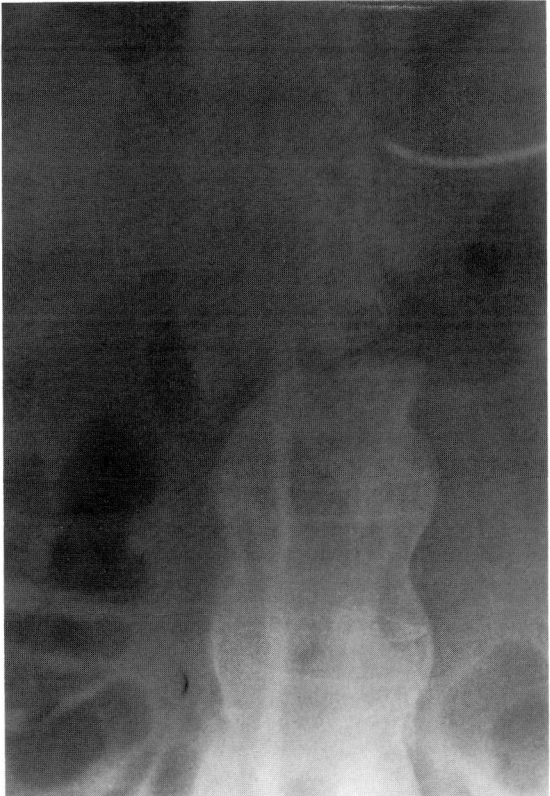

FIGURE 143-4. Anterior x-ray film showing fracture dislocation at T12-L1. The fracture was through the body, pedicles, and lamina of L1. Note the large dilated loops of bowel.

cluded that nonsurgical immobilization was the most successful treatment regimen unless spinal dislocation or bone fragment displacement was present at the fracture site.

No consensus exists on the surgical treatment itself of fractures of the thoracic and lumbar spine. The same is true for the treatment of spondylodiscitis. Many physicians recommend that spondylodiscitis be treated with an external orthotic for several months and believe that the pain deformity can be well managed in this manner.[5, 7, 22, 26] However, Fox and colleagues[16] noted that all of the patients with spondylodiscitis whom they saw failed this conservative regimen and subsequently required internal fixation and fusion. Minimal posterior fusion may be needed if the body fractures are in good alignment and an adequate fixation exists either internally or externally. However, most clinicians would proceed with fusion if internal fixation was being performed.

The choice of using pedicle screws with interconnecting rods or the more simple Luque rectangle has not been clarified, but each has its proponents. Usually, little distraction or compaction is needed, and the rectangle may be sufficient. In either event, an external brace is invaluable for several months after surgery. Nondisplaced fractures can be managed by bed rest. I try to keep patients in a brace, even when they are at bed rest, and continue aggressive physical therapy. This is a long treatment regimen and puts the patient at risk for the complications of immobility. However, it is successful in most patients. When surgery is needed, I prefer to perform internal fixation with pedicle screws and interconnecting rods because I think that this procedure offers a more stable construct; this stability is especially important in these patients, who have a concomitant element of osteoporosis. Fox and coworkers[16] perform a more aggressive procedure for displaced fractures, including posterior and anterior fixation and anterior and posterior fusion. One of the difficulties is determining which spines are unstable, and therefore most should be considered unstable; however, I do not believe that this more aggressive procedure is always required. The principles of treatment are

1. Most of the fractures through the body or disc space should be considered unstable. If, however, they are in anatomic alignment and remain that way, the likelihood that fusion will occur is very high.

2. The purpose of internal fixation is to place and maintain the spine in good alignment. Posterior fusion may not be required in these patients, but in someone who is being operated on for internal fixation, performing an onlay bone graft adds little time or difficulty to the procedure.

3. These patients should be treated conservatively whenever possible.

SPINAL STENOSIS

Because ankylosing spondylitis involves calcification of the ligaments, encroachment of the spinal canal might be anticipated. In fact, this condition is quite uncommon. Luken and associates[27] reported on one patient with claudication and urinary sphincter dysfunction in whom CT scan demonstrated stenosis of the lateral recesses and multiple lumbar spinal foramina. Myelography was decidedly inferior to CT in diagnosing the problem. The response to removing the extensive posterior soft tissue ossification was excellent.

Similar results have been reported by others in small numbers of patients.[16] Luken and associates postulated that the findings in their patient may have resulted from repeated injuries of the spine during the patient's early adult life. Spinal stenosis is an uncommon entity in these patients, but the surgical treatment, which consists of unroofing the foramina and decompressing the affected nerve roots, has afforded relief of symptoms.

CAUDA EQUINA SYNDROME

The cauda equina syndrome[28–30] appears late in the disease and is a different clinical entity from spinal stenosis. Patients may have radicular pain, but generally they have a dull ache in their back and buttocks. However, given their complaints, the degree of sensory loss is greater than would be expected. It is usually confined to the sacral and lower lumbar dermatomes and rarely occurs above the third or fourth lumbar vertebral bodies. Their strength and deep tendon reflexes are rather well preserved, especially when compared with the sensory loss. The most remarkable feature of this process is that over time, all patients will develop a neurogenic bladder and sphincter disturbances at the bladder neck. Overflow incontinence is a major disability for these patients. Unfortunately, some of these patients are treated with a urethral resection that is ineffective and causes them to be incontinent virtually all of the time. The underlying pathology for this problem is particularly surprising. They have arachnoid diverticula, particularly dorsally, in the lumbar and sacral spinal canal. The caudal dural sac is patulous, and there is no suggestion of stenosis of the canal. These cysts may rarely extend above the lumbar region. CT scans demonstrate erosion of the lamina and spinous process that is not well demonstrated on plain x-ray studies. In the sacrum, the dorsal sacrum becomes eroded. MRI does not visualize the bony changes as well as CT but is sufficient to suggest the diverticula. Performing myelography to diagnose these patients is generally unnecessary.

No successful treatment regimen has been reported for cauda equina syndrome in these patients. Steroid and anti-inflammatory drug therapies do not appear to help. Surgical treatments ranging from laminectomies to wide foraminotomies have not been useful and may in fact cause a deterioration in the patient's condition.[8] The process is almost invariably progressive, although very slowly. The differential diagnosis is extensive but includes all compressive lesions of the cauda equina. However, visualizing the distinctive arachnoid diverticula is the key to the diagnosis.

SUMMARY

Ankylosing spondylitis is a disease with protean manifestations. The surgeon must be aware of the systemic, especially cardiopulmonary, disorders that occur in these patients. The spinal deformities are caused by a destructive and sclerotic process that, at its endpoint, leaves the spine as one long continuous bone susceptible to fractures from relatively mild trauma. Fixed spinal deformities in the thoracic and lumbar spine may cause great pain and disability. Surgical treatment generally alleviates pain and improves the vision of the patient. These are fragile patients in whom great care must be taken before, during, and after surgery. The cauda equina syndrome in these patients, which is caused by multiple arachnoid diverticula, should not be treated by spinal surgery.

REFERENCES

1. Calvin A, Elwood J, Rigg S: Ankylosing spondylitis: An analytical review of 1500 patients. The changing pattern of disease. J Rheumatol 15:1234–1238, 1988
2. Savolaine ER, Ebraheim NA, Stitgen S, et al: Aortic rupture complicating a fracture of an ankylosed thoracic spine. Clin Orthop 272:136–140, 1991
3. Fazl M, Bilbao JM, Hudson AR: Laceration of the aorta complicating spinal fracture in ankylosing spondylitis. Neurosurgery 8:732–734, 1981
4. Foo D, Rossier AB: Post-traumatic spinal epidural hematoma. Neurosurgery 11:25–32, 1982
5. Wilkinson M, Bywaters EGL: Clinical features and course of ankylosing spondylitis. As seen in a follow-up of 222 hospital referred cases. Am Rheum Dis 17:209–228, 1958
6. Cruickshank B: Pathology of ankylosing spondylitis. Clin Orthop 74:43–58, 1971
7. Simmons EH: Surgical treatment of ankylosing spondylitis in the spine, in Evarts CM (ed): Surgery of the Musculoskeletal System, Vol 3, 2nd ed. New York, Churchill Livingstone, 1990, pp 2331–2394
8. Weinstein PR, Karpman RR, Gall EP, et al: Spinal cord injury, spinal fracture, and spinal stenosis in ankylosing spondylitis. J Neurosurg 57:609–616, 1982
9. Carter ET, McKenna CH, Brian DD, et al: Epidemiology of ankylosing spondylitis in Rochester, Minnesota: 1935–1974. Arthritis Rheum 22:365–370, 1979
10. Cruickshank B: Pathology of ankylosing spondylitis. Bull Rheum Dis 10:211–214, 1960
11. Masi AT, Medsger TA: A new look at the epidemiology of ankylosing spondylitis and related syndromes. Clin Orthop 143:15–29, 1979
12. van der Linden SM, Valkenburg HA, deJongh BM, et al: The risk of developing ankylosing spondylitis in HLA-B27 positive individuals. Arthritis Rheum 27:241–249, 1984
13. Cawley MID, Chalmers TM, Kellgren JH, et al: Destructive lesions of vertebral bodies in ankylosing spondylitis. Ann Rheum Dis 31:345–358, 1972
14. Simmons EH, Graziano GP, Heffner R: Muscle disease as a cause of kyphotic deformity in ankylosing spondylitis. Spine 16:S351–360, 1991
15. Smith-Peterson MN, Larson CB, Aufranc OE: Osteotomy of the spine for correction of flexion deformity in rheumatoid arthritis. J Bone Joint Surg Am 27A:1, 1945
16. Fox MW, Onofrio BM, Kilgore JE: Neurological complications of ankylosing spondylitis. J Neurosurg 78:871–878, 1993
17. Jeffray D, Becker V, Eisentein S: Closing wedge osteotomy with transpedicular fixation in ankylosing spondylitis. Clin Orthop 279:122–126, 1992
18. Osgood CP, Abbasy M, Mathews T: Multiple spine fractures in ankylosing spondylitis. J Trauma 15:163–166, 1975
19. Graham GP, Evans PD: Spine fractures in patients with ankylosing spondylitis. Br J Accident Surg 22:426–467, 1991
20. Hunter T, Dubo HIC: Spinal fractures complicating ankylosing spondylitis. A long term followup study. Arthritis Rheum 26:751–759, 1983
21. Grisolia A, Bell RL, Peltier LF: Fractures and dislocations of the spine complicating ankylosing spondylitis. A report of six cases. J Bone Joint Surg Am 49:339–344, 1967
22. Matthews WB: The neurological complications of ankylosing spondylitis. J Neurol Sci 6:561–573, 1968
23. Murray GC, Persellin RH: Cervical fracture complicating ankylosing spondylitis. A report of eight cases and review of the literature. Am J Med 70:1033–1041, 1981
24. Woodruff FP, Dewing SB: Fracture of the cervical spine in patients with ankylosing spondylitis. Radiology 80:17–21, 1963
25. Thorngren KG, Liedberg E, Aspelin P: Fractures of the lumbar and thoracic spine in ankylosing spondylitis. Arch Orthop Trauma Surg 98:101–107, 1981
26. Boland EW: Ankylosing spondylitis, in Hollander JE (ed): Arthritis and Allied Conditions. Philadelphia, Lea & Febiger, 1966, pp 633–655
27. Luken MG III, Patel DV, Ellman MH: Symptomatic spinal stenosis associated with ankylosing spondylitis. Neurosurgery 11:703–705, 1982
28. Bartleson JD, Cohen MD, Harrington TM, et al: Cauda equina syndrome secondary to long-standing ankylosing spondylitis. Ann Neurol 14:662–669, 1983
29. Rosenkranz W: Ankylosing spondylitis: Cauda equina syndrome with multiple spinal arachnoid cysts. Case report. J Neurosurg 34:241–243, 1971
30. Russel ML, Gordon DA, Ogryzlo MA, et al: The cauda equina syndrome of ankylosing spondylitis and rheumatoid arthritis. Ann Intern Med 78:551–554, 1973
31. Ahearn J, Hochberg M: Epidemiology and genetics of ankylosing spondylitis. J Rheum 15 (suppl):22–28, 1988
32. Rapp GF, Kernek CB: Spontaneous fractures of the lumbar spine with correction of deformity in ankylosing spondylitis. J Bone Joint Surg Am 56A:1277, 1974
33. Weatherly C, Jeffray D, Terry A: Vascular complications associated with osteotomy in ankylosing spondylitis. A report of two cases. Spine 13:43, 1988

CHAPTER 144

Anterior Cervical Disc Excision in Cervical Spondylosis

Henry H. Schmidek
Donald A. Smith

Over the past decades, operations have been devised in which a direct anterolateral approach is used to gain access to the spine from the base of the skull to the sacrum. The inventiveness has been particularly apparent with regard to the cervical spine, where anterior approaches have undergone constant development and reassessment to treat cervical disc disease, cervical fractures, tumors, and infections. At present, at least a half dozen variations of the anterior approach have been fashioned.[2-9] All allow access to the ventral aspect of the dura, the nerve root sheaths, and the vertebral arteries, and all provide for considerable flexibility in the approach available to remove lesions, or stabilize the cervical spine, or both. These approaches are most commonly employed to decompress cervical roots or the cervical spinal cord compressed by disc material or osteophytes. Because the surgery is performed with the patient in the supine position and with dissection in avascular planes, the low morbidity has resulted in the widespread acceptance of these approaches.

The anterolateral approaches to the cervical spine were applied to cervical disc disease associated with radiculopathy and myelopathy, beginning with the reports of Robinson[7,10,11] and of Cloward.[5,6,12] Since that time, the operation has become a standard part of the neurosurgical armamentarium because the predominant changes associated with cervical spondylosis are situated ventral to neurovascular structures within the spine, and the anterolateral approach allows these structures to be decompressed directly.

SURGICAL INDICATIONS

CERVICAL RADICULOPATHY

Cervical disc disease often involves the C4-C5, C5-C6, and C6-C7 levels of the spine. These herniations, both of the "hard" or "soft" type, are situated centrally, laterally, or anterolaterally. The lateral and anterolateral herniations project into the intervertebral foramina, whereas the central disc herniations may be limited to the midline. As the disc degenerates, its nucleus is affected first and begins to bulge transversely. The patient may then experience neck, shoulder, and arm pain, occipital headache, intrascapular pain, and anterior chest pain. The *painful disc syndrome* produces pain in the neck, shoulders, and arm, often with subjective numbness in a dermatome. In the early stages of the deterioration of the disc, pain may develop when the fibers of the annulus, or anterior and posterior ligaments, are stretched. In these cases, standard radiographic studies are normal. Further degeneration leads to cracks and fissures of the disc. These may extend into the joints of Luschka, and nuclear material may be extruded into these joints beneath or through the posterior longitudinal ligament or through the cartilaginous plates into the vertebral bodies. Changes in the cartilage further interfere with nutrition of the disc, contributing to its further degeneration. Radiographically, there is now a loss of the disc space height. Sliding movements between the vertebrae and alterations in the bone adjacent to the disc develop. The end of the vertebral body mushrooms and expands, and bony outgrowths develop with the periosteal activity provoked by the abnormal direction and stresses on lamellar fibers, forming osteophytes around the lateral margins of the vertebrae. The hard disc is a degenerative spur mainly associated with outgrowth from the uncovertebral joint, but it may be accompanied by spur formation in the immediate adjacent posterior portion of the disc. The radicular symptoms and signs associated with either hard or soft discs are probably the result of neural compression and perineural inflammation.

Surgical decompression is appropriate in cervical radiculopathy with subjective and objective evidence of nerve root compression in which conservative treatment, involving adequate sedation and analgesics, cervical traction, and physical therapy, fails. As mentioned by Scoville and colleagues,[12] unrelenting symptoms usually are present for a 3- to 4-week period, although some patients who experience severe pain and neurologic deficit require surgery almost immediately after their symptoms begin. In these patients, cervical traction often accentuates their discomfort, and, inevitably, a large disc fragment is found to be responsible for their discomfort.

CERVICAL SPONDYLOTIC MYELOPATHY

Cervical spondylotic myelopathy often occurs in patients who have a cervical spinal canal that is narrower than normal (under 14 mm sagittal width) and in whom osteophytes and ligamentous hypertrophy further compromise the size of the canal.[1] The pathogenesis of the disease remains uncertain. Compression of the spinal cord by disc material or traction of the cord against osteophytes is etiologically important, particularly in the case of an acute myelopathy, for example, one associated with traumatic disc protrusion. In chronic myelopathy, however, the factors of disc degeneration, spur formation, foraminal encroachment, and a congenitally narrow canal are probably potentiated by motion, and the motion may result in the progression of signs and symptoms. Whether compromise of radicular vessel is important in some cases of myelopathy is not known. Acute myelopathy secondary to thrombosis of the anterior spinal artery is very rare and does not explain the progression seen in chronic myelopathy. It may be that secondary to the spondylotic distortion and flattening of the cord, distortion of its intrinsic arterioles and compromise of the feeding and intrinsic vessels of the cord occur, leading to vascular insufficiency. Robinson[13] has suggested that the stepwise progression of neurologic deficit characteristically seen in certain cases with cervical spondylotic myelopathy actually represents repeated small infarctions within the cord substance.

Cervical spondylotic myelopathy was characterized as a distinct entity by Clarke and Robinson[14] and was further defined by Gregorius and colleagues[15] as consisting of five distinct syndromes including (1) a transverse lesion syndrome with corticospinal, spinothalamic, and dorsal column involvement; (2) a motor system syndrome with corticospinal tract and anterior horn cell dysfunction; (3) a mixed syndrome with root and cord findings presenting with radicular pain and long tract involvement; (4) a partial Brown-Séquard syndrome; and (5) an anterior cord syndrome with distal arm weakness. They noted that although complete remission was never seen, regression occurred in two patients. Of their 120 cases, 75 percent had a series of episodes with progression, 20 percent were steadily and slowly progressing, and 5 percent had a rapid onset of findings, with plateauing before further deterioration at a later date. Of 22 patients treated nonoperatively, 16 were treated with a neck brace alone. In eight of the 16 patients, walking, the ability to dress, and radicular signs in the arms improved; this improvement was striking in two. Although the remaining patients did not improve, their disease did not progress.

Lees and Turner[16] and Balla[17] also attempted to define the natural history of cervical myelopathy. In Lee and Turner's series, deterioration often ceased after the first few years; other patients experienced remissions lasting for years and then became worse. Progression and recurrence were particularly evident in patients with a congenitally narrow canal. Balla,[17] in a series of 123 patients followed up for up to 10 years, found that without treatment, 52 percent improved, 35 percent remained unchanged, and 13 percent became worse.

DYSPHAGIA ASSOCIATED WITH CERVICAL SPONDYLOSIS

Compression of the esophagus or hypopharynyx by osteophytes had been reported in the literature since 1926. A review published in 1960 reported on 36 cases of dysphagia associated with osteophytes.[18] In 1971, Maran and Jacobson[19] reported on the tenth surgically treated case (Fig. 144–1). These authors advocated interbody fusion in addition to ex-

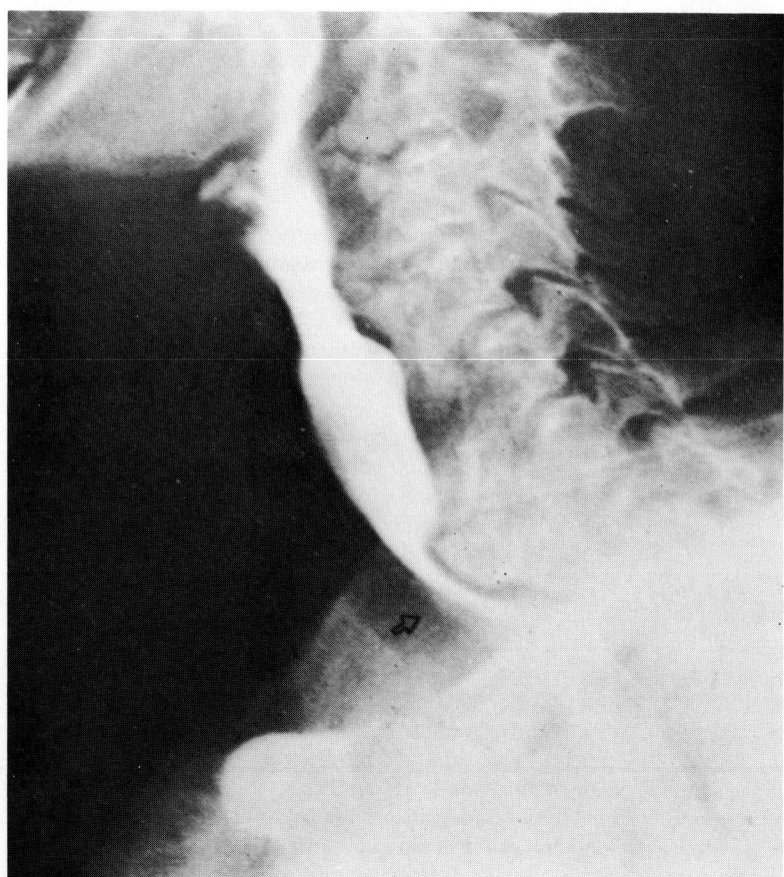

FIGURE 144–1. A cervical osteophyte (arrow) in a patient with dysphagia. (Reprinted from Meeks LW, Renshaw TS: Vertebral osteophytosis and dysphagia. J Bone Joint Surg 55A:197–201, 1973. With permission.)

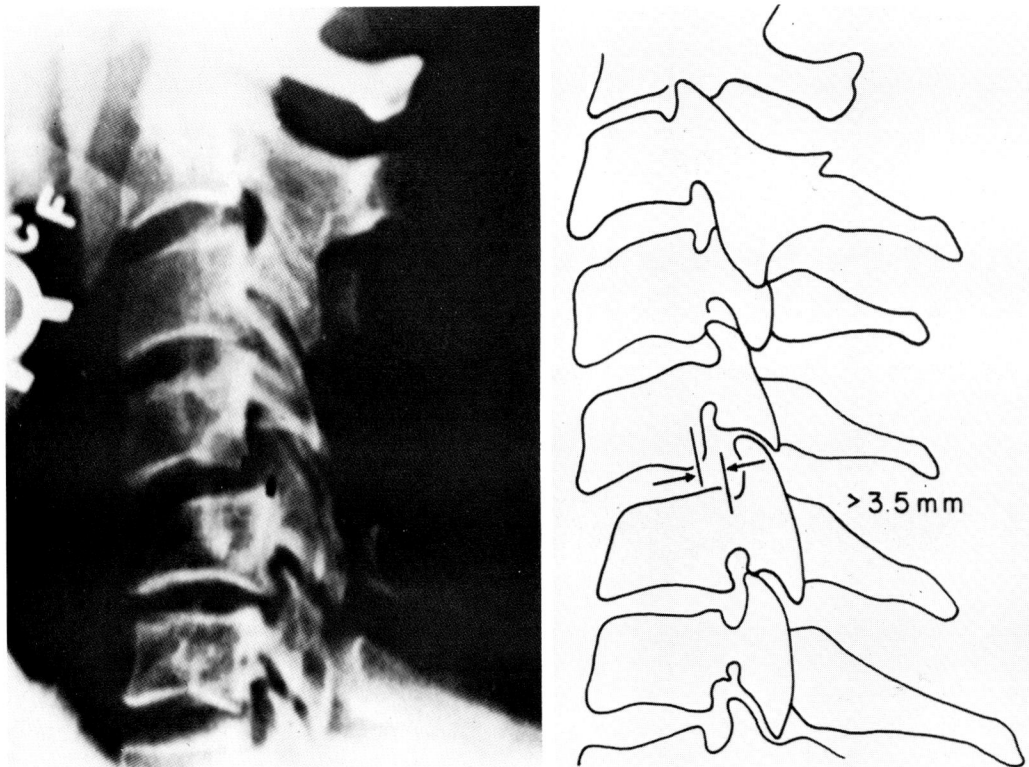

FIGURE 144–2. Biomechanical studies have shown that horizontal motion in excess of 3.5 mm, as demonstrated on plain roentgenograms, indicates instability. (Reprinted from White AA, Johnson RM, Panjabi MM, et al: Biomechanical analysis of clinical stability in the cervical spine. Clin Orthop 109:85–96, 1975. With permission of J. B. Lippincott.)

cision of the osteophyte to prevent recurrent spur formation at the involved level.[20, 21]

Compression of the hypopharynx is experienced as a lump in the throat and is seen with osteophytic compression above C6.

Anteriorly projecting cervical osteophytes have been reported along the entire cervical spine, with the C5-C6 level being the commonest site. In two-thirds of the cases, one level is involved, and in the remaining one-third, osteophytes at several levels contribute to the symptoms. Surgical removal of the exostosis usually is not indicated, although with persistent dysphagia or lump sensation, the lesion can be excised and the surgeon can consider the removal of the involved degenerate disc at that time.

VERTEBRAL ARTERY COMPRESSION ASSOCIATED WITH CERVICAL SPONDYLOSIS

Osteophytes projecting from the uncovertebral joints can intrude into the foramina transversaria and cause vertebral artery compression. To be clinically significant, this compression must impair the flow of blood to the brainstem. Hutchinson and Yates[22] showed that the effect of vertebral artery compression by osteophytes can be enhanced by rotating the head or extending the neck, which may result in giddiness or drop attacks. These symptoms, however, also may occur in the absence of head movement. Primary or secondary lateral extraspinal extrusions may indent or occlude the vertebral artery in its second portion. In two patients with traumatic lateral disc rupture, angiograms showed compression and displacement of the vertebral artery. These patients had radicular pains and motor deficit. Both, however, had normal cervical myelograms, so this investigation sometimes is useful in delineating ruptured cervical disc.[23]

DIAGNOSTIC EVALUATION

Investigations of cervical spondylosis involve standard roentgenograms and flexion and extension views of the spine to obtain evidence of spinal stability. White and associates[24] (Figs. 144–2 and 144–3), in a biomechanical study of adult cadaver spines, showed that the ligaments normally permit very little motion between vertebrae and that horizontal motions (greater than 3.5 mm) of one vertebral body on another, as seen on plain lateral roentgenograms, indicate instability. If the angulation of one vertebral body with respect to another is 11 percent greater than the angulation of adjacent vertebrae and the vertebral body is not compressed, the spine is relatively unstable. A large number of ligaments must be injured to permit motion exceeding these limits. Instability means that the spine will fail under physiologic loads, causing the spine to lose its ability to move without further deformity and excessive pain.

Electromyography and nerve conduction studies provide additional objective evidence of root compression in patients with relatively minor neurologic findings. It is also important in differentiating root, plexus, peripheral nerve, and muscle disorders that may mimic cervical radiculopathy and may help to uncover a second problem that may coexist with the

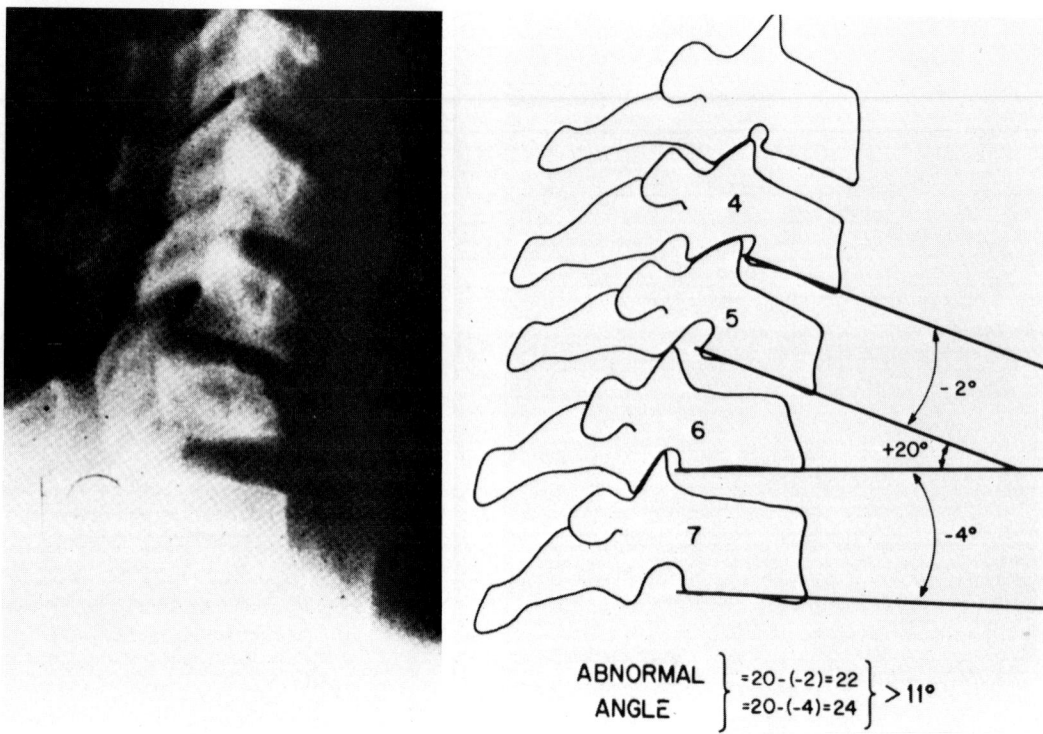

FIGURE 144–3. Biomechanical studies have shown that angulation of one vertebral body of more than 11 degrees with respect to another indicates an unstable spine. (Reprinted from White AA, Johnson RM, Panjabi MM, et al: Biomechanical analysis of clinical stability in the cervical spine. Clin Orthop 109:85–96, 1975. With permission of J. B. Lippincott.)

cervical radiculopathy, such as carpal tunnel syndrome or ulnar neuropathy.

Unenhanced computed tomographic (CT) scan of the spine demonstrates bony changes, spondylotic changes, disc calcification, and foraminal narrowing. However, accurate preoperative delineation of the relationship of the nerve roots and spinal cord to the structures of the cervical spinal canal requires either CT myelography or magnetic resonance imaging (MRI). In a recent study by Perneczky and colleagues[26] of 63 patients prospectively analyzed to establish the relative value of MRI versus cervical myelography in selecting patients for surgery for cervical discs, the MRI in the T1-weighted and gradient modes was associated with a 10 percent error rate and myelography, a 5 percent error rate. MRI tends to miss small, laterally protruding disc fragments and cervical myelography is valuable in cases in which MRI does not satisfactorily agree with the clinical assessment.

MRI has been particularly valuable in the assessment of cervical myelopathy both before and after surgery. Matsuda and associates[27] investigated increased signal intensity on the spinal cord on the T2-weighted images and its relevance to the patient's clinical condition. The exact cause of the increased signal intensity on the T2 images is not known but may represent edema, inflammation, ischemia, or gliosis. The decreased signal intensity diminished postoperatively in patients who improved clinically and remained the same or increased in those who remained the same or worsened after decompression.[28] MRI has also been used postoperatively to evaluate the effectiveness of decompressive procedures. In a study of 22 patients who underwent a decompressive procedure for myelopathy, 12 were judged as adequately decompressed by MRI criteria, 10 exhibited evidence of residual cord indentation and intrinsic cord damage, and one required a second decompressive procedure for residual compression. MRI may be used postoperatively in this manner in patients with residual deficit to assess the adequacy of the operation and the potential need for another procedure.[29]

SURGICAL ANATOMY

The anterior approach is the easiest along the anterior margin of the sternomastoid and medial to the carotid sheath (Fig. 144–4). The incision may be centered by noting the hyoid bone at the level of C3, the thyroid cartilage opposite C4, and the cricoid opposite the level of C6 (Fig. 144–5).

Dissection is carried out in avascular planes, passing through the pretracheal fascia first and then the prevertebral fascia. The longus colli muscles, covering the lateral parts of the vertebral body, the vertebral canal, and the transverse

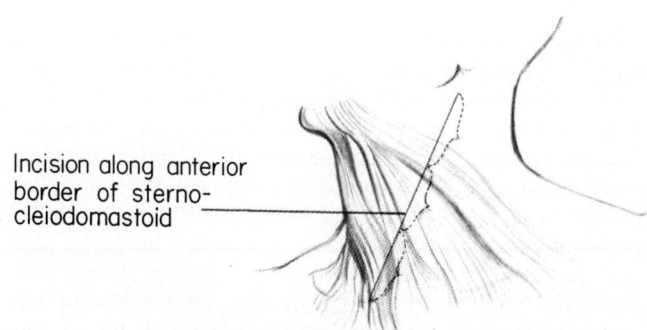

FIGURE 144–4. The line of incision for the anterior approach.

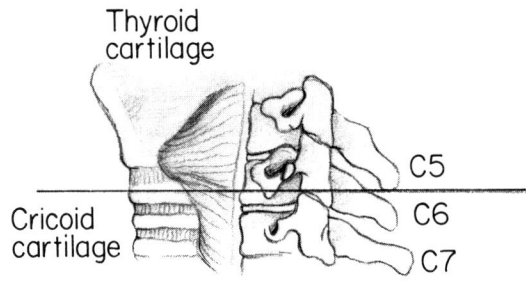

FIGURE 144-5. Points for centering the incision opposite C5 and C6.

processes, then can be seen. These muscles extend from the atlas to the body of T3. No muscle covers the anterior aspect of the vertebrae in the midline. The cervical sympathetic chain lies on the longus colli muscles and extends from C2 to T1. Because Horner's syndrome results from damage to the spinal cord fibers, it is important to retract the longus colli, starting at its medial edge.

The anterior longitudinal ligament is a strong band that extends from the base of the skull to the sacrum. It is thickest in its midportion, tapers laterally, and is bound to the anterior annulus, functioning to limit the extension of the spine. The posterior longitudinal ligament also extends as a thick band from the skull to the sacrum, between the posterior annulus and the dura. Because the ligament does not extend laterally over the nerve roots, its normally thick portion, which prevents disc material from extruding into the spinal canal, is absent, permitting disc material to enter the foramen. Functionally, this ligament limits flexion of the spine. Physiologically, the ligamentum flavum does not compress the dura or spinal cord; however, as elasticity is lost, the ligamentum buckles and may compress the spinal cord.

The left recurrent laryngeal branch of the vagus nerve arises at the level of the aortic arch, loops beneath the arch, and then passes between the trachea and the esophagus to reach the larynx. On the right side, the recurrent laryngeal nerve has an inconstant course. It usually descends within the carotid sheath, looping beneath the subclavian artery to reach the larynx between the trachea and the esophagus. The nerve may follow one of several aberrant courses, leaving the carotid sheath at a higher level. To avoid injury to an aberrant right recurrent laryngeal nerve, it is preferable to operate on the left side of the neck, irrespective of the side of the radicular symptoms.

SURGICAL PROCEDURE

Prophylactic antibiotics are begun preoperatively. The patient is placed in the supine position on an operating table under general anesthesia. The neck is moderately hyperextended by placing a roll beneath the shoulder blades, and a sandbag is placed beneath the hip. The head is turned about 10 degrees to the right. Dissection is carried out with headlight illumination and magnifying loupes of 3.5×. The operating microscope may be used instead of the loupes, especially to perform total removal of osteophytes.

Routinely a left-sided skin incision is used, centered over the anterior border of the sternomastoid muscle and the segment of spine to be exposed (see Figs. 144-3 and 144-4). A vertical incision is preferred because different types of anterior and lateral operations on cervical vertebral bodies and intervertebral discs, transverse processes, and vertebral arteries can be carried out without undue traction.

When the platysma has been exposed, it is grasped with forceps and incised with a scalpel parallel to the anterior margin of the sternomastoid. The underlying sternomastoid muscle then is visible. The anterior border of the sternomastoid must be clearly identified and mobilized throughout the limits of the exposure so that the medial border of the sternomastoid muscle can be retracted laterally to expose the middle layer of the cervical fascia. The omohyoid muscle crosses the field at C5-C6 and may be retracted or transected at its midtendinous segment. An avascular plane is developed through the cervical fascia medial and parallel to the carotid sheath. The carotid sheath and the sternomastoid muscle are retracted laterally. As this is done, the anterior surface of the cervical spine is seen. The esophagus and trachea are retracted medially. The prevertebral fascia is cauterized with bipolar cautery and incised longitudinally in the midline, exposing the anterior longitudinal ligament. The medial aspect of the longus colli muscles is then cauterized for a length corresponding to the discs to be exposed which helps to keep the wound essentially bloodless. Cloward blades are placed beneath the cauterized medial edges of the longus colli muscles. *This is probably the most important maneuver in the operation*: failure to correctly position the blades is responsible for most of the complications associated with this operation. When the vertical incision is used, a single set of blades placed beneath the muscle edges will suffice to give adequate exposure. A spinal needle is placed in the disc space, and a cross-table, cervical-spine roentgenogram is obtained to confirm the level. The retractors need not be removed to obtain this study.

The margins of the disc to be entered are cauterized and the disc is incised. Removing the bony spurs overhanging the disc space from the upper vertebra is often necessary before significant amounts of intervertebral disc can be removed. Once the anterior one-half to two-thirds of the disc and the cartilaginous plates have been removed, the Cloward disc-space spreader is introduced laterally in the disc space. Dissection up to this point is continued under 3.5× loupes or the procedure can be completed at 6 to 15× magnification with the operating microscope. Under magnification, the entire disc is excised to the posterior longitudinal ligament. This structure is characterized by its glistening, white, vertically oriented fibers. The remaining cartilage and disc are removed with fine curettes. Often a defect is visible in the midportion of the posterior longitudinal ligament through which disc material has herniated. The posterior ligament is incised to reach the fragment beneath it, foraminal spurs, or in the presence of severe cord compression. Lateral dissection exposes the uncovertebral joints and the dura, which is not covered by the posterior longitudinal ligament.

Using a 20-degree angled diamond drill the osteophytes above and below the disc space are carefully removed, particularly if the surgeon decides to perform an anterior discectomy without fusion, to prevent subsequent nerve root compression.

If an interbody fusion is to be performed, a horseshoe-shaped tricortical bone graft is taken from the ilium using a reciprocating saw or the Midas drill. The graft is countersunk in the disc space. The wound is irrigated, and a drain is placed above the anterior aspect of the spine and is brought out through the lower end of the incision. The platysma and skin are closed with fine sutures, and the drain is removed 12 hours later. Improvement after surgery for radiculopathy is apparent to many patients soon after they awaken from anesthesia. Percocet or oral meperidine (Demerol) suffices for any pain. The patient is allowed to get out of bed within a day, in a collar fashioned from a bath towel and reinforced by a broad Velcro band. The patient is discharged about 2 days later in a Philadelphia collar. The patient remains immobilized in the Philadelphia collar for approximately 2 months or until there is radiologic evidence of bony fusion.

COMPLICATIONS

Tew and Mayfield[25] summarized a combined experience of possible complications of this operation, and they appear formidable. Lunsford and coworkers[31] also report a complication rate of 13 percent for discectomy alone and a rate of 23 percent overall in their series; however, the complication rate of the procedure in experienced hands is very modest, and serious neurologic injury is rare.

The exception is the reoperative case in which exploration of the neck can be difficult. In this group of patients, serious problems can and do arise.

Retraction-related problems are the commonest form of postoperative morbidity and result in laryngeal edema, hoarseness, dysphagia, or a sensation of a lump in the throat. These problems can be avoided by a vertical incision, preferably on the left side; meticulous placement of the blades of the Cloward retractor beneath the medial aspect of the longus colli muscles; a gentle degree of retraction; and a drain placed prevertebrally at the end of the operation. Should these problems arise, a short course of steroid therapy may provide symptomatic relief. Occasionally, tracheostomy has been necessary because of upper airway obstruction.

Profuse bleeding from the disc space results from either injury to the bone as the cartilaginous endplates are removed, injury to the vertebral body with the disc-space spreader, or venous bleeding. In these cases, the bleeding can be controlled with gentle pressure and Avitene. Injury to the carotid artery has been reported to occur with resultant cerebral ischemia secondary to excessive compression of the vessel by retraction, and to the vertebral artery by dissection carried into the vertebral canal. The complications that result from excessive bleeding can be reduced if the surgeon ensures that if a graft is used, adequate room exists on each side of the graft to allow blood to extravasate away from the spinal canal. In addition, a Jackson-Pratt drain is left in place along the anterior aspect of the spine overlying the operated level to remove blood and irrigating fluid.

Esophageal and tracheal perforation can be prevented by use of the Cloward blades properly, but if an esophageal perforation occurs it should be repaired immediately with interrupted nonabsorbable sutures, and the area is drained. Fusion under these circumstances is contraindicated. In the presence of a complication involving the esophagus, an emergency consultation should be sought from a general or thoracic surgeon while the lesion is amenable to optimal surgical correction, in the operating room.

Graft extrusion and donor-site problems occur in about 2 to 4 percent of cases, and with the interbody technique, fusion failed in 10 percent of Tew and Mayfield's[25] cases. The incidence of failures is higher with the Cloward technique. However, the significant postoperative discomfort that follows discectomy without fusion and is characterized by a nagging neck, shoulder, and intrascapular pain often lasting several months is a significant consideration when the merit of this modification in the treatment of spondylosis is evaluated. Although a recent study[30] reports no difference in results of disc excision with or without fusion, it does not address the very real set of complaints seen in patients on our service in whom fusion has not been performed. This same report finds no difference in results between the Cloward and the Smith-Robinson fusion techniques; however, this information does not correspond with other reported experiences, and we prefer the Robinson technique based on the biomechanical study of Simmons and Bhalla,[31] which demonstrated that the surface area of the rectangular graft is approximately 30 percent more than the surface area of the cylindrical graft of comparable size. Stability studies showed the keystone graft of comparable size and to be more stable than the dowel graft, and that the fusion rate with the keystone graft is 100 per cent.

In patients with advanced spondylosis, degenerative changes affect the supporting structures of the spine, and subluxation often is seen even before surgery. This situation, particularly if associated with cervical myelopathy and buckling of the ligamentum flavum, would not favor eliminating the graft. The significant degrees of angulation seen in up to 20 percent of cases in recently reported series according to the criteria discussed earlier represent spinal instability. This instability may escalate into a series of problems significantly worse than the radiculopathy for which the operation was originally performed.

RESULTS OF ANTEROLATERAL DISC EXCISION

CERVICAL RADICULOPATHY

Since the publication of the first edition of this book in 1982, the results of surgery for cervical radiculopathy have continued to be consistently reported as excellent,[4, 6, 7, 10, 13, 16, 29, 32-34] irrespective of whether an anterior or posterior approach was used to decompress the nerve root. Improvement is seen in over 90 percent of the patients not involved in litigation or Workman's Compensation issues.

Radiculopathy associated with symptomatic disc degeneration at two levels is managed in the same way, although we prefer to complete the disc excision and fusion of the lower level before proceeding to the next level.

When radiographic findings are extensive and suggest alterations in the disc, ligamentous, and bony structures, then disc excision with removal of the annulus, anterior longitudinal ligament, and possibly the posterior longitudinal ligament may potentiate the instability of the cervical spine, and therefore we prefer fusion and postoperative immobilization of the neck.

CERVICAL MYELOPATHY

When cervical spondylosis was first recognized as a cause of myelopathy, it appeared that favorable results should be produced by removal of the mechanical impingement. Allen[35] attempted to remove the protrusions extradurally through a posterior laminectomy with disastrous results. Subsequently, posterior laminectomies and foraminotomies were fashioned to allow the cord to migrate from the spondylotic projections along the anterior aspect of the spine. An evaluation of the various reports and our own review of 45 cases reveals that good-to-excellent results were obtained in approximately 60 percent of patients; another 10 to 15 percent became worse immediately after technically faultless surgery. Long-term follow-up revealed that none of the patients ever again had entirely normal results on neurologic examination. Stoops and King[36] reported on 42 patients who were treated by extensive laminectomy without opening of the dura. These patients were followed up for up to 6 years. Even though 80 percent improved, no prognostic factor could be identified. Crandall, reporting on his long-term study of 55 patients with cervical myelopathy followed up from 2 to 25 years, felt that a deficit for less than 1 year was associated with a better prognosis. In contrast, a poor outcome is predictable among patients with sphincteric disturbances owing to the myelopathy. Among these patients, none improved, irrespective of the type of operation.

The debate concerning the appropriate surgical procedure(s) in the management of cervical myelopathy continues. The operative procedure needs to be tailored to the particulars of the case. Posterior cervical laminectomy has a specific indication in patients with prominent dorsal encroachment on the cord caused by either bony or ligamentous structures. Excessive cervical lordosis may be seen in patients with spondylotic myelopathy; overlapping of the lamina, referred to as shingling, may contribute to the myelopathy. Vertebral subluxation may also be seen and may lead to pinching of the cord, from the posterior, by the laminae and infolded ligamentum flavum. Inaccessibility to a disc space, for example, C2-C3 or C3-C4 in some cases, is an indication for posterior decompressive cervical laminectomy, as is a secondary procedure in the presence of neurologic progression, particularly with posterior column signs, and in some cases with widespread bony changes and spontaneous fusions anterior to the spinal cord. It has been reported in several series that even in the presence of technically faultless surgery, up to 20 percent of patients treated by laminectomy had an increased deficit after surgery.

Dereymaeker and coworkers analyzed two groups of patients with spondylotic myelopathy operated on either by the anterior or posterior approach and followed up for 2 to 6 years. Clinical and radiographic findings showed that of 31 patients with anterior fusion, 20 were improved; of the 12 who had laminectomy with excision of the disc, four were improved. Crandall and Batzdorf reported that of 28 cases of myelopathy treated by anterior discectomy and fusion, 71 percent improved when posterior projections were removed from the floor of the canal and the involved interspaces were stabilized. No patient was made worse by the operation. This experience was reaffirmed in Crandall's report which indicated that none of his patients treated by the Cloward operation was worse postoperatively, but postoperative disability again was increased following decompressive laminectomy. Bohlman has reported his experience with anterior discectomy and interbody arthrodesis in 17 cases of myelopathy. In these cases, no attempt was made to remove the posterior longitudinal ligament or osteophytes. Cartilaginous plates and disc material were removed to the posterior longitudinal ligament. Neural function was not lost in any of the 17 patients treated, and of the 17, 14 improved over their preoperative condition. Bone remodeling, but not resorption, occurred at the fused levels, and the size of the osteophytes decreased with time.

In Lunsford's series of 32 cases of myelopathy, 92 percent had anterior spondylotic deficits, and 13 percent had a sagittal canal width of under 13 mm at one or more levels. Fifty-nine percent had a myelopathy only, and 41 percent had a myeloradiculopathy. Eight patients had a previous posterior cervical decompressive procedure, and one patient a previous anterior operation—so that 24 of the cases address the merits of the anterior approach alone. Surgery involved removal of ventral osteophytes at one or more levels, with two patients having four levels operated on in two stages. One-half of the patients improved, and one-half of the patients were either unimproved or worse. No predictive indices could be identified, although patients over 60 years old and symptomatic for more than 2 years tended to have unsatisfactory results. No difference existed in outcome based on the severity of the myelopathy, the number of levels operated on, or the presence of canal stenosis.

A recent comparative study reviews the experience with 50 cases treated by means of extensive laminectomy, foraminotomy, and excision of osteophytes for cervical myeloradiculopathy. Epstein emphasizes the importance of careful patient selection, adequate laminectomy including two levels above and below areas of significant canal encroachment, and foraminal decompression with removal of only the inner third of the foramen. In this series, 85 percent of patients improved, and 15 percent did not improve after this operation. In a comparison with other forms of posterior operation, this yielded the best results and compared favorably with a 73 percent improved category after anterior cervical discectomy.

Based on our assessment of the reported experiences and our own results, we have adopted the following approaches in the management of neurologic sequelae of spondylotic spinal cord with or without root compression, being constantly aware of the very real possibility of increasing the patient's neurologic deficit even when the operation appears to have been technically faultless. In the case of major ventral compression occurring at a single level, an anterior approach is taken. A Cloward drill is used to remove the bone on either side of the involved disc space. The remainder of the disc, bone, and osteophyte are then removed with a high-speed drill under magnification. The decompression is considered to be complete when the entire ventral aspect of the involved dura is exposed and no compressive element can be identified rostrocaudally or laterally along the nerve roots. Following this extensive decompression an iliac crest bone graft is fashioned and countersunk into position. Postoperatively, the patient is told to ambulate within 1 day, and the neck is immobilized in a Philadelphia collar until bony union has been demonstrated radiographically.

A similar radical ventral decompression is performed

when two contiguous interspaces are involved by severe spondylotic changes resulting in anteriorly situated spinal cord compression. It is often impossible to attribute the neurologic presentation to one or the other level in spite of the information obtained clinically and radiographically. The lower of the two levels is decompressed, and the decompression is then extended rostrally. This involves removal of a trough of bone constituting the center of the vertebral body between the two interspaces. Decompression is carried superiorly through the disc space and into the body above. All ventrally situated disc, osteophytes, and ligament at the two levels are removed. Examination of the surgical field exposes the dura over a length corresponding to the two vertebral bodies. Following decompression, an iliac bone strut graft is fashioned to fill the bony deficit and countersunk into position. Postoperatively, the neck is immobilized for 3 to 4 months in a Philadelphia collar.[38]

When confronted with a severe degree of cervical spondylotic changes at more than two levels, we generally opt for posterior decompressive laminectomy using the Midas air drill to cut the laminae and then removing the laminae plus the spinous processes en bloc. This technique prevents even minimal intraoperative compression of the compromised spinal cord. Unless there is an associated radiculopathy, no attempt is made to decompress the nerve roots. The dura is not opened. Although much has been written in the orthopedic literature concerning instability occurring after decompressive cervical laminectomy, we have not seen this complication except in children, in patients with weakness of the cervical musculature due to their underlying neurologic problem, or those in whom there has been a removal of the facets bilaterally.

The anterior approach has evolved into an operative procedure for cervical spondylotic myelopathy provided that the major compressive elements are situated anterior to the spinal cord. Whether the osteophytes require radical removal in this situation is problematic. It is possible with the operating microscope and diamond drills to remove them without substantial risk, and on our service this is done in conjunction with fusion of the involved interspaces in cases of myelopathy.

REFERENCES

1. Adams CBT, Logue V: Studies in cervical spondylotic myelopathy. 3. Some functional effects of operations for cervical spondylotic myelopathy. Brain 94:587, 1971
2. Aronson NI: The management of soft cervical disc protrusions using the Smith-Robinson approach. Clin Neurosurg 20:253, 1973
3. Bailey RW, Badjley CE: Stabilization of the cervical spine by anterior fusion. J Bone Joint Surg Am 42A:565, 1960
4. Cloward RB: New method of diagnosis and treatment of cervical disc disease. Clin Neurosurg 8:93, 1962
5. Cloward RB: Lesions of the intervertebral disc and their treatment by interbody fusion methods. Clin Orthop 27:51, 1963
6. Smith GW, Robinson RA: The treatment of certain cervical spine disorders by anterior removal of the intervertebral disc and interbody fusion. J Bone Joint Surg Am 40A:607, 1958
7. Murphy MB, Bado M: Anterior cervical discectomy without interbody bone graft. J Neurosurg 37:711, 1972
8. Robertson JT: Anterior operations for herniated cervical disc and for myelopathy. Clin Neurosurg 25:245, 1978
9. Robinson RA, Walker AE, Ferlick DE: The results of anterior interbody fusion of the cervical spine. J Bone Joint Surg Am 44A:1569, 1962
10. Robinson RA: Anterior and posterior cervical fusions. Clin Orthop 35:34, 1964
11. Cloward RB: Treatment of acute fractures and fracture dislocations of the cervical spine by vertebral body fusion. J Neurosurg 18:201, 1961
12. Scoville WB, Dohrmann AM, Corkill AR: Late results of cervical disc surgery. J Neurosurg 45:203, 1976
13. Robinson RA: Personal communication, 1976
14. Clarke, Robinson PK: Cervical myelopathy: Complication of cervical spondylosis. Brain 79:483, 1956
15. Gregorius FK, Estrin T, Crandall PH: Cervical spondylotic radiculopathy and myelopathy: A long-term follow-up study. Arch Neurol 33:618, 1976
16. Lees F, Turner JWA: Natural history and prognosis of cervical spondylosis. Br Med J 2:1607, 1963
17. Roth DA: Cervical analgesic discography: A new test for the definitive diagnosis of the painful disc syndrom. JAMA 235:1713, 1976
18. Hilding DA, Tachdjian MO: Dysphagia and hypertrophic spurring of the cervical spine. N Engl J Med 263:11, 1960
19. Maran A, Jacobson I: Cervical osteophytes presenting with pharyngeal symptoms. Laryngoscope 81:412, 1971
20. Facer JA: Osteophytes of the cervical spine causing dysphagia. Arch Otolaryngol 86:341, 1967
21. Meeks LW, Renshaw TS: Ankylosing vertebral hyperostosis and dysphagia, in Bailey RW (ed): The Cervical Spine. Philadelphia, Lea Febiger, 1974, pp 242–249
22. Hutchinson EC, Yates PO: The cervical portion of the vertebral artery. A clinicopathological study. Brain 79:319, 1956
23. Verbiest H: From anterior to lateral operations on the cervical spine. Neurosurg Rev 1:47, 1978
24. White AA, Johnson RM, Panjabi MM, et al.: Biomechanical analysis of clinical stability in the cervical spine. Clin Orthop 109:5, 1975
25. Tew JM Jr, Mayfield FH: Complications of surgery of the anterior cervical spine. Clin Neurosurg 23:424, 1976
26. Perneczky G, Bock FW, Neuhold A, Stiskal M: Diagnosis of cervical disc disease. MR versus clinical myelography. ACTA Neurochir (Wien) 116:44–48, 1992
27. Matsuda Y, Miyazaki K, Tada K, Yasuda A: Increased MR signal intensity due to cervical myelopathy. Analysis of 29 surgical cases. J Neurosurg 74:887–892, 1991
28. Mehalic TF, Pezzuti RT, Appelbaum BI: MR imaging and cervical spondylotic myelopathy. Neurosurgery 26:217–226, 1990
29. Batzdorf U, Flannigan BD: Surgical decompressive procedures for cervical spondylotic myelopathy. A study using magnetic resonance imaging. Spine 16:123–127, 1991
30. Lundsford LD, Bissonette DJ, Jannetta PJ, et al: Anterior surgery for cervical disc disease. J Neurosurg 53:11, 1980
31. Simmons EH, Bhalla SK: Anterior cervical discectomy and fusion: A clinical and biomechanical study with eight year follow-up. J Bone Joint Surg 51B:225, 1969
32. Aronson N, Bagan N, Filtzer DL: Results of using the Smith-Robinson approach for herniated and extruded cervical discs. J Neurosurg 32:721, 1970
33. Martins AN: AC discectomy with/without interbody bone graft. J Neurosurg 44:290, 1976
34. Riley LH Jr, Robinson RA, Johnson DA: The results of anterior interbody fusion of the cervical spine. Review of 93 consecutive cases. J Neurosurg 30:127, 1969
35. Allen KL: Neuropathies caused by bony spurs in the cervical spine with special reference to surgical treatment. J Neurol Neurosurg Psychiatry 154:20, 1952
36. Stoops WL, King RB: Neural complications of cervical spondylosis: Their response to laminectomy and foraminotomy. J Neurosurg 19:986, 1962
37. Epstein JA, Janin Y, Carras R, Lavine LS: A comparative study of the treatment of cervical spondylotic myeloradiculopathy. Acta Neurochir 61:89, 1982
38. Saunders RL, Bernini PM, Shirreffs TG Jr, Reeves AG: Central corpectomy for cervical spondylotic myelopathy: A consecutive series with long-term followup evaluation. J Neurosurg 74:1632–1670, 1991

CHAPTER 145

Anterior Surgical Approaches in Multisegmental Cervical Spondylosis

Volker Seifert

Surgical treatment of cervical myelopathy resulting from multisegmental cervical spondylosis (MSCS) is performed by either anterior or posterior approaches. The operative procedures that have been employed for this entity include multisegmental anterior fusion, corpectomy and graft placement, and laminectomy and laminoplasty. Considering the complex nature of the underlying disease, which involves more than one cervical segment, as well as the pathobiomechanical features of the spondylotic cervical spine, adequate decompression of the spinal cord and correction of hypermobility should be achieved by surgery in one stage to effect an immediate and long-term benefit for the patient. Because the offending bony lesions, which are largely responsible for the development of the myelopathic process, are located anteriorly in the cervical spinal canal in the overwhelming majority of the patients, neurosurgeons have increasingly used the anterior approach for decompression of the cervical spinal cord. The application of the surgical microscope and of microsurgical techniques is extremely helpful for the atraumatic and radical decompression of the spinal cord. Moreover, recently developed osteosynthetic techniques are now available and can be used for augmentation of the subsequent bony fusion. For these reasons, vertebral body replacement combined with microsurgical decompression and anterior plating has emerged as a viable therapeutic approach for the treatment of MSCS.

PATHOLOGIC CONSIDERATIONS

Although a detailed discussion of the complex pathologic and pathobiomechanical changes responsible for the development of cervical spondylotic myelopathy (CSM) is beyond the scope of this chapter, a brief survey of current concepts is justified. CSM is the result of progression of severe degenerative processes affecting the cervical spinal column and supportive structures, the nerve roots, and the spinal cord itself. The multifactorial etiology of CSM involves mechanical, vascular, and dynamic factors, which are of additive importance for the development of the disease.[1-4] The reduced size of the cervical spinal canal, either of congenital or acquired origin, and the development of anterior osteophytes with further compromise of the canal size are considered to be the major mechanical factors in the pathogenesis of CSM (Fig. 145–1). The normal anteroposterior diameter of the cervical spinal canal shows large variation among individuals, ranging from 16 to 18 mm at C3-C7, and the spinal cord diameter ranging from 8.5 to 11.5 mm.[5] Several authors have reported that in patients with CSM, the average diameter of the lower cervical spine is about 3 mm less than in those with spondylosis without CSM. Wolf and coworkers[6] were able to demonstrate that a canal size of less than 10 mm in anteroposterior diameter was likely to be associated with CSM, whereas the average canal size of patients with CSM evaluated by Adams and Logue[7] was less than 12 mm. These findings have been confirmed by other authors.[8-14] Although compromise of the cervical spinal canal is probably the single most important component in the pathogenesis of CSM, further narrowing of the cervical canal by bony osteophytes, especially when they are located anteriorly, ossification of the posterior longitudinal ligament (PPL),[15,16] and

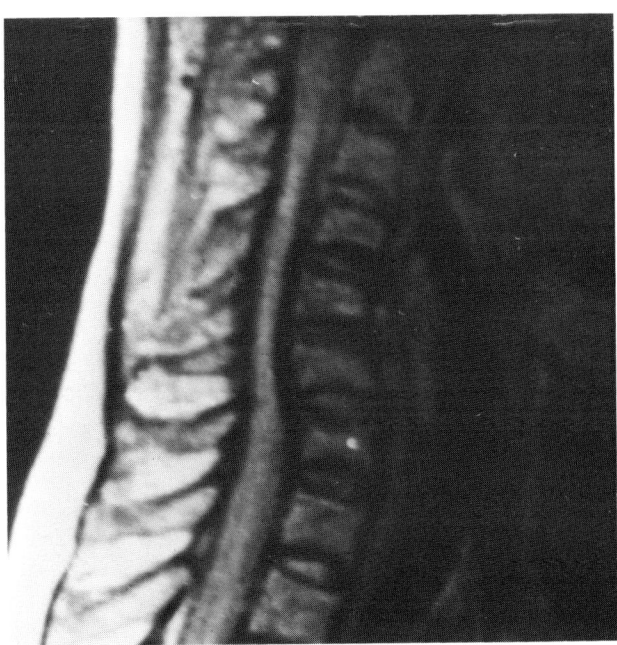

FIGURE 145–1. MRI examination (T2-weighted) demonstrating multisegmental cervical canal stenosis from C4-C6 with anterior compression of the cervical cord.

hypertrophy of the ligamentum flavum[17] result in further deformation and compromise of the cord, aggravating the effects of the narrow canal.[18, 19] Especially under flexion and extension, bony osteophytes may act as a fulcrum over which the spinal cord in motion is stretched.

Some controversy still exists over the contribution of vascular factors to the pathogenesis of CSM.[20] However, the initial hypothesis, put forward by Mair and Druckmann,[21] that ischemic changes in the spinal cord are the result of compression of the anterior spinal artery by anteriorly located osteophytes does not correspond to comparative studies of experimental occlusion of the anterior spinal artery in animals and the histopathologic patterns of ischemic intramedullary changes detected in postmortem studies of patients with severe CSM.[22] Several authors have stressed the importance of compression and occlusion of intramedullary vessels rather than anterior spinal artery compression.[23–26] These are considered to be the result of tensile stresses and central shear forces acting on the intramedullary arteries in the presence of congenital or acquired cervical canal compromise. However, as Hukuda and Wilson[27] have pointed out, the effects of cervical cord compression and repeated ischemia affecting the cervical cord are very likely to be additive for the development of CSM.[28–30] Considering the fact that in severe cervical spondylosis, motion of the cervical cord in flexion and extension leads to aggravation of either spondylotic cord compression or medullary ischemia, increased mobility of the cervical spine represents a significant dynamic factor in the pathogenesis of CSM.[31–33] In this regard, the spinal cord, compromised by spondylotic encroachments, is more vulnerable to adverse tensile stresses that are likely to occur under the condition of pathologic increase of segmental vertebral column motion,[31] resulting in further aggravation of the pre-existing cervical cord injury.

SURGICAL CONSIDERATIONS

Indication for surgery in patients with MSCS is primarily based on the progression of clinical symptoms of advanced cervical myelopathy and on the radiologic detection of multisegmental spondylosis. The clinical diagnosis of CSM is based on the clinical picture, the summary of data derived from radiologic procedures, and the exclusion of other possible nonmechanical causes of long tract alteration.[34] Additional electrophysiologic examinations, such as the recording of somatosensory evoked potentials, may add helpful information for establishing the diagnosis in selected cases[35, 36] but should not be regarded as an alternative for a thorough neurologic examination. The sine qua non for the clinical diagnosis of spondylotic myelopathy is the presence of spastic paraparesis or tetraparesis accompanied by gait abnormality. Severe nuchal, shoulder-arm, or radicular pain as well as sensory deficits or sensations, although present in a large number of myelopathic patients, are not reliable aids to clinical diagnosis.[34, 37] Additionally, the severity of the signs mentioned earlier and symptoms varies considerably among patients, which is why different clinical grading systems have been developed in the past, for example, those of Nurick[38] or Harsh and colleagues.[39] Although these grading systems are far from satisfactory, they are widely used to classify the degree of myelopathy in patients, while allowing comparison of different forms of conservative or surgical treatment.

Once the possibility of the clinical diagnosis of cervical myelopathy has been raised, numerous radiologic procedures can be used to confirm the existence of relevant bony compression and injury of the cervical cord. Over many years, plain x-ray studies and cervical myelography have been used exclusively for the diagnosis of spondylotic myelography, and the diagnostic accuracy of myelography still represents the gold standard against which the sophisticated methods of computed tomography (CT) and magnetic resonance imaging (MRI) must be compared.[40, 41] Despite the wide and rapid availability of CT and MRI, we continue to use cervical myelography in selected cases and for the performance of dynamic studies in flexion and extension of the cervical spine. The virtue of plain CT is that it is still the best radiologic method for demonstrating the presence and amount of bony compression, by clearly showing the pathologic anatomy in regard to anterior osteophytes as well as bony narrowing of the cervical canal. Moreover, this technique can be used postoperatively to document the amount of bony decompression achieved by the surgery.[42] The additional question of the degree of bony impingement of the cervical spinal cord can also be reliably answered by CT myelography, although this has now been largely supplanted by the superior imaging qualities of MRI.[41, 43–48] Additional clinicoradiologic studies have demonstrated that the severity of compressive alteration of the cervical cord can be evaluated by increased MR signal intensity within the cord on T2-weighted images.[49] However, the major advantage of modern imaging techniques, whether CT or MRI, is their ability to clearly demonstrate the pathoanatomic relation between the extent and especially location of the offending compressive bony lesions and the amount of cord compromise, which can then be used to tailor the kind and extent of the operative approach. CT and MRI have impressively confirmed earlier suggestions derived from surgical experience or myelography that in CSM, the relevant bony compression is located anteriorly in more than 75 percent of patients.[22] These findings have called into question the routine application of posterior approaches to the cervical spine in CSM, which have been in use for the treatment of this entity for many years.

Although numerous series have reported outcomes of either the anterior or posterior decompressive approaches, comparative analyses of these procedures are rare.[22, 50–57] A review of these few studies reveals that the anterior approaches have a success rate of approximately 75 percent, compared with 60 percent for posterior approaches. Although in most of these studies, only single-level myelopathic disease has been treated, the question of the appropriate surgical approach becomes more complicated when more than one cervical segment is affected by the spondylotic process. Again, posterior approaches, like multilevel laminectomies, or canal-expansive techniques, like laminotomy or laminoplasty, have been used primarily for the treatment of MSCS.[58–63] Much data have been accumulated from anterior surgery for the treatment of cervical disc disease as well as for tumor and trauma of the cervical spine, with a high percentage of good or excellent results.[54, 64–69] Based on these experiences and the technical problems and results from extensive posterior surgery in patients with MSCS, vertebrectomy combined with radical microsurgical removal of anterior osteophytes has emerged as a highly efficient and relatively atraumatic procedure for the treatment of this disease.[55, 70] The convincing concept of vertebrectomy, for which the terms *corpectomy* and *spondylectomy* are used synonymously, lies in the surgeon's ability to treat the two main pathogenetic factors of cervical myelopathy (bony compression of the cervical cord and multisegmental spinal hypermobility) during a single surgical procedure. Single-level or multilevel corpectomy with removal of the posterior longitudinal ligament and microsurgical osteophytectomy eliminates cord compression, and hypermobility is treated by bone graft fusion and is, according to the preference of the surgeon, augmented by osteosynthesis.

SURGICAL TECHNIQUE

Patients are given prophylactic antibiotics intravenously before skin incision and thereafter every 8 hours for a total of 36 hours. The patient is placed supine on the operating table under general anesthesia. In cases of severe anterior compression, intubation is performed with a fiberoptic device. The head is slightly extended and secured in a three-point skull fixation device. A standardized approach along the medial border of the sternocleidomastoid muscle to the anterior cervical spine is employed. After a transverse skin incision, the subcutaneous fat is separated from the underlying platysma muscle. The platysma is incised and the incision extended vertically in the cranial and caudal directions. Thereafter, the anterior margin of the sternocleidomastoid muscle is mobilized by sharp dissection of the areolar tissue along its medial border. The cleavage plane between the carotid artery and the esophagus is identified and further developed by either blunt or sharp dissection. After the spine is exposed, the avascular tissue covering the vertebral bodies and discs is incised vertically along the anterior aspect of the affected vertebra. By use of intraoperative fluoroscopic control, the disc spaces above and below the planned level of vertebrectomy are identified and marked by an incision of the anterior longitudinal ligament. The medial border of the longus colli muscle is cauterized bilaterally, stripped from the adjacent vertebra, and retracted with a retractor. The Caspar cervical spine instrumentation system (Aesculap Company, Tuttlingen, Germany) is routinely used for the procedure.[65]

The surgical microscope is now introduced, and both cervical discs are removed down to the level of the posterior longitudinal ligament. The ligament is incised and removed until the dura is exposed. When removal of more than one vertebra is planned, the appropriate disc spaces between the segments are also removed. Thereafter, the screws of the vertebral body distractor are inserted into the vertebrae above and below the planned vertebrectomy site, the vertebral body distractor is slipped over the screw shafts, and gradual distraction is performed, which allows excellent and unobstructed view along the exposed disc spaces. The vertebrectomy is performed starting with rongeurs of different sizes and a high-speed drill. The mass of the vertebral body is removed until only the posterior cortical margin remains. These parts of the vertebra and the posterior longitudinal ligament are then removed completely under high magnification with a diamond drill and small biting forceps. Because the dural surface has already been exposed after radical disc space evacuation, this delicate part of the spondylectomy can

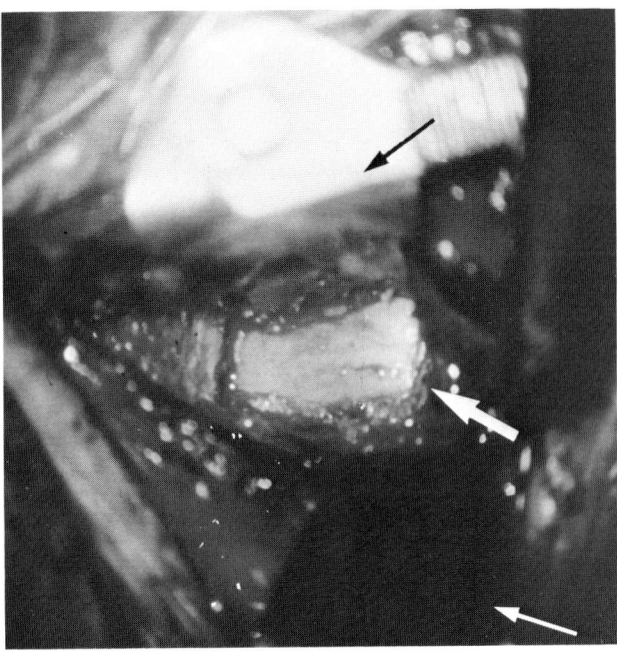

FIGURE 145–2. Intraoperative view after two-level vertebrectomy as seen through the surgical microscope. The dura, which is bulging into the operative defect, is visible in the depth of the operating field.

be performed safely under direct vision of the dura and under the illumination and magnification of the surgical microscope. Lateral resection of the vertebral body and posterior longitudinal ligament is performed to the lateral gutter on both sides. Usually, bleeding occurs from larger epidural veins located in the lateral gutter, but this can be easily controlled with hemostyptic foam and placement of cottonoids. Radical removal of osteophytes at the posterior margin of the remaining vertebrae cranial and caudal to the spondylectomy site is performed with the diamond drill and microrongeurs, which are used in an undercutting technique. Radical decompression of the exposed dural space from all offending bony lesions is absolutely necessary. This can be judged to be complete when the pulsating dura is bulging into the operative vertebrectomy defect (Fig. 145–2). Frequently, the pulsatile movements of the cerebrospinal fluid (CSF) can be observed through the thinned dura.

After radical corpectomy is completed, an appropriate bone graft is harvested from the iliac crest and is shaped to a rectangular size that fits to the vertebrectomy defect by use of a cutting forceps and a high-speed drill. Apart from the rectangular form of the graft, no special configuration is necessary. Even in multisegmental spondylectomy, iliac bone is preferred to a fibular strut graft because it can be more easily contoured according to the lordotic curvature of the cervical spine, which is important if a plating procedure is planned. After vertebral body replacement, the distraction instruments are removed, so that the bone graft is locked in place by the self-retracting forces of the adjacent vertebra (Fig. 145–3). Osteosynthesis is performed with a steel plate of appropriate length. Overlapping of nonfused interspaces should be avoided, because this leads to excessive plate motion and possible plate breakage. If the plate length is chosen correctly, it should allow insertion of the screws approximately into the midportion of the vertebral body at both ends

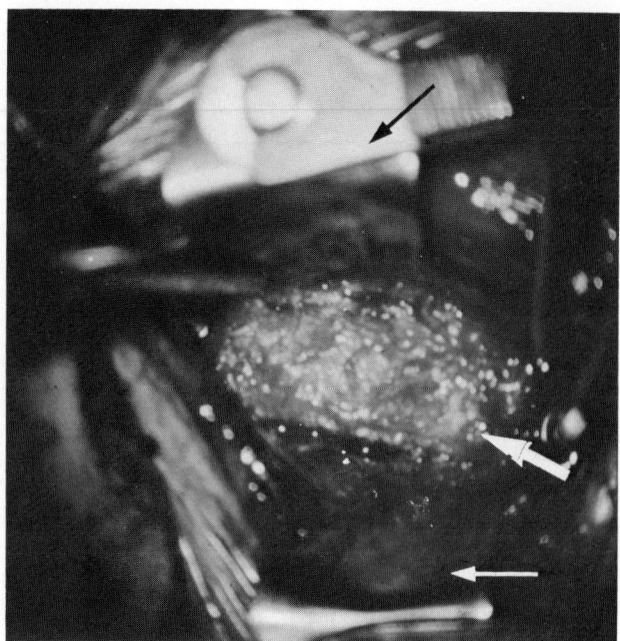

FIGURE 145–3. Same operative field as in Fig. 145–2 after insertion of iliac bone graft.

of the plate. The plate should be prebended before placement so that it fits tightly to the cervical lordosis and to the graft. Under radiologic control, two drill holes measuring 2 mm each are made into the vertebrae above and below the spondylectomy level. This procedure can be performed safely with an adjustable drill guide while advancement of the screw within the vertebral body is observed with fluoroscopy (Fig. 145–4). After the length of the drill canal, which should almost reach the posterior vertebral cortex, has been measured, four 3.5-mm, self-tapping spongiosa screws are inserted that are about 1 mm longer than the measured length of the drill canal. The screw tip should lie in the posterior vertebral cortex or as close to it as possible. In general, the length of the spongiosa screws is 20 to 22 mm in adults. After all four screws are placed, they are tightened in an opposite fashion under fluoroscopic control to safely secure the plate into position. One or two additional screws of 14-mm length can be used for securing the graft in position. After meticulous hemostasis is achieved, a drain is inserted, and the wound is closed in layers. In the case of a single-level vertebrectomy, only a soft collar is used. When more than one vertebra has been removed, a Philadelphia collar–type orthosis is applied and should be worn for 12 weeks. Because of the immediate stability provided by the osteosynthesis, the application of a halo device is not necessary. The day after surgery, the drain is removed, and the patient is mobilized. Seven days after surgery, a control x-ray study of the cervical spine is performed, and the patient is discharged.

RESULTS

In comparison to the extensive literature that exists on the surgical treatment of CSM, larger detailed reports on the use of vertebrectomy and subsequent stabilizing techniques in the treatment of MSCS are scarce and have appeared predominantly in the orthopedic literature. An evaluation of the results of the 13 larger series on corpectomy in MSCS that have been published to date reveals that the percentage of improvement reported ranged from 73 to 100 percent. However, different series on this form of treatment in patients with CSM are difficult to compare. The complex nature of the clinical picture of the myelopathic disease makes evaluation of preoperatively existing signs and symptoms and of postoperative results difficult. Either different descriptions of myelopathic symptoms, or different grading systems of myelopathy, like those of Nurick[38] or Harsh and colleagues,[39] or individual scores are used by the authors, which does not allow for adequate comparison of results. Moreover, the differences in the surgical techniques used are considerable, such as the extent of vertebrectomy and decompression, the use of macrosurgical or microsurgical techniques for removal of compressive epidural structures, type and configuration of the inserted graft, and finally, whether or not an osteosynthetic procedure is performed. In the first published description of this technique, Whitecloud and LaRocca,[71] in their series of 18 patients with symptomatic multisegmental spondylosis, reported an improvement of 100 percent. However, the authors stated that clinical outcome is difficult to tabulate and compare. Despite the fact that excellent results consisting of relief of all preoperative symptoms and improvement in abnormal clinical findings could not be achieved, significant pain relief, functional recovery, and improvement of overall neurologic status, although not further detailed, was noted in all of their patients. Hanai and coworkers,[72] in their study of subtotal vertebrectomy for CSM, used the more specific eval-

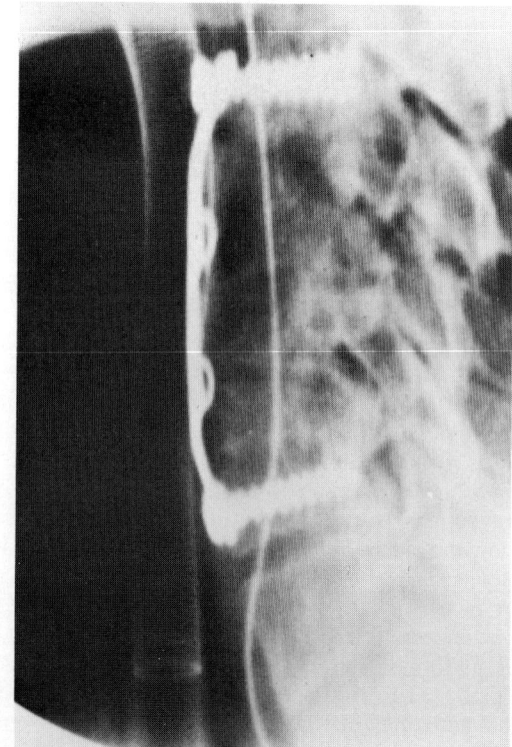

FIGURE 145–4. Example of intraoperative fluoroscopic control demonstrating good positioning of the screws and plate, which fits tightly to the graft. The screws have been inserted into the midportion of the respective vertebra and have been advanced until the posterior vertebral cortex is reached.

uating score of the Japanese Orthopedic Association, in which 17 points are considered normal findings in motor, sensory, and bladder function. The preoperative score for their patients ranged from five to 14 points. Marked improvement was noted shortly after the operation in all patients, with long-lasting relief of symptoms in almost all patients. The postoperative Japanese Orthopedic Association score ranged from nine to 16 points. No patient reported deterioration of the symptoms at the final consultation. Boni and coworkers,[73] who evaluated the results of 29 cases of CSM treated by resection of the central portion of multiple vertebral bodies followed by iliac graft stabilization, reported good results in 53 percent and moderate improvement in 39 percent.

Bernard and Whitecloud[74] evaluated their results in 21 patients with CSM who were treated with aggressive anterior multilevel resection of compressive bony structures and stabilization by autogenous fibular strut graft. Significant improvement was found in 19 of the 21 patients. Doi and coworkers[75] reported on their limited experiences in a small number of six patients with CSM and ossification of the PLL treated by multilevel partial vertebrectomies and stabilization by a vascularized fibular graft. Results were again evaluated by the Japanese Orthopedic Association score and Hirabayashi's Improvement Score, classifying the clinical results into four grades from excellent to poor. The mean preoperative Japanese Orthopedic Association score was 9.6, and the mean postoperative score was 13.9. Five overall good or excellent results and one fair result was found. Comparable satisfactory results in larger groups of anterior multilevel decompression and fusion were reported by Senegas and coworkers,[76] who found 73 percent improvement in 45 cases, by Rengachary and Redford,[77] who had 86 percent improved patients in a group of 22 with CSM, and by Zdeblick and Bohlman,[78] who had a 100 percent improvement in their small series of eight patients with cervical kyphosis and myelopathy. Okada and coworkers[79] reported their results in 37 patients with spondylotic myelopathy treated by partial or subtotal corpectomy followed by strut bone grafting. Patients were graded preoperatively according to the Nurick scale. A satisfactory postoperative result was obtained in 29 patients, or 78 percent. All but one of the 37 patients had improved walking ability after surgery. During follow-up, one patient reverted to the preoperative status after initial improvement, and three patients had deterioration, which was the result of new spondylotic changes associated with stenosis of the cervical spinal canal.

Yonenobu and coworkers[57] evaluated their results of three different forms of surgical treatment in 90 patients with cervical myelopathy. Extensive laminectomy was performed in 24 patients, anterior fusion in 50, and subtotal vertebrectomy and fusion in 21. The results of subtotal vertebrectomy were considered to be significantly better than the other two procedures. Kojima and coworkers[80] reported their results of anterior cervical vertebrectomy and interbody fusion in 45 patients with either multilevel spondylosis, ossification of the PLL, or a combination of both diseases. In their study, results of operation were evaluated by the classification of Harsh and coworkers. Although this classification does not include neurologic symptoms and signs of the upper extremities, it was considered by the authors to be convenient and practical for neurologic symptoms and signs in the lower extremities. Improvement of one grade or more in Harsh's myelopathic scale was classified as a good result. In this regard, 16 of the 19 patients with multilevel cervical spondylosis had good results (84 percent). Eleven of 12 patients (92 percent) with ossification of the PLL had good results, and 12 of 14 patients (86 percent) with both cervical spondylosis and ossification of the PLL had good results.

In two recent studies, Saunders and coworkers[81] and our group[70] evaluated the results of multilevel corpectomy and fusion. In their detailed study, Saunders and coworkers followed up 40 cases over a period ranging from 2 to 5 years. The patient's myelopathic symptoms were graded by Nurick's classification with additional evaluation of resolution of preoperative central cord syndrome.[37, 82] The outcome was defined as a cure if the patient was satisfied with the operation and had no complaints and no signs other than active reflexes or residual minor hand intrinsic atrophy. Improvement was defined as a change of at least two grades in the Nurick classification or resolution of hyperpathia and dysesthesia, or both. Failure was defined as less change than described earlier or regression of improvement. By these criteria, the long-time cure rate was 57.5 percent, and the failure rate was 15 percent. No worsening of myelopathic symptoms was documented. In our initial report, we detailed the results in 22 patients with MSCS treated by spondylectomy, microsurgical decompression, and fusion using iliac bone graft. It is the only study in the series discussed here in which an additional osteosynthetic procedure with metal plates and screws was performed. Additionally, it is the only study in which the postoperative ability to return to work was evaluated. In 19 of the 22 patients, the clinical symptoms consisted of typical signs of advanced myelopathy, including gait disturbance, severe impairment of sensory and motor function, and bladder dysfunction. Pain radiating into the upper extremities as well as into the craniocervical region was present in 15 of these patients. In three patients, incapacitating pain was the most prominent symptom of cervical spondylosis, accompanied by only moderate spastic paresis and hyperreflexia. In 14 patients, one vertebra was removed; in seven patients, two vertebrae were removed; and in one patient, three vertebrae were removed. The level of single vertebrectomy was at C5 in eight patients, at C4 in two patients, at C6 in two patients, and at C3 and C7 in one patient each. Spondylectomy incorporating two vertebrae was performed four times at the C4-C5 level, two times at the C5-C6 level, and one time at the C3-C4 level. In one patient, C4, C5, and C6 were removed. Of the 19 patients with advanced myelopathic disease, 14 patients were symptom-free or had only minor residual symptoms (73.7 percent). Three patients complained of persistent phases of nuchal or cervicobrachial pain, which could be controlled by the temporary use of analgesics or the application of a soft collar. Symptoms of myelopathy were still present in two patients; however, both patients considered the severity of their disease to be less than before surgery, and neither was incapacitated by the myelopathic process. Three patients suffering from excruciating pain secondary to severe cervical spondylosis had significant pain relief. In regard to the socioeconomic results of surgery, of 15 patients who were employed before surgery but were unable to perform regular work because of their disease, 13 patients returned to a full-time job. Radiologic follow-up examinations at different intervals showed solid bony fusion

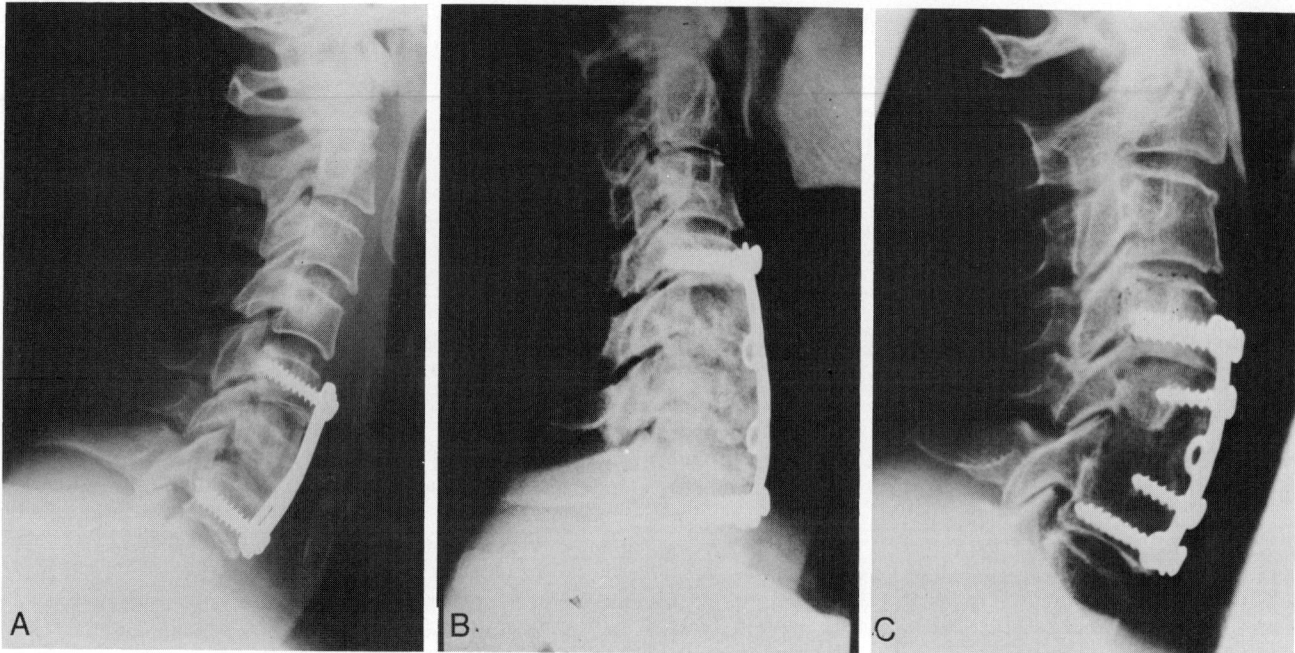

FIGURE 145–5. (A to C) Typical examples of follow-up x-ray studies in three different patients showing good positioning of the inserted iliac bone graft as well as of the osteosynthetic material. In the patient in C, additional screws have been inserted into the graft. However, from a biomechanical point of view, this is not absolutely necessary to achieve a stable and solid bony fusion.

in all patients (Fig. 145–5A to C). These data from our initial study on the use of vertebrectomy, microsurgical decompression, and osteosynthesis have been confirmed by our more recent experiences, which brings the total number of patients with MSCS treated in the described manner to over 50, in whom good or satisfactory results have been found in an overall percentage of 75 percent. By mid-August 1993, 15 more patients had had a spondylectomy and osteosynthesis. Follow-up ranged from 10 months to 4 years for the first 50 patients.

Case Reports

CASE REPORT 1

A 50-year-old Turkish man presented with a 2-year prior history of increasing neck pain with a diffuse distribution into both arms. Chiropractic treatment did not result in any amelioration of symptoms. Within 6 months, the patient's clinical condition deteriorated to Nurick's disability classification grade 4, with gait disturbance, weakness, and paresthesias in both arms. When admitted to our clinic, the patient had severe gait abnormality and needed assistance to walk, and he demonstrated tetraspasticity with exaggerated deep tendon reflexes and positive Babinski's sign. Cervical myelography demonstrated almost complete block of the contrast medium at C5 (Fig. 145–6). Additional CT myelography showed significant compression and obstruction of the epidural space by extensive cervical spondylosis at the C4-C5, C5-C6 and C6-C7 levels (Fig. 145–7). Owing to the multisegmentality of the compression, a two-level spondylectomy of C5 and C6 with microsurgical decompression at all three cervical segments was performed. Within 6 months after surgery, the patient's severe myelopathy showed significant improvement, with almost complete resolution of the preoperative tetraspasticity and paresis, and was classified as Nurick's grade 2. Postoperative plain x-ray studies and CT scans demonstrated good position of the bone graft and implanted osteosynthetic material (Fig. 145–8A and B). CT scan through the spondylectomy area demonstrated complete resection of the midline compressive spondylotic bone with a wide bony decompression (Fig. 145–9).

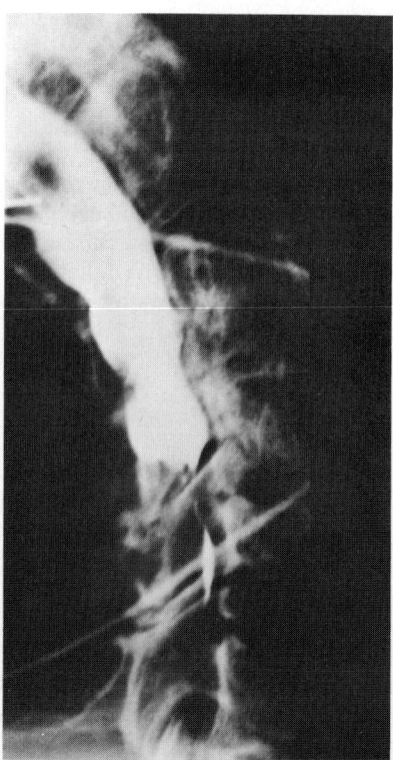

FIGURE 145–6. Case Report 1: Preoperative cervical myelography in a patient with MSCS demonstrating almost complete stop of the contrast media at the C5 level.

Anterior Surgical Approaches in Multisegmental Cervical Spondylosis | 1797

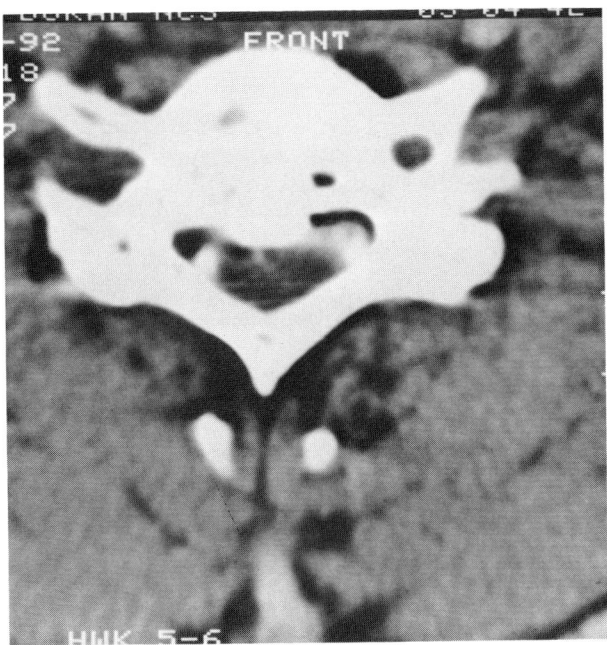

FIGURE 145-7. Case Report 1: Preoperative myelo-CT at the C5 vertebra level demonstrating narrow cervical canal and anterior compression by midline osteophyte.

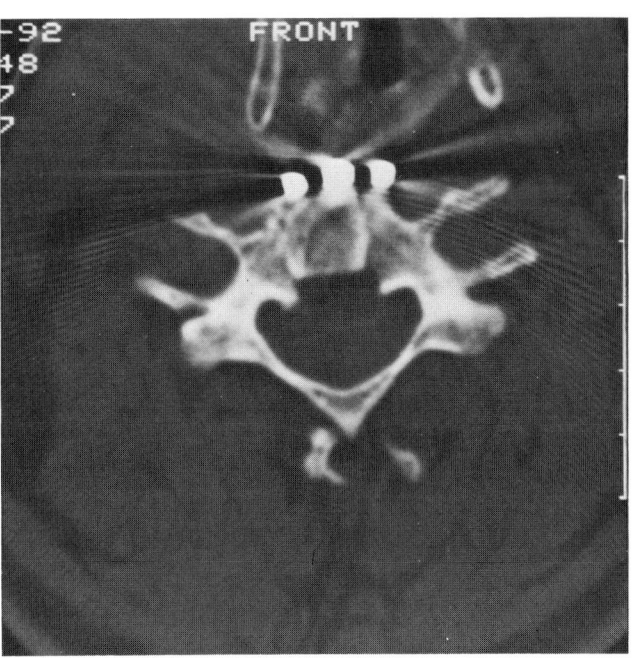

FIGURE 145-9. Case Report 1: Postoperative CT scan through the vertebrectomy and graft area demonstrates wide bony decompression and exact placement of grafted iliac bone.

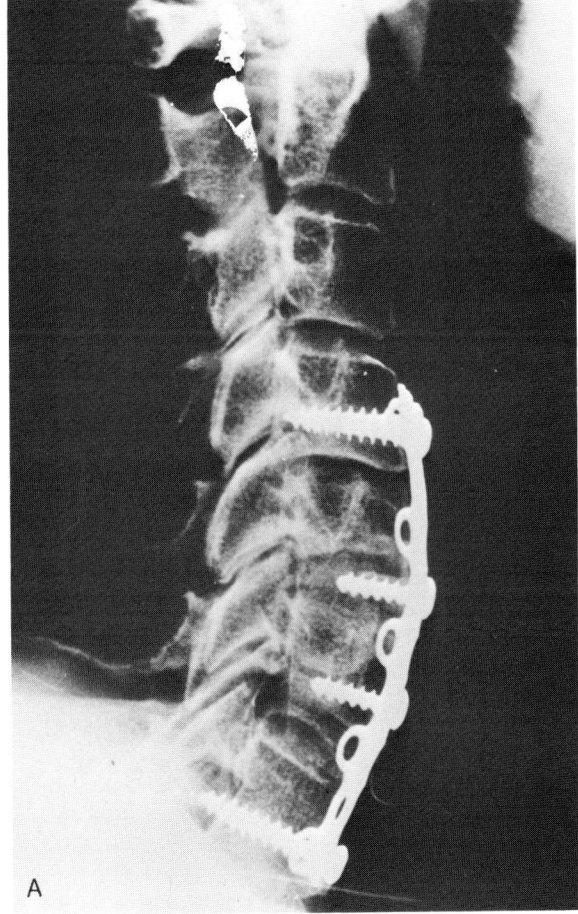

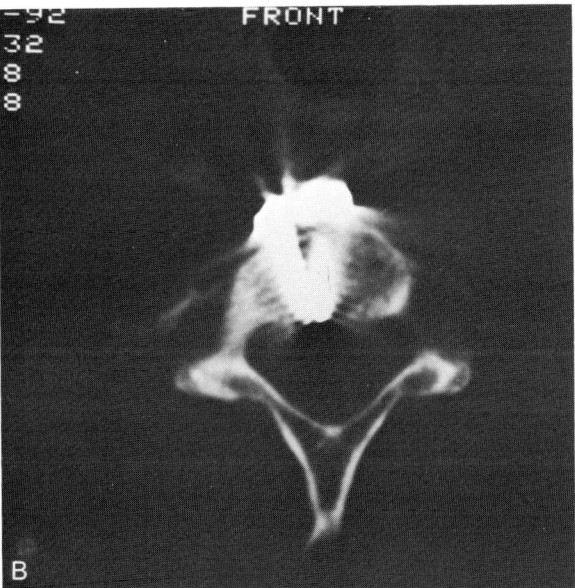

FIGURE 145-8. Case Report 1: (A) Postoperative x-ray study at 9 months after surgery demonstrates good position of inserted graft and osteosynthetic material. Slightly oblique projection gives the impression that screws in C7 have penetrated too far. (B) However, the CT study demonstrates that the screw tips are both placed exactly in the posterior vertebral cortex.

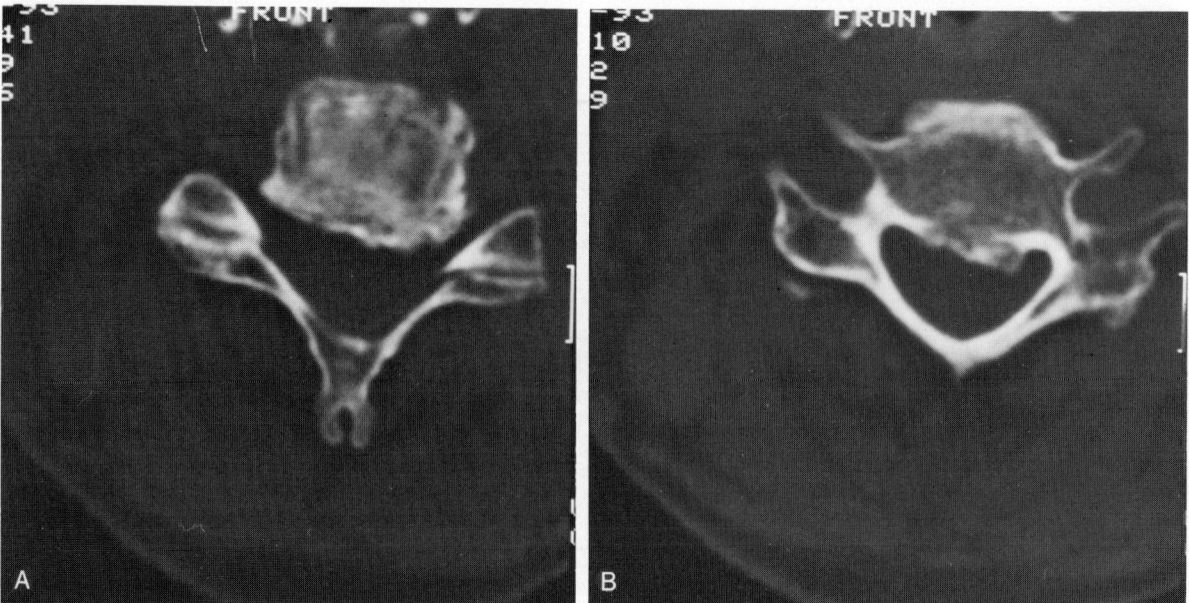

FIGURE 145–10. (A and B) Case Report 2: Preoperative CT scan demonstrates narrow cervical canal and asymmetric bony encroachment of the cervical cord.

CASE REPORT 2

This 64-year-old woman suffered from long-standing rheumatoid arthritis and had already undergone several operations for joint correction at both hands. Gradually, over several years, she developed progressing compromise of the cervical spinal cord and nerve roots. When she was first seen at our institution, she complained of pain in the neck that radiated into the occiput and into both arms. Wearing a soft collar reduced the pain. Plain cervical spine x-ray studies in flexion and extension views demonstrated only slight widening of the atlantoaxial distance. Additionally, radiologic signs of subaxial rheumatoid involvement of the cervical spine were most pronounced at the C3-C4 and C5-C6 levels. Except for exaggerated deep tendon reflexes, there were no signs of spinal cord compression. Over the next few months, the patient's pain became increasingly worse, so that the patient was readmitted to the hospital. Apart from the neck pain, the patient now described bilateral excruciating pain radiating into both arms and exhibited a spastic tetraparesis and gait abnormality. CT scan of the cervical spine at the C3-C4 and C5-C6 segments demonstrated narrowing of the cervical spinal canal by posterior osteophytes at the C4 level and asymmetric cervical canal stenosis at the C5 level (Fig. 145–10A and B). MRI confirmed partially asymmetric cervical canal stenosis with cervical cord compression (Fig. 145–11). Functional studies of the cervical spine in flexion and extension revealed subaxial hypermobility at the C5-C6 level. Because of the multisegmental involvement of cervical canal stenosis at least over two vertebrae and three segments, a corpectomy was performed of vertebrae 4 and 5 with resection of adjacent osteophytes and fusion. Intraoperatively, the posterior longitudinal ligament was found to be thickened because of a rheumatoid pannus, which compounded the effect of the bony compression of the cervical cord. All compressive bony elements, as well as the posterior longitudinal ligament, were meticulously removed, followed by bone grafting and osteosynthesis (Fig. 145–12A and B). Postoperatively, the patient developed a temporary weakness of the right arm, which resolved completely within a few weeks. Although the preoperative excruciating pain subsided almost immediately after surgery, the myelopathic symptoms resolved slowly over the next few months. At follow-up, the patient was still pain-free and ambulatory. Plain CT as well as sagittal CT reconstruction confirmed that wide bony decompression had been achieved by surgery (Fig. 145–13A and B).

COMPLICATIONS

The complications of the procedure described, either experienced by ourselves or reported in the literature, usually result from the traumatic handling of the prevertebral soft

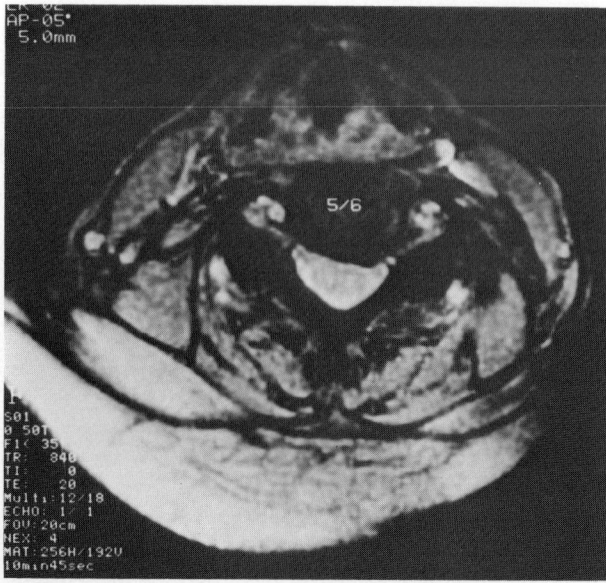

FIGURE 145–11. Case Report 2: Preoperative MRI showing asymmetric bony compression of cervical cord and nerve root.

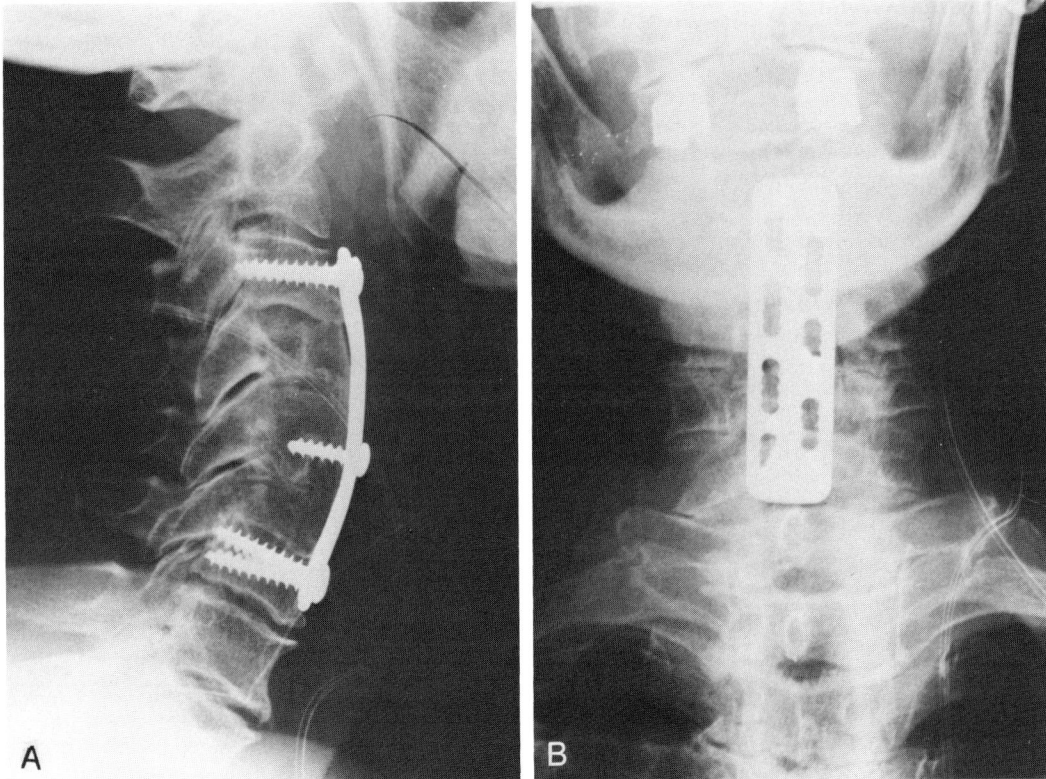

FIGURE 145–12. (A and B) Case Report 2: Early postoperative x-ray examination in lateral and AP projection demonstrates good position of graft and osteosynthetic material.

tissue during the approach to the cervical spine, incomplete decompression, and graft-related problems. In our series of over 90 CSM patients treated with spondylectomy, microsurgical decompression, and osteosynthesis, there was no mortality and no worsening of the preoperative neurologic condition. Complications attributable to the surgical procedure were as follows. Postoperative loosening of a single screw was detectable on follow-up x-ray studies in six patients. In none of these patients did this condition lead to morbidity or loosening of the prosthetic plate. Breakage of a plate after uneventful postoperative follow-up occurred in one patient 12 months after surgery. However, solid bony fusion had occurred at that time, and, because the patient refused plate removal, the plate was left in place without any adverse effects. Transient pain at the donor graft site occurred in 70 percent of the patients but was controllable with oral analgetics. Despite routine placement of a drain, three large hematomas developed at the donor site: two resolved sponta-

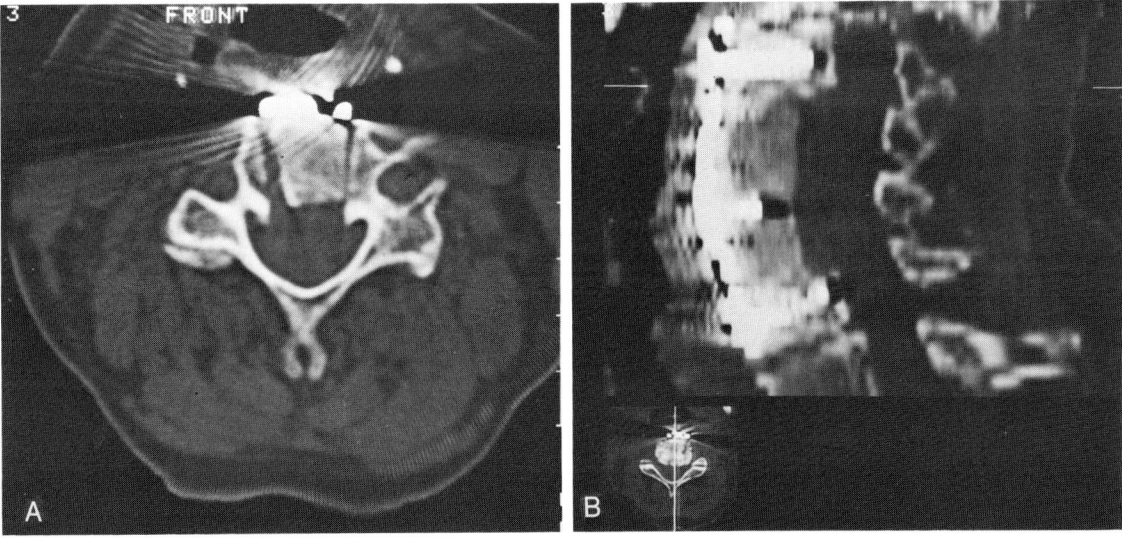

FIGURE 145–13. (A and B) Case Report 2: Postoperative CT scan (A) and CT reconstruction (B) showing wide bony decompression as well as adequate position of bone graft.

neously, and one hematoma had to be surgically evacuated. Transient recurrent laryngeal nerve palsy occurred in four patients but resolved spontaneously after 4, 10, 12, and 14 weeks. One patient had a superficial wound infection at the cervical incision, and another patient had a minor infection at one of the penetration points of the three-point skull fixation device. Both infections healed without specific therapy.

The most severe complication was a prevertebral abscess in one patient secondary to an infection with *Staphylococcus aureus*. Five days after surgery, the patient began to complain of severe cervical pain and dysphagia. A plain x-ray study of the lateral cervical spine revealed extensive widening of the prevertebral soft tissue. With the patient under general anesthesia, the wound was reopened, drained, and irrigated with an antibiotic solution. The plate and the bone graft were left in place. A drain was placed, and the patient was treated with intravenous antibiotics for 2 weeks, followed by oral antibiotic therapy for another 6 weeks. The patient made a complete recovery, with resolution of the preoperative myelopathic symptoms. Several radiographic follow-up examinations demonstrated satisfactory bony fusion without signs of screw or plate loosening. The overall complication rate, including minor complications, was 20 percent. However, no adverse long-term complications attributable to the surgical procedure could be noted. Complications of vertebrectomy and fusion reported in the literature differ widely not only among authors but also among the techniques employed. Comparison of graft-related problems in the literature are difficult because most vertebrectomy studies have consisted of simple graft intrusion without additional osteosynthesis. In their 1976 paper on a series of patients treated with fibular strut graft after spondylectomy and without osteosynthesis, Whitecloud and La Rocca[71] reported graft extrusion in three patients, and in one of these, graft dislodgment recurred four times. Splitting of the graft during insertion occurred in one patient. Postoperative abscess after infection with *S. aureus* occurred in another patient. Hoarseness persisted more than 1 month in one patient, and dysphagia lasting for more than 3 days occurred in three patients. Donor site complications were noted in four patients. In the paper by Hanai and coworkers[72] on subtotal vertebrectomy without osteosynthesis, no severe operative complications were reported. In one patient, laryngeal pain occurred 1 day after the operation, continued for 10 days, and finally disappeared 1 month after the operation. In three patients, the grafted iliac bone showed minimum displacement within 1 week after surgery, but no further displacement occurred thereafter. Kojima and coworkers[80] reported on 45 patients treated with single-level or multilevel vertebrectomy without plating technique. In four patients, the graft extruded anteriorly within 5 days postoperatively, and in one patient the graft extruded 3 weeks after the operation. Dysphagia occurred in one patient, and Horner's syndrome and temporary hoarseness developed in two patients. A transient subcutaneous CSF leak was seen in three patients and was treated with spinal drainage. The most severe complication after vertebrectomy was reported by Emery and coworkers,[83] who reported on seven cases of upper airway obstruction after multilevel corpectomy for myelopathy. All patients had required reintubation, and the early compromise of the upper airway was believed to result from edema. Five patients had no complications, but two died of complications related to the obstruction. Six of the patients had a history of heavy smoking, and one of asthma. The authors point out that extra caution should be used in the postoperative management of the airways when multilevel corpectomy is performed in patients who have these pre-existing conditions. In their study on central corpectomy without osteosynthesis Saunders and coworkers[81] reported an overall complication rate of 47.5 percent, with a 7.5 percent incidence of persistent problems consisting of C5 radiculopathy in one patient, swallowing dysfunction in one patient, and hypoglossal nerve palsy in another patient. Graft-related problems (extrusion and fracture) without complication occurred in two patients. Awasthi and Vorrhies,[84] in their recent technical report on the use of bone-bank fibular strut graft in six patients, reported no surgical morbidity, no mortality, and no graft extrusions, although follow-up in this series was short.

DISCUSSION

In most degenerative diseases involving the cervical spine, the relevant compressive abnormality of discogenic or bony origin is located anterior to the spinal cord. Posterior approaches to the cervical spine, although in use for many years for the treatment of soft disc disease as well as spondylotic processes, have been considered unsatisfactory by many neurosurgeons because of their inability to adequately approach and remove the offending epidural lesions when they are primarily in an anterior location, and because of the inherent possibility of late instability. This is even more true in cases of MSCS. For this entity, either an extensive laminectomy or different forms of laminotomy or laminoplasty procedures have been proposed.[58, 60, 62, 63, 85] However, in both techniques, the anterior compression, resulting either from narrowing of the vertebral bodies themselves, in the case of significant cervical canal stenosis, or from bony osteophytes at multiple segments, cannot be alleviated. Therefore, anterior compression of the medulla remains unchanged, leaving an additional fulcrum for the spinal cord in motion. Moreover, extensive laminectomy procedures in patients with MSCS, by loss of posterior elements, significantly aggravates the already preoperatively existing increased spinal mobility,[86-88] which is regarded as an important dynamic factor in the pathogenesis of CSM. Additionally, the possible risk of scar tissue formation because of exposure of the thecal sac to the dorsal musculature has been mentioned as a potential drawback of this procedure.[62] Although laminotomy or laminoplasty may to some extent prevent or diminish the occurrence of late postoperative instability, these procedures are not easy to perform along the cervical spine and may cause cervical cord injury. The anterior approach to the cervical spine, developed and popularized by Bailey and Badgley,[89] Cloward,[90] Dereymaker and Muller,[91] and Smith and Robinson,[92] has gained wide acceptance among neurosurgeons, especially since the addition of the surgical microscope.[93, 94] The surgical technique for the anterior approach to the spine along the anteromedial border of the sternocleidomastoid muscle and through the areolar prevertebral soft tissue is a standardized procedure that is performed rapidly and relatively atraumatically for the patient.[65, 68, 90, 95, 96] Technical adjuncts, like the instrumentarium developed by Caspar,[65] have greatly facilitated the procedure, allowing for a wide exposure from C2 to T1.

A large amount of data relating to experiences with anterior microsurgical disc excision and removal of osteophytes have been collected on patients with degenerative disease.

The combination of these experiences with those gained from vertebrectomy and plating in patients with cervical tumor and trauma has paved the way for the application of these techniques in patients with MSCS. Additionally, since the advent of MRI, the pathoanatomic relation between the offending multisegmental bony lesion and the extent of spinal cord compression can be precisely demonstrated preoperatively and can be used for proper planning of the surgical strategy. In patients with MSCS, there are two surgical options for the anterior approach. One is to resect the discs at all levels involved, remove the appropriate posterior osteophytes, and perform a Cloward or Smith-Robinson procedure, probably followed by an anterior plating technique that spans the fused segments.[69, 97–101] However, as has been already stressed, in most patients with cervical myelopathy due to severe MSCS, the bony compression does not result only from osteophytic lesions but also, and frequently more relevantly to the development of the myelopathic process, from additional compression resulting from anterior narrowing of the spinal canal by the vertebral body itself. In these cases, a multilevel osteophytectomy would lead to an incomplete decompression of the spinal cord. Additionally, from a biomechanical point of view, a plating procedure crossing several grafted disc spaces is not as stable as when an extensive vertebrectomy and bone graft replacement has been performed.[2, 102–104] Inevitable micromotions along the multiple grafted disc spaces may frequently lead to early screw and plate loosening and consequent instability. Moreover, the pathologic hypermobility along the grafted segments that is still present with this technique consequently leads to new formation and growth of compressive osteophytes.

These drawbacks are avoided in patients with MSCS when the second surgical option, consisting of a single-level or multilevel vertebrectomy followed by graft placement and an appropriate osteosynthesis, is used. The procedure, although apparently complex, is relatively straightforward. From our experience, it is also a safe procedure, especially in regard to the pathology and age group treated. The most severe complication from corpectomy reported in the literature has been upper airway obstruction,[83] which, according to our experience, can be reliably prevented by meticulous dissection and atraumatic handling of the prevertebral tissue during the approach to the cervical spine. However, major complications did not arise in our patients reported on here, and in none of the patients was worsening of the preoperatively existing myelopathic symptoms noted. Moreover, the success rate in terms of recovery from preoperative myelopathy as well as from incapacitating pain is satisfactory, as is the percentage of patients being able to return to work after surgery.

However, a few technical details in regard to the decompressive procedure, choice and configuration of graft material, and the final plating technique are appropriate. We believe that the surgical result in patients with MSCS is directly related to the radicality of epidural decompression, which is furthermore related to the consequent use of the surgical microscope. The high rate of unsatisfactory recovery reported after anterior macrosurgical procedures for cervical myelopathy[8] is largely the result of incomplete removal of all bony lesions. Radical resection of the posterior rim of the vertebral bodies involved as well as of the adjacent cranial and caudal osteophytes by use of different-sized rongeurs down to microrongeurs and small-sized diamond drills is the first and most important step of epidural decompression. Removal of bone should also be performed in the direction of the lateral gutter on both sides. For removal of osteophytes and for lateral decompression, the application of an undercutting technique is usually more effective and safer than the extensive use of a high-speed drill. Radical removal of the PLL has been performed in all our patients with MSCS as part of the decompression. One might argue that removal of the PLL adds a considerable risk to the procedure. However, because we always remove the PLL and expose the dura in the depth of the disc space before vertebrectomy, its complete resection after removal of the vertebral bodies has not been considered extremely difficult or even risky. Although we have not found true ossification of the PLL in our patients, frequent hardening or some sort of sclerotic changes in the PLL, which added considerably to the bony compression, was detected. In rheumatoid patients with subaxial MSCS, ingrowth of compressive pannus in the PLL could be noted also. Moreover, removal of the PLL allows an excellent overview of the spondylectomy region with adequate evaluation of the radicality and completeness of epidural decompression.

In all our patients, an appropriate bone graft has been harvested from the iliac crest and used for vertebral body replacement. We have avoided the use of fibular strut graft because of unsatisfactory earlier experiences using this material. The main reason for exclusive use of iliac bone graft is that the graft can be obtained in almost any length and size wanted. Moreover, the possibility of contouring the bone graft according to the curvature of the cervical spine allows for an almost anatomic remodeling of the cervical lordosis, which is additionally important for the following plating technique. Proper fitting of the graft into the vertebrectomy defect is much easier and especially more rigid when an individually designed iliac bone graft is used, instead of a straight-configured fibular strut graft. Stability of the iliac bone graft in comparison to a fibular strut graft, under clinical circumstances, is underestimated. In none of our patients, some of whom were older or osteoporotic, did compression fracture of the iliac bone graft occur. Because a plating procedure was always employed after graft placement, we did not perform any additional configuration of the graft apart from contouring it according to the spondylectomy defect and the cervical lordosis. When the graft is inserted into the surgical defect, the Caspar retractor is removed, after which the graft is kept in place by the adjacent vertebrae and their self-retracting forces. Extrusion of the graft is reliably prevented by the subsequent plating technique, which spans the graft and keeps it in place. The necessity for special graft configuration, for example, the "keystone" or "dovetailed" graft, or others that have been developed and used to avoid graft extrusion,[55, 84] is thereby avoided. Apart from prevention of graft extrusion, the additional application of an anterior osteosynthetic technique after vertebrectomy and graft placement with a plate and screws adds to the immediate and long-term stability of the fusion. The applicability and validity of an anterior plating procedure of the cervical spine has been established by many recent studies.[65, 66, 67, 105]

Our experiences have been satisfactory in degenerative and traumatic and tumorous diseases in which the Caspar system and either Caspar, Wolter, or rarely, AO (Arbeitsgemeinschaft Osteosynthese) plates have been used.[106] However, the following points concerning the procedure need to be stressed. Correct choice of the plate length is important. The plate should not cover more than two thirds of the adjacent vertebrae, allowing screw insertion almost in the middle of the respective vertebrae. Impingement on the adjacent intact disc spaces or even vertebrae should be avoided. Inevitable motions in these neighboring segments leads to plate movement, with the inherent risk of plate breakage or screw loosening. To avoid extensive traction forces on the inserted screws, the plate should be prebended according to the lordosis of the cervical spine and placed tightly against the spine and the graft. Performing the drill holes and insertion of the screws into the vertebral bodies is probably the part of the procedure that holds the highest potential for cervical cord injury. However, with certain precautions, it can be performed safely and without additional risk to the patient. First of all, continuous fluoroscopic control is absolutely mandatory. The consequent use and correct adjustment of a drill guide, which is routinely purchased with the Caspar system, reliably prevents undue penetration of the drill and injury of the dura and cervical cord. Moreover, almost always in adult patients, a screw length of 20 to 22 mm is sufficient to reach the posterior vertebral cortex. We have never used screws longer than this, and only very rarely shorter ones. One should try to penetrate the posterior cortex, or at least put the screw tip as close as possible to it. However, in our experience from over 300 anterior plating procedures along the cervical spine, posterior cortex puncture is not absolutely necessary to avoid screw loosening. A recent experimental study has substantiated this experience, by showing that the pull-out strength of Caspar screws is not improved by posterior cortical penetration in an isolated vertebral body model.[107] However, it is hoped that future advances in osteosynthetic technology,[108] for example, the development of the hollow titanium locking screw,[105] will further increase the safety and applicability of anterior plating techniques along the cervical spine.

REFERENCES

1. Bohlman HH, Emery SE: The pathophysiology of cervical spondylosis and myelopathy. Spine 13:843–849, 1988.
2. Panjabi M, White AA: Biomechanics of nonacute cervical spine trauma, in Sherk HH (ed): The Cervical Spine, 2nd ed. Philadelphia, JB Lippincott, 1989, pp 91–96
3. Parke WW: Correlative anatomy of cervical spondylotic myelopathy. Spine 13:831–851, 1988
4. Penning L, van der Zwaag P: Biomechanical aspects of spondylotic myelopathy. Acta Radiol 5:1090–1103, 1966
5. Burrows HR: The sagittal diameter of the spinal canal in cervical spondylosis. Clin Radiol 14:77–86, 1963
6. Wolf BS, Khilnani M, Malis L: The sagittal diameter of the bony cervical spinal canal and its significance in cervical spondylosis. J Mt Sinai Hosp 23:283–292, 1956
7. Adams CBT, Logue V: Studies in cervical spondylotic myelopathy: II. The movement and contour of the spine in relation to the neural complications of cervical spondylosis. Brain 94:569–586, 1971
8. Braakmann R: Cervical spondylotic myelopathy, in Krayenbühl H (ed): Advances and Technical Standards in Neurosurgery 6. Wien-New York, Springer, 1979, pp 137–170
9. Edwards WC, La Rocca H: The developmental segmental sagittal diameter of the cervical spinal canal in patients with cervical spondylosis. Spine 8:20–27, 1983
10. Hashimoto I, Tak Y: The true sagittal diameter of the cervical spinal canal and its diagnostic significance in cervical myelopathy. J Neurosurg 47:912–916, 1977
11. Hink VC, Sachdev NS: Developmental stenosis of the cervical spinal canal. Brain 89:27–36, 1966
12. Kessler J: Congenital narrowing of the cervical spinal canal. J Neurol Neurosurg Psychiatry 38:1218–1224, 1975
13. Ogino H, Tada K, Okada K, et al: Canal diameter, anteroposterior compression ratio, and spondylotic myelopathy of the cervical spine. Spine 8:1–15, 1983
14. Payne EE, Spillane JD: The cervical spine. An anatomico-pathological study of 70 specimens with particular reference to the problem of cervical spondylosis. Brain 80:571–592, 1960
15. Murakami N, Muroga T, Sobue I: Cervical myelopathy due to ossification of the posterior longitudinal ligament. A clinicopathological study. Arch Neurol 35:33–36, 1978
16. Nagashima C: Cervical myelopathy due to ossification of the posterior longitudinal ligament. J Neurosurg 37:653–660, 1972
17. Stoltmann H, Blackwood W: The role of the ligamenta flava in the pathogenesis of myelopathy in cervical spondylosis. Brain 87:45–50, 1964
18. Breig A, Turnbull I, Hassler O: Effects of mechanical stress on the spinal cord in cervical spondylosis. J Neurosurg 25:45–56, 1966
19. Cusick JF, Myklebust JB: Biomechanics of cervical spondylotic myelopathy. Contemp Neurosurg 9(5):1–8, 1987
20. Jellinger K: Spinal cord arteriosclerosis and progressive vascular myelopathy. J Neurol Neurosurg Psychiatry 30:195–206, 1967
21. Mair WGP, Druckmann R: The pathology of spinal cord lesions and their relation to the clinical features in protrusions of cervical intervertebral discs. Brain 76:70–91, 1953
22. Cusick JF: Pathophysiology and treatment of cervical spondylotic myelopathy. Clin Neurosurg 37:661–681, 1991
23. Fried L, Aparicio O: Experimental ischemia of the spinal cord. Neurology 23:289–293, 1973
24. Hoff JT, Nishimura M, Pitts L, et al: The role of ischemia in the pathogenesis of cervical spondylotic myelopathy. A review and new microangiographic evidence. Spine 2:100–108, 1977
25. Taylor AR: Vascular factors in the myelopathy associated with spondylotic myelopathy. Neurology 14:62–68, 1964
26. Wilson CB, Landry RM: Experimental cervical myelopathy: I. Blood supply of the canine cervical spinal cord. Neurology 14:809–814, 1964
27. Hukuda S, Wilson CB: Experimental cervical myelopathy, effects of compression and ischemia on the canine cervical cord. J Neurosurg 37:631–652, 1972
28. Gooding MR, Wilson CB, Hoff JT: Experimental cervical myelopathy: Effects of ischemia and compression of canine cervical cord. J Neurosurg 43:9–17, 1975
29. Gooding MR, Wilson CB, Hoff JT: Experimental cervical myelopathy: Auto-radiographic studies of spinal cord blood flow patterns. Surg Neurol 5:233–239, 1975
30. Hukuda S, Ogata M, Katsuura A: Experimental study on acute aggravating factors of cervical spondylotic myelopathy. Spine 13:15–20, 1988
31. Barnes MP, Saunders M: The effect of cervical mobility on the natural history of cervical spondylotic myelopathy. J Neurol Neurosurg Psychiatry 47:17–20, 1984
32. Batzdorf U, Batzdorff A: Analysis of the cervical spine curvature in patients with cervical spondylosis. Neurosurgery 22:827–836, 1988
33. Olsson S: The dynamic factor in spinal cord compression: A study on dogs with special reference to cervical disc protrusions. J Neurosurg 15:306–321, 1958
34. Clark CR: Cervical spondylotic myelopathy: History and physical findings. Spine 13:847–848, 1988
35. Hattori S, Saiki K, Kawai S: Diagnosis of the level and severity of cord lesion in cervical spondylotic myelopathy: Spinal evoked potentials. Spine 4:478–485, 1979
36. Yiannikas C, Shahani BT, Young RR: Short-latency somatosensory evoked potentials from radial, median, ulnar and peroneal nerve stimulation in the assessment of cervical spondylosis. Arch Neurol 43:1264–1271, 1986
37. Crandall PH, Batzdorf U: Cervical spondylotic myelopathy. J Neurosurg 25:57–66, 1966
38. Nurick S: The natural history and the results of surgical treatment of the spinal cord disorder associated with cervical spondylosis. Brain 95:101–108, 1972
39. Harsh GR, Sypert GW, Weinstein PR, et al: Cervical spine stenosis

secondary to ossification of the posterior longitudinal ligament. J Neurosurg 67:349–357, 1987
40. Badami JP, Norman D, Barbaro NM, et al: Metrizamide CT myelography in cervical myelopathy and radiculopathy. Correlation with conventional myelography and surgical findings. Am J Roentgenol 144:675–680, 1985
41. Karnaze MG, Gado MH, Sartor KJ, Hodges FJ: Comparison of MR and CT myelography in imaging the cervical and thoracic spine. Am J Roentgenol 150:397–403, 1988
42. Clifton AG, Stevens JM, Whitear P, Kendall BE: Identifiable causes for poor outcome in surgery for cervical spondylosis. Post-operative computed myelography and MR imaging. Neuroradiology 32:450–455, 1990
43. Brown BM, Schwartz RH, Frank E, Blank NK: Preoperative evaluation of cervical radiculopathy and myelopathy by surface coil MR imaging. Am J Neuroradiol 9:859–866, 1988
44. Czervionke LF, Daniels DL: Degenerative disease of the spine, in Atlas SW (ed): Magnetic Resonance Imaging of the Brain and Spine. New York, Raven Press, 1991, pp 855–864
45. Han JS, Benson JE, Yoon YS: Magnetic resonance imaging in the spinal column and craniovertebral junction. Radiol Clin North Am 22:805–827, 1984
46. Haughton V: MR imaging of the spine. Radiology 166:297–301, 1988
47. Mehalic TF, Pezzuti RT, Applebaum BI: Magnetic resonance imaging and cervical spondylotic myelopathy. Neurosurgery 26:217–226, 1990
48. Modic MT, Hardy RW, Weinstein MA, et al: Nuclear magnetic resonance imaging of the spine. Clinical potential and limitation. Neurosurgery 15:583–592, 1984
49. Matsuda Y, Miyazaki K, Tada K, et al: Increased signal intensity due to cervical myelopathy. Analysis of 29 cases. J Neurosurg 74:887–892, 1991
50. Arnasson A, Carlsson CA, Pelletieri L: Surgical and conservative treatment of cervical spondylotic radiculopathy and myelopathy. Acta Neurochir (Wien) 84:48–54, 1987
51. Henderson CM, Hennessy RG, Shuey Jr HM, Shackelford EG: Posterior-lateral foraminotomy as an exclusive operation for cervical radiculopathy. A review of 846 consecutively operated cases. Neurosurgery 13:504–512, 1983
52. Hukuda S, Mochizuk T, Ogata M, et al: Operations for cervical spondylotic myelopathy. A comparison of the results of anterior and posterior procedures. J Bone Joint Surg Br 67:609–615, 1985
53. Mayfield FH: Cervical spondylosis. A comparison of the anterior and posterior approaches. Clin Neurosurg 13:181–188, 1965
54. Raynor RB: Anterior and posterior approaches to the cervical spinal cord, discs and roots. A comparison of exposures and decompressions, in Sherk HH (ed): The Cervical Spine, 2nd ed. Philadelphia, JB Lippincott, 1989, pp 659–669
55. Saunders RL: Anterior reconstructive procedures in cervical spondylotic myelopathy. Clin Neurosurg 37:682–721, 1991
56. Verbiest H: The management of cervical spondylosis. Clin Neurosurg 20:262–294, 1973
57. Yonenobu K, Fuyi T, Ono K, et al: Choice of surgical treatment for multi-segmental cervical spondylotic myelopathy. Spine 10:710–716, 1985
58. Casatto A, Buoncris P: Posterior approach in cervical spondylotic myeloradiculopathy. Acta Neurochir (Wien) 57:275–285, 1981
59. Fager CA: Management of cervical disc lesions and spondylosis by posterior approaches. Clin Neurosurg 24:488–507, 1978
60. Hirabayashi K, Watanabe K, Wakano K, Suzuki N: Extensive open-door laminoplasty for cervical spondylotic myelopathy. Spine 8:693–699, 1983
61. Jeffreys RV: The surgical treatment of cervical myelopathy due to spondylosis and disc degeneration. J Neurosurg Psychiatry 49:353–361, 1986
62. Kimura I, Ohama M, Shingu H: Cervical myelopathy treated by canal-expansive laminoplasty. J Bone Joint Surg Am 66:914–920, 1984
63. Tsuji H: Laminoplasty for patients with compressive myelopathy due to so-called spinal canal stenosis in cervical and thoracic regions. Spine 7:28–34, 1982
64. Camins MB, Rosenblum BR: Osseous lesions of the cervical spine. Clin Neurosurg 37:722–755, 1991
65. Caspar W, Barbier DD, Klara PM: Anterior cervical fusion and Caspar plate stabilization for cervical trauma. Neurosurgery 25:491–502, 1989
66. Dickmann CA, Sonntag VKH, Marcotte PJ: Techniques of screw fixation of the cervical spine. BNI Q 8:9–26, 1992
67. Goffin J, Plets C, Van den Bergh R: Anterior cervical fusion and osteosynthetic stabilization according to Caspar: A prospective study of 41 patients with fractures and/or dislocations of the cervical spine. Neurosurgery 25:865–871, 1989
68. Hoff JT, Waters D: Anterior approaches to the cervical spine. Clin Neurosurg 30:606–699, 1983
69. Schmidek HH: Anterior cervical disc excision in cervical spondylosis, in Schmidek HH, Sweet WH (eds): Operative Neurosurgical Techniques. New York-London, Grune & Stratton, 1982, pp 1237–1258
70. Seifert V, Stolke D: Multisegmental cervical spondylosis: Treatment by spondylectomy, microsurgical decompression and osteosynthesis. Neurosurgery 29:498–534, 1991
71. Whitecloud TS III, La Rocca H: Fibular strut graft in reconstructive surgery of the cervical spine. Spine 1:33–43, 1976
72. Hanai K, Fujiyoshi F, Kamei K: Subtotal vertebrectomy and spinal fusion for cervical spondylotic myelopathy. Spine 11:310–315, 1986
73. Boni M, Cherubino P, Denaro V, Benazzo F: Multiple subtotal somatectomy. Technique and evaluation of a series of 39 cases. Spine 9:358–362, 1984
74. Bernard TN, Whitecloud TS: Cervical spondylotic myelopathy and myeloradiculopathy. Anterior decompression and stabilization with autogenous fibula strut graft. Clin Orthop 221:149–160, 1978
75. Doi K, Kawai S, Sumiura S, Sakai K: Anterior cervical fusion using the free vascularized fibular graft. Spine 13:1239–1244, 1988
76. Senegas J, Guerin J, Vital JM, et al: Decompression medullaire etendue par voie anterieure dans le traitement des myelopathies par cervicarthrose. Rev Chir Orthop 71:291–300, 1985
77. Rengachary S, Redford J: Partial median vertebrectomy and fibular grafting in the management of cervical spondylotic myelopathy (abstract). J Neurosurg 70:325A, 1989
78. Zdeblick TA, Bohlman HH: Cervical kyphosis and myelopathy. Treatment by anterior corpectomy and strut-grafting. J Bone Joint Surg Am 71:170–182, 1989
79. Okada K, Shirasaki N, Hayashi H, et al: Treatment of cervical spondylotic myelopathy by enlargement of the spinal canal anteriorly, followed by arthrodesis. J Bone Joint Surg Am 73:352–364, 1991
80. Kojima T, Waga S, Kubo Y, et al: Anterior cervical vertebrectomy and interbody fusion for multi-level spondylosis and ossification of the posterior longitudinal ligament. Neurosurgery 24:864–872, 1989
81. Saunders RL, Bernini PM, Shirreffs TG, Reeves AG: Central corpectomy for cervical spondylotic myelopathy: A consecutive series with long-term follow-up evaluation. J Neurosurg 74:163–170, 1991
82. Maroon JC, Abla AA, Wilberger JI, et al: Central cord syndrome. Clin Neurosurg 37:612–621, 1991
83. Emery SE, Smith MD, Bohlman HH: Upper airway obstruction after multilevel corpectomy for myelopathy. J Bone Joint Surg Am 73:544–551, 1991
84. Awasthi D, Voorhies RM: Anterior cervical vertebrectomy and interbody fusion. Technical note. J Neurosurg 76:159–163, 1992
85. Itoh T, Tsuji H: Technical improvements and results of laminoplasty for compressive myelopathy in the cervical spine. Spine 10729–10736, 1985
86. Mikawa Y, Shikata J, Jamamuro T: Spinal deformity and instability after multilevel cervical laminectomy. Spine 12:6–11, 1987
87. Oiwa T, Hirabayashi K, Uzawa M, Ohira T: Experimental study on post-laminectomy deterioration of cervical spondylotic myelopathy: Influences of intradural surgery and persistent spinal block. Spine 10:717–721, 1985
88. Sim FH, Svien HJ, Bickel WH: Swan-neck deformity following extensive cervical laminectomy. A review of twenty-one cases. J Bone Joint Surg Am 56:564–580, 1974
89. Bailey RW, Badgley CE: Stabilization of the cervical spine by an anterior fusion. J Bone Joint Surg Am 42:565–571, 1960
90. Cloward RB: Vertebral body fusion for ruptured cervical discs. Description of instruments and operative technique. Am J Surg 98:722–727, 1959
91. Dereymaker A, Muller J: Nouvelle cure chirurgicale des discopathies cervicales. La meniscotomie par voie ventrale, suivie d'arthrodese par greffe intercorporeale. Neurochirurgie 2:233–234, 1956
92. Smith GW, Robinson RA: The treatment of certain cervical disorders by anterior removal of intervertebral disc and interbody fusion. J Bone Joint Surg Am 40:607–624, 1958
93. Caspar W: A new surgical procedure for lumbar disc herniation causing less tissue damage through a microsurgical approach. Adv Neurosurg 4:74–77, 1977
94. Seeger W: Microsurgery of the Spinal Cord and Surrounding Struc-

tures. Anatomical and Technical Principles. Berlin, Heidelberg, New York, Springer Verlag, 1982
95. Dunsker SB: Anterior cervical discectomy with and without fusion. Clin Neurosurg 24:516–521, 1977
96. Whitecloud TS: Anterior surgery for cervical spondylotic myelopathy. Smith-Robinson, Cloward and vertebrectomy. Spine 13:861–863, 1988
97. Galera RG, Tovi D: Anterior disc excision with interbody fusion in cervical spondylotic myelopathy and rhizopathy. J Neurosurg 28:305–310, 1968
98. Kadoya S, Nakamura T, Kawak R: A microsurgical anterior osteophytectomy for cervical spondylotic myelopathy. Spine 9:437–441, 1984
99. Kadoya S, Nakamura T, Kwak R, Hirose G: Anterior osteophytectomy for cervical spondylotic myelopathy in developmentally narrow canal. J Neurosurg 63:845–850, 1985
100. Mann KS, Koshia VK, Gulati DR: Cervical spondylotic myelopathy treated by single-stage multilevel anterior decompression. A prospective study. J Neurosurg 60:81–87, 1984
101. Yang KC, Lu XS, Cai QL, et al: Cervical spondylotic myelopathy treated by anterior multilevel decompression and fusion. Follow-up report of 214 cases. Clin Orthop 221:161–164, 1987
102. Abumi K, Panjabi MM, Duranceau J: Biomechanical evaluation of spinal fixation device: Part III. Stability provided by six spinal fixation devices and interbody graft. Spine 14:1249–1255, 1989
103. Kaufmann HH, Jones E: The principles of bony spinal fusion. Neurosurgery 24:264–270, 1989
104. White AA, Panjabi M: Biomechanical considerations in the surgical management of cervical spondylotic myelopathy. Spine 13:856–860, 1988
105. Suh PB, Kostuick JP, Esses SI: Anterior cervical plate fixation with the titanium hollow screw plate system: A preliminary report. Spine 15:1079–1081, 1990
106. Seifert V, Zimmermann M, Wiedmayer H, Stolke D: Spondylectomy, microsurgical decompression and osteosynthesis in the treatment of complex disorders of the cervical spine. Acta Neurochir (Wien) 124:104–113, 1993
107. Maiman DJ, Pintar FA, Yoganandan N, et al: Pull-out strength of Caspar cervical screws. Neurosurgery 31:1097–1101, 1992
108. Sonntag VKH, Kalfas I: Innovative cervical fusion and instrumentation techniques. Clin Neurosurg 37:636–660, 1991

CHAPTER 146

Posterior Surgical Approaches for Cervical Disc Herniation and Spondylotic Myelopathy

James C. Collias
Melville P. Roberts

The posterior approach to decompression of the spinal cord and nerve roots is used less frequently since the development of the anterior approach to the cervical spine.[1,2] Laminectomy and foraminotomy, however, have retained their importance in the surgical treatment of lateral cervical disc herniation and spondylotic myelopathy. In most instances, either the anterior or posterior approach can be used with satisfactory results; the choice is determined by the preference of the surgeon. In some situations, the lesion requires a specific approach. For this reason, expertise in both approaches is necessary. This chapter describes the posterior operations used at our institution.

LATERAL CERVICAL DISC HERNIATIONS

Although results with anterior discectomy can be just as gratifying, the posterior approach for lateral disc herniation has certain advantages: it allows immediate mobilization of the neck, the disc structure is preserved, and two or more roots can be explored without additional discectomy. In addition, the morbidity associated with fusions is eliminated, as are the inevitable stresses applied to adjacent interspaces after fusion. The C3-C4 and C7-D1 discs are also more easily approached by the posterior route. In contrast, central soft disc ruptures are more safely approached anteriorly.

Since Scoville's early contributions to cervical disc surgery,[3,4,56,57] laminotomy with foraminotomy has been used to treat most lateral cervical disc herniations at the Hartford Hospital. We now have an operative experience of more than 3000 cases over a period of 50 years.

INCIDENCE

In a review of 2035 of our surgical cases for ruptured cervical discs (Roberts and Collias: Unpublished data), lateral soft disc protrusions occurred in 85 percent, hard disc ruptures in 11 percent, and soft central disc ruptures in 4 percent. The male-to-female ratio was 49:51, and the mean age was 37 years, the oldest patient being 73 years old and the youngest, 21 years. The most frequent roots involved were C6 and C7, and 54 percent of disc ruptures occurred at the C6-C7 level, 35 percent at C5-C6, 6 percent at C7-D1, 5 percent at C4-C5, and only two cases (less than 1 percent) at C3-C4.

There was one instance of extruded fragments found at two adjacent levels on the same side during the same operation. A hard disc protrusion and a soft one at adjacent levels when two discs were explored was more common. Fewer than 20 percent of the patients had a history of trauma. Recurrent disc rupture on the same side at the same level occurred in only one patient, and 19 percent of patients developed disc herniations at other locations.[5] Lumbar disc protrusion requiring surgery occurred 10 times more often than cervical disc protrusion requiring surgery.

CLINICAL MANIFESTATIONS

The classic picture of lateral disc herniation is distinctive and easily recognized. Neck pain occurs, usually without a precipitating event, and subsequently extends to the shoulder, the medial scapula, and down the arm to the hand. Pain also can radiate into the anterolateral chest. In acute cases, the head and neck may be held rigidly, flexed, and rotated away from the side of the rupture. Extension of the neck to the side of the lesion is resisted (Scoville-Spurling test)[3] and increases the pain. Upward neck traction or elevation of the shoulder and elbow may relieve the pain. Hard disc herniations usually cause less acute pain.

Radicular syndromes generally can be recognized easily by dermatomal and myotomal findings. Sensory deficit in overlapping dermatomes without reflex loss or weakness may make differentiating between the C6 and C7 roots difficult. Weakness of the deltoid, infraspinatus, and supraspinatus muscles, with sensory loss over the deltoid, occurs in C5 root involvement. Weakness of the biceps and brachioradialis muscles, with numbness and paresthesias in the thumb and index finger, occurs with C6 root compression in C5-C6 lesions. Weakness of the triceps, wrist, and finger extensors, with diminished triceps reflex and numbness in the index and middle fingers, is present with C7 root involvement in C6-C7 ruptures. Weakness of intrinsic hand muscles and ulnar sensory loss is seen in C8 root compression with a C7-D1 disc rupture.

NONSURGICAL TREATMENT

Initial treatment consists of sedation, analgesics, and traction. Cervical traction with 10 to 15 pounds of weight for 20 to 30 minutes with the patient's neck flexed may help. Traction in extension can exacerbate the pain. Many patients improve without further treatment. Setting a time beyond which nonsurgical treatment should be discontinued and surgery considered is difficult. However, nonsurgical treatment should be continued as long as the patient is improving.

Severe, unremitting pain and profound neurologic deficit usually require immediate surgery. Decreasing pain with increasing neurologic deficit also warrants concern and merits prompt diagnosis and treatment. The patient's vocation, such as surgeon or musician, should be considered, particularly if significant dominant arm or hand weakness is present. Early decompression is frequently indicated so that permanent sensory or motor loss can be avoided. Economic factors may make lengthy nonsurgical treatment impractical. Chronic pain that interferes with sleep and work after an initial period of improvement is usually an indication for surgery.

DIAGNOSTIC STUDIES

Flexion, extension, and oblique-view roentgenograms of the cervical spine are obtained initially. In our series, the results were normal in 50 percent of patients and showed disc space narrowing and degenerative changes at levels other than that of the disc rupture in 20 percent. Computed tomographic (CT) scanning and myelography or magnetic resonance imaging (MRI) are the definitive studies carried out on almost all patients considered for surgery to confirm the size, shape, and location of the lesion and also to rule out unsuspected lesions. In one case (Fig. 146–1), a benign intradural tumor and disc protrusion coexisted and were removed at the same operation.

Multiple minor defects can frequently be seen with spondylosis, but the lesion responsible for the patient's symptoms can usually be identified. In our series, myelography was diagnostic in 99 percent of cases. CT scanning of the cervical spine without contrast is frequently worthless. CT with myelography or MRI is the preferred study. Electromyography is helpful in clarifying confusing root syndromes and in ruling out peripheral nerve lesions. Abnormalities usually cannot be demonstrated by electromyography in acute root lesions before the third week.

PATIENT SELECTION FOR SURGERY

All patients selected for surgery should have radicular signs and symptoms. Although nonsurgical treatment is usually indicated initially, exceptions may occur, and all of the factors previously noted must be considered. Diagnostic studies should demonstrate a defect that correlates with the patient's signs and symptoms; frequently it is a root defect, but larger extradural defects may be seen. Selection of pa-

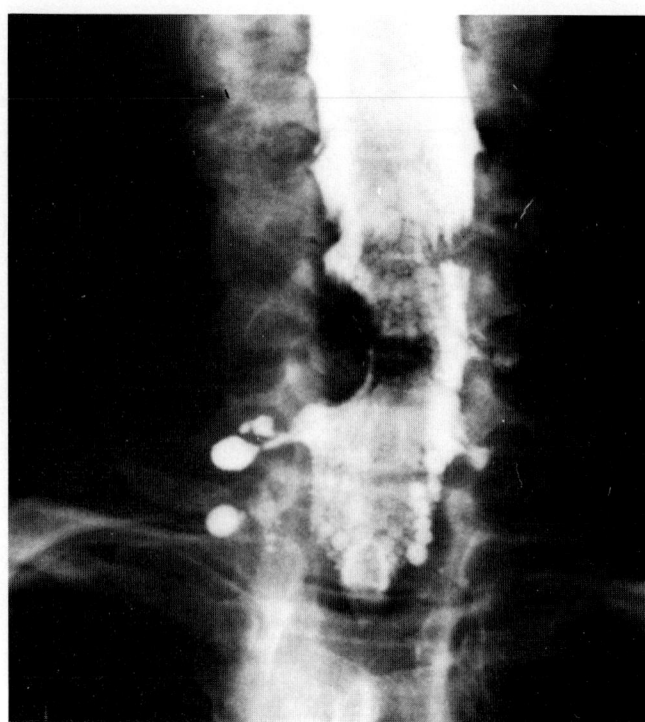

FIGURE 146–1. A myelogram showing a large defect on the left at C6-7 caused by a neurofibroma and a smaller defect on the right at C5-6 caused by a ruptured disc.

tients for surgery is generally not a problem. Surgery is not performed for neck pain alone or when diagnostic study results are normal.

SURGICAL PROCEDURE

Keyhole foraminotomy as described by Scoville[4] is used to treat this condition. If further exposure is necessary, additional portions of the lamina are removed. Extensive laminectomy is rarely necessary.

The procedure is carried out with the patient under general anesthesia in the seated position (Fig. 146–2A and B). The patient's lower extremities are wrapped to midthigh with elastic bandages, and an abdominal binder is applied. The legs and feet are elevated to the level of the heart. The head is slightly flexed and taped to a Mayfield cup headrest or fixed in a Mayfield skull clamp.

A Doppler monitor is placed on the precordium, and a central venous line is passed, generally through the basilic vein, into the superior vena cava. This position allows central venous pressure to be monitored and air to be aspirated, if necessary. End-tidal carbon dioxide and arterial pressure are monitored. During induction, dexamethasone, 10 mg, and an antibiotic such as cefazolin (Ancef) or vancomycin are administered intravenously.

A posterior vertical midline incision is made over the vertebral level involved, and it measures about 2 to 3 inches in length when a single level is to be explored. To aid hemostasis, lidocaine with 1:100,000 epinephrine is infiltrated into the subcutaneous tissue and muscle before the skin incision is made. Exposure is carried down to the ligamentum nuchae, and an incision is made immediately lateral

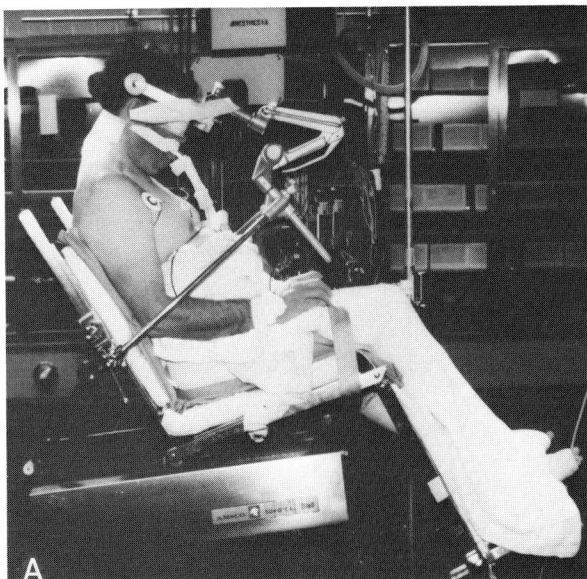 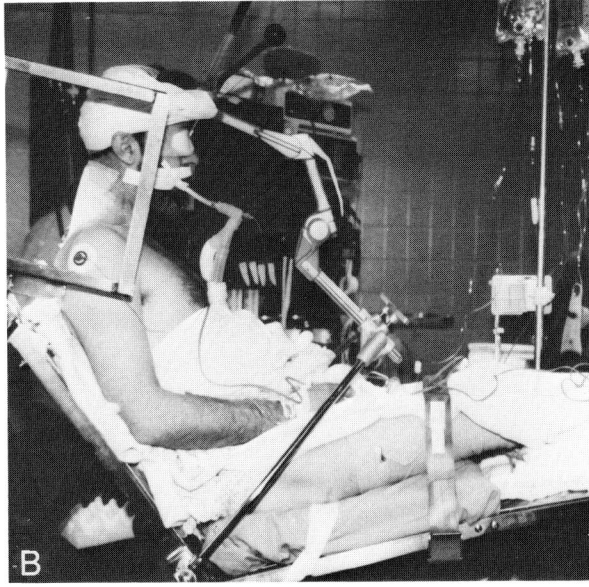

FIGURE 146–2. (A) Incorrect positioning of a seated patient. The legs are dependent, and the neck is excessively flexed. (B) Correct positioning of a seated patient. The legs are elevated and the neck is not excessively flexed. (From Roberts MP. Complications of positioning for neurosurgical operations on the spine, in Tarlov EC (ed): Complications of Spinal Surgery. Park Ridge, Ill, American Association of Neurological Surgeons, 1991, p 5. With permission.)

to the spinous process. An Allis clamp is affixed to the spinous process, and a lateral roentgenogram is obtained for interspace localization. Then, the fascial incision is extended. The periosteum and muscles are dissected from the laminae. A hand-held Meyerding retractor facilitates sharp cutting of ligamentous and muscle attachments to the laminae and facet. Exposure of a portion of the lamina above and below makes lateral retraction easier. A Scoville laminectomy retractor with cross-bar adaptation in the hook to prevent slippage through the interspinous ligament is used to maintain muscle retraction and to expose the lamina and facet.[4] A small pituitary rongeur is used to peel off any remaining tissue from the lamina, interlaminar space, and facet. The lateral extent of the superior lamina and the most medial extent of the facet are clearly defined (Fig. 146–3). The inferior articular process of the superior vertebra generally overhangs the superior articular process of the inferior vertebra. The inferior articular process and then the superior articular process are drilled with an air drill with a small diamond burr and constant irrigation with saline to create a defect in the medial one third or one half of the facet, leaving a thin shell of cortical bone over the foramen and underlying nerve root (Fig. 146–4). The cortical bone is then easily lifted off with small, sharp curettes and delicate sella punches to further expose the extension of the ligamentum flavum, which forms a venous-laden membrane over the nerve root.

A small laminotomy of the superior lamina laterally is carried out with punch rongeurs. The bone where the superior articular facet of the inferior vertebra meets the pedicle is removed with punches to gain access to the axilla of the nerve root, where initial exploration should begin (Fig. 146–5). Loupe magnification may be helpful at this point. A 0.5-cm vertical incision is then made in the ligamentum flavum overlying the dura that covers the lateral spinal cord and just medial to the root origin. A thin, grooved Woodson (dental) dissector is introduced beneath the ligamentum flavum and manipulated laterally (Fig. 146–6); it is pulled backward so that the underlying compressed root is not compressed any further. The thin extension of ligamentum flavum is incised over the dissector as it is moved laterally, in much the same

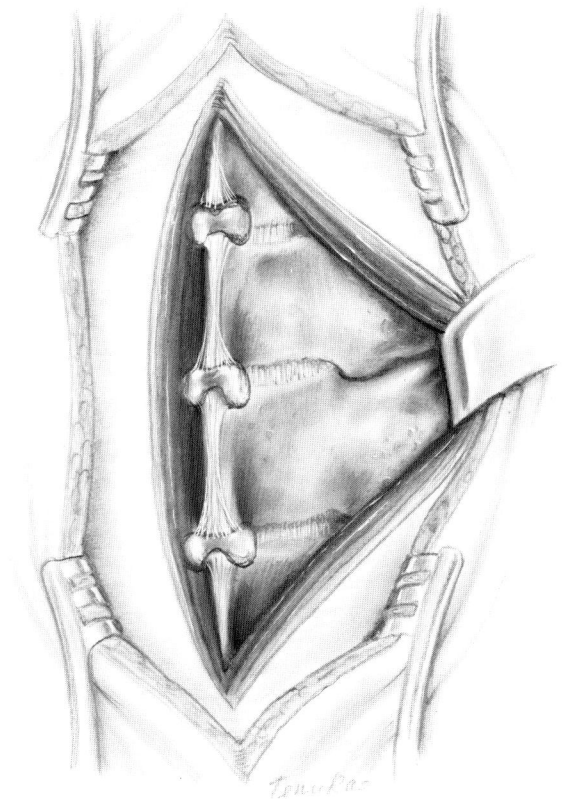

FIGURE 146–3. The initial exposure of laminae and facets.

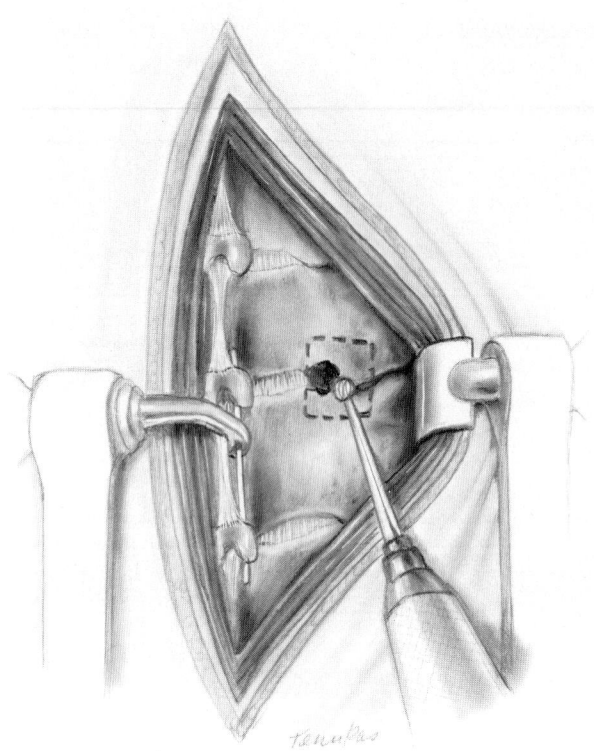

FIGURE 146–4. A diamond burr is used to drill out the medial one third to one half of the facet.

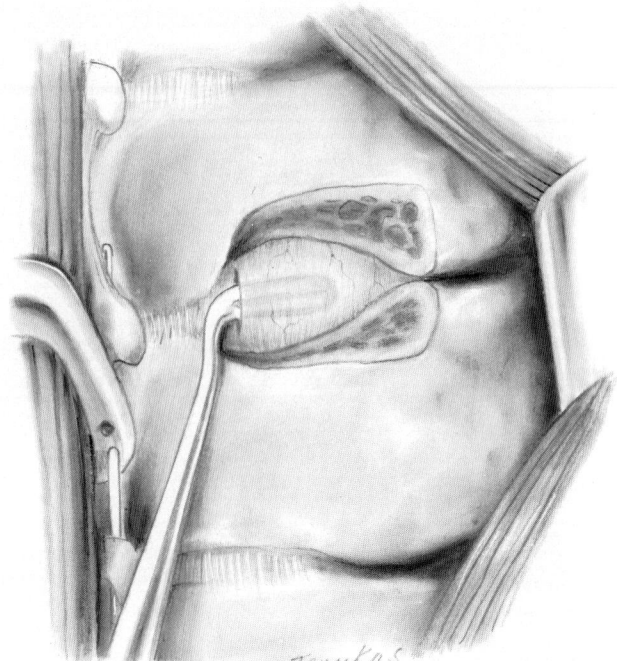

FIGURE 146–6. A thin, grooved Woodson dissector is passed laterally beneath the ligamentum flavum and its lateral extension, allowing safe incision.

way as a dural guide is used. A No. 15 Bard-Parker blade is used for cutting. Bleeding in the superior and inferior edges is controlled with bipolar coagulation and small cottonoids, which can be inserted epidurally and moved about to provide hemostasis while disc fragments are sought and removed. The root has a large sensory component superiorly and posteriorly and a smaller motor portion inferiorly and anteriorly.

The root may be tense if an underlying anterior disc fragment or osteophytic spur is present, and care must be taken not to injure the stretched motor division or to mistake it for a disc fragment. Exploration is initially carried out in the axilla of the root (Fig. 146–7). A blunt Stille hook is an excellent instrument for this purpose. Exploration is continued under the dural sac superiorly, medially, and inferiorly with a swirling motion to deliver fragments from beneath the root (Fig. 146–8). Frequently, the disc is contained within the posterior ligament or annulus, and an incision must be

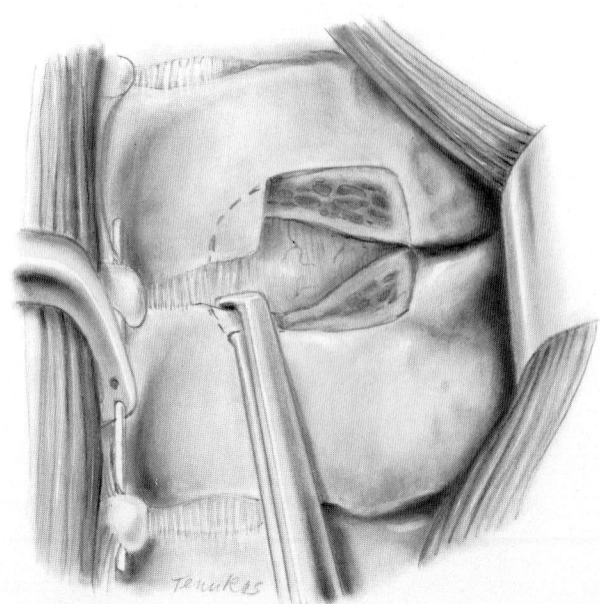

FIGURE 146–5. A punch rongeur is used to remove small bits of pedicle and facet to expose the axilla of the root.

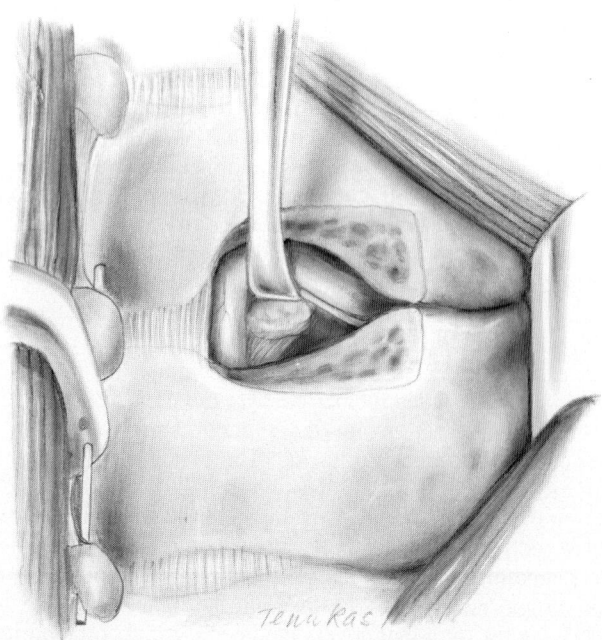

FIGURE 146–7. Nerve root being elevated with a root retractor during exploration.

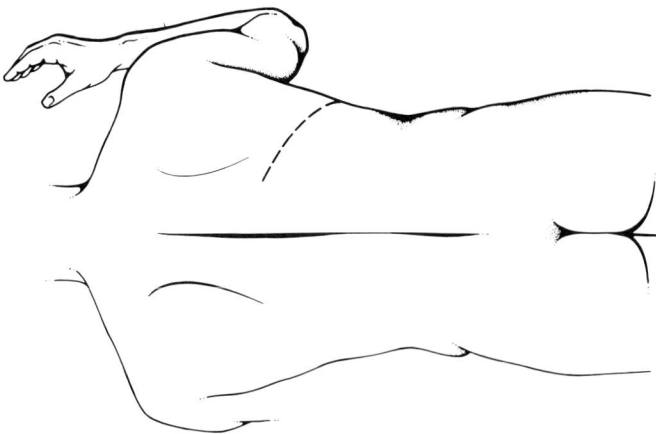

FIGURE 161–10. A standard posterolateral thoracotomy incision is used for exposure of the thoracic segments.

to protect the dura. The resected vertebra is then replaced using the clavicle as a strut graft by impacting it in place under gentle traction. Additional cancellous bone from the sternum is also laid along the strut. Immediate stability can also be achieved by the use of Steinmann pins and polymethyl methacrylate that is allowed to polymerize in situ. Suction drains are placed, and the wound is closed in layers. Postoperatively, a cervicothoracic orthosis is prescribed (generally a Philadelphia collar with thoracic extension). Patients are allowed to ambulate immediately and can begin chemotherapy in a week. If a bone graft is used, radiotherapy should be delayed for 6 weeks. In our experience, all patients usually require a secondary posterior fusion after antitumor therapy.

The transthoracic approach is used for tumors below the third thoracic segment. Patients are positioned in the lateral position on an Olympic Vac-Pac unit, and general endotracheal anesthesia with a double lumen tube is used. A generous skin incision similar to a posterolateral thoracotomy is placed below the scapula (Fig. 161–10). The posterior incision should be parallel to the paraspinal muscles but should not extend to the midline unless a second-stage spondylectomy is planned. After the skin incision is made, we use electrocautery to cut through the chest wall muscles (trapezius, serratus, latissimus, and pectoralis major) to reach the rib cage.

When the interspace is entered, it should be above the body that one has to work with because the ribs turn caudally proximal to the angle. In the lower thoracic segments, at least two spaces above the level of involvement are chosen because of the rising dome of the diaphragm. Only the posterior 5 to 10 cm of rib needs to be removed (Fig. 161–11). Rib resection is performed by using cautery to detach the periosteum of the rib and by using Doyen periosteal elevators to strip the periosteum from the neurovascular bundle. The intercostal bundle should be carefully isolated with right-angled clamps and should then be cleanly ligated or clipped. During the initial phase of tumor resection, the head of the ribs overlies the pedicle and should be kept intact to prevent injury to the cord. A self-retaining thoracic retractor is

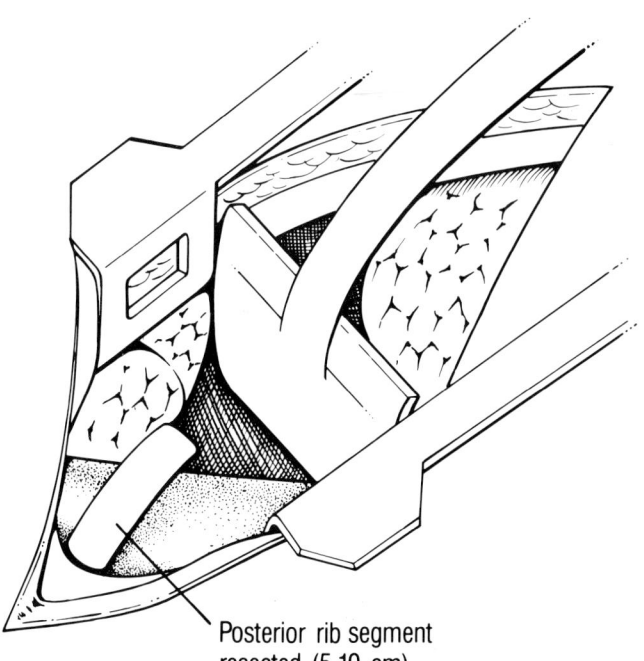

FIGURE 161–11. After the thoracic cavity is opened, self-retaining retractors are positioned. Only the posterior 5 to 10 cm of rib has to be resected as shown.

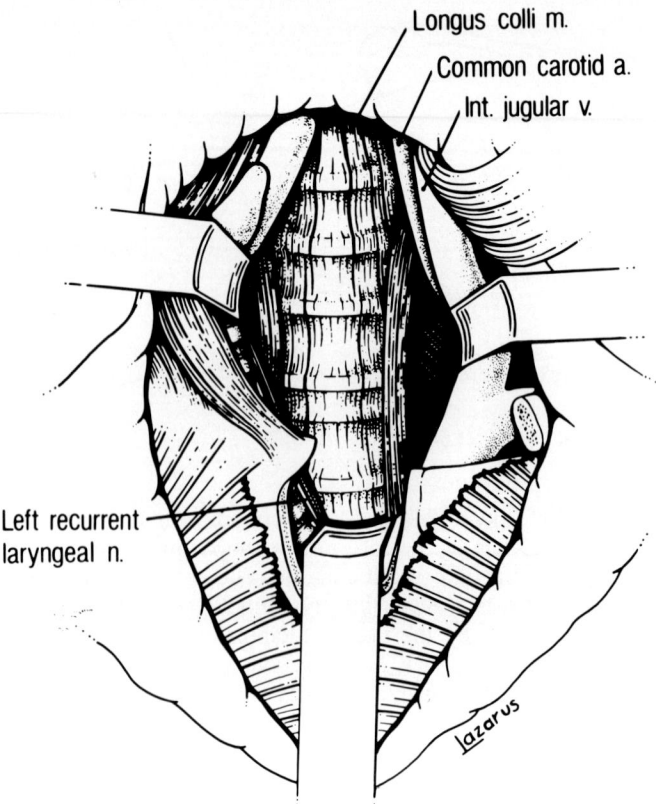

FIGURE 161–8. Following removal of a portion of the manubrium sterni muscle, the trachea and esophagus are retracted medially and the carotid sheath is retracted laterally.

teum. Intact discs above and below the level of involvement are identified. Self-retaining Cloward retractors or an Oberhill retractor (V. Muller, Chicago, Ill) are placed under the longus colli muscles (Fig. 161–9). The involved vertebra is then resected piecemeal with curettes, rongeurs, and osteotomes. If the bone is markedly sclerotic, a high-speed drill can be used. All involved bone and soft tissue tumor and devitalized tissues are removed down to the dura. Meticulous hemostasis is achieved with the bipolar current. After the dura is cleaned of all tumor, a sheet of gelatin sponge is used

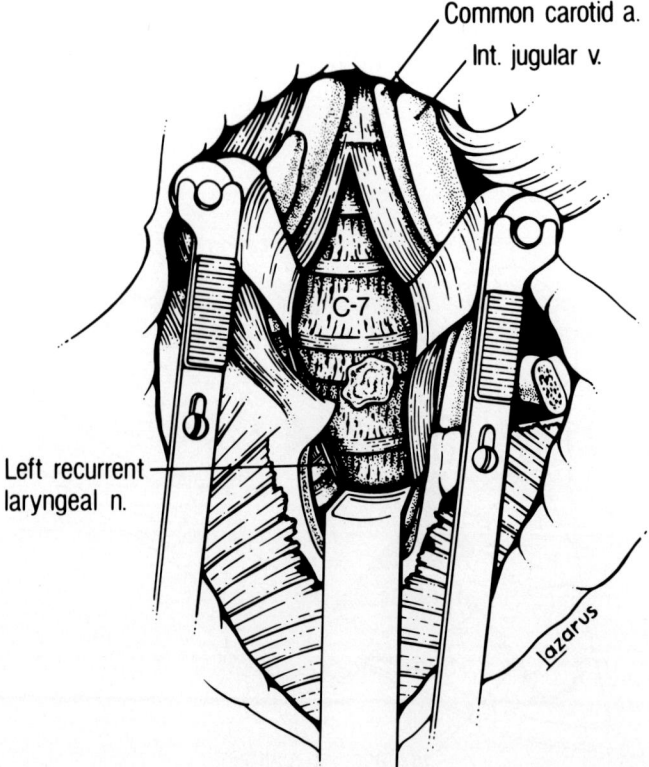

FIGURE 161–9. The longus colli muscles are stripped from the anterior aspect of the spine, and self-retaining Cloward retractors are positioned to expose the bony thoracic inlet posteriorly.

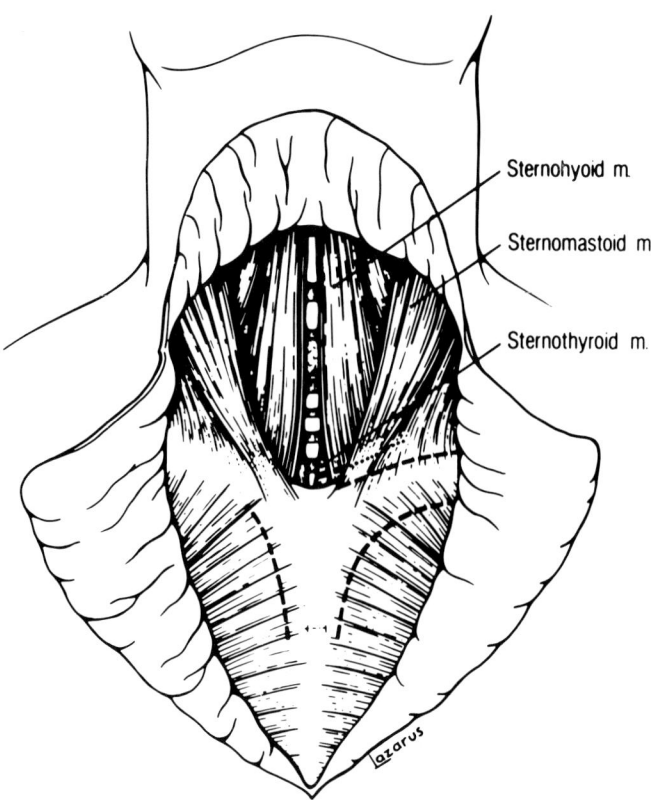

FIGURE 161-6. Surgical exposure of the upper two thoracic vertebrae. Subplatysmal flaps are elevated, and dotted lines indicate muscles that have to be stripped from the clavicle and manubrium (sternomastoid and pectoralis major muscles).

sternum, and the clavicle stripped subperiosteally. The medial third of the clavicle is sectioned with a Gigli saw, and the medial end disarticulated from the sternum. A power drill is used to thin the edges of a rectangular piece of manubrium, which is then cut off with scissors.

Once the periosteum is removed, the vascular structures beneath are exposed. The inferior thyroid veins are ligated, but the innominate vein can be retracted out of the field. The thymus and surrounding fat should be dissected and resected. The avascular plane between the trachea and esophagus medially and the vascular sheath laterally is developed (Fig. 161-8). The recurrent laryngeal nerve should be identified. The prevertebral space is then opened in the midline, and the longus colli muscles are stripped laterally with the perios-

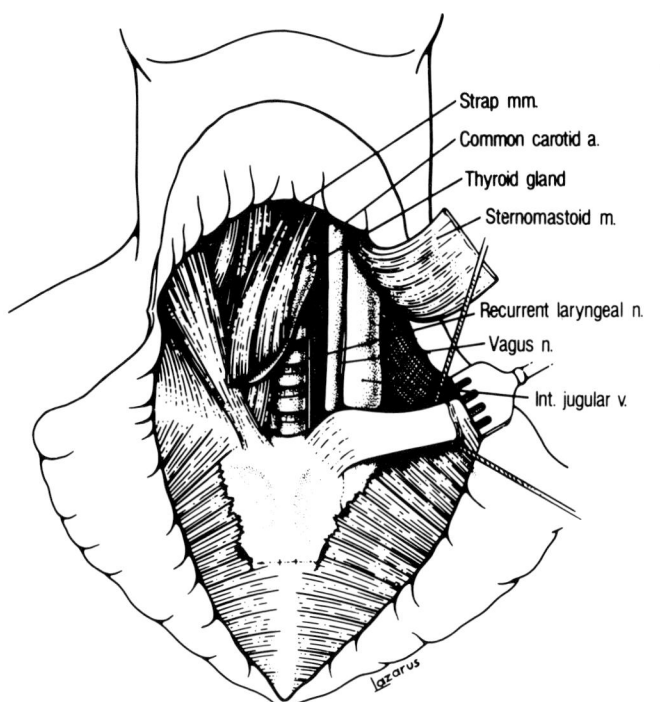

FIGURE 161-7. The sternomastoid muscle is sectioned and retracted laterally; the inferior strap muscles are sectioned and retracted medially; the medial third of the clavicle is removed after subperiosteal stripping.

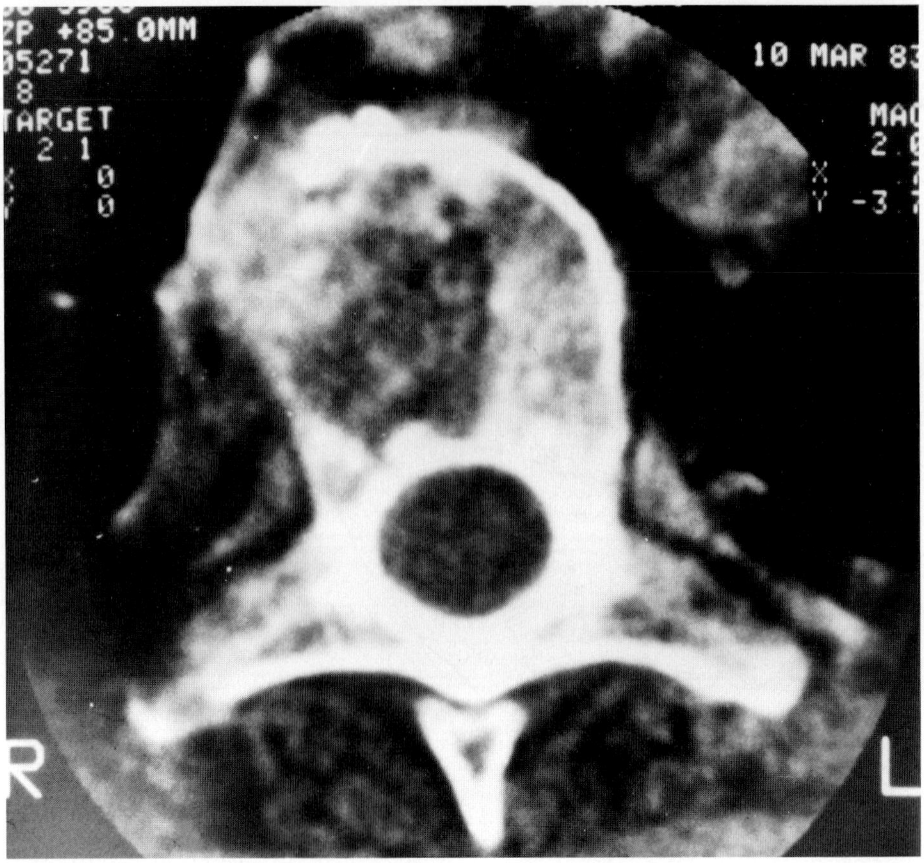

FIGURE 161-4. A CT scan of the spine demonstrating destruction of the vertebral body by metastatic kidney cancer. In patients with solitary foci of relapse, surgical resection is indicated regardless of epidural invasion.

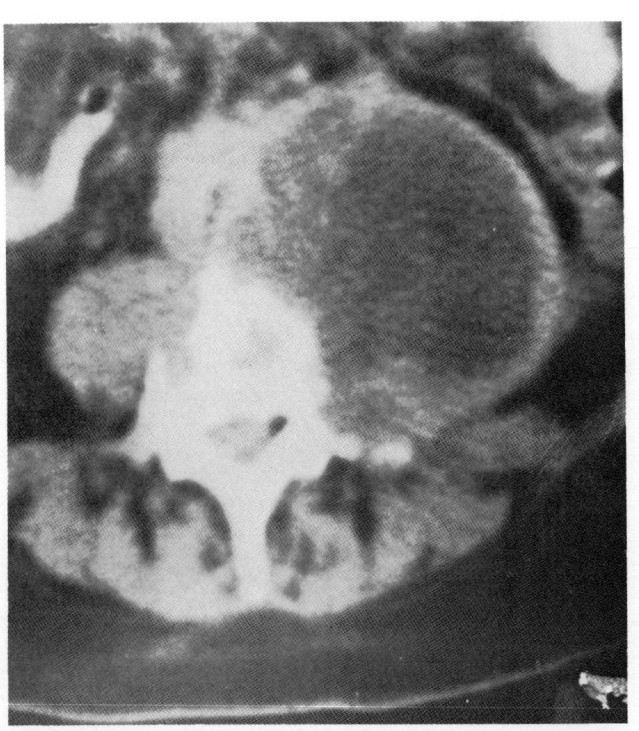

FIGURE 161-5. A CT scan demonstrating paraspinal soft part sarcoma with spine destruction and epidural extension. An anterolateral approach is required for tumor resection.

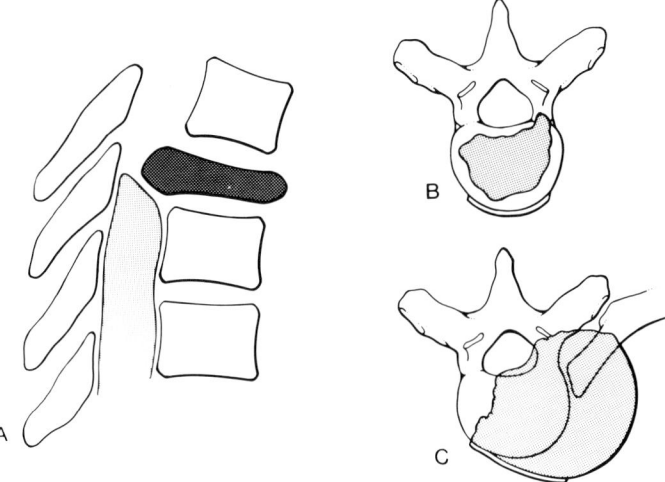

FIGURE 161–2. Radiologic findings that indicate a need for an anterior approach by vertebral body resection: (A) kyphotic deformity secondary to vertebral collapse; (B) anterior osseous destruction by tumor; (C) presence of an anterolateral tumor mass.

in this section, we describe the use of Steinmann pins for anterior fixation of the acrylic.

The anterior spine requires various approaches because of the complex soft part anatomy anterior to the prevertebral space (see Table 161–3). In this review, we focus on the transthoracic approach, which serves as the model for approaches to the other segments. An initial consideration is the side from which an anterolateral exposure should be performed. In most cases, the side that allows maximal tumor resection should be chosen. The side can usually be ascertained by CT. If a CT scan is not available, then either the side of increased pedicle destruction or collapse or the symptomatic side of radiculopathy or plexopathy probably indicates the site of tumor compression. In equivocal cases, a right-sided approach is chosen for thoracic segments, and a left-sided approach for lumbar segments.

The upper two thoracic segments form the posterior border of the thoracic inlet: this region can be exposed by a direct anterior transsternal approach[26] or indirectly by a posterolateral thoracotomy with resection of the upper three ribs for extensive tumors with lateral extension. The transsternal anterior operation is performed with the patient in the supine position with the head extended (the range of extension and flexion is tested with the patient awake before surgery). A T-shaped incision is used. The horizontal limb of the T extends 1 cm above the clavicle and extends past the sternomastoid on either side, and the vertical limb is carried down to the body of the sternum. Subplatysmal flaps are elevated and retained by sutures (Fig. 161–6). Several veins (anterior jugular veins and the jugular venous arch) and the medial supraclavicular nerves cross the field and must be sectioned. The sternal and clavicular heads of the sternomastoid are detached from their bony origins by cautery and are retracted superiorly and posteriorly. The inferior strap muscles (sternohyoid and sternothyroid) are sectioned inferiorly and retracted superiorly and medially (Fig. 161–7). The fatty and areolar tissues in the suprasternal space are cleared. The sternal origin of the pectoralis major is cleared from the

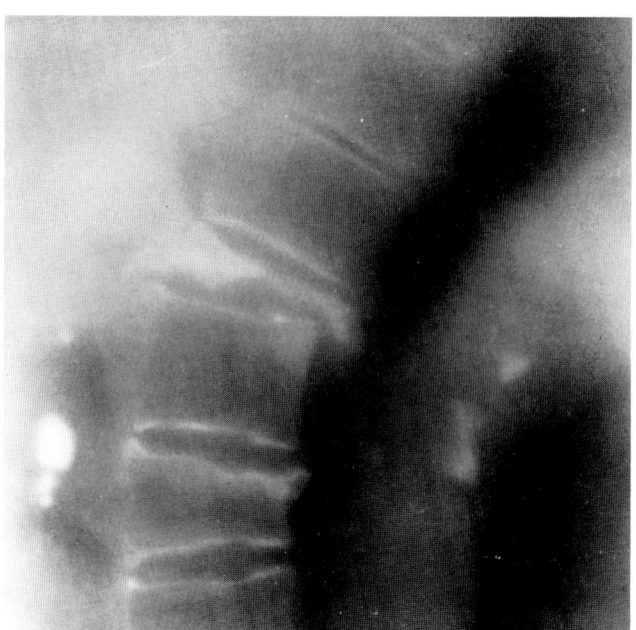

FIGURE 161–3. Localized collapse with kyphosis secondary to breast cancer. The presence of collapse exceeding 50 percent of the vertebral body height indicates instability and requires anterior decompression and stabilization.

on clinical and laboratory criteria, and the desired goal of therapy. If an operation is planned for biopsy of a spinal neoplasm, the incision and execution of the procedure should be such that the tract can be excised later without contamination of tissue planes. Whenever feasible, an anterior approach should be used to obtain biopsy specimens of tumors involving a vertebral body. In addition, we emphasize the usefulness of intraoperative radiography to confirm correct spinal levels and restrict removal of normal bone.

LAMINECTOMY

Laminectomy is indicated for posteriorly placed tumors, for neural decompression and pain relief caused by secondary hypertrophic stenosis, and whenever extensive intradural exploration is indicated. In addition, laminectomy may allow tumor resection within the vertebral body if the pedicles and facet are removed, thus allowing a posterolateral approach to the spine. Our major indications for laminectomy in metastatic cancer are in patients with prostate cancer and lymphoma who relapse after radiation therapy. In patients with primary neoplasms and in those with solitary radioresistant metastases, laminectomy is indicated with posterior instrumentation and bone grafting to complete a staged spondylectomy.

In the thoracic and lumbar region, laminectomies can be performed with the patient in the lateral or prone position; we prefer to use the lateral position on an Olympic Vac-Pac unit because of the ease of patient positioning and because it minimizes intraoperative blood loss. The lateral position also allows extension of the posterior procedure via a lateral osteotomy approach by T-ing the skin incision. In the cervical region, operations are performed in the prone position either with the patient held by the Mayfield skull clamps or the halo apparatus if the head is considered unstable.

A generous midline incision is used after adequate skin preparation and draping with Vi-Drapes and skin towels. We prefer the use of skin staples instead of towel clips on the skin to facilitate intraoperative radiography. The skin incision is infiltrated with local anesthetic (lidocaine [Xylocaine] ½ percent with epinephrine 1:200,000) to minimize bleeding. If the patient has not undergone radiotherapy, we use a midline incision. In previously irradiated patients, an off-midline incision with skin flaps or transverse incisions is suggested. After the dermis is incised, the cautery unit is used to divide the subcutaneous tissue, and the midline located by palpating the spinous processes. The paraspinal muscles are stripped off the spine and lamina, but if the posterior elements are destroyed by tumor, this dissection is best carried out sharply with Cobb elevators or wide-bladed osteotomes to retract the paraspinous muscles. The spinous processes are removed with bone cutters, and the lamina is thinned out with the Adson and Leksell rongeurs. The bone can also be thinned out with a high-speed drill after all ligamentous and soft tissues are stripped away. The final layers of bone are generally removed with curettes and Kerrison punches. The ligamentum flavum should then be removed by sharp dissection. When the epidural space is infiltrated by tumor, normal epidural fat is absent or replaced. Bone removal should be carried out until normal epidural fat is seen, but we emphasize preserving as much normal spine as possible to facilitate either stabilization or instrumentation if required later.

Bleeding from the epidural space can be controlled with bipolar current, and tumor resection is facilitated if the Cavitron ultrasonic instrument is used. Profuse bleeding from the epidural space frequently may be encountered. Enough tumor should be removed to minimize postoperative bleeding, and the tumor bed should be gently packed with hemostatic agents such as microfibrillar collagen (Avitene). Often, repeated gentle packing with cottonoids is required between tumor dissection to control bleeding. In some patients, the tumor may invade the outer sheath of dura or the nerve roots. These can be removed by sharp microdissection. After tumor resection, hemostasis is secured by waxing of all bone edges and coagulating bleeding points. In addition, drainage of the epidural space by suction drains isolated from the dura by gelatin foam (Gelfoam) is often required. If instrumentation or bone fusion is required, it is performed at this juncture. The indications and techniques are described elsewhere.[22]

Closure of the paraspinal muscles is carried out with heavy 2-0 Vicryl or 0 Vicryl sutures, and the subcutaneous tissues with 00 Vicryl sutures. The skin is closed with 000 nylon sutures or staples. In the patient who requires a plaster-of-Paris jacket (after bone fusion), subcuticular stitches and Steri-Strips are used. A sterile dressing is then applied.

Patients are nursed flat with log-rolling maneuvers, and care is taken to prevent pulmonary emboli by the use of Venodyne intermittent pressure stockings or low-dose heparin therapy.

VERTEBRAL BODY RESECTION

In our experience, the anterior approach by vertebral body resection fulfills the basic principles of tumor surgery: it provides extensive exposure, thus allowing complete resection of all gross tumor, and allows adequate access for anterior stabilization (Figs. 161-2 through 161-5). In patients with neoplasms, the importance of immediate stabilization cannot be overemphasized. Stabilization allows immediate ambulation and minimizes pulmonary and embolic complications. In view of the limited life expectancy of cancer patients and the need for postoperative radiation therapy, we believe that polymethyl methacrylate used as an immediate stabilizing agent allows major advantages over bone grafts. Polymethyl methacrylate is an acrylic polymer belonging to the polyolefin group of synthetic plastics. It is commercially available as a liquid monomer (40 ml), which is mixed with the powdered polymer (20 g). Curing, or self-polymerization, occurs through a self-catalytic process and from the addition of agents. During polymerization, intense heat is generated (80° to 100°C) for periods of 5 minutes. The orthopedic polymethyl methacrylate is impregnated with 10-percent barium sulfate and is available from three major sources: Howmedica, Zimmer, and Richards. No bonding occurs at the bone-cement interface, and therefore the brittle acrylic must be kept in place with additional instrumentation. Although various techniques have been described to achieve this, three methods described in the literature require emphasis.[23-25] All three techniques are relatively simple, easy to master, and should be part of the armamentarium of all spinal surgeons;

TISSUE DIAGNOSIS

With current radiologic evaluation, the need for a major procedure to document a diagnosis of malignancy should be rare. The primary site frequently is obvious, that is, on chest x-ray films or abdominal CT scans, or a more accessible site may be seen on radionuclide bone scan. If no site is evident, the diagnosis of malignancy can frequently be established by a CT-guided needle biopsy, especially if a paraspinal soft tissue mass is present. A major indication for operative intervention is to differentiate benign from malignant compression, such as disc disease versus metastatic tumor, or in the occasional intradural lesion in which distinction from a primary intraspinal tumor, such as meningioma versus metastases, must be made. If open biopsy of a tumor is required, the site of laminotomy and the extent of bone removal must be minimized to prevent loss of stability as well as to reduce contamination of tissue planes along the biopsy tract.

PAIN RELIEF

In most patients, resection of tumor and restoration of stability frequently result in pain relief; especially in patients with intractable pain either from local plexus or nerve root invasion, the goal of therapy may be pain relief even though motor deficits are permanent and irreversible. The role of local rhizotomies, cordotomy, and resection of lesions compressing the brachial plexus fall into this category.[20, 21]

PREOPERATIVE EVALUATION AND ASSESSMENT

Many patients with spinal cord compression are referred for neurosurgical evaluation either with an evolving neurologic deficit or after a myelogram has demonstrated a complete block. This may result in a hasty decision to decompress the cord on an emergency basis in an effort to preserve or improve neurologic function. Although such clinical situations cannot always be avoided, we recommend that emergency surgery be considered only in patients with unstable neurologic deficits on steroid therapy. With an initial bolus dose (dexamethasone, 20 to 100 mg given intravenously) and continuous high-dose corticosteroid therapy, most patients stabilize long enough for more complete radiologic assessment. At a minimum, a spinal CT scan should be obtained to determine the proper operative approach.

In patients with a pathologic compression fracture without a prior history of cancer, two diagnostic possibilities exist: (1) a primary cancer is evident on chest x-ray films or abdominal CT scans, or (2) no primary site is seen. Radiologic evaluation should include a radionuclide bone scan; extensive radiologic studies looking for a primary site are not indicated.

Specific laboratory tests that aid in the diagnosis include serum acid phosphatase, serum and urine immune electrophoresis, and carcinoembryonic antigen levels. A bone marrow examination should be performed if myeloma is suspected. Because most patients may require thoracotomy, we believe that preoperative pulmonary function tests should be performed whenever feasible; as a minimum, arterial blood gas studies should be obtained. In patients with chronic obstructive pulmonary disease and those with recent respiratory compromise, therapy with ultrasonic nebulizers a few days before surgery will promote a smoother recovery. In vascular tumors, a complete coagulogram should be performed, and between 4 to 10 units of packed red cells or whole blood should be cross matched for the patient. In view of the need for blood products, such as fresh frozen plasma and platelets, we generally recommend a formal hematologic consultation. A final, most important aspect of preoperative care is to have the patient evaluated for a custom-made or prefabricated orthosis.

CHOICE OF OPERATIVE APPROACH

There are three basic approaches to the spine: (1) posterior approaches by laminectomy, (2) lateral approaches by transverse osteotomy, and (3) anterior approaches by vertebral body resection (Fig. 161–1). In addition, complete spondylectomy can be performed by a combination of an anterior and posterior approach. The choice of surgical approach should be based on the radiographic extent of tumor, the ability of the patient to tolerate the proposed operation based

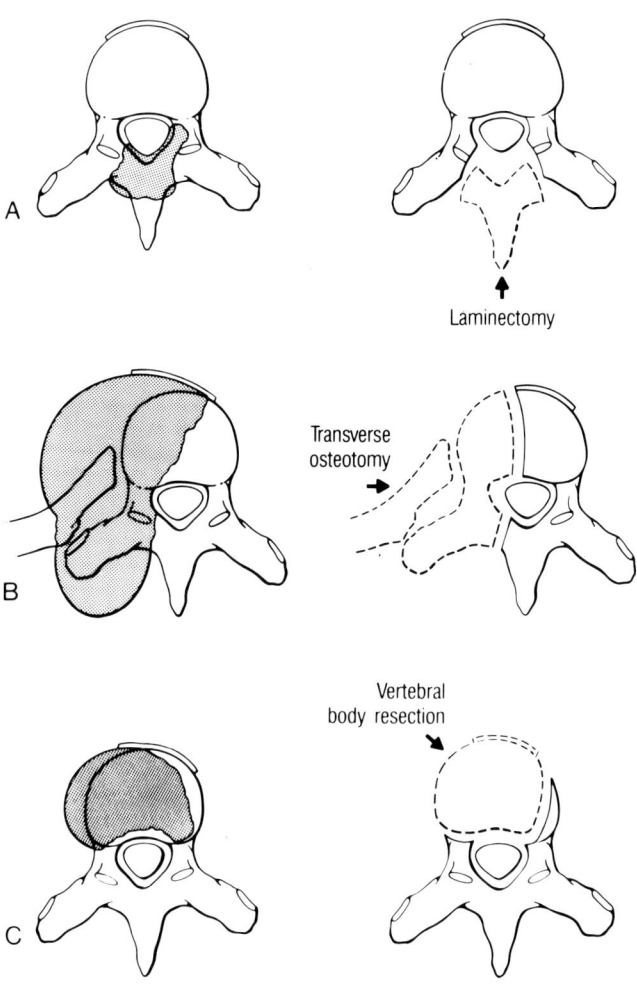

FIGURE 161–1. The three basic approaches to tumor (shaded areas) involving the spine.

better prospects for control by local radiotherapy; whereas patients with grade IIC and IID lesions have a poorer prognosis. In all patients, we believe that spinal CT should follow myelography to determine the actual extent of tumor.

In patients with hypervascular tumors, spinal angiography may be indicated to diminish tumor vascularity, demonstrate feeding vessels, and determine the location of critical spinal arterial supply, such as the artery of Adamkiewicz.[7] Various therapeutic agents can be used for presurgical embolization. Temporary materials (such as autologous clot, gelatin foam, and microfibrillar collagen) are easy to handle, are associated with minimal risk of permanent damage, and are used for temporary embolization until operative resection is scheduled within several days. Permanent materials include polyvinyl alcohol foam (Ivalon) in particulate form, silicone sheeting spheres, silicone polymers, and absolute alcohol. Particles of Ivalon (150–500 μ in diameter) are mixed with solutions of warmed saline and radiographic contrast in proportions designed to produce a liquid slurry of a concentration and viscosity appropriate to the lesion. In our experience, patients with primary tumors, metastases from the kidneys or thyroid, and sarcomas have been safely embolized, resulting in lowered morbidity from intraoperative blood loss. In addition to Ivalon, absolute alcohol can also be used as a sclerosing agent for permanent tumor necrosis before surgery.

INDICATIONS FOR SURGERY

Attempts to define absolute indications for surgery are hampered by the fact that treatment must be individualized in many patients. A knowledge of important prognostic factors may be helpful in the decision-making process. In most series, the site of the primary tumor and histologic type, as well as the pretreatment neurologic deficit are considered the most important pretreatment variables.[8, 9] For optimum results, surgeons therefore should seek intervention in patients who are ambulatory; there is little purpose in subjecting paraplegic or near-paraplegic patients to extensive surgery. Patients who have rapidly evolving deficits (less than 24 hours) probably are destined to have a poor outcome regardless of therapy, especially if the deficits progress on high dose steroid therapy. Patients with structural abnormalities (instability, retropulsed bone fragments, acute collapse of the vertebral body) do not respond to radiotherapy alone, because compression of the neural elements results from bone. The extent of myelographic block (complete versus incomplete) has been noted to be an important factor, but we believe that this is true only if patients with extensive paraspinal masses are excluded. Patients who respond favorably to steroid therapy also are likely to respond to therapy.

Finally, the phase in the cancer patient's illness in which treatment is undertaken is important. Patients with advanced widespread disease and those who have failed previous treatments are much less likely to respond to surgery. With these generalizations, we believe that radiotherapy and steroid therapy are the treatment of choice in the following conditions: (1) patients with advanced systemic metastases such that survival is measured in weeks; (2) patients with lymphoma and other round cell malignancies, such as neuroblastoma and Ewing's sarcoma; and (3) patients with breast and prostate cancer without structural abnormalities of the spine. In all other patients with spinal metastases, neurosurgical evaluation should be sought. Because the goal of therapy in any individual patient may differ, we have classified indications for surgery along five major categories: cancer therapy, stabilization, neurologic salvage, tissue diagnosis, and pain relief.

CANCER THERAPY

In patients with primary osseous neoplasms, localized paraspinal tumors with direct spine involvement, and solitary sites of relapse, local treatment has a major bearing on overall survival.[10, 11] Other patients with pathologic compression fractures and radioresistant tumors, such as kidney cancer with limited systemic disease, also fall into this category. In these patients, the extent of epidural extension and the presence or absence of neurologic deficit have little bearing on the timing of surgery; rather, the goal of surgery should be maximal reduction of tumor bulk.

STABILIZATION

A second but especially major goal of surgery is the restoration or maintenance of stability of the spine involved by tumor. Patients with fracture-dislocations, localized kyphosis, or collapsed vertebrae with retropulsion of a bone fragment may require operative decompression in conjunction with radiotherapy.[12-16] In these patients, the radiosensitivity of the primary tumor has little bearing on the indication for therapy. A major subgroup of patients in this category have segmental instability of the spine that is clinically manifest by pain aggravated by movement, and is usually seen after radiotherapy. Plain roentgenograms may show progressive collapse of the vertebral bodies, or MRI may show retropulsion of bony elements with a local kyphosis. Surgical reduction of movement across this motion segment generally results in prompt relief of pain. This goal can be accomplished by anterior stabilization after vertebral body resection or by posterior stabilization with or without instrumentation.

NEUROLOGIC SALVAGE

For patients who have an acutely evolving deficit, surgery offers the potential of neurologic palliation, even though it may have little impact on overall survival. Similarly, patients who deteriorate while undergoing radiotherapy or those who cannot receive further radiotherapy may be relieved for several months by surgical decompression. In such patients, the goal of therapy is more limited because it is being performed for salvage. Because these patients have received both radiotherapy and prolonged steroid therapy, morbidity from extensive operative procedures may be considerable, and more limited decompression by posterior or posterolateral approaches may be appropriate.[17-19] In our experience, local tumor recurrence is inevitable in almost all patients 1 year after resection.

Table 161-1. SYNDROMES OF SPINAL METASTASES

Clinical Manifestations	Myelographic Findings
Asymptomatic	Varying degrees of intraspinal extension
Back pain, no deficit	Intraosseous or epidural disease
Neurologic deficit; stable on steroids	Varying degrees of epidural block
Neurologic deficit; unstable on steroids	Complete block; unstable spine

Table 161-3. CLASSIFICATION OF ANTERIOR SPINAL APPROACHES

Segment	Levels	Approach
Cervical	C1-C2	Transoral, transmandibular
	C3-C7	Transcervical (Cloward)
Cervicothoracic	C7-T1	Transsternal, transthoracic
Thoracic	T3-T10	Transthoracic, posterolateral thoracotomy
Thoracolumbar	T11-L1	Transthoracic, extrapleural, thoracoabdominal
Lumbar	L2-L4	Retroperitoneal
Lumbosacral	L5-S1	Transabdominal
Sacral	S2-S5	Extra- or intra-abdominal, transperineal

sented earlier, we believe it is useful to classify the various syndromes into four major categories (Table 161-1). Because most patients are promptly treated with high-dose corticosteroid therapy after their diagnosis, the deficits represent assessments made after high-dose corticosteroid therapy and serve as a guide to the need for emergency versus urgent treatment. Tumors in asymptomatic patients with spinal involvement are generally detected during myelography performed for the evaluation of posterior mediastinal or retroperitoneal tumors—for example, neurogenic tumors of the posterior mediastinum, superior sulcus tumors, and paraspinal sarcomas. In patients with solid tumors, radionuclide bone scanning or MRI may identify spine involvement when the study is performed as a routine staging procedure; such spinal involvement may be unifocal or multifocal. Other patients may have back pain alone with minor neurologic deficits, such as radiculopathy. The back pain frequently may resolve on high-dose corticosteroid therapy. At the time of myelography, the major question is whether epidural extension of the tumor is present; currently, patients with purely intraosseous tumors are treated with systemic therapy whenever possible, whereas those with epidural extension are often given emergency radiotherapy. Patients with neurologic deficits may be ambulatory or nonambulatory. We propose that neurologic deficits be classified as stable or unstable on steroid therapy; in view of the current emphasis on ambulation as the major endpoint of therapy, these deficits may be further subclassified on the basis of ambulatory status (Tables 161-2 and 161-3).

RADIOLOGIC EVALUATION

Accurate radiologic assessment of the spinal segments involved, including bone and soft tissue components, as well

Table 161-2. CLASSIFICATION OF NEUROLOGIC DEFICIT

Status	
Ambulatory	Normal neurologic examination
	Radiculopathy
	Plexopathy
Nonambulatory	Pain only, compression fracture, unstable spine
	Radiculopathy
	Plexopathy
	Cauda equina compression
	Paraparesis—mild, moderate, severe
	Other causes—e.g., Brown-Séquard syndrome, ataxia

as the extent of systemic metastases may require several days. To a large extent, the pace of radiologic evaluation should be based on the urgency of treatment, but every effort should be made to obtain as complete an evaluation as possible. Plain roentgenography, involving spot films, should preferably be the initial study. Classic signs of spinal metastases include (1) vertebral collapse, (2) destruction of the pedicle, (3) lytic destruction or focal osteopenia, and (4) malalignment of the spine. In patients with normal x-ray study results, the decision to perform the next procedure is generally based on the evolving neurologic deficit—patients with paraparesis generally undergo myelography, whereas those with pain alone may be further evaluated by MRI, CT, or radionuclide bone scans. Radionuclide bone scans are particularly useful in demonstrating multifocal versus unifocal involvement.

Myelography is recommended in most patients with spinal metastases for several reasons: it is currently the most accurate test for distinguishing intraosseous from epidural disease; discontinuous epidural blocks may be seen in 10 percent of patients, especially those with breast cancer, lymphoma, or prostate cancer; other causes of spinal pain and neurologic deficits in the cancer population may be diagnosed; proper identification of epidural extension allows planning of treatment portals for radiotherapy; and finally, the residual dye can be used for refluoromyelography to assess the effectiveness of therapy. Myelography is not suggested for patients with unstable spines and may be dispensed with for those with adequate demonstration of the subarachnoid space by MRI.[6] If a complete block is identified, the upper limits of the block should be identified by a C1-C2 puncture. Patients with complete block commonly show some degree of neurologic deterioration after lumbar puncture; therefore, all patients with epidural extension of tumor should be treated with an intravenous bolus of dexamethasone (Decadron), 20 to 100 mg, after the myelography procedure; this should be followed by doses every 6 hours of intravenous corticosteroid therapy. Based on myelographic extension, spinal metastases can be classified into varying grades depending on the extent of myelographic block: grade I = intraosseous only; grade IIA = minimal epidural extension (0 to 25 percent); grade IIB = moderate epidural extension (25 to 75 percent); grade IIC = high grade (75 to 100 percent); and grade IID = paraspinal tumor with varying degrees of epidural extension. These subclassifications are offered for two reasons: patients with grade I lesions have

CHAPTER 161

Surgical Management of Primary and Metastatic Tumors of the Spine

Narayan Sundaresan
James E. O. Hughes
George V. DiGiacinto

During the past decade, improvements in neuroradiologic diagnosis by computed tomography (CT) as well as magnetic resonance imaging (MRI), together with the development of effective multidisciplinary treatment have considerably expanded the role of surgery in the treatment of neoplasms of the spine.[1] The goal of surgery previously was limited largely to providing tissue diagnosis as well as palliation of pain and neurologic deficit by decompressive laminectomy. With the radiologic demonstration that most metastases and primary tumors are ventral to the cord, it is obvious that tumor resection requires exposures of the anterior spine that are not generally familiar to most neurosurgeons. The development of anterolateral exposures in the thoracic and lumbar region have now provided the impetus for more attempts at curative rather than palliative surgery. From the standpoint of the surgical oncologist, the goal of surgery is obtaining local tumor control, as is the case at sites elsewhere. The concept of cure requires in addition a multidisciplinary effort to eradicate overt or silent metastases elsewhere by the use of systemic approaches, such as chemotherapy. In addition to tumor resection, a major goal of surgery is the achievement of stability of the spine. Resected segments may be stabilized either by polymethyl methacrylate and spinal instrumentation or by physiologic bone fusion using autologous bone grafts. With the advent of effective instrumentation, removing an entire vertebra (spondylectomy) in either a staged or a single approach is technically feasible.

INCIDENCE

Involvement of the vertebral column is a relatively common feature of many solid tumors. The propensity for some tumors to metastasize selectively to bone has been termed *osteotropism,* and a clearer understanding of this phenomenon may one day allow efforts to prevent the development of bone metastases. At present, clinical data suggest that 20 to 70 percent of patients with metastatic disease from the breast, lung, prostate, and hematopoietic system have involvement of the axial spine.[2] (The vertebral column consists of the true vertebra in the cervical, thoracic, and lumbar regions, as well as the sacrum.) In most series, four primary sites alone account for more than two thirds of all causes of neoplastic cord compression—breast, lung, hematopoietic system, and prostate.[3-5] Clinically, compression of the spinal cord results from extension of a focus to the vertebral body; other possible mechanisms include direct invasion of the spine from a paraspinal tumor, as well as extension through the intervertebral foramina along the perineurium or its lymphatics without bone involvement. Most oncology centers encounter between 40 and 80 patients with this complication every year; in many surgical series of neoplastic cord compression, involvement of the spine may be the initial feature of malignancy in 10 to 40 percent of the patients. In addition to metastases, primary bone tumors and multiple myeloma frequently involve the spinal column; many retroperitoneal tumors (sarcomas, neuroblastomas) also involve the spine by direct extension. Approximately 1000 bone tumors and 5000 soft part sarcomas are diagnosed each year in the United States, of which approximately 10 percent involve the spine. Using extrapolated data, we estimate that spinal neoplasms currently outrank trauma as the major cause of paraplegia.

CLINICAL PRESENTATION

The typical clinical syndrome of neural compression is easily recognized—more than 90 percent of patients have back pain, which may be associated with a referred or radicular component. The median duration of pain is about 6 weeks, and it may be followed by the subacute onset of neurologic deficits. If undiagnosed, the deficit may evolve to complete paraplegia or quadriplegia with bladder and bowel involvement. Unfortunately, despite the emphasis on early diagnosis, up to 50 percent of patients have severe deficits at initial examination, and 10 percent of patients have acute onset of weakness (less than 24 hours), whereas 10 to 20 percent deteriorate either before or shortly after undergoing conservative treatment (radiotherapy).

Because spinal involvement may result in an array of clinical manifestations other than the classical presentation pre-

cord due to missiles, in DeBakey ME, Spurling RG, Woodhall B (eds): American Lecture Series, Publication No. 23. Springfield, Charles C Thomas, 1948, pp 1–64
26. Romanick PC, Smith TK, Kopaniky DR, Oldfield D: Infection about the spine associated with low-velocity missile injury to the abdomen. J Bone Joint Surg Am 67:1195–1201, 1985
27. Tracy PT, Wright RM, Hanigan WC: Magnetic resonance imaging of spinal injury. Spine 14(3):292–301, 1989
28. Barros TE, Oliveira RP, Rosemberg LA, Magalhaes AC: Hemisection of the cervical spinal cord caused by a stab wound: MR findings. AJR Am J Roentgenol 158(6):1413, 1992
29. Moreno-Cabral CE, Mitchell RS, Miller DC: Manual of Postoperative Management in Adult Cardiac Surgery. Baltimore, Williams & Wilkins, 1988
30. Pasteyer J, Signor MB, Honnart F: Anesthesie et reanimation chirurgicale dans la chirurgie du rachis cervical avec troubles neurologiques. Ann Anesthesiol Fr 15:1A–8A, 1974
31. Bracken MB, Shepard MJ, Collins WF, et al: Methylprednisolone or naloxone treatment after acute spinal cord injury: 1-year follow-up data. J Neurosurg 76:23–31, 1992
32. Scarff JE: Injuries of the vertebral column and spinal cord, in Brock S (ed): Injuries of the Brain and Spinal Cord and their Coverings, 4th ed. New York, Springer, 1960, pp 530–589
33. Tindall S, Bierbrauer K: Brain and spinal injuries caused by missiles, in Long DM (ed): Current Therapy in Neurological Surgery, 2nd ed. Philadelphia, BC Decker, 1989, pp 187–190
34. Mariottini A, Delfini R, Ciappetta P, Paolella G: Lumbar disc hernia secondary to gunshot injury. Neurosurgery 15:73–75, 1984
35. Robertson DP, Simpson RK, Narayan RK: Disc herniation due to gunshot wound to the spine. Spine 16:994–995, 1991
36. Braakman R: Traumatic lesions of the spine and spinal cord, in Grossman RG (ed): Principles of Neurosurgery. New York, Raven Press, 1991, pp 447–466
37. Little JW, DeLisa JA: Cauda equina injury: Late motor recovery. Arch Phys Med Rehabil 67:45–47, 1986
38. Ohry A, Rozin R: Acute spinal cord injuries in the Lebanon War. Isr J Med Sci 20:345–349, 1984
39. Rautio J, Paavolainen P: Afghan war wounded: Experience with 200 cases. J Trauma 28(4):523–525, 1988
40. Keane JR, Gamal R: Isolated paraplegia from a remote stab wound. Neurosurgery 33:274–276, 1993
41. Wilson TH: Penetrating trauma of colon, cava, and cord. J Trauma 16:411–413, 1976
42. Hassin G, Johnstone K, Carr A: Bullet lesion of the cauda equina. JAMA 66:1001–1003, 1916
43. Isu T, Iwasaki Y, Sasaki H, Abe H: Spinal cord and root injuries due to glass fragments and acupuncture needles. Surg Neurol 23:255–260, 1985
44. Kanavel A: Old injuries of the spinal cord. Surg Gynecol Obstet 26:601–608, 1918
45. Kihtir T, Ivatury R, Simon R, Stahl WM: Management of transperitoneal gunshot wounds of the spine. J Trauma 31:1579–1583, 1991
46. Benzel EC: Penetrating wounds of the spine, in Rengachary SS, Wilkins RH (eds): Neurosurgical Operative Atlas, vol 1. Baltimore, Williams & Wilkins, 1991, pp 397–403
47. Maiman DJ, Larson SJ: Lateral extracavitary approach to the thoracic and lumbar spine. in Rengachary SS, Wilkins RH (eds): Neurosurgical Operative Atlas, vol 2, 1st ed. Baltimore, Williams & Wilkins, 1992, pp 153–161
48. Seelig JM, Becker DP, Miller JD, et al: Traumatic acute subdural hematoma: Major mortality reduction in comatose patients treated within four hours. N Engl J Med 304(25):1511–1518, 1981
49. Schmidek HH, Smith DA: Anterior cervical disc excision in cervical spondylosis, in Schmidek HH, Sweet WH (eds): Operative Neurosurgical Techniques, 2nd ed. Orlando, Grune & Stratton, 1988, pp 1327–1335
50. Green BA, Klose KJ: Acute spinal cord injury: Emergency room care and diagnosis, medical and surgical management, in Green BA, Marshall LF, Gallagher TJ (ed): Intensive Care for Neurological Trauma and Disease. New York, Academic Press, 1982, pp 249–271
51. Barnett HG, Clifford JR, Llewellyn RC: Safety of mini-dose heparin administration for neurosurgical patients. J Neurosurg 47:27–30, 1977
52. Wolf SM: Delayed traumatic myelopathy following transfixion of the spinal cord by a knife blade. J Neurosurg 38:221–225, 1973

complete deficits immediately after a single bullet wound of the cord above the conus.

INCOMPLETE DEFICITS

At present, no convincing proof exists that surgery improves outcome in patients with incomplete deficits after PSI. In several retrospective, nonrandomized studies, improvement rates were similar regardless of whether surgery was performed.[3, 5, 11, 17] However, the possibility that surgery can reduce the risk of arachnoiditis secondary to the presence of necrotic tissue and blood or can reduce the incidence of chronic pain syndromes has yet to be determined.

CAUDA EQUINA INJURIES

With respect to penetrating injury limited to the cauda equina, including patients with both complete and incomplete deficits, five civilian studies have reported improvement in 47 to 100 percent of surgically treated patients.[2, 5, 6, 11, 17] Cybulski and colleagues[2] found that in a series of 88 civilians with gunshot injuries to the conus or cauda equina, 10 of 29 patients with complete deficits had partial neurologic recovery after laminectomy and debridement. Based on these results, the authors advocate operative intervention for patients with cauda equina injuries, even when they have complete deficits on initial presentation. There seems little doubt that cauda equina injuries have a more favorable prognosis than do other types of PSI.[5, 37] However, how much surgery enhances this improvement remains to be clarified.

COMPLICATIONS

A 5 to 10 percent complication rate has been reported for the surgical management of PSI.[5, 33] Complications include infection, CSF fistulae, pseudomeningocele formation, and iatrogenic worsening of neurologic deficit. Spinal instability and delayed myelopathy following PSI are uncommon but not rare.[9, 52] In three series of civilian PSI, the complication rate was relatively higher in patients subjected to surgery, and 16 to 22 percent of patients developed postoperative meningitis, wound infections, CSF leakage, spinal instability, or pseudomeningocele.[3-5] Postoperative complications may be minimized by strict patient selection, the use of appropriate antibiotics, and careful surgical technique. Three recent civilian series have reported zero percent surgical mortality (defined as death within 30 days of operation).[2, 6, 18]

SUMMARY

The role of surgical intervention in PSI has yet to be examined by a prospective, randomized study. Therefore, the surgeon must depend on personal prejudices, anecdotal data, and retrospective series in management planning. Surgical intervention seems to be beneficial in patients with cauda equina injuries, those with radicular pain due to the presence of bullet or bone fragments, those with spinal instability, and possibly in those with partially preserved neurologic function. In patients with complete cord injuries, the value of surgery is less clear. The overall risk/benefit ratio of surgery in PSI remains to be defined.

Acknowledgment

The authors would like to thank Roberta Abbott for her editorial assistance.

REFERENCES

1. Sights WP: Ballistic analysis of shotgun injuries to the central nervous system. J Neurosurg 31:25–33, 1969
2. Cybulski G, Stone J, Kant R: Outcome of laminectomy for civilian gunshot injuries of the terminal spinal cord and cauda equina: Review of 88 cases. Neurosurgery 24:392–397, 1989
3. Simpson RK, Venger BH, Narayan RK: Penetrating spinal injuries, in Blaisdell FW, Trunkey DD (eds): Craniospinal Trauma. New York, Thieme Medical Publishers, 1990, pp 197–212
4. Heiden JS, Weiss MH, Rosenberg AW, et al: Penetrating gunshot wounds of the cervical spine in civilians: Review of 38 cases. J Neurosurg 42:575–579, 1975
5. Stauffer ES, Wood RW, Kelly EG: Gunshot wounds of the spine: The effects of laminectomy. J Bone Joint Surg Am 61A:389–392, 1979
6. Robertson DP, Simpson RK: Penetrating injuries restricted to the cauda equina: A retrospective review. Neurosurgery 31:265–270, 1992
7. Kraus JF: Injury to the head and spinal cord—the epidemiological relevance of the medical literature published from 1960 to 1978. J Neurosurg 53:S3–S10, 1980
8. Griffin MR, Opitz JL, Kurland LT, et al: Traumatic spinal cord injury in Olmsted County, Minnesota, 1935–1981. Am J Epidemiol 121:884–895, 1985
9. Miller CA: Penetrating wounds of the spine, in Wilkins RH, Rengachary SS (eds): Neurosurgery, vol 2. New York, McGraw Hill, 1985, pp 1746–1748
10. Finuf P: Traumatic spinal cord injuries in Texas: 1991–1992. In: Bureau of Epidemiology, Texas Dept. of Health, 1993:
11. Six E, Alexander E, Kelly DL Jr, et al: Gunshot wounds to the spinal cord. South Med J 72:699–702, 1979
12. Thakur RC, Mittal RS, Khosla VK: Spinal subarachnoid hematoma after stab injury of the cauda equina. S Afr J Surg 28:21–23, 1990
13. Peacock WS, Shrosbee RB, Key AD: A review of 450 stab wounds of spinal cord. S Afr Med J 51:961–964, 1977
14. Cabezudo JM, Carrillo R, Areitio E, et al: Accidental stab wound of the cervical spine from in front. Acta Neurochir (Wien) 53:175–180, 1980
15. Thakur RC, Khosla VK, Kak VK: Non-missile penetrating injuries of the spine. Acta Neurochir (Wien) 113:144–148, 1991
16. Guttmann L: Gunshot injuries of spinal cord, in Guttmann L (ed): Spinal Cord Injuries: Comprehensive Management and Research, 2nd ed. Oxford, Blackwell Scientific Publications, 1976, pp 177–187
17. Yashon D, Jane JA, White RJ: Prognosis and management of spinal cord and cauda equina bullet injuries in sixty-five civilians. J Neurosurg 32:163–170, 1970
18. Benzel EC, Hadden TA, Coleman JE: Civilian gunshot wounds to the spinal cord and cauda equina. Neurosurgery 20:281–285, 1987
19. Lipschitz R: Stab wounds of the spinal cord. Handbook Clin Neurol 25:197–207, 1976
20. Carey ME: Brain and spinal wounds caused by missiles, in Long DM (ed): Current Therapy in Neurological Surgery. Toronto, BC Decker, 1985, pp 114–117
21. Fischer DK, Simpson RK, Narayan RK, Mattox KL: Shielding of the spinal cord by cervical and facial structures. Neurochirurgia (Stuttg) 34:37–41, 1991
22. Venger BH, Simpson RK, Narayan RK: Neurosurgical intervention in penetrating spinal trauma with associated visceral injury. J Neurosurg 70:514–518, 1989
23. Jacobson SA, Bors E: Spinal cord injury in Vietnamese combat. Paraplegia 7:263–281, 1970
24. Lovass ME, Castillo RG, Deutschman CS: Traumatic subarachnoid-pleural fistula. Neurosurgery 17:650–652, 1985
25. Matson DD: The treatment of acute compound injuries of the spinal

At times, dorsal dural defects may require patch grafting for complete closure. In general, it is preferable to use autologous fascia for this procedure. When this material is not readily available, lyophilized dura may be employed. Ventral dural rents, which are inaccessible from the posterior approach, are best left alone. Facet joint integrity should be preserved whenever possible so that spinal stability remains uncompromised.

OTHER APPROACHES

Anterolateral lesions (see Figure 160–6A) and those exclusively involving the ventral dural sac can be approached in several different ways, including the anterior approach to the cervical spine,[49] and the anterior, anterolateral (Fig. 160–9), posterolateral, and lateral extracavitary approaches to the thoracic and lumbar spine (Fig. 160–10). These last approaches are infrequently indicated; furthermore, they offer only suboptimal dural exposure. Therefore, injuries requiring ventral dural closure are relatively complicated and may require a fat pack followed by a fascial repair using fascia lata. A lumbar drain is then used for at least a week.

WOUND CLOSURE

The wound should be closed with absorbable sutures and in multiple layers. A tight closure minimizes the incidence of subsequent CSF leaks. However, the mainstay of treatment for minor CSF leaks is a lumbar drain, which reduces CSF pressure and diverts its flow until the dural defect heals.

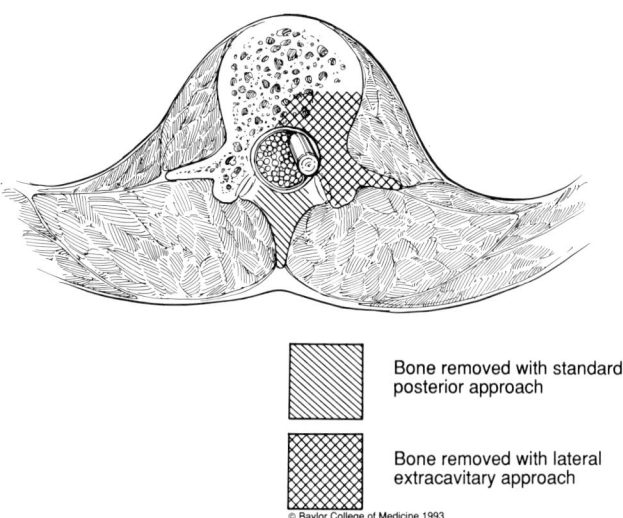

Figure 160–10. A standard posterior laminectomy (single hatch) is appropriate for most dorsal compressive lesions (including those shown in Figures 3A, 3B, and 6B) and some ventrolateral lesions in the lumbar spine. If necessary, extra exposure may be gained by drilling down the pedicle at the level of injury. Alternatively, a lateral extracavitary approach may be used.[46] For the latter, a longitudinal skin incision is made along the lateral margin of the erector spinae muscles, and dissection is carried in an anteromedial direction. The transverse process, pedicle, and apophyseal joint at that level are then removed. Likewise, a standard posterior approach may be used for many penetrating injuries to the thoracic spine. Occasionally, however, for a strictly ventral or ventrolateral lesion, a lateral extrapleural (modified costotransversectomy) approach is indicated. (Copyright © 1993, Baylor College of Medicine.)

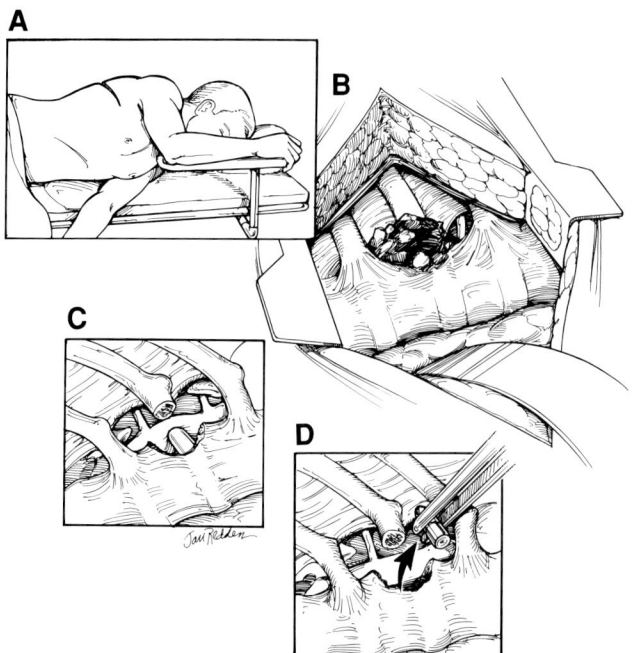

Figure 160–9. (A to D) The anterolateral approach to the thoracic spine first involves placing the patient in the strict lateral position. Starting in the midaxillary line, a skin incision is made and carried posteriorly, centered over the interspace that is one level above the level of interest. A standard thoracotomy is performed. After self-retaining retractors are placed, the lung is collapsed and packed off. After resecting the posterior 5 to 10 cm of the rib at the injured level, the head of the rib is drilled away. The pleura is then opened, and the spine is exposed. (Copyright © 1993, Baylor College of Medicine.)

POSTOPERATIVE MANAGEMENT

All patients with PSI should be followed up carefully to prevent, detect, and treat complications as they arise. A standard care protocol for acute spinal cord injury is used.[50] Special attention is directed to pulmonary, urinary, and skin care in patients with neurologic impairment. In paraplegic or quadriplegic patients, minidose heparin should be considered for the prevention of deep vein thrombosis.[51] Rehabilitation efforts should be initiated as soon as possible in all patients.

RESULTS

After PSI, the prognosis for neurologic recovery correlates highly with the severity of the initial deficit.[4, 11, 17]

COMPLETE DEFICITS

The prognosis is generally poor for patients with immediate, complete deficits following PSI; therefore, these patients are generally not considered to be surgical candidates. In a series by Yashon and coworkers,[17] no marked improvement was observed in either operated or nonoperated civilians with

SURGICAL TECHNIQUES

DORSAL APPROACH

In most PSI cases, a dorsal exposure of the spine is used. At any level of the spine, a vertical midline incision, subperiosteal exposure, and laminectomy are performed (Fig. 160–8A). For a dorsal compressive injury without dural penetration, the offending missile or missiles may be removed after adequate bone removal. If an intradural exploration is indicated, the traumatically incurred dural tear is extended or a longitudinal dural incision is made to expose the injured cord (Fig. 160–8B). If an intramedullary mass and a corresponding neurologic deficit are present, a midline myelotomy is appropriate. When the myelotomy is performed, special care should be exercised to stay strictly in the midline and thereby prevent injury to the posterior columns. Hematoma removal then follows (Fig. 160–8C). Dural closure should be performed without compromise of the intradural contents (Fig. 160–8D). Accessible dural tears should also be closed.

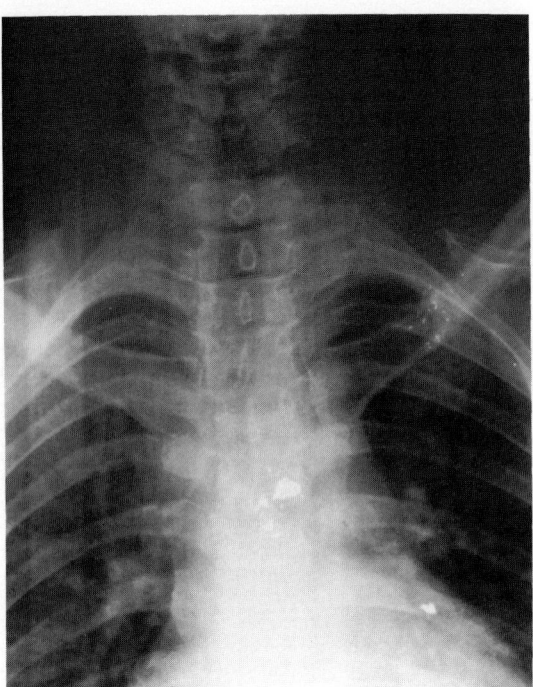

Figure 160–7. Anteroposterior plain radiograph of the lower cervical and upper thoracic spine in a 36-year-old woman who was rendered immediately paraplegic following a gunshot wound to the midthoracic spine. Bullet fragments are present in the midline at the T5-T6 level.

within 3 days of injury did not result in a higher neurologic improvement rate than did surgery performed later.[2] Therefore, some investigators suggest that most surgical candidates undergo delayed surgery, that is, later than 7 days after injury.[46, 47] Contrary to the sentiment supporting delayed surgical intervention for PSI are the data relating to head injury, which support rapid evacuation of intracranial hematomas as the best way to reduce neural injury and to optimize recovery.[48] However, the head injury experience may not be directly applicable to spinal pathophysiology.

AIDS TO SURGERY

NEUROPHYSIOLOGIC MONITORING

Although intraoperative evoked potential monitoring (primarily somatosensory evoked potentials) is believed by some to be useful in certain types of spinal surgery, its value in the management of patients with PSI has not been demonstrated.[46, 47]

INSTRUMENTATION

In the occasional case of spinal instability secondary to PSI, instrumentation-fusion may be indicated. At present, no clear consensus exists as to the timing of this procedure, and each case should be individually considered. In the presence of potential or apparent contamination of the wound, the implantation of foreign material is usually deferred.

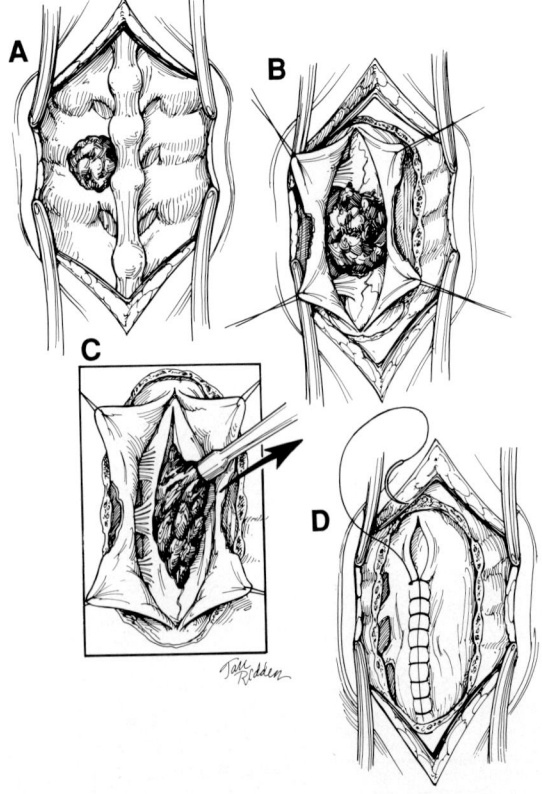

Figure 160–8. (A) The dorsal approach to the cervical region begins with subperiosteal dissection of paraspinous muscles from the laminae, extending a couple of levels above and below the injured level. The normal laminae above and below are exposed first, and then exposure at the level of injury is accomplished with careful dissection. This is to prevent (1) inadvertent injury to herniated neural tissue and (2) bone fragments or surgical instruments from being accidentally pushed into the bony defect. (B) After completing the laminectomy, the dura is opened and the cord is exposed at the level of injury. (C) To adequately expose an intramedullary hematoma, it is often necessary to perform a dorsal midline myelotomy. The clot may then be evacuated. (D) Using continuous sutures, a watertight dural closure is performed. A dural graft may be needed. (Copyright © 1993, Baylor College of Medicine.)

resulted from radicular artery laceration. Eleven months later, the patient was able to ambulate with single-crutch assistance.

Progressive Neurologic Deficit

A worsening result on neurologic examination is an uncommon clinical feature of civilian PSI.[3, 4, 16, 17] When neurologic deterioration does occur, prompt surgical intervention may be indicated.[2, 38, 41] However, in two civilian series, surgery performed for such deterioration did not result in significant postoperative improvement.[4, 17] Despite this lack of success, some authors still consider progression of a deficit to be a surgical indication.[4] If, in this setting, a compressive lesion is demonstrated on imaging studies, surgery is indicated. Conversely, in the absence of a compressive lesion, enthusiasm for surgical intervention is low.

Radicular Pain With or Without Neurologic Deficit

Patients with retained missile or bone fragments may or may not have a significant neurologic deficit but can develop a disabling radicular pain syndrome. In this patient population, several reports, as well as our own experience, have indicated that significant pain relief may follow removal of retained compressive fragments.[6, 42–44] The following case report supports this observation.

Case Report

CASE REPORT 3

A 36-year-old woman suffered complete T7 paraplegia after a gunshot wound to the midthoracic region. Plain radiographs demonstrated intracanalicular bullet fragments at the T5-T6 level (Fig. 160–7) that appropriately corresponded to her complaint of severe bilateral thoracic radicular pain. On the day she was admitted, she underwent T4-T7 laminectomies for debridement. Postoperatively, the severity of her radicular pain was markedly reduced. Nevertheless, she continues to complain of some bandlike dysesthesias and pain 4 years after the injury.

Associated Visceral Penetration

Infections rarely occur in PSI patients when small bowel or stomach is also penetrated. After repair of the visceral injury, these patients should receive a short course of antibiotic therapy. Colonic perforations constitute a somewhat greater risk and require more aggressive antibiotic coverage. Although some authors advocate early debridement of intraspinal bone and bullet fragments in patients with associated colon injuries,[26] others support irrigation of the missile track alone and have found no subsequent spinal or paraspinal infectious complications.[45] We do not favor routine neurosurgical intervention in patients with transperitoneal or transintestinal PSI.

TIMING OF SURGERY

Early surgery (that performed within the first 7 days after injury) is associated with a relatively high complication rate that results primarily from infection and CSF leaks.[46] The former often results from contamination incurred at the time of injury; the latter may result from suboptimal wound closure. Those who favor delayed surgery argue that the bacterial inoculum will have decreased by antibiotic administration and the patient's own defense mechanisms. It has also been suggested that during the period immediately after PSI, tissue friability is increased and results in insufficient wound healing. Delayed surgical intervention may also allow time for hematoma liquefaction, thus facilitating evacuation.[46]

Some data suggest that early surgery does not improve neurologic outcome. In a study of 88 gunshot injuries to the terminal cord and cauda equina, laminectomy performed

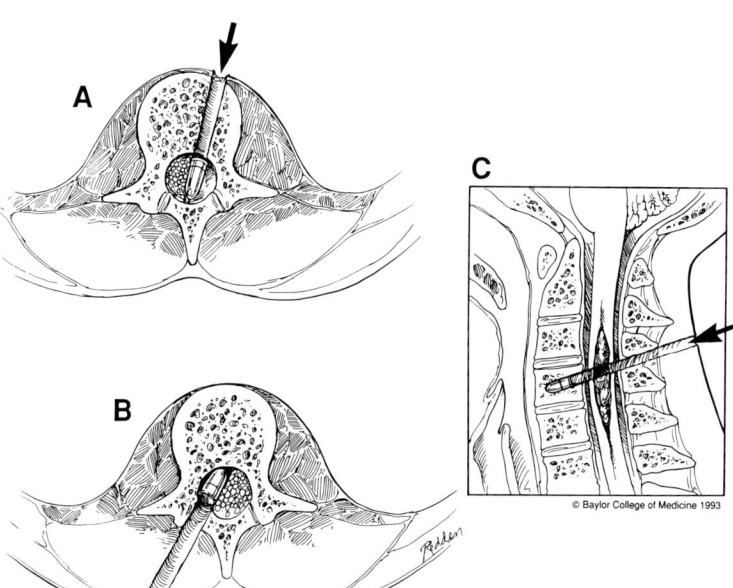

Figure 160–6. (A and B) Gunshot wound to the lumbosacral region resulting in compressive lesions with complete cauda equina deficit. (C) Transection of the cervical spinal cord with an associated intramedullary hematoma following penetrating spinal injury. (Copyright © 1993, Baylor College of Medicine.)

Case Report

CASE REPORT 1

A 28-year-old man suffered complete L1 paraplegia after a high-velocity gunshot wound to the cauda equina. Immediately after the injury, he underwent L1-L2 laminectomies for debridement. Subsequently, he progressively regained lower extremity strength. On his 6-month postoperative examination, he was able to ambulate independently. However, shortly thereafter, he developed an intractable left lower extremity pain syndrome. Myelography and postmyelographic CT scan revealed extensive scarring at the level of injury. After T11-L2 laminectomies with lysis of extradural and intradural adhesions, the severity of pain was significantly reduced. Approximately 18 months later, the patient developed frequent left leg dysesthesias, for which a dorsal column stimulator was placed. This device afforded good pain relief, which was still evident at 3 years when he returned for a battery change.

Although no randomized study has conclusively proved the benefit of surgery in this injury group, there appears to be a consensus on the value of surgery for patients with cauda equina injuries.

Neurologic Deficit without Radiographic Abnormality

Wartime experience has shown that shrapnel and high-velocity missile PSI may cause neural damage by concussive effects without associated canal penetration.[16, 38, 39] Such concussive forces are less likely to occur from weapons typically used for civilian PSI. With such injuries, local wound and supportive care are indicated.

Case Report

CASE REPORT 2

Paraplegia immediately followed a stab wound to a young man's right flank in the posterior axillary line at the T10 level.[40] All sensory modalities were spared. Plain radiography, CT, and MRI of the thoracolumbar spine failed to demonstrate any evidence of canal penetration or nerve root damage. It was presumed that spinal cord infarction

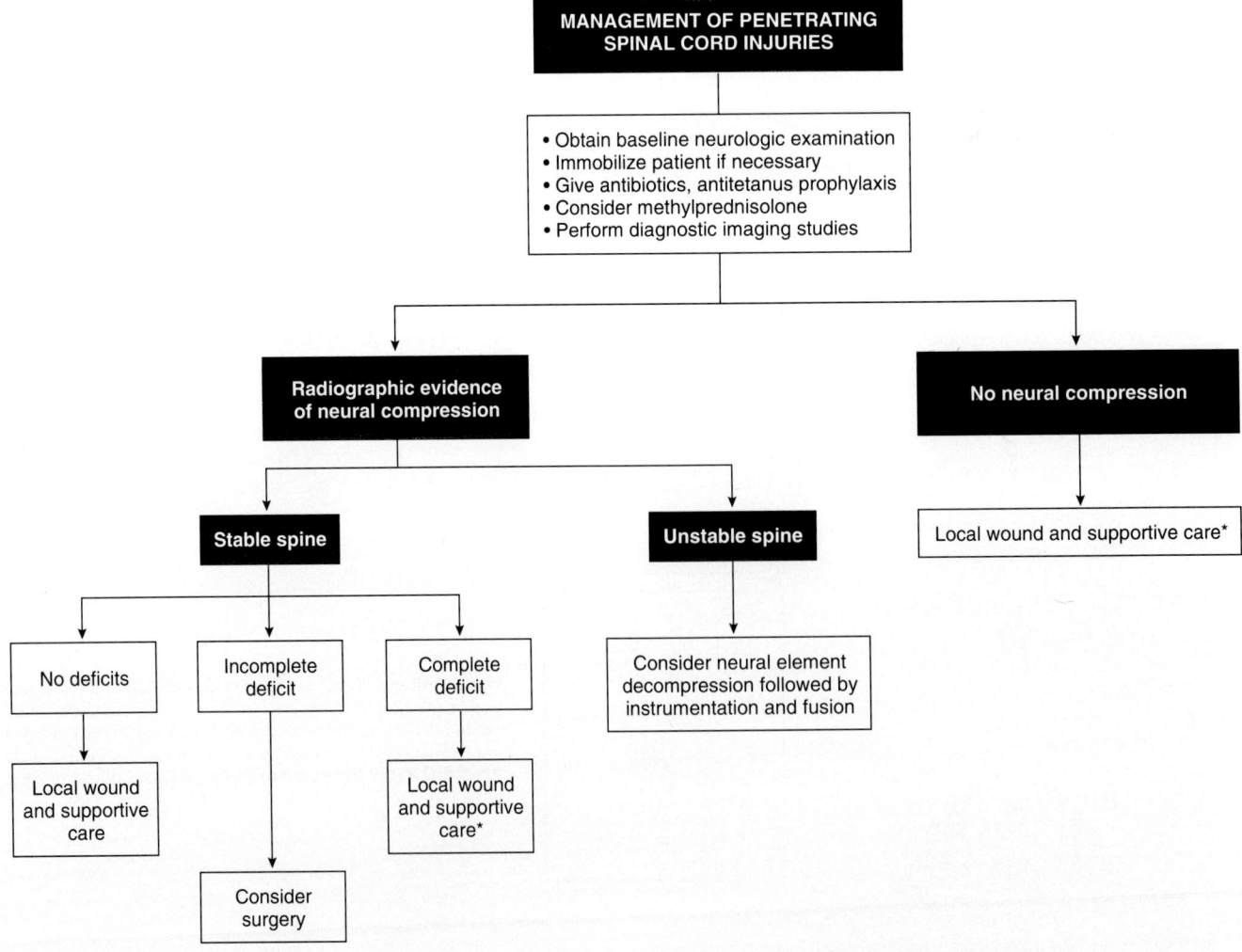

*If neurologic deterioration, CSF leak, or infection occurs, consider repeating imaging studies and/or surgical intervention

Figure 160–5. Management of penetrating spinal cord injury.

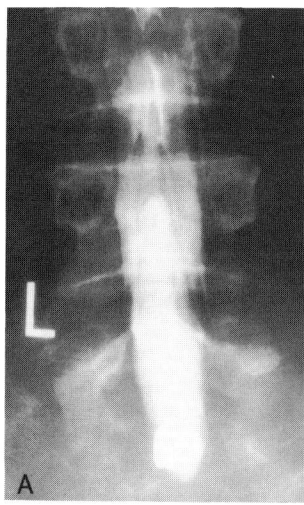
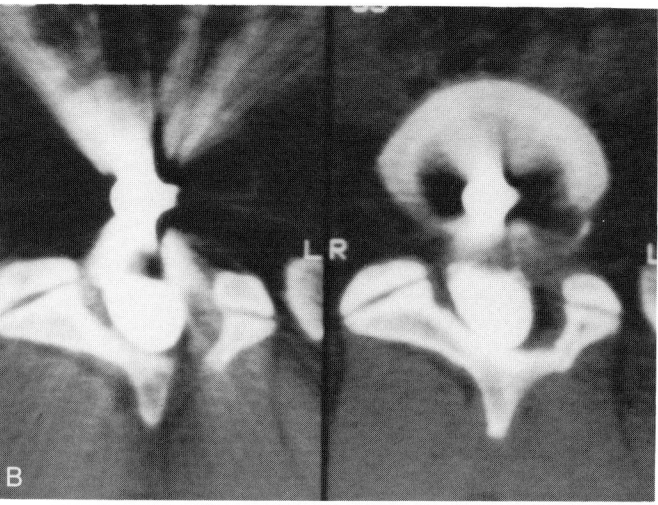

Figure 160–4. (A and B) Myelogram and postmyelogram CT scans of the lower lumbar spine in a 44-year-old man who had left L5 radiculopathy immediately following a gunshot wound. He refused surgical intervention. Seven months after the injury, examination showed continued improvement in his mild radiculopathy.

After intubation is accomplished, the patient is ready for positioning on the operating table. With a cooperative patient, it may be preferable to position with the patient awake, so that subsequent examination may detect any change in neurologic status. For a posterior operative approach, the patient must be turned into the prone position. When a patient with spinal instability is turned, a rigid cervical collar is useful, although it does not afford complete immobility. Therefore, manually applied traction should also be used in such instances. Intraoperatively, adequate spinal cord perfusion, which is primarily dependent on systemic perfusion pressure, must be maintained. Postoperatively, after anesthesia is reversed, immediate extubation should be considered only for patients with

1. Adequate weaning parameters (respiratory rate <30/minutes; vital capacity >10 ml/kg; inspiratory force > −25 mm Hg; PO_2 > 80 mm Hg; PCO_2 < 45 mm Hg)[29]
2. Cord injury at a level below C5
3. Absence of excessive pulmonary secretions
4. Absence of associated head or chest injury[30]

Prophylactic antibiotics are generally administered before and during surgery, and for 24 to 48 hours after surgery, although their efficacy in PSI has never been conclusively established in a randomized trial. Although early administration of high-dose corticosteroids has been effective in treating closed spinal cord injury, no benefit has been specifically documented for PSI, because these patients were excluded from the National Acute Spinal Cord Injury Study II (NASCIS II).[31]

MANAGEMENT DECISIONS

PATIENT SELECTION AND INDICATIONS FOR SURGERY

The purpose of surgery in PSI is to decompress and debride neural tissue, remove bony or metallic fragments, reestablish dural continuity, correct spinal instability, and relieve pain. Although spinal instability is relevant to the decision-making process, it infrequently results from PSI.[9] Spinal decompression is considered when there is extradural or intradural compression from the missile,[11, 25, 32] bone,[11, 33] disc material,[34, 35] hematoma,[11, 33] or indriven foreign bodies.[17] Often, a combination of these conditions are present. PSI may later be complicated by an infectious process, such as osteomyelitis, diskitis, and abscesses, although these are uncommon.[19] If such a process results in neural compression, surgery may be warranted. The following criteria are intended to represent general guidelines rather than absolute standards.

Complete Deficits

Patients with complete deficits are generally not surgical candidates unless they have associated radiographic evidence of neural compression, gross contamination or infection, persistent CSF leak (i.e., >4 days), or an unstable spine (Fig. 160–5).

Incomplete Deficits

Patients with incomplete deficits may be surgical candidates if they demonstrate a ventral or dorsal compressive injury (Fig. 160–6A and B, respectively), partial spinal cord transection (Fig. 160–6C), associated infection, persistent CSF leak, and/or an unstable spine.

Cauda Equina Lesions

Benzel and colleagues reported that nerve root function improves in almost all patients with CE injuries, regardless of management strategies,[18] possibly because of nerve root sparing and recovery processes that are comparable to those seen after peripheral nerve injuries.[36] This finding has led some investigators to recommend only conservative management,[17, 37] whereas others continue to opt for surgical debridement.[9, 11, 20] In general, we favor surgical intervention for patients with PSI to the cauda equina because surgery allows the removal of blood and other necrotic material that may eventually result in scarring and arachnoiditis. It may also reduce the incidence or severity of chronic pain syndromes. Occasionally, other forms of pain control may be employed. The following case report is one example.

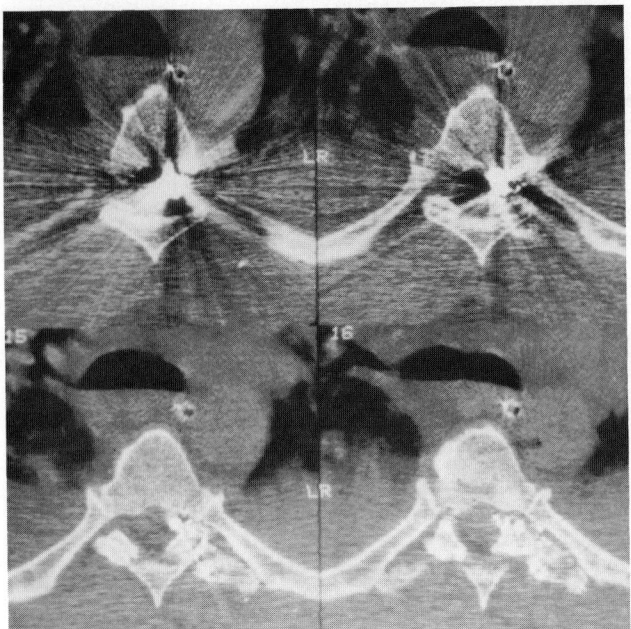

Figure 160–2. Axial CT of the upper thoracic spine that demonstrates intracanalicular bone and bullet fragments. This 54-year-old man was running away from his assailants when he was shot in the back. The bullet entered the interscapular region on the left side at the T5 level, resulting in T6 paraparesis. After a T3-T6 laminectomy with removal of bone and bullet fragments, he had partial, but remarkable, motor and sensory recovery.

1B). These tests may be followed by computed tomography (CT) (Figs. 160–2 and 160–3A and B), myelography (Fig. 160–4A), postmyelographic CT (Fig. 160–4B), or magnetic resonance imaging (MRI).[27, 28] Because of the proximity of the carotid and vertebral arteries to the cervical spine, patients with penetrating injuries in this region should undergo angiography shortly after admission to the hospital. In general, electromyography and nerve conduction studies are not useful diagnostic tools in the acute setting.

PERIOPERATIVE CONSIDERATIONS

Because injury can occur during transport, induction of anesthesia, intubation, or positioning, care should be taken to avoid unnecessary movement of the patient's spine. Patients with cervical injuries may be placed in mechanical traction if instability is present or suspected. In such cases, direct laryngoscopy may result in further neurologic deterioration unless the neck is carefully immobilized. Fiberoptic nasotracheal intubation performed while the patient is awake is the technique of choice whenever cervical spine stability is in question. In patients undergoing emergency surgery, a full stomach is an added hazard during the induction of anesthesia. Factors that predispose to regurgitation include head-down tilt, airway obstruction, intermittent positive-pressure breathing before intubation, and possibly, the use of depolarizing muscle relaxants.

comitant injuries have been reported in approximately 25 percent of civilian cases and in 67 percent of military cases.[23] Indeed, associated neck, chest, or abdominal injuries may take precedence over the spine injury in the initial management of the patient.[5] At times, the diagnosis of an associated abdominal injury may be difficult, especially if the patient is concomitantly intoxicated, head injured, or quadriplegic.

Chest injuries causing hemopneumothorax are the commonest, followed by gastrointestinal and renal lesions. Traumatic subarachnoid-pleural fistulae are uncommon[9, 17, 24] and are generally self-limited. However, they may occasionally require surgical closure of the dural or pleural rent. A missile that has passed through the bowel poses a somewhat higher risk of meningitis, osteomyelitis, or both.[25, 26] Stab wounds to the spine are often aimed haphazardly and occasionally involve other structures. Nonmissile wounds to the lower cervical and thoracic region may penetrate the rib cage and injure the lung, producing a hemothorax, pneumothorax, or hemopneumothorax. Stabs to the lower thoracic or lumbar regions may injure abdominal organs.

PREOPERATIVE EVALUATION

An accurate neurologic examination at admission and subsequent serial observations are of primary importance in the evaluation of a patient with PSI. Before a decision can be made regarding surgical intervention, precise localization of neural and bony injuries is useful. The clinical examination alone, or the observed missile entry and exit points alone, may be misleading. Diagnostic tests begin with plain radiographs of all suspected areas of the spine (Fig. 160–1A and

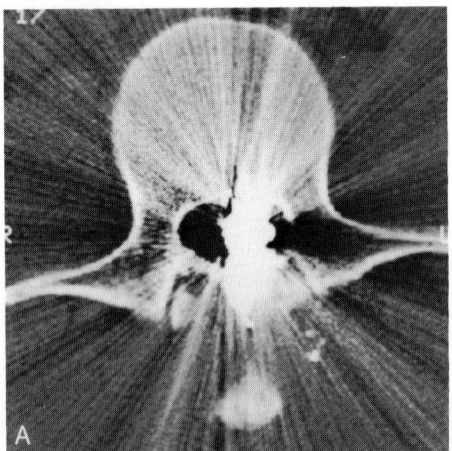

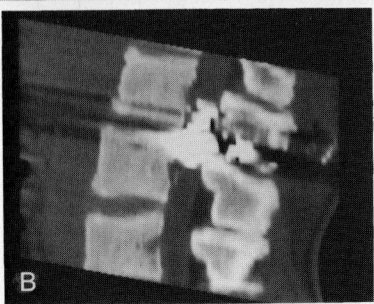

Figure 160–3. (A and B) Axial and sagittally reformatted CT scans of the upper lumbar spine in a 24-year-old man who had a complete L3 paraplegia immediately following penetrating spinal injury. The scans demonstrate the intraspinal location of bone and bullet fragments. After a two-level lumbar laminectomy, removal of indriven fragments, and primary dural closure, the patient regained a unilateral sensory level.

Table 160–1. TYPES OF NEUROLOGIC DEFICITS RESULTING FROM PENETRATING SPINAL INJURIES

Series	Patients (n)	Deficit (%) Complete	Incomplete	CE	Comments
Missile					
Yashon and coworkers[17]	42	88	12	*	Soon after admission, 2 patients deteriorated to develop complete deficits (included in complete group)
Stauffer and coworkers[5]	185	57	43	—	44 of 79 patients with incomplete deficits had injuries to the conus or CE
Six and coworkers[11]	59	49	31	20	—
Benzel and coworkers[18]	35	57	26	17	—
Simpson and coworkers[3]†	142	66	34	—	19% of total patients (M and NM) had lumbosacral or CE injuries
Nonmissile					
Lipschitz[19]	314	33	67	—	Percentage of CE injuries not specified
Peacock and coworkers[13]	450	21	79	—	Percentage of CE injuries not specified
Simpson and coworkers[3]†	18	22	78	—	19% of total patients (M and NM) had lumbosacral or CE injuries

CE = cauda equina; M = missile; NM = nonmissile; PSI = penetrating spinal injury.
*A separate cohort of 23 patients had injuries to the conus or CE.
†Both missile and nonmissile PSI types included in this single series.

wounds to any level of the spine, 49 to 83 percent of patients had complete injuries, 12 to 43 percent had incomplete injuries, and 17 to 20 percent had cauda equina injuries.[3, 5, 11, 17, 18] In separate civilian series of PSI due to nonmissile wounds, only 21 to 33 percent sustained complete injuries, and 67 to 79 percent sustained incomplete injuries (Table 160–1).[3, 13, 19] This comparison of series is limited by the fact that some authors considered injury to the cauda equina as a type of wound location rather than as a distinct type of injury and included these patients under the incomplete and complete deficit group.

CLINICAL FEATURES

WOUND LOCATION

Most missile and nonmissile PSIs involve the thoracic spine, with cervical and lumbosacral levels less frequently affected.[3, 13, 19, 20] This distribution most likely reflects the relative lengths of these cord segments. Factors that determine injury severity include the penetrating object's kinetic energy, the extent of penetration, and the spinal segment involved. The thoracic spine is less mobile than the cervical and lumbar spines and is consequently less likely to become unstable after PSI. In describing four patients who were neurologically intact after penetrating cervical spine trauma, Fischer and colleagues proposed that the cervical spine is somewhat shielded by facial tissues and sinus structures and therefore is relatively less vulnerable to penetrating injuries in the anteroposterior direction.[21]

ASSOCIATED INJURIES

The trajectory of a missile may cause injuries of adjacent musculoskeletal, visceral, or vascular structures.[22] Such con-

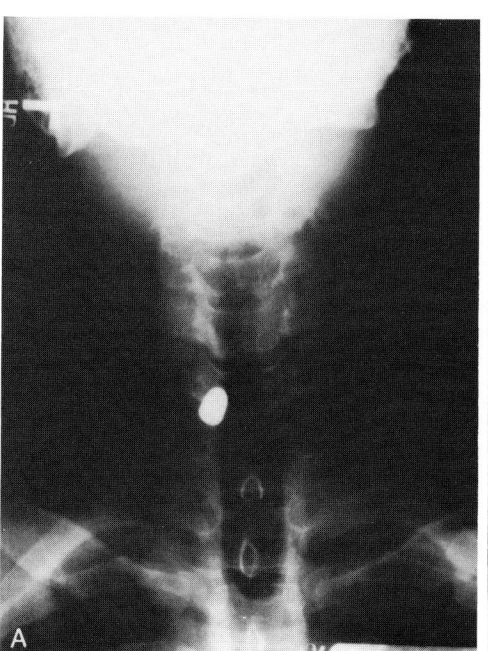
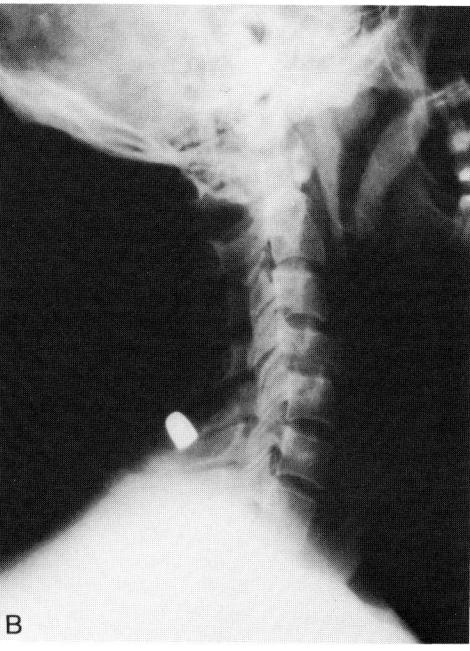

Figure 160–1. (A and B) Anteroposterior and lateral plain radiographs of the cervical spine in a 41-year-old man who was rendered immediately quadriplegic following a gunshot wound to the neck. A large-caliber bullet is present at C5-C6. No surgical intervention was undertaken.

CHAPTER 160

Surgical Management of Penetrating Injuries of the Spine

Cheryl A. Muszynski
Raj K. Narayan

In recent years, the number of penetrating spinal injuries (PSIs) outside of the military arena has increased. In developed countries, most PSIs result from gunshot wounds, and nonmissile injuries are uncommon. Although civilian PSIs have become more commonplace, the optimal treatment in these cases remains controversial. Some authors recommend surgery in most cases, whereas others generally advocate a nonsurgical approach. This dichotomy of opinion stems partly from the fact that PSI is a rather diverse condition, and no single management strategy may be appropriate for every patient. Furthermore, no randomized trial of PSI therapies has ever been conducted, making all of the available data either retrospective or anecdotal.

Since the Korean War, the management of civilian PSI has generally paralleled that of battlefield PSI. Civilian bullets generally have less kinetic energy than high-velocity battlefield missiles, resulting in a lower proportion of concussive-type injuries and a higher percentage of direct cord damage.[1] Military ammunition also causes greater tissue disruption and wound contamination than handgun bullets.[1] However, as the power of civilian weaponry increases, these distinctions between military and civilian PSI are becoming increasingly blurred.

The management controversy is further complicated by the fact that, regardless of the treatment administered, patients with incomplete deficits often experience neurologic improvement, and patients with cord transection rarely show more than a marginal recovery. The potential complications of surgery for PSI are also an important consideration. Some authors have documented the relative safety of surgery for PSI (at least, of the cauda equina),[2] whereas other series suggest a possibly higher complication rate in patients treated surgically.[3-6] When these complications occur, they are generally related to cerebrospinal fluid (CSF) leakage, infection, spinal instability, and iatrogenic neurologic injury.

Thus, the risks and benefits of surgery must be weighed against the potential neurologic improvement expected from conservative management alone. In the absence of a prospective, randomized trial, the relative efficacy of surgical versus nonsurgical therapy in different types of PSI remains unclear. Nevertheless, the following information can help in choosing the optimal management for a given patient.

INCIDENCE

Although reliable nationwide statistics are not available, the annual incidence of spinal cord injuries (SCI) in North America is variously estimated to be 15 to 50 per million population.[7,8] In the United States, approximately 12,000 new cases of SCI occur every year, 50 percent of which result from vehicular collisions and 12 percent from penetrating wounds.[9] These proportions are similar to those of a recently initiated prospective study of traumatic SCI cases in a few key Texas hospitals. Fifty percent of the injuries in the 511 cases recorded in this study resulted from vehicular collisions, and 19 percent resulted from penetrating wounds.[10] As with trauma in general, most patients sustaining PSI are young adults, mostly males aged 21 to 30 years.[3,5,11-13]

Nonmissile PSIs are relatively uncommon in developed countries because of the ready availability of more sophisticated weapons, but they are proportionately commoner in undeveloped countries in which firearms are less accessible.[14,15] While only four cases of stab wounds involving the spinal cord were encountered during a 27-year period at the Stoke Mandeville Spinal Injury Centre in Great Britain,[16] a series of 450 patients with stab wounds of the spinal cord were reported from Cape Town, South Africa, during the 13 years between 1963 and 1976. This latter group of patients with nonmissile PSI comprised over 25 percent of the 1600 patients with SCI admitted during those years.[13]

CLASSIFICATION

Neurologic signs and symptoms relate to the level and severity of the penetrating injury and may include motor or sensory dysfunction with or without loss of sphincter control. Thus, PSI may result in

1. Complete SCI, with loss of sensory, motor and sphincter function below the level of injury
2. Incomplete SCI, whereby some function below the level of injury is spared
3. Cauda equina injuries

In previously reported series of civilians sustaining missile

24. Riseborough EJ: Irradiation induced kyphosis. Clin Orthop 128:101, 1977
25. Smith R, Davidson JK, Flatman GE: Skeletal effects of orthovoltage and megavoltage therapy following treatment of nephroblastoma. Clin Radiol 33:601, 1982
26. Thomas PR, Griffith KD, Fineberg BB, et al: Late effects of treatment for Wilms' tumor. Int J Radiat Oncol Biol Phys 9:651, 1983
27. King J, Stowe S: Results of spinal fusion for radiation scoliosis. Spine 7:574, 1982
28. Daussange J, Rigault P, Renier D, et al: Instability and kyphosis following cervical laminectomy in children. Rev Chir Orthop 66:423, 1980
29. Taddonio RF Jr, King AG: Atlantoaxial rotatory fixation after decompressive laminectomy. A case report. Spine 7:540, 1982
30. Callahan RA, Johnson RM, Margolis RN, et al: Cervical facet fusion for control of instability following laminectomy. J Bone Joint Surg Am 59A:991, 1977
31. Holmes JC, Hall JE: Fusion for instability and potential instability of the cervical spine in children and adolescents. Orthop Clin North Am 9:923, 1978
32. Aung MH: Atlanto-axial dislocation in Down's syndrome. Report of a case with spinal cord compression and review of the literature. Bull Los Angeles Neurol Soc 38:197, 1973
33. Blaw ME, Langer LO: Spinal cord compression in Morquio-Brailsford's disease. J Pediatr 74:593, 1969
34. Brill CB, Rose JS, Godmilow MSW, et al: Spastic quadriparesis due to C1-C2 subluxation in Hurler syndrome. J Pediatr 92:441, 1978
35. Kaplan RJ: Neurological complications of infections of head and neck. Otolaryngol Clin North Am 9:729, 1976
36. Malik GM, Crawford AH, Halter R: Swan-neck deformity secondary to osteomyelitis of the posterior elements of the cervical spine. Case report. J Neurosurg 50:388, 1979
37. McWhorter JM, Alexander E, Davis CH, et al: Posterior cervical fusion in children. J Neurosurg 45:211, 1976
38. Menezes AH, Van Gilder JC, Graf CJ, et al: Craniocervical abnormalities: A comprehensive approach. J Neurosurg 53:444, 1980
39. Nathan FF, Bickel WH: Spontaneous axial subluxation in a child as a first sign of juvenile rheumatoid arthritis. J Bone Joint Surg Am 50A:1675, 1968
40. Sherk HH, Nicholson JT: Rotatory atlanto-axial dislocation associated with ossiculum terminale and mongolism. A case report. J Bone Joint Surg 51A:957, 1964
41. Roy L, Gibson DA: Cervical spine fusions in children. Clin Orthop 73:146, 1970
42. Gilsbach J, Eggert HR: Transoral operations for craniospinal malformations. Neurosurg Rev 61:199, 1983
43. Hall JE, Dennis F, Murray J: Exposure of the upper cervical spine for spinal decompression by a mandible and tongue splitting approach. J Bone Joint Surg 59A:121, 1977
44. Lesoin F, Jomin M, Pellerin P, et al: Transclival transcervical approach to the upper cervical spine and clivus. Acta Neurochir (Wien) 80:100, 1986
45. Hulme A, Dott NM: Spinal epidural abscess. BMJ 1:64, 1954
46. Raimondi AJ, Gutierrez FA, DiRocco C: Laminotomy and total reconstruction of the posterior spinal arch for spinal canal surgery in childhood. J Neurosurg 45:555, 1976
47. Hoffman HJ, Hendrick EB, Humphreys RP: New lumboperitoneal shunt for communicating hydrocephalus. Technical note. J Neurosurg 44:258, 1976
48. Kushner J, Alexander E, Davis CH, et al: Kyphoscoliosis following lumbar subarachnoid shunts. J Neurosurg 34:783, 1971
49. Eisenberg HM, Davidson RI, Shillito J: Lumboperitoneal shunts. Review of 34 cases. J Neurosurg 35:427, 1971
50. Fischer EG, Welch K, Shillito J: Syringomyelia following lumboureteral shunting for communicating hydrocephalus. J Neurosurg 47:96, 1977
51. Welch K, Shillito J, Strand R, et al: Chiari I ''malformation''—an acquired disorder? J Neurosurg 55:604, 1981
52. Hall P, Lindseth R, Campbell R, et al: Scoliosis and hydrocephalus in myelocele patients. J Neurosurg 50:174, 1979
53. Winston K, Hall J, Johnson D, et al: Acute elevation of intracranial pressure following transection of non-functional spinal cord. Clin Orthop 128:41, 1977
54. Moe JH, Winter RB, Bradford DS, et al: Scoliosis and Other Spinal Deformities. Philadelphia, WB Saunders, 1978
55. Drummond D, Guadagno J, Keene JS, et al: Interspinous process segmental spinal instrumentation. J Ped Orthop 4:397, 1984
56. Luque ER: Segmental spinal instrumentation for correction of scoliosis. Clin Orthop 163:192, 1982
57. Cotrel Y, Dubousset J: Personal communication
58. Hall JE, Levine CR, Sudhir KG: Intraoperative awakening to monitor spinal cord function during Harrington instrumentation and spine fusion. Description of procedure and report of three cases. J Bone Joint Surg Am 60A:533, 1978
59. Allen AR, Starr A: Sensory evoked potentials in the operating room. Neurology 27:358, 1977
60. Cohen AR, Young W, Ransohoff J: Intraspinal localization of the somatosensory evoked potential. Neurosurgery 9:157, 1981
61. Machida M, Weinstein SL, Yamada T, et al: Spinal cord monitoring. Electrophysiological measures of sensory and motor function during spinal surgery. Spine 10:407, 1985
62. Mostegl A, Bauer R: The application of somatosensory-evoked potentials in orthopedic spine surgery. Arch Orthop Trauma Surg 103:179, 1984

of the subject can be found in such monographs as that by Moe and colleagues.⁵⁴

The timing of fusion operations is important. Fusion masses do not grow, and deformities may worsen significantly during growth spurts. When a fusion must be performed over many segments, as frequently occurs in patients with idiopathic or paralytic scoliosis, it is often desirable to delay surgery until the patient reaches 10 years of age to allow maximum growth. Attempts to "buy time" with bracing must be monitored closely, and failure to control progression of the deformity is a signal to abandon bracing and recommend surgery, regardless of age. Early operations often are preferable in progressive congenital kyphosis or lordosis because of the possibility of a better result with a limited early procedure, or in radiation-induced kyphosis, in which a high failure rate exists because of poor bone substance. In unilateral defects of segmentation (unilateral bars), no possibility exists of longitudinal growth of the affected segment. Growth of the "normal side" causes only increased deformity, not lengthening of the spine. Serious and progressive spinal deformity and pain frequently follow thoracolumbar fractures that have been subjected to laminectomy without stabilization. Early reduction of deformity and internal fixation by such methods as Harrington instrumentation are considered to give the best chance for root recovery, protection of cord function, and permanent spinal stability.⁵⁴

The type of procedure selected depends on many factors, and more than one procedure may be required. When an anterior compression of the spinal cord is present, as in a sharply angulated kyphosis, anterior decompression is necessary. Anterior release by osteotomy and anterior fusion with inlay grafts is the preferred procedure for treating kyphosis occurring after multiple-level laminectomy and is frequently used in radiation kyphosis, supplemented by Harrington compression rod stabilization posteriorly. Harrington rod instrumentation may be used to provide corrective distraction and may add internal stabilization to many fusions, thereby permitting ambulation in a brace or cast without loss of correction. Lateral curvatures may be corrected by the Dwyer method, which includes lateral compression of the vertebral bodies by a cable apparatus fixed in place with screws, but it is contraindicated in the presence of a kyphosis. The Dwyer method is best used in patients with deficiencies of the posterior spinal elements, as in myelodysplasia.

Recent developments in the stabilization of spinal deformities have included the use of sublaminar or spinous process wires⁵⁵ associated with either Harrington or Luque rods.⁵⁶ The use of these supplemental wires has enabled the operating surgeon to obtain greater stability from the metallic implants, so that many patients can be treated in the postoperative period without outside support by either casts or braces.

An even more recent development from France, known as the Cotrel-Dubousset system of spinal instrumentation, provides even more intrinsic stability and has several types of implants that are useful in the management of idiopathic scoliosis but also in the management of fractures.⁵⁷

It is extremely important that once the deformity has become established or it is apparent that a deformity is inevitable, the orthopedic surgeon who attempts to repair it is familiar with the use of all current methods of instrumentation, because each of them has its merits, and only a surgeon familiar with all of them can decide which is best for any individual patient.

Neurologic deficits can result from Harrington rod distraction in patients with unyielding congenital kyphosis or when the cord is tethered, as in myelomeningocele, diastematomyelia, or thickened filum terminale. A tethered cord must be released before an associated spinal curvature is corrected. Neurologic deficits from operative traction on the spine often can recover to a significant degree if they are considered to be true surgical emergencies, and the traction apparatus is removed immediately. Spinal cord deficits can be detected intraoperatively by awakening the patient to test lower extremity function⁵⁸ or by monitoring posterior column function by cortical or spinal somatosensory evoked potentials.⁵⁹⁻⁶² During anterior operations, neurologic complications can occur because of direct damage to, or subsequent thrombosis of, the anterior spinal artery, or more rarely, because of interruption of the segmental vessels to the cord. If these vessels are ligated in the midline, vascular anastomoses provide adequate collateral circulation. Problems may arise if the final common pathway is interrupted within or near the intervertebral foramen.

REFERENCES

1. Arkin AM, Simon N: Radiation scoliosis, an experimental study. J Bone Joint Surg Am 32A:396, 1950
2. Hass SL: Experimental production of scoliosis. J Bone Joint Surg 21:963, 1939
3. Langenskiold A, Michelsson JE: The pathogenesis of experimental progressive scoliosis. Acta Orthop Scand Suppl 59, 1962
4. Liszka O: Spinal cord mechanisms leading to scoliosis in experimental animals. Acta Med Pol 2:45, 1961
5. Ponsetti IV, Shepard RS: Lesions of the skeleton and of other mesodermal tissues in rats fed sweet-pea (Lathyrus odoratus) seeds. J Bone Joint Surg Am 36A:1031, 1954
6. Schwartzmann JR, Miles M: Experimental production of scoliosis in rats and mice. J Bone Joint Surg 27:59, 1945
7. Caffey J: Pediatric X-Ray Diagnosis, 6th ed. Chicago, Yearbook, 1972
8. Harwood-Nash DC, Fitz CR: Neuroradiology in Infants and Children. St. Louis, CV Mosby, 1976
9. Wolf GL: Safer, more expensive iodinated contrast agents: How do we decide? Radiology 159:557, 1986
10. White RI, Halden WJ Jr: Liquid gold: Low-osmolality contrast media. Radiology 159:559, 1986
11. Tachdjian ME, Matson DD: Orthopedic aspects of intraspinal tumors in infants and children. J Bone Joint Surg Am 47A:225, 1965
12. Audic B, Maury M: Secondary vertebral deformities in childhood and adolescence. Paraplegia 7:11, 1969
13. Cattell HS, Clark GL: Cervical kyphosis and instability following multiple laminectomies in children. J Bone Joint Surg Am 49A:713, 1967
14. Citron N, Edgar MA, Sheehy J, et al: Intramedullary spinal cord tumors presenting as scoliosis. J Bone Joint Surg 66:513, 1984
15. DeSousa AL, Kalsbeck JE, Mealy J, et al: Intraspinal tumors in children. A review of 81 cases. J Neurosurg 51:437, 1979
16. Fraser RD, Paterson DC, Simpson DA: Orthopedic aspects of spinal tumours in children. J Bone Joint Surg Br 59B:143, 1977
17. Lonstein JE: Post-laminectomy kyphosis. Clin Orthop 128:93, 1977
18. Reimer R, Onofrio BM: Astrocytomas of the spinal cord in children and adolescents. J Neurosurg 63:669, 1985
19. Sim FH, Svien HJ, Bickel WH, et al: Swan neck deformity following extensive cervical laminectomy. A review of twenty-one cases. J Bone Joint Surg Am 56A:564, 1974
20. Zajtchuk R, Bowen TE, Seyfer AE, et al: Intrathoracic ganglioneuroblastoma. J Thorac Cardiovasc Surg 80:605, 1980
21. Delinka MK, Mazzeo VR Jr: Complications of radiation therapy. Crit Rev Diagn Imaging 23:235, 1985
22. Katzman H, Waugh T, Berdon W: Skeletal changes following irradiation of childhood tumors. J Bone Joint Surg Am 51A:825, 1969
23. Neuhauser EBD, Wittenborg MA, Berman CZ, et al: Irradiation effects of roentgen therapy on the growing spine. Radiology 59:637, 1952

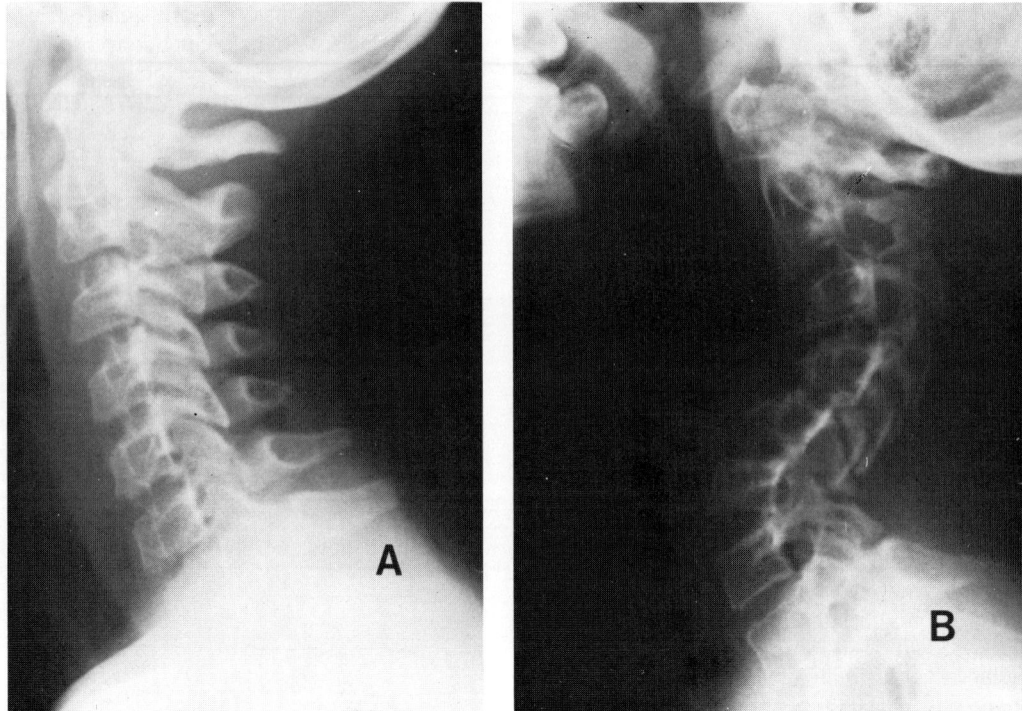

FIGURE 159–2. The cervical spine before (A) and 1 year after (B) laminectomy from C1 through C7, biopsy, and radiation (4860 rad) for a grade II astrocytoma of the cervical spinal cord in an 11-year-old girl. Initially, she had a 3-week history of rapidly progressing, severe left arm and leg weakness that were unchanged after treatment. During the 2 months before detection of the deformity, she developed weakness of the right arm and an increased sensory deficit. The tumor was re-explored and an intramedullary cyst fenestrated. Her neck is supported by a brace, and if tumor growth appears arrested, a fusion will be considered.

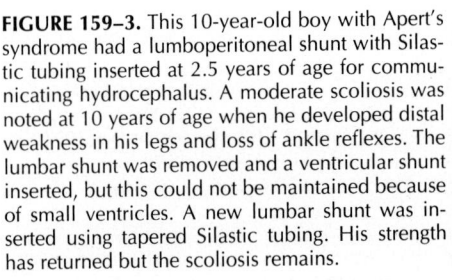

FIGURE 159–3. This 10-year-old boy with Apert's syndrome had a lumboperitoneal shunt with Silastic tubing inserted at 2.5 years of age for communicating hydrocephalus. A moderate scoliosis was noted at 10 years of age when he developed distal weakness in his legs and loss of ankle reflexes. The lumbar shunt was removed and a ventricular shunt inserted, but this could not be maintained because of small ventricles. A new lumbar shunt was inserted using tapered Silastic tubing. His strength has returned but the scoliosis remains.

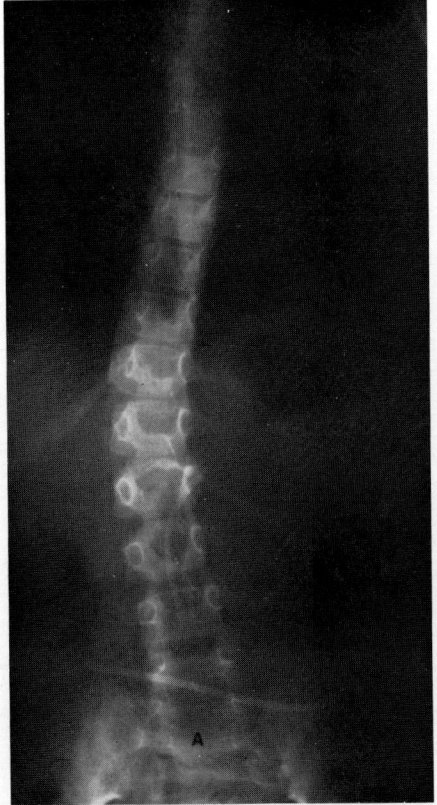
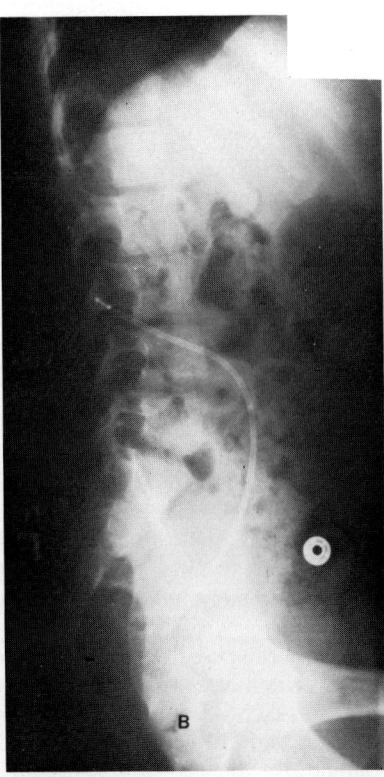

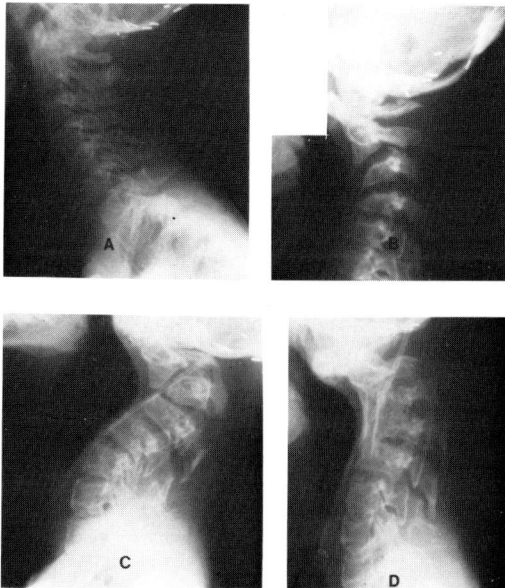

FIGURE 159–1. At 5 months of age, this boy was noted to have communicating hydrocephalus. Because the fourth ventricle could not be filled with air at ventriculography, the posterior fossa was explored, leaving C1 intact. A large cisterna magna was found and it was specifically noted that an Arnold-Chiari malformation did not exist. A lumboureteral shunt was inserted, and the patient did well until 9 years of age, when he developed bilateral spinal accessory nerve palsies, a spastic quadriparesis, and hypalgesia bilaterally in the dermatomes of C2 to C4. Suspecting a tumor, the posterior fossa was re-explored and a laminectomy from C1 to C4 performed. The cerebellar tonsils were found to have descended to the level of C2, and adhesions were present between the spinal cord and dura. Although the upper cervical cord was widened, fluid could not be aspirated from it. It is presumed that the lumbar shunt created a pressure gradient from the intracranial to the spinal compartment, resulting in displacement of the cerebellar tonsils through the foramen magnum, obstruction of the outlets of the fourth ventricle, and a syrinx.[24] His neurologic condition stabilized, but repeated episodes of meningitis and shunt malfunction led to a revision, a ventriculoureteral, and eventually, to a ventriculoperitoneal shunt. Eight years after the second exploration of the posterior fossa and upper cervical laminectomy, he developed increasing weakness, and a severe cervical kyphosis was noted. This was treated by a transoral anterior decompression of C2 through C4 and anterior fusion using iliac bone. He has remained unchanged neurologically over the subsequent 4 years. The figure shows (A) a roentgenogram of the cervical spine 1 year before cervical laminectomy, (B) a roentgenogram 1 year after cervical laminectomy, (C) a roentgenogram 7 years after cervical laminectomy, and (D) a roentgenogram 1 year after anterior decompression and fusion.

PREVENTION OF DEFORMITY AND POSTOPERATIVE MANAGEMENT

Intraoperative measures that may decrease the risk of subsequent deformity include subperiosteal exposure of the posterior elements, which in the very young allows considerable reformation of bone; simultaneous fusion during cervical laminectomy, as mentioned earlier; preservation of facet joints[17]; and en bloc removal and replacement of laminae.[45,46] The last process involves cutting the chosen laminae on either side medial to the facets. The interspinous ligaments above and below the laminectomy are divided in such a way that they can be reapproximated during closure. The interspinous and yellow ligaments between the segments to be removed are preserved. The entire mass is secured in place at the end of the procedure by sutures in the interspinous ligaments above and below and by sutures from the laminae to the lateral masses laterally. The spine is immobilized until fusion of the laminotomy is demonstrated by x-ray study. The extent to which deformities can be prevented or reduced by intraoperative measures remains uncertain, and patients should continue to be followed up closely for subsequent spine deformity regardless of the operative technique used.

Early recognition of developing deformity minimizes eventual treatment, although nonoperative methods are rarely effective. Bracing generally provides only temporary control of curvature and then often at the expense of pressure scores or distorted mandibular growth. In the neck, bracing is particularly ineffective in supporting a paralytic spine or arresting progressive curvature.

SPINAL COMPLICATIONS OF LUMBAR SHUNTS

Spinal deformities and nerve root irritation can occur in as many as 25 per cent of patients after lumboureteral or lumboperitoneal shunts, especially when polyethylene tubing is used.[47,48] The extent of the laminectomy does not seem to be related.[48] The use of silicone tubing may decrease the problem.[47,49] Even with this material, root irritation and spine deformity may occur (Fig. 159–3). Root irritation may subside after the removal or replacement of the lumbar tubing.[49] Syringomyelia presenting as scoliosis also can occur many years after lumbar shunting, probably the result of caudal migration of the cerebellar tonsils because of the pressure gradient created by the shunt between the intracranial and the spinal compartments (see Fig. 159–1), which causes an acquired Chiari I malformation.[50,51] All children with lumbar shunts should be considered to be at risk for syringomyelia and spinal curvature.

SPINAL DEFORMITIES AND HYDROMYELIA IN MYELOMENINGOCELE PATIENTS WITH MALFUNCTIONING SHUNTS

Hall and colleagues,[52] reporting on 11 cases, contended that scoliosis is a common clinical manifestation of hydromyelia in myelomeningocele patients with unshunted hydrocephalus or an otherwise asymptomatic malfunctioning shunt. In seven patients, the curvature improved after shunting. Winston and associates[53] noted the danger of ligating the spinal dura before resecting nonfunctioning spinal cord in the course of kyphosis surgery in meningomyelocele patients. Intracranial pressure may become elevated acutely, and cardiorespiratory arrest may occur if the patient has an asymptomatic malfunctioning shunt and is using the central canal as a conduit for cerebrospinal fluid. The cord should be divided intradurally, and the dura should be closed in a generous pouch over the cut end of the cord.

SURGICAL TREATMENT OF THORACIC AND LUMBAR SPINAL DEFORMITIES

The principles of management of spinal deformities are complex and are beyond the scope of this chapter. Reviews

CHAPTER 159

Spinal Deformities Following Neurosurgical Procedures in Children

Edwin G. Fischer
John E. Hall

Iatrogenic interference with the normal development of the spine is an important consideration in pediatric neurosurgery. Deformities can be induced experimentally by surgical, radiation, or metabolic injury to neural, bony, ligamentous or muscular portions of the spine.[1-6] In children, deformities of the spine can be a major problem either before or after surgery for spinal tumors, trauma, malformations, and syringomyelia or after placement of a lumbar shunt. Seventy-five per cent of patients with myelomeningocele develop kyphoscoliosis. In some, the curvature is the only manifestation of hydromyelia related to untreated hydrocephalus or an obstructed shunt.

RADIOLOGIC EVALUATION

Detailed reviews of radiologic evaluation of the spine of children can be found in the works of Caffey[7] and of Harwood-Nash and Fitz.[8] Posterior arches may appear bifid up until 3 years of age, when the ossification centers of the laminae fuse. Lines of delayed or incomplete fusion of ossification centers may be mistaken for fractures. Bony fusion of the lateral masses to the bodies is not completed until a child is 6 or 7 years old. The odontoid does not fuse with the body of C2 until late childhood. There is also greater mobility of the cervical spine in children than in adults. Up to 3 mm of movement may be seen normally at C2-C3, and up to 3 or 4 mm between the odontoid and C1.

As in adults, the selection of special imaging procedures depends on the nature of the specific problem at hand. Magnetic resonance imaging is of increasing value and availability. Myelography is presently performed with nonionic, water-soluble contrast media[9,10] and polytomographic or computed tomographic scanning. General anesthesia is usually required for children under 10 years of age, and prophylactic anticonvulsants are generally given for 24 hours.

INTRASPINAL TUMORS AND RADIATION THERAPY

Tachdjian and Matson were among the first to draw attention to progressive kyphosis and scoliosis occurring after laminectomy for intraspinal tumors in children.[11] Their observations have been confirmed and elaborated on by others.[12-20] In 117 children, spinal deformities were present in 17 at initial examination and developed in 26 others after laminectomy. Deformities were more likely to occur in children under 2 years of age or when laminectomy was performed over more than three levels. Five patients required fusion. The combination of neurologic deficit, loss of support by posterior elements, and radiation-induced arrest of growth of the vertebral bodies is a triple threat to stability of the spine. If the kyphosis is allowed to progress beyond 50 degrees, combined anterior and posterior stabilization may become necessary.

Fraser did not note an increase in spinal deformity after radiation of spinal tumors in children.[16] Tachdjian and Matson felt it was a significant factor in their patients,[11] however, and it has been well documented that radiation alone and in the absence of neurologic deficit frequently causes changes in vertebral growth that may result in pronounced spinal deformity, especially in children under the age of 2 years.[1,21-26] Spinal fusion may be more problematic after radiation.[27] Bracing is useless in this group of patients, and delay in considering surgery leads to the necessity of more complex procedures to correct and stabilize the spine.

INCREASED RISK OF CERVICAL DEFORMITIES

There is a special propensity for spinal deformity after cervical laminectomy (Figs. 159-1 and 159-2).[13,16,28,29] Some authors have even considered posterolateral cervical fusion at the time of laminectomy in certain patients,[13,30] rather than waiting for the deformity to occur.[31] Cervical and craniocervical instability are also seen without surgery in such conditions as congenital anomalies of the odontoid, direct and nearby infection, mucopolysaccharidoses, Down's syndrome, rheumatoid arthritis, and trauma.[19,31-40] Both anterior and posterior fusions are employed to manage cervical deformities,[13,31,37,41] and in some instances, anterior-transoral or posterior decompression are required.[35,38,42-44]

level. This finding suggests that surgical treatment of asymptomatic but radiographically threatening adjacent levels of stenosis may be helpful to avoid this source of late failure.

Silvers and colleagues[24] reported their experience with a large series of patients (n = 244). Again, the early success rate was high (93 percent pain relief), but the success rate subsequently decreased to 64 percent after a mean follow-up of 4.7 years.

SUMMARY

The successful management of lumbar stenosis requires an extensive knowledge of the complexities of the disease in terms of diagnosis, pathophysiology, and treatment options. Unfortunately, there are few reports of well-controlled prospective studies to help resolve many of the current management controversies.[25] This is no doubt in large part due to the diversity of the patients presenting with this disease. Controversies aside, we believe that the successful management of lumbar spinal stenosis is one of the more gratifying experiences in neurosurgery.

Acknowledgments

The authors thank Cheryl Christensen for manuscript preparation and Stephen Ordway for editorial assistance.

REFERENCES

1. Rydevik B: Neurophysiology of cauda equina compression. Acta Orthop Scand (Suppl) 251:52–55, 1993
2. Porter RW: Central spinal stenosis. Classification and pathogenesis. Acta Orthop Scand (Suppl) 251:64–66, 1993
3. Ooi Y, Mita F, Satoh Y: Myeloscopic study on lumbar spinal canal stenosis with special reference to intermittent claudication. Spine 15:544–549, 1990
4. Takahashi K, Olmarker K, Holm S, et al: Double-level cauda equina compression: An experimental study with continuous monitoring of intraneural blood flow in the porcine cauda equina. J Orthop Res 11:104–109, 1993
5. Onel D, Sari H, Dönmez Ç: Lumbar spinal stenosis: Clinical/radiologic therapeutic evaluation in 145 patients. Conservative treatment or surgical intervention? Spine 18:291–298, 1993
6. Kent DL, Haynor DR, Larson EB, Deyo RA: Diagnosis of lumbar spinal stenosis in adults: A metaanalysis of the accuracy of CT, MR, and myelography. AJR 158:1135–1144, 1992
7. Jönsson B, Strömqvist B: Symptoms and signs in degeneration of the lumbar spine: A prospective, consecutive study of 300 operated patients. J Bone Joint Surg [Br] 75:381–385, 1993
8. McCall IW: Radiology of spinal stenosis. Acta Orthop Scand (Suppl) 251:59–60, 1993
9. Weinstein PR: Decompression of lumbar spinal stenosis, *In* Wilson CB (ed): Neurosurgical Procedures: Personal Approaches to Classic Operations. Baltimore, Williams & Wilkins, 1992, pp 239–253
10. Jinkins JR: Gd-DTPA enhanced MR of the lumbar spinal canal in patients with claudication. J Comput Assist Tomogr 17:555–562, 1993
11. Johnsson K-E, Rosén I, Udén A: The natural course of lumbar spinal stenosis. Acta Orthop Scand (Suppl) 251:67–68, 1993
12. Jönsson B: Patient-related factors predicting the outcome of decompressive surgery. Acta Orthop Scand (Suppl) 251:69–70, 1993
13. Yoshida M, Shima K, Taniguchi Y, et al: Hypertrophied ligamentum flavum in lumbar spinal canal stenosis: Pathogenesis and morphologic and immunohistochemical observation. Spine 17:1353–1360, 1992
14. Postacchini F, Cinotti G, Perugia D, Gumina S: The surgical treatment of central lumbar stenosis: Multiple laminotomy compared with total laminectomy. J Bone Joint Surg [Br] 75:386–392, 1993
15. Yu CS, Tay BK: Wide versus selective decompression in the operative treatment of lumbar spinal stenosis. Singapore Med J 33:378–379, 1992
16. Nakai O, Ookawa A, Yamaura I: Long-term roentgenographic and functional changes in patients who were treated with wide fenestration for central lumbar stenosis. J Bone Joint Surg [Am] 73:1184–1191, 1991
17. Turner JA, Ersek M, Herron L, Deyo R: Surgery for lumbar spinal stenosis: Attempted meta-analysis of the literature. Spine 17:1–8, 1992
18. Deyo RA, Cherkin DC, Loeser JD, et al: Morbidity and mortality in association with operations on the lumbar spine: The influence of age, diagnosis, and procedure. J Bone Joint Surg [Am] 74:536–543, 1992
19. Sanderson PL, Wood PLR: Surgery for lumbar spinal stenosis in old people. J Bone Joint Surg [Br] 75:393–397, 1993
20. Postacchini F, Cinotti G, Gumina S, Perugia D: Long-term results of surgery in lumbar stenosis: 8-year review of 64 patients. Acta Orthop Scand (Suppl) 251:78–80, 1993
21. Postacchini F, Cinotti G: Bone regrowth after surgical decompression for lumbar spinal stenosis. J Bone Joint Surg [Br] 74:862–869, 1992
22. Jönsson B: Vertebral slipping after decompression for spinal stenosis. Acta Orthop Scand (Suppl) 251:76–79, 1993
23. Caputy AJ, Luessenhop AJ: Long-term evaluation of decompressive surgery for degenerative lumbar stenosis. J Neurosurg 77:669–676, 1992
24. Silvers HR, Lewis PJ, Asch HL: Decompressive lumbar laminectomy for spinal stenosis. J Neurosurg 78:695–701, 1993
25. Rydevik B: Spinal stenosis—conclusions. Acta Orthop Scand (Suppl) 251:81–82, 1993

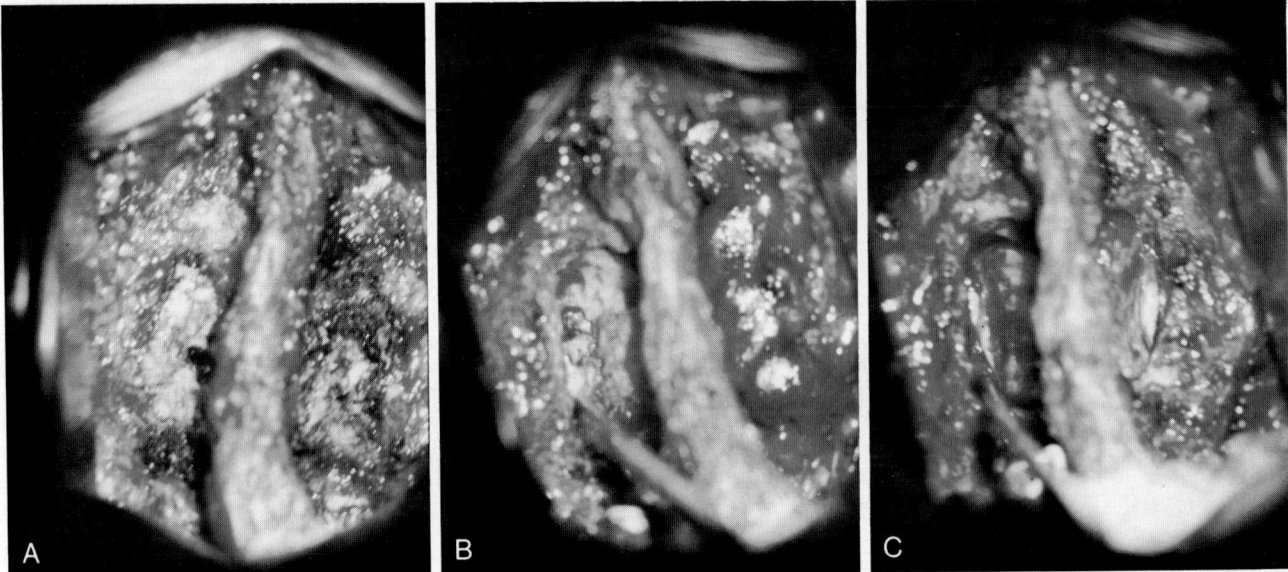

FIGURE 158-4. (A) Operative photomicrograph at low-power magnification demonstrates surgical exposure of the midline supraspinous ligament (preserved) and spinous processes of L4 and L5 in a 62-year-old woman with bilateral L5 radiculopathy due to stenosis of the lateral recess and neural canal at L4-L5. The stenosis was most severe at the disc level and was associated with Grade I degenerative spondylolisthesis, facet osteophytes, and ossification of the ligamentum flavum. The facets are enlarged, reaching toward the midline at the base of the spinous processes, where the lamina are foreshortened. Electrocautery was used to dissect interlaminar muscle and ligament attachments. (B) Photograph showing a laminotomy created on the left by using the power drill to debride caudal L4 lamina and medial inferior facet, as well as rostral L5 lamina and the base of both the L4 and L5 spinous processes. The suction tube points to a large facet capsule osteophyte and nodule of ossified ligamentum flavum that was causing severe anteromedial displacement of the thecal sac and left L5 nerve root. (C) This photograph shows bilateral decompressive laminotomies that have been completed by elevating and totally resecting the ligamentum flavum and its sites of attachment to the interlaminar surfaces of the lamina and facets. The dural sac is fully released from extrinsic compression; both L5 nerve roots are clearly visible and are decompressed as they cross the L4 disc and enter the L5-S1 foramina. Resection of the laminar arches and spinous processes of L4 and L5 was not necessary.

ulous hemostasis is obtained. Dural tears are sutured when possible; in our experience, however, the dura is commonly too fragile to allow repair in patients with severe stenosis. In such cases, fibrin glue or bovine collagen adhesive patches are useful. We promote early mobilization and do not use braces in routine laminectomy performed without fusion.

RESULTS

The most extensive analysis of results for lumbar stenosis decompression was reported by Turner and associates,[17] who reviewed 74 reports. Overall, good to excellent results were found in 64 percent of cases; however, there was a wide variation from study to study, ranging from 26 to 100 percent. No statistically significant difference in outcome based on age or gender, presence of claudication, prior back surgery, associated fusion, or the number of levels decompressed was found. Sanderson and Wood[19] reviewed the results in older patients (mean age, 72.2 years) and found a success rate similar to that in younger patients, without additional morbidity or mortality due to age.

Postacchini and associates[20] reported good to excellent results in 84 percent of patients at up to 6 months, but only 67 percent had good to excellent results after an average of 8 years of follow-up, in their series of 64 patients. This is the longest follow-up period reported to date. These authors also evaluated bone regrowth radiographically after surgical decompression.[21] No regrowth was observed in 5 of 40 patients. Of the 74 levels decompressed, 15 showed no regrowth, 36 showed 11 to 40 percent regrowth, and five showed 71 to 100 percent regrowth. Bone regrowth was greatest at L4-5 and least at L2-3. A significantly greater amount of bone regrowth was observed in patients who had spondylolisthesis either preoperatively or postoperatively and in patients who had narrow laminectomies. Good to excellent clinical results were reported in 80 percent of patients with 40 percent or less regrowth, in 55 percent of patients with 41 to 70 percent regrowth, and in only 40 percent of patients with more than 70 percent regrowth. This suggests that regrowth of bone is at least partly responsible for late surgical failures.

Jönsson[22] prospectively studied 60 consecutive patients who had undergone limited facet removal (less than 50 percent) and total laminectomy. Six of 19 patients with preoperative degenerative spondylolisthesis and 1 of 41 without preoperative spondylolisthesis had an increase in or new onset of subluxation at 1 year. Relief of leg or back pain was not affected by the presence or absence of postoperative slippage.

Caputy and Luessenhop[23] retrospectively analyzed results in 100 patients followed for up to 10 years. They found universal early success but noted failures beginning at 4 months. By 5 years, the total failure rate was 27 percent. Most failures in the back pain category occurred within 3 years, whereas neurologic deterioration was an increasing source of failure throughout the extended follow-up period. Interestingly, of the 16 failures with recurrent neurologic involvement, 8 resulted from new compression at an adjacent

ments, and the midportion of the lamina. We especially prefer this approach in younger patients (in whom postoperative instability is more common), in patients with focal lateral stenosis, and in patients with other risk factors for postoperative instability such as scoliosis or pre-existing spondylolisthesis as well as in patients in whom disc excision is planned (Fig. 158–1).

SURGICAL TECHNIQUE

After intravenous administration of prophylactic antibiotics and placement of sequential compression stockings, the patient is turned to the prone position on a padded laminectomy frame. A midline incision is then made down to the level of the lumbar fascia.

If a total laminectomy is planned, the fascia is opened in the midline, and both lamina are exposed subperiosteally (Fig. 158–3). Care must be taken to avoid fracture of the hypertrophied facets with the periosteal elevator during lateral stripping. A high-speed drill is then used to create bilateral troughs at the medial margin of the facets. Using first a cutting and then a diamond-tip bit, the surgeon can safely drill through the caudal two thirds of the lamina. To avoid dural tears, however, it is best to use the drill only to thin down to anterior cortex of the superior third of the lamina, where there is no protective yellow ligament and where the dura is frequently thinned by severe compression. The remainder of the laminectomy is then performed with a fine 2-mm or 3-mm Kerrison punch.

A Woodson elevator is passed from cephalad to caudad beneath the yellow ligament within the bilateral troughs to dissect the epidural plane. The ligament is divided sharply.

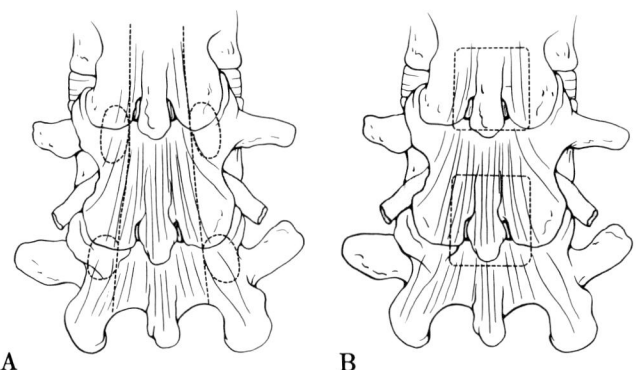

FIGURE 158–3. (A) Drawing of the lumbar spine from L3 to L5 in the posteroanterior plane shows the line of resection (dotted) for decompressive laminectomy in a spinal stenosis patient. The junction between lamina and facets is removed, and the landmark for the lateral extent of decompression is the medial surface of the pedicles. The pars interarticularis and the lateral half of the inferior-superior facet complex is preserved. (B) The margins of bone resection are illustrated at L3-L4 and L4-L5 for interlaminar decompression when limiting the procedure to bilateral laminotomies (dotted line). The entire ligamentum flavum and its bony insertion sites to rostral and caudal lamina as well as to medial facets are resected. The spinous processes, interspinous and supraspinous ligaments, and middle laminar segments are preserved to enhance stability, prevent epidural scarring, and provide bony sites for reattachment of the sacrospinalis muscles. (From Weinstein PR: Decompression of spinal stenosis, in Wilson CB (ed): Neurosurgical Procedures: Personal Approaches to Classic Operations. Baltimore, Williams & Wilkins, 1992, pp 239–253.)

The entire laminar-ligamentous complex can be removed en bloc. The lateral margins of the canal are then widened with a Kerrison punch. Removal of more than the medial third of the facet is rarely required. The lateral recess has not been fully decompressed unless the medial surface of the pedicle and the axilla of each nerve root have been exposed. Foraminotomies are then performed at each level by debriding the rostral tip of each superior facet to allow each nerve root to exit freely.

If selective interlaminar laminotomies are planned, the fascia is opened bilaterally with two vertical paramedian incisions (Fig. 158–3). To gain an unobstructed view, the medial free edges can then be sutured together in the midline if necessary. A high-speed drill, curettes, and rongeurs are then used to perform bilateral laminotomies, medial facetectomies, and foraminotomies at each symptomatic level (Fig. 158–4). The entire ligamentum flavum is removed from beneath the laminar arch, and the arch is undercut as needed to decompress the central canal adequately. The interlaminar approach can be used unilaterally when stenosis and symptoms are limited to one side. As with total laminectomy, devitalized muscle tissue is debrided after the muscle retractors have been withdrawn, and meticulous hemostasis is obtained. The incision is sutured in layers with particular attention to the fascia.

COMPLICATIONS AND THEIR MANAGEMENT

Complication rates are low for lumbar stenosis operations. Turner and associates[17] reviewed 74 articles involving surgical treatment of lumbar stenosis and found an overall average complication rate of 12.6 percent. There was a 0.32 percent mortality rate, a 5.9 percent incidence of dural tears, a 1 percent deep infection rate, a 2.3 percent superficial infection rate, and a 2.78 percent incidence of deep venous thrombosis.

Deyo and coworkers[18] reported a population-based review of the rates of postoperative complications and mortality, as recorded in a hospital discharge registry for the state of Washington. They found that mortality was very low (overall 0.07 percent) but increased significantly with age (0.01 percent in patients younger than 65 years and 0.6 percent in patients older than 74 years). The hospital cost and rate of complications during hospitalization also increased with age (morbidity of 6.4 percent for patients 18 to 40 years and 17.7 percent for patients older than 74 years). Independent of all other variables, arthrodesis resulted in higher costs, longer stay, and higher complication rate (morbidity of 13.9 percent for laminectomy alone versus 19.6 percent for laminectomy and fusion). In contrast, Sanderson and Wood[19] and Turner and associates[17] found no statistically significant increase in complication rates among older patients.

We make several efforts to reduce perioperative complications. All patients receive broad-spectrum antibiotics intraoperatively. All patients are fitted with elastic stockings and sequential compression stockings preoperatively and are required to continue using them until they are fully ambulatory. Subcutaneous heparin (5,000 IU twice a day) is begun on the evening of surgery to prevent postoperative thrombophlebitis or pulmonary embolism. All devitalized muscle tissue is debrided before wound closure to prevent infection, and metic-

conservative management succeeds, the recommendation for surgical intervention is usually justified. Systemic illness and other factors, such as advanced age and osteoporosis, that would tend to increase morbidity would, of course, be relative contraindications. Indications for surgery, therefore, include progression or persistence of neurologic deficits and failure of medical management to relieve intolerable pain that interferes with normal daily activities.

Jönsson[12] studied 160 patients with lumbar stenosis for possible predictors of poor outcome of surgical decompression. The factors evaluated were age, sex, preoperative duration of back pain, time off work, work load, walking distance, and consumption of analgesics. The only preoperative predictor of poor outcome in patients with central stenosis was regular consumption of analgesics; the only unfavorable predictor in those with lateral stenosis was sciatica of long duration. These data support our observation that lumbar surgical decompression can be successful in a wide range of patients.

SURGICAL ANATOMY

To appreciate the surgical anatomy in lumbar stenosis requires an understanding of the pathologic process responsible for the neural compression. In cases of lateral stenosis, compression is usually caused by hypertrophy of the superior articular fact. Central stenosis results whenever the area of the entire canal is reduced, for example by hypertrophy of the inferior articular facet, lamina, and ligamentum flavum or by annular disc bulges. Yoshida et al[13] have emphasized the surgically important point that the ligamentum flavum tends to become hypertrophic at the enthesis (the insertion point of the ligament to the lamina and facet), where loss of elastic fibers and proliferation of type II collagen occurs and subperiosteal osteoneogenesis responsible for osteophyte formation is stimulated. Thus, the major component of neural canal and lateral recess stenosis is situated in the interlaminar space at the level of the hypertrophic ligamentum flavum. Understanding such details of the relevant surgical anatomy makes it possible to select an appropriate surgical approach.

SURGICAL APPROACH

The goals of surgery for lumbar stenosis are to decompress the neural elements and to preserve spinal stability. The current trend is to minimize the amount of bone and soft tissue removed during decompression in an attempt to preserve spinal stability. Although this rationale is appealing, there have been no well-controlled prospective studies documenting the efficacy of techniques of interlaminar decompression in reducing the incidence of postoperative instability. Attempts at studying this issue, however, have been reported. Postacchini and associates[14] prospectively randomized 67 patients into two surgical groups: those to undergo total laminectomy and those to undergo selective bilateral laminotomy. In addition, a third group of patients was described who were initially randomized into the laminotomy group but were found intraoperatively to require total laminectomy. Although this third group introduced a bias, the overall results in the three groups during a mean follow-up of 3.7 years were comparable. Patients undergoing selective laminotomy had significantly more improvement (subjective) in low back pain than the other groups; but they also had higher frequency of nerve root injury and a trend toward less subjective improvement in radicular complaints in comparison with the other groups. No patient in the laminotomy group had postoperative spinal instability. Three patients had instability after total laminectomy; however, two had preoperative scoliosis and one had preoperative spondylolisthesis. The extent of blood loss was similar for the two groups, as was operating time, but only for cases of single-level decompression. There was a statistically significant increase in operating time with the bilateral laminotomy procedures in which a multilevel decompression was performed.

From these findings, Postacchini and associates[14] concluded that selective laminotomy is indicated for developmental stenosis, given that the stenosis is commonly less severe, the patients are typically younger, and disc excision is more frequently necessary. They also concluded that selective laminotomy is indicated for mild-to-moderate degenerative stenosis in older patients, especially when disc excision is planned. They recommended that total laminectomy be performed for severe multilevel combined developmental and congenital stenosis and found that total laminectomy was required for adequate decompression in patients with more than 25 percent spondylolisthesis. The shorter operative time may also be a relative indication for total laminectomy in patients in poor medical condition who require decompression at multiple levels.

Yu and Tay[15] retrospectively reviewed their experience with selective laminotomy versus laminectomy (64 patients) and found no statistically significant difference between the groups in terms of relief of back and leg pain or return to premorbid functional state after a relatively short follow-up of 4 to 26 months. Postoperative spinal stability was not evaluated.

Nakai and colleagues[16] performed a "wide fenestration," described as removal of the medial part of the inferior facet and adjoining ligamentum flavum, in 34 patients with central spinal stenosis. Patients with preoperative spondylolisthesis were excluded. The follow-up period averaged 5.5 years. Early after surgery, 82 percent of patients had good to excellent results, but this proportion decreased to 70 percent 4 years later. Five of 34 patients had radiographic evidence of postoperative instability, which was symptomatic in 2. The authors pointed out that a high percentage of patients with radiographic instability became symptomatic because of failure to remove a sufficient portion of the superior facet. This is a very important observation with respect to understanding the cause of recurrence of symptoms in patients with postoperative spondylolisthesis or instability, because many patients with subluxation after total laminectomy remain asymptomatic. It may be that osseous elements are more likely to be left behind in a selective laminotomy procedure, which results in a greater vulnerability to neural compression in the setting of postoperative instability and therefore a potentially paradoxical increase in the rate of symptomatic instability.

Despite the absence of firm scientific support, it is our current preference to perform selective laminotomies wherever possible, preserving to the maximal extent the posterior elements, including spinous processes, interspinous liga-

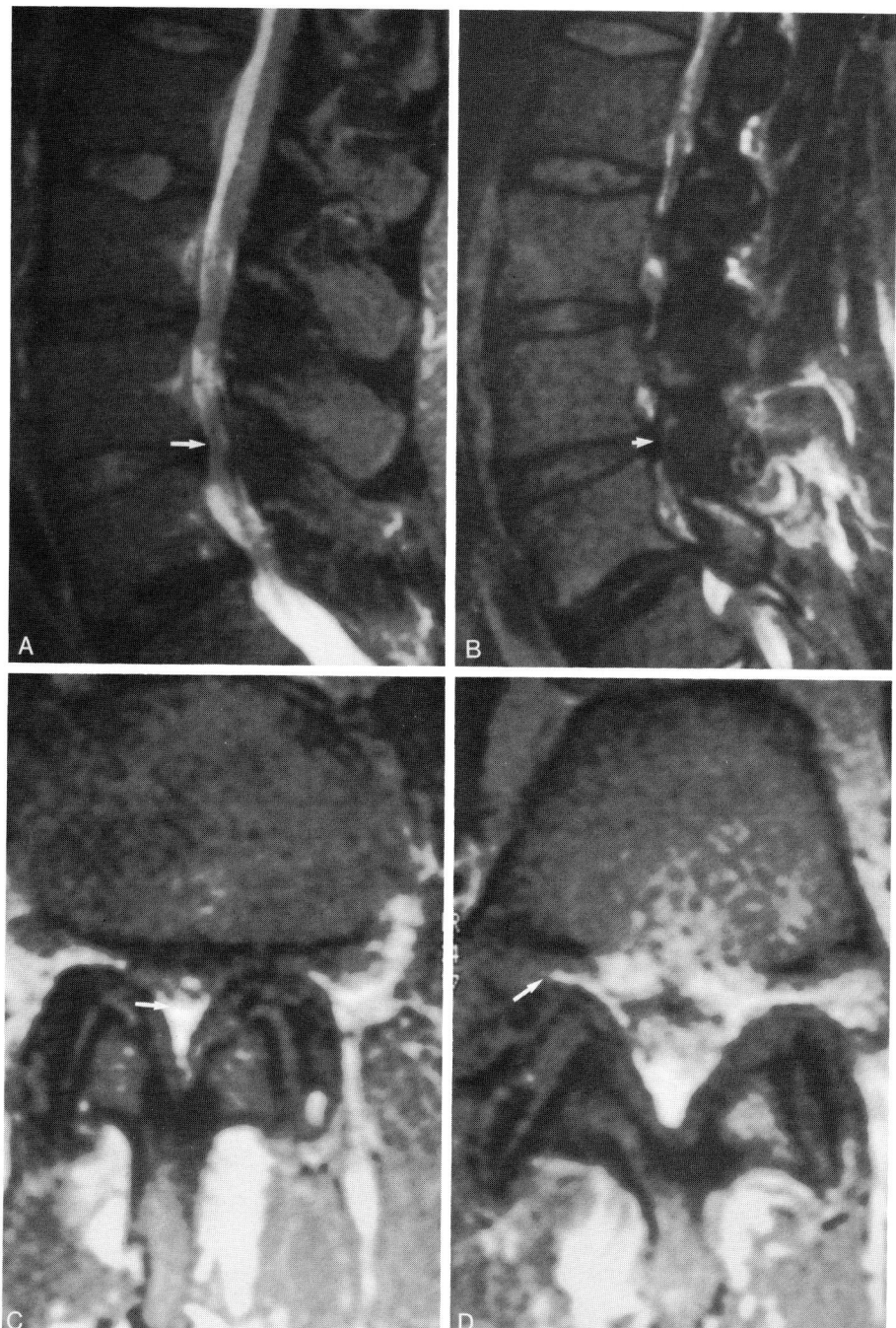

FIGURE 158–2. MRIs of the lumbar spine at the midline (A) and 1 cm to the right (B) in a 45-year-old man with severe bilateral neurogenic claudication in the sciatic distribution demonstrate severe stenosis at the disc level in the midline (large arrow) and lateral recesses (small arrow) at L4-L5 and to a lesser extent at L5-S1 and L3-L4. Features of both developmental stenosis (short pedicles) and acquired stenosis (discogenic osteophytes, facet and ligamentous hypertrophy) are present. (C) Axial MRI shows reduction of the anteroposterior diameter of the thecal sac to approximately 8 mm despite persistence of the posterior epidural fat layer (arrow) at L4-L5. The foreshortened triangular (trefoil) configuration of the neural canal is a classic diagnostic finding. (D) Axial MRI at the L5 midbody level demonstrates moderate stenosis of the neural canal and severe stenosis of the foramen (arrow) beneath the hypertrophic superior facets of L5. Interlaminar segmental decompression would have been technically difficult and probably inadequate in this patient. Laminectomy of L4 and L5 with foraminotomies at L3-L4, L4-L5, and L5-S1 provided excellent relief of postural and ambulation-induced radiculopathy.

therapy, however; the symptoms often recurred. In a natural history study of 27 patients with unoperated spinal stenosis, Johnsson and coworkers[11] found that 19 remained unchanged, 4 improved, and 4 deteriorated during a follow-up period of 10 to 130 months (mean 49 months). These results suggest that even though improvement is unlikely, attempting a trial of medical management is at least safe and perhaps efficacious. There are, however, currently no reports of randomized trials in the literature comparing the outcome of surgery with that of medical management.

Given the high efficacy and low morbidity of surgery for lumbar stenosis and the lack of substantial evidence that

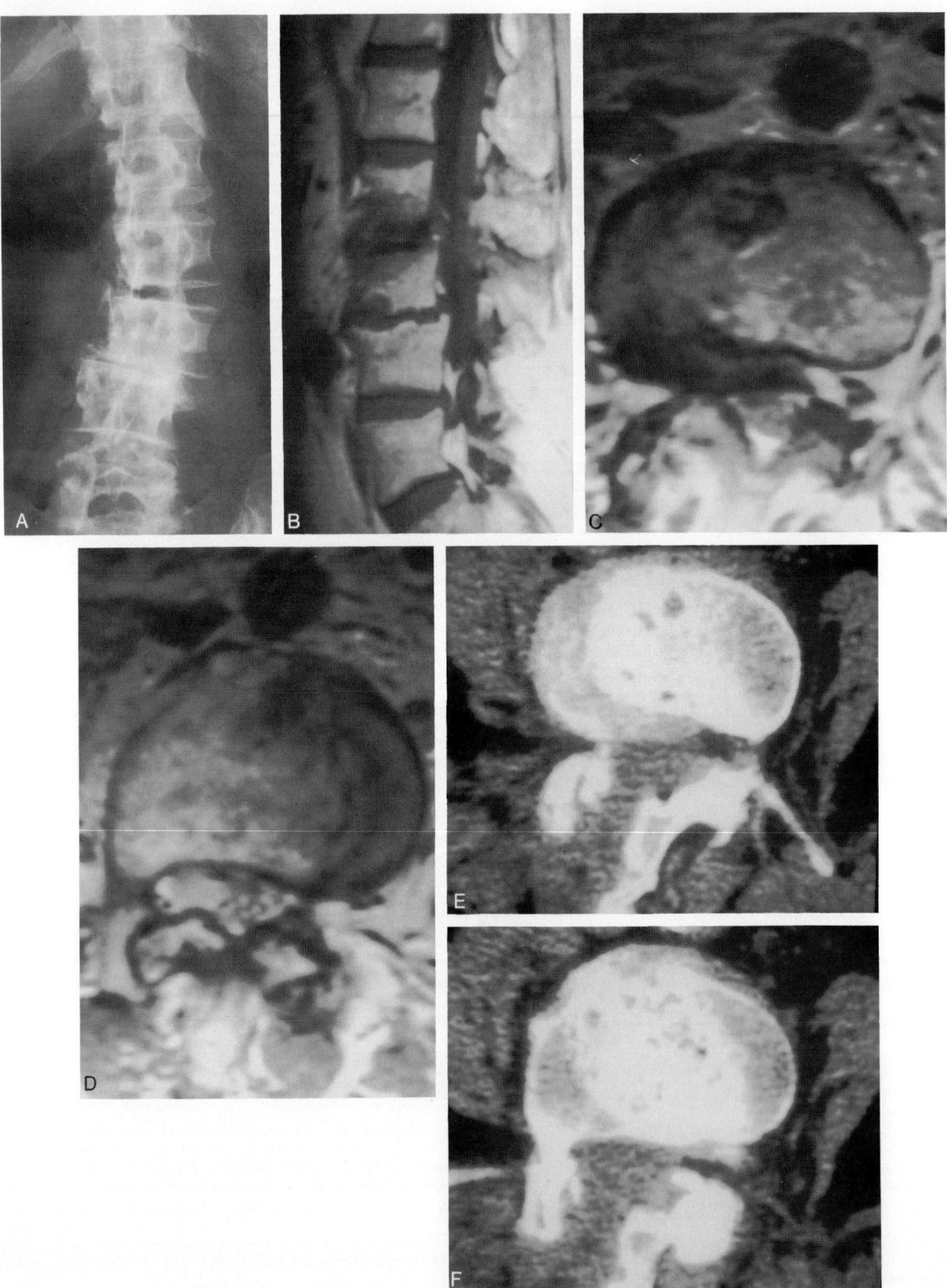

FIGURE 158–1. (A) Anteroposterior radiograph of the lumbar spine in a 54-year-old woman with neurogenic claudication in the right L3 and L4 distribution and a history of long-term steroid therapy for regional enteritis demonstrates rotoscoliosis concave to the left as well as lateral translational subluxation of L3 on L4 and severe spondylosis. Bending films showed no evidence of instability. (B) The sagittal MRI demonstrates scoliosis, stenosis at L2-L3 and L3-L4, and degenerative spondylolisthesis at L2-L3 and L3-L4. (C) Axial MRI at the L3-L4 disc and (D) the upper L4 body levels demonstrate severe focal canal and subarticular stenosis that is worse on the right and is associated with a lateral discogenic osteophyte. Similar findings were observed at L2-L3, but the neural canal diameters were normal at the midbody levels of L3 and L4. Symptoms were substantially relieved by right L2-L3 and L3-L4 laminoforaminotomies. (E) The anatomic results of the surgical decompression of the neural canal and lateral recess are demonstrated by the postoperative axial CT image at the same level as in C, obtained because of persistent dysesthesia in the right thigh. (F) Axial CT scan at the same level as D confirms the decompression of the lateral recess and medial foramen.

tended posture and are relieved by spinal flexion. Therefore, crouching to play tennis or ride a bicycle may be better tolerated than walking. The pain of neurogenic claudication tends to be less severe than that of disc herniation. Typically located in the buttocks and posterior thigh, the pain often radiates into the anterior thigh and groin or posterolateral leg and foot, depending on the levels involved. It may be dull or aching and may be associated with episodes of sharp, shock-like pain. *Vascular claudication* can be distinguished from neurogenic claudication by absence or reduction of the lower extremity pulse, the absence of low back pain, and the relief of pain by rest in the standing position without leaning forward or sitting. Knee buckling due to quadriceps weakness or foot drop due to anterior tibialis and peroneus longus weakness may develop during ambulation. The patellar and Achilles tendon reflexes may be present at rest and absent after ambulation.

The symptoms of *lateral* lumbar stenosis are similar in distribution to those of disc herniation, although pain is more likely to be relieved by lumbar flexion. Radiculopathy predominates, at either single or multiple levels. The symptoms are more likely to be unilateral than those seen with central stenosis.

Jönsson and Strömqvist[7] studied the differences in signs and symptoms of lateral lumbar stenosis, central lumbar stenosis, and lumbar disc herniation. Patients with lateral stenosis and disc herniation were younger than those with central stenosis (mean ages, 41 and 43 years, respectively, versus 65 years), and they more commonly had pain at rest, at night, and with coughing. The straight-leg-raising test was positive in 88 percent of patients with disc herniation, 51 percent of those with lateral stenosis, and 35 percent of those with central stenosis.

PREOPERATIVE EVALUATION

When the clinical history and physical examination suggest lumbar stenosis, radiologic evaluation is indicated. Lateral, anteroposterior, oblique, and flexion-extension radiographs are important to rule out mechanical instability and the presence of a pars interarticularis defect.

Although magnetic resonance imaging (MRI) may be the initial imaging study, computed tomography (CT) after myelography is the "gold standard" for evaluating lumbar stenosis.[8] The classic finding for central lumbar stenosis on myelograms or MRI scans is a thecal sac with a smoothly marginated "waist" or "hourglass" shape. In Weinstein's series,[9] 55 percent of patients with neurogenic claudication had stenosis severe enough to cause a complete myelographic block of the subarachnoid space. Above and below the lesion, there are often redundant serpentine nerve roots that should not be confused with abnormal vessels suggestive of a vascular malformation. Myelography is generally a poor technique for evaluating lateral stenosis; therefore, a post-myelographic CT or MRI scan is needed to make this diagnosis. The axial image defines the contribution of disc protrusion, ligamentous hypertrophy, facet hypertrophy, congenital canal narrowing, congenitally short pedicles, and foraminal stenosis to the overall picture of stenosis. Sagittal reconstructions of the axial images may be obtained to demonstrate constriction of the neural canal, lateral recesses, and foramina. Osseous structures and degenerative ossification may be more clearly demonstrated, especially in anatomically complex cases of rotoscoliosis (Fig. 158–1).

Magnetic resonance imaging is becoming the diagnostic study of choice for patients suspected of having lumbar stenosis (Fig. 158–2). Axial MRI scans of central stenosis typically show a circumferentially narrowed canal, as described for CT. Specifically, hypertrophic bone appears as a dark region of low signal on T1- and T2-weighted images, hypertrophic ligamentum flavum appears as an intermediate signal on T1 and T2 images, and loss of fat in the epidural space (caused by prolonged compression) appears as a loss of high T1 signal. The T2-weighted sagittal images are useful for their myelogram-like representation of the thecal sac. The CSF within the thecal sac below the level of severe stenosis may have an increased T2 signal owing to a reduction in transmission of CSF pulsations. Lateral stenosis is well demonstrated on axial and sagittal views through the lateral recesses and foramina, where it appears as loss of fat signal (best appreciated on T1-weighted images) surrounding the exiting nerve root.

An interesting study by Jinkins[10] examined the appearance of gadolinium-enhanced MRI scans in seven patients with neurogenic claudication who had not previously undergone spinal surgery. Lumbar stenosis was confirmed by CT myelography in all patients who were first evaluated by gadolinium-enhanced MRI. Five patients had abnormal intrathecal enhancement at the level of severe stenosis and extending cephalad to that site. Two patients had epidural and dural enhancement at the sites of stenosis. The author postulated that the enhancement was due either to venous engorgement and congestion or to breakdown of the blood-nerve barrier caused by long-standing compression.

Magnetic resonance imaging and CT each have distinct advantages, but they are comparable in terms of sensitivity and specificity. In an extensive review of the literature, Kent and associates[6] performed a meta-analysis comparing MRI, CT, and myelography. Although the 74 articles they reviewed contained small patient populations, and therefore, possible methodologic flaws, the authors found similar sensitivities and specificities for MRI and CT (with and without intrathecal administration of contrast material). Diagnostic sensitivities of 0.81 to 0.97 for MRI, 0.7 to 1.0 for CT, and 0.67 to 0.78 for myelography alone were reported.

PATIENT SELECTION AND MANAGEMENT DECISIONS

For patients without significant or progressive motor deficits, a trial of conservative management consisting of bed rest, nonsteroidal anti-inflammatory agents, and lumbosacral bracing is indicated. Epidural steroid injections above or below the stenotic levels can also be utilized, especially in patients in poor medical condition, in whom surgery is contraindicated.

Conservative management was found by Onel and colleagues[5] to result in overall clinical improvement, defined as decreased pain, increased walking distances, and reduced neurologic symptoms, that was rated as excellent in 52%, good in 18%, and moderate in 23%. These results appeared to be limited to the period immediately after the intensive

CHAPTER 158

Surgical Management of Lumbar Spinal Stenosis

Richard M. Westmark
Philip R. Weinstein

Lumbar spinal stenosis is a general term used to describe a number of diverse conditions that decrease the total area of the spinal canal, lateral recesses, or intervertebral foramina. Although lumbar stenosis is a common malady, it is important not to underestimate its complexity. Failure to understand the various types of stenosis, underlying pathophysiology, and surgical anatomy is certain to lead to disappointing results. This chapter addresses these issues as well as current controversies in the management of this disease.

PATHOPHYSIOLOGY

The nerve roots of the cauda equina derive their metabolic energy from the cerebrospinal fluid (CSF) via diffusion and from arterial circulation located on the surface of the nerve roots. This anatomic feature has been postulated to place the roots at risk for ischemia in the setting of extrinsic compression as seen in lumbar stenosis. Experimental studies have shown that compression of the cauda equina at pressures similar to those seen in lumbar stenosis can reduce blood flow and impulse conduction in the compressed roots.[1] Blockage of CSF by extrinsic compression that reduces the diffusion of nutrients from the CSF results in further injury. These changes are known to lead to local demyelination and axonal degeneration and thus have been thought by some authors to be the basis of ectopic impulse generation or a lowered threshold to mechanical stimulation responsible for the pain of neurogenic claudication.[1]

Other authors, however, believe that venous congestion is the primary cause of intermittent postural radiculopathy in lumbar stenosis.[2] They point out that myeloscopy reveals congestion rather than ischemia in patients reporting neurogenic claudication.[3] Experiments indicate that compression of 10 mm Hg (a subarterial pressure) at a single level in a porcine cauda equina model has no significant effect, whereas the same compression applied at two levels decreases blood flow by 64 percent.[4] This decrease, they suggest, is caused by reduced venous return in the two-level compression model.

Thus, although the exact mechanism of pain production in patients with lumbar stenosis remains unresolved, it seems likely that both venous and arterial circulatory factors are involved along with mechanical compression of affected nerve roots.

CLASSIFICATION

Lumbar stenosis can be classified both by its etiology and by the location of the stenosis. Etiologically, lumbar stenosis can be divided into two types, developmental/congenital and acquired. *Developmental* stenosis results from inadequate growth of the pedicles and lamina, which leads to formation of a disproportionately smaller neural canal without the vertebral body shortening found in cases of dwarfism. Such stenosis may not be symptomatic unless disc herniation further compromises the space available for the lumbosacral nerve roots. *Acquired stenosis* tends to become symptomatic in older patients; it may be caused by degenerative changes, spondylolisthesis, iatrogenic factors (i.e., after laminectomy and fusion), trauma, or miscellaneous skeletal conditions, such as Paget's disease, diffuse idiopathic skeletal hyperostosis, and ankylosing spondylitis.[5]

Anatomically, stenosis may be classified as central, lateral, or combined, according to radiographic measurements (Table 158–1). It is interesting to note that the vertebral neural canal attains its adult cross-sectional area by 4 years of age.[2]

CLINICAL FEATURES

Degenerative changes can be demonstrated radiographically throughout the spine in 4 to 28 percent of asymptomatic cases.[6] Therefore, surgical planning for treatment of lumbar stenosis relies heavily on the evaluation of clinical signs and symptoms.

The "classic" history of *central* lumbar stenosis is characterized by many years of low back pain followed by the development of neurogenic claudication. *Neurogenic claudication* is the onset or aggravation of pain, with or without motor or sensory deficits or bladder dysfunction with walking. The symptoms are exacerbated by an erect or hyperex-

Table 158–1. NORMAL AND STENOTIC LUMBAR SPINE DIMENSIONS

Dimension	Neural canal (mm)	Lateral recess (mm)
Normal anteroposterior	15–25	3–5
Stenotic anteroposterior	5–10	1–2

to be worse immediately after lumbar surgery even if preoperative pain is diminished. Longer postoperative follow-ups will measure the efficacy of the procedures we carry out.

SUMMARY

I believe that the future of lumbar disc surgery will depend on better and more widespread understanding of the natural history of the degenerative process and on tailoring of surgery to the specific instances in which significant nerve root compression is truly present. The simplest methods to effectively release nerve root compression will no doubt be the ones widely used in the future. At present, the safest, simplest, and most reliable technique is still the open surgery as described here using magnified vision and the gentlest possible neurosurgical techniques.

Acknowledgment

The MOS-SF36 Health Survey is reproduced with permission of The Medical Outcomes Trust, PO Box 1917, Boston, MA 02205, a nonprofit corporation formed to ensure the availability of the SF36 Health Survey while preserving standardization of the content, scoring, and labeling of the instrument. Permission to use the SF36 Health Survey is routinely granted by The Medical Outcomes Trust to individuals and organizations on a royalty-free basis upon receipt of a request. For further information, please contact Trust.

SELECTED REFERENCES

Boden SD, Auris DO, Dina TS, et al: Abnormal magnetic resonance scans of lumbar spine in asymptomatic patients. J Bone Joint Surg 72A:430–408, 1990

Fager CA: Atlas of Spinal Surgery. Philadelphia, Lea & Febiger, 1989

Frymoyer JW, Cots-Baire WL: An overview of the incidences and costs of low back pain. Orthop Clin North Am 22:263–271, 1991

Hood RS: Far lateral lumbar disk herniations. Neurosurg Clin North Am 4:117–124, 1993

Roberts MP: Lumbar disk herniation: Standard approach. Neurosurg Clin North Am 4:91–99, 1993

Robertson JT: The rape of the spine. Surg Neurol 39:5–12, 1993

Schlesinger SM, Fannhauser H, de Tribolet N: Microsurgical anatomy and operative techniques for extreme lateral lumbar disk herniation. Acta Neurochir 118:117–129, 1992

Stewart A: Measuring Function and Well Being: The Medical Outcome Study Approach. Duke University Press, 1992

Tarlov AR: Shattuck Lecture: The increasing supply of physicians, the changing structure of the health services system and the future practice of medicine. N Engl J Med 308:1235–1244, 1983

Tarlov AR, Ware JE, Greenfield S, et al: The Medical Outcomes Study: An application of methods for monitoring the results of medical care. JAMA 262:925–930, 1989

Tarlov E, D'Costa D: Back Attack. Boston, Little Brown, 1985

Tarlov E (ed): Complications of Spinal Surgery. Chicago, American Association of Neurological Surgeons, 1991

Turner JA, Ersek M, Herron L, et al: Patients outcomes after lumbar spinal fusions. JAMA 268:907–911, 1992

Ware JE: SF-36 Health Survey Manual and Interpretation Guide. Boston, The Health Institute, New England Medical Center, 1993

FIGURE 157–17. (A) Health status survey of a 23-year-old, 330-pound nursing home aide who developed sciatica while lifting a patient at work. Studies showed extruded disc at L4-5. The health survey here shows impairment in spheres of physical role functioning, bodily pain, vitality, and mental health areas. In summary, SF 36 shows marked impairment. (B) Health status survey in 54-year-old laborer who underwent surgery for L4-5 disc herniation 4 years previously. He is working fully in a stressful job without apparent limitations. SF 36 shows essentially normal levels of function for his age. Serial measurements before and after surgery would show the effect of intervention. Patient-generated information such as this is in the opinion of this author no more subjective than a surgeon's view that a patient is doing well.

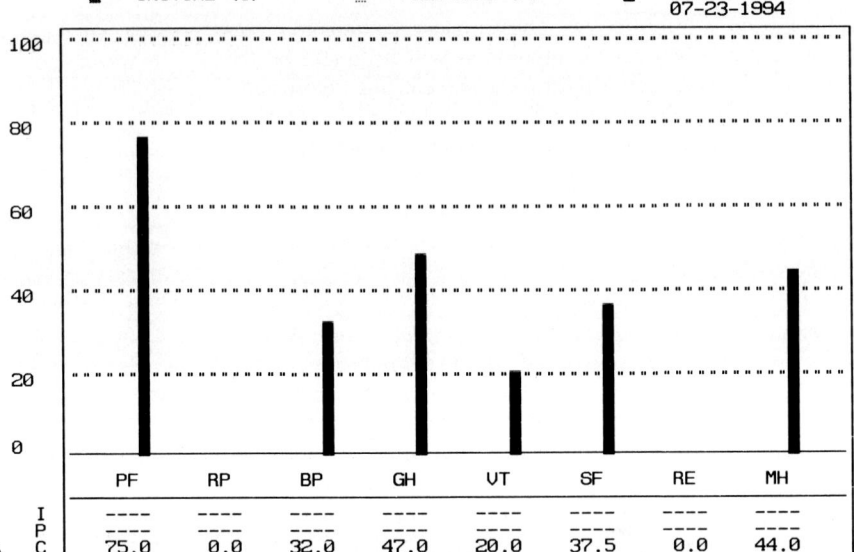

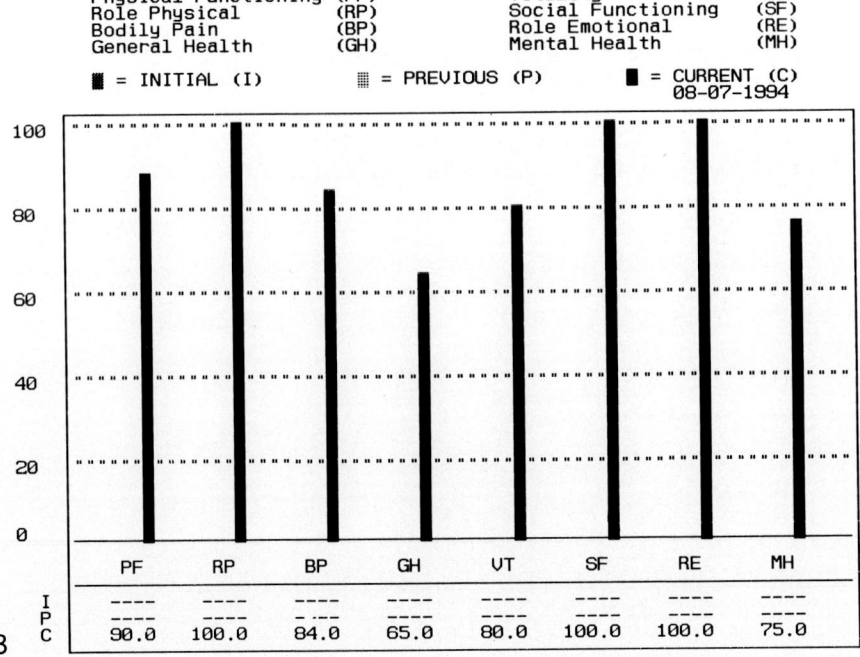

**This is Side 2 of this Questionnaire.
Make sure you complete the OTHER side first.**   SIDE 2

5. During the **past 4 weeks**, have you had any of the following problems with your work or other regular daily activities **as a result of any emotional problems** (such as feeling depressed or anxious)? (Mark one oval on each line.)

	Yes	No
a. Cut down the <u>amount of time</u> you spent on work or other activities	a. ①	②
b. <u>Accomplished less</u> than you would like	b. ①	②
c. Didn't do work or other activities as <u>carefully</u> as usual	c. ①	②

6. During the **past 4 weeks**, to what extent has your physical health or emotional problems interfered with your normal social activities with family, friends, neighbors, or groups? (Mark one oval.)

6. ① Not at all   ④ Quite a bit
   ② Slightly   ⑤ Extremely
   ③ Moderately

7. How much **bodily** pain have you had during the **past 4 weeks**? (Mark one oval.)

7. ① None   ④ Moderate
   ② Very mild ⑤ Severe
   ③ Mild   ⑥ Very severe

8. During the **past 4 weeks**, how much did **pain** interfere with your normal work (including both work outside the home and housework)? (Mark one oval.)

8. ① Not at all   ④ Quite a bit
   ② A little bit ⑤ Extremely
   ③ Moderately

9. These questions are about how you feel and how things have been with you **during the past 4 weeks**. For each question, please give the one answer that comes closest to the way you have been feeling. How much of the time during the **past 4 weeks** . . . (Mark one oval on each line.)

	All of the Time	Most of the Time	A Good Bit of the Time	Some of the Time	A Little of the Time	None of the Time
a. Did you feel full of pep?	①	②	③	④	⑤	⑥
b. Have you been a very nervous person?	①	②	③	④	⑤	⑥
c. Have you felt so down in the dumps that nothing could cheer you up?	①	②	③	④	⑤	⑥
d. Have you felt calm and peaceful?	①	②	③	④	⑤	⑥
e. Did you have a lot of energy?	①	②	③	④	⑤	⑥
f. Have you felt downhearted and blue?	①	②	③	④	⑤	⑥
g. Did you feel worn out?	①	②	③	④	⑤	⑥
h. Have you been a happy person?	①	②	③	④	⑤	⑥
i. Did you feel tired?	①	②	③	④	⑤	⑥

10. During the **past 4 weeks**, how much of the time has your **physical health or emotional problems** interfered with your social activities (like visiting with friends, relatives, etc.)? (Mark one oval.)

10. ① All of the time   ④ A little of the time
    ② Most of the time   ⑤ None of the time
    ③ Some of the time

11. How **true** or **false** is **each** of the following statements for you? (Mark one oval on each line.)

	Definitely True	Mostly True	Don't Know	Mostly False	Definitely False
a. I seem to get sick a little easier than other people.	①	②	③	④	⑤
b. I am as healthy as anybody I know.	①	②	③	④	⑤
c. I expect my health to get worse.	①	②	③	④	⑤
d. My health is excellent.	①	②	③	④	⑤

12a. Which are you? ○ Male   ○ Female

  b. How old were you on your last birthday?
     ○ Less than 35   ○ 65–74
     ○ 35–44   ○ 75–84
     ○ 45–54   ○ 85 and older
     ○ 55–64

13. Have you ever filled out this form before?
    ○ Yes
    ○ No
    ○ Don't remember

Thank you for your time.

14. DO NOT MARK HERE Ⓐ Ⓑ Ⓒ Ⓓ Ⓔ
    NOT LAST CARD   ○

This printed form of the SF-36 Health Status Survey is for use on the RT-2000 Response Terminal made by Response Technologies, Inc. - East Greenwich, RI 02818

B

FIGURE 157–16 *Continued*

SF-36™ HEALTH STATUS SURVEY

INSTRUCTIONS: This survey asks for your views about your health. This information will help keep track of how you feel and how well you are able to do your usual activities.

Answer every question by marking the appropriate oval. If you are unsure about how to answer a question, please give the best answer you can.

Before beginning this questionnaire...
Please pencil in your ID number in the squares to the right and then darken in the appropriate oval below each number.

If you don't know what ID number to use, ask the person who gave you this questionnaire.

Now begin with the questions below.

MARKING INSTRUCTIONS
- Use a No. 2 Pencil ONLY.
- Make dark heavy marks that fill the oval completely.
- Erase unwanted marks cleanly.
- Make no stray marks on this answer sheet.

1. In general, would you say your health is:
   1. Excellent
   2. Very good
   3. Good
   4. Fair
   5. Poor

2. **Compared to one year ago,** how would you rate your health in general now?
   1. Much better now than 1 year ago
   2. Somewhat better now than 1 year ago
   3. About the same as 1 year ago
   4. Somewhat worse now than 1 year ago
   5. Much worse now than 1 year ago

3. The following items are about activities you might do during a typical day. Does **your health now limit you** in these activities? If so, how much? (Mark one oval on each line.)

	Yes, Limited A Lot	Yes, Limited A Little	No, Not Limited At All
a. <u>Vigorous activities,</u> such as running, lifting heavy objects, participating in strenuous sports	①	②	③
b. <u>Moderate activities,</u> such as moving a table, pushing a vacuum cleaner, bowling, or playing golf	①	②	③
c. Lifting or carrying groceries	①	②	③
d. Climbing <u>several</u> flights of stairs	①	②	③
e. Climbing <u>one</u> flight of stairs	①	②	③
f. Bending, kneeling, or stooping	①	②	③
g. Walking <u>more than a mile</u>	①	②	③
h. Walking <u>several blocks</u>	①	②	③
i. Walking <u>one block</u>	①	②	③
j. Bathing or dressing yourself	①	②	③

4. During the **past 4 weeks,** have you had any of the following problems with your work or other regular daily activities **as a result of your physical health?** (Mark one oval on each line.)

	Yes	No
a. Cut down the <u>amount of time</u> you spent on work or other activities	①	②
b. <u>Accomplished less</u> than you would like	①	②
c. Were limited in the <u>kind</u> of work or other activities	①	②
d. Had <u>difficulty</u> performing the work or other activities (for example, it took extra effort)	①	②

PLEASE TURN CARD OVER TO COMPLETE QUESTIONNAIRE

Copyright © 1989 by New England Medical Center Hospitals, Inc. All Rights Reserved

FIGURE 157–16. (A and B) MOS-SF 36 form. Multiple choice questionnaire. This form has been validated worldwide for over a decade in 7.5 million patients in many disease categories. (SF-36 Health Survey, Copyright 1992 Medical Outcomes Trust. All Rights Reserved. Reproduced with permission of the Medical Outcomes Trust.)

Illustration continued on following page

Cerebrospinal fluid (CSF) leak is a potential problem. If this occurs, it is important repair be done early on. Occasionally, a CSF leak is ventral and not accessible. If the area of the leak is reinforced with Surgicel and the deep layers of fascia and skin are well repaired, the leak can heal. If a dural tear is amenable to repair, this procedure is best carried out immediately. Ordinarily, there are no consequences of dural repair, provided that nerve root injury has not occurred.

There are occasional instances in which a dural defect has allowed a root to herniate through it, resulting in incarceration of the root and postoperative radicular pain. Evidence of CSF leak in connection with persistent radicular pain after surgery should alert the surgeon to this possibility. Imaging studies may be unrevealing, and surgery to replace the herniated portion of the root in the dural sac and repair the dura may be helpful.

Failure to relieve symptoms is probably the most common complication. It often results from improper initial diagnosis. It may relate to surgical trauma. Its incidence can be kept down by careful attention to the preoperative diagnosis and to the gentlest possible surgical techniques. This complication probably cannot be avoided completely.

POSTOPERATIVE CARE

Postoperatively, we place few limitations on the patient's activity, relying on the level of pain to regulate it. No normal activity is likely to cause injury to the disc, muscle, or incision. The disc itself is as structurally strong after surgery as it was before. The annulus and the remaining portion of the nucleus support the axial and shearing forces as well after the surgery as before it.

Patients are kept in the hospital for 1 or 2 days postoperatively and then released. They ordinarily can return to work within a short time. There is no medical contraindication to allowing sedentary workers to return to work in a few days. Because of muscular pain, heavily physical laborers may prefer to stay out of work a little longer, but most patients should be back to work within 1 month of surgery and many within a few days or weeks. The mechanisms of disc herniation, as outlined in Figure 157–1 and Table 157–1, render it unlikely that any particular activity will raise the risk of recurrent disc herniation.

OUTCOME ANALYSIS

An important new development in the measurement of health status is the use of a sophisticated patient-based questionnaire to evaluate a patient's functional status, level of pain, and general health. (See reference listings on Medical Outcomes Study and health surveys in ''Selected References.'') Heretofore, health status has been judged on the basis of pathologic findings and the physician's opinion. As new procedures are developed, their proponents have a bias. We are in need of methods to evaluate neurosurgical treatment and to allow it to be compared with the general range of medical and surgical treatments available today.

The Medical Outcomes Study short form, a 36-question survey (MOS-SF36) (Fig. 157–16), has been tested for over a decade in very large populations and in many disease states; the method is just coming into use in neurosurgery. The health status of a patient is assessed by having the patient answer a set of 36 questions. The questionnaire must be filled out by the patient without the help of others. A computerized scoring instrument is used to determine the results. Its use is very simple and does not consume the physician's time. The carefully designed set of questions is weighted and scored to reflect physical functioning, physical role, bodily pain, general health, vitality, social functioning, emotional role, and mental health. The resulting scores can be plotted as a curve and can give an assessment of the patient's status without the bias of the physician.

The MOS-SF 36 is a generic health survey not specific to lumbar surgery but it lends itself very well to evaluating patients with sciatica before and after treatment. Our preliminary studies show that the MOS-SF 36 can be used to assess the impairments of patients with sciatica before and after surgery (Figs. 157–16 and 157–17). The patients are shown

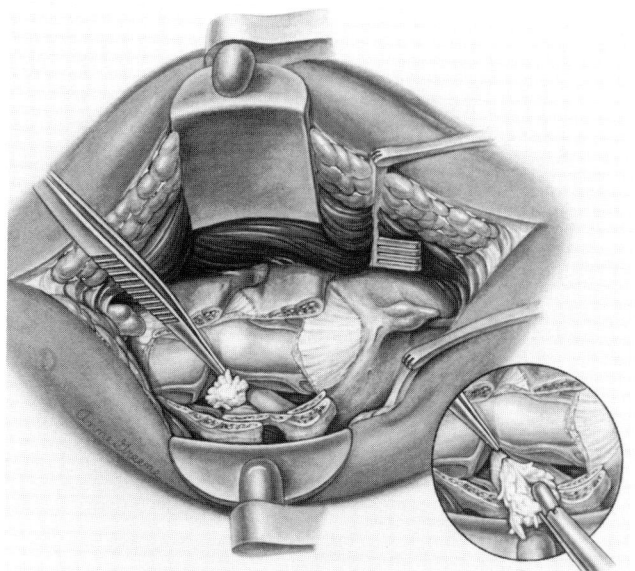

FIGURE 157–15. Facet has been excised to access foraminal extrusion.

of the spinal canal. A larger bony exposure is carried out in such cases, rostrocaudally and across the midline to include a portion of the contralateral lamina. It need not be extended all the way laterally on the other side. In fact, it is better to preserve the facet joint on the other side.

Instability has not been a problem following this operation in our hands. The disc can be removed from the side of the patient's symptoms or, if symptoms are bilateral, from the side of the more severe symptoms. We have almost never carried out fusion in these instances and have not encountered significant postoperative instability in relation to this condition. A wide exposure both rostrocaudally and laterally is helpful in reducing the possibility of neural injury in these large paracentral disc herniations. This is particularly important when cauda equina syndrome is a consideration. Instances of postoperative cauda equina syndrome have occurred when the operative exposure is not wide enough owing to excessive retraction of already compromised nerve roots.

EXTRAFORAMINAL DISC HERNIATION

Far lateral or extraforaminal disc herniation occurs in about 10 percent of instances. It is important to recognize this entity on the preoperative scans. Not diagnosable by plain myelography, it is ordinarily evident on the CT or MRI scan as a mass lateral to the foramen on the axial views.

A purely lateral approach has been devised through a muscle-splitting incision. The arterial branches in the region of the facet must be dealt with in either the purely lateral or the conventional approach. I find it safer to begin dissection medially in the familiar territory of the interlaminar space, widening the standard hemilaminectomy approach laterally so as to have the nerve root well in view. The more lateral approaches do not afford an early exposure of the nerve root. Because the symptoms relate to nerve root compression, it seems to be safest to identify the root medially and, after removing the facet, to follow the nerve root laterally, ensuring removal of the portion of the herniation that is impinging on the nerve root. At L5-S1, the exposure can be difficult in view of the overriding iliac crest. Here, it may be necessary to work from within the interspace itself to draw the herniated portion medially.

REOPERATIONS

Disc herniation recurs in 5 to 10 percent of instances. Obesity may be a risk factor. Although hard physical work can cause back symptoms, it is not clear that recurrent disc herniation is any more common in the physically stressed population than in the general population.

The caveats that apply to primary disc surgery are equally important with recurrent symptoms.

Imaging studies can be difficult to interpret in patients who have previously undergone surgery. If the findings on enhanced MRI or CT scanning are clear and correlate with the patient's symptoms, no further studies are warranted. If the CT and MRI imaging studies are unclear, CT myelography provides definitive results in most cases. Formation of scar tissue is the natural result of any surgery. All too often, scar tissue is implicated as a cause of recurrent symptoms in patients who have previously undergone disc surgery when, in fact, failure of original diagnosis, degenerative spondylosis, or nerve root injury at prior surgery is the cause of continued pain. Arachnoiditis has similarly been inappropriately invoked as a cause of symptoms in many instances. Reoperation for scar alone, or surgery for arachnoiditis, is unlikely to be helpful to the patient. In reoperative surgery, the extensive dissection of scar tissue can be traumatic. If a bona fide recurrent disc herniation has been diagnosed, it is much the safest approach to enter the scar tissue at the site where disc herniation is suspected and to remove the herniated portion of the disc, leaving most of the scar undisturbed. This is important in speeding postoperative recovery and avoiding additional trauma.

INTRADISCAL PROCEDURES

With the advent of laparoscopic cholecystectomy and arthroscopic knee surgery, the public has come to expect that less invasive operations will provide better results. Convincing evidence that this is true for lumbar disc surgery has not been accumulated. A large literature has accumulated relating to theoretically less invasive intradiscal techniques. In actual fact, good results of surgery depend mainly on correct diagnosis and atraumatic manipulation of the tissues.

Percutaneous techniques for disc aspiration have been introduced. These have mainly been applied to the "contained" disc—the disc that has not herniated. Like chymopapain injection, these procedures are directed at the contents of the interspace. The rationale is to remove normal disc tissue, trusting that herniation will reduce itself into the space created within normal disc. No percutaneous technique has been devised to address the extruded fragment directly, and it has not been shown that procedures on the interior of the disc itself provide any better outcome than the natural course of healing.

COMPLICATIONS

Complications have been extensively treated. One of the most catastrophic relates to ventral perforation. Awareness of this possibility is most important. Arterial injury to the iliac arteries can occur if a curette or rongeur is inserted through the interspace and through the anterior annulus. Occasionally, the anterior annulus itself is not patent, and an instrument may pass through it without evident change in resistance. Marking the instruments in such a way as to warn of too-deep penetration has not always been helpful. Ventral perforation has occurred even in the hands of the most experienced neurosurgeons. A sudden drop in blood pressure should alert the surgical team to this possibility. Visible bleeding in the interspace is evident in fewer than 50 percent of cases. With major hypotension, it is important to terminate the operation, place the patient supine on the operating table, and call for the help of a vascular surgeon. If a vascular surgeon is not available, an incision can be made and a hand placed through a midline abdominal incision onto the spine to compress the aorta until help arrives. The rupture ordinarily involves the common iliac artery, and the iliac vein is sometimes injured. Both the artery and the vein can be injured, in which case an arteriovenous fistula may form. There are occasionally injuries to the bowel or ureter, or both; these too require early recognition and corrective surgery.

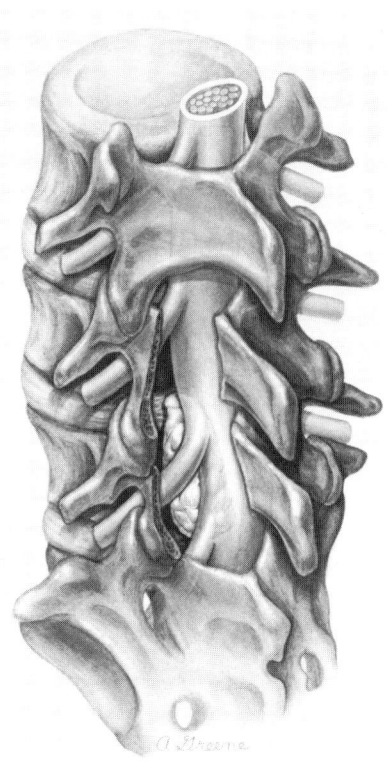

FIGURE 157-13. Wider exposure is necessary for safest removal of paracentral disc herniation. (From Fager CA: Atlas of Spinal Surgery. Philadelphia, Lea and Febiger, 1989.)

Regarding operating on the correct level, it is important to emphasize that if only patients with major disc ruptures are being operated upon, then the correct level is the level with the obvious disc rupture. This is often a free fragment or at least a most obvious major prolapse, what I call grade II or grade III if the patients are well selected.

Several errors must be made for the surgeon to operate on the wrong level. One possible error is to operate on the wrong patient—in other words, to have made the wrong diagnosis. If the patient has no disc rupture, there is no correct level for surgery. This is an error made more often than one might like to think. The same is true for minimally herniated discs. The taking of radiographs in such instances can confirm the level being operated upon, but there is usually a more fundamental problem: No matter what level is operated, the outcome will likely be poor. If a large disc rupture is expected and no disc rupture is found, then one is at the wrong level. If no disc rupture is expected, the operation should probably not have been carried out to begin with.

Regarding the technique of dissection, I prefer to place the muscles on a slight stretch by using a periosteal elevator to retract them laterally and then using the cutting cautery at low setting to divide the attachments of the paraspinous muscles to the spine.

Two Markham retractors are used to maintain the exposure. The Leksell rongeur is used to start the hemilaminectomy. This rongeur has a special feature incorporated into its design; it can be held to cut in a nearly vertical position. Its lower cutting jaw should never be inserted beneath the lamina because of the danger of injury to the underlying nerve root. The initial hemilaminectomy is widened with a thin foot plate Kerrison rongeur. The yellow ligament is carefully excised, being drawn dorsally with toothed forceps as it is cut to avoid dural injury. The Kerrison punch, which may pick up a fold of dura, also must be used with great care to avoid dural or root injury. A dural tear, if recognized and repaired, is usually of no consequence. Bony removal is carried out laterally above and below the level of herniation. The yellow ligament is excised and the root exposed. Bipolar coagulation of the epidural veins is carried out.

The nerve root is gently retracted medially over the dome of the herniation. A conjoined root may be apparent on preoperative studies but may sometimes be recognized only at this stage. Medial retraction of a conjoined root may be difficult, and it may be necessary to work in the limited space beneath the axilla of the root rather than in the safer zone lateral to the shoulder of the retracted root. If a free fragment is present, it is removed from the epidural space at this point. If a herniated fragment is contained within a portion of the annulus, an incision in these thinner annular fibers is made. The therapeutic portion of the operation is removal of the epidural mass. It is safest to limit the operation to this maneuver. It is not clear to what extent curettage of the interspace is helpful, and it raises the level of risk of the operation slightly. Removal of the herniated portion of the disc is likely to be sufficient to provide relief. It has not been shown that recurrence is any less likely if curettage of the interspace is carried out.

PARACENTRAL DISC HERNIATION

Slight central bulging of lumbar discs is common and ordinarily of no clinical significance. The posterior longitudinal ligament forces most disc herniations to a posterolateral position. Occasionally, I estimate in 10 percent of instances, significant disc herniation may occur near the midline. Ordinarily it occurs immediately to one side of the midline. Such a paracentral disc herniation can obstruct the major portion

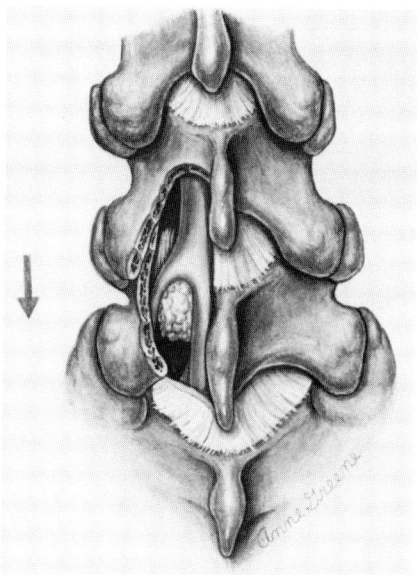

FIGURE 157-14. Caudal migration of fragment requires its removal via axilla of the nerve root. Similar exposure is necessary for conjoined nerve root. (From Fager CA: Atlas of Spinal Surgery. Philadelphia, Lea and Febiger, 1989.)

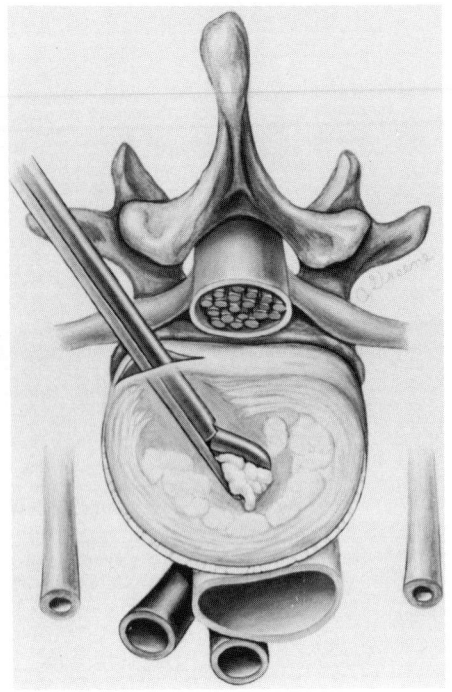

FIGURE 157–11. Proximity of common iliac arteries, iliac veins and ureters to anterior surface of L4-5 annulus. Curettage within the interspace increases the risk of operation and likely has no effect on the incidence of recurrence. The incidence of recurrence is suspected to relate more to degenerative changes in annulus (Fig. 157–1 and Table 157–1). (From Fager CA: Atlas of Spinal Surgery. Philadelphia, Lea and Febiger, 1989.)

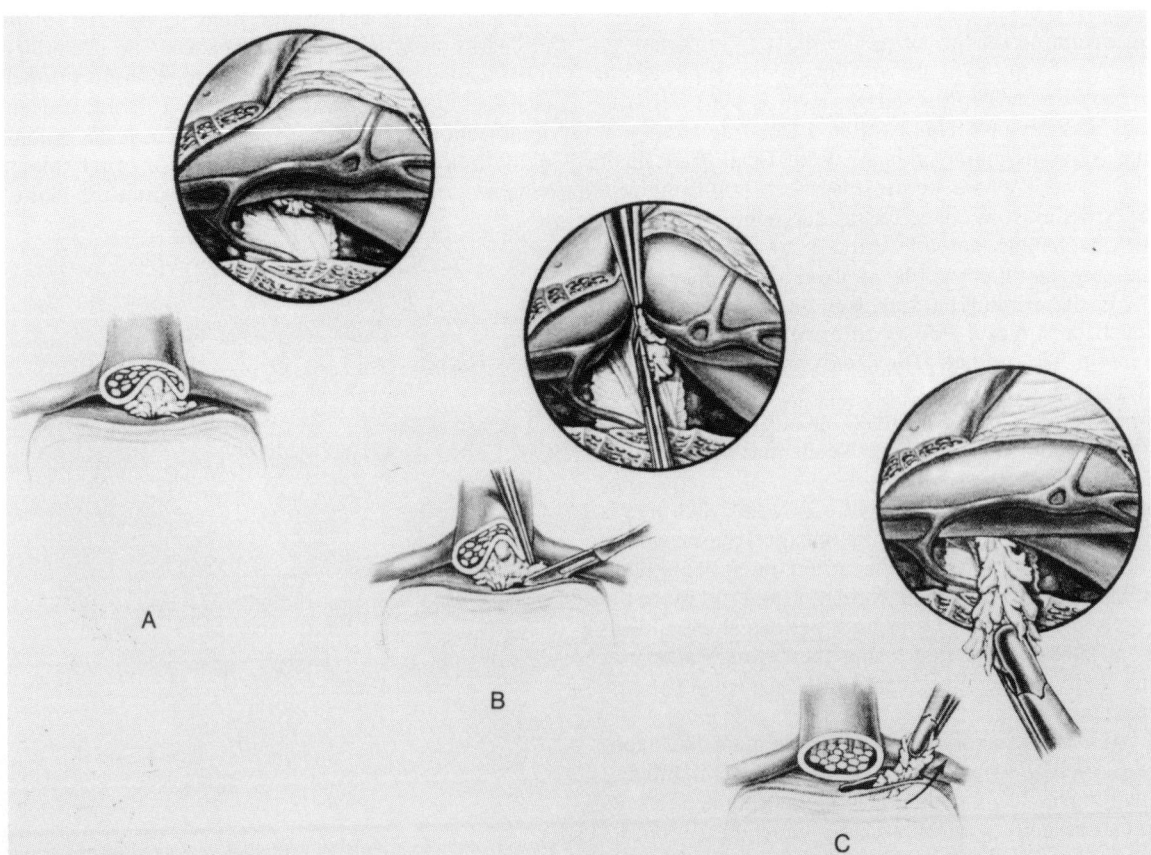

FIGURE 157–12. Steps in gentle retraction of dural sac, in which extruded disc material is drawn laterally. At surgeon's initial view (A), extruded fragment may not be obvious. (From Fager CA: Atlas of Spinal Surgery. Philadelphia, Lea and Febiger, 1989.)

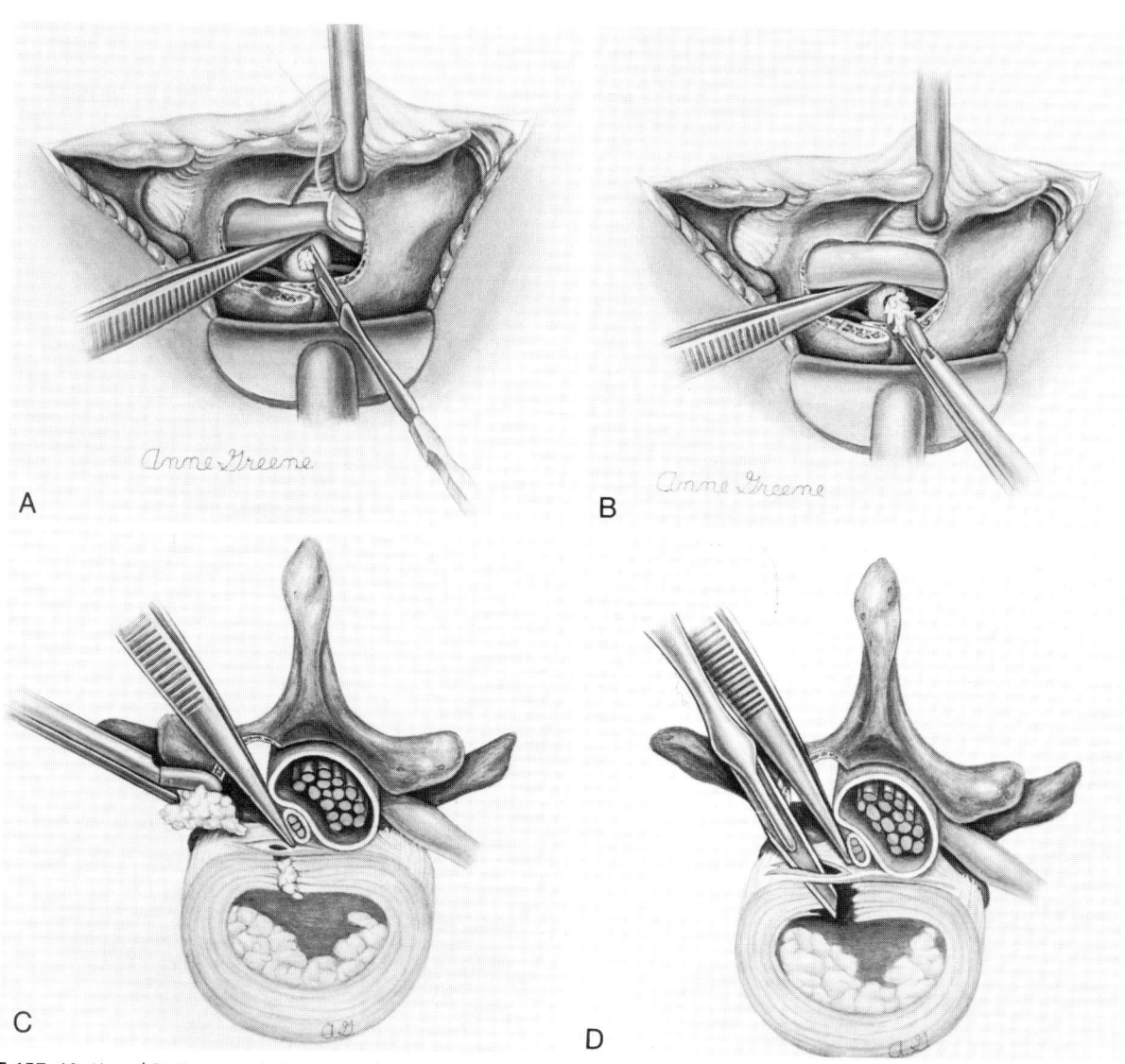

FIGURE 157-10. (A and B) Fragment being grasped. Dissection from a medial to lateral direction avoids increasing pressure on nerve root. (C) Fragment being brought out of epidural space. (D) The annulus is being incised so that interspace can be explored for loose fragments of nucleus. (From Fager CA: Atlas of Spinal Surgery. Philadelphia, Lea and Febiger, 1989.)

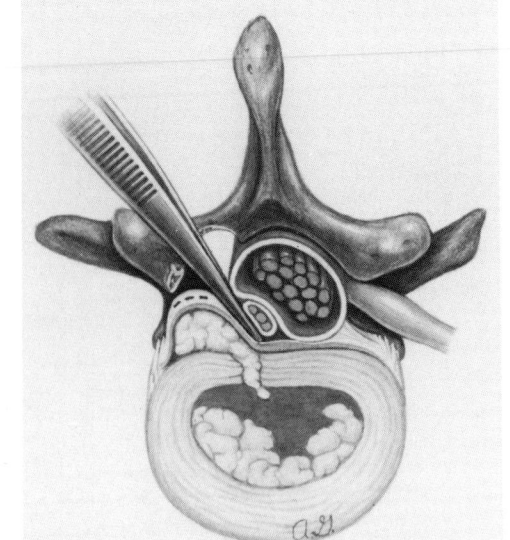

FIGURE 157–8. Extruded fragment seen in the foramen, displacing the root and dural sac medially. (From Fager CA: Atlas of Spinal Surgery. Philadelphia, Lea and Febiger, 1989.)

and the table flexed, is commonly used. My own preference is for the knee-chest position, in which the laminae are spread apart, the depth of the wound is reduced to the absolute minimum, the epidural veins are totally decompressed, and the great vessels in the abdomen must hang away from the spine to some extent. It is important to avoid neck extension during any prone operation, in order to prevent cervical spinal cord injury (see Fig. 157–5).

POSTEROLATERAL DISC HERNIATION

Most herniated discs occur in a posterolateral position (see Fig. 157–4). I estimate that 80 percent of ruptured discs are in this location. A paramedian incision is made on the side of the herniation. Regarding surface landmarks, a surgeon's relaxed hand with the thumb and little finger spread apart corresponds to the size of the sacrum in almost all patients. If the surgeon's little finger is placed on the tip of the coccyx, the thumb of the hand in this relaxed position will lie on the lumbosacral interspace. This has been of greater help to me in localizing the level than any other method.

Intraoperative radiographs are not ordinarily required but should be used in cases of spondylosis and whenever the relationship of the pathology to the level of surgery is in doubt. In most instances, the presence of a large disc herniation is the indication that the correct level is being exposed.

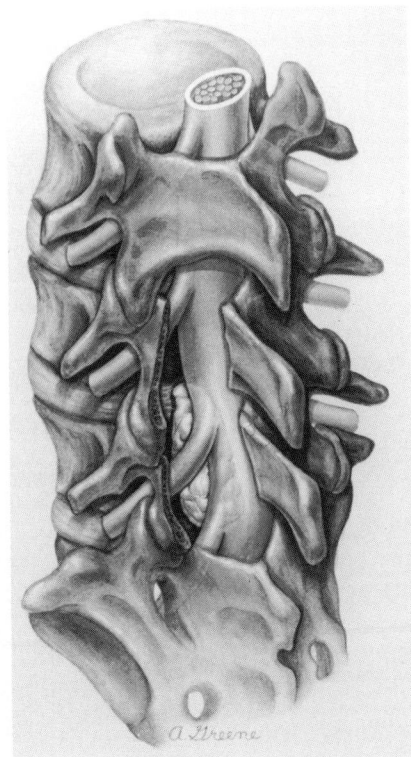

FIGURE 157–9. Large extruded fragment straddling the L5 nerve root. Wider bony exposure is required for safe removal of an extensive lesion. (From Fager CA: Atlas of Spinal Surgery. Philadelphia, Lea and Febiger, 1989.)

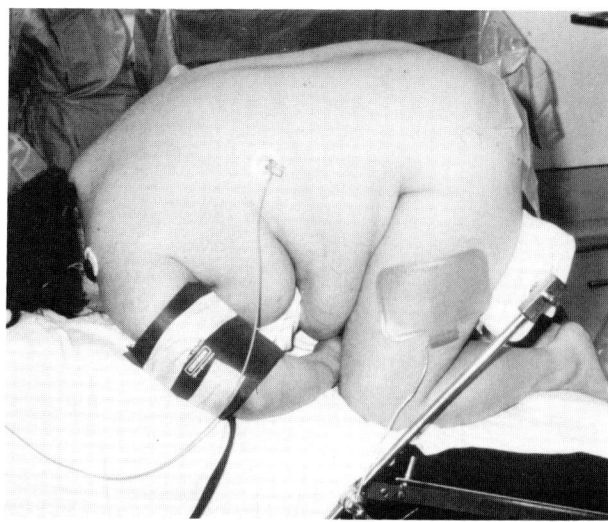

FIGURE 157-5. Knee-chest position. Note that the abdomen is dependent. This lowers the pressure in the epidural veins. Laminae are separated and brought more superficial by the flexed position. The patient's buttocks are supported on a seat. As with any prone position, care is taken to avoid neck extension. Even in an obese patient such as this, operation can be relatively bloodless. (From Fager CA: Atlas of Spinal Surgery. Philadelphia, Lea and Febiger, 1989.)

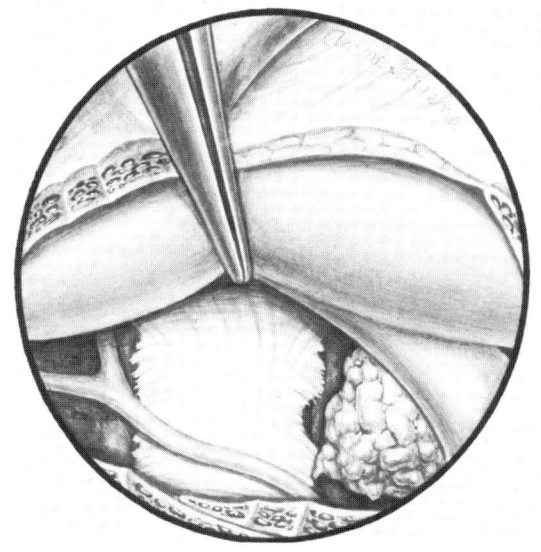

FIGURE 157-6. Left-sided exposure. Dural sac retracted medially. Nerve root seen at right. Extruded fragment of a disc can be seen to have extruded caudally from an interior marginal tear in the annulus. (From Fager CA: Atlas of Spinal Surgery. Philadelphia, Lea and Febiger, 1989.)

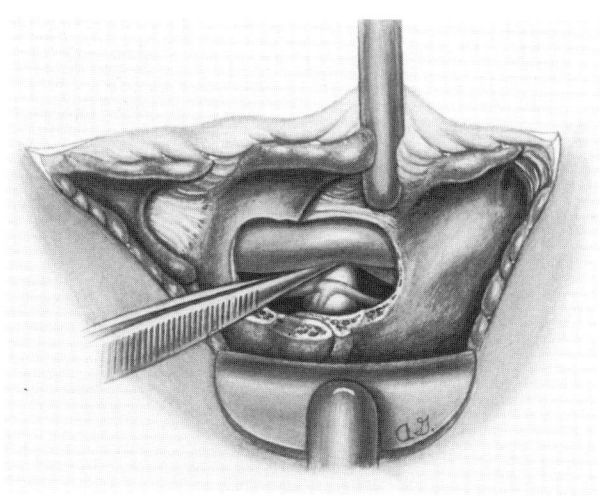

FIGURE 157-7. Extruded fragment is visible beneath the epidural vein at the level of the interspace. (From Fager CA: Atlas of Spinal Surgery. Philadelphia, Lea and Febiger, 1989.)

ment is definitely not an indication for surgery in the absence of diagnosis of bona fide disc rupture. Sometimes included in contraindications to surgery is a first episode of sciatic pain without an adequate trial of conservative management. There are, however, occasional instances in which pain is so severe that it may be worse at bedrest.

It is worth mentioning that now, with widespread use of MRI and CT scanning, the combination of a negative CT or MRI scan with a negative myelogram, or of negative CT and MRI scans makes it extremely unlikely that a surgically remediable disc rupture will be found. For this reason, exploratory lumbar surgery is almost never advisable.

Epidural venography and discography are currently of no value.

TIMING OF SURGERY

Finally, a few points on the timing of surgery. Ordinarily, an operation for removal of a herniated disc is carried out semielectively. I say this because the patient who needs surgery is usually in fairly intense pain, making the operation not totally elective. If, however, there is a disabling neurologic deficit, such as profound foot drop or quadriceps weakness, the chances of good motor recovery are better if the operation is carried fairly promptly. Sometimes, even with immediate surgery, a profound deficit does not recover, but if the deficit is not quite complete, there is a reasonable chance for recovery if the pressure on the nerve root is promptly relieved.

The natural healing process of lumbar disc herniation has been documented. The herniated material absorbs over a long period. We have seen a number of instances in which bona fide disc extrusion has been imaged and, over a period of months or longer, has been shown to resolve spontaneously.

Well-documented cases are unusual. The radiologic findings have not always correlated with the clinical findings. There are instances in which the herniation appears better but the patient's symptoms are worse or vice versa. The remarkable healing process of the spine can lead to reduction in symptoms in most patients. It is only with unremitting sciatic pain and significant disc herniation that surgery is clearly of value.

Risk factors negatively influencing the results of surgery include unclear diagnosis, atypical symptoms, equivocal imaging studies, very long duration of symptoms, workers' compensation claims, litigation, drug dependence including heavy smoking and alcoholism, obesity, and concurrent medical problems. Once all factors have been considered and it has been determined that surgery is likely to be very helpful, the patient should be preoperatively informed of the possibility of death, paralysis, rupture of the abdominal vessels or viscera, and the worst imaginable complications. The physician needs to be reassuring in manner and should if, his or her experience warrants, indicate that such problems are very unlikely to occur.

OPERATIVE TECHNIQUES
(Figs. 157-1 to 157-14)

The primary operation for a patient with herniated lumbar intervertebral disc has been very thoroughly described in previous editions of this volume and elsewhere. The use of fiberoptic illumination and magnifying loupes is well established. The microscope is an option but probably does not add to the efficacy of operation. In fact, at times, visualization of the entire disc fragment may be hindered by inexperienced use of the microscope.

A variety of patient positions have been used. The prone position, with rolls placed under the chest and iliac crests

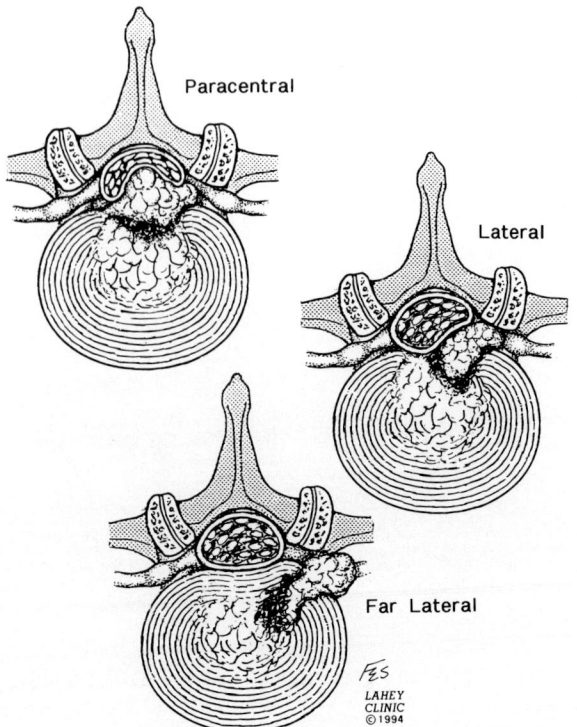

FIGURE 157-4. Position of disc herniation. Most herniations, (estimated at 80 percent) occur in the posterolateral quadrant, compromising spinal canal and medial foramen. Posterior longitudinal ligament forces herniation to one side of midline. An estimated 10 percent of herniations occur in paracentral location, and an estimated 10 percent of herniations occur laterally in the lateral foramen or lateral to foramen, where the root existing above may be compromised. Preoperative recognition of location of herniation helps in operative planning. (From Fager CA: Atlas of Spinal Surgery. Philadelphia, Lea and Febiger, 1989.)

of neurologic examination. If pain is improving, a residual deficit may improve along with it over a slightly longer time. Therefore, if pain is diminishing, a weakness of dorsiflexion of the foot is not in itself necessarily an indication for surgery. A severe foot drop with sciatic pain is an indication for surgery. Even with prompt surgery, recovery from severe foot drop does not always occur.

A cauda equina syndrome can sometimes be difficult to diagnose. The event may be acute. Experienced neurologic consultation may not be available. Sometimes the deficit is more pronounced than the pain. Widespread sensorimotor loss and impairment of bladder function may be present. The condition is unusual. It can result from massive disc herniation. In this situation, urgent surgery is indicated if the diagnosis can be made. Recovery, which may be partial, does not always occur even with prompt surgery.

IMAGING

Once a clinical diagnosis of disc herniation has been made in a patient whose severity of pain is sufficient to warrant surgery, preoperative imaging studies are in order. When no surgery is being contemplated, the expense of imaging, which has become considerable, is probably not warranted. Sometimes, imaging studies are carried out in response to patients' demands that "something" be done. Scanning is theoretically harmless, but the danger of over-diagnosis referred to previously is great, particularly because the radiologist's report may be given to the patient. Then, too, there is a tendency to carry out excessive studies even when a diagnosis is clear on one study. To a large extent, these problems of imaging are reduced when patients and doctors have an incentive to reduce the costs of care by avoiding unnecessary tests.

High-quality CT scanning can clearly demonstrate disc herniation, particularly in patients who are not obese and who have not undergone previous surgery. MRI appears to be approximately equal to CT scanning in terms of accuracy for diagnosis of disc herniation. Both studies tend to be over-interpreted by radiologists, who do not have the opportunity of seeing the patient and the correlating signs and symptoms.

In patients strongly suspected on clinical grounds of having disc herniation and whose CT or MRI scans are unrevealing, it is justifiable to carry out further study by CT myelography. In this test, a small amount of water-soluble intrathecal contrast is instilled, followed by CT scanning. This is still our most accurate diagnostic test. Even when scar tissue is present from previous surgery, an accurate diagnosis of nerve root displacement should be possible in almost all cases. The use of CT scanning permits using smaller quantities of intrathecal contrast agent and a diminution in side effects. In its present form, MRI scanning requires the patient to lie still for a prolonged period. Some patients in severe pain cannot do so even with medication. For some, even CT scanning, which requires less time, is intolerable. For these patients, too, CT myelography, which skillfully carried out can offer more flexibility of positioning, may be the best test. CT myelography may also be more acceptable to patients who are claustrophobic.

It is important to emphasize the pathology of lumbar disc rupture. The strong posterior longitudinal ligaments in the midline cause most disc herniations to occur laterally, in other words, to one side. Disc herniations rarely affect both legs; the painful syndrome is in the vast majority of instances unilateral, e.g., right or left, not both. Midline bulging of discs occurs so commonly that it should hardly be considered pathologic. Lateral views on myelogram as well as CT and MRI scans that demonstrate disc bulging usually do not indicate a likely benefit from surgery.

My colleagues and I use a system of grading disc ruptures to distinguish among free fragments, major disc ruptures, and normal discs with minimal bulging. We consider the disc grade 0 or grade I if there is no bulge or little bulging; grade II if there is a marked herniation with a few fibers of annulus intact; and grade III if there is an extruded free fragment. Grade II and grade III are the pathologic conditions most likely to be helped by surgery. This grading system is illustrated in Figure 157–3.

The importance of true sciatic pain down the back of one leg below the knee cannot be over-emphasized. Atypical variations that are not true sciatica, however, namely pain confined to the buttock or back of the thigh and variable sciatic pain involving both legs, are negative factors and tend to be correlated with poor outcome from surgery.

Progressively worsening neurologic deficit is often included among indications for surgery, perhaps most commonly in orthopedic circles. In fact, it is extremely unusual for disc rupture to cause a progressive neurologic deficit. This condition should be removed from the standard list of surgical indications. Intractable pain is also listed as indication for disc surgery and should also be removed. The pain from disc rupture typically fluctuates, and most motivated patients often do not stop work because of it. In general, injuries that occur in the workplace do not cause disc rupture. The severe twisting, shearing forces that are necessary to rupture the annulus usually do not occur after lifting and after falls in the workplace. The failure of conservative treat-

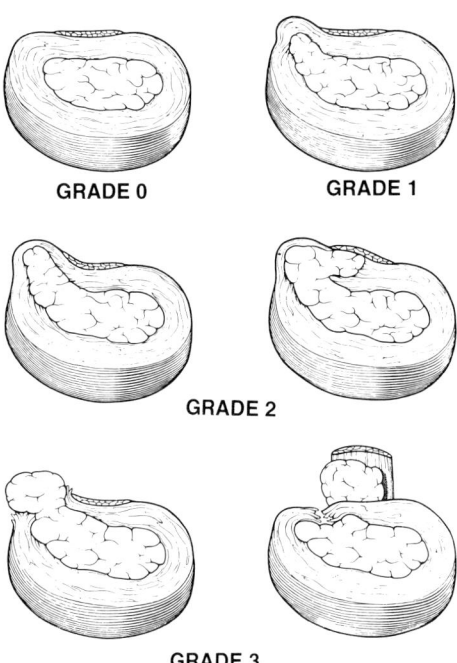

FIGURE 157–3. Gradations of disc bulging and herniation. Normal disc—grade 0. Slightly bulging disc—grade 1. Moderate disc herniation—grade 2. Extruded disc—grade 3.

Table 157-1. DEGENERATIVE CHANGES LEADING TO DISC SPACE NARROWING, VACUUM DISC PHENOMENON, DISC BULGING, AND DISC HERNIATION

Status of Disc	Status of Nucleus and Annulus	Stresses	Comment
Normal disc	Normal annulus, normal nucleus	Stresses proportionately borne by nucleus and annulus	
Degenerated narrowed disc	Loss of substance in both annulus and nucleus	Stresses proportionately borne by nucleus and annulus	
Vacuum disc phenomenon	Disproportionate loss of substance, greater in nucleus	Stresses disproportionately borne by annulus	Gas in interspace
Preherniation of disc	Disproportionate loss of substance	Stresses disproportionately borne by nucleus	Axial forces translated in nucleus to centrifugal forces leading to herniation
Herniated disc		Once herniation has occurred, stresses borne proportionately by remaining nucleus and annulus herniated fragment of nucleus exerts pressure on adjacent root, causing sciatica	
Postoperative herniated disc			May have gas in interspace

and annulus lead only to a loss of height of the interspace. If there is a preferentially greater loss of annulus, however, the axial pressures on the nucleus from the weight of the body and the pull of the paraspinous muscles leads to excessive pressure on the remaining portion of the nucleus, which is unsupported by the degenerated narrowed annulus. This is transferred to centrifugal pressure, which together with shearing forces may produce tearing of the fibers of the annulus, allowing extrusion of nuclear material. After the excess nucleus has herniated, the disc is structurally stable. The forces on the degenerated nucleus and annulus are in balance, and there is no vector force driving further nuclear material out—unless the annulus further degenerates.

Mixed situations may occur in which there is loss of substance in one part of the nucleus, resulting in gas formation, and excessive pressure in another part of the nucleus. In such an instance, a herniation with intradiscal gas may occur (Fig. 157-2).

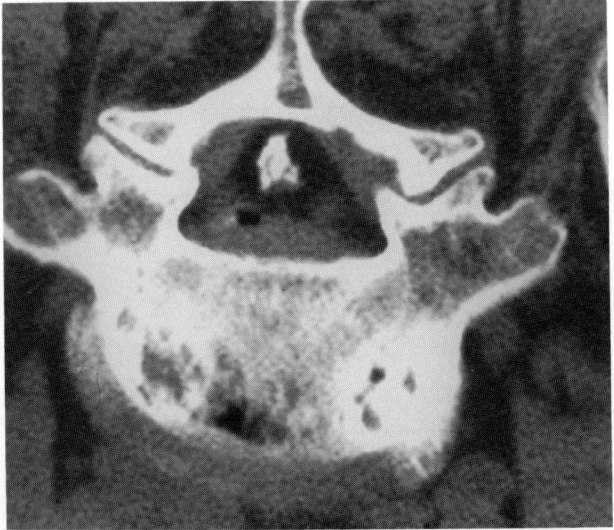

FIGURE 157-2. MRI scan showing extruded disc fragment with gas in the fragment. Prior degenerative changes in the nucleus apparently led to gas formation. Subsequent degenerative changes in the annulus, as outlined in Figure 157-1 and Table 157-1, may lead to herniation of the degenerated nucleus.

CLINICAL EVALUATION: INDICATIONS FOR IMAGING AND SURGERY

The most common indication for lumbar surgery to excise the herniated portion of a lumbar intervertebral disc is persistent severe pain in a sciatic distribution together with imaging findings clearly indicating a disc herniation in a patient who is likely to be helped by the operation. Patients with severe sciatic pain in whom a bona fide disc herniation has clearly been demonstrated usually have good results from surgery. Disc herniation ordinarily occurs as an isolated event at one level. It is extremely unusual to have more than one bona fide disc herniation at the same time. A diagnosis of multiple disc herniations is usually incorrect. Judging the severity of a patient's pain can be difficult. There is obviously no quantitative method of doing so. A very severe pain for a short period may be tolerable, whereas a less severe pain persisting for a long period may be intolerable. Patients' tolerances of pain vary widely. Often, it requires all of the physician's cognitive skills and intuition to make a wise judgment in this area.

Workers' compensation laws are a severe deterrent to health. Bona fide disc herniation rarely occurs in the workplace, but muscular and ligamentous strain is common. All too often, the patient injured in the workplace is subjected to excessive testing, over-diagnosis, and over-treatment, all of which can lead to loss of confidence and disability. Patients with workers' compensation issues must be judged especially carefully and a very clear diagnosis ensured before any surgery is contemplated.

In the last edition of this volume, Finneson discussed the fallibility of the neurologic examination. The usual lateral disc herniation at L4-L5 compresses the L5 root. The usual lateral disc herniation at L5-S1 compresses the S1 root. Occasionally, a more medial disc herniation at L4-L5 may compress the S1 root, and a far lateral herniation at L5-S1 may compress the L5 root. The same principles apply at higher levels of the lumbar spine. A deficit may not be present. Although there may be weakness of the extensor hallucis longus with involvement of the L5 nerve root, it is quite common, even with a very large disc rupture at L4-L5, to have no obvious neurologic deficit because of the overlapping distribution of adjacent roots. This, too, is a limitation

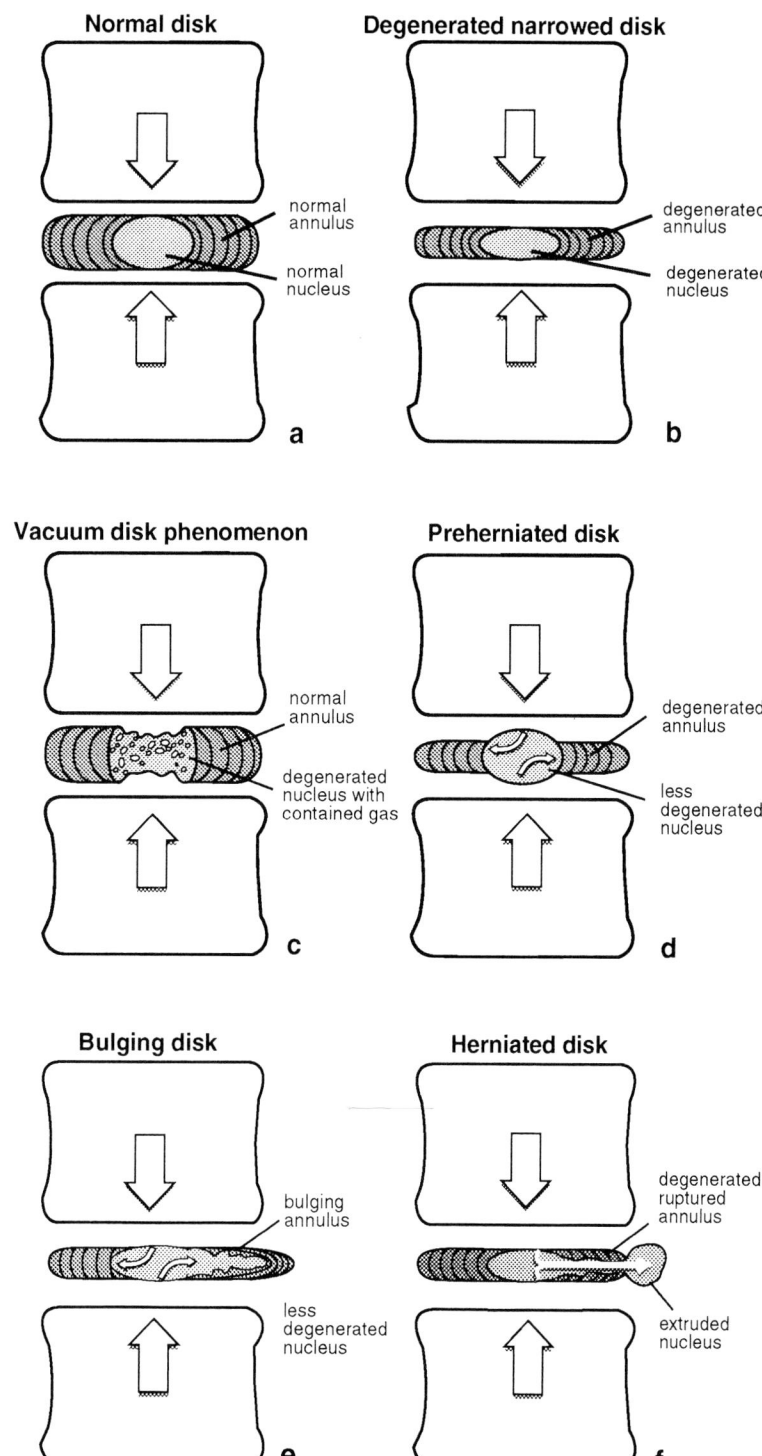

FIGURE 157-1. Exploded views of vertebrae and disc in axial section. Theoretical diagrams of changes in the lumbar discs leading to disc herniation and extrusion. (A) Normal annulus and nucleus. Axial forces (arrows) balanced by elastic properties of nucleus and annulus. (B) Degenerated disc. Annulus and nucleus have proportionately narrowed. Axial forces still balanced by elastic properties of the disc. Some flexibility may be lost due to loss of height of disc. (C) Degenerated disc with vacuum disc phenomenon. Annulus relatively preserved. Relatively more degenerative change has occurred in the nucleus, leading to loss of substance in the nucleus. Axial forces are mainly borne by the annulus. There is no pressure on the nucleus. Gas is seen in the nucleus due to loss of substance of involuted nucleus. (D) Preherniated disc. Annulus has degenerated more than nucleus. Bulk of remaining nucleus, unsupported by degenerated axially narrowed annulus, is now under increased pressure. Axial forces are now translated to centrifugal forces within the nucleus (small arrows) that can lead to disc herniation. (E) Bulging disc. Some fibers of annulus on the right in the diagram of disc are stretched or incompetent, allowing elevated intranuclear pressure to displace disc material from the interspace into the epidural space. (F) Frank disc extrusion. Incompetent fibers of the annulus have ruptured. Shearing forces can be the final event leading to this problem either in the midportion of the annulus or at the margin of annulus. Axial pressures translated to centrifugal forces (small arrows seen in D lead to extrusion of disc material into the epidural space.

CHAPTER 157

Surgery of Ruptured Lumbar Intervertebral Disc

Edward C. Tarlov

*L*umbar and sciatic pain are among the symptoms for which patients most commonly seek medical advice. Because these symptoms are so widespread in the general population and are increasing, the care of patients with lumbar and sciatic pain forms and will continue to form the majority of most neurosurgical practice. Only a small proportion of symptomatic patients benefit by operation. In the referral practice at the Lahey Clinic, about 10 percent of the patients we see require operation. The remainder are best treated by conservative programs of exercise, by brief courses of physiotherapy, by encouragement to return to their normal activities, and by the tincture of time.

The title of this chapter emphasizes the importance of confining surgical treatment to those instances in which a lumbar disc is found clinically and on imaging studies to have ruptured. Magnetic resonance imaging (MRI) and computed tomography (CT) scanning are being used increasingly. Radiologists who interpret these studies, because they usually do not have an opportunity to correlate the patients' symptoms, have a tendency to over-interpret the images. A report of "normal for this patient's age" almost never appears. In spite of advanced imaging technology, the onus of correct diagnosis rests more than ever on clinical judgment, correlating the patient, the symptoms, and the imaging studies. Better imaging has done little to improve the outcome of surgery. Many asymptomatic patients have abnormal imaging studies.

The natural history of degenerative and spondylitic changes in the lumbar spine is gradually progressive over the years. Facet arthropathy is ubiquitous in the population and is seen on the CT scans of most adult spines. CT with its bone detail shows these changes even more clearly than MRI. Disc degeneration, also ubiquitous, is demonstrated in its earliest stages by changes seen best on MRI. Most degenerated discs remain confined to the intervertebral space with slight to moderate bulging. As part of the degenerative process in discs, if the annulus degenerates relatively more than the nucleus, herniation of a part of the nucleus can occur, compressing the adjacent nerve root or roots. This process is described later. It is not commonly enough recognized that disc and facet degeneration can cause referred pain in the buttock and down the thigh. All too often, it is assumed that if there is leg pain there must be nerve root compression. This not the case. This important point cannot be overemphasized. True sciatica radiating down the back of the thigh, below the knee and involving the calf, may indicate nerve root compression by herniated disc. Less well-defined pains, particularly those predominantly involving the buttock or thigh without radiation in a full sciatic distribution, bilateral pain in buttocks or thighs, and pains that vary from side to side are most likely to be referred pain from facet arthropathy or disc degeneration. In general, patients with these pains will not be helped by surgery—almost no matter what myelograms or scans are believed to demonstrate. In other words, patients with back pain alone are unlikely to be helped by surgery even if scans, as they often do, demonstrate disc protrusions. Also, there are patients with typical sciatica and intense disabling pain in whom high-quality imaging studies demonstrate no nerve root compression. In these patients, no surgery is advisable. In time, the symptoms usually subside.

MECHANISM OF DISC HERNIATION AND NATURAL HISTORY

A better understanding of the forces that lead to disc herniation may help in advising patients about activity, including work. There has been a tendency for physicians to be overly cautious in this regard, often advising limitation of activity or work and thus promoting an outlook that is detrimental to a patient's feeling of health and economic well-being. In fact, the back is beautifully engineered and quite strong. The forces leading to disc herniation result, I suspect, in the relative proportion of degeneration and loss of vertical height of the annulus and nucleus. From observation of the distortion of neural elements resulting from a disc herniation, there is considerable force involved. The extruded disc fragment most commonly is forced to pass to one side of the posterior longitudinal ligament by the confining effect of the posterior longitudinal ligament itself. From clinical observations, it seems likely that the sequence leading to disc herniation is that shown in Table 157–1 and Figure 157–1.

During the normal course of life, dehydration and degenerative changes lead to a loss of height of the lumbar intervertebral discs. This loss usually occurs at the expense of both annulus and nucleus. In some patients, a disproportionate loss of nuclear material with relative preservation of the annulus leads to the *vacuum disc phenomenon,* with gas at the center of the interspace resulting from relative loss of nuclear material and inability of the degenerated nucleus to collapse owing to the support of the relatively less degenerated annulus. Ordinarily, the degenerative changes of nucleus

Occasionally, a patient develops a CSF leak postoperatively. The first step to solving this problem is immediately oversewing of the wound. Once a seal is obtained, the wound usually heals. Leaks that persist more than a short time require reopening and repairing of the fistula.

FUSION DURING REOPERATION

The techniques of fusion are described elsewhere in detail. The fusions used in reoperation are not different from those employed in any other situation. The important question is: when is fusion required? In the past, simply employing fusion as a part of a second or third operation was common practice in the hope that this procedure would improve the outcome of reparative surgery. I believe that most failures of lumbar reoperation are not secondary to unrecognized instability but rather are a combination of failure to select patients on the proper grounds and failure to correct the underlying compressive abnormalities. Fusion should be performed for two reasons: demonstrated instability and preoperative studies showing transient or permanent subluxation or clear disruption of zygapophyseal joints. The final decision for fusion is always made in the operating room after exposure.

When fusion is an issue, exposure of bone on all sides of the laminectomy defect is required so that careful exploration of the pars and zygapophyseal joints can occur. Pars fracture, disruption of capsular ligaments, anatomic disruption of the joints, and subluxation all can be indications for fusion. A great deal of controversy still exists over universal indications for the use of fusion.

Once the bone is exposed, the surgeon has a much better idea of posterior stability. Then the decision for or against fusion can be made. Our preference is to err on the side of conservatism and fuse only for obvious instability.

The techniques of fusion include the standard posterolateral approaches and any of the many forms of instrumentation available. The actual techniques of fusion are described in other sections. However, one variation may be useful and is appropriately described here.

LOCAL POSTERIOR FUSION

During laminectomy, all bone removed should be saved, cleansed of all soft tissue, and then morselized. Small pieces of no more than 8 to 10 mm with exposed cancellous surfaces are desirable. All the posterior area of bone is then exposed and roughened with a high-speed drill. The usual indication for this procedure is a disrupted zygapophyseal joint. The joint itself should be entered, and the cartilaginous surfaces should be drilled away until some areas of cancellous bone are showing through the cortical bone in an irregular pattern. The joint is packed with bone, and the remaining pieces of bone are packed to cover the exposed surfaces. The wound is then closed without unusual precautions. The patient is immobilized in a chairback brace or its equivalent for 3 months. We do not have definitive studies indicating that this technique is comparable to more formal fusions, and we do not employ it except when there appears to be disruption of a single segment of joints that does not result in subluxation. My impression of the bony healing that occurs is that it is comparable to that seen in more radical forms of fusion and useful when some instability exists but indications for major fusion are not obvious.

SUMMARY

Reoperation on the lumbar spine for persistent symptoms after disc surgery requires precise anatomic definition of the abnormalities and equally precise surgery for their correction. It is just as important to be certain that the attendant comorbidities have not influenced a decision for surgery improperly and are treated in their own right.

REFERENCES

1. Long DM: Reoperation on lumbar spine, in Long DM, McAfee PC (eds): Atlas of Spinal Surgery. Baltimore, Williams & Wilkins, 1992, pp 23–57
2. Long DM: Laminotomy for lumbar disc disease, in Watkins RG, Collis JS (eds): Lumbar Discectomy and Laminectomy. Rockville, Md, Aspen Publishers, 1987, pp 173–178
3. Long DM: Surgical decision-making in the chronic back syndrome, in Hardy RW Jr (ed): Lumbar Disc Disease, 2nd ed. New York, Raven Press, 1993, pp 285–291

is to be obtained. In that case, obtaining the decompression is more important than attempting to preserve the joint intact.

REOPENING OF LAMINECTOMY

The patient may have been treated by laminectomy at one or more levels and still have persisting pain. The usual problems in this situation are persisting cauda equina compression from inadequate decompression or scar, unrelieved foraminal compression, and recognized instability. Just as with the more limited operations, the imaging studies should clarify the anatomic abnormalities so that the corrective surgery is planned to repair all potential symptomatic problems. These problems will include the extent of the laminectomy, whether superior, inferior, and lateral; the number of foraminotomies and their nature; and the need for fusion. The degree of compressive scar must be assessed to guide removal.

REOPERATIVE LAMINECTOMY

General anesthesia is used with the patient in the prone position. The previous skin incision should be opened at least one segment above and below the planned laminectomy. Intact bone above and below the laminectomy should be identified, and the muscles should be dissected free from spines and laminae, exposing normal territory both above and below the previous operation. Judging the location of the lateral margins of the laminectomy is then possible, and the dissection can be safely carried down the midline to approximately this level. Sometimes the thecal sac bulges back into the laminectomy defect. This phenomenon can be judged by previous imaging studies and the depth of the midline exposure estimated correctly. Once the midline incision is approximately at the level of the posterior margin of the dura with a few millimeters of scar left over the dura, the direction of the dissection is changed to proceed laterally to the bony margin. If this procedure is performed effectively, the bone should be exposed circumferentially, and a scar approximately the thickness of the laminae should be left over the dura.

Scar is then removed from the bone until normal bony surfaces are exposed at all margins of the laminectomy. The scar is freed from bone laterally, superiorly, and inferiorly until the epidural space is exposed. Removing a small amount of bone above and below may be necessary for the normal dura to be seen. Once the dura is exposed, a semisharp instrument, such as an Adson periosteal elevator, is used to develop a plane superiorly between scar and dura. This plane is then gradually developed in the midline, sweeping laterally to free the scar back to the bony margin. The scar is incised in the midline over the dissector and then cut away sharply by use of a small knife. The incision then proceeds from the midline toward the lateral margin of the scar. In this way, the scar is totally removed over the exposed segment. The process is then repeated, and scar is dissected away from dura. The scar is often very densely adherent to the dura, and sometimes a false plane must be created to leave a small amount of scar over the dura for strength. Occasionally, the dura has been entered by the previous surgeons and the adherence is extremely difficult to free. In this case, leaving noncompressive scar is better than losing cerebrospinal fluid (CSF). When the CSF is evacuated, epidural bleeding increases and the protective effect of the CSF is lost during dissection of the dural sac and the nerves. Therefore, when a leak occurs, it should be repaired immediately whenever possible.

Removal of the scar continues until the bottom of the laminectomy is reached. When the laminectomy is complete, the dural sac should be nearly free of scar, and no posterior compression should exist.

The adherence of the dural sac should then be separated circumferentially from overlying bone, which allows the laminectomy to be extended laterally until all canal compression is gone. The lateral recess compression of the sac and nerves is a significant problem. By use of punches or small chisels, the laminectomy should be undercut laterally down to the junction of the pedicle with vertebral body. This process allows the canal to be opened satisfactorily.

Then, the necessary foraminotomies should be performed, as described earlier. Foraminotomies must be carried out at every necessary level until all potentially involved roots are decompressed. Once the procedure is complete, assessment for stability should be performed. If no fusion is contemplated, the wound can be closed.

A 2- to 3-mm-thick fat graft, which will cover the entire posterior dura, should be harvested. In my experience in many reoperations, the fat graft is protective and reduces the degree of epidural scar. It need not be more than 3 mm thick and should be harvested in a place where healthy fat is available. Usually, harvesting can be performed by simply undercutting the margins of the wound and proceeding laterally. Making a new incision is not necessary to find unscarred fat. Then the wound is closed by approximation of the lumbar fascia without muscular sutures. Subcutaneous and skin stitches complete the closure.[1]

INTRAOPERATIVE CEREBROSPINAL FLUID LEAK

In my experience, the dura is torn in about 5 percent of reoperations. Dural laceration is not a serious complication but does need to be repaired whenever possible. Leaving a little dura-thickening scar is one way to prevent laceration. However, if the dura is torn, then primary repair using fine sutures is the best alternative. The laceration should be inspected carefully to be certain that no adherent nerve roots are caught in a suture.

When direct repair is not possible, a patch may be used. Local tissue, fascia lata, or one of the available dural substitutes may be employed as a patch and sutured in place in a watertight fashion.

Sometimes the dura cannot be repaired directly. In these cases, packing the area of the dural leak with fresh fat is usually satisfactory. Plasma clot also works well, if available. A blood patch is an acceptable way to obtain a plasma clotlike substitute. At the time of closure, with the area packed well with fat, the blood can simply be allowed to accumulate over the area, or a small amount can be deliberately used to cover the fat and its margins with the dura. Then closure of the wound to obliterate dead space is usually satisfactory to provide a watertight seal.

may be reduced by means of chisels or drills. A laser is an atraumatic way to remove these tissues that simultaneously provides good hemostasis. The surgeon must ensure that the compressed nerve root is completely decompressed.

Once this stage is completed, the anatomy of the interspace should be very close to normal, with all scar removed. Then the interspace should be entered by use of standard discectomy techniques, and as much degenerated disc material as possible should be removed.[1]

No certain method exists to prevent scar from recurring, but my experience with many reoperations suggests that the use of a thin, insulating fat graft is valuable. At this point, I harvest a graft of 2 to 3 mm in thickness that will surround the nerves and cover the dural sac. It is tucked into place so that it completely separates roots and dural sac from the potential scarring that will develop in the wound. The wound is then closed by simple reapproximation of the lumbar fascia and closure of subcutaneous tissues and skin.

ADDITION OF FORAMINOTOMY TO THE LOCAL PROCEDURE

When foraminotomy is required, the procedure is performed in the same way as described in the preceding section. However, when the roots are adequately visualized and the bony margins are clearly delineated, performing a foraminotomy may be necessary to adequately decompress the nerve root. If the patient has been studied with three-dimensional CT techniques or high-resolution MRI, the need for foraminotomy is usually identified in advance. If not, it may become obvious that the procedure is necessary because decompressing the root adequately is not possible without removal of bone.

The key to successful foraminotomy is understanding the anatomy of the foramen. The imaging studies and inspection should be adequate to determine what bone is compressive and what needs to be removed. When the interspace collapses, the downward migration of the pedicle most likely produces the compressive force. Facet arthropathy produces overgrowth of the superior articular process and produces posterior compression. The root may be trapped in a diminished lateral recess, and there may be anterior compression from lateral disc bulge or bony spurring. The foraminotomy needs to be planned carefully to alleviate whatever is causing the compression without disruption of the pars interarticularis or the zygapophyseal joint, if possible.

FORAMINOTOMY

Once the bone has been exposed and the extradural scar removed so that the root can be mobilized, the foraminotomy can be performed. This procedure can be performed either before or after excision of any anterior compressive mass. The foraminotomy is usually safer once the root has been decompressed, but sometimes retracting the root effectively is not possible until the foraminotomy has been performed.[1] There is no way to prescribe which should be done first.

The goal of the foraminotomy is to remove bony compression from the nerve. The surgeon may determine what must be removed on the basis of the imaging studies. The instruments used in the removal are crucial. If large punches are employed, the nerve root may be injured and the joint will probably be entered. The goal is to ream out the foraminal canal from the inside out, not to remove the articular process above. Sometimes, adequately decompressing a root is not possible without removing the facet at least partially, but the goal should always be to perform the surgery without entering the joint space. Small punches are useful for this purpose. I prefer to use delicate chisels because they allow precise removal of bone under direct vision. A guarded drill may also be used.

The first surgical step is to remove the remnants of the lamina completely to the lateral margin. The canal is often trefoil, and compression in the lateral recess may be present. By use of chisels, small punches, or the guarded drill, the lateral aspect of the lamina and the overhanging pedicle should be removed until the lateral recess is completely exposed and no compression exists in that area. Then the relationship of the pedicle to the root should be examined. The lower margin of the pedicle often is deforming the root, which is hooked around it. To take tension off the root, removing the lower portion of the pedicle is necessary. A punch cannot be used for this purpose because there is no overhanging lip. By use of using a guarded drill or small chisels, the lower third of the pedicle can be removed from the posterior vertebral surface to the articular processes. The removal needs to be in a lateral direction so that no root compression is possible. A small instrument should be maneuverable around the superior margin of the root between the root and bone, and no tension should be present superiorly when this maneuver is complete.

Then the posterior wall must be removed. Punches are useful here, but chisels or drill are more precise. The overhanging undersurface of the superior articular process needs to be removed, angling laterally at 30 to 45 degrees so that the joint space is not entered. Again, the removal must be carried far enough out into the foramen so that no compression exists. Decompressing what can be easily seen in the medial part of the foramen is of no value if a markedly stenotic lateral exit is left uncorrected. The decompression must be through the entire foraminal canal, and the success of the process must be proved by passage of a small instrument on all sides of the root. The foraminotomy is not complete until the instrument easily passes into the paravertebral space.

The anterior surface must now be inspected. The surgeon should ensure that no lateral disc protrusion needs to be removed. Removal of any anterior compressive mass, such as spur or overgrown ligament, is difficult and dangerous to the root. Usually, the foraminotomy provides adequate decompression of the root. If compression is still present anteriorly, then the anterior mass must be removed as described earlier. Laser, knife, and disc rongeurs are all useful for recurrent disc, scar, or ligament, and bone can be removed by curettes and disc rongeurs. At the end of the procedure, the root should be identified circumferentially, and no compression should be present. Otherwise, the foraminotomy is not satisfactory.

The surgeon should not thin the pars interarticularis, thereby making it susceptible to fracture, and should not enter the joint itself, if possible. Of course, in some circumstances, the joint must be opened if adequate decompression

ARACHNOIDITIS

A small number of patients with persisting symptoms will have developed arachnoiditis. There is no specific clinical syndrome for this disorder, and the diagnosis is made with certainty only on CT myelography. Determining whether the observed arachnoiditis is related to the persisting symptoms is often difficult. Direct surgery on the arachnoiditis is rarely indicated and is a separate issue.

PATIENT EXAMINATION

Evaluation of the patient provides the information needed to design an appropriate operation. The key to successful reoperation is definition of the anatomic abnormalities to be repaired. The history of the pain usually localizes the problem well, and when the description of the pain is not in a specific anatomic area, a focal abnormality is unlikely to be found. The physical examination may confirm the problem but frequently reveals no specific abnormality. Imaging studies are extremely important: a combination of MRI and three-dimensional CT usually demonstrates a correctable abnormality. In the absence of specific definable pathology, surgery is unlikely to be of any value.

The imaging studies must be examined in great detail. Simply seeing an abnormality is not sufficient to plan an appropriate reparative procedure; any compressive mass must be defined. The surgeon must know where it is, what it is, and how it affects specific nerve roots to be absolutely certain that decompression will be satisfactory. Because finding a nerve root in dense scar can be difficult, identification before the exposure is very important. The spinal canal must be examined so that the extent of the laminectomy required can be estimated both longitudinally and transversely. The neural foramina must be studied in great detail, and the cause of foraminal compression must be defined so that the surgeon knows what part of the foramen to enlarge. The pedicle, the anterior surface, and the posterior surface all must be assessed if an appropriate foraminotomy is to be performed without entering the zygapophyseal joint. The width of the pars interarticularis is also an important feature. Surgical disruption of the pars or excessive thinning is a common error.

At the same time, the surgeon must know about instability so that a decision for or against fusion can be made. The extent of facet arthropathy should also be known because it will influence laminectomy, foraminotomy, and fusion.

THE FINAL DECISION FOR SURGERY

Although all these anatomic abnormalities are important, in themselves their discovery does not constitute an indication for surgery. The abnormalities must be commensurate with the complaints, the claimed disabilities must be reasonable, and the comorbidities must be addressed if reasonable outcomes are to be obtained. In my experience, failure of reparative surgery is more often related to the comorbidities that affect the patient than to lack of ability to correct anatomic abnormalities. However, if the patient is a suitable candidate for surgery, reparative operations on the spine have much to offer.[3]

REOPERATION FOR ROOT COMPRESSION FROM RECURRENT DISC OR LOCALLY COMPRESSIVE SCAR

The operation is carried out with the patient under general anesthesia and in the prone position. Infiltration of a long-acting local anesthetic in the skin and paravertebral muscles reduces postoperative pain. The old skin incision is opened, and the paravertebral muscles are dissected from the adjacent spinous processes and laminae to expose the area of previous surgery. I always take an x-ray film to be certain of localization in reoperations. Up to this point, the operation is the same as that carried out for simple discectomy.[2] However, now the exposure becomes more difficult because of the previous scar. The bony margins should be identified circumferentially; then the dissection should be carried further out to expose the zygapophyseal joint. The surgeon should be certain not to disrupt the ligaments unnecessarily. Then the scar is dissected free from the bony margins circumferentially. Using a semisharp dissector, such as the Adson periosteal elevator, the surgeon tries to free the scar from the undersurface of the laminae above and below. It is usually worthwhile to remove a little more bone above or below in order to see normal dura. Then the scar can be removed from the dura. I usually remove the scar sharply with a knife because less chance of tearing the dura exists while an adherent scar fragment is being pulled. Once the scar is removed and the dura is exposed circumferentially, the surgeon can proceed laterally into the gutter above the involved nerve root. The preoperative images should be studied to ascertain the location of both the exiting nerve and the nerve in passage. These areas may be difficult to identify in the scar, and it is much better to have visualized where they are in the interspace so they can be located deliberately rather than by chance.

The surgeon follows the exiting nerve out into the neural foramen and frees it from the pedicle and from the overlying surface of the superior articular process. Then the scar can be removed from the posterior surface of the nerve and its inferior margin identified. Once the entire nerve is identified, dissecting along the lateral surface of the dural sac and the nerve in passage is easier. These maneuvers allow removal of all the posterior scar and identification of both of the nerves and the dural sac. Then the compressive mass must be identified in the same way that an underlying disc would be seen. The nerves may be retracted medially or laterally, depending on what produces least root tension. The approach used should provide the least retraction possible to expose mass beneath the nerve.

Removal of the mass is quite different than removal of a simple disc. Even when the problem is a recurrent disc, there is often enough scarring so that the root is difficult to free from the nerve. I prefer to free the root sharply with a knife to decrease traction on the root. Then all of the mass of scar, recurrent disc, bulging ligament, and bone must be removed to provide complete decompression of the nerve. The technique of removal is not particularly important. The mass may be cut away with a knife down to bony spurs, and the bone

CHAPTER 156

Management of Persistent Symptoms Following Lumbar Disc Surgery

Don M. Long

The surgical management of the patient with persistent or new symptoms after lumbar disc surgery is straightforward and rarely presents any difficulty if approached logically with a clear understanding of what is correctable and what is not. By contrast, the overall evaluation and management of patients whose symptoms are not relieved after disc surgery are among the most complex in medicine and require definition of not only the anatomic abnormalities but also all of the serious comorbidities that may mediate the ongoing complaint of pain.[3]

IDENTIFICATION OF THE CAUSE OF PERSISTENT PAIN

A limited number of identifiable and correctable abnormalities exist. Surgery is effective for only two conditions, root compression and instability, and reoperation is to be undertaken only when one or both are demonstrated. The first step in the evaluation of these patients is always a clear definition of underlying spinal pathology, with emphasis on abnormalities that are correctable.

PERSISTING ROOT COMPRESSION

The original operation may have failed to relieve root compression permanently. A fragment of disc may have been missed, or incomplete removal of degenerated disc from the interspace may have led to a recurrence. Ligamentous and bony deformities may still compress the root, foraminal stenosis with or without canal stenosis may be responsible for the ongoing compression, or a lateral disc fragment may have been overlooked. All of these diagnoses can be made directly, and the presence or absence of root compression is usually discernible. Magnetic resonance imaging (MRI) and three-dimensional computed tomography (CT) reconstructions are usually satisfactory to visualize the roots and neural foramina and to define the spinal canal. Root compression can usually be seen by these methods. Occasionally, CT myelography is required when noninvasive studies are not determinant.

SPINAL INSTABILITY

Painful instability may be segmental or may involve one zygapophyseal joint unilaterally. Flexion extension films usually show segmental movement. CT with three-dimensional reconstruction allows accurate visualization of facet arthropathy and surgical defects. Occult abnormalities, such as fractures of the pars interarticularis, can also be seen.

ROOT INJURY

Root injury is a relatively common cause of persisting radiculopathy—the original disc herniation surgery has simply injured the root. Such patients have classic radiculopathy or radiculitis that persists in the absence of demonstrated compression. Electromyography may be confirmatory but cannot distinguish between ongoing compression and injury. However, in the absence of demonstrated compression, electromyography may be diagnostic. Relief of pain by root blockade also suggests that nerve root injury is the diagnosis. No surgical treatment exists for this problem, and we employ spinal stimulation for these individuals.

DISC SPACE INFECTION

Most disc space infections are associated with systemic signs of the infection, and the differential diagnosis is not difficult. Occasionally, however, a low-grade infection can be very indolent and difficult to identify. Imaging changes usually signal the diagnosis. The treatment of disc space infection is a separate issue.

EPIDURAL SCAR

Root compression secondary to epidural scarring is said to be less amenable to surgical decompression than recurrent disc herniation. This, however, has not been my experience. I believe that the existence of root compression itself is more important than its cause, as long as the subsequent decompression is satisfactory. However, no evidence exists that removal of noncompressive epidural scar is of value.

33. Faubert C, Caspar W: Lumbar percutaneous discectomy. Neuroradiology 33:407–410, 1991
34. Kambin P, Schaffer JZ: Percutaneous lumbar discectomy—Prospective review of 100 patients. Clin Orthop 188:24–34, 1989
35. Davis GW, Onik G: Clinical experience with automated percutaneous discectomy. Clin Orthop 238:98–103, 1989
36. Heikkinen ER: "Whole body" stereotaxy: Application of stereotactic endoscopy to operations of herniated lumbar discs. Acta Neurochir Suppl(Wien) 54:89–92, 1992
37. Ascher PW, Holzer P, Choy DSJ, Jury H: Percutaneous nucleus pulposus denaturation and vaporization of protruded discs, in Proceedings of the 9th International Congress of Neurologic Surgery. New Delhi, October 8–13, 1989, pp 145
38. Fan M, Ascher PW: KTP/532 laser as a new laser source for percutaneous nucleus pulposus vaporization (NPV)—An experimental study, in Spinelli P, Dal Fante M, Marchesini R (eds): Photodynamic Therapy and Biomedical Lasers. Amsterdam, Elsevier Science Publishers BV, 1992, pp 363–365
39. Ascher PW: Disc disease treated with the laser through a needle. Abstracts Seara Medica Neurochir 3:S36, 1986
40. Ascher PW, Clarici G, Holzer P: Therapie des Bandscheibenleidens mit Chymopapain und durch Nucleus Pulposus Vaporization, in Singer F, Smerak O (eds): Rehabilitation bei Veränderungen des Discus intervertebralis und der Spondylolithese. Wien, Verl. Brüder Hollinek, 1988, pp 242–245
41. Ascher PW, Sutter B, Holzer P: Nucleus pulposus denaturation in protruded lumbar disks. Proceedings of 5th International Congress of the European Laser Association. Graz, November 8–10, 1990, p 72
42. Ascher PW, Fan M, Sutter B: Nucleus pulposus vaporization of protruded lumbar discs, in Spinelli P, Dal Fante M, Marchesini R (eds): Photodynamic Therapy and Biomedical Lasers. Amsterdam, Elsevier Science Publishers BV, 1992, pp 366–369

(5 to 6 mm) for the percutaneous mechanical and percutaneous suction methods.

All of the methods discussed earlier can be carried out on an outpatient basis with the patient under local anesthesia. In reality, however, the only procedure performed under these conditions is laser vaporization.

We have never endoscopically observed these procedures at our clinic. Instead, we judge the effect of the procedure by constant communication with the patient and the change in neurologic signs. We do not carry out a discography to judge the effect of the improvements.

Postoperative examinations are routinely conducted 1 week, 1 month, 3 months, and 6 months after the procedure and yearly thereafter. X-rays studies and other radiographic procedures, such as CT scan, MRI and CT myelography, are conducted only if the patient has new or recurrent complaints.

All of the percutaneous methods lessen treatment costs because of the absence of long hospitalization and the extra personal costs for surgery and clinical postoperative care, as well as the reduction in costs for treatment supplies. These costs differ, however, from method to method. For the suction methods and the various laser methods, disposable equipment is available, which raises costs.

To keep costs for laser treatment low, we had probes and needles manufactured that can be sterilized and reused. In addition, our goal has been to move away from developments that require specialized laser equipment to ones that use the standard laser equipment available in neurosurgery departments. In this regard, we have usually succeeded.

FUTURE DIRECTIONS

In the future, we would like to make the laser procedures even safer and simpler. To this end, we are trying to apply our experimental results with the carbon dioxide laser to future clinical use by adapting the laser system and our puncture materials. These advances should allow us to quantitate the amount of disc volume evaporated per unit of time with certain energy levels. Therewith, it should also be possible to quantitatively establish whether or not the procedure is successful. Today, we can offer minimally invasive neurosurgery for 10 to 20 percent of all cases requiring operative treatment for disc protrusion. By improving the technique, we will try to apply these methods to more patients in the future.

Acknowledgments

The author would like to thank Dr. Fan Ming for his experimental studies and Dr. Catherine Ojakangas Friehs for her translation of this chapter into understandable English.

REFERENCES

1. Nachemson AL: The lumbar spine: An orthopaedic challenge. Spine 2:59–71, 1976
2. Kelsey JL, White AA: Epidemiology and impact of low back pain. Spine 5:133–142, 1980
3. Harris AI: Handicapped and impaired in Great Britain: Part 1: Social survey division. London, Office of Population Census and Surgery. Her Majesty's Stationary, 1971
4. Kambin P: Arthroscopic microdiscectomy: Minimal intervention in spine surgery. Baltimore-Munich, Urban & Schwarzenberg, 1991, pp 3–6
5. Goldthwait JE: The lumbosacral articulation: An explanation of many cases of ''lumbago,'' ''sciatica'' and paraplegia. Boston Med Surg J 164:365–372, 1911
6. Elsberg CA: Pain and other sensory disturbances in diseases of the spinal cord and their surgical treatment. Am J Med Sci 149:337–339, 1915
7. Putti V: The Lady Jones lecture: Pathogenesis of sciatic pain. Lancet ii:53–60, 1927
8. Dandy WE: Loose cartilage from intervertebral disc simulating tumor of the spinal cord. Arch Surg 19:660–672, 1929
9. Mixter WJ, Barr JS: Rupture of the intervertebral disc with involvement of the spinal canal. N Engl J Med 211:210–215, 1934
10. Williams W: Microlumbar disectomy: A conservative surgical approach to the virgin herniated lumbar disc. Spine 3:175–182, 1978
11. Wilson DH, Harbaugh R: Microsurgical and standard removal of the protruded lumbar disc: A comparative study. Neurosurgery 8:422–427, 1981
12. Maroon JC, Alba A: Microdiscectomy versus chemonucleolysis. Neurosurgery 16:644–649, 1985
13. Caspar W: A new surgical procedure for lumbar disc herniation causing less tissue damage through microsurgical approach. Adv Neurosurg 4:74–77, 1977
14. Yasargil MG: Microsurgical operation for herniated lumbar disc. Adv Neurosurg 4:81, 1977
15. Saunders RL: Microsurgical lumbar disectomy: A dissenting view, in Schmidek HH, Sweet WH (eds): Operative Neurosurgical Techniques, vol 2. Orlando, Grune & Stratton, 1982, p 1399
16. Smith L: Enzyme dissolution of the nucleus pulposus in humans. JAMA 187:137–140, 1964
17. Smith L, Brown JE: Treatment of lumbar intervertebral disc lesion by direct injection of chymopapain. J Bone Joint Surg Br 49B:502–519, 1967
18. Hijikata SA: A method of percutaneous nuclear extraction. J Toden Hosp 5:39, 1975
19. Kambin P, Gellman H: Percutaneous lateral discectomy of the lumbar spine: A preliminary report. Clin Orthop 174:127–132, 1983
20. Onik G, Helms C, Ginsberg L, et al: Percutaneous lumbar discectomy using a new aspiration probe: Porcine and cadaver model. Radiology 155:251–252, 1985
21. Ascher PW: Laser trend in minimal invasive treatment: Atherosclerosis, disk herniations. J Clin Laser Med Surg 9:49–57, 1991
22. Choy DSJ, Ascher PW, Saddekni S, et al: Percutaneous laser disc decompression. A new therapeutic modality. Spine 17:949–956, 1992
23. Finneson BE: Lumbar disc excision, in Schmidek HH, Sweet WH (eds): Operative Neurosurgical Techniques, vol 2. Grune & Stratton, Orlando, FL, 1988, pp 1375–1392
24. McCulloch JA: Chemonucleolysis. J Bone Joint Surg Br 59B:45–52, 1977
25. Kambin P: Arthroscopic microdiscectomy: Minimal intervention in spine surgery. Baltimore-Munich, Urban & Schwarzenberg, 1992, pp 67–100
26. Schreiber A, Yoshinori S, Leu H: Does percutaneous nucleotomy with discoscopy replace conventional discectomy? Eight years' experience and results in treatment of herniated lumbar disc. Clin Orthop 238:35–42, 1989
27. Mayer H, Brock M, Berlien HP, et al: Percutaneous endoscopic laser discectomy (PELD). A new surgical technique for non-sequestrated lumbar discs. Acta Neurochir Suppl(Wien) 54:53–58, 1992
28. Ball RO: Needle aspiration biopsy. J Tenn Med Assoc 27:203, 1934
29. Valls J, Ottolenghi C, Schajowicz F: Aspiration biopsy in diagnosis of lesions of vertebral bodies. JAMA 136:376–382, 1948
30. Craig FS: Vertebral body biopsy. J Bone Joint Surg Am 38A:93–95, 1956
31. Schweigel J: Compression of chemopapain and percutaneous discectomy, in Onik G, Helms CA (eds): Automated Percutaneous Lumbar Discectomy. San Francisco, Radiology Research and Education Foundation 199:85–92, 1988
32. Mooney V: Percutaneous and suction discectomy, in Frymoyer JW (ed): The Adult Spine: Principles and Practice. New York, Raven Press, 1991, pp 1751–1763

Table 155–4. THE PARAMETERS OF DIFFERENT LASERS AND ADJUNCT OPTIC FIBERS USED FOR 515 PLNPV PROCEDURES

Lasers and Fibers	Procedures	Parameters		
		Power (W)	Pulse (sec)	Energy/(J) (Mean)
1.06/ND:YAG (BF)	19*	20–35	0.25–1.0	589 (400–800)
1.06/Nd:YAG (FT)	23	20–40	1.0	1826 (999–2561)
1.32/Nd:YAG (BF)	235/(before Oct 1989)	20–30	1.0	1152 (800–1703)
	218/(after Oct 1989)	20–30	1.0	1819 (800–3006)
KTP/532 (BF)	20	17	0.5 and 1.0	1437 (1087–2286)

BF = bare fiber; FT = frosted tip; KTP = potassium titanyl phosphate; Nd:YAG = neodymium: yttrium-aluminum-garnet; PLNPV = percutaneous laser-assisted nucleus pulposus vaporization.
*First 19 patients were treated with inadequate energy.

has a high water content. Normally, the patients were able to leave the operating room independently after the procedure, and in most cases, the procedures were conducted on an outpatient basis. Before 1990, some patients were admitted for 1 to 3 days. In a few cases, localized pain was reported at the injection site for 2 to 3 days.

After 1 week, a routine examination usually reveals that the neurologic symptoms have disappeared. However, in many cases, a dysesthesia is present at the diseased level. At the beginning of the study, an x-ray study of the lumbar spine was routinely performed after the procedure. These examinations showed a narrowing of the intervertebral space. With CT scan, a full restitution of the protrusion was seen in some cases, and MRI revealed a change in water content of the disc. Neurologically, 75 percent of the patients had no further complaints. For the 25 percent of patients who did have complaints, and whose neurologic symptoms had not improved, an open operation was performed. In half of these patients, an explanation for the continued discomfort was found. The conditions of these patients were usually not clear, and there were free or subligament herniations, narrow spinal canals, spondylolisthesis, and similar complications.

The intervertebral spaces L3-L4, L4-L5, and L5-L6 are easier to reach than L5-S1 and L6-S1. At these levels, problems ensue, especially when the transverse process and the joint facets are very pronounced. In approximately 8 to 12 percent of the punctures at this segmental level, we had to stop the procedure and opt for conventional microsurgery. The procedures at levels L3-L4, L4-L5, and L5-L6 lasted an average of 15 to 20 minutes, with maximum x-ray exposure of 1 minute and maximum laser exposure of 2 minutes.

Of the 509 patients, one complication (discitis) occurred right after the procedure. The patient had an elevated erythrocyte sedimentation rate preoperatively, to which we did not attend. We believe, therefore, that the percutaneous laser-assisted nucleus pulposus vaporization triggered a latent infection and discitis. The patient was treated with antibiotics and had a complete recovery after 6 weeks.

COMPARISON OF MODERN METHODS OF DISCECTOMY

Common to all of the discussed methods is that they require strict indications to be successful. Only 10 to 20 percent of neurosurgical patients are suitable candidates for these procedures. These methods can be performed with the patient under local anesthesia, which saves the patient the risks of general anesthesia. Furthermore, the percutaneous methods do not usually produce a scar, as do operative procedures. All percutaneous methods have the advantages of needing no skin incision, muscle damage, or bone removal, and the patient has therefore only minimal local complaints after the procedure. Thus, these procedures can be carried out on an outpatient basis. The dural sac and the peripheral nerve root are not manipulated; thus, dural injuries and nerve root irritations are avoided. In contrast, Choy sometimes punctures the disc through the dural sac at segmental level L5-S1. Since we began to offer minimally invasive neurosurgery, we have tried to find the most efficient way to manage the patient's complaints, the physician's time and effort, and society's costs. A review of statistics from other authors and our own experiences reveals a long-term success rate of approximately 60 to 70 percent with these methods (as defined by no complaints for at least 2 years).

The differences between the individual percutaneous techniques can be compared with regard to time and equipment expenditures. Slight technical differences also exist. For the endoscopic mechanical and automatized suction method of discectomy, the same amount of time is required as for a skilled surgeon to perform an open operation. However, the advantage of the percutaneous technique is that a scar is not created by this procedure. The time expenditure for lasering is about 80 to 120 seconds, depending on the laser source used. A skilled surgeon can perform the technique with an x-ray exposure time of less than 1 minute for segmental levels L4-L5 or L3-L4. Eighty percent of cases at segmental levels L5-S1 or L6-S1 can be completed in the same time period. We have already mentioned that in 20 percent of patients, anatomic anomalies of lumbosacral discs exist that preclude puncture. These cases are usually excluded from this treatment. Naturally, with this lumbosacral segmental level the above-mentioned three other methods are at a disadvantage and are more difficult to perform because of the thicker instruments used.

The instruments required for each method have also been described. Although for the laser procedures we use an 18-gauge needle, we need instruments that are usually over ½ cm

Table 155-2. VOLUMES OF LESIONS VAPORIZED BY DIFFERENT LASERS AND ADJUNCT FIBERS

Energy/(J)	Volume of Vaporized Lesion/(mm^3)		
	1.06/Nd:YAG/ (FT) (20/W, 1.0/sec)	1.32/ND:YAG/ (BF) (20/W, 1.0/sec)	KTP/532/(BF) (17/W, 1.0/sec)
300	3.75	23.57	22.92
400	19.71	40.73	30.17
500	20.54	42.38	42.91
1000	35.82	99.14	90.50
1500	77.06	106.06	188.55

BF = bare fiber; FT = frosted tip; KTP = potassium titanyl phosphate; ND:YAG = neodymium: yttrium-aluminum-garnet.

shape. However, with the 1.32 Nd:YAG laser, the lesion was irregular, and microscopic analysis revealed a delicate necrotic margin around the vaporized area. Sometimes, this necrotic margin also reached the perichondrium and the bone, and it always did so when more than 500 J of total energy was used.

The carbon dioxide laser required the shortest treatment time and the least amount of total energy for vaporization of the nucleus pulposus. The KTP/532 and the 1.32 Nd:YAG lasers had a stronger vaporization effect than did the 1.06 Nd:YAG laser, which stood out clinically and experimentally because of the smoke and steam that escaped through the guide needle.

CLINICAL STUDIES

The technique of percutaneous laser-assisted nucleus pulposus vaporization is the same as that described for the other percutaneous methods. This procedure is performed with the patient under local anesthesia and without sedation to ensure good communication between patient and surgeon. The patient is turned onto one side with the diseased side facing upwards. We try to puncture the patient from the opposite side at the L5-S1 level only when a very prominent transverse process and a short distance to the sacral bone exist. The entrance point for the skin puncture is 8 cm lateral to the spinous process at the height of the iliac crest for L4-L5 (see Fig. 155-1). For L5-S1, the entrance point is shifted 1 cm caudally and medially from that for L4-L5.

Local anesthesia with 1% procaine in an 18-gauge needle with trocar (Aesculap, Germany) is introduced into the intervertebral space by aid of the image intensifier. The insertion occurs at a 50- to 60-degree angle, and the needle is pointed directly at the disc and thereby reaches the facet, after which it is directed laterally to bypass the facet. The angle must not be too small or the nerve root will be punctured, and the patient will experience pain. The disc is reached by a trajectory between the nerve root laterally and the facet joint medially. When the annulus is cut through, a resistance is felt, after which the needle is shifted to the center of the disc, and its position is verified with the image intensifier in two planes.

This puncture technique consistently succeeds at the L3-L4 and L4-L5 levels; however, problems can arise with the L5-S1 level. Puncturing the disc at this level is possible only in approximately 80 percent of cases. Although Choy describes a puncture of this disc transdurally, we reject this method because of the unavoidable cerebrospinal fluid leakage and headaches that will occur. For the remaining 20 percent of patients, we recommend an open operative procedure.

After placement of the instruments, the trocar is removed, and the laser fiber, whose length is equal to that of the trocar, is introduced. The different adjustments for the nucleus pulposus denaturization on the diverse laser systems are depicted in Table 155-4. We conduct the first check of the procedure after about 300 J has been administered. During this check, the laser fiber is removed and the tip examined, and the patient's leg-raising sign is tested. In almost all cases, after an average of 12 to 18 bursts, the leg-raising sign is normal and the patient experiences pronounced relief. At every 500- to 600-J interval, the tip of the needle is slightly shifted or pulled back to denature the back portions of the nucleus pulposus as well. At the end of the procedure, the laser fiber is removed first and its tip checked once more. Subsequently, the guide tube is removed. A sterile bandage is applied, and the patient can leave the operating table and the hospital without assistance.

RESULTS

Since February 1986, we have treated 509 patients with this procedure.[21, 39-42] Fifty-eight percent (296) were men, and 42 percent (213) were women. The youngest patient was 17 years old and the oldest 88 years old. Four hundred fourteen patients presented with a documented herniated disc. Six patients who had disc injury at two segmental levels were treated at both levels on the same day. We have conducted a total of 515 such procedures. The first 19 patients were treated with the bare-fiber Nd:YAG 1.06 laser system; 22 patients, with the Nd:YAG laser system with the frosted tip; 20 patients, with the KTP/532 laser system; and 448 with the 1.32 Nd:YAG laser with the bare tip. The first 250 patients consisted of 56 percent men (142) and 43 percent (108) women and were treated between February 26, 1986 and October 19, 1989. These patients had follow-up examinations for more than 3 years. So far, the longest postoperative follow-up is 80 months, and the average follow-up is 40 months.

In most cases, the patient reported a significant relief from the symptoms after 300 J of total energy during the procedure. The leg-raising sign changed during the procedure to variable extent. Smoke and steam from the guide tube were seen mostly with young patients, whose nucleus pulposus

Table 155-3. CARBON DIOXIDE LASER PARAMETERS THAT VAPORIZED THE ENTIRE NUCLEUS PULPOSUS (105 mm^3) OF SWINE CADAVER LUMBAR NUCLEUS PULPOSUS

Power/(W)	Exposure Time/ (sec)	Total Energy/(J)
10	90	900
15	45	675
20	30	600
25	20	500
30	15	450

procedure while at the same time making it more expensive and partly negating its rationale. Because of the difficulties that sometimes arise at the L5-S1 level, a special surgical set has been designed for the lumbosacral disc. Kambin and Schaffer[34] reported on a very comprehensive series in which satisfactory results were achieved in 25 percent of the cases. Davis and Onik[35] had similar results.

PERCUTANEOUS STEREOTACTIC DISCECTOMY

The methods discussed here involve a combination of stereotactic techniques and the microsurgical operative technique of Caspar. The goal of this procedure is to treat herniated as well as protruded discs.

INDICATIONS AND TECHNIQUE

For this treatment, nine patients were chosen to have nucleotomy performed with possible removal of the herniated disc.[36] The patients were first examined by CT scan. Then, under either general or local anesthesia with sufficient sedation, the patient was placed in the prone position. Next, a mark was drawn with a radio-opaque marking pencil parallel to the midline at the level of the diseased disc. After the stereotactic frame (Laitinen) was positioned, a skin incision was made and the disc sited and punctured with a percutaneous nucleotomy set (Mayer and Brock; Aesculap). The operative incision was widened with dilators, the posterior longitudinal ligament was perforated, and the nucleotomy was performed. This procedure succeeded in all nine cases without complication. In five cases, a herniated disc was successfully identified from endoscopy and was removed in one piece. In four cases a subsequent open operative discectomy had to be performed.

In conclusion, percutaneous mechanical discectomy, percutaneous suction technique for discectomy, and percutaneous stereotactic discectomy involve considerable expense and do not ensure removal of the herniated disc. The microsurgical procedures like that of Caspar do not present a significantly larger increased stress.

PERCUTANEOUS LASER-ASSISTED DISCECTOMY (Fig. 155–6)

EXPERIMENTAL STUDIES

Four different laser systems and optical fibers were used in our experiments:
1. The 1.06-μm neodymium:yttrium-aluminum-garnet (Nd:YAG) laser (Medilas 2, MBB Germany) with a bare fiber[37]
2. The 1.32 Nd:YAG laser (Medilas 2, Germany) and a 600-μm silicon fiber, likewise bare
3. The 1.06 Nd:YAG laser with a 600-μm silicon fiber with frosted or hemispheric tips (Sharplan, Israel)
4. The potassium titanyl phosphate (KTP/532) laser with a 600-μm bare fiber (Laserscope, United States)
5. A carbon dioxide laser with 10.6-μm wavelength with a so-called hollow wave guide used for light transmission

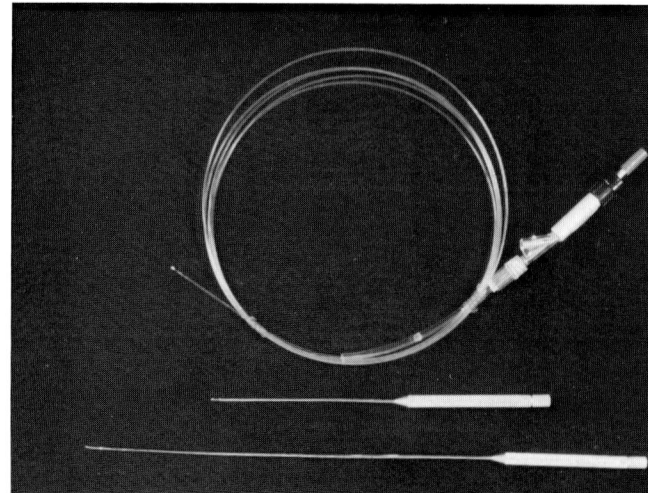

FIGURE 155–6. Two needles and laser fiber with spherical tip for percutaneous laser-assisted discectomy.

The different parameters of the various laser systems are shown in Table 155–1.

For these experiments, we used porcine lumbar discs. An 18-gauge needle with trocar was placed in the center of the nucleus pulposus. The trocar was removed and replaced with the laser, which protruded 5 mm from the end of the guide tube. The laser vaporization took place in steps. We checked the fiber periodically and retracted and cleaned it before placing it again in the nucleus pulposus. This care is necessary because with local overheating of the laser tip, the superficial tissue begins to char, and the laser fiber begins to melt. Consequently, the light conduction of the fiber can be impaired. After successful lasering, the disc was fixed in formalin, and the lasered areas were photographed, measured, and prepared for histologic examination.[38]

The bare fibers of the KTP/532 and the 1.32 Nd:YAG were periodically checked for quality of light conduction. Only when a circular emission of light was seen was the laser used repeatedly. If this was not the case, the laser tip was cleaned and newly cut.

Lesion sizes produced by the various energy levels used with the 1.06 Nd:YAG laser with the frosted tip, or with the 1.32 laser and the KTP/532 with bare fiber, are depicted in Table 155–2. Table 155–3 shows the vaporization effect, which was dependent on the energy:time ratio, from the carbon dioxide nucleus pulposus was vaporized. The lesion produced by different laser systems is usually elliptical in

Table 155–1. PARAMETERS OF DIFFERENT LASERS AND FIBERS USED IN EXPERIMENTS

Lasers and Fibers	Parameters		
	Power (W)	Pulse (sec)	Energy (J)
1.06/Nd:YAG (FT)	20–40	0.5 and 1.0	300–1500
1.32/Nd:YAG (BF)	20–40	0.5 and 1.0	300–1500
KTP/532 (BF)	10–17	0.5 and 1.0	300–1500
CO_2 (HW)	10–30	CW	300–900

BF = bare fiber; CO_2 = carbon dioxide; CW = continuous wave; FT = frosted tip; HW = hollow wave guide; KTP = potassium titanyl phosphate; Nd:YAG = neodymium-yttrium-aluminum-garnet.

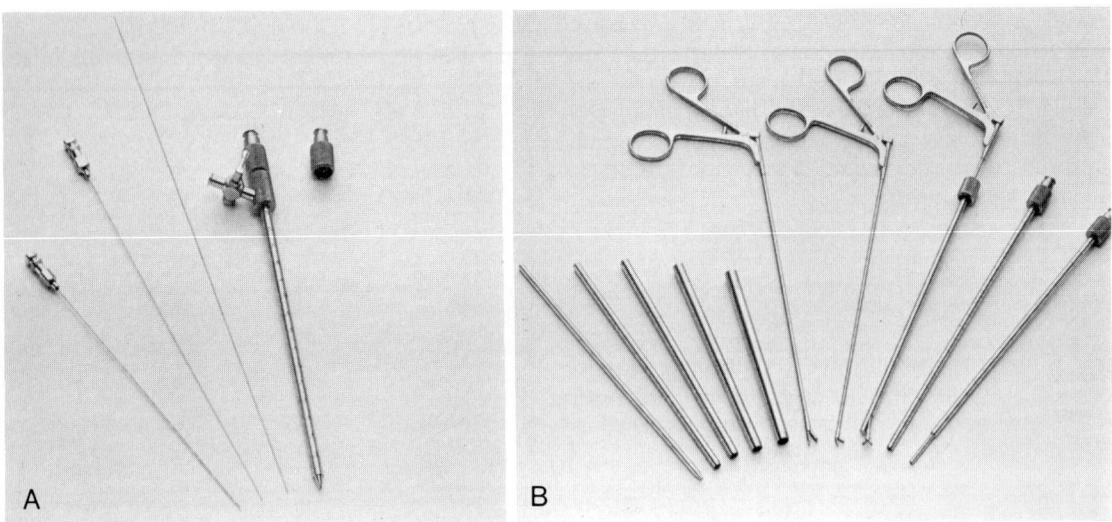

FIGURE 155–4. (A) Cannula, guiding wire, and trocar sleeve. (B) Trephines and forceps.

ened with use of dilators of gradually increasing size; four to six such dilators are pushed over the original needle. After installation of the last dilator, which is guided to the outer side of the annulus fibrosus, the annulus fibrosus is opened and the dilator removed. After fenestration of the annulus, an x-ray study is performed to confirm the correct position of the instruments before the different sharp spoons and rongeurs are introduced. The size of the ronguer is restricted because of the 4- to 5-mm diameter of the working channel. The disc is taken out piecemeal with continuous radiographic control.

Schreiber and coworkers[26] and Mayer and coworkers,[27] conduct this procedure under endoscopic control; however, this method requires a two-sided percutaneous approach for the nucleotomy. This procedure, first described by Hijikata, is also conducted with the patient in the prone position. Then, the freely moving disc tissue can be removed under visual control from the opposite side.

Since the early procedures of Ball in 1934,[28] Valls and Ottolenghi[29] in 1948, and Craig in 1956,[30] many different instruments have been developed and refined for this purpose. Modified Craig instruments, Hijikata instruments, Balgrist percutaneous nucleotomy sets, and a set from the Aesculap Company are available (Fig. 155–4A and B). Our own experience in this area is limited, and we have performed this procedure in only a few cases. Schweigel[31] has reported a success rate of 78 percent with percutaneous discectomy in 300 cases. In other studies, Ooi reported a success rate of 83 percent in 30 patients; Choy, 65 percent with 49 patients; Cotta, 74 percent with 137 patients; Hijikata, 72 percent with 50 patients[34]; and Kahanovitz, 55 percent with 39 patients.[32] Faubert and Caspar[33] conducted successful treatments in 64.3 percent of their 28 patients.

PERCUTANEOUS SUCTION TECHNIQUES FOR DISCECTOMY

The technique of puncture is similar to that already discussed. A lateral or prone position is used, and monitoring ensues with the aid of an image intensifier. The procedure is conducted with the patient under local anesthesia. The difference between this technique and others is that the surgical instruments for this procedure are offered as a disposable set from several companies (Fig. 155–5), which simplifies the

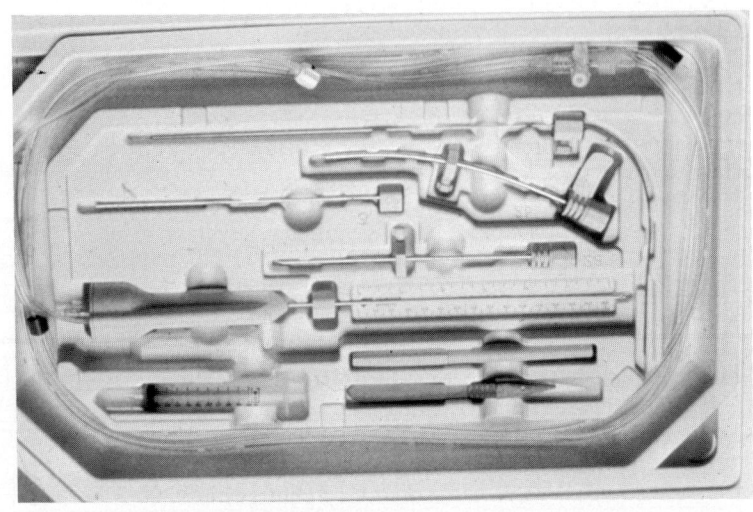

FIGURE 155–5. Disposable puncture set for percutaneous suction technique.

conservative treatment. Patients who respond well to conservative treatment but who have recurrences are the ideal candidates for this type of treatment.

Percutaneous discectomy is not indicated in the following instances:

1. A persistent herniated disc with some of the disc external to the posterior longitudinal ligament or free in the spinal canal
2. Osteophytes and exostoses
3. A narrowing of the intervertebral foramen, narrowing of the intervertebral disc space, and a narrow spinal canal
4. The presence of air within the disc, as detected by MRI or CT, because in these cases the nucleus pulposus is often already herniated
5. Spondylolisthesis
6. An increased erythrocyte sedimentation rate, which suggests an infection in the spinal column
7. Hemorrhagic diathesis

GENERAL TECHNIQUES FOR PERCUTANEOUS DISCECTOMY

All of these procedures are conducted with the patient under local anesthesia. If the procedures are performed on an outpatient basis, a local anesthetic is applied to site of puncture (10 ml of 1-percent lidocaine [Xylocaine]) around the region of the intervertebral joint. With inpatients who require endoscopic or stereotactic procedures, a sedative can be administered. The patients' intraoperative help is essential because their reactions to the procedure provide an indication of its success or failure. Expressions of pain by the patient during the procedure may also signal the occurrence of complications.

We usually conduct the procedure with the patient lying on one side with the painful side facing up (Fig. 155–1). The patient lies with chest and pelvis sideways, supported by a flat pillow. The knees are pulled up, and a pillow is placed underneath the shoulders, chest, and head. Patients who require entry from both sides, for example, as is required for endoscopic discectomy, can be placed in the prone position (Fig. 155–2). With this position, support of both hips and shoulders is required, so that the patient does not tire during the procedures.

We have had much experience with lateral positioning, which makes the localization of the L4-L5 level extremely simple. The point of intersection of a parallel line 8 to 10 cm away from the spinous process as, that is, from the midline with a line drawn connecting the two iliac crests is the injection point for L4-L5 disc after the point of McCulloch (Fig. 155–3). The landmarks for the puncture to L5-S1 are 1

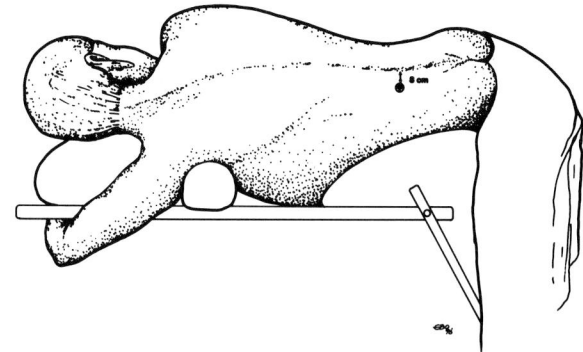

FIGURE 155–2. Prone position.

cm medial and caudal to the point of McCulloch. The L3-L4 and higher disc spaces can be identified by moving two to three fingerwidths per segment cranial from the puncture point for the L4-L5 disc.

This process is performed and controlled in two planes with the use of an image intensifier. With practice, the irradiation time can be limited to a few seconds.

We use the following techniques:

1. Percutaneous mechanical discectomy with different, specially developed microinstruments (with and without endoscopic control)
2. Percutaneous automatized suction discectomy
3. Other stereotactic techniques for discectomy
4. Percutaneous laser-assisted discectomy (nucleus pulposus denaturation or vaporization)

PERCUTANEOUS MECHANICAL DISCECTOMY

The technique of percutaneous mechanical discectomy varies among surgeons and depends on the instruments used. Kambin's[25] method for percutaneous lumbar discectomy and decompression by means of endoscopic microdiscectomy is carried out with the patient in the prone position. The disc is punctured dorsolaterally about 10 cm parallel to the midline, from the affected side, and the angle must be very carefully chosen so that the puncture runs purely through the paravertebral musculature. The final placement of the needle in the nucleus pulposus is important and must be in the middle of the disc. Subsequently, the punctured opening is slowly wid-

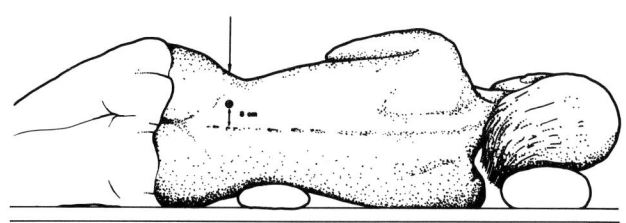

FIGURE 155–1. Lateral position.

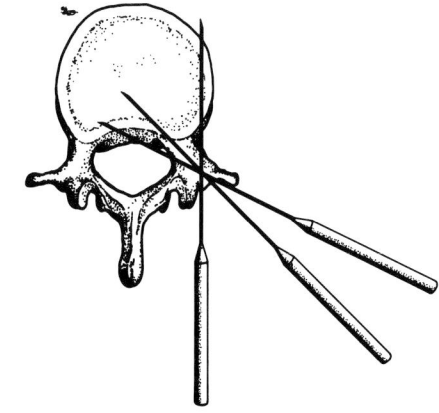

FIGURE 155–3. Puncture angle. Middle needle positioned exactly.

CHAPTER 155

Percutaneous Lumbar Discectomy

Peter W. Ascher

Back pain is one of society's costliest medical problems, both socially and economically. Approximately 80 percent of all people will suffer from back problems at least once in their lives,[1] and regardless of the nation's health care system, back problems precipitate many lost working days. Regardless of whether they are operated on or not, back problems are the most common cause of early retirement. Professions most susceptible to back problems are construction and sedentary occupations.

According to an American study published in 1980, 2.5 million Americans, and 2% of all workers, suffer from back problems. Because of this, 28.6 working days per 100 employees are lost each year, that is, 17 million working days per year. In addition, 1.2 million adults are unable to perform their jobs because of back problems on any given day.[1,2] In England, one of 25 people per year changes profession because of backache,[3] and two thirds of all those who retire early in Austria do so because of back problems.

The connection between disease and injury of the spinal column and the sciatic nerve was already historically noted at the time of the Assyrians (1665 B.C.). Hippocrates (460 to 370 B.C.) described the sciatic nerve, as did the Persians and Arabs in the ninth century A.D., when they finally conveyed this knowledge to the Europeans. Despite this early knowledge of the connection between backache from injury or disease of the spinal column and spinal column anatomy, no therapeutic attention was paid until the twentieth century.[4] The first laminectomies for back pain were performed by Goldthwait in 1911.[5] However, he attributed the problems solely to a narrow spinal canal. After many other studies,[6–8] a study by Mixter and Barr[9] finally led to the conclusion that a laminectomy with decompression and extraction of the herniated lumbar disc could improve the suffering caused by sciatic pain. Since this time, an ever-increasing number of patients have been operated on because of this disorder.

The microsurgical approach to the spinal column has been promoted since the early 1970s. Williams,[10] Wilson and Harbaugh,[11] Maroon and Albar,[12] Caspar,[13] Yasargil,[14] Saunders,[15] and many others recommend microsurgery because it is more exact and less stressful than larger surgical procedures. Consequently, many authors have tried to develop early alternative methods to replace the classic conservative treatment methods while avoiding larger operations. The purpose of this chapter is to present and compare these methods and to weigh their value. Every method's goal is to reduce the volume of the nucleus pulposus, thereby minimizing the stress on the nerve root.

Smith[16] tried to accomplish this goal by using intradisc injection of chymopapain to dissolve the nucleus pulposus, and he published the first clinical study on this technique in 1967.[17] Hijikata[18] and Kambin and Gellman[19] developed the percutaneous mechanical discectomy using specially developed instruments in 1975 and 1983, respectively, and this development was followed by the introduction of the automatized percutaneous discectomy by Onik and colleagues.[20] For this purpose, special partly disposable instruments were developed. In 1985, Ascher[21] began using the percutaneously introduced laser for this operation (at the suggestion of Choy[22]) to denature the nucleus pulposus. These methods are now being employed by an increasing number of orthopedic surgeons and neurosurgeons.

INDICATIONS

The percutaneous methods are minimally invasive neurosurgical procedures, and they fall somewhere between conservative treatment and operative procedures. They are best employed as the last conservative, minimally invasive step or as the first minimally invasive operative procedure. In the previous edition of *Operative Neurosurgical Techniques*, Finneson[23] stated, "The first disc-operation is relatively easy. The repeat operative procedure, however, presents a problem both in technique and even more in satisfactory outcome. The recommended solution to this problem is to avoid the first operation...."

In spite of the fact that these procedures are minimally invasive and are associated with minimal risk, the indications for them must be stringent and are as follows:

1. Signs of clear-cut compression, that is, muscle weakness at the compromised segmental level with corresponding reflex reduction or loss, a positive jugular vein sign (Naffziger's), a positive symmetrical or crossed straight-leg-raising sign, as well as sensory loss appropriate to the level of the affected segment.

2. Confirmation of neurologic findings with computed tomography (CT), magnetic resonance imaging (MRI), CT myelography or discography.*

3. Treatment with conservative measures for an appropriate length of time, to exclude the possibility of a cure with

---

*The editors and author think that discography has become obsolete in view of its pain, the uncertainties, its interpretation, and the great superiority of the CT and MRI procedures cited.

sive neurologic deficit. Thus, I suggest removing this indication from the list. Intractable pain is also listed as an indication for disc surgery and should also be removed. The pain from typical disc rupture typically fluctuates, and motivated patients do not stop work because of it in most instances. Injuries that occur in the work place do not usually cause disc rupture. Failure of conservative treatment is also not an indication for surgery in the absence of diagnosis of disc rupture.

Finneson has listed among contraindications to surgery a first episode of sciatic pain without an adequate trial of conservative management. There are, however, occasional instances in which pain is so severe that it may be worse at bed rest. However, I do agree that pain on the wrong side means that a correct diagnosis has not been reached, and that if the patient significantly improves after conservative treatment, surgery is not indicated.

The combination of either a negative CT or MRI result with negative results on myelography makes a surgically remediable disc rupture extremely unlikely. For this reason, exploratory lumbar surgery is almost never advisable. Finneson also mentions the use of epidural venography and discography in disc herniation. However, at this time, these studies are of no value at all.

Regarding the technical aspects of surgery, the use of fiberoptic illumination and loupes is well established. The microscope may be used but probably does not add to the efficiency of the operation. In fact, visualization of the entire disc fragment may be hindered at times by inexperienced use of the microscope.

Numerous patient positions have been used in surgery for lumbar disc herniation. My own preference is for the knee-chest position, in which the laminae are spread apart, the depth of the wound is reduced to the absolute minimum, the epidural veins are totally decompressed, and the great vessels in the abdomen must hang away from the spine. Neck extension must be avoided during any prone operation so that cervical spinal cord injury is prevented.

Regarding surface landmarks, I would add only that the relaxed hand with the thumb and little finger spread apart corresponds to the size of the sacrum in almost all patients, and that if the little finger is placed on the tip of the coccyx, the thumb with the hand in this relaxed position lies on the lumbosacral interspace. This method has been of greater help to me than any other in localizing the level.

I would like to make a few points regarding operating on the correct level. If only patients with major disc ruptures are being operated on, the correct level is the level with the obvious disc rupture, most often a free fragment or an obvious major prolapse—what we call grade II or grade III if the patients are well selected. Several errors must be made for the surgeon to operate on the wrong level. One possible error is an incorrect diagnosis. If the patient has no disc rupture, there is no correct level. This error is made more often than one might like to think. The same is true for minimally herniated discs. The taking of x-ray studies in such instances can confirm the level being operated on, but a more fundamental problem exists—no matter what level is operated on, the outcome will be poor.

If a large disc rupture is expected and no disc rupture is found, then the surgeon is operating at the wrong level. If no disc rupture is expected, the operation should probably not have been carried out.

Regarding the technique of dissection, I prefer to place the muscles on a slight stretch by using a periosteal elevator to retract laterally and then using cutting cautery at a low setting to divide the attachments of the paraspinous muscles to the spines. Rather than using the rongeur in the manner depicted in Figure 121–13, the Leksell rongeur has a special feature incorporated in its design. It can be held to cut in a position that is nearly vertical. The lower cutting jaw of the instrument should never be inserted beneath the lamina in the manner depicted in this picture because of the likelihood of injury to the underlying nerve root.

The points made about avoiding injury to the nerve root at the yellow ligament are very important, and the danger of using the Kerrison punch, which may pick up the edge of the dura, should also be emphasized. Once the fragment has been removed, my method is to use a curved curette to remove residual loose disc material from the interspace. Nerve root anomalies and wound closure have been well discussed in the chapter.

The use of the operating microscope in lumbar disc surgery has been discussed. The experienced neurosurgeon should carry out lumbar disc excision with the aid of the microscope, if he or she prefers to do so. This technology allows a neurosurgeon to keep his or her microsurgical skills honed. In experienced hands, the use of a very small incision has occasionally led to excessive retraction and neural injury, which must be carefully avoided.

Since Finneson's chapter was written, we have become aware of the occurrence of lateral or extraforaminal disc herniation in the foramen itself or lateral to it. This phenomenon can be imaged only on CT scanning or MRI. It is not shown on conventional myelography. Surgery to remove a herniated disc in the foraminal or extraforaminal location is best carried out by following the nerve root out from the conventional or medial approach. Through a more lateral muscle splitting approach, the surgeon can come down directly on the lateral part of the foramina. The arterial branches in the region of the facet need to be dealt with whether a linear or lateral approach is used, but I believe that localization of the correct level and avoidance of extensive muscle dissection make the more medial approach preferable. Sacrifice of the facet joint on the side of the lesion has never been a problem in my experience.

Finally, a few points should be made on the timing of surgery. Ordinarily, an operation for removal of a herniated disc is carried out semielectively, meaning that the patient who needs surgery is usually in fairly intense pain, making the operation not totally elective. However, if a disabling neurologic deficit is present, such as a profound foot drop or quadriceps weakness, the chances of good motor recovery are better if the operation is carried out on an urgent basis. Sometimes, even with immediate surgery a profound deficit does not recover, but if the deficit is not quite complete, a reasonable chance exists for recovery if the pressure on the nerve root is promptly relieved.

CHAPTER 154

Surgical Management of Primary Lumbar Disc Herniation—Commentary

Edward C. Tarlov

Two fundamentally different kinds of pathologic conditions can occur in lumbar discs as a result of the combination of trauma and aging. Disc degeneration is the commonest problem and is nearly ubiquitous in the population. The fact that disc degeneration can cause referred pain in the buttock and down the thigh is not commonly enough recognized. All too often, clinicians assume that if leg pain is present, nerve root compression must exist. This is not the case. True sciatica radiating down the back of the thigh, below the knee, and involving the calf may indicate nerve root compression by herniated disc. Less well-defined pains, particularly those predominantly involving the buttock or thigh, without radiation in a full sciatic distribution; bilateral buttock or thigh pain; or pains that vary from side to side are most likely to be referred pain from disc degeneration. These conditions are not helped by surgery, regardless of what myelograms or computed tomographic (CT) scans are felt to demonstrate.

Finneson discusses the fallibility of the neurologic examination and the relationship of the location of a disc herniation to the lumbar nerve roots and plexus, all of which are important points. The commonest disc herniation, which occurs at the L4-L5 level, typically affects the L5 nerve root. Although weakness of the extensor hallucis longus with involvement of the L5 nerve root may occur, the absence of obvious neurologic deficit, even with a very large disc rupture at L4-L5, is quite common. This limitation of the neurologic examination should be added to those listed by Finneson.

Once a clinical diagnosis of disc herniation has been made in a patient whose severity of pain is sufficient to warrant surgery, preoperative imaging studies should be performed. When no surgery is being contemplated, the expense of imaging, which has become considerable, is not warranted. Clinicians tend to carry out excessive studies, even when a diagnosis is clear from one study. In most instances, the results of one study, either magnetic resonance imaging (MRI) or CT myelography, should allow a definitive diagnosis. Since Finneson's chapter was written, myelography has been carried less frequently. High-quality CT scanning can clearly demonstrate disc herniation, particularly in patients who are not obese and who have not undergone previous surgery. MRI appears to be equal to CT scanning for accuracy of disc herniation diagnosis, and MRI is now a well-established method for diagnosing disc herniation in many cases. Both studies tend to be over interpreted by radiologists, who do not have the opportunity to see the patients and to correlate signs and symptoms. In patients strongly suspected on clinical grounds of disc herniation and whose CT scan or MRI is unrevealing, an additional study should be performed.

An understanding of the pathology of lumbar disc rupture is essential for diagnosis. The strong posterior longitudinal ligaments in the midline cause most disc herniations to occur unilaterally. Midline bulging of discs occurs so frequently that it should hardly be considered pathologic. Lateral views on myelogram as well as CT scans and MRI that demonstrate disc bulging usually do not indicate a need for, or a likely benefit from, surgery.

We have used a system of grading disc ruptures to differentiate free fragments, major disc ruptures, and normal discs with minimal bulging. In grade 0 or grade I discs, there is no bulge or little bulging; in grade II, there is a marked herniation with a few fibers of the annulus intact; and grade III, an extruded free fragment. Grades II and III are the pathologic conditions most likely to be helped by surgery.

Finneson's lumbar disc surgery predictive score card is a graphic way to draw attention to negative risk factors. However, from the practical viewpoint, its value is somewhat questionable. For example, in the list of positive factors, a neurologic examination demonstrating a single root syndrome that indicates a specific interspace is given 25 positive points. As mentioned earlier, a major disc rupture at L4-L5, which is the commonest level at which disc rupture occurs, may not be associated with an identifiable neurologic deficit. Does this mean that a major disc rupture at L4-L5 carries a less favorable prognosis than one at L5-S1? Obviously not. I suggest that in addition to the positive factors listed, the importance of true sciatica in diagnosis be emphasized and that a number of points be given if the pain is typical, in other words, down the back or in one leg below the knee. On the other hand, atypical variations that are not true sciatica, namely pain confined to the buttock or back of the thigh, variable pain, and variable nonsciatic pain involving both legs, are negative factors and tend to be correlated with a poor outcome from surgery.

Progressively worsening neurologic deficit is often included in indications for surgery, perhaps most often in orthopedic circles. In fact, disc rupture rarely causes a progres-

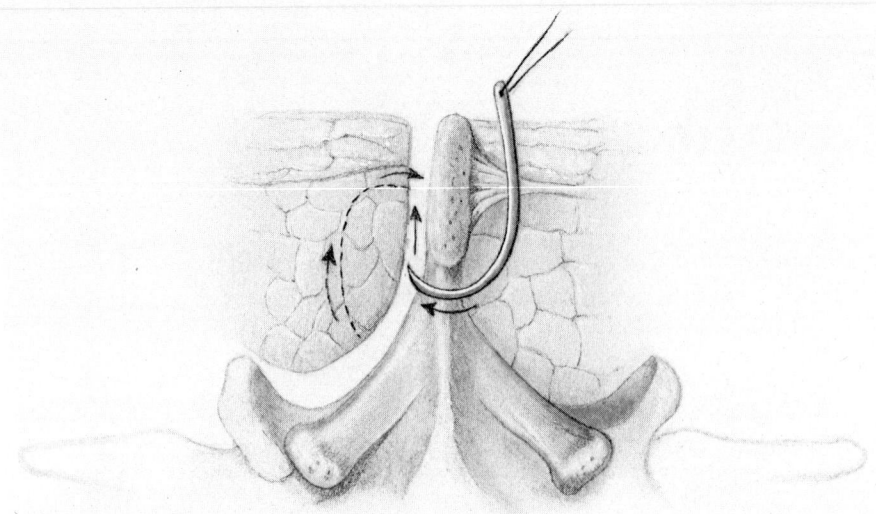

FIGURE 153–21. Muscle closure to eliminate "dead space." (Reprinted from Finneson BE: Low Back Pain, 2nd ed. Philadelphia, J.B. Lippincott, 1981. With permission.)

WOUND CLOSURE

The suture material of personal preference is 2-0 chromic gut for muscle and fascia, 3-0 plain gut for subcutaneous tissue, and monofilament nylon for skin.

An important, but often overlooked, hemilaminectomy closure technique is the elimination of the dead space, which may fill with clot and contribute to postoperative discomfort (Fig. 153–21). This is accomplished with 2-0 chromic suture passed through the interspinous ligament and then into the paraspinal muscles to approximate the paraspinal muscles against the laminae and spinous processes. This hemostatic suture should not be tied so tightly that it causes muscle necrosis.

REFERENCES

1. Finneson BE: A lumbar disc surgery predictive score card. Spine 3:186, 1978
2. Barr JS, Mixter WJ: Posterior protrusion of the lumbar intervertebral discs. J Bone Joint Surg 23:444, 1941

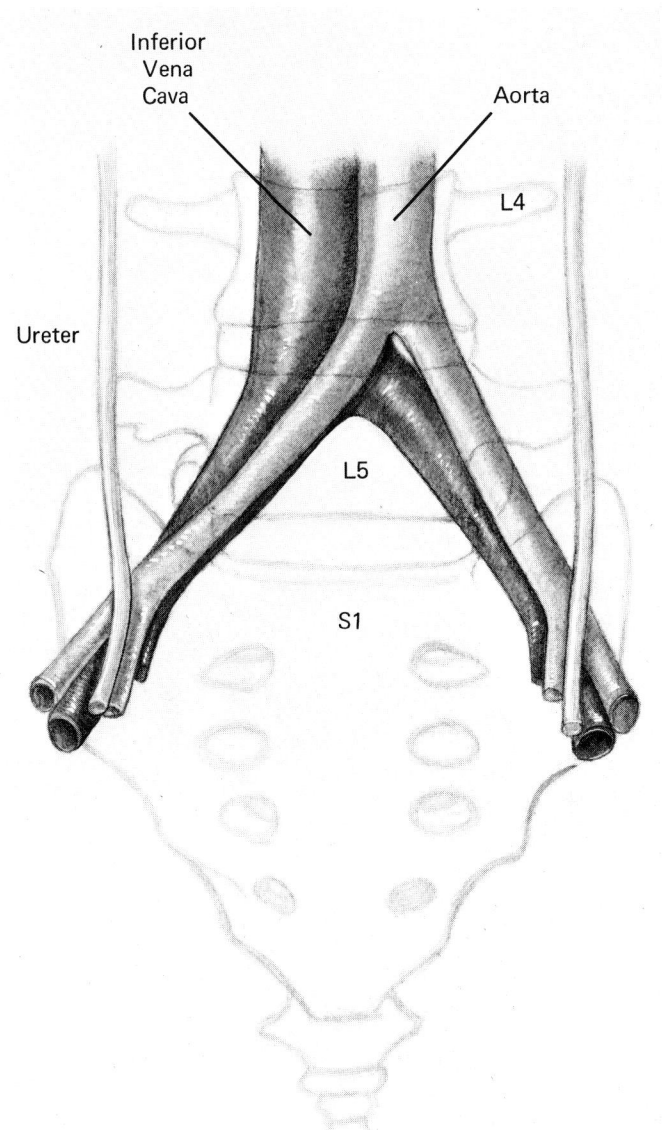

FIGURE 153–20. The major vessels and ureters and their relationship to the anterior lumbar spine. (Reprinted from Finneson BE: Low Back Pain, 2nd ed. Philadelphia, J.B. Lippincott, 1981. With permission.)

deviation is not significant unless the surgeon happens to carry out a rather extensive lateral interlaminar exposure. Because the surgeon's attention is focused on the nerve root under direct vision, he or she may be unaware of an equally vital neural structure that is partially hidden by the lateral reflection of the yellow ligament. Even more rarely, two nerve roots may exit from the same foramen. When the dura and its nerve root is exposed, a second root is present just lateral to the first root. If it is recognized as a nerve root, there is no problem, but occasionally the laterally positioned root is mistaken for a bulging disc, and attempts are made to excise it. In doing so the root may be injured beyond repair. There is no substitute for good lighting and magnification. In addition, the operation should always be done carefully, because the surgeon is working through a "keyhole," and identification of structures is extremely important.

After the protruded intervertebral disc has been adequately excised, the operating room table or spinal rest is flattened, so that the original flexed position is now a relatively straight one. This change in position places the root under less tension, narrows the posterior intervertebral disc space, and increases the depth between the skin surface and the interlaminar space. The interspace then is re-explored, and occasionally several additional fragments of disc material can be removed with the posterior vertebral bodies closer together. At the termination of the procedure, the nerve root should be under no pressure whatsoever, either anteriorly from the intervertebral disc or from bony constriction within the intervertebral foramen, which should have been partially opened during the bony dissection.

Bleeding from epidural veins should be carefully controlled before closure of the wound. Occasionally, a small pledget of absorbable gelatin sponge is required to control venous bleeding.

A No. 11 blade is used to make a rectangular slab-shaped window through the annulus, and through this opening, an adequate subtotal excision of disc contents is performed. This window extends from the most medial exposure of the annulus to the lateral limits of the bony exposure and comprises the entire width of the intervertebral disc, which is bounded by the bodies of the superior and inferior vertebrae (Fig. 153–19). Pituitary forceps of various sizes and shapes, as well as a curette, can be used to free up loose fragments of disc material. Excision of a rectangular slab of annulus may prevent the remaining shell of annulus from buckling as the disc space narrows. This buckling is to be prevented because it may fibrose and provide a source of root compression a year or two postoperatively. Some reduction of the intervertebral space will occur, and patients with long-standing disc disease who have not had surgery often demonstrate interspace narrowing.

When intervertebral disc rongeur forceps are used within the intervertebral space, great care is necessary to avoid penetrating the instrument through the anterior annulus fibrosus and the anterior longitudinal ligament. Such penetration is precarious and may result in laceration of one of the great vessels located anterior to the vertebral space (Fig. 153–20). Experienced and competent lumbar disc surgeons have suffered this calamity, and when working deep within the intervertebral space, the surgeon must remain alert to the possibility of this mishap. Degenerative changes affecting an intervertebral disc are generalized and may cause softening of the anterior annular fibers and anterior longitudinal ligament. These structures, when reasonably firm, usually offer resistance to instrument penetration, but when they are softened, the surgeon may unknowingly poke through the anterior annular fibers with disc rongeur forceps. After such inadvertent penetration, the iliac artery may be grasped and torn by the forceps. Various methods have been advocated to avoid this problem, including marking the instruments 1½ inches from the tip as a visual reminder of depth penetration. Good lighting and magnification aid in the depth perception and in visualization of the interior of the disc space.

FREE DISC FRAGMENTS

Occasionally, the protruded disc is in the axilla between the dural sac and the nerve root. A most meticulous dissection of this extruded fragment is necessary, and care should be taken when this fragment is grasped with an intervertebral disc rongeur forceps to avoid damage to the adjacent laterally displaced nerve root. Recognizing a completely free extruded fragment within the axilla is sometimes difficult. It may resemble epidural fat, and in some cases, only the tip of the extruded fragment presents dorsally, with the bulk of it not being visible and indenting the inferior portion of the dural sac medially. The surgeon, unaware of this large extrusion, may retract the nerve root and dural sac medially together with the free fragment and expose a bulging or protruding annulus. The disc protrusion is then excised and the interspace evacuated as thoroughly as possible by the usual methods, including curettage and the use of the intervertebral disc forceps. The offending free fragment that is causing root pressure, however, is inadvertently left untouched. The lack of free nerve root mobility may be an indication that such a

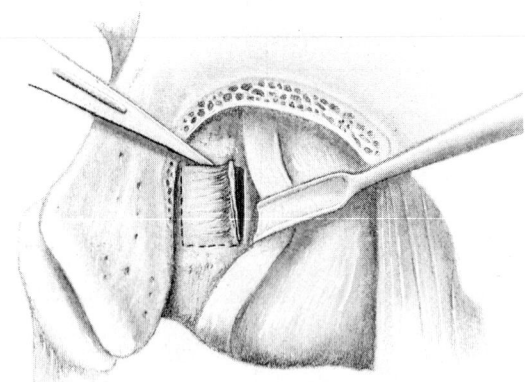

FIGURE 153–19. Incision of rectangular window through the annulus fibrosus. (Reprinted from Finneson BE: Low Back Pain, 2nd ed. Philadelphia, J.B. Lippincott, 1981. With permission.)

fragment is present. When the nerve root is not free, further inspection is necessary.

A free disc fragment may extrude beneath the posterior spinal ligament and occasionally produces a sizable mass that is capable of producing symptoms that are not evident on casual inspection. Palpation over the posterior spinal ligament with a thin elevator discloses this extrusion, and it can be "milked" laterally to expose an amount of disc tissue sufficient enough to be grasped with the intervertebral disc forceps and removed.

SURGICAL JUDGMENT

In patients in whom no gross protrusion of the disc but rather a slightly humped-up annulus exists, the surgeon must use judgment in deciding whether to excise the high annulus and curette the intervertebral disc space, or to be content with posterior bony decompression of the nerve root by means of a foraminotomy.

A disc should not be violated unless it can be seen to be causing nerve root pressure. Once the disc is violated, however, thorough disc excision is probably advisable. A bulging annulus does not have to be removed, particularly if the nerve root can be adequately decompressed. The root can easily go over a slight hump as long as there is no bony counterpressure above it. Sometimes a generous foraminotomy alone is adequate. In equivocal cases, injection of saline into the disc with a 10-ml syringe may be helpful. If the bulging disc does not take more than 1 or 2 ml of saline without a great deal of pressure, it might be tempting to limit the approach to a decompressive foraminotomy. On the other hand, if the entire 10 ml of the saline can be injected into the intervertebral disc space without a great deal of difficulty, the disc could be considered more pathologic.

NERVE ROOT ANOMALIES

Occasionally, the nerve root exiting from the foramen above the surgically exposed interspace descends medially beneath the facets of the next lower interspace. This minor

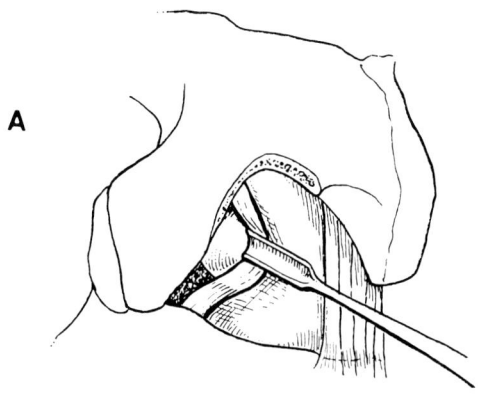

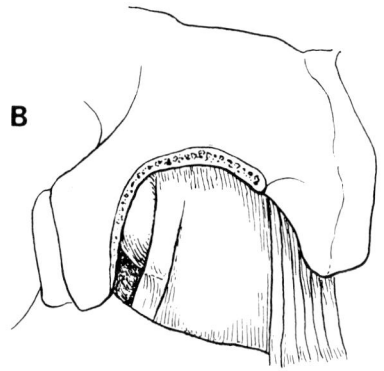

FIGURE 153-18. (A) Overstretched root and dural sac with an inadequate lateral bony exposure. (B) Very little root retraction is necessary with adequate lateral bony exposure. (Reprinted from Finneson BE: Low Back Pain, 2nd ed. Philadelphia, J.B. Lippincott, 1981. With permission.)

forceps can be used to separate the fat from the underlying dura and nerve root. To preserve the fat, it should be peeled medially to form a retractable flap that can be tucked back into place around the root after disc excision. Only after exposure of the nerve root can blood vessels within the epidural fat be safely cauterized without danger of damage to the root by cautery current. The Malis bipolar coagulator with bipolar forceps allows current to flow only from one forceps tip to the other. This isolated current, which produces much less heat, reduces the likelihood of inadvertent nerve root irritation or damage.

INTERLAMINAR SURGERY

Although the interlaminar space is rather small, the minute anatomy of this area varies considerably. It is always amazing to see how much can be hidden within this tiny space. An orderly and systematic approach to the area is paramount to successful disc surgery.

INSPECTION

The field should be dry at this stage. If bleeding remains a problem, decreasing lumbar flexion to a flatter position may reduce abdominal pressure and so reduce engorgement of the lumbar epidural veins. If this change in position is effective in controlling epidural venous bleeding, the surgeon should proceed with surgery in the flatter position.

Is the root elevated or is it flat? Does the root appear swollen or hyperemic, or is it the same color as the rest of the dura?

In patients who have had long-standing symptoms, adhesions between the nerve root and the posterior longitudinal ligament are occasionally quite dense. Very careful dissection of the root and the dura may be necessary to allow free retraction and exposure of the protruding disc.

ROOT TENSION

It should be possible to retract medially, without resistance, a root that is under no pressure by use of a narrow blunt retractor. The typical protruding disc is apparent when the root is retracted medially and manifests itself by slight elevation of the root and by increased pressure on medial retraction. At this stage of the procedure, considerable care must be taken to avoid stretching a compromised root. When the disc protrusion is extensive, it is best not to retract the root too vigorously over it so that excessive stretching of the root does not occur. When the root is under too much pressure to be retracted medially with ease, the root should not be retracted but should be decompressed by working laterally to it.

If extruded disc fragments are free within the canal, they usually can be manipulated laterally, grasped with the pituitary forceps, and gently removed. If the disc is not extruded but is bulging so much that the nerve cannot be moved medially easily, the surgeon should work lateral to the disc, introduce the pituitary forceps into the intervertebral disc space, and remove disc fragments piecemeal until the root can be retracted more easily over the partially decompressed annular shell.

The major error at this point comes under the heading of "grandstanding." There is a temptation to demonstrate the pathology to any and all present in the operating room. The root is retracted medially and maintained in an overstretched position while residents, interns, nurses, and visitors are invited to inspect the protruding disc. This is not the time to "entertain the troops," and a herniated disc is not a very spectacular sight in any event. Retraction of such a swollen, inflamed nerve is best kept to a minimum to avoid adding to the irreversible damage already caused by the disc protrusion.

Sometimes, a disc protrusion is a bit more medial, and the nerve root does not appear elevated or under pressure. On attempting to retract the nerve root medially, however, an obstruction is encountered. The surgeon then must be careful to lift the root and dura to determine whether or not a medially protruding disc is present.

INTERVERTEBRAL DISC EXCISION

Once the disc has been partially excised, the root can be retracted medially with little difficulty. A nerve root retractor then can be used to expose the disc space more completely.

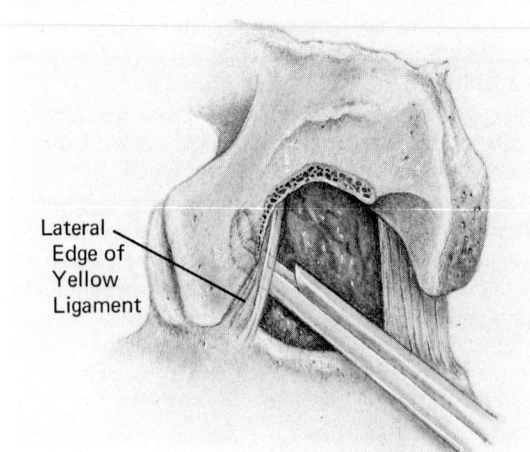

FIGURE 153-16. In widening the interspace, do not mistake the rolled-up lateral edge of yellow ligament for the root. (Reprinted from Finneson BE: Low Back Pain, 2nd ed. Philadelphia, J.B. Lippincott, 1981. With permission.)

glistening piece of tissue, resembling spaghetti, comes out, followed by bloody spinal fluid. These errors are classifiable as surgical tragedies and usually can be avoided by proper hemostasis, good visualization, and a cautious pace at this point in the operation.

A thin edge of bone is removed from the superior edge of the inferior lamina by use of a laminectomy punch that is not angled downward. The 40-degree angled jaw is helpful in working on the superior lamina and laterally but may produce a dural tear at the inferior lamina (Fig. 153-17). A slight fold of dura may bulge and be pinched and torn in the jaws of the bone-biting instrument. Most of the fibers in the dura are longitudinal (running up and down); if the instrument catches a fiber and the surgeon pulls without adequate visualization, to quote that outstanding spinal surgeon George Ehni, "The dura will rip open like a seam." Just a small bite of bone easily can cause a tear an inch long in the dura. If the dura is opened inadvertently, a small hole is usually easier to close than a large one. Dissection should therefore proceed cautiously on the inferior lamina. A bite of bone should not be taken with the rongeur and ripped out. The instrument should be closed carefully and the bone eased out very slowly, so that if the dura is tugged even slightly, the surgeon is able to visualize the tenting of the dura and can then release the instrument and inspect the area carefully before proceeding further. This type of complication always occurs before an adequate exposure has been obtained. Cerebrospinal fluid may fill the wound suddenly, becoming tinged with blood, so that it is impossible to see the damaged area. There is a tendency to try to close this opening immediately, but this is a mistake. It is also a mistake to try to visualize the damage by putting a sucker directly into the wound, because the roots may float out of the dural tear with the escaping spinal fluid, catch on the tip of the sucker, and sometimes be severely damaged. Instead of direct suction, a cottonoid should be inserted into the opening, and suction should be applied only on the cottonoid until the structures can be seen. Then a square of absorbable gelatin sponge (Gelfoam) can be placed over the dural tear and a cottonoid can be placed on top of the gelatin sponge square. The table should be tilted head-down so that spinal fluid pressure decreases in the lumbar region. If the table or laminectomy frame is flexed, it should be flattened. The surgeon then can proceed as though the dura had not been opened. After the disc has been excised and the root has been decompressed, full attention can be given to the torn dura. Before the dural tear is closed, both sides and both ends of the tear must be exposed. Dural closure must be watertight; 4-0 or 5-0 suture material should be used.

For a lateral bony exposure, a partial excision of the facet may be necessary for exposure of the lateral margin of the nerve root. This does not cause pain or an unstable spine when performed unilaterally. Bilateral facet excision and disc excision at that level may produce spinal instability and pain.

An adequate intervertebral lateral exposure may be of value for three reasons:

1. It facilitates satisfactory disc excision because less danger exists of overstretching the nerve root and dural sac as these structures are retracted medially. With an adequate lateral exposure, much less root retraction is necessary to afford good access to the disc (Fig. 153-18A and B).

2. A satisfactory lateral exposure is the first step of a foraminotomy that provides bony decompression of the involved root and almost always manifests some degree of edema and swelling.

3. In the years after surgery, hypertrophic osteoarthritic bony spurring, in association with postoperative epidural and perineural scarring, will be less likely to lead to root compression symptoms in the presence of a generous lateral exposure and foraminotomy.

After an adequate bony exposure, the epidural fat is visible. If the nerve root is obscured by the fat, two Cushing

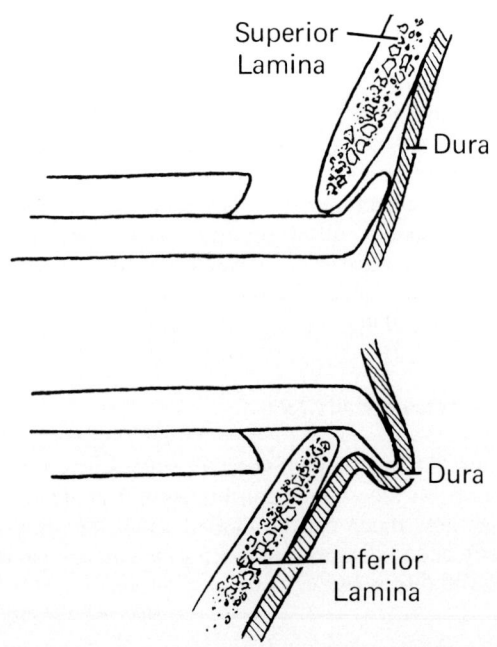

FIGURE 153-17. The laminectomy punch with a 40-degree angled jaw is helpful when working on the superior lamina, but it is not suited for the slope of the inferior lamina and may produce a dural tear. (Reprinted from Finneson BE: Low Back Pain, 2nd ed. Philadelphia, J.B. Lippincott, 1981. With permission.)

a small stamp of subcutaneous fat can be placed over the dura and nerve root as a free fat graft. Subsequent dissections and explorations have demonstrated a reasonably high rate of "take" of this type of graft.

The goal of surgery is adequate decompression of the root, as well as gentle and safe handling of the root. At this stage of the surgery, nerve root damage may occur in two ways. One occasional error is to mistake the lateral reflection of the yellow ligament immediately over the root for the root itself. Sometimes, after excision of the medial portion of the yellow ligament, the lateral portion rolls up on itself, creating a cylindrical appearance that may be quite deceptive (Fig. 153–16). If this cylinder is retracted medially, the underlying root may be mistakenly identified as a bulging disc, which is then attacked with vigor. Another error may occur when the interlaminar exposure is extended laterally and the lateral reflection of yellow ligament and bone is trimmed. This portion of the exposure must be performed under good visualization, with care being taken to hug the inferior bony and ligamentous surface with the jaws of the Schlesinger punch. If the tip of this rongeur is inserted too deeply, it may grasp a bit of the root along with the edge of the yellow ligament and bone. As the surgeon tugs on the instrument, a fairly long,

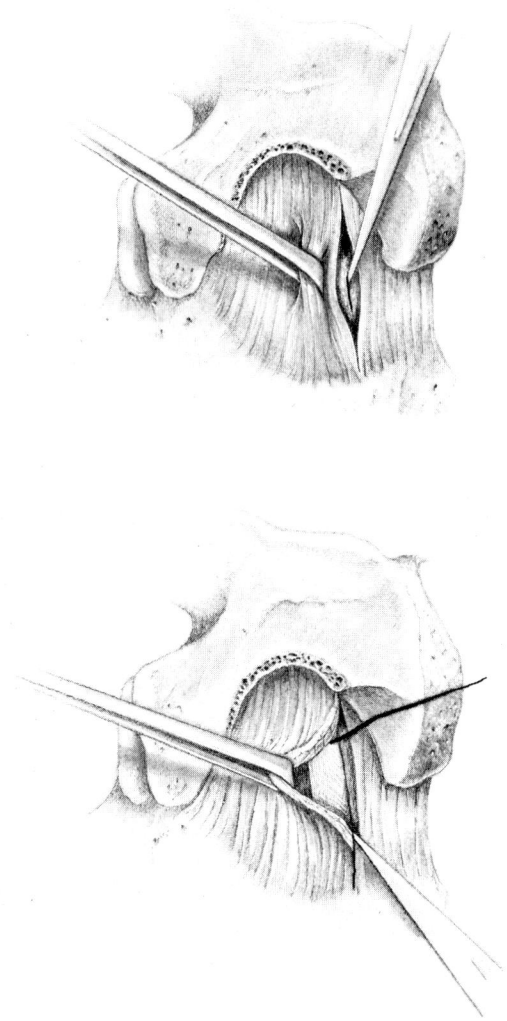

FIGURE 153–14. The yellow ligament is cut. (Reprinted from Finneson BE: Low Back Pain, 2nd ed. Philadelphia, J.B. Lippincott, 1981. With permission.)

recently has developed into a conjectural issue. It is now generally agreed that preservation of a layer of epidural fat, especially around the nerve root, is helpful in preventing subsequent encasement of the root within the dense epidural scar tissue that forms after an interspace exploration. For this reason, surgeons attempt to carry out disc excision without disturbing the epidural fat. This fatty layer, however, almost always obscures the dura and nerve root. In this laudable effort to prevent future damage of the root by postoperative scar tissue, the surgeon may create immediate, and possibly persisting, injury to the root during surgery because of his or her inability to visualize this structure adequately.

Frequently, a flap of epidural fat can be retracted so that good visualization of the root and dura is obtained. After completion of this procedure, the epidural fat can be tucked back into position around the root. If satisfactory root identification and visualization are not possible with preservation of the fat, however, it should be excised. A surgeon is not able to protect a structure that cannot be adequately visualized, and I am aware of two recent postoperative nerve root injuries that two separate surgeons attributed to their desire to preserve epidural fat. If the epidural fat has been removed,

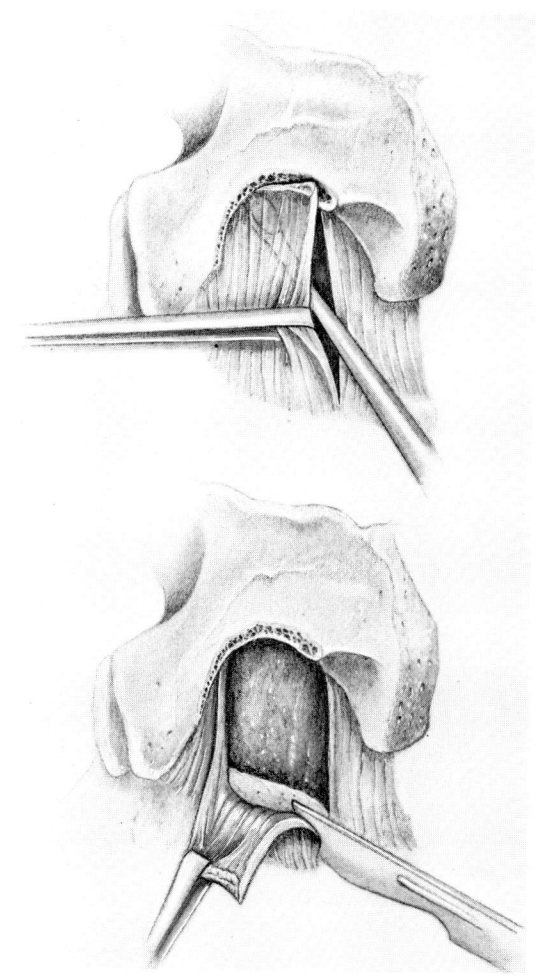

FIGURE 153–15. The yellow ligament is curetted. (Reprinted from Finneson BE: Low Back Pain, 2nd ed. Philadelphia, J.B. Lippincott, 1981. With permission.)

ization has been established, he or she can place the hemilaminectomy retractors in position (Fig. 153–12A). Many hemilaminectomy retractors are available, the simplest being the Taylor spinal retractor, which consists of a right-angled metal ribbon with a slightly hooked tip that can be inserted laterally and cephalad to the articular facet. The great disadvantage is that it has to be either hand-held by the assistant or tied to the base of the operating table or to the foot of the surgeon. Also, it has the unfortunate propensity to slip out of place occasionally—invariably at the worst possible moment of the procedure. Most surgeons prefer to use a self-retaining hemilaminectomy based on the many modifications of the Hoen hemilaminectomy retractor (Fig. 153–12B).

When the hemilaminectomy retractors are positioned, the shortest blades possible should be used to achieve adequate exposure, so that the flange of the blades rest flush against the skin surface. If the flange projects above the skin, it increases the depth through which the surgeon must work. The spinous process blade of the retractor should fit between the spinous interspaces, with the hook or hooks embedded into the interspinous ligaments. The muscle blade should rise above the hump of the articular facet (Fig. 153–12C). An occasional error is made by impinging the tip of the muscle blade against the facet, which causes the exposure to be needlessly narrow. If the paraspinal muscles are placed under tension, the retractors will stop most muscle bleeding. After the retractors are in place and the exposure is deemed satisfactory, any remaining muscle bleeding is controlled with cautery.

The remainder of the surgery takes place in that small keyhole of interlaminar space, and any skin, fascia, or muscle bleeding funnels directly into the work area. If the assistant must provide suction to remove the blood, his or her head will be in the way, which will obstruct the surgeon's vision, or the assistant will be poking the suction tip into the wound blindly, which also has its disadvantages. The other alternative is for the surgeon to hold the suction in one hand and operate with the other; this option also is not really satisfactory. Control of bleeding at this stage is therefore necessary for smooth, safe surgery.

DEVELOPING THE INTERSPACE

The laminae vary greatly in width, angulation, and position relative to each other, so that occasionally the interlaminar space is sufficiently wide to permit exposure and removal of a protruding intervertebral disc without removal of any, or very little, bone. This widened interlaminar space is seen most commonly between the L5–S1 levels and less frequently above the interspace.

The more strenuous bone work of the operation is followed by relatively delicate dissection of the soft tissue interspace involving yellow ligament, nerve root, and dura. This strenuous manual work tends to create a hand tremor that is distressingly obvious when the surgery is being performed with magnification techniques, such as loupes or an operating microscope. Air-powered rongeurs can be used for much of the bone work in the hope of reducing a postexertion tremor that may develop while the nerve root and other soft tissues are manipulated within the interspace.

When an interspace of normal dimensions is present, any rongeur, including duckbilled, Leksell, or Kerrison, can be used to remove the overhanging, inferior edge of the superior vertebrae (Fig. 153–13). If the L5-S1 interspace is being worked on, this would be the inferior edge of the L5 lamina. Some surgeons prefer rongeuring away the inferior half of the superior lamina, which exposes the superior border of the yellow ligament. This can be grasped with an Allis tissue forceps and the remainder of the ligament excised by sharp dissection with a scalpel. I prefer to remove only the inferior third of the superior lamina so that the edge of the yellow ligament is not exposed. Bone wax is used to control all bone bleeding from the rongeured edge of the lamina. After the one-third overhang of the superior lamina has been removed, an ample area of the ligamentum flavum will be exposed to view. A No. 11 blade on a long handle then is used to make a shallow incision in the ligamentum flavum along the direction of its fibers. The edge of the incision is grasped with an Allis forceps and tugged laterally to spread the incision. This maneuver allows the No. 11 blade to be used to incise the entire thickness of the yellow ligament down to the epidural fat (Fig. 153–14). After a small, moistened cotton patty has been introduced beneath the ligamentum flavum to separate it from the dura, this incision is extended from the superior lamina to the inferior lamina. Care should be taken to insert merely the tip of the blade beneath the ligament to avoid accidentally cutting into the dura. A second Allis forceps is used to get a firmer grasp on the full thickness of yellow ligament. A curette is introduced below the yellow ligament against the inferior surface of the superior vertebra, which permits a flap of yellow ligament to be curetted laterally while the remainder is left attached to the dorsal surface of the inferior lamina. This attachment then can be safely excised with a scalpel or scissors (Fig. 153–15).

EPIDURAL FAT AND NERVE ROOT DAMAGE

Once the yellow ligament has been excised, the epidural fat can be clearly visualized. Treatment of the epidural fat

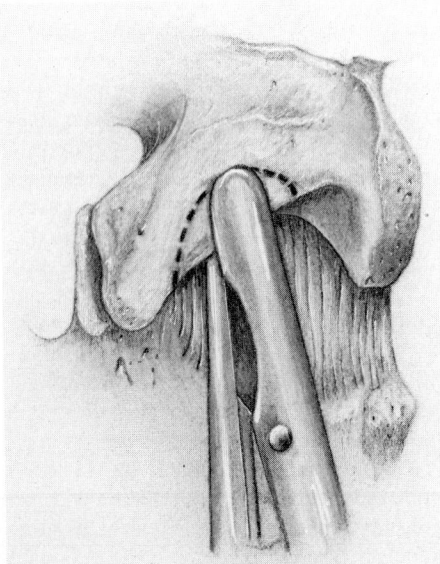

FIGURE 153–13. The overhanging edge of the superior lamina is rongeured. (Reprinted from Finneson BE: Low Back Pain, 2nd ed. Philadelphia, J.B. Lippincott, 1981. With permission.)

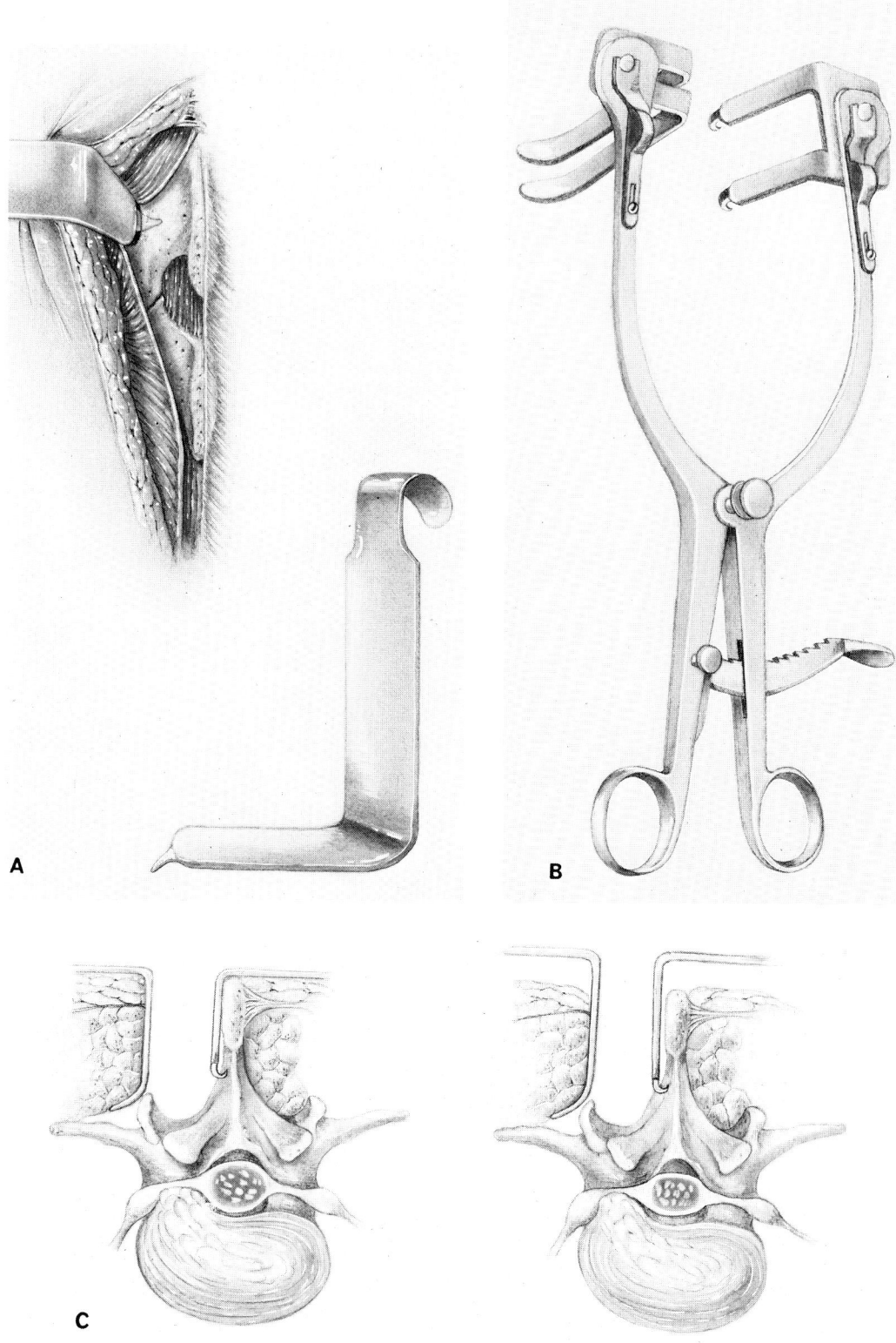

FIGURE 153-12. (A) Taylor hemilaminectomy retractor. (B) Hoen hemilaminectomy retractor. (C) If the hemilaminectomy retractor blades are longer than necessary, the depth through which the surgeon must work is increased. (Reprinted from Finneson BE: Low Back Pain, 2nd ed. Philadelphia, J.B. Lippincott, 1981. With permission.)

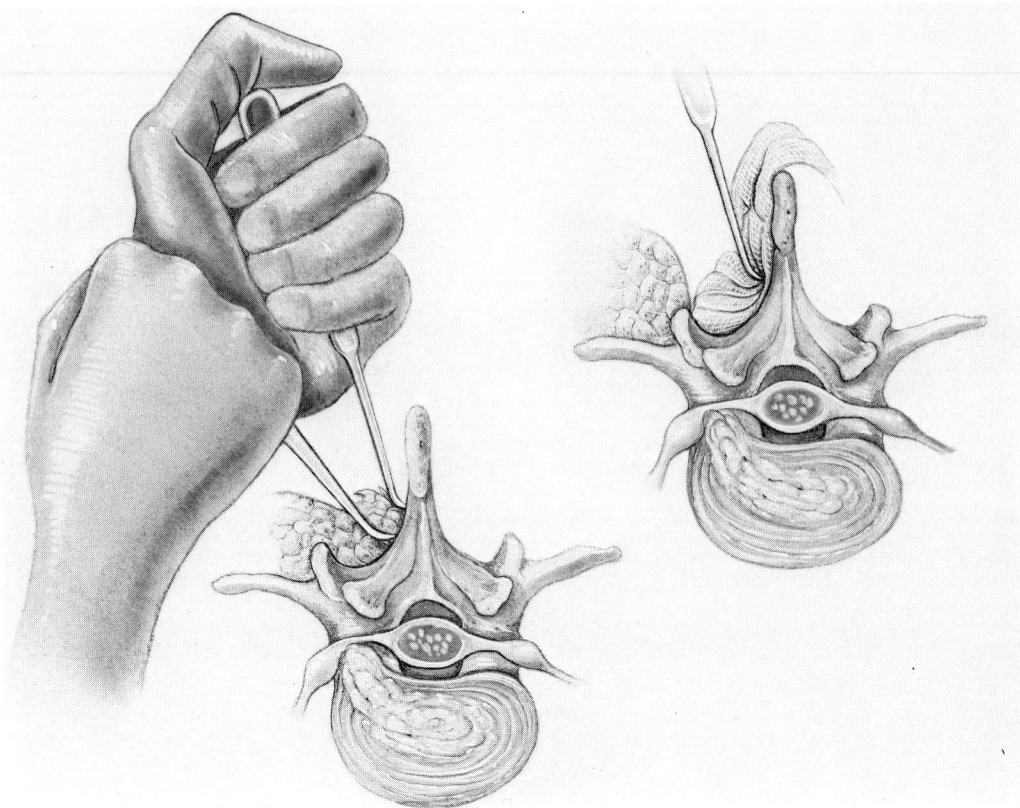

FIGURE 153–11. Subperiosteal dissection technique. (Reprinted from Finneson BE: Low Back Pain, 2nd ed. Philadelphia, J.B. Lippincott, 1981. With permission.)

pressed against the edge of the spinous process and to cut directly against the lateral edge of the spine. In this manner, the posterior spinous ligament or supraspinal ligament, which is a strong fibrous cord that extends without interruption along the tips of the spinous processes from C7 to the median sacral crest and which is continuous with the interspinal ligaments, is preserved. It is valuable to preserve this structure and so avoid unnecessary weakening of the spinal supporting ligaments. To prevent unnecessary tissue destruction and scarring, a scalpel rather than a cutting cautery should be used to incise the fascia. The muscles are best stripped from the spinous processes and lamina with the bimanual two-periosteal-elevator method. One periosteal elevator is used to retract the muscle mass laterally, while the other is used to perform a careful subperiosteal dissection. The periosteum should be peeled as cleanly as possible from the spinous process and lamina without penetrating the muscle which, if torn, may be a source of troublesome bleeding.

After the subperiosteal dissection has been accomplished under direct vision, a sponge extended to its full length is used to strip the bone of any remaining fragments of muscle and fascia. As bone is cleaned with the sponge, it should be allowed to accumulate within the incision to act as a tamponade and prevent muscle bleeding. Any bleeding occurring from the cut edge of the fascia is controlled with cautery. The subperiosteal muscle dissection is carried out laterally to expose the articulation between the superior and inferior articular processes.

After all surface bleeding has been controlled, the sponges are removed, and the desired interspace is localized by the time-honored method of palpating the sacrum and then counting up from it. This localization should be checked against the plain x-ray films of the spine to be sure that the patient does not have a lumbarized first sacral segment or sacralized fifth lumbar segment. Skeletal localization then should be correlated with the myelographic defect.

If the sacrum cannot be adequately palpated, or if for some other reason the surgeon is not totally satisfied with the identification of the anatomic level, surgery should be stopped at this point and a definite interspace confirmation obtained with a lateral lumbar spine roentgenogram.

One topic not likely to be discussed at length in the medical literature is the frequency of interspace misidentification at surgery. I occasionally find such an error in a referred patient, and I am aware of two occasions when I myself made such a mistake. Both of my mishaps occurred in the 1950s, when I was less aware of my fallibility and much too decisive to slow up my surgery for an "unnecessary x-ray film." This error is most likely to occur in either grossly obese patients or patients whose partial lumbarization of the first sacral segment dorsal element confuses the surgeon.

When in doubt, a roentgenogram should be obtained, not only for the surgeon's peace of mind but also to be absolutely certain that the interspace being worked on is the proper one. When a pathologic situation is not apparent at first inspection, such knowledge may provide additional incentive for a most thorough and meticulous interspace exploration and decompression, including a generous foraminal decompression.

Once the surgeon is completely satisfied that proper local-

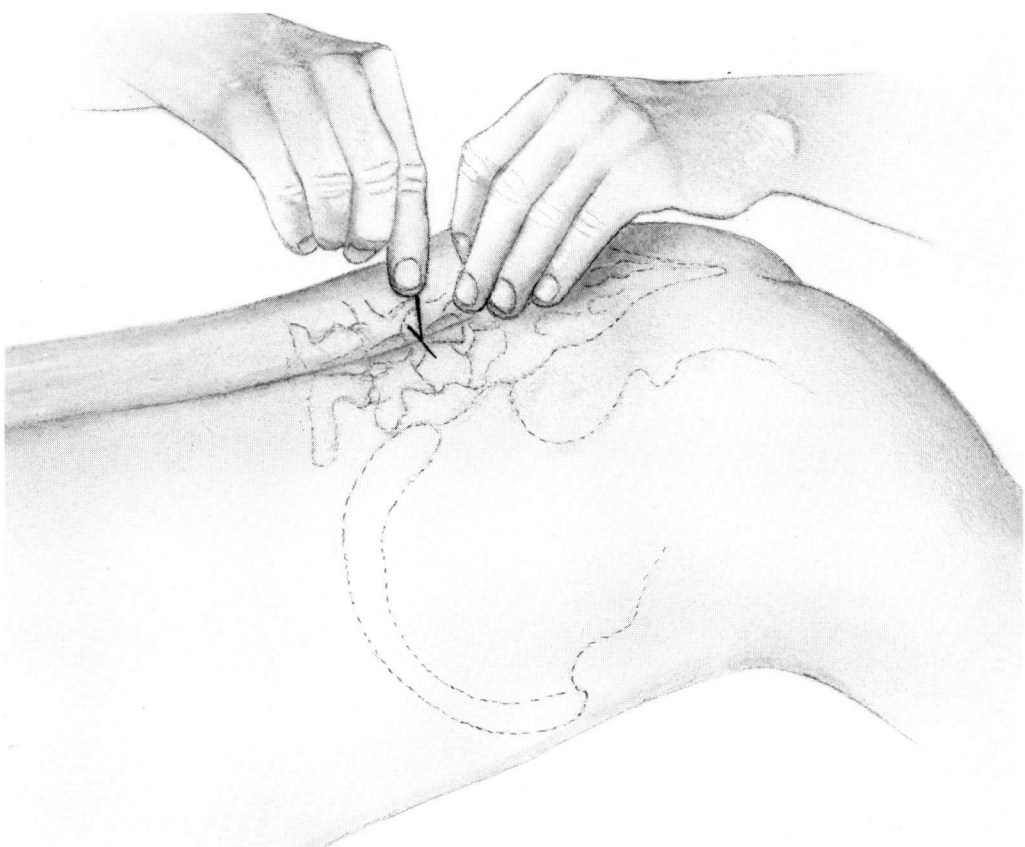

FIGURE 153–10. The skin is scratched at the "involved" interspinous space. (Reprinted from Finneson BE: Low Back Pain, 2nd ed. Philadelphia, J.B. Lippincott, 1981. With permission.)

sidered the short incision an ego trip on the part of the surgeon. Further experience has changed my opinion, and I presently believe that the short incision is beneficial to the patient's postoperative recovery.

There is no question that patients feel immeasurably better in the immediate interval after a short-incision operation than after a large- or standard-incision operation. Of greater importance is the fact that the long incision, which extends over several spinous processes, produces a band of scar that extends from the skin and attaches to the spinous processes and laminae along the length of the incision. This scar tissue is not as supple as nonscarred muscle and fascia. The lack of elasticity and suppleness is not conducive to a nicely distributed lumbar curvature after the wound has healed. This nonsupple lumbar spine probably makes the patient more vulnerable to recurrent low back dysfunction in the future. When a small incision is made, the precise location of the involved interspace is crucial, as described under the section "Surface Landmarks."

When the small incision is used, fiberoptic lighting and magnification are a necessity. The fiberoptic lighting and operating loupes or the operating microscope are of great advantage. These instruments aid greatly in ensuring that tissue is handled delicately, and they help to prevent nerve root damage. I consider them an integral and essential aid to the surgery.

Various methods are used to control skin bleeding, including Michel clips, Kolodney clamps, and mosquitoes. Weitlaner self-retaining retractors, which place the skin under tension, stop most of the minor skin bleeding; the several remaining subcutaneous vessels are easily controlled by cautery. Blood vessel cauterization should not be performed with a hemostat because its use invariably results in considerable tissue destruction. When carried out near the surface of the skin, hemostat cauterization may result in a full-thickness skin burn, and the resulting skin slough or necrosis may eventuate into a wound infection. To properly control skin bleeding with cautery, an assistant should use fine-toothed forceps to evert the skin edge, while the surgeon employs suction to locate the bleeding vessel precisely and then uses a fine-tipped Cushing forceps to cauterize only the vessel, taking care to avoid cautery spread to surrounding tissue.

A second knife ("clean knife") should be used to incise through fat to the fascia. If the patient is extremely obese, the Weitlaner retractors may have to be reset more deeply. Additional bleeding can be controlled with the use of the cautery. When performing the initial incision, the surgeon should not be obsessive about sweeping the fat cleanly away from the fascia. He or she must remember that a surgical procedure is being carried out, not an anatomic exposure. Such a maneuver can only serve to increase the blood loss and, even more serious, to create a false space that may fill with blood in the postoperative period.

SUBPERIOSTEAL DISSECTION

The subperiosteal muscles can be dissected by various methods (Fig. 153–11). I prefer to use a periosteal elevator

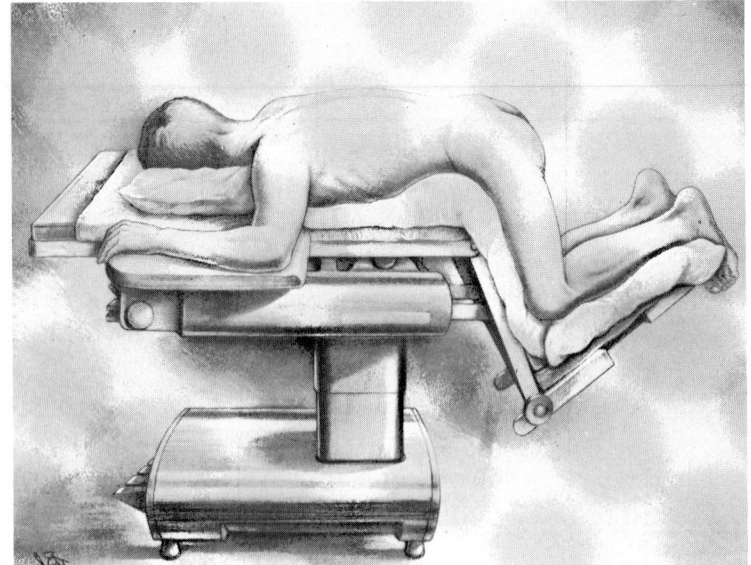

FIGURE 153-8. Modified prone position. (Reprinted from Finneson BE: Low Back Pain, 2nd ed. Philadelphia, J.B. Lippincott, 1981. With permission.)

level are obscured. For this reason, preparing a surface guide to interspace identification before draping is necessary. Personal preference is the cutaneous tatoo, which is made at the level of the disc protrusion with fluoroscopic guidance after completion of the myelogram. If this is not part of the surgeon's routine, other aids can be employed.

If a myelogram has been performed recently, the lumbar puncture mark on the skin can be used as a landmark for the spinal level. For example, if the lumbar puncture needle is seen on the myelogram films to be at the L3-L4 interspace, this will serve as an excellent surface guide for identification of the underlying vertebrae. If a myelogram has not been carried out recently, the first interspace at or immediately below the iliac crest can be considered L3-L4 (Fig. 153–9). Using this as a starting site, the surgeon can count down to the involved interspace and scratch a crosshatch in the skin at that level with a sterile hypodermic needle subsequent to cleansing the skin with an alcohol sponge (Fig. 153–10).

When surface guides are used, the elasticity of the skin must be kept in mind, particularly with obese patients. This elasticity may permit a surface marking to shift to the extent of an interspace as a result of the distortion caused by the use of retractors and alterations in the degree of lumbar flexion during surgery.

INCISIONS

For many years, my routine incision extended over approximately three spinous processes to allow for interspace localization and for adequate illumination, with the ends of the incision permitting overhead lighting to funnel in. I con-

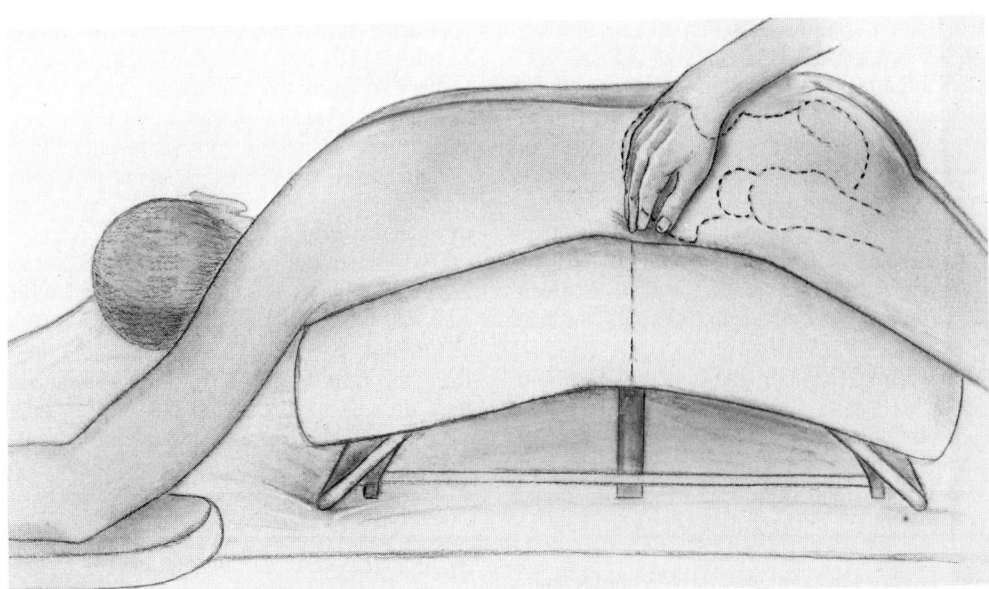

FIGURE 153-9. Flexion "break" in table or frame at level of iliac crest. (Reprinted from Finneson BE: Low Back Pain, 2nd ed. Philadelphia, J.B. Lippincott, 1981. With permission.)

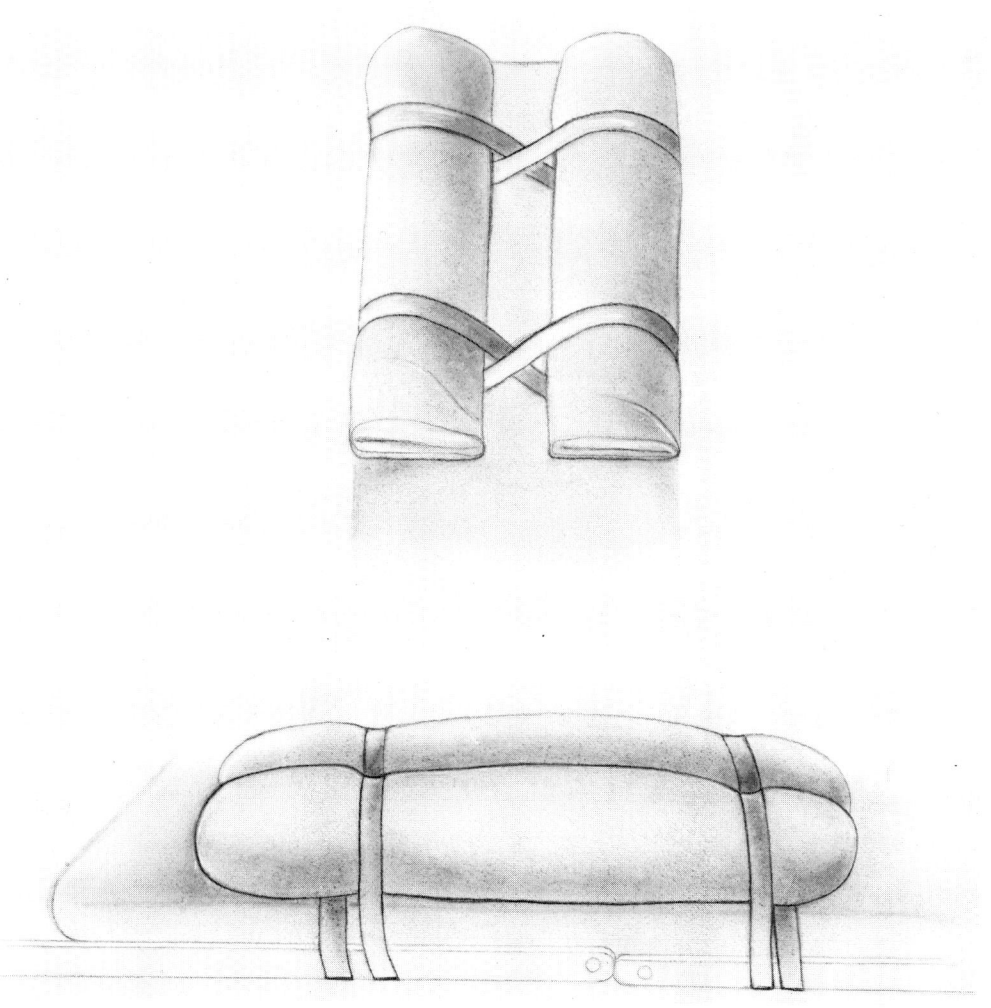

FIGURE 153-6. Blanket rolls taped in place. (Reprinted from Finneson BE: Low Back Pain, 2nd ed. Philadelphia, J.B. Lippincott, 1981. With permission.)

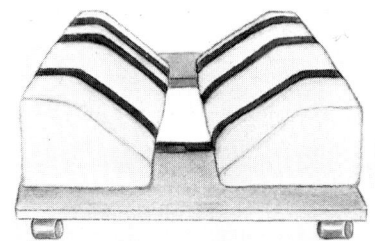

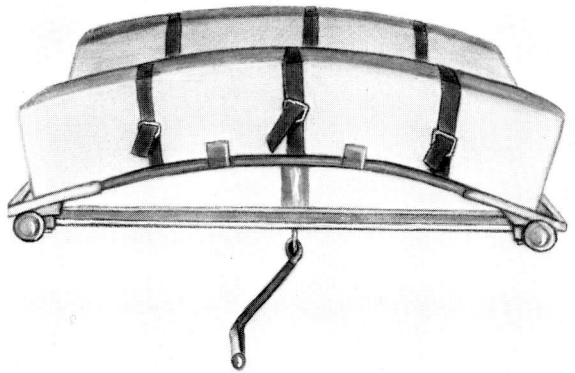

FIGURE 153-7. Prone position frame. (Reprinted from Finneson BE: Low Back Pain, 2nd ed. Philadelphia, J.B. Lippincott, 1981. With permission.)

Before the induction of anesthesia, the patient should always be asked to indicate the painful leg. Of course, the painful side is noted on the chart, and the radiologic studies also are labeled appropriately.

ANESTHESIA

Many surgeons prefer the use of spinal anesthesia, employing a hypobaric solution; epidural anesthesia also has some advocates. Intravenous sodium pentothal supplemented with halothane, nitrous oxide, and oxygen administered through an endotracheal tube is the anesthesia of my personal choice and is probably used by most clinics in lumbar disc surgery.

PATIENT POSITION

Various positions have been used for operation on patients with protruded lumbar discs.

For the unilateral disc excision, many surgeons prefer to use the lateral position (Fig. 153–5). This is the position of choice from the point of view of anesthesia because it does not hamper respiratory excursions as much as the prone position. The principal surgical advantage is that the lateral position allows the abdomen to be relatively free, which reduces pressure on the great veins and, in turn, reduces epidural venous distention and bleeding. This position does not allow blood to pool within the depths of the wound, and it promotes posterior lumbar flexion. Another technical advantage is that the surgeon can spread the uppermost interlaminar space laterally by positioning the patient on the table, so that the disc space involved is above the flexion break in the table, and then flexing the table.

The disadvantage of this position is increased difficulty on the part of the assistant in holding the root retractor or in performing other necessary functions. Those who are not experienced with this position may find it technically unsatisfactory.

Most lumbar disc surgeons prefer the prone position, in which the patient is intubated on a litter. After the endotracheal tube has been taped securely in place, the patient is rolled onto the operating table, which has previously been prepared either with blanket rolls or a prone position frame (Figs. 153–6 and 153–7).

A modification of the prone position can be obtained by flexing the hips and knees 90 degrees, with no effort made to flex the lumbar spine itself. Flexing the hip affords satisfactory flexion of the lumbar spine comparable to the other positions, and it may be associated with somewhat less abdominal pressure. To achieve this position, a minor adjustment of the operating table is accomplished by removing the adjustable headrest and fitting it to the footrest so that it will provide adequate support for the legs (Fig. 153–8).

The thin patient with a flat belly does well either with the prone position frame or with blanket rolls. Such a position, however, is poorly tolerated by the obese individual because neither the frame nor the blanket rolls adequately accommodate a large, protuberant abdomen. Abdominal compression is apt to increase lumbar epidural venous distension, and the resulting hemorrhage is an impediment to satisfactory visualization. In the presence of copious epidural bleeding, the surgeon may have difficulty concentrating on the prime objective of disc excision and adequate nerve root decompression because the major efforts are then directed at controlling the hemorrhage. Such an irritating environment may lead to a mishap and is not conducive to the calm and deliberate atmosphere so helpful to safe and smooth surgery.

Several positions have evolved in which the abdomen is completely free and unencumbered. Usually, some sort of operating table attachment is required to secure and immobilize the hips and thighs. This support is usually assembled by a hospital maintenance machinist or a handy surgeon.

SURFACE LANDMARKS

After the patient is draped, the iliac crests and other bony landmarks that provide approximate relationships to spinal

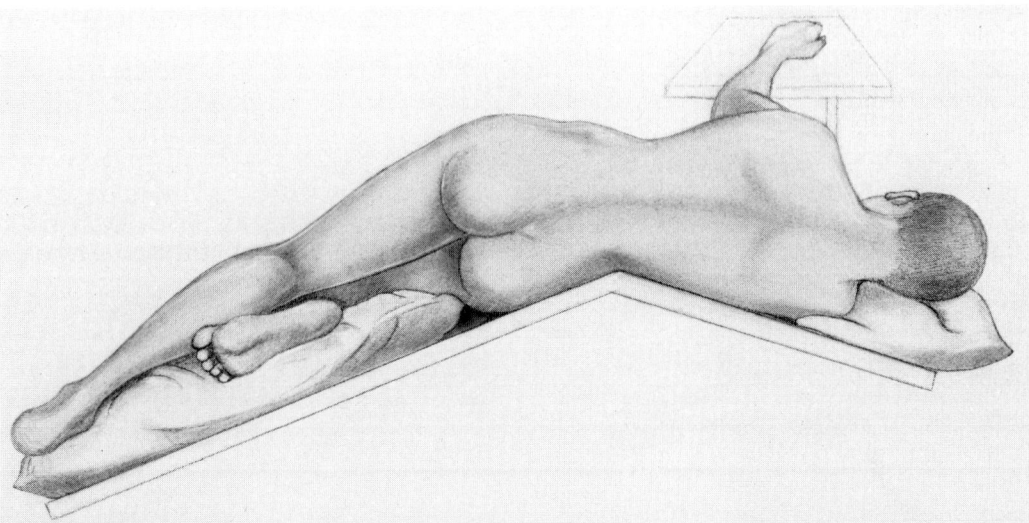

FIGURE 153–5. Lateral position for lumbar disc surgery. (Reprinted from Finneson BE: Low Back Pain, 2nd ed. Philadelphia, J.B. Lippincott, 1981. With permission.)

SURGERY

HISTORICAL DEVELOPMENT

Fifty years ago, an occasional laminectomy was performed for lumbar disc disease, and the extruded disc fragments were identified as "chondromata." Some question existed regarding the exact nature of these lesions, although many surgeons did recognize them as consisting of displaced intervertebral disc material. The surgical technique used in the removal of such lesions invariably involved an extensive bilateral laminectomy. This usually was followed by opening of the dura in the midline, separating of the nerve roots to either side, and palpating of the anterior spinal canal by means of a narrow probe until the underlying protrusion was identified. The anterior dura was then incised over the most eminent portion of the protrusion, and, through this very limited anterior dural opening, the protruding portion of the disc was exposed and removed.

The entire concept of ruptured intervertebral discs changed after the classic paper of Barr and Mixter.[2] They conclusively and unequivocally demonstrated the origin of these lesions, laid to rest any lingering doubt that they were neoplasms, and documented their etiology as protrusions of the nucleus of an intervertebral disc. They delineated the lumbar disc syndrome and the indications for surgical treatment of this condition. Shortly after the appearance of this paper, the surgical technique for protruding lumbar intervertebral discs underwent an important change, with the dura being left intact and the protruding disc being removed extradurally, although the extensive bilateral laminectomy was continued. Further surgical refinements followed, including the hemilaminectomy, which leaves the spinous process and lamina intact on the pain-free side. Twenty-five or 30 years ago, it became common practice to carry out disc surgery in most cases by means of the unilateral interlaminar approach.

In the past 6 or 7 years, the combined use of a fiberoptic headlight and 2.5 to 4.5× operating loupes has been accepted by an increasing number of disc surgeons. The fiberoptic lighting is helpful not only in providing dependable illumination to the depths of the incision but also in eliminating the technical necessity for the rather long laminectomy incision that extends over three interspaces (although the actual disc surgery was confined to an interlaminar space measuring approximately ½ inch). The lengthy skin and muscle incision was required to allow the standard overhead operating room lighting to illuminate the apex or depth of the operative field. With the brighter beam of light made available by fiberoptic techniques, a much smaller incision is possible. The magnification provided by the operating loupes aids greatly in ensuring delicate handling of tissue and helps prevent nerve root damage. Increasing the magnification to 25× with the use of an operating microscope has led to the development of a specific microsurgical discectomy technique involving a distinct departure from prior surgical concepts. A much more limited removal of disc material is performed. This technique avoids laminectomy, curettement of the disc space, and removal of epidural fat, and it avoids incision of the annulus fibrosis with a scalpel; instead, it employs a blunt probe to perforate this surface.

With advances in knowledge and equipment, continued technical changes can be anticipated.

CHOICE OF OPERATIVE PROCEDURE

Once the decision has been made that surgery is indicated, the surgeon must determine which operative procedure is most suitable for the patient's particular low back dysfunction.

Is a disc herniation producing a clear single-root syndrome? If so, interlaminar disc excision is the procedure of choice.

Is it primarily a stenotic lumbar spinal canal syndrome associated with sciatica produced by foraminal impingement and secondary to a bony spur? Attempting to treat this condition with an interlaminar disc excision often is technically difficult and is likely to have a disappointing clinical result. The operation of choice for a stenotic lumbar spinal canal is decompressive laminectomy and foraminotomy at the appropriate level.

If the symptoms are unilateral and the myelographic defect is bilateral, should surgery be confined to the side of the pain or should a bilateral interlaminar disc excision be performed? This is often a gray area and may be open to controversy. As a basic principle, performing the minimal amount of surgery that can adequately relieve the symptoms is preferred over attempting prophylactic surgery of symptoms that have not yet developed. Any decision made in this situation can be wrong. After a bilateral interlaminar operation, the patient may awaken from the anesthesia with postoperative pain in the previously painless leg. Surgery can be confined to the painful side, and in the near or distant future, pain may develop on the nonoperated side.

Should disc excision be followed by a fusion? We do not routinely perform a combined disc excision and spinal fusion but reserve this combined procedure for unusual situations.

DOUBLE-CHECKING THE SIDE OF LESION

Performing an operative procedure on the "wrong side" is not a common mishap, but it can occur when surgery is performed on any structure that is paired. Patients who have undergone herniorrhaphies, hip surgery, cataract surgery, or carpal tunnel decompressions occasionally have awakened from anesthesia and have been surprised to find the surgical dressing and the incisional discomfort at an unanticipated site. Because the patient undergoing lumbar disc surgery is in the prone position with his "sides reversed," this error may occur with greater frequency than is likely to happen in the supine position. The best way to preclude this blunder is for the surgeon to remain alert to such a possibility and to establish a preventive behavior pattern.

When reviewing spine x-ray films, the surgeon should make a point of placing the films on the view box as though the patient were in the prone position, with the left marker on the left side. Radiologists, who are trained to visualize films as though the patient is in the anatomic position, may look with mild disfavor at this heresy. It is not the radiologist, however, who will be sued for operating on the wrong side. This practice reinforces a mental image of the patient in the prone position.

Another helpful aid to lateralization is the small tatoo that is routinely made at the completion of a myelogram. This permanent mark is radiologically localized at the level of the lesion and is placed laterally on the side of the pain.

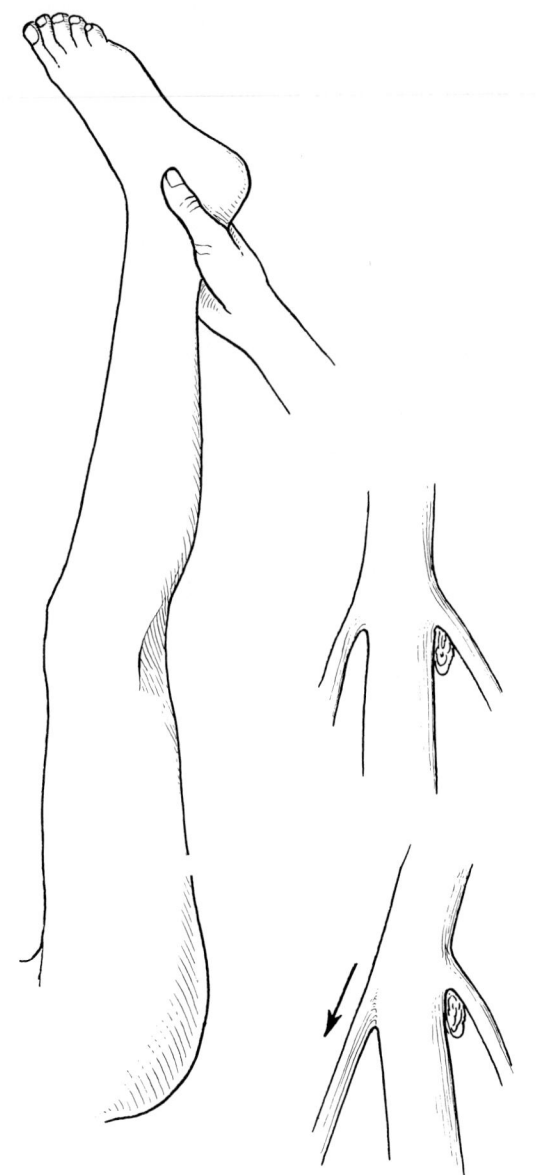

FIGURE 153–4. The well leg-raising test of Fajerstajn. (Reprinted from Finneson BE: Low Back Pain, 2nd ed. Philadelphia, J.B. Lippincott, 1981. With permission.)

with a high incidence of less than satisfactory results. With these factors in mind, four indications for surgery exist:

1. Intractable pain
2. Progressively worsening neurologic deficit
3. Intractable recurrence of pain
4. Cauda equina syndrome

With the exception of cauda equina syndrome, each of these indications is relative and depends on how well the patient tolerates the symptoms, on the extent of the neurologic deficit, and on the psychological and sociologic background of the patient.

CONTRAINDICATIONS TO SURGERY

Five important contraindications to surgery exist:

1. A first episode of low back and sciatic pain without an adequate trial of conservative management.

2. Intermittent low back pain associated with occasional pains of an equivocal nature, extending into one or the other lower extremity, and equivocal results on myelography.

3. A prolonged history of intermittent low back pain and equivocal results on myelography.

4. Low back and intermittent sciatic pain with a myelogram demonstrating a lesion on the "wrong," or pain-free, side. (I have seen two patients on whom disc surgery was performed with "a contralateral myelogram," and the two surgeons who elected to proceed on the basis of this information were divided in choosing the side of surgery on which to operate. The one who operated on the painful side used as his justification myelographic evidence of disc dysfunction at a specific interspace; because the pain was on the opposite side, he decided it would be best to decompress the nerve root on the side of the pain rather than on the side of the myelographic defect. The surgeon who elected to operate on the side of the myelographic defect rather than on the side of the pain felt that the disc protrusion might cause a shift of the cauda equina enclosed within its dural sac, which would press the opposite root against the lamina and produce radicular symptoms. Both patients fared poorly after surgery.)

5. Improvement of the patient. In the presence of significant motor weakness, if some slight improvement in the pain occurs, it may be justifiable to proceed with surgery. If pain is the primary symptom, however, improvement is an indication to cancel surgery. (I adhere to this principle and have canceled many scheduled cases on the day of surgery after being told that the patient no longer had pain or that the pain was markedly improved.) Pain surgery performed during an interval of improvement may result in patient dissatisfaction, despite an adequate postoperative result. The patient may be less willing to accept residual symptoms, even of a relatively minor nature, and is more apt to question in retrospect how pressing and indispensable the need was for surgery. If, in the face of improvement, the patient is discharged and subsequently readmitted for surgery with an exacerbation of pain, occasional residual symptoms may be tolerated more kindly. When lumbar disc surgery is contemplated, the indications must be clear to the patient as well as to the surgeon.

EXPLORATORY LUMBAR DISC SURGERY

Ten years ago, the patient with persisting sciatica and a normal myelographic result and who failed to respond to conservative treatment often was considered by many surgeons to be a suitable candidate for exploratory lumbar disc surgery. Usually, the L5-S1 and L4-L5 levels were explored on the symptomatic side. Although some patients possibly benefited by this approach, a significant number either were not improved or were worse after surgery. At this time, with the additional diagnostic help provided by MRI scans and CT scans of the lumbar spine, surgeons are able to assess intraspinal areas that previously may have been hidden. Given these new diagnostic tools, a suitable indication for a blind exploration based purely on the persistence of pain is inconceivable. The likelihood of finding a surgically treatable lesion if myelographic, MRI scans, and CT scan results are all normal is so poor that the era of exploratory lumbar disc surgery is best brought to a close.

LUMBAR DISC SURGERY PREDICTIVE SCORE CARD

This questionnaire is of predictive value when limited to candidates for excision of a herniated lumbar disc who have not previously undergone lumbar spine surgery. It is not designed to encompass candidates for other types of lumbar spine surgery such as decompressive laminectomy or fusion.

Positive Points	POSITIVE FACTORS	NEGATIVE FACTORS	Negative Points
5	1. Low back and sciatic pain severe enough to be incapacitating.	1. **Back pain primarily**	15
15	2. Sciatica is more severe than back pain.	2. **Gross obesity**	10
5	3. Weight bearing (sitting or standing) aggravates the pain; bedrest (in some position) eases the pain.	3. **Nonorganic signs and symptoms**—entire leg numb; simultaneous weakness of flexion and extension of toes; extension of pain into areas not explainable by an organic lesion.	10
25	4. Neurologic examination demonstrates a single root syndrome indicating a specific interspace.	4. **Poor psychologic background**—attempted suicide, unrealistically high expectations from surgery; previous admissions for nonorganic symptoms—hyperventilation—unexplainable chest pains and abdominal pains—intractable incisional pain; alcoholic; not happy with job; physical demands of present occupation excessive; hostility to environment–employer–spouse; much time off from work for medical reasons (man out of work 6 months—woman out of work 16 months).	15
25	5. MRI scan defect corroborating the neurologic examination		
10	6. Positive straight-leg-raising test.		
20	Crossed-straight-leg-raising test.		
10	7. Patient's realistic self-appraisal of future life style.		
		5. **Secondary gain**—work-connected accident; vehicular accident; medico-legal adversary situation; near retirement age—eligible for disability pension if symptoms persist.	20
		6. **History of previous lawsuits** for medico-legal problems.	10

Positive Total ☐

Negative Total ☐

Subtract negative total from positive total ☐ for predictive number.

SCORING
75 & over . . . . good
65—75 . . . . fair
55—65 . . . . marginal
below 55 . . . . poor

FIGURE 153–3. A sample Lumbar Disc Surgery Predictive Score Card.

there are surgeons. All medical judgments relating to therapy are made by assigning positive and negative relative values to various aspects of the clinical picture, and the final decision is made by mentally balancing out these relative values. A numerical value system is not commonly used, but such a system may allow surgeons to communicate more easily about this complex problem.

A review of the various clinical factors that play a role in surgical decision making was carried out in 200 postsurgical patients who had a good result and were compared with 96 postsurgical patients who had a poor result.[1] This clinical review was employed as a base on which to list the major positive and negative factors involved in preoperative selection and to assign these factors positive and negative numerical values. Employment of such a system provides a "predictive number" indicating the likely outcome of surgery. In an effort to make the system usable by almost all physicians involved in lumbar disc surgery, only criteria that have broad acceptance and that are generally employed were included. Studies that have less widespread use, such as electromyography, discography, lumbar venography, and special psychological studies, were purposely excluded. The result of this study was a Lumbar Disc Surgery Predictive Score Card (Fig. 153-3).

POSITIVE SCORE CARD FACTORS

The positive predictive score card lists seven positive factors with a total of 115 possible points.

FACTOR 1. The key word is incapacitating. If pain is not severe enough to hamper activities of daily living, the patient often is likely to be unsatisfied with the results of surgery.

FACTOR 2. Excision of a herniated lumbar disc usually relieves nerve root pain. If sciatica is not the major symptom and surgery provides relief of sciatica but no improvement of the back pain, the unhappy patient may well ignore the disappearance of the minor sciatica and concentrate on the persisting predominant back pain.

FACTOR 3. Body position should affect a lumbar disc syndrome if it is indeed a mechanical problem. Sciatic syndromes that are unaffected by changes in body position are often nonmechanical in nature and are not alleviated by the mechanical removal of pressure.

FACTOR 4. A neurologic examination that demonstrates a single root syndrome indicating a specific interspace obviously increases the possibility of a successful outcome.

FACTOR 5. The MRI scan defect must corroborate the results of the neurologic examination. Various reports indicate abnormal lumbar myelographic results in (low back) symptom-free patients in percentages varying from 25 to 30 percent.

FACTOR 6. The straight-leg-raising test is a good predictive factor. The crossed-straight-leg-raising test (the nonpainful leg is raised, which produces aggravation of pain radiating into the painful leg) is twice as effective (Fig. 153-4).

FACTOR 7. The patient's realistic appraisal of future life style is an important factor that easily may be ignored by the surgeon. The only way to appreciate the patient's postoperative expectations is to spend some time listening to the patient.

NEGATIVE SCORE CARD FACTORS

The negative score card lists six negative factors with a total of 80 possible points.

FACTOR 1. Back pain primarily is the reverse of positive factor 2.

FACTOR 2. Although grossly obese people initially seem to do about the same as those patients with a more normal habitus, after 1 or 2 years the recurrence rate is somewhat higher.

FACTOR 3. Simultaneous weakness in flexion and extension of the great toe cannot be explained by pressure on a single root, and unless some neurologic explanation can be offered for this finding, it should be considered nonorganic.

FACTOR 4. Poor psychological background is an ambiguous label, but any of these factors should cause the surgeon to be cautious. The alcoholic, for example, may have demonstrated a very steady work history in the past and may never have been hospitalized previously. However, alcoholics arise every morning and set about their tasks only with great effort and difficulty. Any break in their routine may produce a behavior reversal.

FACTOR 5, secondary gain, and **FACTOR 6,** history of lawsuits, are self-explanatory.

By adding the positive scores and adding the negative scores and subtracting the negative total from the positive total, the surgeon can derive a predictive number and compare it against the scoring table (see Fig. 153-3) to determine the likely outcome of disc surgery.

PREDICTIVE FACTORS

The four most important factors in determining a satisfactory outcome for surgery are
1. Sciatic pain more severe than the back pain
2. An abnormal MRI scan that correlates with the clinical picture
3. Positive Leségue sign
4. Neurologic deficit

The crossed Leségue sign is probably the most specific test for lumbar disc herniation. If all four of these factors are present, technically adequate surgery is likely to produce a satisfactory result. If one of them is absent, the surgeon should be very satisfied with the accuracy of the other three factors before proceeding. Surgery considered when only one or two of these factors are present is likely to be associated

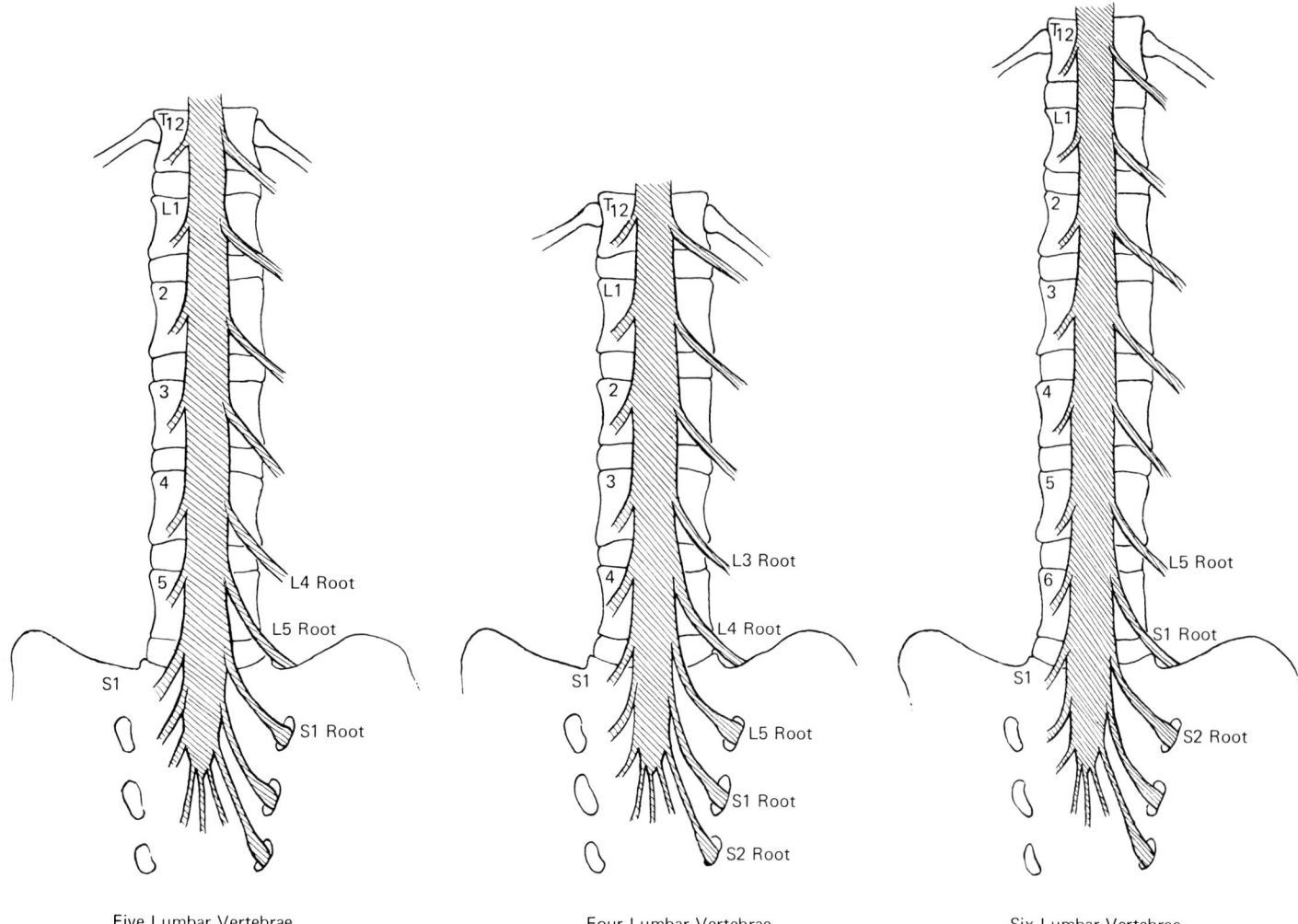

FIGURE 153-2. Transitional lumbosacral vertebral and root function. (Reprinted from Finneson BE: Low Back Pain, 2nd ed. Philadelphia, J.B. Lippincott, 1981. With permission.)

3. Temporal changes. As the patient grows older, degenerative changes within the discs occur in a progressively cephalad direction. This phenomenon is well documented by discography, which demonstrates that degenerative changes usually occur first at the L5-S1 level; some years later, they advance to the L4-L5 interspace, and with advancing age, they advance progressively cephalad. For this reason, an individual over the age of 50 who has severe sciatica associated with an Achilles reflex and a narrow L5-S1 disc space could be suffering from an acute lesion at the level of L4-L5. The absent Achilles reflex may be a residual finding from a previously protruded lesion at the level of L4-L5. The absent Achilles reflex may be a residual finding from a previously protruded lesion at the level of L5-S1 that has long since fibrosed, leaving less mobility at that level, and is no longer a source of pain. The new painful disc lesion at the level of L4-L5 may not have been present long enough to establish hard neurologic findings.

RADIOLOGIC CONFIRMATORY STUDIES

CT lumbar scans, MRI scans, or lumbar myelography should be performed on all patients before lumbar disc surgery. These studies are used principally to confirm clinical localization and to determine if more than one disc herniation is present. They also help to rule out possible lumbar spinal tumors, which can very easily simulate herniated lumbar discs. At one time used mainly as a preoperative test, the noninvasive MRI and CT scans are increasingly performed on patients who have not fared well with an adequate course of conservative management and in whom significant uncertainty exists regarding the nature of their complaints. None of these studies are infallible and are associated with a significant incidence of both false-negative and false-positive results. Most false-negative results are noted at the L5-S1 level, where there is a large space between the anterior dural edge and the posterior bony spine. This space is less wide above the L5-S1 level, so the incidence of false-negative results is much lower from the level of L4-L5 upward. The incidence of false-positive results is greater in patients over the age of 55 because of the hypertrophic osteoarthritic degenerative changes associated with advancing years.

LUMBAR DISC SURGERY PREDICTIVE SCORE CARD

Any surgical judgment that is based primarily on such a subjective symptom as pain can have as many variables as

CHAPTER 153

Lumbar Disc Excision

Bernard E. Finneson

CAVEAT DISC SURGEON

The first disc operation is relatively easy. The repeat operative procedure, however, presents a problem in technique and, even more, in satisfactory outcome. The recommended solution to this problem is to avoid the first operation that is apt to lead to a less than satisfactory result and thus not create a clinical condition that requires repeat disc surgery.

PATIENT SELECTION

The most important consideration affecting the outcome of lumbar disc surgery is patient selection. What factors help predict whether or not a patient will benefit from surgery? The surgeon who can select a patient who will benefit from surgical intervention has won half the battle before the incision is made. It is perhaps even more important for the surgeon to be able to predict which individuals will not benefit from surgery. The surgeon who operates on this type of patient is handicapped before he or she starts; a satisfactory clinical result is not likely even with the finest, most meticulous surgical technique. The most that can reasonably be expected is that the patient will not be too discernibly worse after surgery. The lack of response to nonsurgical treatment is not, in itself, an indication for surgery. All too often the patient with low back pain who is not readily cured with nonsurgical management is brought to the operating room under the banner of "we must do something for this poor suffering patient." This "something" often produces new, and sometimes irreversible, surgically produced signs and symptoms, which are superimposed on the original complaints. The surgeon should remember that no matter how severe and intractable the pain is, it can always be made worse with surgery.

FALLIBILITY OF THE NEUROLOGIC EXAMINATION

Neurosurgeons, in comparison to their orthopedic colleagues, are perhaps a bit more prone to rely on neurologic examination to identify the level of disc protrusion. Of course, certain general findings, such as severe paraspinal muscle spasm in the lumbar area or poor mobility of the lumbar spine, are common to most disc syndromes at any level and are not considered of localizing value. The classic findings of a diminished or absent Achilles reflex and numbness along the lateral aspect of the foot in the presence of sciatic pain generally is accepted as representing an L5-S1 disc protrusion. If the lumbar spine films demonstrate a narrow disc space at the level of L5-S1, some disc surgeons might forego a magnetic resonance imaging (MRI) or computed tomography (CT) scan and proceed with surgery. In most cases, they would be right, and a surgically treatable lesion would be found at the L5-S1 level. Three factors can be responsible for neurologic changes, however, that may mislead the surgeon as to the involved interspace.

1. Location of the disc protrusion (Fig. 153–1). The disc fragment may extrude laterally into the foramen so that it compresses the exiting root from the interspace above. Such a laterally located fragment at the L5-S1 foramen may produce an L4-L5 syndrome.

2. Neuroanatomic changes (Fig. 153–2). A partially lumbarized first sacral segment, which may be dismissed as being of no clinical significance, might be associated with a postfixed plexus. In such a situation, an L5-S1 disc protrusion may produce weakness of the great toe and numbness over the dorsum of the foot within the L5 dermatome and might be identified as a L4-L5 protrusion at the level of L4-L5 on the basis of the neurologic examination.

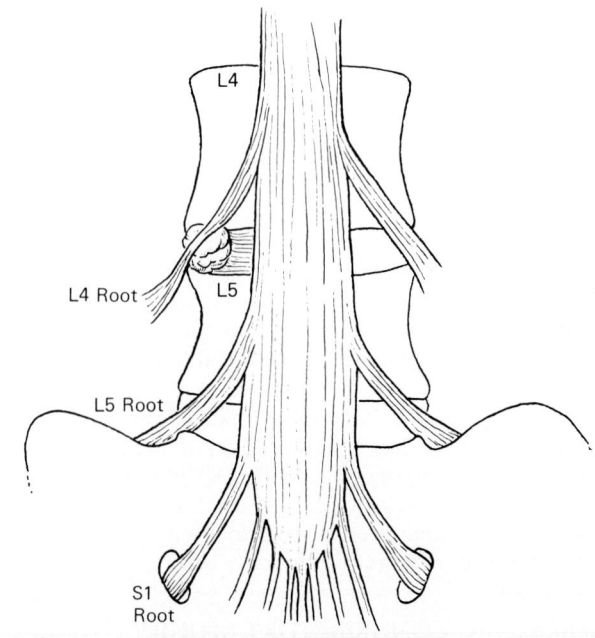

FIGURE 153–1. Foraminal root compressive syndrome. The laterally situated L4-L5 disc protrusion will extend into the intervertebral foramen impinging upon the L4 root and simulate an L3-L4 syndrome. (Reprinted from Finneson BE: Low Back Pain, 2nd ed. Philadelphia, J.B. Lippincott, 1981. With permission.)

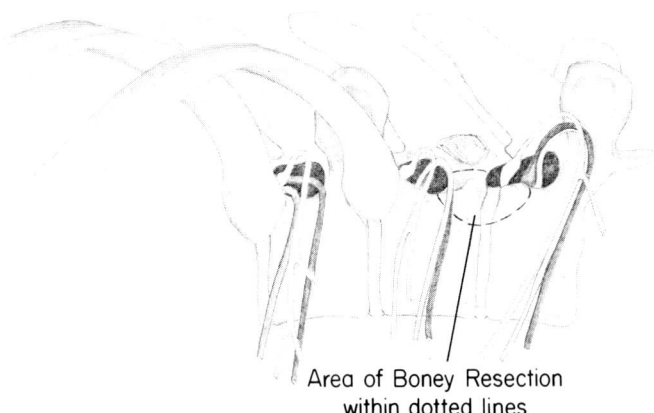

FIGURE 152–18. Area of Boney Resection within dotted lines

paraplegia is in the past, as are the days when the surgeon would take a vacation and pass a patient with a thoracic disc to a colleague!

REFERENCES

1. Awwad EE, Margin DS, Smith KR, Baker BK: Asymptomatic versus symptomatic herniated thoracic discs: Their frequency and characteristics as detected by computed tomography after myelography. Neurosurgery 28(2):180–186, 1991
2. Williams MP, Cherryman GR, Husband JE: Significance of thoracic disc herniation demonstrated by MR imaging. J Comput Assist Tomogr 13(2):211–214, 1989
3. Stillerman CB, Weiss MH: Management of thoracic disc disease. Clin Neurosurg 38:325–352, 1992
4. El-Kalliny M, Tew JM Jr, van Loveren H, Dunsker S: Surgical approaches to thoracic disc herniations. Acta Neurochir (Wien) 111:22–32, 1991
5. Brown CW, Deffer PA, Akmakjian J, et al: The natural history of disc herniation. Spine 17 (6 suppl):S97–102, 1992
6. Sundaresan N, Shah J, Feghali JG: A trans-sternal approach to the upper thoracic vertebrae. J Neurosurg 61:686–690, 1984
7. Kumar R, Buckley TF: First thoracic disc protrusion. Spine 11(5):499–501, 1986
8. Kumar R, Cowie RAC: Second thoracic disc protrusion. Spine 17:120–121, 1992
9. Simeone FA, Rashbaum R: Transthoracic disc excision, in Schmidek HH, Sweet WH (eds): Operative Neurosurgical Techniques, 2nd ed. New York, Grune & Stratton, 1987, pp 1367–1374
10. Patterson RH, Arbit E: A surgical approach through the pedicle to protruded thoracic discs. J Neurosurg 48:768–772, 1978
11. Carson J, Gumpert J, Jefferson A: Diagnosis and treatment of thoracic intervertebral disc protrusions. J Neurol Neurosurg Psychiatry 34:68–77, 1971
12. Hulme A: The surgical approach to thoracic intervertebral disc protrusions. J Neurol Neurosurg Psychiatry 23:133–137, 1960
13. Capener N: The evolution of lateral rhachotomy. J Bone Joint Surg Br 36B:173–179, 1954
14. Larson SJ, Holst RA, Hemmy DC, et al: Lateral extracavitary approach to traumatic lesions of the thoracic and lumbar spine. J Neurosurg 45:628–637, 1976
15. Maiman DJ, Larson SH, Luck E, El-Ghatit A: Lateral extra-cavitary approach to the spine for thoracic disc herniation: Report of 23 cases. Neurosurgery 14:178–182, 1984
16. Otani K, Manzoku S, Shibasaki K, Nomachi S: The surgical treatment of thoracic and thoracolumbar disc lesions using the anterior approach. Spine 2(4):266–275, 1977
17. Otani K, Nakai S, Fujimura Y, et al: Surgical treatment of thoracic disc herniation using the anterior approach. J Bone Joint Surg Br 64B:340–343, 1882
18. Denis F: The three column spine and its significance in the classification of acute thoracolumbar spinal injuries. Spine 8(8):817–831, 1983
19. Crafoord C, Hiertonn T, Lindblom K, Olsson SE: Spinal cord compression caused by a protruded thoracic disc. Report of a case treated with antero-lateral fenestration of the disc. Acta Orthop Scand 28:103–107, 1958
20. Perot P, Munro DD: Transthoracic removal of midline thoracic disc protrusions causing spinal cord compression. J Neurosurg 31:452–458, 1969
21. Ransohoff J, Spencer F, Siew F, Gage L: Transthoracic disc protrusions causing spinal cord compression. J Neurosurg 31:459–461, 1969

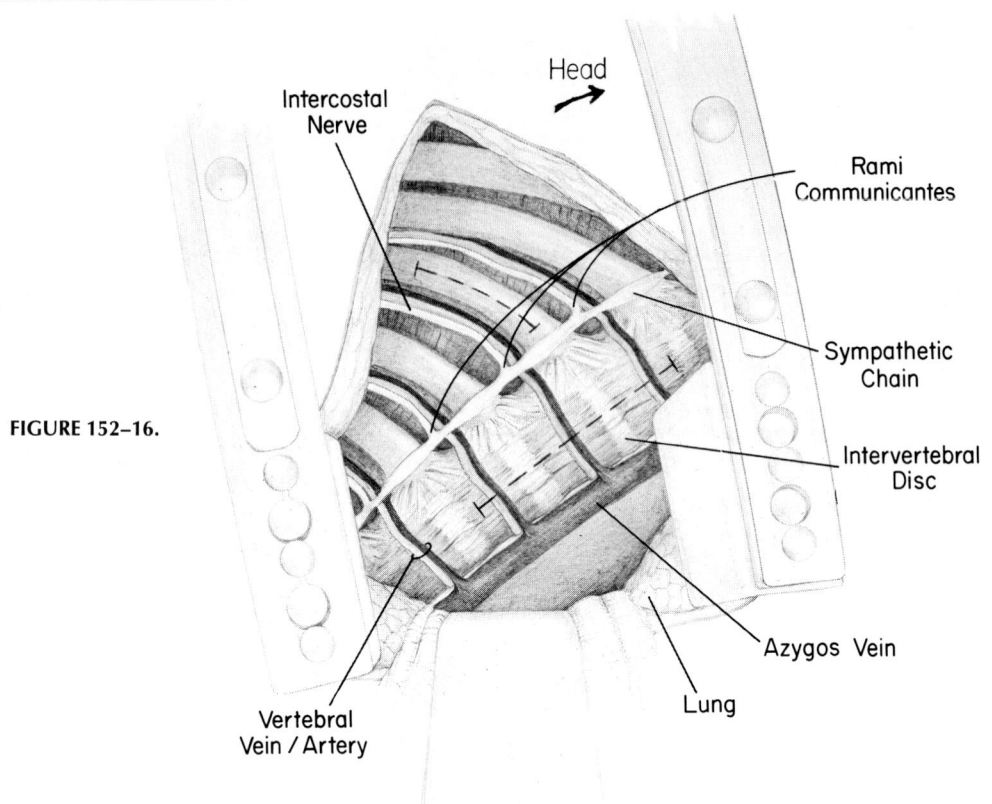

FIGURE 152–16.

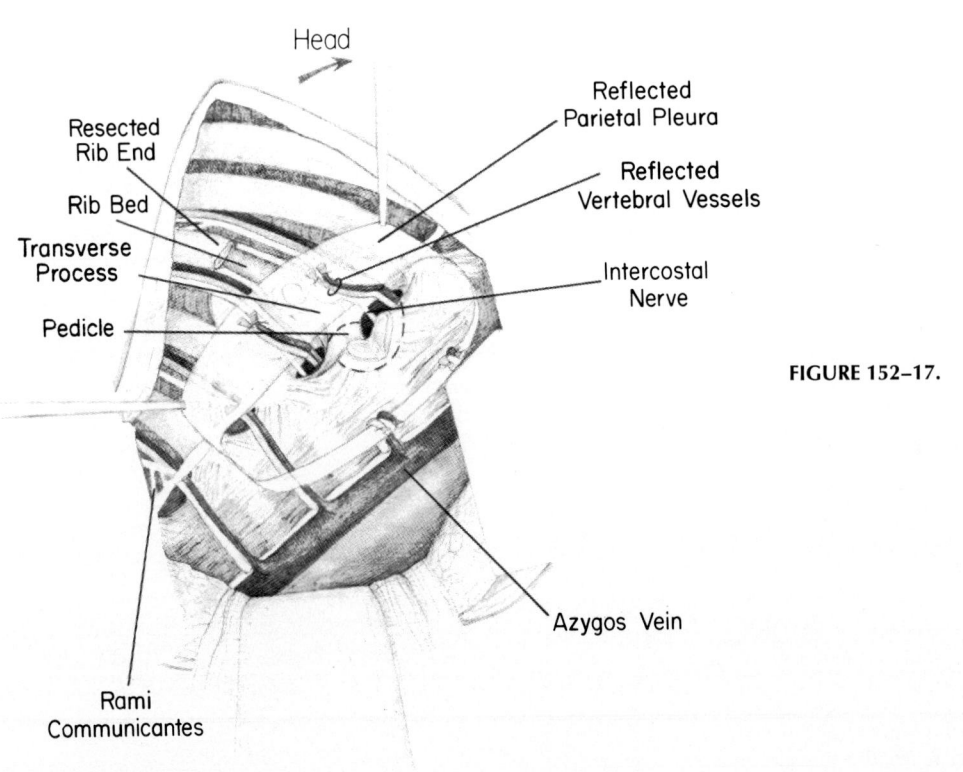

FIGURE 152–17.

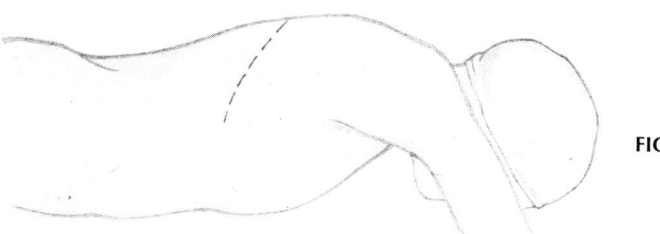

FIGURE 152–14.

The operative site is thoroughly irrigated, and the chest wound is closed in layers in a routine fashion after the lungs are inflated. The extrapleural space is drained by use of a closed suction drainage. A thoracotomy drain is usually not required unless a large pleural tear has occurred. Because the anterior and posterior columns remain intact, the middle column has been removed in part, and the spine is stable, fusion and bone grafting are usually not required.[18] However, if more bone has been removed from the vertebral body, as may be necessary when this approach is used for indications other than disc herniation, rib struts may be impacted into place. After fusion, a thoracolumbar molded brace is required for about 12 weeks. A postoperative chest x-ray study is performed to observe for evidence of pneumothorax and, if present, is followed by serial x-ray studies until resolution. Early ambulation and incentive spirometry are encouraged.

TRANSTHORACIC TRANSPLEURAL DISC EXCISION

In 1958, Crafoord and associates[19] performed anterolateral fenestration but did not excise the intraspinal herniated thoracic disc. In 1969, Perot and Munro[20] and Ransohoff and colleagues[21] described excision of thoracic disc by the transpleural approach. The patient's pulmonary evaluation must be complete before surgery because single lung ventilation will be required during the operation. Potential postoperative pulmonary complications are also greater with this approach.

The patient is intubated with a Carlens tube. A standard right thoracotomy incision is made, to avoid the artery of Adamkiewicz (as noted earlier) (Figs. 152–14 and 152–15). In young patients, entry into the thoracic cavity is through the costal interspace because the ribs are sufficiently mobile, and the rib spreaders maintain the exposure. In older patients, rib resection is required. The rib to be removed is one or two levels superior to the disc to be excised. An x-ray study is performed at this stage to identify the correct interspace. For the T8-T9 disc, the parietal pleura is reflected off T8 and T9 vertebral bodies and the head of the T9 rib (Fig. 152–16). The segmental artery and vein are ligated and divided. The T9 rib head is removed (Fig. 152–17). With the aid of an operating microscope and a high-speed drill, the pedicle of the T9 vertebra and adjacent parts of the bodies of T8 and T9 vertebral bodies are excised to expose the dura. The posterior half of the intervertebral disc is removed (Fig. 152–18). The herniated disc is then dislodged anteriorly and removed. The epidural veins are coagulated, as noted earlier. The posterior longitudinal ligament is incised to explore the epidural space and remove any sequestrated disc fragment. As the anterior and posterior columns remain intact, fusion is rarely indicated.

Closure is performed by suture of the parietal pleura over the vertebral bodies. An apical dependent chest drain is inserted through a separate stab incision. The thoracotomy is closed in a routine fashion.

Pulmonary complications are the commonest and result from atelectasis, contusion, and pneumonia. A chest drain is required for 2 to 3 days, and pneumothorax usually clears by this time. Hemothorax, however, necessitates re-exploration. Chronic pleural effusion, bronchopleural fistula, and empyema are rare.

SUMMARY

Various operative approaches to herniated thoracic discs allow decompression to be performed safely by choosing the correct route and taking care to provide bony decompression before introducing any instrument in the tight spinal canal. If an approach that allows good visualization is chosen, blind dissection is avoided, and meticulous hemostasis is achieved with bipolar cautery, without need for packing with hemostatic agents. It is hoped that the great fear of postoperative

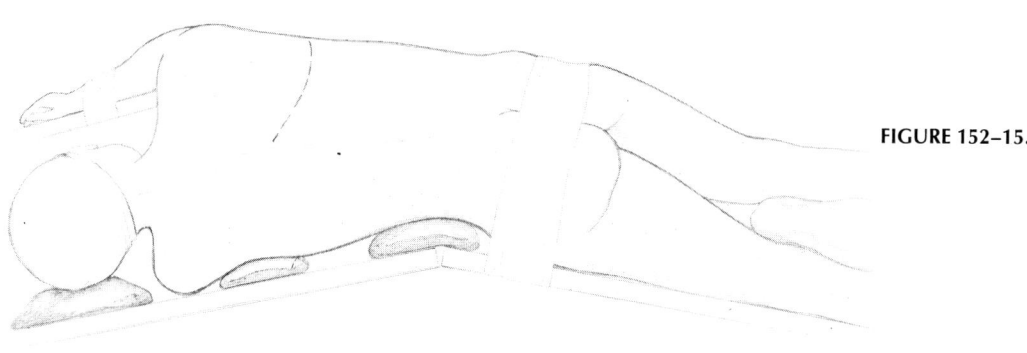

FIGURE 152–15.

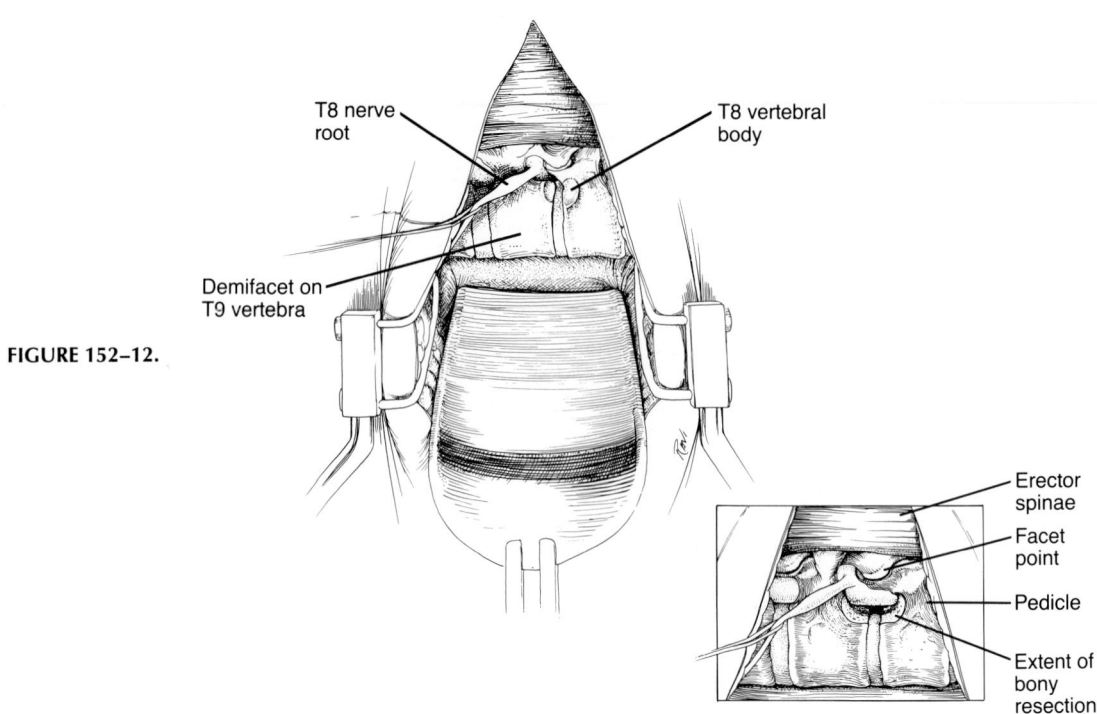

FIGURE 152–12.

leads to the pathologic T8-T9 disc between the T8 and T9 pedicles. The nerve may be gently retracted superiorly by a rubber band.

By blunt dissection, the parietal pleura, which is thicker in the posterior than in the anterior half of the thorax, is separated from the ribs above and below and from the spinal column. Damage to the thoracic duct and lymphatics near the left side of the spine occasionally lead to a chyle fistula. This problem may be prevented by use of bipolar coagulation before section of suspicious-looking "bands," which may be large lymphatic trunks. A self-retaining Balfour retractor is set up, and a third malleable blade is used to retract the pleura previously covered with a lap sponge (Fig. 152–12). Approach to the T12-L1 space is achieved by resection of the twelfth rib, and by blunt extrapleural dissection, the crux of the diaphragm is identified. This structure is detached from its vertebral attachment, thereby exposing T12-L1 level. Division of the diaphragm is thus avoided.

At this time, the surgeon changes position and stands in front of the patient. This new position provides better visualization of the anterior aspect of the spinal canal. The operating microscope is now brought in. With a high-speed air drill, the superior part of the T9 pedicle is drilled off. The bony dissection is continued into the posterior 1 cm of the vertebral body adjacent to the disc, and a thin shell of the posterior cortex is kept intact to avoid epidural venous bleeding at this stage. We remove the posterior one third or one half of the disc and the posterior one third of the vertebral body adjacent to the disc, but at this stage, we leave the posterior longitudinal ligament intact. The depth of bony dissection across the vertebral body is estimated from axial CT or MRI and is the distance from the outer aspect of the vertebral body at the pedicle level to the inner limit of the spinal canal on the far side (Fig. 152–13). Thus, adequate room is created to allow inspection of the anterior face of the spinal canal. The thin, bony shell of the posterior cortex is

dislodged anteriorly into the defect so created. Troublesome bleeding from the anterior epidural veins is prevented by coagulation with bipolar cautery. One lip of the forceps is placed in the epidural space, and the other is placed anterior to the posterior longitudinal ligament. The posterior longitudinal ligament is then incised and displaced anteriorly, both above and below the herniated disc. Packing is avoided, but a thin layer of Surgicel and thrombin spray may be required to control persistent venous bleeding. The herniated disc can now be dislodged anteriorly and removed. The epidural sequestrated fragments, if any, are then removed, and the decompression is completed.

In rare instances of intradural disc rupture, the dura may be opened anterior to the nerve root, and intradural disc fragments may be removed. Interrupted closure of the dura is performed. Postoperative closed spinal drainage is then instituted for 1 to 2 days.

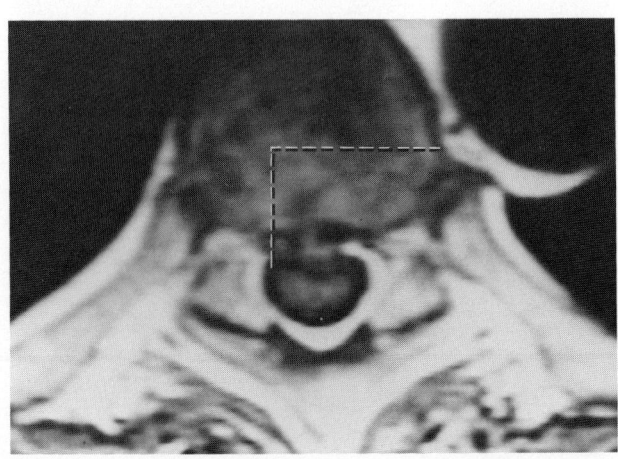

FIGURE 152–13.

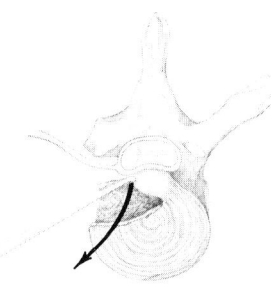

Direction of removal

FIGURE 152-9.

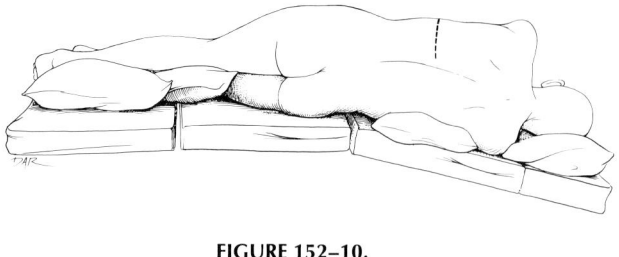

FIGURE 152-10.

described by Capener[13] in 1954, who called it "lateral rachotomy." Larson and coworkers,[14] in 1976, described a similar approach for traumatic lesions of the thoracic and lumbar spine and termed it the *lateral extracavitary approach*. This posterolateral approach provides a view better than that afforded by costotransversectomy. However, to visualize the anterior aspect of the spinal canal, a mirror is required (Larson SJ: Personal communication). The nerve root overlying the disc may need to be sectioned to allow greater room for adequate decompression. Because this is also a posterolateral approach, intradural exploration is not possible.

The procedure is similar to that of the costotransversectomy approach. The skin incision is along the rib to be resected, but rib resection is undertaken more laterally, up to the posterior axillary line. After disc excision, anterior interbody fusion is performed with rib grafts. Postoperatively, a bivalve body jacket is worn for 8 to 10 weeks.[15]

ANTEROLATERAL EXTRAPLEURAL DISC EXCISION

The anterolateral extrapleural approach provides direct visualization of the entire anterior aspect of the spinal canal and dura without the morbidity of a transpleural approach. It also avoids the disadvantages of the extracavitary approach noted earlier. In particular, fusion is rarely required, unlike in the description by Otani and associates,[16, 17] who routinely perform interbody fusion.

The operation is performed with the patient under general anesthesia and intubated with a Carlens tube, so that each lung may be intubated separately, if required. The procedure is usually accomplished without entrance into the plural cavity. Even with a tear in the parietal pleura, single lung deflation is rarely required. The patient is placed in the lateral position, the side facing up being dictated by the pathology. The artery of Adamkiewicz, which enters on the left side in 80 percent of cases, is a concern, but we believe we should have access to the side of greater cord compression. An axillary roll is placed, and the patient is positioned over the table break or kidney rest to laterally flex the patient for increased exposure.

The surgeon initially stands behind the patient's back. The skin incision used is similar to that used for a posterior thoracotomy but is less oblique. It begins from 1 inch lateral to the midline and extends over the T8 rib (Fig. 152-10). The skin incision is cephalad to the rib to be resected, so that the skin does not hang over the exposure; the skin can be easily slid down to remove the T9 rib. Each rib head straddles the disc space and bears the number of the vertebral body at its lower limit, except the twelfth rib, which articulates only with the body of the T12 vertebra. Hence, to approach the T8-T9 level, the surgeon should resect approximately 20 cm of the posterior part of the T9 rib. At the T11-T12 interspace, the angulation of the twelfth rib often makes access to the interspace more difficult. At this level, if a markedly angled twelfth rib is followed to the intervertebral disc, the surgeon will be trying to look into the interspace from an inferior position or over the unresected eleventh rib. In patients with markedly angled ribs, this practice can be avoided by resection of the eleventh rib and the head of the twelfth rib or by resection of the eleventh and twelfth ribs.

The skin incision is then deepened through the subcutaneous tissues, latissimus dorsi, and serratus anterior muscles and is retracted with self-retaining retractors. The fascia immediately lateral to the erector spinae is divided along its length, and the muscle is dissected off the rib anterior to it, with the dissection proceeding medially to the transverse process. The erector spinae is retracted medially, and if necessary, its lateral part is cut to expose the transverse process. The periosteum over the rib is incised along its exposed length with cautery, stripped off the rib with Alexander and Doyen elevators, and transected laterally. Medially, sharp dissection is required to section the capsular and costotransverse ligaments to disarticulate the rib head, and occasionally, the transverse process may need to be resected to accomplish this. The neurovascular bundle associated with the rib leads to the space one level below the area of interest (Fig. 152-11). In this instance, the neurovascular bundle at the lower border of the T9 rib leads under the T9 pedicle to T9-T10 disc. The T8 neurovascular bundle under the T8 rib is identified and followed medially. The T8 intercostal nerve

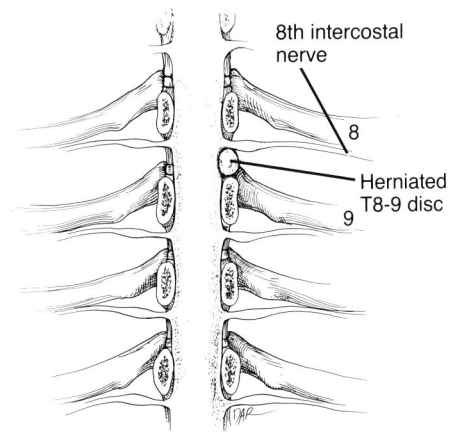

FIGURE 152-11.

Surgical Management of Thoracic Disc Herniations | **1899**

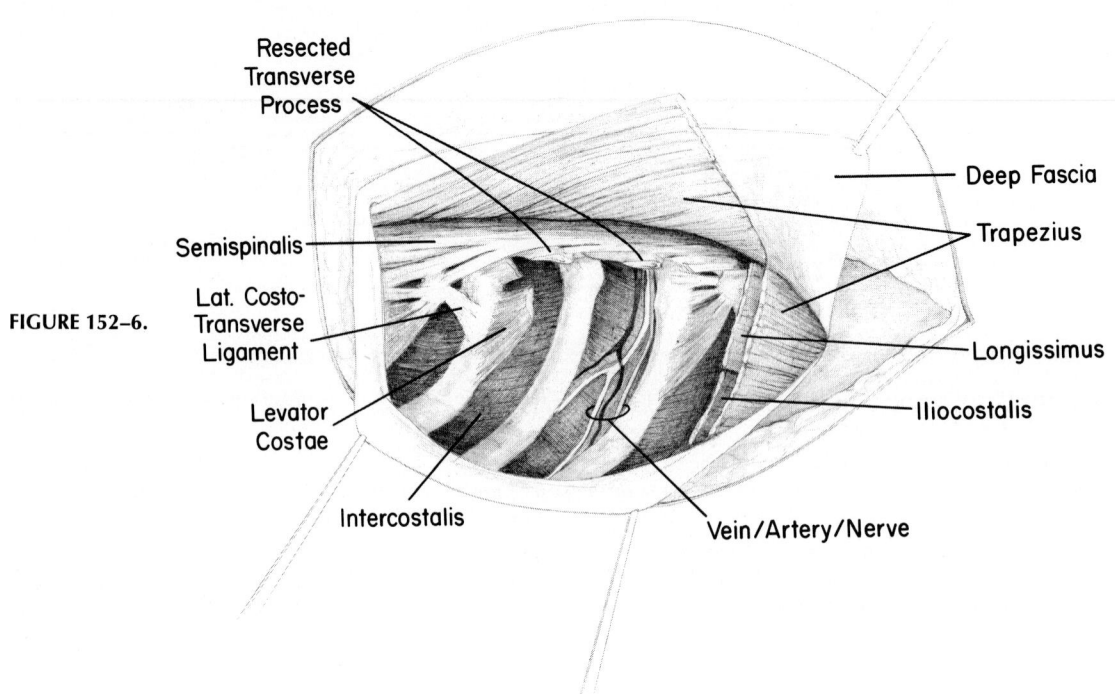

FIGURE 152–6.

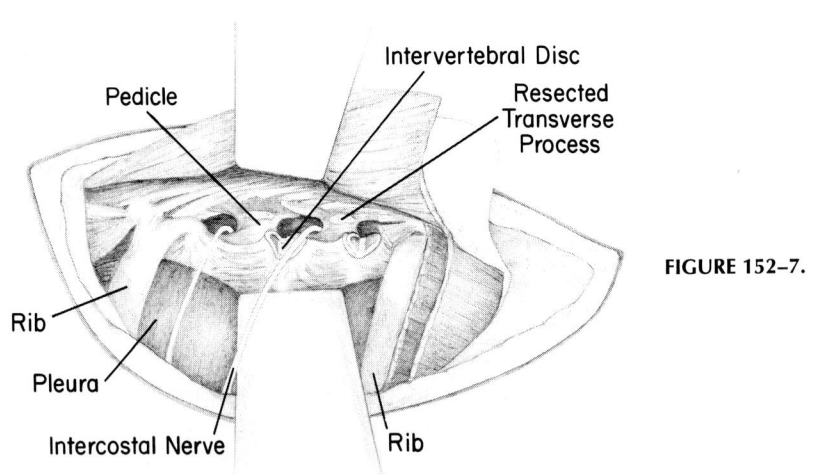

FIGURE 152–7.

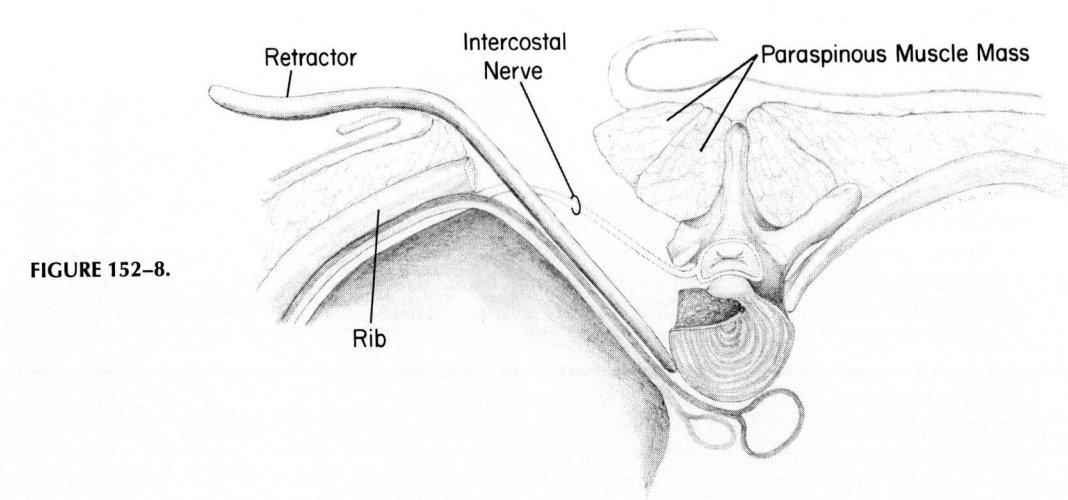

FIGURE 152–8.

tus position. A midline incision is made centered over the disc space of interest. The deep fascia is incised along the entire length in the midline. Dissection is performed on the affected side only, and the erector spine muscle is dissected subperiosteally and retracted laterally to the lateral aspect of the facet joints. The pedicle inferior to the disc, the T9 pedicle, is identified. We prefer to use the operating microscope and a high-speed air drill. The superior half of the T9 pedicle and the T8-T9 facet superior to it are drilled (Fig. 152–4A and B). The lateral parts of the T8 and T9 laminae are also drilled to expose the lateral limit of the theca and the T8 nerve root. The laterally herniated disc is removed and the disc space entered lateral to the theca. The disc space is then cleared of its contents. Only after a cavity has been created in the disc space can ventrally herniated disc material be dislodged into this space and removed. Hemostasis from epidural veins is achieved with bipolar cautery and/or Surgicel and thrombin spray.

COSTOTRANSVERSECTOMY AND DISC EXCISION

Costotransversectomy and disc excision for the removal of a herniated thoracic disc was first used by Hulme[2] in 1960, with good results. The patient is placed in the lateral oblique position (Fig. 152–5), the side facing up being dictated by the lesion. The surgeon stands in front of the patient.

After confirmation of the level by x-ray study, a long curved incision is made that extends up to the posterior axillary line and spans three levels above and below the herniated disc. The skin is reflected medially in one layer with the deep fascia and the trapezius muscle (Fig. 152–6). The erector spinae is dissected off the posterior aspect of the ribs until the transverse processes are seen and reflected medially. The lateral part of this muscle may be divided, if required, to improve the exposure. To approach the T8-T9 disc, the transverse process of T9 is removed with a rongeur. Subperiosteal resection of the T9 rib, laterally to the limit of the exposure and medially by disarticulation of the rib head, is performed. The parietal pleura is separated from one rib above and below and from the lateral aspect of the spinal column and is held by a malleable blade. The T8 nerve, in the neurovascular bundle one level superior to the resected

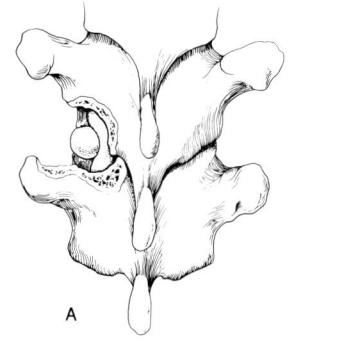
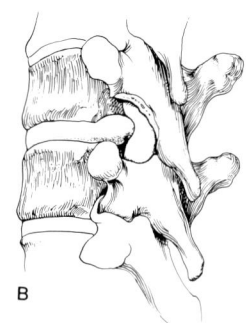

FIGURE 152–4.

rib, is identified and traced medially to the intervertebral foramen (Fig. 152–7).

By use of the operating microscope and a high-speed drill, the T9 pedicle is drilled off, thereby exposing the lateral aspect of the dura and the herniated disc. The epidural veins are coagulated, and the laterally herniated disc is removed. The posterior half or posterior third of the disc space on the exposed side is cleared, starting laterally (Fig. 152–8). Ventrally herniated disc may then be dislodged into the cavity that has been created in the intervertebral space and may then removed (Fig. 152–9). A dissector is used to palpate the posterior longitudinal ligament for retained or sequestrated fragments. Because this is a posterolateral approach, intradural exploration is not possible.

Closure is performed after inspection of the pleura for tears through positive-pressure ventilation. A chest drain is not required in most instances. The tissues are reconstituted in layers, and a closed suction drain is left in the surgical bed for about 24 hours.

LATERAL EXTRACAVITARY APPROACH AND DISC EXCISION

The lateral extracavitary approach and disc excision, also called the posterolateral extrapleural approach, is a modification of the costotransversectomy approach and was first

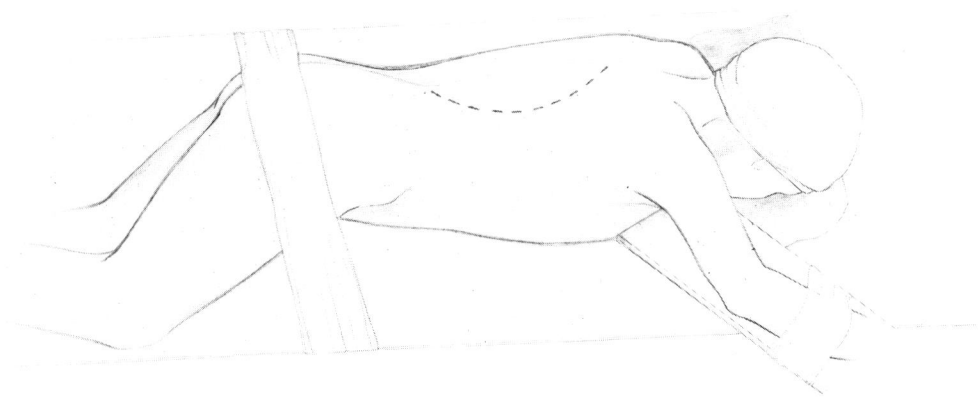

FIGURE 152–5.

plications and greater morbidity of this approach make this route unattractive. Access by the posterior route, akin to cervical laminectomy, foraminotomy, (see Chapter 146) and removal of the herniated disc fragment from the front of the nerve root, has provided good results.[7, 8]

The approach to the herniated disc is determined by evaluation of the laterality of the herniation and the extent of the deformity of the spinal cord from the displaced disc. Vertical migration of the disc fragment in itself is not a consideration in the decision of which approach to use. The ability to visualize the herniated disc without retraction of the already deformed spinal cord is the key issue. Even a small amount of additional deformation, caused by retraction of the cord that is already compromised, may lead to increased neurologic deficit, if not paraplegia. This is precisely why this problem is called the "most devastating of all disc lesions."[9] Figure 152–1 demonstrates the extent of the medial and dorsal view that may be achieved by the different approaches without retraction of the cord. Visualization of the anterior aspect of the spinal cord is usually determined by how far laterally the skin incision is situated (Fig. 152–2). The approaches are shown in order of increasing medial and anterior view as well as increasing morbidity of the procedure.

In cases of multiple disc herniation, when each herniated disc is situated laterally in the canal, the transpedicular route may be appropriate. The transthoracic route provides access to more than one level and is preferred in other situations.

SURGICAL TECHNIQUE

A pitfall common to all the approaches is identification of the correct level before and during surgery. On MRI, level count is often from C2 down to the level of the disc. At operation, the surgeon usually counts upward from L5 or the last rib, assuming this to be twelfth rib. This approach can cause an error. To avoid this, we perform a preoperative x-ray study of the whole spine. The number of the last visualized rib is noted and is used as a reference during surgery. Different methods of identifying the correct disc level at operation exist, but we find that affixing a paper tape with paper clips aligned in different directions to the midline of the back to be most satisfactory. An anteroposterior chest x-

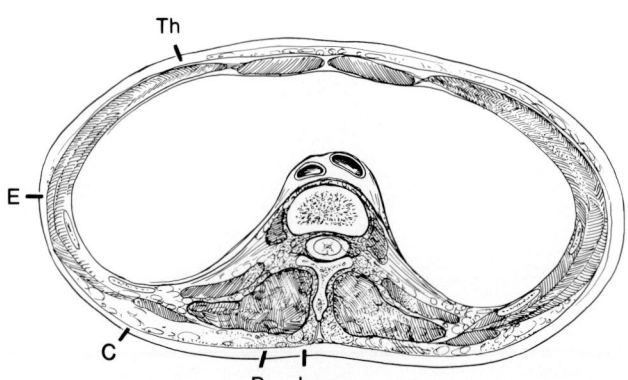

FIGURE 152–2. L=Laminectomy, P=transpedicular approach, C=costotransversectomy, E=anterolateral extrapleural approach, Th=transthoracic transpleural approach.

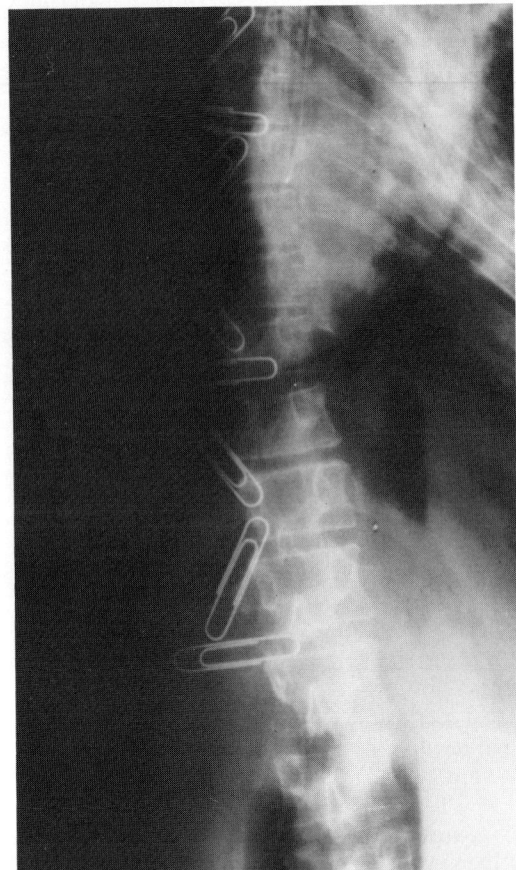

FIGURE 152–3.

ray study is performed, and the disc level is counted upward from the last visualized rib. The appropriate paper clip localizes the level on the patient (Fig. 152–3). Later, in the operation, another x-ray study is performed with a needle inserted into the pedicle or transverse process to confirm the correct level.

All operations are performed with the patient under general anesthesia. We do not use muscle relaxants, or if they have been used initially, then their effect is reversed before work begins near the spinal canal. We prefer to monitor somatosensory evoked potentials during the procedure. We use a high-speed Midas Rex air drill with a cutting burr for bony dissection. With other types of drills, a diamond burr may be needed near the dura.

In all of the following operative details, we describe the approach for the T8-T9 disc, unless otherwise specified.

TRANSPEDICULAR DISC EXCISION

Patterson and Arbit[10] first described the transpedicular approach for disc excision in 1978. This approach was a modification of the lateral gutter approach described by Carson and associates[11] in 1971. Patterson and Arbit achieve anterior disc removal and decompression of the theca before laminectomy and if indicated, anterior intradural exploration by rotation of the cord. The transpedicular approach is performed in the prone position, though some prefer the lateral decubi-

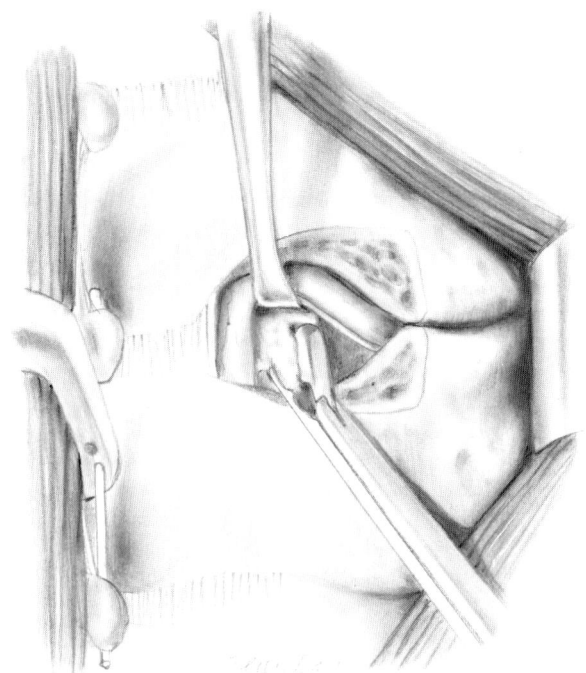

FIGURE 146-8. Fragment of disc being removed from beneath the nerve root.

made to deliver the fragments. Exploration must be thorough above, below, and medial to the root to ensure that all fragments are removed. The fragments generally are small, compared with those seen in the lumbar region. Retained fragments are the commonest cause of failure of surgery to cure the patient. The dura or cord is not retracted, and the interspace is not entered. If an osteophytic spur is encountered, a soft disc fragment should be sought because the two are often associated. We have not found chiseling off the osteophyte necessary; root and foraminal decompression alone have been adequate. Small pledgets of absorbable gelatin sponge (Gelfoam) and bipolar cautery are used to control venous bleeding.

After hemostasis is achieved in the muscles, the ligamentum nuchae, subcutaneous fascia, and skin are closed in layers with nonabsorbable sutures. Proper closure leaves an inconspicuous scar. Wound dehiscence has not been a problem. A soft cervical collar is generally applied for the immediate postoperative period but is removed on the following day, and flexion, extension, and rotation exercises are started. Most patients achieve a full range of neck motion by the time they are discharged. Dexamethasone is continued at 4 mg every 6 hours postoperatively and is then tapered over a 3- to 4-day period. We believe that this regimen contributes to a smoother, less painful postoperative course. The possibility of postoperative gastritis can be reduced by the use of a competitive inhibitor of histamine H_2 receptors, such as famotidine. Patients with a history of peptic ulcer or hiatal hernia and those receiving steroid therapy should be given famotidine or a similar drug until they are out of the hospital and are taken off of steroid therapy.[6] Prophylactic antibiotics are not continued postoperatively unless a specific reason exists to do so. Patients can begin ambulation on the evening of surgery and are discharged 24 to 48 hours after surgery. Sutures or staples are removed 5 to 7 days after surgery.

Results and Complications

The results from this procedure are gratifying. In our series of 2032 patients (Roberts and Collias: Unpublished data), 96 percent had a good-to-excellent result; approximately 4 percent obtained no benefit from the procedure. The radicular pain and root deficits may improve dramatically immediately after the procedure. Recurrences are rare, occurring only in one patient in our series. In a series of 381 cases reported by Scoville and associates[5] and included in our present series, one third of the patients returned to work or former activity within 2 weeks, and the average resumption of activity time was 4.2 weeks. Ninety-six percent of men returned to their previous job. Nineteen percent of patients with lateral disc rupture developed other cervical (8 percent) or lumbar (11 percent) disc herniations that required surgery. Other authors have also reported excellent results with this operation.[7–9] Murphey, Simmons, and Brunson[10] reported on 653 cases, with 96 percent exhibiting excellent results and all but 4 percent of the patients returning to their previous job.

The morbidity in our series was 0.2 percent, including transient increased root deficits. This complication is more apt to occur when more than one root is exposed. Wound dehiscence or infections rarely occurred. Two cases of paradoxical air emboli with severe brain damage indicate the potential risks of the sitting position. Both instances occurred in the early years of the experience, when local and regional anesthesia were used and before the advent of Doppler monitoring. With Doppler monitoring during the past 18 years, no significant complications from air emboli have occurred. The risk of paradoxical air embolism can be greatly reduced or eliminated by preoperative screening of patients by use of echocardiography to rule out potential right-to-left shunting of air through a patent foramen ovale. If a shunt is detected, the patient should be positioned prone rather than sitting.[11]

Two patients developed major postoperative neurologic deficits directly related to the surgery. In one patient, a resident plunged a periosteal elevator through the interlaminar space, causing cord injury with permanent residual Brown-Séquard syndrome. In the other patient, the deficit was secondary to cord retraction and injury when a transdural approach was added to an extradural approach for a herniated disc that extended medially. This hazardous approach for central disc herniation is no longer used; central soft disc herniations are now approached anteriorly.

The posterior approach, keyhole laminectomy and foraminotomy, provides a reliable, safe, and very effective procedure for the treatment of lateral cervical disc protrusions. Failures generally occur because of errors in diagnosis or disc fragments that are missed. If severe radiculopathy persists unchanged postoperatively, these errors should be considered, and the patient should be re-examined after a reasonable period of time.

A patient with a lateral cervical disc herniation can be told that the procedure affords him or her a 96 percent chance of improvement or cure. There is a 4 percent chance of no benefit and less than a 1 percent chance of an adverse effect. Murphey, Simmons, and Brunson[10] called the results the most gratifying of any neurosurgical procedure except perhaps those for trigeminal neuralgia.

SPONDYLOTIC MYELOPATHY

Decompressive laminectomy is commonly used to treat cervical spondylosis with spinal cord compression. Eighty-four patients operated on during a 20-year period were reviewed (Collias and Roberts: Unpublished data). This group does not include 39 cases previously reported on by Scoville and associates.[5]

INCIDENCE AND PATHOGENESIS

Cervical spondylotic myelopathy is the commonest disease of the spinal cord in middle age and later. Of 84 patients in our series, the mean age was 59 years, and the oldest patient was 84 years, and the youngest, 27 years. More than half of the patients were in the sixth and seventh decades of life. The male-to-female ratio was 1:2.

The cause of the myelopathy is a narrow cervical spinal canal that is further narrowed by a ventral osteophyte, hypertrophic facets, and a thickened, infolding ligamentum flavum. The changes result in compression of the spinal cord, with flattening in its sagittal diameter. The most commonly involved level is C5-C6, with one or more of the adjacent levels also affected. Two-level involvement is commoner than single-level involvement. Multilevel involvement also occurs, usually between C3 and C7. Congenitally blocked vertebrae occurred in 10 percent of patients in one series.[12]

The normal sagittal cervical canal diameter averages 17 mm (at a tube-to-film distance of 6 feet), and the spinal cord diameter averages 10 mm. Any sagittal diameter of the cervical canal that measures less than 12 mm can be associated with cord compression, and cord compression is certain if the cervical canal is less than 10 mm at any level. Spinal canal diameters of 13 mm or greater make spondylosis an unlikely cause of myelopathy.[13]

Although the pathogenesis of myelopathy in cervical spondylosis is imperfectly understood, it is generally accepted that both mechanical and vascular abnormalities are responsible. Flexion and extension movements cause compression and distortion of the spinal cord, creating axial tensions and hemodynamic disturbances that produce ischemic lesions. This hypothesis is supported by histologic studies that show ischemic changes in the cord.[14, 15] Structural changes of the vessels are not seen. During surgery, Allen[16] noted pallor of the spinal cord associated with spondylosis that increased with passive flexion of the neck.

Prolonged and repeated episodes of compression can lead to added effects that culminate in small areas of cord infarction. The lesions are found most prominently in the lateral columns, the ventral gray matter, and the posterior columns. Early, potentially reversible lesions may in time become fixed. The timing of decompressive surgery must take these facts into consideration. The results of decompression are apt to be better if surgery is performed early in the course of the disease.

Degenerative changes resulting in subluxations[17] and kyphotic deformities cause further injury. Kahn[18] suggested that the denticulate ligaments tether the cord against the ventral osteophytes, preventing dorsal movement and producing increased stresses on the lateral columns. He later abandoned the hypothesis. Reid's[19] studies have shown that the denticulate ligaments do not restrict dorsoventral movement of the cord but do restrict cephalocaudad movement.

CLINICAL MANIFESTATIONS

Brain, Northfield, and Wilkinson[20] aptly described the clinical symptoms and findings in this condition as protean, polymorphic, and without features that distinguish them from other neurologic disorders. The onset is generally insidious, except with acute trauma, and the course is intermittent and variably progressive. Long periods of remission can occur. Although improvement can occur, function rarely returns to normal.

Spastic weakness of the lower extremities, clonus, and Babinski's sign are the commonest manifestations. Ataxia, in part caused by involvement of the spinocerebellar tracts, is also noted. Weakness, atrophy, and clumsiness of the hands with associated stereoanesthesia can occur alone or in combination with spasticity and hyperreflexia in the lower extremities. With upper extremity involvement, distinguishing myelopathy from associated radiculopathy is difficult at times. Fasciculations are uncommon and, when present, are limited to the involved myotomes.

Neck and arm pain are uncommon except when radiculopathy is present. Lhermitte's sign may be present. Severe sensory loss is not a prominent feature. Hypalgesia may be present as a result of spinothalamic tract involvement. Posterior column dysfunction is less common than spinothalamic deficit. The bladder and bowel sphincters are usually spared but may be involved as a late manifestation and generally indicate a poor prognosis.[21] Various syndromes may be seen, including transverse cord syndrome (corticospinal, spinothalamic, and posterior column dysfunction), Brown-Séquard syndrome, and central cord syndrome, particularly after trauma.

Cervical spondylotic myelopathy is frequently confused with other neurologic disorders, including amyotrophic lateral sclerosis (ALS), multiple sclerosis, combined systems disease, spinal cord tumor, and syringomyelia. With the predominance of motor signs and symptoms occurring in cervical spondylotic myelopathy, it is not surprising that it is commonly confused with ALS. Widespread fasciculations in ALS (including the tongue) and an increased jaw jerk indicate a lesion above the cervical cord. The absence of sensory findings also provides a strong clue to the diagnosis. Cervical spondylosis should not be presumed to be responsible for symptoms attributable to lesions of the spinal cord unless it is confirmed by CT with myelography or MRI. Errors in diagnosis are common causes of the failure of surgical therapy.

DIAGNOSTIC STUDIES

Flexion, extension, and oblique-view x-ray films of the cervical spine are obtained to assess abnormalities of movement and kyphotic deformities. CT with myelography and MRI are now the definitive studies. Both produce excellent visualization of the subarachnoid space and areas of cord compression, and both permit accurate measurement of the sagittal diameter of the spinal canal. T2-weighted MRI permits detection of abnormal cord signals that may indicate underlying pathology, which might have prognostic significance for recovery of function after surgical decompression. Electromyographic studies are useful in recognizing peripheral nerve lesions and widespread fasciculations (favoring the diagnosis of ALS), and in differentiating radiculopathy from myelopathy. Spondylotic myelopathy and ALS are relatively common disorders and may coexist.

NONSURGICAL TREATMENT

Nonsurgical therapy for this disease includes neck immobilization and physical therapy. Continuation of such treatment over a long period is appropriate for elderly patients with long-standing fixed lesions and a poor surgical prognosis. It is also indicated for patients with severe medical problems in whom a major surgical procedure is contraindicated and for those who decline surgical therapy.

INDICATIONS FOR SURGERY

Decompression should be performed when there is progression in the myelopathy and documented compression of the spinal cord. Delay should be avoided because symptoms of short duration correlate positively with improved results. Age has no such correlation, and an older person with a short history of symptoms has a good chance of significant improvement.

SURGICAL CONSIDERATIONS

Two general approaches are used in the surgical treatment of cervical myelopathy. The posterior operative procedure commonly employed to decompress the spinal cord consists of laminectomy with or without foraminotomy. Partial removal of anterior bony ridges through a posterolateral approach is used by some surgeons. The anterior procedure consists of discectomy and fusion or corpectomy and strut graft fusion. Both approaches may give satisfactory results in the restoration of neurologic function or the arrest of the progression of the disease. In most instances, statistics do not favor one approach over the other.

Many surgeons use the anterior approach only in patients with one- or two-level involvement when no diffuse narrowing of the spinal canal exists.[12, 21-24] Kyphotic angulation or major subluxations require the decompression and stabilization afforded by the anterior approach.

The posterior approach has wide application and can be used for single-level involvement as well as for multilevel involvement. It permits decompression of the extremes of the cervical spine, which are out of reach through an anterior approach. It is the preferred approach if intradural exploration might be necessary or if the diagnosis is in doubt. It is the procedure of choice in congenital spinal narrowing associated with myelopathy.

Combined procedures may be necessary at times. The anterior approach may be required if the result of posterior decompression is not satisfactory and significant anterior compression persists. Instability, kyphosis, and swan neck deformity after a posterior operation with coexisting regression in neurologic function may require anterior stabilization.

Posterior Approaches

The aim of decompressive laminectomy is to enlarge the spinal canal by removal of posterior compressing elements, thereby allowing the dural tube and spinal cord to migrate posteriorly away from the compressing ventral osteophytes. It also relieves posterior compression caused by infolding and hypertrophy of the ligamentum flavum.

Since Horsley's successful case, reported by Taylor and Collier,[25] decompressive laminectomy has been used to treat spinal cord compression caused by ventral osteophytes. Limited laminectomies gave results that were no better than those obtained with nonsurgical treatment.[26-29] Total first cervical to first dorsal laminectomy[30] or extensive laminectomy[31-36] improved results. Some surgeons include intradural section of the denticulate ligaments[31, 37, 38] to further untether the cord.[18] Reid,[19] however, has shown that contact between the cord and ventral protrusions is not reduced when the denticulate ligaments are sectioned and that these specific structures do not restrict the dorsoventral movement of the cord. Piepgras,[39] in a study of two comparable groups of patients with and without denticulate ligament section, found no difference in surgical results or neurologic recovery. However, there is an increased risk of damage to the cord and a slightly higher morbidity associated with opening the dura. Some surgeons[32-36, 40-42] combine laminectomy with foraminotomy and facetectomy bilaterally at as many as three levels to decompress the nerve roots. They are convinced that results of this procedure are superior and suggest that freeing the roots enables the cord to move posteriorly. No substantial evidence exists to indicate that decompression of the nerve roots involved with epidural fibrosis associated with spondylosis and osteophytic spurs untethers the cord. Reid[19] found no evidence that the roots tethered the cord anteriorly. Epstein and Janin[36] have added a "global decompression" by curetting the lateral portions of the ventral bar after carrying out foraminotomy at involved levels. Most surgeons are hesitant to remove ventral bars through a posterolateral extradural approach for fear of cord damage.

We have found that laminectomy extending above and below the areas of maximum involvement and carried out widely to expose the posterolateral aspects of the dural sac has been effective. The dura is not opened, and only the medial portion of the facet is removed. Foraminotomies are carried out only if radiculopathy is present.

Surgical Procedure

The spinal cord in this disease is highly vulnerable and requires protection. Extreme flexion or extension during intubation for general anesthesia can cause irreparable ischemic cord damage. Determining the limits of neck motion before induction of anesthesia and not exceeding them is most important.

During positioning of the patient, the head and neck should be supported manually in the neutral position to avoid flexion or extension and cord damage. The surgeon must be present during intubation and positioning. Ischemic cord damage can result from hypotension. Experimental work

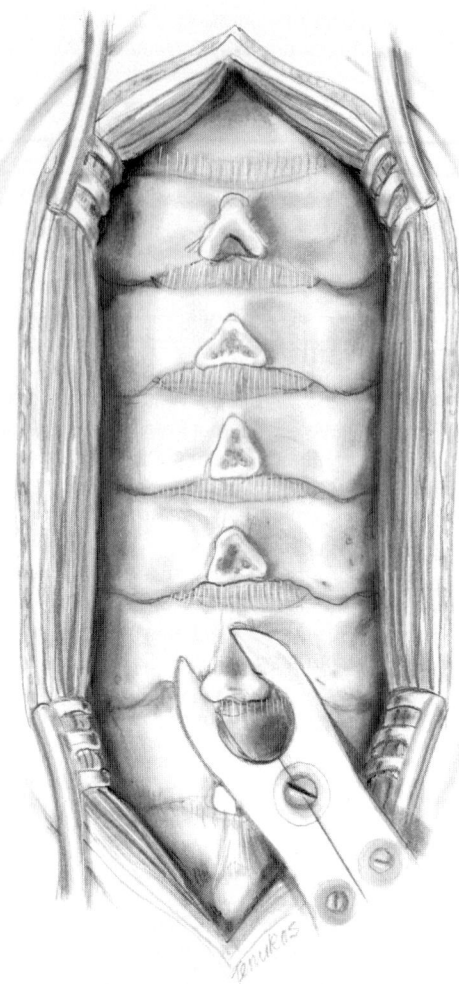

FIGURE 146–9. The initial removal of a spinous process during laminectomy for spondylotic myelopathy.

taken for localization. The spinous processes of the laminae to be removed are exposed, and the muscles are sharply dissected from the lamina and facets with a broad periosteal elevator, starting inferiorly and working superiorly, first on one side and then the other. A hand-held Meyerding retractor is helpful in the dissection of the muscular and ligamentous attachments to the laminae and facets.

If foraminotomies are to be performed, they are carried out at this stage by use of a Scoville retractor, with the spinous processes and laminae kept intact, and by the technique previously described. It is safer to perform the foraminotomy before the spinous processes and lamina are removed so that the dura and spinal cord are protected. The spinous processes are then removed (Fig. 146–9). Small, sharp curettes are used in separating the ligamentum flavum from the anterior surface of the lamina at each level (Fig. 146–10).

The laminectomy can be carried out as an en face or an en bloc procedure[31, 36] (Fig. 146–11). Both procedures require cutting longitudinal channels laterally in each lamina with small punch rongeurs or an air drill and removing the laminae as a single unit. We prefer to perform a piecemeal excision of the laminae with flat-heeled rongeurs (Fig. 146–12). Leksell rongeurs with a shallow inferior lip or Schlesinger and Cloward rongeurs with ground-down inferior lips are useful for removing laminae in this way. A high-speed air drill may be used to thin down excessively heavy laminae before rongeuring begins.

suggests loss of autoregulation and sensitivity to carbon dioxide in the anesthetized and ischemic cord, and blood flow is dependent on adequate pressure.[43]

Although the procedure is not technically difficult, a careful and unhurried approach is necessary. Rongeurs should have flat heels, and care should be taken not to wedge any instrument into the already crowded epidural space.

The sitting position is optimal because it allows better exposure and improved venous drainage, and it aids hemostasis. However, it unquestionably increases the potential for air embolus. Patients with vascular instability or cardiac disease may do better in the prone position. If the sitting position is used, bone wax should be used on the denuded bone, along with copious irrigation and meticulous hemostasis, to reduce the risk of air embolus. The operating table should be set so that it can be quickly brought to the horizontal position in case of a drop in blood pressure or development of a significant air embolus.

General endotracheal anesthesia and the sitting position are used as described for foraminotomy for cervical disc rupture. The neck is placed in the neutral position. Central venous catheters and monitoring devices are used as previously described.

The incision is made vertically in the midline. A spinous process is isolated, a marker is placed, and an x-ray film is

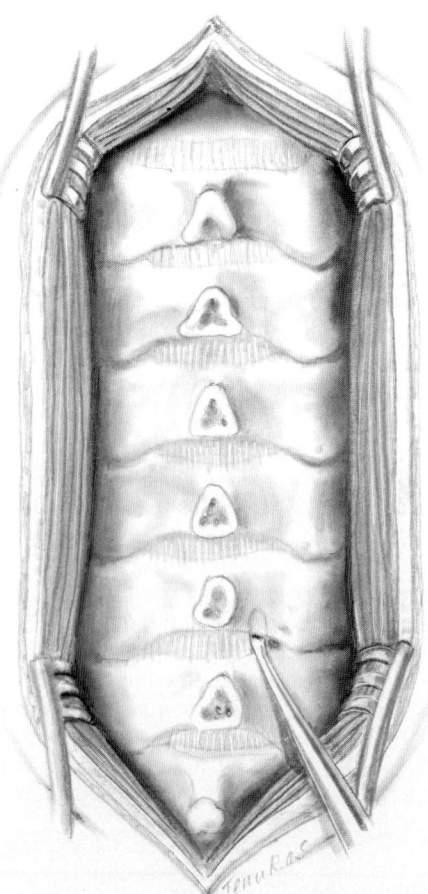

FIGURE 146–10. A curette is used to separate the ligamentum flavum from the inferior surface of a lamina.

Posterior Surgical Approaches for Cervical Disc Herniation and Spondylotic Myelopathy | 1813

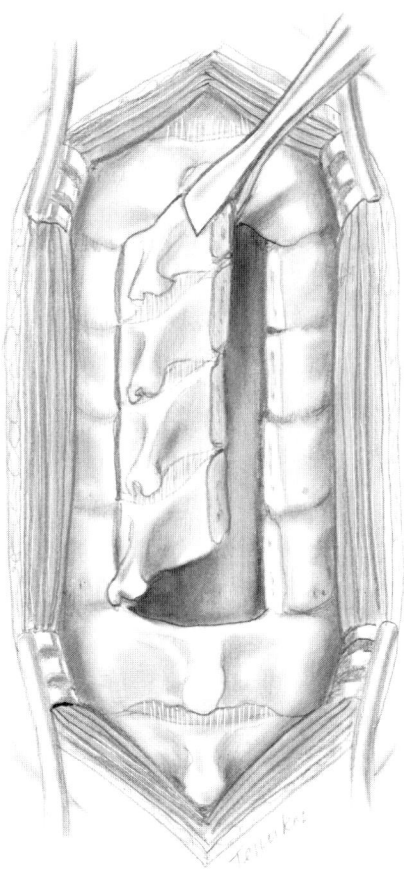

FIGURE 146-11. A laminectomy being carried out en bloc.

The laminectomy is extended to the most lateral edge of the dura (Figs. 146-13 and 146-14). Portions of the medial facets are removed to barely expose the emerging nerve roots. Complete facetectomy is not required and may result in an unstable cervical spine. The thickened ligamentum flavum is excised, and if the laminectomy is adequate, the dural sac should balloon posteriorly and pulsate normally. Including C2 in the laminectomy is generally not necessary, because the canal at that level is quite generous unless craniocervical junction stenosis is present. The lamina and spinous process of C2 frequently obscures the upper extent of the C3 lamina, and a portion may have to be removed to ensure complete removal of the C3 lamina.

Bipolar cautery, pledgets of gelatin sponge soaked in thrombin, or oxidized cellulose is used to obtain thorough epidural hemostasis. The dura is not opened. A thin layer of gelatin sponge strips is placed over the dura, and the muscle, fascia, subcutaneous tissue, and skin are closed in layers with nonabsorbable sutures. Prophylactic antibiotic therapy is continued for 24 hours postoperatively. Dexamethasone (4 mg every 6 hours and tapered over 3 to 5 days) reduces postoperative pain.

A soft collar is applied and worn for the first week or two. Lateral flexion and extension x-ray films are obtained to ascertain that no postoperative instability exists. Gentle ''yes and no'' neck exercises are begun during the second week. The patient can get out of bed on the day of surgery and is discharged 3 to 5 days after surgery. Sutures or staples are removed 5 to 7 days after surgery.

Complications

The complications of this procedure are generally less severe than those reported for the anterior procedure.[44–47] Ten complications related to surgery occurred in our 84 cases; none of these was associated with significant neurologic sequelae. Three mild subluxations, one superficial wound infection, and one extradural hematoma occurred; the hematoma was evacuated promptly without significant sequelae. No deaths or significant air emboli occurred. Three errors in diagnosis did occur: one patient had a cerebral thrombosis, one an intramedullary spinal cord tumor, and one had ALS coexisting with spondylotic myelopathy.

Transient worsening occurred in a few patients, but none was permanently worse. In two patients who were considered worse postoperatively, errors in diagnosis had occurred.

In the 39 cases previously reported on by Scoville and coworkers,[5] five cases had minor adverse residua. No infections and no deaths occurred. One patient required further decompression, and one patient had wound dehiscence. Three incorrect diagnoses occurred: one patient had multiple sclerosis; the second, a congenital anomaly of the odontoid; and the third, a vascular occlusion.

Air embolus was not a significant problem. There were few patients in series for whom the sitting position was used.[5, 31, 36] In the one instance of postoperative extradural hematoma in our series, the patient awoke from anesthesia with quadriparesis and was immediately returned to the op-

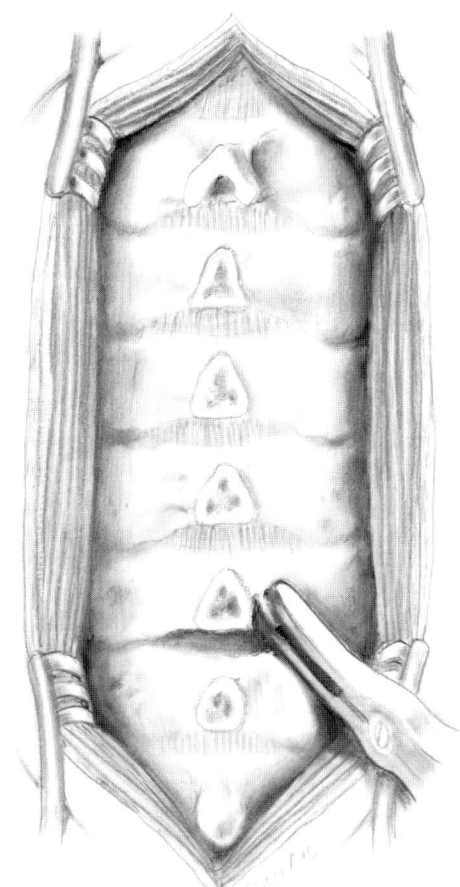

FIGURE 146-12. Piecemeal excision of a lamina with a Leksell rongeur with a shallow inferior lip.

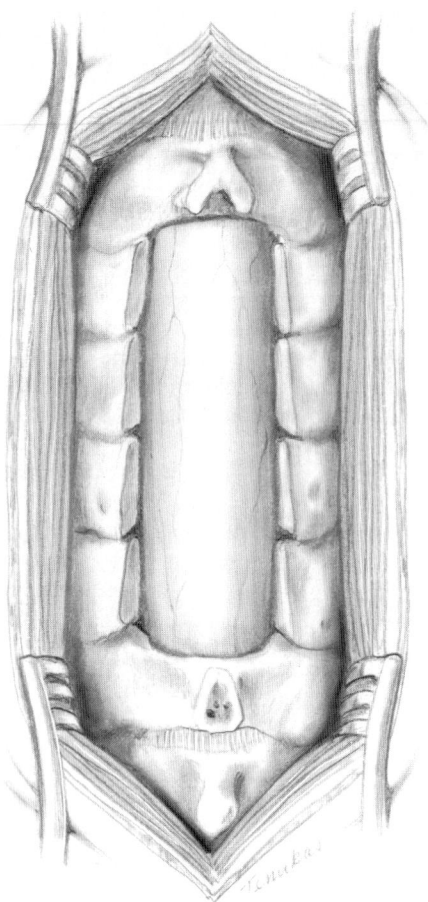

FIGURE 146–13. Completed decompression with four-level laminectomy and medial facetectomy.

seven, two were over 70 years of age, and five had had symptoms for a year or less.

Three errors in diagnosis occurred, and two of these patients were worse after surgery. One had ALS, and one had an astrocytoma of the spinal cord. All three had regressed after a previous anterior operation. Fifty-one patients (60 percent) returned to work or equivalent activity.

Scoville and associates[5] reported on 39 patients treated by decompressive laminectomy two laminae above and two laminae below the areas of involvement. Bilateral facetectomies were performed in 31 patients, and unilateral facetectomies were performed in seven. Good-to-excellent results were noted in 64 percent of cases, and clinical cure occurred in three. All patients showed an arrest of their disease, and none was worse after surgery. The two series from our institution suggest that no substantial benefit can be derived from the addition of facetectomy or foraminotomy to laminectomy.

In the series of Stoops and King,[33] the dura was not opened. In 83 percent of their patients, conditions improved. Remarkably, five quadriparetic patients returned to normal or near normal. No correlation existed between postoperative improvement and age, sex, duration of symptoms; severity of symptoms; myelographic findings; or number of osteophytes decompressed.

erating room and the hematoma removed. The quadriparesis cleared immediately and completely. Other causes of quadriparesis, such as cord ischemia from positioning or hypotension, intubation injury, or surgical trauma, require no further surgical therapy, but if a hematoma is strongly suspected, prompt reopening of the wound is indicated. If the situation appears less urgent, a CT scan may be helpful in the diagnosis.

Instability of the spine, reported to be one of the drawbacks of the posterior operation,[22, 48, 49] is probably exaggerated,[38] and an incidence of 10 percent has been noted.[43] Two kyphotic deformities, one of which required anterior fusion, occurred in our series. Scoville, Dohrmann, and Corkill[5] performed bilateral facetectomies in 39 cases and saw no instability. Epstein and Janin[36] found no postoperative instability after foraminotomies in 50 cases. Stoops and King[32, 33] reported on 42 patients who underwent laminectomies and foraminotomies, as many as six for a single patient, and had not one instance of instability.

Results

Our 84 patients were followed up from 3 months to 15 years; the average follow-up was more than 2 years. Sixty-nine and one-half percent of the patients improved, 28.5 percent remained unchanged, and 2 percent were worse after the procedure. Seven patients had excellent results. Of the

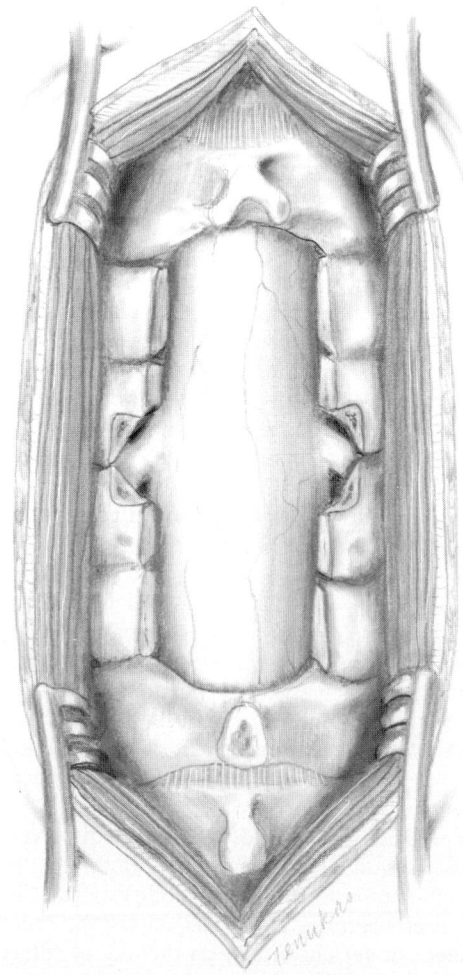

FIGURE 146–14. Completed four-level laminectomy with single-level bilateral facetectomy and foraminotomy to relieve root compression.

Epstein and Janin[36] studied 1355 patients treated for cervical spondylotic myelopathy. Of 114 patients not treated surgically, 36 percent improved, and 64 percent did not improve. Of 353 who underwent an anterior cervical procedure, 73 percent improved, and 27 percent did not improve. The remainder of the 1355 patients had extensive or limited laminectomies with or without foraminotomy, denticulate ligament sectioning, or dural grafting. In these patients, 60 to 85 percent were improved, with the higher figure (85 percent) representing patients with extensive laminectomy, foraminotomies, and excision of osteophytes. Age and sex had no specific effect on the results, but no patient over the age of 70 years had an excellent result. Epstein and Janin suggested that removal of the ventral osteophyte through a posterolateral approach improved the results significantly, but even if the osteophytes were not removed, a satisfactory result could be obtained in most patients.

Symon and Lavender[50] studied 41 patients who underwent extensive laminectomy without foraminotomy. Seven had the denticulate ligaments sectioned, and 70 percent of the 41 patients improved. Ten patients were unchanged, and two were worse. The authors believed that improved results were related to the extent of the laminectomy rather than to section of the denticulate ligaments or foraminotomy.

Gorter[51] reviewed a series of patients undergoing an anterior procedure as well as total laminectomies and laminectomies with denticulate ligament section or opening of the dura. Of 345 patients treated with an anterior approach, 73.4 percent were cured or improved, 18.7 percent were unchanged, 6.9 percent were worse, and 1 percent died. Of 184 patients who underwent total laminectomy from C2 to D1, 70.3 percent were cured or improved, 18.2 percent were unchanged, 7.5 percent were worse, and 4 percent died. Of 567 patients treated with laminectomy and section of the denticulate ligaments or opening of the dura, 57.4 percent were improved, 22.7 percent were unchanged, 14.8 percent were worse, and 4.7 percent died. Surgical results were poorer for procedures in which the dura was opened.

Fager[31] reported on 35 patients who had extensive laminectomies with opening of the dura and section of the denticulate ligament. Twenty-four percent improved, nine had their disease arrested, and five of the eight most severely afflicted patients improved. Two worsened postoperatively during a follow-up period of 1 to 6 years. Piepgras[39] reported on two groups of patients, both of which underwent extensive laminectomies. In one group, the dura was opened, and the denticulate ligaments were sectioned; in the other, they were not. No significant difference existed between the results of the two groups.

Saunders and associates[52] reported on a consecutive series of 40 patients with cervical spondylotic myelopathy treated by central vertebrectomy and strut grafting. The follow-up period was 2 to 5 years. The long-term cure rate was 57.5 percent, and the failure rate was 15 percent. There was no worsening of the myelopathy. The perioperative complication rate was 47.5 percent, with a 7.5 percent incidence of persistent sequelae. Decompressive laminectomy is a simpler and safer procedure, particularly for older patients and for those with associated serious medical problems.

Gregorius, Estrin, and Crandall[21] observed that some patients with myelopathy had late deterioration after initial improvement. Deterioration can occur 6 to 8 years later. There were six such cases in their series; two had pseudomeningocele, and three had a retained laminar arch of C3 under an elongated spinous process of C2. One developed spondylosis above the site of decompression.

In our study of 84 patients, six regressed. Three patients regressed within 1 year, two within 3 years, and one after 14 years. One patient had an anterior surgical fusion at two spaces after regressing, only to have further deterioration 2½ years later.

Hokuda, Machizoki, Ogata, et al[23] studied 269 patients with cervical spondylotic myelopathy; 191 were followed up for 1 to 12 years. One hundred fifty-six of the patients had a Cloward procedure, and 38 had a laminectomy. Fifteen recurrences occurred in 14 patients (5.2 percent). Eleven recurrences occurred in the group undergoing an anterior procedure, and four occurred in the group undergoing a posterior procedure. A constricting membrane was the cause in one patient. Spinal instability after laminectomy occurred in three patients. Progression of the spondylosis occurred in nine patients in the anterior group. Two patients who had unrecognized stenosis of the canal before their anterior operation required laminectomy. Reports of other series have noted such regressions and illustrate the need for long-term follow-up for accurate assessment of results.[27, 30, 38, 41, 53]

Routine postoperative myelography was not carried out in our patients. Six of the 84 patients who underwent myelography showed improvement in their myelographic picture. There was no significant compressive lesion in five, and one showed persistent anterior compression that required anterior discectomy. Of the series of Scoville and colleagues[5] 12 patients had complete or nearly complete relief of their block on follow-up myelography.

In two series[54, 55] in which preoperative and postoperative MRI was carried out, the abnormally increased cord signal intensity, if present preoperatively, diminished postoperatively in the patients who improved clinically and remained the same or increased in those worse or unchanged after decompression. The favorable signals may represent intramedullary ischemic changes that resolve after decompression.

The commonest causes of failure of surgery are related to patient selection, errors in diagnosis, and inadequate decompression. Laminectomy with adequate decompression in properly selected patients gives satisfactory results in restoring neurologic function or at least in arresting progression of the disease. The duration of symptoms appears to be the most important prognostic factor and is an argument for surgery as soon as it is convenient. Patients with symptoms for less than 6 months do best. Age and severity of symptoms have less prognostic value and do not militate against a beneficial result. An elderly patient with severe myelopathy may have significant recovery, provided that the surgery is performed at an early stage.

REFERENCES

1. Cloward RB: New method of diagnosis and treatment of cervical disc disease. Clin Neurosurg 8:93, 1962
2. Robinson RA, Smith GW: Anterolateral cervical disc removal interbody fusion for cervical disc syndrome. Bull Johns Hopkins Hosp 96:223, 1955

3. Spurling RG, Scoville WB: Lateral rupture of the cervical intervertebral discs. Surg Gynecol Obstet 78:350–358, 1944
4. Scoville WB: Cervical disc: Classification, indications and approaches with special reference to posterior keyhole operation, in Dunsker SB (ed): Cervical Spondylosis. New York, Raven Press, 1981, pp 155–167
5. Scoville WB, Dohrmann GT, Corkill G: Late results of cervical disc surgery. J Neurosurg 45:203–210, 1976
6. Roberts MP: Complications of lumbar disc surgery, in Hardy RW (ed): Lumbar Disc Disease, 2nd ed. New York, Raven Press, 1993, pp 161–170
7. Raaf JA: Surgical treatment of patients with cervical disc lesions. J Trauma 9:327, 1969
8. Odom GL, Finney W, Woodhall B, et al: Cervical disc lesions. JAMA 166:23, 1958
9. Fager C: Management of cervical disc lesions and spondylosis by posterior approaches. Clin Neurosurg 24:488, 1977
10. Murphey F, Simmons J, Brunson B: Ruptured cervical discs: 1939 to 1972. Clin Neurosurg 20:9, 1973
11. Roberts MP: Complications of positioning for neurosurgical operations on the spine, in Tarlov EC (ed): Complications of Spinal Surgery. Park Ridge, IL, American Association of Neurological Surgeons, 1991, pp 1–13
12. Crandall PH, Batdorf U: Cervical spondylotic myelopathy. J Neurosurg 25:57, 1966
13. Wolf BS, Khilnani M, Malis L: Sagittal diameter of bony cervical spinal canal and its significance in cervical spondylosis. J Mt Sinai Hosp 23:283, 1956
14. Mair WGP, Druckman R: The pathology of spinal cord lesions and their relation to the clinical features in protrusion of cervical intervertebral discs. Brain 76:70, 1953
15. Brain R, Wilkinson M: Cervical Spondylosis. London, Heineman, 1967
16. Allen KL: Neuropathies caused by bony spurs in the cervical spine with special reference to surgical treatment. J Neurol Neurosurg Psychiatry 15:20, 1952
17. Penning L: Some aspects of plain radiography of the cervical spine in chronic myelopathy. Neurology 12:513, 1962
18. Kahn EA: The role of the dentate ligaments in spinal cord compression and the syndrome of lateral sclerosis. J Neurosurg 4:191, 1947
19. Reid JD: Effects of flexion-extension movements of the head and spine upon the spinal cord and nerve roots. J Neurol Neurosurg Psychiatry 23:214, 1960
20. Brain WR, Northfield DWC, Wilkinson M: The neurological manifestations of cervical spondylosis. Brain 75:187, 1952
21. Gregorius FK, Estrin T, Crandall PH: Cervical spondylotic radiculopathy and myelopathy. Arch Neurol 33:618, 1965
22. Verbeist H: The management of cervical spondylosis. Clin Neurosurg 20:262, 1973
23. Hokuda S, Mochizoki T, Ogata M, et al: Operations for cervical spondylotic myelopathy, a comparison of the results of anterior and posterior procedures. J Bone Joint Surg Br 67B:609–615, 1985
24. Koyama T, Handa J: Cervical laminoplasty using apatite beads as implants: Experiences in 31 patients with compressive myelopathy due to developmental canal stenosis. Surg Neurol 24:663, 1985
25. Taylor J, Collier J: The occurrence of optic neuritis in lesions of the spinal cord, injury, tumour, myelitis (an account of twelve cases and one autopsy). Brain 24:532–551, 1901
26. Haft H, Shenkin HA: Surgical end results of cervical ridge and disk problems. JAMA 186:312, 1963
27. Bradshaw P: Some aspects of cervical spondylosis. Q J Med 26:177, 1957
28. Lees F, Turner JWA: Natural history of prognosis of cervical spondylosis. Br Med J 2:1607–1610, 1963
29. Nurick S: The natural history and the results of surgical treatment of the spinal disorder associated with cervical spondylosis. Brain 95:101, 1972
30. Aboulker J, Metzger J, David M, et al: Les myelopathies cervicales d'origine rachidienne. Neurochirurgie 11:87–198, 1965
31. Fager CA: Results of adequate posterior decompression in the relief of spondylotic cervical myelopathy. J Neurosurg 38:684, 1973
32. Stoops WL, King RB: Chronic myelopathy associated with cervical spondylosis: Its response to laminectomy and foramenotomy. JAMA 192:281, 1965
33. Stoops WL, King RB: Neural complications of cervical spondylosis: Their response to laminectomy and foramenotomy. J Neurosurg 19:986, 1962
34. Epstein JA, Carras R, Lavine LS, et al: The importance of removing osteophytes as part of the surgical treatment of myeloradiculopathy in cervical spondylosis. J Neurosurg 30:219, 1969
35. Epstein J: Management of cervical spinal stenosis, spondylosis, and myeloradiculopathy. Contemp Neurosurg 7:18
36. Epstein JA, Janin Y, Carras R, Lavine LS: A comparative study of the treatment of cervical spondylotic myeloradiculopathy: Experience with 50 cases treated by means of extensive laminectomy, foraminotomy, and excision of osteophytes during the past 10 years. Acta Neurochir (Wien) 61:89–92, 1982
37. Hunt W: Cervical spondylosis: Natural history and rare indications for surgical decompression. Clin Neurosurg 27:466, 1979
38. Bishara SN: The posterior operation in the treatment of cervical spondylosis with myelopathy. J Neurol Neurosurg Psychiatry 34:393, 1971
39. Piepgras D: Posterior decompression for myelopathy due to cervical spondylosis: Laminectomy alone versus laminectomy with dentate ligament section. Clin Neurosurg 24:500–515, 1977
40. Phillips DG: Surgical treatment of myelopathy with cervical spondylosis. J Neurol Neurosurg Psychiatry 36:879, 1973
41. Northfield DWC: Diagnosis and treatment of myelopathy due to cervical spondylosis. BMJ 2:1474, 1955
42. Scoville WB: Cervical spondylosis treated by bilateral facetectomy and laminectomy. J Neurosurg 18:423, 1961
43. Hoff JT, Wilson C: The pathophysiology of cervical spondylotic radiculopathy and myelopathy. Clin Neurosurg 24:474, 1977
44. Tew JM Jr, Mayfield FH: Complications of surgery of the anterior cervical spine. Clin Neurosurg 23:424, 1975
45. Mann KS, Khosla V, Gulati DR: Cervical spondylotic myelopathy treated by single stage multilevel anterior decompression. J Neurosurg 60:81, 1984
46. Aronson N: The management of soft cervical disc protrusions using the Smith-Robinson approach. Clin Neurosurg 20:253, 1973
47. Lunsford LD, Bissonette DJ, Zorub D: Anterior surgery for cervical disk disease: Part II. Treatment of cervical spondylotic myelopathy in 32 cases. J Neurosurg 53:12, 1980
48. Mayfield FH: Complications of laminectomy. Clin Neurosurg 23:435, 1975
49. Mayfield FH: Cervical spondylosis: Observations based on surgical treatment of 400 cases. Postgrad Med Oct:72–75, 1965
50. Symon L, Lavender P: The surgical treatment of cervical spondylotic myelopathy. Neurology 17:117, 1967
51. Gorter K: The influence of laminectomy on the course of cervical myelopathy. Acta Neurochir (Wien) 33:265, 1976
52. Saunders RL, Bernine PM, Shirreffs TG, Reeves AG: Central corpectomy for cervical spondylotic myelopathy: A consecutive series with long-term follow-up evaluation. J Neurosurg 74:163–170, 1991
53. Scoville WB, Aronson N, Simeone FA: Viewpoint: Soft cervical disc neurosurgery. Neurosurgery 2:80, 1978
54. Mehalic TF, Pezzuti RT, Applebaum BI: Magnetic resonance imaging and cervical spondylotic myelopathy. Neurosurg 26:217–227, 1990
55. Wilberger JE, Chedid MK: Acute cervical spondylotic myelopathy. Neurosurgery 22:145, 1988
56. Scoville WB, Whitcomb BB, McLaurin R: The cervical ruptured disk: Report of 115 operative cases. Transactions of the American Neurology Association 76th Annual Meeting, 1951, pp 222–224
57. Scoville WB, Whitcomb BB: Lateral rupture of the cervical intervertebral disc. Postgrad Med 39:174, 1966

CHAPTER 147

Surgical Management of Ossification of the Posterior Longitudinal Ligament

Takao Asano
Nobuyuki Tsuzuki

Ossification of the posterior longitudinal ligament (OPLL) was first described by Key in 1838.[1] It then remained unnoticed for a long time until Tsukimoto reported on an autopsy case presenting the syndrome of compression of the spinal cord owing to ossification within the cervical spinal canal.[2] As the occurrence as well as the pathogenetic significance of OPLL was confirmed by the succeeding reports in Japan[3-7] and in other countries,[8-12] OPLL has gradually become established as a disease entity that is distinguishable from ankylosing spinal hyperostosis,[13] ankylosing spondylitis, and diffuse idiopathic skeletal hyperostosis (DISH).[14] Meanwhile, the Investigation Committee on OPLL of the Japanese Ministry of Public Health and Welfare was organized in 1974, and the annual reports of the Committee have served as milestones in every aspect of research on OPLL in Japan.[15]

PREVALENCE

According to the Committee Report on the 2162 patients registered for clinical analysis,[15] the radiographic prevalence of OPLL in Japanese adults has been estimated to be around 2 percent. However, the incidence of asymptomatic OPLL increases markedly with advancing age and is as high as 3.2 percent in people over 50 years of age.[16] Nakanishi and associates[17] reported that asymptomatic OPLL was found in 11 percent of persons in the sixth decade when the cervical spine was examined by lateral tomography. Histologic evidence of OPLL was observed in 20 percent of the 350 autopsied cases without previous history of OPLL.[18] Although the incidence of OPLL in East Asiatic countries was about the same as in Japan (1.4 percent), it was as low as 0.16 percent among whites.[15] However, a recent review of 1000 consecutive radiographs of the spine in adults over 20 years of age in New York City revealed OPLL in 0.7 percent,[19] and in 1.7 percent in a similar study in Italy.[20] In this regard, nearly 50 percent of patients with DISH had concomitant OPLL on cervical roentgenograms.[14, 21] Because the prevalence of DISH is 3 percent in adults over 40 years of age[22] and 12 to 15 percent in patients over 65 years of age,[14, 23] OPLL may be a much commoner entity among whites than previously believed.

PATHOLOGY

The posterior margin of the vertebral body, where the posterior longitudinal ligament is attached firmly to the spine, is the common site of occurrence of OPLL. From there, ossification proceeds rostrally and caudally along the ligament. Histopathologically, enchondral ossification has been found in most specimens, and in some cases of massive OPLL, intramembranous ossification has been found as well (Fig. 147–1A and B). Whether or not OPLL is preceded by hypertrophy of the ligament remains controversial, but hypertrophy or ossification of the ligament has been demonstrated in the vicinity of the prolapsed disc material in some cases. Therefore, the prolapsed nucleus pulposus may exert some influence on the nearby ligament, leading to induction of bone formation.[24] Proliferation of small vessels in the ligament was observed at the initial stage of ossification.[18] The origin of bone-forming cells is believed to be the undifferentiated mesenchymal cells in the ligaments. Results of recent histochemical investigation indicate that some bone-inducing substances, such as transforming growth factor–β and bone morphogenetic protein, are involved in the progression of OPLL.[25]

A genetic study of 1030 relatives of probands with cervical OPLL in 347 families revealed OPLL in 26.2 percent of the parents and 28.9 percent of the siblings of the probands.[26] Although these prevalences were significantly higher than in the general population, the possibility of polygene inheritance was ruled out. Insomuch as OPLL is likely a disorder controlled by autosomal dominant inheritance, its genetic aspect has become a target of intensive research using molecular biologic techniques.

CLINICAL FEATURES

Like cervical spondylosis, the clinical manifestation of OPLL is radiculopathy, myelopathy, or both. In the 2162 registered patients discussed earlier, the commonest initial symptom of OPLL was pain or dysesthesia in the upper extremities (48 percent), followed by neck pain (42 percent), pain or dysesthesia in the lower extremities (19 percent),

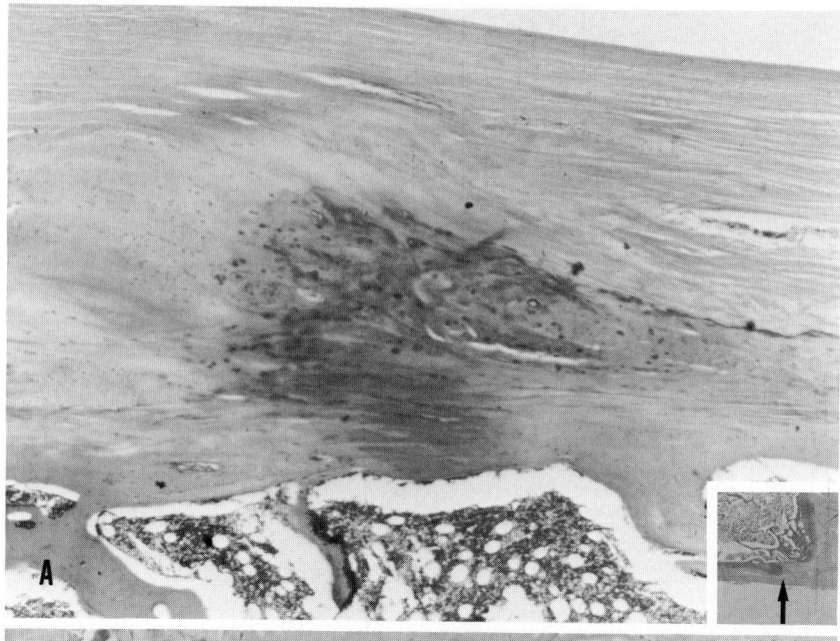

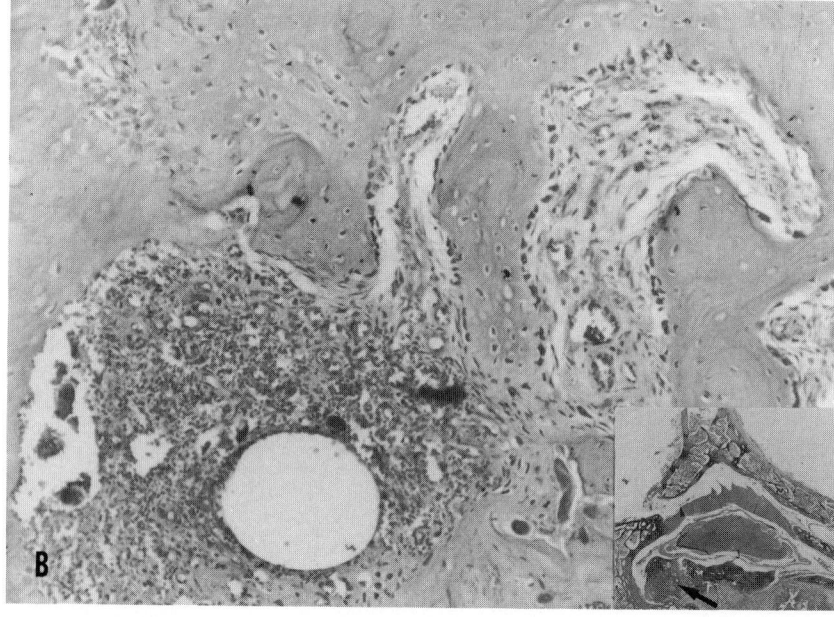

FIGURE 147–1. Types of ossification processes of OPLL. (A) Enlarged view of the area indicated by an arrow in the inlet. An enchondral ossification process of the posterior longitudinal ligament in its initial stage was observed at the upper posterior edge of C6 vertebral body (HE stain, × 25). Forty-six-year-old man with C4 segmental type of OPLL. (B) Enlarged view of the area indicated by an arrow in the inlet. An intramembranous ossification process of the posterior longitudinal ligament was observed at the anterior aspect of a massive OPLL at C4 level (HE stain, × 25). Sixty-five-year-old man with C2-C5 continuous type of OPLL.

motor dysfunction in the lower extremities (15 percent), motor dysfunction in the upper extremities (10.4 percent), and bladder disturbance (1 percent).[15] Those symptoms developed insidiously at the age of around 50 years in both sexes, without any particular cause in 85 percent of the patients. However, an acute development or aggravation of tetraparesis after minor trauma was noticed in 21 percent. The downward development of symptoms from the upper to the lower extremities was commoner than the reverse. Acute aggravation of neurologic deficits within a year or two after the onset was particularly common in relatively young patients (30 to 40 years of age).[27] Although the presenting symptoms or signs usually correspond to the cervical level where the cord compression is most pronounced, cervical OPLL is frequently accompanied by lesions in the thoracolumbar region. The possibility of multiple lesions calls for special attention in the neurologic evaluation of patients with cervical OPLL.

PREOPERATIVE EVALUATION

LABORATORY EXAMINATIONS

Routine laboratory results, including blood cell counts, serum protein, serum calcium, phosphorus, and alkaline-phosphatase levels, C-reactive protein, RA test, and erythrocyte sedimentation rate, were shown to be within normal limits. Human leukocyte antigens, such as BW40 and SA5, were relatively commoner among OPLL patients, but A27, which was very frequently positive in patients with ankylosing spondylitis, was negative in those with OPLL.[15] OPLL is common in obese persons, who often have glucose intolerance, indicating a close relation between the ossifying tendency of the ligaments and glucose metabolism. OPLL is a common complication of metabolic or hereditary diseases, such as acromegaly, hypoparathyroidism, vitamin D–resistant rickets, constrictive muscular dystrophy, and spondyloepiphyseal dysplasia tarda.[28]

DIAGNOSTIC PROCEDURES

Most OPLL can be easily diagnosed by lateral roentgenography of the cervical spine. Because a small OPLL is apt to be overlooked in the roentgenogram, sagittal tomography or computed tomography (CT) should be obtained in suspected cases. According to its shape in lateral roentgenography, cervical OPLL has been classified into segmental, continuous, mixed, and localized types (Fig. 147–2),[29] which occupied 39, 27, 29, and 8 percent of the registered cases, respectively.[15] OPLL was most frequently observed at C5, and the number of vertebral bodies involved was an average of 3.1. The narrowing ratio of the spinal canal, which is calculated as the ratio of the maximum anteroposterior (AP) thickness of the ossified ligament to the AP diameter of the spinal canal in the mixed, continuous, segmental, and localized types, was 42, 41, 25, and 30 percent, respectively. Patients with OPLL frequently show concomitant ossification of the anterior longitudinal ligament (62 percent), the posterior longitudinal ligament in the thoracolumbar region (37 percent), and the yellow ligament (37 percent).[30] The association with ankylosing spinal hyperostosis or DISH was significantly commoner in the mixed or continuous type than in the segmental type. Hence, a radiologic survey of the entire spine is mandatory in every patient with cervical OPLL.

Follow-up of the natural course of the disease for more than 10 years[31] revealed that an increase in either the length or thickness took place in approximately 76 percent of patients with cervical OPLL. Marked (> 2 mm) growth was observed in 40 percent of patients. In patients with the segmental type, the growth was less marked than in those with the other types, but transformation to the mixed or the continuous type was observed in about half of the cases. Interestingly, growth of OPLL has been shown to be markedly accelerated by laminectomy,[30] a result that is partly ascribed to increased mobility to the cervical spine. Regrowth of OPLL is much less frequent after laminoplasty or the anterior approach.[32]

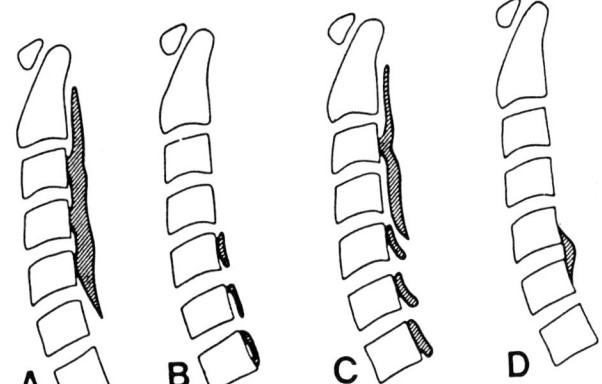

FIGURE 147–2. Classification of the cervical OPLL on lateral roentgenogram. (A) Continuous, (B) segmental, (C) mixed, and (D) localized. Reprinted with permission from Investigation Committee on OPLL.

Myelography usually reveals that OPLL causes a longitudinal, rodlike filling defect in the anterior aspect of the cervical spinal cord. This defect is easy to find in the posteroanterior projection but is often difficult to identify in the lateral view because the contrast material present in the patent subarachnoid space lateral to the compressed cord obviates the filling defect near the midline. More exact information can be obtained by carrying out CT immediately after myelography.

Because OPLL mostly consists of ossified mass, CT is the most reliable method for its identification in the cervical and the thoracolumbar regions. In conjunction with myelography, it clearly demonstrates the sizes and shapes of both the OPLL and the cord, as well as the spatial relationship between them. Commonly, the initial symptom of the OPLL located near the midline is myelopathy, and that of the more laterally located OPLL is radiculopathy with or without some features of lateral cord compression.

Although CT provides better osseous detail, magnetic resonance imaging (MRI) offers superior soft tissue resolution. Because MRI cannot depict ossification, OPLL is demonstrated as a low-signal intensity band between the bone marrow of the vertebral body and the dural sac on T1- and T2-weighted images (Fig. 147–3).[33] Although detectability of OPLL by MRI is inferior to that afforded by CT, MRI provides invaluable information about the underlying pathology of cord damage and of the OPLL. In this regard, a surge of interest has focused on the clinical significance of increased signal intensity on T2-weighted images within the compressed spinal cord.[34-37] Such an increased signal intensity was found in 11.7 percent of patients with cervical spondylosis and in 16.1 percent of those with OPLL, and its frequency was proportional to the severity of clinical myelopathy as well as to the degree of spinal canal compression.[33, 37] Insomuch as the pathophysiologic basis of such an abnormality was presumed to be myelomalacia or cord gliosis secondary to a long-standing compressive effect,[35] how it corresponds to the various pathologic changes within the spinal cord[38] requires further study. In the MRI images of OPLL, a band of intermediate or high signal intensity surrounded by a thick area of hypointensity was frequently found. This signal was considered to represent bone marrow within areas of ossification.[33] Recently, attention has been directed toward detection by MRI of the calcification front (the enthesis) as well as the hypertrophic posterior longitudinal ligament. In the future, such information will greatly contribute to prognostication of the disease.

In the past, electrophysiologic investigation on the compressed cervical spinal cord has been undertaken to determine the site of the lesion responsible for the neurologic symptoms, particularly in cases of OPLL with multilevel distribution. Potentials evoked by electrical stimulation, applied either on the peripheral nerve or directly on the spinal cord, were recorded at the spinal level or at the head level. Injury potentials, which indicate the site of cord damage, have been recorded by direct recording from the spinal cord.[39] However, the drawback of the previous electrophysiologic examinations was that they could not detect lesions of the motor pathway in a selective fashion. The advent of magnetic stimulation made direct stimulation of the cortical motor area possible. By the use of this method, the conduction velocity within the motor pathway at the cervical level

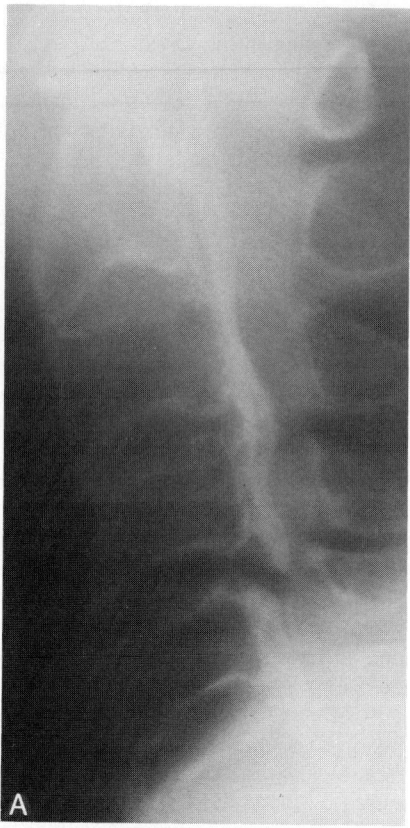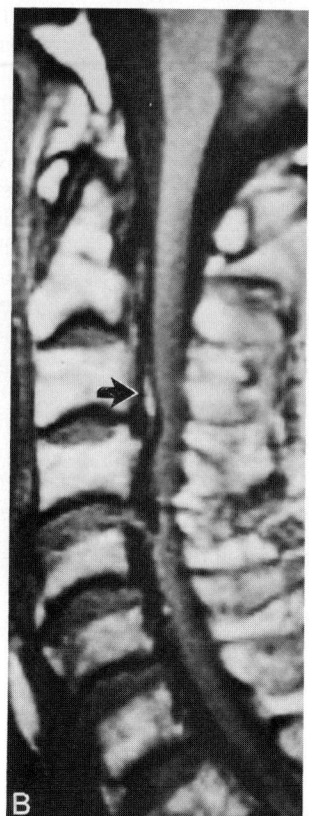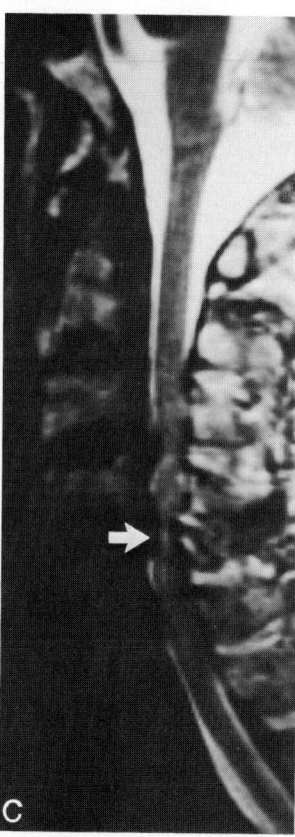

FIGURE 147–3. Lateral tomogram and MR images of the mixed type of OPLL. (A) Lateral tomogram, (B) T1-weighted MRI. The OPLL extends from C2 to C7, exerting maximal compression on the spinal cord at the level of C4-C5 interspace. The arrow indicates the area of high intensity within the OPLL, namely the bone marrow. (C) T2-weighted MRI. The arrow indicates the small areas of high intensity at the level of C4-C5.

was shown to be significantly reduced in patients with cervical myelopathy.[40] This technique may be useful in determining the level of cord injury resulting from OPLL.

CORRELATION BETWEEN THE NEUROLOGIC STATUS AND THE FINDINGS OF DIAGNOSTIC PROCEDURES

The advent of various modern diagnostic methods has enabled us to clearly illustrate the size and location of the OPLL together with the status of cord compression. How these findings correlate with the patient's neurologic condition or prognosis has been a matter of great concern. It has widely been admitted that a narrowing ratio of more than 40 percent as estimated from the plain roentgenogram, CT, or MRI is generally associated with a high incidence of neurologic deficits.[27, 29] Frequently, however, a patient with a greater narrowing of the spinal canal remains relatively asymptomatic.[15, 17] Furthermore, in patients with a narrowing ratio of greater than 40 percent, the type of ossification, the extent of OPLL, the narrowest level of the available spinal canal, and the minimum AP diameter did not have a significant correlation with the severity of clinical symptoms.[41] Although the contour of compressed spinal cord is clearly delineated by CT myelography, no correlation was revealed between the degree of cord transformation (the ratio of the transverse diameter of the cord to its AP diameter) and the severity of preoperative clinical symptoms.[42, 43] The only significant correlation revealed is that between the postoperative Japan Orthopedic Association score (vide infra) and the preoperative cross-sectional area of the cervical spinal cord as measured by CT myelography.[42, 43] Complete recovery after decompressive surgery cannot be expected when the cross-sectional area of the cervical cord is less than 50 percent of normal.[43]

PATIENT SELECTION

CONSERVATIVE THERAPY

Because mobility of cervical spine is a major factor influencing the development of symptoms, strict bed rest with or without skull traction has been the representative mode of conservative therapy for symptomatic OPLL. This therapy is effective, particularly in patients with modest symptoms.[15] As long as the cord is persistently compressed by the OPLL, however, relief of the symptoms is neither complete nor long lasting. Because recurrence or aggravation of symptoms is likely without decompressive measures, conservative therapy has only a limited role in the treatment of OPLL. Surgical treatment should not be so delayed that irreversible cord damage occurs.

INDICATION FOR SURGICAL TREATMENT

The most widely accepted view is that surgical treatment is indicated for patients who have neurologic deficits hindering activities of daily life despite the conservative treatment.[32] However, there is a trend toward a more radical view that patients who have radiologic evidence of severe cord compression should undergo prophylactic decompressive operation regardless of the severity of symptoms. Insomuch as the issue is still controversial, difficulty in establishing strict criteria for surgical indication stems from the fact that no single diagnostic method that exactly predicts the outcome exists. Therefore, all patients with OPLL are potential candidates for surgical treatment, although indiscriminate surgery should be condemned.

For the sake of decompression, the most reasonable and straightforward method is to remove the OPLL itself. Although the anterior approach can achieve this goal, it is not only more invasive than the posterior approach but it is also accompanied by the risk of complications. In the past, pros and cons of these approaches have been debated without resolution. To maintain balance in this respect, each approach is described by each of the authors according to his personal experience.

SURGICAL TECHNIQUES

ANTERIOR APPROACH

The anterior approach by the Cloward technique was applied to OPLL for the first time by Onji and colleagues,[4] with reportedly disastrous results. For a considerable period after this report, the anterior approach had been only occasionally employed in the treatment of OPLL and aimed merely at the removal of the concurrent ruptured disc or the stabilization of the mobile portion of the cervical vertebrae. The technique of corpectomy (vertebrectomy) and strut bone graft, which has been employed in cases of trauma, infection,[44] or multiple-level cervical spondylosis,[45] was also employed for the resection of OPLL in Japan. Through the pioneering works at various institutes,[43, 46–50] the feasibility of the anterior approach for OPLL has come to be widely recognized. One of the authors (T.A.) has also employed the anterior approach for the treatment of OPLL and multiple-level cervical spondylosis since 1978. Because the general procedure of anterior approach is described in detail elsewhere,[44, 51] the author discusses only the techniques that are particularly relevant to OPLL.

With the patient in the supine position, the operating table is slightly flexed, and the head and the neck are elevated to lower the intravenous pressure. The head is held in slight extension. Patients with instability of the cervical spine due to trauma or prior laminectomy, with marked cord compression, or with the plan of postoperative halo-vest immobilization, are equipped with the halo and are subjected to skull traction. The left iliac crest, from where the graft is obtained, is elevated by a pad underneath. Either a longitudinal skin incision along the anterior border of the sternomastoid muscle or a transverse skin incision is used, depending on the number of consecutive interspaces to be operated on. When the lower part of C2 needs to be exposed, a horizontal incision in the submandibular area may be added at the top of the longitudinal incision, especially in a stout, short-necked patient. Special maneuvers[52] are required to develop the surgical plane above C2. After the prevertebral fascia is reached,

the cervical level is determined by intraoperative lateral roentgenography. The plane is widened as much as necessary, and the prevertebral fascia is incised in the midline. The medial insertion of the bilateral longus colli muscles are coagulated and separated from the underlying vertebral bodies. The blades of the Cloward retractor should always be placed under the reflected longus colli muscle to avoid inadvertent damage to the esophagus, the carotid artery, and the other surrounding structures. Then, the intervertebral discs are removed together with the cartilaginous plate until the posterior half of the annulus fibrosus is exposed.

The area of corpectomy is determined by the findings of preoperative CT. In principle, the corpectomy should allow enough access to the lateral border of the attachment of the OPLL to the vertebral bodies. The wider the area of corpectomy, the easier the procedure. However, resecting too much of the vertebral body should be avoided because fusion of the bone graft with the remaining lateral surface or surfaces of the vertebral body increases the postoperative stability of the cervical spine. A longitudinal groove of 10- to 15-mm width is first made in, or a little lateral to, the midline, according to the width and the location of the OPLL. Through the emptied interspaces above and below, the vertebral body is resected by use of a Leksell rongeur. At this step, the cortical bone in the posterior aspect of the vertebral body is left unresected. The obtained bone chips are preserved for later use.

Then, the operating microscope is introduced. At each interspace, the remaining disc material, the annulus, and the adjacent fibrous tissue is removed by use of small, angled curettes or a miniature bone punch, until the anterior surface of the OPLL is exposed. The lateral margins of the OPLL are confirmed at each interspace, and the groove is enlarged posteriorly by oblique excision of the posterior half of the vertebral bodies by use of an air drill with a diamond burr (Fig. 147–4). The cortical bone in the posterior aspect of the vertebral bodies is usually contiguous with the OPLL. This part of the OPLL is only flattened, and the drilling is advanced toward the epidural space abutting the lateral border of the OPLL. In this procedure, the optical axis must be kept in the right direction. Both the microscope and the operating table should be frequently manipulated to obtain an adequate visual field. Because a narrow visual field tends to lead to incomplete removal of OPLL, further widening of the groove should be performed without hesitation, if it is felt necessary. If the drilling within the vertebral body has proceeded in the right direction, the epidural space is opened. Subsequent bleeding from the venous plexus can be easily controlled by packing with small pieces of thrombin-soaked absorbable gelatin sponge (Gelfoam). If the incision has gone medially, the dura attached to the posterior surface of the OPLL is exposed. When the dura is tightly adherent to the OPLL, it may be torn during the drilling, and the underlying arachnoid space and the cord may be seen. This indicates that the drilling must be directed more laterally.

After the above-mentioned procedure, the whole OPLL is bilaterally isolated from the vertebral bodies (Fig. 147–5A). Then, attention is directed toward the caudal end of the OPLL. The posterosuperior edge of the vertebral body, which is usually contiguous with the OPLL, is resected by the use of an air drill. Because the thickness of the OPLL is diminished near the rostral and caudal margins, ample space

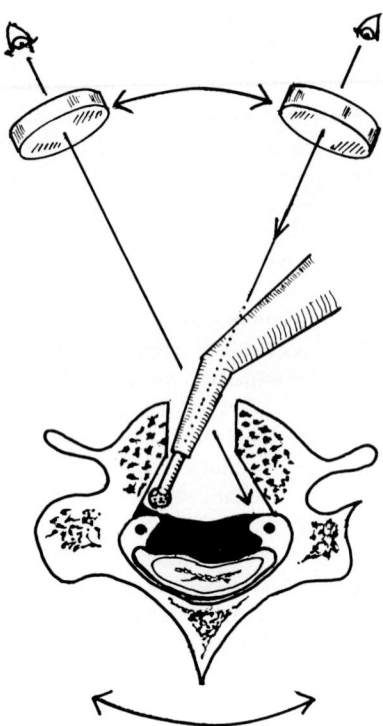

FIGURE 147–4. The technique of widening of the posterior half of the gutter. The drilling is directed toward the epidural space lateral to the OPLL (the black area), minimizing the danger of cord damage. The closed circles indicate the epidural space with the engorged venous plexus. To obtain an adequate visual field, the angle of microscope as well as the position of operating table must be adjusted frequently.

usually exists between the OPLL and the dura to allow the use of small curettes and bone punches. The underlying dural sac is exposed between the dural sleeves. The OPLL is completely isolated from the vertebral bodies if a similar maneuver is carried out with the rostral end.

If the OPLL is to be removed, its rostral end is drilled thin so that it can bend like a hinge. Then, the caudal end of the OPLL is gradually elevated by use of a small, curved bone curette as a lever, while the dura is separated from the OPLL (Fig. 147–5B). If the OPLL is completely isolated, either end is firmly grasped by an instrument so as not to allow its downward movement while the other end is elevated. As the space between the dura and the OPLL is widened, a small bone punch may be used to reduce the size of the OPLL. This step helps to identify the area of dural adhesion, which can be separated by blunt dissection in most cases. The dura that cannot be separated from the OPLL may be excised, thereby leaving the arachnoid membrane intact. In this way, the OPLL can be lifted up from the dura and removed in toto. A defect of the dura is covered by fascial patch, which is fixed to the dura by a few stitches. Alternatively, the OPLL may be resected by the use of an air drill, leaving a paper-thin layer of bone attached on the dura.[48] In the author's view, this technique is time consuming and is no less risky than the isolation-elevation technique described earlier because drilling must be carried out all over the posterior surface of the OPLL in close proximity to the underlying dura and the spinal cord.

Although the OPLL can be successfully resected by this procedure in most cases, a large OPLL with a wide area of dural adhesion presents a special problem. The larger the OPLL, the more difficult its removal becomes, particularly when a wide area of dural adhesion is present. In the past, it has been recommended not to remove the part of the OPLL that is tightly adherent to the underlying dura.[43, 46, 47, 49] Going a step farther, Yamaura[43] advocated not removing but merely isolating the OPLL (the anterior floating method). If adequate space anterior to the dural sac was created, the OPLL isolated from the vertebral bodies was shown to migrate anteriorly because of cerebrospinal fluid (CSF) pressure, resulting in sufficient decompression of the cord. The long-term result of this operation compared favorably with the preceding ones, and further growth of the isolated OPLL has been observed in only one of the 33 cases during the follow-up period of over 5 years.[53] Because the risk of OPLL removal is not negligible, this operation certainly appears to deserve a trial.

Regardless of whether the OPLL is removed or merely isolated, decompression of the root sleeves should then be carried out. This procedure can be performed by use of an air drill and other instruments, using the same technique employed in the resection of osteophytes around the joint of Luschka. A generous corpectomy may be added in the lateroposterior part of the vertebral body to ensure complete decompression of the root sleeves at every interspace involved (Fig. 147–5C). During this procedure, attention should also be paid to the residual OPLL, which might be present in the lateral aspect of the dural sac. Together with the residual OPLL, the adjacent ligament is resected as completely as possible to curtail regrowth of OPLL.

After the spinal cord and the root sleeves are completely decompressed (Fig. 147–6), hemostasis is secured, and a bone graft is resected from the iliac crest. A bone graft as long as 8 to 9 cm can be obtained from the iliac crest, and this length usually suffices to fill a groove extending over as many as four consecutive interspaces. A longer bone graft, when necessary, can be obtained from the tibia or fibula. Then, the bone graft is fashioned with keys at either end, and troughs are made in the endplates of the adjacent vertebrae to prevent anterior or posterior extrusion of the graft (Fig. 147–6A).[44] The bone graft is further shaped to fit the groove and is tamped into place while the skull is longitudinally retracted. The interspaces and the slit between the graft and the vertebral bodies are amply filled with the bone chips previously harvested. Then, an intraoperative lateral cervical roentgenogram is obtained to confirm that the graft is correctly positioned. The operative field is thoroughly irrigated with saline that contains antibiotics, and the wound is closed in layers. The author uses the halo vest when more than three interspaces are involved, which is usually the case in patients with OPLL. However, for a day or two after the operation, those patients are put on mild skull traction on the bed, using the already equipped halo so that any immediate postoperative complications could be readily dealt with. The halo is furnished with the vest after the patient's condition is stabilized. Ambulation or a rehabilitation program is started within about a week. The halo vest immobilization is continued for several weeks, and then a cervical collar is used for the next month.

Results

In the preceding papers reporting favorable results of the anterior approach,[46–50, 54] various scales were employed to

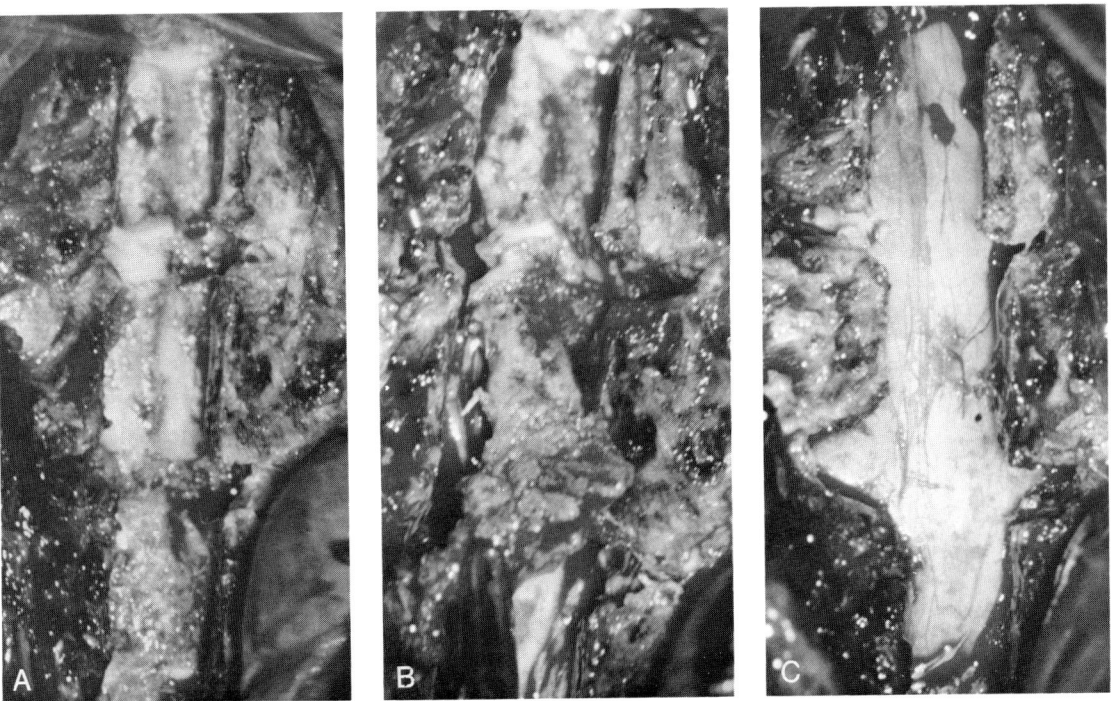

FIGURE 147–5. Intraoperative photographs. (A) The extent of corpectomy. (B) Elevation of the isolated OPLL from its lower end. (C) Complete decompression of the cord and the root sleeves.

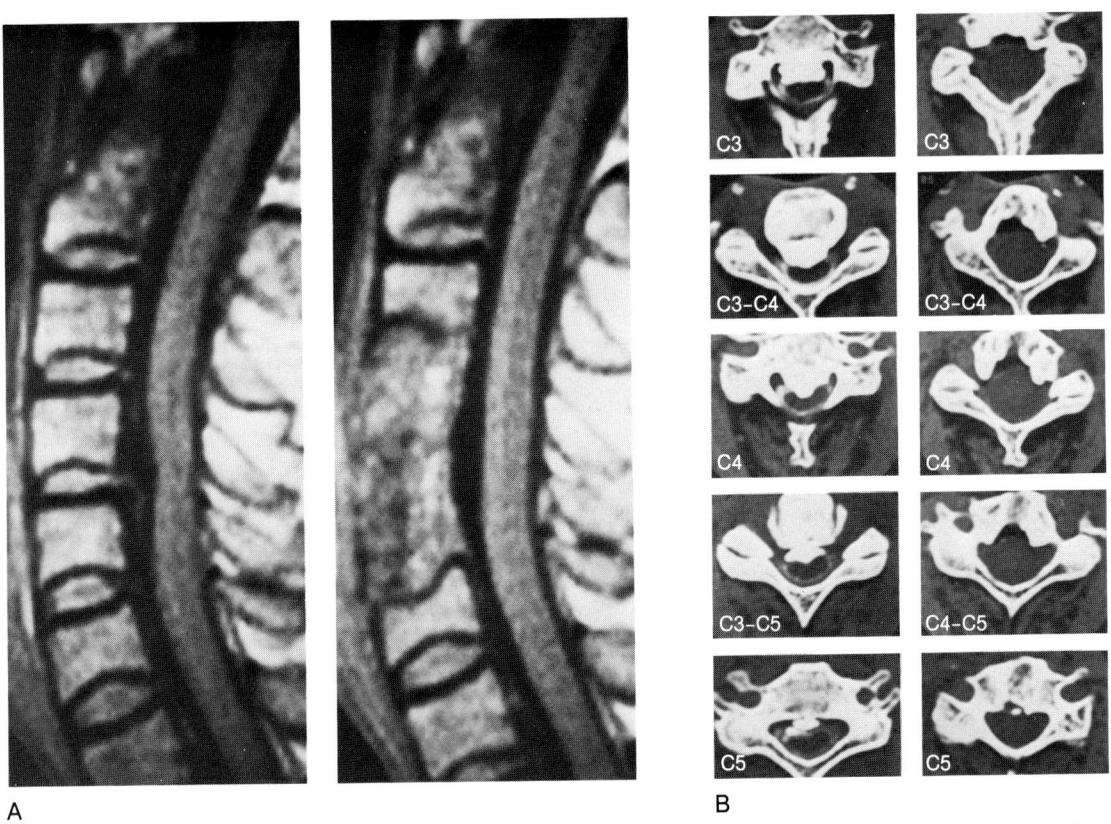

FIGURE 147–6. Preoperative and postoperative MR images and CT. (A) Left: the preoperative MRI showing the OPLL extending from C3 to C6; Right: the postoperative MRI of the same patient. Note complete decompression of the cord and the positioning of iliac bone graft. (B) Left: the preoperative CT myelography of the OPLL extending from C2 to C6; Right: the postoperative CT of the same patient. Note the extent of corpectomy and resection of the OPLL at each level. There is complete, bilateral union between the bone graft and the vertebral bodies.

evaluate the patient's preoperative and postoperative neurologic status. To compare the surgical results in an unbiased manner, however, the use of a common scale is indispensable. The criteria for evaluation of the operative results of patients with cervical myelopathy formulated by the Japan Orthopedics Association have been widely used for this purpose in Japan (Table 147–1). Postoperative improvement is expressed as the recovery rate:

$$\frac{\text{postoperative condition} - \text{preoperative condition}}{17 - \text{preoperative condition}} \times 100$$

In Satomi and Hirabayashi's series,[32] the average recovery rate after the anterior approach ($n = 16$) was 57.7 percent, whereas that occurring after the expansive laminoplasty ($n = 54$) was 62.8 percent. Yamaura reported that 83.3 percent of a total of 71 patients with OPLL who underwent the anterior approach had a good outcome (recovery rate > 25 percent).[43] Kamikozuru[53] showed that in 33 cases, the percentages of excellent (>80 percent), effective (50 to 79 percent), improved (20 to 49 percent), unchanged (zero to 19 percent), and worse (<0 percent) groups were 33.3, 30, 24.2, 12.1, and zero percent, respectively. In the author's consecutive series, ongoing since 1978, 60 percent (12 of 20) had an excellent outcome; 35 percent (seven of 20) had an effective outcome; 5 percent (one of 20) were unchanged; and zero percent were worse according to the same scale. The average preoperative Japan Orthopedic Association score was 9.6, and the postoperative score, 15.0, yielding an average recovery rate of 77.5 percent. Insomuch as mere comparison of the presented values may be of little significance because the operative outcome depends on various preoperative factors, such as age, duration of symptoms, and extent of cord atrophy, the generally favorable results of the anterior approach support its feasibility and effectiveness as a therapy for cervical OPLL.

Complications

Multifarious complications have been reported with the anterior approach for OPLL or other lesions, including extrusion or fatigue fracture of the bone graft, palsy of the recurrent laryngeal or the hypoglossal nerve, hematoma, wound infection, esophagocutaneous fistula, CSF fistula, stress ulcer, swallowing dysfunction, pseudarthrosis, and aggravation of neurologic deficits. Among these, extrusion of the bone graft is common. In the author's series, one patient required repositioning of the graft because of complete extrusion of the inferior end, and another required reoperation because of the fatigue fracture of the graft. Severe C5 radicular pain occurred in one patient, but the pain disappeared a few weeks later. Postoperative aggravation of neurologic deficits occurred in one patient with a large OPLL of continuous type from C2 to C6 who had been bedridden for more than a year because of progressive tetraparesis. After resection of the OPLL from C4 to C6 by the anterior approach, tetraparesis became complete. Because this effect partly resulted from insufficient decompression at the C3 level, emergent expansive laminoplasty from C2 to C6 was carried out. A few months later, tetraparesis was gradually reduced to the level of the preoperative condition. In two other cases, postoperative CT revealed a remaining mass of OPLL behind the vertebral bodies. Although the patient's myelopathy was markedly improved, some radicular symptoms persisted at the corresponding level. Local regrowth of OPLL at the lateral margin of the corpectomized area took place in two patients.

Restrictions on the Indications

For technical reasons, several restrictions should be placed on the indications for the anterior approach. First, because the anterior approach is generally more invasive than the posterior approach, it should be withheld in patients with advanced age or in poor physical condition. Second, OPLL in the C1-C2 level cannot be treated by the conventional anterior approach. Because decompression of the cord at this level can be easily achieved by the posterior approach, carrying out an extensive exposure[52] would be unrewarding in those cases, unless it is otherwise indicated. Third, the longitudinal extent of OPLL resection is somewhat limited in the anterior approach. Although the anterior floating method involving as many as six interspaces has been safely carried out with the fibular graft,[43] complications certainly increase as the range of OPLL resection, namely, the length of the bone graft, becomes greater. Presently, the maximal range of OPLL that can be safely treated by the anterior approach is considered to be four consecutive interspaces. In fact, the anterior approach is sufficient for most patients with OPLL because the number of vertebral bodies involved is 3.1 on average.[15] Fourth, the anterior approach might increase the danger of cord damage in patients with an extremely narrowed spinal canal. In consideration of the preceding reports of operative results, there is no indication that the anterior approach generally carries more risk than the posterior approach. Nonetheless, an attempt at removal of a very large

Table 147–1. THE JAPAN ORTHOPEDIC ASSOCIATION (JOA) SCORE FOR EVALUATION OF CERVICAL MYELOPATHY

I. Motor function
 Upper extremity: feeding oneself with chopsticks or a spoon
 (0) Total disturbance: unable to feed oneself
 (1) Severe disturbance: unable to use chopsticks, but able to use a spoon
 (2) Moderate disturbance in the use of chopsticks
 (3) Mild disturbance in the use of chopsticks
 (4) Normal
II. Motor function
 Lower extremity: gait
 (0) Total disturbance: unable to walk
 (1) Severe disturbance: need aid on flat ground
 (2) Moderate disturbance: need aid on stairs
 (3) Mild disturbance: need no aid on stairs but unstable
 (4) Normal
III. Sensory function
 Upper extremity, lower extremity, and trunk
 (0) Apparent sensory loss or paresthesia
 (1) Mild sensory loss or paresthesia
 (2) Normal
IV. Bladder function
 (0) Total disturbance: complete retention or complete incontinence
 (1) Severe disturbance: Incomplete retention, incomplete incontinence, or straining
 (2) Mild disturbance: frequency or hesitation
 (3) Normal

percent of the preoperative range of flexion-extension movement was lost. Because this became a major cause of discomfort and poor quality of activities of daily living, one of the authors (N.T.) developed the tension-band laminoplasty, which aimed to minimize postoperative contracture of the neck.

TENSION-BAND LAMINOPLASTY

The tension-band laminoplasty is based on the following mechanistic principle. Unilateral reflection of the laminae in the open-door fashion causes stretching of the spinous ligaments and ligamenta flava when these are kept intact. They

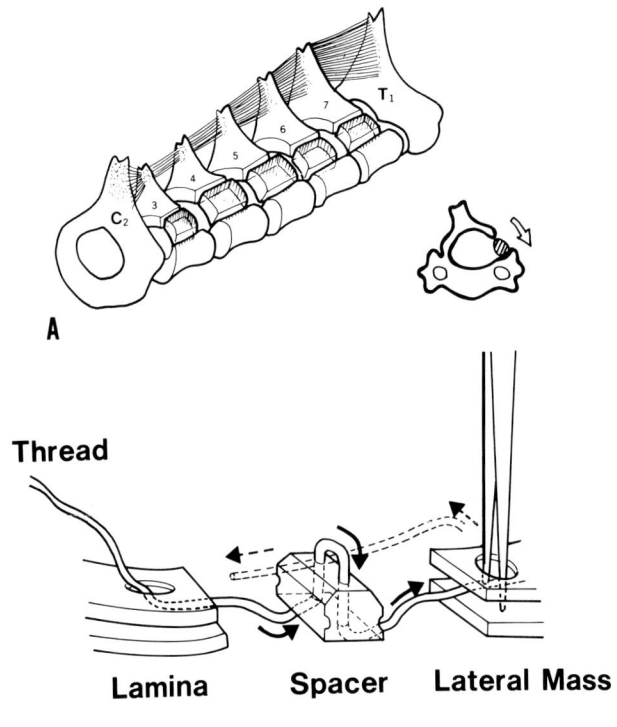

FIGURE 147-7. (A) Mechanistic principle of the tension-band laminoplasty. (B) Technique of threading a spacer. The tip of a thread is hardened by a surgical skin-adhesive material, which makes it easier to pass a thread through holes in bones and a spacer.

OPLL carries an undeniably significant risk of cord damage. Either isolation of the OPLL (the anterior floating method) or the posterior approach seems to be the procedure of choice for such cases.

POSTERIOR APPROACH

Posterior decompression for OPLL can be successfully carried out by laminectomy in the traditional fashion, namely piecemeal excision of the laminae, if it is performed very carefully.[55] However, partial decompression is always accompanied by bulging of the dural sac, which may lead to angulation and subsequent damage of the cord. To prevent such a complication, Kirita developed an "extensive, simultaneous laminectomy," in which the laminae are drilled paper-thin before they are simultaneously excised. Later, facet fusion was added to this technique to stabilize the spine.[56] Since then, various methods of expansive laminoplasty[56-60] have been devised to secure the postoperative stability of the cervical spine, afford the osseous protection of the spinal cord, and minimize the invasion of scar tissue into the spinal canal. The surgical results of those posterior decompressive methods were generally favorable, and the postoperative stability of the cervical spine as well as the osseous covering of the spinal cord were well maintained. Compared with laminectomy, laminoplasties have shown a lower incidence of regrowth of OPLL, presumably because of postoperative stiffness of the neck. Because of contractures of the posterior elements accompanied by ectopic bone formation, however, the postoperative stiff neck was so severe that 30 to 50

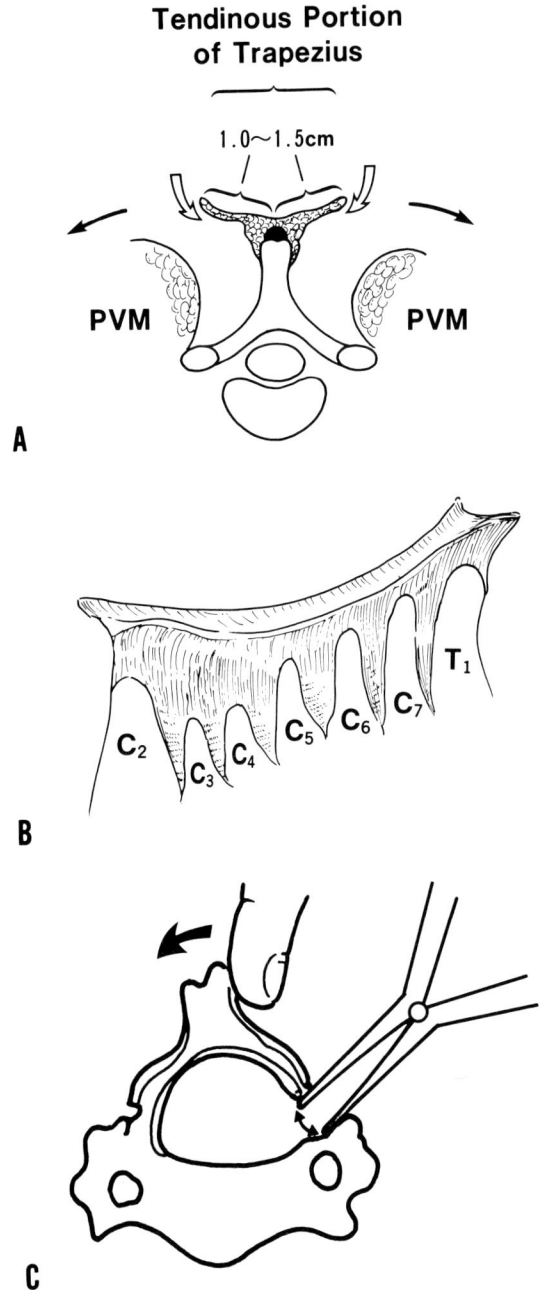

FIGURE 147-8. (A) Approaches to preserve the spinoligamentous complex. (B) Oblique view of the preserved spinoligamentous complex after exposure. (C) Technique of opening a lamina.

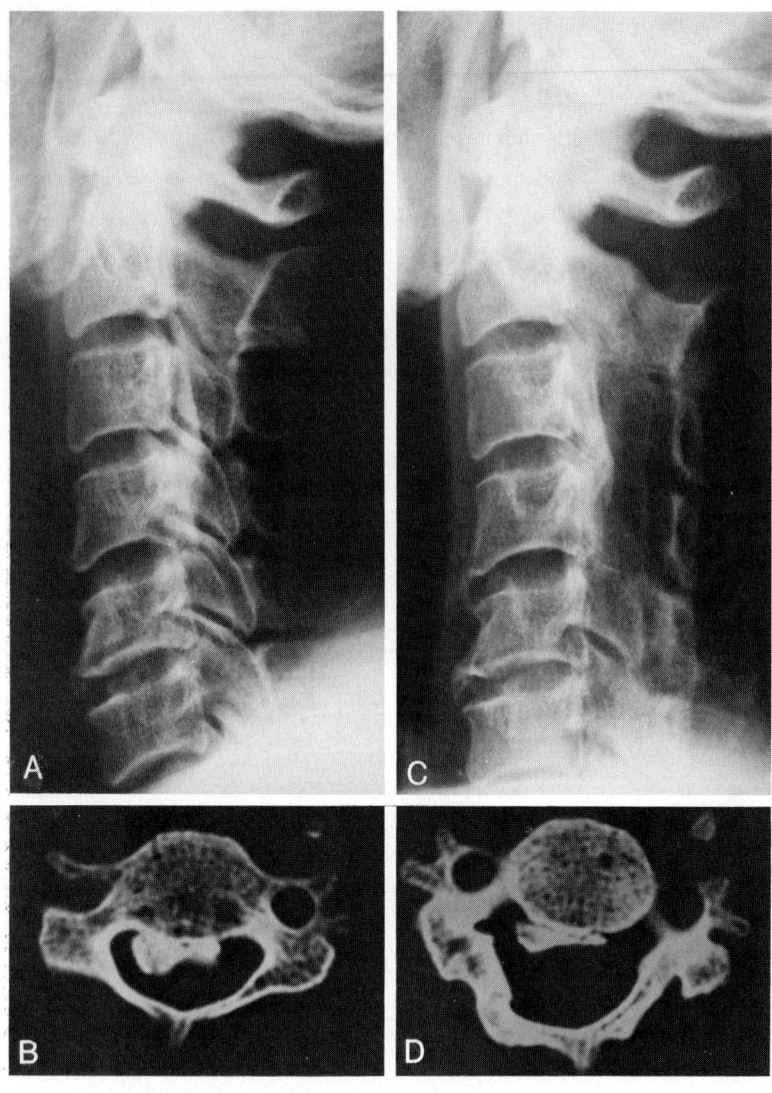

FIGURE 147–9. A case of C2-C7 tension-band laminoplasty with autograft in a 57-year-old man with a preoperative JOA score of 6 points. Tension-band laminoplasty from C2 to C7 was carried out with posterior fusion from C2 to C6 using a long iliac graft. One year after operation, the patient had complete neurologic recovery. (A, B, C, and D) Lateral views in the roentgenogram and CT (C4 level) (A and B) before operation; (C and D) 4 years after operation.

behave like a tension band, exerting force on the laminae to close the opened space (Fig. 147–7A). This compressing force stabilizes the spacers inserted into the opened space when the cervical spine is in the neutral position. Furthermore, every neck movement only adds to the compressing force on the spacers as follows: (1) flexion increases the tension-band effect of ligaments; (2) extension causes overlapping of the laminae, which then generates force to close the opened space; (3) on lateral bending or rotation, overlapping of both the laminae and facets acts in combination with the tension-band effect of the spinous ligament to further compress the spacers; and (4) a circumductory movement of the neck is a combination of these movements. Consequently, the spacers remain stable even before union takes place; hence, early postoperative mobilization of the cervical spine is enabled.

After the patient is placed in the prone position, the head is fixed in slight flexion by the use of a three-pin skull fixator. The posterior aspect of the laminae of the cervical spine is exposed through the middorsal approach. While the paravertebral muscles are detached and retracted bilaterally from the laminae, the whole spinoligamentous complex is kept intact. The supraspinous ligament together with the tendinous attachment of trapezius muscle is preserved as a wide band that is 1 to 1.5 cm wide on each side, so that the blood supply to the ligaments is maintained (Fig. 147–8A). In the high cervical region, the funicular and laminar portions of the nuchal ligament are also preserved (Fig. 147–8B). In principle, the spinal canal is enlarged from one above to one below the longitudinal extent of anterior impingement resulting from OPLL. A longitudinal groove of 3 mm in width is made by an air drill along the lamina-facet junction line on each side of the laminae, leaving the cancellous portion and the inner cortical layer. Then, the inner cortical layer of the longitudinal groove of the opening side is drilled thin, and together with the underlying ligamenta flava, it is severed longitudinally by a Kerrison punch with a 1-mm-wide blade.

The laminae are opened while the neck is kept in a neutral position. At first, the spinous process is pushed by a finger that feels its resistance (Fig. 147–8C). If hard resistance is felt, the groove in the hinge side is deepened slightly with an air drill. This procedure is repeated until the lamina is opened wide enough to insert a spacer of required width. From our experience, a spacer up to 10 mm in width can be inserted under good compressive force. The force resulting from the tension-band effect of ligaments and that resulting from elasticity of the lamina at the site of greenstick fracture act in combination to hold the spacer in place. As measured on the lateral roentgenogram obtained with a tube-film distance of 1 m, the insertion of a spacer of 8 mm width enlarges the AP diameter by 3 to 5 mm, and that of 10 mm width by 6 to 7 mm. A metal spacer is temporarily inserted until hole-making procedures for thread fixation are completed (see Fig. 147–7B). Thereafter, a permanent spacer is used that may be either an autograft or ceramic. When more than two facet joints need to be fixated in a continuous fashion, a spacer of adequate length is used. If necessary, the lamina of C2 can also be enlarged in the same manner described earlier. In this instance, however, the bone at the bottom of the groove in the hinge side must be kept as thick as possible to secure postoperative stability of the lamina. Generally, the AP diameter of the spinal canal at C5 can be enlarged up to 1.5 times in case of C3-C7 enlargement. If more enlargement is required, the canal of C2 should be included (Fig. 147–9). Such an enlargement of the spinal canal is considered to provide ample space for the spinal cord to comply with the future growth of OPLL, which might be accelerated by preservation of mobility of the cervical spine. After the insertion of spacers, the erector muscles are reattached firmly to the corresponding spinous processes. On the day after the operation, the patient is allowed to sit up in bed wearing a cervical collar, and on the second postoperative day, to walk. Exercise of the neck without the cervical collar is started soon after hemostasis within the wound is confirmed. The cervical collar is discarded by the end of the third postoperative month, or somewhat later if facetectomy was carried out.

Results

Since 1987, a total of 50 patients (49 to 80 years of age; average, 58 years) with OPLL underwent the tension-band laminoplasty. The follow-up period ranged from 6 to 60 months. The mean preoperative and postoperative Japan Orthopedic Association scores were 8.1 and 13.0, respectively, which is comparable to results of other types of laminoplasties. Union of autograft spacers took place within 3 months. With the ceramic spacers, which were of the bioactive type with a porosity of 40 percent (Apaceram, Asahi Optical Company, Tokyo), the occurrence of union could not be judged by postoperative roentgenography because no dependable criteria exist. So far, all the ceramic spacers have remained stable. About 70 percent of preoperative range of motion of the neck was regained by the end of the fourth postoperative week. During follow-up, the stability of the neck has been preserved without deformity, postoperative ankylosis of laminae at the site of the grooves, or ectopic bone formation around the ligaments. The mean ratio of postoperative to preoperative range of motion of the neck was 75 percent on flexion and 50 percent on extension (Fig. 147–10). No aggravation of neurologic symptoms has been noticed except for C5 and C6 radiculopathies, which occurred in 3 percent of patients.

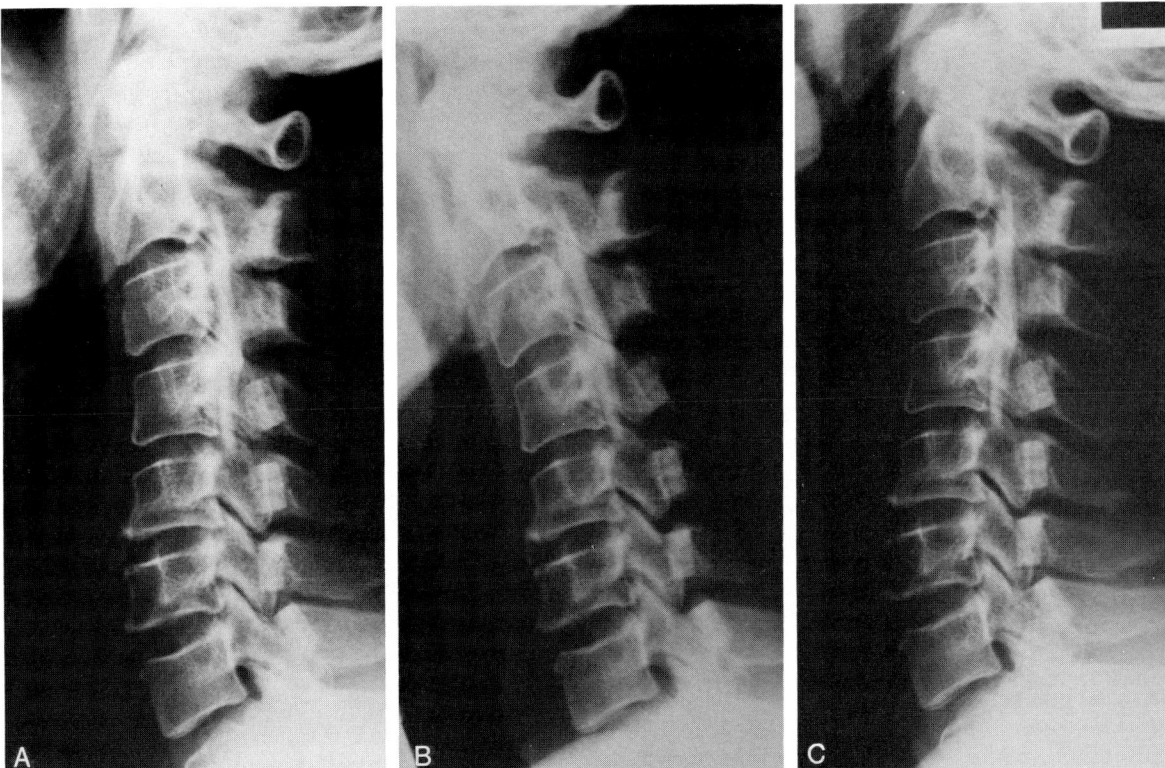

FIGURE 147–10. A case of C2-C7 tension-band laminoplasty with ceramic spacers. Fifty-two-year-old male with a preoperative JOA score of 8 points. Tension-band laminoplasty from C2 to C7 was carried out using ceramic spacers. Two years postoperatively, the JOA score was 15 points and the range of motion of his neck showed preservation of 90 percent on flexion and 50 percent on extension of the preoperative ranges. (A, B, C) Lateral views of the cervical spine 2 years after operation. (A) neutral, (B) flexion, and (C) extension.

SUMMARY

For every new patient with symptomatic OPLL, the surgeon must choose between the anterior and the posterior approaches. Here, the relevant issue is not which of the two approaches is generally better or worse, but which can better cope with the particular type of OPLL the patient has. The advantages of the posterior approach over the anterior approach are as follows: (1) it is technically easier and has a lower probability of damaging the spinal cord; (2) the stability of the spine immediately after operation is better, which makes postoperative management easier; and (3) some degree of spinal movement is maintained, even after an extensive decompression. However, complete decompression of the cord and the root can hardly be achieved by the posterior approach when there is a severe degree of anterior impingement resulting from the OPLL, particularly of the segmental or localized type. Thus, the primary target of the anterior approach is OPLL of the segmental or localized type, and the target of the posterior approach, OPLL of the continuous or mixed type. However, this categorization by no means poses absolute restrictions on the indication of either approach because the anterior floating method can be safely employed even in the large, continuous OPLL. Furthermore, the influence of regrowth of OPLL on the outcome remains to be determined. Presently, the roles of these two approaches in the therapy of OPLL may better be regarded as complementary to each other rather than mutually exclusive. If the outcome of the initial approach is unsatisfactory, a second-stage operation by the other approach can be performed. Although the scheme of a two-stage operation is justifiable, selection of the initial approach belongs to the realm of the surgeon's experience and clinical judgment.

REFERENCES

1. Key CA: On paraplegia depending on disease of the ligaments of the spine. Guys Hosp Rep 3:17–34, 1838
2. Tsukimoto H: On an autopsied case of compression myelopathy with a callus formation in the cervical spinal canal. Arch Jpn Chir 29:1003–1007, 1960
3. Terayama K, Maruyama S, Miyashita J, et al: Ossification of the posterior longitudinal ligament in the cervical spine. Seikei Geka 15:1083–1095, 1964
4. Onji Y, Akiyama H, Shimomura Y, et al: Posterior paravertebral ossification causing cervical myelopathy. A report of eighteen cases. J Bone Joint Surg Am 49A:1314–1328, 1967
5. Okamoto Y, Yasuma T: Ossification of the posterior longitudinal ligament of cervical spine with or without myelopathy. J Jpn Orthop Assoc 40:1349–1360, 1967
6. Yanagi T: Ossification of the posterior longitudinal ligament. A clinical and radiological analysis of 46 cases. No To Shinkei 22:909–921, 1970
7. Nakanishi T, Mannen T, Toyokura Y, et al: Symptomatic ossification of the posterior longitudinal ligament of the cervical spine. Neurology 24:1139–1143, 1974
8. Minagi H, Gronner AT: Calcification of the posterior longitudinal ligament: A cause of cervical myelopathy. AJR Am J Roentgenol 105:365–369, 1969
9. Breidahl P: Ossification of the posterior longitudinal ligament in the cervical spine. "The Japanese disease" occurring in patients of British descent. Autralas Radiol 13:311–313, 1969
10. Bakay L, Cares HL, Smith RJ: Ossification in the region of the posterior longitudinal ligament as a cause of cervical myelopathy. J Neurol Neurosurg Psychiatry 33:263–268, 1970
11. McAfee PC, Regan JJ, Bohlman HH: Cervical cord compression from ossification of the posterior longitudinal ligament in non-orientals. J Bone Joint Surg Br 69B:569–575, 1987
12. Trojan DA, Pouchot J, Pokrupa R, et al: Diagnosis and treatment of ossification of the posterior longitudinal ligament of the spine: Report of eight cases and literature review. Am J Med 92:296–306, 1992
13. Forestier J, Lagier R: Ankylosing hyperostosis of the spine. Clin Orthop 74:65–83, 1971
14. Resnick D, Guerra J, Robinson CA, Vint VC: Association of diffuse idiopathic skeletal hyperostosis (DISH) and calcification and ossification of the posterior longitudinal ligament. AJR Am J Roentgenol 131:1049–1053, 1978
15. Tsuyama N: The ossification of the posterior longitudinal ligament of the spine (OPLL). Report of the investigation committee on OPLL of the Japanese Ministry of Public Health and Welfare. J Jpn Orthop Assoc 55:425–440, 1981
16. Ohtsuka K, Terayama K, Yanagihara M: A radiological population study on the ossification of the posterior longitudinal ligament in the spine. Arch Orthop Trauma Surg 106:89–93, 1987
17. Nakanishi T, Mannen T, Toyokura Y: Asymptomatic ossification of the posterior longitudinal ligament of the cervical spine: Incidence of roentgenographic findings. J Neurol Sci 19:375–391, 1973
18. Tsuzuki N: Ossification of the posterior longitudinal ligament (OPLL) of the cervical spine. Its incidence and histopathology. Japanisch Dtsch Med Berichte 32:11–22, 1987
19. Firooznia H, Benjamin VM, Pinto RS, et al: Calcification and ossification of posterior longitudinal ligament of spine: Its role in secondary narrowing of the spinal canal and cord compression. NY State J Med 82:1193–1198, 1982
20. Terayama K, Ohtsuka K, Berlini L, et al: Ossification of the spinal ligament: A radiographic reevaluation in Bologna, Italy. J Jpn Orthop Assoc 61:1373–1378, 1987
21. Arlet J, Pujol M, Buc A, et al: Role de l'hyperostose vertébrale dans les myélopathies cervicales. Rev Rhum 43:167–175, 1976
22. Julkunen H, Heinonen OP, Knekt P, Maatela J: The epidemiology of hyperostosis of the spine together with its symptoms and related mortality in a general population. Scand J Rheumatol 4:23–27, 1975
23. Boachie-Adjei O, Bullough PG: Incidence of ankylosing hyperostosis of the spine (Forestier's disease) at autopsy. Spine 12:403–405, 1987
24. Tsuzuki N, Imai T, Hotta Y: Histopathological findings of the ossification of the posterior longitudinal ligament of the cervical spine and their significance. J Jpn Orthop Assoc 55:387–397, 1981
25. Kawaguchi H, Kurokawa T, Hoshino Y, et al: Immunohistochemical demonstration of bone morphogenetic protein-2 and transforming growth factor-β in the ossification of the posterior longitudinal ligament of the cervical spine. Spine 17:S33–S36, 1992
26. Terayama K: Genetic studies on ossification of the posterior longitudinal ligament of the spine. Spine 14:1184–1191, 1989
27. Kirita Y, Miyazaki K, Hayashi T, et al: The clinical aspects and the therapeutic results of ossification of the longitudinal ligament of the cervical spine. Rinsho Seikei Geka 10:1077–1085, 1975
28. Terayama K: Ossification of the posterior longitudinal ligament of the spine, in Suzuta T, Yamauchi Y (ed): Rheumatology-SEAPAL, 1988. Amsterdam, Elsevier Science Publishers BV, 1989, pp 33–37
29. Seki H, Tsuyama N, Hayashi K, et al: Clinical study on the 185 patients with ossification of the longitudinal ligaments of the cervical spine. Seikei Geka 25:704–710, 1974
30. The Investigation Committee on OPLL: The follow-up study for more than five years of ossification of the spinal ligament, in The report of the Investigation Committee on OPLL of the Japanese Ministry of Health and Welfare—1983, 1984, pp 85–96
31. The Investigation Committee on OPLL: The follow-up study for more than ten years of ossification of the spinal ligament, in The report of the Investigation Committee on OPLL of the Japanese Ministry of Health and Welfare—1985, 1986, pp 71–77
32. Satomi K, Hirabayashi K: Ossification of the posterior longitudinal ligament, in Rothman RH, Simeone FA (eds): The Spine, 3rd ed. Philadelphia, WB Saunders, 1992, pp 639–654
33. Yamashita Y, Takahashi M, Matsuno Y, et al: Spinal cord compression due to ossification of ligaments: MR imaging. Radiology 175:843–848, 1990
34. Hackney DB, Asato R, Joseph PM, et al: Hemorrhage and edema in acute spinal cord compression: Demonstration by MR imaging. Radiology 161:387–390, 1986
35. Takahashi M, Sakamoto Y, Miyawaki M, Bussaka H: Increased MR signal intensity secondary to chronic cervical cord compression. Neuroradiology 29:550–556, 1987
36. Ramanauskas WL, Wilner HI, Metes JJ, et al: MR imaging of compressive myelomalacia. J Comput Assist Tomogr 13:399–404, 1989

37. Takahashi M, Yamashita Y, Sakamoto Y, Kojima R: Chronic cervical cord compression: Clinical significance of increased signal intensity on MR images. Radiology 173:219–224, 1989
38. Hashizume Y, Iijima S, Kishimoto H, Yanagi T: Pathology of spinal cord lesions caused by ossification of the posterior longitudinal ligament. Acta Neuropathol (Berl) 63:123–130, 1984
39. Shinomiya K, Furuya K, Sato R, et al: Electrophysiologic diagnosis of cervical OPLL myelopathy using evoked spinal cord potentials. Spine 13:1225–1233, 1988
40. Iizuka T, Azuma H, Tanaka H, et al: Magnetic transcutaneous stimulation of the motor pathway in spinal cord disorders, in Simoji K, Kurokawa T, Tamaki T, Willis WD Jr (eds): Spinal Cord Monitoring and Electrodiagnosis. Berlin, Springer-Verlag, 1991, pp 253–260
41. Kawaguchi H, Kurokawa T, Machida H, et al: Roentgenological manifestation of ossification of the posterior longitudinal ligament in the cervical spine causing severe spinal canal stenosis—A group comparison with and without marked spinal cord dysfunction. J Jpn Orthop Assoc 65:173–180, 1991
42. Fujiwara K, Yonenobu S, Ebara S, et al: An analysis of cervical myelopathy due to cervical spondylosis or ossification of posterior longitudinal ligament by CT myelography. Rinsho Seikei Geka 23:419–424, 1988
43. Yamaura I: Anterior approach (anterior floating method) and its surgical results for cervical myelopathy caused by ossification of the posterior longitudinal ligament (OPLL). J West Pac Orthop Assoc 27:47–55, 1990
44. Southwick WO, Robinson RA: Surgical approaches to the vertebral bodies in the cervical and lumbar regions. J Bone Joint Surg Am 39A:631–644, 1957
45. Pansini A, Lore F: Une nouvelle technique: la somatotomie médiane longitudinale dans les myélopathies par discarthroses cervicales. Neurochirurgie 1:189–202, 1972
46. Sakou T, Miyazaki A, Tominura K, et al: Ossification of the posterior longitudinal ligament of the cervical spine: Subtotal vertebrectomy as a treatment. Clin Orthop 140:58–65, 1979
47. Manabe S, Nomura S: Anterior decompression for ossification of the posterior longitudinal ligament of the cervical spine. Neurol Surg 5:1253–1259, 1977
48. Abe H, Tsuru M, Ito T, et al: Anterior decompression for ossification of the posterior longitudinal ligament of the cervical spine. J Neurosurg 55:108–116, 1981
49. Hanai K, Inouye Y, Kawai K, et al: Anterior decompression for myelopathy resulting from ossification of the posterior longitudinal ligament. J Bone Joint Surg Br 64B:561–564, 1982
50. Harsh GR IV, Sypert GW, Weinstein PR, et al: Cervical spine stenosis secondary to ossification of the posterior longitudinal ligament. J Neurosurg 67:349–357, 1987
51. Schmidek HH, Smith DA: Anterior cervical disc excision in cervical spondylosis, in Schmidek HH, Sweet WH (eds): Operative Neurosurgical Techniques. Indications, Methods and Results, 2nd ed, vol 2. Orlando, Grune & Stratton, 1988, pp 1327–1342
52. McAfee PC, Bohlman HH, Riley L, et al: The anterior retropharyngeal approach to the upper part of the cervical spine. J Bone Joint Surg Am 69A:1371–1383, 1987
53. Kamikozuru M: Significance of the anterior floating method for cervical myelopathy due to the ossification of the posterior longitudinal ligament. J Jpn Orthop Assoc 65:431–440, 1991
54. Kojima T, Waga S, Kubo Y, et al: Anterior cervical ossification of the posterior longitudinal ligament. Neurosurgery 24:864–872, 1989
55. Nagashima C: Cervical myelopathy due to ossification of the posterior longitudinal ligament. J Neurosurg 37:653–660, 1971
56. Miyazaki K, Kirita Y: Extensive simultaneous multisegment laminectomy for myelopathy due to the ossification of the posterior longitudinal ligament in the cervical region. Spine 11:531–542, 1986
57. Tomita K, Nomura S, Umeda S, Baba H: Cervical laminoplasty to enlarge the spinal canal in multilevel ossification of the posterior longitudinal ligament with myelopathy. Arch Orthop Trauma Surg 107:148–153, 1988
58. Iwasaki H: Expansive laminoplasty. Seikei Geka 2(Suppl):228–233, 1987
59. Hirabayashi K, Watanabe K, Wakano K, et al: Expansive open-door laminoplasty for cervical spinal stenotic myelopathy. Spine 8:693–699, 1983
60. Itoh T, Tsuji H: Technical improvements and results of laminoplasty for compressive myelopathy in the cervical spine. Spine 10:729–736, 1985

CHAPTER 148

Surgical Management of Injuries of the Cervical Spine and Spinal Cord

Daniele Rigamonti
Aizik L. Wolf
Stuart E. Mirvis

EPIDEMIOLOGY

The prevalence of spinal cord injury is estimated to be 906 cases per million population, affecting approximately 250,000 individuals in the United States.[1] Each year, between 5000 and 10,000 persons in the United States suffer spinal cord injury; 20 to 35 persons per million survive until hospital admission.[1] Spinal cord injury occurs most frequently among males between 15 and 20 years of age. The most common mechanisms of injury are motor vehicle accidents, falls, water sports accidents, and penetrating injuries due to gunshot or knife wounds. Approximately 60 percent of spinal injuries involve the cervical region. A recent review of a large number of cases confirms the high incidence of injuries in the third decade,[2] with a second peak in the sixth and seventh decades. A recent review from Northwestern University shows the highest incidence of cervical spine injury occurs at the C5 and C6 levels.[3] Injuries to C3-T1 gradually decrease with age, and the incidence of fractures of C1 and C2 gradually rises because of odontoid fractures in the elderly.

PREHOSPITAL EVALUATION AND CARE

The final outcome in any case of spinal cord injury depends on the degree of reversible damage to the cord because damage to neurons and fiber tracts is irreversible, and no therapeutic intervention results in spinal cord regeneration and increased functional recovery. In the absence of a therapeutic modality proved to induce regeneration, the best treatment of cord injury is the prevention of secondary injury and begins at the accident scene with personnel trained in safe and expeditious evacuation of these patients to a hospital capable of providing for their definitive care. Cervical spine injury presents a significant hazard to the injured patient because of the possibility of inducing or aggravating spinal cord damage in the presence of an unstable neck injury. This complication occurs in an estimated 3 percent of the patients who enter the emergency medical system. The prevention of such a complication can preserve residual neurologic function and is the main management goal of acute spinal cord injury.

At the scene of the accident, the victim's head and neck must be immobilized until formal evaluation can rule out a fracture-dislocation. The initial evaluation should include inspection of the head and neck area—especially the forehead and occiput—for abrasions or contusions. Tenderness of the spine strongly suggests the likelihood of a spinal cord injury, as does any significant trauma at or above the level of the clavicle. Unconscious and uncooperative patients pose special hazards. The victim of high-impact injury should be assumed to have sustained a cervical injury until proved otherwise. Once a patient with a potential spinal cord injury is identified, respiratory and cardiovascular stabilization must follow immediately after adequate stabilization. Many effective and simple alternative methods of transportation have been identified, but because aspiration and shock are the major causes of morbidity and mortality in these patients, transporting patients in 30 degrees of Trendelenburg's position is the best prophylactic measure. Optimally, spinal cord–injured victims should be moved by the log-rolling maneuver, which minimizes the chances of secondary neurologic injury.

If the patient requires extrication, the entire spine should be kept immobilized, with the neck in a neutral position. Immobilizing the neck with hard collar alone is inadequate. We do not advocate cervical traction without radiologic control, because this method may exacerbate a spinal deformity and worsen a neurologic deficit. If life-saving resuscitative measures are necessary, extreme care must be taken to minimize motion of the neck. Nasotracheal intubation may provide the least amount of motion.

Paramedics at the accident scene can provide valuable information by use of a standard neurologic assessment scheme. Assessment of motor and sensory levels can accurately pinpoint the level and nature of spinal cord or nerve injury. The motor level of a spinal cord injury is defined as the lowest level of significant motor function. A quick assessment of the patient's ability to breathe (diaphragmatic function) can be followed by a quick screening of the patient's ability to move his or her head and each of the extremities, as well as the feet and toes. This process provides a quick assessment of a spinal cord injury. In the unconscious or impaired patient, proximal and distal motor response can be assessed in each extremity by use of noxious stimuli to ascertain gross motor function. In the alert patient, a systematic examination of the major motor groups of the upper and lower extremities, proceeding rostrally to caudally, provides a baseline examination for determination of improvement or deterioration (which, in certain cases, may necessitate a change in therapeutic management). At the accident scene, we advocate the grading of motor function as follows: 0 = no palpable contraction; 1 = strength sufficient to move the joint; 2 = strength against gravity; and 3 = full strength against resistance. More subtle grading scales are of no help in the field setting.[4]

EMERGENCY ROOM EVALUATION AND MANAGEMENT

Evaluation and management of a cervical cord injury patient requires an understanding of the pathophysiology of the injury; a knowledge of complicating factors, such as cardiovascular instability and the coexistence of blunt trauma; and prompt radiologic assessment and intervention.

TRACTION

Immobilization should be maintained until a lesion is documented or excluded radiologically. In the emergency room, immobilization should be supplemented by skeletal traction.

Traction immobilizes the fracture, and when it succeeds in reducing the fracture, it helps provide initial decompression of the spinal cord. If traction does not succeed in reducing a fracture-subluxation within a reasonable period of time, operative reduction is considered. The timing of surgery remains a controversial point. Some authors argue that early operation is associated with significant morbidity or, at best, is hazardous.[5] Others feel that early intervention is not associated with a higher incidence of complications.[6]

In our series of 403 spinal cord–injured patients, 143 patients (35 percent) required realignment of the cervical spine because of unilaterally or bilaterally locked facets or fracture-subluxation.[7] At the Maryland Institute for Emergency Medical Services Systems, we attempt closed reduction immediately at the patient's arrival in the hospital[8-10] because as an acute measure, reduction reconstructs the spinal canal and reduces compression of the spinal cord. As a chronic measure, reduction affords an improved spinal alignment for fusion and, subsequently, less pain. Unfortunately, the original tissue destruction induced by the forces causing the subluxation is not altered by reduction. The reversal of bony compression may alter two factors responsible for irreversible spinal cord injury, namely, ischemia and further tissue destruction.

Closed reduction can be accomplished either with Gardner-Wells tongs (Codman) or magnetic resonance imaging (MRI)–compatible tongs (PMT, Minneapolis, MN) made of a graphite composite with titanium pins. Halo rings may be the appropriate track-reduction device when halo vest stabilization is used for a given fracture.

The site for the Gardner-Wells tongs placement is determined primarily by one of three desired effects: straight in-line traction, as in burst or some chip features; flexion traction, for reduction of unilateral or bilateral locked facets; or the less likely extension traction, for flexion fractures with angulated retroluxations.

Traction pin placement should be below the equator of the skull, typically, 1 cm above the pinna. This is extremely important when higher weights are necessary to reduce bilaterally locked facets. The possible complications of a slipped pin include significant scalp laceration, skull fracture, and more importantly, neurologic deterioration from too rapid a resubluxation of the cervical spine. For straight in-line traction, tongs are placed on an auditory meatal line drawn from the inferiorly, external auditory meatus through the most anterosuperior edge of the pinna. Flexion traction is accomplished by placing Gardner-Wells pins 2 cm behind the anterior meatal line. This point is located directly above the mastoid process. The rate and speed in reducing locked facets, often with lower reduction weights, is significantly improved with this pin placement.

Because of the relatively low incidence of retroluxations, extension traction is less commonly employed. Extension via tong placement alone is possible but often requires anterior displacement of the shoulders when the commonly employed Stryker or Roto-Rest bed is used. This is because the downward or extension direction of traction is mechanically limited by the integral traction configurations on these beds. Placement of the tongs anterior to the anterior meatal line should be limited to 1 cm; because of the much thinner squamous temporal bone, the risk of skull fracture and epidural hematoma increases, as does the patient's discomfort from temporalis muscle involvement.

The amount of weight permitted for closed reduction of the cervical spine is a matter of debate.[9-12] The initial weight for traction typically has been stated as 5 lb/vertebra to the level of injury. Some centers limit the total weight to 10 lb/vertebra. For example, a bilaterally locked facet at C5-C6 is limited to 50 pounds. Other centers, including our own, have used weights of up to two thirds of the patient's body weight with success and without significant complication.[10,12] Others have used up to 140 lb without any complications.[12] Distraction is the commonest untoward result in closed reduction. Most often, distraction is not a complication, however, because some degree of distraction is required to reduce the jumped facet, and immediate reduction in weight usually reverses the distraction.

Radiologic guidance should be employed when closed reduction of the spine is attempted.[9-12] As much of the cervical spine as possible should be imaged during the reduction procedure; maximum imaging reduces the potential distraction of an unrecognized injury. Evidence of distraction, particularly when heavier weights are used, must be identified as soon as possible. In most instances, standard plain film radiography is technically acceptable, but it may have some significant disadvantages. The first disadvantage is the additional radiation exposure. When a total of 100 lb is used in 5-lb increments, with corresponding standard radiographs, up to 30 films can be taken. (With judicious use of fluoroscopy, however, the amount of radiation is diminished by nearly half.) The second disadvantage is the increased time and personnel required to perform standard radiography; an x-ray technician is not always available for a sequence of reduction films with each increase in weight. If the institution is busy when a patient with a cervical spine subluxation arrives, the amount of time between films and the total time of the reduction procedure is greatly increased. With the evidence that functional recovery may depend on rapid reduction, prolonged reductions requiring 8 and 12 hours are not consistent with diminution of further damage. Before the advent of closed reduction, when fluoroscopic guidance under neurosurgical control was used, longer reduction procedures were common. Presently, each 5-lb increase in weight is imaged. The endpoints of increasing weight are as follows:

1. Successful reduction, which is followed by a prompt decrease in weight, particularly in cases of high weight applied for bilaterally locked facets. A postreduction maintenance weight for spine injury is typically 20 to 25 lb.

2. New or increased neck pain, or evidence of a worsening deficit.

3. Unsuccessful reduction at weights of up to two thirds of the body weight.

4. Exceeding a 4-hour limit for reduction.

In cases of unsuccessful reduction, the weights are reduced to one third of the attempted weight, and muscle relaxants, typically diazepam, are administered.[11] Because diazepam is a respiratory depressant when given at higher doses, it must be used with caution in patients who have pulmonary compromise as a result of the loss of their intercostal muscle function. The sequence of increasing weight is then repeated to two thirds of the body weight.

If the reduction procedure is still unsuccessful, progression to medical paralysis after elective awake intubation is an option for the patient with a complete neurologic deficit.[10] This procedure is performed after the weight is reduced—usually to approximately 25 lb. The drawbacks to performing reductions under medical paralysis are the potential complications of the intubation and mechanical ventilation, as well as the loss of the patient's response (i.e., pain) to the reduction or to the worsening clinical status. For these reasons, intubation-paralysis is reserved for the functionally transected patient.

The 4-hour time limit for reduction is self-imposed: in our experience, rapid reduction with the aid of fluoroscopy has improved the functional recovery in a small number of completely paralyzed patients. In the best scenario, the 4-hour time limit includes the total time elapsed from the time of injury. Delays in patient transfer significantly limit reduction attempts within an hour from the time of arrival. If all attempts at closed reduction are unsuccessful, expedient preparations should be made for open reduction and fusion.

A study of a recent Maryland Institute for Emergency Medical Services Systems series of patients who underwent closed reduction within 4 hours of injury or had open reduction revealed that three patients (10 percent) who had clinically complete cervical spinal cord defects with associated physiologic parameters of spinal shock (including hypotension, bradycardia, and priapism) improved to a functional level after the procedure. A significantly larger number who had a complete motor deficit and some sensory sparing (without the associated physiologic parameters of spinal shock) also regained a functional status, and some patients even improved during the actual reduction.[10, 12]

CARDIOVASCULAR CONSIDERATIONS

Acute hypotension can result from cervical spinal cord injury, and experimental models demonstrate that elevating the blood pressure improves spinal cord blood flow and improves outcome.[13] The "sympathectomy" response and autonomic imbalance that occurs during the acute phase that follows spinal cord injury is generally thought to parallel the signs of complete neurologic injury in the cervical cord. The pulmonary vasculature response is altered in spinal cord injury. Patients with a complete spinal cord injury manifest a reduced response to conventional volume challenge within the pulmonary vasculature: data from our institute show an intense reduction of the peripheral vascular resistance, supporting the hypothesis that the pulmonary vascular bed is very sensitive to the sympathectomizing effect of an acute complete cervical cord injury.

Rapid restoration of cardiac output and tissue perfusion is necessary during the acute phase of spinal cord injury.[14] Because proper fluid resuscitation may be complicated by overload, invasive patient monitoring is necessary. Aggressive hemodynamic monitoring includes pulmonary and peripheral arterial catheters. Pulmonary artery monitoring optimizes tissue perfusion by manipulating cardiac output and vascular reactivity.

On our service, all patients receive invasive monitoring through arterial and Swan-Ganz pulmonary artery catheters. The hemodynamic profile of the patient is recorded immediately after placement of the invasive lines, and other measurements are taken every 12 hours thereafter. Cardiac index is determined at the bedside by the thermodilution method. The initial goal of replacement therapy, which uses balanced salt solution, is a mean arterial blood pressure above 90 mm Hg. Parameters from the hemodynamic profile are assessed to prevent further deterioration of the cardiac output and to maintain adequate oxygen consumption and delivery.

Optimum cardiac output is determined at the point which the oxygen consumption plateaus in the face of rising oxygen delivery (and paralleled rising cardiac output). We achieve optimal cardiac output by both fluid and vasoactive agent administration. Because constant measurement of cardiac output (and hence oxygen delivery) and extraction is not feasible, optimal perfusion is arbitrarily set at a mean arterial pressure of at least 90 mm Hg. This value is calculated with the pulmonary artery catheter measurements and adjusted when other mean arterial pressure values correlate with optimum perfusion.

Dopamine and dobutamine are the most commonly used agents for altering vascular reactivity in spinal cord injury. Recently, dopamine receptor activity has been found in the pulmonary vascular tree, and early reports suggest that these agents may favorably affect the intrapulmonary shunting seen in spinal cord injury. Although most patients respond to dopamine, or dobutamine, or both, some require the use of phenylephrine (Neo-Synephrine). Tachycardia, which can result from the higher levels of dopamine and dobutamine occasionally required for the additional vasoconstrictive effect necessary to maintain optimal perfusion, is one indication for the use of phenylephrine. Phenylephrine may be the more physiologically correct agent to use in neurogenic shock, particularly in young, healthy patients: it is an exclusive alpha agent that returns vascular tone. The argument against the use of phenylephrine is based on its unbalanced effect on the cardiovascular system and the difficulty in titrating the desired systemic vascular resistance. Also, phenylephrine does not affect associated bradycardia and may adversely affect cardiac function by increasing outflow resistance in patients with underlying cardiac disease. Concomitant low-dose dopamine should be used with phenylephrine as a precaution against renal ischemia. On our service, dopamine was used in low doses (2 to 10 mg/kg/min) for a mean duration of 5.3 days and at a mean dose of 6.0 mg/kg/min. Dobutamine was used in a dose of 2 to 10 mg/kg/min for a mean duration of 5.7 days and at a mean dose of 5.4 mg/kg/min.

Epinephrine, like dopamine and dobutamine, has a balanced effect on the cardiovascular system; like phenylephrine, however, it has a small therapeutic window, which complicates the cardiovascular manipulation and limits its therapeutic index, particularly in the elderly or in those with underlying heart disease.

We set the duration of hemodynamic manipulation at 5 days, based on edema formation peaking 48 to 72 hours after the injury: 5 days of therapy allow a 48-hour margin beyond this peak. Patients with more labile responses to vasoactive stimulation may require longer courses of therapy while being weaned off hemodynamic support.

We consider early surgery a second insult to the spinal cord and thus extend hemodynamic manipulation of the patient for an additional 4 to 5 days postoperatively. The possibility of neurologic regression in the face of tapering vasoactive agents is another reason to extend the length of therapy. Orthostatic hypotension, which normally is self-limiting, occurring in the subacute and rehabilitation phases, is treated with thromboembolic disease hose, Ace leg wraps, or some other compressive stocking and, occasionally, with fluid boluses.

COEXISTENT BLUNT TRAUMA

The early treatment of patients who sustain a combination of blunt trauma and cervical spinal cord injury presents a unique challenge. Time-consuming diagnostic tests are often performed in lieu of a careful physical examination to determine if the etiology of hemodynamic instability is hemorrhage or spinal cord injury-induced sympathectomy. The incidence of blunt intra-abdominal trauma in patients with cervical cord injury is low (7.6 percent), and in only 1.43 percent of cases (five of 350 patients) did these patients require surgical repair to stop the hemorrhage.[15] Our experience thus suggests that intra-abdominal injury as the cause of hemorrhagic shock is rarely seen in patients who suffer blunt trauma to the cervical cord, and when it is present, it results from a major injury, such as pelvic-ring disruption, femoral fracture and dislocation, intrathoracic injury, and abdominal wall injury.[15] For patients without these associated injuries but with clinical signs of spinal shock, invasive diagnostic tests, such as diagnostic peritoneal lavage, needlessly delay appropriate management.[15]

DIAGNOSTIC IMAGING OF THE CERVICAL SPINE

Imaging of the injured cervical spine has significantly evolved over the years as a result of the advent of newer technology. These different techniques are complementary, and their discriminate use is cost effective.

PLAIN FILMS

Indications for cervical spine radiographs have generally included the following: a significant mechanism of injury, an unreliable history or an altered mental status, complaint of neck pain or neurologic symptoms, and a positive physical examination, including pain on palpation of the neck and neurologic signs.[16, 17] Recently, the criteria for obtaining cervical spine radiographs have been criticized as expensive and of low yield, and for causing unnecessary radiation exposure to the patient.[18] The need for balancing cost effectiveness and the risk of missing a cervical spine fracture has been recently stressed.[19] A high index of suspicion should be maintained (especially in high-risk patients) and cervical spine roentgenograms should be performed to prevent the oversight of an unstable, occult cervical spine fracture.[19]

The cross-table, horizontal, lateral-view x-ray study should be initially performed to exclude a fracture or significant soft tissue injury. A high-quality, lateral cervical spine radiograph can be accurate in 70 to 90 percent of cases.[20, 21] The next radiograph to be taken is the cervical anteroposterior view. In a cooperative patient, visualization of the atlantoaxial articulation is obtained with the opened-mouth odontoid view. Although the sensitivity and accuracy of each view alone is inadequate, the sensitivity of the cervical spine series has been estimated at 93 percent and the accuracy at 84 percent in diagnosing fracture dislocations.[20] An oblique view best depicts the uncinate processes, pedicles, inferior and superior facets, and laminae. The C7-T1 relationship may be determined in this view and may negate the need for a swimmer's view.[22] Lateral flexion-extension views are important to assess the integrity of the ligaments in the cooperative patient.

COMPUTED TOMOGRAPHY

The use of contiguous or overlapping thin sections with reformatting in different planes greatly increases our ability to demonstrate subtle fractures and intraspinal pathology not detected by plain radiographs (Fig. 148–1A and B).[23] Posterior arch fractures (Fig. 148–2), fractures and subluxations of the articular facets (Fig. 148–3), C1 and C2 fractures (Fig. 148–4), and intraspinal bone fragments (Fig. 148–5) are best visualized by computed tomography (CT). CT is also very useful for the visualization of the craniocervical and cervicothoracic junctions.

MAGNETIC RESONANCE IMAGING

At our institution, the cervical spine MRI is performed with a Siemens 1.5-T magnet scanner (Siemens Medical Sys-

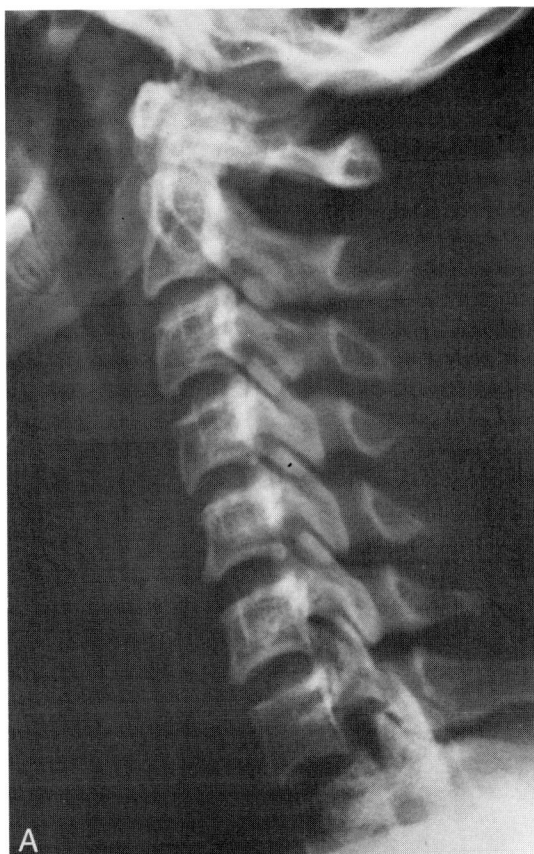
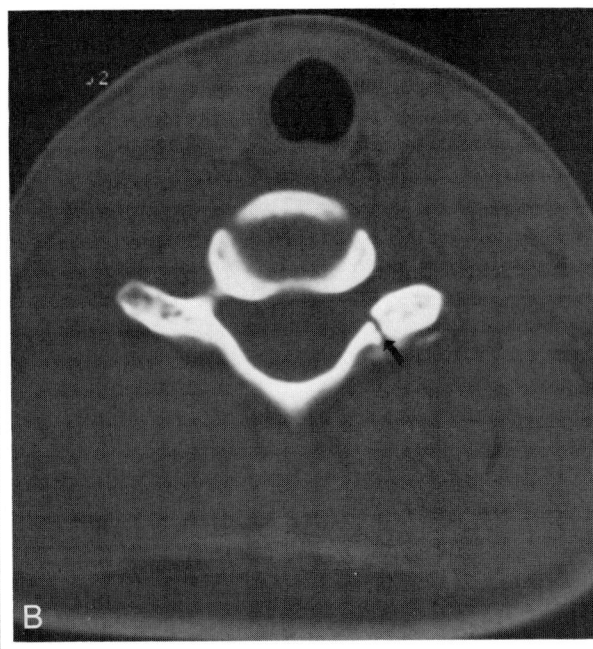

FIGURE 148–1. CT detection of subtle cervical spine fracture. (A) This lateral cervical spine radiograph obtained in a trauma patient with lower cervical pain is normal. (B) A C7 left laminar-articular mass junction fracture is detected by CT (arrow).

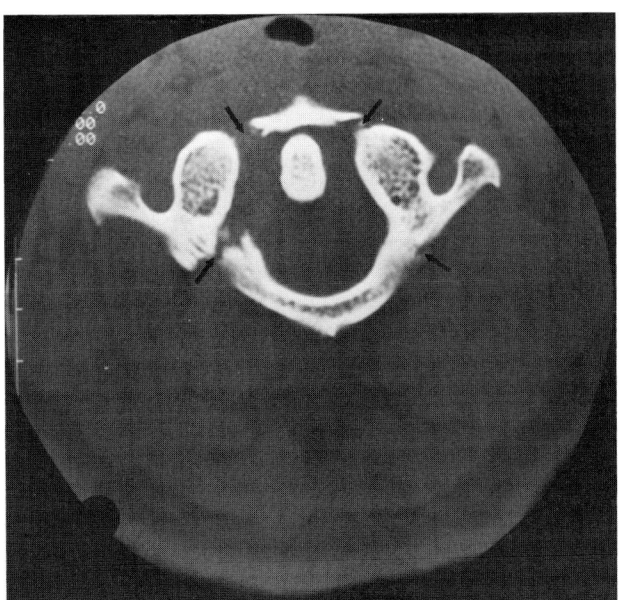

FIGURE 148–2. CT of a Jefferson fracture. Axial image reveals four-part fracture of C1 ring (arrows). Usually, anterior arch fractures are not seen by radiography.

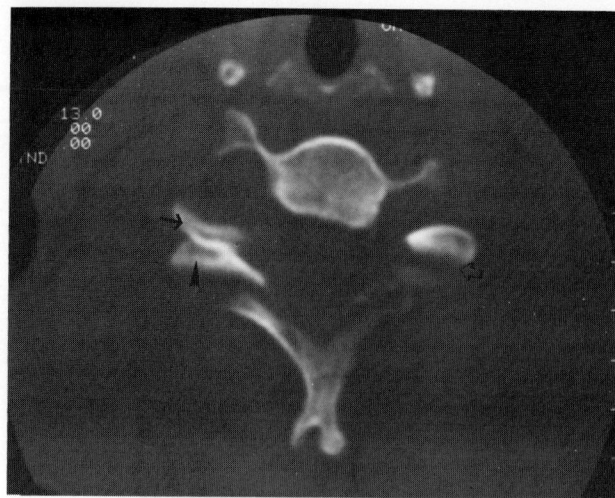

FIGURE 148–3. CT of unilateral facet fracture. Axial image reveals dislocation of right inferior facet (arrow) anterior to superior facet (arrowhead) of the vertebral body below. Note diastasis of contralateral left facetal joint (open arrow) and rotation of vertebral body.

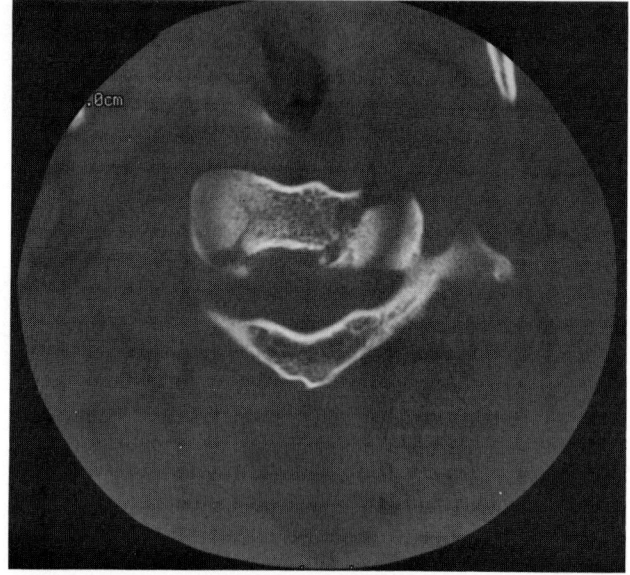

FIGURE 148–4. CT of type III odontoid fracture. Axial image reveals comminution of C2 body and narrowing of spinal canal due to anterior displacement of C1 secondary to transverse alar ligament injury.

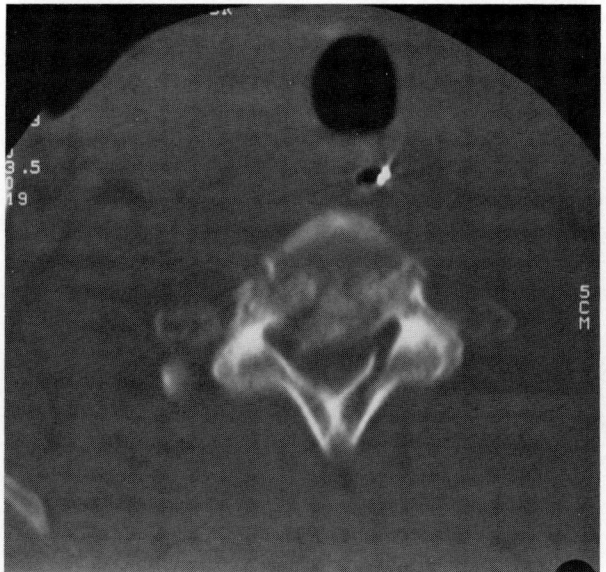

FIGURE 148–5. CT of vertebral burst fracture. Axial image shows markedly retropulsed posterior fragment from the C7 vertebral body encroaching on the spinal canal. A left lamina fracture is also seen.

tems, Iselin, NJ) or a General Electric 1.5 Signa system (General Electric Medical Systems, Milwaukee, WI). Our current MRI protocol performed on the General Electric Signa system includes the following sequences: (1) T1-weighted spin-echo sagittal images, (2) fast spin-echo T2-weighted sagittal images with fat suppression, (3) gradient echo (small flip angle of 10 to 15 degrees) sagittal images, (4) three-dimensional gradient echo volumetric axial images, and (5) T1-weighted spin-echo axial images. This examination requires 25 to 30 minutes to perform, and most patients are immobilized in a rigid collar (Philadelphia Collar Company, Westville, NJ) with plastic fasteners for the MRI.[24, 25]

Two cervical immobilization devices that permit acceptable MR image quality include a PMT halo cervical orthosis (PMT Corporation, Chanhassen, MN) and an MR-compatible Bremer halo system (Bremer Medical Corporation, Jacksonville, FL).

When cervical traction immobilization is required to maintain reduction, in-line cervical traction can be achieved with either MRI-compatible graphite tongs and a series of nonferrous pulley and water bags or a Sokhoff board and plastic traction weights. Ventilatory support, if required, is provided by a Siemens SY-900 servo ventilator (Siemens-Elema, Iselin, NJ) placed at least 1.2 m from the magnet. A 12-foot, low-compliance pediatric circuit connects the ventilator to the patient's endotracheal tube. This system provides all standard modes of respiratory support without detectable deterioration in image quality.[24]

Although information derived from plain radiographs and CT is usually sufficient to plan appropriate surgical or non-surgical management, in our institution, MRI is performed on any patient with incomplete neurologic deficit after cervical cord injury, provided that the patient is hemodynamically stable and has no contraindication to an MRI examination.

MRI can best assess whether the spinal cord is being compressed before attempts at reduction of cervical spine, and it is also used to detect root compression or avulsion within the intervertebral foramen. MRI also is used to clarify if a mechanical basis can explain a delayed increase of neurologic deficit, or in cases in which a level of deficit does not correlate with the level of injury of the osseous spine.

The limitations of plain roentgenograms and CT become particularly obvious in the patient with clinical evidence of spinal cord injury and no evidence of bone injury on either the plain radiographs or on the CT scan of the neck.[26, 27]

Compression of the cervical spinal cord may result from epidural hematomas (Fig. 148–6), dislocated vertebrae, displaced fragments (Fig. 148–7), osteophytes, or ossification of the posterior longitudinal ligament. Fracture-dislocations are underdiagnosed by MRI, when compared with CT, in up to 50 percent of cases;[28] however, disc protrusions are more easily recognized by MRI than by CT (Fig. 148–8). In a series of 33 patients studied with both modalities, only 27 percent of disc protrusions seen on MRI were visualized by CT.[28] Epidural hematomas may develop acutely after trauma, in a delayed fashion, or after open or closed reduction of the spinal column (Fig. 148–6). The MRI appearance of a hematoma changes over time—an acute hematoma will have a low signal on T2-weighted images because of intracellular deoxyhemoglobin and will have a progressively increasing signal on T1-weighted images, as extracellular methemoglobin content increases.

Even more dramatic is the difference between the abilities of CT and MRI to recognize direct cord injury (Fig. 148–9A and B and Fig. 148–10): In one study, MRI could identify such changes in 13 cases of cord injuries, compared with none visualized on CT.[28] MRI has proved particularly useful in demonstrating the structural changes associated with an acute central cord syndrome. In this situation, a hyperintense signal is seen within the parenchyma of the cervical spinal cord on gradient echo MRI without features characteristic of

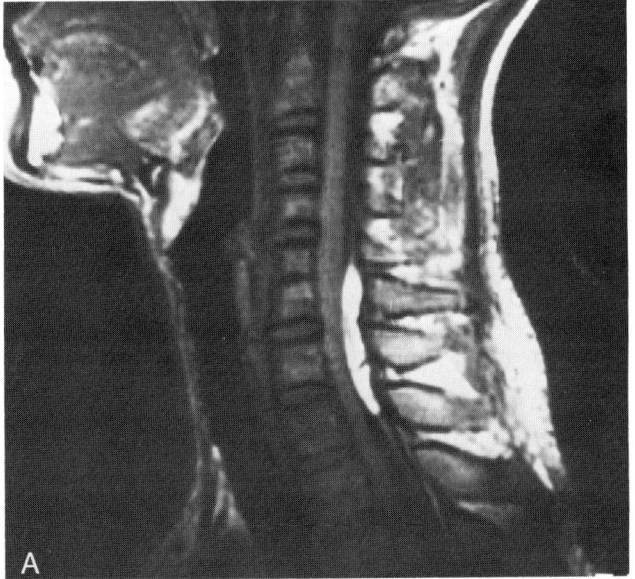 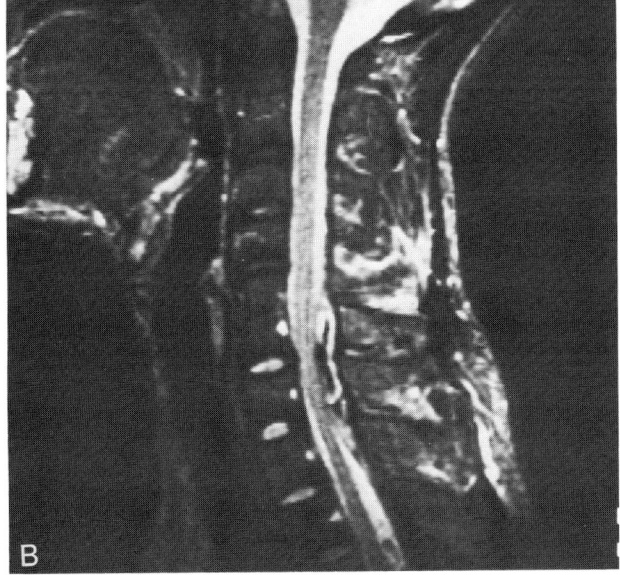

FIGURE 148–6. MRI of epidural hematoma. (A) T1-weighted MR image shows high signal intensity in the posterior epidural space at C5 to C7 level. The spinal cord is compressed. (B) T2-weighted sequence shows a low signal center compatible with intracellular hemoglobin, with bright surrounding area compatible with extracellular methemoglobin. (Reprinted with permission from Mirvis SE, Young JWR: Cervical spine trauma, in Mirvis SE, Young JWR (eds): Imaging in Trauma and Critical Care. Baltimore, Williams & Wilkins, 1992, pp 291–379.)

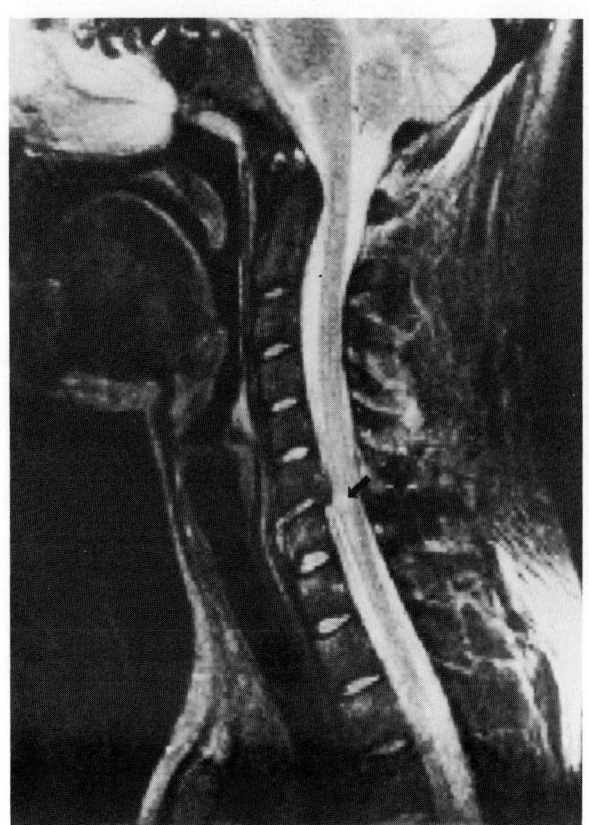

FIGURE 148-7. MRI of cord compression. Sagittal T2-weighted image shows retropulsion of posterior bone fragment from C6 impacting the cord. A contusion (bright signal) is observed in the cord adjacent to the fragment (arrow). The C6-7 intervertebral disc is extruded anteriorly. Titanium posterior fixation allows follow-up MR imaging without significant artifact. (Reprinted with permission from Mirvis SE, Young JWR: Cervical spine trauma, in Mirvis SE, Young JWR (eds): Imaging in Trauma and Critical Care. Baltimore, Williams & Wilkins, 1992, pp 291–379.)

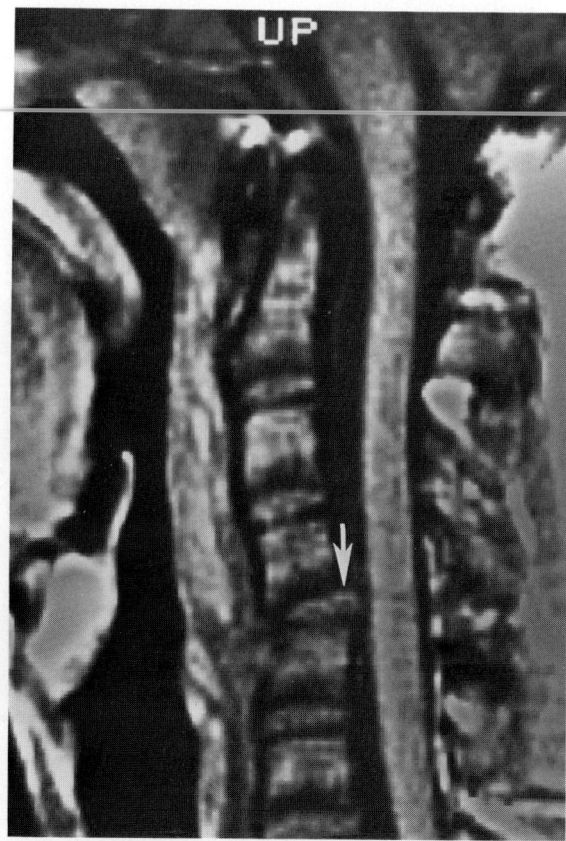

FIGURE 148-8. MRI of traumatic disc herniation. Sagittal T1-weighted image shows hyperflexion sprain at C4-5 with herniation of intervertebral disc (white arrow) at this level. The cord is not indented by the disc. (Reprinted with permission from Mirvis SE, Young JWR: Cervical spine trauma, in Mirvis SE, Young JWR (eds): Imaging in Trauma and Critical Care. Baltimore, Williams & Wilkins, 1992, pp 291–379.)

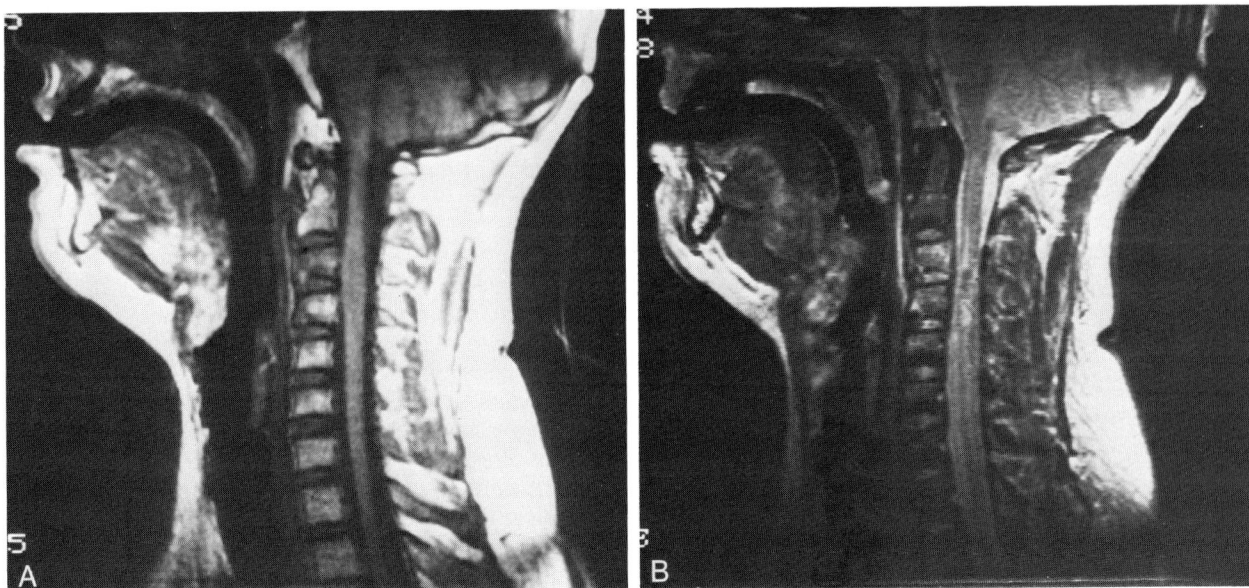

FIGURE 148-9. MRI of cord contusion. (A) Sagittal T1-weighted image in quadriplegia patient after blunt trauma reveals some widening of the spinal cord at C3 and C4. There is a C3 anterior compression fracture. (B) On the T2-weighted sequence, there is a bright signal at C3-4, with a central low signal suggestive of central blood and surrounding edema. C3 and C4 compression fractures are observed.

hemorrhage in either T1- or T2-weighted images. Pathologic correlation in necropsy specimens showed no evidence of blood within the cord parenchyma, but diffuse disruption of axons, especially within the lateral columns in the region occupied by the corticospinal tracts.[29] However, that more severe trauma is likely to be accompanied by tissue destruction, mostly in the anterior horn area.[30]

The ability of MRI to directly image the spinal cord not only makes it a more sensitive diagnostic test but theoretically could provide important prognostic clues in the early phases of treatment. Initial limited studies at the University of Texas and at the University of Maryland suggest that MRI information obtained in the acute period can provide information on the potential for recovery of neurologic function.[31, 32] In this study, three different MRI patterns existed in 57 patients with acute cervical spine injuries and were associated with a major neurologic deficit: (1) intramedullary hematoma, (2) intramedullary edema over more than one spinal segment without hemorrhage, and (3) intramedullary edema involving one spinal segment or less.[33] Not unexpectedly, patients with intramedullary hematomas had motor scores at admission that were significantly lower than those of the other two groups and significantly lower motor recovery rates than the other two groups (9 percent versus 41 percent and 72 percent, respectively).[33] This study is important because it shows that the MRI pattern observed in the acute phase after injury is prognostically important and also because it provides a basis for the homogeneous grouping of patients undergoing different treatment protocols.

MRI is also useful in the demonstration of ligament injuries, which helps in establishing the mechanism of trauma in the course of evaluating damage to the spinal cord.[34] MRI demonstrates ligaments as regions of low signal intensity. Injured ligaments manifest increased signal on T2-weighted sequences because of edema, and disrupted ligaments demonstrate a discontinuity in the normal continuous low signal intensity of the ligament (Figs. 148-11 and 148-12).

Cervical vascular injury may accompany blunt force injury to the neck. This type of injury can result in overstretching, excessive torsion, direct impact, or laceration of the major arteries, which can result in the absence of a flow void (spin echo) or of increased signal (gradient echo), indicating a vascular injury. More recently, MR angiography has been applied to the diagnosis of cervical vascular injuries (Fig. 148-13A to C).

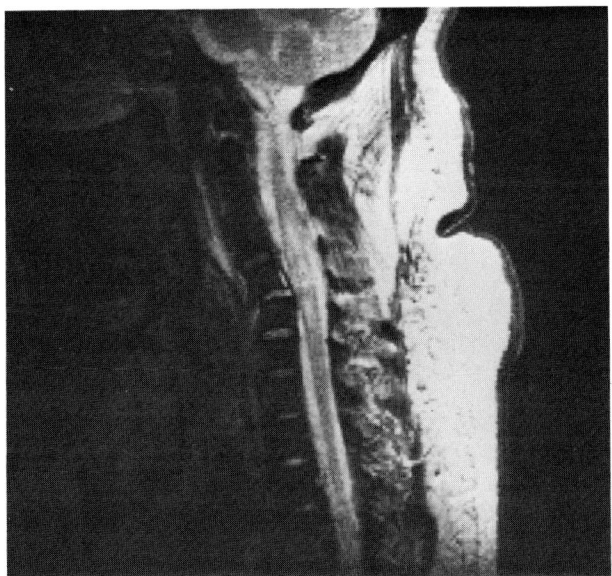

FIGURE 148-10. MRI of cord contusion. Sagittal T2-weighted image obtained in quadriplegic patient shows C4 on C5 anterior subluxation with stripping of the posterior longitudinal ligament from C3. A spindle-shaped region of increased signal spreads distally from the impact site indicating edema. (Reprinted with permission from Mirvis SE, Young JWR: Cervical spine trauma, in Mirvis SE, Young JWR (eds): Imaging in Trauma and Critical Care. Baltimore, Williams & Wilkins, 1992, pp 291-379.)

1840 | *Surgery of the Craniovertebral Junction and Spine*

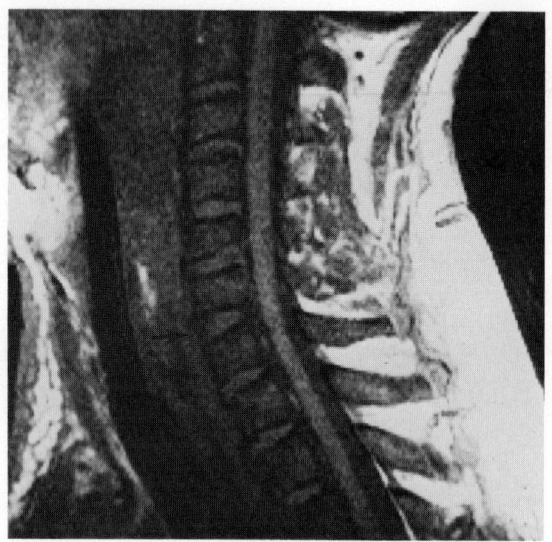

FIGURE 148–11. MRI of ligament disruption. Sagittal image shows loss of low signal stripe at C6-7 (arrow) and widening of corresponding anterior disc space. The finding is compatible with hyperextension injury with anterior longitudinal ligament and anterior annulus fibrosis injury. (Reprinted with permission from Mirvis SE, Young JWR: Cervical spine trauma, in Mirvis SE, Young JWR (eds): Imaging in Trauma and Critical Care. Baltimore, Williams & Wilkins, 1992, pp 291–379.)

THERAPY

The knowledge that an injury triggers a chain of events at the cellular level of the spinal cord is fundamental to sound pharmacologic management. Even after realignment of a dislocated spine, spinal cord compression may persist and be deleterious, possibly because of increased vascular permeability to albumin in the acute and chronic phases of spinal cord compression, or because of the effects of direct physical injury to neural membranes.

HYPOTENSION. Spinal cord function is profoundly affected by hemodynamic changes that follow spinal cord injury and may compound the effect of the initial injury.

ISCHEMIA. A decrease in spinal cord blood flow and ischemia develop soon after injury, adding to the deleterious effect of compression.

Ischemia also leads to mitochondria dysfunction, lysosomal accumulation, membrane lipid perioxidation, and free radical production. Because of the loss of autoregulation and the eventual loss of tissue oxygen tension, the initial ischemia does not trigger any protective response, which further impairs cord metabolism.

PHARMACOLOGIC TREATMENT

The goal of medical treatment in acute spinal cord injury is to restore adequate spinal cord perfusion and oxygenation. This effect is accomplished by providing adequate volume replacement, atropine to treat bradycardia, and vasopressors to support the blood pressure if fluid resuscitation alone does not restore adequate tissue perfusion.

The degree of bradycardia occurring after cord injury may be aggravated by hypoxia and tracheal suctioning, which may trigger a vagal response not balanced by any sympathetic reflex.

Early preventive treatment of gastric dilatation is also useful in the prevention of acute hypoxia resulting from poor ventilation or delayed hypoxia occurring after aspiration or sepsis.

Corticosteroids remain the cornerstone in the current medical treatment of acute spinal cord trauma. The National Acute Spinal Cord Injury Study, or NASCIS-1, did not demonstrate a statistically significant difference in the rates of neurologic recovery between naloxone- and methylprednisolone-treated groups of patients; however, other data from animal studies suggested that the dose of methylprednisolone used in the NASCIS-1 study was below the theoretical therapeutic threshold. The NASCIS-2 study was undertaken to study the effects of higher doses of methylprednisolone, and this study demonstrated that patients with acute spinal cord injury treated with methylprednisolone at higher doses have a better neurologic recovery than the control group if treated within the first 8 hours after the injury.[35] The 1-year follow-up study of NASCIS-2 confirmed that improvements in patients treated with high-dose methylprednisolone continued at 1 year.[36] The NASCIS-2 trial raises a considerable degree of skepticism about the value of naloxone in the management of acute spinal cord injury and shows that frequently, encouraging results from animal data cannot be translated to humans.

Thyrotropin-releasing hormone improves neurologic outcome in experimental studies of cervical cord injury,[37] but no

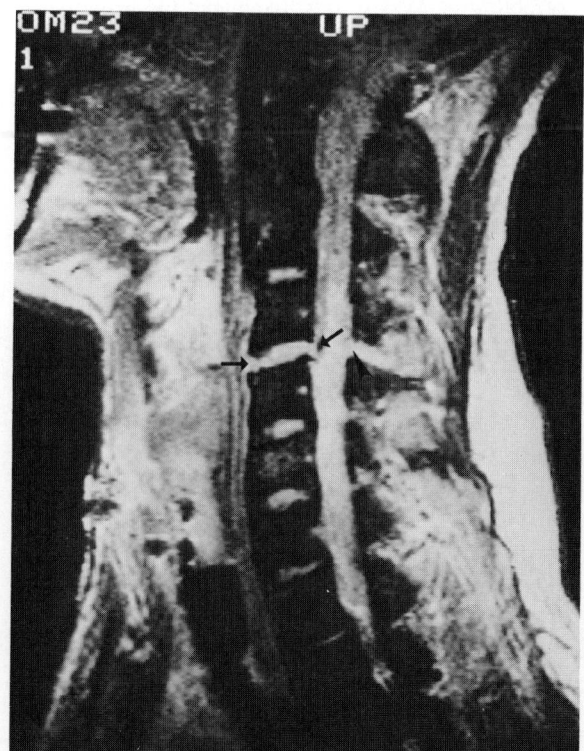

FIGURE 148–12. MRI of ligament injury. Sagittal T2-weighted gradient echo image in acutely quadriplegic patient shows complete disruption of the anterior and posterior longitudinal ligaments (arrows) as well as the posterior ligamentum flavum (arrowhead).

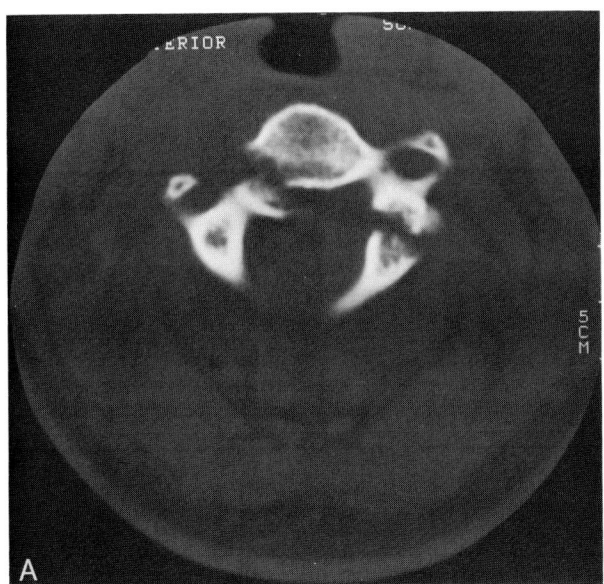
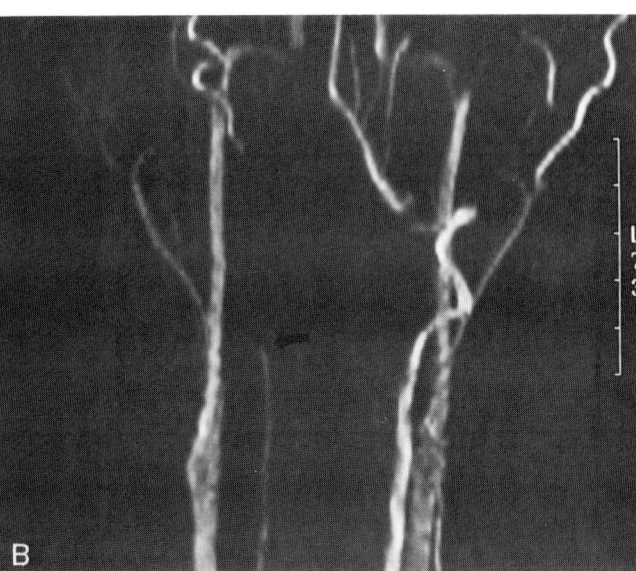
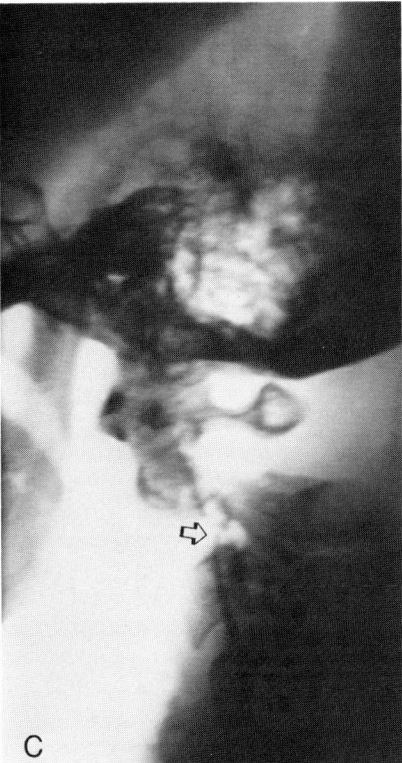

FIGURE 148-13. MR angiogram of cervical vascular injury. (A) Axial CT image shows a Hangman type fracture at C2 extending into the right vertebral artery foramen. (B) MR angiogram (two dimensional, time-of-flight) shows complete occlusion of the right vertebral artery (arrow) at the C2 level. (C) Lateral view of the neck from digital arteriogram confirms complete interruption of the vessel just below the fracture site (open arrow). The patient remained asymptomatic.

proof exists of its efficacy in humans in clinical trials.[13] Recently, gangliosides have been reported to enhance functional recovery of damaged neurons in animals. Gangliosides, present in high concentrations in central nervous system cells, form a major component of the cell membrane. A small study in humans that was recently published suggests that the use of gangliosides improves recovery of neurologic function after 1 year, and at present, a multicenter study is underway to confirm on a larger scale the efficacy of the new pharmacologic agent.[38]

USE OF ORTHOTIC DEVICES IN CERVICAL SPINE TRAUMA

Orthotic devices are used either as postoperative adjuncts, to reduce motion and promote the healing of disrupted osseous and ligamentous structures in the nonsurgical patient, or as a treatment for the pain of muscle spasm.[39]

The selection of an orthotic device depends on the degree of immobilization desired. A comparison of different types of orthosis was made by Johnson and coworkers:[40, 41] the cervical collar, the Philadelphia collar, the Yale brace, the sterno-occipitomandibular immobilization brace, and the halo vest were tested in flexion-extension and lateral bend as well as in axial rotation. This study concluded that the longer and stiffer devices offer more immobilization, and that the non-halo orthoses somewhat restrict flexion-extension and lateral bending but not rotation. The best, although by no means absolute, immobilization of the upper cervical spine is provided by the halo vest.[39] Immobilization of the lower cervical spine is not provided adequately by any one orthosis, including the halo.[39]

The soft collar provides minimal immobilization, and we limit its use to the treatment of pain caused by muscle spasm, after more serious osseous or ligamentous injuries have been ruled out. The Philadelphia collar provides more immobilization and support than the soft collar, especially in flexion-extension movement. We often use the Philadelphia collar in the early postoperative course, after internal fixation. The Yale brace is used as a postoperative adjunct after some fixation procedures and provides a better immobilization than the Philadelphia collar because it extends along the length of the sternum anteriorly and along the thoracic spine posteriorly.

The halo brace provides the most reliable control of motion, especially in the high cervical spine.[39] We use the halo brace extensively, especially in the nonoperative management of high cervical fractures. However, the halo vest does not prevent motion in either the normal or the injured spine. Lateral radiographs taken with the patient in the supine and upright positions have shown evidence of intervertebral motion. At the noninjured level, the degree of motion can amount to 3.9 degrees of angulation, with the greatest motion occurring between occiput and C1.[42] At the injured level, sagittal plane angulation can average 7.0 degrees, and translation can average 1.7 mm between the two positions.[42] This information is the basis for obtaining supine and upright radiographs of the cervical spine after the application of the halo device. Furthermore, any observation of excessive motion should immediately suggest that an alternative method of treatment be considered.

SURGERY

A cervical spine fracture-dislocation may be stabilized by various internal fixation techniques. The surgical approach (anterior, posterior, or combined) depends on the level of instability and the mechanism of injury. The goal of internal fixation is to immobilize the spine until a bony arthrodesis occurs,[43] to reduce the deformity, to restore a stable spine, and to achieve neural decompression. Operative intervention of the unstable spine has the advantage of

1. Providing the optimal mechanical environment for neurological recovery[10]
2. Facilitating early mobilization and avoiding the adverse effects of prolonged bed rest
3. Creating the opportunity for an earlier start of the rehabilitation process.

OCCIPITO–C1-C2 ARTHRODESIS. The ligamentous instability of the C1-C2 complex secondary to transverse ligament rupture may be corrected through either C1-C2 or occipital-C2 wiring and fusion, depending on the integrity of the arch of C1.[44–48] The primary indication for an occipital-cervical fusion is gross occipitoatlantal joint instability or atlantoaxial instability in the absence of a structurally deficient posterior atlantal arch (Fig. 148–14A and B). Occipital-atlantal instability is most often associated with trauma, and treatment is directed toward reduction and stabilization by external fixation, followed by internal arthrodesis. Several methods have been advocated, including placing a simple inlay of bone graft using corticocancellous bone placed between the occiput and C2, wiring cancellous bone to the posterior arch of the atlas, or wiring the second cervical vertebra to the adjacent occiput through an adjacent occipital burr hole. Other options include placing anatomically conforming occipitocervical loops fashioned from a Wisconsin or Luque rod or a large, threaded Steinmann pin with associated cancellous bone chips into the lateral gutters.[45, 49, 50] A standard 39-mm fragment T-plate bent backward at its head-shaft junction and sewed to the occiput and the spinous process of C2 by fixation screws has also been described.[51]

Fractures of the dens have been classified into three types: type I, involving the tip of the odontoid process, which in our experience is extremely uncommon; type II, which extends through the base of the odontoid process; and type III, which extends into the C2 body. Odontoid fractures are best visualized radiographically by a combination of the opened-mouth odontoid projection and the lateral projection. If nondisplaced, odontoid fractures may be difficult to appreciate by radiographs, and might require tomography or CT. When CT is used, axial images must be closely spaced in 1.5- or 2-mm sections to avoid volume averaging a fracture within the CT slice. A high incidence of nonunion has been described with type II odontoid fractures that reaches nearly 100 per cent when fractures remain displaced by more than 5 mm. Type III fractures occur through the C2 body and generally proceed to good fusion with immobilization. Because of the rarity of type I dens fractures, these injuries have been more recently divided into high (type II) and low (type III) fractures.

Numerous procedures have been described for atlantoaxial arthrodesis.[45, 46, 48, 50, 52, 53] We favor a tricortical iliac crest graft wedged between the laminae of C1-C2. By use of a

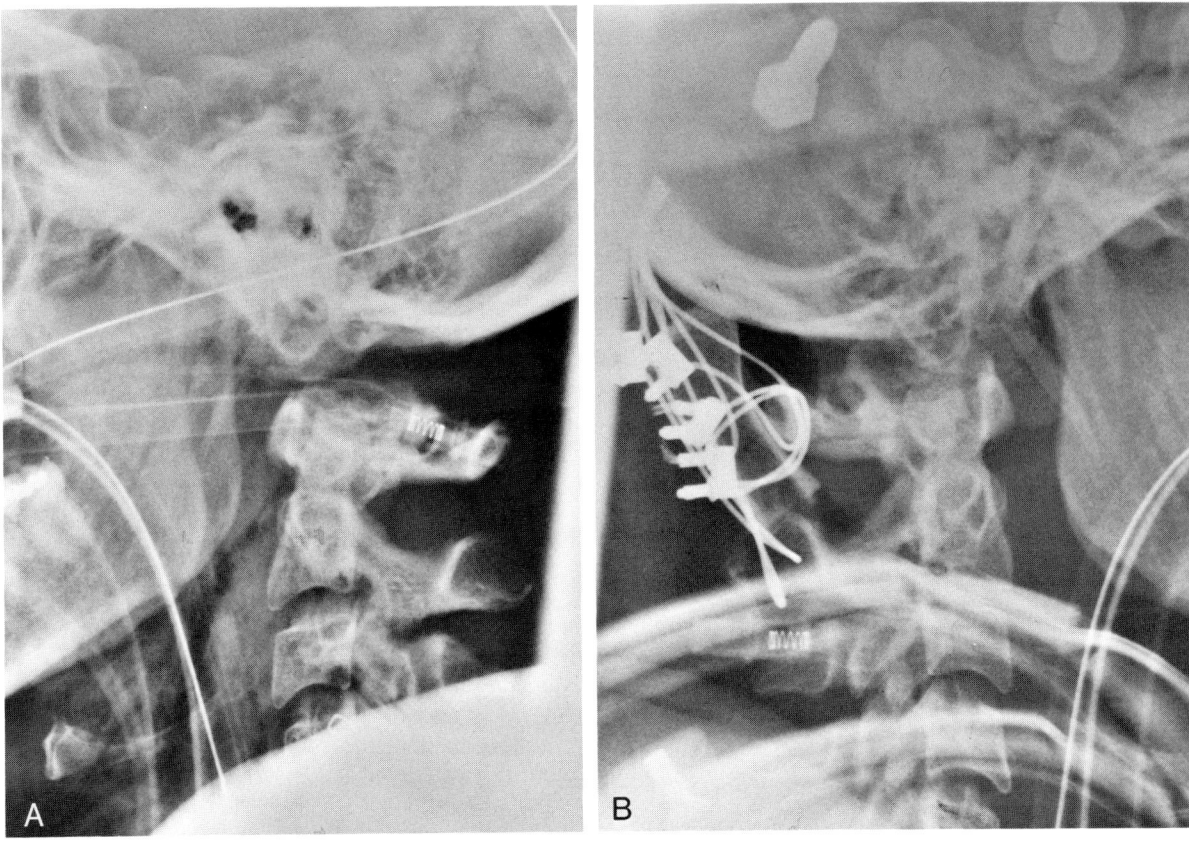

FIGURE 148–14. Atlanto-occipital fusion. (A) Lateral radiograph obtained in trauma patient reveals anterior dislocation of the occiput and disarticulation of the occipital condyles the atlas. (B) Tension band wiring and bone graft span from the occiput, through posterior C1, and into the C2 spinous process to obtain fixation.

flexible-cable system[48] threaded beneath the arch of C1 for lamina-to-spinous process fusions, the cable is then passed through or otherwise anchored to the strut graft (Fig. 148–15).

A posterior atlantoaxial facet screw fixation approach has been described[47, 54, 55] that allows for the placement of screws (3.5-mm diameter) through the C2 pedicle, across the C1-C2 facet, and into each lateral mass of the atlas. The atlas and axis become rigidly coupled, and when the articular surfaces of C1-C2 are prepared, a solid fusion across the facet joint is accomplished. Although some advocate an interspinous C1-C2 wiring and fusion,[46] a recent report provides evidence for a high degree of fusion without halo immobilization or C1-C2 interspinous wiring.

Anterior odontoid screw fixation is best reserved for the patient with an acute type II odontoid fracture, an intact transverse ligament, or a subluxation greater than 6 mm, or in patients in whom posterior fractures of the C1 ring or C2 spinous process preclude posterior fusions (Fig. 148–16A and B). Although numerous reasons have been given for an increased incidence of nonunion in type II odontoid fractures (including amount of displacement, direction of displacement, and patient age), the advantages of direct fixation are immediate stabilization, restoration of normal spine biomechanics, sparing of the normal rotation between C1 and C2, and no external arthrosis. The major limitations are the surgeon's inability to add bone graft to enhance fusion and the procedure's contraindication in transverse atlas ligament disruption.[44, 56, 57]

Anterior C1-C2, tranfacetal screw fixation is similar to odontoid screw fixation. Operative exposure is identical, and intraoperative C-arm fluoroscopic visualization is necessary in both the anteroposterior and lateral dimensions for the transfacetal approach, and the facet joints are decorticated with an angled curette to enhance fusion. The screws are placed into the C2 vertebral body in the groove between the body and the superior C2 facet. The angle of drilling is adjusted in a superolateral direction to allow for the passage of the drill through the lateral mass of C2, across the C1-C2 joint space, and into the lateral mass of C1. Either cortical or self-tapping cancellous screws may be used. Unlike a transodontoid screw, the technique sacrifices all motion of C1-C2.[54]

C3-T1 ARTHRODESIS. The anterior approach to the cervical spine has been advocated for the management of cervical spine injuries since 1961. Since that time, authors have advocated various anterior approaches to stabilize the cervical spine, including the use of metal plates and interbody fusions with the iliac crest bone grafts or fibular strut grafts.[58–65] Several anterior plating systems have been advocated[60–62] that use osteosynthetic metal plates and instrumentation designed specifically for this technique.

In the presence of anterior and posterior column injury,

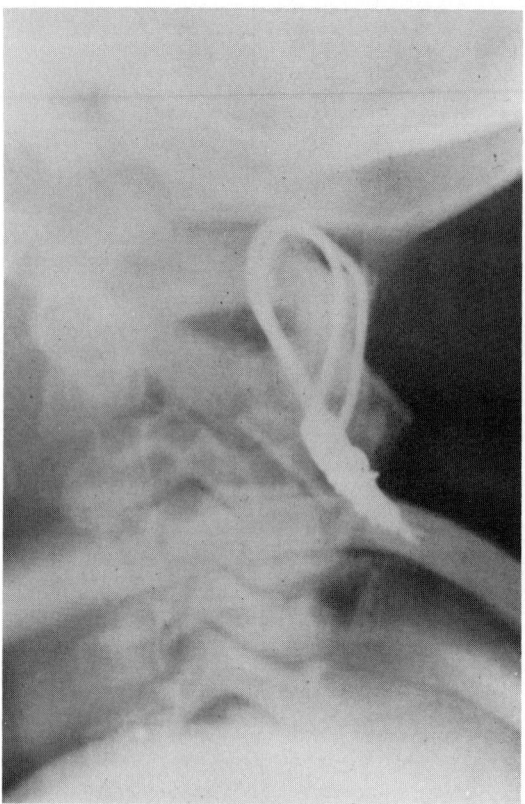

FIGURE 148–15. Lateral cervical radiograph showing C1-2 wire and bone graft posterior arthrodesis.

anterior fusion without internal fixation may result in bone graft displacement, angulation across the unstable motion segment, or resubluxation.[10, 66] Anterior plate fixation systems were developed to avoid such complications and to avoid the need for a combined anterior and posterior fusion or an anterior fusion followed by prolonged, external orthotic immobilization.

We believe that anterior plates are useful when vertebrectomies or discectomies are necessary to stabilize or decompress an unstable spine.[45, 54, 64, 67] These systems permit neural decompression and spinal fusion in a single-staged surgical procedure. We reserve the anterior approach for cases in which compromise of the canal anteriorly by bone or disk has been documented unequivocally along with posterior instability. Plating provides immediate stabilization, thus permitting the safe performance of all nursing maneuvers intended to reduce patient morbidity.[63, 64] It also provides early mobilization unencumbered by a halo vest.[58, 63–65, 68] By temporarily reducing micromobility and holding the bone graph under compression (without migration), bone healing is facilitated.

Many plating systems have been designed. The earlier anterior plating systems required bicortical engagement of the bone screws for optimal plate fixation; therefore, the use of intraoperative fluoroscopy was preferred during the placement of these plates to minimize the risk of injury to the dura and spinal cord. With such precautions, these early anterior fixation systems quite effectively stabilized the traumatized spine.[60, 63, 64]

A new addition to anterior plating systems is the MRI-compatible osteosynthesis plating system by Synthes (Waldenberg, Switzerland) (Fig. 148–17).[65, 69] We prefer this system to the Caspar system because it does not require bicortical engagement of the screws; therefore, it avoids potential complications to the spinal cord and the necessity of intraoperative fluoroscopy. The Synthes screws lock in a triangular fashion into a plate that resists pullout. The insertion of a second screw, a ''locking screw,'' into the head of the anchor screw expands the anchor screw head. The locking screw compresses the anchor screw against the plate hole and locks

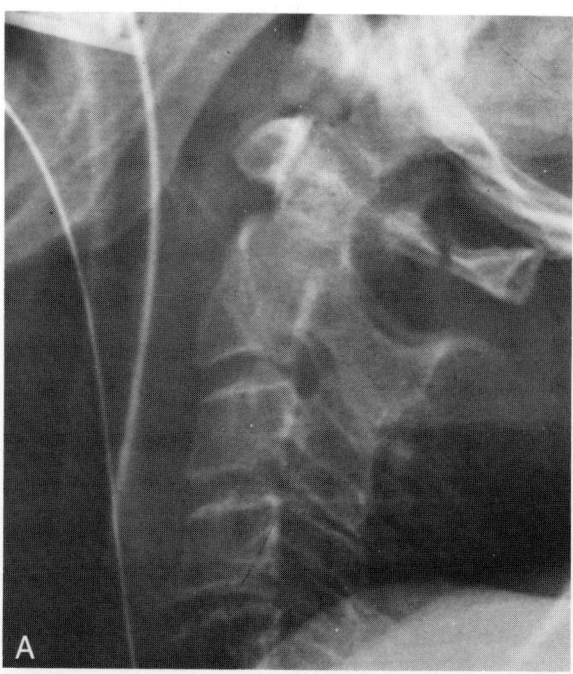
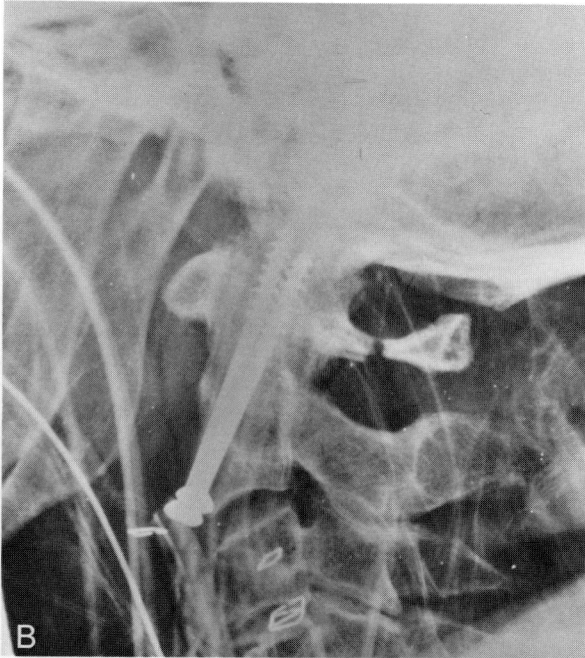

FIGURE 148–16. Anterior odontoid screw fixation. (A) Lateral cervical radiograph in trauma patient reveals a posteriorly displaced type III odontoid fracture and posterior C1 ring fracture. (B) Postoperative radiograph shows anterior odontoid screw placement fixating fracture.

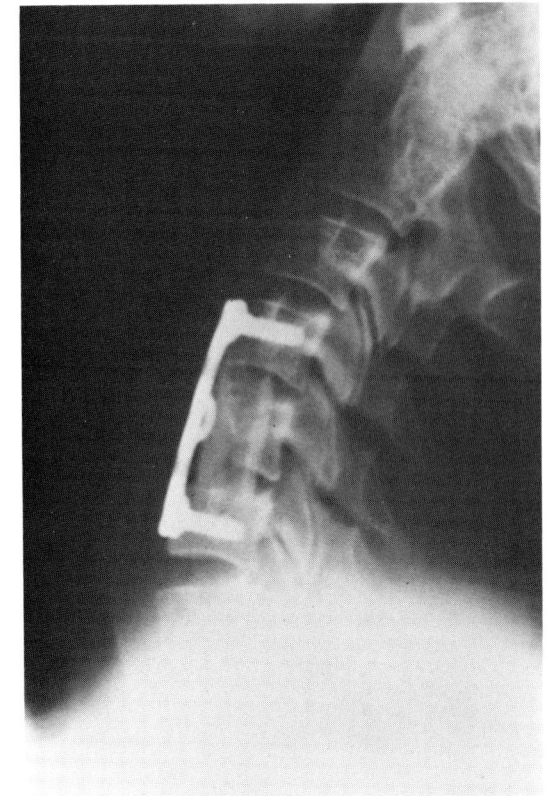

FIGURE 148–17. Synthes plate fixation. Postoperative study obtained with Synthes plate fixation anteriorly from C4 to C6 and interbody bone grafts in the intervertebral disc spaces.

the screws to the plate.[65] Like all anterior cervical operative procedures, recurrent laryngeal nerve injury, arterial injury, and esophageal injury are among the known complications, although they are rare.[54, 56, 63–65, 68, 70, 71]

With the rare exception of documented traumatic disc herniation, facet injuries should be approached posteriorly because the posterior ligamentous complex is disrupted by flexion, distraction, and rotational forces so that the only structure maintaining some integrity at this level is the anterior spinal ligamentous complex. Surgical intervention should not disrupt the intact structures and increase the instability and stress on a fixation construct.

Many surgical options are available for posterior stabilization,[8, 10, 46, 48, 52, 54, 59, 66, 72–75] but the interspinous process wiring and bone grafting approach proposed by Rogers in 1942 is the most commonly used.[66] We believe, however, that despite the fact that it provides adequate stabilization against translational forces, interspinous wiring alone does not provide stability against rotational forces. We prefer the bilateral facets-to-spinous process approach, with iliac bone graft fusion using a flexible-strand titanium cable system (Songer Cable System, Danek Medical, Memphis, TN) (Fig. 148–18).[48] We have found the technique to be very effective in stabilizing the cervical spine in bilateral-locked facets.[10] If one or both facets are disrupted, or if laminae or spinous processes are missing or incompetent, we prefer to use posterior cervical screw plates for the lateral masses (Fig. 148–19).[74, 75] A contoured universal bone plate system (AME, Dallas, TX) has been designed for lateral mass fixation to restore the normal lordotic curvature of the cervical spine. Indications for this plating system include cervical subluxation without fracture, postlaminectomy instability, bilaminar and spinous process fractures precluding use of cable, recurrence of subluxation, or angulation despite halo immobilization.[52]

Appropriate techniques must be employed to avoid injury to the vertebral artery and nerve root during bicortical penetration necessary to insure adequate screw fixation to the lateral masses. Caution should be used when lateral mass screws are placed in C7 because of the transitional morphology of this vertebra. The C7 facets and lateral masses are thin,[76] and posterior compression of adjacent nerve roots complicate their use.[76, 77] We advocate bone grafting into the facet joint at this level.

Interlaminar clamps (Halifax Clamp, Codman, Boston, MA) should be used for cervical subluxation secondary to posterior ligamentous injury with minimal or no posterior body element fracture,[52, 54] but they should probably not be used in the presence of significant vertebral body injury.

We do not advocate the use of sublaminar wiring to immobilize the cervical spine below C2. Because of the relatively small size of the canal in relation to the spinal cord, blindly passing wire under the laminae is hazardous, and in addition, when the wire is passed under three laminae, the wire tends to bow anteriorly, thereby compromising the neural canal and encroaching on the dura and spinal cord.[66] Operative manipulation and tension adjustment of the stainless steel wire used in such a fusion is often difficult, suboptimal, and subject to a degree of malleability. Although others have advocated the use of methyl methacrylate with combinations of Kirschner pins, wire mesh, and sublaminous wiring, we feel the disadvantages of acrylic (i.e., it does not bind to bone, it weakens with time, and it remains as a permanent foreign body) outweigh its benefits.[66]

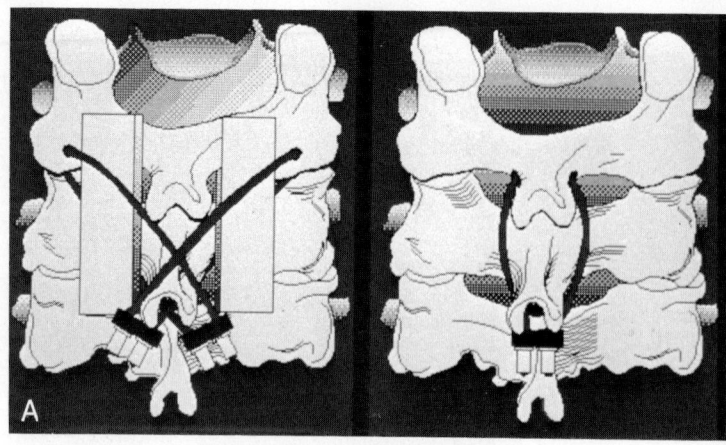

FIGURE 148–18. Facet to interspinous posterior fixation. (A) Schematic drawing of facet to spinous process with the iliac bone graft fusion and interspinous fusion. (B) Lateral radiograph showing combined facet to spinous process and interspinous wiring.

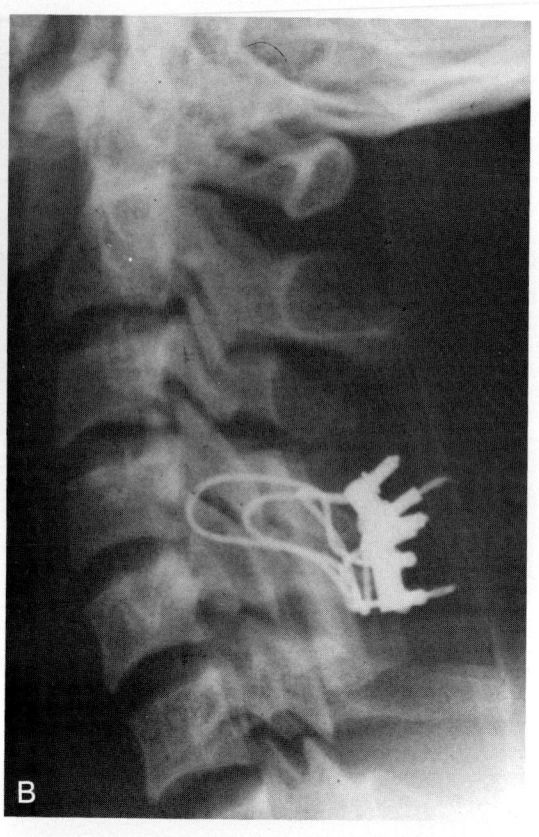

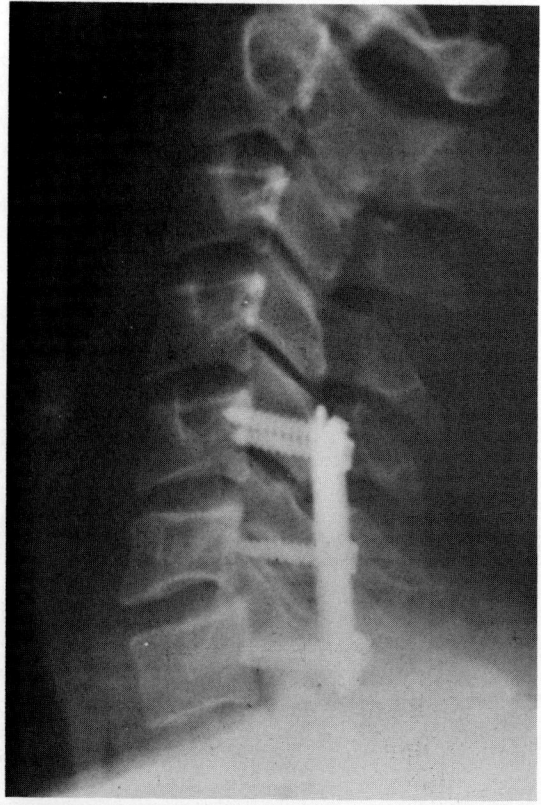

FIGURE 148–19. Posterior lateral mass fixation plating.

Unilateral facet injuries also are better treated by surgery: halo traction is inadequate for obtaining and maintaining anatomic reduction in unilateral facets injuries, nonanatomic reduction and cervical translation are associated with late pain and stiffness, and the best means for obtaining and maintaining anatomic reduction is operative intervention.[10] We think that surgical stabilization offers the best chance for prevention of late spinal instability and pain from pseudoarthrosis in bilateral facet dislocations as well.[10]

In spite of the improvements in management, the mortality rate during the first few months after a cervical spinal cord injury remains high—20 percent in some series. For patients who survive the early period after injury, the mortality is then relatively low. The life expectancy for a spinal cord injured patient is 30 to 40 years, and most deaths occurring during the acute phase result from respiratory problems, whereas those occurring in the chronic phase result from renal failure or factors unrelated to the injury, such as cardiovascular disease and cancer. The treatment of incomplete injuries, which occur in most patients, is far more rewarding because the degree of recovery can be as high as 70 percent of the lost neurologic function.

REFERENCES

1. DeVivo MJ, Fine PR, Maetz HM, Stover SL: Prevalence of spinal cord injury: A re-estimation employing life table techniques. Arch Neurol 37:707–708, 1980
2. Ryan MD, Henderson JJ: The epidemiology of fractures and fracture-dislocations of the cervical spine. Injury 23(1):38–40, 1992
3. Meyer PR, et al: Spinal cord injury. Neurol Clin 9(3):625–661, 1991
4. Wolf AL: Initial management of brain- and spinal-cord-injured patients. Emerg Med Serv 18(6):35–41, 1989
5. Marshall LF, Knowlton S, Garfin SR, et al: Deterioration following spinal cord injury. J Neurosurg 66:400–404, 1987
6. Levi L, Wolf A, Rigamonti D, et al: Anterior decompression in cervical spine trauma: Does the timing of surgery affect the outcome? Neurosurgery 29(2):216–222, 1991
7. Dunham CM, Cowley RA, Gens DR, et al: Methodologic approach for a large functional trauma registry. Md Med J 38:227–233, 1989
8. Hadley MN, Fitzpatrick BC, Sonntag VKH, Browner CM: Facet fracture-dislocation injuries of the cervical spine. Neurosurgery 30:661–666, 1992
9. Sabiston CP, Wing PC, Schweigel JF, et al: Close reductions of the lower cervical spine. J Trauma 28:832–835, 1988
10. Wolf A, Levi L, Mirvis S, et al: Operative management of bilateral facet dislocation. J Neurosurg 75:883–890, 1991
11. Star AM, Jones AA, Cotler JM, et al: Immediate closed reduction of cervical spine dislocations using traction. Spine 15:1068–1072, 1990
12. Cotler JM, Herbison GJ, Nasuti JF, et al: Closed reduction of traumatic cervical spine dislocation using traction weights up to 140 pounds. Spine 18(3):386–390, 1993
13. Arias MJ: Treatment of experimental spinal cord injury with TRH, naloxone, and dexamethasone. Surg Neurol 28:335–338, 1987
14. Piepmeier JM, Lehman KB, Lane JG: Cardiovascular instability following acute cervical spinal cord trauma. Centr Nerv Syst Trauma 2(3):153–160, 1985
15. Albuquerque F, Wolf A, Wagner R, et al: Frequency of intra-abdominal injury in cases of blunt trauma to the cervical spinal cord. J Spinal Disord 5(4):476–480, 1992
16. Knopp RK: Evaluation of the cervical spine: Unresolved issues. Ann Emerg Med 16:819–820, 1987
17. Ringenberg BJ, Fisher AK, Urdaneta LF: Rational ordering of cervical radiographs following trauma. Ann Emerg Med 17:792–796, 1988
18. Spain DA, Trooskin SZ, Flancbaum L: The adequacy and cost effectiveness of routine resuscitation area cervical spine radiographs. Ann Emerg Med 19(3):276–278, 1990
19. Mace SE: The unstable occult cervical spine fracture: A review. Am J Emerg Med 10:136–142, 1992
20. Streitwieser DR, Knopp R, Wales LR: Accuracy of standard radiographic views in detecting cervical spine fractures. Ann Emerg Med 12:538–542, 1983
21. Berquist TR, Cabancia ME: The spine, in Berquist TR: Imaging of Orthopedic Trauma and Surgery. Philadelphia, WB Saunders, Co, 1986, pp 91–180
22. Murphey MD, Batnizky S, Batnizky JM: Diagnostic imaging of spinal trauma. Radiol Clin North Am 27:855–872, 1989
23. Keene JS, Goletz TH, Lilleas F: Diagnosis of vertebral fractures: A comparison of conventional radiography, conventional tomography, and computed axial tomography. J Bone Joint Surg 64:586–594, 1982
24. Mirvis SE, Borg U, Belzberg H: MR of ventilator-dependent patients: Preliminary experience. AJR Am J Roentgenol 149:845–846, 1987
25. Mirvis SE, Wolf AL: MRI of acute cervical spine trauma. Appl Radiol 21(12):15–22, 1992
26. Dachling P, Pollack IF: Spinal cord injury without radiographic abnormality in children: The SCIWORA syndrome. J Trauma 29:654–663, 1989
27. Kowalski HM, Cohen WA, Cooper P: Pitfalls in the CT diagnosis of atlantoaxial rotary-subluxation. AJNR Am J Neuroradiol 8:697–702, 1987
28. Levitt MA, Flanders AE: Diagnostic capabilities of magnetic resonance imaging and computed tomography in acute cervical spinal column injury. Am J Emerg Med 9:131–135, 1991
29. Quencer RM, Bunge RP, Egnor M: Acute traumatic central cord syndrome: MRI-pathological correlations. Neuroradiology 34:85–94, 1992
30. Martin D, Schoenin J, Lenelle J: MRI-pathological correlations in acute traumatic central cord syndrome: Case report. Neuroradiology 34:262–266, 1992
31. Kulkarni MV, McArdle CB, Kopanicky D: Acute spinal cord injury: MR imaging at 1.5T. Radiology 164:837–843, 1987
32. Mirvis SE, Geisler FH, Jelinek JJ: Acute cervical spine trauma: Evaluation with 1.5T MR imaging. Radiology 166:807–816, 1988
33. Schaefer DM, Flanders AE, Osterholm JL: Prognostic significance of magnetic resonance imaging in the acute phase of cervical spine injury. J Neurosurg 76:218–223, 1992
34. Harris JH, Yeakley JW: Hyperextension-dislocation of the cervical spine: Ligament injuries demonstrated by magnetic resonance imaging. J Bone Joint Surg Br 74(B):567–570, 1992
35. Bracken MB, Shepard MJ, Collins WF: A randomized, controlled trial of methylprednisolone or naloxone in the treatment of acute spinal cord injury. N Engl J Med 322:1405–1411, 1990
36. Bracken MB, Shepard MJ, Collins WF: Methylprednisolone or naloxone treatment after acute spinal cord injury: 1-year follow-up data. J Neurosurg 76:23–31, 1992
37. Faden AI, Jacobs TP, Holaday JW: Thyrotropin-releasing hormone improves neurologic recovery after spinal trauma in cats. N Engl J Med 305:1063–1067, 1981
38. Geisler FH, Dorsey FC, Coleman WP: Recovery of motor function after spinal cord injury: A randomized, placebo-controlled trial with GM-1 ganglioside. N Engl J Med 324(26):1829–1838, 1991
39. Sears W, Fazl M: Prediction of stability of cervical spine fracture managed in the halo vest and indications for surgical intervention. J Neurosurg 72:426–432, 1990
40. Johnson RM, Hart DL, Simmons EF, et al: Cervical orthosis: A study comparing their effectiveness in restricting cervical motion in normal subjects. J Bone Joint Surg Am 59(A):332–339, 1977
41. Johnson RM, Owen JR, Hart DL, et al: Cervical orthoses: A guide to their selection and use. Clin Orthop 154:34–45, 1981
42. Anderson LD, D'Alonzo RT: Fractures of the odontoid process of the axis. J Bone Joint Surg 56:1663–1674, 1974
43. Kaufman HH, Jones E: The principles of bony spinal fusion. Neurosurgery 24:264–270, 1989
44. Geisler FH, Cheng C, Poka A, Brumback RJ: Anterior screw fixation of posteriorly displaced type II odontoid fractures. Neurosurgery 25:30–38, 1989
45. Dickman CA, Douglas R, Sonntag VK: Occipitocervical fusion. Posterior stabilization of the craniovertebral junction and upper cervical spine. BNI Q 6:2–14, 1990
46. Dickman CA, Sonntag VKH, Papadopoulos SM, Hadley MN: The interspinous method of posterior atlantoaxial arthrodesis. J Neurosurg 74:190–198, 1991

47. Grob D, Dvorak J, Panjabi M, et al: Posterior occipitocervical fusion: A preliminary report of a new technique. Spine 16:S17–S24, 1990
48. Huhn SL, Wolf AL, Ecklund J: Posterior spinal osteosynthesis for cervical fracture/dislocation using a flexible multistrand cable system: Technical note. Neurosurgery 29(6):943–946, 1991
49. Fielding JW: The status of arthrodesis of the cervical spine. J Bone Joint Surg Am 70A:1571–1574, 1988
50. Ransford AO, Crockard HA, Pozo JL, et al: Craniocervical instability treated by contoured loop fixation. J Bone Joint Surg Br 68B:173–177, 1986
51. Heywood AWB, Learmonth ID, Thomas M: Internal fixation for occipitocervical fusion. J Bone Joint Surg Br 70B:708–711, 1988
52. Aldrich EF, Crow WN, Weber PB, et al: Use of MR imaging-compatible Halifax interlaminar clamps for posterior cervical fusion. J Neurosurg 74:185–189, 1991
53. Holness RO, Huestis WS, Howes WJ: Posterior stabilization with an interlaminar clamp in cervical injuries: Technical note and review of the long term experience with the method. Neurosurgery 14:318–322, 1984
54. Dickman CA, Sonntag VKH, Marcotte PJ: Techniques of screw fixation of the cervical spine. BNI Q 8(2):9–26, 1992
55. Hanson PB, Montesano PX, Sharkey NA, et al: Anatomic and biomechanical assessment of transarticular screw fixation for atlanto-axial instability. Spine 15:1141–1145, 1990
56. Apfelbaum RI: Anterior screw fixation for odontoid fracture: Disorders of the cervical spine, in Camins MB, O'Leary PF (eds): Disorders of the Cervical Spine. Baltimore, Williams & Wilkins, 1992, pp 603–608
57. Montesano PX, Anderson PA, Schlehr F, et al: Odontoid fractures treated by anterior odontoid screw fixation. Spine 16 (3 suppl):33–37, 1991
58. Cabanela ME, Ebersold MJ: Anterior plate stabilization for bursting teardrop fractures of the cervical spine. Spine 13:888–891, 1988
59. Capen D, Garland D, Waters R: Surgical stabilization of the cervical spine: A comparative analysis of anterior and posterior spine fusions. Clin Orthop 196:229–237, 1985
60. Caspar W, Barbier D, Klara P: Anterior cervical fusion and Caspar plate stabilization for cervical trauma. Neurosurgery 25:491–502, 1989
61. Lesoin F, Cama A, Lozes G, et al: The anterior approach and plates in lower cervical posttraumatic lesions. Surg Neurol 21:581–587, 1984
62. Oliveira JC: Anterior plate fixation of traumatic lesions of the lower cervical spine. Spine 12:323–329, 1987
63. Tippets R, Apfelbaum R: Anterior cervical fusion with the Caspar instrumentation system. Neurosurgery 22:1008–1113, 1988
64. Randle MJ, Wolf AL, Levi L, et al: The use of anterior Caspar plate fixation in acute cervical spine injury. Surg Neurol 36:181–189, 1991
65. Suh PB, Kostuik JP, Esses SI: Anterior cervical plate fixation with the titanium hollow screw plate system. Spine 15(10):1079–1081, 1990
66. Sonntag VKH, Kalfas I: Innovative cervical fusion and instrumentation techniques. Clin Neurosurg 37:636–660, 1990
67. Tuite GF, Papadopoulos SM, Sonntag KH: Caspar plate fixation for the treatment of complex hangman's fractures. Neurosurgery 30(5):761–765, 1992
68. Caspar W, Barbier DD, Klara PM: Anterior cervical fusion and Caspar plate stabilization for cervical trauma. Neurosurgery 25(4):491–502, 1989
69. Smith TJ: In vitro spinal biomechanics. Experimental methods and apparatus. Spine 16:1204–1210, 1991
70. Goffin J, Plets D, Van den Bergh R: Anterior cervical fusion and osteosynthetic stabilization according to Caspar: A prospective study of 41 patients with fractures and/or dislocations of the cervical spine. Neurosurgery 25:865–871, 1989
71. Cooper PR: Stabilization of fractures and subluxations of the middle and lower cervical spine. Contemp Neurosurg 10:1–6, 1988
72. Bengol EC, Keslerson L: Posterior cervical interspinous compression wiring and fusion for mid to low cervical spinal injuries. J Neurosurg 70:893–899, 1989
73. Maiman DJ, Barolat G, Larson SJ: Management of bilateral locked facets of the cervical spine. Neurosurgery 18:542–547, 1986
74. Cooper PR, Cohen A, Rosiello A, Koslow M: Posterior stabilization of cervical spine fractures and subluxations using plates and screws. Neurosurgery 23:300–306, 1988
75. Cherny WB, Sonntag VKH, Douglas RA: Lateral mass posterior plating and facet fusion for cervical spine instability. BNI Q 7(2):2–11, 1991
76. An HS, Gordin R, Renner K: Anatomic considerations for plate-screw fixation of the cervical spine. Spine 16(10):S548–S551, 1991
77. Heller JG, Carlson GD, Abitbol JJ, et al: Anatomic comparison of the Roy-Camille and Magerl techniques for screw placement in the lower cervical spine. Spine 16(10):S552–S557, 1991

CHAPTER 149

Surgical Techniques for the Stabilization of the Cervical Spine

Curtis A. Dickman
Volker K. H. Sonntag

The art and science of surgical fixation of the cervical spine have undergone rapid evolution. Techniques have been developed for rigid, segmental vertebral fixation. Instrumentation devices can often restore spinal stability immediately and can ultimately promote bone fusion. The development of new techniques and instrumentation requires that surgeons continually develop their skills, their understanding of pertinent anatomy and biomechanics, and their knowledge of the merits and limitations of each instrumentation system. This chapter is devoted to techniques for stabilization of the cervical spine. The surgical procedures, rather than the operative indications, are emphasized.

Surgical procedures must be used judiciously and are indicated only when nonoperative therapy has failed, or when it is unlikely to be successful. Careful planning is necessary to achieve the mechanical goals, restore stability, and protect the spinal cord, while preserving the normal motion of the spine. Each surgeon must assess the individual clinical situation and answer several questions: Is surgery needed or can the patient heal with just external cervical immobilization alone? Is spinal reconstruction or neural decompression needed? Which fixation devices are mechanically best and have the lowest risks?

The term *spinal instability* is often used to denote pathologic hypermobility of the spine, which usually requires surgery to internally fixate the spine. Stability and instability, however, are not absolute phenomena and may occur along a continuum of anatomic and functional changes. Instability does not necessarily occur instantaneously but may develop slowly and progressively.[1-3]

White and Panjabi[4] provide an inclusive definition of spinal stability: "under physiological loads to the spine there is no pain, deformity, or neurological injury." Other authors suggest anatomic definitions that divide the spine into functional "columns" and suggest criteria for stability.[5] The osseous and ligamentous interrelationships of the vertebral column are not simplistic and are not explained fully by a single conceptual model.

INDICATIONS FOR SURGERY

Defining "cookbook" criteria for surgery is impossible; the approach to each patient's problem must be individualized. Neural decompression, spinal reconstruction, and spinal stabilization all may be required in a given patient. Operative decisions must reflect the patient's medical condition, the specific spinal levels involved, the extent of neurologic signs and symptoms, the radiographic abnormalities, and the individual pathology. The mechanism of injury, extent of spinal deformity, architectural bone compromise, ligament integrity, and bone strength influence how extensive a fusion is needed, which techniques can be applied safely, and whether a postoperative orthosis is needed.

The cervical vertebrae are complex geometric, multiarticular structures whose movements are strongly coupled.[4] Rotation and translation can occur simultaneously about three-dimensional axes that are determined by the articular and ligamentous interfaces.[2,4,6,7] Ligaments serve as elastic tension bands that facilitate normal motion but limit excessive motion of the vertebrae.[4,6,8] Discs provide shock-absorbing capabilities and rotational and translational interfaces; they also decrease the energy transmitted directly to the bones.[4] The bones provide structural support and scaffolding, protect the neural elements, and interface to limit and facilitate movement.[4] The neural and muscular systems coordinate the integrated movements of the spine. All anatomic components are arranged to protect the spinal cord and nerve roots and allow smooth, coordinated motions to occur.[2,7] Injury to any of the components of the vertebral column can cause instability. Excessive motion can have many causes, including trauma, tumors, arthritis, infections, and congenital pathology.

SELECTION OF A SURGICAL APPROACH

Once instability of the cervical spine is detected, the immediate goals of treatment are to reduce pathologic subluxations, to maintain vertebral column alignment, and to brace the spine externally until internal fixation can be achieved.

Many anterior or posterior techniques can be used for cervical spine stabilization (Table 149-1). Several decisions are required for the successful planning of surgery. The surgeon must determine whether the neural elements need to be decompressed, whether the spinal architecture needs to be rebuilt, and whether instrumentation is necessary. All of

Table 149–1. OPERATIVE TECHNIQUES FOR STABILIZATION OF THE CERVICAL SPINE

Type of Fixation	Anterior Approaches	Posterior Approaches

Atlantoaxial	Ventral odontoid screw fixation
	Ventral atlantoaxial facet screw fixation
		Wiring and bone grafts
		    Interspinous technique
		    Gallie technique
		    Brooks technique
		Halifax clamps
		Posterior atlantoaxial facet screw fixation

Occipitocervical	Transoral arthrodesis
	High cervical retropharyngeal arthrodesis
		Wiring and bone grafts
		Metal implant fixation
		    Steinmann pin
		    Luque rectangle
		    Ransford loop
		Screw-plate fixation

Subaxial (C2–C7)	Ventral interbody bone grafts
	Screw-plate fixation
	Methacrylate
		Wiring and bone grafts
		    Facet wiring
		    Laminar wiring
		    Spinous process wiring
		Halifax clamps
		Hook-plate fixation
		Screw-plate fixation
		Methacrylate

these goals should be achieved with a single operative approach whenever possible.

When the spine is unstable, bone grafts and fixation with wire or instrumentation should be used to restore stability. Onlay fusions and nonfixated bone grafts do not provide immediate spinal stability; stability is fully achieved only after the bone heals solidly, which in the cervical spine usually takes 12 weeks or more. Onlay fusions should be avoided unless the bone is so osteoporotic or so extensively destroyed that wires or instrumentation cannot be used. When onlay fusions are performed, a supplemental halo brace should be used until the bone heals satisfactorily.

Methyl methacrylate does not promote fusion and should not be used routinely.[9, 10] Its use should be reserved for patients who have reduced life expectancies, such as those with cancer, in whom temporary structural support is needed. Because methacrylate is a foreign body, it is not incorporated into the bone healing process and actually reduces the surface area of bone available for healing. It can also fatigue, loosen, and become infected. An osseous union should be pursued whenever possible.

Individuals with spinal instability and reducible pathology can be treated solely with internal fixation. Patients with neurologic deficits from irreducible cervical subluxations or persistent compression require decompression, reduction, and arthrodesis. The decompression should be performed first because using instruments in a stenotic spinal canal can cause neurologic injury. When decompression of the neural elements is planned, the pathology should be attacked directly. Anterior compression should be treated by anterior operative exposures, and posterior compression, by posterior exposures.

In anterior cervical operative approaches, a transverse or oblique incision is made along the medial border of the sternocleidomastoid muscle (Fig. 149–1). The patient is positioned supine on the operating table with the neck in a neutral or slightly extended position.

A transverse incision made within a skin crease is cosmetically preferable and permits adequate exposure for the middle and lower cervical spine. The incision is centered directly over the level of the pathology. The C4-C5 level is usually at the cricothyroid junction. Access to multiple vertebral levels is facilitated by wide undermining of the platysma and opening of the fascial planes. The fascial plane separating the carotid sheath from the trachea and esophagus is dissected, thereby avoiding injury to the recurrent laryngeal nerve. The longus colli muscles are cauterized and dissected from the anterior surface of the vertebral bodies.

An oblique neck incision is used when the neck is very short or when extensive or very high cervical exposure is needed. Access to the upper cervical spine (occiput, C1, and C2) is difficult to obtain from an anterior cervical exposure and requires mobilization of the digastric muscle and hypoglossal nerve and division of branches of the external carotid artery.[11] A direct transoral approach is an alternative for access to C1-C2; this approach, however, violates the pharyngeal mucosa and risks infection of bone grafts.[1, 12–14]

Anterior approaches are performed while an adjustable headrest supports the head. The Caspar headrest and neckrest facilitates radiographic visualization of the lower cervical spine during anterior operations (Fig. 149–2).[15, 16] This headrest immobilizes the head and neck with an elastic chin strap and permits traction to be applied with skull tongs, if needed. An adjustable neck support can be used to push the cervicothoracic junction anteriorly, causing the shoulders to fall away. Gauze straps can be applied to the wrists to pull the shoulders out of the way when radiographs are taken.

Posterior operative approaches to the cervical spine are performed with the patient in a prone position on the operating table while the head is fixed with a Mayfield skull clamp. A horseshoe-shaped headrest can be used if traction is needed intraoperatively. If the patient can tolerate flexion of the head, access to the cervical spine from a posterior approach is easier. A midline sagittal posterior incision is made from the external occipital protuberance to the C7 spinous process. The nuchal fascia is divided in the midline where

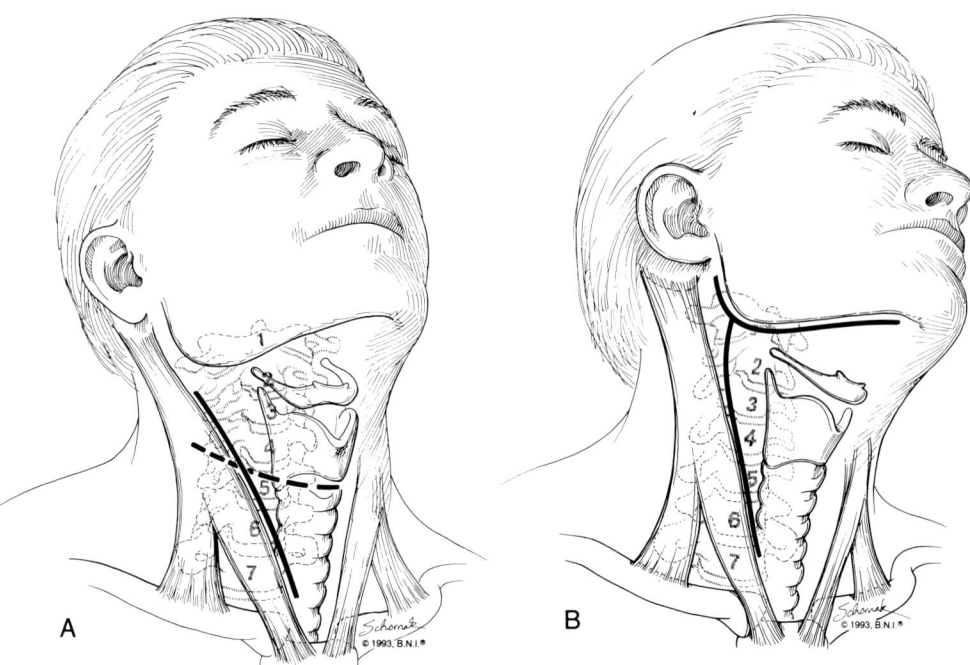

FIGURE 149–1. Incisions for anterior exposure of the cervical spine. (A) a transverse skin incision is used to access C3 to C7 (dotted line). Wide exposure can be achieved by undermining the platysma muscle. The C4-C5 level is usually adjacent to the cricothyroid junction. An oblique skin incision (solid line) is used for wide exposure or high cervical access. (B) Exposure of the atlas and axis by a retropharyngeal approach requires mobilization of the branches of the external carotid artery, hypoglossal nerve, and digastric muscle. (© 1993, Barrow Neurological Institute. Used with permission.)

the dissection plane is relatively avascular and the involved vertebrae are exposed by use of subperiosteal dissection. The muscles are detached from the spinous processes and swept laterally by use of broad-surfaced, lightweight periosteal elevators. Uninvolved segments are not exposed. Subperiosteal dissection of adjacent vertebrae can cause inadvertent fusion, called a ''creeping fusion,'' which is frequently seen in children.

If the spine is grossly unstable, a halo brace is applied preoperatively. The brace reduces the risk of a subluxation or neurologic injury when the patient is positioned on the operating table. The anterior or posterior bars or vest plates of the halo brace can be partially removed, if needed, to gain access to the neck or the iliac crest. The halo brace can be used during anterior or posterior operations. The brace is supported on the operating table with stacked traction weights or with a Mayfield adaptor for the halo ring (Fig. 149–3).

OPERATIVE ADJUNCTS

Intraoperative electrophysiologic monitoring of spinal cord function helps detect complications. Somosensory evoked potentials measure the activity of the dorsal columns of the spinal cord. If the posterior fossa is exposed (as in occipito-cervical fusion), then brainstem auditory evoked potentials can be monitored. Motor evoked potential monitoring has great clinical potential but needs to be developed and refined.

Radiographic visualization of the cervical spine intraoperatively serves several purposes. Fluoroscopy can be used to verify the correct level of exposure, to monitor the progress

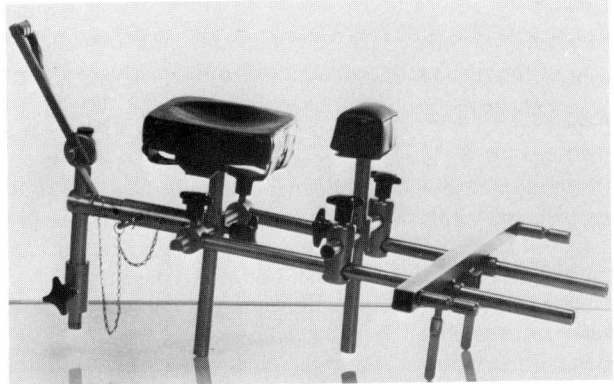

FIGURE 149–2. An adjustable headrest and neckrest allows intraoperative radiographic visualization for anterior cervical screw-plate fixation. (© 1993, Barrow Neurological Institute. Used with permission.)

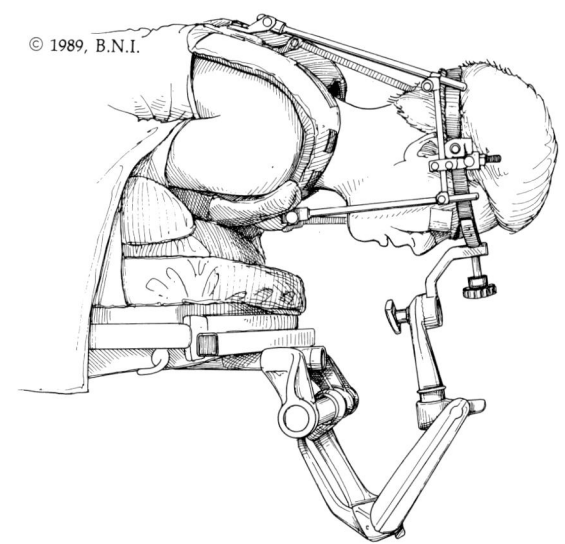

FIGURE 149–3. The Mayfield fixation device can be attached to the halo brace to fixate patients to the operating table. (© 1989, Barrow Neurological Institute. Used with permission.)

of a decompression, to judge the depth of drilling, and to visualize the precise placement of instrumentation. During decompressive procedures, a vertebral body defect can be filled with a contrast medium to judge the depth or width of exposure.

A fluoroscopic C arm with an image intensifier is required when screw or screw-plate procedures are performed. This instrument provides on-line visualization of the surgical maneuvers. Radiographic monitoring allows a precisely directed drill and screw trajectory. The C arm allows the surgeon to fit the plate correctly, to position the screws correctly, and to avoid complications from screw malpositioning or overdrilling.

BONE GRAFT TECHNIQUES

The goals of spinal internal fixation procedures are to achieve anatomic alignment, to protect the neural elements, and to stabilize the spine, while preserving the motion of normal spinal segments. These goals may be attained only by a satisfactory arthrodesis.

It is most important to recognize that instrumentation provides only temporary spinal fixation. Wires, cables, screws, clamps, and metallic plates are susceptible to fatigue and can break. Instrumentation may fail, even after a fusion has formed.[17, 18] Only a solid osseous union ensures long-term spinal stability.

Autogenous bone grafts are preferred for fusion because live bone contains the active cellular and structural components needed for fusion, bone remodeling, and new bone formation.[19] Autogenous grafts have a significantly higher fusion rate than allograft when used for multilevel cervical fusions.[20, 21]

Iliac crest bone grafts, obtained as corticocancellous struts, provide versatility. Cortical bone is compact, can provide immediate structural support, and resists tensile and compressive forces much better than cancellous bone.[4] By comparison, cancellous bone is porous, becomes rapidly vascularized, and promotes fusion better than cortical bone.[4, 19, 22, 23] A mixture of cortical and cancellous structure provides the ideal reconstruction graft. Cancellous bone fragments are especially useful for covering adjacent bone surfaces that one wishes to fuse. When structural support or struts are needed, cortical or corticocancellous grafts are used.

Allograft bone is reserved for cases in which the patient's bone stock is inadequate or diseased. Allograft fibular struts can be useful if a multilevel cervical corpectomy has been performed, or if a very long bone graft is needed. Caution should be used when reconstruction is performed with allograft because allograft bone is slowly resorbed and replaced by new bone,[19] and allograft struts weaken as they are resorbed and remodeled. In addition, collapse of an allograft strut graft can occur several months after surgery.[4] When allograft fibular struts are used for vertebral body reconstruction, the fusion can be augmented by filling the hollow center of the fibular graft with autogenous bone, which is obtained during the vertebrectomy.

Bone that is placed under compressive or tensile stress undergoes remodeling. This principle is known as *Wolff's law*[4] and implies that bone is laid down where stresses require its presence, and that bone is absorbed where stresses do not require it. This law has been misinterpreted to mean that bone is formed when it is loaded in compression and is absorbed when it is loaded in tension. This is not true. Tensile *or* compressive loading of bone can stimulate osteogenesis.[4]

Stress shielding is an important concept in spinal fixation. Rigid fixation of vertebrae can shield the bones from physiologic stresses and can cause relative osteoporosis. However, rigid instrumentation significantly improves fusion rates in both clinical and experimental models.[17] The beneficial effects of rigid spinal instrumentation on fusion rates clearly outweigh the potential disadvantages of instrument-related osteoporosis. The ideal rigidity of a spinal instrument system has not yet been defined.

Proper bone preparation is critical for successful fusion,[19, 22, 23] and the bone grafts and the recipient bed are equally important. All periosteum and soft tissue must be meticulously removed from the bone graft and fusion bed because soft tissue can provide a fibrous interface where a nonunion can form. When adjacent laminae and facets or bone surfaces are to be fused, the bone should be segmentally decorticated with a high-speed drill to expose bleeding cancellous bone surfaces. Pits are made in the cortical surface with a small burr. However, excessive drilling should be avoided because it can weaken the bone. Instead, atraumatic dissection technique should be used. Cautery should be used judiciously to avoid devascularization of the bone. The articular cartilage should be removed from articular surfaces. Curettes or drills can be used to roughen the bone surfaces adjacent to the disc or facet joints to promote arthrodesis across joint surfaces.

Bone grafts should fit precisely to maximize the surface area for bone-to-bone contact. Grafts should be compressed against the recipient bed, and rigid, segmental fixation of the vertebrae and the grafts is desirable. Dead space within the fusion bed should be obliterated by filling defects with cancellous bone, and bone should fill the entire fusion site. A margin is preserved adjacent to the dura to prevent neural compression.

Autologous bone grafts may be obtained from the anterior or posterior iliac crest (Fig. 149–4). Anteriorly, bone grafts should be obtained at least 4 cm behind the anterior superior iliac spine to avoid an avulsion fracture of the remaining bone anteriorly. Careful dissection should be performed subperiosteally to avoid injury to the ilioinguinal nerve, the lateral femoral cutaneous nerve, or the blood vessels and viscera.[3]

Posteriorly, bone grafts are obtained from the medial 6 to 8 cm of the iliac crest. A lateral exposure can cause buttock numbness or painful neuromas from injury to the superior cluneal nerves.[3] Tricortical grafts, cortical strips, or cancellous bone can be harvested posteriorly (Fig. 149–5).

Bone grafts should be obtained carefully from the posterior iliac crest with sharp osteotomes, saws, curettes, or bone gouges. These tools should be used precisely, and all bone and soft tissue dissection should be performed under direct visualization to prevent complications.[3] Dissection of the bone surfaces should remain subperiosteal to avoid major arteries. If the gluteal arteries are torn or cut, they can retract into the muscle and cause profuse bleeding. Ureteral injury can occur if retroperitoneal perforation occurs. The sacroiliac

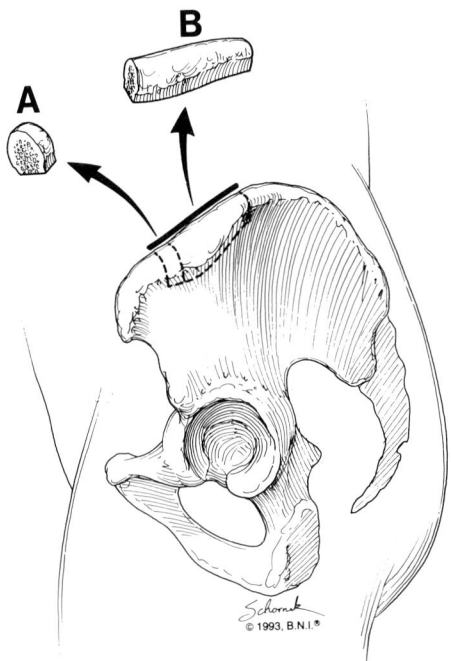

FIGURE 149–4. Bone grafts obtained from the anterior iliac crest should be harvested 4 or 5 cm behind the anterior iliac spine to avoid an avulsion fracture. (A) Single level tricortical graft. (B) Strut graft for vertebral body replacement. (© 1993, Barrow Neurological Institute. Used with permission.)

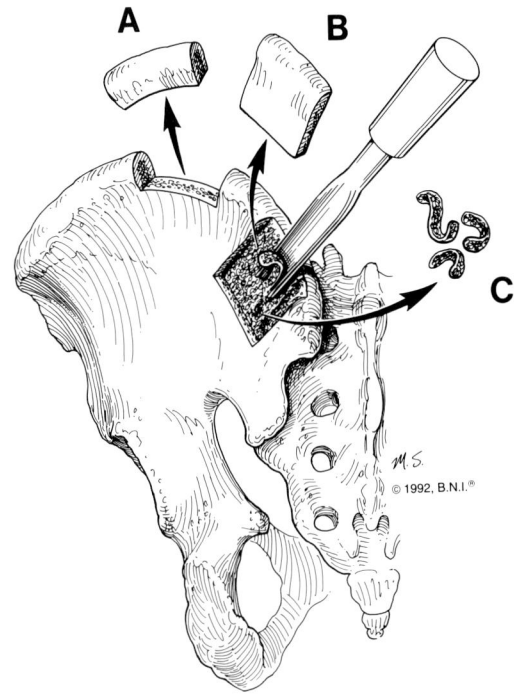

FIGURE 149–5. Bone grafts harvested from the posterior iliac crest should be obtained from the medial 8 cm of the iliac crest to avoid injuring the superior cluneal nerves. (A) Tricortical bone strut. (B) Unicortical bone plate. (C) Cancellous bone strips. (© 1992, Barrow Neurological Institute. Used with permission.)

joint and the sciatic notch should be avoided during the dissection, and the sacroiliac ligaments should be preserved to avoid sacroiliac joint instability.

After bone grafts are harvested, meticulous hemostasis should be obtained with bone wax or absorbable gelatin sponge (Gelfoam). Suction drains are placed if any oozing from the graft site remains. All periosteal and fascial layers are closed to obliterate dead space, to prevent herniation of abdominal contents, and to reduce postoperative pain.

CERVICAL WIRING TECHNIQUES

Historically, posterior cervical internal fixation was initially achieved by cerclage with suture, and subsequently, with wire.[22, 24–32] Wire fixation is used posteriorly, but not anteriorly, for cervical stabilization. The spinous processes, the laminae, the facets, and the occiput can be wired. Wire should not be used without bone grafts because wire can fatigue and break. In addition, when used alone, wire does not guarantee fusion.

Surgical wires are made of stainless steel or titanium. Titanium wire is compatible with magnetic resonance imaging (MRI) but is notch sensitive, more susceptible to fatigue, and more easily broken than steel wire.[33, 34] Monofilament wire, double-stranded twisted wire, Drummond buttons, or multistranded braided cables can be used for cervical fixation.

Eighteen or 20-gauge monofilament wires are suitable for cervical fixation. When monofilament wire is tightened, both ends of the wire should be grasped and pulled upward, thereby directing tension away from the fusion site to remove slack. Alternatively, the wire can be twisted bilaterally to evenly distribute tension (Fig. 149–6). Wires should be twisted uniformly and not kinked or bent in an acute angle, because bends, notches, and excessive twisting weaken wire and may cause it to break. Excessive twisting also causes secondary turns to appear in the wire. Caution should be used when wire is tightened; overtightening causes wire to pull through soft, osteoporotic bone.

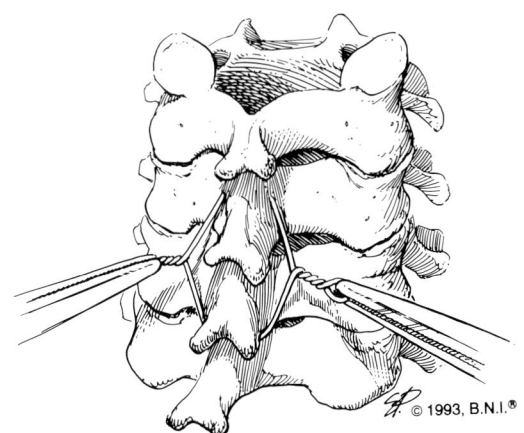

FIGURE 149–6. Eighteen- or twenty-gauge monofilament wire is relatively stiff. Bilateral wire twisting evenly distributes tension in the wire for spinous process fixation. (© 1993, Barrow Neurological Institute. Used with permission.)

Double-stranded wire, with two or three turns per centimeter, is stronger and more flexible than single-stranded, monofilament wire of a comparable diameter.[35] Double-stranded wire for cervical fusion is easily made with two strands of 24-gauge monofilament wire: and the ends of a pair of wires are inserted into the shaft of a hand-held twist drill, and the other ends of the wires are held with a Kocher clamp. The drill is used to pull the wires taut, and they are then twisted uniformly.

Multistranded, braided cables were developed as an alternative to monofilament or double-stranded wires.[33, 36] Cables are stronger, more flexible, and more fatigue resistant than monofilament wire; however, they are also considerably costlier. The flexibility of cable reduces the risk of neurologic injury during wire placement or wire removal.

Braided cables are tightened by use of an instrument with a specific, predetermined tension and are fixated with a crimp (Fig. 149–7). The cable's flexibility reduces kinking, makes removing slack easy, and prevents overtightening. Generally, 8 to 12 inch-pounds of torque is recommended for normal adult bone,[33] but less torque should be used for osteoporotic or thin bone to prevent the cables from pulling through the bone. Titanium or stainless steel braided cables are available. The steel braided cables are stronger.[33]

Biomechanically, the strength of a wire or fixation device depends on the distance of the wire fixation from the instantaneous axis of rotation of a vertebrae.[4] A longer lever arm increases the moment applied to the vertebrae (Fig. 149–8). For posterior cervical fixation, spinous process wiring should have a stronger fulcrum than laminar or facet wiring when there is a fixed instantaneous axis of rotation, which is usually located in the vertebral body.[4] If the facets are fractured, the vertebral bodies crushed, or the anterior spinal ligaments disrupted, then multidirectional rotation and translation of vertebrae can occur without a fixed axis of rotation. Wires are inadequate to fixate these three-columned spinal injuries (Fig. 149–9).

A biomechanical comparison of wiring techniques that used cadaveric cervical spines demonstrated that spinous process wires were strong and that facet wires were weak when compared with sublaminar wires.[37] Posterior cervical wiring techniques prevented flexion but poorly inhibited neck extension, axial rotation, and lateral bending.[37] The wire fixations did not restore normal strength to the injured spine. Posterior wire stabilization can be improved by positioning segmentally fixated bone grafts or H grafts between the spinous processes to resist extension.[4, 25, 38–40]

Spinous process wires can be used to fixate single- or multiple-motion segments (Fig. 149–10).[24, 41–43] A hole is made in the center of the base of the spinous process with a drill, and the hole is then completed with a towel clip. A wide margin of bone is preserved adjacent to the hole to resist wire pullout. The wire is looped beneath the inferior adjacent spinous process or passed through a hole in the base of the adjacent spinous process. A "figure-eight" or loop of wire can be created to wire the segments together. The inter-

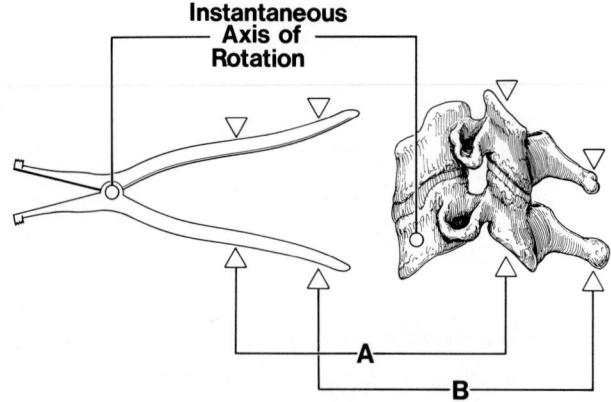

FIGURE 149–8. Spinous process fixation has a mechanical advantage to laminar or facet fixation because of a longer fulcrum. (Modified from White AA, Panjabi MM: Clinical Biomechanics of the Spine. 2nd ed. J.B. Lippincott, 1975, p 533.)

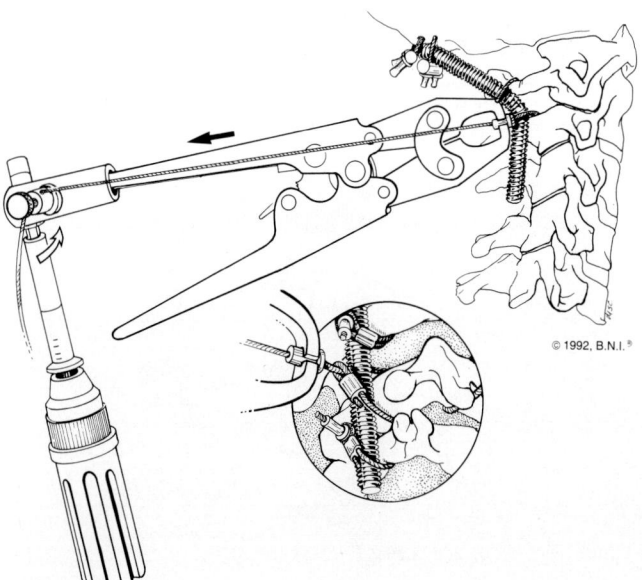

FIGURE 149–7. Songer cables are fixated with a crimping mechanism (inset). Tension is applied to the cable using a torque wrench. (© 1992, Barrow Neurological Institute. Used with permission.)

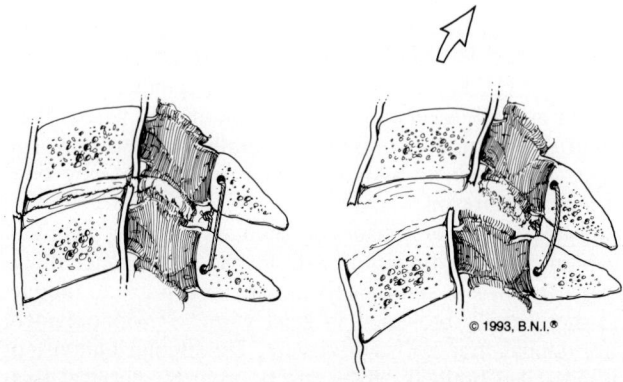

FIGURE 149–9. Three-column injury of the cervical spine. Circumferential ligament disruption occurs with a loss of the tension band fixation of the ligaments. Posterior cervical wiring alone is inadequate to restore spinal stability in this injury. (© 1993, Barrow Neurological Institute. Used with permission.)

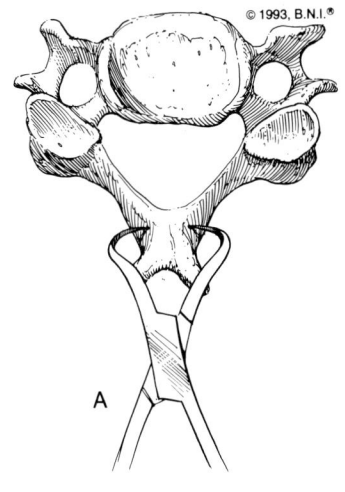
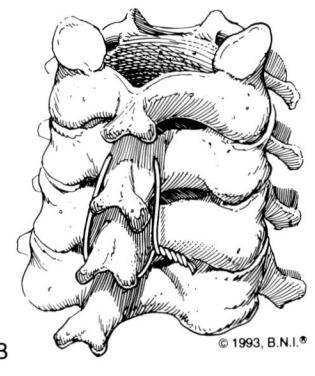
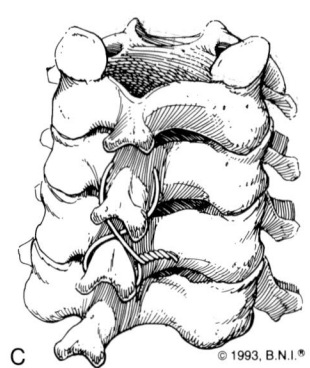
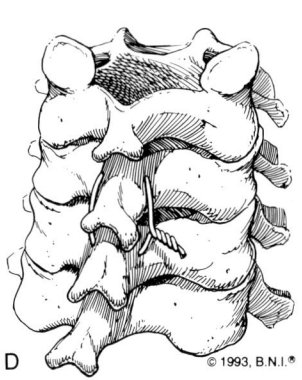
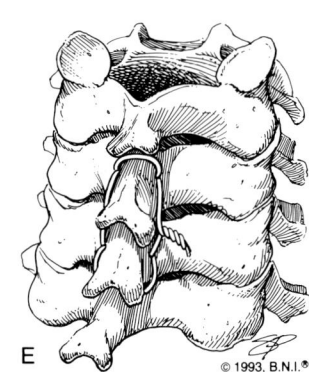

FIGURE 149–10. Spinous process wiring. (A) Drill holes are made in the base of the spinous processes. The hole is completed with a towel clip. Several wiring configurations can be used. (B) The wire is looped beneath the adjacent inferior spinous process. (C) Figure-eight configuration. (D) The wire is passed through a hole in the base of the adjacent spinous processes. (E) The wire encircles the spinous processes after being passed through holes in the spinous processes. (© 1993, Barrow Neurological Institute. Used with permission.)

spinous and supraspinous ligaments are preserved at levels adjacent to the fused segments.

Spinous process wires are safe, easy to use, and strong, and with their use, sublaminar instrumentation can be avoided. However, they do not resist extension and cannot be used after a laminectomy has been performed.

Facet wires are an excellent alternative after a laminectomy and can be used to fixate bone struts or metal implants to the vertebrae. Facet wires are placed into the lateral masses.[43–45] The facet joint surface is opened with a small currette and is held open with a Penfield dissector (Fig. 149–11). A drill hole is placed through the inferior facet into the facet joint. Facet-spinous process wiring can also be performed.[43]

Facet wires have several drawbacks. Because the facets are relatively thin, wires can be pulled out of the facets if enough force is applied or if the wires are overtightened. Facet wires are weaker than sublaminar or spinous process wires. If facet wires are used, an orthosis may be needed to supplement the wiring until fusion occurs.

Sublaminar wires can be used to fixate adjacent motion segments or to wire struts or implants to the vertebrae (Fig. 149–12).[33, 43, 46–51] Sublaminar wires carry a risk of neurologic injury, especially at the middle and lower cervical levels.[51]

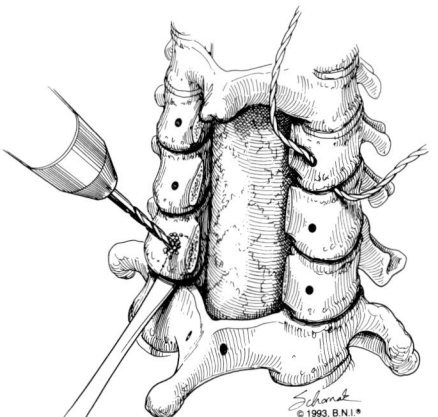
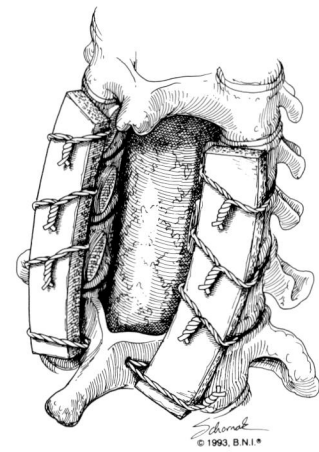

FIGURE 149–11. The facets are wired after removing the articular cartilage from the facet joints. (A) The joint is held open with a dissector, and a drill hole is made into the facet joint. (B) Bone grafts (or metal implants) can be wired to the facets to achieve internal fixation. (© 1993, Barrow Neurological Institute. Used with permission.)

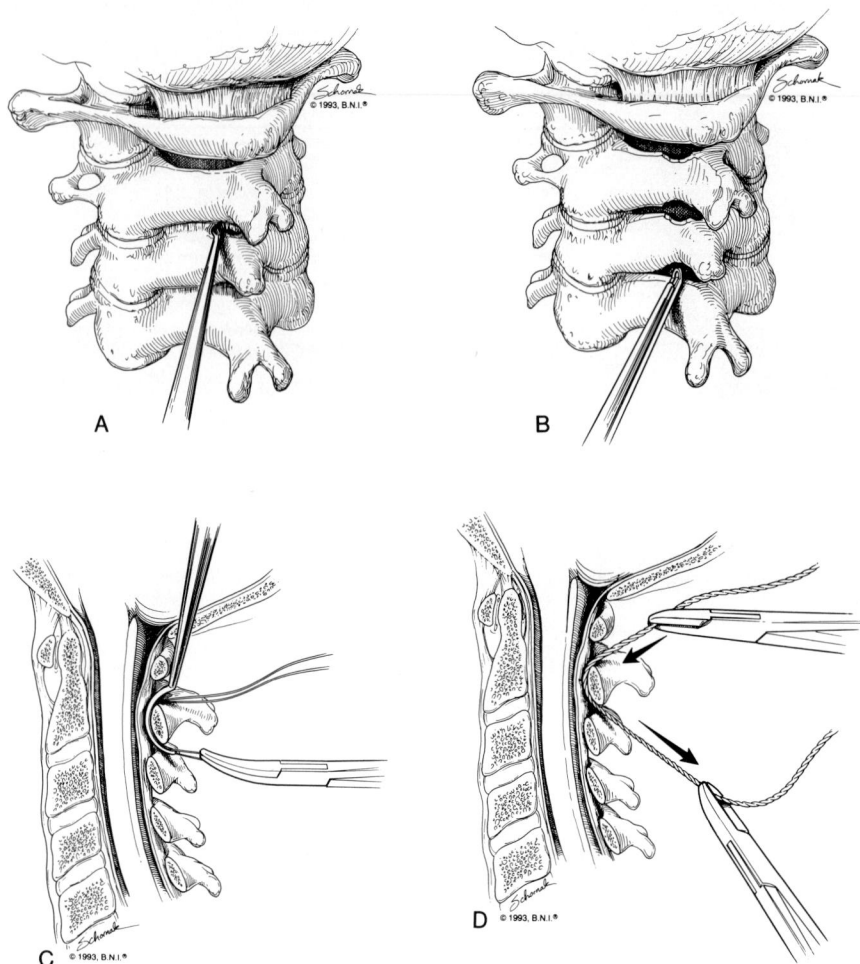

FIGURE 149–12. Sublaminar wires. (A and B) The ligamentum flavum is removed, and laminotomies are performed to visualize the dura. (C) A wire passer or suture is used to guide the wire along the undersurface of the bone. (D) Precise technique is required to avoid wire displacement and neurologic injury. The wire is fed and pulled using a two-handed technique. (© 1993, Barrow Neurological Institute. Used with permission.)

Precise technique and cautious maneuvers are required to avoid complications. The dura should be directly visualized before sublaminar wires are passed. The ligamentum flavum should be removed from the upper and lower surfaces of the laminae. Small laminotomies are made in the edge of the medial laminae to facilitate wire passage; however, weakening of the bone with an extensive laminotomy should be avoided.

A wire passer or heavy silk suture can help position and guide the wire beneath the undersurface of the lamina. A sublaminar wire should be passed with a two-handed process in which the wire is simultaneously fed and pulled to avoid displacement of the wire or the vertebrae. The wire is bent to conform to the shape of the laminae.

ATLANTOAXIAL WIRING TECHNIQUES

INTERSPINOUS FUSION[25]

A routine posterior exposure of C1 and C2 is performed, and the soft tissues are meticulously removed from the bone surfaces to facilitate fusion. The ligamentum flavum and posterior occipitoatlantal membrane are removed from the posterior margins of the atlas and axis by use of sharp curettes, and all soft tissue is removed from the superior and inferior margins of C1 and from the superior margin of C2. The C2-C3 interspinous ligament is also removed. The bony surfaces that will contact the cancellous bone of the graft are decorticated with a high-speed drill or a Kerrison rongeur to expose cancellous bone. To seat the wire, notches are made bilaterally in the inferior surfaces of the C2 laminae, where they join the C2 spinous process (Fig. 149–13).

An autologous, curved, tricortical bone graft (4 cm long × 3 cm high) is obtained from the posterior iliac crest. The rounded upper cortical edge of the graft is removed with a Lexsell rongeur to create a bicortical curved strut graft. The strut graft is precisely fitted between C1 and C2 to recreate the normal C1-C2 height. The curve of the graft approximates the curve of the ring of C1, and the inferior margin of the bone graft is notched in the midline to match the contour of the spinous processes of C2. The graft is temporarily removed to allow wire placement.

A braided cable or double-stranded, twisted, 24-gauge surgical wire is halved, looped, and passed beneath the posterior arch of C1 in the midline and is directed superiorly. The graft is replaced into position between the atlas and the axis, and the loop of wire is passed over the ring of C1, behind the graft, and is secured beneath the base of the C2 spinous process. The free ends of the wire are positioned anterior to the graft and are passed beneath the spinous process of C2. The wires are tightened into position, thereby compressing the bone between the posterior arches of C1 and C2. The graft is fixed by wire anteriorly and posteriorly and compressed between C1 and C2.

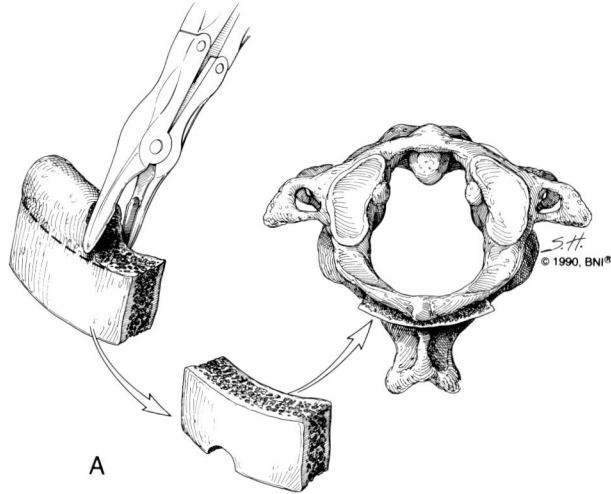

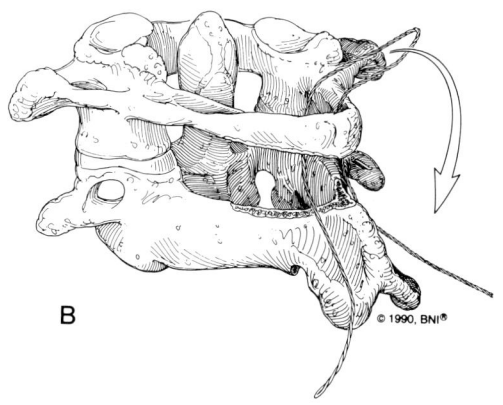
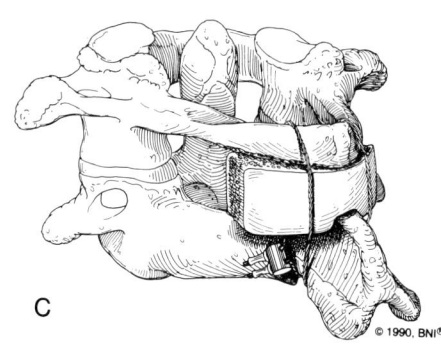

FIGURE 149-13. Interspinous atlantoaxial fusion. (A) A curved autologous bicortical iliac crest strut is positioned between C1 and C2 and sized to recreate the normal C1-C2 anatomic distance. (B) A wire or braided cable is halved and passed sublaminar beneath C1 directed cephalad. The loop is secured beneath the C2 spinous process. (C) The free ends of wire are passed beneath the C2 spinous process and positioned anterior to the graft. The strut is entrapped by wire anteriorly and posteriorly and is compressed between the posterior arches of C1 and C2. (© 1990, Barrow Neurological Institute. Used with permission.)

The posterior arches of C1, C2, and the bone graft are segmentally decorticated with a high-speed drill. Fragmented cancellous bone is compressed against the fusion surfaces. A rigid or semirigid orthosis is used postoperatively.

Unlike other methods of C1-C2 wiring, the interspinous method for atlantoaxial arthrodesis can be used when C1 is dislocated posteriorly. This method avoids sublaminar wire passage at C2, minimizes the risk of neural injury, and provides excellent translational and rotational stability.[52] A fusion rate of 86 percent has been obtained in 74 patients treated with this technique.

GALLIE FUSION

Gallie[30, 53] referred to the principle of cervical fusion using wires and bone grafts, but he did not publish the details of his wiring technique. Several authors have referred to a midline wiring technique for C1-C2 fusion and have called this the Gallie fusion (Fig. 149-14).[4, 26, 27, 52] A unicortical plate of bone (5 to 8 mm thick) is harvested from the iliac crest and shaped into a modified H. The graft is positioned dorsal to the C1 arch, and the notch of the H is fitted to straddle the C2 spinous process. Wire or braided cable is halved, looped, and passed sublaminar at C1 and is directed superiorly. The loop is secured beneath the C2 spinous process. The graft is positioned, and the free ends of the wire are wrapped dorsally to affix the graft into position. A routine wound closure is then performed.

The Gallie fusion technique is simple, but it cannot be performed when C1 is posteriorly dislocated. This construct does not resist translation and rotation as well as other wiring techniques for C1-C2 fixation.[4, 52, 54]

BROOKS FUSION

In 1978, Brooks and Jenkins[28] described a wedge compression method of C1-C2 fixation, and since then, a modification of their technique, which employs sublaminar wire passage at C1 and C2, has become popular (Fig. 149-15).[29] This modified technique provides better rotational fixation than that afforded by the Gallie wiring.[52, 54] In the modified method, the atlas and axis are exposed by use of routine techniques, and two sublaminar wires are passed bilaterally beneath C1 and then beneath C2. The dura is visualized to prevent injury during wire passage. Two rectangular corticocancellous wedges of autologous iliac crest bone are harvested and positioned bilaterally between the C1 ring and C2 laminae. The bone grafts are wedged into the interlaminar

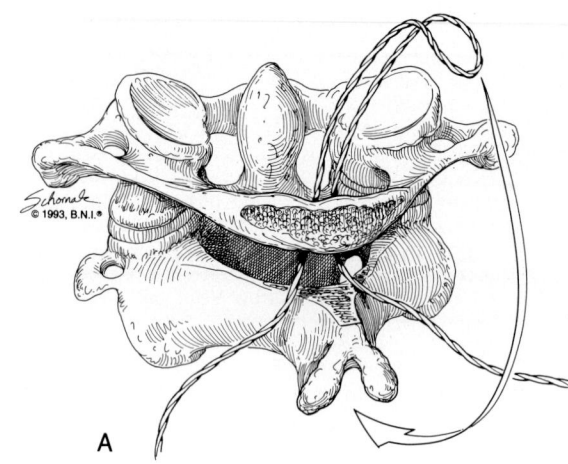

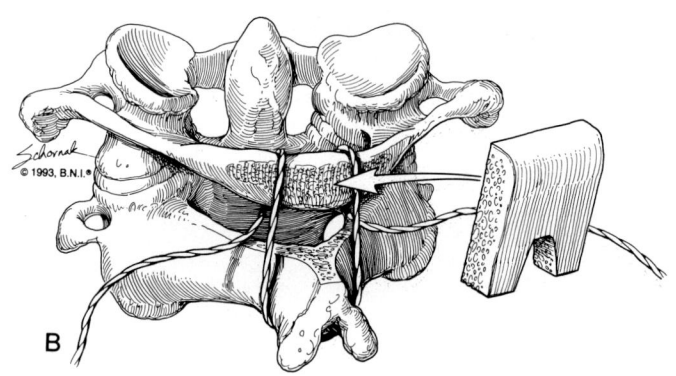
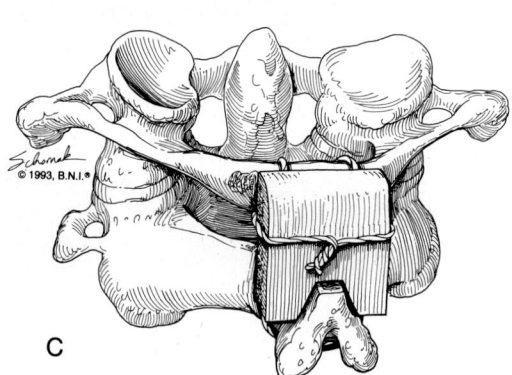

FIGURE 149–14. Gallie fusion. (A) A loop of wire is passed beneath C1. The loop is fixated beneath the C2 spinous process. (B) A notched unicortical bone graft is fitted over the C2 spinous process and positioned behind the C1 ring. (C) The free ends of the wire are wrapped behind the graft. (© 1993, Barrow Neurological Institute. Used with permission.)

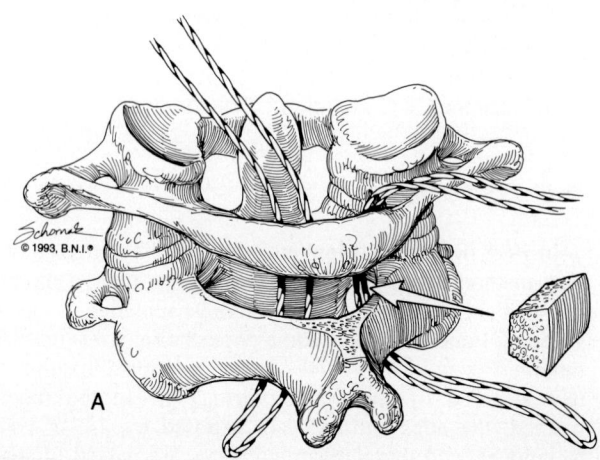
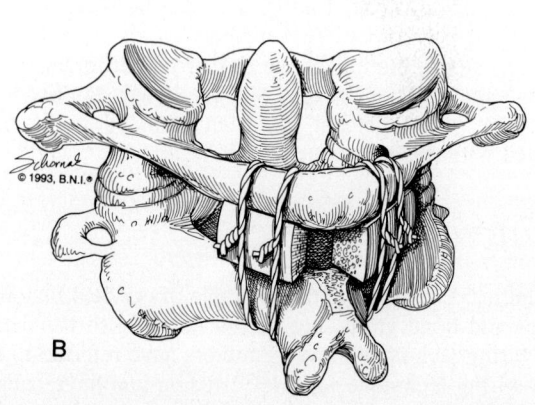

FIGURE 149–15. Brooks fusion. (A) Loops of wire are passed sublaminar at C1 and C2. Wedge-shaped bone grafts are positioned bilaterally between the arches of C1-C2. (B) Each graft is fixated by two wires. (© 1993, Barrow Neurological Institute. Used with permission.)

space on each side, and the wires are tightened behind the grafts, thereby securing them into position. After routine wound closure, a postoperative orthosis is used.

OCCIPITOCERVICAL WIRING

Occipitocervical fixation requires more extensive osseous dissection, which exposes the occipital squamosa, the rim of the foramen magnum, and the cervical levels to be fused. The occiput should be wired where the bone is thick: near the foramen magnum, at the nuchal line, or along the midline crest. Laterally, the occipital squamous is thin, and wires can easily pull out.

To wire the bone adjacent to the foramen magnum, the posterior lip of the foramen magnum is enlarged with a Kerrison rongeur (Fig. 149–16). Two burr holes are placed into the occipital bone, 0.5 cm superior to the rim of the foramen magnum. The dura is separated from the inner table of the skull, and wire is passed between each burr hole and the foramen magnum.

Midline wiring of the occiput can be performed by positioning burr holes bilaterally, adjacent to the midline crest. The dura is separated, and the thick midline crest is wired. Care must be taken to avoid injury to the cerebellum and cerebral venous sinuses. Alternatively, the midline crest can be wired by use of tangential holes drilled into the crest (Fig. 149–17A).[55]

Stabilization is achieved by wiring of the bone struts or metal struts to the occiput, spinous process, cervical laminae, or facets. Rib or iliac crest struts are directly wired against the bone (Fig. 149–17B).[13, 48, 55] The struts provide immobilization and bone for fusion. Because bone struts are relatively weak and can fracture, a rigid or semirigid orthosis is usually needed postoperatively until fusion occurs.

Metal fixation devices are used to achieve immediate segmental fixation; however, they should be used with autogenous bone grafts to ensure fusion. Metal contoured loops (Ransford loop), rectanglar rods (Luque rectangle), threaded Steinmann pins, and other metal fixation devices can be used for occipitocervical stabilization.*

To overcome the settling allowed by the smooth surfaces

---

*See references 12, 13, 41, 47, 49, 50, and 56–59.

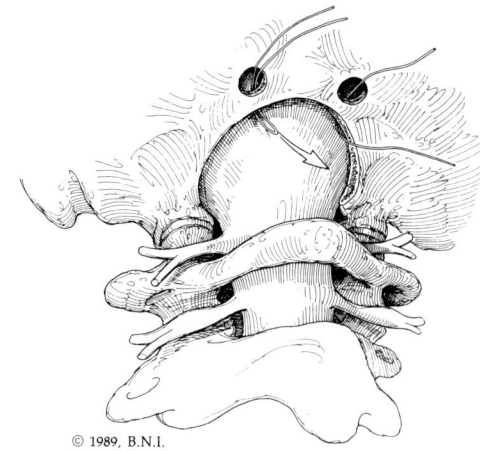

FIGURE 149–16. The occiput can be wired after enlarging the rim of the foramen magnum and positioning burr holes in the adjacent occipital bone. The dura is elevated to ensure safe wire passage. (© 1989, Barrow Neurological Institute. Used with permission.)

of other metal rods, we developed a technique for occipitocervical fusion using a threaded Steinmann pin.[46, 47] A wide diameter, threaded, 5/32-inch-diameter Steinmann pin is bent into a U shape and fashioned to fit the contour of the occipitocervical region (Fig. 149–18A). Secondary bends are placed in the U-shaped Steinmann pin to match the lordotic contour of the occipitocervical region. The curves of the pin should be smooth because sharp angles create stress risers where the pin can fracture. The ends of the pin, when cut, should not extend beyond the fused segments.

The Steinmann pin is wired against the occiput and cervical lamina or facets, contacting the bone surfaces at each level to achieve a rigid fixation. Gaps between the pin and the bone surfaces loosely fixate the vertebrae and result in excessive motion.

The wide diameter and smooth bends of the Steinmann pin are needed to minimize postoperative pin breakage. A threaded pin is essential because the threads of the pin prevent vertical settling of the construct.

The occiput and posterior arches of the cervical levels to be fused are segmentally decorticated, and cancellous bone fragments are compressed against the levels to be fused. If a suboccipital craniotomy or cervical laminectomy has been

FIGURE 149–17. Occipitocervical fixation. (A) The occiput can be wired using tangential drill holes placed in the midline crest. The C1 ring and C2 spinous processes can be wired for segmental vertebral fixation. (B) The wires are threaded through bone struts. The wires are twisted to compress the grafts against the fusion surfaces. (© 1993, Barrow Neurological Institute. Used with permission.)

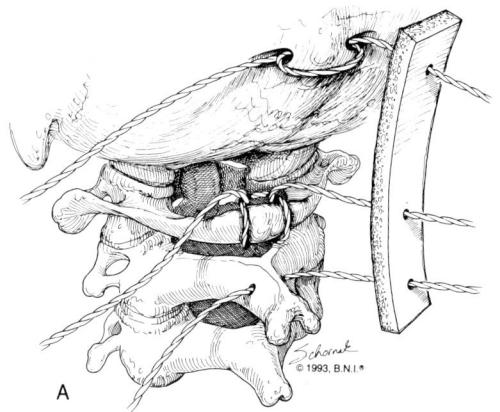
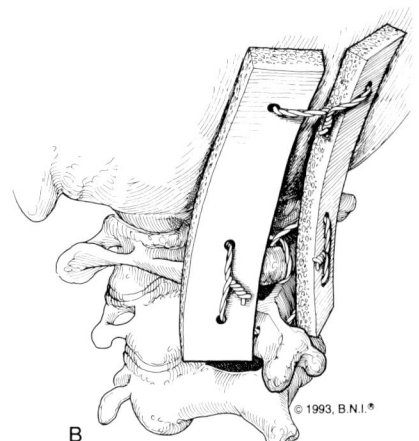

A   B

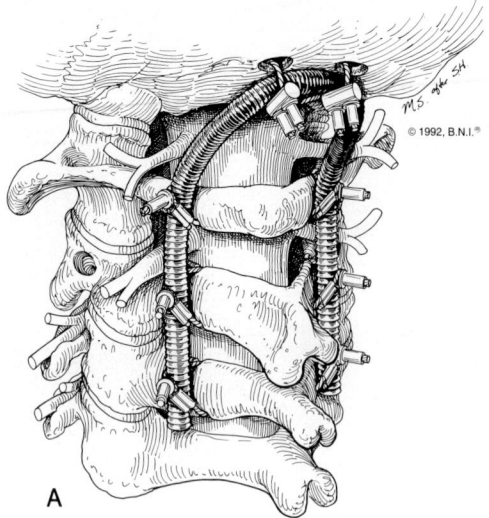
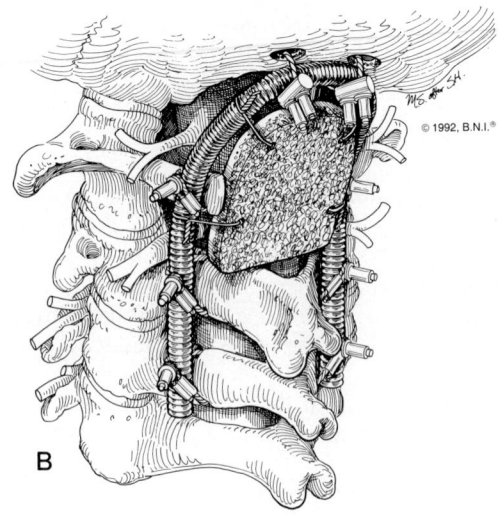
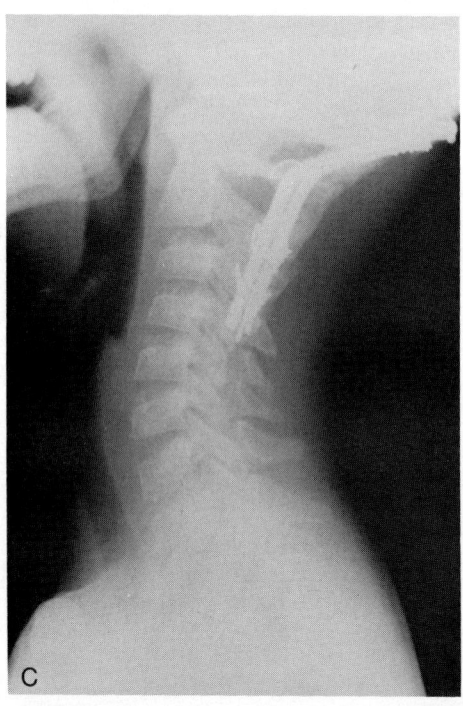

FIGURE 149–18. Occipitocervical fixation with a threaded Steinmann pin. (A) Smooth bends are created to avoid stress risers and fatigue of the pins. The rod is secured to the occiput and cervical laminae with braided cables or wires. The threads of the pin prevent settling of the fixation. (B) A bone plate is wired to the central region of the pin after a decompressive craniectomy or laminectomy is performed. (C) Postoperative lateral cervical radiograph demonstrates a well-formed fusion mass. (A and B, © Barrow Neurological Institute. Used with permission.)

performed, a cortical iliac crest bone plate can be wired to the central portion of the Steinmann pin (Fig. 149–18B). This bone plate provides a template for the fusion to develop and preserves the dural decompression. A routine multilayered wound closure is then performed.

SUBAXIAL WIRING TECHNIQUES

Methods for facet, laminae, and spinous process wiring have been reviewed. These procedures can be used for fixation of the subaxial cervical spine using bone grafts or metal implants. Different subaxial wiring techniques are depicted in Figures 149–19 through 149–21.

The Rogers wiring technique uses loops of wire in a loop or a figure-eight configuration passed through holes in the spinous process, then passed beneath the spinous process of the adjacent inferior level.[43, 60] When multiple levels are fixated, the process is repeated for each adjacent level to create interlocking linkages (Fig. 149–19A).

The Bohlman triple-wiring technique segmentally fixates bone struts that reinforce spinous process wires (Fig. 149–19B).[37, 42, 43] The spinous processes are wired together with 20-gauge wire or 24-gauge, double-stranded, twisted wire. Additional wires are passed through holes in the spinous processes and are threaded through holes in bone struts. The wires are tightened to compress the bone struts against the spinous processes and laminae (Fig. 149–19C). The bone

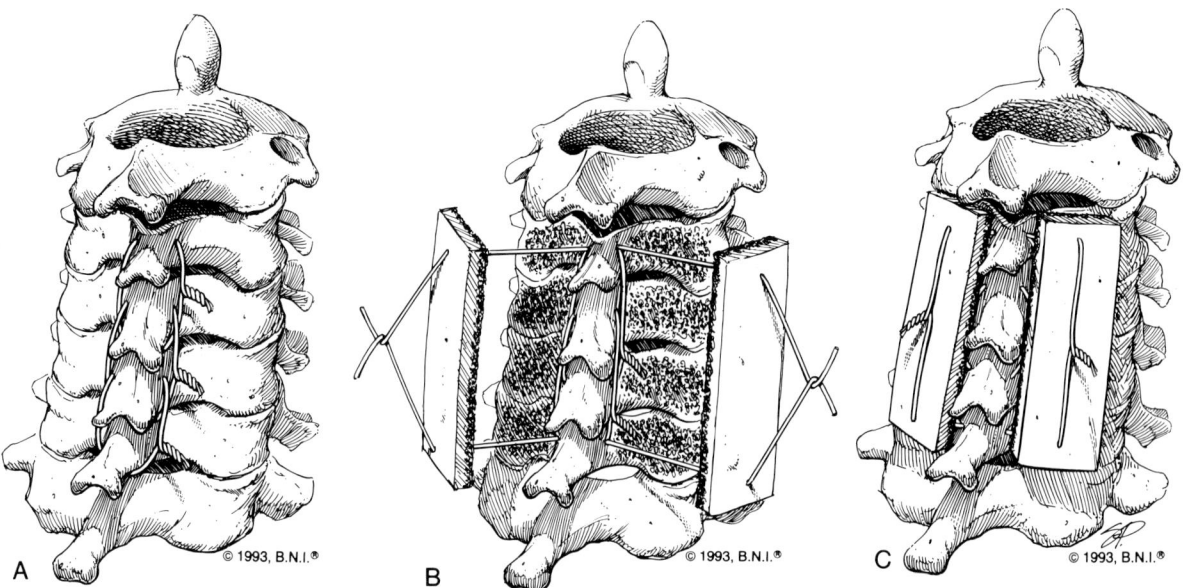

FIGURE 149–19. Subaxial wiring fixation techniques. (A) Separate wires are used to create interlocking links at adjacent levels. (B) The Bohlman triple-wiring technique uses interspinous wires. Bone struts are wired to the spinous processes. (C) The grafts are compressed against the bone surfaces, which adds mechanical stability to the spinous process wires. (© 1993, Barrow Neurological Institute. Used with permission.)

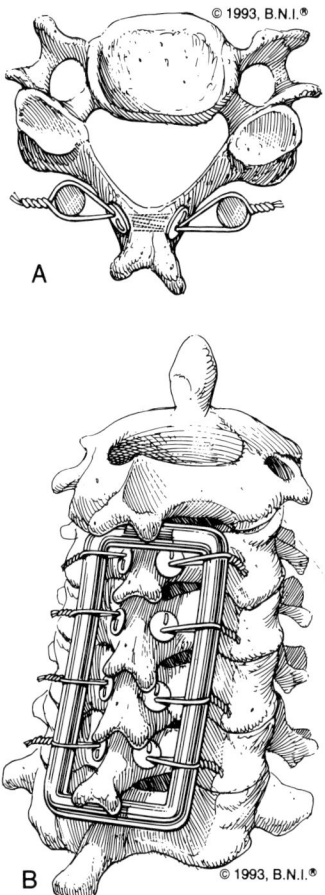

FIGURE 149–20. (A) Drummond wires are passed through a hole in the base of the spinous process. The wires are threaded through buttons, which are positioned against the spinous process to reinforce the fixation. (B) Drummond buttons can be used to attach a Luque rectangle for cervical or occipitocervical fixation. (© 1993, Barrow Neurological Institute. Used with permission.)

grafts promote fusion and inhibit flexion, extension, and axial rotation,[4, 37] adding significant stability to the spinous process wires.[4, 37, 43]

Drummond wires, which are used to secure bone grafts or metal rods, have buttons at their base to reinforce the fixation (Fig. 149–20). These wires are passed through holes in the spinous processes and are interlocking. To prevent wire pull-out, holes in the spinous processes should be created at the junction of the spinous process and laminae, where the bone is thick. Metal rods or bone struts can also be wired to the laminae or facets.

The Dewar posterior cervical fusion technique uses Kirschner wires (K-wires), 2 mm in diameter, to fixate the spinous processes.[61] K-wires are drilled into adjacent spinous processes, and cortical bone grafts are fitted and skewered by the K-wires. Wire is wrapped around the K-wires and spinous processes to compress the bone grafts against the spinous process and laminae (Fig. 149–21). This technique creates segmental stabilization that resists flexion, extension, lateral bending, and axial rotation.[4, 43]

Callahan devised a cervical facet fusion that uses autologous bone struts (Fig. 149–11).[26, 43, 44] Facet fusion can also be performed by use of a facet-to-spinous process wiring technique (Fig. 149–22).[26, 43]

INTERLAMINAR CLAMPS

Halifax interlaminar clamps may be used for posterior atlantoaxial or subaxial cervical stabilization.[39, 62, 63] These clamps were developed by Tucker and reported on by Holness and colleagues in 1984.[62] Several different clamp sizes and shapes are available, and they can be manufactured to conform to the shape of the laminae. The C1 clamps have a semicircular profile, and the subaxial clamps have a hooklike profile. The clamp is preassembled with a screw and is mounted on the clamp applicator forceps (Fig. 149–23).

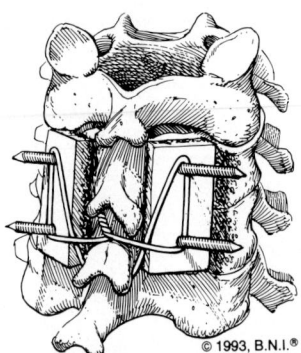

FIGURE 149-21. Dewar fusion. Kirschner wires (2-mm diameter) are drilled into the spinous processes and are used to "skewer" bilateral bone struts. Wires are wrapped around the Kirschner wires and beneath the spinous process. (© 1993, Barrow Neurological Institute. Used with permission.)

Clamp application is relatively simple. A standard posterior cervical exposure is performed, and the upper clamp is sized to fit around the upper laminae or posterior ring of C1. A lower clamp is fitted beneath the inferior laminae of the adjacent vertebrae. Laminotomies are performed, and the ligamentum flavum is removed to permit the clamps to seat properly against the bone.

After the bone surfaces are prepared and the clamps are sized, bone grafts are fitted. At C1-C2, an interspinous strut graft or two wedges of bone are positioned between the posterior arches to prevent extension and rotation. At subaxial levels, an H graft is used to prevent hyperextension. The clamps are tightened sequentially with a 90-degree-angled locking adjustment wrench. The site should be inspected to ensure that the clamps engage the lamina securely and that the hooks are seated properly. Because the clamps hug the undersurface of the laminae, care must be taken to avoid neural compression. After the screws are tightened into their final position, the distal threads of the screws can be stripped, or a locking mechanism can be used to prevent screw loosening.

At C1-C2, Halifax clamps provide mechanical stability comparable to that of the Brooks wiring technique.[54] The clamps have a broad surface area that distributes forces over

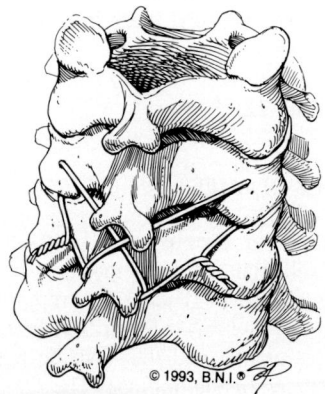

FIGURE 149-22. Facet to spinous process wiring. (© 1993, Barrow Neurological Institute. Used with permission.)

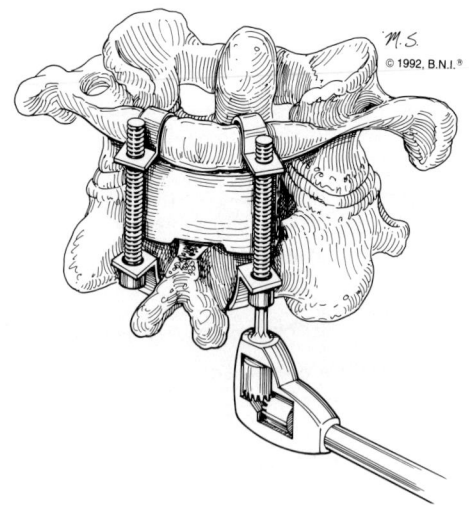

FIGURE 149-23. Halifax interlaminar clamps. The clamps have different profiles to conform to the shape of the laminae. A bone strut is positioned between adjacent vertebrae to add stability and prevent overreduction. A 90-degree angled wrench is used to tighten the screws. (© 1992, Barrow Neurological Institute. Used with permission.)

a wide bone surface. Theoretically, the clamps are less likely than wire to pull through osteoporotic bone. Bone struts are necessary to reinforce the fixation of the clamps, to limit extension and rotation, and to prevent overreduction. Halifax clamps are best suited for a single motion-segment. Spanning multiple motion segments should be avoided because no fixation is provided at intermediate levels. Unilateral clamps should also be avoided. Bilateral clamps are needed to achieve rotational stability, but the clamps should not be used if the facets are fractured or if significant destruction of the vertebral body exists. Screw loosening and loss of fixation have been reported with the clamps, but the clamp design has since been modified to prevent screw loosening.

SCREW FIXATION OF THE CERVICAL SPINE

PRINCIPLES OF VERTEBRAL SCREW FIXATION

Screw fixation has been used extensively for long bone fractures,[32] and during the past 20 years, screw techniques have been developed for vertebral fixation as well. Screw methods are used to obtain immediate rigid fixation of bone fragments and to apply plates to bone for fixation of adjacent segments.

A screw is composed of a head, a shaft, and a threaded portion. The major diameter refers to the widest diameter of the screw (i.e., outer diameter of the threads). The minor screw diameter, also called the core or inner diameter, refers to the diameter of the shaft beneath the threads. Screws can be characterized as cortical or cancellous, lag, self-tapping or non–self-tapping, cannulated or noncannulated, solid or hollow, or locking.

Screw sites are initially prepared by penetrating the cortical bone with a bone awl or high-speed drill. A cylindrical bone drill is then used to create a pilot hole into the bone for screw insertion.

SELF-TAPPING AND NON–SELF-TAPPING SCREWS

Self-tapping and non–self-tapping screws are differentiated by the design of their threads and require different surgical techniques for insertion (Fig. 149–24).[64] Both types of screws require the drilling of a pilot hole in the bone to create a tract for the screw. The diameter of the pilot hole should match the minor diameter of the screw. Self-tapping screws have sharp threads that cut into the bone as they are inserted. They are simply screwed into the tract. The threads of non–self-tapping screws are less sharp than those of self-tapping screws. Before non–self-tapping screws are inserted, the screw thread pattern is cut into the bone adjacent to the pilot hole by use of a tap. The width and pitch of the tap's threads correspond to the thread characteristics of the screw.

Non–self-tapping screws can be removed and reinserted without a high risk of creating a new tract, whereas reinserting self-tapping screws can create a new screw tract, and a wide, inadequate hole. The threads of non–self-tapping screws bite deeper into the adjacent bone than do those of self-tapping screws, giving non–self-tapping screws a slightly stronger purchase in bone than that afforded by self-tapping screws, at least theoretically. However, there is no proven biomechanical advantage to support tapping a screw site.[65,66]

CORTICAL AND CANCELLOUS BONE SCREWS

Cortical bone screws are non–self-tapping screws that are threaded along their entire length. They are available in numerous diameters and lengths, and each size has its corresponding drill bit and tap. The diameter of the drill bit corresponds to the minor diameter of the screw; the diameter of the tap corresponds to the major diameter of the screw.

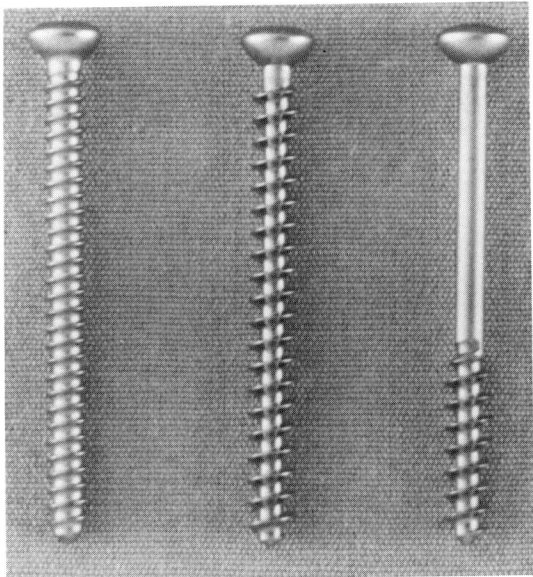

FIGURE 149–24. Screw thread profiles. (Left) Non–self-tapping cortical bone screws have a dull, narrow, thread profile. (Middle, Right) Self-tapping cancellous bone screws have a sharp, wide thread profile.

Cancellous bone screws are self-tapping screws. Their minor diameter is narrow, and their thread is wide and deep. These wide thread dimensions increase the holding power of the screw in trabecular bone. Cancellous bone screws have either partially or fully threaded shafts.

LAG SCREWS

Lag screws place adjacent bone fragments under compression and facilitate healing. The threads of a lag screw should engage a distal, but not a proximal, bone fragment. When the threads engage only the distal fragment, the bone fragments can be reduced and compressed. As the screw is tightened, the lag effect (i.e., compression) is generated as long as the functioning screw threads do not cross the fracture line or joint surface (Fig. 149–25).

Screw purchase in the proximal bone is avoided by one of two mechanisms. Either the proximal screw shaft must have no threads, or the hole in the proximal bone must be drilled wider than the major diameter of the screw. The latter approach is used with fully threaded screws. Such a wide proximal hole is called the *gliding hole*.

Partially threaded screws with threads confined to their distal portion provide one method for lag screw fixation. Lag screw fixation can also be achieved by use of a double-threaded compression screw.[67] The pitch of the proximal and distal screw threads differs, so that the distal fragments are compressed as the screw is tightened.

When possible, fractures should be reduced and alignment restored before a lag screw is placed. Lag screws should be inserted at a right angle to the fracture line[64]; otherwise, shearing forces can shift the bone fragments when the screw is tightened. Oblique fractures of the odontoid are particularly susceptible to this problem.[38]

CANNULATED SCREWS

Cannulated screws can be used for odontoid screw fixation or for atlantoaxial facet screw fixation. Cannulated screw systems consist of a long K-wire, a drill guide, a hollow tap, a hollow screw driver, and hollow screws (Fig. 149–26).[64,68] The thin (1.2-mm), threaded K-wires guide the placement of the screws. The K-wires are inserted with a drill to the desired depth and trajectory in the vertebrae. The drill, instruments, and screws are threaded sequentially over the K-wire so that they maintain the intended trajectory into the bone. Cannulated non–self-tapping or self-tapping screws can be used.

Cannulated screw systems permit screws to be placed precisely within bone. If the K-wire is misdirected, it can be repositioned easily without affecting the screw purchase site. In comparison, a wide screw hole that is malpositioned can destroy the purchase site if the bone adjacent to the screw site is weakened. The major risk associated with cannulated screws is migration of the K-wire. Inadvertent advancement of the K-wire intradurally could cause neural injury. Surgical maneuvers must be carefully observed fluoroscopically to avoid this complication.

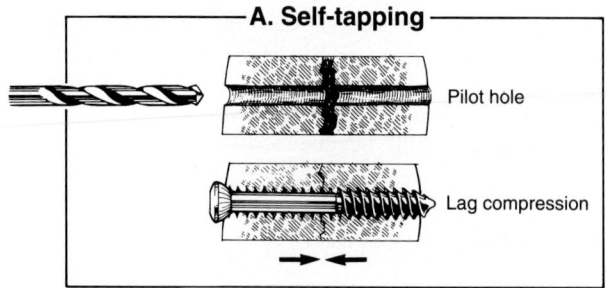
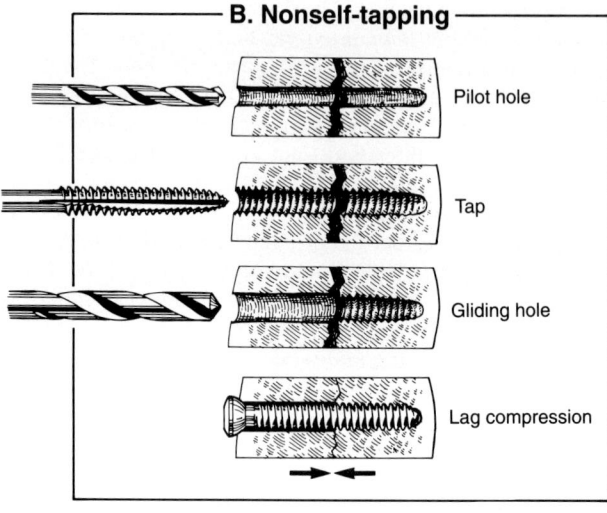
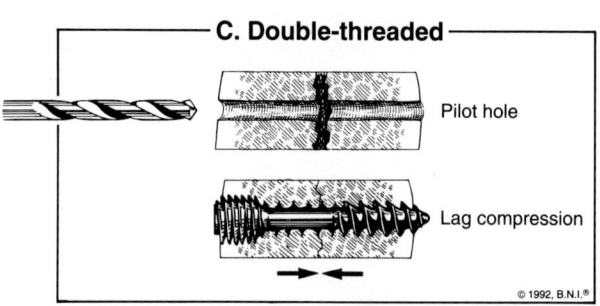

FIGURE 149–25. Lag screw fixation compresses adjacent bone surfaces together. (A) A partially threaded screw is inserted into a pilot hole. The screw threads should not cross the fracture line or compression will not be generated. (B) A lag effect can be achieved with a fully threaded screw if a wide hole is drilled in the proximal bone (i.e., gliding hole), so the proximal screw threads are not functional. (C) A double-threaded compression screw generates compression because the pitch of the proximal and distal threads differ. (© 1992, Barrow Neurological Institute. Used with permission.)

HOLDING POWER OF SCREWS

Bone screws are usually composed of stainless steel, titanium, or titanium alloys. Metal screws are more than 10 times harder than bone.[4, 28] Because metal is so much stronger than bone, when screws fail, they usually loosen and shear the bone from beneath the screw threads.[4, 69] Screw fixation strength within bone is determined by the area of bone beneath the screw threads.[69] The length of the screw, the width of the threads, and the density of the bone determine the pullout strength of the screw.[38, 65, 69]

Screws bend, fatigue, and can break during repetitive cyclic loading.[4, 65] Failure typically occurs at the junction of the shaft and the first screw thread. A screw's bending strength is determined by the composition of its metal and by the minor diameter (i.e., the diameter of the shaft beneath the threads). The bending strength of a screw is proportional to the third power of the minor screw diameter.[4, 38, 65] Thus, small changes in minor screw diameter can greatly alter bending strength.

Fixation will be inadequate if the bone adjacent to a screw is diseased, fractured, softened, or weakened. Screws that purchase thick, cortical bone are more rigidly fixed than screws in cancellous, trabecular bone.[38, 64, 66, 69]

Excessive heating of the bone during drilling damages the bone and can cause bone resorption around the screw. Thorough irrigation during drilling cools the bone and helps minimize subsequent screw loosening.

Screws in the cervical spine should be "finger tight" (i.e., use only two fingers to grasp the screwdriver). Overtightening strips the screw hole and results in an inadequate screw purchase. If a screw hole becomes stripped, a wider-diameter "rescue screw" can be used, or the hole can be filled with cancellous bone or methyl methacrylate to recover a screw purchase.

ANTERIOR ODONTOID SCREW FIXATION AND ANTERIOR ATLANTOAXIAL FACET SCREW FIXATION

Odontoid or atlantoaxial facet screw fixation may be performed by an anterior operative approach.[11, 38, 68, 70–72] These techniques are suitable for unstable odontoid fractures or for atlantoaxial instability in which the posterior arches of C1-C2 cannot be directly incorporated into a fusion (Fig. 149–27).

Both methods of screw fixation are performed through an identical operative exposure with the patient in a supine position. Lateral and anteroposterior fluoroscopic guidance is necessary to provide precise intraoperative visualization of the upper cervical spine. Preoperative computed tomographic (CT) studies are required to determine the position of the

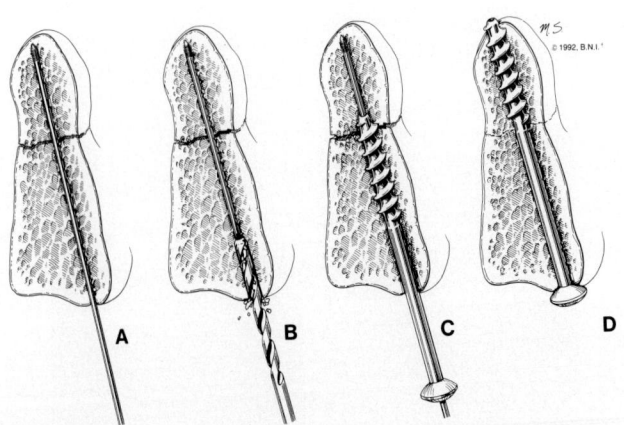

FIGURE 149–26. Cannulated screws. (A) A 1.2-mm Kirschner wire (K-wire) is drilled into the odontoid bone. (B) A 5-mm deep pilot hole is drilled into the body of C2 under fluoroscopic visualization. (C) A hollow screw is threaded over the K-wire, and inserted into the bone. (D) The screw threads should engage only the distal bone fragment. (© 1992, Barrow Neurological Institute. Used with permission.)

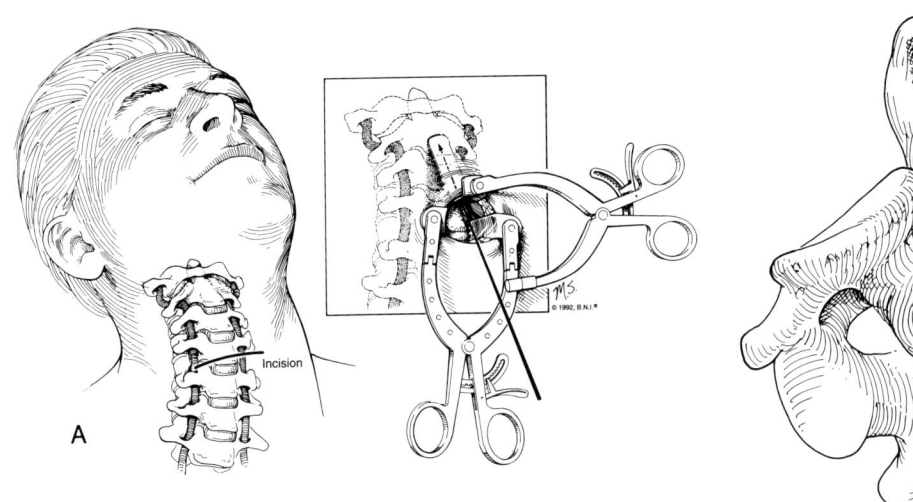

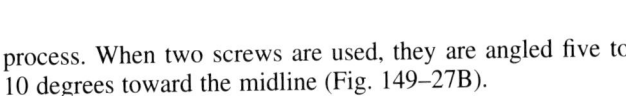

FIGURE 149–27. (A) The neck is extended for odontoid or anterior C1-C2 facet screw fixation. The Apfelbaum self-retaining retractor system (inset) helps maintain a drill trajectory parallel to the surface of the spine. (B) One or two lag screws are used to fixate the dens. When two screws are used, the dens must be wide. The screws are angled 5 to 10 degrees medially. (© 1992, Barrow Neurological Institute. Used with permission.)

vertebral arteries, to evaluate the bony architecture, and to assess for abnormalities that would preclude screw placement.

Odontoid screw fixation is ideal for fixating acutely unstable odontoid fractures because it preserves normal C1 motion. This technique can be employed only if the transverse atlantal ligament is intact. If the transverse ligament is disrupted, fixating the odontoid does not stabilize the atlas. The integrity of the transverse atlantal ligament can be directly assessed with MRI.[73] Odontoid screw fixation can be problematic for odontoid fracture nonunions. It is difficult to remove the scar tissue from a nonunion and to reduce the fracture to facilitate a bony union.

Odontoid screw fixation is performed with the patient positioned supine on the operating table with the head extended (Fig. 149–27). A transverse or oblique anterior cervical incision is made at the level of the cricothyroid junction. To facilitate exposure, the platysma muscle is widely undermined. The dissection is deepened to the level of the anterior cervical vertebrae and extended cephalad directly over the anterior longitudinal ligament to expose the inferior aspect of the C2 vertebrae. The longus colli muscles are elevated from the C2-C3 interspace to permit placement of self-retaining retractors and a drill guide. Apfelbaum retractors and instrumentation were developed specifically to facilitate anterior upper cervical screw fixation (Aesculap, San Francisco, CA).

Under fluoroscopic guidance, a drill guide is positioned at the C2-C3 interspace, and the drill is inserted at the anteroinferior body of C2 and angled parallel to the body of C2. The drill is directed into the tip of the dens. Odontoid screw fixation is performed with one or two lag screws, 3.5 mm in diameter (Fig. 149–27). A single screw can reduce and fixate an odontoid fracture satisfactorily. Two screws provide better rotational control, but the dens must be large enough to satisfactorily accommodate both screws. The internal diameter of the dens should be measured preoperatively with CT scans to determine if it can accommodate two screws. The screw tip should barely penetrate the tip of the odontoid process. When two screws are used, they are angled five to 10 degrees toward the midline (Fig. 149–27B).

Self-tapping, non–self-tapping, or cannulated screws may be used in this procedure. A lag effect is needed to compress the odontoid fragment to facilitate healing. Partially threaded, cancellous, self-tapping screws minimize the number of surgical steps. A pilot hole is drilled through the C2 body into the dens. The depth of the hole is measured, and a self-tapping screw is then inserted directly into the pilot hole. If a fully threaded screw is used, a proximal gliding hole must be drilled. When a cannulated screw system is used, a 5-mm-deep pilot hole is drilled over the K-wire into the proximal bone of C2, and a self-tapping, partially threaded screw is then inserted directly over the K-wire (see Fig. 149–26).

Anterior atlantoaxial facet screw fixation is similar to odontoid screw fixation. The operative exposure is identical; however, the screw insertion and trajectory differ. Before the screws are placed, the facet joints are decorticated with a bone curette to enhance fusion. Screws enter the C2 vertebral body in the recess between the vertebral body and the superior C2 facet. The screws are directed rostrally into the lateral masses of C1 (Fig. 149–28). The screws are shorter (i.e., 20 to 25 mm) than those used for odontoid fixation.

A pilot hole is made with a 2.5-mm-diameter drill beginning in the groove between the C2 vertebral body and the C2 superior facet. A single, 3.5-mm-diameter screw, either non–self-tapping or self-tapping, is placed into each facet under fluoroscopic guidance. A lag effect is preferred so that the C1-C2 facets will be compressed. This technique stabilizes C1-C2 rigidly but sacrifices all C1-C2 motion.

The anterior operations for C1-C2 facet or odontoid screw fixation are limited by the difficulties caused by high cervical exposure and soft tissue retraction and by the inability to add grafts to enhance fusion. Anterior upper cervical screw fixation is technically more demanding than posterior cervical fixation.

Anterior upper cervical screw fixation requires a thin-body habitus and extension of the head to facilitate screw placement. The trajectory of the drill must be almost parallel to

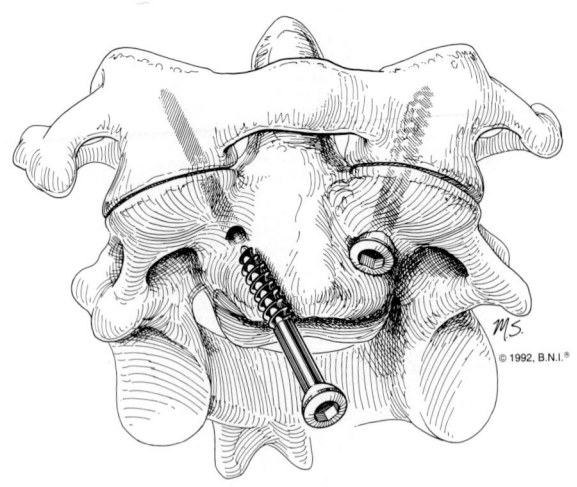

FIGURE 149–28. Anterior atlantoaxial facet screws are directed rostrally through the C2 superior facet into the C1 lateral mass. The drilling begins in the groove that separates the body and the superior facet. (© 1992, Barrow Neurological Institute. Used with permission.)

the anterior surface of the cervical spine. Short necks and barrel-shaped chests hinder operative access. These techniques should only be performed if C1-C2 aligment can be restored before screw insertion; otherwise, the fixation will be malaligned.

POSTERIOR ATLANTOAXIAL FACET SCREW FIXATION[74–77]

Before posterior atlantoaxial screw fixation is attempted, the morphology of the atlas and axis must be studied with CT. Comminuted fractures of C1 or C2 or an anomalous course of the vertebral artery contraindicates posterior atlantoaxial screw fixation. Atlantoaxial subluxations must be reduced and the superior facet joints of C2 and lateral masses of C1 must be realigned to obtain an adequate screw purchase.

Intraoperatively, the proper trajectory for insertion of drills and screws can be obtained through controlled flexion of the patient's neck (Fig. 149–29). The patient's head is affixed with a Mayfield skull clamp, and the patient is placed in a prone position. Lateral fluoroscopic visualization with a C arm is used to monitor atlantoaxial alignment during positioning and to guide screw placement. A posterior cervical incision is made to gain access to the atlas and axis and should extend to the C7 spinous process. The skin preparation should extend to the upper thoracic levels in case a longer incision or percutaneous access is required for drilling.

The atlas and axis are realigned by manual reduction after the vertebrae are exposed subperiosteally. With anterior atlantoaxial subluxations, C2 can be gently displaced anteriorly, and C1 can be pulled posteriorly. Opposite forces are applied for posterior subluxations. A wire can be placed around the ring of C1 for traction and subsequent fixation of a bone graft. An Allis clamp attached to the C2 spinous process can be used to retract the C2 spinous process toward the occiput to obtain an improved trajectory for drilling.

The ligamentum flavum adjacent to the C2 laminae and pedicles must be removed. The C2 pedicle and the C1-C2 articular surfaces are exposed and directly visualized. A thin K-wire or a No. 4 Penfield dissector is placed directly along the surface of the C2 pedicle into the atlantoaxial facet joint. The C2 nerve root and veins are retracted superiorly to allow direct visualization of the C2 pedicle and the facet joint during drilling.

With lateral fluoroscopic monitoring, the drill trajectory is aimed toward the dorsal cortex of the anterior arch of C1 (Fig. 149–30), and the screw is placed through the central axis of the C2 pedicle on an axial trajectory of zero to 10 degrees medially. The drill enters the posterior C2 cortex 2 to 3 mm above the C2-C3 facet and 2 to 3 mm lateral to the medial border of the C2-C3 facet. The posterior cortical bone of C2 is penetrated with a high-speed drill or bone awl to precisely direct the drill insertion for the pilot hole.

The pilot hole can be prepared by use of a 2.5-mm-diameter drill or a 2.4-mm-diameter, 9-inch-long, calibrated, end-threaded guide pin. The guide pin is used if percutaneous access is needed to obtain the proper drill trajectory (see Fig. 149–29). A 3.5-mm-diameter cortical bone screw is inserted into the pilot hole. As the screw crosses the joint space into C1, the atlas and axis become rigidly coupled. Satisfactory fixation can be achieved with a minimum number of operative steps by inserting the screw directly into the hole without tapping the hole. Cannulated, self-tapping, or non–self-tapping screws can be used depending on the surgeon's preference, but lag screws are recommended to compress the facet joints together to facilitate arthrodesis.

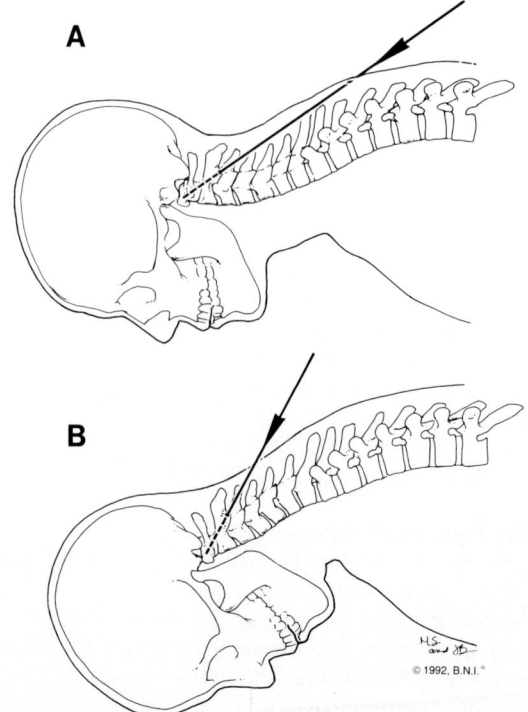

FIGURE 149–29. Posterior atlantoaxial facet screw fixation. (A) Percutaneous drilling must be performed when the patient's neck cannot be flexed. (B) Neck flexion permits direct drilling through the incision used to expose C1 and C2. (© 1992, Barrow Neurological Institute. Used with permission.)

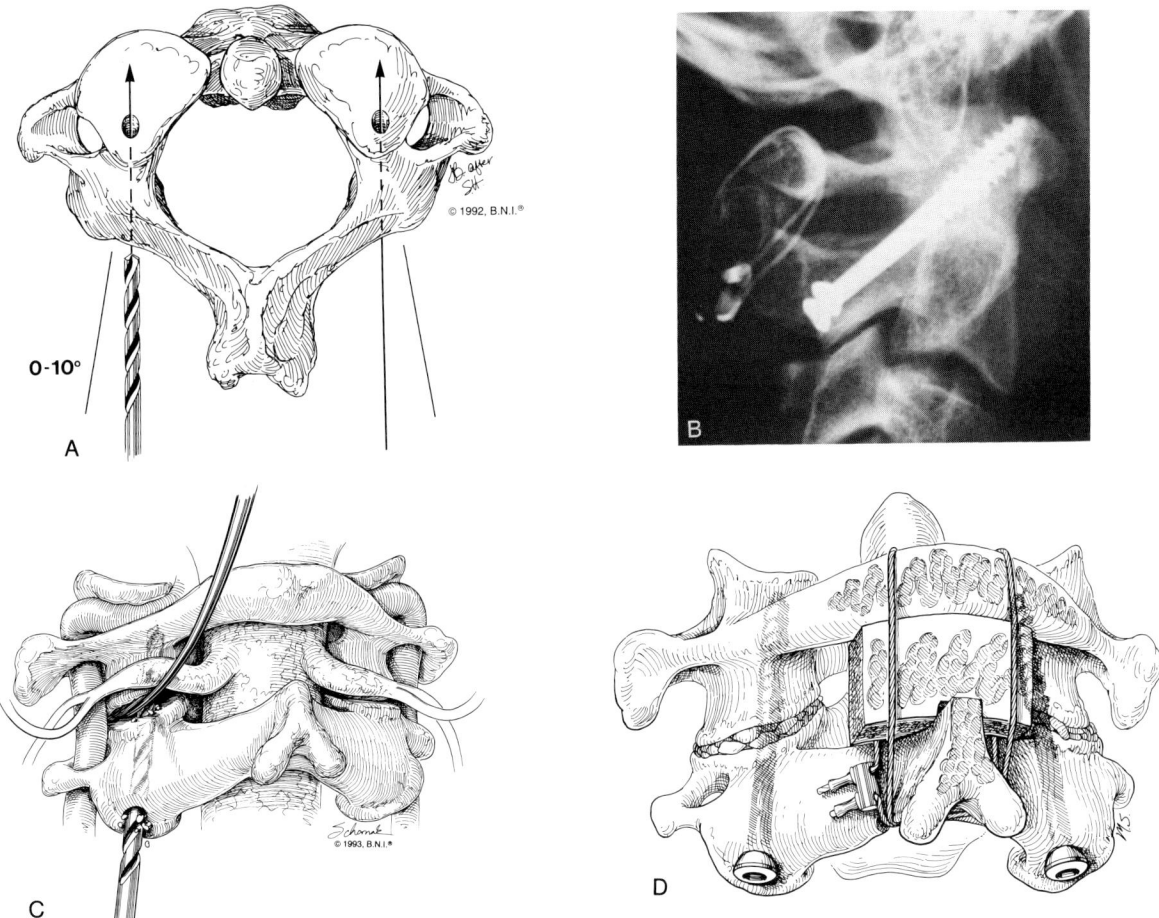

FIGURE 149–30. Posterior atlantoaxial facet screws. (A) An axial trajectory of 0 to 10 degrees medially is used to position the screw through the central axis of the C2 pedicle. A lateral trajectory is avoided to preserve the vertebral artery. (B) Screws are directed toward the dorsal cortex of the anterior arch of C1 on lateral fluoroscopic imaging. (C) The screws enter the C2 inferior facet 2 to 3 mm above the C2-C3 facet joint. The C2 nerve root and venous plexus are retracted upward during drilling. (D) An interspinous bone strut is wired to C1-C2 to provide three-point stabilization and to facilitate fusion. (A, C, and D, © 1992, 1993, Barrow Neurological Institute. Used with permission.)

The C1-C2 facet screws are supplemented with an interspinous wiring and fusion unless the posterior arches of C1 or C2 are fractured (Fig. 149–30D).[25] This three-point fixation of C1-C2 provides greater mechanical stability than either technique used alone.[74] The bone graft, which is compressed between the posterior arches of the C1 and C2, facilitates formation of a solid fusion.

Posterior screw fixation rigidly couples the facets of C1 and C2 to obtain immediate internal fixation. Because of the rigid coupling of C1 and C2, a postoperative halo brace is unnecessary.

Posterior atlantoaxial facet screw fixation can be used even when the posterior ring of the atlas is fractured or incompetent. This technique provides the most rigid form of internal fixation available for the atlantoaxial joint. It is biomechanically superior to wire or Halifax clamps for prohibiting atlantoaxial rotation and translation.[54, 74] Atlantoaxial facet screws can also be combined with metallic plates for fixation of the occiput or adjacent cervical segments.[56, 57]

Posterior atlantoaxial facet screw fixation is an excellent technique, but it is potentially dangerous. However, it can be performed safely if meticulous attention is paid to detail. A precise screw trajectory and preoperative CT studies are essential to avoid neural or vertebral artery injury. Among 25 patients treated with this technique, we have had no major complications and no failures of treatment.

SCREW-PLATE FIXATION

Bone plates, like screws, are usually composed of stainless steel or titanium. Metal plates are manufactured in various configurations for anterior or posterior cervical fixation, and hook plates, Y plates, and lateral mass plates are available.[38, 39, 57, 78–80] Plates may be contoured to restore the normal curvature of the cervical spine; however, excessive bending weakens the plate and should be avoided.

Plates should fit flush against the surfaces of the bone so that the fixation forces are evenly distributed. Anterior cervical plates are used to fixate vertebral bodies, and posterior plates are used for lateral mass or occipitocervical fixation.

Screw plates can serve mechanically as a tension band and as a buttress to resist vertical and horizontal translation of the spine.[4, 38, 75, 81] Anterior cervical screw plates provide an anterior tension band that resists extension.[4, 72, 81] However, with three-column spinal injuries, anterior cervical plates

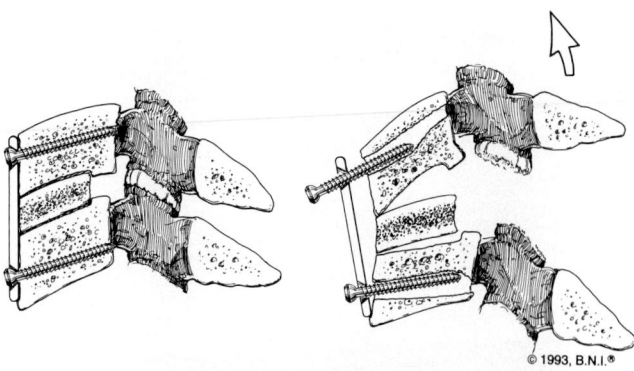

FIGURE 149–31. Anterior cervical screw plates provide an anterior tension band and buttress effect that strongly resists neck extension. In three-column cervical spine injuries, anterior screw plates weakly resist flexion or rotation. A hinge effect can occur causing the fixation to fail. (© 1993, Barrow Neurological Institute. Used with permission.)

weakly resist flexion or rotation (Fig. 149–31).[81, 82] In comparison, posterior cervical plates or wires strongly resist flexion of the neck but poorly resist extension or rotation.[81, 83] Posterior fixation can fail when the vertebral bodies are incompetent or when extreme ligament injuries coexist. Consequently, in three-column injuries of the cervical spine, anterior or posterior cervical plate fixation should be supplemented with a halo brace or with additional internal fixation.[4, 82]

Although plates and screws can increase the rigidity of injured spinal segments, they do not always restore normal strength to the spine.[4, 81, 84, 85] This is an important caveat. The uninjured spine is often much stronger than the internally fixated injured spine[4, 37, 40, 81, 84, 85]; therefore, surgeons should not exclusively or excessively depend on internal fixation. Instrumentation can fail if enough stress is applied to the destabilized spine, and instrumentation should be supplemented with an external orthosis appropriate for the type of injury and the method of internal fixation used.[86]

ANTERIOR SCREW PLATES

Anterior cervical screw plates fixate vertebral bodies and may be used to treat instability of the C2-C7 segments. Anterior screw plates cannot be used to fixate the occiput or C1 because of morphologic differences at the craniovertebral junction. Anterior plates can, however, provide stability after vertebrectomies or discectomies are performed. These systems permit neural decompression, reconstruction, and spinal stabilization to be accomplished in a single-stage surgical procedure. Anterior cervical plates can provide rigid segmental fixation and improve the fusion rates associated with anterior cervical fusion.[15, 16, 87, 88] They are useful for reducing spinal deformities and for preventing bone-graft migration.

Many plating systems have been used. Bicortical screws or unicortical locking screws can be used to fixate plates to the vertebrae (Fig. 149–32). Operative access for anterior cervical fusion is obtained by an anterior transcervical retropharyngeal approach.

Decompression and grafting are performed with standard techniques. A precision fit of bone grafts maximizes the surface area of bone apposition and thereby promotes fusion. The bone graft should be compressed between the vertebrae; such compression can be facilitated with traction or with an interspace distractor during placement of the bone graft. Osteophytes and the anterior longitudinal ligament should be removed from the surfaces of the vertebral bodies so that the plates fit flush against the bone.

Plates and screws are placed under fluoroscopic guidance to prevent complications. The plate is fitted along the anterior portion of the vertebrae and sized so that it does not extend across the adjacent disc spaces. The size of the plates should allow screw placement into the midvertebral bodies. If the plates are too long and extend beyond the fused segments or if the screws extend into the disc spaces, the screws and plate can loosen. Holes are drilled into the vertebrae to accommodate fixation screws, and a drill guide is used to control the depth and trajectory of the advancing drill. Screws can also be placed into the bone graft for fixation.

Bicortical systems are fixated with non–self-tapping, cortical bone screws (Fig. 149–32A).[15, 16, 57, 88, 89] Screw holes are drilled, the depth of the holes are individually measured, and the holes are tapped. The drill holes and screws are directed at an angle of 15 to 20 degrees toward the midline. The tips of the cortical fixation screws engage the posterior vertebral body cortices to secure the plate into position.[89] Screw plates can be contoured individually to fit abnormal curvatures. Slotted plates permit a choice of screw sites and allow screw repositioning, if needed (Fig. 149–32C).

Unicortical anterior cervical locking screw plates (Synthes) have screws that lock into a plate in a triangular configuration to resist pullout (Fig. 149–32B).[64, 87] A locking screw is inserted into the head of the anchor screw to expand the anchor screw head. The locking screw compresses the anchor screw against the plate hole and locks the screw to the plate, thereby providing rigid fixation.

Screw trajectory is predetermined and cannot be altered without altering the locking mechanism. All screws are angled 20 degrees medially. An arrow on the surface of the plate indicates the upper plate position. On lateral fluoroscopic imaging, the upper two screws are angled 10 degrees superiorly, and the lower screws are placed perpendicular to the bone (Fig. 149–32B, C, and D).

Screw heads are countersunk into the recessed holes in the plate and have a flat profile. Solid or hollow, fenestrated, anchoring screws (16 mm long, 4.0 mm wide) are used for this purpose. The hollow, fenestrated screws theoretically enhance bone growth into the screws and are designed for osteoporotic bone. However, the hollow screws are significantly weaker than solid screws and can break.

The major advantage of the locking screw system is that it avoids the risk of neurologic injury that can occur from penetration of the posterior vertebral body with the screw. The locking screw plates can be contoured, but bends should not be made near the locking mechanisms. A drawback of the locking screws is that screws cannot be removed easily once they are locking into position.

POSTERIOR CERVICAL SCREW PLATES

Posterior cervical screw plates are more versatile than anterior plates. Screws can be used to fixate the occiput, C2

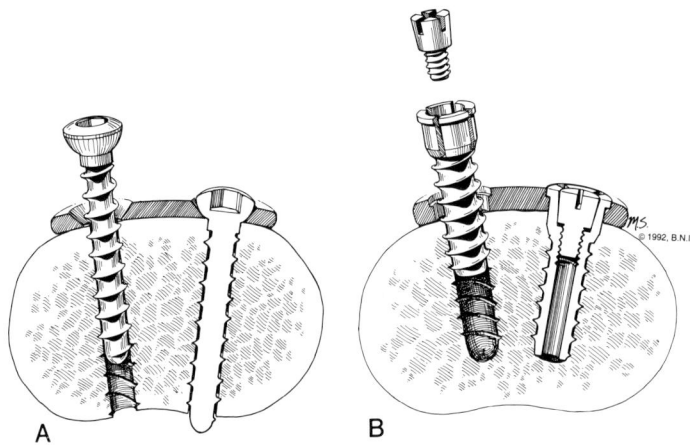

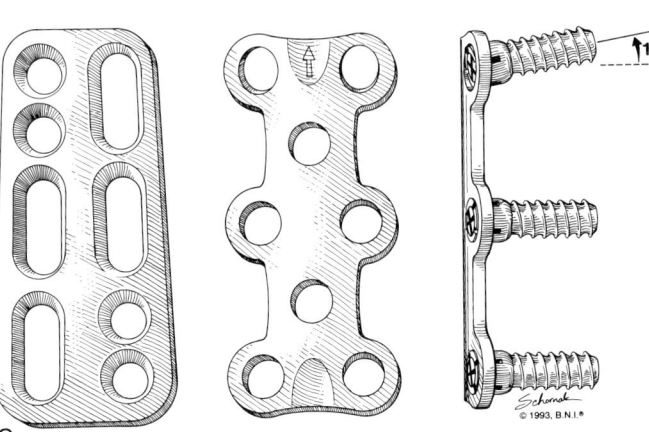

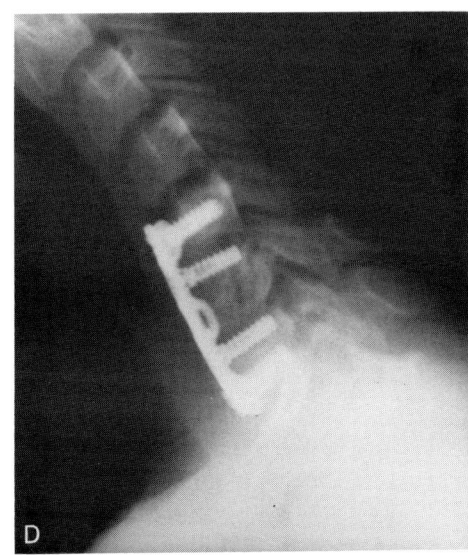

FIGURE 149–32. Anterior cervical screw plates. (A) Bicortical screws penetrate through the posterior cortex of the vertebral body. (B) Unicortical locking screws. A locking screw is inserted into the head of the anchor screw. The head of the anchor screw expands and is compressed against the plate. The screws converge medially to avoid plate pull-out. (C) Anterior view of Caspar (left) and Synthes (middle) screw plates. The upper screws of the locking plate are angled 10 degrees superiorly (right). (D) Postoperative lateral flexion radiograph of a locking cervical screw plate. (A to C, © 1992, 1993, Barrow Neurological Institute. Used with permission.)

pedicles, C1-C2 facets, or C3 to C7 lateral masses. Lateral mass plates, occipitocervical Y plates, or laminar hook-screw plates are available.[56, 57, 59, 78, 79, 90] Posterior cervical screw plates are excellent alternatives to wiring and are especially useful when the laminae or spinous processes are missing or incompetent.

LATERAL MASS SCREWS[54, 79, 90, 91]

Lateral mass screw plates, which are available in several sizes, can span one to four adjacent motion segments. They are placed via a standard midline posterior cervical operative exposure. Subperiosteal dissection is performed to expose the lateral edges of the lateral masses to receive the instruments. Subluxations are reduced, and the facet joints are curetted to remove the articular cartilage and to decorticate the facets. Thin wedges of autologous bone are compressed in the facet joints to facilitate fusion.

For the placement of lateral mass screws from C3 to C7, the landmarks for the center of the lateral mass are identified by use of the lateral and medial facet margins and the rostral and caudal aspects of the facets (Fig. 149–33). Screw placement is begun 1 mm medial to the center of the lateral mass. A bone awl is used to pierce the cortical bone to mark the starting point and to ensure a good drill purchase. For C3 through C7, the drill is angled 20 to 30 degrees laterally and 20 to 30 degrees rostrally. The trajectory must follow these guidelines to avoid the vertebral artery and the nerve root.[91, 92]

Several plate sizes are available and can span one to four adjacent motion segments. The lateral mass plates are fitted to the reduced vertebrae. Distal holes are drilled first, and the holes at intermediate levels are drilled after the end screws are placed. Bicortical penetration of the lateral masses is recommended to ensure adequate screw fixation. Self-tapping screws (16 mm × 3.5 mm) are placed into the lateral masses with trajectories identical to that of the drill. The screws are tightened sequentially to affix the plates.

Screws should not be placed in a level with a lateral mass fracture because they can easily pull out of a fractured facet. Lateral mass screws should be cautiously placed in C7 because the morphology of this vertebrae is transitional, and its facets and lateral masses are thin. Screws placed into the C7 lateral mass can potentially compress adjacent nerve roots.

C2-PEDICLE SCREWS

Posterior C2-pedicle screws are versatile and can be combined with lateral mass plates or with various other plates for cervical or occipitocervical fusion.[38, 78] A C2 screw is di-

1870 | *Surgery of the Craniovertebral Junction and Spine*

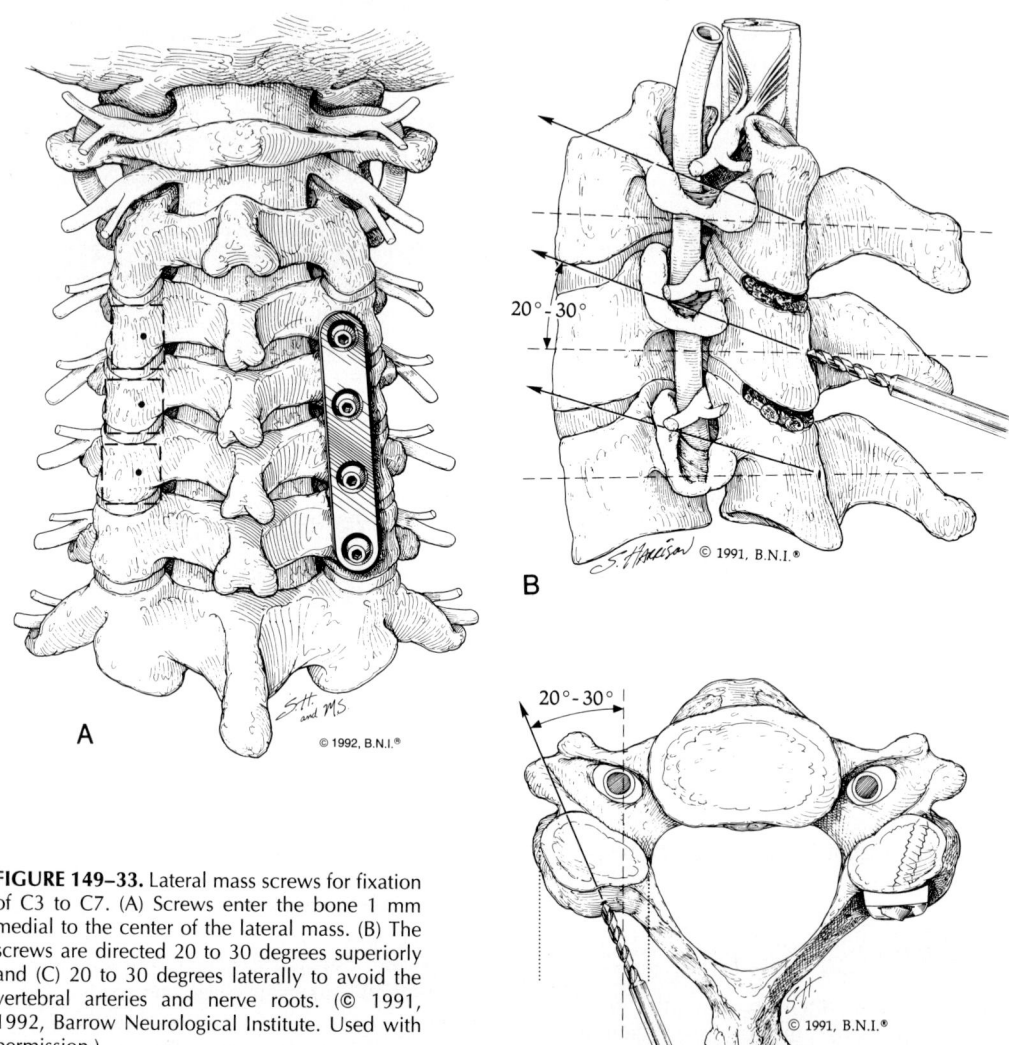

FIGURE 149–33. Lateral mass screws for fixation of C3 to C7. (A) Screws enter the bone 1 mm medial to the center of the lateral mass. (B) The screws are directed 20 to 30 degrees superiorly and (C) 20 to 30 degrees laterally to avoid the vertebral arteries and nerve roots. (© 1991, 1992, Barrow Neurological Institute. Used with permission.)

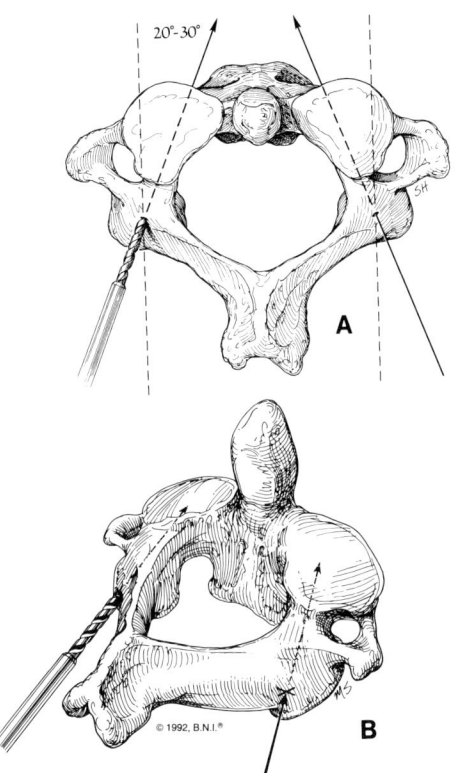

FIGURE 149–34. (A) C2 pedicle screws are directed 20 to 30 degrees medially and (B) 20 to 30 degrees superiorly. The screws enter the C2 inferior facet 2 to 3 mm above the C2-C3 facet joint. (© 1992, Barrow Neurological Institute. Used with permission.)

rected into the central axis of the C2 pedicle by angling of the drill 20 to 30 degrees rostrally and 20 to 30 degrees medially (Fig. 149–34). The ligamentum flava adjacent to the C2 pedicle and laminae are removed. Direct visualization

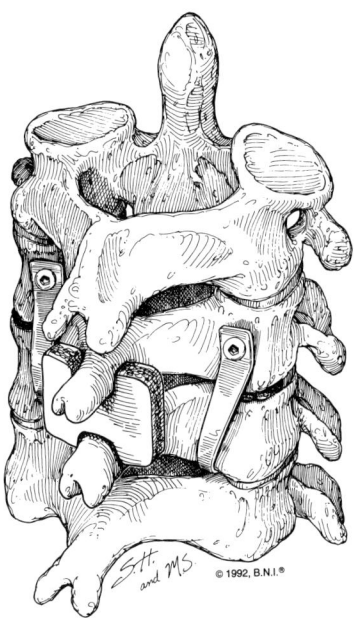

FIGURE 149–35. Magerl hook-plates should be used with an H graft to prevent hyperextension and to facilitate fusion. (© 1992, Barrow Neurological Institute. Used with permission.)

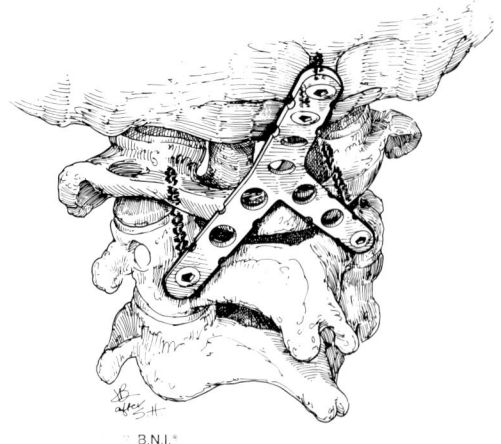

FIGURE 149–36. Occipitocervical fixation with a Y-shaped screw plate. Midline screws fixate the plate to the occiput near the nuchal line. The plate is secured to the cervical spine with bilateral posterior atlantoaxial facet screws. (© 1992, Barrow Neurological Institute. Used with permission.)

of the C2 pedicle and fluoroscopic monitoring ensure an accurate screw trajectory. The vertebral artery and penetration of the anterior body of C2 must be avoided.

OTHER SCREW-PLATE DESIGNS

Posterior cervical or occipitocervical fixation can be achieved with other types of plates secured with lateral mass screws, atlantoaxial facet screws, or C2-pedicle screws.

Magerl and coworkers[75, 80] developed laminar hook-screw plates that fixate the cervical laminae and lateral masses (Fig. 149–35).[38, 78] Screws are placed into the pedicle at C2 or into the lateral masses at lower cervical levels. The hook hugs the undersurface of the lamina of the adjacent inferior vertebral level. An H graft is fitted and compressed between the spinous processes of the fixated levels. The bone graft prevents overreduction and hyperextension and facilitates fusion. Hook plates require intact lamina and lateral masses for successful fixation.

An inverted Y-shaped screw plate has been used for occipitocervical fusion (Fig. 149–36).[56] Screws are placed through the Y plate into the midline of the occiput and into the C1-C2 facet joints bilaterally. The screw plate is supplemented with cancellous bone grafts. The C1-C2 facet screws obliterate atlantoaxial motion. When the Y plate is used, the thickness of each patient's occipital bone must be precisely measured with CT scans. The midline crest near the nuchal line has an average thickness of 14 mm (range, 10 to 18 mm). Short screws with limited pullout strengths must be used in the occiput. A risk of cerebellar or venous sinus injury is present if the occipital screws are too long or if they are malpositioned.

SUMMARY

Several mechanically advantageous techniques are available for internal fixation of the spine. The use of these techniques requires skill, judgment, technical precision, and a thorough knowledge of vertebral anatomy. Wiring techniques are reasonably safe and effective but have mechanical limitations and are not universally applicable. Screw fixation is an alternative to wiring. Screw techniques can be used when wiring is impossible, when anterior decompression and stabilization are needed, when wiring is inadequate to stabilize the spine, or when a rigid implant is indicated.

The effective surgical treatment of instability of the cervical spine depends on a thorough knowledge of each patient's pathology. Operative strategies are directed at decompressing neural structures, fixating unstable segments directly, attaining an osseous union, and preserving as much normal cervical mobility as possible.

Stringent criteria must be applied to the selection of the appropriate operative approach to ensure a successful outcome. The method affording the greatest likelihood of attaining internal fixation and fusion, while minimizing the risk to the patient, should be employed. This standard cannot be overemphasized. Techniques should be implemented based on the surgeon's knowledge and technical expertise, the available resources, and the patient's pathology. The financial and biologic costs of surgery should be minimized and the likelihood of attaining a solid fusion maximized.

REFERENCES

1. Dickman CA, Locantro J, Fessler RG: The influence of transoral odontoid resection on stability of the craniovertebral junction. J Neurosurg 77:525–530, 1992
2. Panjabi MM: The stabilizing system of the spine: Part I. Function, dysfunction, adaptation, and enhancement. J Spinal Disord 5(4):383–389, 1992
3. Kurz LT, Garfin SR, Booth RE Jr: Harvesting autogenous iliac bone grafts. A review of complications and techniques. Spine 14(12):1324–1331, 1989
4. White AA III, Panjabi MM: Clinical Biomechanics of the Spine. Philadelphia, JB Lippincott, 1978
5. Denis F: The three column spine and its significance in the classification of acute thoracolumbar spinal injuries. Spine 8(8):817–831, 1983
6. Frank C, Amiel D, Woo SL, et al: Normal ligament properties and ligament healing. Clin Orthop 196:15–25, 1985
7. Panjabi MM: The stabilizing system of the Spine: Part II. Neutral zone and instability hypothesis. J Spinal Disord 5(4):390–397, 1992
8. Dvorak J, Schneider E, Saldinger P, et al: Biomechanics of the craniocervical region: The alar and transverse ligaments. J Orthop Res 6:452–461, 1988
9. McAfee PC, Bohlman HH, Eismont FJ, et al: Failure of methylmethacrylate stabilization of the spine: A retrospective analysis of 24 cases, in Cervical Spine Research Society (ed): The Cervical Spine, 2nd ed. Philadelphia, JB Lippincott, 1989, pp 838–849
10. McAfee PC, Bohlman HH, Ducker T, et al: Failure of stabilization of the spine with methylmethacrylate. A retrospective analysis of twenty-four cases. J Bone Joint Surg Am 68A:1145–1157, 1968.
11. Lesoin F, Autricque A, Franz K, et al: Transcervical approach and screw fixation for upper cervical spine pathology. Surg Neurol 27:459–465, 1987
12. Crockard HA, Pozo JL, Ransford AO, et al: Transoral decompression and posterior fusion for rheumatoid atlanto-axial subluxation. J Bone Joint Surg 68(3):350–356, 1986
13. Menezes AH, VanGilder JC, Graf CJ, et al: Craniocervical abnormalities. A comprehensive surgical approach. J Neurosurg 53:444–455, 1980
14. Spetzler RF, Dickman CA, Sonntag VKH: The transoral approach to the anterior cervical spine. Contemp Neurosurg 13(9):1–6, 1991
15. Caspar W: Anterior stabilization with the trapezial osteosynthetic plate technique in cervical spine injuries, in Kehr P, Weidner A (eds): Cervical Spine I. New York, Springer-Verlag, 1987, pp 198–204
16. Caspar W, Barbier DD, Klara PM: Anterior cervical fusion and Caspar plate stabilization for cervical trauma. Neurosurgery 25(4):491–502, 1989
17. McAfee PC, Farey ID, Sutterlin CE, et al: Device-related osteoporosis with spinal instrumentation. Spine 14(9):919–926, 1989
18. Dickman CA, Fessler RG, Macmillan M, et al: Transpedicular screw-rod fixation of the lumbar spine: Operative technique and outcome in 104 cases. J Neurosurg 77(6):860–867, 1992
19. Prolo DJ: Biology of bone fusion. Clin Neurosurg 36:135–146, 1988
20. Zdeblick TA, Ducker TB: The use of freeze-dried allograft bone for anterior cervical fusion. Spine 16(7):726–729, 1991
21. Fernyhough JC, White JI, LaRocca H: Fusion rates in multilevel cervical spondylosis comparing allograft fibula with autograft fibula in 126 patients. Spine 16(10 Suppl):S561–S564, 1991
22. Fielding JW: The status of arthrodesis of the cervical spine. J Bone Joint Surg 70(10):1571–1574, 1988
23. Kaufmann HH, Jones E: The principles of bony spinal fusion. Neurosurgery 24:264–270, 1989
24. Murphy MJ, Southwick WO: Posterior approaches and fusions, in Cervical Spine Research Society (ed): The Cervical Spine, 2nd ed. Philadelphia, JB Lippincott, 1989, pp 775–791
25. Dickman CA, Sonntag VKH, Papadopoulos SM, et al: The interspinous method of posterior atlantoaxial arthrodesis. J Neurosurg 74:190–198, 1991
26. Robinson RA, Southwick WO: Surgical approaches to the cervical spine, in American Academy of Orthopedic Surgeons (ed): Instructional Course Lectures, vol 17. St. Louis, CV Mosby, 1960, pp 299–330
27. McGraw RW, Rusch RM: Atlanto-axial arthrodesis. J Bone Joint Surg 55(3):482–489, 1973
28. Brooks AL, Jenkins EB: Atlanto-axial arthrodesis by the wedge compression method. J Bone Joint Surg Am 60A(3):279–284, 1978
29. Griswold DM, Albright JA, Schiffman E, et al: Atlanto-axial fusion for instability. J Bone Joint Surg Am 60A(3):285–292, 1978
30. Gallie WE: Fractures and dislocations of the cervical spine. Am J Surg 46:495–494, 1939
31. Fielding JW, Hawkins RJ, Ratzan SA: Spine fusion for atlanto-axial instability. J Bone Joint Surg Am 58A:400–407, 1976
32. Mixter SJ, Osgood RB: Traumatic lesions of the atlas and axis. Ann Surg 51:193–207, 1910
33. Songer MN, Spencer DL, Meyer PR Jr, et al: The use of sublaminar cables to replace Luque wires. Spine 16 (8 suppl):S418–S421, 1991
34. Geisler FH, Mirvis SE, Zrebeet H, et al: Titanium wire internal fixation for stabilization of injury of the cervical spine: Clinical results and postoperative magnetic resonance imaging of the spinal cord. Neurosurgery 25:356–362, 1989
35. Taitsman JP, Saha S: Tensile strength of wire-reinforced bone cement and twisted stainless-steel wire. J Bone Joint Surg 59(3):419–425, 1977
36. Huhn SL, Wolf AL, Ecklund J: Posterior spinal osteosynthesis for cervical fracture/dislocation using a flexible multistrand cable system: Technical note. Neurosurgery 29:943–946, 1991
37. Pelker RR, Duranceau JS, Panjabi MM: Cervical spine stabilization. A three-dimensional, biomechanical evaluation of rotational stability, strength, and failure mechanisms. Spine 16(2):117–122, 1991
38. Dickman CA, Sonntag VKH, Marcotte PJ: Techniques of screw fixation of the cervical spine. Barrow Neurol Inst Q 8(2):9–26, 1992
39. Moskovich R, Crockard HA: Atlantoaxial arthrodesis using interlaminar clamps. An improved technique. Spine 17(3):261–267, 1992
40. Ulrich C, Woersdoerfer O, Kalff R, et al: Biomechanics of fixation systems to the cervical spine. Spine 16 (3 suppl):S4–9, 1991
41. MacKenzie AI, Uttley D, Marsh HT, et al: Craniocervical stabilization using Luque/Hartshill rectangles. Neurosurgery 36:32–36, 1990
42. McAfee PC, Bohlman HH: One-stage anterior cervical decompression and posterior stabilization with circumferential arthrodesis. A study of twenty-four patients who had a traumatic or a neoplastic lesion. J Bone Joint Surg Am 71A(1):78–88, 1989
43. Abdu WA, Bohlman HH: Spinal trauma management update. Techniques of subaxial posterior cervical spine fusion: An overview. Orthopedics 15(3):287–294, 1992
44. Callahan RA, Johnson RM, Margolis RN, et al: Cervical facet fusion for control of instability following laminectomy. J Bone Joint Surg Am 59A:991–1002, 1977
45. Garfin SR, Moore MR, Marshall LF: A modified technique for cervical facet fusions. Clin Orthop 230:149–153, 1988
46. Sonntag VKH, Dickman CA: Operative management of occipitocervical and atlantoaxial instability, in Holtzman RN, Farcy J, McCormick P (eds): Spinal Instability. Berlin, Springer-Verlag, 1993, pp 255–294

47. Dickman CA, Douglas RA, Sonntag VKH: Occipitocervical fusion: Posterior stabilization of the craniovertebral junction and upper cervical spine. Barrow Neurol Inst Q 6(2):2–14, 1990
48. Grantham SA, Dick HM, Thompson RC Jr, et al: Occipitocervical arthrodesis. Indications, technic and results. Clin Orthop 65:118–129, 1969
49. Ransford AO, Crockard HA, Pozo JL, et al: Craniocervical instability treated by contoured loop fixation. J Bone Joint Surg 68(2):173–177, 1986
50. Sakou T, Kawaida H, Morizono Y, et al: Occipitoatlantoaxial fusion utilizing a rectangular rod. Clin Orthop 239:136–144, 1989
51. Geremia GK, Kim KS, Cerullo L, et al: Complications of sublaminar wiring. Surg Neurol 23:629–634, 1985
52. Hanley EN Jr, Harvell JC Jr: Immediate postoperative stability of the atlantoaxial articulation: A biomechanical study comparing simple midline wiring, and the Gallie and Brooks procedures. J Spinal Disord 5:306–310, 1992
53. Gallie WE: Skeletal traction in treatment of fractures and dislocations of cervical spine. Ann Surg 106:770–776, 1937
54. Grob D, Crisco JJ III, Panjabi MM, et al: Biomechanical evaluation of four different posterior atlantoaxial fixation techniques. Spine 17:480–489, 1992
55. Wertheim SB, Bohlman HH: Occipitocervical fusion. Indications, technique, and long-term results in thirteen patients. J Bone Joint Surg 69(6):833–836, 1987
56. Grob D, Dvorak J, Panjabi M, et al: Posterior occipitocervical fusion. A preliminary report of a new technique. Spine 16 (3 suppl):S17–S24, 1991
57. Weidner A: Internal fixation with metal plates and screws, in Cervical Spine Research Society (ed): The Cervical Spine, 2nd ed. Philadelphia, JB Lippincott, 1989, pp 404–421
58. Hamblen DL: Occipito-cervical fusion. Indications, technique and results. J Bone Joint Surg 49(1):33–45, 1967
59. Heywood AW, Learmonth ID, Thomas M: Internal fixation for occipitocervical fusion. J Bone Joint Surg 70(5):708–711, 1988
60. Rogers WA: Fractures and dislocation of the cervical spine. An end-result study. J Bone Joint Surg 39:341–376, 1957
61. Davey JR, Rorabeck CH, Bailey SI, et al: A technique of posterior cervical fusion for instability of the cervical spine. Spine 10(8):722–728, 1985
62. Holness RO, Huestis WS, Howes WJ, et al: Posterior stabilization with an interlaminar clamp in cervical injuries: Technical note and review of the long term experience with the method. Neurosurgery 14(3):318–322, 1984
63. Aldrich EF, Crow WN, Weber PB, et al: Use of MR imaging-compatible Halifax interlaminar clamps for posterior cervical fusion. J Neurosurg 74:185–189, 1991
64. Muller ME, Allgower M, Schneider R, et al: Manual of Internal Fixation. Techniques Recommended by the AO-ASIF Group. Berlin, Springer-Verlag, 1991
65. Krag MH: Biomechanics of thoracolumbar spinal fixation. A review. Spine 16 (3 suppl):S84–S99, 1991
66. Schatzker J, Sanderson R, Murnaghan JP: The holding power of orthopedic screws in vivo. Clin Orthop 108:115–126, 1975
67. Knoringer P: Double-threaded compression screws for osteo-synthesis of acute fractures of the odontoid process, in Voth D, Glees P (eds): Diseases in the Cranio-Cervical Junction. Anatomical and Pathological Aspects and Detailed Clinical Accounts. New York, de Gruyter, 1987, pp 127–136
68. Etter C, Coscia M, Jaberg H, et al: Direct anterior fixation of dens fractures with a cannulated screw system. Spine 16:S25–S31, 1991
69. Brod JJ: The concepts and terms of mechanics. Clin Orthop 146:9–17, 1980
70. Barbour JR: Screw fixation in fracture of the odontoid process. South Aust Clin 5:20–24, 1971
71. Borne GM, Bedou GL, Pinaudeau M, et al: Odontoid process fracture osteosynthesis with a direct screw fixation technique in nine consecutive cases. J Neurosurg 68:223–226, 1988
72. Geisler FH, Cheng C, Poka A, et al: Anterior screw fixation of posteriorly displaced type II odontoid fractures. Neurosurgery 25:30–38, 1989
73. Dickman CA, Mamourian A, Sonntag VKH, et al: Magnetic resonance imaging of the transverse atlantal ligament for the evaluation of atlantoaxial instability. J Neurosurg 75:221–227, 1991
74. Hanson PB, Montesano PX, Sharkey NA, et al: Anatomic and biomechanical assessment of transarticular screw fixation for atlantoaxial instability. Spine 16(10):1141–1145, 1991
75. Magerl F, Seemann P-S: Stable posterior fusion of the atlas and axis by transarticular screw fixation, in Weidner PA (ed): Cervical Spine I. New York, Springer-Verlag, 1987, pp 322–327
76. Jeanneret B, Magerl F: Primary posterior fusion C1/2 in odontoid fractures: Indications, technique, and results of transarticular screw fixation. J Spinal Disord 5:464–475, 1992
77. Grob D, Jeanneret B, Aebi M, et al: Atlanto-axial fusion with transarticular screw fixation. J Bone Joint Surg Br 73B(6):972–976, 1991
78. Roy-Camille R, Saillant G, Mazel C: Internal fixation of the unstable cervical spine by a posterior osteosynthesis with plates and screws, in Cervical Spine Research Society (ed): The Cervical Spine, 2nd ed. Philadelphia, JB Lippincott, 1989, pp 390–403
79. Cooper PR, Cohen A, Rosiello A, et al: Posterior stabilization of cervical spine fractures and subluxations using plates and screws. Neurosurgery 23:300–306, 1988
80. Magerl F, Grob D, Seemann P: Stable dorsal fusion of the cervical spine (C2-Th1) using hook plates, in Kehr P, Weidner A (eds): Cervical Spine I. New York, Springer-Verlag, 1987, pp 217–221
81. Sutterlin CE III, McAfee PC, Warden KE, et al: A biomechanical evaluation of cervical spinal stabilization methods in a bovine model. Static and cyclical loading. Spine 13(7):795–802, 1988
82. Cybulski GR, Douglas RA, Meyer PR Jr, et al: Complications in three-column cervical spine injuries requiring anterior-posterior stabilization. Spine 17(3):253–236, 1992
83. Montesano PX, Juach EC, Anderson PA, et al: Biomechanics of cervical spine internal fixation. Spine 16 (3 suppl):S10–S16, 1991
84. Maiman DJ, Yoganandan N: Biomechanics of cervical spine trauma. Clin Neurosurg 37:543–570, 1991
85. Yoganandan N, Larson SJ, Pintar F, et al: Biomechanics of lumbar pedicle screw/plate fixation in trauma. Neurosurgery 27:873–881, 1990
86. Johnson RM, Hart DL, Simmons EF, et al: Cervical orthoses. A study comparing their effectiveness in restricting cervical motion in normal subjects. J Bone Joint Surg Am 59A:332–339, 1977
87. Suh PB, Kostuik JP, Esses SI: Anterior cervical plate fixation with the titanium hollow screw plate system. A preliminary report. Spine 15(10):1070–1081, 1990
88. Tippets RH, Apfelbaum RI: Anterior cervical fusion with the Caspar instrumentation system. Neurosurgery 22:1008–1013, 1988
89. Maiman DJ, Pintar FA, Yoganandan N, et al: Pull-out strength of Caspar cervical screws. Neurosurgery 31:1097–1101, 1992
90. Cherny WB, Sonntag VKH, Douglas RA: Lateral mass posterior plating and facet fusion for cervical spine instability. Barrow Neurol Inst Q 7(2):2–11, 1991
91. An HS, Gordin R, Renner K: Anatomic considerations for plate-screw fixation of the cervical spine. Spine 16(10):S548–S551, 1991
92. Heller JG, Carlson GD, Abitbol J-J, et al: Anatomic comparison of the Roy-Camille and Magerl techniques for screw placement in the lower cervical spine. Spine 16(10):S552–S557, 1991

CHAPTER 150

Surgical Approaches to the Cervicothoracic Junction

Richard G. Fessler
Donald D. Dietze

Surgical access to the cervicothoracic junction has traditionally been divided into anterior, posterior, and posterolateral techniques. Posterior approaches, such as laminectomy and pediculectomy, are performed easily, quickly, and frequently and are well known to all neurosurgeons. However, these approaches provide poor exposure of the anterior vertebral elements and, thus, are limited in their usefulness. When performed for vertebral body disease, laminectomy has a lower probability of success and a higher probability of complication.[1, 2] Furthermore, when anterior disease results in unstable anterior and middle columns, laminectomy may be totally destabilizing.

Fortunately, pathologic processes in this region are relatively uncommon. However, up to 10 percent of spinal metastases are seen in the region of T1 to T4. Other pathologic processes involving this area are listed in Table 150–1.

The necessity to approach this region surgically, and the limitations imposed by purely posterior approaches, resulted in the development of several anterior and posterolateral approaches to the vertebral elements. The first detailed posterolateral approach to the anterior elements of the spine was the costotransversectomy.[3] Although this approach gave adequate exposure of the middle and low thoracic spine, it was limited in its usefulness in the upper thoracic region by the scapula, levator scapulae, rhomboid, and trapezius musculature. A more extensive posterolateral approach, the lateral rachiotomy, was described by Capener in 1954.[4] In 1976, Larson and colleagues[5] reported on a modification of the lateral rachiotomy, the lateral extracavitary approach, which provided improved exposure of the middle and lower thoracic spine and had lower morbidity. Both the lateral rachiotomy and the lateral extracavitary approaches, however, were still limited in their usefulness for the upper thoracic spine and cervicothoracic junction by the scapula and the trapezius and rhomboid musculature. A modification of the lateral extracavitary approach, the lateral parascapular extrapleural approach, eliminated those obstructions, however, and has yielded excellent exposure of the thoracic vertebrae up to the inferior endplate of C7.[6]

Purely anterior approaches to the cervicothoracic junction were independently described by Jonnesco[7] and Brunig[8] in 1923. These were supraclavicular approaches and were later used by Royle for spastic paralysis[9]; Gask, for Raynaud's disease[10]; and Ochsner and DeBakey, for thoracic sympathectomy.[11] Because the clavicle was left intact, however, exposure of the thoracic area was limited. A modification of this approach, the transmanubrial and transclavicular approach, was described by Sundaresan and associates[12] in 1984 and was modified by Birch and associates[13] in 1990. These modifications removed the medial third of the clavicle as well as a portion of the manubrium and significantly increased the exposure of the upper thoracic vertebrae.

The third major approach to the anterior vertebral elements of the thoracic spine was first described by Hodgson and coworkers.[14] This approach, the anterolateral thoracotomy, involved resection of the third rib and required transpleural mobilization of the lung as well as ligation and division of the intercostal arteries, veins, and hemiazygos vein.

The following sections evaluate the clinical presentation of disease at the cervicothoracic junction and preoperative evaluation of the disease. Thereafter, the relevant surgical anatomy is reviewed, with specific reference to each surgical approach. Anesthetic techniques important for surgery in this region of the spine are then considered. Finally, the three major surgical approaches to the anterior vertebral elements in this region are described in detail.

CLINICAL FEATURES

The differential diagnosis of disease processes in this region is listed in Table 150–1. Depending on the exact location of the lesion, disease processes in this region can present as pain without hard neurologic signs, thoracic myelopathy, C7 or T1 radiculopathy, or a combination of these signs and

Table 150–1. DIFFERENTIAL DIAGNOSIS OF LESIONS OF THE CERVICOTHORACIC JUNCTION

Metastatic tumors
Primary tumors of bone
Primary lymphoma
Intradural, extramedullary tumors
Intradural, intramedullary tumors
Bacterial infections
Tuberculous infections
Vascular malformations
Pathologic fracture (primary metabolic disease of bone)
Connective tissue or skeletal disorders
Traumatic vertebral fractures
Disc herniations

Table 150–2. SIGNS AND SYMPTOMS AT PRESENTATION OF 17 PATIENTS WITH C7-T4 PATHOLOGIC PROCESSES

Signs and Symptoms	Patients with Signs or Symptoms (%)
Back pain	83
Radicular pain	33
Leg weakness	58
Decreased sensation	92
Hand weakness	35
Bowel or bladder dysfunction	17
Ataxic	25
Babinski's sign	58

symptoms. Table 150–2 presents the percentage of patients presenting with various signs and symptoms from our series of patients with pathologic processes located between C7 and T4.

PREOPERATIVE EVALUATION

RADIOLOGIC EVALUATION

Radiologic evaluation of this area of the spine begins with anteroposterior and lateral plain x-ray studies. These x-ray studies may demonstrate traumatic or pathologic vertebral fractures, infections, evidence of metabolic bone disease, and primary or metastatic tumors. Pathologic and traumatic fractures are demonstrated by malalignment, vertebral collapse, and widening of the pedicles on anteroposterior x-ray study. The earliest and most constant radiographic findings in osteomyelitis or discitis is narrowing of the disc space, which is present in 74 percent of patients at presentation.[15] After 3 to 6 weeks, destructive changes in the body can be noted. These changes usually begin as lytic areas in the anterior aspect of the body adjacent to the disc and endplate. Active bone formation and sclerosis are present in 11 percent of patients on presentation. Approximately 30 to 70 percent of the bone must be destroyed before osteomyelitic metastases are visible on plain x-ray study.[16] Several classic signs, however, do suggest the presence of vertebral metastases. These signs include vertebral collapse, unilateral erosion of a pedicle, "fish mouthing" (cephalad and caudal endplate concavity within the vertebral body), and osteoblastic lesions.

Radionuclide bone scintigraphy is very sensitive in detecting metastatic disease to the spine, infections, and fractures, although it is not specific for any of these.[17, 18] False-negative results have been reported with very aggressive lesions, such as lung cancer, renal cell carcinoma, and myeloproliferative diseases, as well as in areas of regional ischemia and in leukopenic patients.[19–21]

The use of myelography is primarily to evaluate the patency of the subarachnoid space. It can demonstrate the level of a metastatic lesion in the thoracic spine by indentation or complete blockade of the myelographic contrast column as it flows through the thoracic spinal canal. In addition, it can demonstrate the presence of intradural extramedullary or intramedullary tumors, thoracic disc herniations, retropulsed vertebral fragments from pathologic or traumatic fractures, and vascular malformations.

Computed tomographic scanning performed after myelography aids in the evaluation of metastatic disease to the thoracic spine and can detect the exact location of intradural tumors, thoracic disc herniations, and the presence of vascular malformations. In addition, it is helpful in determining the extent of paraspinal soft tissue involvement for staging of metastatic tumors, as well as in determining the extent of bone destruction. Finally, it may be helpful in distinguishing between osteoporosis and tumor.

Magnetic resonance imaging (MRI) is the most important new diagnostic tool for the evaluation of disease in the thoracic spine. MRI permits early diagnosis of infection and recognition of paravertebral or intraspinal abscesses without the risk associated with myelography.[22] MRI is also effective in demonstrating the extent of metastatic disease, primary tumors of bone, primary lymphoma, intradural tumors, thoracic disc herniations, and vertebral fractures, and it may be helpful detecting in spinal vascular malformations. It has been found to be at least as sensitive and accurate as gallium and bone scanning combined.[23]

METABOLIC EVALUATION

Routine metabolic evaluation of pathology in the cervicothoracic junction should include complete blood count with platelets and differential as well as kidney profile (electrolyte, blood urea nitrogen and creatinine values), liver profile, and erythrocyte sedimentation rate. Other metabolic evaluations include calcium, phosphorus, alkaline phosphatase analyses, serum protein electrophoresis, and serum transferrin analysis. Antinuclear antibody and rheumatoid factor analyses may help evaluate for rheumatoid arthritis, and bone marrow aspirate may be helpful in the diagnosis of blood-borne dyscrasias. Finally, specific antigen markers that may contribute to the diagnosis of a specific tumor include carcinoembryonic antigen for liver and pancreatic tumors, serum acid phosphatase, and prostate-specific antigen for prostatic carcinoma.

REGIONAL SURGICAL ANATOMY

LATERAL PARASCAPULAR EXTRAPLEURAL AND ANTEROLATERAL THORACOTOMY APPROACHES

The following sections briefly describe the anatomy relevant to each of the three surgical approaches discussed in this chapter. In view of the relative unfamiliarity of many neurosurgeons with the anatomy of the upper torso, many may find it useful to use an anatomic atlas to supplement the illustrations provided. The illustrations in this chapter emphasize those points of the anatomy relevant to each surgical approach.

The lateral parascapular extrapleural approach to the cervicothoracic junction is an extreme posterolateral approach that allows nearly lateral access to the vertebral bodies. The transthoracic approach through the third rib is an anterolateral approach to the upper thoracic vertebrae that allows access to the anterior and lateral aspects of the vertebrae and control of mediastinal vasculature. Because of the extensive overlap of anatomy relevant to these two approaches, they are considered together and may be summarized in three major areas: (1) scapula and parascapular anatomy, (2) posterior thoracic cage, and (3) retromediastinal space and spinal anatomy.

Scapula and Parascapular Anatomy

Posterolateral access to the thoracic cage and vertebral elements is hindered by the scapula and the parascapular shoulder musculature (Fig. 150–1). Mobilization of the scapula anterolaterally is necessary and requires the disruption of the posteromedial shoulder musculature.

The first muscle encountered after skin incision is the trapezius muscle, which originates along the superior nuchal line and external occipital protuberance and on each spinous process (via the ligamentum nuchae) from C1 through T12. The insertion of the trapezius muscle is divided into upper, intermediate, and lower divisions, which pass to the lateral third of the clavicle, the acromion, and the scapular spine, respectively. The lower fibers form an aponeurosis that inserts on the tubercle of the lower lip of the scapular spine. These insertions enable the trapezius muscle to function in stabilization and abduction of the shoulder. The trapezius muscle is supplied by the spinal accessory nerve, which arises from C1-C5, and directly via the ventral rami of C3 and C4. The spinal accessory nerve lies deep to the trapezius muscle but superficial to the levator scapulae. Its arterial supply is from branches of the dorsal scapular artery.

Immediately deep to the trapezius muscle lie the rhomboid major, rhomboid minor, and levator scapulae muscles. The rhomboid major originates on the ligamentum nuchae of the spinous processes T1 through T4, and the rhomboid minor originates similarly on the spinous processes of C6 and C7. Both of these muscles insert along the vertebral edge of the scapula, the rhomboid minor above, and the rhomboid major below, the scapular spine. The innervation and arterial supply of the rhomboid muscles come from the dorsal scapular nerve and artery. Nervous supply to the levator scapulae muscle is via branches from C3, C4, and C5. Arterial supply to the levator scapulae is also from branches of the dorsal scapular artery. Both of these structures lie deep to the bodies of the muscles and are located somewhat medially under the scapula. Thus, in a routine exposure, neither the dorsal scapular nerve nor the dorsal scapular artery or vein are directly exposed.

Immediately deep to the trapezius muscle from C6 through approximately T2 lies the serratus posterosuperior muscle. Ventral to this, the splenius arises from the ligamentum nuchae and upper thoracic spines and divides into two parts, the splenius capitis and splenius cervicis. The splenius capitis inserts with the sternocleidomastoid muscle on the superior nuchal line and the mastoid process. The splenius cervicis joins the levator scapulae to insert on the transverse processes of C1 through C4. These muscles function in stabilization and rotation of the skull.

In the initial dissection for exposure of the cervicothoracic junction, the spinous process insertions of the trapezius, rhomboid, serratus posterosuperior, splenius capitis, and splenius cervicis muscles are taken down as a single group for lateral retraction. As these muscles are taken down, the scapula is released from its attachments to the spinous processes and rotates anteriolaterally out of the operative field. This maneuver exposes the posterior and posterolateral rib cage for the remainder of the procedure. During this rotation, all neural and arterial supply rotates with the scapula and is at no risk of injury.

Posterior Thoracic Cage

The muscles of the next group encountered are the deep, or intrinsic, muscles (Fig. 150–2) and include the erector spinae muscles and the transversospinalis muscles. The erector spinae muscles originate as a dense aponeurotic band from the sacrum and divide into three columns below the last rib. The iliocostalis muscle is located most laterally of these three and is inserted into the angles of the ribs and into the cervical transverse processes from C4 through C6. This insertion is achieved through a series of related bundles of muscles that extend over about six segments each. Where one muscle is inserted, another arises on its medial side and extends cephalad. The longissimus muscles (thoracis, cervicis, and capitis) are inserted into lumbar and thoracic transverse processes and nearby parts of the ribs between T2 and

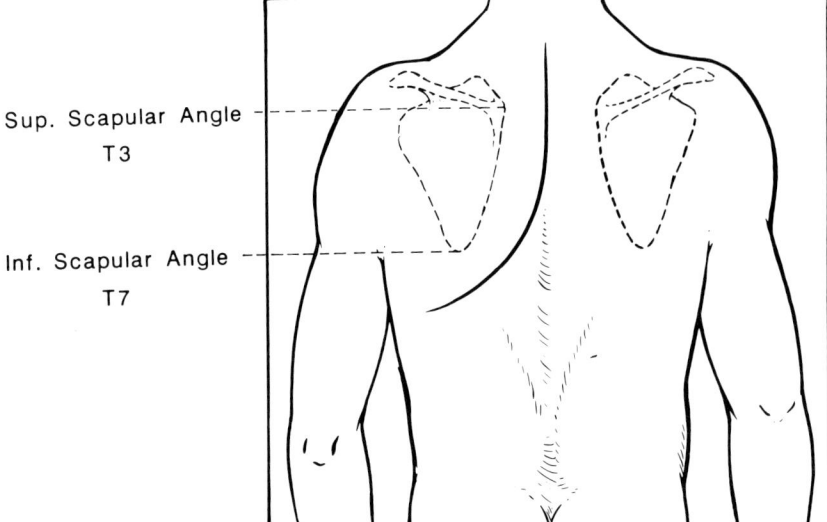

FIGURE 150–1. Relation of scapula to incision and surgical approach to the cervicothoracic junction via the lateral parascapular extrapleural approach.

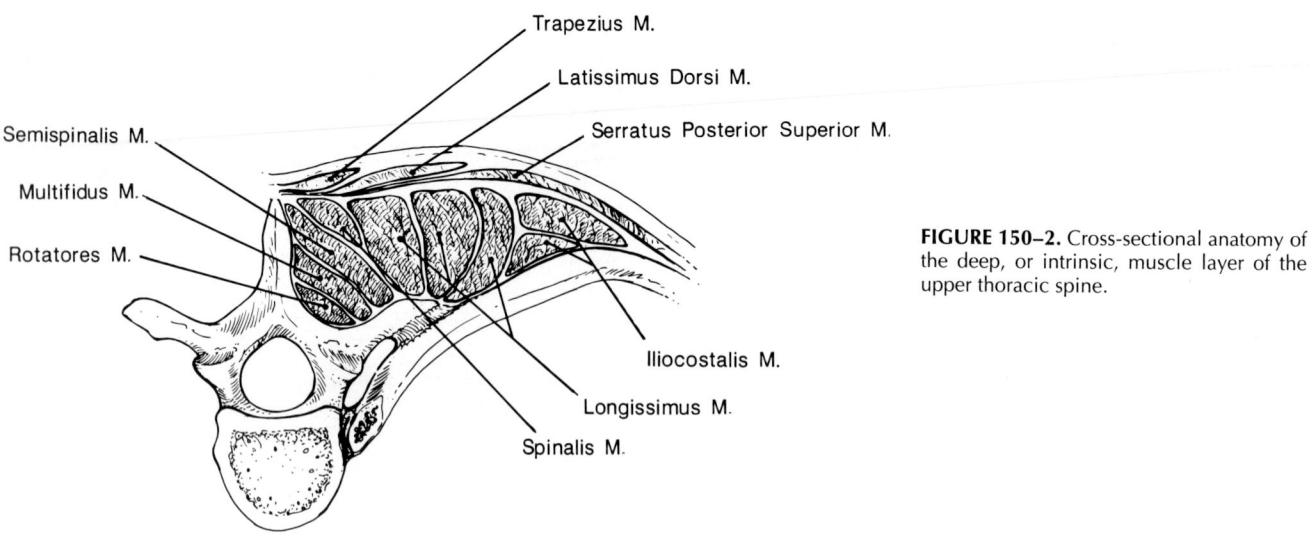

FIGURE 150–2. Cross-sectional anatomy of the deep, or intrinsic, muscle layer of the upper thoracic spine.

T12. Muscle bundles arising medial to these, from T1 through T4, are relayed to the cervical transverse processes from C2 through C6. Other bundles arising medial to these insertions extend as a broad, fleshy band and attach to the mastoid process deep to the splenius capitis and sternocleidomastoid muscles. These insertions make the longissimus the only erector spinae muscle to reach the skull. The spinalis muscle is largely aponeurotic and extends from the upper lumbar to the lower cervical spinous processes.

The transversospinalis group of muscles passes obliquely cephalad from the transverse processes to the spinous processes immediately deep to the erector spinae muscles. These muscles fall into three layers. The most superficial layer, the semispinalis, arises near the tips of the transverse processes and inserts near the tips of the spinous processes approximately five vertebral levels cephalad. In the upper thoracic and lower cervical spine, most of this muscle is comprised of the semispinalis capitis, which passes from the upper thoracic transverse processes and lower cervical articular processes (C4 through T5) to the occipital bone between the superior and inferior nuchal lines. Its fibers run nearly vertically, and its medial border is free, separated from its contralateral partner by the ligamentum nuchae. The intermediate layer, the multifidus, arises from the dense aponeurosis of the overlying erector spinae muscle, and from all transverse processes up to C4, and inserts into the lower border of each spinous process. This muscle generally spans about three levels. Finally, the deepest muscles of this group, the rotatores, are small muscles that bridge one interspace. They pass from the root of one transverse process to the root of the spinous process immediately above. The actions of these muscles extend the vertebral column, or, acting individually on one side, bend and rotate the vertebrae. The entire group of erector spinae muscles and transversospinalis muscles can be dissected off the spinous processes, laminae, facets, and transverse processes as a single muscular mass. Control of the musculature in this way exposes all vertebral elements from the tip of the spinous processes to the tip of the transverse processes, as well as the costotransverse ligaments and joints and the ribs.

Each rib articulates with its own vertebral body, the vertebra above, and the intervertebral disc between them (Fig. 150–3). In the upper thoracic spine, the only exception to this general rule is the first rib, which articulates only with its own vertebral body. The tubercle of each rib also articulates with the transverse process of its own vertebra. Each of these articulations forms separate synovial joints. Those formed with the posterolateral surfaces of each vertebral body are separated by an intra-articular ligament, which is attached to the intervertebral disc. These joints are surrounded by an articular capsule and are attached to the vertebral body anteriorly by the radiate ligament. The third synovial joint of this complex, the costotransverse joint, is also surrounded by an articular capsule, which is strengthened laterally by the lateral costotransverse ligament and the costotransverse ligament. In addition, the superior costotransverse ligament joins the neck of the rib to the transverse process immediately above. The canal formed between this ligament and the vertebral column transmits the dorsal ramus of the spinal nerve and the dorsal branch of the intercostal artery. The ribs are also attached to each other through the intercostal musculature, which originates medially on each superior rib and inserts laterally on its immediately inferior rib.

After blunt dissection of the intercostal muscles and costotransverse and radiate ligaments, each rib can be resected, which isolates a strip of intercostal musculature between each rib. This strip of musculature contains the intercostal nerve, artery, and vein as they pass laterally between the internal intercostal membrane and the pleura, and then between the internal intercostal membrane and the innermost intercostal muscles. Although a great deal of interweaving exists between nerve, artery, and vein, most frequently, the intercostal vein is most cephalad and the intercostal artery is close, but caudal, to it. The intercostal nerve is frequently found separate from these structures and is located most caudal of the three. Immediately ventral to the intercostal bundle and the intercostal muscles lies the pleura.

Retromediastinal Space and Spinal Anatomy

With blunt dissection, the pleura can be separated from these structures to expose the lateral vertebral elements. The neural foramen can be identified by following the intercostal bundle medially. Within the neural foramen, the dorsal root ganglion can be identified along with the gray and white

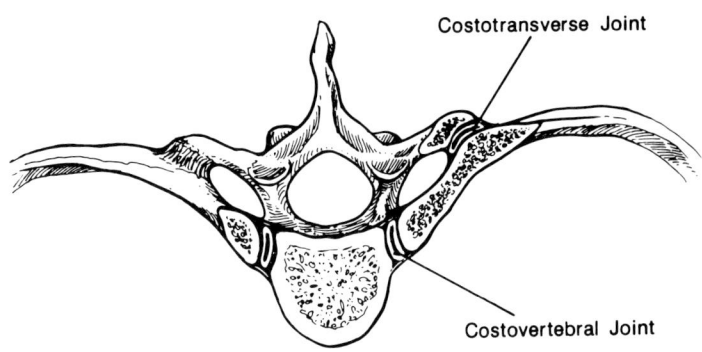

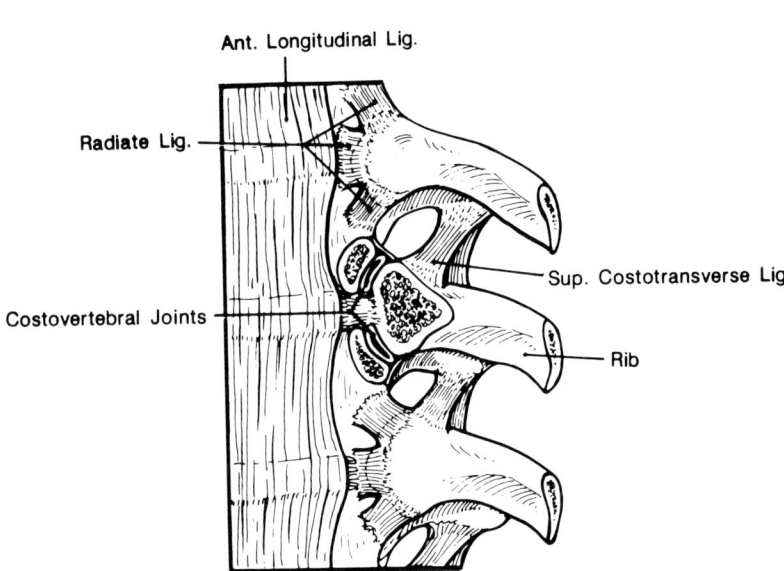

FIGURE 150-3. Relation of each rib and rib head with the transverse process, vertebral bodies, and intervertebral disc. Note that each rib articulates not only with its own transverse process and vertebral body but also with the vertebral body immediately above it.

rami communicantes, which course ventral to the sympathetic chain and ganglia. The sympathetic chain is contained within a fascial compartment formed by fusion of the mediastinal and prevertebral fascia over the juxtovertebral articulation.

Because the aortic arch does not extend to the top of the thoracic cavity, the arterial supply to the chest wall in this region has become somewhat specialized. The first two intercostal spaces are supplied by branches of the costocervical trunk through the highest intercostal artery. This artery descends anterior to the ventral rami of the eighth cervical and first thoracic nerves on the necks of the first two ribs. The remaining intercostal arteries arise from the posterior surface of the thoracic aorta. Because the aorta is displaced downward and to the left, the upper four aortic posterior intercostal arteries ascend to reach intercostal spaces three through six. Each intercostal artery stretches obliquely across each vertebral body from caudal to cephalad in direct apposition to the periosteum of the vertebral body and is located deep to the azygous or hemiazygous vein, the thoracic duct, and the sympathetic trunk.

The major portion of the ventral ramus of the first thoracic nerve passes cephalad across the neck of the first rib to join the eighth cervical nerve in the brachial plexus. A small intercostal branch runs across the inferior surface of the first rib to enter the first interspace close to the costal cartilage. The ventral ramus of the second thoracic nerve also usually sends a small branch to the brachial plexus. Occasionally, this branch is very large, in which case, the lateral cutaneous branch of the second intercostal nerve is small or absent. Although the intercostal nerves below T1 can usually be sacrificed to facilitate exposure, T1 and C7, which frequently are exposed during this procedure, cannot be sacrificed without causing severe neurologic deficit affecting hand function. Therefore, working around the inferior portion of the brachial plexus in this exposure is occasionally necessary.

TRANSMANUBRIAL APPROACH

The transmanubrial approach is an anterior approach that allows direct access to the vertebral bodies and the pathologic processes contained within them. This approach can also be divided into three major steps: (1) the thoracic inlet, (2) the visceral and vascular compartments of the superior mediastinum, and (3) the retromediastinal space.

Thoracic Inlet

The superior mediastinum is defined anteriorly by the manubrium, which corresponds to the T2-T3 level at the suprasternal notch and the T4-T5 level at the sternal angle and lies only 5 cm anterior to these structures. The sternohyoid muscle runs from the ventrocaudal aspect of the hyoid bone to the dorsal surface of the manubrium, also attaching to the sternoclavicular joint capsule. The sternothyroid muscles attach along the dorsal midline of the manubrium. These muscles are supplied by the ventral rami of C1-C3 via the hypoglossal nerve and the ansa cervicalis. The sternocleidomastoid muscle arises on the mastoid process and superior nuchal line and attaches to the manubrioclavicular joint. Its nervous supply is from the accessory nerve and its arterial supply branches from the superior thyroid artery. Careful dissection of the fascial planes enables safe removal of the manubrium and medial third of the clavicle without injury to the brachiocephalic or subclavian veins. Such dissection reveals the pleural apices, which are covered by an extension of the transthoracic fascia, called Sibson's fascia.

Vascular and Visceral Compartments of the Superior Mediastinum

The visceral fascia circumscribes the trachea, esophagus, and thyroid gland defining a visceral compartment, and the carotid sheath circumscribes the carotid arterial system, internal jugular vein, and vagus nerve, thereby defining a neurovascular compartment. These adjacent compartments create a potential space (the viscerocarotid space) that extends from the base of the skull to C7-T4, depending on the location of fusion between the visceral and the alar fascia.

In the upper thorax, the visceral compartment continues down to the bronchi, where the fascia fuses with the parietal and visceral pleurae. Between the visceral and parietal pleurae exists a potential intrapleural space. The carotid sheath extends down to the subclavian vessels, where it fuses into the axillary sheath. In the superior mediastinum, the vascular compartment is not circumscribed by its own well-defined fascial sheath but is defined secondarily by independent surrounding fasciae. Ventrally is the prevertebral fascial extension, the transthoracis fascia; caudally is the visceral fascia; laterally are the parietal pleurae; and inferiorly is the pericardium.

The venous structures consist of the brachiocephalic veins with their branches. These veins descend from the neck into the superior mediastinum just posterior to the thymus gland or its remnants. The right brachiocephalic vein is formed just posterior to the medial end of the right clavicle and descends vertically into the superior mediastinum. The left brachiocephalic vein is formed just posterior to the medial end of the left clavicle and descends diagonally to join the right brachiocephalic vein just posterior to the right first costal cartilage to form the superior vena cava. Tributaries draining into the brachiocephalic veins are the vertebral and first posterior intercostal veins in the neck, and the internal thoracic, thymic, and inferior thyroid veins in the superior mediastinum. On the left, the superior intercostal vein (which drains the second and third intercostal spaces) also drains into the left brachiocephalic vein.

The arterial structures consist of the aortic arch, and the brachiocephalic, left common carotid, and left subclavian arteries with their branches. The aortic arch initially ascends posterior to the superior vena cava but also turns diagonally posterior, then inferior just anterior and to the left of the vertebral column. A second concave turn occurs as the arch curves around the anterolateral visceral compartment to reach the vertebral column. The brachiocephalic artery is the first branch off the aortic arch and ascends vertically and slightly rightward to branch into the right common carotid and subclavian arteries posterior to the right sternoclavicular joint. The left common carotid artery arises next off the arch and ascends vertically into the carotid sheath without branching in the superior mediastinum. The left subclavian artery is the third branch and ascends superiorly and leftward to curve around the thoracic inlet and into the axillary sheath without branches in the superior mediastinum.

The carotid sheath is a circumferential sheath of fused middle and deep fascial layers around the carotid arterial system and internal jugular vein and vagus nerve. At the thoracic inlet, the carotid sheath merges with the subclavian vasculature to form part of the axillary sheath. The esophagus and trachea are encompassed in the visceral fascia, which extends throughout the superior mediastinum. Between these two adjacent compartments lies the viscerocarotid space. Blunt dissection of this space exposes the alar fascia and the retropharyngeal space. In the superior mediastinum, the left brachiocephalic vein runs obliquely from left inferior to right superior. Caudally, the field is limited by the aortic arch and its branches, which obstruct access to T3 and T4 vertebrae. Major structures potentially crossing this retropharyngeal and retromediastinal space are the right recurrent laryngeal nerve and the lymphatics terminating in the thoracic duct. The left recurrent laryngeal nerve branches off the vagus in the superior mediastinum, loops around the ligamentum arteriosum, and ascends within the visceral fascia between the esophagus and the trachea. The right recurrent laryngeal nerve, however, can cross the retropharyngeal or retromediastinal space anywhere from C7 to T3.

The thoracic duct runs dorsal and to the left of the esophagus between the visceral and alar fascia in the superior mediastinum and ascends to the C7 level, where it lies laterally in a plane dorsal to the carotid sheath. It then courses caudal and ventral to the branches of the thyrocervical trunk and phrenic nerve to terminate at the junction of the left internal jugular and subclavian veins. A lymphatic trunk located on the right side follows a similar course to the thoracic duct.

Retromediastinal Space

By incision of the alar and mediastinal fascia, the median compartment of the retromediastinal space is entered. The prevertebral fascia covers the vertebral bodies and envelops the longus colli muscles. Autonomic branches to the cardiopulmonary plexi may be seen in this region and can be sacrificed, if necessary.

CHOICE OF SURGICAL APPROACH

Appropriate choice of surgical approach to the cervicothoracic junction depends on the exact location of the pathologic process. The transmanubrial approach exposes the vertebral bodies directly anteriorly and allows excellent exposure of the lower cervical vertebrae and of T1 and T2. Depending on anatomic variations, T3 may also be accessible. Exposure of T4, however, is rarely possible, and to obtain this exposure, dissection of the vascular compartment of the superior mediastinum is required. The exposure is limited by the anatomic positions of the left brachiocephalic vein, subclavian veins, aortic arch, and the great vessels and the degree of thoracic kyphosis. Potential anatomic risks are injury to the carotid sheath structures, trachea, esophagus, recurrent laryngeal nerves, aortic arch and its branches, vertebral arteries, brachiocephalic and subclavian veins, sympathetic trunk and stellate ganglion, spinal cord, and the pleural apices. The most significant advantage of this approach is the simultaneous excellent exposure of both the cervical and upper thoracic spine. The disadvantages are that the corpectomy is performed blindly with regard to the thecal sac, and posterior spinal stabilization cannot be performed without repositioning of the patient or as a second procedure. However, anterior plates may be applied easily through this approach down to T2, and occasionally T3, and may obviate posterior stabilization.

The transthoracic approach exposes the vertebral bodies anterolaterally after extensive mobilization of the scapula. Excellent exposure of T3 and T4 can be achieved, but access to T1 and T2 is limited by the narrowing of the thoracic inlet. Lower cervical vertebrae are not accessible through this approach. To obtain this exposure, the intrapleural space is dissected to reach the paramedian compartment of the retromediastinal space. Potential anatomic risks include injury to the neurovascular supply to the shoulder musculature, the lungs, superior mediastinal structures (aorta and its branches, trachea, esophagus, thoracic duct), sympathetic trunk and stellate ganglion, lower trunk and posterior cord of the brachial plexus, and the intercostal, long thoracic, and thoracal dorsal nerves. Advantages of this approach include rapid exposure of the anterior spinal elements and excellent control of intercostal segmental arteries. Disadvantages of this approach to the cervicothoracic junction are the transmuscular mobilization of the scapula, the intrapleural dissection, the long depth of field, and the inability to obtain exposure of the lower cervical vertebrae.

The lateral parascapular extrapleural approach is an extended posterolateral approach that allows direct lateral exposure of the vertebral bodies. Excellent exposure of T1-T4 vertebral bodies can be obtained, and the inferior portion of C7 may be exposed under the T1 nerve root. To obtain this exposure, the thoracoscapular space is dissected after anatomic mobilization of the scapula, and the paraspinal musculature is mobilized to open directly into the paramedian compartment of the retromediastinal space. Potential anatomic risks include injury to the dorsomedial parascapular musculature, pleura and lungs, superior mediastinal structures, sympathetic trunk and stellate ganglion, and spinal cord. Advantages of this approach are decompression of neural tissue under direct visualization, a totally extrapleural dissection, simultaneous exposure of C7 through T4, and the ability for simultaneous posterior stabilization through the same incision and patient position. Disadvantages of this approach are a more tedious paraspinal muscle dissection, and the fact that it does not allow simultaneous exposure of any cervical vertebrae beyond the inferior-most aspect of C7.

ANESTHETIC CONSIDERATIONS

General anesthesia has been used for all patients undergoing any of these three surgical approaches. In general, we prefer a combined protocol of enflurane (Ethrane) inhalant and intravenous sufentanil. Three types of intubation have been used in patients undergoing surgery of the cervicothoracic junction: (1) routine single-lumen endotracheal intubation, (2) double-lumen endotracheal intubation, and (3) single-lumen endotracheal intubation with high-frequency ventilation. Routine, single-lumen endotracheal intubation is the most rapidly performed but requires that the ipsilateral lung expand and contract within the surgical field during anterolateral thoracotomy or lateral parascapular extrapleural surgical procedures. Double-lumen intubation is a much longer procedure but allows unilateral deflation of the lung during the critical periods of corpectomy and spinal cord decompression. Single-lumen intubation with high-frequency ventilation also can be performed very rapidly and enables the lung to be retracted out of the surgical field with minimal reinflation during corpectomy and decompression; however, it allows simultaneous ventilation of the remainder of the ipsilateral lung. We have found this to be the ideal ventilatory technique for anterolateral or posterolateral procedures of the upper thoracic spine. Single-lumen intubation with standard ventilation is adequate for transmanubrial-transclavicular procedures.

SURGICAL TECHNIQUES

LATERAL PARASCAPULAR EXTRAPLEURAL APPROACH

The posterior aspect of the neck and back from the nuchal line to the sacrum is sterilely prepared and draped for surgery. The incision begins midline three spinous processes above the intended surgical area and is brought to three spinous processes below before curving gently to the surgical side of approach. A myocutaneous flap is then developed by incising the deep fascia at the spinous processes and dissecting them off sharply to expose the trapezius muscle. The trapezius and rhomboid muscles are then dissected off the spinous processes, and the plane of loose areolar tissue located between these muscles and the paraspinal muscles is identified. By development of this plane, the skin and the trapezius and rhomboid muscles can be reflected together toward the medial border of the scapula (Fig. 150-4). The inferior fibers of the trapezius muscle must be transsected to reflect this flap, and care must be taken to leave an identifiable cuff of muscle for reapproximation. Aggressive dissection of the levator scapulae muscles in the cervical region maximizes exposure of the cervicothoracic junction. Mobilization of the myocutaneous flap in this fashion enables the scapula to fall laterally out of the surgical field, a maneuver that provides wide exposure of the lower cervical region, upper dorsal rib cage region, and dorsal vertebral elements.

The deep cervical fascia and thoracolumbar fascia cover the splenius and erector spinae muscles. Dissection of this paraspinal muscle mass from the spinous processes and dorsal spinal elements enables retraction of this muscle mass medially to the contralateral side, thereby exposing the entire dorsal rib cage and dorsal vertebral elements from the tip of the spinous process to the transverse process.

Subperiosteal dissection of the appropriate ribs can then be performed to free the neurovascular bundles and intercostal muscles. The costotransverse and costovertebral ligaments are then incised and the rib removed from its costovertebral tip to the posterior bend of each rib. The intercostal neurovascular bundles are next dissected free of the intercostal

1882 | *Surgery of the Craniovertebral Junction and Spine*

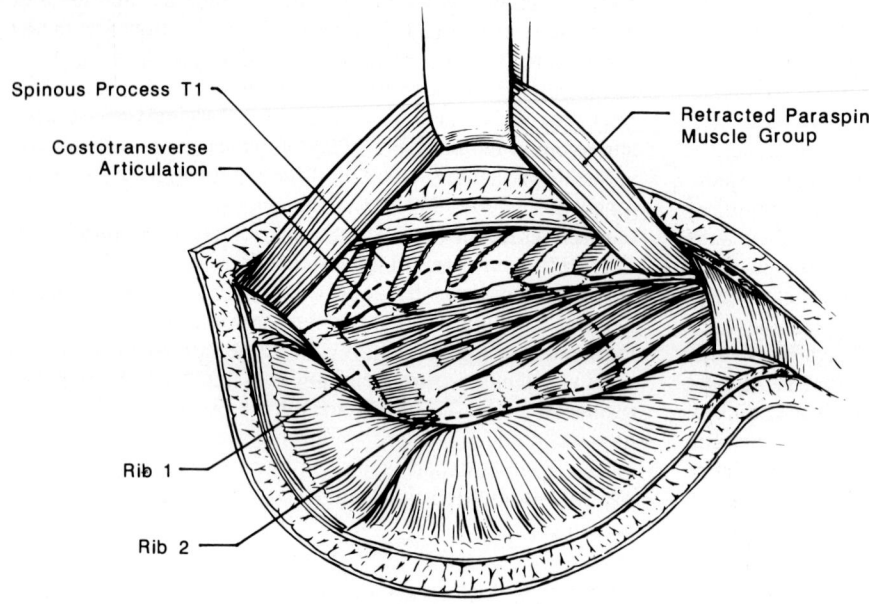

FIGURE 150-4. Reflection of the trapezius and rhomboid muscles laterally and paraspinal muscle mass medially to expose the dorsal and lateral spinal elements and ribs.

FIGURE 150-5. Operative field after corpectomy and neural decompression.

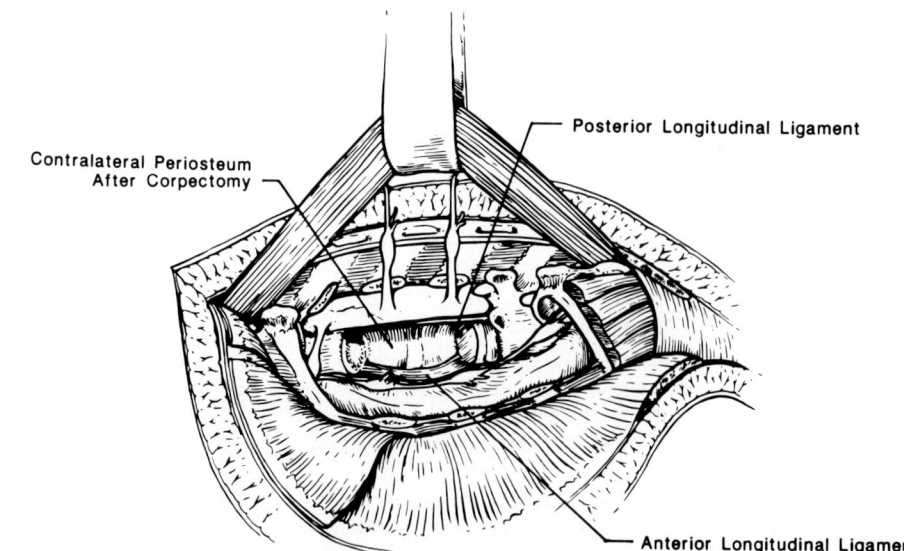

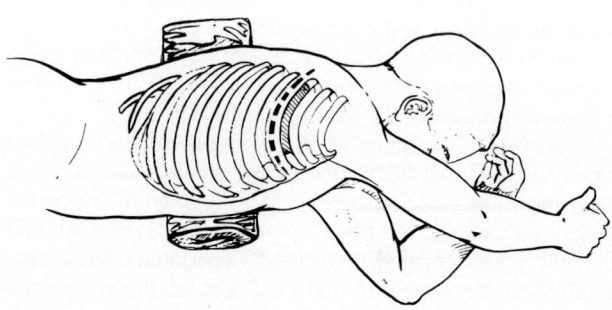

FIGURE 150-6. Patient position and skin incision for right anterolateral transthoracic approach to the upper thoracic spine.

muscles, and the intercostal arteries are ligated and transsected. For exposure of the intervertebral disc, the intercostal nerves can be retracted out of the surgical field. To resect a vertebral body, however, one or more intercostal nerves must be resected for adequate exposure.

The intercostal nerve can be traced for identification of the vertebral foremen. The sympathetic chain can then be identified on the lateral vertebral surface. The rami communicantes are transsected, and the intercostal arteries are ligated and transsected as well. Displacing the sympathetic chain anterolaterally via subperiosteal dissection reveals the vertebral body, pedicle, and foremen. Removal of the transverse process, lamina, and pedicles by use of either a high-speed drill or a Kerrison punch (using the intercostal nerve as a guide) exposes the lateral thecal sac. Direct visualization of the neural elements, therefore, is available during the remainder of decompression. Corpectomy can then be performed with either a high-speed drill or curette, as described earlier. The anterior longitudinal ligament, and if possible, the posterior longitudinal ligament, are preserved to serve as protective barriers to the thecal sac and superior mediastinal structures (Fig. 150–5). Vertebral reconstruction is performed with a rib graft or fibular allograft strut. If the pathological process is malignant, Steinmann pins and methyl methacrylate are used.

Any sacrificed nerve roots are then ligated proximal to the dorsal root ganglion, and the remainder of the nerve is removed. Appropriate posterior spinal fixation is then performed.

Before wound closure, the operative field is filled with saline to check for evidence of an air leak. If an air leak is present, a small (22 or 24 F) chest tube is placed into the wound and brought out through a separate stab wound below the incision. Two Hemovac drains are then placed, and a layered wound closure is performed.

ANTEROLATERAL TRANSTHORACIC APPROACH

For the anterolateral transthoracic approach to the cervicothoracic junction, the patient is placed in the lateral decubitus position with the appropriate side up. The skin is incised from the paraspinous area at approximately T1, and the incision is taken distally along the medial border of the scapula to the seventh rib (Fig. 150–6). This incision is continued first laterally, then anteriorly, then medially to the costal cartilage of the third rib. The trapezius, latissimus dorsi, rhomboid major, and serratus posterior muscles are divided, after which the third rib is identified. The scapula is then retracted cephalad and medially by use of a scapular retractor. The fact that the first rib is located somewhat medial to the second rib helps in the identification of the third rib. Confirmation of location frequently can be made by identification of the attachment of the scalenus anticus or medius muscles on the second rib. A subperiosteal dissection of the third rib is then performed, and the rib is resected from its angle to the costal cartilage. The chest spreader can then be inserted and opened, thereby exposing the pleura and underlying lungs, aorta, and spine.

The parietal pleura can then be opened by incision of the pleura from the costochondral cartilage to the midvertebral body. After the lung is deflated and retracted, the spine is clearly exposed (Fig. 150–7). The pleura can then be incised cephalad and caudad to expose the pathologic vertebrae. This maneuver enables clear identification of the intervertebral discs and the intercostal arteries and veins that lie in the midvertebral body. Appropriate intercostal arteries and veins are dissected, ligated, and cut. Vertebrectomy can then be performed as described earlier.

After resection of the pathologic vertebral elements and vertebral reconstruction, closure is begun by first inserting a chest tube and bringing it to water seal. The ribs are reapproximated with "figure of eight" 0 stainless steel wires. Each muscle layer is independently reapproximated with 0 Vicryl stitches, and subcutaneous 2-0 Vicryl stitches and skin staples are used to close the wound.

TRANSMANUBRIAL-TRANSCLAVICULAR APPROACH

The patient is positioned supine with the head turned slightly to the side contralateral to the approach. A T-shaped incision is made with the transverse limb of the incision located in a skin crease 1 to 2 cm above the clavicle and extending from the contralateral sternocleidomastoid to 2 to 3 cm lateral to the ipsilateral sternocleidomastoid (Fig. 150–8). The vertical portion of the incision extends in the midline midway down the sternal body. The platysma muscle is divided in the line of the skin incision, and a wide mobilization of the platysma is performed cephalad and caudad to the incision. The external jugular vein is identified and divided, and supraclavicular nerves are identified and protected where possible. Medial branches of these nerves frequently are sacrificed.

The sternocleidomastoid muscle is next identified and dissected free from deeper structures, and the medial half of the clavicle and the manubrium are freed from the pectoralis major muscle by subperiosteal dissection. Careful dissection of the superficial and middle layers of the deep cervical fascia allows safe reflection of the sternocleidomastoid, sternohyoid, and sternothyroid muscles from the manubrium and clavicle with preservation of their neurovascular supply. Opening the suprasternal space of Burns (a suprasternal midline space created by a leaflet split in the superficial layer of deep fascia) allows subperiosteal dissection of the manubrium, leaving the periosteum along with an anterior extension of the transthoracic fascia for protection of the brachiocephalic veins. Next, the omohyoid muscle is divided between identifying sutures, and the anterior aspect of the internal jugular vein and common carotid artery are identified.

After appropriate protection of the deeper structures, the ipsilateral two thirds of the manubrium is cut by a high-speed drill. Similarly, the first costal cartilage is divided, and the clavicular manubrial joint is left intact. After holes are drilled for the eventual application of a fixation plate, the clavicle is divided at its midpoint. The manubrium, sternoclavicular joint, and medial half of the clavicle are then elevated on the pedicle of the sternocleidomastoid muscle. This maneuver exposes the infrahyoid muscles, trachea, brachiocephalic veins and tributaries, brachiocephalic artery and branches, subclavian and common carotid arteries, scalenus anterior

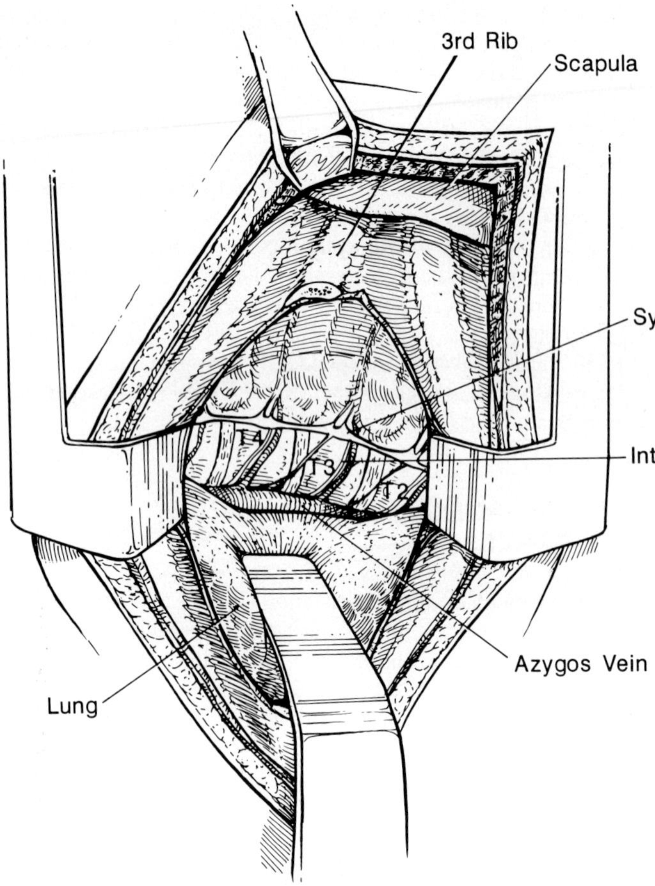

FIGURE 150–7. Operative exposure of the upper thoracic spine through a T3 anterolateral transthoracic approach.

muscle, phrenic nerve, brachial plexus, and part of the first rib. Blunt dissection can then be performed medial to the carotid sheath to expose the alar and mediastinal fasciae. Incision of these fasciae enters the retromediastinal space and exposes the prevertebral fascia that covers the vertebral bodies and longus colli muscles (Fig. 150–9).

After placement of appropriate retractors, removal of the pathologic process can then be performed by many techniques. Soft tumors can be removed through curettage and suction, and bony elements can be removed with a high-speed drill and Kerrison punch.

After complete decompression of the spinal cord, reconstruction is begun with either autologous or allograft bone. Tricortical iliac crest or fibula are adequate for grafts. After bony reconstruction, stabilization can be achieved through placement of an anterior plate screwed to the intact vertebrae above and below the pathologic levels, or by use of a halo brace.

The wound is then closed in layers over vacuum drainage. If the pleura has been opened, a chest tube is inserted through a separate stab wound, threaded into the pleural space, and connected to an underwater seal. The osseomuscular flap is then returned to its appropriate position. The manubrium is reattached by use of wires, and the clavicle is reattached by use of plate and screws.

DISCUSSION

The anatomic relationships of the upper thoracic spine have made surgical access to this region challenging. Attempts to approach this area have frequently used procedures designed for approaching the vertebral elements of the lower thoracic region and thoracolumbar junction (e.g., costotransversectomy, lateral rachiotomy [laminectomy], and lateral extracavitary). Unfortunately, the exposure provided by these procedures is limited by the scapula and by the trapezius,

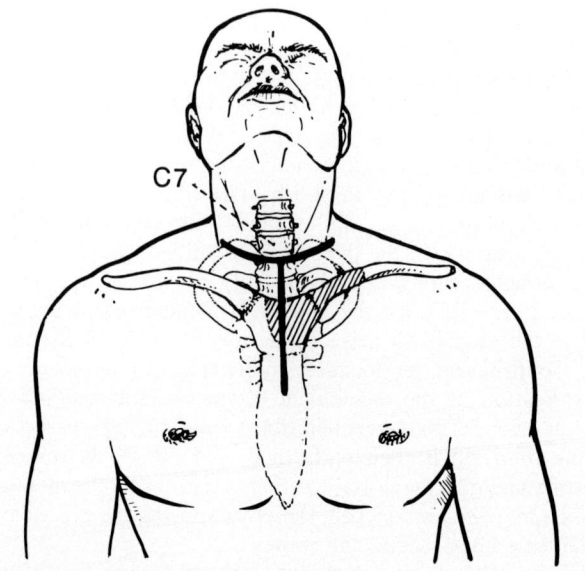

FIGURE 150–8. Patient position and skin incision for transmanubrial and transclavicular approach to the cervicothoracic junction.

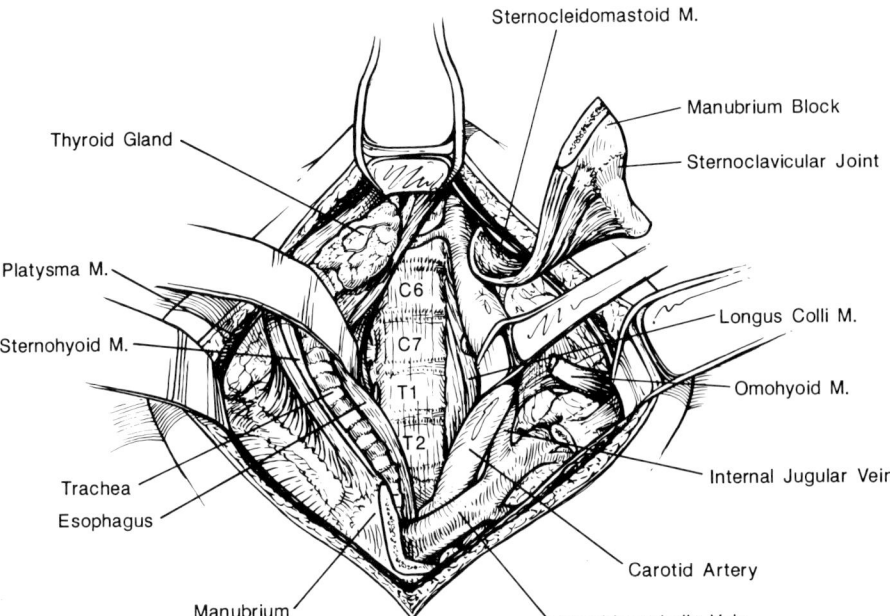

FIGURE 150-9. Operative exposure of the cervicothoracic junction via the transmanubrial and transclavicular approach.

rhomboid, and levator scapulae muscles. Approaches designed specifically for this region include the transmanubrial-transclavicular, the anterolateral thoracotomy, and the lateral parascapular extrapleural approaches.

Among these approaches, the transmanubrial-transclavicular approach of Sundaresan and coworkers[12] provides the best approach for pathologic processes that include both the lower cervical and the upper thoracic region. It gives excellent access from the lower cervical region to T2, and occasionally, to T3. To obtain this exposure, dissection of the vascular compartment of the superior mediastinum is required to reach the median compartment of the retromediastinal space. The exposure is limited by the anatomic positions of the left brachiocephalic vein, subclavian veins, aortic arch, and the great vessels, as well as the degree of thoracic kyphosis. Potential risks include injury to the carotid sheath structures, trachea, esophagus, recurrent laryngeal nerves, aortic arch, vertebral arteries, sympathetic truck and stellate ganglion, spinal cord, and the pleural apices. The advantage of this approach is the simultaneous exposure of the cervical and thoracic spine. The disadvantages are that the corpectomy is performed blindly until the thecal sac can be identified, and posterior stabilization cannot be performed without a second procedure.

The transthoracic approach through the third rib exposes the vertebral bodies from an anterolateral approach but requires extensive mobilization of the scapula and a relatively long surgical depth of field. Exposure of T3 and T4 vertebral bodies is generally adequate, but access to T1 and T2 is limited by the narrowing of the thoracic inlet. The intrapleural cavity is opened to reach the paramedian compartment of the retromediastinal space. Potential risks include injury to the neurovascular supply of the shoulder musculature, lungs, superior mediastinal structures, sympathetic trunk and stellate ganglion, lower trunk and posterior cord of the brachial plexus, and the intercostal, long thoracic, and thoracodorsal nerves. Advantages of this approach include excellent access to superior mediastinal vasculature, if necessary for control. Disadvantages of this approach are the extensive mobilization of the scapula, intrapleural dissection, long depth of field, inability to reach T1 and T2, and inability to perform posterior stabilization in the same procedure.

The lateral parascapular extrapleural approach is an extended posterolateral approach that allows excellent exposure of T1-T4 vertebral bodies but limited exposure of C7. To obtain this exposure, the thoracoscapular space is dissected to partially mobilize the scapula, and the paraspinal musculature is mobilized to open directly into the paramedian compartment of the retromediastinal space. Potential anatomic risks include the dorsal medial parascapular musculature, pleura and lungs, superior mediastinal structures, sympathetic trunk and stellate ganglion, and spinal cord. The advantage of this approach is that decompression of neural tissue is performed under direct visualization at all times, with minimal manipulation of the thecal sac. Simultaneous exposure of C7 to T4 is easily achieved. In addition, posterior stabilization can be performed simultaneously through the same incision. Disadvantages are that only the inferior aspect of C7 is available through this approach, and that is partially obstructed by the T1 nerve root and rami communicantes to the stellate ganglion.

SUMMARY

Three surgical approaches to the cervicothoracic junction exist. Depending on the location and extent of pathology,

Table 150-3. RECOMMENDED SURGICAL APPROACHES ACCORDING TO PATHOLOGY

Transmanubrial-transclavicular
  Pathology extends from C6 or C7 to T1 or T2 but not below T2
Lateral parascapular extrapleural or anterolateral thoracotomy
  Pathology limited to T3 and/or T4
Lateral parascapular extrapleural
  Pathology extends up to but not beyond C7-T1 disc

one or another may be more appropriately used. Considerations for selection of the most appropriate surgical approach are listed in Table 150–3.

REFERENCES

1. Siegal T: Surgical decompression of anterior and posterior malignant epidural tumors compressing the spinal cord: A prospective study. Neurosurgery 17:424–432, 1985
2. Sundaresan N, DiGiacinto GV, Hughes JEO, Krol G: Spondylectomy for malignant tumors of the spine. J Clin Oncol 7:1485–1491, 1989
3. Menard V: Etude Pratique sur le Mal de Pott. Paris, Masson, 1900
4. Capener N: The evolution of lateral rachiotomy. J Bone Joint Surg 36:173–179, 1954
5. Larson SJ, Holst RA, Hemmy DC, Sances A: Lateral extracavitary approach to traumatic lesions of the thoracic and lumbar spine. J Neurosurg 45:628–637, 1976
6. Fessler RG, Dietze DD, MacMillan M, Peace D: Lateral parascapular extrapleural approach to the upper thoracic spine. J Neurosurg 75:349–355, 1991
7. Jonnesco T: Le sympathique cervico-thoracico. Paris, Masson, 1923
8. Brunig F: Technik der kombinierten Resektionsmethode samtlicher sympathischen Nervenbaum am Halse. Zentralbl Chir 50:1056–1059, 1923
9. Royle ND: Observations on the alteration of the circulation of the brain by surgical means in diseases of the central nervous system. BMJ 1:1063–1068, 1932
10. Gask GE: The surgery of the sympathetic nervous system. Br J Surg 21:113–130, 1933.
11. Ochsner A, DeBakey M: Peripheral vascular disease. Surg Gynecol Obstet 70:1058–1072, 1940
12. Sundaresan N, Shah J, Foley KM, Rosen G: An anterior surgical approach to the upper thoracic vertebrae. J Neurosurg 61:686–690, 1984
13. Birch R, Bonney G, Marshall RW: A surgical approach to the cervicothoracic spine. J Bone Joint Surg Br 72B:904–907, 1990
14. Hodgson AR, Stock FE, Fang HSY: Anterior spinal fusion: The operative approach and pathological findings in 412 patients with Pott's disease of the spine. Br J Surg 48:172–178, 1960
15. Sapico BL, Montgomerie JZ: Vertebral osteomyelitis in intravenous drug abusers: Report of three cases and review of the literature. Rev Infect Dis 2:196–206, 1980
16. Edelstyn GA, Gillespie PJ, Grebbel FS: The radiological demonstration of osseous metastases. Clin Radiol 18:158, 1967
17. O'Mara RE: Bone scanning in osseous metastatic disease. JAMA 229:1915, 1974
18. Butler EG, Dohrmann PJ, Stark RJ: Spinal subdural abscess. Clin Exp Neuro 25:67–70, 1988
19. Galasko CSB: Skeletal metastases. Clin Orthop 210:18, 1986
20. Schlaeffer F, Mikolich DJ, Mates SM: Technetium Tc 99m diphosphonate bone scan. False normal findings in elderly patients with hematogenous vertebral osteomyelitis. Arch Intern Med 147:2024–2026, 1987
21. Staab EV, McCartney WH: Role of gallium 67 in inflammatory disease. Semin Nucl Med 8:219–234, 1978
22. Bruns J, Maas R: Advantages of diagnosing bacterial spondylitis with magnetic resonance imaging. Arch Orthop Trauma Surg 108:30–35, 1989
23. Pauschter DM, Modic MT, Masaryk J: Magnetic resonance imaging of the spine: Applications and limitations. Radiol Clin North Am 23:551–562, 1985

CHAPTER 151

Surgical Approaches to the Thoracic and Thoracolumbar Spine for Decompression and Stabilization

Lawrence F. Borges

The neurosurgeon treating a pathologic process within the thoracic or thoracolumbar spine is faced with a wide range of surgical options (Table 151–1). The major difference between these procedures is the anatomic locus of the spine for which they provide exposure. This chapter reviews these surgical approaches and provides the criteria for selecting the different surgical procedures.

Because the surgical procedures differ in anatomic exposure of the spine, the neurosurgeon must first determine the precise anatomic position of the pathologic process. Clinical studies[1] and experimental studies using somatosensory evoked potentials[2] and angiography[3] demonstrated that ventral compression of the thoracic spinal cord is not relieved by posterior decompression, such as laminectomy. Therefore, the neurosurgeon should select a surgical procedure that addresses the offending compression directly.

POSTERIOR APPROACH: LAMINECTOMY

Laminectomy is the most commonly performed neurosurgical procedure. The first successful laminectomy is credited to Alban G. Smith, a general surgeon in Kentucky.[4] In 1828, Smith was called to attend a young man who had been thrown from a horse and was paralyzed. Smith explored the abnormal area of the spine and removed a lamina that had been fractured and pushed into the spinal cord. Some recovery ensued. As surgical care improved with the introduction of anesthesia and antisepsis, spinal exposures also improved. Bickham[5] introduced the technique of osteoplastic laminectomy in 1905. Subsequently, laminectomy became the exposure of choice for most spinal pathology.

The surgical techniques used to perform laminectomy are well known to neurosurgeons. My preference is to use a high-speed diamond drill to drill lateral troughs along either side of the lamina, cut the ligamentum flavum sharply, and remove the lamina as a single piece. This technique avoids placing any instrument deep to the bone that could injure a compromised spinal cord. Thoracic laminectomy alone is a rare procedure in my practice. Although a thoracic laminectomy provides good access to the middorsal aspect of the thoracic spine, very few pathologic processes are limited to the middorsal thoracic spine, and I usually combine laminectomy with a unilateral excision of the facet joint and pedicle to gain access to the dorsal and lateral thoracic spinal canal. The lateral access provided by facet and pedicle resection increases the safety of a laminectomy, whether it is performed for intradural tumors or extradural metastases. Laminectomy alone is not indicated for ventrally placed lesions, such as thoracic disc herniations and ventral extradural tumors.

Stabilization of the thoracic and thoracolumbar spine is very straightforward after posterior exposures. The instrumentation systems designed for posterior implantation are usually based on a system of rods that are secured to the laminae with hooks, sublaminar wires, or wires passed through the base of the spinous processes. These rods can also be attached to the spine by pedicle screws, although the small size of most thoracic pedicles may limit the use of thoracic pedicle screws. The rods are made from ¼-inch stainless steel and provide a rigid system of fixation that is stronger than most systems used for anterior spine stabilization. These systems can be implanted to produce distraction, compression, or in situ stabilization. Typically, one rod is implanted on either side of the spine, and several methods are available for cross linking the two rods to prevent rotation of the spine. In most situations, posterior instrumentation

Table 151–1. SURGICAL APPROACHES TO THE THORACIC AND THORACOLUMBAR SPINE

Posterior
   Laminectomy
Posterolateral
   Costotransversectomy
   Lateral rachiotomy
   Lateral extracavitary
   Transpedicular
Anterolateral
   Thoracotomy
   Thoracoabdominal exposure
Anterior
   Median sternotomy

provides the strongest, most rigid stabilization construct in the thoracic spine.

POSTEROLATERAL APPROACHES

COSTOTRANSVERSECTOMY

Costotransversectomy was described originally by Menard in 1894[6] as a method of decompressing a tubercular abscess of the spine. The original operation was performed through a midline incision and was accompanied by resection of 2 inches of medial rib as well as the transverse process of the vertebrae. This approach provided limited exposure to the lateral vertebral body. Although the approach was satisfactory for draining an abscess, it did not provide sufficient exposure of the vertebral body to directly address ventral pathology.

Seddon[7] improved on this exposure by moving the incision laterally and resecting a longer segment of several adjacent ribs. The lamina, transverse process, and pedicles of the adjacent vertebral process were resected. These maneuvers provided a longer, wider exposure of the lateral vertebral body and were the impetus for the lateral "rhachotomy" proposed by Capener in 1954.[8]

The lateral rhachotomy extended the costotransversectomy to also excise the fixed dorsal kyphotic bony angulation of the spine that frequently developed after Pott's disease. After exposing the lateral spinal canal by the bone removal method just described, Capener transected the intercostal nerve and used it to rotate the spinal cord and dura away from the dorsal vertebral body. This action provided enough exposure ventral to the dura such that the sharp, dorsally projecting angle of vertebral body could be resected with an osteotome. The tension with which the spinal cord was drawn across this angulation was illustrated by Capener's description of the "sharp spasms of the leg" that accompanied exposure of the bony spur in his patient.

Although costotransversectomy is still used by neurosurgeons, its popularity has been eclipsed by the lateral extracavitary approach and by thoracotomy.[9,10] Costotransversectomy provides access to the posterolateral spine and the lateral vertebral body. It can be used for removal of fractured bone fragments, decompression of vertebral infection, or removal of a herniated thoracic disc. Its primary advantage over more direct anterolateral procedures is that costotransversectomy avoids a thoracotomy; however, it does not always avoid a pneumothorax. This procedure can be attractive when the surgical goal is limited, as in obtaining a biopsy to aid in treatment planning.

Costotransversectomy has several limitations. As it is classically performed, costotransversectomy involves a plane of approach lateral to the erector spinae muscles. Because the motor innervation to the erector spinae muscle enters it laterally, this incision and approach are likely to denervate the paraspinal muscles over several segments. Reinnervation of these muscles is not always complete, and some individuals experience a permanent replacement of much of the muscle by fibrous tissue. Furthermore, the neurovascular bundles (nerve root and intercostal artery) are interposed between the surgeon and the lateral vertebral body. Sometimes, two to three neurovascular bundles must be sectioned to gain exposure to the lateral vertebral body. Dividing these structures with a thoracotomy is not always necessary. Even after the neurovascular bundles are sectioned, the exposure to the ventral spine is limited. This approach provides exposure to the lateral ventral body, but resection of the ventral vertebral body, especially immediately ventral to the dura, is not performed under direct vision. Occasionally, the surgeon must use a drill or curettes in this area in a semiblind fashion. This aspect of the procedure adds an element of risk that is avoided by thoracotomy. Another drawback is that costotransversectomy in its classic form provides little exposure to the spine for instrumentation. The posterior laminae are typically not exposed, thereby eliminating the possibility of posterior instrumentation, and the limited exposure of the lateral vertebral bodies makes placement of plates, screws, or rods problematic. Therefore, obtaining immediate postoperative stability is difficult with the classic costotransversectomy approach.

Costotransversectomy is performed with the patient under endotracheal anesthesia and in a semiprone position. The patient is placed prone on padded blanket rolls of asymmetric height such that the side of approach is elevated 30 to 60 degrees, depending on the body habitus and the level of the spine being exposed. A straight or curved longitudinal incision is made 2 to 3 inches lateral to the spinous processes in the groove just lateral to the erector spinae muscles. The incision is centered over the pathologic area that requires decompression. The incision is deepened through subcutaneous tissue, trapezius, latissimus dorsi, and lumbodorsal fascia until the angle of the ribs is reached. The paraspinal muscles are dissected subperiosteally from lateral to medial, away from the proximal rib angles and transverse processes. The ribs to be removed are skeletonized subperiosteally. Care must be taken to avoid injuring the pleura, which would result in pneumothorax.

If simple biopsy or drainage is the goal, resection of a single rib may be sufficient. More commonly, however, two to three ribs and their associated transverse processes must be removed. After the ribs are skeletonized approximately 3 inches lateral to the transverse process, the transverse process itself is removed, thereby exposing the head of the rib. During removal of the transverse process, the costotransverse ligaments are resected, and the rib is transected with a rib cutter lateral to the angle of the rib. The rib can be subsequently removed piecemeal with a rongeur, or as a single piece after the costovertebral ligaments are transected with a knife or periosteal dissector. Additional exposure to the lateral vertebral body is facilitated by resection of additional rib laterally. After the rib head is removed, the lateral anatomy of the vertebrae should be identified, particularly the pedicle. Emerging just caudal to the pedicle is the nerve root and associated arteries and veins. The ventral ramus of the root becomes the intercostal nerve. If possible, the dissection should proceed between two adjacent intercostal nerves by exposing the lateral pedicle and then subperiosteally moving from the lateral pedicle to the upper lateral vertebral body. Subperiosteal dissection is continued along the lateral vertebral body until its ventral aspect is reached. During this maneuver, the radicular vessels from the aorta are being lifted off of the midlateral vertebral bodies. Nutrient branches penetrating from these vessels into the bone are disrupted and must be controlled with bipolar cautery laterally and with bone wax medially. The pedicle emerges from the rostral posterior aspect of the vertebral body immediately caudal to the adjacent disc space. At this point, the surgeon may be able to accomplish the surgical goals by the limited exposure afforded between the two adjacent intercostal neurovascular bundles. If this exposure is insufficient, the neurovascular bundles may be transected for additional exposure. The neurovascular bundles may be followed medially to maintain orientation of the position of the intraspinal contents. Further bone removal may be performed, depending on the precise pathologic process under attack. A high-speed drill may be used to remove the pedicle, which will give exposure to the lateral spinal canal such that the floor of the spinal canal can be identified readily. Once identification of the floor of the spinal canal is made, additional bone or disc removal may be performed ventral to the dura. After the decompression is completed, bone graft struts may be placed in the cavity created by vertebral body removal. The necessity for such an anterior fusion is based on whether or not instability is part of the pathologic process and the extent to which ventral and dorsal bone is removed.

Before closure, the surgical area is filled with saline and assessed for air leaks from the adjacent pleura. Pleural defects are sutured, if possible, and a chest tube is placed if pneumothorax is seen. The incision is closed in layers over an external drain. A chest x-ray is obtained in the recovery room to assess for pneumothorax. Postoperative nursing decisions and mobilization are based on the extent of spinal instability.

LATERAL EXTRACAVITARY APPROACH

Two major problems with the costotransversectomy operation have been (1) lack of exposure of the posterior lamina, which prevents implantation of indwelling instrumentation that can provide immediate stabilization and (2) limited exposure of the ventral vertebral body. Larson and colleagues[11] made modifications to the costotransversectomy operation to overcome these problems and first published his experience with this lateral extracavity approach applied to traumatic lesions in 1976. Subsequently, this approach has been applied to other pathologic processes, including persistent spinal instability[12] and thoracic herniations.[13] A succinct account of these modifications, as well as some additional modifications, was published by Benzel, one of Larson's students, in 1989.[14]

In the lateral extracavitary approach, the patient is positioned into a three-quarter prone position on the operating table on blanket rolls and secured with 3-inch tape. The incision, centered over the pathologic area, is begun in the midline and is gently extended into a hockey-stick shape caudal to the side of the exposure. The incision extends 8 to 10 cm laterally from the midline at its caudal-most point. A gentle angle to the hockey stick minimizes ischemic injury to the skin flap. A skin flap is then raised above the thoracodorsal fascia, which is then incised in the shape of a T. The underlying erector spinae muscles are separated from the ribs and intercostal muscles in the thoracic region or the quadratus lumborum muscle in the lumbar region. The soft tissues are separated away from the medial 6 to 10 cm of one to three ribs, and the ribs are skeletonized subperiosteally. The ribs are transected laterally and removed after the costotransverse and costovertebral joints are separated and saved for subsequent interbody or posterior grafting. The intercostal nerves are sacrificed, and the nerve roots are followed medially to their foramina. After the pedicle is identified, the pedicle or the vertebral body, or both, are removed with a high-speed drill to decompress the offending pathology and create a ventral trough for placement of a strut graft. After decompression, the spinous processes and lamina are exposed by a standard midline subperiosteal exposure over the appropriate levels, thereby allowing for the placement of standard posterior stabilizing instrumentation. Once the instrumentation is placed, the original operative site is re-exposed, and a ventral strut graft of bone is placed in the defect created by drilling of the vertebral bodies. Wound closure and postoperative management are similar to that described earlier for costotransversectomy.

The lateral extracavitary approach has been used to treat a wide range of pathologic processes and has yielded generally good results and few complications. One series reported a 13-percent incidence of postoperative pneumothorax, an eight-percent incidence of superficial wound infection, an eight-percent incidence of postoperative atelectasis, and a four-percent incidence of anesthesia dolorosa related to a sectioned thoracic root.[13] One problematic area for the lateral extracavitary approach has been the upper thoracic spine because the scapula and shoulder muscles complicate and limit the exposure at these levels. Fessler and coworkers[15] addressed these issues and described a lateral parascapular extrapleural approach to the upper thoracic spine that preserves innervation to the shoulder muscles while allowing exposure for decompression and fusion. These procedures are often lengthy and can involve significant blood loss.

TRANSPEDICULAR APPROACH

In contradistinction to the two previous posterolateral approaches, which begin the exposure by actually approaching the spine posterolaterally, the transpedicular approach begins with a direct midline posterior approach through a midline incision. After the spinous processes are encountered, the paraspinal muscles are stripped subperiosteally on either side. On the side of the planned pedicle resection, the paraspinal muscles are stripped until they are 2 to 3 cm lateral to the tips of the transverse processes bracketing the pathologic level. The lamina, facets, and pedicle are removed unilaterally with a combination of rongeurs and a high-speed diamond drill. The medial transverse process is also removed as it attaches to the lateral pedicle, and the pedicle is drilled until it is flush with the vertebral body. Additional removal of ventral vertebral bodies or discs may be performed, depending on the pathologic process encountered. This approach allows excellent access to the ventral epidural space without the risk of pneumothorax or injury to intercostal nerves or nerve roots. However, much of the ventral epidural decompression is performed by passing instruments blindly ventral to the dura. Therefore, this approach is satisfactory for decompressing ventral soft tissue that is not significantly adherent to dura or invading the dura. I have found this approach to provide very satisfactory ventral and lateral decompression for infection and metastatic tumors in the thoracic spine.[16] Metastatic tumors can usually be separated easily from the dura with a dental instrument and curetted from under the dura with long foot plate curettes.

A disadvantage to this procedure is that the surgeon cannot visualize whether or not all tumor tissue has been resected. Because most operations are followed by radiotherapy, this disadvantage is not of major clinical significance when metastatic tumors are being treated. I do not use this surgical approach with primary sarcomas of the spine: sarcomas can be adherent or invade the dura. Also, I prefer to surgically remove all sarcoma tissue; therefore, I prefer a direct thoracotomy when I am treating a sarcoma.

The transpedicular approach has also been used to treat thoracic disc herniations.[17, 18] Le Roux and associates[17] recognized that this surgical approach does not allow good visualization of the ventral epidural space; therefore, they supplement their exposure by examining the epidural space endoscopically. Most of their 20 patients improved after surgery, including those with myelopathy. I have used the transpedicular approach in selected patients with lateral thoracic disc herniations. However, because some of these lesions can penetrate the dura, I prefer to approach thoracic disc herniations via a thoracotomy.

A major advantage to the transpedicular approach is that the posterior laminae are exposed, thereby facilitating the implantation of posterior stabilizing instrumentation. Conversely, the ventral exposure provided by this approach is not usually large enough to place a ventral strut graft of bone. If the anterior vertebral column fails to heal solidly, late kyphotic deformity and failure of posterior instrumentation may occur. This problem is seen most commonly when thoracolumbar burst fractures are managed by transpedicular decompression and posterior stabilization alone.

ANTEROLATERAL APPROACH

THORACOTOMY

The anterolateral approach to the thoracic spine is the posterolateral thoracotomy, which when extended into a thoracoabdominal exposure, can expose the thoracolumbar and lumbar spine. Hodgson and Stock[19] first used thoracotomy to decompress and stabilize a tubercular abscess of the thoracic spine. Since that initial use of thoracotomy, its use has been expanded to treat many pathologic problems of the thoracic and thoracolumbar spine, including infections, trauma, disc herniations, and tumors.[1, 20–29] The past decade has seen more neurosurgeons using thoracotomy to decompress and stabilize ventral compressive lesions because it provides better direct visualization of the ventral spinal canal than do the approaches discussed previously. In addition, the devices available for anterior internal stabilization of the spine have improved and in many instances can be used alone rather than with a subsequent posterior stabilization.

Because the anterolateral approach transgresses the thoracic cavity, many neurosurgeons perform this procedure with the help of a thoracic surgeon. The thoracic surgeon must understand the reason for the thoracotomy so that the chest is opened at the correct level and on the correct side. The standard thoracotomy performed by most chest surgeons for intrathoracic pathology is through the bed of the fifth rib, which provides them with exposure to the lung hilus, which is their usual focus. The thoracotomy performed for spinal surgery is more variable and must be based on the spinal level and the side of the pathology. Because the ribs slope downward, entering the chest one level above the pathology is preferable. For example, exposure of a disc herniation at T7-T8 is best accomplished by entering the chest through the bed of the seventh rib, which articulates posteriorly with the T6-T7 disc. Because of the slope of the ribs, this method positions the surgeon such that he or she is directly over the T7-T8 disc. Usually, the ribs slope downward more steeply at the lower levels. Therefore, entering the chest two ribs above the pathologic level is often necessary when the lower thoracic spine is being exposed. Conversely, the upper thoracic spine is usually exposed by a thoracotomy through the bed of the fourth or fifth rib. The apex of the chest may be gained by extension of the posterior incision upward medial to the scapula and cutting of additional ribs posteriorly. Careful communication between the neurosurgeon and the thoracic surgeon ensures that the appropriate spinal level is exposed.

Neurosurgeons with experience in these procedures may elect to perform these operations without the assistance of a thoracic surgeon. We generally perform uncomplicated thoracotomies for herniated disc, spinal fractures, infections, and localized tumors without involving a thoracic surgeon. However, we always involve a thoracic surgeon when the chest has been opened before, when the pathologic process extends to the lung or mediastinum, or when a double-lumen endotracheal tube is used. The first two indications are obvious. For the third, accurate placement of a double-lumen endotracheal tube almost always requires bronchoscopy to check placement; therefore, a thoracic surgeon is needed. An additional indication for involving a thoracic surgeon is a very sick patient who may require postoperative bronchoscopy to mobilize secretions and to treat atelectasis. The neurosurgeon should not hesitate to involve a thoracic surgeon and to scrub with him or her during the opening to increase his or her knowledge and clinical experience.

Many textbooks suggest that opening the chest from the patient's left is preferable because it avoids the vena cava. A simple perusal of an anatomy book reveals the inaccuracies in this statement. In the chest, the vena cava is within the structures of the mediastinum and has no direct relationship to the bony spine. The azygous vein runs along the ventrolateral bony spine in the right side of the chest, and the hemiazygous vein occupies a similar position in the left side. These structures are variable in size and position but may be ligated and divided if exposure is required to a vertebral body. Therefore, the surgeon should approach the area on the side where the pathologic process is localized. An exception to this statement occurs in the thoracoabdominal approach, which is most easily performed from the patient's left side because retraction on the right side can be impaired by the bulk of the liver.

In addition to the standard preoperative preparations for surgery, patients undergoing thoracotomy should also have pulmonary function studies, an arterial blood gases assessment, and a chest x-ray that delineates exactly how many ribs the patient has. The x-rays are an important aid in the intraoperative localization of the surgical level (see later). Furthermore, preoperative preparation with bronchodilators and preoperative teaching about deep breathing and incentive spirometry help to prevent postoperative atelectasis. Patients must also be told about the possibility of the postthoracotomy pain syndrome, although it has occurred rarely in my experience.

Thoracotomy for spinal exposure is performed with the patient in the lateral decubitus position. An arterial line is placed in the radial artery of the dependent arm, which allows monitoring of arterial pressure and blood gases during the procedure. Placing the arterial line in the dependent arm allows the anesthesiologist to monitor the arterial wave form and ensures that the dependent axilla is not compressed or distorted. Frequently, a foam pad is placed between the dependent chest wall and the operating table to give room for the axilla. I prefer to perform most thoracotomies for spinal exposure with a single-lumen endotracheal tube, which avoids the small but definite risk of tracheal injury that accompanies the use of double-lumen endotracheal tubes. Because the spine is the most posterior structure within the thoracic cavity, even the expanded lung can usually be easily retracted away from the spine. The Thompson-Farley spinal retractor provides excellent exposure of the spine while the lung remains expanded during these procedures.

As discussed earlier, the incision is centered over a rib that takes into account the downward slope of the chest wall. The incision usually begins along the anterior axillary line and extends posteriorly along the rib to the angle of the rib, from where it curves upward just lateral to the paraspinal muscles. After opening the subcutaneous tissue, the latissimus dorsi muscle is divided in the line of the incision. After the latissimus dorsi muscle is divided, the posterior edge of the serratus anterior muscle is undermined rostrally and caudally. Undermining the serratus anterior muscle allows it to be retracted anteriorly and eliminates the need for division of any of its fibers. Keeping this muscle intact greatly reduces postoperative ipsilateral shoulder discomfort and obviates specific postoperative shoulder physical therapy. Undermining of the serratus anterior rostrally is continued until the avascular plane under the scapula is reached. A scapula retractor is placed, and this space is opened bluntly with fingers. Blunt finger dissection is continued rostrally along the outer chest wall until the first rib is encountered. Palpating the first rib can be difficult and requires practice. The intercostal space between the second and third ribs is wider than the intercostal space at other levels. Conversely, the intercostal space is usually narrow between the first and second ribs. Remembering these relative intercostal space widths prevents the surgeon from mistakenly identifying the second rib as the first rib. Once the first rib is identified, the ribs are counted downward until the appropriate rib area is found from which to enter the chest. This rib is skeletonized subperiosteally to the angle of the rib and removed with a rib cutter. For thoracic disc operations, in which no bone graft is used, the rib is simply removed. If a ventral bone strut will be required after the decompression, the rib is cut anteriorly but left uncut posteriorly, and the vascular pedicle is left attached to the rib. At the conclusion of the decompression, the vascularized rib graft is placed into the bony defect. Although no controlled study has been performed regarding the use of these vascularized rib grafts, our clinical impression is that they heal faster and are especially well tolerated in an infected area.

Once the chest is entered, the ribs are counted from inside the chest, beginning with the first rib rostrally, which is now more easily identified. The best means of localizing the correct spinal level in this operation is by counting the ribs intraoperatively—both outside the chest wall and again inside the chest. This method is far more accurate than attempting to interpret the multiple overlying shadows that are seen on intraoperative radiographs. It is *very* important that the surgeon realize, therefore, that intraoperative localization of the pathologic level is based on the count from T1 downward. For this reason, preoperative localization of the pathologic level must also be based on computed tomography or magnetic resonance imaging (MRI) studies that count downward from T1. Preoperative studies that count upward from the sacrum can lead to mislocalization in patients with an abnormal number of ribs or lumbar vertebral bodies.

After the appropriate pathologic level is determined by rib count, a chest spreader is placed and opened to approximately 4 to 5 cm. The lung is retracted with a hand-held or table-based retractor. The parietal pleura is reflected medially off the vertebral body or disc level to be exposed. The radicular vessels travel across the middle of the vertebral bodies; therefore, if a vertebral body is to be resected, the radicular vessel is ligated and divided away from the neural foramen. If the exposure is for disc excision, dividing radicular vessels is not usually necessary. The sympathetic chain runs lateral to the head of the rib and can be divided. Similarly, the azygous and hemiazygous vein may be ligated and divided, if necessary. The head of the rib is removed to expose the lateral pedicle and to allow identification of the underlying neural foramen. A high-speed diamond drill is used to resect pedicle and vertebral bodies as needed to gain access to the spinal canal. Epidural venous bleeding can be problematic in these exposures because it obscures spinal canal anatomy. Therefore, removing the ventral aspect of the pedicle and gaining access to the lateral epidural space is best. The epidural tissues can be divided bluntly and coagulated until the dura is encountered. Once the lateral dura is identified, the ventral epidural tissues can be coagulated with a bipolar forceps and divided to completely expose the ventral spinal dura. If the pathologic process penetrates into the dura, as is sometimes encountered in calcified disc herniations, opening the dura or even excising a small ventral patch of dura may be necessary. Such dural openings are closed best by direct suturing with a small piece of fascial graft.

After the ventral pathology is decompressed, the surgeon must decide whether or not to place bone graft or stabilizing instrumentation. If the bony defect is small and substantial ventral or lateral vertebral body remains, neither bone graft nor instrumentation is necessary. We do not place bone graft or instrumentation after thoracic disc excisions. However, if a large resection has been performed or significant instability exists, then both bone graft and instrumentation are used. The first choice for bone graft is a piece of vascularized rib. If the rib is too small or not available, then autologous iliac crest is used. Large-tumor resections can produce large defects that can be bridged only by allograft humerus or femur. When allograft is used, the central marrow cavity is cleaned out and packed with autograft from the patient's rib or iliac crest.

Numerous instrumentation systems have been used to stabilize the anterior thoracic spine.[22, 30-34] Many of these systems are still being used, whereas others, such as the Dunn device, are no longer available because they were associated with late injury to vascular structures. The early devices were constructed from stainless steel. Although strong, these devices precluded subsequent use of MRI to assess the spinal canal near the instrumentation area. Many of the universal instrumentation systems, including the Texas Scottish Rite Hospital system, Cotrel-Dubousset systems, and Synthes systems, have bone screws that can be implanted anteriorly into the thoracic vertebral bodies and fixed to rods. Some of these components are available in titanium. Two manufacturers (Danek and Synthes) offer titanium plate systems in which large titanium plates are fixed to the lateral thoracic vertebral bodies above and below the decompressed region with cancellous bone screws. These plates are affixed after a ventral bone graft is placed into the decompressed region. Each of these instrumentation systems have unique advantages and disadvantages. They continue to be improved each year. The neurosurgeon planning an anterior stabilization procedure should review the systems available and select one that provides the most rigid fixation and lowest profile and can be implanted the most expeditiously.

THORACOABDOMINAL EXPOSURE

The thoracoabdominal exposure is simply an extension of the thoracotomy exposure into the retroperitoneal space so that exposure of the lateral thoracic spine may be combined with exposure of the lumbar spine. Through this approach, the lumbar spine may be exposed caudally to the upper sacrum. This exposure has been used for many years by orthopedic surgeons for anterior stabilization and fusion of scoliosis. In recent years, it has become more popular with neurosurgeons for decompression and stabilization of tumors, herniated discs, and burst fractures in the thoracolumbar spine.

For a thoracolumbar exposure, the patient is in the lateral decubitus position, and then is rotated dorsally until the patient is approximately 20 to 30 degrees from a full lateral position. An incision is made over the tenth rib posteriorly and carried forward until the costal margin is reached. If only the first lumbar vertebral body is to be exposed, the incision need not be any larger. However, if more exposure of the lumbar spine is needed, then the incision should continue along the lateral margin of the rectus abdominus muscle as far caudally as needed. The tenth rib is skeletonized subperiosteally and removed. If it will be needed for a bone graft, the vascular pedicle may be left intact. The pleural cavity is entered through the bed of this rib. After the diaphragm is identified, dissection is continued through the costal margin and underlying abdominal muscles until the underlying retroperitoneal space is reached. With a sponge, the retroperitoneal space is developed below the diaphragm as far caudally as required. The diaphragm is divided circumferentially with electrocautery, leaving a 1-cm cuff of diaphragm laterally that is used to suture the diaphragm closed at the end of the case. The superficial part of the diaphragm is marked with two sutures to facilitate closure. As the opening in the diaphragm extends toward the spine, it is divided down to the midbody of its insertion onto the L1 vertebral body. The periosteum is opened between the diaphragm insertion and the upper insertion of the psoas muscle. Then, the diaphragm is swept medially off of the spine subperiosteally. This method of exposure is different than the exposure typically used by vascular surgeons to expose the aortic hiatus. In their exposure, the lateral crus of the diaphragm is left attached to the lateral vertebral body, and the plane of dissection is through the fibers of the crus into the aortic hiatus. However, this vascular approach leaves the lateral crus of the diaphragm attached to the lateral vertebral body, from which it must still be removed to decompress or stabilize the spine. Leaving the lateral crus relatively intact and subperiosteally sweeping it away from the spine leaves more tissue to enhance healing in this area. The remainder of the spine exposure, decompression, and stabilization follows the principles described earlier in the thoracotomy exposure section.

Closure of the diaphragm is accomplished with interrupted 0 silk sutures, beginning near the crus and continuing circumferentially until the diaphragm is closed. A chest tube is placed, and the chest and abdomen are closed in the standard fashion.

ANTERIOR APPROACH: MEDIAN STERNOTOMY

The only true direct anterior approach to the thoracic spine is the median sternotomy, which is used to provide access to the upper thoracic spine T1-T3. Because pathologic lesions at this level are uncommon, this surgical approach is used rarely. My preference is to begin this incision along the medial border of the left sternocleidomastoid muscle, gain the midline at the sternal notch, then continue along the midsternum. The length of the sternotomy varies with the bony exposure. However, because the upper thoracic spine projects dorsally, and because of the presence of the great vessels, satisfactory exposure below T3 is rare. After the skin incision is made and the platysma is divided in the line of its fibers, the avascular plane between the sternocleidomastoid muscle laterally and cervical strap muscles medially is developed. As this plane is opened toward the sternum, the sternothyroid muscle is divided such that the upper sternum is exposed. The sternum is divided with a sternal saw or Lebsche knife and opened with a self-retaining retractor. The great vessels are gently depressed caudally with a retractor, and the upper thoracic spine is encountered after blunt dissection along the left lateral border of the trachea and esophagus. Although the thoracic duct can be injured on the left side, injuring the recurrent laryngeal nerve from a similar exposure in the right neck is commoner. Therefore, a left-sided exposure is preferred.

Once the thoracic spine is encountered, bony decompression is performed with a high-speed diamond drill. Bone grafts may be placed in the decompressed area. Internal stabilization can be accomplished with the Caspar or Morscher plate systems designed for anterior cervical spine stabilization. When these plates are used at the cervicothoracic junction, the plate should be placed with the arrow pointing caudally instead of rostrally. When placed in this direction, the upper screws follow more closely the orientation of the thoracic curve.

SUMMARY

Although virtually all pathology in the thoracic and thoracolumbar spine was approached surgically by laminectomy in the early history of neurosurgery, modern imaging studies have changed our perspective on how to best manage problems in this area of the spine. Neurosurgeons have realized that ventral compression of the thoracic spinal cord is often made worse by laminectomy. As neurosurgeons have developed a better appreciation for how to apply other surgical exposures to the thoracic spine, the outcomes for these problems have improved. Today, the neurosurgeon must be able to approach the thoracic and thoracolumbar spine through posterior, posterolateral, anterolateral, or anterior surgical approaches tailored to the pathology being treated.

REFERENCES

1. Perot PL Jr, Munro DD: Transthoracic removal of midline thoracic disc protrusions causing spinal cord compression. J Neurosurg 31:452–458, 1969
2. Bennett MH, McCallum JE: Experimental decompression of spinal cord. Surg Neurol 8:63–67, 1977
3. Doppman JL, Girton M: Angiographic study of the effect of laminectomy in the presence of acute anterior epidural masses. J Neurosurg 45:195–202, 1976
4. Patchell RA, Tibbs PA, Young AD, et al: Alban Smith and the beginnings of spinal surgery. Neurology 37:1683–1684, 1987
5. Bickham WS: Technique of exposure of the spinal cord and canal: Osteoplastic resection and laminectomy. Ann Surg 41:372–398, 1905
6. Menard V: Causes de la paraplegie dans le mal de pott. Rev Orthop 5:47–64, 1894
7. Seddon HJ: Pott's paraplegia—Prognosis and treatment. Br J Surg 22:769–774, 1935
8. Capener N: The evolution of lateral rhachotomy. J Bone Joint Surg Br 36B(2):173–179, 1954
9. Garrido E: Modified costotransversectomy: A surgical approach to ventrally placed lesions in the thoracic spinal canal. Surg Neurol 13:109–113, 1980
10. Overby MC, Rothman AS: Anterolateral decompression for metastatic epidural spinal cord tumors: Results of a modified costotransversectomy approach. J Neurosurg 62:344–348, 1985
11. Larson SJ, et al: Lateral extracavitary approach to traumatic lesions of the thoracic and lumbar spine. J Neurosurg 45:628–637, 1976
12. Benzel EC, Larson SJ: Operative stabilization of the posttraumatic thoracic and lumbar spine: A comparative analysis of the Harrington distraction rod and the modified Weiss spring. Neurosurgery 19(3):378–385, 1986
13. Maiman DJ, Larson SJ, Luck E, et al: Lateral extracavitary approach to the spine for thoracic disc herniation: Report of 23 cases. Neurosurgery 14(2):178–182, 1984
14. Benzel EC: The lateral extracavitary approach to the spine using the three-quarter prone position. J Neurosurg 71:837–841, 1989
15. Fessler RG, Dietze DDJ, Millan MM, et al: Lateral parascapular extrapleural approach to the upper thoracic spine. J Neurosurg 75:349–355, 1991
16. Shaw B, Mansfield FL, Borges LF: One-stage posterolateral decompression and stabilization for primary and metastatic vertebral tumors in the thoracic and lumbar spine. J Neurosurg 70:405–410, 1989
17. Le Roux PD, Haglund MM, Harris AB: Thoracic disc disease: Experience with the transpedicular approach in twenty consecutive patients. Neurosurgery 33(1):58–66, 1993
18. Patterson RH Jr, Arbit E: A surgical approach through the pedicle to protruded thoracic discs. J Neurosurg 48:768–772, 1978
19. Hodgson AR, Stock FE: Anterior spinal fusion: A preliminary communication on the radical treatment of Pott's disease and Pott's paraplegia. Br J Surg 44:266–275, 1956
20. Lobosky JM, Hitchon PW, McDonnell DE: Transthoracic anterolateral decompression for thoracic spinal lesions. Neurosurgery 14(1):26–30, 1984
21. Sundaresan N, Bains M, McCormack P: Surgical treatment of spinal cord compression in patients with lung cancer. Neurosurgery 16(3):350–356, 1985
22. Dunn HK: Anterior stabilization of thoracolumbar injuries. Clin Orthop 189:116–124, 1984
23. Harrington KD: Anterior cord decompression and spinal stabilization for patients with metastatic lesions of the spine. J Neurosurg 61:107–117, 1984
24. Sundaresan N, Digiacinto GV, Hughes JE, et al: Treatment of neoplastic spinal cord compression: Results of a prospective study. Neurosurgery 29(5):645–650, 1991
25. Lord CF, Herndon JH: Spinal cord compression secondary to kyphosis associated with radiation therapy for metastatic disease. Clin Orthop 210:120–127, 1986
26. Ransohoff J, Spencer F, Siew F, et al: Case reports and technical notes: Transthoracic removal of thoracic disc. J Neurosurg 31:459–461, 1969
27. Bohlman HH, Zdeblick TA: Anterior excision of herniated thoracic discs. J Bone Joint Surg Am 70A(7):1039–1047, 1988
28. Paul RL, Michael RH, Dunn JE, et al: Anterior transthoracic surgical decompression of acute spinal cord injuries. J Neurosurg 43:299–307, 1975
29. Otani K, Nakai S, Fujimura Y, et al: Surgical treatment of thoracic disc herniation using the anterior approach. J Bone Joint Surg Br 64B(3):340–343, 1982
30. Dunn HK: Anterior spine stabilization and decompression for thoracolumbar injuries. Orthop Clin North Am 17(1):113–119, 1986
31. Kaneda K, Abume K, Fujiya M: Burst fractures with neurologic defects of the thoracolumbar-lumbar spine: Results of anterior decompression and stabilization with anterior instrumentation. Spine 9:788–795, 1984
32. Kostuik JP: Anterior fixation for burst fractures of the thoracic and lumbar spine with or without neurological involvement. Spine 13:286–293, 1988
33. Rezaian SM, Dombrowski ET, Ghista DN: Spinal fixation for the management of spinal injury: The mechanical rationale. Eng Med 12:95–99, 1983
34. Yuan HA, Mann KA, Found EM: Early experience with the Syracuse I-plate, an anterior spinal fixation device. Spine 13:278–285, 1988

CHAPTER 152

Surgical Management of Thoracic Disc Herniations

Rakesh Kumar
Stewart B. Dunsker

A thoracic disc is herniated if focal extension of disc material exists beyond the vertebral margin that abuts, deforms, or displaces the spinal cord. Disc herniations in the thoracic spine are rare, representing 0.25 to 0.57 percent of all symptomatic disc herniations in the spine. Because of the popularity of magnetic resonance imaging (MRI) and computed tomography (CT) with myelography, asymptomatic thoracic disc herniations, some rather large and the spinal cord, are recognized in up to 15 percent of patients.[1, 2] Awwad and associates analyzed different factors of the herniated disc, including the frequency at various levels, laterality, size, multiplicity, and calcification, to try to determine features that separate asymptomatic from symptomatic thoracic discs.[1] One finding correlated with the symptomatic herniated discs, and it was present only some of the time: the absence of cerebrospinal fluid, both anterior and posterior to the cord, indicated that mechanical compression of the spinal cord existed between the herniated disc and the posterior elements.

CLINICAL FEATURES

Localized back pain is a common initial symptom that is present in 60 percent of all symptomatic disc herniation. Neurologic features in decreasing order of frequency are weakness in one or both lower limbs, sensory loss, bladder or bowel dysfunction, and radicular pain. Patients with a painless neurologic deficit are at the greatest risk of misdiagnosis.[3]

PREOPERATIVE EVALUATION

MRI is the screening test of choice, and it has an accuracy of greater than 95 percent in our experience.[4] Myelography, combined with postmyelographic CT can also be used. However, obtaining a sagittal view with the diagnostic accuracy seen in the MRI is more difficult and therefore more subject to error. Myelography has other disadvantages. It is invasive, involves radiation, and carries a risk of complications related to the spinal tap and instillation of contrast medium. In spite of these disadvantages, it often provides complimentary information. Myelography is particularly helpful in defining osteophytes from soft discs and may therefore help the surgeon in the operation.

PATIENT SELECTION AND MANAGEMENT DECISIONS

Myelopathy, radiculopathy, or both, resulting from disc herniation are the primary indications for thoracic disc excision. Recalcitrant cases of back pain and thoracic radiculopathy localized to the herniated disc level may also benefit from disc excision and root section. Asymptomatic cases, however, may be treated by observation and repeat MRI because they may not progress or may even regress. Lower thoracic disc herniations more often lead to myelopathy. In a retrospective study of the natural history of symptomatic thoracic disc herniations, Brown and colleagues[5] noted that 40 of 48 (83 percent) disc herniations from T3-T4 through T8-T9 were managed by a regimen of rest, administration of nonsteroidal anti-inflammatory drugs, and physical therapy. Of these 40 patients managed nonsurgically, only 12 (30 percent) returned to their previous level of activity. Our understanding of the natural history of thoracic disc herniation, both symptomatic and asymptomatic, is still incomplete. The decision to perform surgery should be made from the patient's clinical signs, correlated by imaging studies. Persistent thoracic back pain is also an indication for operation in the presence of herniated disc with cord or root deformity, even in the absence of neurologic signs, because the patient may return to an unrestricted life style. Occasionally, we find patients who are asymptomatic who show considerable spinal cord deformity. Whether they will develop myelopathy is unknown. We have also seen patients who present with myelopathy many years after an injury that probably caused the herniated disc. It is difficult to imagine that the spinal cord can be significantly compromised in a young person for a long time without producing myelopathy in later years. With advanced imaging and with more experience, we will probably be able to select those patients at risk for early surgical intervention.

CHOICE OF SURGICAL APPROACH

The factors to consider in the decision of which of the different approaches is most suitable include
1. Level of disc herniation
2. Laterality of the herniation
3. Whether the disc herniation is single or multiple (Table 152–1)

Table 152–1. GUIDELINES FOR APPROACHES TO THORACIC DISC*

Approach	Indication and Notable Features	Disc Levels
Posterolateral		
Laminectomy and foraminotomy	Lateral disc herniation. No cord deformity.	T1–T2 and T2–T3
Transpedicular	Lateral or centrolateral disc herniation with minimal cord deformity.	At any level
Costotransversectomy	Centrolateral disc herniation with moderate-to-severe cord compression.	At any level
Lateral extracavitary	Same as in costotransversectomy. Provides better visualization.	At any level
Anterolateral		
Anterolateral extrapleural (transthoracic extrapleural)	Central disc herniation. The deformed spinal cord hangs over the herniated disc. Removal of such a disc by the above approaches can be accomplished only by cord retraction or by blindly passing instruments between the disc and the theca. Anterior intradural exploration may be performed.	T4–T5 to T12–L1
Transthoracic (transthoracic transpleural)	Used for any type of thoracic disc herniation but has the highest morbidity and prolonged hospitalization. Should be reserved for multiple thoracic discs.	T4–T12
Transsternal	Large central disc at upper thoracic level only.	T1–T2 to T3–T4

*We recognize that a particular approach may be used for removing different types or extents of herniated thoracic discs.

Thoracic disc herniations occur most frequently at the lower third of the thoracic spine, less frequently at the middle third, and rarely in the upper third. Disc herniations at levels T3-T4 through T12-L1 may be accessed by any approach detailed in this chapter. All of these procedures are designed to provide some access to the anterior part of the spinal canal.

Laminectomy alone, however, has a much higher risk of paraplegia. At T1-T2 and T2-T3 levels, disc herniations are rare and are reported to be located laterally. They present with medial brachialgia, sometimes with associated Horner's syndrome. Though these herniations may be approached anteriorly by use of a transsternal approach,[6] the potential com-

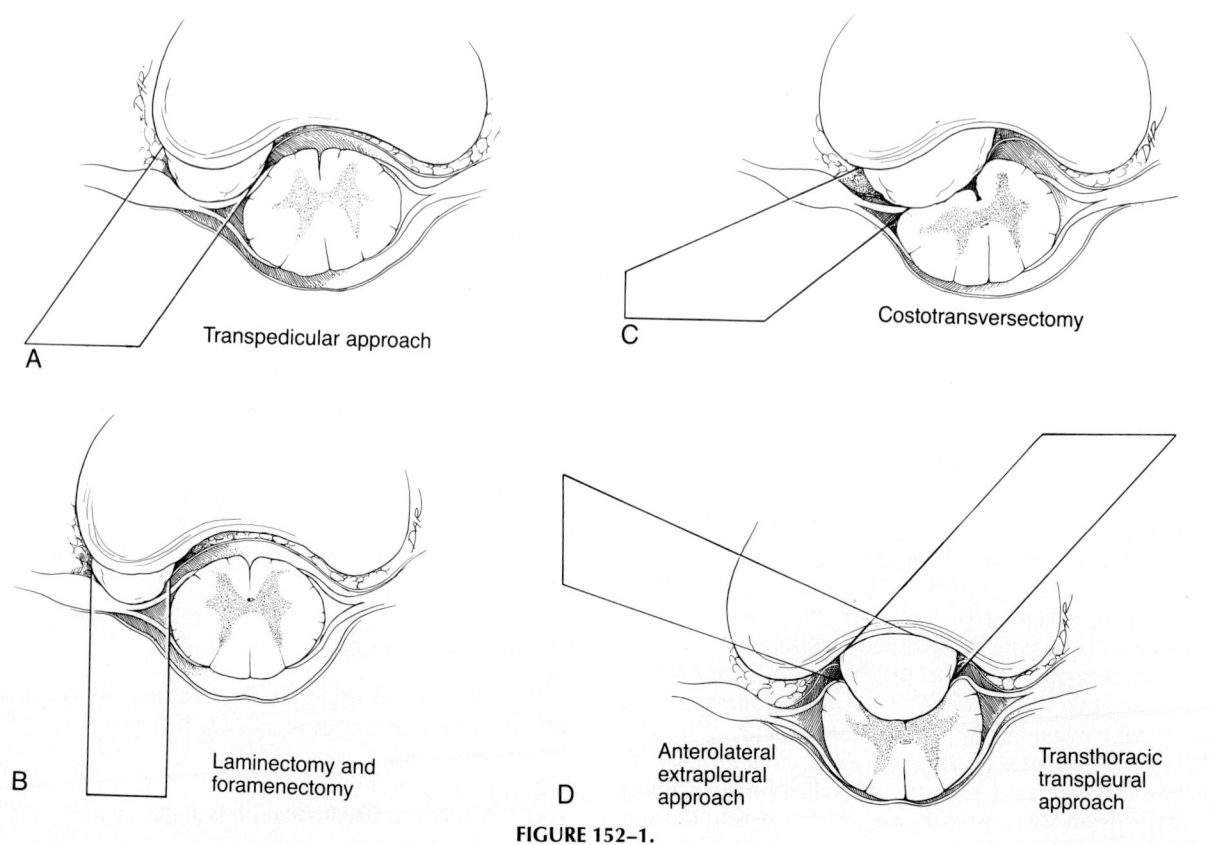

FIGURE 152–1.

placed, and the lung is held out of the field with a malleable Hurson retractor. The anterior spine is then exposed by retraction of the lung, which can be gradually deflated if required. To expose the spine, the pleura is then reflected in the form of a window. Intercostal vessels (which are direct tributaries of the aorta or vena cava) are carefully identified and ligated as well as clipped. This maneuver also allows mobilization of the major vessels over the surface of the vertebra. All soft tissues anterior to the vertebra are dissected off (including the sympathetic ganglia). The isolated segments are packed off with lap pads, and if a prevertebral tumor is identified, we can be reasonably sure of the proper location of the segment to be resected. If no tumor is evident on the surface, the correct level must be established not only by counting the ribs from within the chest but also by obtaining an intraoperative roentgenogram.

Before work begins on the spine, the anterior surface of the vertebral body is cleared by periosteal elevators. Intact disc structures above and below the level of involvement are identified (Fig. 161–12); the discs are incised with a No. 15 blade, and the vertebral segments are removed with rongeurs, curettes, and osteotomes. Tumor resection should be complete, and the posterior longitudinal ligament should be removed. In patients who have not received prior radiation, this resection is relatively easy to accomplish. In radiated patients, the bone and tumor may be fibrotic and the posterior longitudinal ligament densely adherent to the dura. By tracing the epidural tumor posteriorly, it is possible to decompress the dura laterally and posteriorly by performing a facetectomy and removing the pedicle. To allow additional posterior decompression, a hemilaminectomy can be performed at this time. The anterior longitudinal ligament is left intact if it is not destroyed. A high-speed drill is then used to drill out the opposite half of the body until a thin cortical shell is left. If a curative resection is contemplated, every effort must be made to remove all bone and soft tissue so that the spondylectomy can be completed by a second-stage posterior approach. We emphasize the importance of complete tumor resection, even to the extent of using a Cavitron ultrasonic tumor aspirator to remove all gross tumor. After tumor resection, all soft tissues on the endplates above and below are removed to provide the broadest possible support for the polymethyl methacrylate reconstruction. Hemostasis is secured by the use of the fine-tipped bipolar current and hemostatic agents, such as microfibrillar collagen or gelatin sponge pledgets. Before stabilization, the surgeon must be sure that all vertebral segments involved by tumor have been resected because fixation of the acrylic to a diseased vertebra results in postoperative displacement. In half the patients, more than one vertebra has to be removed; we have resected up to four vertebrae, including the involved chest wall in the thoracic region, with little morbidity.

The next phase of the operation is stabilization. Steinmann pins varying in size from 5/64 to 19/64 inch in diameter are selected and cut to straddle the bony defect (Figs. 161–13 and 161–14). We prefer to use the smooth pins instead of the threaded ones. The pins are bent at each end in the shape of hockey sticks and introduced with two heavy sternal needle holders. These pins should straddle the resected segments and be securely in place to the vertebrae above and below. Once the pins (generally two) are secured, polymethyl methacrylate is injected into the space and molded to re-create the resected bodies. At the same time, Penfield dissectors and tongue blades are used to keep the hardening acrylic away from the dura, which is protected by strips of gelatin sponge. Copious irrigation with saline is used to dissipate heat during

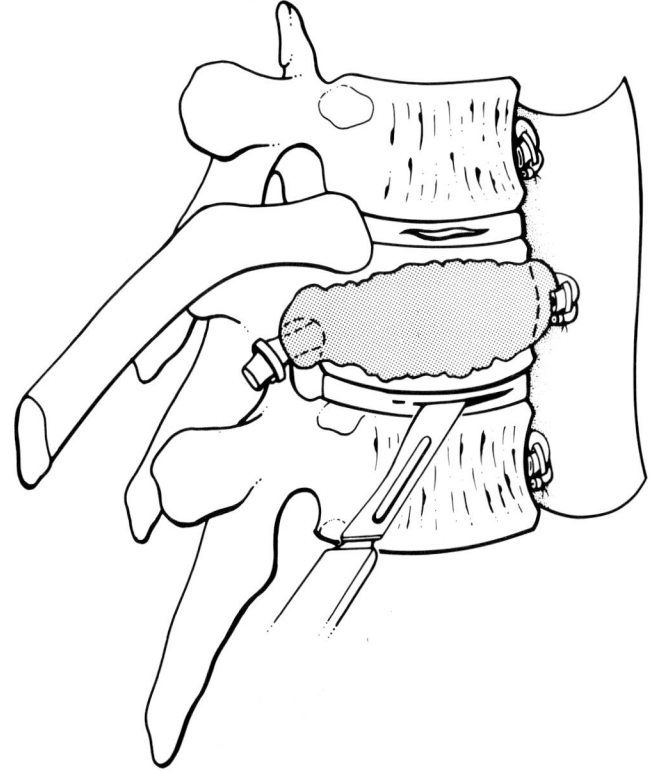

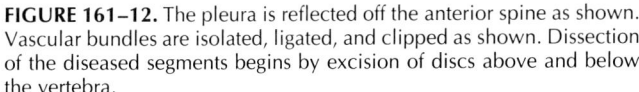
FIGURE 161–12. The pleura is reflected off the anterior spine as shown. Vascular bundles are isolated, ligated, and clipped as shown. Dissection of the diseased segments begins by excision of discs above and below the vertebra.

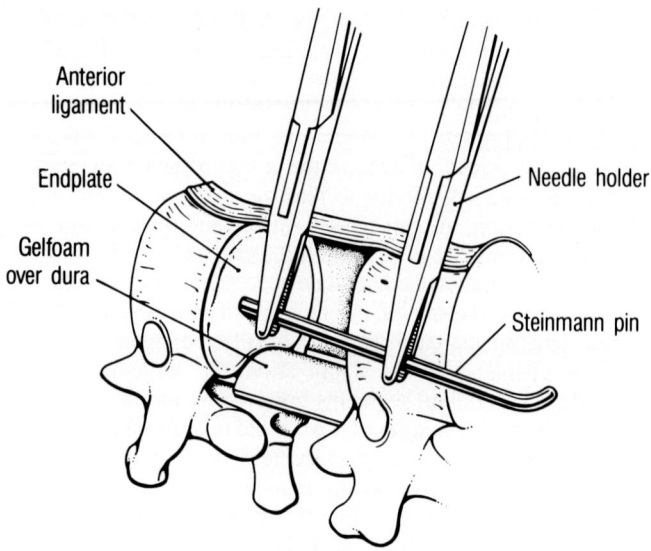

FIGURE 161-13. Following tumor resection, the endplates are carefully cleaned with curettes and Steinmann pins bent at each end introduced with heavy needle holders.

the polymerization process. The epidural space should be kept free of all trapped fluid, and no effort should be made to pack this space tightly. The resected rib can be placed adjacent to the bodies and tied in position with Vicryl sutures as a lateral fusion mass (Fig. 161–15). If the angulation of the spine or technical difficulties do not allow safe introduction of Steinmann pins, we use anterior distraction devices, such as Knodt or Harrington rods. The anterior distraction devices are then incorporated within the acrylic construct.

The chest cavity is drained by chest tubes, and the closure is that of a standard thoracotomy. Postoperatively, patients are kept in intensive care for a few days, and the chest tube drainage is monitored. When less than 100 ml is drained over 24 hours, it is removed. Extensive chest tube drainage over a week suggests a cerebrospinal fluid leak into the pleural cavity. To minimize respiratory complications, we allow early ambulation. A Knight-Taylor brace or a Prenyl jacket is used for patient comfort. Broad-spectrum antibiotics are used routinely during the operation and for 48 hours after surgery. A repeat fluoromyelogram is generally performed to check clearing of the block and alignment of the spine (Fig. 161–16). If postoperative radiation therapy is decided on, it is begun after a week.

ANTERIOR APPROACH TO LOWER THORACIC AND UPPER LUMBAR SEGMENTS

Numerous approaches are available for the thoracolumbar region because the diaphragm separates this region into two cavities. The lower thoracic approach can also be performed by a completely extrapleural procedure, but the widest exposures are obtained by a transthoracic approach with detachment of the diaphragm.

The diaphragm is a dome-shaped muscle that is muscular around its periphery and tendinous centrally. Anteriorly, it arises from the xiphoid and cartilaginous portions of the lower six ribs, and posteriorly, it originates from the crura that are attached to the anterior longitudinal ligament; superiorly, the crura of the diaphragm arise from the medial and lateral arcuate ligaments, which are attached to the transverse processes of the first lumbar and the twelfth rib. The widest

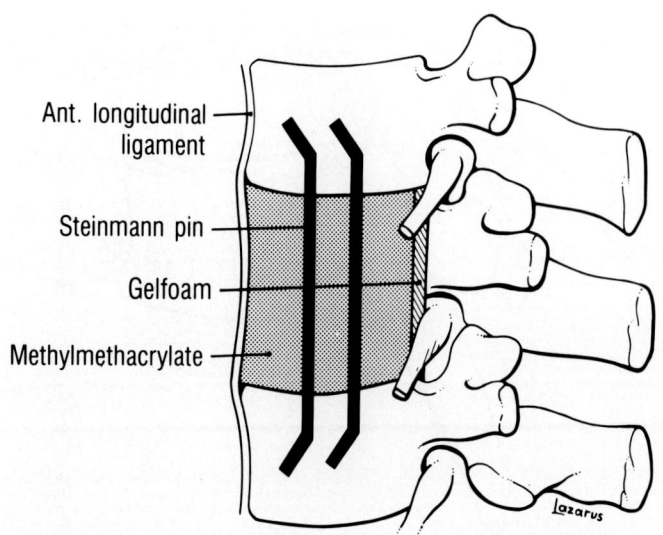

FIGURE 161-14. The Steinmann pins should straddle the resected segments and are incorporated within the methyl methacrylate construct; during the heat of polymerization, saline irrigation is used and a sheet of Gelfoam protects the dura.

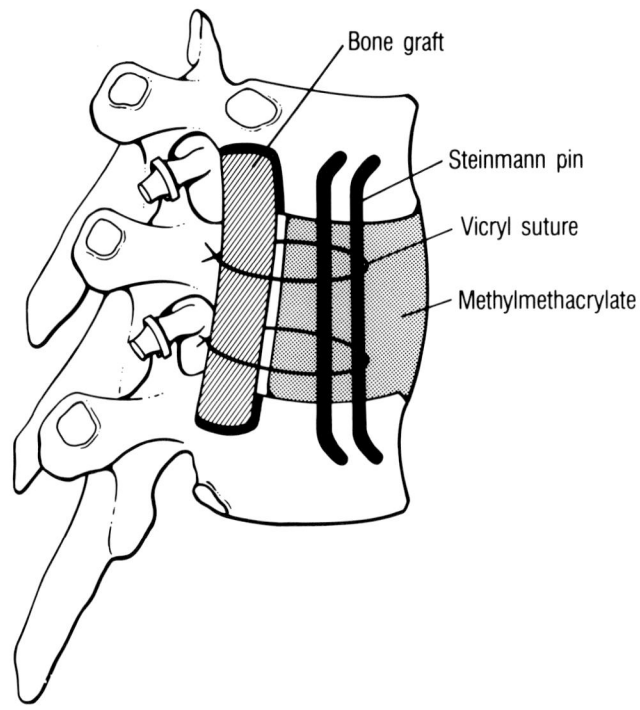

FIGURE 161–15. The rib segment may be used as a lateral fusion mass as shown; it is held in place by Vicryl sutures and tied to the Steinmann pins before insertion of the semisolid acrylic cement.

exposures are obtained by resecting the tenth or eleventh ribs, and detaching the muscle from the costal articulations as well as the arcuate ligaments.

For the widest and most direct anterior exposure to the thoracoabdominal spine, a long skin incision centered on the tenth or eleventh ribs is required. Posteriorly, the incision should extend to the paraspinous muscles. The latissimus dorsi and serratus anterior muscles are divided, and the ribs to be resected are identified. The oblique muscles are detached from the rib with cautery or cut in the intercostal

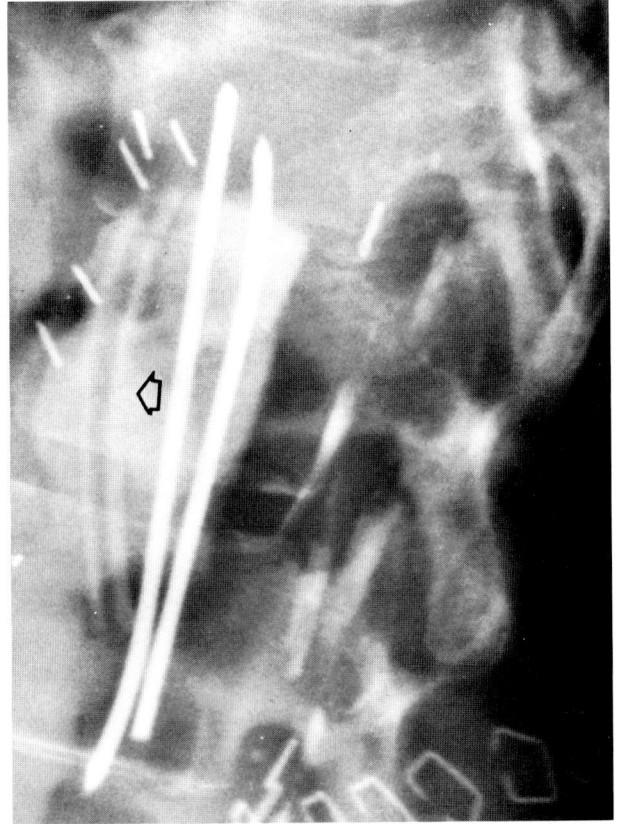

FIGURE 161–16. A postoperative lateral roentgenogram demonstrates normal alignment of the spine and clearing of myelographic block. Arrow indicates rib graft.

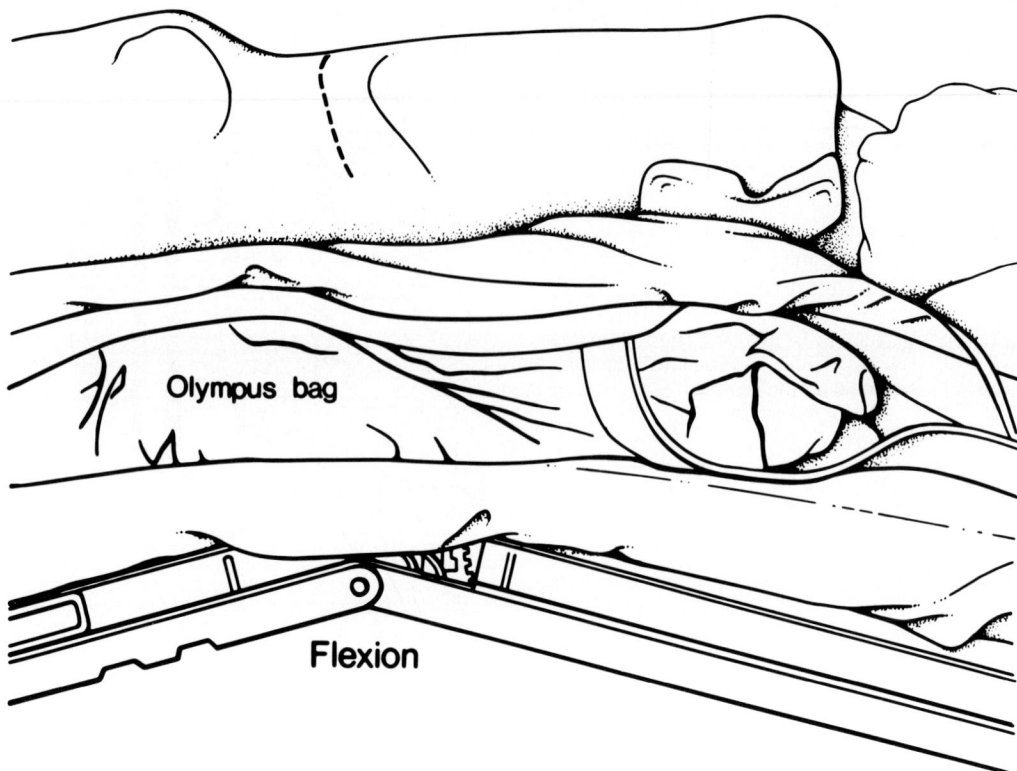

FIGURE 161–17. For exposures of the lumbar segments, a retroperitoneal flank approach is used. The patient is positioned on an Olympic Vac-Pac unit, and the table is flexed to allow a subcostal exposure.

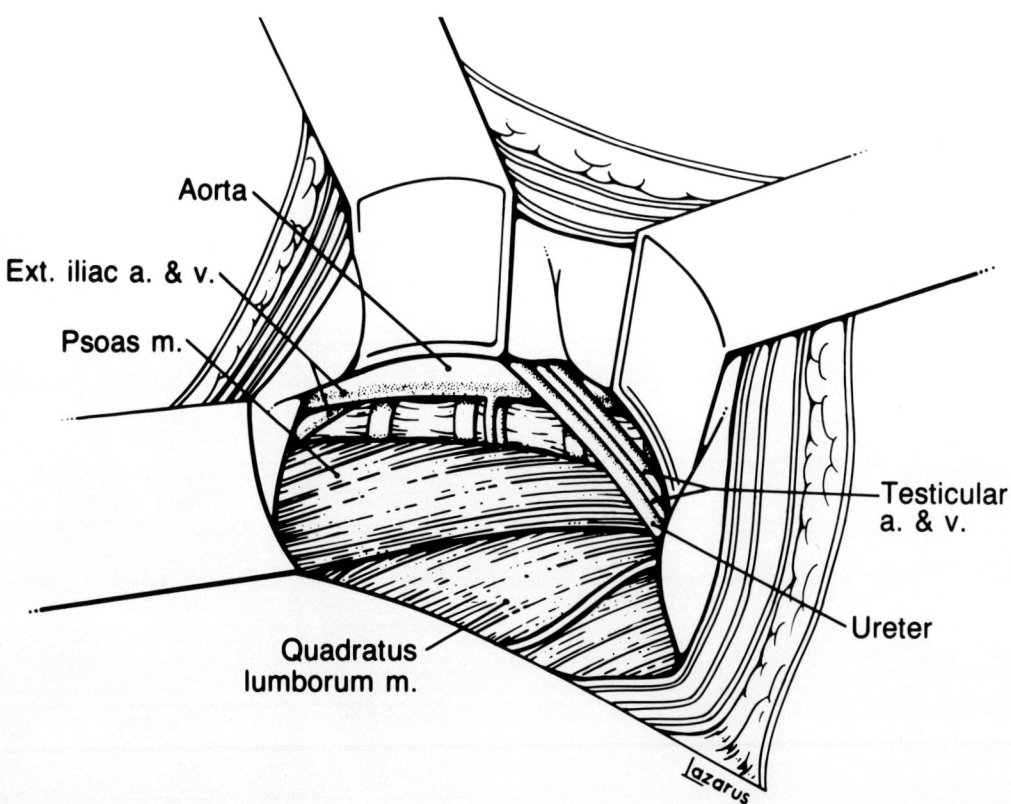

FIGURE 161–18. For exposures of the lumbar segments, the retroperitoneal approach with anterior displacement of the kidney and ureter is used. Note that exposure is anterior to the psoas major muscle.

space. The endothoracic fascia and parietal pleura are opened and the ribs spread. The diaphragm is then put under tension by retraction and is circumferentially detached toward the arcuate ligaments. The retroperitoneal space is gradually enlarged by blunt dissection, and the spleen is retracted downward. The sympathetic trunk and the areolar tissue around the aorta are cleared. Segmental intercostal vessels are carefully ligated and cut. The anterior surface of the thoracolumbar spine is then exposed and the soft tissues cleared to expose the cortical surface. Tumor resection then proceeds as described earlier in this chapter. After tumor resection and stabilization, repair proceeds by closure of the diaphragm and insertion of chest tubes. The muscles and skin are then closed in routine fashion.

To approach the lumbar spine from the second to the fourth segments, an oblique retroperitoneal flank approach is used (Figs. 161–17 and 161–18). The twelfth rib is resected subperiosteally, and the retroperitoneal space behind the fascia transversalis is developed. The kidney and ureters are displaced anteriorly, and the space is kept open by a Balfour retractor. It is important to identify the relatively avascular space behind the peritoneum and Gerota's fascia, and to approach the lumbar spine anterior to the psoas major and quadratus lumborum muscles. A helpful anatomic guide to this region is the crural attachment of the diaphragm, which generally is seen only to the second lumbar segment. The sympathetic chain should be retracted laterally and preserved whenever possible. To remove tumors involving the fifth lumbar vertebra, a retroperitoneal approach is inadequate, and an anterior transabdominal approach should be used. In this segment, Knodt rods are useful because Steinmann pins are difficult to place.

LATERAL OSTEOTOMY APPROACH

The spine can also be approached from the side by the lateral osteotomy approach, which is performed by cutting through the transverse process of the vertebra and fracturing the osteotomized portion of the paraspinal structures anteriorly. The major indications for this procedure are superior sulcus tumors or other lung cancers with chest wall involvement, as well as large paraspinous sarcomas with both anterolateral and posterolateral components. The skin incision can be oblique, as in the thoracic region, or a T with the shorter limbs of the T in the midline. Initially, the paraspinal tumor mass is dissected free from the lateral and anterior attachments, including the intra-abdominal and intrathoracic vessels; secondly, it is freed superiorly and inferiorly by resection of the chest wall or the paraspinous muscles. Finally, the paraspinous muscles are cut over the transverse processes and the main mass of the tumor fractured forward. Nerve roots are carefully isolated and clipped. If the intraspinal extensions of tumor are noted, the spinal resection should include a partial hemilaminectomy and facetectomy. No additional reconstruction is required after such lateral osteotomy procedures. After extensive chest wall resection, extensive skeletal defects may require reconstruction with a Marlex mesh prosthesis.

POSTOPERATIVE MANAGEMENT AND DISCUSSION

Patients undergoing anterior spinal surgery and stabilization procedures require monitoring in the intensive care unit because of the potential for respiratory complications in addition to the other common postoperative problems, such as ileus, venous thrombosis, and infection. Despite their apparent magnitude, these procedures are well tolerated by most cancer patients, and the morbidity is lower than that of decompressive laminectomy. We allow early ambulation and recommend rapid tapering of steroid therapy. In our experience, patients who have received recent radiation therapy as well as high-dose steroid therapy for more than a month are particularly likely to develop perioperative complications.

In our experience with the first 160 patients, the 30-day mortality was 6 percent, and an additional 15 percent developed surgical complications. However, the mortality for patients undergoing de novo operation was 4 percent, and the morbidity was 10 percent. No serious permanent neurologic defect was encountered, and all other complications were effectively treated without sequelae. The neurologic improvement rate exceeded 80 percent, and 80 percent of patients with spinal pain experienced pain relief. In long-term survivors, the long-term ambulation rate exceeded 80 percent at 1 year, although repeat anterior or posterior decompressions were necessary in 20 percent of patients. These figures are superior to those reported for external radiotherapy and steroid therapy alone. In patients with potentially curable tumors, we believe that this operation is indicated even before cord compression has developed, such as in patients with intraosseous disease. For primary malignant neoplasms of the spine, a two-stage approach is required: vertebral body resection as the initial debulking procedure, followed by posterior resection and stabilization. With such aggressive surgery, long-term disease-free survivors and cures may be anticipated with malignant spine tumors. The concept that these patients cannot be cured because the spine has been considered an inaccessible site is no longer valid. Our results suggest that the logic of treating malignant bone tumors elsewhere can now be applied equally successfully to lesions involving the spine.

REFERENCES

1. Sundaresan N, DiGiacinto GV, Hughes JEO: Surgical treatment of spinal metastases. Clin Neurosurg 33:503, 1986
2. Boland PJ, Lane JM, Sundaresan N: Metastatic disease of the spine. Clin Orthop 169:95, 1982
3. Constans JP, De Vitiis E, Donzelli, et al: Spinal metastases with neurological manifestations. J Neurosurg 59:111, 1983
4. Gilbert RW, Kim JH, Posner JB: Epidural spinal cord compression from metastatic tumor: Diagnosis and treatment. Ann Neurol 3:40, 1978
5. Stark RJ, Henson RA, Evans SJW: Spinal metastases: A retrospective survey from a general hospital. Brain 105:189, 1982
6. Krol G, Heier L, Becker R, et al: MRI and myelography in the evaluation of epidural extension of primary and metastatic tumors, in Volk J (ed): Neuroradiology 1985–1986. Amsterdam, Elsevier, 1986, pp 91–97
7. Russell EJ, Berenstein A: Neurological applications of interventional radiology. Neurol Clin 2:873, 1984
8. Barcena A, Lobato RD, Rivas JJ, et al: Spinal metastatic disease:

Analysis of factors determining functional prognosis and choice of treatment. Neurosurgery 15:820, 1984
9. Tang SG, Byfield JE, Sharp TR: Prognostic factors in the management of metastastic epidural cord compression. J Neuro-oncol 1:21, 1981
10. Sundaresan N, Scher H, Yagoda A, et al: Surgical treatment of spinal metastases in kidney cancer. J Clin Oncol 1986, in press
11. Sundaresan N, Hilaris BH, Martini N: The combined neurosurgical-thoracic management of superior sulcus tumors. Arch Surg 1986, in press
12. Sundaresan N, Galicich JH, Lane JM: Treatment of odontoid fracture in cancer patients. J Neurosurg 52:187, 1981
13. Sundaresan N, Galicich JH, Lane JM: Harrington rod stabilization for pathological fractures of the spine. J Neurosurg 60:282, 1984
14. Harrington KD: Anterior cord decompression and spinal stabilization for patients with metastastic lesions of the spine. J Neurosurg 61:107, 1984
15. Flatley JJ, Anderson MH, Anast GT: Spinal instability due to metastatic disease. J Bone Joint Surg Am 66(A):47, 1984
16. Clark CR, Keggi KJ, Panjabi MM: Methyl methacrylate stabilization of the cervical spine. J Bone Joint Surg Am 66(A):40, 1984
17. Martenson JA, Evans RL, Lie MR: Treatment outcome and complications in patients treated for malignant cord compression. J Neuro-oncol 3:77, 1985
18. Overby MC, Rothman AS: Anterolateral decompression for metastatic epidural spinal cord tumors. J Neurosurg 62:344, 1985
19. Macedo N, Sundaresan N, Galicich JH: Decompressive laminectomy for metastatic cancer: What are the current indications? Proc Am Soc Am Oncol 4:287, 1985
20. Foley KH: The treatment of cancer pain. N Engl J Med 31:84, 1985
21. Sundaresan N, DiGiacinto GV: Antitumor and anti-nociceptive approaches to cancer pain. Med Clin North Am 71:329, 1987
22. Siegal T, Siegal T: The management of malignant epidural tumors compressing the spinal cord, in Schmidek H, Sweet W (eds): Operative Neurosurgical Techniques, ed 2. Orlando, Grune & Stratton, 1987
23. Siegal T, Tikva P, Siegal T: Vertebral body resection for epidural compression by malignant tumors. J Bone Joint Surg Am 67A:375, 1985
24. Sundaresan N, Krol G, Hughes JEO: Treatment of malignant tumors of the spine, in Youmans J (ed): Neurological Surgery. Philadelphia, WB Saunders, 1987
25. Sundaresan N, Galicich JH, Lane JM, et al: Treatment of neoplastic epidural cord compression by vertebral body resection and stabilization. J Neurosurg 63:676, 1985
26. Sundaresan N, Shah J, Feghali JG: A trans-sternal approach to the upper thoracic vertebra. Am J Surg 148:473, 1986

CHAPTER 162

Surgical Management of Malignant Epidural Tumors Compressing the Spinal Cord

Tzony Siegal
Tali Siegal

The management of malignant tumors that induce neurologic deficits secondary to involvement of the spinal column and the epidural space has been the subject of debate for many years. The past two decades have witnessed significant shifts in therapeutic approaches, ranging from urgent laminectomy to a combination of laminectomy and radiotherapy to nonsurgical treatment by radiotherapy alone. More recently, attention has been directed toward radiotherapy or to anterior surgical decompression as preferred treatment modalities.[1] Some attempts have been made to compare various management methods, but the absence of satisfactory controlled trials still leaves no clear consensus on management. A synopsis of the current knowledge and concepts related to various therapeutic measures and prognostic factors is presented in this chapter.

Malignant tumors of the spine can be either primary or metastatic. An extensive review of the literature on primary and secondary tumors of the vertebral column revealed that metastatic tumors occur three to four times more frequently than primary malignant neoplasms[2] and that even solitary vertebral lesions are often metastatic.[3]

INCIDENCE

The skeletal system is the third commonest site of cancer metastases after the lung and the liver, and among skeletal metastases, the vertebral column is the commonest site.[4-6] In autopsy series, 30 to 60 percent of patients dying of neoplasia were found to have spinal and epidural metastases.[2, 6, 7] Approximately 50 percent of cases of metastatic epidural compression in adults arise from breast, lung, or prostatic cancer.[1, 8-10] Other common primary cancers include lymphoma, renal cancer, sarcoma, and multiple myeloma,[1, 8-11] and in 9 percent of cases, the origin of the metastases cannot be identified. The tendency of some tumor types to metastasize to the spine is relatively high: in an autopsy series of 704 cancer patients, multiple myeloma had the highest propensity to spinal metastases, followed by prostatic carcinoma.[12] In breast cancer, the spine is the commonest site of bony metastases.[5]

All patients with vertebral metastases are at potential risk of developing spinal cord compression (SCC), but its frequency is unknown. The term SCC includes cauda equina compression, unless otherwise noted. Retrospective clinical studies calculated that 2 to 20 percent of patients with vertebral metastases develop myelopathy secondary to SCC.[6, 13] An autopsy study estimated that 5 percent of cancer patients develop spinal epidural tumor deposits,[12] although a proportion of these may not become clinically evident. Although spinal metastases generally occur in patients with known malignancy, in about 8 percent of patients with SCC, this is the initial symptom of cancer.[10, 11]

The clinical incidence of SCC in children is about 5 percent, but the commonest tumor types are different from those encountered in adults and include sarcomas, neuroblastomas, and lymphomas.[1, 14, 15] Sarcoma and neuroblastoma comprise more than 80 percent of all cases of pediatric SCC, and Ewing's sarcoma has the highest propensity for epidural extension. Most pediatric tumors invade the spinal canal via the neural foramen rather than via vertebral metastases.

TUMOR LOCATION

LEVEL OF SPINAL CORD COMPRESSION

Most investigators agree that the thoracic spine is the commonest site of SCC.[11, 16] If the involvement of any area of the spine by metastatic deposits relates roughly to the number of vertebrae contained therein,[11] the expected rate of SCC in the cervical and lumbar regions is 27 and 19 percent, respectively (coccygeal region excluded). In a review of 2977 cases of SCC described in various clinical series, cervical region involvement occurred at a lower than expected rate (11 to 13 percent versus 27 percent), whereas involvement in the lumbar and thoracic areas was close to the predicted figures.[16] The lower incidence of SCC in the cervical spine is probably related to two major factors: (1) the total bone volume of the cervical spine is smaller than that of other regions, and therefore hematogenous vertebral colonization by a metastatic tumor is less likely to occur; and (2) the spinal canal is more capacious in the upper cervical area relative to the thoracic canal, allowing more space for an expanding epidural tumor and thus diminishing the proportion of epidural deposits that become clinically evident.

LOCATION OF EPIDURAL TUMOR IN RELATION TO THE SPINAL CORD AND THE YIELD OF DIAGNOSTIC IMAGING

Epidural SCC usually results from metastases to one of three sites: the vertebrae, the paravertebral tissue, or the epidural space itself. Extension of the tumor into the spinal canal may produce variable involvement of the anterior (ventral) compartment, the lateral gutters, the posterior compartment, or any combination of these sites (Fig. 162–1).

The vertebral column is the commonest site from which metastases may cause epidural SCC. It is therefore not surprising that spinal radiography is predictive of epidural disease[17] and that an epidural mass is identified at 86 percent of symptomatic spinal segments and 43 percent of asymptomatic segments with an abnormal radiographic result. Vertebral collapse of more than 50 percent is associated with epidural deposits in 85 percent of cases in which the distinction between symptomatic and asymptomatic segments is not made.[17] However, radiographic results require 30 to 70 percent bony destruction before they become positive.[18] A magnetic resonance imaging (MRI) study has recently demonstrated that although an absent pedicle is often the first radiographic sign of metastatic disease, the pedicle is involved by direct extension from either the vertebral body or the posterior elements and is therefore a late occurrence in the disease process.[19] The region of the vertebral column that is most often involved is the vertebral body, probably be-

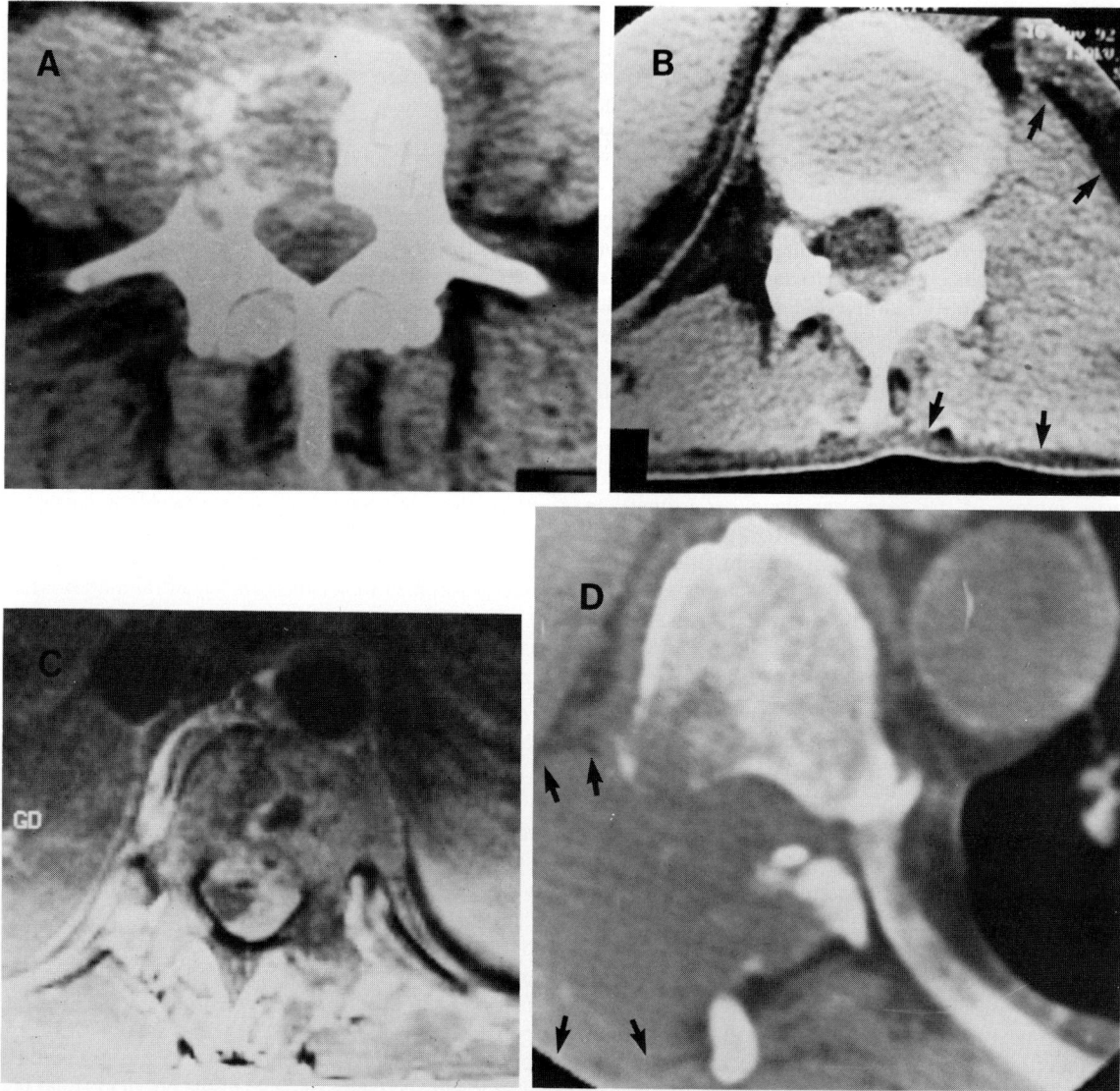

FIGURE 162–1. Location of epidural tumor in relation to the spinal cord. Epidural metastases usually arise from extension of metastases located in the adjacent vertebral column into the spinal canal (A and C) or from paravertebral masses penetrating through the intervertebral foramina (B). The extension of the tumor into the spinal canal produces variable involvement of the anterior (ventral) compartment (A, CT scan of breast cancer), the lateral gutter (B, contrast-enhanced CT scan of Hodgkin's lymphoma), the posterior compartment (C, CT scan of colon carcinoma) or any combination of these conditions (D, MRI with gadolinium of non-Hodgkin's lymphoma: involvement of the anterior, lateral and posterior compartments). Arrows indicate the extent of the paravertebral tumor.

cause of its extensive vascular supply; thus, most epidural tumors arise in a vertebral body and invade the epidural space anteriorly.[12, 16, 20]

Normal spinal roentgenograms do not exclude epidural metastases. Paravertebral tumors may invade the epidural space through the intervertebral foramina rather than via vertebral extension. This is more commonly seen in renal cell cancer, superior sulcus tumors (Pancoast's syndrome), neuroblastoma, and lymphoma. The precise frequency of this mode of epidural invasion is unknown, but it is estimated to comprise approximately 10 percent of all SCC.[21] One study demonstrated that on myelography, 36 percent of patients with paraspinal tumor had epidural metastases.[22] With the advent of computed tomographic (CT) scanning and MRI, which adequately demonstrate the paravertebral soft tissues, these lesions are being more frequently recognized. Pure epidural lesions alone are rare, and their incidence is about 5 percent.[8]

The location of the extradural metastases within the vertebral canal has important surgical implications. Accurate definition of the epidural mass as either posterior, lateral, cuff, or anterior requires the combination of CT myelography or a noninvasive MRI study. Although myelography has until recently been the procedure of choice for definitive imaging of the spinal canal to diagnose epidural compression, MRI is reported to be equally sensitive in most cases.[23] Several investigators found MRI equal to myelography in detecting epidural disease and superior in detecting vertebral metastases and paravertebral masses.[1, 23, 24] In centers in which MRI is readily available, it has become the preferred imaging method. Myelography (combined with CT) should be performed, however, when diagnosis and treatment are delayed by the inability to perform MRI in a timely fashion, when patients are unable to undergo MRI (because of pacemakers or claustrophobia), or when a technically adequate MRI cannot be obtained (e.g., in the presence of spinal instrumentation at the investigated level or extreme obesity).

SYMPTOMS AND SIGNS

The onset of symptoms of SCC may be acute or insidious, and the duration of symptoms varies widely before diagnosis. Pain is usually the initial symptom (in 96 percent of cases), preceding other symptoms by 5 days to 2 years (median, 7 weeks).[11, 20, 25] The pain can be localized close to the site of the lesion or can be radicular. Pain generally results from nerve root compression or infiltration, compression fractures, segmental instability, displacement of the dura, or dural invasion. In cancer patients with symptoms and signs of spinal metastases, distinguishing those with vertebral metastases alone from those with SCC is often difficult. No clinical parameters can accurately tell them apart[26]; thus, each patient with symptomatic spinal metastases must be viewed as at risk for SCC.

Although the patient's pain should alert the clinician to the diagnosis, delay in diagnosis frequently results because pain may be nonspecific or referred to other sites. This is especially true in patients who do not have a known history of cancer. By the time of diagnosis, neurologic signs are common[1, 11, 20] and include various degrees of muscle weakness in 76 percent of cases, bladder and bowel dysfunction in more than 50 percent, and sensory symptoms in about 50 percent. Nearly half of severely affected patients develop a complete deficit (no residual spinal cord function) after diagnosis and before undergoing any treatment, and 28 percent of paraparetic patients become paraplegic less than 24 hours before treatment.[27] Therefore SCC must be treated as soon as possible, and early diagnosis is crucial because outcome largely depends on neurologic function before treatment.[11, 20, 27, 28]

Apart from the typical manifestations of the syndrome of SCC, several unusual clinical presentations may be seen. Patients may present with an atypical Brown-Séquard syndrome, with ataxia secondary to posterior column dysfunction, or with herpetic rash along the affected dermatomes.[1, 20, 29]

PATHOPHYSIOLOGY

The pathophysiologic mechanisms involved in neoplastic SCC were investigated in experimental animal tumor models.[30–42] The mechanism of spinal cord injury induced by the expanding extradural tumors is complex and probably multifactorial (Fig. 162–2). The enlarging extradural tumor causes early obstruction of the spinal epidural venous plexus and enhances production of a vasogenic type of edema. The edema involves initially the white matter and eventually the gray matter in the late stage of compression. In the end stage, a rapid decrease in spinal cord blood flow occurs at the site of compression. The ischemia may play the final deleterious role, leading to irreversible loss of function if the compression is not promptly alleviated. Abnormalities in spinal somatosensory evoked responses preceded neurologic signs of myelopathy in an animal model of SCC.[34] The conduction block may be related to myelin destruction that has been demonstrated by an electron microscopic study.[34] The disruption of myelin is probably caused by both mechanical compression and ischemia. Although demyelination can occur at sites of spinal compression,[43, 44] remyelination may take place after transient compression,[45] thereby providing a possible morphologic correlate for recovery of function after prompt surgical decompression.

Local production of substances such as prostaglandins may mediate promotion of vasodilation, plasma exudation, and edema formation. In fact, elevation in prostaglandin E_2 synthesis is demonstrated in the compressed segments concomitantly with the development of spinal cord edema. In keeping with that concept, a rapid antiedema effect is achieved only when partial or marked reduction of prostaglandin E_2 synthesis is accomplished either by steroidal or by nonsteroidal anti-inflammatory drugs (e.g., indomethacin).[35–38] In addition, a marked increase in the utilization of serotonin is present in the compressed cord segments. Inhibition of serotonin receptors results in attenuated vascular permeability and a protracted clinical course toward paraplegia, similar to the favorable effect produced by steroids or nonsteroidal anti-inflammatory agents.[41, 42] Therefore, receptor-activated serotonergic mechanisms may participate in the disruption of the blood–spinal cord barrier in the subacutely developing compression injury.

In the end stage, when conduction block and ischemia are present, cytotoxic edema may also develop. A recent report demonstrated that the noncompetitive glutamate receptor an-

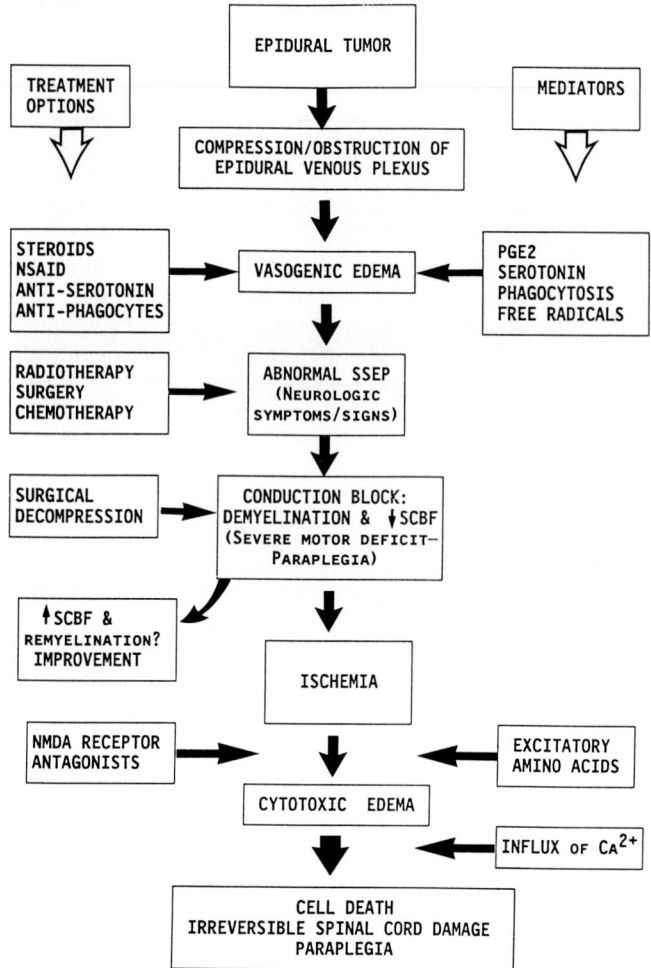

FIGURE 162–2. An algorithm of the recognized mechanisms involved in the pathophysiology of spinal cord compression. Treatment options represent possible pharmacologic interventions that may reduce neural tissue damage. Most of the data related to pharmacologic manipulations are derived from investigation of animal models of neoplastic spinal cord compression. The relationship of the currently used therapeutic modalities in humans (corticosteroids, radiotherapy, surgery, and chemotherapy) to the specific stage of spinal cord injury is demonstrated as well.

tagonists ketamine and MK-801 produce an antiedema effect in SCC, which is not associated with inhibition of prostaglandin synthesis and from reduction of the vascular permeability. These results mean that cytotoxic edema may be present and that excitotoxins (such as glutamate) probably mediate in its evolution.[39, 40]

These experimental findings indicate that early pharmacologic intervention may offer the potential to delay neurologic deterioration and may thus attenuate neuronal damage. However, although such experimental studies may offer new therapeutic approaches in the future, in face of the complexity of the involved pathophysiologic mechanisms, pharmacologic manipulations should first be carefully assessed in animal models before their extrapolation to human clinical studies.

SURVIVAL AND SPINAL CORD COMPRESSION

The magnitude of the clinical problem of spinal epidural metastases is usually evaluated at less than the actual figure. The estimated annual incidence of cancer-induced spinal injury in the United States of America is 8.5 per 100,000.[46] This calculated incidence exceeds the annual rate of traumatic spinal cord injury (three to five per 100,000). However, the socioeconomic impact of neoplastic SCC is much less than that of the traumatic injury because of the relatively high mortality (50 to 70 percent at 1 year) in such patients. In spite of the overall grim prognosis of the disease, treatment is warranted in many cases[1, 11, 47] and is aimed at preserving or restoring ambulation and continence, or at alleviating intractable pain. SCC in itself is not generally fatal, except when it occurs in the upper portion of the cervical spine. The overall survival in SCC is related to the natural history of the systemic malignancy, and only about 30 percent of patients are expected to survive beyond 1 year, and rarely as long as 4 to 9 years.[10, 48]

FACTORS INFLUENCING RECOVERY OF FUNCTION

Some of the following factors have been considered to be important determinants of functional prognosis in patients with SCC and therefore deserve a critical review.

TUMOR BIOLOGY AND CELL TYPE

The biologic activity of the primary neoplasm determines both systemic and local aggressiveness, which are represented, respectively, by the rates of posttreatment survival and therapy success.[27, 49] Patients with myeloma, lymphoma, Ewing's sarcoma, neuroblastoma, or carcinoma of the breast have a favorable prognosis for recovery of function. The outlook for patients with metastatic bronchogenic carcinoma is generally poor. However, exceptions to these results make it difficult to prognosticate in individual cases. In general, high tumor radiosensitivity is significantly related to a favorable prognosis, and the contrary is true for radioresistant tumors.[11, 20, 25, 27]

RESPONSE TO HIGH-DOSE DEXAMETHASONE ADMINISTRATION

The use of steroids in the treatment of SCC is widely accepted.[11, 20, 25, 27, 50-52] The scientific basis for steroid use stems from animal models of SCC, in which reduction of spinal cord edema and delayed onset of paraplegia were observed after treatment with dexamethasone.[30, 31, 33, 36] Greenberg and coworkers[25] recommended the use of high-dose steroids based on their experience of rapid symptom relief in some patients receiving initial doses of 100 mg of dexamethasone. However, they were unable to demonstrate an outcome superior to that of their historic group, who had received lower doses of steroids. In a recent prospective study, patients with SCC were randomly assigned to receive an initial treatment with either high-dose dexamethasone (100 mg) or a conventional dose (10 mg intravenous bolus), followed by 16 mg/day orally.[52] No dose effect was observed on neurologic function or outcome, but the substantial effect on pain noted within 24 hours was similar. Several other investigators observed a dramatic resolution of symptoms after treatment with steroids alone.[50, 53, 54] Such steroid-related improvement was closely related to the type of tumor and probably represented a direct oncolytic effect,[50] as occurs in lymphomas and leukemias. Therefore, the response to steroids has no proven intrinsic prognostic value.

PRETREATMENT NEUROLOGIC STATUS

The outcome of SCC relates to the patient's neurologic status at the time of treatment, and a positive correlation exists between the pretreatment motor status and the functional outcome.[1, 5, 8, 11, 20, 27, 55] Seventy percent of the patients who can walk at the time of diagnosis retain that ability after treatment, 35 percent of those who are initially paraparetic become ambulatory, and only 5 to 7 percent of paraplegic patients regain the ability to walk. These success rates show no significant difference between treatment with radiotherapy alone or unselective laminectomy followed by radiotherapy.[27, 28] The success rate achieved by all therapies in paraplegic patients is different, depending on whether the patient has complete functional cord transection or whether there is preservation of some neurologic function (motor most significant). The fact that only 2 percent of the former patients recovered, compared with 20 percent of the latter, indicates the strong prognostic significance of residual neurologic function. Complete paraplegia carries a bad functional prognosis, regardless of the mode of therapy employed. The value of early diagnosis is clear; therefore, it is discouraging that only 25 percent of patients are diagnosed while still being able to walk.[11, 20, 25, 28, 51]

PROGRESSION RATE OF SYMPTOMS

Some investigators have claimed that rapid onset and progression of neurologic symptoms are associated with a worse prognosis than that of gradual onset and slow progression.[20, 49] However, these results also should be analyzed in relation to completeness of spinal cord damage. If this factor is taken into account, then in rapidly developing symptoms (in less than 24 hours), the neurologic grade itself may have a greater influence on prognosis than the symptom progression rate.[27] Thus, 20 percent of paraparetic patients with a rapidly evolving deficit recovered, compared with none of the paraplegic patients. A recent report emphasized the importance of progression rate of symptoms.[56] In this study, of 15 paraplegic patients who were treated by radiotherapy, five regained ambulation after a delay of 3 months or more. The median time from the initial motor symptoms to total paralysis was longer (45 days) in those who recovered than in the permanently paralyzed patients (9 days).

The rapidity of neurologic deterioration may be related to other prognostic variables, such as tumor biology or topography within the spinal canal. It is therefore unclear whether this factor should be considered as an independent prognostic parameter. However, residual cord function should be taken into account in the rapidly evolving deficit as an important prognostic variable. Once paraplegia has set in, the duration of paralysis does have prognostic significance, although recovery has been reported even after periods of 4 to 8 weeks.[56]

LOCATION OF TUMOR WITHIN THE SPINAL CANAL

Some investigators have claimed that tumor position within the spinal canal carries an intrinsic prognostic significance because a positive correlation exists between tumor location and the response to surgical treatment.[8, 49, 57] Furthermore, some authors stated that vertebral collapse reduced the chances of neurologic recovery.[28, 49] These statements are based on success rates obtained by indiscriminate use of laminectomy performed in patients with ventrally located tumors. After laminectomy, only 9 to 16 percent of these patients maintained ambulation. These figures are considerably lower than the overall rates of 30- to 50-percent ambulation occurring in patients with tumors located posterolaterally.[27, 28, 57]

When the epidural tumor is situated anterior to the spinal cord, the accessibility of the tumor to surgical removal by laminectomy is limited. Accordingly, an alternative approach to the spine by way of an anterolateral route has recently been reported.[51, 55, 58–62] The anterior approach yielded favorable results: 70 to 80 percent of the patients regained or maintained ambulation. In only two studies was the surgical approach for decompression selected prospectively according to tumor topography in the spinal canal.[51, 62] The success rate was 80 percent for the ventrally located tumors when they were decompressed by an anterior approach but was only 39 percent for the posteriorly located tumors decompressed by laminectomy.[51] Although the figure for posterior compartment tumors seems inferior, the results should not be considered discouraging, because only 8 percent of the patients with posterior compression were ambulatory at presentation. We conclude that with proper tailoring of the operative approach, no evidence exists that tumor position within the spinal canal is an important or an independent prognostic factor.

PRINCIPLES OF MANAGEMENT

Although metastases to the spine from systemic cancer represent the commonest spine tumor encountered,[2] the management of this problem continues to be controversial.[11, 27, 28, 47, 63] Controversy stems from the lack of controlled clinical studies directly comparing various treatment modalities and from an absence of standard criteria for evaluation of response. Patients with metastatic SCC have, by definition, tumors that have spread from a primary site and thus are no longer curable by local measures. The therapeutic modalities of surgery and radiotherapy are only palliative, and preservation or restoration of ambulation and bladder control are the criteria of successful therapy. Pain relief is also an important, but secondary, goal. Because the treatment is not curative, it emphasizes the importance of considering also the effect of treatment on the quality of further survival.

The therapeutic modalities currently available for the treatment of patients with epidural SCC are listed in Table 162–1. Figure 162–3 illustrates an algorithm of treatment selection in the various categories of SCC.

Table 162–1. THERAPEUTIC MODALITIES IN SPINAL EPIDURAL METASTASES

Pharmacotherapy
   Specific (antineoplastic)
   Nonspecific (antiedema, analgesia)
Radiation Therapy
   External
   Internal (brachytherapy)
Surgery
   Laminectomy (posterior decompression) ± spinal stabilization
   Vertebral body resection (anterior decompression) + spinal stabilization
   Combined anterior and posterior decompression + spinal stabilization (may be staged as sequential procedures)

PHARMACOTHERAPY

SPECIFIC CHEMOTHERAPY

Epidural metastases arising from primary tumors that show good chemotherapeutic response are likely (but not certain) to respond to chemotherapy, like the rest of the systemic tumor, particularly early in the course of the disease. Unfortunately, this effect has drawn little investigative interest. The response of certain spinal lymphomas to corticosteroid treatment[50] may serve as an example. Because corticosteroids are used in almost all patients as nonspecific chemotherapy, their occasional specific effect may be undistinguishable from the effect of radiotherapy.

The usual policy is not to use specific chemotherapy alone as the primary treatment of patients with SCC because of the uncertainty of its response and the irreversibility of severe spinal cord dysfunction. Whenever possible, specific chemotherapy is combined with other therapeutic modalities. Nevertheless, several reports suggest that good recovery of neurologic function can be obtained by chemotherapy alone in chemosensitive neoplasms, such as lymphoma, myeloma, or neuroblastoma.[64] However, published experience with such a therapeutic approach is still limited to a few patients per report, and not even one large scale study is available.

NONSPECIFIC PHARMACOTHERAPY

CORTICOSTEROIDS. In humans, glucocorticoids rarely, if ever, produce the dramatic relief of neurologic disability derived from SCC that they produce in brain metastases. When high doses of corticosteroids are used in the treatment of SCC, most patients experience dramatic relief of pain.[25, 52] Some experience an arrest of progressively deteriorating neurologic function, and a few actually improve from the use of corticosteroids alone. Many clinicians use high doses of steroids in SCC, although no clear-cut advantage over conventional doses has been demonstrated.[25, 52] Therefore, the associated side effects that can arise with the use of corticosteroids should be kept in proper perspective.

The incidence of serious steroid-related complications in neuro-oncology patients has been the subject of recent studies.[65, 66] Fifty-one percent of the patients developed at least one steroid-related toxicity, and 19 percent required hospital admission. Both the duration of steroid therapy and the total dose predicted toxicity. A significant increase in severe complications, including fatal sepsis, was noted when dexamethasone was used for more than 40 days to treat SCC.[67] In addition, intestinal perforation occurred as frequently as gastrointestinal bleeding, and significantly more rectosigmoid perforation occurred in neurologic (nononcologic) patients manifesting steroid toxicity.[65] Patients with SCC present fewer signs and symptoms of peritonitis than non–steroid treated patients with intestinal perforation. Because major complications occur in patients who receive steroids for more than 1 month, they must be used judi-

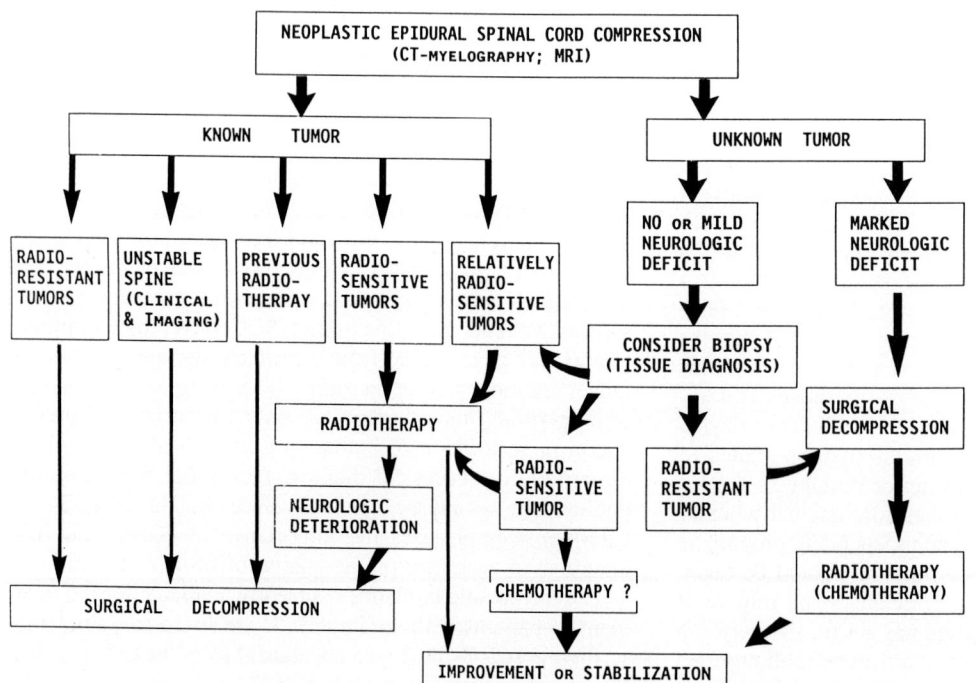

FIGURE 162–3. An algorithm for evaluation and selection of the preferred therapeutic approach in patients with neoplastic spinal cord compression.

ciously, and their use should be discontinued as rapidly as possible or tapered down to the lowest possible level that is compatible with clinical benefit.

ANALGESIA. Because pain is the presenting symptom in over 95 percent of patients with epidural SCC,[11, 20, 25] the principles of good analgesic management must be applied. In most patients, treatment with either radiotherapy alone or resection of tumor and restoration of stability frequently results in pain relief.[1, 16] Exceptionally, in patients with intractable pain either from plexus or nerve root invasion, neurosurgical procedures directed at pain control (e.g., cordotomy, rhizotomy) may be considered mainly for patients with limited life expectancy.[68]

RADIATION THERAPY

EXTERNAL BEAM IRRADIATION

Table 162-2 summarizes the results of radiation therapy in patients suffering from various metastatic tumors. Between 35 and 50 percent of patients so treated either regain or maintain ambulation at the end of therapy, and of those who survive 1 year, 50 percent maintain that improvement.[20, 25] Studies that have addressed the question of pain relief indicate that more than half of patients with pain have pain relief by radiation therapy alone.[1, 16] The efficacy of radiation therapy depends on the radiosensitivity of the tumor, on the patient's neurologic status at the time radiation therapy is undertaken, and on maintenance of spinal stability. Patients with highly radiosensitive tumors (such as lymphoma, Ewing's sarcoma, neuroblastoma, seminoma, and myeloma) are far more likely to regain or maintain ambulation than those with less radiosensitive tumors (60 to 80 percent versus 40 percent).[16, 20, 27, 51, 54, 64] Even in patients harboring a radiosensitive neoplasm, improvement from radiotherapy begins a few days after initiation of therapy. This result is cause for concern because 28 percent of severely paraparetic patients are expected to become paraplegic within 24 hours.[27] Thus, radiotherapy is most clearly indicated for radiosensitive tumors, but it is also the primary therapy for moderately radiosensitive neoplasms, such as breast carcinoma. In the latter, the need for surgical intervention should be critically reviewed for each patient. We have no doubt that in stable patients who are ambulatory or paraparetic on presentation, radiotherapy should be tried first. However, in severely paraparetic patients, surgical decompression should be considered because radiotherapy may cause an irreversible delay in the reduction of spinal cord damage. If surgery is contraindicated, such as in patients with a poor general medical status, patients with multiple compression levels, and those with longstanding paraplegia, radiotherapy alone should be employed.

The indication for radiotherapy is less clear for tumors generally regarded as radioresistant; even in these, however, radiotherapy should be tried as a primary modality if the patient's neurologic deficit is not severe and if the rate of progression of the deficit is such that there would be time to resort to surgical decompression should radiotherapy fail. In situations in which surgery is the primary therapy, postoperative radiation should generally be employed in the hope that it may help suppress residual tumor and contribute to pain relief.

No controlled studies have compared various dose and fractionation schedules of radiation therapy, but if the studies reported in the literature are compared (Table 162-2), neither the dose nor the fractionation schedule appears to have a major effect on outcome.

BRACHYTHERAPY

The major theoretical advantage of brachytherapy is that high doses of radiation can be delivered to the tumor without endangering the surrounding normal structures. The major disadvantages are the difficulties in treating a large tumor volume and the fact that an operation is required to place the radioactive seeds or the afterloading catheters for internal radiation. The published experience of brachytherapy in SCC is very limited, and it appears to have its most practical advantage in the treatment of paravertebral tumors that cannot totally be removed by surgical resection. Brachytherapy may also be considered in relapse of SCC previously treated by radiation therapy, when surgical decompression is recommended. In patients so treated, although the numbers are small, the results appear comparable with, but no better than, the results of treatment by surgical decompression alone.[69]

SURGERY

The oldest approach to the treatment of neoplastic SCC has been decompressive laminectomy, with or without postoperative radiation therapy. As Table 162-3 indicates, ambulation is maintained or regained in between 35 to 50 percent of the patients, a result similar to that achieved by radiation therapy (Table 162-2). Several studies indicate that pain is improved in 50 to 70 percent of patients after laminectomy, results similar to those of radiation therapy. Pa-

Table 162-2. RESULTS OF TREATMENT FOR SPINAL CORD COMPRESSION: RADIOTHERAPY ALONE

Authors	Year	Patients (n)	(%) Improved*	(%) Worse
Brady and colleagues[76]	1975	19	47	—
Mones and colleagues[77]	1966	41	41	—
Khan and colleagues[78]	1967	82	42	—
Cobb and colleagues[13]	1977	18	50	22
Gilbert and colleagues[20]	1977	130	49	—
Marshall and Langfitt[54]	1977	29	41	—
Greenberg and colleagues[25]	1980	83	57	7
Stark and colleagues[79]	1982	31	35	—
Constans and colleagues[8]	1983	108	39	26
Obbens and colleagues[80]	1984	83	28	23
Harrison and colleagues[81]	1985	33	27	36
Bach and colleagues[10]	1990	149	35	18
Mean		—	41	22
Total		806	—	—

*Improvement was judged by criteria of motor function.

Table 162–3. RESULTS OF TREATMENT FOR SPINAL CORD COMPRESSION: LAMINECTOMY AND RADIOTHERAPY

Authors	Year	Patients (n)	(%) Improved*	(%) Worse	Operative Mortality (%)
Hall and MacKay[57]	1973	129	30	—	—
Brady and colleagues[76]	1975	90	61	—	—
Merrin and colleagues[100]	1976	22	22	0	0
Cobb and colleagues[13]	1977	26	46	23	—
Gilbert and colleagues[20]	1977	65	45	—	—
Marshall and Langfitt[54]	1977	17	29	—	—
Gianotta and Kindt[101]	1978	33	30	18	12
Kleinman and colleagues[82]	1978	20	15	5	15
Livingston and Perrin[83]	1978	100	58	—	0
Baldini and colleagues[84]	1979	140	30	19	0
Gorter[102]	1979	31	39	—	13
Dunn and colleagues[85]	1980	104	33	23	10
Levy and colleagues[86]	1982	39	82	15	8
Stark and colleagues[79]	1982	84	37	—	—
Constans and colleagues[8]	1983	465	46	13	—
Klein and colleagues[87]	1984	194	54	16	—
Kollmann and colleagues[88]	1984	103	56	—	—
Garcia-Picazo and colleagues[89]	1990	53	41	—	—
Bach and colleagues[10]	1990	91	59	11	—
Landmann and colleagues[9]	1992	127	58	2	—
Mean		—	44	13	7
Total		1933	—	—	—

*Improvement was judged by criteria of motor function.

tients treated by radiotherapy can deteriorate neurologically in the same way as surgical patients (Tables 162–2 and 162–3), but they are spared the other adverse effects of surgery, namely operative morbidity and mortality. Approximately 25 percent of patients ambulatory on presentation deteriorate neurologically, and of those paraparetic before surgery, about 20 percent get worse. It is therefore not surprising that current oncology texts favor initial management with radiotherapy in all patients and relegate surgery to a purely salvage or diagnostic role. However, the fact that the only surgical procedure used as a basis for comparison was laminectomy is generally ignored. This midline posterior approach is technically easy and safe and allows for tissue diagnosis but provides adequate decompression only when the tumor mass lies dorsolateral to the dura. Laminectomy also destabilizes the spine if the vertebral body and the pedicles are destroyed by tumor and allows very little access to tumor lying ventral to the cord. Thus, the important reasons for surgical failures in the past can be summarized as follows: (1) nonselective use of one single surgical approach, (2) inadequate tumor resection, (3) ineffective stabilization, and (4) poor patient selection.

INDICATIONS FOR SURGICAL INTERVENTION

Some trends have emerged regarding surgical indications. Figure 162–3 specifies the circumstances in which surgery should be considered, and although some of them are clear-cut, others still need further evaluation.

DIAGNOSIS IN DOUBT. In 8 percent of patients with neoplastic SCC, spinal involvement is the initial presentation of cancer.[11, 20] When the etiology of the spinal lesion is in doubt, surgical decompression is considered to establish a tissue diagnosis and to achieve rapid decompression. With current radiologic evaluation, the need for a major procedure to document a diagnosis of malignancy should be rare. If no primary site or a more accessible location is evident, the diagnosis of malignancy can frequently be established by needle biopsy,[70] especially if a paraspinal soft tissue mass is present. However, if the neurologic status is unstable, with rapidly evolving signs, surgical decompression is advisable to achieve a prompt diagnosis and to initiate treatment without delay.

SPINAL INSTABILITY OR BONE COMPRESSION. A major goal of operation is the restoration or maintenance of stability of the spine. The determination of spinal instability is of paramount importance in choosing the appropriate form of management for patients with metastatic disease of the spine. Unfortunately, no validated system exists for making this determination.

CRITERIA FOR SPINAL STABILITY IN NEOPLASTIC DISEASE. In trauma, the accepted biomechanical model for thoracolumbar fractures is the three-column concept of the spine (Fig. 162–4).[71] The anterior column consists of the anterior half of the vertebral body, the anterior longitudinal ligament, and the anterior annulus fibrosus; the middle column includes the posterior longitudinal ligament, the posterior half of the vertebral body, and the posterior annulus; and the posterior column consists of the neural arch (laminae and pedicles) facets, the ligamentum flavum, and the supraspinous and interspinous ligaments. The spine is considered unstable if two of the three columns are disrupted. Spinal fractures are classified according to the mechanism of injury and involvement of the columns. In neoplastic destruction of the spine, these concepts may not always be applicable, because trauma and tumors are quite different conditions in terms of the disruption of bone, disc, and ligament; the qual-

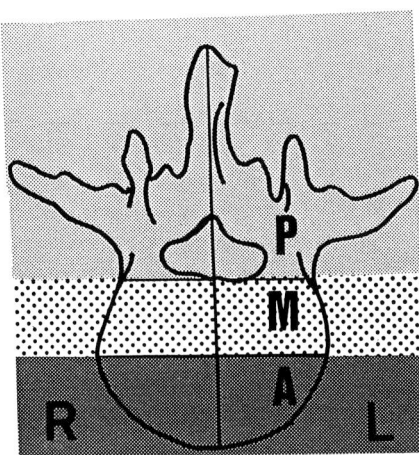

FIGURE 162–4. Classification systems for the evaluation of spinal stability. The three-column system of Denis has been devised for assessment of spinal cord stability in trauma and divides the spine into the anterior (A), middle (M), and posterior (P) columns. The spine is considered unstable if two of the three columns are disrupted.
The six-column system of Kostuik and Errico is devised for the evaluation of stability in spine tumors. The three columns, as defined by Denis, are subdivided into left (L) and right (R) halves. The spine is unstable if three to four of the columns are destroyed.

sis and extrusion of bone, tumor, or disc into the spinal canal with neural compromise. Tumor involvement of the middle and posterior column may produce forward shearing deformity. In addition, segmental instability is assumed to be present when the clinical syndrome is characterized by pain aggravated by movement (in the absence of significant neural encroachment) that is associated with progressive collapse of vertebral bodies or localized kyphosis on imaging studies.

A systematic approach to determine the clinical instability of the spine should include anatomic, biomechanical, clinical, and therapeutic considerations.[73, 74] Apart from the neuroimaging studies that define anatomic details used in the three-column spinal model (Fig. 162–4), the concept of clinical instability should be taken into account. Clinical instability is defined as "loss of the ability of the spine under physiologic loads to maintain relationships between vertebrae in such a way that there is either damage or subsequent irritation to the spinal cord or nerve roots, and in addition there is development of incapacitating deformity or pain due to structural changes."[74] Thus, symptoms and signs should direct therapeutic consideration. Patients with fracture-dislocation, localized kyphosis, collapsed vertebra with retropulsion of a bone fragment, or segmental instability may require operative decompression and stabilization if either pain or neurologic symptomatology are present. Not every case defined by the criteria for unstable spine requires surgical intervention. If the tumor is relatively radiosensitive, a course of radiotherapy may result in satisfactory axial settling and pain relief over a period of weeks or months. These patients should be carefully followed up because they are potentially unstable. Surgery is reserved only for symptomatic cases because preventive surgery is probably unjustified in the management of metastatic disease of the spine.

When the anterior and middle columns are destroyed by tumor, treatment considerations should include decompression by the anterior approach to the spine as well as restoration of stability by vertebral body replacement constructs. If the posterior column structures are involved, then the treatment plan is to replace or substitute for the support role of these structures by posterior decompression (laminectomies) combined with posterior instrumentation for maintenance of stability. Tables 162–4 and 162–5 summarize the results of

ity of surrounding bone stock; and the ability of the spine to heal.

Kostuik and Errico[72] created a set of criteria specifically for spine tumors that still needs to be validated. In their system, the spine is divided into six columns: the three columns as defined by Denis[71] subdivided into left and right halves (Fig. 162–4). The spine is considered to be stable if fewer than three of the six columns are destroyed, is unstable if three to four of the columns are destroyed, and is markedly unstable if five to six of the columns are involved. Angulation of 20 degrees or more adds to the consideration of instability.

Instability does not usually occur when involvement is limited to the vertebral spongy bone core or to the anterior column. When the posterior half (middle column) of the vertebral body is also involved (cortical bone included), pathologic compression fracture can occur, producing kypho-

Table 162–4. RESULTS OF TREATMENT FOR SPINAL CORD COMPRESSION: LAMINECTOMY (POSTERIOR DECOMPRESSION) AND STABILIZATION*

Authors	Year	Patients (n)	(%) Improved†	Improved Pain (%)	(%) Morbidity	Operative Mortality (%)
Brunon and colleagues[90]	1975	20	—	100	—	—
Hansebout and Blomquist[91]	1980	82	84 amb	100	1	—
Miles and colleagues[92]	1984	23	65	100	—	—
DeWald and colleagues[93]	1985	17	45	65	12	6
Overby and Rothman[94]	1985	12	75	—	—	—
Solini and colleagues[95]	1985	33	73	—	3	3
Heller and colleagues[96]	1986	33	70	79	21	—
Sherman and Waddell[97]	1986	23	92 amb	55	13	—
Perrin and McBroom[98]	1987	200	65 amb	80	4	8
Mean		—	66	83	9	6
Total		443	—	—	—	—

amb = ambulatory.
*Before or after radiotherapy.
†Improvement was judged by criteria of motor function.

Table 162-5. RESULTS OF TREATMENT FOR SPINAL CORD COMPRESSION: VERTEBRAL BODY RESECTION (ANTERIOR APPROACH) AND STABILIZATION*

Authors	Year	Patients (n)	(%) Improved†	Improved Pain (%)	(%) Morbidity	Operative Mortality (%)
Slatkin and Posner[69]	1982	29	56	60	41 (6)	7
Harrington[58]	1984	52	55	77	8 (2)	4
Siegal and Siegal[51]	1985	61	80 amb	91	11 (2)	6
Sundaresan and colleagues[55]	1985	101	80 amb	80	10 (1)	6
Fidler[99]	1986	18	93	94	—	6
Ominus and colleagues[59]	1986	36	72	97	—	6
Perrin and McBroom[98]	1987	21	76	90	—	5
Mean		—	73	84	18 (3)	6
Total		318	—	—	—	—

amb = ambulatory.
*Before or after radiotherapy.
†Improvement was judged by criteria of motor function.

surgical treatment in which decompression is combined with spinal stabilization. The criteria for patients' selection varied, as did the methods of stabilization. Current recommendations for selection of patients and optimal methods of decompression and stabilization are undergoing constant development. The criteria of spinal instability that should bring about consideration for spinal stabilization are summarized in Table 162-6.

PREVIOUS RADIATION EXPOSURE. When radiotherapy cannot be used, surgical decompression is indicated as the primary therapeutic modality, even in highly radiosensitive tumors, because of the risk of exceeding spinal cord tolerance by adding further irradiation. Surgery is warranted for relapse occurring months or even years after a successful previous treatment in hopes of preserving neurologic function.

RADIORESISTANT TUMORS. In radioresistant tumors, decompressive surgery might be considered as the primary mode of therapy. Postoperative radiotherapy is administered with the hope of retarding tumor regrowth. However, this indication is not generally accepted, and sometimes, especially in neurologically stable patients, radiotherapy may be tried first.

NEUROLOGIC DETERIORATION DURING RADIOTHERAPY. Neurologic deterioration that occurs during radiotherapy of a relatively radiosensitive tumor should prompt early consideration for surgical decompression. The decline in neurologic function may reflect radioresistancy, progressive spinal instability, or bone compression secondary to vertebral collapse, all of which may be most effectively treated by spinal decompression and stabilization.

There has been concern that radiation therapy may result in neurologic deterioration, presumably by inducing radiation edema in the tumor, spinal cord, or both. So far, experimental studies do not support this concept;[47] therefore, deterioration represents treatment failure, prompting consideration of surgery as the alternative treatment.

SELECTION OF SURGICAL APPROACH

The goal of surgery is optimal removal of the compressing epidural mass and restoration and maintenance of spinal stability. Therefore, the selection of the surgical approach should be determined by variables such as the location of the tumor inside and outside the spinal canal, the main cause of instability, and feasible options for stabilization. Table 162-7 details the preoperative assessment required for determination of surgical approach. Most authors agree that the location of epidural compression should dictate the approach for decompression. Based on tumor location, McLain and Weinstein[75] classified primary spinal tumors according to zones of involvement and used this information to determine the optimal surgical approach (Fig. 162-5). These guidelines are also applicable to metastatic spine lesions. Zone 1 includes the spinous process to the pars interarticularis and inferior facets and is best approached posteriorly. Lesions that involve the superior articular facets, transverse process, and pedicle are classified as zone 2 and may be resected via a posterior or posterolateral approach. Zone 3 tumors are located in the anterior three quarters of the vertebral body and are best approached anteriorly. Zone 4 is the most inaccessible region of the spine—the posterior fourth of the body, and a combined anterior and posterior approach is recommended for these lesions. However, in patients with metastatic spine disease and limited life expectancy, radical excision of the vertebral tumor is not always the main goal; therefore, selection of surgical approach requires further consideration in addition to the zone of vertebral involvement. In patients with progressive kyphosis without anterior cord compression or in patients with thoracic or lumbar pathologic fracture or

Table 162-6. CATEGORIES OF SPINAL INSTABILITY IN METASTATIC DISEASE THAT REQUIRE CONSIDERATION FOR SPINAL STABILIZATION*

Anterior + middle column involvement or >50% collapse of vertebral body height
Middle + posterior column involvement or shearing deformity
Three-column involvement
Involvement of same column in two or more adjacent vertebrae
Iatrogenic
  Laminectomy in face of anterior and/or middle column disease
  Resection of >50% of cut surface of the vertebral body

*Definition of potential instability relies on imaging studies and is valid only if the vertebral cortical shell is involved.

Table 162–7. PREOPERATIVE ASSESSMENT OF TUMOR LOCATION AND EXTENT OF PATHOLOGY IN NEOPLASTIC INVOLVEMENT OF THE SPINE

Bone involvement (CT, MRI)
   Vertebral body and pedicles, posterior elements, or a combination of both
   Number of vertebrae involved
   Percentage of bone mass loss of the vertebral cut surface
Epidural mass (CT myelography, MRI)
   Epidural mass related or unrelated to the bone lesion
   Number of spinal levels involved
   Position of the epidural mass: anterior, lateral, posterior, and/or encircling
Spinal stability (spinal radiography + CT and/or MRI)
   Involvement of two or more adjacent vertebrae
   Involvement of two or more spinal columns as well as the vertebral cortical shell
   Loss of more than 50% of the vertebral width
   Shearing deformity
   Any combination of the above
Retroperitoneal and/or paravertebral mass (CT, MRI)
   Location
   Extent
   Involvement of adjacent structures or organs (kidneys, uterus, large vessels)
   Involvement of posterior chest or abdominal wall

CT = computed tomography; MRI = magnetic resonance imaging.

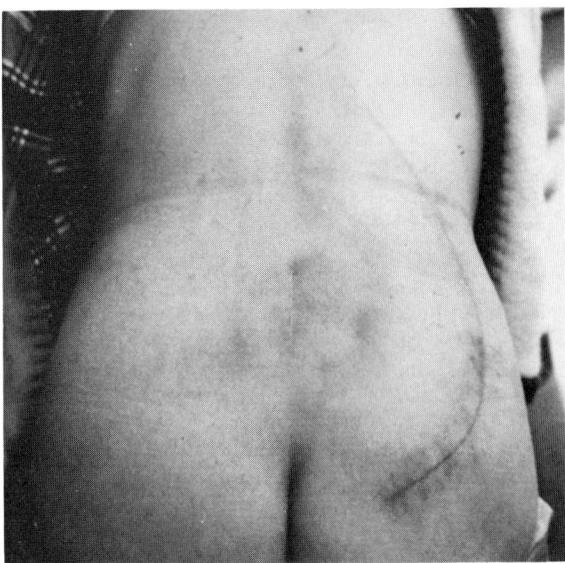

FIGURE 162–6. Planning the skin incisions. The incision is placed in healthy nonirradiated tissues. The midline irradiated area, which can be recognized by the skin discoloration or by loss of subcutaneous fat or both, is circumvented by a laterally placed incision, creating a large flap.

dislocation without significant soft tissue or bony neural compromise, posterior realignment and stabilization may relieve most cord impingement. In patients in whom the anterior approach is not feasible for technical reasons, poor medical status, or widespread disease, partial decompression (via a posterior approach) and stabilization may be a useful palliative procedure.[103]

OPERATIVE TECHNIQUE

The anterior and posterior surgical approaches to the spine at every level have been covered in depth in other chapters of this book. To avoid redundancy, the technical notes herein are restricted to issues specific to malignancies in the spinal column.

Posterior Decompression and Instrumentation

Laminectomy for decompression of the posterior aspect of the spinal canal is indicated when the compressive tumor is in a posterior or posterolateral location. It can also be required as a second-stage procedure at the end of an anterior decompression in patients with residual tumor left beyond the equator of the dura.

The intubated patient is placed face down on a spinal frame to prevent increased intra-abdominal pressure and to lessen epidural bleeding during surgery. If a frame is not available, the patient is placed on rolls, leaving the abdomen and lower chest free for breathing movements. The head is positioned on a horseshoe headrest, which allows free access to the connections of the anesthesia apparatus. After the field is prepared, draping of the back is wide to allow for large skin flaps and possible lengthening of the incision.

Skin incisions through radiation portals must be avoided at all costs. Some of these surgical wounds can dehisce, and some take many months to heal, being further complicated by chronic discharge. Therefore, the area of intended decompression is reached through an incision placed laterally in healthy tissue, circumventing the irradiated area (Fig. 162–6). Thus, a generous skin flap is created to be elevated and retracted. The extent of the lateral placement of the incision is dictated by the width of the radiation portal, which can usually be determined by discoloration of the skin, or in inveterate cases, by the loss of the subcutaneous fat. The incision is usually placed 8 to 10 cm lateral and parallel to the midline, long enough to allow exposure of four to five spinal segments above and below the planned area of decompression, in anticipation of the use of spinal instrumen-

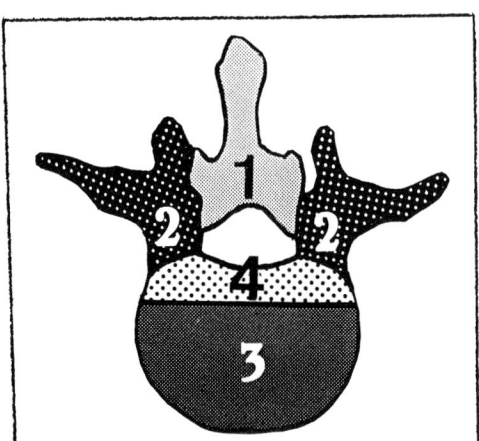

FIGURE 162–5. Classification system of McLain and Weinstein suggested for determination of the optimal surgical approach for resection of spinal tumors. The spine is divided into four zones of possible tumor involvement. Zone 1 is best approached posteriorly. Zone 2 tumors may be resected via a posterior or posterolateral approach. Zone 3 tumors are best approached anteriorly. Zone 4 is the most inaccessible region for which a combined anterior and posterior approach may be recommended.

tation (Fig. 162–6). The incision is carried down to the fascial plane, and the full-thickness flap is elevated toward the midline to reach the spinous processes and 5 cm beyond. Moderate and careful traction on the flap is applied by sutures in the subcutaneous tissue with hemostats on their ends. Wet gauze protects the upturned flap.

The fibrous caps of the spinous processes are split in the midline with diathermy, and subperiosteal dissection of the paravertebral soft tissues is carried out. Possible involvement of the posterior arch elements with tumor dictates caution. Tissues even mildly resistant to dissection are released by cautery. In most cases, involvement of a posterior arch indicates the level in need of decompression. However, detecting tumor deposits at other levels that may have been designated for anchorage of the stabilizing instrumentation is not unusual. This situation necessitates exposure of additional segments to ensure firm ground for placement of implants.

Identification of the spinal levels by an intraoperative x-ray study is mandatory to determine the extent of the laminectomy. For exact reference, the x-ray study must include an anatomic landmark (e.g., cervicothoracic, thoracolumbar, or lumbosacral junction) that is close to the area of the intended decompression. A towel clip is attached to the base of a spinous process close to its superior margin in that area. If so placed, the location of the tongs of the towel clip on the posteroanterior x-ray study corresponds to the midportion of the vertebral body at the same level. The x-ray study is compared to the preoperative study of the same region, and the spinous process is nicked for further reference.

Laminectomy is begun one level distal to the caudal margin of the compressing mass, and decompression is continued cephalad. Only after the proximal and distal tumor borders have been exposed is tumor removal considered. Because neurologic deterioration as a direct result of laminectomy in cancer patients is common (Table 162–3), every effort must be made to minimize possible iatrogenic insult. Magnifying loupes or an operating microscope may be needed in some cases.

The neoplasm is most conveniently approached from its distal margin. In the area adjacent to the tumor, the epidural fat is split in the midline to reach the normal dura underneath. The split is advanced until the tumor margin is encountered. A dissection plane is sought by gentle elevation of the tumor edge from the dura. Some tumors present no problem at removal because they are flexible, friable, or easily detachable. Other tumors are of firm consistency; elevating one end may cause the other to impinge on the dura, requiring piecemeal removal with sharp instruments. The tumors that adhere tenaciously to the dura (e.g., osteoblastoma, lung carcinoma) deserve special notice. They are also excised piecemeal, but here the surgeon must accept neoplastic residua on the dural surface. Caution must be exercised not to violate the dura when the tumor is scraped off its surface. The malignant remnants are treated by postoperative irradiation only if spinal cord tolerance is not exceeded.

In many cases, the tumor encircles the dura. In these cases, the tumor is elevated off the dura and then incised in the midline from its undersurface up either by sharp incision or by bipolar diathermy. This process is continued until the cut margin of the tumor can be grasped. It then can be gently peeled laterally. The segmental nerves are sought, and, if possible, the tumor is peeled off them as well. In the lateral compartment, the overlying tumor is removed with sharp instruments, preferably sharp curettes of appropriate size. These cut the tumor against the local bone elements and thus allow evacuation without pulling on the dura or the tumor itself.

The dura matter is usually an effective barrier to tumor penetration. The segmental nerves are protected by the dural sleeves to their point of exit at the intervertebral foramen. Distally, however, tumor invasion of the nerves may and does occur. This phenomenon is one of the causes of the intractable pain often encountered in these unfortunate patients. A thoracic segmental nerve involved with tumor is ligated and severed. In the lumbar or cervical regions, gentle peeling of the tumor off the nerves is attempted to preserve motor function.

Intraoperative bleeding can be very significant and is controlled by application of either absorbable gelatin foam (Gelfoam) or Surgicel with gentle pressure on the bleeding surface. Vascular feeders of the tumor mass are difficult to control from the posterior aspect of the spine. The tumor vessel walls may be devoid of contractile components and may thus lack the ability to contract. The continuous gentle pressure is to encourage coagulation. Excess blood should be removed only by suction; rubbing an oozing tumor surface removes the already formed clots.

When removal of the tumor is complete or optimal for the specific case, the bare dura and roots are routinely covered with free fat grafts harvested from the available subcutaneous tissue at the incision site. The fat grafts are fixed to soft tissues with a few sutures to prevent displacement.

Evaluation of residual spine stability is performed at this stage. A sound policy is to aim for a firmly stable spine. When decompression may have led to an unstable spine, the surgeon should proceed with spine stabilization. A stable spine maximizes neurologic function and saves the patient the severe intractable pain of instability. The surgeon can choose any of the major double-rod posterior instrumentation systems in current use (e.g., Cotrel-Dubousset, Texas-Scottish-Rite-Hospital, or Isola). We prefer to use the Isola double-rod system supplemented by segmental sublaminar wiring because it satisfies the main requirements for reestablishing spinal stability: distraction, reconstitution of sagittal contour, and excellent fixation. The gradual distraction obtained by the Isola instrumentation causes optimal tension in the spinal and paraspinal soft tissues (ligaments, joint capsules, muscles), thereby reducing the slack that accompanies vertebral compression. It can also correct local deformity (kyphosis), restore lost vertebral height, and lessen compression at the level of the intervertebral foramina. When Isola instrumentation is coupled with sublaminar wiring, which fixes the spine segmentally to the parallel rods, it results in a firm and solid internal fixation system with instant spinal stability (Figs. 162–7 to 162–9). No external appliances, such as braces or jackets, are required.

The technique entails placement of a closed Isola hook in the thoracic apophyseal joint under the inferior facet on both sides of the fourth vertebra above the laminectomy area. On the transverse process of the same vertebra, another hook is placed that faces distally. Approximating and closing these two hooks on the Isola rod causes an excellent hold on the vertebra, usually referred to as a claw arrangement (Fig. 162–8). This hold may be enhanced by adding another upgoing

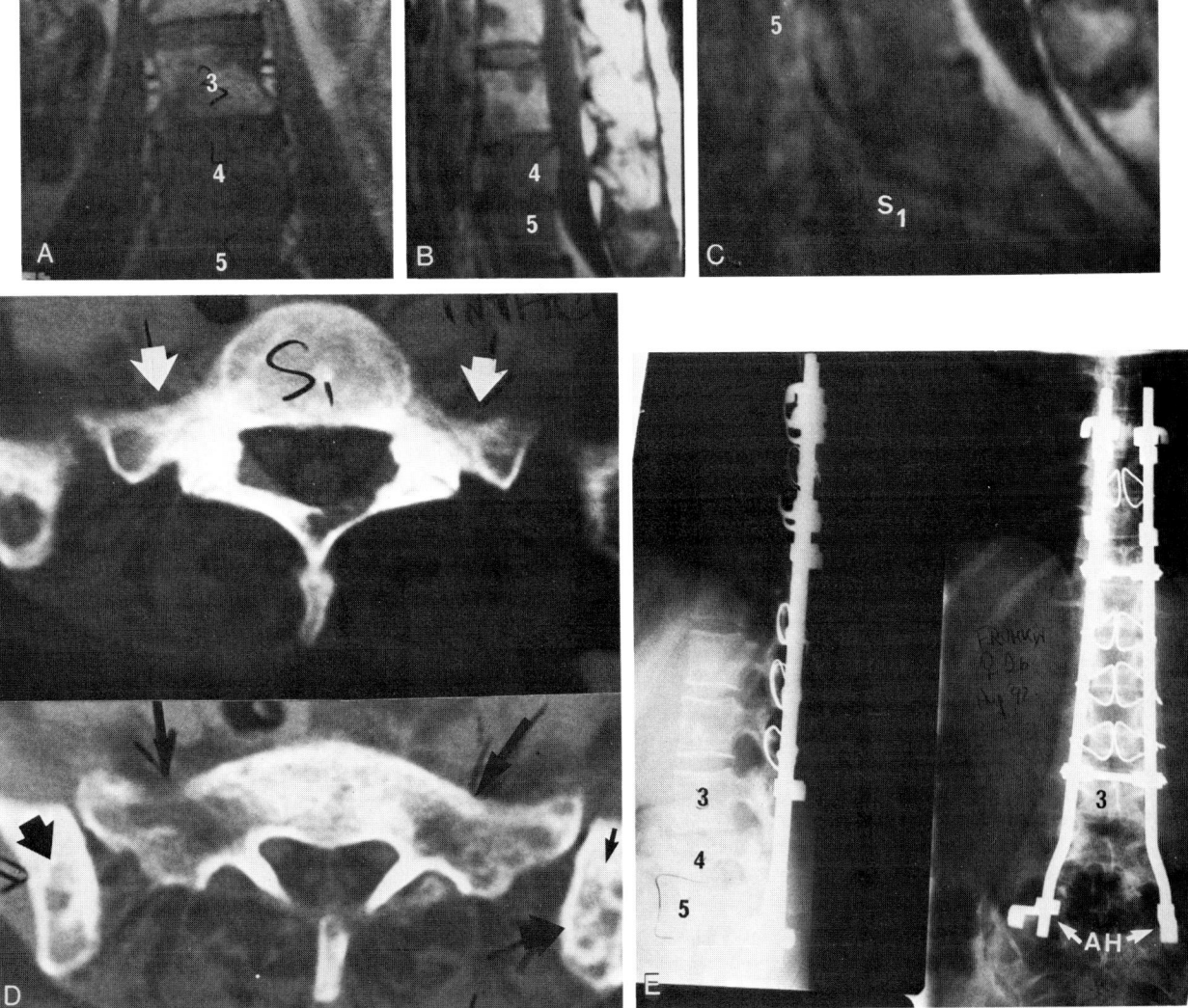

FIGURE 162–7. Posterior instrumentation for spine stabilization and avoidance of pathologic compression fractures of affected vertebral bodies. (A and B) Widespread spine involvement in a 31-year-old teacher with breast carcinoma without neurologic deficit but with severe back pains. (C and D) Involvement of the sacrum precluded use of transpedicular screws. The CT scan shows that the upper alar bone was intact (white arrows point to the intact superior alar cortex, while the black arrows show that both the sacrum and the posterior iliac bones were riddled with tumor). (E) Therefore, for the distal foundation of the instrumentation, the Isola sacral alar hooks (AH) were used and adequate stabilization was attained using the double-rod Isola system combined with segmental sublaminar wire fixation. This rendered the patient's spine painless and she went back to teaching.

hook one or two levels below. Placement of the caudal hooks is more elaborate: the lamina designed as the seat of the distal claw is prepared by removal of the coronal edge of the vertebra with its ligamentum flavum and the distal flavum.

These details are important: the lumbar lamina has an inclination that brings the proximal rim of the lamina in close contact with the dura, while its distal edge is at some distance. Taking off some of the proximal lamina allows space

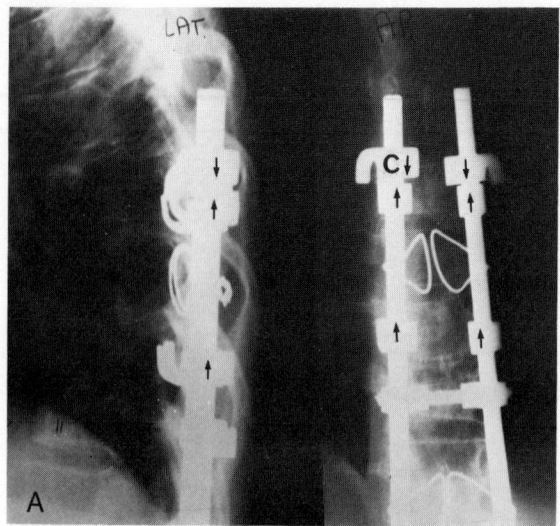
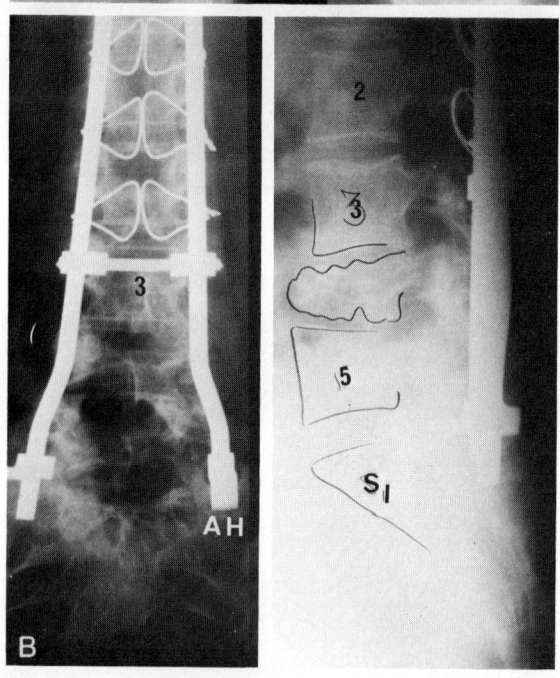

FIGURE 162–8. Foundations for posterior spine–stabilizing instrumentation. (A) Claw arrangement of hooks in the thoracic area for the proximal foundation of the instrumentation. The upper hook pointing distally is riding on the transverse process, while the immediately adjacent hook is insinuated into the joint facet and points rostrally. When they are brought close together on the rod and their set screws tightened, a stable grasp on that spinal level is obtained. Further support can be added by placing yet another up-pointing hook into a facet joint two levels distally (c - claw; the arrows show the direction of the hook blades, which, when brought together, embrace posterior vertebral elements in a firm claw). (B) Detail of the distal foundation showing the Isola sacral alar hooks (AH) in place.

for the seat of the hook without causing a localized iatrogenic stenosis. The inclination of the lumbar lamina must be taken into account when the claw hooks are placed. An upgoing short blade hook is fitted on the distal laminar margin, and a longer blade hook, facing distally on the proximal edge. The Isola rod in this area is given a bend to conform with the natural lordosis (Fig. 162–9); otherwise, the patient is left with a flat lumbar spine and a forward-bent uncomfortable gait. In the upper spine, the Isola rods are bent to accommodate the thoracic kyphosis.

For surgeons versed in transpedicular screw fixation, an excellent distal foundation for the Isola rods can be obtained by Steffee transpedicular screws, which are then bound to the Isola rods by special slotted connectors. We prefer to use this method to get a solid purchase on the distal instrumented spinal segments (Fig. 162–10).

Laminae between the proximal and distal claws that are free of hooks are used for sublaminar wiring. Passing of the sublaminar wires bilaterally is preceded by incision of the ligamenta flava above and below the lamina. If spinous processes are in the way, their overhang is osteotomized. Isola stainless steel sublaminar wires are gently bent so that the hairpin end can be passed under the lamina. It is usually introduced under the caudal edge of the lamina and surfaces cephalad. As it is pulled out, the wire ends are crossed on the lamina to prevent the wire from wandering and pushing against the dura during further instrumentation endeavors.

When the sublaminar wires have been passed above and below the laminectomy site, the distance between the upper and lower hooks is measured. Two Isola rods 3 cm longer than the measured distance are contoured to fit the sagittal alignment of the operated spine and positioned in the hooks. The hooks of the distal claw are approximated on the rod and fixed by firm closure of the set screws. When transpedicular screws are used, the slotted connectors are applied to the screws, and the Isola rods, which are located within, are firmly fixed by closure of the set screws. The upper claw hooks are moved up on the rods until optimal tension is reached for both rods. They are then fixed by firm closure of their screws. The wires are then fixed by crossing the ends forcefully across the rod and are then tightened by a wire twister. Excess twisting is avoided to prevent wire breakage. The wire ends are cut, and the braids are bent toward the rod shaft to avoid future discomfort.

Rigidity of the internal instrumentation is greatly enhanced by the use of two transverse connectors, which are applied close to the claw sites (see Fig. 162–7). The system is highly reliable, and patients may walk the very next day.

Bone Grafting

Before wound closure, the advisability of bone grafting to achieve bony arthrodesis must be considered. This practice is controversial. Orthopedic surgeons have traditionally regarded bone grafting as an integral part of spine fusion with internal fixation because experience has shown that single or even double Harrington rodding can end in rod breakage if solid bone arthrodesis has not been obtained, especially in young, active people. However, most patients with primary or metastatic spinal deposits are not young, and with the advent of segmental instrumentation, rod breakage is a rare occurrence. In many cases, activity is restricted by neurologic deficit, pain, or a less-than-optimal medical status. It is therefore reasonable to assume that in these conditions, modern spinal instrumentation alone will provide satisfactory and durable stability.

When the addition of bone grafts is considered, time must also be taken into account. If bone autografts are employed, the time required for spinal arthrodesis to occur is about 6 months, and 6 more months are needed for the arthrodesis to mature. When bank bone (allografts) is used, the time required is longer, especially if postoperative irradiation is

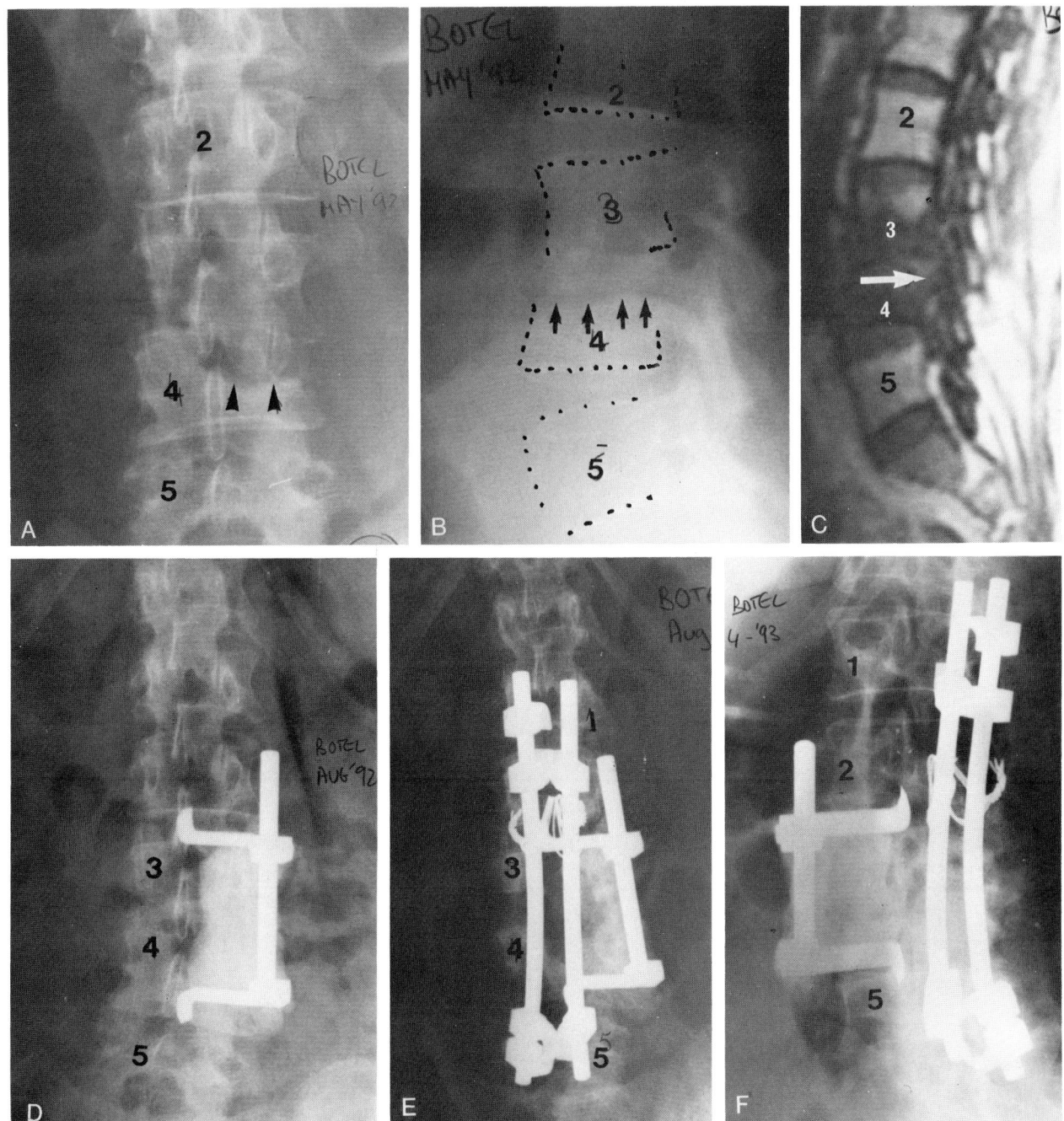

FIGURE 162-9. Two-stage anterior and posterior decompression and reconstructive instrumentation in the lumbar spine. Unknown primary metastatic carcinoma in a 56-year-old woman. (A and B) Lytic lesions at L3-L4 with obvious instability. (C) MRI demonstrating compression of the cauda equina. (D and E) Two-stage anterior and posterior stabilization. (F) The distal foundation of the posterior instrumentation is a claw placed on the lumbar lamina. The lumbar lamina is prepared by performing flavectomies above and below the lamina, followed by partial resection of the cephalad portion of the lamina that is closest to the dural sac. This approach allows placement of the laminar hook without causing a localized iatrogenic stenosis. The rods are bent to preserve lumbar lordosis.

scheduled. The median survival of patients with spinal cord compression caused by metastatic spread is 12 to 18 months. Therefore, our main indication for adding iliac cancellous bone grafts is a benign or slow-growing tumor in children and young adults (e.g., osteoblastoma, giant cell tumor, or aneurysmal bone cysts).

There are three additional arguments against bone grafting: (1) it requires a separate incision and therefore increased operating time and morbidity in patients with active disease, (2) the iliac bone graft can be microscopically involved with tumor, and (3) inhibition of bone graft incorporation by postoperative radiotherapy will probably occur.

When bone grafts are used, either autologous grafts or allografts, decortication is limited to the transverse and spinous processes because access to the lamina is obstructed by the presence of rods and segmental wiring. An ample quan-

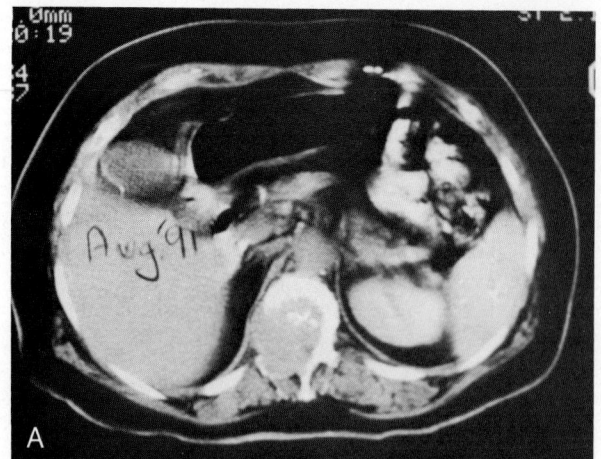
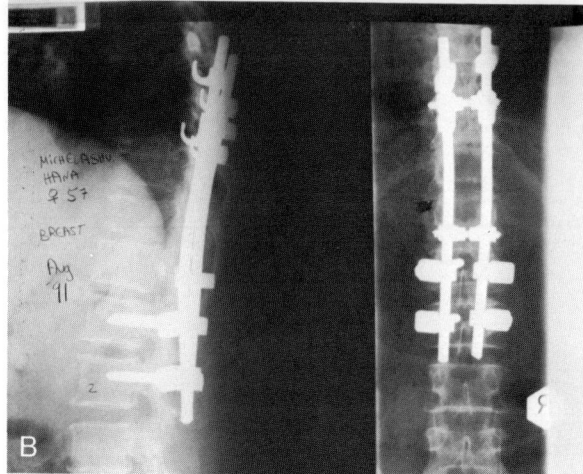

FIGURE 162-10. Posterior stabilization at the thoracolumbar junction using the transpedicular Steffee screws for the distal foundation of the instrumentation. (A) Breast carcinoma in a 58-year-old woman with progressive severe paraparesis. On the CT scan, the metastatic deposit is compressing the spinal cord at D11 in a posterior and right lateral location. (B) Following posterolateral decompression of the spinal cord, posterior stabilization is by the Isola double-rod system, with transpedicular screw fixation in the lower segments (lumbar) and hooks in the thoracic segments. The spinal column was rendered stable and painless, and the patient regained the ability for unaided ambulation.

tity of grafts is applied to the decorticated areas in continuity. If internal fixation obtained by instrumentation is adequate, external appliances are not needed.

We used posterior spine stabilization with rods and segmental sublaminar wiring without bone grafting in 23 cancer patients. Stabilization was satisfactory in all of them. The instrumentation did not dislodge, nor did any mechanical failure occur. Hook cut-out or dislodgement was encountered before the institution of segmental wiring and use of claw arrangement of hooks. Eighteen patients were followed up for 6 months or more, 13 of them for more than 1 year. The longest follow-ups were 134 and 121 months for thyroid carcinoma and giant cell tumor, respectively. Three of the earlier cases were complicated by skin breakdown because the skin incision was placed in irradiated areas. We have abandoned the occasional use of bone cement for fixation in the posterior approach because of significant sterile serous accumulation, which had to be evacuated by repeated percutaneous puncture. We conclude that with proper technique, the Isola double-rod instrumentation coupled with segmental wiring provides a reliable corrective posterior fixation for cancer patients with unstable spines after posterior decompression.

Postoperative bleeding from the residual tumor or the tumor bed may account for the neurologic deterioration observed after surgery. Therefore, we cover the dura and segmental nerves with a free fat graft and then place a large-bore noncollapsible drain next to one of the Isola rods near the decompression area. Care is taken to ensure that the rod separates the fat graft from the drain because the free fat graft may dislodge with suction, obstruct the drain, stop the evacuation of the hematoma, and leave the dura bare. Further care is taken to position the drain so that it does not get caught in the wire ends on removal. The drain exit is lateral (posterior axillary line) and not through irradiated tissue.

Meticulous technique is used in wound closure. The paravertebral muscles are closed in a watertight fashion over the rods. The skin flap is brought down by sutures in sequential rows to cause the flap to adhere to its bed and eliminate potential spaces. The sutures also release tension on the flap edges, having the skin on both sides of the incision lean toward each other to a touch. No skin overriding is accepted. Skin sutures are used only for alignment of the skin flap and therefore need not be tight. Because sutures are routinely left in place for at least 14 days, a tight suture may submerge, knot and all, under the skin.

Postoperative Care

The patient is kept flat on his or her back for a least 10 hours. The heels and sacrum are protected from weight-bearing contact with the mattress. Even for paraplegics, turning frames are not used because patients find them very uncomfortable. Regular beds are used, and after the initial 12 postoperative hours, free turning in bed is allowed.

Perioperative antibiotics are discontinued on the third postoperative day, unless otherwise indicated. The patient is allowed to sit up and walk on the first postoperative day if he or she is able to do so. The drain is usually removed on the second postoperative day. Radiotherapy, when indicated, can be administered on the fourth postoperative week, provided that healing of the surgical wound is per primum. Before discharge, standing and supine x-ray films of the spine are obtained to evaluate stability.

Most instrumentation systems are made of stainless steel alloys, which rules out follow-up imaging (CT and MRI) in cases of recompression of the spinal cord anywhere along the instrumented area. In these cases, CT myelography is indicated to delineate the extent of a recurring compressing mass and to precisely locate the upper and lower tumor borders.

Anterior Decompression of the Spine and Vertebral Body Replacement

Most operations for resection of tumors located anterior to the spinal cord are performed in the thoracic spine. Most of the principles of the anterior surgical approach to the thoracic spine (e.g., patient positioning, intraoperative identification of the level for decompression, exposure of the vertebral bodies, tumor removal, and vertebral body replacement) apply as well to other anatomic areas of the spine. Therefore, we present in detail the technical measures for the transthoracic approach and limit the description in the other areas to the variations in the technique dictated by differences in anatomy.

Thoracic Spine (T3-T11)

The transthoracic approach to the spine is by thoracotomy, right- or left-sided, according to the preoperative assessment of tumor location and bone destruction. Induction of general anesthesia occurs with the patient on a stretcher, and the patient is intubated with a double-lumen endotracheal tube. This approach enables the anesthesiology team to deflate the lung at thoracotomy and enhances the exposure. The midsection of the operating table is bent (Fig. 162–11), and the anesthetized patient is rolled onto the table and placed in the right or left lateral decubitus position. The midthoracic level is positioned over the acute bend in the table, which stretches the side of the chest facing the surgeon. This is an important technical detail that greatly facilitates exposure; when thoracotomy is in progress, retraction is almost unnecessary.

The actual location of the thoracotomy is determined after patient positioning and before preparation. To determine the thoracotomy level, we consult the x-ray films of the chest, the thoracolumbar junction, and the thoracic spinal segments awaiting decompression. Entry into the chest is obtained by a partial rib resection. The anteroposterior chest x-ray study reveals the slant of the ribs. If the ribs are horizontally aligned, then the rib to be excised is the one that articulates with the diseased vertebral body. If the rib cage is drooped, the downward inclination of the ribs will interfere with visualization. Therefore, the rib selected for removal is one or two levels above the upper level of the vertebral bodies to be exposed. Locating the selected rib is easy; inspection of the anteroposterior thoracolumbar x-ray film reveals which is the lowest palpable rib, either a long twelfth rib or the eleventh rib in cases of a hypoplastic twelfth rib. By palpating and counting rostrally, the desired rib is reached and the skin overlying it is marked.

The skin incision over the rib is placed from just lateral to the bulk of the paraspinal muscles, all the way ventrally to the costochondral junction. The incision is deepened by cautery down to the rib and is carried along the rib. By subperiosteal dissection, the anterior two thirds of the rib is freed of soft tissues. For expediency, an opened gauze is passed under the rib, and by successive pulls of the gauze to each side, a fast and thorough soft tissue stripping is obtained. The rib is cut ventrally close to the costochondral junction, and dorsally, close to the lateral border of the paravertebral muscles. These muscles should not be incised, because bleeding is usually profuse. Cutting through them does not improve the surgical exposure, and when intact, they contribute to spine stability. The proximal one third or one quarter of the rib is usually not removed unless it is involved with the tumor. If intact, the costovertebral joints contain ligamentous structures that contribute considerably to the stability of that spinal segment. In addition, because the head of the rib is situated astride the intervertebral disc, it firmly binds the two adjacent vertebral bodies. Other stabilizing components worth preserving are the costotransverse, costovertebral, and costocostal ligaments.

Entry into the pleural cavity is gained through the rib bed. The lung is inspected for metastatic spread and for tumorous adhesions of the visceral pleura to the chest wall or spinal column. In most cases, the pleural adhesions are good indicators of the location of the metastatic deposit in the spinal column. These adhesions can be separated by blunt dissection, and the associated bleeding is easily controlled. Rarely, separating the adhesions off the spine can be tedious, and ligation of feeding vessels should be undertaken before the blunt dissection. When the lung is free and mobilized, warm wet towels are applied to both sides of the incision, an automatic chest retractor is positioned, and gentle retraction of the ribs is obtained. A wet towel is applied to the lung, and a malleable retractor is placed on it, the toe of which is located in the angle between the pulsating aorta and the spinal column.

The spine is inspected for paravertebral mass, deformation, discoloration, or change in consistency. Normally, the circumference of the vertebral body is significantly smaller than that of the intervertebral disc, causing it to appear as a depression between the bordering discs. The segmental arteries and veins make their way along the narrow midportion of the vertebral body. Most tumors appear as a swelling of the vertebral midportion, with a reddish or blue tint (or black, in melanoma) localized to one or more vertebral bodies. The swelling may be soft or rubbery and must be palpated for pulsation. The pulsating tumor is a certain bleeder with substantial vascular feeders that must be located and ligated.

The parietal pleura overlying the anterolateral aspect of the vertebrae to be decompressed is cut longitudinally with a No. 15 blade. The pleura is peeled off the disc by gentle blunt dissection. This stage is usually bloodless. The longitudinal structures usually encountered are sympathetic nerves, which can be cut or preserved at the discretion of the surgeon.

Bleeding is minimized by ligation of the vascular bundles as they follow the waists of the vertebral bodies. The vertebral waist, covered by areolar tissue, is examined for the segmental bundle, which sometimes may show through. The tip of a long curved hemostat is brought down on the bone close to one disc. It is swept toward the other disc with its tip close to the bone surface. As it emerges near the other

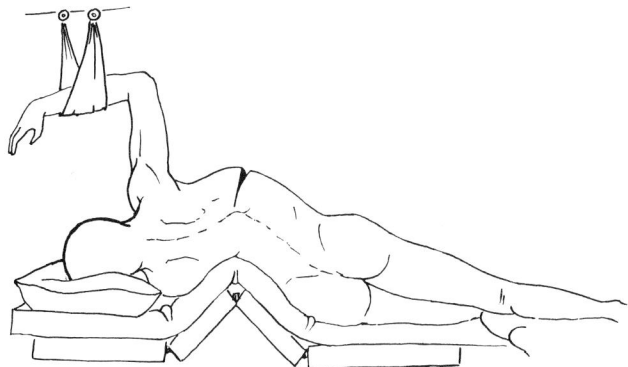

FIGURE 162–11. Patient positioning for anterior decompression of the thoracic spine. Correct patient positioning is important. The acute bend of the operating table is placed under the area intended for decompression. It stretches the side of the trunk facing the surgeon and keeps the surgical wound wide, minimizing the need for retraction and greatly facilitating exposure. It significantly shortens operating time.

disc, the vascular bundle is elevated on the jaws of the hemostat. Opening the instrument stretches the vessels across the jaws and so allows clipping or ligating on both sides of the instrument. No effort is made to separate the segmental artery from the vein, and both are contained in the same ligature. The two ligatures are placed as far away from each other as possible. The vascular bundle is then cut midway between the ligatures. The procedure is repeated at each level of interest. With the segmental vessels ligated, a thorough subperiosteal dissection is carried out anteriorly across the midline of the vertebral bodies, displacing the aorta or vena cava and protecting it with a malleable retractor inserted between it and the spine. In some instances, the segmental vessels may have been obliterated by the chronic localized pressure of the tumor. In other cases, the vessel is embedded within the tumor capsule. Every effort is made to localize and ligate these vessels, although a torn segmental artery can be controlled. The dissection is continued laterally, and all soft tissues are elevated off the vertebral bodies and discs to the anterior margin of the intervertebral foramina. Dissection is not carried onto the pedicles unless need exists for lateral decompression as well.

At this stage, the tumor-bearing vertebrae are easily identified, but if the tumor is contained within the vertebral body and no localizing deformation can be perceived, then the level to be decompressed is located according to the preoperative radiologic studies. In the operative field, the vertebra is identified by the rib to which it is connected by palpation and counting of the ribs on the inner aspect of the chest wall, starting either from the almost circular first rib down, or from the twelfth rib up. The surgeon must remember that the head of the rib is located on the superior disc (e.g., the seventh rib is situated on the intervertebral disc T6-T7).

Because of the possibility of serious bleeding, all participants, especially the anesthesiology team, are alerted when excision of the tumor has begun. If the tumor is contained within the vertebral compact bone, decompression is started by chiseling of a generous opening with a straight chisel and hammer. In a vertebra soft with tumor, large curettes are appropriate for expedient removal of large lumps of tissue; this practice provides the pathologist with better, uncrushed specimens for examination. The vertebral body is removed all the way back to the posterior longitudinal ligament. If evidence exists of tumor in the spinal canal, the ligament, if still present, must be removed to visualize the dura and decompress it. Pulsations of the dura, if present, signify opening of the myelographic block. Safe reaching of the epidural space can be achieved by following the segmental nerve exit at the intervertebral foramen, decompressing it there, and, once in epidural space, introducing a curved, No. 2 curette into the space with the active edge hugging the posterior wall of the vertebral body. By slow rotation of the curette, the rounded blunt end gently peels off the soft tissue adhering to the bone. When the surgeon is confident of the dissection, a short controlled pull dislodges the bone segment forward. Care must be taken not to pull on the segmental nerve.

The segmental roots may be encased in tumor tissue. In the thoracic area, these nerves are dispensable. Releasing the nerves may be time consuming, and the release may be incomplete. There is also a possibility of direct penetration of the nerve root by the tumor, which may lead to intractable pain. Therefore, the thoracic nerve root is ligated close to its outlet to avoid cerebrospinal fluid (CSF) leakage and is then amputated.

When the main bulk of the tumor has been removed, the anatomy is assessed. Because bleeding may interfere with the inspection, palpation should proceed posteriorly for correct location of the decompressed dura. Passing a piece of thin rubber tubing above and below the decompressed area is an innocuous method of assessing the patency of the epidural space. When necessary, more vertebral segments are decompressed in the same fashion.

The blood loss during anterior decompression of the spine is usually 1500 ml or less, but in some cases (carcinoma of the thyroid, hypernephroma, multiple myeloma), it can be profuse. The bleeding can originate from overlooked major vascular feeders of the tumor; from pathologic vessels within the tumor, which do not contract when severed; from spongy vertebral bone; or from the epidural venous plexus. We have not experienced accidental tears of large vessels. Expeditious removal of the tumor is recommended because after a major debulking, the bleeding is likely to lessen, more so in cases of complete excision. When bleeding continues, we usually apply absorbable gelatin sponge or Surgicel on a gauze to the bleeding area and wait for the anesthesiology team to compensate with fluid replacement. With bleeding under good or even partial control, decompression is completed, and vertebral body replacement is considered.

Vertebral body replacement is a spine-stabilizing procedure. We have attempted to define instability of the spine involved with neoplasm (see Table 162–6); however, there are obstacles to reaching a comprehensive definition because neoplasm-induced instability cannot be judged by the same criteria as traumatic vertebral instability. Any classification is valid only if the integrity of the vertebral cortical bone is taken into account (see Table 162–6). Adequate decompression of the spinal cord, correction of deformity, and stabilization of the spinal column are inherent to the technique and, if obtained, maximize spinal cord function. The optimal technique for vertebral body replacement has yet to be devised. We believe that the vertebral body replacement method should be reliable, simple to use, economical on operating time, and include elements well known and in wide use by most spinal surgeons. We have reported on our experience with vertebral body replacement in which components of the Harrington instrumentation system were used, namely threaded rods, nuts, and hooks.[51, 60] With the advent of the Isola instrumentation system, the Isola alar hooks seem adequate, handy, and easy to use on a short Isola rod for creation of a sturdy vertebral body construct. In our hands, it has proved efficient and durable and has the additional advantage of not enlarging the surgical armamentarium.

Of all vertebral body replacements, thoracic replacement is the most often performed and the easiest to master, and replacements in other areas of the spine are adaptations of the same technique. Therefore, a detailed account of the steps of the technique is given here.

Vertebral Body Replacement

The Isola system offers rods with a diameter of 6.35 mm (¼ inch, adult set) and of 5 mm (pediatric set). High in the thoracic spine, where the vertebral bodies are of smaller dimensions, the surgeon may choose to use implants of a reduced size, whereas lower down in the thoracolumbar area, a larger-sized construct is appropriate. The alar hooks are made to meet these requirements (Fig. 162–12A).

An Isola rod is cut about 1.5 inches longer than the distance to be spanned by the vertebral replacement construction. On one end of the rod, an Isola alar hook is fastened in place by fastening of the screw set (Fig. 162–12B). This is the **fixed hook**. Another alar hook is added that faces the other way, but its set screw is not fastened. This is the **mobile hook**. Hook clamps (Fig. 162–12C) are applied to both hooks to allow insertion of the assembly into the spinal gap in a coronal plane, with the rod of the construct running parallel to the spinal canal (Fig. 162–12D). The assembly is positioned at the widest vertebral diameter, with the blades of the hooks reaching across the midline of the intact vertebral bodies, above and below. Distracting the hooks on the rod causes their blades to sink into the vertebral bodies. After the initial manual positioning of the assembly with the hook ends touching the vertebral bodies above and below, a large lamina spreader is positioned between and in direct contact with the hook blades rather than the hook clamps. Opening the spreader gently drives the sharp hooks into the vertebral bodies (Fig. 162–12D and E). The gentle distraction is performed in stages to ascertain that the distraction forces are correctly directed and do not dislodge the assembly. Special care is also taken to avoid impingement on the spinal canal. When optimal height of replacement has been obtained and the kyphosis corrected, the mobile hook is fastened (Fig. 162–12E), and the spreader and hook clamps are removed (Fig. 162–12F). Testing of the stability of the inserted assembly is carried out by a controlled manual pull on the rod. Instrumentation time of this stage is usually 20 minutes or less. A thorough rinsing with warm saline is followed by packing of gauze into the decompressed area.

A long-standing kyphosis (Fig. 162–13) resists correction because of ligamentous or bone tethers. To overcome this, the anterior longitudinal ligament is sectioned, and the residual vertebral shell on the opposite side of the decompression may have to be removed as well. Radiopaque polymethyl methacrylate (bone cement) is used to reconstruct the excised vertebral bodies. The material is inserted into the gap while still soft and applied around and over the metal instrumentation (Fig. 162–12G). The cement covers the sharp edges of the rod and hooks to prevent direct contact with the large vessels or lungs. Special care is taken not to exert any pressure on the dura mater. While hardening, the cement is kept at a distance from the dura with a Freer elevator, and thus a cleft is formed (Fig. 162–12G) leading from the epidural space into the pleural cavity, allowing free drainage of postoperative epidural bleeding. Excess bone cement is removed. When the polymethyl methacrylate has set, the area is rinsed again. If possible, the construct is covered with parietal pleura, although this step is not absolutely necessary. In most of our cases, coverage was not attained. After lavage of the pleural cavity, one or two large-bore thoracic drains are inserted in the midaxillary line, preferably distal to the thoracotomy incision. The operating table is straightened, the wound edges are brought together, and closure occurs in layers. The skin is meticulously approximated and sutured without tension, and the drains are connected to a suction system. The patient is transferred to the intensive care unit and extubated a few hours later. Extubation is usually delayed when paraplegia is high thoracic or cervical in origin.

Postoperative Care

Turning in bed is not restricted. In paraplegic patients, the patient is turned every 3 hours, and the turns are so noted on the bed chart. Intravenous antibiotic administration is continued for 48 hours postoperatively. Dexamethasone is tapered by 30 percent every day, as tolerated, starting on the day after surgery. Chest x-ray films are obtained daily with the patient in the sitting position to check on the draining efficacy. When the amount drained per 24 hours is less than 100 ml, the drain is removed. The wound is covered again and left undisturbed until the tenth postoperative day. Sutures are then alternately removed. If wound dehiscence is probable or edge necrosis begins to show, suture removal is delayed. The patient is allowed to sit up on the first postoperative day, and ambulation is considered the day after the chest drain is removed. Corsets, plaster jackets, or any other external fixation devices are not needed. Evaluation of stability at the site of the vertebral body replacement is accomplished by spine x-ray films (Fig. 162–14) taken with the patient standing and supine. Assessment of patency at the site of the preoperative compression site can be evaluated by CT (see Figs. 162–12G and 162–13), despite the metal induced artifacts, but not by MRI.

Excision of the Thoracic Wall

Neoplastic involvement of the posterior thoracic wall contiguous with the thoracic spine requires resection of that area. The tumor usually destroys or encases a few adjacent ribs and extends medially into the spinal column and canal.

The patient is positioned in the lateral decubitus position, as with the transthoracic approach, and the skin incision is planned as in anterior decompression of the spine. The ribs to be excised are identified, and the intact overlying muscles are dissected free. The osteotomy of the ribs is placed 5 cm ventral to the tumor margin. The rib ends are elevated, the neurovascular bundles are ligated and cut, and the entire segment of the posterior thoracic wall containing the tumor is pulled up and then detached from the spine by severing of all structures, especially the segmental nerves at their point of exit from the spine. The surgeon must ensure that these nerves extending into the resected segment are cut to avoid inadvertent pulling on the compressed spinal cord. Once the partial chest wall resection is completed, the exposure of the spinal canal is wide and comfortable, and access to residual epidural tumor is prompt.

The chest wall is reconstructed with a synthetic fabric. The resulting paradoxic breathing movement of the chest wall lessens with time as a result of scar tissue formation. The postoperative management and follow-up are the same as for transthoracic decompression of the spine.

High Thoracic Spine (T1-T3)

The approach to a vertebral body in the high thoracic area (T1-T3) is through a costotransversectomy. The patient is positioned face down in the knee-chest position, with the head on a horseshoe cerebellar frame. The upper extremities

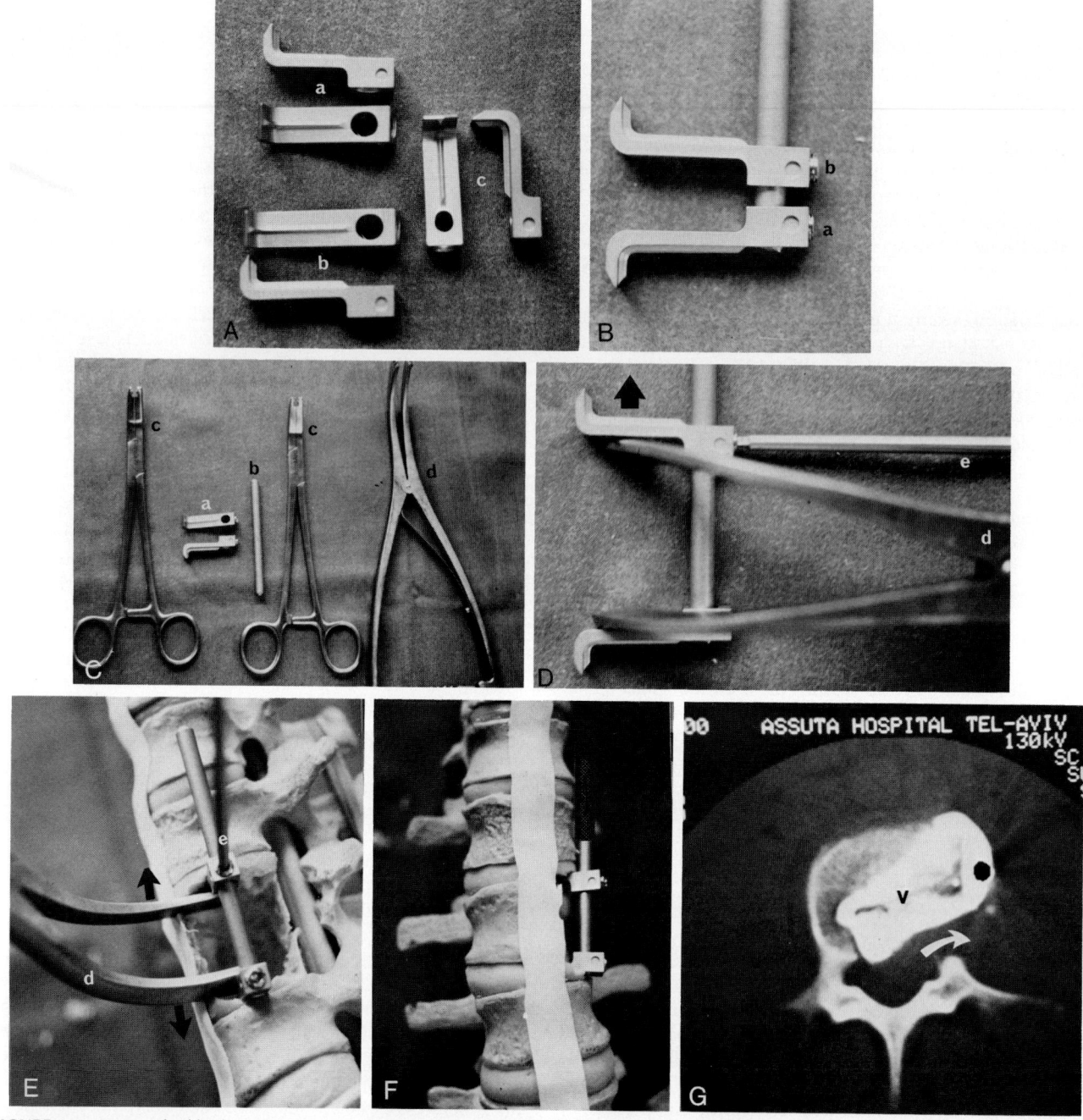

FIGURE 162–12. Vertebral body replacement construct using the Isola sacral alar hooks on an Isola rod and polymethyl methacrylate. (A) The sacral alar hooks available cover most vertebral dimensions: **a.** Alar hooks suitable for thoracic vertebral body replacement. These fit the adult (¼ inch) rod; **b.** Long blade alar hooks suitable for lumbar vertebral body replacement, fitting on a ¼ inch rod; **c.** Alar hooks that fit on the pediatric size rod intended for use in the upper thoracic area and the occasional pediatric patient. All hooks are ribbed so that once they are embedded in the vertebral bodies above and below, an increased torsional stability is obtained.

(B) Two alar hooks on a rod are the components of the vertebral body construct: **a.** The **fixed** hook is tied down to the end of the rod by tightening the Isola set screw; **b.** The **mobile** hook is facing the other way, the screw stays untightened.

(C) The required instruments for the vertebral body replacement construct: **a.** alar hooks; **b.** an Isola rod cut to measure; **c.** Isola hook clamps; **d.** a large lamina spreader.

(D) The principle of fixation: The blades of the hooks are spread apart by the large lamina spreader (d). The mobile hook moves along the rod. By gently increasing the distraction forces, the sharp blade ends become embedded into the vertebrae above and below the decompressed area. When the optimal construct height has been reached, the mobile hook is fixed as well by the hexagonal screw driver (e).

(E) The rod-and-hooks assembly in place on a model. Note that in the lateral aspect the position of the rod is parallel to the spinal cord. The lamina spreader drives apart the blades of the hooks and so embeds them into the neighboring vertebrae. It is important to correct kyphosis and so take out the slack from the ligaments, joint capsules, and surrounding the muscles. It also generates compressive forces on the construct, which will avoid dislodgement.

(F) The anterior view of the construct in place. The implants will all be covered by bone cement (polymethyl methacrylate) to avoid direct contact with the large vessels.

(G) Postoperative CT of a 16-year-old boy with osteogenic sarcoma of the pelvis metastasizing to the lumbar spine. The vertebral construct (v) is all covered by polymethyl methacrylate. While hardening, a fissure was formed by just keeping the bone cement away from the dura. Through this fissure, any epidural bleeding that may occur will drain into the pleural cavity or retroperitoneal space (white arrow) and the spinal cord will be spared the compression.

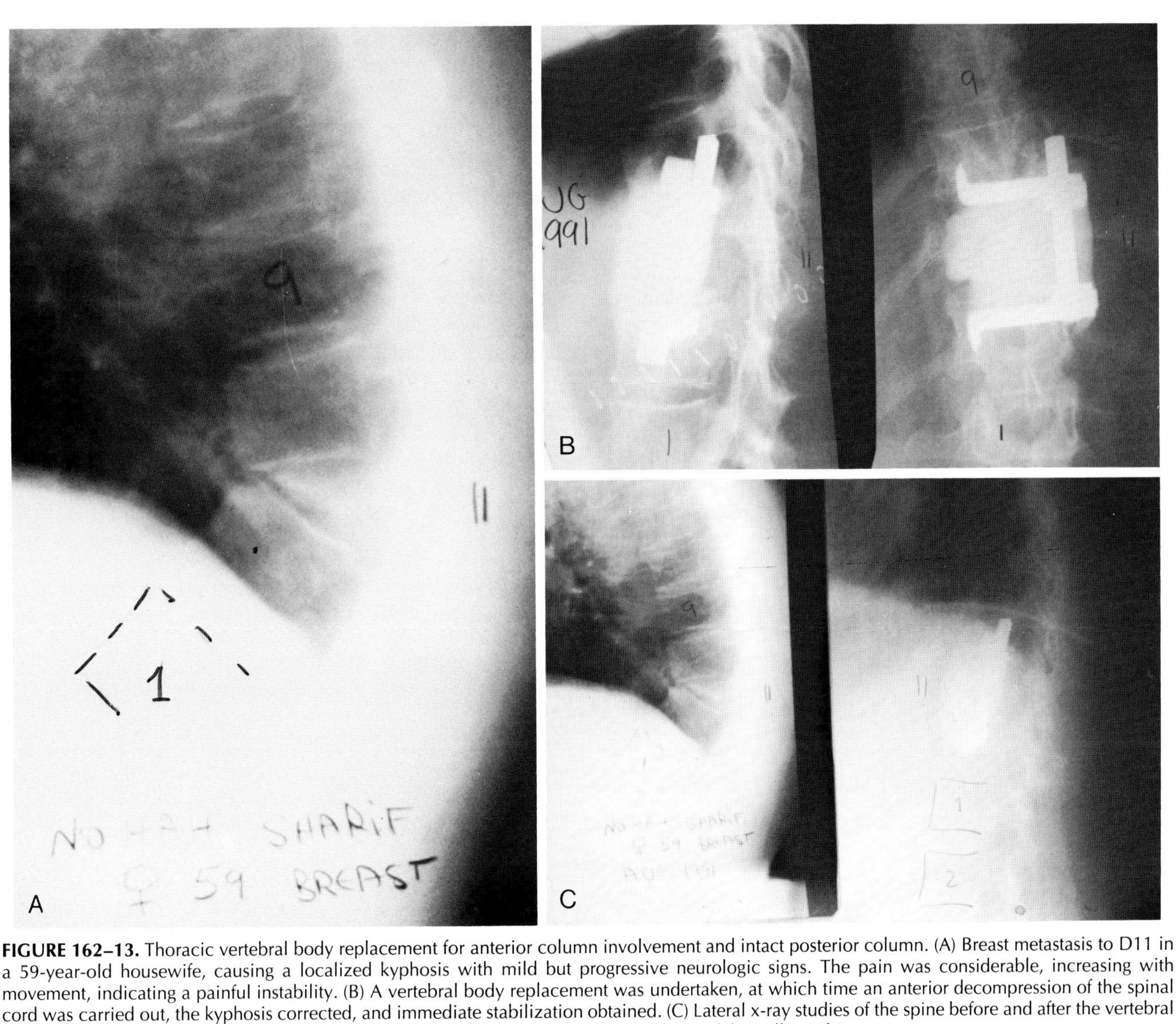

FIGURE 162–13. Thoracic vertebral body replacement for anterior column involvement and intact posterior column. (A) Breast metastasis to D11 in a 59-year-old housewife, causing a localized kyphosis with mild but progressive neurologic signs. The pain was considerable, increasing with movement, indicating a painful instability. (B) A vertebral body replacement was undertaken, at which time an anterior decompression of the spinal cord was carried out, the kyphosis corrected, and immediate stabilization obtained. (C) Lateral x-ray studies of the spine before and after the vertebral body replacement at D11. Observe the satisfactory correction of the kyphosis at the site of the collapsed D11.

are brought forward to pull the scapulae away from the midline. The skin incision is placed parallel and 6 to 8 cm lateral to the spine. The incision is deepened to the fascia of the paravertebral muscles. Undermining medially at this level creates a flap with its base along the spinous processes.

The paravertebral muscles are incised longitudinally with diathermy in a line parallel to the spine and 5 to 6 cm lateral to it. Deepening the incision reveals the transverse processes. The muscles are subperiosteally peeled off the laminae and transverse processes two levels above and two below the level of required decompression. The ribs are denuded in a similar manner 7 to 8 cm lateral to spinous processes. The subperiosteal stripping is extended all around the proximal quarter or third of the ribs, with care taken not to violate the pleural space. The entire procedure is extrapleural. When circumferential rib stripping has been completed, a rib cutter is introduced 8 cm lateral to the midline, and the ribs are osteotomized at least one level above and one below the intended level of decompression. The proximal rib segments are elevated at the osteotomy end, and the soft tissue stripping is completed on their undersurface, including the costovertebral joint and the head of the rib. Cutting the transverse processes leaves the rib connected to the vertebral body by the irradiate ligament. Before the proximal rib segment is freed from this joint by simple twisting, the surgeon must

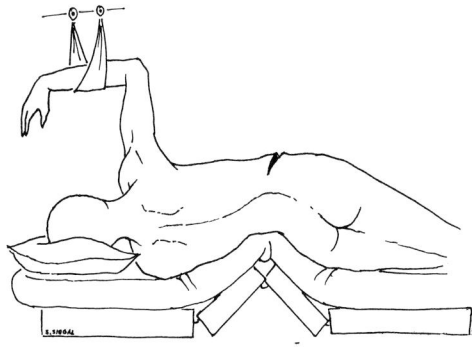

FIGURE 162–14. Patient positioning for anterior decompression of the lumbar spine. The acute bend in the table is placed under the lumbar region of the patient, who is positioned in a lateral decubitus position.

ensure that the segmental nerves are totally detached from the rib and are not pulled inadvertently. A rib attached to the site of pathologic involvement is easy to detach and constitutes an affirmative indication to the site of prospective decompression. Often, the head of the rib is involved with tumor and may break on twisting. The remaining rib fragment can be removed with curettes.

At this point, the soft tissues are gently peeled off the anterolateral and anterior aspects of the vertebral bodies, and the field is open for decompression. The tumor is scooped out with curettes. If the segmental root is followed medially, it safely indicates the position of the intervertebral foramen and leads to the epidural space. If feasible, the T1 and T2 roots are preserved to maintain ulnar functions. Removal of the compressing tumor is performed as described in the transthoracic approach.

Once the extrapleural removal of tumor is completed, the dura is free and pulsating, and bleeding is reduced, reconstruction of the vertebral segments is considered. The upper thoracic vertebrae are smaller than the lower thoracic or lumbar vertebrae. Vertebral body replacement requires the smaller Isola alar hooks with an intervening 5-mm (pediatric) Isola rod (see Fig. 162–12A, item c). After a thorough lavage to provide optimal exposure of the dura, the assembly is inserted with the fixed hook being manually pushed into the spongy bone of the caudal vertebra in the gap. Caution is taken when the rostral hook is positioned because when the patient is in the prone position the upper thoracic spine takes a downward dip to follow the normal thoracic kyphosis. This process requires positioning of the vertebral construct on a slope, with its rostral end pointing downward.

Placement of the instrumentation is accompanied by repeated visual and palpatory examination to avoid unintentional impingement on the spinal canal. When the direction has been ascertained, the lamina spreader is placed on the hook blades, and gradual distraction is applied; the spine is observed constantly to ascertain that the distraction is performed in the correct axis. When optimal distraction has been obtained, the set screw of the mobile hook is fastened, and construction stability is checked by manual testing.

Once the instrumentation is firmly placed, polymethyl methacrylate reconstruction is carried out as described for thoracic vertebral body replacement. After a final lavage, a large-bore chest drain is placed on the cement-covered construction, and the wound is closed in layers. The route of drain insertion should not pass through irradiated skin but should proceed laterally at a distance from the midline. If the pleural space has not been violated, no additional drain is necessary. Postoperative care and follow-up are as for the transthoracic approach.

Thoracolumbar Spine (T11-L1)

The transition zone at the thoracolumbar junctions is somewhat more difficult to expose, but otherwise, all other steps of spinal decompression and vertebral body replacement are identical to those used in the thoracic or lumbar regions. To approach the T11-L1 area, the surgeon must displace not only the lungs and the abdominal contents, but also the diaphragm. The insertion of the diaphragm is at L2, but the slope of its dome obstructs the approach to the lower thoracic spine.

The intubated patient is placed in the lateral decubitus position with the low thoracic area positioned over the acute bend in the operating table. The approach is through the bed of the tenth rib. After the skin over the anterior two thirds of this rib is incised, the incision is carried obliquely to the lateral aspect of the rectus abdominis on the same side, then down to the bone and continued to the costochondral junction. The distal two thirds of the rib is excised at the junction after the usual subperiosteal stripping of soft tissues. The thoracic cavity is entered with care because it is much narrowed at this level by the ascent of the dome of the diaphragm. Now, the chondral end of the tenth rib is longitudinally split, and at this point, the surgeon can localize the anterior border of the diaphragm at its insertion. Blunt dissection separates the peritoneum from the undersurface of the diaphragm, the lateral and posterior abdominal walls, the iliopsoas muscle, and the upper lumbar spine. With the abdominal contents and the lung retracted forward, the diaphragm is well visualized. From the split end of the tenth rib, the diaphragm is cut along its insertion line, leaving a 2-cm-wide strip attached to the chest wall. Long sutures are placed every 4 or 5 cm on both sides for later precise approximation of the diaphragmatic edges during wound closure. The crus is detached as well, and vertebral body excision and replacement are carried out as outlined in the transthoracic approach. Before closure, large-bore drains are positioned both in the chest cavity and in the retroperitoneum. Interestingly, although the diaphragm is sutured back over the synthetic vertebral construct and there is no chance of any biologic adhesion between the two, we have not encountered symptoms of transdiaphragmatic herniation.

Lumbar Spine (L2-L5)

The intubated patient is placed in the right or left lateral decubitus position, according to the tumor location as assessed from the preoperative studies. The lumbar area is positioned over the acute bend of the table (see Fig. 162–14). The incision is started at the lateral border of the paravertebral muscle group at the midlumbar level and is carried laterally and ventrally to the lateral border of the rectus abdominis. The incision is deepened by cautery to the peritoneum. By blunt manual dissection, the peritoneum is peeled off the lateral abdominal wall, extending the dissection to the iliopsoas posteriorly. In the same manner, the peritoneum is detached from the undersurface of the diaphragm. No intentional dissection is performed to reveal the ureter or kidney. When the peritoneum has been entirely dettached off the diaphragm, the posterior abdominal wall, the iliopsoas, and the spine, the abdominal contents fall forward, thereby opening the way for surgery on the vertebral bodies. If the patient has been conveniently placed over the bend of the operating table, the incised lateral abdominal wall stays widely open, necessitating minimal retraction.

The iliopsoas muscles cover the lateral and anterolateral aspects of the lumbar spine, and between them is the anterior longitudinal ligament, which runs as a strong white strip in the midline that is segmentally elevated by the bulge of the intervertebral discs. Intraoperative location of the diseased vertebrae is performed in much the same way as in the thoracic spine. The surgeon inspects the iliopsoas muscle for a swelling, which would indicate an underlying or infiltrating paravertebral tumor. In addition, discoloration or bulging of the anterior longitudinal ligament, the presence of frank anterior penetrating tumor, or an abnormally short interdiscal distance are all good localizing signs of the area to be decompressed. If the tumor is contained within the vertebra and its level is difficult to identify, an intraoperative anteroposterior film can be obtained of the lumbar spine with a heavy intravenous needle hammered lightly into the lateral aspect of a vertebra. To expose the lumbar spine, a round-ended retractor is placed under the medial border of the iliopsoas, kept in close contact with the vertebral bodies, and pulled laterally to the intervertebral foramina.

The vertebral waist, covered by areolar tissue, is now examined to locate the segmental vascular bundle. The tip of a long, curved hemostat is positioned on the bone close to one disc and is swept toward the other disc with its tip close to the bone surface. As it emerges near the other disc, the segmental vascular bundle is elevated on the hemostat's jaws. Opening the instrument stretches the vessels to allow clipping or ligating on both sides (for details of the technique, see transthoracic anterior decompression of the spine, discussed earlier).

Regardless of the number of vertebrae to be replaced, the steps of anterior instrumentation of the spine (vertebral body replacement) are the same. The lumbar vertebrae are the largest; therefore, the large Isola alar hooks on the quarter-inch rod are adequate for a sound purchase across the vertebral bodies (see Fig. 162–12A, item b, and Fig. 162–15). The technique of replacement was described earlier. However, a few points deserve special notice. The lumbar spine at its lower segments is in close contact with the bifurcations of the aorta and vena cava, and the lateral aspects of L5 are in close relation to the iliac artery and vein. Careful manipulation and retraction therefore are indicated, and the vertebral replacement construction should not be in the way of the pulsating large vessels. We have not experienced vascular complications, such as tears of the vena cava or iliac veins or late occurrence of iatrogenic aneurysms. Here, as elsewhere along the spinal column, the rod and hooks are covered by poly-methyl methacrylate cement, which also fills the gap left after excision of the diseased vertebrae. While hardening, the cement is kept from pressing on the dura. At the same time, a cleft is fashioned between the dura and the cement, leading into the retroperitoneum to allow free drainage of postoperative epidural bleeding (see Fig. 162–12G). After thorough lavage with warm saline, a noncollapsible large-bore drain is introduced into the retroperitoneum close to the outlet of the cleft. The drain exit is distal to the incision wound and in the posterior axillary line. The acute bend in the operating table is straightened, and the wound is meticulously closed in layers. The approximation tension in the tissues at the incision wound are carried by the fascial and subcutaneous layers. The skin sutures are intended only to maintain alignment of wound edges and must not be tightened. Postoperative care and follow-up are similar to those outlined for transthoracic decompression.

Cervical Spine (C2 to D1)

The available systems for posterior cervical instrumentation are not designed to act in the modes of the scoliosis instrumentation systems, namely to obtain rigid fixation, allow distraction or compression, control sagittal alignment (maintain cervical lordosis), and make use of transverse connecting members. The surgeon-friendly double-deck posterior cervical system (AcroMed b.v., Rotterdam, The Netherlands) is therefore presented (Fig. 162–16). One of the main indications for its use is either the acquired cervical instability induced by neoplastic vertebral lesions or cervical spine destabilization following excision of such lesions. It was designed to replace the problematic halo systems and the current inadjustable screw and plate assemblies.

The cervical skeleton is characterized by its paucity of bone when compared with the other spine areas. The articular mass is the bulkiest of the posterior elements and is not adjacent to neural and vascular structures. It is an adequate site for placement of instrumentation.

The system consists of cervical facet hooks (Fig. 162–16A) and longitudinal and transverse connecting members of 1.6-mm stainless steel wires (Fig. 162–C). Anchorage of the double-deck system is solely to the cervical articular masses. Attempts to position the facet hooks in a sublaminar location are dangerous to the patient's neurologic integrity. The system's design is anatomically contoured to fit the cervical articular masses only.

The double-deck hook houses the longitudinal member in the lower deck (Fig. 162–16A to C). The transverse member has been placed in the higher upper deck to allow clearance, when needed, of the dura or posterior elements. This is the first cervical system to employ transverse fixation, which imparts considerable rigidity to the posterior scaffolding. The double-deck system may stabilize the cervical spine as a first-stage procedure performed before anterior decompression when stability may be difficult to establish. It may also be employed as a second-stage procedure performed when postoperative stability is less than optimal after anterior decompression or stabilization.

Instrumentation

1. X-ray and imaging studies determine levels of instability and areas of bone loss or bone weakness resulting from destabilizing surgery or presence of tumor or infection. Cord compression is best visualized by MRI studies. Presurgery planning should consider maintenance of a normal sagittal alignment. Flexion and extension x-ray studies demonstrate mobility of the facets to be instrumented and illustrate arthrotic nonmobile joints, into which hook insertion can be difficult.

2. The patient is placed in any position with which the surgeon is most familiar, but the surgeon must have the option of restoring cervical lordosis at the end of the decompression stage. If the patient has not been irradiated, a midline incision carried down to the spinous processes allows a bilateral subperiosteal dissection out to the lateral aspects of the cervical articular masses, from C2 down to D1. A laterally placed skin incision should be used in patients who have been subjected to irradiation so that a large skin flap is created.

3. Posterior or posterolateral decompression is carried out through formal laminectomies. Release of individual roots is undertaken when required.

4. Instrumentation is started by insinuation of the blade of the starter into the joint slit (Fig. 162–16B). The reverse hand

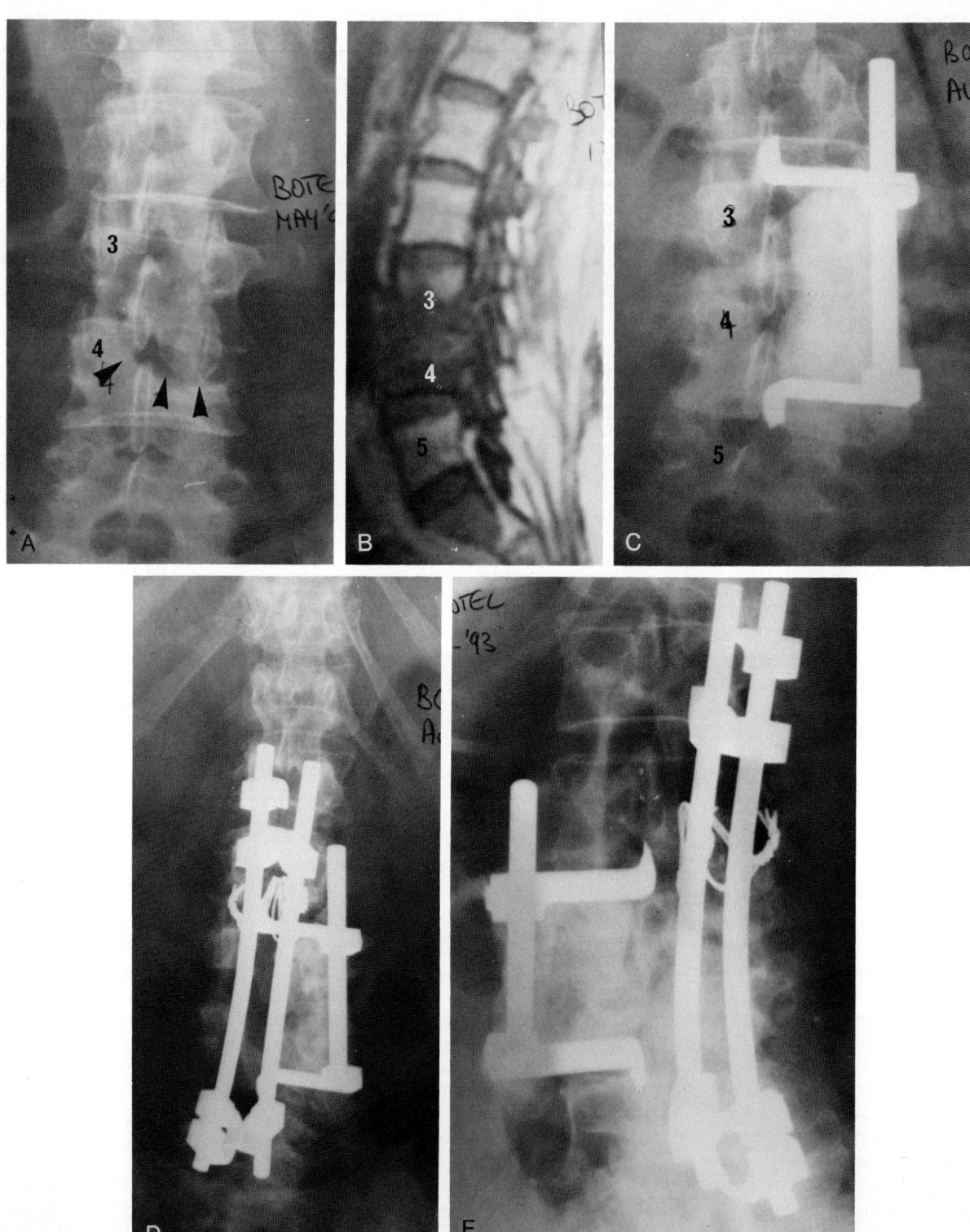

FIGURE 162–15. Two-stage anterior and posterior decompression and stabilization of the lumbar spine. (A) Unknown primary adenocarcinoma in a 58-year-old woman infiltrating the third and fourth lumbar vertebral bodies with obvious instability. (B) The MRI shows retropulsion of vertebral body contents and compression of the thecal sac mainly by the sequestrated disc. (C) Following an anterior decompression and excision of most of the vertebral bodies and the intervening disc, a vertebral body replacement construct was introduced. Two months later, the pain returned. (D) A posterior Isola instrumentation did away with most of her problems. Note the superior and inferior claws. (E) An oblique view showing the prebending of the rods to restore the natural lumbar lordosis. Failing to do so results in a tiring and ungainly forward bent gait, which will seriously hinder the patient's convalescence and future activities.

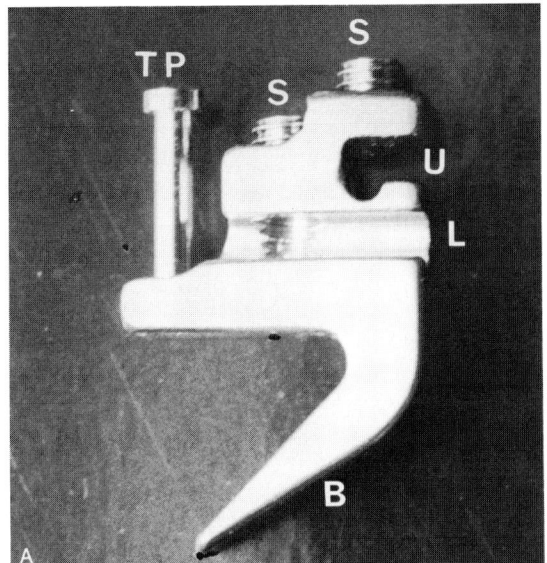
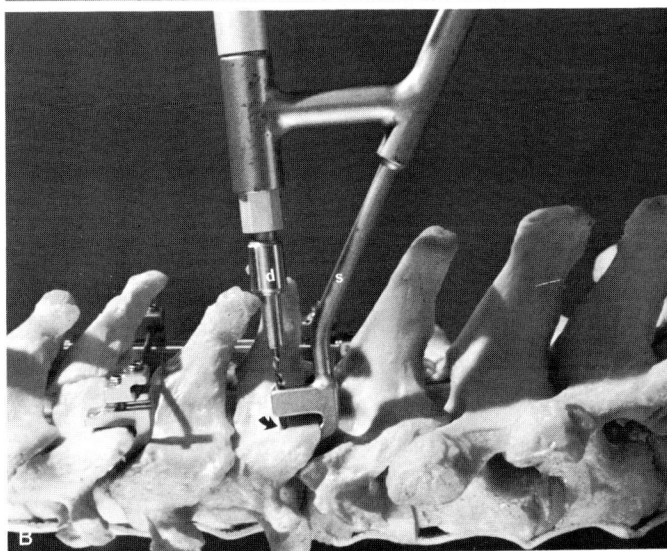
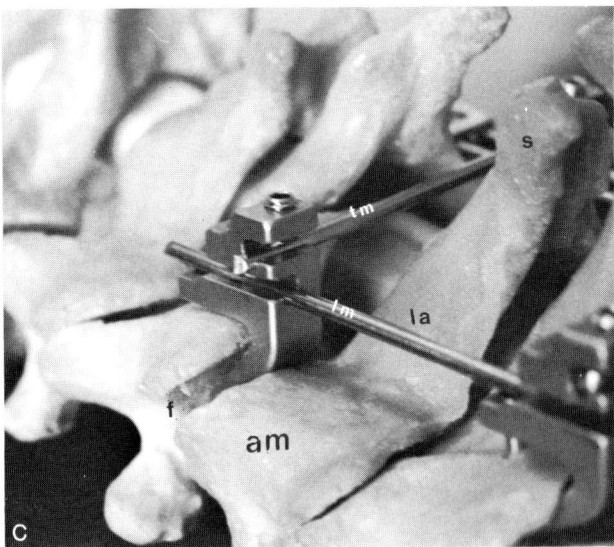

FIGURE 162–16. The double deck posterior cervical instrumentation system. (A) The double deck cervical facet hook. B = The straight blade of the hook for insertion into the cervical joint; TP = the transfixing pin penetrates the dorsal aspect of the cervical articular mass at an angle to the hook blade, creating a solid grasp on the bone; S = the set screws when tightened will fix the longitudinal or transverse members within the upper or lower decks; U = upper deck for the transverse member; L = lower deck for the longitudinal member. (B) The starter (s) is introduced in the cervical facet joint to establish the path of insertion for the hook blade. Once located, the reverse hand drill (d) is introduced to prepare the hole for the transfixing pin to drop in through the dorsal aspect of the articular mass. (C) The hook is in place: The blade is located in the facet joint (f) between two articular masses (am). The longitudinal member (lm) located in the lower deck is somewhat longer to ensure that it does cover the head of the transfixing pin to prevent the pin from backing out and loosening. The transverse member (tm) is situated in the upper deck to clear the dura. It may be necessary to put an omega-like bend in it to place it farther away dorsally from the dura.

drill driven through the starter prepares with precision the pin hole through the dorsal aspect of the articular mass. The double-deck hook is then perched on the hook holder and inserted into the site prepared by the starter. The transfixing pin is then lowered into the pin hole. When the hooks on one side are mounted, the longitudinal wire, either straight or prebent, is positioned within the lower decks through the side openings and secured by tightening of the set screws (Fig. 162–16A and B). Attention is paid to the complete coverage of the pin heads by the longitudinal members to avoid pin backout and loosening of the system. The procedure is repeated on the other side.

5. The transverse members are positioned in the higher deck for clearing the dura in cases of laminectomy. When clearing is still difficult to obtain, the dorsally prebent omega-shaped wire can be used. After tightening of the set screws in the upper decks, all screws are revisited. In this way a rigid scaffolding has now been obtained (Figs. 162–17 and 162–18).

6. The double-deck instrumentation leaves ample space laterally for placement of bone grafts, which are harvested from one of the posterior superior iliac spines (the laminectomy fragments should not be used because the local bone may be involved with tumor as well). The components of the system create a protective fence to avoid medial migration of bone fragments onto the bare dura.

7. Closure occurs in layers, and use of protective collars or braces is at the surgeon's discretion. Ambulation is encouraged the very next day. Perioperative antibiotic administration is continued for 3 days.

Complications registered among the 18 patients on whom this procedure was performed consisted of one case of severe left C6 radicular pains, which took 2 months to subside. To date, no infections, instrumentation pullout, or neurologic worsening have been encountered.

Cervicothoracic Stabilization

The double-deck instrumentation system may be employed by itself to negotiate the cervicothoracic junction. Another possibility would be to treat two or three adjacent cervical levels with the double-deck instrumentation, cephalad to the area of instability. Then, any double-rod system could be

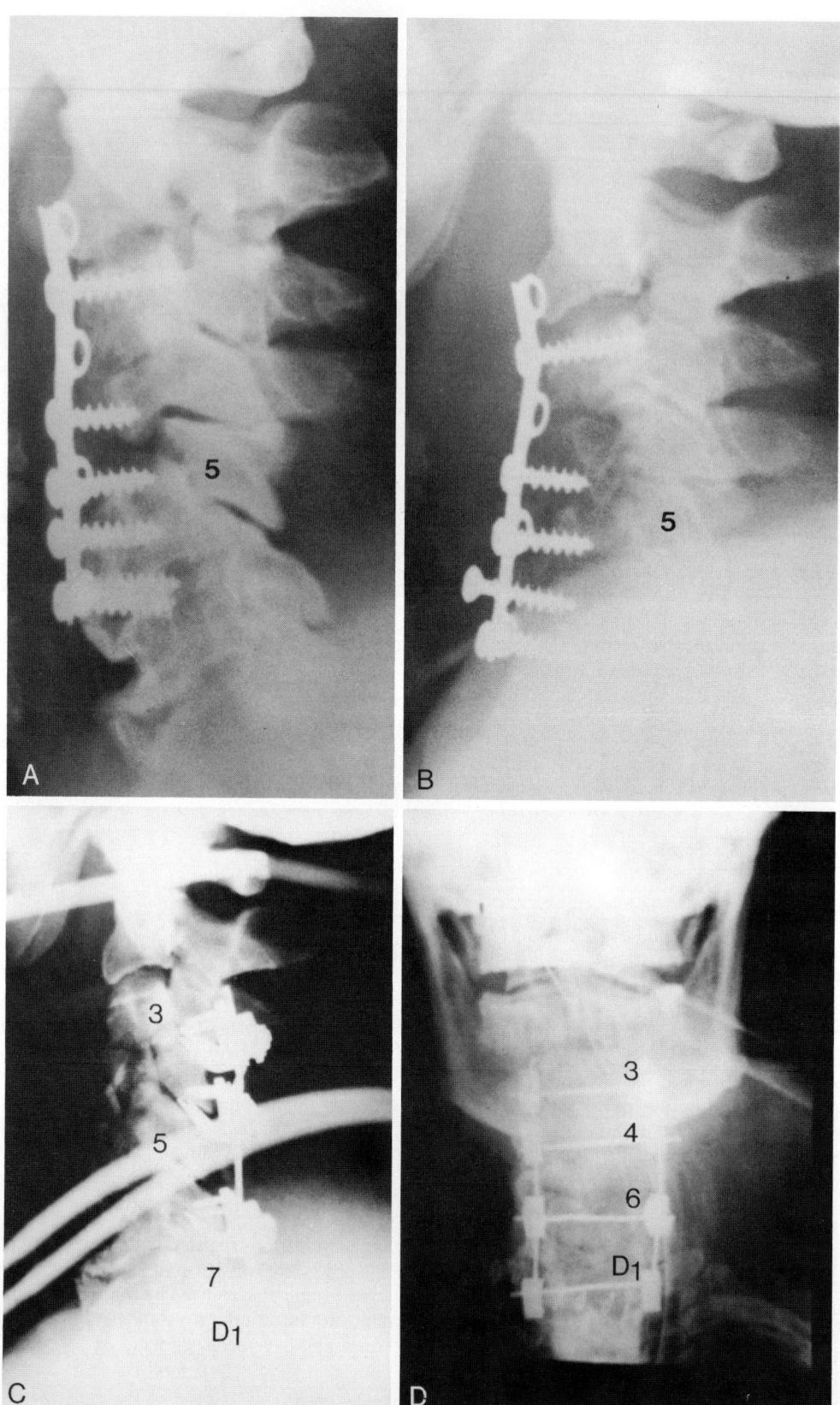

FIGURE 162-17. Posterior cervical instrumentation for massive destruction of cervical elements, loss of stability, and incomplete quadriplegia. (A) Direct extension of thyroid carcinoma to C5, after a destabilizing laminectomy and an attempt at stabilization by anterior cervical plating. (B) Retropharyngeal abscess formation causing loosening of anterior cervical plate and resulting in total instability and severe quadriplegia. (C and D) Posterior cervical stabilization from C3 down to D1, removal of anterior cervical plate, and drainage of abscess. The neurologic improvement was dramatic. The patient was able to sit the next day and walked with aid a couple of days later.

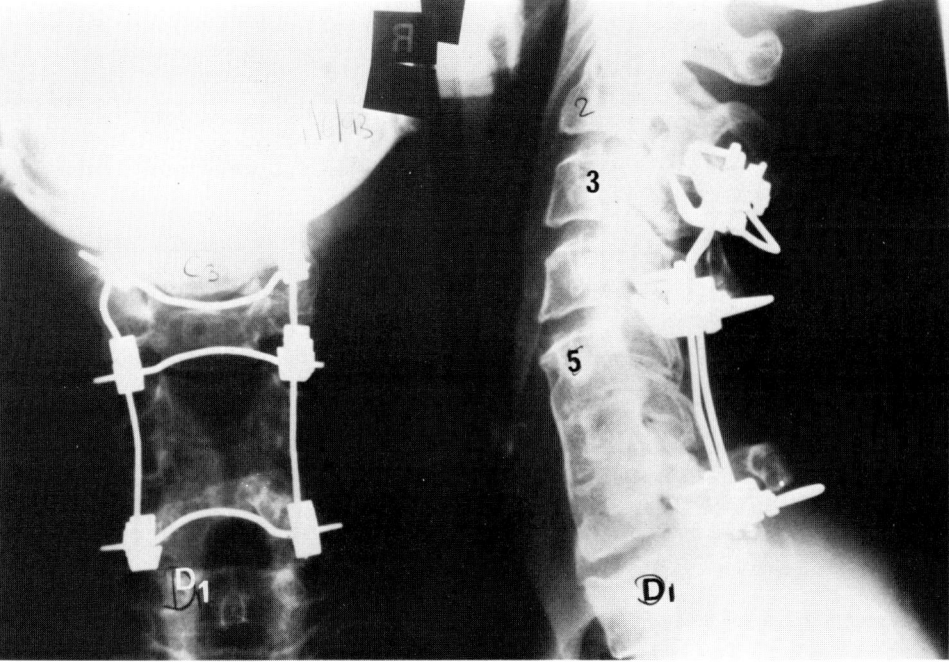

FIGURE 162–18. Preserving cervical lordosis (sagittal alignment). The longitudinal members are bent to conform to the cervical lordosis, and transverse wires can be given a dorsal omega-shaped bend to clear the dura or the posterior elements. (Courtesy of Dr. P. Pavlov, Nijmegen, Holland).

attached to the thoracic spine below to bridge over the problematic cervicothoracic junction and then tied above to the cervical double system by wires at the level of the upper transverse connecting bar. We have not had the chance to implement this option.

COMPLICATIONS

RADIOTHERAPY. Most papers dealing with radiotherapy alone do not comment on complications of therapy or mortality. Death in the first month after radiotherapy is likely to result from the primary disease: in one series, 70 percent of patients considered severely ill at the time of diagnosis of SCC died within 30 days after diagnosis.[51]

SURGICAL COMPLICATIONS. MORTALITY. The incidence of death within the first month after decompressive laminectomy ranges from 3 to 15 percent with an average mortality rate of 7 percent (see Tables 162–3 and 162–4). Surgical mortality rate after vertebral body resection falls within the same range (see Table 162–5).

MORBIDITY. The risk of neurologic deterioration as a result of surgery is a major concern in patients who present while still able to walk. It occurred in 5 to 23 percent of patients undergoing laminectomy, with a mean of 13 percent (see Table 162–3). After vertebral body resection, neurologic worsening is rare and occurs in only 2 to 6 percent of patients (see Table 162–5).

In patients undergoing laminectomy combined with radiotherapy, nonneurologic complications include wound infection, wound dehiscence, spinal epidural hematoma, CSF leak, and spinal instability. The frequency of these complications ranges from 8 to 42 percent, with a mean of 11 percent.[11, 28] Only a few authors specifically mentioned the problem of instability,[20, 49] reporting its occurrence in about 9 percent of cases. The incidence of nonneurogenic complications is similar in vertebral body resection and in laminectomies. However, the operation and instrumentation techniques require considerable expertise: these procedures should be undertaken by a surgeon familiar with the techniques of spinal posterior and anterior instrumentation with different options to suit specific levels along the spine.

SUMMARY

This chapter is a plea for early diagnosis and treatment of neoplastic SCC. A high index of suspicion is essential, especially in patients known to harbor a neoplastic process. Wider acceptance and judicious use of modern and novel surgical techniques for spinal decompression and stabilization may improve the quality of life of many patients too often denied such treatment.

REFERENCES

1. Byrne NT: Spinal cord compression from epidural metastases. N Eng J Med 327:614–619, 1992
2. Paillas J-E, Alliez B, Pellet W: Primary and secondary tumors of the spine, in Vinken PJ, Bruyn GW (eds): Handbook of Clinical Neurology, vol 20. Amsterdam, North-Holland Publishing, 1976, pp 19–54
3. Cohen DM, Dahlin DC, MacCarty CS: Apparently solitary tumors of the vertebral column. Mayo Clin Proc 39:509–528, 1964
4. Galasko CSB: The anatomy and pathways of skeletal metastases, in Weiss L, Gilbert HA (eds): Bone Metastases. Boston, GK Hall, 1981, pp 49–63
5. Miller F, Whitehall R: Carcinoma of the breast metastatic to skeleton. Clin Orthop 184:121–127, 1984
6. Schaberg J, Gainor BJ: A profile of metastatic carcinoma of the spine. Spine 10:19–20, 1985
7. Abrams HL, Spiro R, Goldstein N: Metastases in carcinoma. Analysis of 1000 autopsied cases. Cancer 3:74–85, 1950
8. Constans JP, De Divitiis E, Donzelli R, et al: Spinal metastases with neurological manifestations: Review of 600 cases. J Neurosurg 59:111–118, 1983

9. Landmann C, Hunig R, Gratzi O: The role of laminectomy in the combined treatment of metastatic spinal cord compression. Int J Rad Oncol Biol Phys 24:627–631, 1992
10. Bach F, Larsen BH, Rohde K, et al: Metastatic spinal cord compression. Occurrence, symptoms, clinical presentations and prognosis in 398 patients with spinal cord compression. Acta Neurochir (Wien) 107:37–43, 1990
11. Black P: Spinal metastases: Current status and recommended guidelines for management. Neurosurgery 5:726–746, 1979
12. Barron KD, Hirano A, Araki S, Terry RD: Experiences with metastatic neoplasms involving the spinal cord. Neurology 9:91–106, 1959
13. Cobb CA III, Leavens ME, Eckles N: Indications for nonoperative treatment of spinal cord compression due to breast cancer. J Neurosurg 47:653–658, 1977
14. Raffel C, Neave VCD, Lavine S, McComb JG: Treatment of spinal cord compression by epidural malignancy in children. Neurosurgery 28:349–352, 1991
15. Klein SL, Sanford RA, Muhlbauer MS: Pediatric spinal epidural metastases. J Neurosurg 74:70–75, 1991
16. Siegal T, Siegal T: Spinal epidural metastases from solid tumors. Clinical diagnosis and management, in Twijnstra A, Keyser A, Ongerboer de Visser BW (eds): Neuro-Oncology. Primary Tumors and Neurological Complications of Cancer. The Netherlands, Elsevier Science Publications, 1993, pp 283–305
17. Portenoy RK, Galer BS, Salamon O, et al: Identification of epidural neoplasm. Radiography and bone scintigraphy in the symptomatic and asymptomatic spine. Cancer 64:2207–2213, 1989
18. Edelstyn GA, Gillespie PJ, Grebbel FS: The radiological demonstration of osseous metastases: Experimental observations. Clin Radiol 18:158–163, 1967
19. Asdourian PL, Weidenbaum M, DeWald RL, et al: The pattern of vertebral involvement in metastatic vertebral breast cancer. Clin Orthop 250:164–170, 1990
20. Gilbert RW, Kim JH, Posner JB: Epidural spinal cord compression from metastatic tumor: Diagnosis and treatment. Ann Neurol 3:40–51, 1978
21. Posner JB: Spinal metastases: Diagnosis and treatment, in Posner JB (ed): Neuro-Oncology Course at Memorial Sloan-Kettering Cancer Center. New York, 1981, pp 42–54
22. Graus F, Krol G, Foley KM: Early diagnosis of spinal epidural metastases: Correlation with clinical and radiological findings. Proc Am Soc Clin Oncol 4:269, 1985
23. Carmody RF, Yang OJ, Seeley GW, et al: Spinal cord compression due to metastatic disease: Diagnosis with MR imaging versus myelography. Radiology 173:225–229, 1989
24. Colletti PM, Dang HT, Deseran MW, et al: Spinal MR imaging in suspected metastases: Correlation with skeletal scintigraphy. Magn Reson Imaging 9:345–355, 1991
25. Greenberg HS, Kim J-H, Posner JB: Epidural spinal cord compression from metastatic tumor: Results with a new treatment protocol. Ann Neurol 8:361–366, 1980
26. Bernat JL, Greenberg ER, Barret J: Suspected epidural compression of the spinal cord and cauda equina by metastatic carcinoma. Cancer 51:1953–1957, 1983
27. Barcena A, Lobato RD, Rivas JJ, et al: Spinal metastatic disease: Analysis of factors determining functional prognosis and the choice of treatment. Neurosurgery 15:820–827, 1984
28. Findlay GFG: Adverse effects of the management of malignant spinal cord compression. J Neurol Neurosurg Psychiatry 47:761–768, 1984
29. Hainline B, Tuszynski MH, Posner JB: Ataxia in epidural spinal cord compression. Neurology 42:2193–2195, 1992
30. Ushio Y, Posner R, Posner JB, Shapiro WR: Experimental spinal cord compression by epidural neoplasms. Neurology 27:422–429, 1977
31. Ikeda H, Ushio Y, Hayakawa T, et al: Edema and circulatory disturbance in the spinal cord compressed by epidural neoplasms. J Neurosurg 52:203–209, 1980
32. Kato M, Ushio Y, Hayakawa T, et al: Circulatory disturbance of the spinal cord with epidural neoplasm in rats. J Neurosurg 63:260–265, 1985
33. Delattre JY, Arbit E, Thaler HT: A dose-response study of dexamethasone in a model of spinal cord compression caused by epidural tumor. J Neurosurg 70:920–925, 1989
34. Siegal T, Siegal T, Sandbank U, et al: Experimental spinal cord compression: Evoked potentials, edema, prostaglandins light and electron microscopy. Spine 12:440–448, 1987
35. Siegal T, Siegal T, Shapira Y, et al: Indomethacin and dexamethasone in experimental neoplastic spinal cord compression: Part I. Effect on water content and specific gravity. Neurosurgery 22:328–333, 1988
36. Siegal T, Shohami E, Shapira Y, Siegal T: Indomethacin and dexamethasone in experimental neoplastic spinal cord compression: Part II. Effect on edema and prostaglandin synthesis. Neurosurgery 22:334–339, 1988
37. Siegal T, Siegal T, Shohami E, Shapira Y: Comparison of soluble dexamethasone sodium phosphate with free dexamethasone and indomethacin in the treatment of experimental neoplastic spinal cord compression. Spine 13:1171–1176, 1988
38. Siegal T, Siegal T, Shapira Y, Shohami E: The early effect of steroidal and non-steroidal anti-inflammatory agents on neoplastic epidural cord compression. Ann N Y Acad Sci 559:488–490, 1989
39. Siegal T, Siegal T, Shohami E, Lossos F: Experimental neoplastic spinal cord compression: Effect of ketamine and MK-801 on edema and prostaglandins. Neurosurgery 26:963–966, 1990
40. Siegal T, Siegal T: Experimental neoplastic spinal cord compression: Effect of anti-inflammatory agents and glutamate receptor antagonists on vascular permeability. Neurosurgery 26:967–970, 1990
41. Siegal T, Siegal T: Participation of serotonergic mechanisms in the pathophysiology of experimental neoplastic spinal cord compression. Neurology 41:574–580, 1991
42. Siegal T, Siegal T: Serotonergic manipulations in experimental neoplastic spinal cord compression. J Neurosurgery 78:929–937, 1993
43. Blight A: Morphometric analysis of experimental spinal cord injury in the cat: Relationship of injury intensity to survival of myelinated axons. Neuroscience 19:321–341, 1986
44. Waxman SG: Demyelination in spinal cord injury. J Neurol Sci 91:1–14, 1989
45. Gledhill RF, McDonald WI: Morphological characteristics of central demyelination and remyelination: A single-fibre study. Ann Neurol 1:552–560, 1977
46. Murray PK: Functional outcome and survival in spinal cord injury secondary to neoplasia. Cancer 55:197–201, 1985
47. Siegal T, Siegal T: Current considerations in the management of neoplastic spinal cord compression. Spine 14:223–228, 1989
48. Podd TJ, Carpenter DS, Baughan CA, et al: Spinal cord compression: Prognosis and implications for treatment fractionations. Clin Oncol (R Coll Radiol) 4:341–344, 1992
49. Brice J, McKissock W: Surgical treatment of malignant extradural spinal tumors. BMJ 2:1341–2344, 1965
50. Posner JB, Howieson J, Cvitkovic E: "Disappearing" spinal cord compression: Oncolytic effect of glucocorticoids (and other chemotherapeutic agents) on epidural metastases. Ann Neurol 2:409–413, 1977
51. Siegal T, Siegal T: Surgical decompression of anterior and posterior malignant epidural tumors compressing the spinal cord: A prospective study. Neurosurgery 17:424–432, 1985
52. Vecht CHJ, Haaxma-Reiche H, van Putten WLJ, et al: Initial bolus of conventional versus high-dose dexamethasone in metastatic spinal cord compression. Neurology 39:1255–1257, 1989
53. Clarke P, Saunders M: Steroid-induced remission in spinal canal reticulum cell sarcoma. Report of two cases. J Neurosurg 42:346–348, 1975
54. Marshall LF, Langfitt TW: Combined therapy for metastatic extradural tumors of the spine. Cancer 40:2067–2070, 1977
55. Sundaresan N, Galicich HJ, Lane JM, et al: Treatment of neoplastic epidural cord compression by vertebral body resection and stabilization. J Neurosurg 63:676–684, 1985
56. Helweg-Larsen S, Rasmusson B, Sorensen PS: Recovery of gait after radiotherapy in paralytic patients with metastatic epidural spinal cord compression. Neurology 40:1234–1236, 1990
57. Hall AJ, Mackay NNS: The results of laminectomy for compression of the cord or cauda equina by extradural malignant tumors. J Bone Joint Surg Br 55B:497–505, 1973
58. Harrington KD: Anterior cord decompression and spinal stabilization for patients with metastatic lesions of the spine. J Neurosurg 61:107–117, 1984
59. Ominus M, Schraub S, Bertin D, et al: Surgical treatment of vertebral metastases. Spine 11:883–891, 1986
60. Siegal T, Siegal T: Vertebral body resection for epidural compression by malignant tumors. Results of forty-seven consecutive operative procedures. J Bone Joint Surg Am 67A:375–382, 1985
61. Moore AJ, Uttley D: Anterior decompression and stabilization of the spine in malignant disease. Neurosurgery 24:713–717, 1989
62. Sundaresan N, DiGiacinto GV, Hughes JEA, et al: Treatment of neo-

plastic spinal cord compression: Results of a prospective study. Neurosurgery 29:645–650, 1991
63. Cybulski GR: Methods of surgical stabilization for metastatic disease of the spine. Neurosurgery 25:240–252, 1989
64. Siegal T, Siegal T: Spinal epidural involvement in haematological tumors: Clinical features and therapeutic options. Leuk Lymphoma 5:101–110, 1991
65. Fadul CE, Lemann W, Thaler HT, Posner JB: Perforation of the gastrointestinal tract in patients receiving steroids for neurologic disease. Neurology 38:348–352, 1988
66. Weissman DE: Glucocorticoid treatment for brain metastases and epidural cord compression: A review. J Clin Oncol 6:543–551, 1988
67. Martenson JA, Evans RG Jr, Lie MR, et al: Treatment outcome and complications in patients treated for malignant epidural spinal cord compression. J Neurooncol 3:77–84, 1985
68. Sundaresan N, DiGiacinto GV: Antitumor and antinociceptive approaches to control cancer pain. Med Clin North Am 71:329–348, 1987
69. Slatkin NE, Posner JB: Management of spinal epidural metastases. Clin Neurosurg 30:698–716, 1982
70. Fyfe I, Henry APJ, Mulholland RC: Closed vertebral biopsy. J Bone Joint Surg Br 65B:140–143, 1983
71. Denis F: Spinal instability as defined by the three-column spine concept in acute spinal trauma. Clin Orthop 189:65–76, 1984
72. Kostuik JP, Errico JN: Differential diagnosis and surgical treatment of metastatic spine tumors, in Frymoyer JW (ed): The Adult Spine: Principles and Practice, vol 1. New York, Raven Press, 1991, pp 861–888
73. Bradford DS: Spinal instability: Orthopedic perspective and prevention. Clin Neurosurg 27:591–610, 1980
74. White AA III, Panjabi MM: Clinical Biomechanics of the Spine. Philadelphia, JB Lippincott, 1987, pp 191–276
75. McLain RF, Weinstein JN: Tumors of the spine. Semin Spine Surg 2:157–180, 1990
76. Brady LW, Antoniades J, Prasasvinichai S, et al: The treatment of metastatic disease of the nervous system by radiation therapy, in Seydel HG (ed): Tumors of the Nervous System. New York, John Wiley and Sons, 1975, pp 176–189
77. Mones RJ, Dozier D, Berrett A: Analysis of medical treatment of malignant extradural spinal cord tumors. Cancer 19:1842–1853, 1966
78. Khan FR, Glicksman AS, Chu FC, Nickson JJ: Treatment by radiotherapy of spinal cord compression due to extradural metastases. Radiology 89:495–500, 1967
79. Stark RJ, Henson RA, Evans SJW: Spinal metastases: A retrospective survey from a general hospital. Brain 105:189–213, 1982
80. Obbens EAMT, Kim J-H, Thaler H, et al: Metronidazole as a radiation enhancer in the treatment of metastatic epidural spinal cord compression. J Neurooncol 2:99–104, 1984
81. Harrison KM, Muss HB, Ball MR, et al: Spinal cord compression in breast cancer. Cancer 55:2839–2844, 1985
82. Kleinman WB, Kiernan HA, Michelsen WJ: Metastatic cancer of the spinal column. Clin Orthop 136:166–172, 1978
83. Livingston KE, Perrin RG: The neurosurgical management of spinal metastases causing cord and cauda equina compression. J Neurosurg 49:839–843, 1987
84. Baldini M, Tonnarelli GP, Princi L, et al: Neurological results in spinal cord metastases. Neurochirurgia (Stuttg) 22:159–165, 1979
85. Dunn RC, Kelly WA, Wohns RNW, Howe JF: Spinal epidural neoplasia. A 15-year review of the results of surgical therapy. J Neurosurg 52:47–51, 1980
86. Levy WJ, Latchaw JP, Hardy RW, Hahn JP: Encouraging surgical results in walking patients with epidural metastases. Neurosurgery 11:229–233, 1982
87. Klein HJ, Richter HP, Schafer M: Extradural spinal metastases. A retrospective study of 197 patients. Adv Neurosurg 12:36–43, 1984
88. Kollmann H, Diemath HE, Strohecker J, Spatz H: Spinal metastases as the first manifestation. Adv Neurosurg 12:44–46, 1984
89. Garcia-Picazo A, Ramirez PC, Rivas PP, Garcia de Sola R. Utility of surgery in the treatment of epidural vertebral metastases. Acta Neurochir (Wien) 103:131–138, 1990
90. Brunon J, Sautreaux JL, Sindau M, Fischer G: Posterior osteosynthesis in the treatment of spinal cord tumors. Neurochirurgie 21:435–446, 1975
91. Hansebout RR, Blomquist GA Jr: Acrylic spinal fusion. A 20-year clinical series and technical note. J Neurosurg 53:606–612, 1980
92. Miles J, Banks AJ, Dervin E, Noori Z: Stabilization of the spine affected by malignancy. J Neurol Neurosurg Psychiatry 47:897–904, 1984
93. DeWald RL, Bridwell KH, Prodromas C, Rodts MF: Reconstructive spinal surgery as palliation for metastatic malignancies of the spine. Spine 10:21–26, 1985
94. Overby MC, Rothman AS: Anterolateral decompression for metastatic epidural spinal cord tumors. Results of a modified costotransversectomy approach. J Neurosurg 62:344–348, 1985
95. Solini A, Paschero B, Orsini G, Guercio N: The surgical treatment of metastatic tumors of the lumbar spine. Ital J Orthop Traumatol 11:427–442, 1985
96. Heller M, McBroom RJ, MacNab T, Perrin R: Treatment of metastatic disease of the spine with posterolateral decompression and Luque instrumentation. Neuroorthopedics 2:70–74, 1986
97. Sherman RPM, Waddell JP: Laminectomy for metastatic epidural spinal tumors. Posterior stabilization, radiotherapy and postoperative assessment. Clin Orthop 207:55–63, 1986
98. Perrin RG, McBroom RJ: Anterior versus posterior decompression for symptomatic spinal metastases. Can J Neurol Sci 14:75–80, 1987
99. Fidler MW: Posterior instrumentation of the spine. An experimental comparison of various possible techniques. Spine 11:367–372, 1986
100. Merrin C, Avellanosa A, West C, et al: The value of palliative spinal surgery in metastatic urogenital tumors. J Urol 115:712–713, 1976
101. Gianotta SL, Kindt GW: Metastatic spinal cord tumors. Clin Neurosurg 25:495–503, 1978
102. Gorter K: Results of laminectomy in spinal cord compression due to tumors. Acta Neurochir (Wien) 42:177–178, 1978
103. Shimizu K, Shikata J, Lida H, et al: Posterior decompression and stabilization for multiple metastatic tumors of the spine. Spine 17:1400–1404, 1992

CHAPTER 163

Surgical Management of Spinal Cord Tumors and Arteriovenous Malformations

Kalmon D. Post
Bennett M. Stein

INTRAMEDULLARY SPINAL CORD TUMORS

Although von Eiselsberg totally excised a neurofibrosarcoma from the spinal cord in 1907 and Cushing operated on an 8-year-old child and completely removed an intramedullary ependymoma extending from C1 to T2 in 1924,[1] the first well-documented surgical effort to remove an intramedullary tumor was reported by Elsberg[2] in 1925. Of the 13 tumors he reported on, 3 were totally removed and the remainder were partially removed. Elsberg stressed that because some of these tumors were infiltrating, they defied removal; nevertheless, he emphasized that the surgeon must search out those tumors with well-defined cleavage planes that permit total removal of the neoplasm. Considering his lack of magnification techniques and previous surgical experience with such tumors, these results were remarkable. When a definitive plane between the tumor and the spinal cord was not visible, Elsberg proposed a second operation in which the tumor might present through the myelotomy, making total removal possible. Later, Matson[3] also advocated this technique. With the exception of these reports, little experience with two-stage removal has been published. Following Elsberg's early reports, others[1, 3–9] have described successful removal of intramedullary tumors. Successful surgical removal of these tumors was mounted on a firm foundation when Greenwood[5] presented his experience with 10 intramedullary tumors, primarily ependymomas, which he totally removed with no deaths. These results, with useful survival, justified his enthusiasm for an aggressive surgical approach to these lesions. He also emphasized the use of magnification techniques and microsurgical instrumentation.

Guidetti[6] published his experience with a large group of intramedullary tumors and noted the difficulty in totally removing astrocytomas. In the presence of intramedullary ependymomas and other tumors, however, he believed that every effort should be made to achieve total removal, although only a line of cleavage between the normal spinal cord and the tumor would make this possible. Once a cleavage was established, gentle dissection separated the tumor from the normal spinal cord on each side; then the tumor could be lifted carefully by one end and slowly removed from its bed. Blood vessels were severed close to the tumor by bipolar cautery with irrigation. Guidetti achieved an overall total removal of 24 of 71 tumors, representing a wide variety of histologic types, with a 10 percent operative mortality.

In the famous case of Horrax and Henderson,[7] an intramedullary ependymoma extending the entire length of the spinal cord was totally enucleated during a series of operations, resulting in recovery and long-term survival.

Our series comprises 40 cases of intramedullary tumor.[4, 10] A range of histology is represented, with astrocytoma and ependymoma the most common tumors and teratomatous types less common. No lipomas are included in this group.

Some patients had undergone previous treatment, including decompressive laminectomy, tapping of cysts associated with the tumors, and radiotherapy. The effects of treatment other than total removal are difficult to evaluate. It is clear, however, that the degree of neurologic deficit caused by the disease process before surgery often determined the postoperative result.

CLINICAL PRESENTATION

Although intramedullary tumors occur most commonly in adults,[2, 4–6, 10] a significant incidence has been reported in children.[3, 11, 12] The symptomatology in the two age groups is similar. It is quite amazing at times to see an extensive tumor filling the majority of the intramedullary space yet causing few symptoms. Often, however, an endpoint is reached when compensatory ability fails, and marked neurologic deterioration occurs rapidly. Persistent pain involving the dorsal root dermatomes in the area of tumor involvement is often the signature of an intramedullary neoplasm. Dysfunction of the posterior column may occur in a progressive fashion, with sensory dysesthesias in the arms, torso, and legs, depending on the site of the intraspinal neoplasm. Sacral sparing may or may not be present and is not an invariable finding with intramedullary neoplasms. Lower motor neuron symptomatology and signs usually occur at the level of the tumor. Well-defined central cord syndromes, as seen in syringomyelia, with disassociated sensory loss and the classic signs of anterior horn cell involvement, may be lacking. Children often have a scoliosis. The symptomatology generally is progressive with few remissions or exacerbations. Symptoms are usually bilateral, but in rare instances, neurologic abnormalities are confined to one extremity. The duration of symptoms generally is measured in years, although some neoplasms may have histories of 6 months or less.

DIAGNOSTIC EVALUATION

The radiologic demonstration of intramedullary tumors depended on myelography with either iohexal, a nonionic water-soluble agent, or iophendylate.[13] A fusiform dilatation of the cord in the region of the tumor usually was seen, but a complete block was not generally present (Fig. 163–1). If a block was present, dye was also instilled from the opposite end of the spinal canal to define the complete extent of the tumor. Since the introduction of water-soluble contrast agents, radiologic definition has been significantly improved. Dilated venous channels at the caudal aspects of small intramedullary tumors may suggest the differential diagnosis of a vascular malformation. Making this distinction is rarely a problem, and spinal angiography has not been of diagnostic value except for the identification of an intramedullary hemangioblastoma. The exception is the intramedullary arteriovenous malformation (AVM), which can mimic a vascular intramedullary tumor.

Routine computed tomographic (CT) scanning of the spinal canal has not been of practical use in the diagnosis of these neoplasms. We have retrospectively scanned a number of patients with large tumors and failed to visualize the tumors. CT scanning with water-soluble contrast agents aids in the diagnosis of a wide spinal canal. It also assists in the definitive diagnosis of syringomyelia. CT scanning has shown metrizamide leaking into the fluid within a syrinx,[14, 15] particularly with a 6-hour delayed scan. The use of magnetic resonance imaging (MRI) has facilitated the localization of tumors and the identification of cysts (Fig. 163–2). It relies on a quiescent patient and will fail to define these lesions if there is movement. The thoracic region has been particularly difficult. A presurgical histologic diagnosis of the lesion cannot be made from MRI scans, other than the fact that it may or may not be associated with a cyst. Manipulation of different pulse sequences and additional surface coils may improve tumor characterization.

Angiography has been carried out in the presence of dilated vessels and has been helpful in the diagnosis of hemangioblastoma and AVMs.[9] A point should be made here about radiologic changes that appear to be unique to the hemangioblastoma. We have observed, in four or five cases of hemangioblastoma, extensive widening of the spinal cord in either direction from the primary lesion, which in these cases has been discrete and confined to one or two spinal segments. At operation, we have not been able to define the nature of this widening as seen on myelograms. It does not appear to be due to a cyst extending from the tumor or to multiple hemangioblastomas. We have been perplexed as to the nature of the widening and assume it is due to congestion and edema of adjacent spinal cord secondary to the high vascularity of these lesions. Follow-up myelography done in two of these cases shows that the spinal cord has returned to normal size following removal of the primary lesion.

Percutaneous cord puncture and myelocystography have been reported[16] and were performed once in our series. This patient underwent percutaneous puncture to distinguish a cord tumor from a syrinx rather than for relief of symptoms.

SURGICAL PATHOLOGY

Intramedullary spinal cord tumors account for one third of primary intraspinal neoplasms.[2, 6, 8, 10] Astrocytomas and ependymomas constitute the largest group of intramedullary tumors and occur with about equal frequency. They are generally low grade and extend over many segments of the spinal cord. Astrocytomas most commonly appear in the cervical and thoracic regions of the spinal cord, whereas ependymomas have a higher incidence in the caudal regions because of their prevalence in the conus medullaris and filum terminale.[17]

Tumors that occur less commonly include dermoids, epidermoids, teratomas, oligodendrogliomas, hemangioblastomas, and either primary or metastatic malignant tumors. Lipomas, common in children, have different growth patterns and therapeutic implications and are not discussed further.

Intramedullary ependymomas often have a distinct plane between the neoplasm and spinal cord tissue. These tumors generally are soft and solid and have a pseudocapsule. They are not highly vascular and may have necrotic areas. Astrocytomas usually are infiltrative with an ill-defined margin between the neoplasm and the normal spinal cord tissue. Where a well-defined margin between the neoplasm and the normal spinal cord exists, a pseudocapsule is found. This variety is similar to cerebellar astrocytoma, which has a uniformly soft consistency and minimal vascularity sometimes associated with cysts containing yellow fluid high in protein.

At times, astrocytomas may appear to have a plane between the tumor and the normal cord tissue, yet pathologically they demonstrate infiltration (Fig. 163–3). The pathologic grade may also vary in different parts of the tumor, just as it does within brain tumors. Astrocytomas and ependymomas produce a fusiform enlargement of the spinal cord, often without any indication of their presence on the surface of the cord other than an occasional dilated vein at the caudal end of the tumor. In some cases, the dorsal surface of the cord will be so thin that it will be transparent. Glioblastomas produce a discoloration of the cord and are associated with a plethora of enlarged arterialized veins and obvious feeding arteries. Ependymomas of the conus or filum terminal region often grow in an exophytic fashion from the intramedullary locus into the cauda equina, displacing and sometimes adhering to the nerve roots. Because of the expanding nature of these neoplasms, structural changes in the osseous spinal canal may be produced.

Teratomas and dermoid tumors have varying amounts of grumous material in their central portions, are commonly variegated, and have a capsule that is adherent to the surrounding spinal cord tissue; often there is a pedicle of fibrous tract involving the dura and overlying bone and soft tissues. Radiographic defects may be present in the overlying bone if a fibrous tract is present.

Intramedullary tumors receive their blood supply from perforating branches of the anterior spinal artery that enter the ventral aspect of the tumor. These vessels are small and are

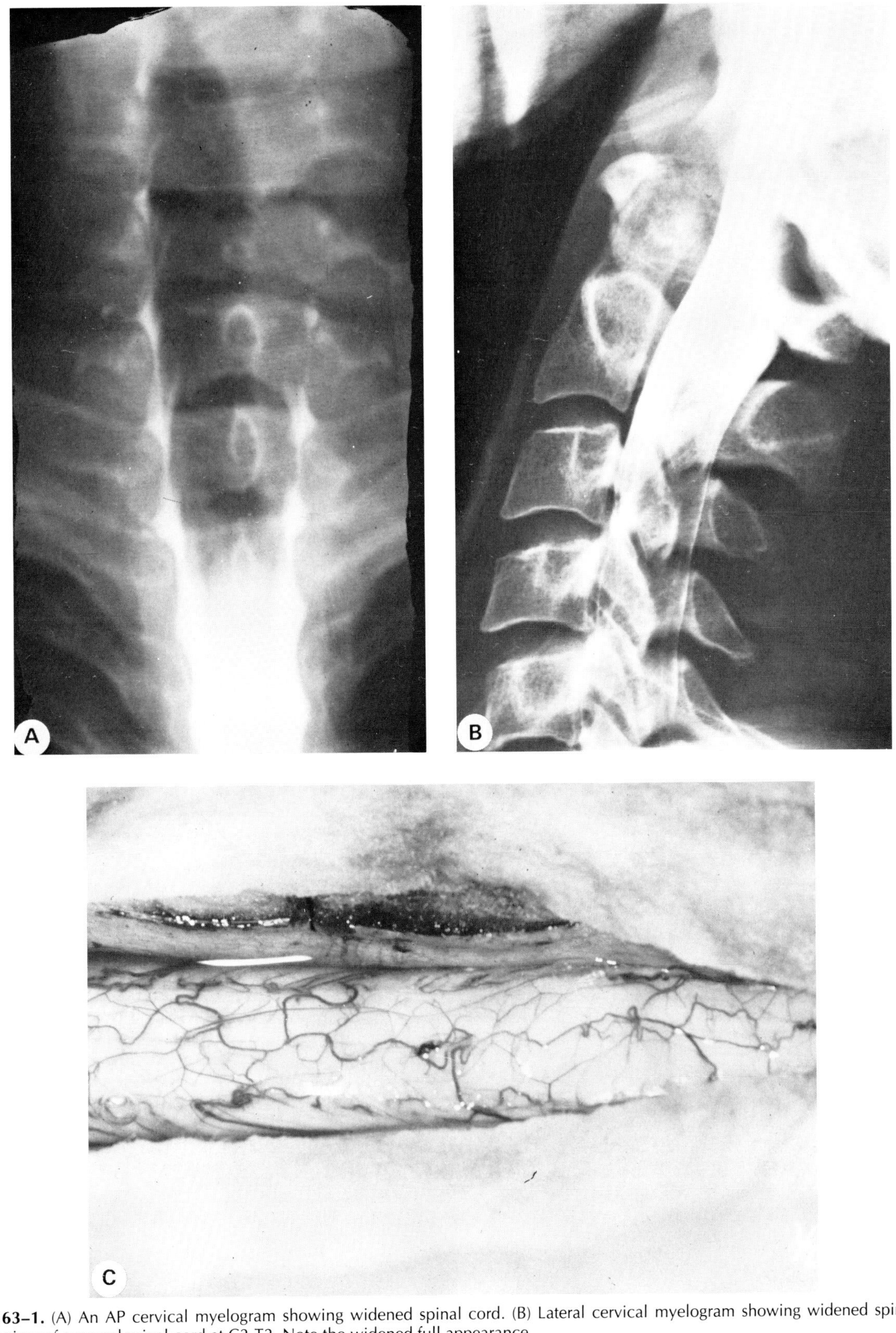

FIGURE 163–1. (A) An AP cervical myelogram showing widened spinal cord. (B) Lateral cervical myelogram showing widened spinal cord. (C) Operative view of exposed spinal cord at C2-T2. Note the widened full appearance.

Illustration continued on following page

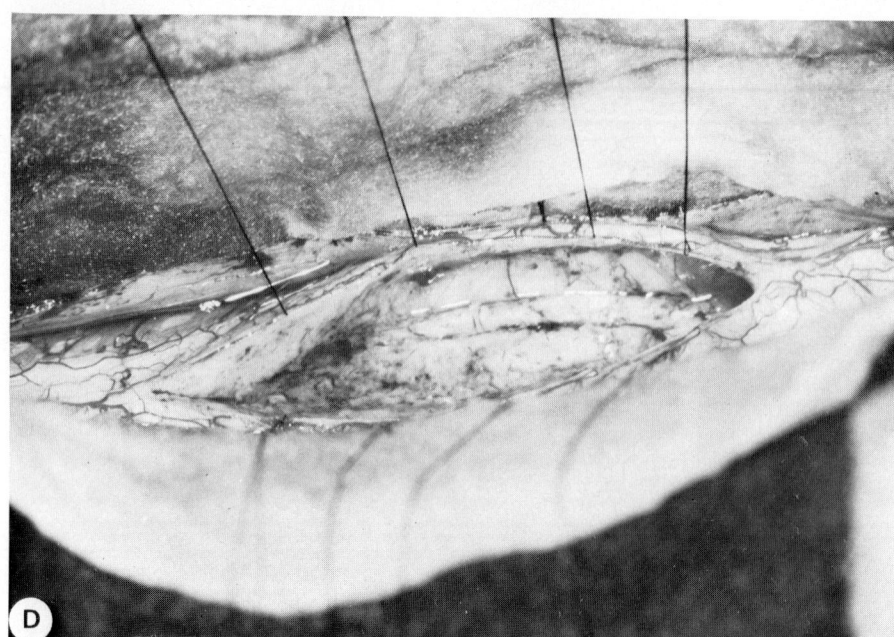

FIGURE 163–1 Continued (D) Operative view of spinal cord after cystic ependymoma was removed.

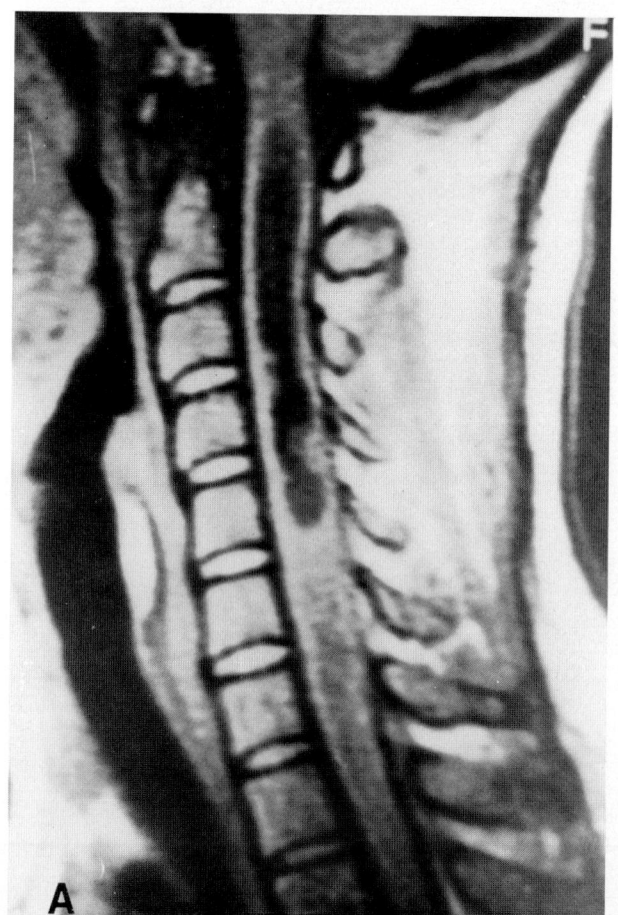
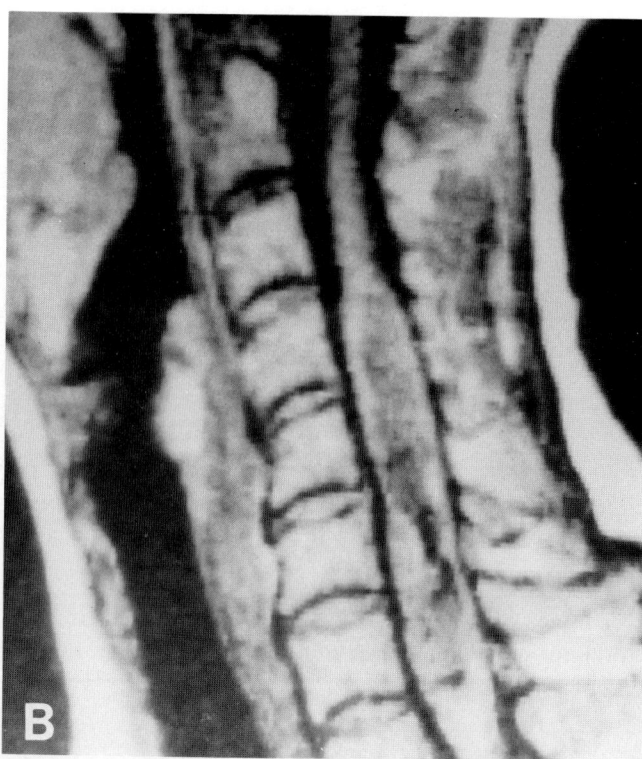

FIGURE 163–2. (A) Sagittal MRI scan demonstrating cyst within the cervical spinal cord and a mural hemangioblastoma at the C4-5 level. (B) Sagittal MRI scan demonstrating a wide cervical spinal cord with an intramedullary tumor.

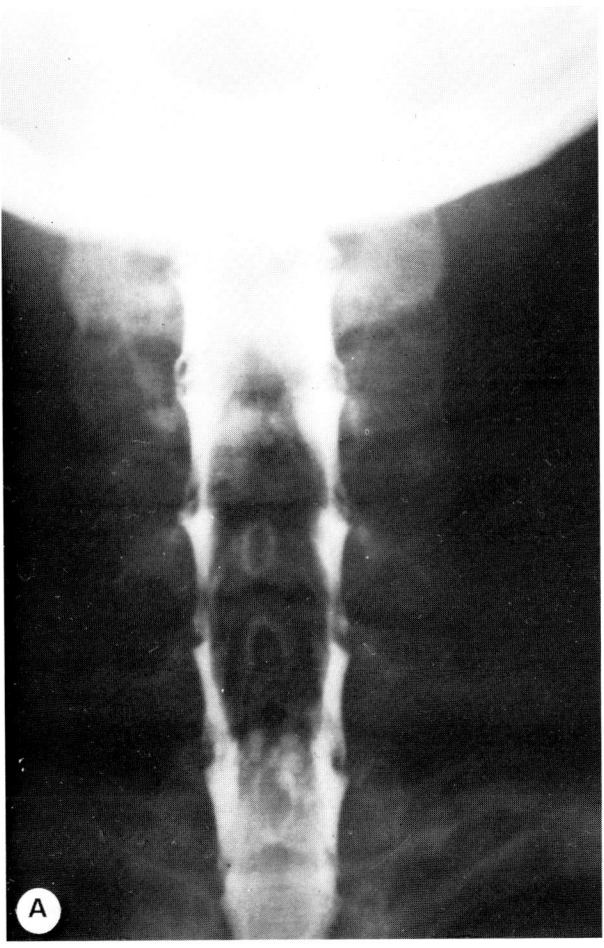
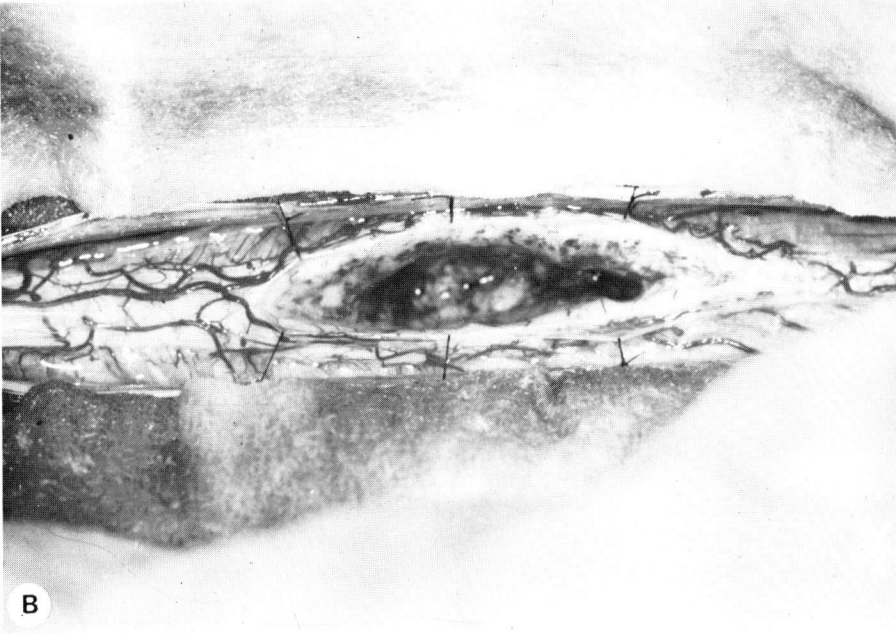

FIGURE 163-3. (A) AP view of cervical myelogram showing widened spinal cord. (B) Operative view of exposed spinal cord during first operation.
Illustration continued on following page

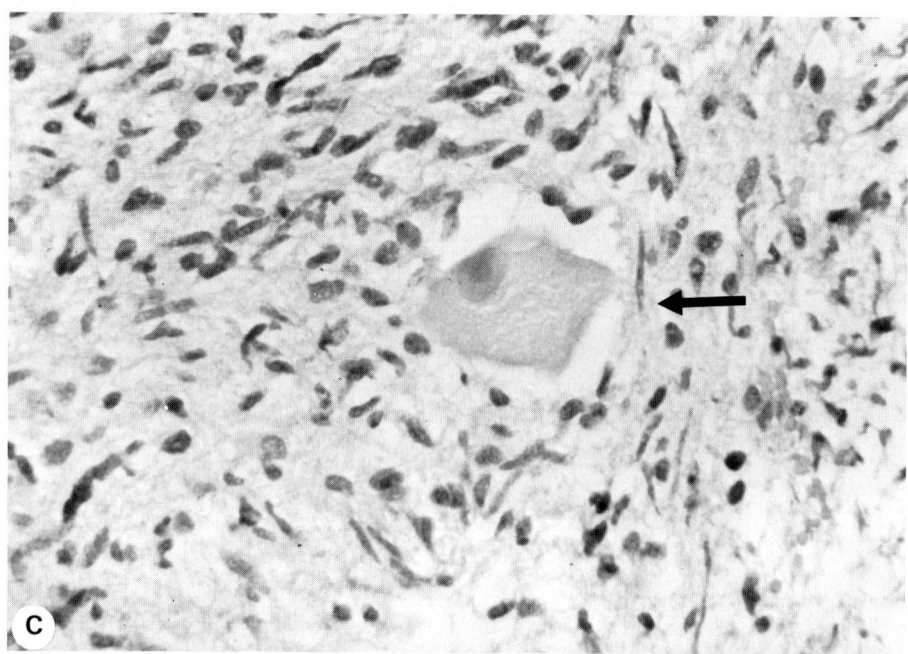

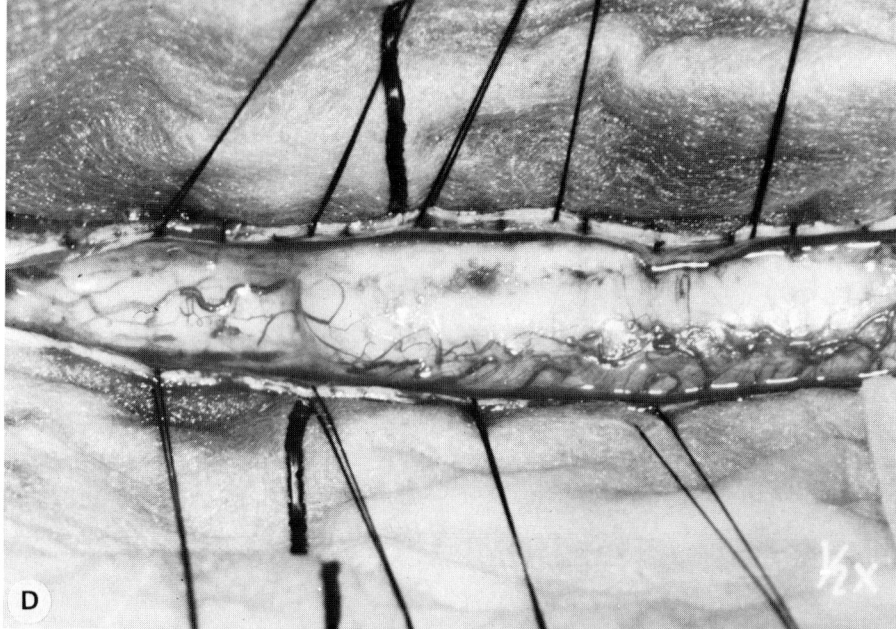

FIGURE 163–3 *Continued* (C) Microscopic picture of tissue removed during first operation. Pathology was mixed ependymoma-astrocytoma grade II. Note invasion with the tumor surrounding a neuron. (D) Operative view of exposed spinal cord during second operation. Note extreme fullness of spinal cord.

not associated with a high degree of vascularity within the tumor. Small vessels also enter the tumor from the dorsal and lateral positions of the spinal cord. The tumors tend to be eccentric and located in the more dorsal portion of the spinal cord. Invariably, there is a thin layer of compressed spinal cord tissue overlying the dorsal surface of these tumors, which rarely present directly on the surface of the cord.

In our series, 80 percent of the tumors were divided almost equally between astrocytoma and ependymoma.[10] Fortunately, only three of the astrocytomas were glioblastoma. There were five cases of hemangioblastomas, a relatively rare intramedullary tumor. Four of the hemangioblastomas involved the cervical thoracic region, and one involved the thoracolumbar region. Teratomas generally occurred in the lumbosacral region. A cavernous malformation occupied the lumbar region and gave rise to a 21-year history. A rare intramedullary pigmented neurofibroma, extending from the mid-cervical region to the obex of the medulla was successfully removed from an elderly patient.

SURGICAL TECHNIQUE

Turnbull[1] stated: "A surgeon exploring a spinal cord for a suspected intramedullary tumor must be prepared to face a formidable problem and also have the courage of conviction to make every attempt to remove the tumor. Anything less than this, with a cursory inspection of the spinal cord or aspiration thereof, can only create problems of a more com-

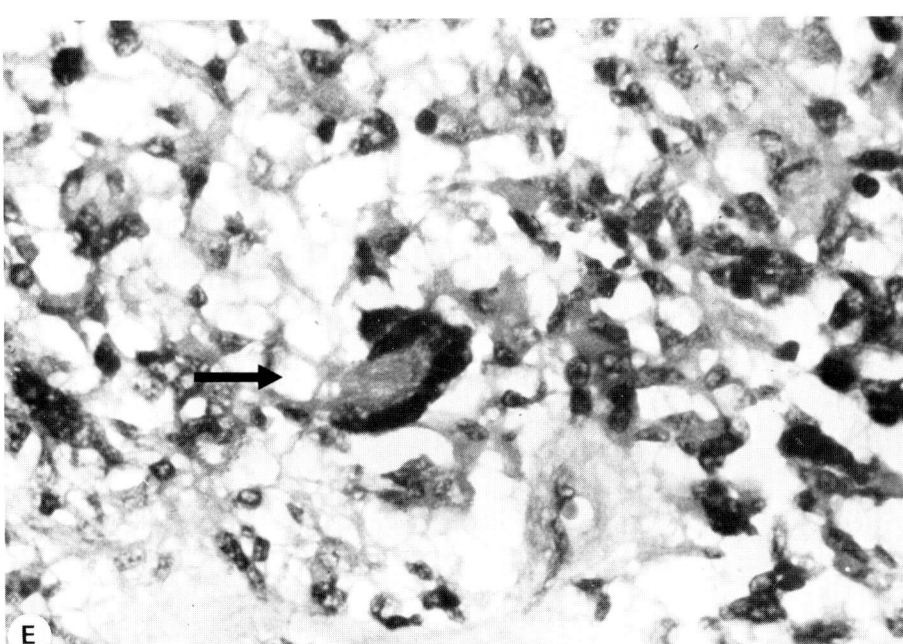

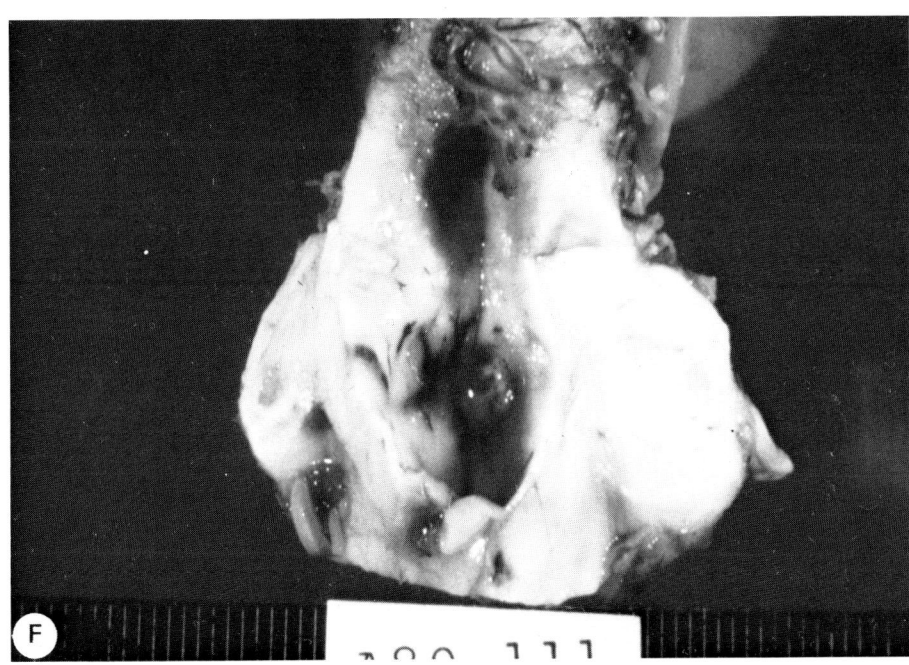

FIGURE 163–3 *Continued* (E) Microscopic picture of tissue removed during second operation. Pathology was glioblastoma. Note giant cell. (F) Pathologic specimen, postmortem. Note metastatic nodules along the floor of the fourth ventricle.

plex nature for the subsequent surgical effort to remove such tumors."

Surgery is the primary treatment for intramedullary tumors. Radiotherapy has little to offer even for malignant tumors.[10, 12, 17, 18] Surgery should be planned as soon as possible after diagnosis. There is nothing to be gained by allowing the tumor growth to devastate the patient while withholding surgery. The surgical results are generally predicated on the preoperative condition of the patient, no matter how large the tumor. If the patient preoperatively has minimal neurologic findings, then the postoperative course should be gratifying, especially if the tumor can be resected in toto. Those patients who arrive for surgery in a wheelchair or with severe paralysis or sensory loss may regain little of this function even after a successful operation.

The prone position is generally used now for all intramedullary cord tumors, although early in our experience, the sitting position was used for some cervical cord cases. The prone position is preferred because it decreases the potential for vasomotor collapse, which can be significant when the autonomic pathways are compromised by the tumor or surgery; this position also allows the assistant to take a more active role in the operation, providing traction, irrigation, or assistance with the dissection.

All operations are carried out with evoked potential monitoring of dorsal column function. This has been of some use in guiding the operation, although we prefer to rely on observations through the operating microscope as to the extent of dissection. In the future, we hope to utilize with greater efficiency recordings from the corticospinal tract. General anesthesia with endotracheal intubation is always used, and the endotracheal tube is commonly left in place for 24 to 48 hours after surgery on more extensive cervical intramedullary tumors.

The full extent of the tumor must be known before the operation. This usually is demonstrated on a myelogram, often taken from above as well as from below. In the case of a suspected hemangioblastoma, the vasculature should be demonstrated by arteriography to aid in the surgical removal. A wide laminectomy then is performed over the entire extent of the tumor, extending to levels above and below it. The dura must be opened carefully, because the pia-arachnoid of the enlarged spinal cord often adheres to the underside of the dura. It is important to prevent any injury to the cord vasculature; hemorrhage during this phase of the operation would otherwise obscure all landmarks and significantly compromise the surgical effort. In a patient who has undergone previous surgery, particularly if the dura has been left open, this early dissection is tedious, but care must be taken to reestablish all anatomic landmarks. In our patients with and without previous surgery, the initial appearances of the cords generally were similar; the cords appeared widened, often

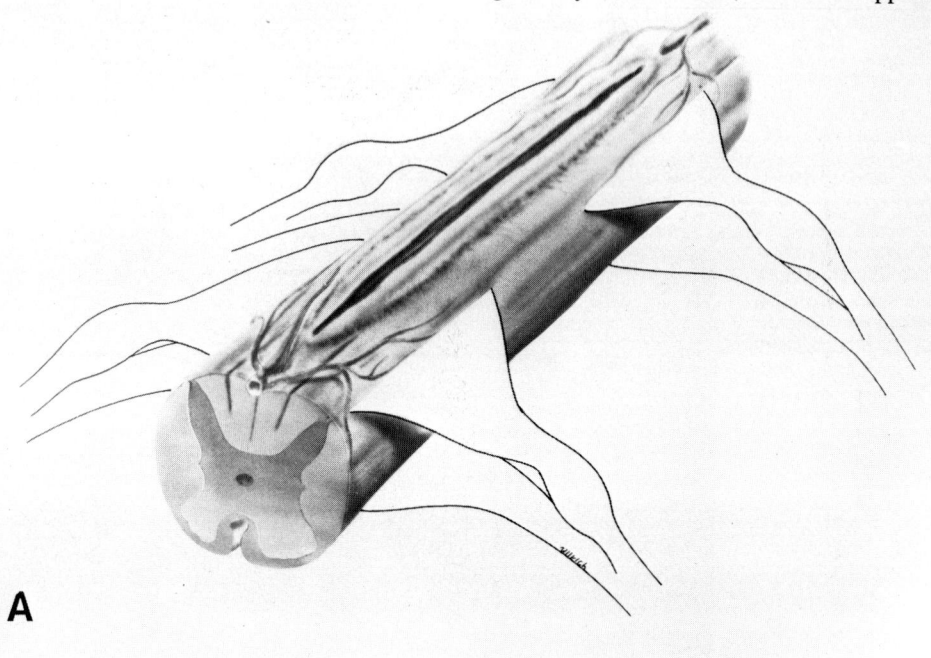

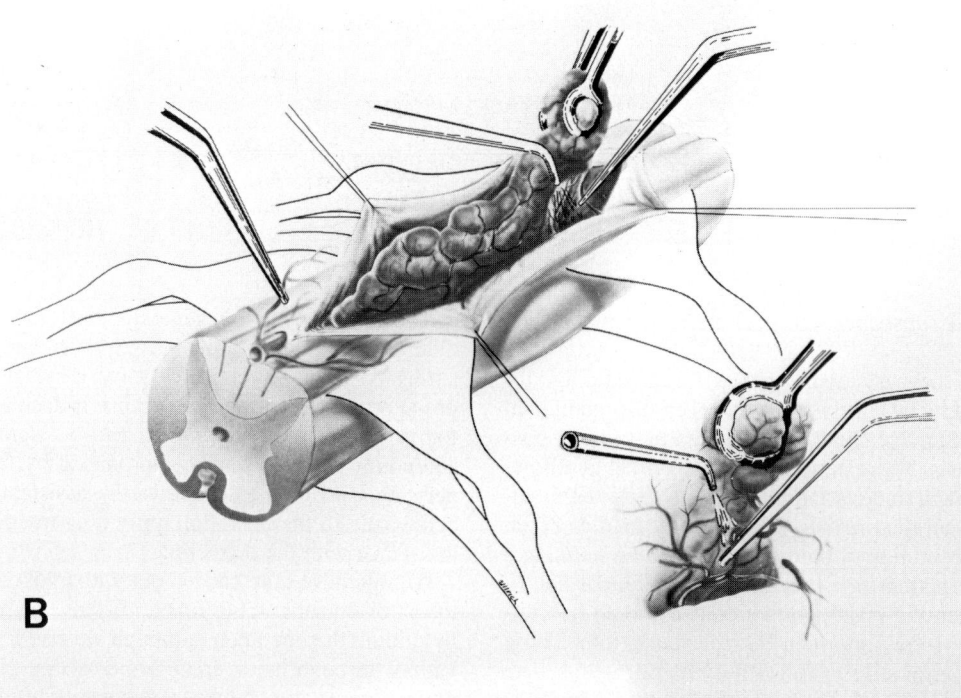

FIGURE 163–4. (A) Myelotomy over an intramedullary tumor. (B) Removal of an intramedullary tumor.

without evidence of tumor on the surface. The widening of the spinal cord and the presence of dilated veins at the caudal end of the tumor site were indications of the underlying pathologic process. When observing a widened spinal cord, the surgeon must not be misled in those rare instances of anterior extramedullary lesion in which the cord is splayed out over the lesion.[19]

The dorsal surface of the cord at the area of greatest enlargement then is inspected for the site of the myelotomy. Generally, myelotomies are performed in the midline with a preference for the thinnest and most avascular areas; at times, however, it is more expeditious to use a paramedian approach (Fig. 163–4).

Some of the vasculature must be sacrificed during this myelotomy. An initial incision of approximately 1 to 2 cm is performed over the greatest enlargement of the spinal cord to evaluate the plane between the tumor and the spinal cord tissue. In some instances, the presence of a cyst associated with the tumor may be easily noted; if so, additional room may be gained by aspirating some of the cystic contents through a small-bore needle. To facilitate dissection, however, these cysts should not be completely evacuated. Once it is determined that the neoplasm is cystic or has well-defined planes, the myelotomy is lengthened over the extent of the tumor. With a teratoma, a stalk between the cord and the dura should be removed as an integral part of the lesion. With an ependymoma extending from the conus, the extra-axial portion in the cauda equina may be removed first, to provide adequate decompression and visualization of the residual tumor involving the intramedullary portion of the conus. The draining veins of intramedullary hemangioblastomas must be left to the latter part of the surgical resection.

Following the myelotomy, 6-0 or 7-0 traction sutures are placed through the pial margins on either side to expose the interior of the spinal cord (Fig. 163–4). Generally, the tumor is visible a few millimeters under the dorsal surface of the spinal cord. There is often a soft gliotic interface between the tumor and the spinal cord proper. With the operating microscope and microsurgical techniques, using bipolar cautery, small suction tubes, and various dissectors, a plane is developed around the margin of the tumor, with care being taken to retract primarily on the tumor and not on the spinal cord. The surgeon works to one or the other end of the tumor. At the pole where the tumor is the narrowest, it may be possible to grasp the end and gently extract it from the interior of the cord. All the fine vascular adhesions to the spinal cord, especially on the ventral aspect of the tumor, should be cauterized with bipolar cautery and sharply divided. No blunt dissection should be carried out in areas where vascular channels connect the tumor to the spinal cord. Most tumors are amazingly avascular and present no threat of hemorrhage or the loss of control of large blood vessels. It is important to keep the operative field meticulously dry so that the plane between the tumor and the spinal cord may be readily identified (Fig. 163–4).

If the tumor is too large to remove in toto or necessitates too much retraction on the spinal cord, its interior may be decompressed. We prefer to use the CUSA unit (Cavitron ultrasonic surgical aspirator; Cooper Medical, Stamford, Conn) to debulk the tumor, facilitating dissection around its capsule and its removal. This maneuver has a minor disadvantage of spilling the contents of the tumor into the dissection plane or obscuring the dissection plane by bleeding. In most instances, however, the tumors are relatively avascular and bleeding is not a major problem even with the use of the CUSA. Gradually, the entire tumor may be removed. For those tumors (usually astrocytomas) that are infiltrating, a debulking procedure is valuable, especially in children. The CO_2 and argon lasers have also been utilized for this maneuver.[20]

Cystic collections at the margins of the tumor, as in the case of astrocytomas, facilitate the tumor resection. We make

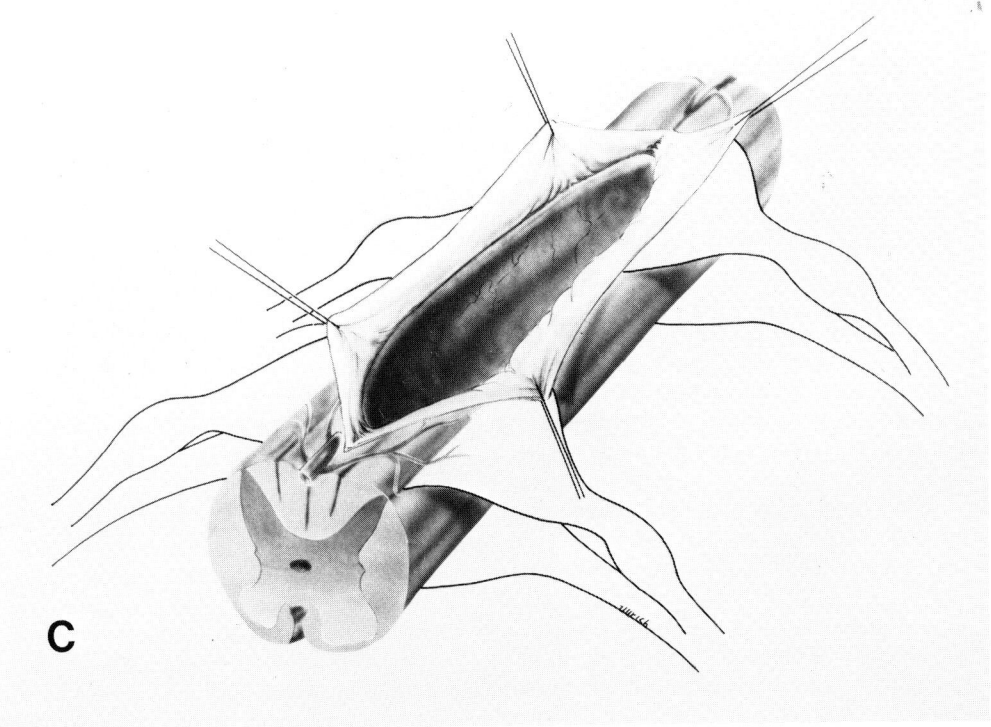

FIGURE 163–4 *Continued* (C) The open cord after removal of an intramedullary tumor.

no attempt, however, to remove the wall of the cyst, which is thin and nonneoplastic. If there is any doubt about the totality of removal, small biopsy specimens may be obtained from the margin of the resection and evaluated by frozen section during surgery. In most instances, the margins are well defined and there is no question about the removal of the tumor (see Figs. 163–4 and 163–6). Malignant tumors such as the glioblastoma respond poorly to surgery and do not appear to respond to radiation therapy; these are usually hopeless cases.

In children, the syndrome of holospinal cord widening is associated with extensive astrocytomas or localized astrocytomas and extensive cysts.[12] Here we must localize the tumor through either clinical or radiologic evaluation and remove it while only draining the cyst. A subtotal radical removal with the CUSA or laser appears to pay dividends in such children with long-term remission of the disease process. Although these astrocytomas are histologically identical to those in adults, they may have different growth behavior related more to the child's development than to the histologic appearance.

Special attention is given to the removal of hemangioblastomas. These are highly vascular tumors, and if they are decompressed or cut into, the bleeding not only will obscure the anatomic planes but also may result in catastrophic problems. Therefore, even in large hemangioblastomas, we work around the margin of the tumor, interrupting the feeding arteries and finally the primary draining vein as the tumor is rolled out on the last venous pedicle. Often these tumors are associated with a cyst, facilitating their removal. They are identified by their characteristic orange-red appearance and in all instances extrude from the pial surface. Their presence is also identified by large dilated arterialized veins that often surround them. This will mimic an AVM on the myelogram and occasionally on spinal angiography. In some instances, hemangioblastomas may be multiple, and additional tumors may be removed if they are accessible. In rare instances, they are associated with cranial tumors or the von Hippel–Lindau syndrome.

In cases in which the tumor has been treated with radiation previously, we have noted intense intramedullary gliosis on biopsy, distinctly separate from the margin of the tumor, usually at the caudal or rostral interface. It is assumed that the gliosis is an adverse effect of preoperative radiation. Previous surgery with aspiration of a cyst but without definitive removal of the intramedullary tumor has provided transient benefits and allowed for reaccumulation of the cyst fluid.

In teratomas, the border of the tumor, although well defined, may be densely adherent to the surrounding spinal cord. Every attempt should be made to remove this capsule, which is a potential source of regrowth. There may be extensive involvement of central areas of the spinal cord, and the tumors may extend from the posterior to the anterior surface. Teratomatous tumors also may have a dumbbell configuration within the substance of the spinal cord, and the surgeon must be careful not to miss satellite portions of the primary tumor.

When the margins of the cord are allowed to fall back into position, the remarkable decompressive effect of tumor removal is quite apparent. The dorsal columns are often thin to the point of being transparent. If there has been minimal retraction on the cord, these fiber tracts function in a satisfactory way and will show progressive functional recovery. Rarely has the function of the spinal cord been made permanently worse by this dissection. Gentleness of dissection may be gauged by the vascular pattern on the dorsal surface of the cord at the completion of tumor resection. Distended veins that were present before removal, usually at the caudal end of the tumor on the surface of the spinal cord, will not be less prominent. No attempt has been made to sew the pial surfaces of the spinal cord together. The dura is closed in a watertight fashion; it is rarely necessary to use a fascial graft except in those cases in which the dura was left open after previous surgery. If total removal of an intramedullary tumor is not feasible, the dura should be reconstructed, preferably with a fascial graft, to facilitate subsequent surgical endeavors.

The most important factor determining the ease of the operation is the presence and nature of previous operations. In patients who have had previous surgery and in whom the dura mater was left open, the initial exposure of the tumor and the dissection of adjacent tissues from the spinal cord have prolonged the operation and made exposure more difficult. In those cases in which radiation was administered previously, gliotic areas in the dorsocentral portion of the spinal cord have been verified by biopsy. There have been no histologic changes in the tumor that were attributed to radiation. Similarly, none of the tumors previously irradiated showed malignant changes. Problems with wound healing also were encountered frequently in those cases in which radiotherapy was used previously.

POSTOPERATIVE TREATMENT

Steroids are routinely used preoperatively and postoperatively in high doses (dexamethasone, 10–20 mg IV q4h) with a slow taper depending on the neurologic condition. Prophylactic antibiotics are used intraoperatively and for 48 hours postoperatively. If the operation involved extensive areas of the cervical region, the endotracheal tube is left in place for at least 24 hours, regardless of the patient's condition at the termination of surgery.

Radiation therapy is considered postoperatively for children with astrocytomas, but we generally defer such therapy in adults and consider re-operation if the tumors recur.

Careful orthopedic follow-up and possible bracing are necessary for the pediatric patients.

RESULTS

Removal of large intramedullary tumors can be performed with a fair degree of safety (Table 163–1) and can offer significant neurologic improvement in many situations. Generally, those patients with only mild to moderate neurologic deficit before surgery did extremely well, regardless of the size of the tumor. The total removal of these tumors offers a much improved outlook for patients whose tumors show no response to previous decompressive laminectomy and radiotherapy. Our follow-up in the astrocytoma and ependymoma group has been too short to draw definite conclusions regarding a recurrence rate, although many patients have lived 5 years or more postoperatively without evidence of recur-

Table 163–1. INTRAMEDULLARY SPINAL CORD TUMORS*

Case No.	Patient Age	Location of Tumor	Histology	Extent of Removal	Result	Follow-Up
1	26	C	Ependymoma	T	I	3 mos.
2	24	Conus	Ependymoma	T	I	1½ yrs.
3	49	C	Ependymoma	T	I	5 yrs.
4	28	C-D	Ependymoma	T	S	4½ yrs.
5	38	C	Ependymoma	T	S	4½ yrs.
6	45	Conus	Ependymoma	T	S	2 yrs.
7	35	Conus	Ependymoma	T	S	2 yrs.
8	20	Conus	Ependymoma	T	S	2 yrs.
9	35	C	Ependymoma	T	I	1½ yrs.
10	12	C	Astrocytoma	P	S	6 mos.
11	60	C-D	Astrocytoma	90%	S	6 yrs.
12	13	D-L	Astrocytoma	T	S	4 yrs.
13	3	C-D	Astrocytoma	95%	I	4 yrs.
14	48	C	Astrocytoma	T	I	4½ yrs.
15	38	C	Astrocytoma	T	I	5 yrs.
16	7	C	Astrocytoma	T	I	1½ yrs.
17	5	C-D-L-S	Astrocytoma	50%	S	1 yr.
18	14	C	Malignant glioma	P	W	1 yr. (died)
19	20	C	Malignant glioma	P	W	6 mos. (died)
20	13	D	Teratoma	T	I	4½ yrs.
21	12	Conus	Dermoid	T	I	11 yrs.
22	4 mos.	Conus	Epidermoid	T	I	11 yrs.
23	28	D-L	Mixed	P	W	2 yrs.
24	52	D	Metastatic	P	S	1 mo. (died)
25	57	C	Hemangioblastoma	T	I	2 mos.

*C = cervical; D = dorsal; L = lumbar; T = total; P = partial; I = improved; S = same; W = worse.

rence. Experience would indicate that the recurrence rate should be low following total removal.[2, 5, 7, 8, 21, 22]

CASE REPORT

A 35-year-old woman was asymptomatic until 6 months before admission, when she developed sharp pains radiating around the right breast as well as progressive numbness in a suspended pattern over the right side from the nipple line to the umbilicus level. Subsequently, she developed numbness in the right V2 distribution as well as around the shoulders. Minimal weakness was present in the upper arms.

Examination showed hypalgesia in the right V1 and V2 distribution. Strength was uniformly good except for minimal weakness of the left biceps muscles. Sensory examination showed a marked suspended sensory level loss from T1 to T8 with a lesser loss extending up to C2. Posterior column function was good. Reflexes were decreased in the left biceps but slightly increased in the lower extremities. Babinski signs were absent.

Myelography demonstrated a widened cord extending from T2 to C2 (see Fig. 163–1). Subsequently, a laminectomy from C2 through T2 was performed, with myelotomy and total removal of a cystic ependymoma (Fig. 163–1). Follow-up examination at 4½ years postoperatively showed the patient to be functioning extremely well at home. She noted some numbness under the right breast and tingling in her left fingers. Examination showed full muscle power with a decreased left biceps and triceps reflex. Joint position sense and vibratory sensation were decreased in the lower extremities but normal in the uppers.

Radicular pain in the distribution of the nerve roots associated with the tumor has been a distressing postoperative problem. This pain has a burning quality, severely disturbing to the patient and extremely difficult to control. Derangement of the physiologic pathways for pain at the dorsal route entry zone has been postulated as the cause. Unfortunately, we have not had satisfactory results in the treatment of such postoperative dysesthetic or pain syndromes.

Our experience[4, 10] and that of others[5, 6] indicate that a decompressive laminectomy, whether or not a tumor cyst has been evacuated, and with or without radiotherapy, has had little beneficial effect on the course of most intramedullary spinal cord tumors. Some reviews[6, 23] of the effects of radiation on these tumors are clouded by incomplete knowledge of the pathology, the natural course of these tumors, and the number of associated variables, including decompression and partial surgical removals.

One report by Schwade and colleagues[24] retrospectively reviewed 34 cases, 25 of which had confirmed histology. They recommended conservative surgery to remove as much tumor as safely possible. Postoperative radiation therapy was given, at 4500 to 5000 rad in 5 to 6 weeks, through portals that cover the tumor generously. All 12 patients with ependymomas were alive without recurrence after a minimum follow-up of 3 years. Five of 6 patients with low-grade astrocytomas survived longer than 3 years. Although these results are encouraging, longer follow-up may be needed to evaluate this fully. In most reports, there has been little objective follow-up evaluation of reduction in tumor size following radiation therapy. A significant number of reports indicate that surgical removal is the treatment of choice.[3–6, 8–12] Improvement in the patient's condition or at least an arrest of the neurologic deterioration may be anticipated in most cases following surgery. Postoperative result is determined by the degree of preoperative neurologic involvement. Many surgeons have reported difficulty in totally removing astrocytomas. In our series, we were able to totally remove about half the astrocytomas with no more significant problems than those encountered in the removal of ependymomas.

Through the use of microsurgical techniques and strict attention to postoperative pulmonary function, negligible mortality and morbidity rates can be expected, even with removal of extensive tumors in the cervical region.

We have not used postoperative radiation for intramedullary tumors that have been totally removed, and we do not advocate postoperative radiation for benign intramedullary tumors that have been incompletely removed, except occasionally in children. The patient's course should be monitored closely, facilitated by the use of water-soluble contrast agents and CT and MRI scanning. A second surgical attempt should be made to remove the tumor at the time of recurrence. Following this operation, radiation may be considered.

SPINAL CORD ARTERIOVENOUS MALFORMATIONS

Arteriovenous malformations of the spinal cord are relatively rare, being only one tenth as common as cerebral AVMs and one tenth as common as primary spinal neoplasms. They appear more commonly in males (4:1) and generally occur in an older age group than AVMs of the brain. Eighty percent occur in the thoracolumbar spinal cord, although they may involve the entire cord from cervical to sacral levels.[25, 26]

ANATOMY

There are two arterial systems of the spinal cord: an anterior one and a posterior one. These are supplied by the anterior and posterior radiculomedullary arteries, respectively. The anterior spinal artery usually is a well-defined single artery running in the anterior-median fissure and supplying approximately the anterior two thirds of the spinal cord.[27] The posterior arteries, although paired on either side of the midline, are variable and often are represented by numerous interlacing smaller arteries. They supply the posterior one third of the cord.[27] The largest and most important radicular artery supplying the cord is the artery of Adamkiewiez (great anterior medullary artery, which arises most frequently on the left side between T8 and L4.[28] After entering the spinal canal, it ascends and makes a hairpin turn, with its largest branch directed caudally and its smaller branch cephalad. It anastomoses caudally with the artery accompanying the first sacral root. The posterior arteries have rich anastomoses with the anterior ones around the circumference of the cord.[27, 29, 30] Because the dorsal arteries enter at almost every level, forming a very complete collateral network, they are much smaller than the ventral arteries and are normally demonstrated angiographically only with difficulty. The venous system is similar to the arterial in that it is paired and more diffuse over the dorsal aspect than it is on the anterior aspect. Those vascular malformations that are primarily located intramedullary receive the bulk of their arterial supply from median and paramedian penetrating branches of the anterior spinal artery. Their venous drainage is either dorsal or ventral.

The artery of Adamkiewiez often contributes to spinal AVMs, because it supplies the most commonly involved area of the spinal cord. The intercostal arteries, the dorsal segmental arteries, and the lumbosacral radicular arteries also may contribute blood supply to an AVM. In the cervical region, the vertebral arteries and the costocervical or thyrocervical trunks of the subclavian artery may also supply an AVM. Because such AVMs tend to be dorsal, a majority are supplied by the dorsal radicular arteries. In some instances, however, the anterior spinal artery sends perforating branches to supply portions of the AVM in the central or dorsal portion of the cord. The feeding arteries often are limited to a few radicular arteries, but on occasion, there may be multiple small twigs at numerous levels shunting into an extensive venous draining system. These lesions primarily involve the pial surface of the cord rather than the parenchyma, but at times, a portion of the malformation or a venous aneurysm may extend into the center of the spinal cord.[31] Because of the dorsal pial position, their surgical removal is often feasible.

In the past, such terms as "cavernous angioma" and "racemose angioma," both arterial and venous, were often used descriptively.[32, 33] With the advent of spinal angiography, however, and the operating microscopic exposure, a more practical scheme has been developed.[34–36]

The majority of these lesions represent arteriovenous communications of varying extent and degree. The communication between arteries and veins develops primarily between the dorsal radicular arteries and the dorsolateral veins of the spinal cord. The classification of Ommaya and colleagues[35] is useful in the surgical evaluation of these lesions. Ommaya's type 1, the most common, represents an extensive, single-coiled vessel with one or two arterial feeders entering at various levels. (These small arteries are not visualized at arteriography and are difficult to see without the operating microscope.) The flow is slow, and the blood supply appears distinct from that of the cord.

The lesion appears at the pial level of the cord, rarely penetrates the cord, and may extend laterally but is usually dorsal in location. The ligation of major arterial feeders to these lesions often significantly decreases the flow in the malformation and leads to stasis, but small arterial contributions at numerous other levels keep the malformation "alive." These latter arteries, however, may be insignificant. The major feature of these malformations is a well-identified arterial contribution at the one or two levels.

Type 2 is a glomus or nidus type of malformation. The lesion is angiographically and surgically well visualized and well defined[37] (Figs. 163–5 and 163–6). It is generally a discrete coil of arteriovenous vessels supplied by well-identified arteries at the margin of the glomus or nidus. A subgroup of this type is the intramedullary vascular malformation.[31] The intramedullary type has been reported in the cervical region by Malis[38] and has been seen at many other regions of the spinal cord, including the conus. These malformations are generally high pressure and can be well demonstrated by arteriography. They can be resected discretely. Venous aneurysms are commonly associated with this type of malformation, especially when intramedullary.

Type 3, the so-called juvenile type, most commonly seen in children, is a more diffuse, comprehensive arteriovenous lesion of the cord, which often encircles it in a cuirass configuration (Fig. 163–5). A better term is diffuse intramedullary

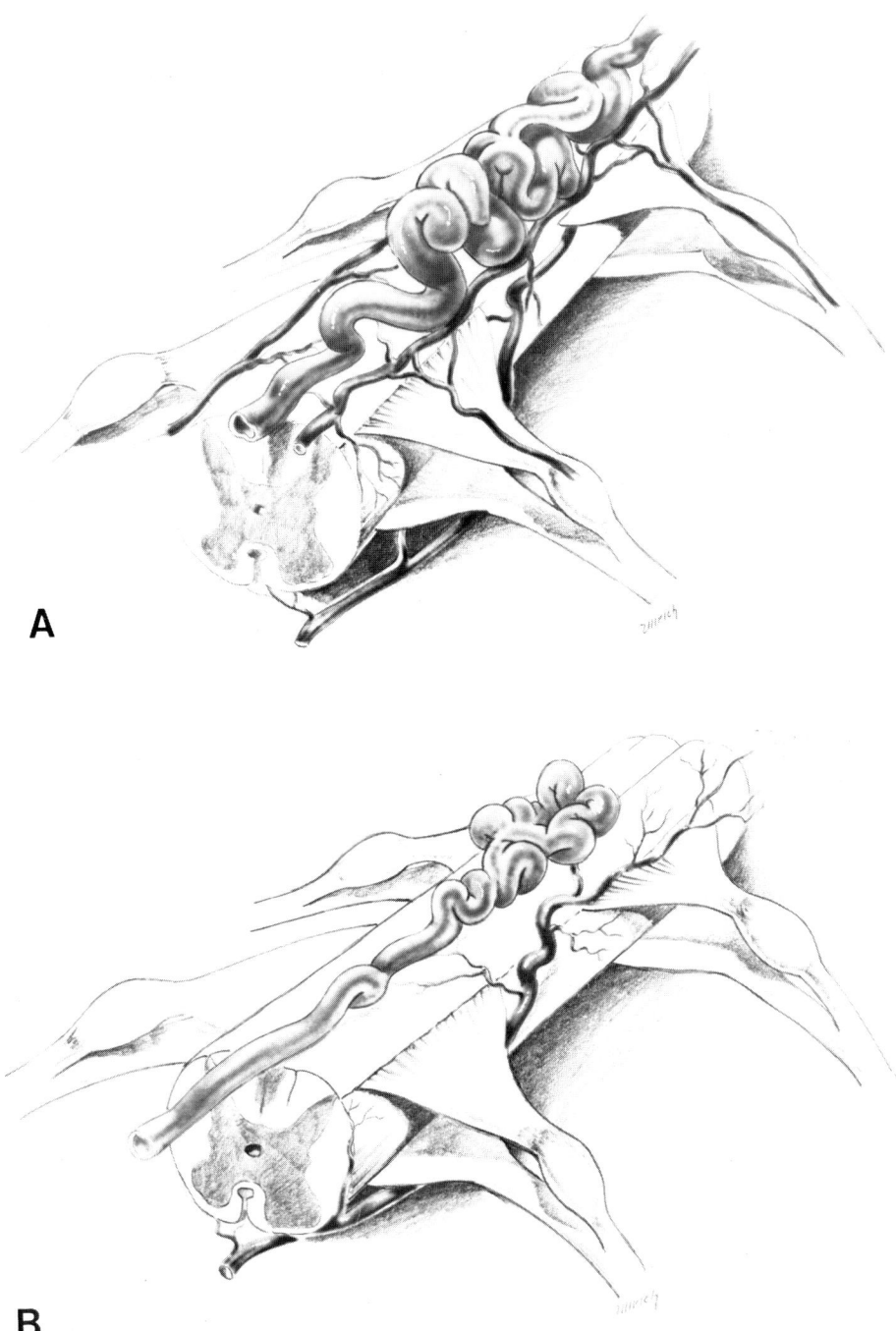

FIGURE 163-5. AVMs of the spinal cord. (A) Abnormal arterialized tortuous veins cover the dorsal aspect of the cord (lighter and larger vessels). These are fed by numerous arterial branches at multiple levels (smaller and darker vessels). (B) A nidus with a feeding artery (dark vessel) and a localized tangle of abnormal draining veins (lighter and larger vessels).

Illustration continued on following page

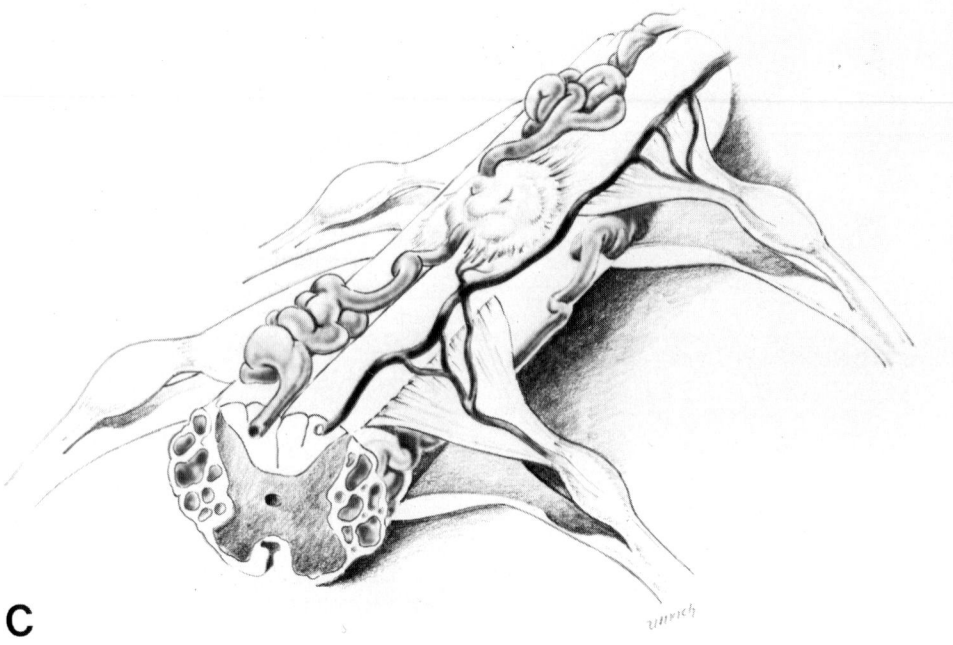

FIGURE 163–5 Continued (C) This AVM lies both within and on the surface of the spinal cord. It consists of large cavernous channels and multiple arteriovenous shunts. (Reprinted with permission of Baker HL Jr, Love JG, Layton DD Jr: Angiographic and surgical aspects of spinal cord vascular anomalies. Radiology 88:1078–1085, 1967. © Radiological Society of North America.)

and extramedullary AVM, because these lesions permeate the spinal cord, making their obliteration impossible (Fig. 163–5). They have varying degrees of arterial contributions that may or may not be visualized at arteriography. Flow is rapid, and the blood supply of the AVM and the cord may be closely related. Doppman[37] emphasizes the "nidus" concept in regard to some of these lesions. In these cases, angiography demonstrates discrete arteriovenous communications with limited involvement of the rostrocaudal extent of the spinal cord. A detailed picture of the vascular anatomy is therefore essential when one is considering the extent of laminectomy and whether or not a lesion can be totally removed. Ventral lesions are most difficult to treat surgically.

The lesions that do not have arteriovenous communications and that represent pure venous or arterial abnormalities are exceedingly rare and have not been demonstrated by arteriography. The concept that such lesions exist is primarily based on data from autopsy specimens. Whether this concept has any validity in the present-day evaluation of spinal cord AVMs is open to question.

CLINICAL PRESENTATION AND NATURAL HISTORY

Spinal AVMs tend to occur in males (male-to-female ratio of 2-4:1), 30 to 70 years old, primarily at the thoracolumbar levels.[25] Frequently, AVM is not suspected, and a diagnosis of tumor or disc disease is made. In the planning of therapy, which may involve procedures of considerable risk, the natural history of these lesions must be considered. Aminoff and Logue,[39, 40] in an extensive review of 60 cases, reported that the vast majority had an insidious onset with progressive deterioration, and that 50 percent of patients were severely disabled within 3 years of the onset of the disorder. Only 20 percent of the cases had an acute onset, and subsequently many of these had progression of symptoms. Subarachnoid hemorrhage occurred at one time or another in 10 percent of the cases but was an initial symptom in only 5 percent. Herdt et al[41] found that only 6 percent of patients had definite proof of subarachnoid hemorrhage. Tobin and Layton,[25] reviewing the Mayo Clinic experience with 71 patients, found a slowly progressive course in 73 percent and an abrupt onset with subarachnoid hemorrhage in 10 percent. The symptom complex of leg weakness, sensory loss, pain, and early sphincteric involvement was the most common presentation. The prognosis once the lesion becomes symptomatic generally is poor; a progressive and disabling disease ensues. In a small number of cases, the threat of instantaneous neurologic disaster is present. In such instances, the onset may be devastating, with all the manifestations that go with a ruptured intracranial aneurysm.

Subarachnoid hemorrhage with the sudden onset of neurologic symptomatology is unusual, however, except in patients under 30 years of age.[42] An insidious, progressive course is most common; it is accentuated by pain of radicular origin, depending on the location of the lesion. The location of the pain, however, is often not a reliable indication of the levels of involvement.[25] Progressive upper or lower motor neuron involvement is the rule, with spasticity or absence of reflexes, depending on location. Involvement of the dorsal columns with paresthesias, loss of position, and other sensory modalities is also part of the progressive picture.

Spinal AVMs appear to produce symptoms because of ischemic changes in the spinal cord secondary to a vascular steal and the mass effect of the lesion.[36, 43, 44] On occasion, the arterialized veins that compose these malformations are layered four to five deep on the surface of the spinal cord (Fig. 163–7). When the lesions are removed, grooves from the dilated vascular channels can be noted on the surface of the spinal cord. Many of the symptoms associated with spinal AVMs may relate to increased venous pressure altering the

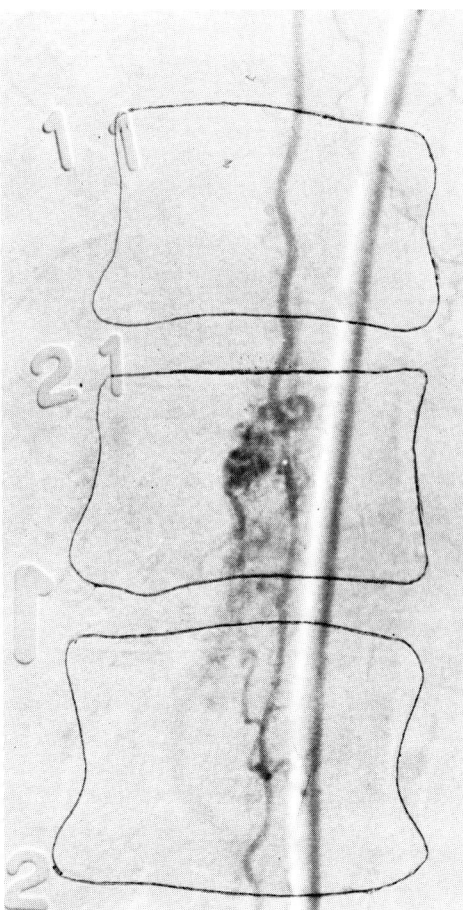

FIGURE 163-6. Anteroposterior spinal cord arteriograms with subtraction technique. The nidus of the AVM is seen at the small arrows. The feeding artery is present at the open arrow. (Reprinted with permission of Kasdon DL, Wolpert SM, Stein BM: Surgical and angiographic localization of spinal arteriovenous malformations. Surg Neurol 5:279-283, 1976.)

dynamics of blood flow within the spinal cord, leading to venous congestion and infarction within the substances of the spinal cord.

DIAGNOSIS

On examination, two signs are helpful if present. A bruit over the spine is virtually diagnostic,[45] and the presence of a cutaneous angioma helps diagnostically and also in localizing the level of the lesions.[46] Plain films of the spine generally are noncontributory. Cerebrospinal fluid evaluation shows some abnormality in 75 percent of cases, protein elevation and pleocytosis being most common.[25, 47]

Spinal myelography with iophendylate was often diagnostic in the series reported by Aminoff and Logue.[39, 40] Because most of these lesions occurred on the dorsal surface of the cord, it was necessary to insert the iophendylate, turn the patient supine, and run the contrast agent up the dorsal surface of the spinal cord. Often the webbing or trabeculation of the dorsal arachnoid led to the erroneous diagnosis of a vascular malformation, and occasionally, tortuous nerve roots, spinal metastases, and dilated vessels associated with intramedullary tumors could produce a false-positive diagnosis (Fig. 163-8).

Myelography is now performed with nontoxic contrast agents that are water soluble and nonelectrolyte and that will coat the spinal cord. It is easier to study the dorsal as well as other aspects of the spinal cord and visualize the malformations. The diminished density of these agents and the refined detail also facilitate the diagnosis. A CT scan may also augment these studies.[48] Often, myelography indicates the longitudinal extent of the malformation and then spinal angiography can be helpful in pinpointing the arterial anatomy.

Spinal angiography with selective injection of the relevant arteries and a serial study with subtraction technique are important. In the cervical region, selective injection of the subclavian branches, including the vertebral, thyrocervical, and costocervical trunks, should be done. Spinal angiography must be comprehensive. If there is no myelographic clue to the location of the AVM, the surgical procedure is extremely laborious and tedious.

Unfortunately, a lesion must represent a significant arteriovenous shunt in order for arteriography to be successful in the demonstration of all of the ramifications of the lesion. Opacification of the posterior spinal arteries is rare, whereas the thoracic anterior spinal artery is small and often hard to visualize under normal circumstances.

It should be understood that there is a certain risk in performing spinal angiography, because the catheter is commonly wedged into the feeding artery and the cord becomes temporarily ischemic during the injection. Flexor spasms have occurred during the injection, especially when a pathologic process is present and collateral circulation is comprised.

A flush of the aorta may show a flash filling of the lesion but is contraindicated because of spinal cord toxicity. Selective arteriography must be done at individual levels to demonstrate spinal arteriovenous malformations properly. In some instances, arteriography may fail to define the arterial contribution to an extensive malformation of dilated arterialized veins extending over multiple segments of the spinal cord. In other instances, in which a nidus exists, it may be difficult to tell on angiography whether the lesion is intramedullary or extramedullary.[49]

The variability of the position of the spinal cord in the anteroposterior plane within the spinal canal plays a major role in the difficulty of precise localization. Displacement of the spinal cord by thrombosed portions of malformations, which are not visualized with contrast material, is an additional source of error in localization by spinal angiography. A CT scan of the spine with intravenous contrast enhancement may hold some promise for screening and follow-up of patients with spinal AVMs. The axial-transverse view of the lesion may permit a better appraisal of the anatomic relationships of the extrathecal extension of the malformation.[48]

Evoked potentials have been most useful during surgery and radiologic procedures.[50] As clinical tools prior to operation, these methods have not shown great promise, especially in definitively locating and diagnosing the presence of a spinal AVM. It is unlikely that MRI will lead to as detailed an evaluation as angiography often accomplishes.

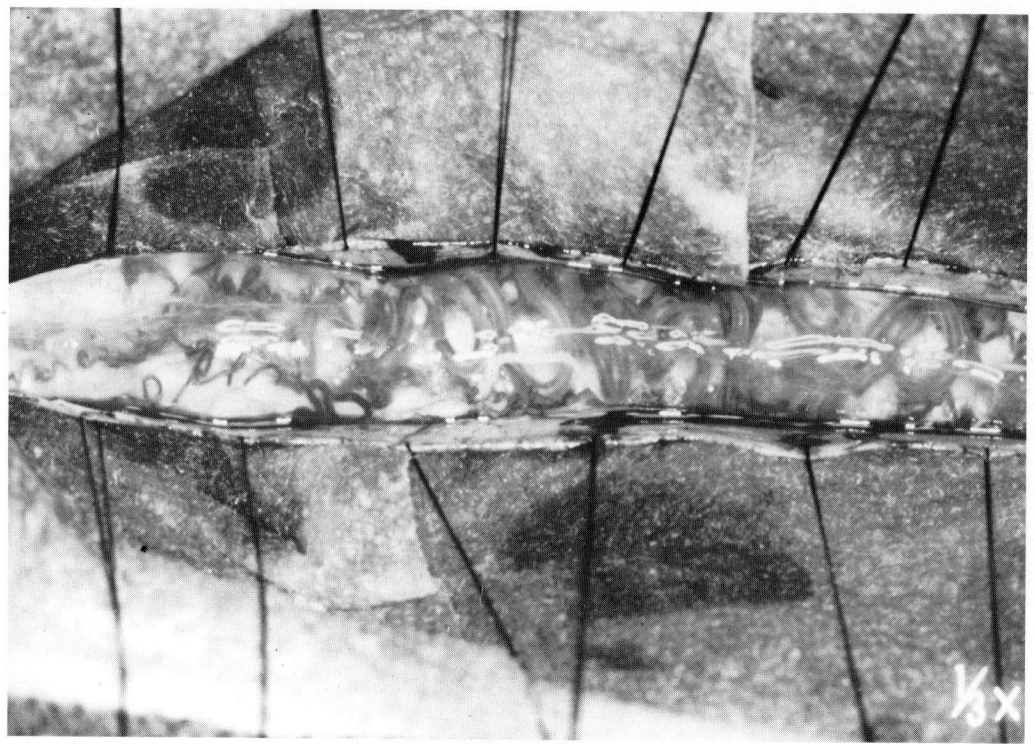

FIGURE 163–7. Operative exposure of a large AVM of the spinal cord composed principally of tortuous, distended, arterialized veins.

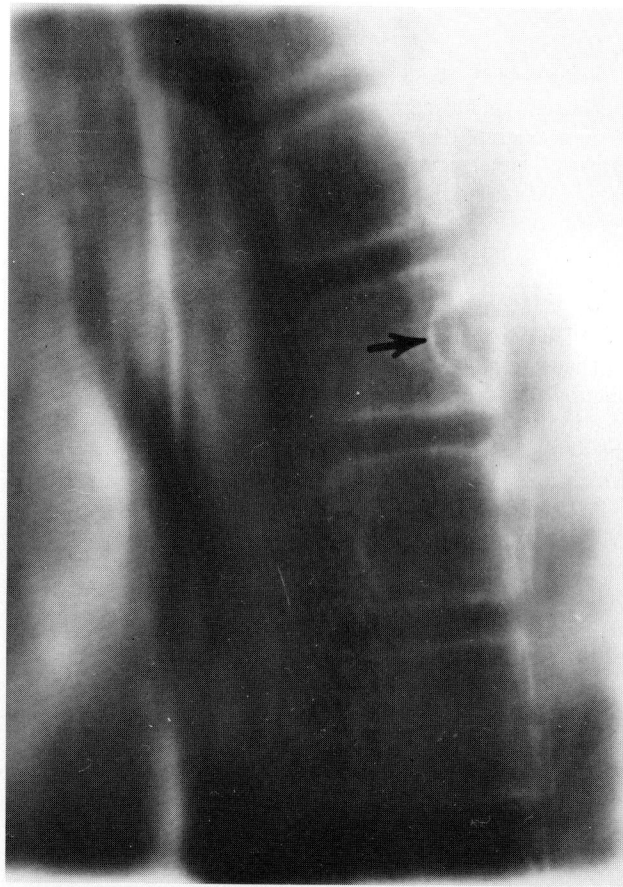

FIGURE 163–8. Lumbar thoracic myelogram demonstrating tortuous shadows suggestive of abnormal vascular channels but representing redundant nerve roots (arrows). (Reprinted with permission of Stein BM: Arteriovenous malformations of the brain and spinal cord, in Practice of Surgery, Hagerstown, MD, Harper & Row, 1979.)

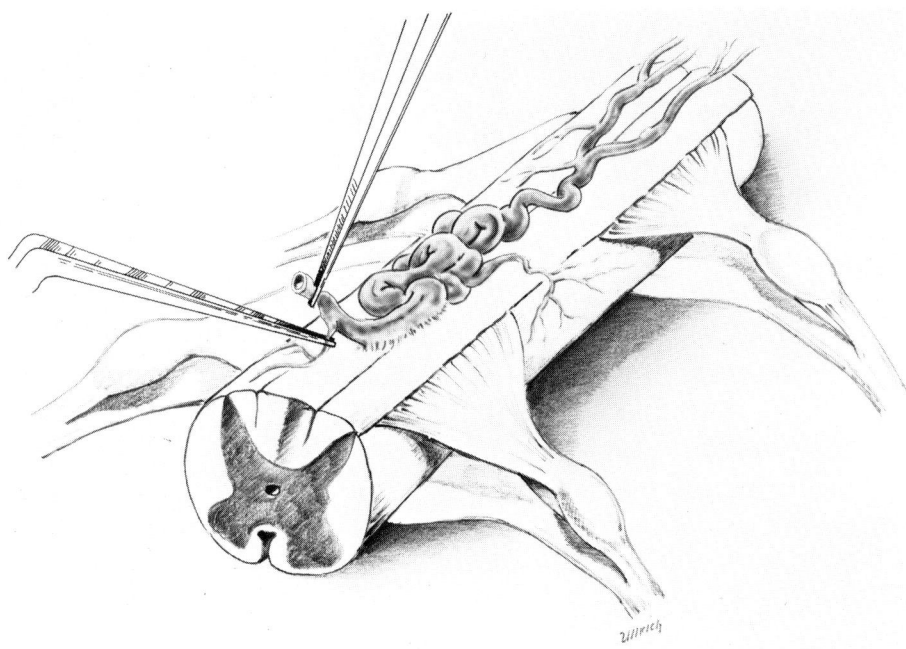

FIGURE 163–9. The surgical resection of an AVM showing meticulous cautery of the feeding arteries and gradual peeling away of the abnormal venous channels from the surface of the spinal cord. (Reprinted with permission of Stein BM: Arteriovenous malformations of the brain and spinal cord, in Practice of Surgery, Hagerstown, MD, Harper & Row, 1979.)

TREATMENT

Because the prognosis is poor for patients with spinal arteriovenous malformations that are untreated or simply decompressed, we believe that surgical exploration to assess resectability is important. Exploration should be carried out in spite of an angiographic appearance suggesting a largely intramedullary location of the malformation.

The only completely satisfactory treatment for spinal AVMs is total obliteration or excision. Thus far, the usefulness of embolization has been limited.

Embolization

Various embolization techniques have been used, including silicone emboli that are placed via catheter into the feeding arteries.[51–53] This technique is limited because of the small size of the feeding arteries and the fact that these arteries, which are proximal to the lesion, may be significant contributors to the normal spinal cord circulation. Furthermore, in lesions with comparatively low blood flow, there is an additional hazard of inadvertent embolization of normal vessels.

Surgical Excision

The cornerstone of treatment for spinal AVMs is microsurgical obliteration.[34–36, 42, 49, 54–56] The lesions lend themselves to surgery because the vast majority lie on the dorsal surface of the spinal cord and are thereby accessible (Figs. 163–7, 163–9, and 163–10). They also represent low-flow and low-pressure systems in which there is a limited arterial contribution with a significant venous component that is readily visualized on the surface of the spinal cord. Uncommonly, an AVM invades portions of the spinal cord. Even in such instances the AVM occasionally may be removed microsurgically with satisfactory results.[31]

The axiom that the preoperative neurologic status is often related to the postoperative outcome is particularly pertinent in these lesions. Surgery should be accomplished early in the disease, before major neurologic deficits develop. Function is unlikely to improve in a patient who already is severely incapacitated.

The patient is prepared with dexamethasone prior to surgery. Malis[38] prefers to use the sitting position for those lesions located in the upper thoracic, cervical, and cervicomedullary region. This position creates a certain degree of hypotension, which may be useful. It also minimizes respiratory movement artifact. In lesions located at the lower levels, Malis[38] prefers an oblique position so as to limit respiratory excursions. Both of these positions preclude the effective use of an assistant during the operation, which we consider a major disadvantage. We prefer to operate on all AVMs with the patient in the prone position, leaving the patient's abdomen and chest free for respiratory excursions. The surgeon and assistant work together across the operating table. The extent of the lesion, as identified by myelography and spinal angiography, determines the exposure. The laminectomy should be moderately broad, and the dura opened widely with preservation of the arachnoid until the extent of the lesion is determined by visualization through the arachnoid. The operating microscope is always used from the point of dural opening. The arachnoid is then opened widely with small scissors or an arachnoidal knife. It may be necessary to rotate the cord, cutting the dentate ligament and grasping it, to see the lateral supply to the malformation. In many cases of long dorsal AVMs, the malformation may extend over different regions of the spinal cord, and a few cases have been described in which the lesion extends the entire length of the spinal cord. As reported by Oldfield and

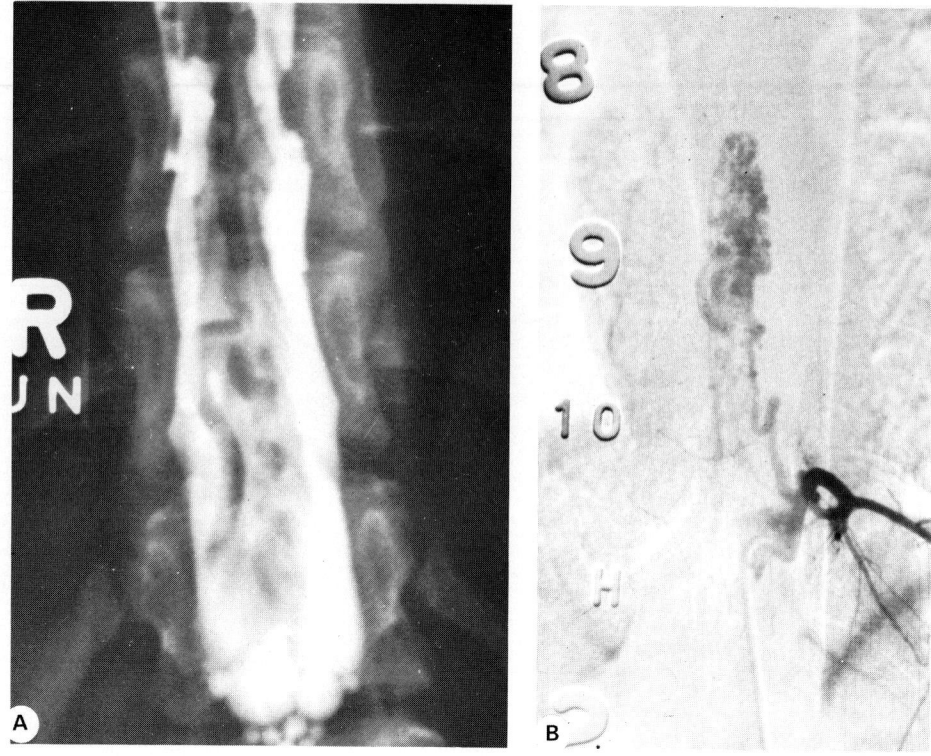

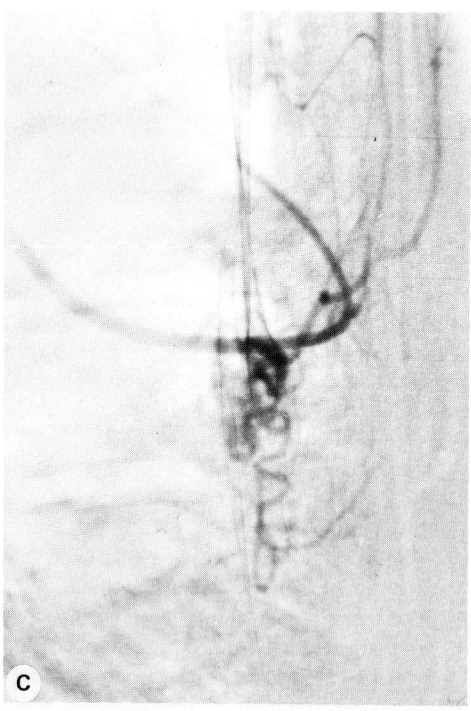

FIGURE 163–10. (A) A low thoracic myelogram (AP projection) demonstrating serpiginous filling defect suggestive of an AVM. (B) A selective spinal arteriogram (AP view) demonstrating spinal AVM opposite T8-T10. (C) A selective spinal arteriogram (lateral view) demonstrating spinal AVM with components appearing dorsal, ventral, and possibly within the spinal cord.

associates,[57] it may not be necessary to remove the entire malformation. Interrupting the fistula between the major arterial supply and the arterialized venous system may suffice.[57] There may be minor arterial contributions, however, and in such cases, the malformation may remain turgid, with the veins containing arterialized blood under pressure. It may be necessary to remove the entire arterialized venous system in one or multiple stages, interrupting even the smallest arterial contribution.

Those lesions of the juvenile variety or lesions that permeate the spinal cord can be easily identified by visualization of the dorsal, dorsolateral, and ventrolateral portions of the spinal cord. Lesions that are primarily intramedullary may be identified as a local bulge of the spinal cord with draining

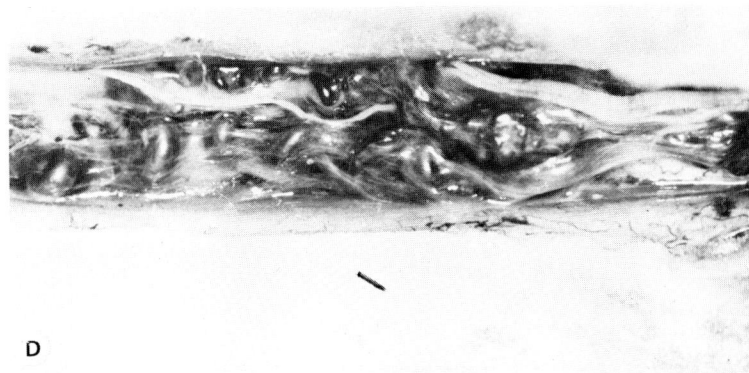

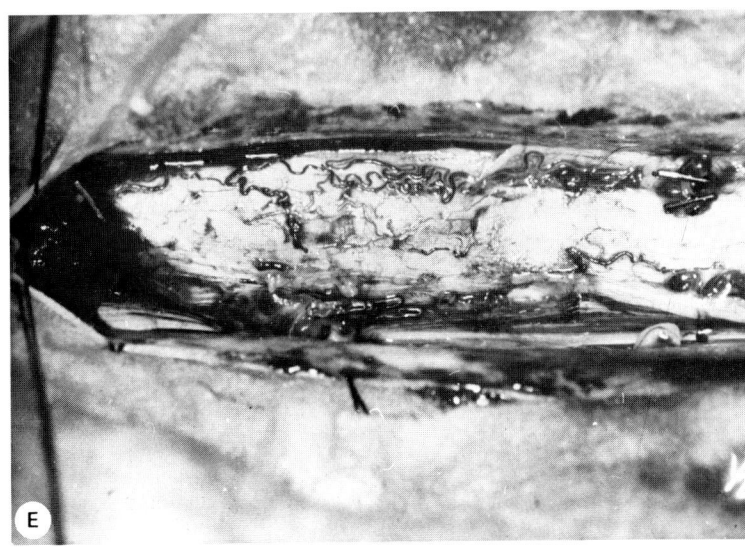

FIGURE 163–10 *Continued* (D) Operative exposure of spinal cord from T7-T11 with extensive AVM. (E) Operative view after dorsal and lateral portions of the AVM were removed.

veins coming out over the dorsal surface of the spinal cord. Occasionally, discoloration due to old hemorrhage or thrombosis within the lesion is seen. These are treated by myelotomy and techniques similar to those used in intramedullary tumor surgery.

Microbipolar cautery is utilized under constant moisture during the occlusion of the AVM vessels. Only the largest vessels are clipped; from a practical point of view, this usually means none, one, or two arteries. It is extremely difficult to use the standard metallic clips in the removal of an intramedullary lesion, which must be accomplished by bipolar cautery. We prefer to approach the lesions from the arterial side first. The venous flow, even though arterialized, is often slow and can be managed easily should rupture occur on the venous side. We see no advantage in attacking the lesion primarily from the venous side, if definitive arterial contributions are easily visualized. The lesion is generally peeled away from the spinal cord while additional arterial contributions are coagulated and divided (Fig. 163–9). In general, malformations located within the spinal cord are associated with large venous aneurysms, often partially thrombosed. These are rather dangerous "bombs," and we do not want to threaten the venous drainage or the aneurysm more than necessary to collapse it so that it may be removed safely from within the spinal cord. We have not been using hypotension during the removal, especially if the patient is in the sitting position. In the prone position, hypotension is not necessary because of the low flow in these systems. The dura is always closed, no matter what has been accomplished at the time of the operation.

Lesser surgical procedures, such as decompressive laminectomy with or without opening of the dura, appear to have little or no merit in the treatment of these malformations. In fact, such operative "explorations" may be detrimental, in that they make future definitive surgery more difficult. If the lesion is found to be inoperable and all that can be offered is decompression with opening of the dura, then the dura should be closed with a patch graft of fascia to prevent adhesions to the surface of the spinal cord. If there is a possibility that surgery will be performed in the future, it is mandatory to close the dura, because the adhesions that will otherwise form will preclude subsequent, definitive surgical ventures.

SPECIAL CONSIDERATIONS

Long Dorsal AVM

There is no question that these large coiled arterialized veins are fed by one or two primary arteries that are part of the dorsal radiculomedullary arteries. Anyone who has resected the entire coil of veins will also note small arterial contributions at numerous levels. If a segment of the malformation is isolated from its major blood supply, it will still bleed from the contribution of these small arterial feeders. It has been general practice to gradually sweep the entire malformation off the dorsal aspect of the cord, interrupting all arterial feeders to it until the venous system turns blue.

Oldfield and coworkers[7] reaffirmed the suggestion of others[35, 58, 59] that only the major arterial contribution be interrupted. These studies suggest a significant reduction in the flow of the malformation but not complete obliteration following this maneuver. They also point out that this fistula may occur at the dura where the radicular arteries enter the dural root sleeve. Postoperative arteriographic studies have shown no visualization of the AVM in such cases. Because the residual arterial feeders are tiny, however, they are not ordinarily shown by arteriography. Clinically, this limited procedure has led to dramatic improvement in many cases. It remains to be seen what will be accomplished over the long term. It is quite possible that the malformation will reactivate with time. That has been the case with many cerebral malformations that were partially treated by obliteration of the major feeders.

We recommend that observations at surgery be considered in determining the extent of the operation and that the major coils of veins that remain arterialized should be obliterated. This may also be accomplished by selective cautery rather than by stripping of the entire dorsal venous system. There is some evidence that this stripping procedure may cause compromise of the normal cord blood supply and ischemic changes beyond the area of the malformation. After the stripping of large coiled veins from the dorsal surface of the cord, it appears significantly devascularized (Fig. 163–10). In those cases in which we have interrupted the major arterial fistula and then selectively cauterized portions of the remaining dorsal venous system, the circulation has a more appealing appearance. Long-term follow-up is lacking to determine which is the correct procedure, however.

Glomus AVM

Arteriovenous malformation in the form of a nidus or glomus is the easiest to comprehend and treat. Such lesions produce symptoms of mass hemorrhage or venous thrombosis. They can be circumscribed by interruption of their feeding arteries at the exact margin of the glomus. Interrupting the major venous drainage first may jeopardize the operation by creating intolerable intraluminal forces within the malformation, resulting in hemorrhage.

Malformations that are primarily intramedullary are usually glomus in configuration. A rare type of malformation is associated with a long dorsal type of lesion in conjunction with the primary intramedullary lesion. We have had an unusually high incidence of intramedullary lesions—approximately 20 percent of all spinal cord AVMs.[1] Management consists of removing a glomus from the dorsal or dorsolateral surface of the cord with the additional considerations akin to removal of an intramedullary tumor. The locus of the lesion is visualized as the cord is exposed. A myelotomy is made in a longitudinal direction from the polar aspects of the lesion, allowing visualization of the rostral and caudal margins of the lesion. Dissection is carried carefully around the appropriate margin, depending on the anatomy of the venous drainage and arterial supply as determined from angiograms and intraoperative observations. These lesions are preferably approached from the arterial side, with bipolar cautery used for interruption of the arterial feeders while the malformation is rolled toward the venous pedicle. In some occasions, the venous pedicle is in direct relationship to the major supply from the anterior spinal artery. It should be possible to approach the lesion from the arterial side, and once the arterial connection is interrupted, the venous pedicle is easy to manage. Clips are rarely used. Sharp dissection is always preferred in the removal as opposed to blunt or a tearing type of dissection technique. These lesions are frequently associated with a large aneurysmal dilatation, often partially thrombosed but still active and thin-walled, predisposing to intraoperative hemorrhage secondary to excessive manipulation. Careful use of a broad bipolar tip under irrigation may be utilized to shrink venous aneurysms, but care must be taken that the wall is not violated. In many cases, the venous aneurysm may be gently teased out of the cord intact. The venous aneurysm is often on the edge of the shunt component of the malformation. The cavity left by removal of such lesions is similar in size and configuration to that left by the total removal of a large intramedullary tumor. It is remarkable how thin the surrounding cord structure can be and still result in a functional neurologic state.

Juvenile or Diffuse AVM

Diffuse and juvenile arteriovenous malformations are the most difficult lesions to treat. They permeate the cord, and histologic examination indicates functional neural tissue interspersed with vascular channels of the malformation. It is obvious that they do not have well-defined margins permitting resection and that they comprehensively involve both the interior and exterior of the spinal cord over many segments. It is our opinion that confirmation of these lesions must be left to surgical exploration and that definitive knowledge as to their presence, which would preclude intraoperative interventions, cannot be obtained by the usual radiographic studies. Perhaps MRI will answer this question in the future. Although these are nonresectable lesions, in one instance under evoked potential monitoring, we were able to clip a major radicular artery and witness a rather remarkable clinical improvement in an individual who had been plagued by progressive deterioration of spinal cord function. In most cases, these lesions can be treated with little more than a decompressive procedure and perhaps, in exceptional cases, selective ligation of arteries under evoked potential monitoring. These maneuvers are of questionable benefit.

RESULTS

In those patients in whom surgical obliteration or resection of a spinal cord AVM has been accomplished, good results in terms of an improved or arrested neurologic status are seen in approximately 80 to 90 percent of the patients.*
Unfortunately, the results are often predicated on the preoperative condition of the patient, so that those with neurologic devastation or severe, advanced disease are less apt to make gratifying recoveries following successful resection of the lesion. On the other hand, individuals who have mild or modest neurologic deficits before surgery will receive the

---

*See references 35, 36, 38–40, 42, and 55.

most benefit and often return to normal or near normal neurologic status. Resection of these malformations precludes the possibility of devastating neurologic deficit from subsequent hemorrhage.

Luessenhop and Dela Cruz[34] reported, in a broad review of the literature, that decompressive procedures resulted in improvement in 19 percent and deterioration in 81 percent of cases, whereas ligation of some feeders resulted in improvement in 34 percent and worsening in 66 percent. When these figures are compared with those of surgical resection, it is clear that the latter procedure, if feasible, is preferable. Radiation plays no role in the therapy of these lesions and may even be deleterious, producing scar tissue that would make subsequent definitive operative procedures difficult or impossible.

A postoperative arteriogram may or may not be obtained to define the completeness of resection. We do not believe that postoperative angiography is as important in these cases as in the treatment of cerebral AVMs, because one is better able to gauge the effectiveness of resection while at the same time realizing the limitations of spinal arteriography in fully defining the lesions.

MENINGEAL AND PARAMENINGEAL ARTERIOVENOUS MALFORMATIONS

In addition to the AVMs that directly involve the spinal cord, some exist in the meninges or parameningeal areas. These are often represented by enormous arteriovenous communications involving the intercostal or cervical arteries and involving not only the dura and sometimes the spinal cord but also often extensively the muscles and surrounding soft tissues. These are associated with bruits and may not manifest with the spinal cord syndrome so familiar for true AVMs of the spinal cord. Unfortunately, these lesions, being extensive with large shunts between arteries and veins, are difficult to treat by embolization, surgery, or both. In many instances, emboli transverse the fistula and enter into the systemic venous circulation. Because of the extensive nature of these lesions, it is often impossible to remove them entirely, even with thoracotomy and massive resection. They are similar to cirsoid aneurysms of the scalp and some of the soft-tissue AVMs that involve the face and tissues at the base of the skull.

REFERENCES

1. Turnbull F: Intramedullary tumors of the spinal cord, in Clinical Neurosurgery, vol 8. Baltimore, Williams & Wilkins, 1962, pp 237–247
2. Elsberg CA: Tumors of the Spinal Cord. New York, Paul B. Hoeber, 1925, pp 206–239
3. Matson DD: Neurosurgery of Infancy and Childhood. Springfield, IL, Charles C Thomas, 1969, pp 647–688
4. Garrido E, Stein BM: Microsurgical removal of intramedullary spinal cord tumors. Surg Neurol 7:215–229, 1977
5. Greenwood J Jr: Surgical removal of intramedullary tumors. J Neurosurg 26:276, 1967
6. Guidetti B: Intramedullary tumors of the spinal cord. Acta Neurochir 17:7, 1967
7. Horrax G, Henderson DG: Encapsulated intramedullary tumor involving whole spinal cord from medulla to conus: Complete enucleation with recovery. Surg Gynecol Obstet 68:814, 1939
8. Malis LI: Intramedullary spinal cord tumors. Clin Neurosurg 25:512, 1978
9. Yasargil MG, Antic J, Laciga R, et al: The microsurgical removal of intramedullary spinal hemangioblastomas: Report of twelve cases and a review of the literature. Surg Neurol 6:141, 1976
10. Stein BM: Spinal intradural tumors, in Wilkins RH, Rengachary SS: Neurosurgery. New York, McGraw-Hill, 1985, pp 1048–1061
11. Rand RW, Rand CW: Intraspinal Tumors of Childhood. Springfield, IL, Charles C Thomas, 1960
12. Epstein F, Epstein N: Surgical treatment of spinal cord astrocytomas of childhood: A series of 19 patients. J Neurosurg 57:685, 1982
13. Tievsky AL, Davis DO: Radiology of spinal cord neoplasia, in Wilkins RH, Rengachary SS: Neurosurgery. New York, McGraw-Hill, 1985, pp 1039–1048
14. Vigneud J, Aubin MD, Jardin C: CT in 40 cases of syringomyelia (abstract). AJNR 1:112, 1980
15. Kan S, Fox AJ, Vineula F, et al: Delayed CT metrizamide enhancement of syringomyelia secondary to tumor. AJNR 4:73, 1983
16. Quencer RM, Tenner MS, Rothman LM: Percutaneous spinal cord puncture and myelocystography. Radiology 118:637, 1976
17. Fischer G, Mansuy L: Total removal of intramedullary ependymomas: Follow-up study of 16 cases. Surg Neurol 14:243, 1980
18. Guidetti B, Mercuri S, Vagnozzi R: Long-term results of the surgical treatment of 129 intramedullary spinal gliomas. Neurosurgery 54:323, 1981
19. Stein BM: Case records of the Massachusetts General Hospital—case 26. N Engl J Med 293:33, 1975
20. Powers SK, Edwards SB, Boggan JE, et al: Use of the argon surgical laser in neurosurgery. J Neurosurg 60:523, 1984
21. Greenwood J Jr: Intramedullary tumors of the spinal cord: A follow-up study after total surgical removal. J Neurosurg 20:665, 1963
22. Love JG, River MH: Thirty-one year cure following removal of intramedullary glioma of cervical portion of spinal cord: Report of case. J Neurosurg 19:906, 1962
23. Wood EH, Berne AS, Taveras JM: The value of radiation therapy in the management of intrinsic tumors of the spinal cord. Radiology 63:11, 1954
24. Schwade JG, Wara WM, Sheline GE, et al: Management of primary spinal cord tumors. Int J Radiat Oncol Biol Phys 4:389, 1978
25. Tobin WD, Layton DD: The diagnosis and natural history of spinal cord arteriovenous malformations. Mayo Clin Proc 51:637, 1976
26. Krayenbuhl H, Yasargil MG: Die Varicosis spinalis und ihre Behandlung. Schweiz Arch Neurol Psychiatr 92:74, 1963
27. Doppman JL, DiChiro G, Ommaya AK: Selective Arteriography of the Spinal Cord. St. Louis, Warren Green, 1969
28. DiChiro G, Doppman J, Ommaya AK: Selective arteriography of arteriovenous aneurysms of spinal cord. Radiology 88:1065, 1967
29. Djindjian R, Faure C, Houdart R, et al: Exploration angiographique des malformations vasculaires de la moelle épinière. Acta Radiol (Diagn) 5:145, 1966
30. Djindjian R: Arteriography of the spinal cord. Am J Roentgenol 107:461, 1969
31. Cogen P, Stein BM: Spinal cord arteriovenous malformations with significant intramedullary components. J Neurosurg 59:471, 1983
32. Bergstrand A, Hook O, Lidvall H: Vascular malformations of the spinal cord. Acta Neurol Scand 40:169, 1964
33. Wyburn-Masson R: The Vascular Abnormalities and Tumors of the Spinal Cord and Its Membranes. London, Krimptom, 1943
34. Luessenhop AJ, Dela Cruz T: Surgical excision of spinal intradural vascular malformations. J Neurosurg 30:552, 1969
35. Ommaya AK, DiChiro G, Doppman, JL: Ligation of arterial supply in the treatment of spinal cord arteriovenous malformations. J Neurosurg 30:679, 1969
36. Krayenbuhl H, Yasargil MG, McClintock HG: Treatment of spinal cord vascular malformations by surgical excision. J Neurosurg 30:427, 1969
37. Doppman JL: The nidus concept for spinal cord arteriovenous malformations: A surgical recommendation based on angiographic observations. Br J Radiol 44:758, 1971
38. Malis LI: Microsurgery for spinal cord arteriovenous malformations. Clin Neurosurg 26:543, 1979
39. Aminoff MJ, Logue V: Clinical features of spinal vascular malformations. Brain 97:197, 1974
40. Aminoff MJ, Logue V: The prognosis of patients with spinal vascular malformations. Brain 97:211, 1974
41. Herdt JR, DiChiro G, Doppman JL: Combined arterial and arteriovenous aneurysms of the spinal cord. Radiology 99:589, 1971

42. Houdart R, Djindjian R, Hurth M: Vascular malformations of the spinal cord: The anatomic and therapeutic significance of arteriography. J Neurosurg 24:583, 1966
43. Kaufman HH, Ommaya AK, DiChiro G, et al: Compression vs. "steal": The pathogenesis of symptoms in arteriovenous malformations of the spinal cord. Arch Neurol 23:173, 1970
44. Djindjian M, Djindjian R, Hurth M, et al: Steal phenomenon in spinal arteriovenous malformations. J Neuroradiol 5:187, 1978
45. Matthews WB: The spinal bruit. Lancet 2:1117, 1959
46. Doppman JL, Wirth FP Jr, DiChiro G, et al: Value of cutaneous angiomas in the arteriographic localization of spinal cord arteriovenous malformations. N Engl J Med 281:1440, 1969
47. Yasargil MG: Diagnosis and treatment of spinal cord arteriovenous malformations. Prog Neurol Surg 4:355, 1971
48. DiChiro G, Doppman JL, Wener L: Computed tomography of spinal arteriovenous malformations. Radiology 123:351, 1977
49. Kasdon DL, Wolpert SM, Stein BM: Surgical and angiographic localization of spinal arteriovenous malformations. Surg Neurol 5:279, 1976
50. Berenstein A, Young W, Ransohoff J, et al: Somatosensory evoked potentials during spinal angiography and therapeutic transvascular embolization. J Neurosurg 60:777, 1984
51. Doppman JL, DiChiro G, Ommaya AK: Percutaneous embolization of spinal cord arteriovenous malformations. J Neurosurg 34:48, 1971
52. Hilal SK, Sane P, Michelson WJ, et al: The embolization of vascular malformations of the spinal cord with low-viscosity silicone rubber. Neuroradiology 16:430, 1978
53. Djindjian R: Embolization of angiomas of the spinal cord. Surg Neurol 4:411, 1975
54. Kunc Z, Bret J: Diagnosis and treatment of vascular malformations of the spinal cord. J Neurosurg 30:436, 1969
55. Yasargil RW, DeLong WB, Guarnaschelli JJ: Complete microsurgical excision of cervical extramedullary and intramedullary vascular malformations. Surg Neurol 4:211, 1975
56. Latchaw TW, Harris RD, Chou Sn, et al: Combined embolization and operation in the treatment of cervical arteriovenous malformations. Neurosurgery 6:131, 1980
57. Oldfield EH, DiChiro G, Quindlen EA, et al: Successful treatment of a group of spinal cord arteriovenous malformations by interruption of dura fistula. J Neurosurg 59:1019, 1983
58. Bailey WL, Sperl MP: Angiomas of the cervical spinal cord. J Neurosurg 30:560, 1969
59. Baker HL Jr, Love JG, Layton DD Jr: Angiographic and surgical aspects of spinal cord vascular anomalies. Radiology 88:1078, 1967

CHAPTER 164

Surgical Management of Cerebrospinal Fluid Leakage After Spinal Surgery

Stephen R. Freidberg

In 1954, Mixter[1] wrote that "After the operative work is finished comes the question of closing the wound . . . the dura is closed tightly with a continuous fine silk stitch. . . . If there is a dural defect, it is patched with a fascial graft carefully applied. . . . This careful closure is to prevent any cerebrospinal fluid leak which is always fraught with danger."

Most, although not all, authors[2-6] agree with Mixter's observation. In this chapter, methods of prevention, diagnosis, and treatment of patients with leakage of spinal cerebrospinal fluid (CSF) are discussed.

ETIOLOGY AND PREVENTION

The presence of spinal dural CSF leakage can change a well-performed operation into one with a serious complication: a dural cutaneous fistula can lead to meningitis, a meningocele can disrupt the muscle as well as the skin closure and may cause spinal cord or nerve root compression, and CSF leakage increases morbidity and the length of hospital stay. Leakage and the formation of a collection of CSF can be noted after the purposeful opening or resection of dura and with the tearing of dura during laminectomy or dural puncture, or after spinal trauma. Each of these situations presents specific technical problems that are addressed in this chapter.

Repair of a midline or paramedian dural opening fashioned in the course of intradural exploration should involve a straightforward repair. The dural incision separates dural fibers that, when retraction on them is released, have a natural tendency to fall together. Assuming that the spinal cord need not be decompressed, the incision can be sutured easily in a watertight fashion. The difficulty in elective dural opening arises, for example, when it is necessary to resect dura in the course of removing a tumor, such as a meningioma. When the dural resection is dorsally situated, the defect can be repaired easily with a patch of fascia; however, when the defect in the dura is ventrally situated or is in the axilla of the nerve root, sutured dural repair may not be possible. Other measures, described later, may be necessary to prevent CSF leakage.

Inadvertent CSF leakage during an elective extradural operation can frequently be avoided if the surgeon adheres to careful technique. In my experience, dural laceration occurs most commonly with the use of a Kerrison punch when the dura has not been separated adequately from the overlying bone or ligament in the presence of severe lumbar spinal stenosis or during an operation for recurrent disease. Laceration of the dura may also occur in the course of routine lumbar disc excisions.

When the patient's spine is being operated on for the first time, the dura must be separated from the overlying tissue with a fine dissector before the foot plate of a rongeur is placed in the epidural space. Heavy bone should be removed with a Leksell rongeur or a high-speed drill so that the more delicate Kerrison instrument is not required to perform this task. If a drill is used to thin the bone, the motion of the drill must be medial to lateral so that if any slippage occurs, it is away from the dura. An effort should be made to operate superficial to the ligamentum flavum because this structure will protect the dura. After bone removal is completed, the ligament should be cut sharply and not torn with a rongeur.

Another source of dural tear and CSF leakage is the sharp bone spicule,[7] which may cause a dural laceration and CSF leakage days after the operation. A similar situation can occur with a medially placed pedicle screw, which tears the dura.[8] In both situations, CSF leakage can develop in an occult fashion. Bone edges must be smooth, and screws and other hardware must be well placed before final closure.

In a patient who has had previous surgery at the site of reoperation, one must identify normal dura by extending removal of bone rostrally and caudally from the margins of the previous laminectomy or hemilaminectomy. Then, the plane of the normal dura must be identified so that dissection can proceed safely through the scar to free the dura and the nerve root or roots. When the scar readily separates from the dura, dissection with a blunt dissector is satisfactory. However, when the scar is firmly adherent to the dura, sharp dissection is necessary to prevent dural tear. When the repeated operation is for a lateral lesion, such as recurrent lumbar disc herniation, bone and scar lateral to the nerve root must be removed. The plane lateral and ventral to the nerve root and dura can then be dissected with minimal retraction and with less chance of dural injury.

CEREBROSPINAL FLUID LEAKAGE AFTER ANTERIOR SPINAL SURGERY

Prevention of dural injury during anterior spinal surgery requires the same attention to surgical principles as does laminectomy. The plane of the dura must be identified and the dura separated from the overlying tissue before further bone, ligament, or tumor is removed. In the cervical spine, cervical corpectomy in patients with ossification of the posterior longitudinal ligament (OPLL) deserves special mention.[9] At times, the lesion from ossification of the posterior longitudinal ligament invades dura, making resection of dura inevitable. Smith and colleagues[10] recommend the use of autogenous fascial or muscle graft and lumbar subarachnoid shunting in this situation. They stress the need to prevent sudden increases in CSF pressure with its resultant vomiting and coughing. At other times, the posterior longitudinal ligament can be dissected from the dura. The dissection should be performed with the knife parallel to the fibers of the dura. Should a laceration occur, suture repair may be possible. When the laceration is perpendicular to the dural fibers, the defect gaps and the sutures pull out.

Anterior vertebral resection at thoracic or lumbar levels of the spine for tumor, degenerative disease, or herniated disc should follow the same principles described previously. Should a dural tear occur and CSF be seen during operation at these levels, sufficient room exists to drill bone to adequately expose the leak and deal with it by direct suture or a patch. A CSF drain may be necessary.

With nonsurgically managed spinal trauma, a CSF leakage under the skin or into a body cavity is unlikely unless the patient has sustained a penetrating injury. If surgery is required for the injury, severe disruption of the dura may be found that requires repair with a fascial graft using a suture technique, if possible, or fibrin glue. Diversion of CSF to reduce the pressure on the repair is then necessary.

The use of spinal instrumentation at any level of the spine can be a cause of dural laceration. Leakage of CSF has been reported[11] with sublaminar wires and with pedicle screws, especially when they are placed more medially than is appropriate. Great care must be taken with the use of these instruments and devices. Dura must be stripped from the overlying bone and ligament before sublaminar wires are passed. The surgeon who uses any spinal instrumentation must be well trained and careful so that the screws are of appropriate length and are placed at the correct angles.

A CSF fistula in an operative field in which radiotherapy had previously been delivered usually is an extremely difficult problem to manage. The tissues are firm and, when brought together, do not conform to the cavity created by the operation. Sutures do not hold well; they must be tied with excess force to bring the rigid tissues together. Most importantly, the irradiated tissue has a poor blood supply caused by the characteristic vascular changes of radiation, which include hyaline thickening of blood vessel walls.

DIAGNOSIS

INTRAOPERATIVE CEREBROSPINAL FLUID LEAKAGE

Leakage of CSF during operation is usually obvious. When the dura has been opened on purpose, it should be repaired. When the tear is accidental, CSF usually appears in the operative field. The source of the leakage must be found and, if possible, repaired. Untreated CSF leakage during the operation invites postoperative complications.

POSTOPERATIVE CEREBROSPINAL FLUID LEAKAGE

Leakage of CSF during the postoperative period presents in two clinical patterns. The first is that of the low-pressure, posture-related headache that is similar to the common postlumbar puncture headache. The patient experiences headache and often nausea, light-headedness, and sweating when

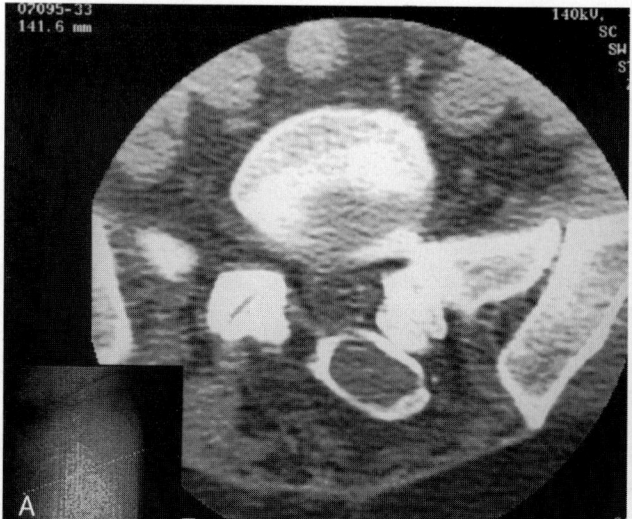
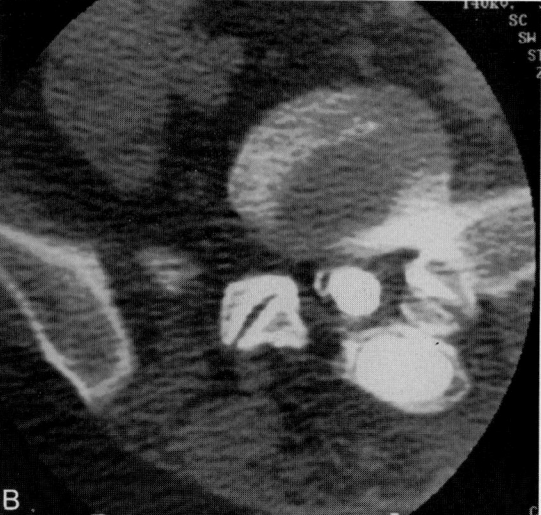

FIGURE 164–1. Computed tomographic view through the lumbar spine at L5-S1. (A) Status after laminectomy with fusion. An ovoid mass with rim calcification is present in the laminectomy defect to the left of the midline. (B) Myelogram after administration of iopamidol shows contrast material in the thecal sac and filling into the previously demonstrated ovoid mass, the pseudomeningocele.

he or she assumes a vertical posture. These symptoms are somewhat relieved by lying down. The second clinical pattern relates to the wound. A laminectomy wound bulges, and CSF leakage occurs at the suture line. Continual leakage of CSF prevents the incision from healing and increases the possibility of infection. When the nature of wound drainage is in doubt, glucose-oxidase paper is a reliable test for glucose. Although other body fluids may contain some glucose, a strongly positive result is diagnostic of CSF, and no further diagnostic tests are necessary to establish that CSF is passing from the incision.

A collection of CSF after anterior spinal surgery can present as a fluid-filled mass in the anterior neck. Thoracic leakage can result in CSF coming out of a chest tube or a significant collection of pleural fluid, and lumbar CSF leakage can result in a pelvic collection.

After it has been established that CSF leakage exists, the site of leakage must be localized. Various techniques have been used to accomplish this: fluorescein, 5 percent, and methylene blue, injected intrathecally, have been used to demonstrate the site of such leakage. Both of these agents are neurotoxic and should therefore not be used.[12, 13] The radioisotope ^{99m}Tc-diethylaminetriaminepenta-acetic acid (DTPA) can be used to demonstrate CSF leakage either by routine scanning or by single photon–emission computed tomography.[14, 15] With its ability to perform three-dimensional reconstruction, single photon–emission computed tomography provides better localization than does biplanar scanning. Magnetic resonance imaging (MRI) demonstrates the CSF collection, which has low signal characteristics on T1 imaging, low signal intensity on proton density, and increased signal on T2-weighted pulse sequences. The best method of demonstrating the exact anatomic location of the leakage, however, is the use of water-soluble positive-contrast myelography followed by computed tomography (CT) (Fig. 164–1).[16] The exact site of the fistula tract in relation to the adjacent bony anatomy can be clearly shown, as can the leakage of the contrast agent into the soft tissues or into a pseudomeningocele.

TREATMENT

Most authors,[2, 3] including myself, believe that with confirmation of the diagnosis of persistent spinal CSF leakage, the appropriate treatment is prompt re-exploration of the wound and repair of the dural defect. Not all authors agree. One should not be dogmatic about this problem. Clearly, some minor leakage heals with nonoperative treatment. Should a soft subcutaneous bulge occur in a well-healed incision in a patient with no symptoms of postural headache, a waiting period is certainly justified. Conversely, early operation must be considered in a patient with a tense or enlarging subcutaneous mass, especially when the incision appears to be breaking down. The morbidity and uncertainty associated with a prolonged nonoperative course of treatment of CSF leakage is not justified.

With a small series of patients, Waisman and Schweppe[5] advocated nonoperative treatment of postoperative leakage. They reported good results with watertight skin closure, the Trendelenburg position, daily subcutaneous taps, and administration of antibiotics. In their series, all wounds cleared within 10 to 28 days. Rosenthal and coworkers[4] described the use of multilayered watertight soft tissue closure in situations in which the dura cannot be closed. They advocated the use of mannitol, 20 g every 4 hours, and nursing supervision to ensure that the patient's head is not raised for 7 days.

The ideal method of dural repair, either as prevention during the primary operation or as treatment of the complication, is watertight suture of the dural defect. The choice of suture material and method of suture closure are important. Because the suture line is rarely exposed to stress, fine suture material, such as a 5-0 or 6-0 braided, coated synthetic, or monofilament, can be used. The needle should be swedged to minimize the size of the suture hole. Leakage of CSF can occur from needle holes in the dura. My preference is to suture dura with closely spaced interrupted sutures. This repair is slower and more tedious than a running stitch, but it avoids the unraveling of the entire suture line when the tension is not perfect or when the suture breaks.

The surgical techniques are shown in Figures 164–2 through 164–5. The ability to perform these techniques depends, to some extent, on the character of the dura itself. When the dura is thin and friable, as sometimes occurs in ossification of the posterior longitudinal ligament or severe lumbar stenosis or when the defect is ventrolateral, a creative, individualized solution is necessary. When the dural defect is at the margin of bone, the laminectomy must be enlarged to gain access to the entire dural defect. Magnification and bright headlight lighting improves the surgical technique.

When the dural defect is linear, a simple suture repair is possible. However, when the dura is thin or slightly irregular or when CSF is leaking from the suture holes, the sutures should be tied over a thin pledget of muscle. All of the sutures are placed, the muscle is placed over the defect and is held by an assistant, and the sutures are tied (see Figs. 164–2 and 164–3).

When a large dural defect is present, the dura must be patched (Fig. 164–4). The graft is anchored at the corners and then sutured with closely spaced interrupted sutures. The

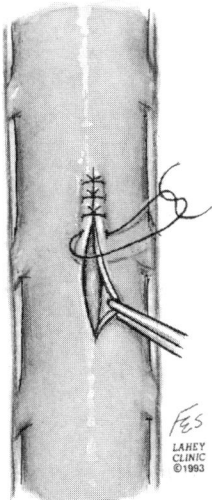

FIGURE 164–2. A linear incision in the dura is repaired with interrupted closely placed 5-0 sutures. (Reprinted by permission of the Lahey Clinic, Burlington, MA.)

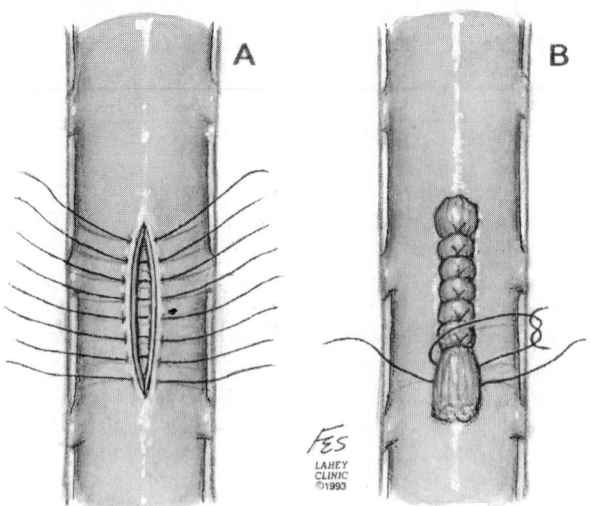

FIGURE 164-3. The sutures are placed, the muscle is placed in the defect, and all sutures are tied. (Reprinted by permission of the Lahey Clinic, Burlington, MA.)

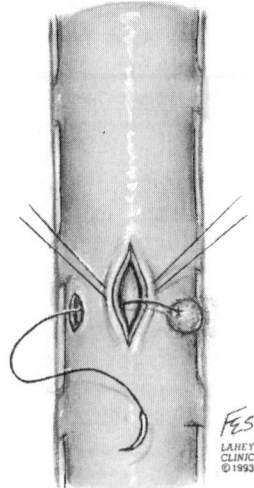

FIGURE 164-5. A pledget of muscle is tied to a suture, which is drawn intradurally and is fastened to plug the hole. (Modified from Mayfield FH, Kurokawa K: Watertight closure of spinal dura mater. J Neurosurg 43:639, 1975. Reprinted by permission of the Lahey Clinic, Burlington, MA.)

graft is then trimmed to fit with minimal redundancy. A minimal overlap of approximately 1 mm at the suture edge provides adequate tissue to plug the leakage. Excess tissue interferes with the suture line. Heavy fascia is readily available for use in grafting from the tissues superficial to the paraspinal muscles, which can be harvested easily on an as-needed basis and trimmed to fit the dural defect. When such paraspinal fascia is not readily available, fascia lata may be used. Although commercially prepared cadaver dura is available for grafting, we do not use it. This preparation is expensive, and transmission of Creutzfeldt-Jakob disease has been reported with its use.[17, 18]

Mayfield and Kurokawa[19] described a method of plugging small dural holes that are difficult to suture. This repair is performed through a midline durotomy. A suture is tied to a piece of fat or muscle, and the suture is passed from the durotomy through the dural defect. This suture can then be tied firmly. The graft located on the inside of the dura seals the leakage (see Fig. 164-5).

It is not always possible to suture a dural defect directly. Most commonly, this situation occurs with anteriorly situated or anterolaterally situated defects, defects involving nerve root sleeves, or thin friable dura. This is a special problem during corpectomy when placing sutures is not possible. In such situations, tissue adhesives have been used in conjunction with fascial or muscle patches and sometimes as an adjunct to partial suturing. The use of CSF drainage may be required to reduce the hydrostatic pressure on the dural defect until healing takes place. This process needs to be combined with meticulous multilayered soft tissue closure if the repair is to succeed. Wiesel[20] believes that the use of wound drains may cause fistulae. We have used drains freely in the presence of dural tear and removed them when no further bleeding is observed. CSF fistula has not been a problem.

Although the cyanoacrylates[21, 22] alkyl-2 and isobutyl-2 have been used with patch grafting to accomplish a biologic seal, these substances are no longer sanctioned by the Food and Drug Administration[23] for this purpose, and the common biologic adhesive in current use is fibrin glue.[24, 25] The commercial preparation is made from pooled plasma and therefore has the risk of transmission of acquired immunodeficiency syndrome. We use fibrin glue made by the hospital's blood bank from the patient's own blood. Preparing the glue takes 24 hours; therefore, its use must be anticipated. The glue must be used in a dry surgical field for the muscle or fascial graft to adhere to the dura. The graft can then be covered by a layer of absorbable fabric and again anchored with the fibrin adhesive (Fig. 164-6).

In the patient with a difficult suture line or with an adhesive repair or a persistent CSF leakage, the CSF dynamics may be altered, a condition that does not permit the defect to seal.[21] Reduction of the CSF pressure with lumbar CSF drainage for 4 or 5 days is frequently sufficient to permit the leakage to seal. The external lumbar drainage is to a closed collection system.[26] We obtain daily CSF cultures and protect

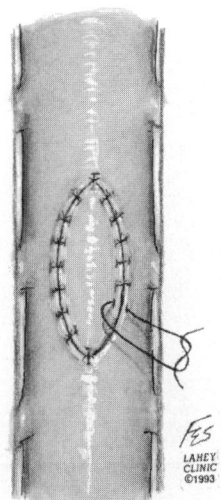

FIGURE 164-4. The patch is held in place with sutures at either end. It is then sutured with interrupted sutures. (Reprinted by permission of the Lahey Clinic, Burlington, MA.)

the patient with broad-spectrum antibiotics while the drain is in place. Instead of the external drainage systems, lumbar peritoneal shunts have been used to provide drainage.[27] However, we have not used a permanent, implanted system to treat what is usually a transient phenomenon.

The use of myocutaneous flaps to cover dura in operative fields in which tissue has been irradiated has been invaluable. Irradiated tissue has poor blood supply and, therefore, poor healing potential.[28] A flap of muscle or muscle and skin with its vascular pedicle and excellent blood supply can be rotated from an uninvolved area to the poorly vascularized defect and then sutured to well-vascularized surrounding tissue. This technique has the benefit of not only permitting the skin to heal but also providing healthy soft tissue that will fill in and mold itself to a cavity and seal a hole in the dura. The well-vascularized flap is resistant to bacteria and can therefore be used in the presence of infection.[29, 30]

Postlumbar puncture CSF leakage has been the commonest cause of procedure-related symptoms associated with low CSF pressure after diagnostic lumbar puncture, spinal anesthesia, or myelography. Classically, a headache develops when the patient assumes the vertical position, and this symptom is relieved when the patient is supine. The cause is the persistent leakage of CSF through a dural rent. This symptom usually clears with nonoperative treatment, rest, and hydration. Before the 1980s, when myelography was performed with iophendylate and a 19-gauge needle, CSF was commonly encountered in the wound during laminectomy performed within a few days of myelography. When the site of the needle puncture was unroofed, a nerve rootlet was seen herniating through, preventing the hole from closing and allowing the leakage to persist. It was necessary to reduce the nerve root hernia and to suture the dura (Fig. 164–7). At times, it was necessary to enlarge the dural defect to reduce the root. Excellent relief of low-pressure symptoms has been reported[31] with an autologous blood patch injected in the epidural space near the site of the puncture. Szeinfeld and associates[32] demonstrated that 12 to 15 ml of blood spreads over eight to 10 spinal segments. The spread is easier in a cephalad direction. Therefore, the injection should be caudad to the lowest interspace in cases of multiple punctures. Although most blood patches have been placed in the lumbar area, Waldman and associates[33] used this technique successfully in the cervical spine with the injection of 8 ml of blood.

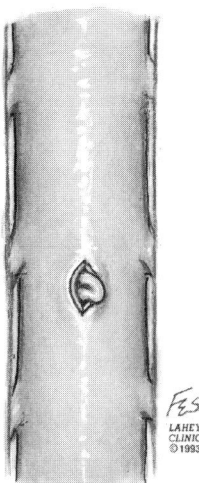

FIGURE 164–7. A nerve rootlet is herniated through a small hole in the dura. (Reprinted by permission of the Lahey Clinic, Burlington, MA.)

SUMMARY

Postoperative CSF leakage should be treated aggressively. Failure to stop the leakage can lead to infection of the wound and meningitis, inability to heal the wound, and prolonged hospitalization and morbidity. It is reasonable to attempt nonoperative treatment for a short while, but when the response is not prompt, the wound should be re-explored and the dura repaired.

REFERENCES

1. Mixter WJ: Spinal column and spinal cord: Laminectomy, in Lewis D (ed): Practice of Surgery, vol XII. Hagerstown, MD, WF Prior Company, 1954, p 29
2. Agrillo U, Simonetti G, Martino V: Postoperative CSF problems after spinal and lumbar surgery: A general review. J Neurosurg Sci 35:93–95, 1991
3. Eismont FJ, Wiesel SW, Rothman RH: Treatment of dural tears associated with spinal surgery. J Bone Joint Surg Am 63A:1132–1136, 1981
4. Rosenthal JD, Hahn JF, Martinez-G J: A technique for closure of leak of spinal fluid. Surg Gynecol Obstet 140:948–950, 1975
5. Waisman M, Schweppe Y: Postoperative cerebrospinal fluid leakage after lumbar spine operations: Conservative treatment. Spine 16:52–53, 1991
6. Dagi TF, George ED: The management of cerebrospinal fluid leaks, in Schmidek HH, Sweet WH (eds): Operative Neurosurgical Techniques, 2nd ed. New York, Grune & Stratton, 1988, pp 57–70
7. Horwitz NH, Rizzoli HV: Laminectomy: General complications, in Horwitz NH, Rizzoli HV (eds): Postoperative Complications of Extracranial Neurological Surgery. Baltimore, Williams & Wilkins, 1987, pp 2–29
8. Olerud S, Sjöström L, Karlström G, Hamberg M: Spontaneous effect of increased stability of the lower spine in cases of severe chronic back pain: The answer of an external transpedincular fixation test. Clin Orthop 203:67–74, 1986
9. Harsh GR IV, Sypert GW, Weinstein PR, et al: Cervical spine stenosis

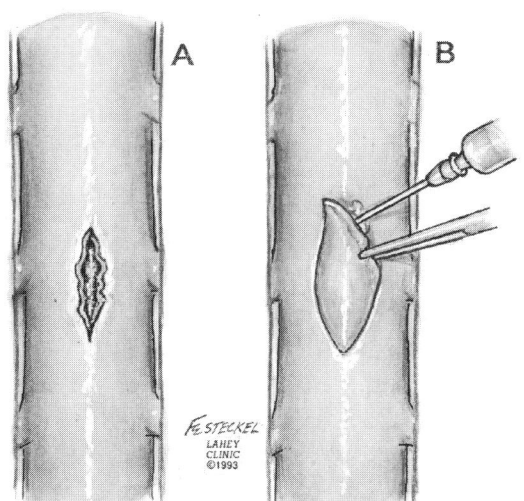

FIGURE 164–6. The patch is held in place with fibrin glue. (Reprinted by permission of the Lahey Clinic, Burlington, MA.)

secondary to ossification of the posterior longitudinal ligament. J Neurosurg 67:349–357, 1987
10. Smith MD, Bolesta MJ, Leventhal M, Bohlman HH: Postoperative cerebrospinal-fluid fistula associated with erosion of the dura: Findings after anterior resection of ossification of the posterior longitudinal ligament in the cervical spine. J Bone Joint Surg Am 74:270–277, 1992
11. Georgis T Jr, Rydevik B, Weinstein JN, Garfin SR: Complications of pedicle screw fixation, in Garfin SR (ed): Complications of Spine Surgery. Baltimore, Williams & Wilkins, 1989, pp 200–210
12. Wallace JD, Weintraub MI, Mattson RH, Rosnagle R: Status epilepticus as a complication of intrathecal fluorescein: Case report. J Neurosurg 36:659–660, 1972
13. Evans JP, Keegan HR: Danger in the use of intrathecal methylene blue. JAMA 174:856–859, 1960
14. Kadrie H, Driedger AA, McInnis W: Persistent dural cerebrospinal fluid leak shown by retrograde radionuclide myelography: Case report. J Nucl Med 17:797–799, 1976
15. Lewis DH, Graham MM: Benefit of tomography in the scintigraphic localization of cerebrospinal fluid leak. J Nucl Med 32:2149–2151, 1991
16. Patronas NJ, Jafar J, Brown F: Pseudomeningoceles diagnosed by metrizamide myelography and computerized tomography. Surg Neurol 16:188–191, 1981
17. Thadani V, Penar PL, Partington J, et al: Creutzfeldt-Jakob disease probably acquired from a cadaveric dura mater graft: Case report. J Neurosurg 69:766–769, 1988
18. Gummerlock MK, Kaufman HH, Narayan RK: FDA panel discussion on cadaver dura. J Neurosurg 73:310, 1990
19. Mayfield FH, Kurokawa K: Watertight closure of spinal dura mater: Technical note. J Neurosurg 43:639–640, 1975
20. Wiesel SW: Neurologic complications of lumbar laminectomy: A standardized approach to the multiply operated lumbar spine, in Garfin SR (ed): Complications of Spine Surgery. Baltimore, Williams & Wilkins, 1989, pp 64–74
21. Lehman RA, Hayes GJ, Martins AN: The use of adhesive and lyophilized dura in the treatment of cerebrospinal rhinorrhea: Technical note. J Neurosurg 26:92–95, 1967
22. Papadakis N, Mark VH: Repair of spinal cerebrospinal fluid fistula with the use of a tissue adhesive: Technical note. Neurosurgery 6:63–65, 1980
23. Samson D: Isobutyl-2-cyanoacrylate (letter). Neurosurgery 19:885, 1986
24. Dresdale A, Rose EA, Jeevanandam V, et al: Preparation of fibrin glue from single-donor fresh-frozen plasma. Surgery 97:750–755, 1985
25. Shaffrey CI, Spotnitz WD, Shaffrey ME, Jane JA: Neurosurgical applications of fibrin glue: Augmentation of dural closure in 134 patients. Neurosurgery 26:207–210, 1990
26. Kitchel SH, Eismont FJ, Green BA: Closed subarachnoid drainage for management of cerebrospinal fluid leakage after an operation on the spine. J Bone Joint Surg Am 71A:984–987, 1989
27. Spetzler RF, Wilson CB: Management of recurrent CSF rhinorrhea of the middle and posterior fossa. J Neurosurg 49:393–397, 1978
28. Azizkhan RG, Roberson JB Jr, Powers SK: Successful use of a vascularized intercostal muscle flap to seal a persistent intrapleural cerebrospinal fluid leak in a child. J Pediatr Surg 26:744–746, 1991
29. Mathes SJ, Nahai F: Classification of the vascular anatomy of muscles: Experimental and clinical correlation. Plast Reconstr Surg 67:177–187, 1981
30. Chang N, Mathes SJ: Comparison of the effect of bacterial inoculation in musculocutaneous and random-pattern flaps. Plast Reconstr Surg 70:1–10, 1982
31. DiGiovanni AJ, Galbert MW, Wahle WM: Epidural injection of autologous blood for postlumbar-puncture headache: II. Additional clinical experiences and laboratory investigation. Anesth Analg 51:226–232, 1972
32. Szeinfeld M, Ihmeidan IH, Moser MM, et al: Epidural blood patch: Evaluation of the volume and spread of blood injected into the epidural space. Anesthesiology 64:820–822, 1986
33. Waldman SD, Feldstein GS, Allen ML: Cervical epidural blood patch: A safe effective treatment for cervical post-dural puncture headache. Anesthesiol Rev 14:23–24, 1987

CHAPTER 165

Surgical Management of Meningoceles and Myelomeningoceles

A. L. Amacher

During the past decade, the incidence of myelomeningocele and anencephaly has been declining.[1] In the United States, the incidence fell to 0.32/1000 live births by 1990. Although regional differences persisted in the early 1980s, perhaps reflecting residual pools of ethnic genetic vulnerability, by 1990 little difference existed between incidences for whites, blacks, and Hispanics in the United States. People of Asian or Pacific Island descent still enjoyed the lowest rates. A similar decline in incidence has been noted in Scotland, from 3.0 to 0.58/1000 live births by 1988[2] for myelomeningocele. Such an ebbing of influx of new cases is welcome for pediatric neurosurgeons. I have observed that the severity of the deformity has declined as well.

Whether or not significant environmental factors are implicated in the incidence of myelomeningocele remains moot, although there seems to be clear indictment of valproic acid and carbamazepine[3, 4] when these agents are taken during early pregnancy. A diet high in folic acid (4.0 mg/day or more) appears to exert a protective effect for women who have borne an affected child,[1] and overall better nutrition may in fact be a major factor in the decline in incidence of this disorder. Screening of amniotic fluid for alpha-fetoprotein remains a useful endeavor that has the practical limitations of any screening program.

The financial burden of myelomeningocele for any society remains significant. In the United States, annual medical and surgical costs for persons with spina bifida exceed $200 million (1985 dollars).[1] Nevertheless, the quality of life enjoyed by an increasing proportion of myelomeningocele survivors has increased dramatically in the past 2 decades. Although family stresses remain high, many more facilities and agencies exist for the support of involved families. Well-equipped and well-staffed centers for the rehabilitation of children with handicaps are widely available, and they often provide educational opportunities and integration into normal schools. Early and long-term control of hydrocephalus, which becomes symptomatic in at least 80 percent of myelomeningocele survivors, has contributed significantly to the educability and eventual self-sufficiency of children with this disorder.

Over the past 2 decades, substantial improvements have been made in our ability to correct and prevent significant disease of the upper and lower renal tract, the relentless progression of which was until recently a major cause of late morbidity and mortality. Urodynamic evaluation of newborns with myelodysplasia and other spinal dysraphic states has a predictive value for the risk of upper tract deterioration; dyssynergia of detrusor–external sphincter coordination is an early warning signal of later trouble.[5] When indicated, early institution of an intermittent catheterization protocol is usually effective in preserving renal function.

Continuing developments in corrective orthopedics and orthopedic appliances are making it feasible for more afflicted children to become and remain ambulatory. McLone reported that 47 percent of patients from an unselected series were ambulatory within the community (not wheelchair bound) 3.5 to 7 years after closure of the lesion.[6]

SURVIVAL DATA

Recent reports of long-term follow-up of children with myelomeningocele emphasize both the seriousness of the condition and the hopeful outlook for certain patients. Nelson and colleagues[7] stated that based on more than 800 unselected patients with myelomeningocele operated on, 2 percent die during initial hospitalization; 15 percent are dead by the age of 10 years; 32 percent will have serious hindbrain dysfunction, of whom 38 percent will die; 27 percent will have an intelligence quotient of less than 80; and a like number will have an intelligence quotient of more than 100. Fifty percent of all myelomeningocele survivors have a learning disability. Thirty-seven percent of survivors show motor improvement after repair—my own experience is 50 percent. Eighty-five percent of survivors achieve social sphincter continence.

Hunt[8] found that 38 percent of survivors are severely disabled, retarded, and dependent. High sensory levels were associated with mortality of 52 percent, whereas 26 percent of patients with sensory levels below L3 died by age 16. Findings among survivors included diabetes mellitus in 4 percent, precocious puberty in 33 percent, and obesity in 33 percent; visual disturbances and pressure sores were common. Twelve percent had normal gait and intelligence.

Steinbok and associates[9] reported a mortality of 18 percent by age 9. Fifty-eight percent were grade appropriate in normal schools, and 75 percent were socially continent of urine,

86 percent for stool. Eighty-five percent had shunts, with a revision rate after 2 years of 10 percent/year.

THE SELECTION CONTROVERSY

Between the extremes of opinion relating to the moral and ethical issues raised in the treatment of children with myelomeningocele, many pediatric neurosurgeons employ some system of selection criteria in determining whether or not to initiate therapy. From the Sheffield[10] experience, initial findings associated with an adverse physical or mental outcome, or both, included associated major congenital anomalies, such as congenital heart disease or renal tract defects; megalencephaly present at birth; severe orthopedic problems, such as pronounced gibbus at the site of the rachischisis; dislocated hips and ankles; and total paraplegia.

In their retrospective analysis of predictors of outcome, Stein and coworkers[11] found that poor outcome was predicted most reliably by the presence of at least two more of the above-mentioned adverse findings and lückenschädel. This German word means "holes in the skull," which describes the congenital status of gaps in the cranial vault. However, some infants with big holes in the skull have normal mental abilities, as do a few with almost any combination of adverse criteria.

The group at the Children's Hospital of Philadelphia made valuable observations in their report on their selected series.[12] They emphasized that no difference for such criteria as the development of ventriculitis, developmental delay, or paresis existed between children whose myelomeningoceles were closed within 48 hours and those operated on between 2 and 7 days after birth or even later. No untreated child lived for more than 10 months. Their point was that if selection criteria are to be used, there is time to consider all of the factors.

Recent enactment of Baby Doe legislation has been accepted by some as justification for jettisoning any decision making in these situations. Such attitudes are not in the best interest of the patient or the family, to say nothing of being a surrender of professional standards and responsibility in response to legislation, an action for which dangerous precedents exist.

Some have suggested that special selection committees should be established for the triage of congenitally handicapped infants. A report of such a process and a severe critique of the committee and its actions have appeared in the literature.[13, 14] Apart from the potential hazards of allowing such committees (which would be made up of various assortments of "socially conscious" people) to assume a triage role in any field of medicine, the person best equipped to assess the potential and the treatment requirements for such children is the one on whom falls the responsibility for the initial decision regarding therapy. In this difficult area, the conscientious, self-searching, and compassionate surgeon who will spend the next several years caring for the child is the best guarantee the public can have against irresponsibility.

O'Korie and coworkers[15] have suggested that delayed myelomeningocele closure in severely affected children may in fact yield better outcomes for such survivors, particularly for children not requiring a shunt. However, small numbers compromise the reliability of their findings.

EARLY CARE OF CHILDREN WITH MYELOMENINGOCELES

The presence of myelomeningocele is usually discovered prenatally. My long-time view that such pregnancies, if not terminated by parental choice, should be followed up closely by ultrasonography and should be allowed to progress to 36 to 38 weeks before delivery can be supported.[16] Further, no evidence exists that cesarean section improves initial presentation or outcome.[17] The suggestion extrapolated from an experimental fetal rat myelomeningocele model that exposure to amniotic fluid in utero may induce placode and root injury preventable by intrauterine coverage of the lesion merits further investigation.[18] Extrapolations from animal models to a complex human situation are fraught with problems, however.

POSTNATAL CARE

No evidence exists that immediate or urgent closure of a myelomeningocele improves neurologic function or reduces the risk of infection.[12] Parents approached within minutes or hours after the birth of an afflicted child can be stampeded into signing uninformed consent documents by such statements as "If we don't close it right away, the baby may end up paralyzed." Such attitudes are mischievous, as is a prolonged delay once a treatment plan has been reached. Forrest defined the issue precisely when he said ". . . initial action or delay need in no way prejudice later decisions about management, and is not the most important factor determining survival."[19]

Lower extremity function or rectal tone increases during the first few postnatal days, regardless of whether the lesion is closed, as though delivery induces a state of spinal shock that begins to recede rather quickly. A delay of a few days in closing the rachischisis allows proper initial evaluation of the child and proper briefing of the parents as well as of the total care team and is perfectly safe if certain precautions are taken.

The infant should be nursed on his or her belly with soft rolls placed beneath the hips and ankles. The sac, even if leaking, can be maintained in a sterile state by use of changes of saline and antibiotic dressings twice daily. Contamination of the site by stool and urine is easily avoided.

When the parents and the surgeon agree on the desirability of operative treatment, the child should be operated on at the next convenient time. Parents should be made to realize that they have played a part in the decision making, but only rarely can the final decision be theirs entirely. Whatever the initial decision, continuing support for the parents and their realization that early treatment decisions may be reversed or modified by later events are essential aspects of the overall approach to the child and the family.

An untreated infant with an open rachischisis is unlikely to survive for more than a few weeks, but some will for several years. One cannot ask nurses or parents to provide suboptimal care for the infant to promote his or her demise. Under such circumstances, the situation must be reassessed and, often, initial decisions reversed.

TECHNICAL ASPECTS

POSITIONING

The lesion should be protected against pressure during intubation. Frequently, a baby with a myelomeningocele requires a smaller endotracheal tube than may be apparent from the weight of the child.

Once the baby is in the prone position, soft rolls should be placed under the shoulders, hips, and ankles. The dressing should remain in place until the skin is ready to be prepared. A mild aqueous preparation is satisfactory and safe. If extensive skin undermining or preparation of rotation or myocutaneous flaps is anticipated, a wide preparation of the skin and field is necessary.

DISSECTION

Figure 165–1 is a montage of commonly seen myelomeningocele defects. Anticipating the type of skin closure that can be achieved is almost always possible, and using skin along the edge of a tense sac as closure material becomes much more likely once sac tension is released.

The dissection is begun at a site covered by the thinned leptomeninges. Only bipolar coagulation is permissible, and nothing less than 4.5 power loupes should be used. All epidermal elements must be removed from the placode: I have had one epidermoid tumor arise within a retubulated spinal cord when a scrap of skin was left on the placode, an experience echoed by Scott and colleagues.[20] The placode requires special attention. *Placode* is the name given to a plate of embryonic epithelial cells constituting a primordial grouping from which a structure arises, in this instance, the spinal cord.

Extreme care must be taken at the upper end of the placode, especially when this abuts directly against the skin. The cord lies directly beneath the placode at this point, and removing its very outer edge with the skin to avoid leaving skin behind is safe. The large, tortuous veins in the leptomeninges can be sacrificed, but rootlet arterioles must be preserved.

Once the placode is circumcised from its tetherings (Fig. 165–2), closure may be planned. Figure 165–3 indicates the potential layers available for closure. It is possible to retubulate the placode with a fine running suture, but I have abandoned this maneuver because it is unnecessary. A leptomeningeal layer can be raised from off the deep fascia; the mobilization is begun just medial to the facet bulges. Almost always, a watertight closure can be obtained, and a tubulated cord can be produced in the process (Fig. 165–4).

Before the dura is closed, a gentle lifting of the placode demonstrates the sensory (lateral) and motor (medial) rootlets (Fig. 165–5). Undue lifting and jerking of the placode must be avoided at all stages of the dissection. In some of the large saccular types of myelomeningoceles, with redundant skin and elongated rootlets, the placode and some of the roots are adherent to skin and scar tissue. A nerve stimulator is useful here to avoid damage to functional neural tissue. Damage to functioning lower sacral rootlets can be avoided by a combination of nerve stimulation and placement of an indwelling catheter attached to a water manometer (an operating cystometrogram).

A good fascial layer frequently can be raised from off the paraspinal muscles and closed over the spinal cord. A larger fascial flap can be raised from the thoracic wall, simply rotated down on its inferior pedicle. I have never regretted eschewing the muscle-bone covering of the canal. If this technique is used, considerable blood loss should be anticipated.

SKIN CLOSURE

Figure 165–6 outlines some strategies for skin closure. With experience, the surgeon will find it possible to close an increasing percentage of lesions by direct suture. The figure of 25 percent stated by Paterson and Till[21] as being uncloseable by direct suture is much higher than my current experience. Claims that primary closure has no role in myelomeningocele repair are arbitrary and unwarranted.

In the case of large defects, surgeons unfamiliar with the techniques of raising viable rotation flaps should enlist the assistance of a plastic surgeon. Shaving down the bony excrescences of a gibbus to allow easier and looser approximation of skin edges is quite safe. When the skin edges are undermined, as much subcutaneous tissue as possible should be left with the skin, and button holing of the flap must be avoided.

A rotation flap should have a length:base ratio of 1:1. The infant usually supports a flap, even one that crosses the midline, that has a ratio of 1.5:1. Venes[22] described a method of assessing skin edge vascularity with systemic fluorescein injection that may be most helpful in assessing flap viability. The suggestion that nitroglycerin paste rubbed onto a suture line may salvage dubious closures has not been evaluated in a standard model.[23] Bipedicle flaps may be useful in some situations, with the resulting elliptic defects closed by further undermining of the donor edges or by split-thickness skin grafts.

Double-Z rhomboid flaps and latissimus dorsi or gluteus maximus myocutaneous flaps may be necessary for some large defects. Ramirez and colleagues[24] described this technique in 1987 and indicated that lateral relaxing incisions, delayed rotations, and split-thickness grafts are unnecessary. When split-thickness grafts are used, they should be cut with sufficient thickness (0.011 of an inch or more) to ensure durable coverage. I have occasionally used secondary split-thickness grafting on small areas of flap necrosis with good success.

"Dog ears" frequently occur at the distal corners of incisions after direct suture or flap rotation. Only the larger redundant ones need be trimmed; the smaller ones mold out with time.

Skin edges that are white and strained at the end of closure do not survive; those that are blue usually do. The subcutaneous closure layer is the most important, and such closure should be performed with interrupted sutures. Skin-edge approximation must be conducted loosely, with as few sutures as possible. Skin-edge approximation strips are excellent aids in this situation.

Figure 165–7 illustrates direct suture closures corresponding to defects A, B, and C of Figure 165–1. Even round defects 6 to 7 cm in diameter are amenable to closure by direct suture if careful undermining techniques are used.

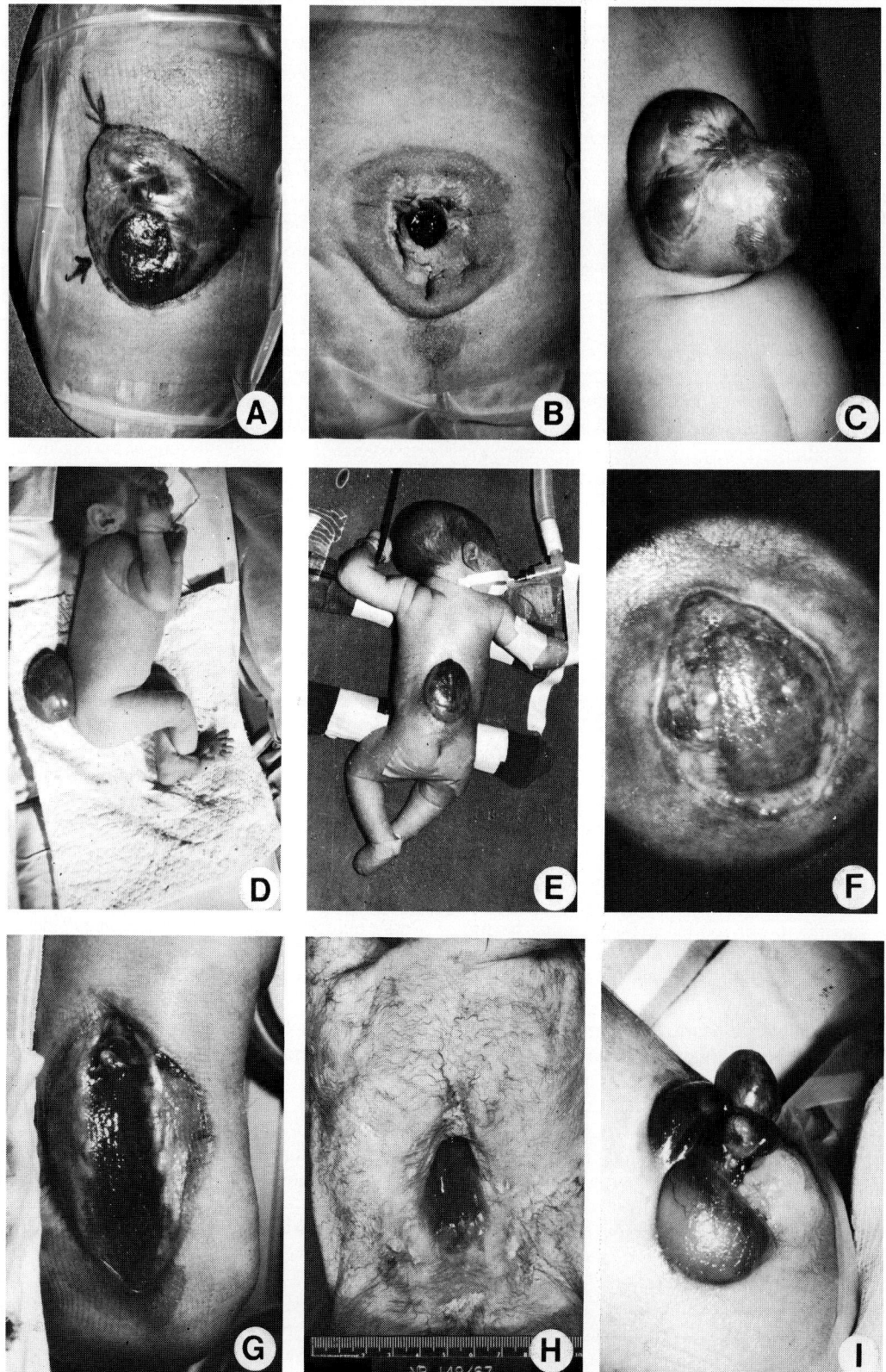

FIGURE 165–1. (A to I) Examples of configurations of myelomeningoceles preoperatively.

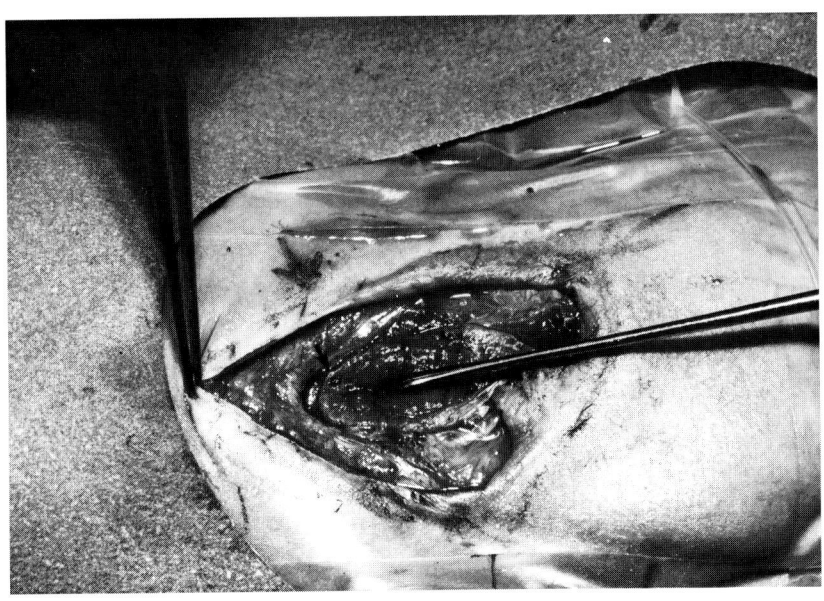

FIGURE 165–2. The neural placode is trimmed (the arrow marks the edge).

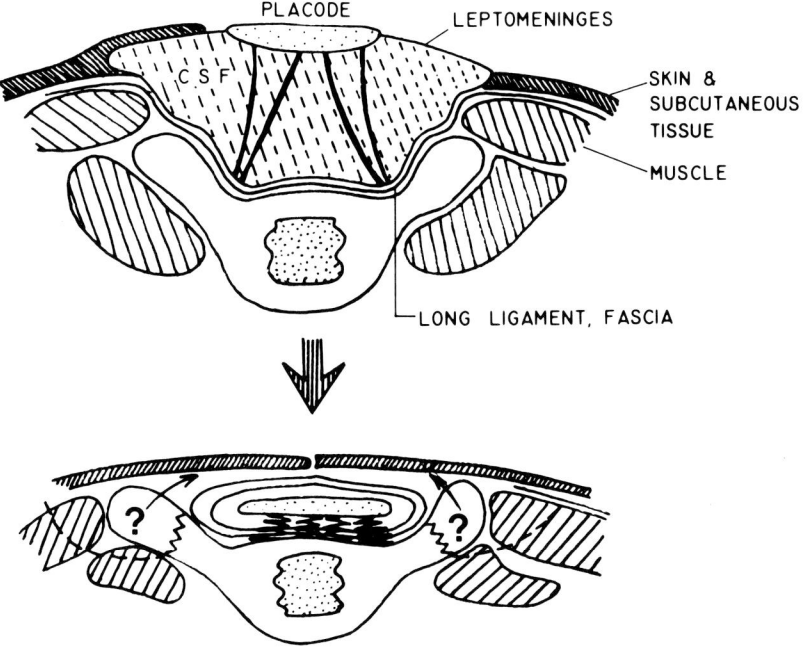

FIGURE 165–3. Layers available for closure of myelomeningoceles.

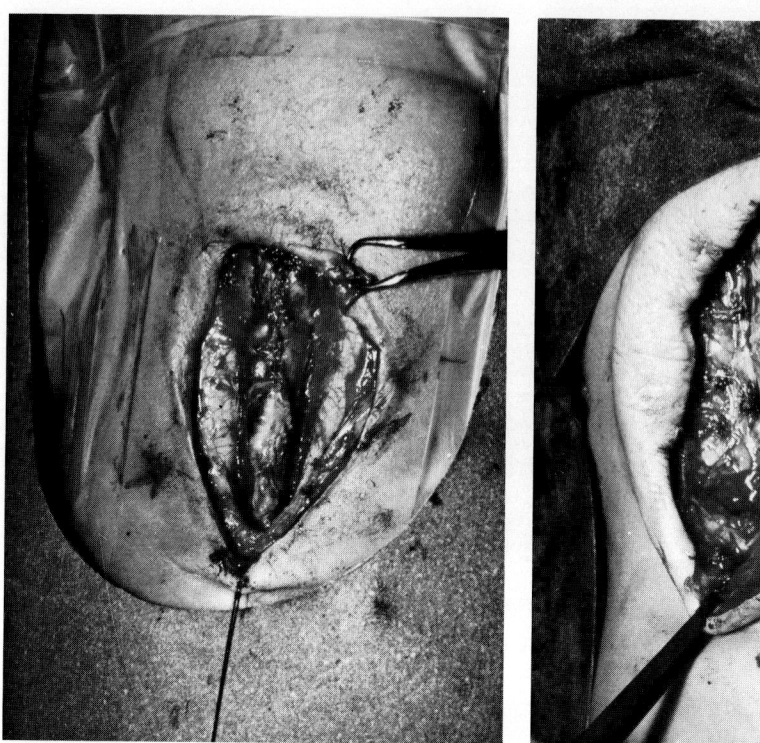

FIGURE 165-4. Examples of dural tubes after closure.

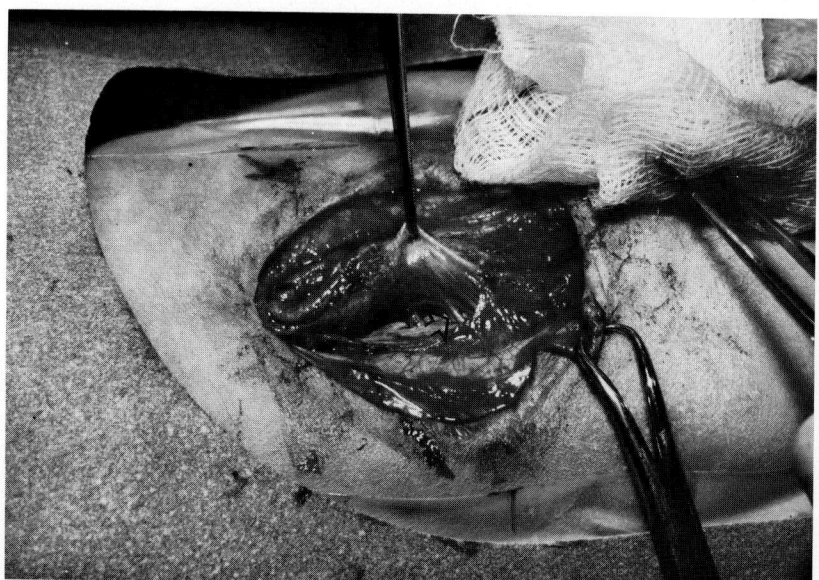

FIGURE 165-5. Motor and sensory roots exiting from the placode (arrow).

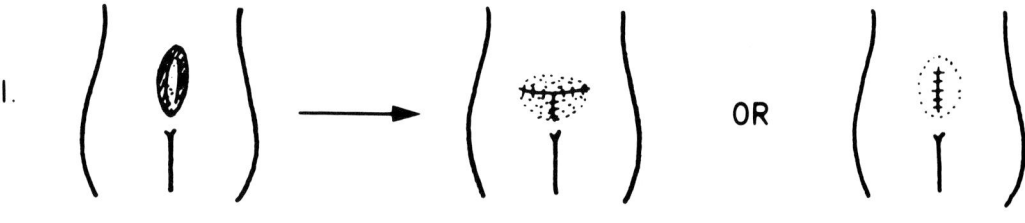
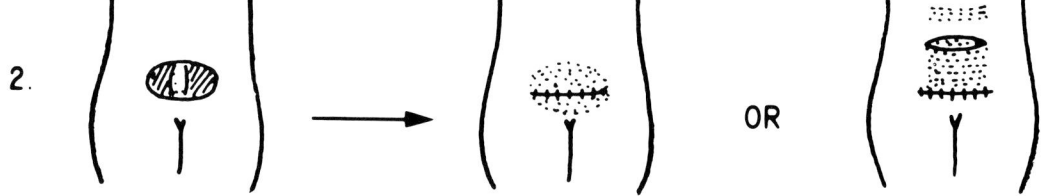

FIGURE 165–6. Strategies for skin closure.

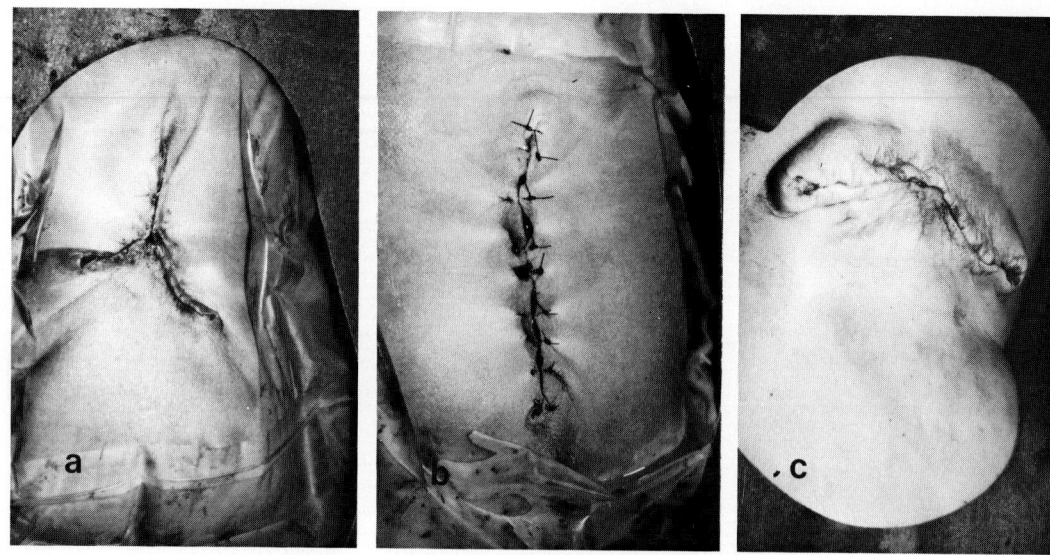

FIGURE 165–7. (A to C) Completed incisions corresponding to the myelomeningoceles in Figure 165–1. a = Figure 165–1A; b = Figure 165–1B; c = Figure 165–1C.

POSTOPERATIVE CARE

The baby must be kept off his or her back until wound healing is secure. Newborns tolerate the prone position very well, and if soft rolls are kept beneath the hips and ankles and a small sheepskin mat beneath the child, skin irritation is minimized. Collections of serous exudate or cerebrospinal fluid (CSF) beneath the closure should be evacuated if tension of the suture line is produced. I have not found suspending the baby's abdomen in a soft sling necessary, although this maneuver may help reduce lateral suture-line tension. Once the incision is obviously stable and healthy, the baby can be nursed on its sides as well. Recently, I have encouraged the picking up and cuddling of these children as soon as possible.

Any required physiotherapy or corrective casting of the lower extremities can begin immediately. Dressings should be changed frequently, and the viability of the closure should be assessed. A necrotic closure should be revised quickly to forestall serious infection of the closure site.

Progressive hydrocephalus or persistent CSF collection at the closure site should be treated by shunting. The question of whether or not myelomeningocele closure increases the likelihood of progressive hydrocephalus is moot,[25] but because a small percentage of children with myelomeningocele do not require shunting, preclosure or concurrent insertion of a shunt should be performed only for rigid indications. Mapstone and associates[26] presented evidence that children with myelomeningocele who do not require a shunt exhibit higher mean intelligence quotients later on than do their shunted cohorts.

Hyperbaric oxygen therapy may salvage an ischemic closure,[27] but it should not be relied on to do so as an alternative to the use of myocutaneous flaps. Neurosurgeons not trained in the planning and preparation of rotation or myocutaneous flaps or rapid tissue expansion techniques should routinely enlist the participation of a plastic surgeon. To fail to do so is a disservice to one's patient.

About 10 percent of infants with myelomeningocele develop laryngeal stridor of sufficient severity to require decompression of the posterior fossa and upper cervical cord several days to several weeks after birth. Occasionally, such manifestations of lower brainstem dysfunction (stridor, swallowing dyssynergia, pseudobulbar vocalization) may be delayed for months, even years. In a significant number of children or infants, decompression of the posterior fossa and upper cervical cord does not alleviate the problem, the etiology of which may reside in the brainstem nuclei themselves.

LATER MAJOR CLOSURE SITE PROCEDURES

For proper seating and bracing, removing a prominent lumbar gibbus may be necessary. The technique has been described by Hall and Poitras[28] and can be safely performed by early to midchildhood.

UNUSUAL SCENARIOS

Panel I of Figure 165–1 shows a lesion that contained anomalous sheets of cartilage, osteoid, isolated cysts, and a diastematic peg. When diastematomyelia coincides with myelomeningocele, it should be resected at the initial procedure.

Gupta and Deodhar[29] described a split notochord syndrome wherein a myelomeningocele was associated with a dorsal enteric fistula. My own experience includes a child with diplomyelia below the thoracic level with a typical placode and exiting roots on one of the cord halves only. The ipsilateral leg had an L4 motor level, and the contralateral one was normal.

Loder and coworkers[30] have pointed out that the aorta bridges thoracolumbar kyphoses associated with severe high myelomeningoceles, and that the upper renal poles may be nearly in the midline. Both structures may be at risk during kyphectomy.

LATE TETHERING

Recently, considerable discussion has arisen about late, or secondary, tethering in myelomeningocele patients. Sagittal magnetic resonance images (MRIs) always show a low conus-placode and apparent tethering of roots. Certainly, performing survey MRIs in children without symptoms of tethering provides reasonable baseline information. Other lesions found routinely include terminal syrinxes, lipomas, epidermoids, dermal sinuses, and diastematomyelias.[31, 32] Tumors and lesions with potential for growth should probably be removed, but advocating prophylactic detethering of placodes and roots based on MRI findings is unwarranted. Of more than 300 infants with myelomeningoceles whose lesions I have repaired personally, symptoms clearly related to late tethering have arisen in fewer than 10 percent of cases.

SUMMARY

Precise closure techniques for myelomeningocele provide the maximum potential for rehabilitation of the little victims of this disorder. Only surgeons who are willing to participate fully in the continuing care of such children should presume to expertise in this field.

POSTERIOR SPINAL MENINGOCELES

Cystic lesions anywhere along the spinal axis and not containing neural elements usually are straightforward insofar as closure is concerned. Often, an associated spinal anomaly or hemivertebra exists, such as spina bifida occulta or segmentation defect. Dissection along the neck of the sac with dural closure usually is accomplished easily, as is skin closure. There is a significant caveat, however; the likelihood of an intradural anomaly (cyst, diastematomyelia, bone spur, extradural or intradural lipoma, dermoid tumor, or short and thick filum) is very high.[33] These children should have MRI or metrizamide myelography at 12 to 18 months of age to rule out residual tethering of the spinal cord.

McLone and Naidich[34] have drawn attention to the entity labeled *terminal myelocystocele*. An intrasacral or retrosacral cyst representing an expanded central canal is associated with cloacal exstrophy and sacral spina bifida occulta. A meningocele is usually present as well. The extrasacral cyst may present very low, as a bizarre overhang to the perineal area.

ANTEROLATERAL SPINAL MENINGOCELES

Meningoceles that emerge from the spinal column to lie anteriorly or laterally are very rare. Of Matson's total series of 1381 meningoceles and myelomeningoceles, only 0.43 percent were anterior or lateral.[35] Many anterolateral sacs, however, remain asymptomatic well into adult life; thus, the known prevalence of such meningoceles increases with age.

Both thoracic and sacral anterior meningoceles have been discussed with increasing frequency over the past 2 decades. A fairly definitive description now can be given of the manifestations and treatment of such lesions.

CERVICAL MENINGOCELES

If the lesion is present at birth as a swelling in the posterior cervical triangle, a diagnosis of cystic hygroma may be made.[36] Multiple cervical meningoceles have been seen in association with neurofibromatosis.[37] An example of a cervical meningocele above the clavicle occurring after nerve root avulsion was reported by Jakobsen and associates.[38]

Delashaw and coworkers[39] described four cases of cervical meningocele with a compendium of associated anomalies, including hydrocephalus, Chiari's malformation, hydromyelia, lipomyelomeningocele, tethered cord, filum-thickening diastematomyelia, Klippel-Feil syndrome, thoracic hemivertebrae, and subluxation of C1 on C2. Any combination of these lesions can be encountered with any case of meningocele of the spine.

The very rare situation of an anterior basioccipital meningocele causing airway obstruction in a neonate has been described by Azizkhan and colleagues.[40] They resected the lesion transorally with good outcome.

THORACIC AND LUMBAR MENINGOCELES

Most thoracic and lumbar meningoceles are probably asymptomatic until they are encountered in the course of routine or other examinations. A rounded soft tissue density in the superior or posterior mediastinum on a routine chest x-ray film frequently heralds the meningocele. Occasionally, radicular pain in the thorax or abdomen or aching of the arm has been noted. Very occasionally, a myelopathy has been described, but such cord compression is usually ascribable to an associated spinal pathologic condition. Headache of a paroxysmal nature, frequently associated with exercise or with prolonged upright posture, may occur because of pooling of CSF in large sacs.

Increasingly, an association of thoracic meningoceles with von Recklinghausen's disease (neurofibromatosis) has been reported.[41, 42] A posterior or superior mediastinal mass in a patient with neurofibromatosis is likely to be either a dumbbell neurofibroma or a meningocele. Sometimes, both are found. In addition, such patients may have multiple lesions. These patients in particular may have kyphoscoliosis or gibbus formation of a degree sufficient to cause chronic cord compression. Intrathoracic meningoceles may exert sufficient chronic pressure to erode both bodies and lateral elements, rendering the spine unstable.[43]

Galzio[44] reported on a unique case in which a giant lumbosacral meningocele opened into the abdominal cavity from a tiny neck that perforated the L5-S1 disc. The patient also had multiple congenital anomalies of the urogenital system and intracranial meningiomas.

The very rare lumbar anterior meningocele is usually discovered incidentally as an abdominal or loin mass in children or adolescents. It occasionally produces back or loin pain,[45] and neurofibromatosis is commonly associated. Usually, the sac emerges from an enlarged intervertebral foramen (Fig. 165–8), but rarely it may come straight forward through a disc or a vertebral body. When a kyphoscoliosis is present, the sac is seen most frequently on the convex side of the deformity.[45]

The capsule comprises an amalgam of parietal pleura,

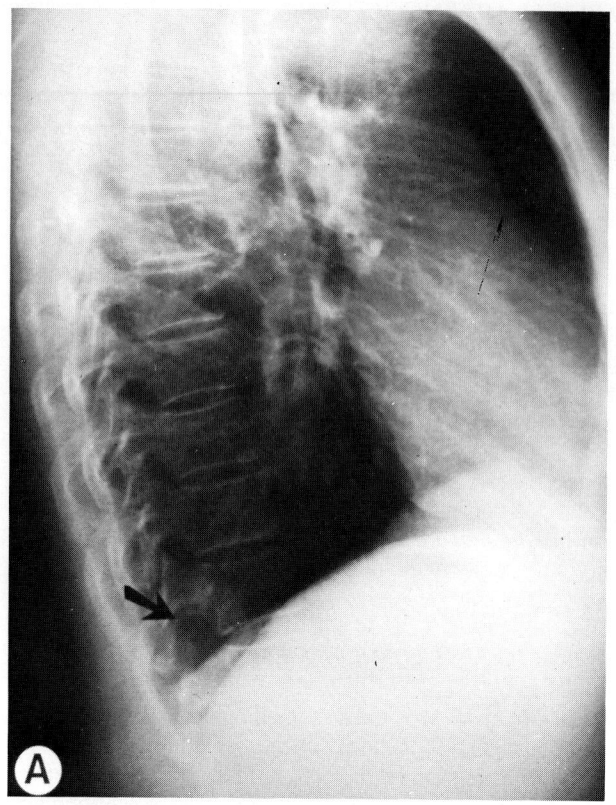

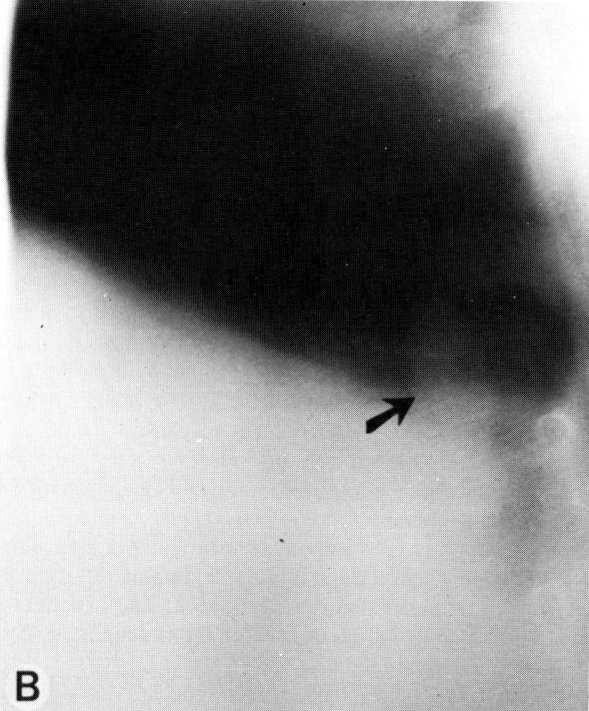

FIGURE 165–8. (A) A lateral chest x-ray film showing an enlarged intervertebral foramen (arrow). (B) A lateral tomogram of the thoracic spine showing an enlarged intervertebral foramen and the shadow of a lateral thoracic meningocele.

retropleural connective and fibrous tissue, and dura. It is tough and resilient and holds sutures well. The sacs may enlarge with time.

The sac seems to originate from the root sleeve in front of the motor rootlet, emerging as a narrow stalk that balloons out into its sac. The segmental nerves and small vessels occasionally are stretched over the sac, as are splayed-out epidural veins. A neurofibroma rarely may be seen in the wall of the sac. Almost always, the communication of CSF between the sac and the subarachnoid space is unimpeded, but not invariably.

RADIOLOGY AND DEFINITIVE DIAGNOSIS

As with dumbbell neurofibromas, the hallmark of an anterolateral thoracic or lumbar meningocele is the finding of an enlargement of the intervertebral foramen on plain x-ray films (Fig. 165–8). In addition, fused or hemivertebrae, posterior body scalloping, fused foramina, and kyphoscoliosis may be seen.

Myelography has been the commonest method of defining the nature of the mass. At present, ultrasonography, MRI, and CT scanning should be performed first because these may provide a reliable answer without resorting to invasive methods. When contrast-enhanced CT scanning is performed, delayed images may be required to demonstrate the communication of the cyst and the subarachnoid space.

TREATMENT

Attacking an asymptomatic anterolateral cervical, thoracic, or lumbar meningocele is purposeless unless it is known to be enlarging. If pain or proven expansion are present, a posterior or posterolateral approach is advisable, with simple transfixation of the neck. The sac should be collapsed, but it need not be removed. Near the thoracolumbar junction, preoperative angiography is essential in locating the notoriously nomadic artery of Adamkiewicz. If this vessel is involved with the neck of the sac, it must be preserved at all costs. Hemilaminectomy may facilitate neck exposure, but pediculectomy or facetectomy are unnecessary.

INTRASACRAL AND ANTERIOR SACRAL MENINGOCELES

Since our report and search of the literature on anterior sacral meningocele (ASM) in 1968,[46] accounts of ASM and intrasacral meningoceles (ISM) have accumulated slowly.[47] In recent years, the spectrum of presentations has been confirmed and widened,[48–51] and a consensus for treatment has emerged.

SYMPTOMATOLOGY

The incidence of ASM and ISM is unknown. Most seem to come to attention in adult women; because the discovery of ASM in children appears to be likely equally in boys and girls, a sex preponderance is improbable at any age.

Among the commonly reported symptoms are headache, either because of excessive CSF pooling in the sac or reflux of CSF into the subarachnoid space; enuresis and encopresis, particularly in children; abdominal masses, usually discovered incidentally with or without vague abdominal complaints; pelvic masses discovered during labor or during routine rectal examinations; pain in the low back or pelvis, occasionally in a sacral nerve distribution; and constipation and difficult defecation. Occasionally, lax sphincters and reduced perineal sensation may be discovered. An ASM presenting as a groin mass has been reported.[52] Acute flexion injury to a sacrum ballooned out by an ISM may produce a transverse fracture of the sacrum, perhaps with neurologic findings.

Of greater import is the potential for infection in the subarachnoid space in the presence of a rectomeningeal fistula, with either ASMs or ISMs. Such fistulas may occur spontaneously, after childbirth, or after attempted aspiration or needle biopsy of a presacral mass.[45, 47] In the report of Brihaye and associates,[53] a fistulous, presumably congenital, tract was discovered between the rectum and an ISM in two cases.

ASMs have been reported in association with presacral teratoma, intrasacral and presacral neurofibroma, von Recklinghausen's disease, intrasacral lipoma, and bony evidence of spinal dysraphism, particularly in the lumbar spine. Quigley and colleagues[54] reported on the case of a young woman who suffered repeated bouts of aseptic meningitis because of a dermoid tumor associated with an ASM. Very rarely, a family incidence has been noted, as have anomalies in other organ systems.[45] Yates and coworkers[55] chronicled the remarkable occurrence of 11 members of one family pedigree with sacral bony defects, ASMs, and presacral teratomas. They suggested that these lesions may be transmitted as an autosomal dominant trait.

The Currarino triad consists of a complex of anal-rectal anomalies, sacral bony abnormality (scimitar sacrum), and presacral ASM, teratoma, or enteric cyst. The anorectal anomalies range from stenosis or ectopia to imperforation. Transmission is autosomal dominant of variable expression. A high risk of gastrointestinal-CSF fistulous connections exists.[56]

PATHOLOGIC ANATOMY

Because of the associated bony abnormalities found in full measure in children as well as adults, both ASMs and ISMs likely represent a congenital anomaly of the bone and the meninges. The sacs are thick walled and contain elements of dura, leptomeninges, connective and fibrous tissue, epidural veins, and, occasionally, incorporated nerve fibers. They probably enlarge with time, perhaps because of hydrostatic forces.

RADIOLOGY AND DEFINITIVE DIAGNOSIS

The ISM produces a distinctive ballooning of the intrasacral canal, with thinning of posterior elements, scalloping of the posterior vertebral body, and expansion of the sagittal

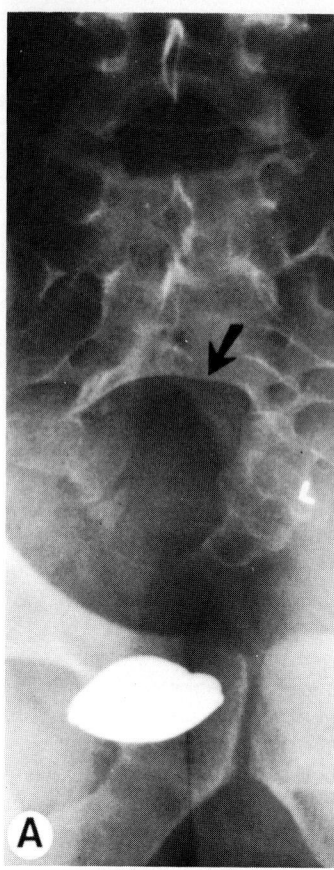
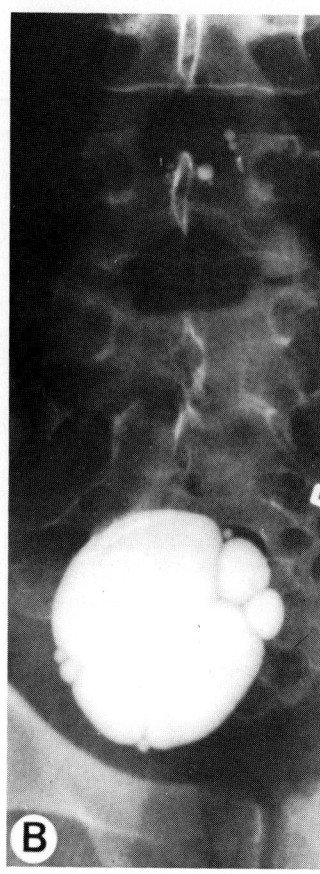

FIGURE 165-9. (A) A posteroanterior sacral myelogram showing a scimitar sacrum (arrow). (B) A posteroanterior sacral myelogram with contrast falling to the anterior aspect of the sac.

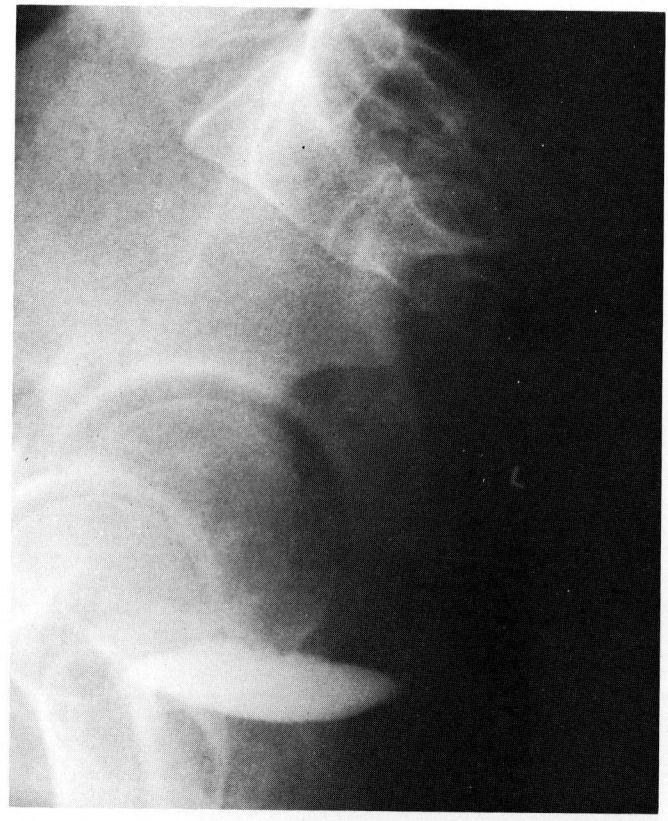

FIGURE 165-10. The true size of an ASM is revealed by this lateral x-ray film. The patient is in the erect position.

diameter of the sacrum. Intervertebral foramina may be enlarged, but usually only to a moderate degree.

The ASM may be associated with complete agenesis of the lower sacrum and with marked enlargement or fusion of one or more intravertebral foramina. The most characteristic finding, however, is the so-called scimitar sacrum (Fig. 165–9A).

The sac itself can be delineated by contrast myelography, sonography, CT, and, of course, MRI. Unless such measures have been used to rule out the presence of an ASM, needle aspiration of a presacral mass via a transrectal or perineal approach must never be performed because introduction of infection into an ASM is extremely serious. The sac may be huge, filling the pelvis and extending into the abdomen (Figs. 165–9B and 165–10).

TREATMENT

Little can be done for an ISM. If sacral pain or ingravescent or paroxysmal neurologic deficits occur, a cystoperitoneal shunt is advisable.

There are two approaches to treating ASMs. Most should be approached by sacral laminectomy with plication of the neck, and care should be taken to avoid damage to nerves in the wall of the sac. The neck of the meningocele may be much larger than anticipated from a myelogram or it may extend through more than one foramen.

The anterior approach to ASMs has a very bad reputation,[45] but it is a safe and useful approach when huge abdominal sacs are encountered.[47] With the sac in direct view, a great deal of operating space can be developed by sac aspiration and blunt dissection along the sac wall and in the retrorectal space. Before the neck is ligated, the sac must be opened and any neural elements in the wall preserved.

REFERENCES

1. Centers for Disease Control: Spina bifida incidence at birth—United States, 1983–1990. MMWR 41:497–500, 1992
2. Davis CF, Young DG: The changing incidence of neural tube defects in Scotland. J Pediatr Surg 26:516–518, 1991
3. Omtzigt JG, Los FJ, Grobbee DE, et al: The risk of spina bifida aperta after first-trimester exposure to valproate in a prenatal cohort. Neurology 42 (4 suppl 5):119–125, 1992
4. Rosa FW: Spina bifida in infants of women treated with carbamazepine during pregnancy. N Engl J Med 324:674–677, 1991
5. Bauer SB, Hallett M, Khoshbin S, et al: Predictive value of urodynamic evaluation in newborns with myelodysplasia. JAMA 252:650, 1984
6. McLone DG: Results of treatment of children born with a myelomeningocele. Clin Neurosurg 30:407, 1983
7. Nelson MD, Bracchi M, Naidich TP, et al: The natural history of repaired myelomeningocele. Radiographics 8:695–706, 1988
8. Hunt GM: Open spina bifida: Outcome for a complete cohort treated unselectively and followed into adulthood. Dev Med Child Neurol 32:108–116, 1990
9. Steinbok P, Irvine B, Cochrane DD, et al: Long-term outcome and complications of children born with meningomyelocele. Childs Nerv Syst 8:92–96, 1992
10. Lister I, Zachary RB, Brereton R: Open myelomeningocele—a ten year review of 200 consecutive closures. Prog Pediatr Surg 10:161, 1977
11. Stein SC, Schut L, Ames ML: Selection of early treatment of myelomeningocele: A retrospective analysis of selection procedures. Dev Med Child Neurol 17:311, 1975
12. Charney EB, Weller SC, Sutton LN, et al: Management of the newborn with myelomeningocele: Time for a decision-making process. Pediatrics 75:58, 1985
13. Gross RH, Cox A, Tatyrek R, et al: Early management and decision-making for the treatment of myelomeningocele. Pediatrics 72:450, 1983
14. Freeman JM: Early management and decision making for the treatment of myelomeningocele: A critique. Pediatrics 73:564, 1984
15. O'Korie NM, MacKinnon AE, Lonton AP, et al: Late back closure in myelomeningoceles—better results for the more severely affected? Z Kinderchir 42 (suppl I):41–42, 1987
16. Hogge WA, Dungan JS, Brooks MP, et al: Diagnosis and management of prenatally detected myelomeningocele: A preliminary report. Am J Obstet Gynecol 163:1061–1064, 1990
17. Bensen JT, Dillard RG, Burton BK: Open spina bifida: Does cesarean section delivery improve prognosis? Obstet Gynecol 71:532–534, 1988
18. Heffez DS, Aryanpur J, Hutchins GM, et al: The paralysis associated with myelomeningocele: Clinical and experimental data implicating a preventable spinal cord injury. Neurosurgery 26:987–992, 1990
19. Forrest DM: Spina bifida: Some problems in management. Proc R Soc Med 70:233, 1977
20. Scott RM, Wolpert SM, Bartoshesky LE, et al: Dermoid tumors occurring at the site of previous myelomeningocele repair. J Neurosurg 65:779–783, 1986
21. Paterson TJS, Till K: The use of rotation flaps following excision of lumbar myelomeningoceles. An aid to the closure of large defects. Br J Surg 46:606, 1959
22. Venes JL: The use of intravenous fluorescein in the repair of large myelomeningoceles. Technical note. J Neurosurg 47:126, 1977
23. Lehman RAW, Page RB, Saggers GC, et al: Technical note: The use of nitroglycerin ointment after precarious neurosurgical wound closure. Neurosurgery 16:701, 1985
24. Ramirez OM, Ramasastry SS, Granick MS, et al: A new surgical approach to closure of large lumbosacral meningomyelocele defects. Plast Reconstr Surg 80:799–807, 1987
25. Linder M, Nichols J, Sklar F: Effect of myelomeningocele closure on the intracranial pulse pressure. Childs Nerv Syst 11:176, 1984
26. Mapstone TB, Rekate HL, Nulsen FE, et al: Relationship of CSF shunting and IQ in children with myelomeningocele. A retrospective analysis. Childs Nerv Syst 11:112, 1984
27. Dillon BT, Warford LR, Vogel RG: Hyperbaric oxygen therapy in a newborn infant. J Ark Med Soc 83:325–326, 1987
28. Hall JE, Poitras B: The management of kyphosis in patients with myelomeningocele. Clin Orthop 128:33, 1977
29. Gupta DK, Deodhar MC: Split notochord syndrome presenting with meningomyelocele and dorsal enteric fistula. J Pediatr Surg 22:382–383, 1987
30. Loder RT, Shapiro P, Towbin R: Aortic anatomy in children with myelomeningocele and congenital lumbar kyphosis. J Pediatr Orthop 11:31–35, 1991
31. Just M, Schwarz M, Ludwig B, et al: Cerebral and spinal MR findings in patients with post repair myelomeningocele. Pediatr Radiol 20:262–266, 1990
32. Balasubramaniam C, Laurent JP, McCluggage C, et al: Tethered-cord syndrome after repair of meningomyelocele. Childs Nerv Syst 6:208–211, 1990
33. Chaseling RW, Johnson IH, Besser M: Meningoceles and the tethered cord syndrome. Childs Nerv Syst 1:105, 1985
34. McLone DG, Naidich TP: Terminal myelocystocele. Neurosurgery 16:36, 1985
35. Matson DD: Neurosurgery of Infancy and Childhood, 2nd ed. Springfield, IL, Charles C Thomas, 1969
36. Shore RM, Chun RWM, Strother CM: Lateral cervical meningocele. Clin Pediatr 21:430, 1982
37. O'Neill P, Whatmore WJ, Booth AE: Spinal meningoceles in association with neurofibromatosis. Neurosurgery 13:82, 1983
38. Jakobsen H, Roder OC, Bojsen-Moller: Large paracervical meningocele due to lesion of cervical spinal nerve roots. Acta Chir Scand 149:537, 1983
39. Delashaw JB, Park TS, Cail WM, et al: Cervical meningocele and associated spinal anomalies. Childs Nerv Syst 3:165–169, 1987
40. Azizkhan RG, Cuenca RF, Powers SK: Transoral repair of a rare basioccipital meningocele in a neonate. Neurosurgery 25:469–471, 1989
41. Dolynchuk KN, Teskey J, West M: Intrathoracic meningocele associated with neurofibromatosis: Case report. Neurosurgery 27:485–487, 1990
42. Sarkar PK, Fagan AM: Intrathoracic meningocele in a patient with neurofibromatosis. Respir Med 85:163–165, 1991

43. Kornberg M, Rechtine GR, Dupuy TE: Thoracic vertebral erosion secondary to an intrathoracic meningocele in a patient with neurofibromatosis. Spine 9:821, 1985
44. Galzio RJ: Giant anterior lumbosacral meningocele associated with intracranial meningiomas and multiple congenital malformations. Surg Neurol 18:419, 1982
45. Wilkins RH, Odom GL: Anterior and lateral spinal meningoceles, in Vinken PJ, Bruyn GW (eds): Handbook of Clinical Neurology, vol 32. New York, North Holland, 1978, pp 198–230
46. Amacher AL, Drake CG, McLachlin AD: Anterior sacral meningocele. Surg Gynecol Obstet 126:986, 1968
47. Amacher AL: Surgical management of meningoceles and myelomeningoceles, in Schmidek HH, Sweet WH (eds): Operative Neurosurgical Techniques: Indications, Methods, and Results, 2nd ed. Orlando, FL, Grune & Stratton, 1988, pp 151–162
48. Mellion BT, George RE, Fischer DK, et al: Anterior sacral meningocele and tuberculous spondylitis of the sacrum in a patient with neurofibromatosis. Neurofibromatosis 2:299–308, 1989
49. Bayar MA, Yidiz B, Buharali Z: Management problems in cases with a combination of asymptomatic occult intrasacral meningocele and disc prolapse. Acta Neurochir (Wien) 108:67–69, 1991
50. North RB, Kidd DH, Wang H: Occult, bilateral anterior sacral and intrasacral meningeal and perineurial cysts: Case report and review of the literature. Neurosurgery 27:981–986, 1990
51. Doty JR, Thomson J, Simonds G, et al: Occult intrasacral meningocele: Clinical and radiographic diagnosis. Neurosurgery 24:616–625, 1989
52. Dyck P, Wilson CB: Anterior sacral meningocele. Case report. J Neurosurg 53:548, 1980
53. Brihaye J, Gerard A, Kiekens R, et al: Rectomeningeal fistulae in dysraphic states. Surg Neurol 10:93, 1978
54. Quigley MR, Schinco F, Brown JT: Anterior sacral meningocele with an unusual presentation. J Neurosurg 61:790, 1984
55. Yates VD, Wilroy RS, Whitington GL, et al: Anterior sacral defects. An autosomal dominantly inherited condition. J Pediatr 102:239, 1983
56. Kirks DR, Merten DF, Filston HC, Oakes WJ: The Currarino triad: Complex of anorectal malformation, sacral bony abnormality, and presacral mass. Pediatr Radiol 14:220, 1984

CHAPTER 166

Surgical Management of Occult Spinal Dysraphism

Paul H. Chapman

The term *spina bifida* is generally understood to connote a wide variety of congenital pathologic conditions of the spine. Such dissimilar entities as myelomeningocele, dermal sinus with or without tumor, spinal lipoma, tethered filum terminale, and diastematomyelia have been variously included under the heading of spina bifida.[1] The common denominator is, as implied, a congenital defect in the posterior elements of one or more vertebral segments. Such a grouping on the basis of a single pathologic feature, however, has led to confusion about the relationship between these various conditions with regard to clinical presentation, course, and treatment. The major difficulty results from a juxtaposition of myelomeningocele (or meningocele, spina bifida cystica, spina bifida aperta, myeloschisis) and so-called spina bifida occulta and its associated conditions. Myelomeningocele, with its attendant problems, is a common and widely recognized entity. In such cases, there is characteristically a dorsal protrusion of more or less severely malformed spinal cord elements and their coverings between the bifid bony elements on the surface of the back. Neurologic deficits in the lower extremities are often severe, with associated loss of bladder or bowel control. These deficits are present at birth and usually are unchanging. The Arnold-Chiari malformation of the cerebellum and brainstem is usually present, as are lesser deformities of the forebrain. Progressive hydrocephalus is common.

On the other hand, a group of congenital lesions of the caudal spinal canal and its overlying tissues exists that involve the spinal cord to produce progressive neurologic deficits. Because spina bifida is associated with these lesions, they are often discussed under the designation *spina bifida occulta*. Use of the term *spinal dysraphism* to designate them as a group is also common.[2-5] Pathologically, these lesions are not consistently associated with Arnold-Chiari malformation, hydrocephalus, or other cerebral anomalies, and no clear pattern of heritability exists. The degree of spinal cord dysplasia is relatively minor compared with that found in the typical case of myelomeningocele. Likewise, the dysplasia of overlying tissues, in particular the skin, is usually minor, although it is extremely valuable in suggesting the presence of underlying difficulty. Occult spinal dysraphism typically causes progressive neurologic deterioration, whether of bladder, bowel, or lower extremity sensorimotor function. The deficits initially are often minor and may or may not occur in the context of pre-existing fixed deformities of the lower extremities, such as talipes or unequal size of the feet or legs. Finally, approximately two-thirds of the patients are female, whereas in myelomeningocele, no clear sex predilection exists.

PATHOLOGY

The intraspinal pathologic features of spinal dysraphism are quite diverse. Certain common features, however, underlie this diversity. In most cases, the congenital abnormality exerts an immobilizing influence on the spinal cord, usually at its distal extremity. The use of the term *tethered spinal cord* reflects this feature. Occasionally, expanding lesions, such as intraspinal dermoid tumors or lipomas, produce neurologic symptomatology by direct compression of the adjacent spinal cord or nerve roots. Even in these cases, however, the presence of an ancillary immobilizing influence must be considered. In conjunction with tethering, the conus medullaris is found to lie at an abnormally low level within the spinal canal, as is demonstrable either during surgery or by myelography, and constitutes an important feature in diagnosis. During fetal development, gradual relative ascent of the conus occurs within the spinal canal because of the disparate rate of longitudinal growth of the spinal cord and spine.[6,7] At 17 weeks' gestation, the spinal cord ends opposite the L4 vertebral level. At term, the mean level of termination is at the lower border of L2. Several months postnatally, it has reached the level of the L1-L2 interspace. No further ascent occurs. Therefore, if the conus terminates at the level of L3 or below after 5 to 6 months of age, it can be considered to be abnormally low.

In spinal dysraphism, the conus is not only low but also tends to be situated posteriorly within the spinal canal (see Fig. 166–4). With caudal fixation of the conus, the lumbosacral lordosis tends to bring it into a posterior position. Another factor, which is discussed later, may be actual fixation of the conus to the posterior dura by a thickened filum, lipomatous mass, or fibrous bands.

Aside from these general considerations, the spinal pathology usually assumes one of several forms. An understanding of the pathologic anatomy of these lesions is necessary for their proper recognition and surgical management. Intraspinal lipoma is a common pathologic entity (Fig. 166–1A). Emery and Lendon[8] studied its various forms in detail. A term that is synonymous with intraspinal lipoma in the literature is *lipomyelomeningocele*. The lipomatous mass is usu-

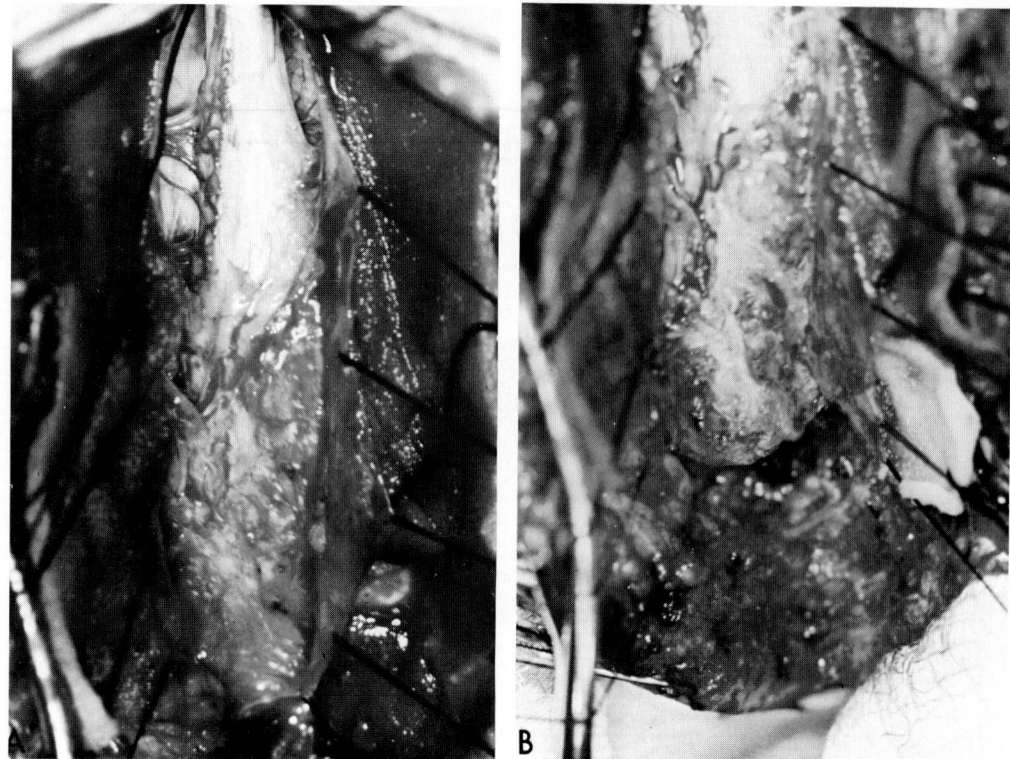

FIGURE 166–1. (A) An intradural lipoma confluent with the conus medullaris. Note the horizontal direction of the exiting nerve roots. (B) A closer view of the lipoma shown in Figure 166–1A after subtotal resection. Surgery resulted in improved bladder function.

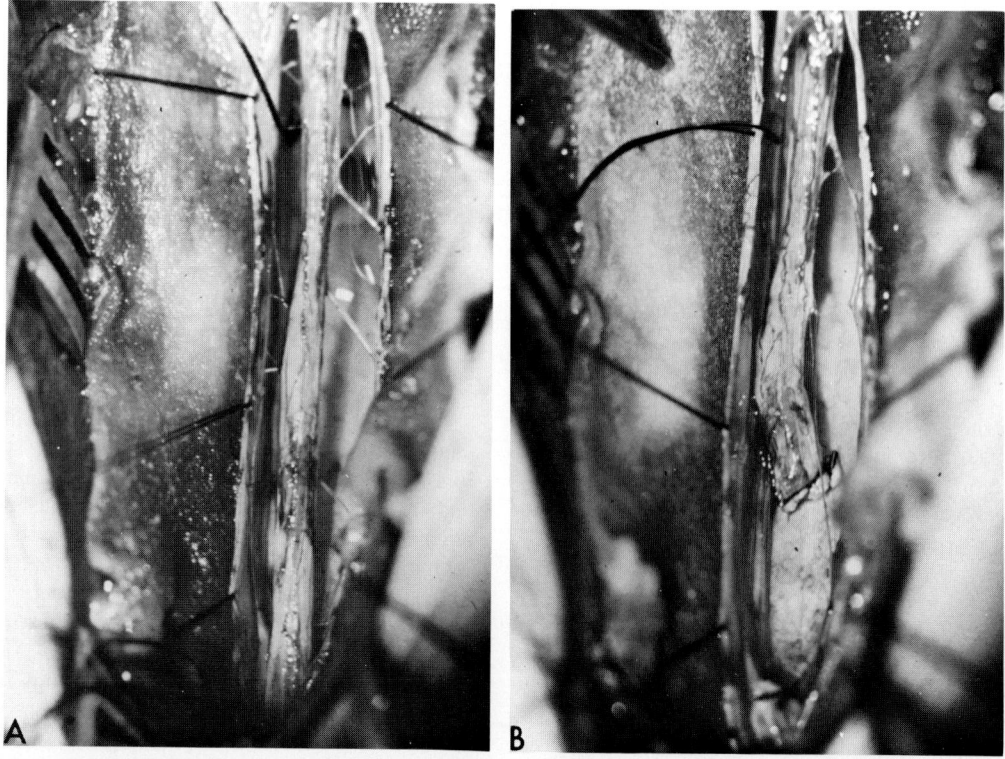

FIGURE 166–2. (A) A thick filum with a low conus medullaris (top). (B) The filum shown in Figure 166–2A after division. Note the distance between the divided ends of the filum and the more vertical direction of the nerve roots, indicating upward migration of the conus and proximal filum after division of the filum.

ally situated in the caudal extremity of the spinal canal and is coextensive with the conus medullaris. The connection with the conus may be a stalklike fibrolipomatous structure, or the lipoma may gradually merge with the conus in such a way that extensive intermingling of fatty and neural tissues occurs at a rather indistinct interface. Careful histologic examination of the lipoma may, in fact, reveal a wide variety of mesodermal and ectodermal tissue elements including, on rare occasions, epithelium-lined cysts.[9] This finding does not have any special significance with respect to management or prognosis.

The site of fixation of the lipoma to the conus is important surgically and separates these lesions into two general categories.[10] On the one hand, the fatty mass may insert into the dorsal aspect of the conus. In this circumstance, the lesion typically extends from the subcutaneous space into the spinal canal through widely bifid bony elements and a congenital posterior dural defect. This has been designated a *leptomyelolipoma* by Emery and Lendon.[8] The interface between the lipoma and the conus usually lies just posterior to the point of emergence of sensory rootlets so that neither these nor the more anteriorly situated motor rootlets are within the substance of the lipoma. On the other hand, the lipoma may insert into the distal extremity of the conus, in which case the fatty mass may be entirely intraspinal or, more commonly, may extend through a dural defect caudally to present as a subcutaneous mass. In this second type of lesion, nerve roots are encountered running to their foramina of exit within the substance of the lipoma. These features are obviously important surgically and are discussed further in the section on operative technique.

A simpler type of abnormality is the short, thickened filum terminale (Fig. 166–2A). The filum terminale is normally a threadlike structure that represents a nonneural continuation of the conus medullaris. The filum inserts at the distal end of the dural sac and generally contains a microscopic continuation of the central canal of the spinal cord. In its abnormal state, the filum is thickened to a diameter of 3 to 5 mm. It is shorter than normal by virtue of the low position of the conus and lies posteriorly within the dural sac, often in contact with the posterior dura. A lipoma in continuity with it may be present, particularly at the point of distal insertion of the filum. The thickened filum may insert posteriorly in the dura, proximal to the termination of the dural sac. Microscopically, the abnormal filum is collagenous, with a centrally placed core of ependymal cells representing the remnant of the central canal. Small islands of fatty tissue may be present within the collagenous substrate.

Occasionally, fibrous bands may be found. These arise from the conus and insert on the dura posteriorly, laterally, or even anteriorly. Such bands may continue through the dura to end in relation to overlying bony elements or within subcutaneous tissue. At times, these have the appearance of aberrant nerve roots with dorsal root ganglia present. Stimulation typically reveals no motor function. Lassman and James[11] have devised the term *meningocele manqué* for cases with adhesions of the conus, filum, or cauda equina rootlets to the inner aspect of the posterior dura, usually in the lumbosacral area.

Diastematomyelia is a less common form of spinal dysraphism. The pathologic features consist of a bony or fibrocartilaginous spur that traverses the spinal canal in an anteroposterior direction in the midline (see Fig. 166–6).[12–14] It is attached anteriorly to the vertebral body and posteriorly to the arch of bone that constitutes the back of the spinal canal. The spur may incompletely span the canal, in which case it might be based either anteriorly or posteriorly. Abnormalities such as small or hemivertebrae, disc-space narrowing, fusion of anterior or posterior elements, or transverse widening of the canal generally occur at that level. The spur characteristically divides the spinal canal in a midsagittal direction, thus effectively skewering the divided cord, the halves of which rejoin above and below the spur. The spur may occur at any point along the spine but is commonest in the lower thoracic and lumbar area, with a peak incidence at L2.[15] The term *diastematomyelia* implies a division of the spinal cord into two halves. Uncommonly, one may in fact be dealing with actual duplication of the spinal cord or diplomyelia. Because these two conditions are indistinguishable clinically, the term diastematomyelia has been adopted by convention. Finally, diastematomyelia may occur without an associated spur or septum.

Dermal sinus, with or without a related intraspinal dermoid tumor, is found in association with occult spina bifida. The tumor is often situated partially within the substance of the spinal cord, particularly in the region of the conus. In such cases, it cannot be totally extirpated. Microscopically, these tumors consist of dermal elements, including appendages such as hair follicles with hair, sweat, and apocrine glands. Epidermoid tumors occur as well.

Although these various lesions have been described as discrete entities, the pathologic state often is more complex than such a description would indicate. There is a tendency for more than one type of lesion to occur in a single case (Fig. 166–3). Thus, one occasionally finds a short, thick filum; fibrous bands; or intraspinal lipoma in the presence of diastematomyelia. Alternately, lipoma, tethering bands, and a thickened filum may occur in varying combinations. Finally, the lesions encountered are not strictly limited to those just described. Lesions such as occult meningocele and hydromyelia also have been observed, either singly or in combination with the commoner lesions, especially lipomas or diastematomyelia.[16] Despite the occasional lesion associated with Arnold-Chiari malformation, this hindbrain deformity generally has not been found in cases of spinal dysraphism, where it has been specifically sought.[17]

The mechanism by which these diverse pathologic conditions produce neurologic impairment is unclear. Except when a mass lesion or fibrous bands exert obvious pressure on neural elements, the common denominator appears to be the immobilizing effect of the lesion on the distal spinal cord and, possibly, the nerve roots (see Fig. 166–2B). It has been suggested that this prevents normal ascent of the conus with growth of the spinal cord in the canal, and that the traction thus exerted results in progressive neurologic deficits. Although the conus remains at the same vertebral level after several months of age, subsequent to that age, longitudinal growth of the vertebral column is relatively greater than that of the spinal cord. In cases of caudal spinal cord tethering, this has the effect of subjecting the cord to increasing tension, particularly during growth spurts of childhood and adolescence. In addition, a degree of mobility of distal spinal cord elements in response to changes in position may be important. Some mobility can be demonstrated at myelogra-

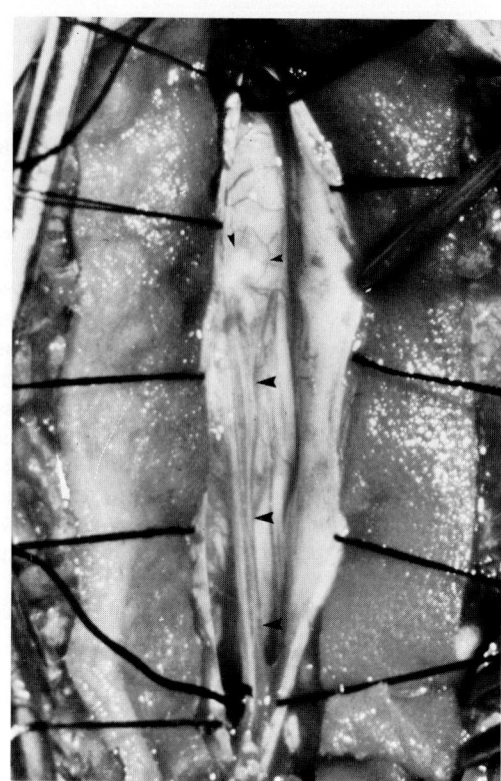

FIGURE 166-3. Fibrous bands (large arrows, lower) attaching to the conus posteriorly in the region of an associated small intramedullary dermoid tumor (small arrows, upper). No sinus tract was demonstrated pathologically.

phy, although this technique alone has not provided a clear differentiation between normal and pathologic conditions. Immobilization of neural elements may prevent normal protective accommodative movements in response to changes in position during activity. The possibility of vascular insult, as a result of cord immobility, also has been considered.[18, 19] In this regard, Yamada and associates[20] have demonstrated reversibly impaired oxidative metabolism in the tethered cord, both experimentally and clinically.

SPINE ABNORMALITIES

The presence of spina bifida occulta is, as the name implies, an important feature in the diagnosis of this condition. Some confusion may arise in that a substantial proportion of the normal population harbors an occult spina bifida without intraspinal pathologic features. When spina bifida is a normal variant, the split element is generally at S1 and occasionally at L5. This degree of bifida has its highest incidence in early life and is commoner in males. The incidence appears to vary with different racial groups.[21-24] In symptomatic spina bifida occulta associated with spinal dysraphism, spinal segments other than L5 and S1 usually are involved, they often multiply, and the degree of diastasis is more pronounced. Although spina bifida may be the only demonstrable bony abnormality, other defects do occur. Examples of these were enumerated briefly in the discussion of diastematomyelia. Pang and Hoffman[25] have called attention to the possible existence of spinal cord tethering in cases of sacral agenesis.

Although uncommon, this is of particular significance because the sensorimotor and sphincter disturbances associated with this condition generally have not been considered amenable to surgery.

Although a general geographic relationship exists between the site of bony abnormality and the underlying intraspinal lesion, this relationship is not exact. The two lesions may be separated by several segmental levels. This fact assumes importance in the proper recognition of the site of an intraspinal pathologic condition at surgical exploration. It also emphasizes the need for careful preoperative radiographic evaluation.

SKIN ABNORMALITY

Cutaneous stigmata are often present and may provide a valuable clue to the problem. These abnormalities usually occur in the middle or lower back in the midline and, like the bony deformity, may not correspond to the segmental level of the intraspinal lesion. The nature of the skin lesion varies. It may consist of a circumscribed area of hyperpigmentation or capillary hemangioma. The latter is common as a normal variant over the inferior occipital area and is of no concern there. If such a lesion is found in the thoracic or lumbar midline region, unseen difficulties should be anticipated. There may be a hairy patch of skin, either with or without associated abnormal skin pigmentation. Hair growth can be extremely luxuriant, constituting what is aptly called a *fawn's tail*. A subcutaneous lipoma may be present. As indicated previously, such fatty masses are usually coextensive with intraspinal lipomas or other dysraphic anomalies. Other lesions associated with a subcutaneous lumbosacral mass that can be confused with lipoma include meningocele, myelocystocele, and sacrococcygeal teratoma. Myelocystocele represents a combined meningocele and focal hydromyelia. It tends to occur in association with omphalocele, bladder exstrophy, and imperforate anus.

A midline skin pore is common in association with intraspinal dermoid tumors. It represents the opening of a sinus tract that extends inward and attaches to the tumor. This tract is directed rostrally so that the skin pore lies caudal to the level of the tumor. It is important to distinguish between a true dermal sinus pore and a simple pilonidal dimple. The latter, which lies more inferiorly, usually at the tip of the coccyx, is of no consequence in the present context.

CLINICAL PRESENTATION

About two-thirds of patients with spinal dysraphism are females. Although symptoms may arise at any age, most occur initially in children. In most cases, the presenting problem reflects neurologic impairment of the lower extremities or of bladder function. Gait disturbance is common and may represent simple weakness or postural deformity of one or both lower extremities, particularly distally. Equinus deformities are also common. In addition, shortening or wasting of the involved foot or leg may occur. Orthopedic deformities are present at birth in some instances. Further neurologic impairment then may be superimposed on this pre-existing disability. In this context, it may be difficult to detect progressive functional impairment at an early stage, especially in younger children. The problem might manifest itself, for instance, only as repeated failure of orthopedic corrections. A significant percentage of patients initially have urinary incontinence, which can be minor or severe. This problem may become apparent only when the child is well past the usual age of training, despite the disorder's presence from infancy. In infancy, patients often come to medical attention because of concern regarding the skin lesion alone, especially in cases of subcutaneous lipomas and hairy patches. At this time, no neurologic abnormality exists. If the skin lesion is disregarded, the child may return later as a deficit appears, as sphincter disturbance is unmasked, or as he or she verbalizes discomfort. This shifting pattern of presenting features is well described for spinal lipomas[26] and diastematomyelias.[15] In most cases of tethered cord, the bladder dysfunction reflects partial denervation with hypotonicity and preserved sensation, although an atonic bladder can also occur.[27, 28]

Although the foregoing covers the principal modes of presentation, occasionally other problems prompt initial concern. Impaired sensation in the lower extremities can result in trophic ulceration of the involved part. Septic meningitis, especially if recurrent or caused by an unusual organism, should elicit careful examination for the presence of a dermal sinus tract. Back pain may be the chief concern. This pain is characteristically exacerbated by movement or exercise, and the child limits his or her activity, even though he or she may not complain about it specifically.[29] At one time, symptomatic dysraphism was felt to be exclusively a problem of childhood and adolescence. It is now recognized that symptoms may first appear in adulthood and even late life.[30] Figure 166–4 shows the magnetic resonance imaging (MRI) of a woman with a thick filum who initially presented at the age of 60 years with recent onset of urinary incontinence, leg weakness, and low back pain.

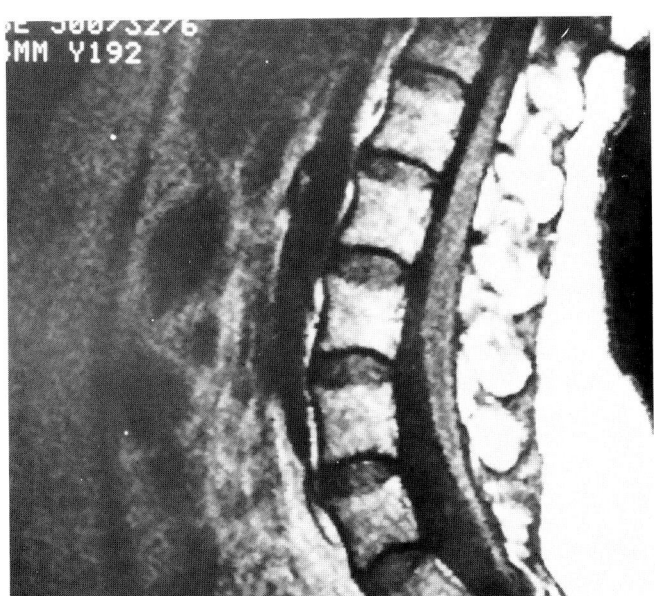

FIGURE 166–4. A magnetic resonance scan of a 60-year-old woman with a thick filum terminale and recent onset of back pain, motor disturbance, and bladder dysfunction. The symptoms were relieved by surgical untethering.

DIAGNOSTIC ASSESSMENT AND INDICATIONS FOR SURGERY

The initial assessment of these children requires a careful history and examination designed to detect what might be minor degrees of neurologic impairment. Any suspected case should be studied further. Also, a child with dermal sinus should be handled similarly, regardless of neurologic status. In the latter instance, the high incidence of associated intraspinal tumor or potential communication with the subarachnoid space, with its attendant risk of meningitis, demands surgical intervention. An element of controversy arises regarding the proper management of patients with clinical and radiologic stigmata of spinal dysraphism but without evidence of deterioration or neurologic deficit. In cases of spinal lipoma, delayed neurologic deterioration is well documented, both in childhood[26, 31-34] and in adulthood.[35, 36] This common phenomenon reflects our own experience. Because of such cases, we feel that the presence of a lumbosacral lipoma per se is an indication for further investigation and surgery. This opinion is shared by others,[26, 36] including Till,[4] who further felt that any child with clinical and radiologic stigmata of spinal dysraphism should undergo myelography, regardless of neurologic status. If radiographic studies show either a specific lesion or a low conus, then surgical exploration is warranted. This view represents an extension of the concept of prophylactic surgery for all patients with spinal dysraphism. It is based on the observation that neurologic deficits that occur, even under close follow-up, cannot predictably be reversed by subsequent surgery. Implied is the fact that surgery, when properly executed, has a sufficiently low risk to warrant such action. Till[37] reviewed his own extensive experience with regard to the question of prophylactic surgery. In a detailed review of 65 cases of diastematomyelia, Kennedy[15] reached similar conclusions with respect to that condition. These considerations regarding preventive surgery do not apply to adults, in whom surgery should be considered only on indication of progressive symptomatology.

SPECIAL RADIOGRAPHIC STUDIES

Because of the diverse and often complex intraspinal pathologic features associated with spinal dysraphism, it is important to gain maximum information from radiographic studies before surgical exploration. To do so requires a technique that clearly defines the structures within the caudal spinal canal. Iophendylate (Pantopaque, Lafayette Pharmaceuticals) introduced by the lumbar route frequently has been used[17, 36] but has several disadvantages. Because it is a dense contrast medium, structures such as fibrous bands, tracts, or a thickened filum may be poorly visualized. The level of termination of the conus may not be apparent. The position of the conus is important. A low-lying conus represents a more or less constant pathologic concomitant of spinal dysraphism and may be the only abnormality found on a myelogram. Puncturing the spinal canal in an area where displaced neural tissue may be situated logically presents the risk of injury to these structures. Finally, it may be difficult to enter the subarachnoid space, especially if a lipoma is present. Introducing the contrast by cisternal tap[17] presents problems in retrieving the substance.

Air myelography[4] represented a partial solution to these problems but has been superseded by computed tomographic scanning with intrathecal water-soluble contrast agents and, most recently, by MRI. Conventional myelography with water-soluble contrast agents can also be performed but gives less anatomic detail, which may be important in the surgical approach to complex cases (Fig. 166–5 through 166–7). Computed tomography and MRI techniques also have the advantage of providing axial as well as sagittal and coronal projections (Fig. 166–8).[38, 39] High-resolution MRI scanning is noninvasive and gives detailed three-dimensional information. With improved availability, it will undoubtedly supplant other types of radiographic studies.

SURGICAL TECHNIQUE

Successful surgery of spinal dysraphism depends on a detailed knowledge of the pathologic anatomy that will be encountered, especially when lesions are complex or multiple. In spite of preoperative studies, however, one often must rely on surgical observation to clarify the anatomic details. Intraoperative nerve stimulation is an important adjunct in this regard. It is of considerable help in identifying and avoiding injury to important neural structures, particularly in cases in which anatomic relationships are seriously distorted. The patient is draped to allow examination of the feet and legs during stimulation. Electronic twitch monitors can also be placed on the toes to detect slight movement in response to stimulation. Manometric monitoring of bladder tone in response to stimulation may be helpful. At present, we also monitor bladder and rectal sphincter electromyographic responses using a ring electrode catheter and surface needle electrodes, respectively. The anesthetic technique should

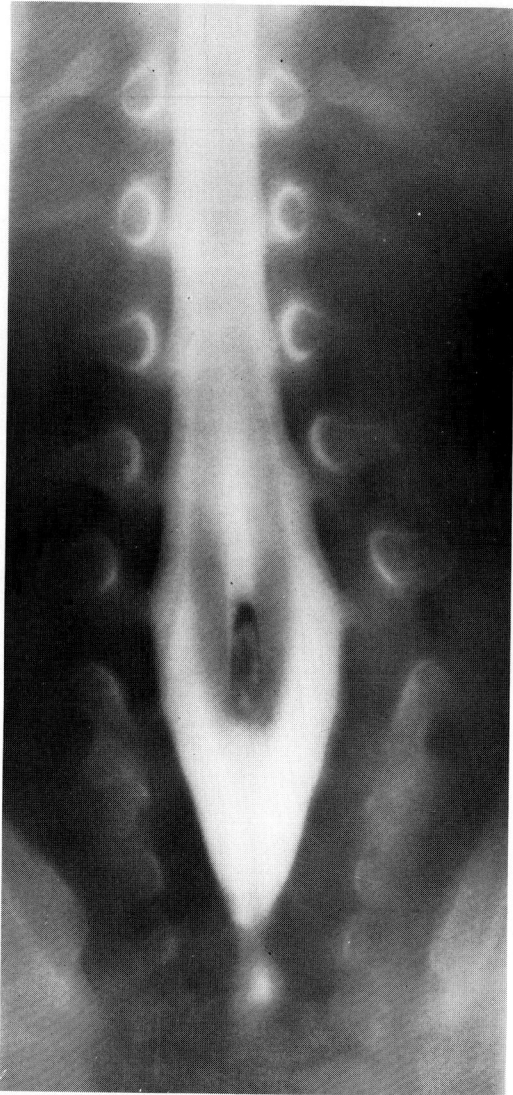

FIGURE 166–6. Diastematomyelia of the lower lumbar region demonstrated by metrizamide-enhanced myelography.

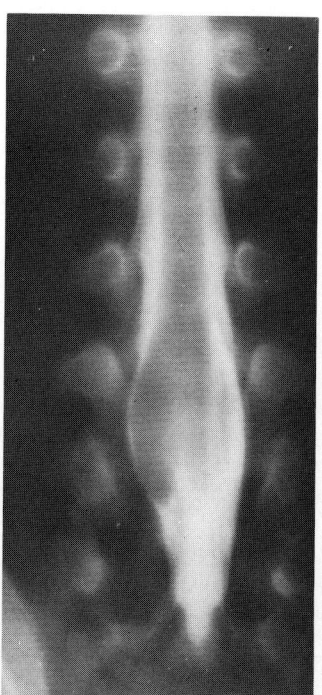 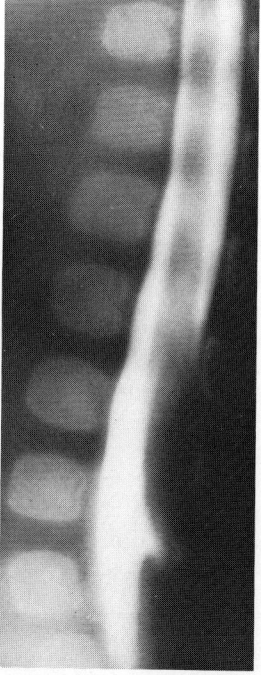

FIGURE 166–5. An intraspinal lipoma with dorsal attachment to the conus medullaris.

avoid the use of muscle relaxants, which might mask motor responses. In addition to nerve stimulation, we have occasionally used intraoperative recording of either cortical or spinal epidural evoked potentials. Such recording is useful principally to assess the effects of surgical manipulations rather than to identify neural elements. In view of the importance of accurate operative observations, we feel that microsurgical techniques should be used routinely.

The principle of surgery is usually to relive the mechanical constraint exerted by the intraspinal lesion on the conus or nerve roots. In its simplest form, such surgery involves merely dividing a thickened filum or the tethering bands (see Fig. 166–2). The filum should be sectioned well caudal to the point of emergence of the lowermost nerve roots. If the attenuated conus extends far distally, dividing the stalk virtually at its point of insertion into the dural cul-de-sac may be necessary. Often, a small lipoma exists in continuity with the stalk at this point. The tethering bands of a *meningocele manqué* may be divided quite easily, or they may represent substantial displaced neural elements attached to the posterior dura, in which case, they should be freed by actually

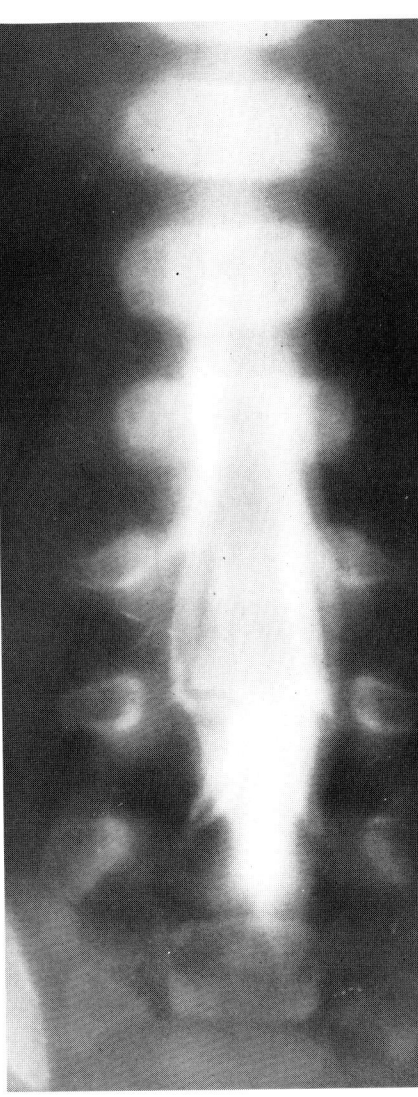

FIGURE 166–7. An intraspinal lipoma with a major artery to the conus medullaris demonstrated by myelography. The vascular nature of the structure was confirmed at surgery.

sectioning the dura itself. Occasionally, one finds the conus and filum adherent to the inner aspect of the posterior dura over a considerable distance. Freeing neural elements in this circumstance represents a formidable and tedious surgical task. It is probably wisest, if possible, to excise the dura circumferentially about the point of attachment to free the conus. Dural closure then will require a watertight graft.

In cases of diastematomyelia, the bony or fibrocartilaginous septum at the midline is excised along with the dural sleeve. Closing the anterior dural defect is not necessary. With spurs in the lumbar area, one may find small, aberrant nerve roots, occasionally with dorsal root ganglia, entering the dural sleeve at the midline from the medial aspect of each hemicord. These nerve roots may end blindly or may re-enter the dura distally. Sacrificing these structures to eliminate the midline septum is generally necessary. Finally, one must be alert to the fact that diastematomyelia at any point along the spine may be associated with caudal tethering of the conus because of a thickened filum or a lipoma in continuity with the conus. This should be detected on preoperative myelo-

grams. If overlooked, it can cause functional deterioration at a later date, even though the bony spur has been dealt with successfully. Depending on the level of the diastematomyelia, it may be necessary to correct the caudal tethering in a second operation.

Dermoid tumors, along with their associated dermal sinus tracts, should be excised in toto where possible in view of their propensity to recur. They may, however, be intimately associated with the conus (see Fig. 166–3), making attempts at total excision inadvisable. Intraspinal lipoma represents a special problem.[10] The interface of the lipoma with neural tissue is often complex and indistinct, and nerve roots of the cauda equina may traverse its substance. The goal of surgery remains, however, to relieve the restraining influence the lipoma exerts on the distal spinal cord. This process requires freeing the conus from the mass of the lipoma by dividing its fibrofatty attachment within the spinal canal (see Fig. 166–1). In doing this, it is not necessary to completely eliminate the lipoma from the cord substance; in fact, attempts to do so are unnecessarily hazardous. Merely excising the extradural mass without freeing the conus intradurally does not relieve the problem and leaves the patient with a risk of subsequent neurologic deterioration. As previously described, the lipoma may insert into the posterior aspect of the conus via a dural defect (Fig. 166–9). This attachment usually is quite fibrous in its central portion and may contain substantial blood vessels. The edge of the dural defect is fused circumferentially to the conus-lipoma interface, and the posterior rootlets lie just ventral to the line of fusion. Initially one opens the dura just rostral to the lipoma and identifies the conus. The dural opening is then continued caudally on either side of the point of entrance of the lipoma stalk so that the lipoma-conus interface can be identified. This attachment then is divided rostrocaudally, and the posterolateral line of attachment is progressively divided as well, first on one side, then on the other. The posterior rootlets provide a useful orientating landmark during this process. Care must be taken to completely transect the caudal point of fixation of the conus to achieve a satisfactory result (Fig. 166–10A,B).

If a lipoma attaches to the distal extremity of the conus (Fig. 166–11) and emerges from the dura caudally in the cul-de-sac or laterally to either side, one can expect nerve roots to traverse its substance. This circumstance presents a more serious surgical challenge and requires sparing all but the most caudal, rudimentary rootlets while progressively transecting the lipoma. Substantial arteries that might be critical to the blood supply of the conus should be sought and spared (see Fig. 166–7). The conus should be circumferentially freed of all fibrous attachments to the lipoma as well as the adjacent dura before the mass is transected as far caudally as possible (Fig. 166–12). Often, one finds an admixture of the two lipoma types. Rostrally, the lipoma attaches to the posterior aspect of the conus so that the emerging rootlets are outside of its substance. As one proceeds caudally, however, elements of the fatty mass are found to insert into the distal or lateral dura in the region of the neural foramina, with nerve roots traversing the mass accordingly (Fig. 166–13). This situation can be anticipated by a careful study of the preoperative radiographs, with attention given to the relationship of the lipoma to the conus within the spinal canal. Surgically, such a lesion is approached as described above by adapting technique to the circumstances (Fig. 166–14).

2076 | *Surgery of the Craniovertebral Junction and Spine*

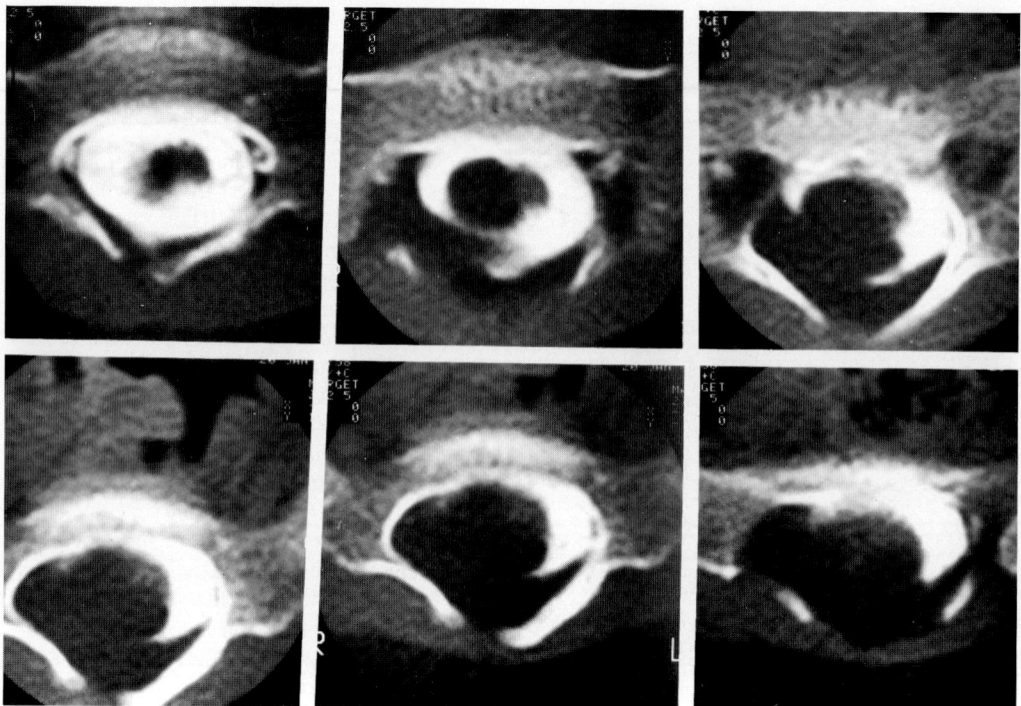

FIGURE 166–8. Axial CT scans with intrathecal contrast showing the complex anatomic relationships of an intraspinal lipoma. (Reprinted from Raimondi AJ [ed]: Concepts in Pediatric Neurosurgery, Volume 3. Basel, S. Karger AG, 1983, p 187. With permission.)

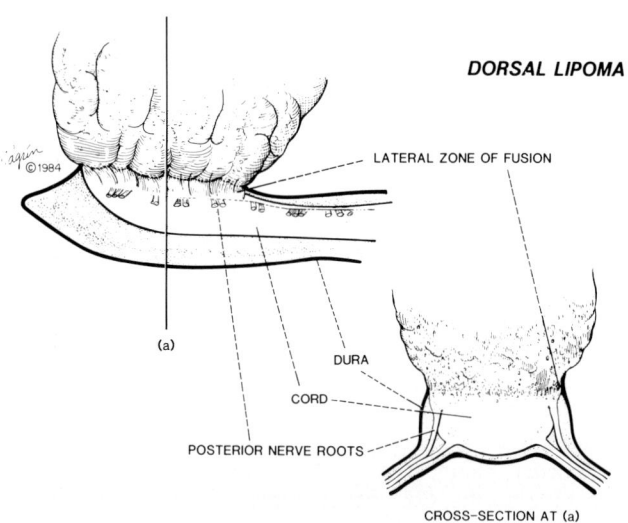

FIGURE 166–9. Diagram of a dorsal lipoma.

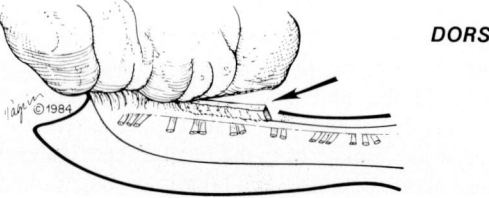

FIGURE 166–10. Surgical steps in untethering a dorsal lipoma. Detaching the subcutaneous mass and releasing the circumferential zone of fusion at the edges of the dorsal defect.

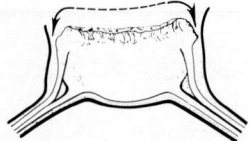

Surgical Management of Occult Spinal Dysraphism | 2077

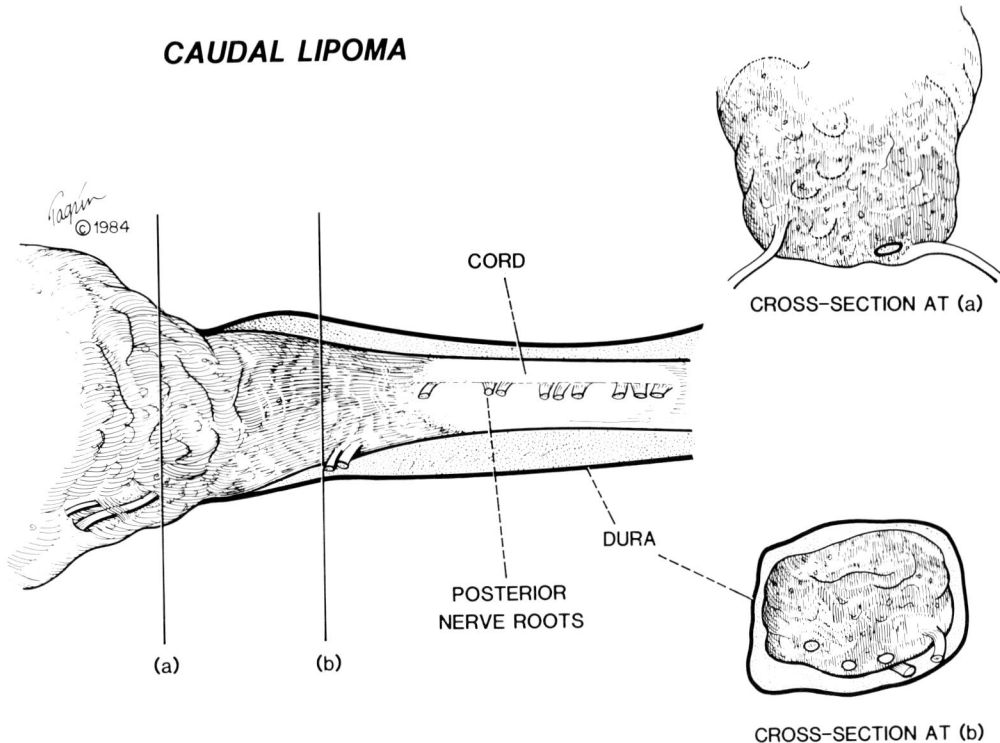

FIGURE 166–11. Diagram of a caudal lipoma.

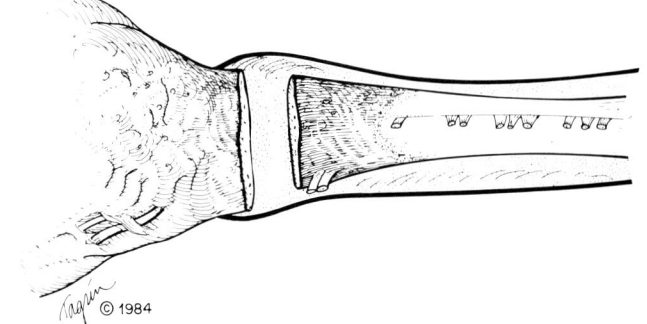

FIGURE 166–12. Surgical detachment of a caudal lipoma.

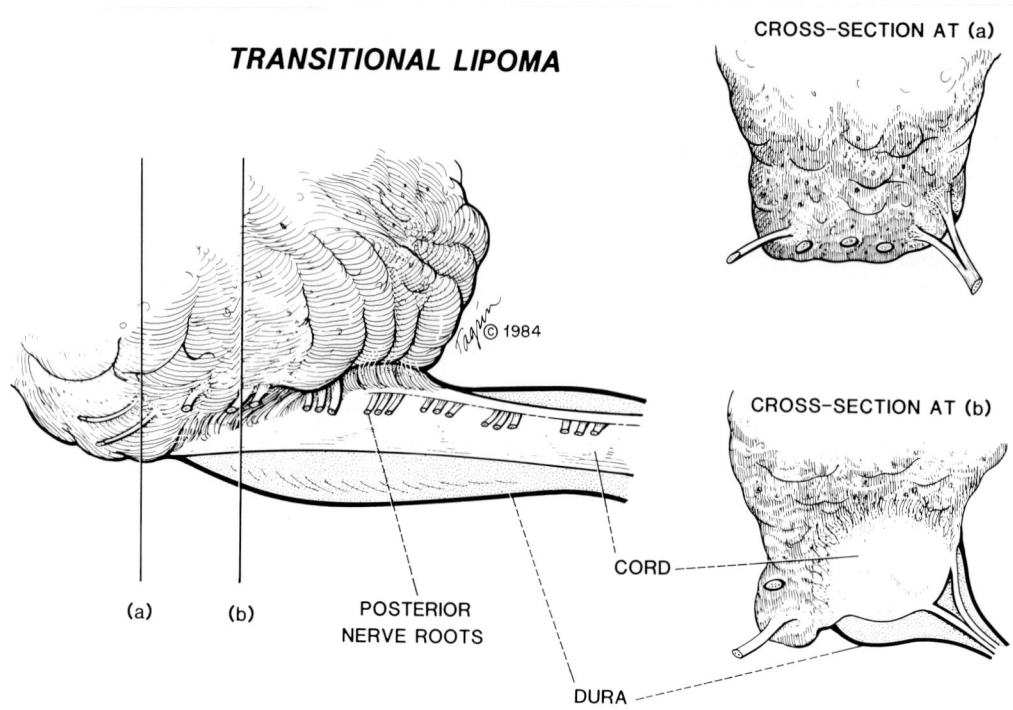

FIGURE 166-13. Diagram of a transitional form of lipoma with features of both the dorsal and caudal varieties. Note the axial asymmetry of this lesion.

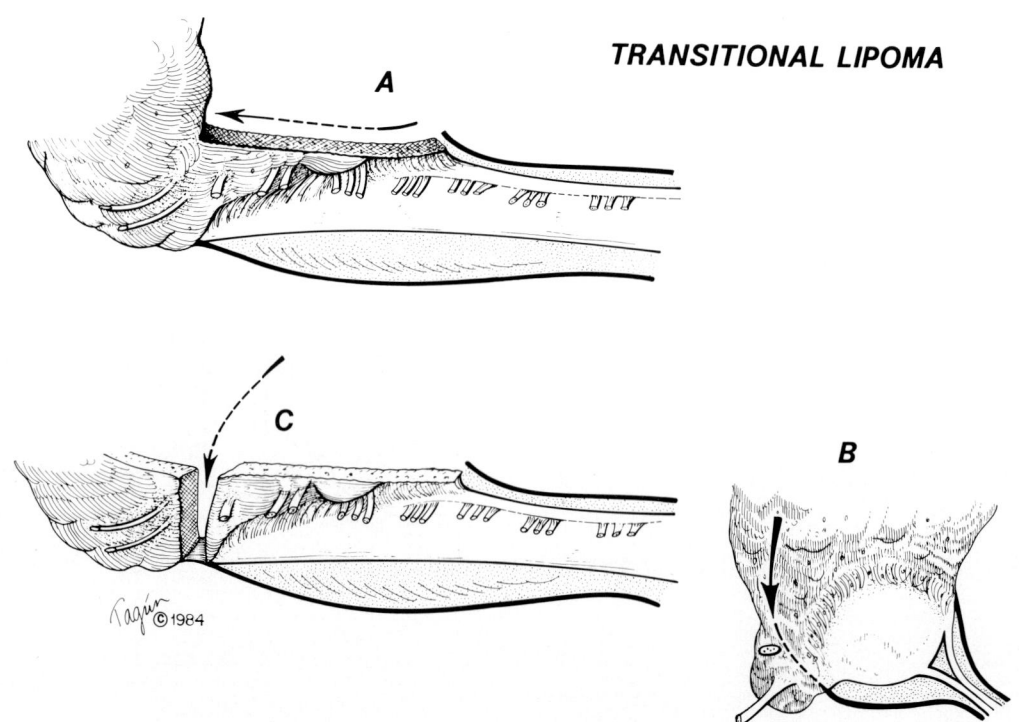

FIGURE 166-14. Surgical steps in the release of a transitional lipoma.

Once the conus has been successfully untethered, it will relax anteriorly in the spinal canal and usually will migrate upward somewhat as well. During the dissection, any bulk of fatty tissue that is contiguous with the conus can be removed if necessary. The carbon dioxide laser and ultrasonic aspirator are quite useful for this purpose.

Cerebrospinal fluid leak is the commonest complication of surgery and is facilitated by the congenital absence of dura, particularly in cases of spinal lipoma. Careful attention must be given to obtaining a relaxed watertight dural closure, using a dural graft if necessary. It is useful, during the initial exposure, to spare tissues that later can serve to buttress a tight wound closure.

RESULTS AND FOLLOW-UP

Most authors report some cases of improved sphincter or sensorimotor function after surgery. However, surgery should not be undertaken in anticipation of achieving neurologic improvement. Rather, it should be performed to prevent further deterioration. As stated previously, the rationale for prophylactic surgery rests, in part, on this fact. It also implies that surgery should not be delayed once any degree of progressive impairment of sphincter or limb function is recognized in patients chosen for follow-up without initial studies. Finally, occasional instances of delayed postoperative deterioration in function have been reported. The deterioration may be the result of a previously undetected lesion, such as a thickened filum accompanying a treated diastematomyelia. Such cases warrant reinvestigation. In isolated instances of intraspinal lipoma, one may find further worsening of a pes cavus foot deformity, which had been progressive preoperatively. This can occur after seemingly satisfactory cord untethering. Despite one's best surgical efforts, retethering can occur, especially in the case of extensive lipomas of the transitional variety. In such circumstances, reoperation may be required to relieve progressive symptoms.

SUMMARY

In summary, successful management of the patient with spinal dysraphism demands proper regard for the underlying problem. This requires, in the first instance, recognition of the true nature of the difficulties, which, at first glance, may appear to be orthopedic, urologic, or cosmetic. Early attention to lesions that will cause progressive deficits is vital. Finally, the surgeon dealing with these lesions must respect their often complex nature and the technical difficulties implicit in surgery. In such cases, a thorough understanding of the pathologic anatomy, aided by appropriate preoperative studies, is necessary.

REFERENCES

1. Ingraham FD: Spina Bifida and Cranium Bifidum, Cambridge, Harvard University Press, 1944
2. James CCM, Lassman LP: Spinal dysraphism. An orthopedic syndrome in children accompanying occult forms. Arch Dis Child 35:315, 1960
3. James CCM, Lassman LP: Spinal Dysraphism. Spina Bifida Occulta. London, Butterworths, 1972
4. Till K: Spinal dysraphism. A study of congenital malformations of the lower back. J Bone Joint Surg Br 51B:415, 1969
5. Anderson FM: Occult spinal dysraphism: A series of 73 cases. Pediatrics 55:826, 1975
6. Reimann AF, Anson BJ: Vertebral level of termination of the spinal cord with report of a case of sacral cord. Anat Rec 88:127, 1944
7. Barson AJ: Vertebral level of termination of spinal cord during normal and abnormal development. J Anat 106:489, 1969
8. Emery JL, Lendon RG: Lipoma of the cauda equina and other fatty tumors related to neurospinal dysraphism. Dev Med Child Neurol 20(suppl):62, 1969
9. Walsh JW, Markesbery WR: Histological features of congenital lipomas of the lower spinal canal. J Neurosurg 52:564, 1980
10. Chapman PH: Congenital intraspinal lipomas. Anatomic considerations and surgical treatment. Childs Nerv Syst 9:37, 1982
11. Lassman LP, James CCM: Meningocoele manqué. Childs Nerv Syst 3:1, 1977
12. Naidich TP, Harwood-Nash DC: Diastematomyelia: Hemicord and meningeal sheaths; single and double arachnoid and dural tubes. AJNR 4:633, 1983
13. Houd RW, Riseborough EJ, Nehme AM, et al: Diastematomyelia and structural spine deformities. J Bone Joint Surg Am 62A:520, 1980
14. Guthkelch AN: Diastematomyelia with median septum. Brain 97:729, 1974
15. Kennedy PR: New data on diastematomyelia. J Neurosurg 51:355, 1979
16. Linder M, Rosenstein J, Sklar FH: Functional improvement after spinal surgery for the dysraphic malformation. Neurosurgery 11:622, 1982
17. Gryspeerdt GL: Myelographic assessment of occult forms of spinal dysraphism. Acta Radiol 1:702, 1963
18. Fitz CR, Harwood-Nash DC: The tethered conus. AJR Am J Roentgenol 125:515, 1975
19. Beyerl B, Ojemann R, Davis KR, et al: Adult cervical diastematomyelia. Case report. J Neurosurg 62:449, 1985
20. Yamada S, Zinke DE, Sanders D: Pathophysiology of "tethered cord syndrome." J Neurosurg 54:494, 1981
21. Fawcitt J: Some radiological aspects of congenital anomalies of the spine in childhood and infancy. Proc R Soc Med 52:331, 1959
22. Lorber J, Levick K: Spina bifida cystica. Incidence of spina bifida occulta in parents and in controls. Arch Dis Child 42:171, 1967
23. Manley CB, Frech RS: Urinary tract infections in girls: Prevalence of spina bifida occulta. J Urol 103:348, 1970
24. Sutow WW, Pryde AW: Incidence of spina bifida occulta in relation to age. Am J Dis Child 91:211, 1956
25. Pang D, Hoffman HJ: Sacral agenesis with progressive neurologic deficit. Neurosurgery 7:118, 1980
26. Bruce DA, Schut L: Spinal lipomas in infancy and childhood. Childs Nerv Syst 5:192, 1979
27. Pavlakis AJ, Siroky MG, Goldstein I, et al: Neurologic findings in conus medullaris and cauda equina injury. Arch Neurol 40:570, 1983
28. Borzyskowski M, Neville BGR: Neuropathic bladder and spinal dysraphism. Arch Dis Child 56:176, 1981
29. Hoffman HJ, Hendrick EB, Humphrey RP: The tethered spinal cord. Its protean manifestations, diagnosis, and surgical correction. Childs Nerv Syst 2:145, 1976
30. Pang D, Wilberger JE: Tethered cord syndrome in adults. J Neurosurg 57:32, 1982
31. Swanson HS, Barnett JC Jr: Intradural lipomas in children. Pediatrics 29:911, 1962
32. Dubowitz V, Lorber J, Zachary RB: Lipoma of the cauda equina. Arch Dis Child 40:207, 1965
33. Yashon D, Beatty RA: Tethering of the conus medullaris within the sacrum. J Neurol Neurosurg Psychiatry 29:244, 1966
34. Hoffman HJ, Taecholarn C, Hendrick EB, et al: The management of lipomyelomeningoceles: Experience at the Hospital for Sick Children, Toronto. J Neurosurg 62:1, 1985
35. Loeser JD, Lewin RJ: Lumbosacral lipoma in the adult. Case report. J Neurosurg 29:405, 1968
36. Villarejo FJ, Blazquez MG, Gutierrez-Diaz JA: Intraspinal lipomas in children. Childs Nerv Syst 2:361, 1976
37. Till K: Occult spinal dysraphism. The value of prophylactic surgical treatment, in Recent Progress in Neurological Surgery. Amsterdam, Excerpta Medica, 1973, pp 61–66
38. Naidich TP, Harwood-Nash DC, McClone DG: Radiology of spinal dysraphism. Clin Neurosurg 30:341, 1982
39. Naidich TP, McClone DG, Mutluer J: A new understanding of dorsal dysraphism with lipoma (lipomyeloschisis). Radiologic evaluation and surgical correction. AJNR 4:103, 1983

CHAPTER 167

Surgical Management of Spinal Injuries in Children

Derek A. Bruce

Traumatic injury to the vertebral column, with or without accompanying spinal cord injury, is unusual in children. The true incidence of such injuries is not known because of the tendency for minor injuries to be underreported. The population incidence of spinal injury has been reported at 53.4/1,000,000:[1] 64/1,000,000 in patients 20 to 24 years of age, and 2/1,000,000 in patients under 19 years.[2] The incidence is lowest in children younger than 8 years of age. Depending on the age at which patients are declared children, spinal injury in children accounts for from 1 to 10 percent of all spinal injuries,[1–4] and the lower figures are for children under 13 years of age. The incidence of spinal injury greatly increases after age 13 years,[5] and only 25 percent of spinal injuries occurring in patients under age 19 years occur in children 12 years old or younger. In children younger than 9 years, the male:female ratio is 60:40, whereas in children over 13, the ratio is 70:30. The reported incidence of multiple spinal column injuries varies from 10 to 30 percent.[6–8] In most reports of pediatric spinal trauma, 50 to 70 percent of the children have no neurologic deficit. This effect seems to be age related, with 75 percent of those under 9 years having associated spinal cord injury. Overall, 40 to 50 percent of children with spinal cord injury present with a complete lesion. The mortality rate for those reaching the hospital alive ranges from 3 to 30 percent,[5, 7, 9] and recovery from partial lesions is high, with 75 percent showing improvement and 50 percent or more making a full recovery. However, for those with complete lesions, only 10 percent or less demonstrate any significant functional recovery below the level of the injury.[3–8] A recent population study in Canada that examined the incidence of spinal injury in children dying from trauma reported a mortality rate of 28 percent for children under 17 years versus 11 percent for adults. Ninety percent of the children's deaths occurred at the accident site, although only 13 percent of these deaths were the result of the spinal cord injury, and most deaths were the result of multiple trauma.[7] The human and financial costs are enormous. The solution is clearly prevention of the injury, and efforts are being made at the public health level to increase awareness and decrease the incidence of spinal injuries.

The commonest cause of injury is motor vehicle accidents, occurring in 50 percent of cases; however, in children under 9 years, the commonest cause of injury is a fall, and when an automobile is involved, the child is usually a pedestrian. In infants, child abuse is a common cause of upper cervical and medullary injury.[10] Other causative factors are sports injuries,[11] bicycle and motor bike accidents, gunshots, and other penetrating trauma.

Cervical spine injuries are the most commonly seen at all ages and account for 40 to 50 percent of injuries: 30 percent are thoracic, and 20 to 30 percent are lumbar.[9, 12, 13] In children under 9 years, the upper cervical spine, occiput to C2, accounts for 60 to 70 percent of all cervical spine injuries, whereas injuries at this level in older children account for fewer than 20 percent of the cervical injuries. The reasons for this high incidence of occipitocervical injuries has been explained on the basis of (1) a disproportionately large head with poor neck musculature, (2) spinal column hypermobility, (3) partially cartilaginous vertebrae, (4) incomplete ossification, and (5) weakness at the attachments of the growth plates. The spinal column hypermobility is heightened by excessive ligamentous laxity, wedge-shaped vertebral bodies, horizontal facet joints, absent uncinate bodies, and relatively weak paraspinous musculature. Around the age of 8 years, the vertebral column assumes a more mature anatomy and after 15 years is similar to the adult spine. In the child under 9 years, 20 to 60 percent of spinal cord injuries at all levels occur in the absence of any bony abnormality (SCIWORA: spinal cord injury without radiographic abnormality).[14–17] In children over 8 years, the distribution of injury is similar to that in adults, and the lower cervical spinal segments sustain most of the injuries. SCIWORA accounts for only 10 percent of injuries in children over 9 years of age.

Classification of the injury is usually based on the radiographic abnormality (fracture only, fracture with subluxation, subluxation only, and SCIWORA) and the severity of the myelopathy as determined by the Frankel classification.[17a] For summary and reporting purposes, neurologic injuries are generally recorded as complete or incomplete. Children under 9 years have a lower incidence of fractures (26 percent) than older children (50 to 60 percent). Fracture with subluxation occurs in 25 percent of younger children and in 30 percent of older children, whereas subluxation alone is uncommon at all ages, varying from 2 to 10 percent, depending on the series. SCIWORA accounts for 20 to 60 percent of injuries in children under 8 years but only 10 to 15 percent in older children. In most reports 50 percent of children hospitalized with a spinal injury have no neurologic damage, 25 percent have incomplete injuries, and 25 percent have complete injuries. This figure again varies with age, as discussed earlier, and complete injuries are commoner in children under 9 years.

In an effort to better classify spinal cord injuries, the American Spinal Injury Association has proposed a new classification to clarify the clinical pathophysiology, and they use this classification to evaluate the results of treatment and outcome:

Level of injury
Type and degree of spinal column disruption
Type and degree of neurologic deficit
Type and degree of parenchymal injury

These entries can be further refined by the results of electric studies, somatosensory evoked potentials, and motor-evoked responses. By better defining the injury, comparison of the results of new therapeutic interventions will be more easily seen and will be separated by type of spinal cord lesion.

CLINICAL FEATURES

In most cases, even those associated with head injury and altered consciousness, spinal cord injury can be recognized from neurologic examination, appropriate x-ray studies, and if necessary, more sophisticated studies, such as magnetic resonance imaging (MRI) and evoked potentials. Before the initial examination, a thorough history of the accident should be obtained. The incidence of head injury is about 200 times that of spinal injury in children; therefore, the type of trauma often helps define how likely a spinal injury is. High-speed motor vehicle accidents, high falls, diving accidents, and child abuse all carry a higher risk of spinal injury than lower-velocity injuries. Lap belt injuries in children are probably the commonest cause of lumbar injury, and a history of seat belt use should be established.

In the awake child, complaints of neck or back pain are always warning signs of potential spinal injury and must not be ignored. The resting position of the extremities can give a clue to the level of spinal cord injury. The neurologic examination should always include comparisons of proximal to distal movements and sensation as well as side-to-side comparison, and sphincter tone should be evaluated. In the infant, a complete digital insertion is unnecessary because of the risk of producing a mucosal tear; it is adequate practice to observe the anus, check the anal wink, and evaluate tone with the tip of the small finger. Muscle tone and reflex activity complete the examination. The prognosis is very different for complete and incomplete lesions, and every effort should be made to conduct as complete an examination as possible. Full evaluation of other organ systems is mandatory. The standard ABCs (apnea, bradycardia, and cyanosis) of resuscitation are always the first step, with insertion of intravenous lines and fluid resuscitation, if necessary. If the spinal injury is above the thoracic area, hypotension results from loss of sympathetic tone, and a sympathomimetic agent may be required to attain an adequate blood pressure for the patient's age. The blood pressure can also be raised by leg elevation. If associated head injury or chest injury is present, endotracheal intubation may be urgently required and should be carried out without hyperflexion or hyperextension of the neck. The stomach must be decompressed via a nasogastric tube or orogastric tube, and once the perineum is cleared of urethral injury, a Foley catheter should be inserted.

RADIOLOGIC STUDIES

Plain x-ray studies of the spine are the primary radiologic examination and are obtained for any area of the spine that is at risk for injury in each individual case. Typically, the cervical area is at greatest risk, but after major trauma, thoracic and lumbar x-ray studies may be indicated. Multiple levels of injury can occur in 11 to 16 percent of children.[5, 9, 18] The x-ray studies demonstrate bony alignment (subluxation or dislocation), bone structure (fracture), and evidence of paravertebral soft tissue swelling. Cervical x-ray studies are typically obtained with the neck in the neutral position. However, this position can lead to realignment of any cervical subluxation and a failure to diagnose the lesion, particularly at the C1-C2 level. However, in children, physiologic subluxation can occur at C2-C3, and less commonly at C3-C4, and the x-ray studies can easily be overread. Because of children's multiple growth centers, wedge-shaped vertebrae, and physiologic subluxations, reading of cervical x-ray films in children can be very difficult.[19-24] If there is any question of an abnormality, it is safer to place the child's neck in a neutral immobilized position until further studies can be obtained. Tomography is helpful to evaluate questionable fractures but is rarely appropriate in an emergency setting and now is usually replaced by computed tomographic (CT) scan and three-dimensional reconstruction.

COMPUTED TOMOGRAPHY. The CT scan supplements plain x-ray studies, allowing better evaluation of the vertebrae, intervertebral discs, pedicles, and facet joints and spinal canal, and with three-dimensional reconstruction, dislocation or subluxation is better evaluated. CT myelography may be required to evaluate the degree of bony or soft tissue encroachment in the spinal canal and the degree and location of any mass causing cord compression.

MAGNETIC RESONANCE IMAGING. MRI, although it does not show the bony structures as well as CT, gives the best visualization of the spinal cord, nerve roots, cerebrospinal fluid (CSF), discs, and ligaments and muscles in the area of injury. The very sensitivity of the MRI may occasionally provide misleading information about the need for surgery, and more experience in acute spinal cord trauma needs to be obtained (Fig. 167–1). However, MRI may also have predictive value for recovery in patients with neurologic deficits.[25]

Any or all of these studies may be necessary before the surgeon decides that surgical intervention is necessary. In addition, complete evaluation of the child for the presence of other injuries is always necessary, and the presence of such injuries may modify the decision to operate or alter the timing of surgical intervention.

CANDIDATES FOR SURGERY

Only 25 percent of children with injury to the spinal cord or column require surgical intervention other than external immobilization. Progressive loss of neurologic function while under observation always raises the question of progressive spinal cord compression, and CT, CT myelography, or MRI should be obtained if not already available to look for a surgically correctable cause of the progressive func-

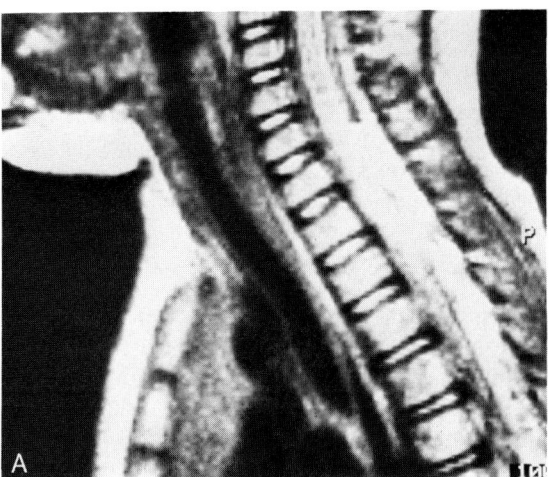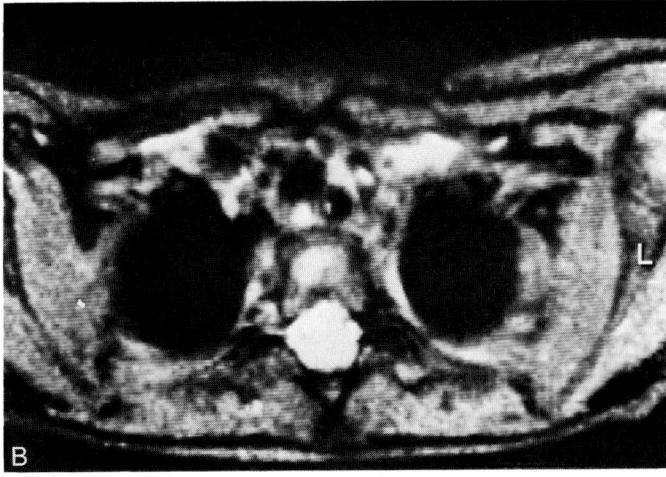

FIGURE 167–1. (A) Sagittal and (B) axial T2-weighted image of cervical and upper thoracic spine in a 2-year-old child suffering from a hyperextension injury, probably resulting from child abuse. Immediate paraplegia with progressive motor loss in the hands occurred several hours after admission. MRI was interpreted as showing a probable epidural hematoma, and thus, surgery was performed. Surgical findings were a totally disrupted dural sac and spinal cord, with epidural, intradural, and intramedullary hemorrhage. The surgery was obviously not helpful and probably should not have been performed.

tional loss. In children with SCIWORA in whom surgery is rarely indicated, 20 to 25 percent have a delayed loss of function over hours to days; thus, automatic exploration of the spinal canal when deterioration occurs is not indicated. Children with impingement of bone, cartilage, or blood into the spinal canal that produces spinal cord compression are most likely to require urgent surgery. Those with a stable neurologic examination result and vertebral malalignment are initially treated with external immobilization, or traction, or both, to re-establish the normal vertebral relationships if possible.* Children who demonstrate unstable fractures despite external immobilization or deterioration of neurologic function during reduction are candidates for internal stabilization to ensure stability, limit further spinal cord damage, and permit early mobilization of the child and the commencement of rehabilitation.

Jumped or locked facets are one cause of failure and may be an indication for surgery once the child is stable systemically and neurologically. Similarly, when the spinal cord is compressed by disc, bone fragments, or epidural hematoma, surgical decompression accompanied by spinal fusion, is often indicated. A recent study[26] suggested that 14 percent of teenagers with flexion injuries of the cervical spine had a late kyphotic deformity. These investigators suggest that surgical stabilization may be a more appropriate therapy. This dilemma requires further study, but as pointed out earlier, once children reach their teen years, they are treated similarly to adults, and information from adult studies can be applied to help make a decision for or against surgery.

Thoracic and thoracolumbar injuries are uncommon in children under 14 years except for lap belt injury and flexion distraction injury.[13, 29–33] These injuries are usually unstable as a result of disruption of the interspinous and posterior longitudinal ligaments and are often missed because of the accompanying abdominal trauma.[34–36] They need elective bony fusion in most cases.[35, 36] These injuries and their treatment are in contradistinction to the simple compression fracture, which can usually be treated conservatively. A significant burst component to a flexion distraction injury often requires an anterior and posterior fusion.[35] Burst fractures of the spine are uncommon in children under 14 years. In the older children, the treatment does not differ from that of adults and depends on the type of fracture.[34] Current evidence suggests that type A fractures require anterior as well as posterior fusion because of the frequency with which late kyphosis develops.[37–39]

Many developmental anomalies occur at the cervicomedullary junction, and these can be confused with traumatic injuries. In addition, many of them, such as os odontoideum and Down's syndrome predispose to injury from minor trauma.[40] Thus, the treating physician must have a full understanding of these anomalies and the diseases of childhood that predispose to spinal anomalies.

PENETRATING TRAUMA. The cause of penetrating injuries to the spine in children are often bizarre and result from play. The objects producing the injury are usually unsterile and often are contaminated by earth. Most penetrating injuries require exploration, debridement, and irrigation. A CT myelogram is often helpful to demonstrate the tract of the leakage and define the point of dural injury, thus limiting the laminectomy or laminotomy that is required. Most bullet wounds of the spine do not require immediate exploration.

SURGICAL ANATOMY

The route for cervical, thoracic, and lumbar surgery in children is posterior or posterolateral (in the thoracic area). The extent of surgical trauma is diminished by avoidance of body cavities in children (pleural and peritoneal spaces), and the frequency of associated thoracic or abdominal trauma further excludes the use of the anterior approach. In children under 8 years (the younger they are the more this rule applies), the vertebral bodies have a lot of cartilage and are poor recipients for anterior bone grafts, making the posterior

---
*See references 3, 5, 6, 8, 9, 12, and 26–28.

approach the best approach if a fusion is required. Depending on the age of the child, the laminae may still be partly cartilaginous. In addition, in the cervical region, bifid laminae may be present, especially in the arch of C1, and the presence of a fracture or subluxation may make the spinal column very unstable. Also, age-related changes in the vertebrae with flat pedicles and wedged bodies and the hypermobile ligaments make the spinal column easy to distort during the exposure. The ligamentum flavum is continuous rather than segmented, and especially in the very young child, if a dural tear has occurred (leading to CSF anterior to the ligament), the ligament can be easily mistaken for the dura; if no epidural fat is present, the surgeon can spend some time defining the actual dura, which can lead to confusion and prolongation of the operation. The distance between the spinous processes and the laminae is greater than in the adult, and dissection can occur between the spinous processes or lamina, and the spinal canal can be entered inadvertently.

In the upper cervical region, many large veins are present that can result in significant hemorrhage and possible air embolism. These veins are located at the lateral margin of the foramen magnum and just anterior to the ligamentum flavum, which is very thin at the C1-C2 level. Avoidance of these veins makes the surgery much smoother and less bloody. Far lateral dissection at C1 is rarely necessary, but because of the smaller distances in children's anatomy, the vertebral artery is not far away and must be avoided.

In the thoracic area, the rib heads are prominent, and the interpedicular portions of the laminae are short, making it easy to injure the pedicle joint. Thus, care must be taken during the laminectomy not to rongeur bone too laterally. At all levels, because the lateral masses are small in children and do not take screws, laminectomy, if necessary, should be kept as narrow as possible and should leave lamina laterally to facilitate any required instrumentation and laminar wiring. In addition, any laminectomy should be limited to the fewest possible laminae. Laminotomy can be considered if underlying spinal cord compression is not present.

ANESTHESIA AND PATIENT POSITION

Because surgery is usually being performed because of spinal instability or to relieve spinal cord compression, a plan for stable positioning during endotracheal intubation and surgery is the first requisite. In the older child in pin traction, this goal is rarely a problem, but in the child younger than 3 to 4 years of age and certainly in the child younger than 2 years, this goal can be difficult to attain. Fortunately, endotracheal intubation in the child is performed with the child in the sniffing position, which places the head in a neutral position, negating the need for hyperextension of the neck. If a difficult intubation is suspected or encountered, the use of a pediatric-sized flexible bronchoscope is very helpful for minimizing neck distortion and directing the endotracheal tube into the trachea. In children up to age 6, cuffed tubes are not used because of concern about airway size, and a range of uncuffed tubes is necessary if anesthesia is to be performed in small children. The actual anesthetic technique depends on the presence of other injuries, such as cerebral trauma; whether or not evoked responses are to be used; and the general status of the patient. A narcotic, muscle paralyzing, low-dose inhalation technique is used. Monitoring involves the use of an arterial line, an oxygen saturation monitor, end-tidal carbon dioxide and central temperature measurement, and Foley catheter. The younger the child the greater the concern about heat loss, hence the need for heating blankets and warming of the inspired gases. Loss of temperature is not only detrimental to the anesthesiologist's ability to reverse the anesthetic but can also change the evoked potentials if monitoring is in use.

Adequate padding to prevent areas of pressure from producing skin injury must be balanced against adequate chest movement and potential exposure of areas for the harvesting of bone grafts. The use of silicon-filled rolls for chest support in the prone position and placement of the head either in pins or a horseshoe headrest (depending on the level of the fracture) avoids excess pressure on the chest or hips. The knees also need padding. In the child under 12 years, oscillating pressure stockings are not necessary unless the child is particularly obese. If a horseshoe headrest is used, the eyes must be protected both from pressure from the headrest and from preparatory solution running down and pooling at the forehead or eyes because this can produce burns of the skin or cornea.

The prone or lateral position is preferred to the sitting position: the former minimizes the risk of air embolism, makes keeping the child warm easier, decreases the risk of hypotension, and allows for much better control of traction on the cervical spine. Routine use of intraoperative motor or sensory evoked responses is neither necessary nor helpful. It can prolong the operating time and can inhibit the surgeon's aim of perfect alignment because of persisting changes in the evoked responses, the functional importance of which is not known.

Evoked responses can be helpful under specific circumstances. If evoked responses have been used preoperatively to define deteriorating function due to progressive cord compression, their use intraoperatively can help demonstrate relief of the compression, as shown by improvement or return to normal of the responses. This information can be especially helpful when an anterior approach is used and only a short segment of dura is exposed. The problem with relying on this information is that even with complete decompression, the evoked responses may not recover immediately or indeed may never recover, and the surgeon may get only increased worry and no real help from the electrophysiologic information. Evoked responses can also be helpful when a significant malalignment of the vertebrae is present before surgery and needs to be corrected after the induction of anesthesia. The evoked responses are recorded before induction of anesthesia, are repeated after induction, and are then repeatedly recorded during positioning and surgical fixation. Any significant change during correction is used as a signal to either stop repositioning at that time or to allow some small degree of return to the malaligned position to see if the evoked responses recover. Once again, the surgeon may be faced with the dilemma of whether to persist to attain the best anatomic position despite changes in the evoked responses or to accept a lesser degree of alignment because of the risk, as yet unknown, that the altered response predicts clinical deterioration. When a response disappears with positioning and then recovers with relaxation on a repeated basis, it is most sensible to accept the poorer alignment: whether or not this is true of subtler changes in the evoked responses, such as prolongation of the response, is unclear, and the surgeon must use his or her own experience to make a decision. Under these circumstances, I usually try to attain the best alignment. Other surgical events that can affect evoked responses are drop in the arterial pressure, changes in the anesthetic level, changes in body temperature, and irrigation with solutions of varying temperature. This last event is avoided by using warmed irrigation solutions in children.

In preteenagers and especially in children below 8 years of age, the use of metal instrumentation is kept to a minimum. The limitation to the use of rigid metal fixation is the many areas of cartilage that still exist in the spine. These areas are easily disrupted by pulling the laminae away from their attachment to the vertebral bodies and thus making the fixation useless. Pedicular screws are poorly accepted by the cartilaginous vertebrae, and the size of the vertebrae is also a problem. The use of interlaminar clamps, although reported in children, is not recommended unless no other alternative exists because of the anatomy of the injury and any predisposing disease.[41] At the occipitocervical region for occiput to C2 fusion, when the arch of C1 is either absent, fractured, or deficient, a Steinmann pin, tantalum plate, or similar device can be bent to conform to the occipital and cervical curves and used to attain immediate stability with sublaminar and cranial wiring. Bone grafts are also used. Many spinal fusion instrumentations[42, 43] are available for use in the thoracic or lumbar areas. The least length of spine that can be fused to obtain the desired stability should be used to allow for the maximum possible growth of the remainder of the spine. Bony fusion should always accompany instrumentation whenever possible. Much of the segmental instrumentation is bulky, and attention should be paid to its encroachment on the spinal canal. The use of flexible cables for fusion helps to avoid bulging into the canal, but tissue reaction may be greater to multistrand than to single-strand wire. For lesions in the cervical region, the fluoroscope can be of great help to monitor the adequacy of the reduction. In small children, it is often easier to take individual x-ray studies because the small areas in which the surgeon can work cannot accommodate the fluoroscope.

Choosing a site for an autologous bone graft is a problem in children. Ribs are thin and rarely make a good graft. The iliac crest is ideal, but in the younger child, much cartilage is present, and care must be taken to avoid injuring it. Usually only the outer cortex and the cancellous bone are taken separately, and the inner cortex is left intact. This practice avoids the risk of injury to the abdominal cavity and leaves a site for reattachment of the muscles. The fibula in the very small child can be used for anterior grafting, and full- or split-thickness cranial bone is readily available. The skull bone can usually be split by age 3 years; the best area for this procedure is usually the high parietal area. If an external fixation device, such as a halo or collar, is to be used postoperatively, the device needs to be available before the start of the surgical procedure. In children for whom a halo is used, the greatest number of pins possible (up to 10) should be used. Pressure on the pins is usually 2 pounds in children 4 years and older and just finger tight in younger children.[28, 44–47]

The halo is usually applied at the start of the operation and is used to stabilize the head during the procedure. The use of a halo attachment to the standard head holder prevents excess traction that can easily be applied to the young patient if a pulley system is used.

SURGICAL TECHNIQUE

CERVICAL REGION

For surgery at all levels of the spine, the basic technique is the same. The skin and subcutaneous tissues are injected with 0.5 percent lidocaine (Xylocaine) with 1/200,000 epinephrine before patient preparation to give the epinephrine a chance to work. The skin incision is made with a scalpel; thereafter, the remainder of the dissection is made with the Colorado needle connected to the Valley Lab electrocautery, which should be placed on the lowest setting that gives satisfactory tissue splitting, usually 8 on the coagulation current. The setting may be as low as 5 or 6 once the muscle layer is encountered in the infant. After the midline avascular plane is incised, because the muscle thins out superiorly at the nuchal line of the occipital bone, it is useful to open the superior part of the muscle in a Y shape, which permits a better closure. If cranial bone is to be used as a graft, the skin incision is extended off to one side of the midline well above the muscle attachment to expose the parietal bone. The bone graft can be used as a full-thickness graft, and a second matching area can be removed, split, and used to replace the full-thickness bone, or depending on the thickness of the bone, a split cranial graft can be used. Great care must be taken not to move the head while the graft is being taken, and the position of the reduction should be checked after the graft is taken. For a C1 fusion, a full-thickness graft should be taken of skull, and it should be split after it has been removed rather than in situ.

The muscles are dissected off the spinous processes and laminae in the subperiosteal plain by use of sharp dissection. They should not be stripped with the periosteal elevator for the reasons discussed earlier. Sharp dissection is continued laterally if a lateral fusion or rods are to be placed. Full exposure of the transverse processes is best performed after the spinal canal has been explored and at least partially stabilized. The posterior arch of C1 is often incomplete or still cartilaginous, and care must be taken not to enter the spinal canal during the early dissection. When surgery is being performed for a C1-C2 injury, the arch of C1 is often anteriorly displaced; thus, after the avascular midline fascia is incised, the muscle must be gently lifted posteriorly to avoid injury to the atlanto-occipital membrane and potentially the underlying cord and dura as the muscle is freed from the arch of C1, the lamina of C2, and the occipital bone. The C1 vertebra is often extremely mobile and must not be pushed anteriorly during the dissection to avoid cord injury. It is better not to put traction on the arch of C1 to reduce it until the sublaminar wires must be passed. This method avoids repeatedly moving the ring posteriorly and then running the risk of it moving anteriorly again; it also minimizes the risk of breaking the arch of C1 in the very small child by putting too much traction on it. The periosteum of C1 is left intact and the plane of dissection is be-

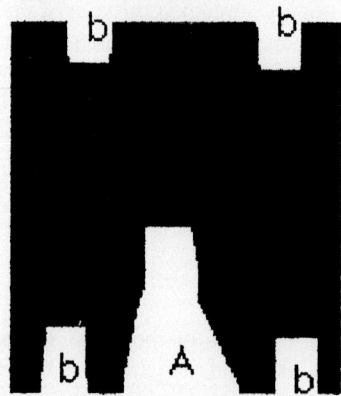

FIGURE 167-2. Drawing of H-shaped graft used for cervical fusion. Spinous process of C2 inserts at A and the fusion cable is kept from slipping by grooves (b).

tween the periosteum and the atlanto-occipital membrane. A fine, right-angled dental tool or Fraser elevator allows this step to be performed with minimal anterior compression of the ligament and dura. The separation is continued laterally to ensure that the loops of wire that go around the lamina are kept lateral and do not migrate to the center of the arch at C1 or the base of the spinous process at other levels. This is particularly true at the C1 level because the weakest part of the arch is in the midline, and the surgeon should avoid having all the stress at this point because of the risk of the wire cutting through the arch of C1 (Fig. 167-3A).

If the occiput is to be included in the fusion, a small drill is used to make two holes approximately 1 to 1.5 cm apart on both sides of the midline of the occipital bone to use for passing the wires. The holes should be several centimeters superior to the foramen magnum where the bone is thick and should be at least 2 to 3 cm from the midline to avoid the midline dural sinus and the very thick bone in this area. In infants and toddlers, the bone of the posterior fossa is very thin, and efforts to decorticate it can lead to penetration of the inner table and therefore are not usually made.

The spinous process of C2 must be completely dissected to allow passage of the fusion wire as anteriorly down the spinous process as possible to prevent slippage. Unless no substantial spinous process exists at C2, freeing the lamina of C2 for sublaminar wiring is not necessary. Once again, efforts to decorticate the bone of the laminae is not recommended because of the thinness of the bone and the risk of weakening it. Bony fusion is rarely a problem after acute trauma in children, and indeed, a greater concern is producing a "creeping fusion" that extends over several segments and can include the muscle. For this reason, only the laminae to be fused are exposed, and disturbance of the anatomic plane of adjacent areas is kept to a minimum.

As the ring of C1 is freed from the underlying ligament and dura, it should be held in place posteriorly, usually not by holding the center of the arch, which is the weakest area, but by supporting it more laterally. This step is often best performed after the sublaminar wire is passed and pushed laterally on the arch and used to support the position of C1. Whatever site is selected for the bone graft, an H-shaped graft is fashioned (Fig. 167-2) as shown. The graft is not inserted between the laminae of C1 and C2 but posterior to them with the superior margin at the level of the superior portion of the arch of the atlas. A loop of wire or flexible cable is passed under the arch of C1 and looped around the base of the spinous process of C2. The wire around the arch of C1 is kept lateral by the superior grooves in the H graft, and the free ends of the wire or cable are brought anterior to the graft, through the inferior grooves of the graft, and are secured over the posterior surface of the graft. If the spinous process of C2 is thick enough, a Kirschner wire is passed through the skin laterally and through the base of the C2 spinous process. It is then cut off with a small lateral projection to either side of the midline. As the wire or cable is tightened, the atlas is pulled posteriorly without the two laminae being approximated. This process keeps the loop of wire or cable from becoming dislodged from its position on C2 and makes for a very rigid fixation (Fig. 167-3). Cancellous bone is packed around the graft, and care is taken not to cover only the laminae being fused. The incision is then irrigated with antibiotic solution and closed typically in sev-

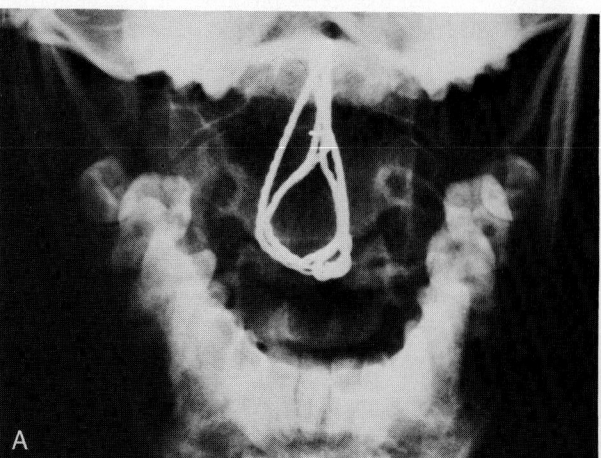 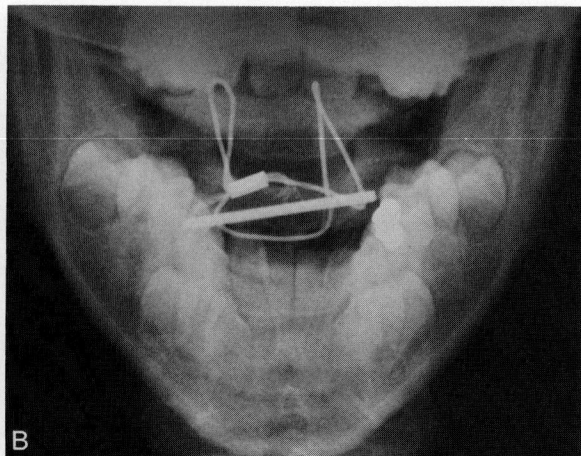

FIGURE 167-3. (A) AP cervical spine x-ray study showing wires holding a C1-C2 fusion have migrated to the center of the posterior arch of C1. This is not a good position because the center of the arch is the weakest point and may indeed be absent in children. (B) AP cervical spine x-ray of a cervical fusion using the H-graft technique shown in Fig. 167-2. The wires round the arch of C1 are well lateral, and the Kirschner wire through the spinous process is shown.

eral layers with absorbable suture, such as Vicryl. The skin is closed with subcuticular absorbing suture and Steri-Strips.

The technique for posterior cervical fusion at other levels depends on the pathology of the lesion. A technique similar to C1-C2 fusion is appropriate if only one level of instability exists and the lamina is intact. The use of the flexible cables diminishes the risk of sublaminar wiring by minimizing the possible protrusion of the wire into the vertebral canal. The Songer cable system has an easier mechanism for crimping the cable in the depth of the wound or in a small space. Increased concern exists about infection or metallic interaction with the tissue as a result of using a braided wire, but over the course of 2 to 3 years, this has not been a problem. As noted earlier, the use of plates and screws is not recommended in children, but in the teenager with fully developed vertebrae, the techniques are similar to those used in adults.[48] No strong evidence exists that screws are any more effective than the classic techniques.[49]

In children under 8 years, because of the relatively horizontal alignment of their facets, locked facets can be reduced with minimal bone removal, and fusion should again include the least number of levels necessary to achieve stability. If anterior compression of the spinal cord exists because of blood clot, disc, bone, or epiphyseal plate, an anterior approach is necessary in the cervical region. In the thoracic area, a posterolateral approach is usually satisfactory and allows posterior fusion at the same time with less surgical trauma.

If rod systems, such as the Texas-Scottish-Rite-Hospital system are required, the minimum segmental fusion that will achieve stability, usually 2 segments above and one below, is performed with associated bone grafting to allow as much truncal growth as possible. The major limiting factor to the use of metallic, rigid fixation in children under 10 years of age is that the joints of the spine are cartilaginous and the pressures applied by the instrumentation risk disrupting the cartilage-bone interface such that many segments have to be included in the fusion. Simple bony fusion and laminar wiring with or without external fixation are usually better alternatives.

In penetrating injuries, the intradural space requires irrigation, exploration for cord or root injury, and dural repair, if possible. Often, the injury is lateral, making dural suture impossible. The use of a fascial graft or suturing of the dura to the inferior margin of the muscle with the addition of tissue glue results in a satisfactory dural seal.

Case Reports

CASE REPORT 1

An 8-year-old girl fell from the top of an eight-foot fence. That evening, she complained of neck pain and was seen in her local emergency room. X-ray studies of the cervical spine were obtained. Apart from pain below the occiput, the neurologic examination was reported to be intact. The films were read as normal (Fig. 167–4A). The patient was sent home in a soft collar. On a visit to her pediatrician a week later, she had stopped wearing the collar despite some continued pain and was started on physical therapy to ease the neck pain and encourage movement. One week into the therapy, she developed acute neck pain and her mother noticed that her ''neck seemed shorter.'' A CT scan of the spine revealed a complete anterior dislocation of the dens on C2, with the dens sitting completely anterior to the body of C2 (Fig. 167–4B). At this time, she was referred to pediatric neurosurgery. Her neurologic examination results were still normal, except for possible minimal weakness of the left distal upper extremity. She was placed in halter traction with her head in mild extension, initially with 1 pound, then 2 pounds (Fig. 167–4C), and eventually 3 pounds. At this weight, the dislocated dens reduced, and the dens was situated on top of the body of C2. However, with the least reduction in weight, the dens subluxed anteriorly. It was felt that a fusion was indicated because of the extreme instability of this injury. A CT scan showed that C1 and the relationship to the occiput were intact and that a C1-C2 fusion was all that was required. Postoperatively, the patient was placed in a halo device for 8 weeks. An excellent fusion at C1-C2 was obtained (Fig. 167–4D), and at 3 months from the occurrence of the injury, the dens was starting to fuse.

CASE REPORT 2

A 4-year-old girl was an unrestrained passenger in an automobile accident. She was found unconscious with agonal respirations. She was resuscitated, intubated in the field, and transferred to Parkland Trauma Center. On arrival she had no eye opening, poor spontaneous ventilation, no pupil responses, and calorics were intact; no motor response could be elicited—thus, the Glasgow coma score was 3, although part of this clearly resulted from her spinal injury. After intubation and stabilization, a cervical spine, crosstable lateral x-ray study and her initial CT scan showed an abnormal amount of subluxation of C2 on C3, with disruption of the posterior cervical line (Fig. 167–5A). An intracranial pressure (ICP) monitor was inserted, the patient was placed in a collar, and methylprednisolone was given. Her ICP was easy to control with hyperventilation, but repeat x-ray studies of the spine showed increased slippage and rotation of C2 on C3. A halo traction was applied on the fourth day. She showed rapid recovery from her head injury and was eye opening and obeying commands with her eyes by the seventh day. She demonstrated no evidence of recovery of spontaneous ventilation and continued to have slippage of C2 on C3. On the fourteenth day after the injury, she was taken to the operating room. A tracheostomy, and then an exploration of the C2-C3 region, were performed. A unilateral fractured and jumped facet was found on the right side with marked instability of C2 on C3. The remainder of the spinal canal appeared stable, and a C2-C3 fusion was performed with iliac crest bone and Songer cables. The halo was left in place for 2 months. She had no return of neurologic function and remained ventilator dependent. However, she developed a solid stable fusion but with a mild angulation still present at C2-C3 (Fig. 167–4B). Rigid immobilization was delayed because of her head injury. Whether or not earlier halo application would have prevented further subluxation and healing without surgery is unlikely because the patient had a highly unstable fracture. In addition to her neurologic deficit, the risk of long-term spinal deformity would have been very high if fusion had not been performed.

CASE REPORT 3

A 15-year-old boy was thrown from a car during an impact accident. He was only briefly unconscious but had

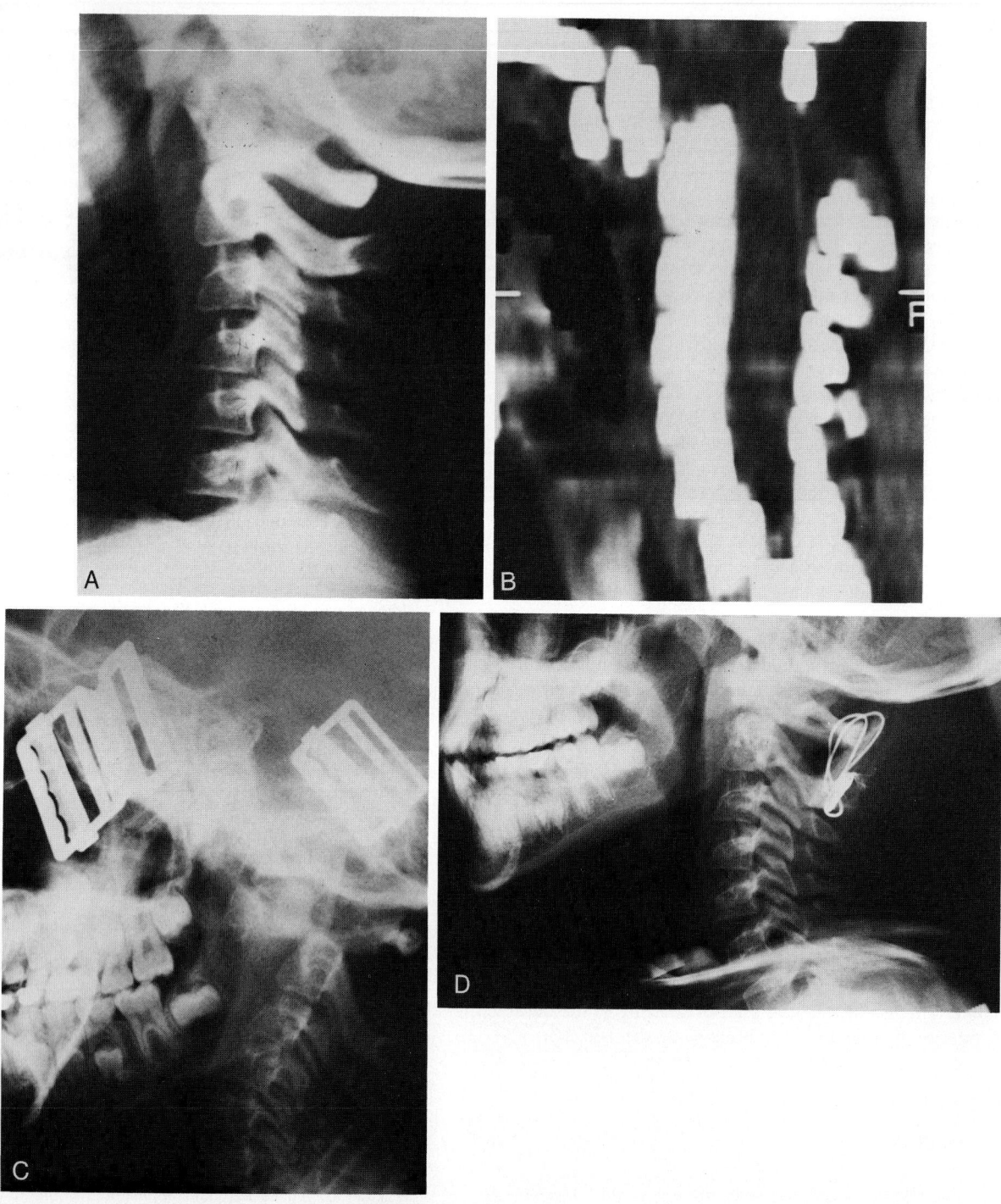

FIGURE 167-4. (A) Lateral cervical x-ray study in the neutral position demonstrating a defect between the dens and the body of C2 at the level of the normal synchondrosis taken 14 hours after the patient fell from 10 feet. No flexion extension films were obtained. (B) CT reconstruction 2 weeks after x-ray study in A. The patient now reports severe neck pain and minimal left arm weakness. The dens is sitting anterior to the body of C2, with marked narrowing of the cervical canal. (C) Lateral x-ray study with 2 pounds of halter traction; the neck is extended. There is minimal improvement in the position of the dens. (D) Lateral cervical x-ray study 4 weeks after C1-C2 fusion using the H-graft technique showing that the dens is now in its normal relationship to the body of C2; the neck is in the neutral position.

FIGURE 167–5. (A) Lateral cervical x-ray study in halo traction after flexion injury that resulted in subluxation of C2 on C3 and disruption of the posterior cervical line. (B) Lateral cervical x-ray study following bony fusion with the addition of Songer cables from C2 to C3. Extension and neutral showing residual slight kyphosis at C2 on C3.

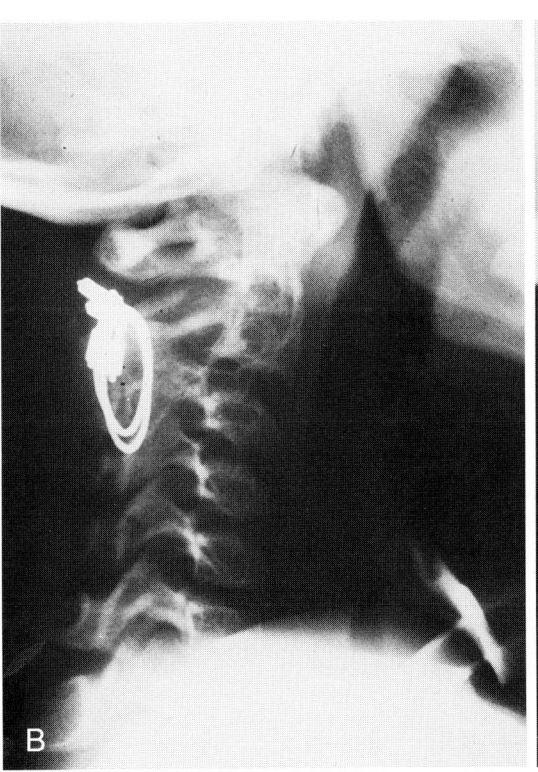
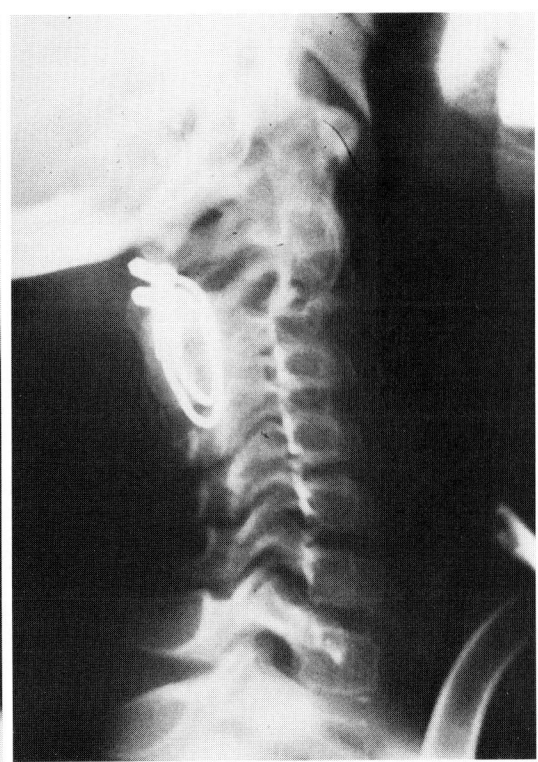

no function in his legs from the time of the injury. When he arrived in the emergency room, he had pain and tenderness in the midthoracic area, no sensation below T9, no voluntary movement in the lower extremities, and flaccid tone and absent deep tendon reflexes. Some rectal sphincter tone was preserved. His head CT scan result was normal, and his spine x-ray studies showed that he had sustained a compression fracture of T7 with disruption of all three columns and anterior dislocation of T6 on T7 (Fig. 167–5A). He became hypotensive soon after arrival, and abdominal CT showed free fluid and air in the abdomen. CT of the spine demonstrated the T6-T7 injury with encroachment of bone into the spinal canal and compression of less than 50 percent. He was taken for laparotomy, at which a bowel perforation and liver laceration were found (methylprednisolone was given). He was positioned in a Roto-Restbed in a hyperextended position. Once he was stable and had recovered from his laparotomy, x-ray studies were repeated and an MRI scan performed (Fig. 167–6C). The studies showed continued encroachment on the spinal canal with dislocation. The patient was taken to the operating room and underwent a posterolateral approach for decompression

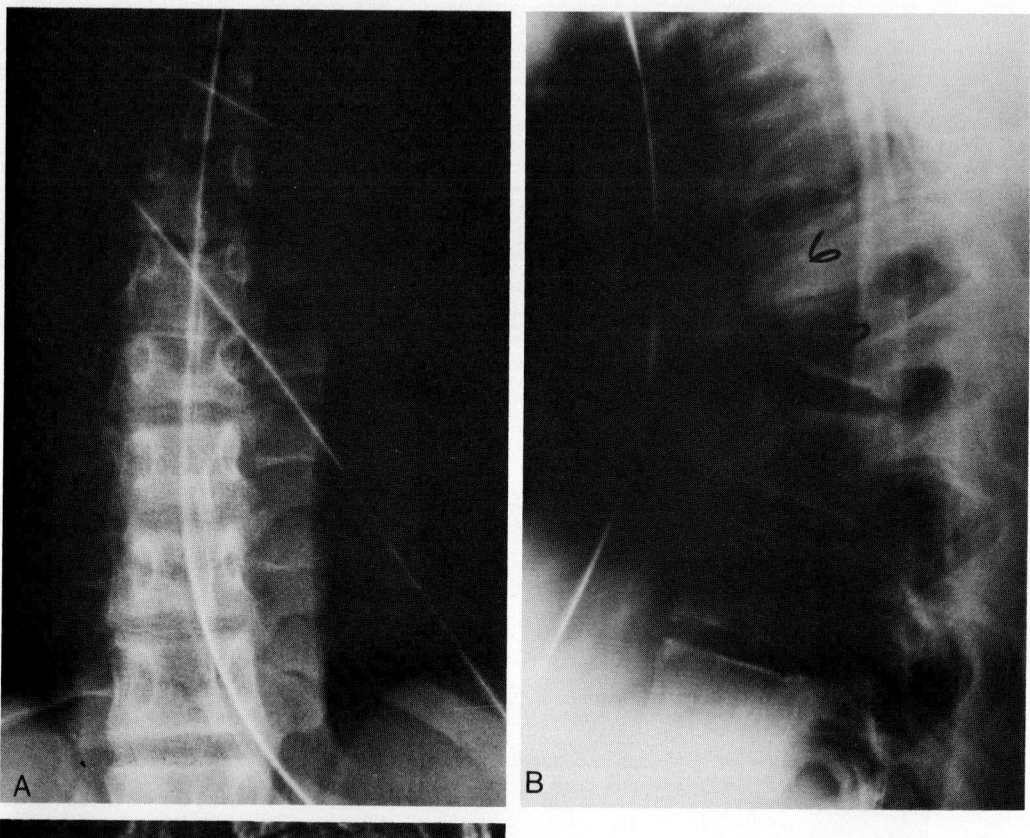

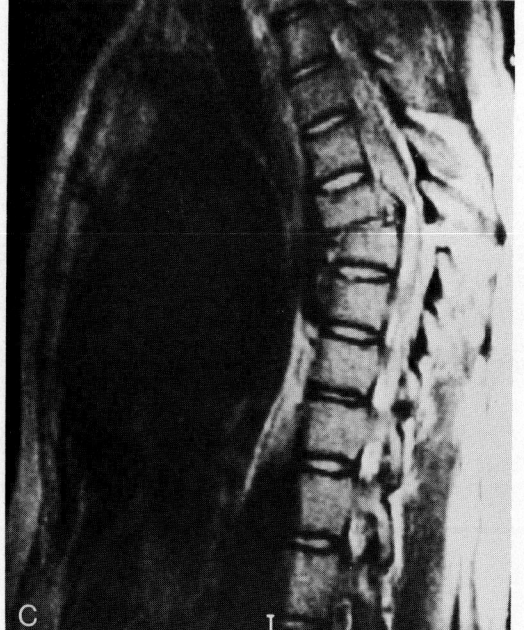

FIGURE 167–6. (A) AP x-ray study of thoracic spine showing loss of disc space between T6 and T7. (B) Lateral thoracic x-ray study showing compression of T6 and T7, increased kyphosis, and probable burst fracture of T7. (C) Sagittal MRI showing fracture subluxation of T6 on T7, with encroachment into the spinal canal of bone and disc and possible intramedullary hemorrhage or edema in the spinal cord below the injury.

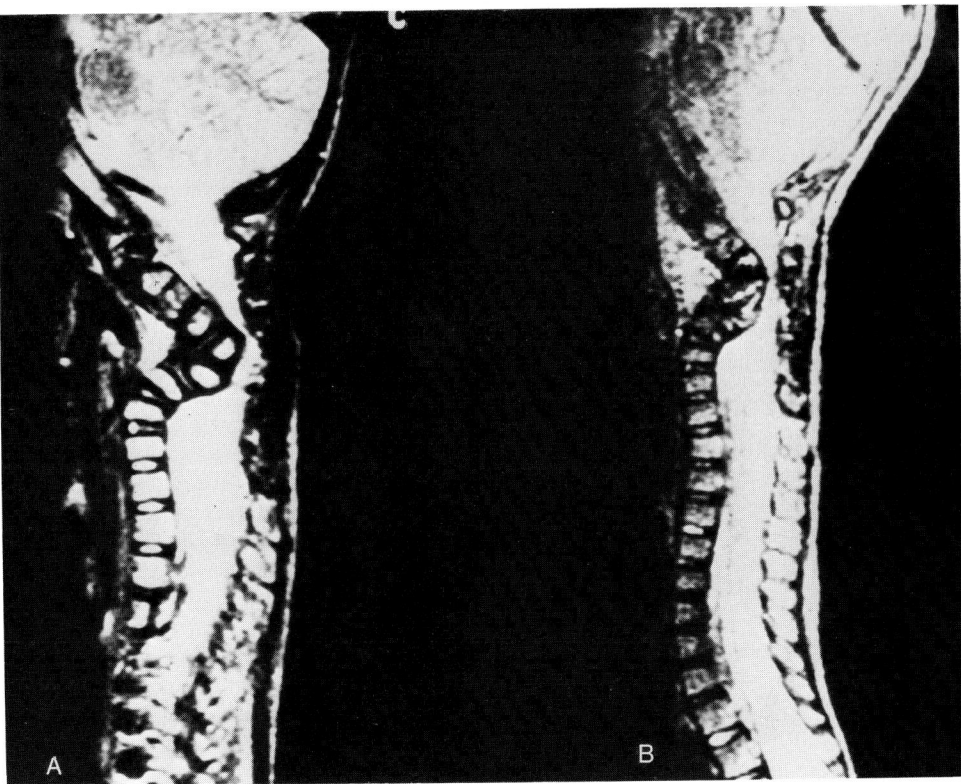

FIGURE 167–7. Sagittal MRI scans with T2-weighting in an 18-month-old child with Larson's syndrome: the child fell from her high chair. The image on the left was taken before surgery and, on the right, after resection of the bodies of C3 and C4 and insertion of a fibular graft. The canal remains narrow, but it is wider than it was before surgery.

of his spinal canal, followed by bony fusion and Texas-Scottish-Rite instrumentation, which had to carry three segments superiorly and three inferiorly to establish stability. He was mobilized immediately and is now in a wheelchair without any significant neurologic recovery. An argument could have been made for immediately decompressing his fracture after his laparotomy. Because of the immediate onset of paralysis with a complete lesion, the less than 50 percent encroachment on the spinal canal, and the severity of his abdominal injuries, it was felt appropriate to treat the spinal injury nonsurgically until he had recovered from his laparotomy.

CASE REPORT 4

The presence of pre-existing disease in the child can significantly complicate the approach to spinal trauma. An 18-month-old girl with Larsen's syndrome and known abnormalities of the cervical spine fell backward in her highchair, striking her occiput. She was not knocked unconscious, but her parents noted that she did not appear to be using her arms or hands. On arrival in the hospital, the examination showed adequate ventilation, good gag and swallow reflexes, but minimal spontaneous activity in the upper extremities, increased deep tendon reflexes in the arms, and some spontaneous activity in the lower extremities, 3/5 at best, with hyperactive reflexes. Plain x-ray studies showed multiple bony abnormalities, and MRI showed dramatic narrowing of the cervical canal C4-C6. She was placed in a halo with eight-pin fixation and gentle 1-pound traction. Any efforts at traction worsened the neurologic examination, and after 2 weeks in the halo, she had increased weakness to 1/5–2/5 in the upper extremities. Because of her worsening state, she underwent anterior decompression with corpectomies of C4 and C5 and fibular grafting and continued halo external stabilization. Postoperative MRI showed resection of the bodies of C3 and C4 and when measured for width of CSF space, the minimum width had doubled (Fig. 167–7). The surgical exposure was easy in this very small child, but positioning and maintenance of stability without traction on the cord was difficult. Somatosensory evoked potentials were used to monitor function but were very delayed before surgery. They served only to ensure that with position and manipulation, no deterioration occurred. Most of the bodies of the cervical vertebrae were cartilaginous, and finding a bony surface above and below on which to place the graft was very difficult. The child recovered to the functional level that was present immediately after the trauma and continued to show slow improvement in neurologic function 1 year later. The spinal alignment remained stable.

INTRAOPERATIVE COMPLICATIONS

The occurrence of intraoperative complications depends on the level of the surgical intervention. At all levels, the complications can be considered in three categories: the surgical exposure, the maintenance of exposure during surgery, the actual treatment of the operatively correctable lesion, or the taking of the bone graft.

During posterior exposure of the cervical spine, problems of surgical exposure are

1. Dissection not in the subperiosteal plane, leading to excessive blood loss and muscle damage

2. Distortion and displacement of the cervical vertebrae resulting from blunt dissection of the paraspinous muscles, possibly resulting in further or new spinal cord injury

3. Injury to the vertebral arteries as they pass from C1 to the intradural space or injury to the large epidural veins that lie deep to the ligamentum flavum

4. Injury to the dura or spinal cord by passing through an incompletely fused arch of C1 or through the thin ligamentum flavum between C1 and the foramen magnum of C1 and C2

These complications are all avoidable if the surgeon uses sharp dissection and stays in the appropriate surgical planes. Taking time to identify the different structures avoids inadvertent injury; the distances are small in children and the vertebrae mobile, and therefore technique and knowledge of the anatomy are required to avoid complications. Bleeding from the epidural veins at the C1-C2 or C1 foramen magnum level can be very brisk and, depending on the surgical position, almost always carries a risk of air embolization. The first step is to gently compress the vein with a wet cottonoid, which stops the bleeding transiently and prevents air aspiration. If the vein is visible, then bipolar coagulation generally suffices. If the vein retracts laterally or is not sufficiently well visualized to coagulate, then compression of the vein in the vertebral canal with Avitene stops the bleeding. The smallest piece of Avitene that will work must be used because stuffing any hemostatic agent into the canal can cause spinal cord compression and can aggravate injury. The Avitene is followed by a small cottonoid with minimal compression and is held in place until the bleeding stops. Patience is required, and the desire to stop the bleeding faster by packing more hemostatic agent into the canal must be avoided. Rarely is dissection under the lateral portion of the ligamentum flavum necessary, and usually bleeding from these veins represents an error in technique. Similarly, if hemorrhage from the vertebral artery is encountered, the first response is compression with a cottonoid for several minutes. If this does not work, then application of a hemostatic agent, such as Avitene, Gelfoam, or Surgicel, on the vessel wall, followed by gentle pressure, is tried. If the hole in the vessel is large and the hemorrhage cannot be stopped, then dissection of the vessel and suture of the hole may occasionally be necessary. The vessel should not be blindly coagulated because of the danger of increasing the size of the hole or occluding the vessel. If the only way to stop potentially fatal hemorrhage is to occlude the vessel, then this procedure may have to be performed. If so, it is necessary to ensure that the end of the vessel within the vertebral canal intradurally is not bleeding.

Because of the relatively large subarachnoid space at the upper cervical region, inadvertent opening of the dura during the dissection usually does not result in damage to the spinal cord. Any dural opening must be exposed and sutured after checking for intradural injury. The presence of a CSF leak interferes with bone healing and predisposes to an external CSF leak and an increased risk of infection.

The second period of potential surgical injury is the maintenance of retraction. If the head and body are well positioned before the procedure, maintaining retraction is rarely a problem. At C1-C2 especially, but at any cervical level at which positioning is limited by a flexion injury and therefore requires the head to be held in a neutral or slightly extended position for the beginning of the surgery, placement of retractors can increase the flexion in the child, and any change in position of the head or spine must be noted. If necessary, the position must be checked by fluoroscopy or x-ray study.

During the actual repositioning of the displaced vertebrae, unlocking of locked facets, and passing of the wires to obtain stability, the greatest risk for spinal cord injury exists. Proper dissection of the undersurface of the laminae from the ligamentum must be performed before passage of the wire. If the vertebrae are displaced anteriorly when the surgery is performed from posteriorly, pulling the arch of the displaced vertebra posteriorly and holding it in this position are necessary. Repeated anteroposterior movements of the vertebra can result in repeated small traumas to the spinal cord; thus, a method to prevent this phenomenon is necessary. In older children with thick bony laminae, this is rarely a problem, and the arch or lamina can be held with various instruments. In smaller children, it is better to free the lamina, pass the wire, and then after the wire is separated laterally on the arch or lamina, use the wire to produce the posterior pull to reposition the bones and hold them in place. This process minimizes the risk of fracture of the lamina. If the lamina of C1 is too thin, is fractured, or gets fractured during dissection, the age of the patient determines the next step. In younger children, the only option may be to proceed to an occiput-to-C2 fusion. The other alternative is to perform a bony fusion of C1 to C2 lateral masses (facet screws are too large, and the bone and cartilage of children's spines do not hold them well) with external fixation. In the lower cervical and thoracic areas, with a posterior midline approach the only real intraoperative complications are those related to further damage to the spinal cord that result from manipulation of the bones to gain exposure or to reduce any malalignment. The best way to avoid these complications is by careful sharp dissection of the paraspinous muscles and slow, controlled realignment. If internal fixation is used, no significant impingement must be present on the spinal canal.

If the dura is torn and the cord damaged, great care must be taken not to aspirate inside the softened spinal cord because it is easily sucked up, and even though such softened necrotic cord is unlikely to recover, it should not be removed. Whenever possible, the dura should be closed, with a graft if necessary, to prevent CSF from coming into contact with the bony fusion. When no lateral dura has been preserved as a result of the injury, the paraspinous muscles can be sutured directly to the dura above and below the level of loss to establish a relatively watertight closure. In the thoracic area, if a posterolateral approach is used, recognition of pleural injury and drainage of any pneumothorax is necessary. However, pneumothorax rarely occurs because positive-pressure ventilation helps prevent it.

At all levels, care must be taken to avoid overtightening of any fixation because of the risk of distraction of the spine at the many cartilage-bone interfaces. Before spinal surgery is performed, the decision must be made about the relative stability of the spinal injury and whether or not external fixation will be necessary. In the child, custom-built appliances are usually necessary and must be prepared before the procedure. High cervical lesions usually require some external immobilization device, halo, collar, or Minerva or Proplast jacket. The decision of which device to use depends on the age of the child and the degree of perceived instability. The halo produces the greatest restriction of movement, but in the small child, concern exists about the thinness of the skull and the risk of skull perforation by the pins. In children under 2 years of age, if a halo is used, the maximum number of pins (up to six to ten) should be used with only finger tightening. A lightweight plaster or Proplast jacket split to form two half shells is a suitable alternative in the infant younger than 2 years. If a solid fusion is obtained, a cervical collar may suffice. The dangers of using the collar are that the collar often impinges on the occiput at the level of the upper pole of the incision and can produce pressure necrosis and wound dehiscence. Thus, careful evaluation and, if necessary, modification of the collar are necessary to prevent this effect. Collars that rub on the chin are also a problem in small children because of the soiling by food and constant rubbing that can easily produce skin irritation and breakdown. Lighter collars that support the angle of the jaw are better tolerated, but in an active child, they may not withstand the demands placed on them, and if worn for a long time, they can interfere with mandibular growth. These potential problems may sway the surgeon to use a halo to avoid contact with the skin of the neck and face.

In the thoracic area, a lightweight vest is often used when the child is mobilized to prevent excessive flexion. In the lumbar area, external fixation devices work poorly.

POSTOPERATIVE PAIN CONTROL

Before surgery, child life services should prepare the patient and family for the surgical ordeal, including pain control. The surgery is rarely required at an hour's notice, and whenever possible, the support services should be used to begin to allay the anxiety that causes so much of the postoperative problem both for the child and the family.

Before the skin is closed, injection of 0.25 percent bupivacaine (Marcaine) into the surrounding muscles can help minimize early spasms and muscle pain. In addition, an intraoperative dose of Ketorolac tromethamine (Toradol), whose dose depends on the patient's weight, is given to help minimize postoperative pain. In children older than 7 years (depending on level of maturity), a patient-controlled analgesia pump with morphine is used. In younger children, a continuous infusion of fentanyl, beginning at 2μ g/kg/hour and increased or decreased as necessary to achieve adequate pain control, is a good way to treat pain occurring during the first 48 postoperative hours. This agent requires an oxygen saturation monitor as well as cardiac and respiratory monitoring and is most safely administered in the pediatric or other intensive care unit. Antispasmodic agents may be useful in older children, but little information exists on their use in young children. For restlessness or anxiety diphenhydramine (Benadryl) or lorazepam (Ativan) is helpful. In addition, an intensive care unit that is quiet, the presence of the parents, a reunion with favorite toys, and the playing of music or of favorite television shows all help to comfort the child as much as medication and should not be neglected. Depending on the presence or absence of spinal cord injury, a variable-pressure mattress or special bed may be required to avoid skin breakdown. In children under 6 years, this measure is rarely necessary because frequent turning is easily performed.

Chest physical therapy should begin soon after surgery, even in infants, to prevent atelectasis and pneumonia. Postoperative intravenous fluid requirements will depend on the site and presence of other injuries, e.g., head or abdomen. Normal saline at maintenance, plus 2 mEq/100 ml potassium chloride, is adequate. If an associated head injury is present, the serum osmolality should be kept above 290 milliosmols if possible. Careful fluid balance and hourly monitoring of intake and output are necessary to prevent or identify changes in fluid balance that may result from third-space pooling, if soft tissue or abdominal injuries are present; inappropriate antidiuretic hormone secretion resulting from the head injury; or reaction to surgery and postoperative narcotics. In preteenagers, venous thrombosis and pulmonary emboli are rare, and low-dose heparin or variable-pressure stockings are usually not required unless the child is especially obese. In teenagers, venous thrombosis is common, and variable-pressure stockings are started in the operating room or earlier if surgery is not performed as an emergency procedure. The use of nonsteroidal anti-inflammatory agents after the first 48 hours helps control pain and helps inhibit platelet adhesion. Bladder control is initially maintained with an indwelling catheter. As soon as possible, this stage is reduced to intermittent catheterization in children with spinal cord injury. Bowel training begins as soon as oral intake starts, with stool softeners and, if necessary, suppositories to establish a routine for bowel evacuation. Ranitidine (Zantac) or a similar agent is used for protection of gastric mucosa in an attempt to avoid stress ulceration and reflux. Antibiotics, if used for prophylaxis during surgery, are usually continued for 24 hours postoperatively. In patients with a penetrating injury, antibiotics are continued until the results of intraoperative cultures are available. Then, depending on the degree of contamination of the wound, antibiotics may be discontinued, or a full course of 10 to 14 days may be given.

Physical therapy is begun as soon as the patient is comfortable in the postoperative period, initially passive and then active. Similarly, social services support and, if necessary, psychiatric and psychological support is begun to help the child and family begin to cope with any loss of function and begin recovery.

The results of surgical decompression are dependent on the neurologic state of the patient. No evidence exists that surgery alters the neurologic outcome. Children with incomplete spinal cord injury are likely to show recovery in 75 percent of cases, with recovery to normal function in 50 percent. Children with complete lesions do no better than adults, and fewer than 10 percent have a single grade of recovery.

Completion of the bony fusion and stabilization almost always occur in children. Complaints of neck pain or some limitation of movement occur in 25 percent. Late kyphosis occurs in 25 percent of flexion injuries in teenagers with just external immobilization, and some degree of late kyphosis is common with thoracic and lumbar injuries. The late spinal deformities are much commoner in children with severe neurologic damage, and this should be remembered when the question of surgical stabilization is considered and is one of the reasons for careful long-term follow-up of these children.

REFERENCES

1. Kewalramani LS, Kraus JF, Sterling HM: Acute spinal cord lesions in a pediatric population: Epidemiological and clinical features. Paraplegia 18:206–219, 1980
2. Bracken MB, Freeman DH Jr, Hellenbrand K: Incidence of acute traumatic hospitalized spinal cord injury in the United States, 1970–1977. Am J Epidemiol 113:615–622, 1981
3. Anderson JM, Schutt AH: Spinal injury in children. A review of 156 cases seen from 1950 through 1978. Mayo Clin Proc 55:499–504, 1980

4. McGrory BJ, Klassen RA, Chao EY, et al: Acute fractures and dislocations of the cervical spine in children and adolescents. J Bone Joint Surg Am 75A:988–995, 1993
5. Hamilton MG, Myles ST: Pediatric spinal injury: Review of 174 hospital admissions. J Neurosurg 77:700–704, 1992
6. Dickman CA, Rekate HL, Sonntag VKH, Zabramski JM: Pediatric spinal trauma: Vertebral column and spinal cord injuries in children. Pediatr Neurosurg 15:237–256, 1989
7. Hamilton MG, Myles ST: Pediatric spinal injury: Review of 61 deaths. J Neurosurg 77:705–708, 1992
8. Hadley MN, Zabramski JM, Browner CM, et al: Pediatric spinal trauma. Review of 122 cases of spinal cord and vertebral column injuries. J Neurosurg 68:18–24, 1988
9. McPhee IB: Spinal fractures and dislocations in children and adolescents. Spine 6:533–537, 1981
10. Hadley MN, Sonntag VKW, Rekate HL, et al: The infant whiplash-shake injury syndrome. A clinical and pathological study. Neurosurgery 24:536–540, 1989
11. Bruce DA, Schutt CL, Sutton LN: Brain and cervical spine injuries occurring during organized sports activities in children and adolescents. Clin Sports Med 1:495–514, 1982
12. Ruge JR, Sinson GP, McLone DG, Cerullo LJ: Pediatric spinal injury: The very young. J Neurosurg 68:25–30, 1988
13. Hubbard DD: Injuries of the spine in children and adolescents. Clin Orthop 100:56–65, 1974
14. Pang D, Wilberger JE Jr: Spinal cord injury without radiographic abnormalities in children. J Neurosurg 57:114–129, 1982
15. Osenbach RK, Menezes AH: Spinal cord injury without radiographic abnormality in children. Pediatr Neurosurg 15:168–175, 1989
16. Pang D, Pollack IF: Spinal cord injury without radiographic abnormality in children—the SCIWORA syndrome. J Trauma 29:654–664, 1989
17. Cheshire DJE: The pediatric syndrome of traumatic myelopathy without demonstrable vertebral injury. Paraplegia 15:74–85, 1977
17a. Frankel HL, Hancock DO, Hyslop G, et al: The value of postural reduction in the initial management of closed injuries of the spine with paraplegia or tetraplegia. I. Paraplegia 7:179–192, 1969.
18. Keenan TL, Anthony J, Benson DR: Non-contiguous spinal fractures. J Trauma 30:489–491, 1990
19. Bulas DI, et al: Traumatic atlanto-occipital dislocation in children. Radiology :155–158, 1993
20. Cattell HS, Filtzer DL: Pseudosubluxation and other normal variations in the cervical spine in children. J Bone Joint Surg Am 47A:1295–1309, 1965
21. Bailey DK: The normal cervical spine in infants and children. Radiology 59:712–719, 1952
22. Sullivan CR, Bruwer AJ, Harris LE: Hypermobility of the cervical spine in children: A pitfall in the diagnosis of cervical dislocation. Am J Surg 95:636–640, 1958
23. Swischuk E: Anterior displacement of C2 in children: Physiologic or pathologic? Radiology 122:759–763, 1977
24. Swischuk LE, Swischuk PN, John SD, et al: Wedging of C3 in infants and children: Usually a normal finding and not a fracture. Radiology 188:523–526, 1993
25. Schaefer DM, Flanders AE, Osterholm JL, Northrup BE: Prognostic significance of magnetic resonance imaging in the acute phase of cervical spine injury. J Neurosurg 76:218–223, 1992
26. Evans DL, Bethem D: Cervical spine injuries in children. J Pediatr Orthop 9:563–568, 1989
27. Birney TJ, Hanley EN Jr: Traumatic cervical spine injuries in childhood and adolescence. Spine 14:1277–1282, 1989
28. Mandabach M, Ruge JR, Hahn YS, McLone DG: Pediatric axis fractures: Early halo immobilization, management and outcome. Pediatr Neurosurg 19:225–232, 1993
29. Anderson PA, Rivara FP, Maier RV, Drake C: The epidemiology of seatbelt-associated injuries. J Trauma 31:60–67, 1991
30. Johnson DL, Falci S: The diagnosis and treatment of pediatric lumbar spine injuries caused by rear seat lap belts. Neurosurgery 26:434–441, 1990
31. Reid AB, Letts RM, Black GB, et al: Pediatric chance fractures: Association with intra-abdominal injuries and seatbelt use. J Trauma 30:384–391, 1990
32. Stylianos S, Harris BH: Seatbelt use and patterns of central nervous system injury in children. Pediatr Emerg Care 6:4–5, 1990
33. Green DA, Green NE, Spengler DM, Devito DP, et al: Flexion distraction injuries to the lumbar spine associated with abdominal injuries. J Spinal Disord 4:312–318, 1991
34. Dennis F: The three column spine and its significance in the classification of acute thoracolumbar spinal injuries. Spine 8:817–831, 1983
35. Gertzbein SD, Court-Brown CM: Flexion distraction injuries of the lumbar spine. Clin Orthop 227:52–60, 1988
36. Gertzbein SD, Macmichael D, Tile M, et al: Harrington instrumentation as a method of fixation in fractures of the spine: A critical analysis of deficiencies. J Bone Joint Surg Br 64:526–529, 1982
37. Kaneda K, Abumi K, Fujiya M, et al: Burst fractures with neurological deficits of the thoracolumbar-lumbar spine. Spine 9:788–795, 1984
38. Farcy JP, Weidenbaum M, Glassman SD, et al: Sagittal index in management of thoracolumbar burst fractures. Spine 15:958–965, 1990
39. Greenwald TA, Keene JS: Results of Harrington instrumentation in type A and type B burst fractures. J Spinal Disord 4:149–156, 1991
40. Menezes AH, VanGilder JC: Anomalies of the craniovertebral junction, in chap. 45, pp 1359–1420
41. LeDoux MS, Naftalis RS, Aronin PA: Stabilization of the cervical spine in spondyloepiphyseal dysplasia congenita. Neurosurgery 28:580–583, 1991
42. McAfee PC, Werner FW, Glisson RR: A biomechanical analysis of spinal instrumentation systems in thoracolumbar fractures. Comparison of traditional Harrington distraction instrumentation with segmental spinal instrumentation. Spine 10:204–217, 1985
43. Panjabi MM, Abumi K, Duranceau J, Crisco JJ: Biomechanical evaluation of spinal fixation devices: II. Stability provided by eight internal fixation devices. Spine 13:1135–1140, 1988
44. Letts M, Kaylor D, Gouw G: A biomechanical analysis of halo fixation in children. J Bone Joint Surg Br 70B:277–279, 1988
45. Johnson RM, Owen JR, Hart DL, Callahan RA: Cervical orthoses. A guide to their selection and use. Clin Orthop 154:34–45, 1981
46. Mubarak SJ, Camp JF, Vuletich W, et al: Halo application in the infant. J Pediatr Orthop 9:612–614, 1989
47. Bucholz RD, Cheung KC: Halo vest versus spinal fusion for cervical injury: Evidence from an outcome study. J Neurosurg 70:884–892, 1989
48. Sonntag VKH, Kalfas I: Innovative cervical fusion and instrumentation techniques, in Black PM (ed): Clinical Neurosurgery, Vol. 37. Baltimore, Williams & Wilkins, 1989
49. Gill K, Paschal S, Corin J, et al: Posterior plating of the cervical spine. A biomechanical comparison of different posterior fusion techniques. Spine 13:813–816, 1988

CHAPTER 168

Surgical Management of Intramedullary Spinal Cord Tumors

Shlomo Constantini
Fred Epstein

Although ependymomas of the cauda equina region have long been successfully removed, intramedullary astrocytomas and other gliomas have not been viewed with surgical optimism. Little impetus has existed to modify the approach of biopsy, dural decompression, and radiation therapy, despite the recognition that after a relatively short remission, serious disability or death ensues. This traditional attitude was based on the assumption that carrying out extensive removal of tumors from within the center of the spinal cord is not feasible without a great likelihood of inflicting additional neurologic injury.[1,2] This is particularly unfortunate because most of these neoplasms are low-grade gliomas and are microscopically identical to their "sister" tumors, which occur in the cerebellum and are surgically curable.[3,4]

This chapter describes the overall approach to patients with intramedullary spinal cord tumors, primarily astrocytomas and ependymomas. The content of this chapter is based on the senior author's (FE) experience with radical excision of around 350 intramedullary spinal cord tumors from 1980 to 1992.[5-8] This chapter addresses intramedullary spinal cord tumors in both children and adults because most surgical principles apply to both groups. Differences in epidemiology and specific points of interest are included.

EPIDEMIOLOGY AND PATHOLOGY

Spinal cord tumors are relatively rare neoplasms, accounting for only 4 to 10 percent of central nervous system tumors. Although in adult life, intramedullary tumors comprise only about 25 percent of all intraspinal neoplasms, most pediatric spinal cord tumors are intramedullary.[9-11] The glioma family account for the vast majority of intramedullary spinal cord tumors.

Among 226 patients (of all ages) with intramedullary spinal cord tumors operated on in our service between 1985 and 1992, 30 percent had astrocytomas; 29 percent, ependymomas; 14 percent, gangliogliomas; 7 percent, other gliomas; and 20 percent, other lesions (e.g., hemangioblastomas, primitive neuroectodermal tumors, lipomas, and ganglioneurocytomas). Astrocytomas and gangliogliomas were especially prevalent in younger patients, whereas ependymomas were commoner in older patients. The incidence of histologically malignant versus benign tumors was stable at 30 to 35 percent throughout the different age groups.

CLINICAL PRESENTATION

In most cases, the clinical evolution was indolent, and, almost invariably, parents became aware of the problem long before objective signs of neurologic dysfunction were present. In a significant number of patients, the onset of symptoms was related to some apparently trivial injury, whereas in others, parents described exacerbations and remissions.

The commonest early symptom was local pain along the spinal axis. Other symptoms included motor disturbance, radicular pain, paresthesias, dysesthesias, and rarely, sphincter dysfunction.

Weakness of the lower extremities is usually first manifested as an alteration of a previously normal gait, which was often extremely subtle and only obvious to a parent who noted a tendency of the child to fall more frequently or to walk on the heels or toes. In young children, there was commonly a history of being a "late walker," and in the youngest (under 2 years), there was often a history of motor regression, such as starting to crawl again instead of walking or refusing to stand.

Seventy percent of patients experienced severe pain along the spinal axis that was most acute in the bony segments directly over the tumor. Characteristically, the pain was worse in the recumbent position because venous congestion further distended the dural tube and resulted in typical night pains. Patients commonly had been on long-standing analgesic therapy, including narcotics, after a nondiagnostic orthopedic evaluation.

Radicular pain occurred in about 10 percent of cases and was usually limited to one or two cervical, thoracic, or lumbar dermatomes, similar to root pain from various disease processes. Painful dysesthesias occurred in about 10 percent of cases and were generally described as painful hot or cold sensations in one or more extremities. In rare circumstances, these dysesthesias were the primary symptom and were not associated with objective signs of neurologic dysfunction.

Paresthesias were occasionally associated with the dysesthetic pain, and both of these symptoms were commoner with neoplasms in the cervical than with those in the thoracic spinal cord.

Mild spasticity, increased reflexes, and extensor plantar signs, with or without clonus, occurred relatively early in the neurologic course in patients with either cervical or thoracic tumors.

In the relatively rare malignant astrocytomas of childhood, symptoms were similar in quality but had a shorter duration and an increased intensity.

With cervical tumors, the commonest early symptoms were nuchal pain and head tilt with torticollis. Mild upper extremity monoparesis was the next commonest symptom and was often extremely subtle during the early stages of the illness. Very often, in young children, the first manifestation of weakness was switching handedness in right- or left-handed patients. Neoplasms in the caudal cervical spinal cord commonly caused weakness and atrophy of the intrinsic muscles of the hand, in contradistinction to tumors rostral to C5, which were less likely to cause significant weakness until relatively late in the clinical course. Interestingly, weakness of the lower extremities evolved months or, rarely, 2 to 3 years after the first symptoms, and bowel and bladder dysfunction was rarely present at the time of primary diagnosis.

Sensory abnormalities were generally limited to one upper extremity, and a discrete sensory level was noted only very late in the course of the disease, and, then only in association with severe neurologic disability. Patients with cervical ependymomas characteristically present with bilateral and symmetrical dysesthesias.

Mild scoliosis was the commonest early sign of an intramedullary thoracic cord neoplasm. Pain and paraspinal muscle spasm commonly occurred before objective signs of neurologic dysfunction were present and were commonly assumed to be secondary to the evolving scoliosis. Insidious progressive motor weakness in the lower extremities was first manifested by awkwardness and, only later, by frequent falls and an obvious limp. Early sensory abnormalities were uncommon, although dysesthesias and paresthesias were occasionally present.

Sphincter laxity is a very late sign, except in patients with tumors that originate in the conus-cauda area. Patients with higher tumors, even with cystic components extending into the conus, rarely present with sphincter abnormalities.

NEURODIAGNOSTIC TECHNIQUES

Intramedullary spinal cord tumors may be either focal or diffusely elongated. Holocord widening occurred in about 60 percent of children and was often manifested by expansion of the entire spinal cord from the medulla or cervicomedullary junction to the conus. Neoplasms extending for such long distances are most often cystic astrocytomas in which the solid component of the neoplasm spans a variable length of the cord and is associated with huge, nonneoplastic rostral and caudal cysts that expand the central canal above and below the tumor.

PLAIN FILMS

Plain spine x-ray studies commonly disclosed a diffusely widened spinal canal with relatively localized erosion or flattening of pedicles. Although the former was secondary to long-standing expansion of the entire spinal cord, the latter usually occurred only adjacent to the solid component of the neoplasm. Scalloping and scoliosis are also common manifestations of holocord intramedullary spinal cord tumors on plain films.

COMPUTED TOMOGRAPHIC SCANNING AND MYELOGRAPHY

Myelogram and computed tomographic (CT) scans were primary investigational tools for many years. Two major problems were associated with the interpretation of these assessments. First, in cases of a complete block (most tumors), a C1-C2 puncture was initially indicated to verify the rostral extent of the tumor. It was subsequently recognized that metrizamide almost invariably trickles past the block and is obvious on the immediate or delayed spinal CT scan and therefore delineates the rostral extent of the expanded cord. The second interpretation problem was that holocord expansion caused by a spinal cord tumor or cyst may be confused with hydromyelia. This differential diagnosis needs to be firmly established before surgery (Fig. 168–1).

MAGNETIC RESONANCE IMAGING

Magnetic resonance imaging (MRI) has relegated most invasive neurodiagnostic studies to history.[12] MRI provides an excellent image of intramedullary neoplasms and usually renders other studies unnecessary. Performing a myelogram might be still necessary in patients with severe scoliosis, when obtaining the mandatory mid-sagittal images is impossible or when an artificial implant produces magnetic artifacts.

The T1-weighted image is the most informative, and it discloses the presence of rostral and caudal cysts (Fig. 168–2), intramedullary cysts, and the solid component of the tumor. T2-weighed images give a myelographic appearance to the cerebrospinal fluid (CSF) and cysts. Injection of gadolinium is mandatory to image all spinal cord tumors.[13, 14] Gd-DTPA (gadolinium diethylenetriaminepenta-acetic acid) usually enhances the solid component of the tumor and helps delineate it from surrounding edema.

RADIOGRAPHIC DIFFERENTIATION BETWEEN ASTROCYTOMAS AND EPENDYMOMAS

In the presence of a very focal expansion of the spinal cord (one to two segments), the tumor was more likely to be an ependymoma than an astrocytoma.[15] In patients with very diffuse spinal cord widening, with or without associated cysts, astrocytoma was present in 90 percent and ependymoma in 10 percent. However, in children under 10 years of age, an intramedullary spinal cord tumor above the conus has a 75 percent likelihood of being either an astrocytoma or a ganglioglioma and only a 10 percent likelihood of being an ependymoma, which is in contradistinction to patients over 20 years of age, in whom there is an approximate 60 percent chance an ependymoma exists.

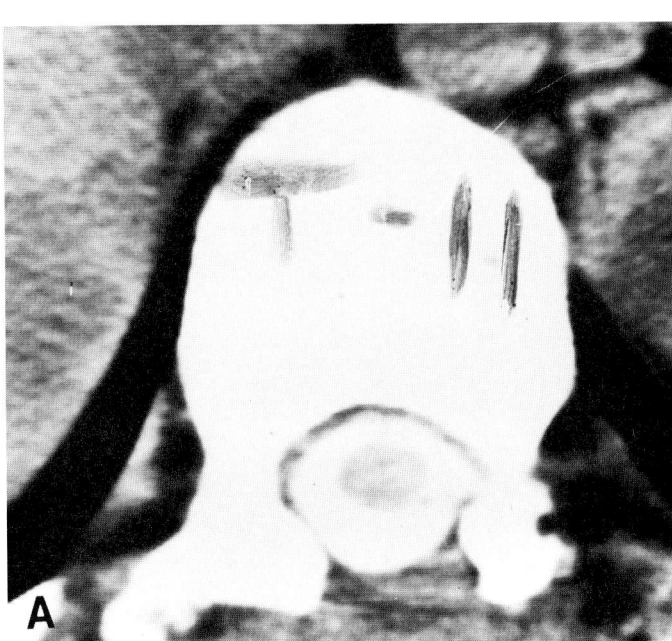 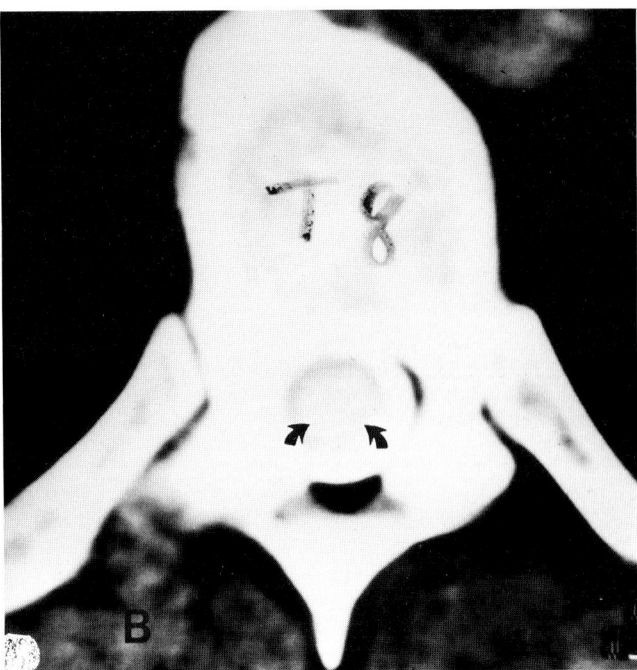

FIGURE 168–1. (A) CT scan obtained immediately after a myelogram, and (B) a CT scan obtained 12 hours later demonstrating an intramedullary cyst (arrows).

All ependymomas enhance brightly and homogeneously (Fig. 168–3), whereas gliomas may or may not enhance heterogeneously. The symmetrical location for spinal cord ependymomas, combined with their enhancement pattern, are quasi-pathognomonic.

SURGERY

SURGICAL INSTRUMENTATION (ULTRASONIC ASPIRATOR AND THE CARBON DIOXIDE LASER)

Spinal cord astrocytomas are relatively firm, occasionally contain microscopic foci of calcium, and only rarely have a cleavage plane to facilitate an en bloc resection. In the overwhelming majority of cases, it is necessary to remove the tumor from inside out until the glia-tumor interface is recognized as a change in color and consistency between the tumor and adjacent normal neural tissues. The principle of an initial central debulking applies also for ependymomas, although they invariably have a discrete cleavage from the surrounding white matter.

In the past, neurosurgeons were limited to traditional suction-cautery techniques for removal of neoplasms and, whereas this method was often satisfactory for brain tumors, it was extremely hazardous in the spinal cord. This danger arose because of the transmitted heat and movement through the tumor to the adjacent normal spinal cord, which was invariably firmly adherent to it. As a result of these technical limitations, a significant morbidity was associated with intramedullary spinal cord tumor surgery.

The development and application of the Cavitron ultrasonic aspirator (CUSA) system was a significant improvement over the conventional systems and made a major contribution to spinal cord surgery.[16, 17] The ultrasonic aspirator is the ideal instrument to rapidly debulk and remove all but residual fragments of a spinal cord neoplasm.

The neurosurgical laser is equally ideal to remove the residual fragments because it may be employed with great precision along the length of the glia-tumor interface. Although the laser may be employed in place of the CUSA, it is extremely tedious and time-consuming to use when directed toward a very voluminous intramedullary neoplasm. In addition, the resulting laser char makes recognizing the glia-tumor interface (Fig. 168–4) difficult and mandates frequent interruptions of the ongoing dissection as the blackened tissues are gently removed with small-caliber suction.

SURGICAL TECHNIQUE

A limited laminectomy should be carried out over the solid component of the neoplasm, but it should not unnecessarily be extended rostrally or caudally. In our first surgical experience with holocord widening, a total laminectomy from C1-T12 was carried out. It was subsequently recognized that exposing the spinal cord over the rostral and caudal cysts was not necessary, and for this reason, the location of the solid component of the neoplasm vis-à-vis the cysts must be defined as accurately as possible.

Even after careful consideration of the results of the clinical and neuroradiologic examination, it is not possible to be certain that the laminectomy is of sufficient length to expose the entire solid component of the neoplasm. For this reason, transdural ultrasonography is used to further define the location of the tumor vis-à-vis the bone removal.[18] Therefore, after laminectomy is carried out, the wound is filled with saline, and the head of the transducer probe is placed into gentle contact with the dura. With this technique, the spinal

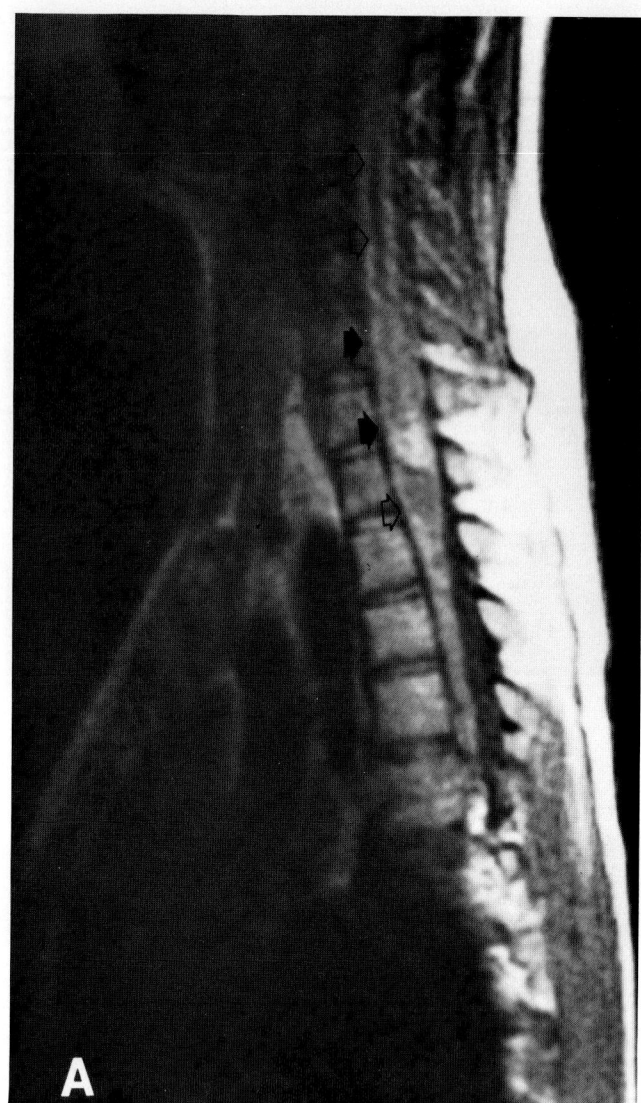
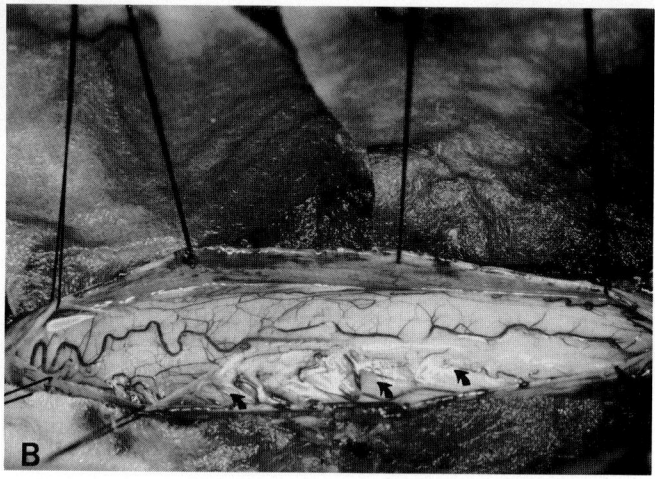

FIGURE 168-2. (A) A preoperative MRI scan showing cysts (open arrows) and solid tumor (arrows). (B) The corresponding photograph of the surgical field. Note the expanded spinal cord that is rotated to expose left dorsal roots (arrows).

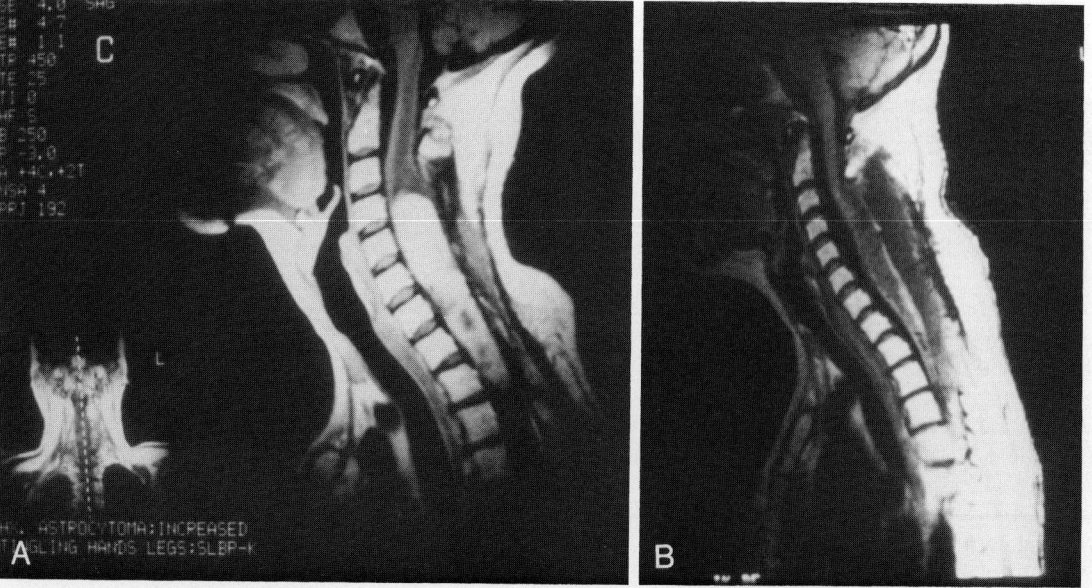

FIGURE 168-3. MRI scan of an adult patient with a cervical ependymoma before (A) and after (B) surgery. Note the bright homogeneous enhancement.

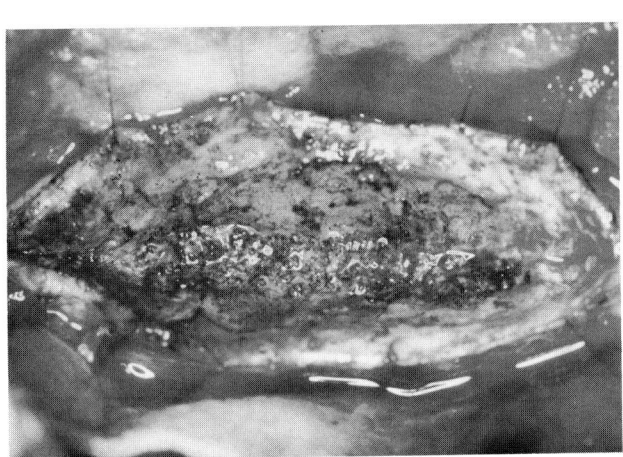

FIGURE 168–4. An intramedullary astrocytoma at the end of an inside-out evaporation with the CO_2 laser. Note the char, which makes it difficult to recognize the correct interface.

cord is viewed in both sagittal and transverse sections. The rostral and caudal limits of the tumor, as well as the presence or absence of associated cysts, are immediately obvious. Ependymomas are commonly homogeneously hyperechogenic vis-à-vis adjacent tissues, and, for this reason, the tumor mass may be completely visualized. In the presence of astrocytomas, the cord and tumor usually have the same acoustic property, but the cord appears to be diffusely widened over the bulk of the tumor and tapers at the rostral and caudal poles. If the laminectomy is not sufficiently long to expose the entire solid component of the neoplasm, it is lengthened, segment-by-segment, until the ultrasound discloses that the entire tumor mass is exposed.

In patients who have not been previously operated on and need bony opening of more than two segments, we use a high speed drill to perform an osteoplastic laminotomy. This procedure permits replacement of the bone, which is a nidus for subsequent osteogenesis, posterior fusion, and protection against future local trauma (see discussion on postoperative scoliosis).

At this juncture, the dura is opened to overlay the expanded spinal cord—it is not extended rostrally or caudally over normal spinal cord. In addition, in the presence of a rostral or caudal cyst, opening the dura widely over the cyst is not necessary, because the cysts are easily drained as the solid component of the neoplasm is excised.

The expanded spinal cord is commonly rotated and distorted (see Fig. 168–2), and careful inspection must identify normal landmarks before the myelotomy is placed. Because the posterior median raphe is always obliterated, the only sure way of recognizing the posterior midline is by identification of the dorsal root entry zones bilaterally. Rotation of the cord may occasionally make this identification difficult, and even surprising, in terms of the distorted location of the midline. However, this step is important because otherwise the myelotomy may be placed away from the median raphe and sever multiple nerves as well as the ipsilateral dorsal column along the dorsal root entry zone.

In the presence of holocord widening associated with rostral and caudal cysts, the ultrasound will have clearly defined the junction of cyst and neoplasm over the rostral and caudal poles of the tumor (Fig. 168–5). Intratumor cysts must not be mistaken for rostral and caudal cysts, because the surgeon may then terminate tumor removal prematurely because of misidentification of tumor poles.

The carbon dioxide laser is an ideal instrument for placing the myelotomy because it allows the cord to be incised and hemostasis to be obtained simultaneously. Although neurosurgeons are loathe to interrupt blood vessels on the surface of the spinal cord, preserving these vascular channels is tedious and time-consuming and not essential to the preservation of neurologic function, and they are almost inevitably disrupted during the course of the procedure, even if they are primarily preserved.

After the cyst is entered, inspection of the cavity localizes the rostral or caudal neoplasm that extends into it. In most cases, the myelotomy need not be extended over the cyst, because it is easily drained as either pole of the neoplasm is identified and removed. Because the cyst fluid is produced by the tumor, it is unlikely to reaccumulate after gross total excision of the neoplasm. After the rostral and caudal cyst-tumor junctions are identified, the myelotomy is continued

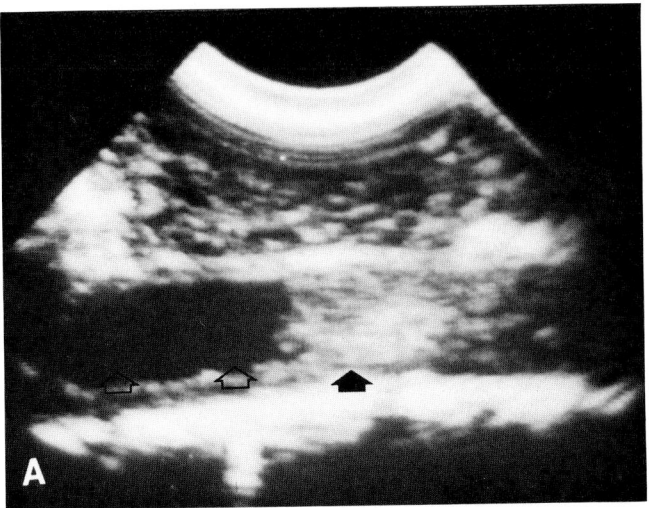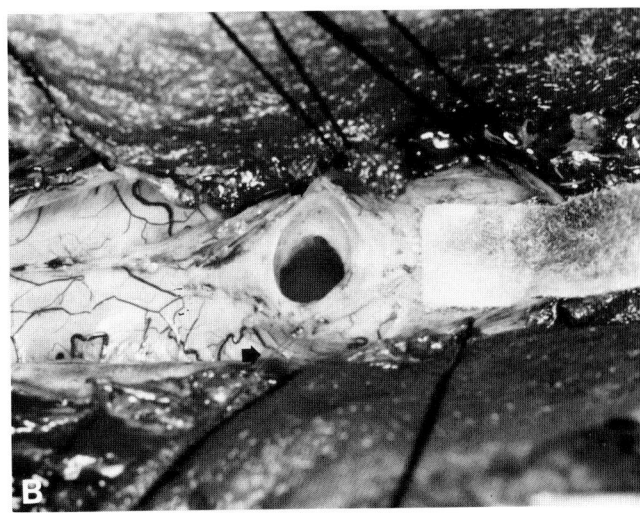

FIGURE 168–5. (A) An intraoperative ultrasonogram (obtained before dural incision) demonstrates the tumor (solid arrow) and a cyst (open arrow). (B) Myelotomy is started over the rostral pole of the tumor exposing the cyst. Note the pial traction sutures (arrows).

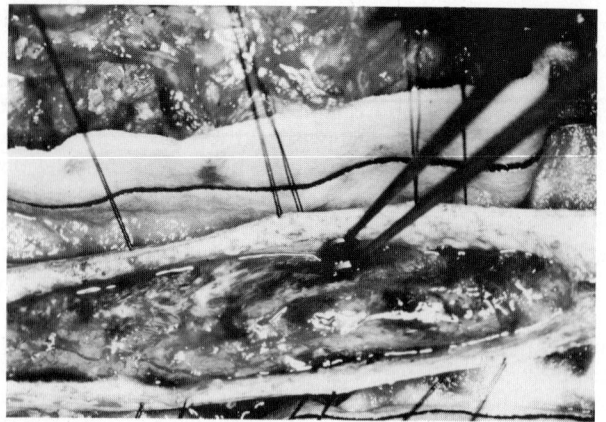

FIGURE 168–6. The plated bayonet is used to define the tumor–white matter interface. Note the pial traction sutures.

over the midline of the cord between the previously placed incisions.

After the myelotomy is completed, 1 to 2 mm of white matter usually overlies the neoplasm and is removed with laser or bipolar cautery and very fine suction. The normal tissue is now splayed to the sides by use of the plated bayonet (Fig. 168–6) (Codman and Shurtleff, CD#5256). This tool is a modification of a simple bayonet in which the tips were replaced with spherical thin plates.[19] It is used by placing the plated tips between the tumor and the adjacent tissues and by gently releasing the instrument. The tension is equally distributed over a relatively wide surface area, and there is no danger of perforating the tissues.

Most astrocytomas are gray and may be distinguished from adjacent white matter. Ependymomas are red or very dark gray and have a clear margin around the tumor. Pia traction sutures are used to open the myelotomy incision and further expose the intramedullary tumor (see Fig. 168–5). Any fine suture material may be used, and we simply hang small clamps on the sutures rather than suture the pia to adjacent tissues.

In the presence of an astrocytoma, no effort must be made to define a plane of cleavage around the tumor. These neoplasms must be removed from inside out until a glia-tumor interface is recognized by the change in color and consistency of the adjacent tissues (Fig. 168–7). A true plane of dissection rarely exists, and futile efforts to define its presence only result in unnecessary retraction and manipulation of functioning neural tissue.

In the presence of a cystic holocord neoplasm, tumor removal is initiated either at the rostral or the caudal pole of the neoplasm in the region of the tumor-cyst junction. As tumor excision continues, it is helpful to recognize that the anterior extent of the neoplasm is very rarely ventral to the anterior wall of the cyst. The bulk of the tumor is most often in the posterior two thirds of the spinal cord (as viewed on cross-section ultrasound) (Fig. 168–7), and the general dimensions of the tumor may be roughly conceptualized after inspection of the rostral and caudal cyst.

Excision of the solid noncystic astrocytoma is initiated in the mid portion rather than at the rostral or caudal pole of the neoplasm because there is no clear rostral or caudal demarcation of the tumor as occurs in rostral and caudal cysts. In addition, the poles of the neoplasm are the least voluminous, and, for this reason, removal of this part of the neoplasm may be the most hazardous because normal neural tissue may be easily disrupted. The last fragments of the rostral and caudal segments of the tumor are removed by working within the myelotomy and distracting the residual neoplasm into the surgical cavity without extending the myelotomy. This is an essential technical point because the tumors characteristically taper, and normal neural tissue is most vulnerable to injury in these areas. Intraoperative ultrasound is very helpful to monitor the progress and to clearly identify the rostral and caudal extent of the tumor. In many cases, the surgeon will have the impression that the anterior pia is

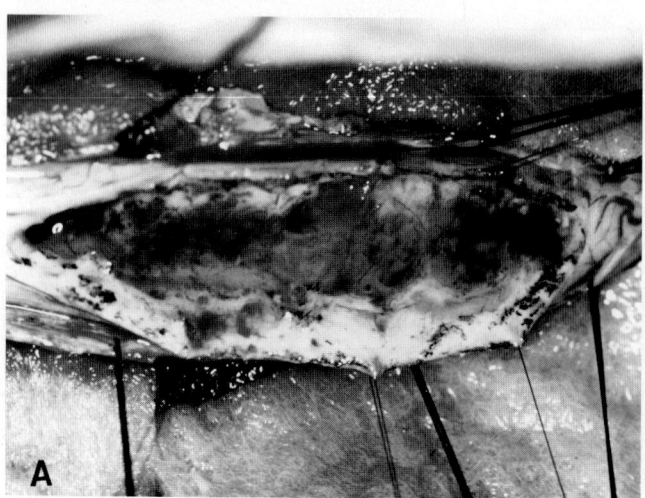
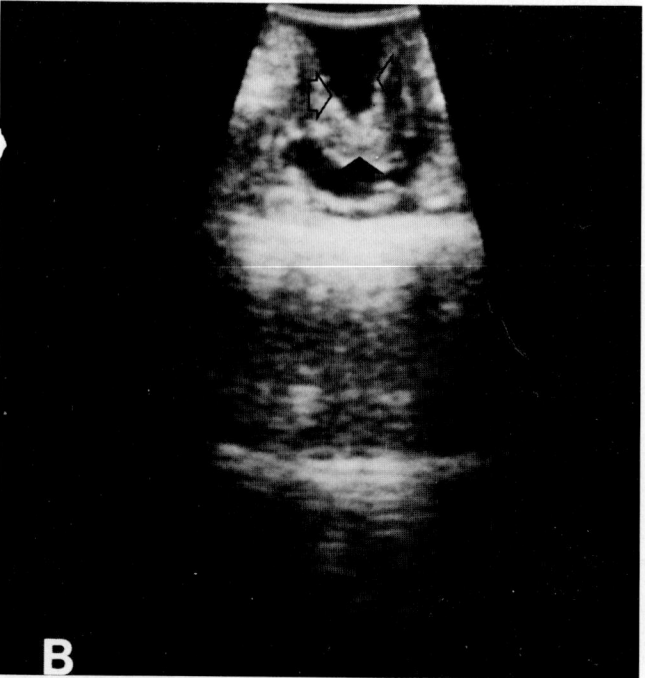

FIGURE 168–7. (A) Tumor resection is completed. (B) A transverse ultrasound image. Note the spinal cord (solid arrow) and the cavity (open arrow) remaining after tumor resection.

visible and that tumor excision must be abandoned. In these situations, ultrasound may be invaluable in cross section by conveying a very precise image of the tumor cavity and its relationship to the anterior subarachnoid space.

The CUSA is used to remove the bulk of the neoplasm, after which, the carbon dioxide laser or suction with bipolar coagulation is employed to vaporize the visible remaining fragments.

Ependymomas almost invariably have a true cleavage plane between the tumor and adjacent neural tissue (see Fig. 168–6).[15] Although this plane contributes to total excision of these neoplasms (see Fig. 168–3), it is also a potential hazard because it encourages the surgeon to attempt an en bloc resection and to remove the entire mass in one or two large pieces. If this type of removal is attempted, excessive and unnecessary manipulation of normal neural tissue will occur; under no circumstances should this be permitted. Rather, the ependymoma must be debulked as an astrocytoma, and only when the center of the tumor has been removed should the surgeon develop the plane of cleavage between the tumor and adjacent tissues. This cleavage may be accomplished by retraction of the remaining tumor tissue into the residual cavity—not retraction of the spinal cord from the tumor. Usually, an area of variable length lies along the anterior extension of the tumor, where it is adherent to the anterior median raphe. These tumor fragments must be removed in pieces, under high magnification, and with sharp dissection (no pulling or tugging) to avoid injury to the anterior spinal artery.

Conus, Filum Terminale, and Cauda Equina

In most cases, these tumors expand the filum terminale, which appears like a sausage-shaped mass that displaces the normal nerve elements of the cauda equina circumferentially around it. In these cases, the tumor en bloc may be removed simply by dividing the distal filum terminale caudal to the tumor, displacing the entire mass out of the cauda equina, and then incising the remainder of the tumor just below the conus. In many cases, the entire mass is within the filum, and pursuing tumor fragments rostrally into the conus is not necessary. However, occasionally, this last step may be mandatory to obtain a surgical cure, but it is essential that no neural tissue in the conus be manipulated in any way and that the tumor fragments be extracted from below.

A few ependymomas of the cauda equina seem to have grown from the region of the conus and to have erupted out of the filum, with tumor tissue filling the entire thecal sac below the conus. In these cases, the normal neural elements of the cauda equina are not displaced circumferentially around the mass but, rather, run through the tumor tissue. In these cases, the tumor must be removed bit by bit between and around the neural elements until all of the neoplastic tissue is removed. In these cases, remaining tumor fragments commonly must be extracted from the conus. However, it is important that the neural tissue be undisturbed and tumor fragments must be removed by working through the area throughout which the tumor has grown into the thecal sac.

WOUND OPENING AND CLOSURE

Patients who have previously undergone irradiation are at high risk for wound dehiscence and spinal fluid fistula. In the first 14 patients who previously underwent irradiation who were operated on in this series, nine had problems with wound healing, and five developed meningitis. Since that experience, we have used plastic surgical expertise.

The skin is scratched superficially with a scalpel and further opened to the fascia by use of cutting monopolar cautery with a needle attached to it. The fascia is opened also with the monopolar cautery. Closure after tumor removal involves several principles.[20, 21] First, at least one layer must have no CSF leaks. Second, permanent colored sutures are always used for the CSF-tight layers. These stitches provide a midline direction in case reoperation is required, especially in scoliotic patients. Third, drainage is always used for the subcutaneous space. Finally, the skin is usually closed in three layers: a deep subcutaneous layer, a superficial layer, and skin stitch. We pay special attention to the fascia because this is usually the watertight layer. The fascia and muscle are released both superficially from the subcutaneous tissues and deeply from the bony elements. If this release is not enough to achieve closure with no tension, relaxing incisions are performed. The musculofascial layer is closed with figure-8 Novofil or Prolene sutures and is tightly knotted. If any doubt exists regarding the seal of the closure, it is tested with fluid injection under pressure (Fig. 168–8).

EVOKED POTENTIALS MONITORING

The information provided by somatosensory evoked potentials (SEPs) is sufficient for the assessment of the functional integrity of the motor system in procedures in which insults usually affect sensory and motor pathways simultaneously. During operations for intramedullary spinal cord tumors, the motor tract may be damaged independently of the sensory system. In addition, the SEPs are often lost after midline myelotomy is performed. We therefore routinely monitor motor evoked potentials (MEPs).[22] We use the Sentinel-4 evoked potential/electroencephalographic analyzer (Axon Systems, Hauppauge, NY) as a mobile unit for recording, analyzing, and storing all operative evoked potentials. After laminectomy is performed, rostral and caudal epidural electrodes are placed. The electrode proximal to the stimulus serves as a control, and the distal one, a monitor for the

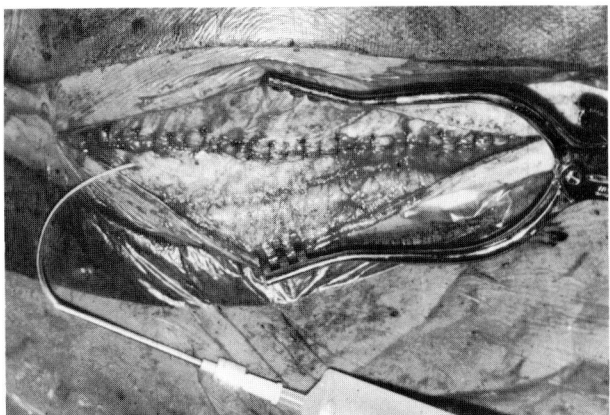

FIGURE 168–8. The watertight quality of the fascial closure is challenged with fluid forced through a subfascial Silastic catheter.

operation. For anesthesia, we use a combination of propofol and narcotics.

Some basic principles apply for both SEPs and MEPs. First, information needs to be immediately available and used by the surgeon to modify the operative dissection. Second, data should be continuously updated and communicated to the surgeon. Third, criteria for significant changes should be set and tailored for each patient, according to the pathology and the baseline potentials.

Several clinical correlations have been made. Midline myelotomy and the placement of pia traction sutures commonly result in transient decrements in the amplitude of SEPs, which probably occur as a result of movement of the posterior columns. Usually, the potential recovers within a few minutes. If it does not, the suture is removed and placed in another location under less tension.

When the laser is employed for more than 20 seconds at one time, an adverse, probably thermal, effect often occurs manifested by a decrease in amplitude and an increase in latency. When this effect occurs, the dissection is temporarily interrupted and the cord irrigated with cool Ringer's solution. In most cases, electrical activity returns to baseline within 30 to 90 seconds.

In some cases, deterioration of evoked potentials occurs as the dissection is directed toward tumor removal in specific locations. When such deterioration occurs, the manipulation is temporarily interrupted and the electrical activity permitted to recover. The procedure is commonly started and stopped many times during the course of tumor removal.

Perhaps the most important observation has been that if the dissection was inadvertently extended beyond the poles of the tumor, as is possible when no rostral caudal cyst is present, dramatic decrease in amplitude and an increase in latency of the evoked potential occurred over the caudal and rostral poles of the neoplasm. This phenomenon is indicative of tapering and warns the surgeon against extending the myelotomy. It is most likely secondary to manipulation of the posterior columns that are in their normal anatomic position and indicates that a normal cord is being disrupted.

Improved electrical conductivity after tumor removal was invariably associated with a benign postoperative course. Impaired activity as compared to the preoperative baseline was common, and it was not necessarily associated with neurologic morbidity. Nevertheless, most patients with deteriorated activity have had transiently greater neurologic dysfunction, although, in most circumstances, this dysfunction has ultimately recovered. In patients with impaired proprioception preoperatively, obtaining baseline SEPs for monitoring was rarely possible.

In several cases, the baseline SEPs were normal or near normal and disappeared completely and permanently as the tumor dissection continued. Although this event inevitably causes the surgeon great anxiety, it must not be construed as an indication for abandoning the surgery. The sensory pathways that conduct the SEPs are via the dorsal columns and, therefore, are not always correlated with motor function. Although the surgeon may be reassured and encouraged by stable or improving SEPs, he or she must not be discouraged by the reverse.

To elicit MEPs we use transcortical electrical stimulation[23] and epidural recording, which is a very reliable intraoperative technique that monitors the upper motor neuron without synapses on the way. It has the disadvantage of not differentiating between left and right.

The MEPs were most helpful during the removal of tumor at the most anterior and lateral aspects of the tumor cavity. Although the threshold for motor recovery has never been scientifically determined in such a set-up, we do not push dissection beyond a 50 percent fall in MEPs. If such a decline occurs, we stop manipulating the cord in this area and wait for recovery of the potentials.

SURGICAL COMPLICATIONS

INCREASED NEUROLOGIC DYSFUNCTION

Patients with malignant tumors are at much greater risk of sustaining a surgical injury. Also, patients with severe preoperative disability and extensive noncystic tumors are very likely to deteriorate as a result of surgery. The incidence of significant motor morbidity in intact patients is below 5 percent. Therefore, patients with known intramedullary spinal cord tumors must be operated on before significant neurologic dysfunction evolves.

Impaired position sense, even in the presence of normal motor function, is a serious functional disability that mandates extensive physical therapy to learn to compensate for it. On the basis of our experience, we emphasize this potential complication in our preoperative discussion with patients and parents. The risk of injury to deep sensation is significantly smaller during operations for childhood astrocytoma than during those for adult ependymoma. In children with congenital tumors, the posterior columns are displaced away from the midline, whereas in adults with centrally located lesions like ependymomas, manipulation of, and occasionally injury to, the posterior columns during the midline myelotomy are almost unavoidable.

Surgery was beneficial in the presence of advanced quadriparesis only when rostral, caudal, or intratumor cysts were drained with little manipulation of neural tissue. In these patients, minor but significant improvement in upper extremity function occurred. Interestingly, a similar degree of improvement in the lower extremities had less functional significance, and for this reason, evacuation of a cystic thoracic tumor in the presence of advanced disability in the lower extremities is rarely indicated.

Parents commonly inquire about the removal of a thoracic tumor in the presence of paraplegia, usually because they fear that the tumor will grow rostrally and ultimately result in quadriplegia and death. This concern directed us to an analysis of patients with long-standing tumors to make some assessment of whether or not the tumor ascended the neural axis over an extended time period. Benign, noncystic astrocytomas caudal to T4 do not usually extend rostrally—they expand and destroy the spinal cord locally but do not seem to threaten upper extremity function. The same tumor occurring above T4 is more likely to threaten upper extremity function because it does not require a great deal of rostral extension to impair hand function. Therefore, tumors closer to the cervical thoracic junction should be removed to preserve function in the hands and arms. All thoracic tumors with a rostral cyst extending into the cervical cord must also be removed because expansion of the cyst (syrinx) ultimately results in significant deterioration in motor function in the upper extremities.

CORRELATION OF POSTOPERATIVE NEUROLOGIC MORBIDITY AND SEGMENTAL LOCATION

Postoperative neurologic morbidity may be correlated with segments of spinal cord that are involved with neoplasm. Although an extensive dissection may be carried out with little risk to segments of spinal cord that are largely white matter, this does not seem to be the case in the lowest segments where gray matter is most abundant.

Dissections within the cervical spinal cord are associated with little morbidity, although some anterior horn cell dysfunction, as manifested by atrophy of one or more muscle groups of an upper extremity, is often present. When this phenomenon has occurred, it has been permanent. Dissections extending from the junction of the cervical and thoracic regions to T9 are also associated with remarkably little neurologic morbidity.

Tumors that are located in the lower spinal cord segments from T9 to T12 have the greatest incidence of significant postoperative neurologic morbidity. This is because neoplasms in the conus compress or infiltrate gray matter, whereas tumors in more rostral regions of the spinal cord compress white matter tracts; therefore, the resultant signs and symptoms are based on pathologic anatomy and pathophysiology that is specific to the segmental location of the neoplasm.

Significant preoperative sphincteric dysfunction suggests that the tumor extends into the conus because such dysfunction rarely occurs if the tumor is rostral to T12. Conversely, the absence of bowel and bladder problems suggests that the tumor does not extend into the conus, although it may be asymptomatically expanded by a caudal cyst. If no preoperative bowel and bladder dysfunction is present, it will occur postoperatively if the conus is disrupted. Therefore, the myelotomy must not be extended over the conus because this process invariably results in sphincter dysfunction that may be permanent.

The patient should be advised that at least a temporary increase in neurologic dysfunction is to be expected with surgery in this area, and that we assume that the long-term or permanent morbidity will also be significant.

ANTERIOR SPINAL ARTERY INJURY

One patient with a cervical astrocytoma and normal preoperative motor function was permanently paraplegic following surgery. The tumor resection extended from C4 to C8, whereas the motor defect was only in the lower extremities and was associated with preservation of sensation. The dissection had likely damaged the anterior spinal artery or an anomalous vascular collateral with the resultant injury. One other patient with a mild preoperative paraparesis and an 18-cm thoracic glioma was paraplegic, but sensation was preserved. The anterior spinal artery had been visualized during the tumor resection, and part of it may have been inadvertently coagulated. We now routinely monitor the progress of the tumor resection with ultrasound to avoid inadvertent injury to the anterior spinal artery.

MISSING ROSTRAL OR CAUDAL TUMOR FRAGMENT

In cases in which the entire spinal cord was expanded (holocord astrocytomas), the neoplasm was consistently associated with a rostral and caudal cyst that extended up and down the central canal but did not contain neoplasm. In three cases, a large, intratumor cyst was confused with a rostral cyst, and the tumor removal was prematurely terminated on the assumption that the superior part of the tumor had been removed. In these cases, the symptoms recurred 3 months, 6 months, and 18 months postoperatively as the cysts reformed. The symptoms were rapidly evolving scoliosis in two patients, and paraspinal and cervical pain in one. In all of these cases, re-exploration disclosed only residual tumor, which had been neglected as a direct result of misinterpretation of a large tumor cyst for a rostral or caudal cyst. When cysts are identified over the poles of the tumor, they must be opened up widely enough to ensure that the cyst extends above or below the tumor and is not a cyst within the tumor. The former are lined by white matter, whereas the latter are lined by tumor tissue.

Intraoperative ultrasound also helps differentiate rostral and caudal cysts from intratumor cysts. The former symmetrically expand the cord, occupy two thirds of the diameter, and are smooth walled. The latter are eccentric and asymmetric, are of varying volume, and often have irregular walls.

ANTERIOR SUBARACHNOID SPINAL FLUID LOCULATION

In eight patients, dramatic posterior extrusion of the spinal cord through the dural opening occurred during the tumor dissection. This event was associated with a deterioration of evoked potentials, and we initially misinterpreted this as acute spinal cord swelling. We now recognize that spinal fluid often becomes loculated anterior to the spinal cord and results in its posterior displacement. This problem is effectively dealt with by retraction of the lateral margin of the spinal cord and puncturing of the cyst. This intraoperative problem has occurred only in patients who have had previous surgery, and in whom there are dense adhesions between the lateral spinal cord and the dural tube. The anterior subarachnoid space seems to not communicate freely with the posterior subarachnoid space, a phenomenon that may be responsible for the hydrodynamics that prompt this occurrence. One patient in this series had a huge tumor in the lower thoracic cord, and although immediately neurologically stable, the patient became paraplegic 1 week after surgery. The CT scan disclosed that the spinal cord had extruded from the spinal canal, and, at surgery, a huge anterior loculation of spinal fluid had displaced the spinal cord posteriorly through the dural decompression, and the cord had become incarcerated on the rostral and caudal dura, with secondary infarction. Retrospectively, the dura had apparently been excised at the time of the first operation, and it had not been closed at the time of the tumor resection. This permitted the trapped anterior subarachnoid compartment to displace the cord out of the spinal canal, and infarction subsequently occurred. As the result of this experience, we do not leave the dura open under any circumstances, and if it has been previously excised, a suitable dural substitute is used.

POSTOPERATIVE SPINE DEFORMITY

Scoliosis and kyphosis commonly evolve after surgery. In severe cases of kyphosis, the deformity may be of a sufficient magnitude to cause spinal cord compression and progressive myelopathy.[24] In these patients, a diagnosis of a recurrent tumor should always be considered before the deformity is identified as being responsible for the neurologic dysfunction. This entity must be understood because treatment and prognosis are obviously very different for bony versus tumoral compression. Scoliosis usually does not cause spinal cord compression, although it obviously potentiates an existing neurologic disability.

All children must be closely followed up by an orthopedic surgeon who is experienced in caring for kyphosis and scoliosis. We recommend that the surgical indication for spinal fusion be regarded as more urgent in this group of patients than in those with idiopathic deformity.

In a recent retrospective study of 45 patients who had surgery for intramedullary spinal cord tumors, we compared the influence of osteoplastic laminotomy with that of a simple laminectomy on the incidence of progressive postoperative kyphoscoliosis in children. Progressive postoperative kyphoscoliosis, during a mean follow-up time of 3.4 years, occurred in three of 20 patients in the osteoplastic laminotomy group and occurred significantly more frequently, in nine of 25 patients, in the laminectomy group. All three patients in the osteoplastic laminotomy group who developed progressively postoperative kyphoscoliosis experienced recurrent disease. We therefore concluded that replacement of the bone in osteoplastic laminotomy is superior to a simple laminectomy, although it does not prevent the postsurgical evolution of spinal deformity if the tumor recurs.

HYDROCEPHALUS

Fifteen patients developed hydrocephalus that was occasionally fulminating in its presentation.[25, 26] Twelve of these patients had an astrocytoma, an associated rostral cyst, or both, and in each case, the tumor extended into the cervical cord, and obvious thickening of the leptomeninges overlying the cervicomedullary junction existed. This lymphomeningeal thickening likely caused obstruction of the outlets of the fourth ventricle. The presence of hydrocephalus associated with an astrocytoma caudal to the cervicothoracic junction strongly suggests a malignant tumor, with secondary dissemination and obstruction of spinal fluid pathways. The hydrocephalus that occurred in patients with an astrocytoma was not associated with a significantly elevated CSF protein level rostral to the block.

This finding was in contradistinction to the hydrocephalus that was associated with ependymomas (in three patients), in which cases the tumors were commonly in the thoracic cord and were associated with massively elevated CSF protein levels rostral to the block. Therefore, in the presence of an ependymoma, the protein-rich viscous fluid apparently obstructs the spinal fluid circulation.

MALIGNANT TUMORS

Most malignant astrocytomas and ependymomas had an atypical clinical course, as compared with "benign" neoplasms.[27, 28] Although children with low-grade neoplasms were symptomatic for a minimum of many months and often years, those with malignant tumors became symptomatic over a few weeks. In addition, patients with low-grade tumors had relatively trivial symptoms vis-à-vis MRI or myelogram, which disclosed massive spinal cord expansion. In contradistinction to this finding, patients with malignant tumors had rapidly evolving and advanced disability that was often associated with less dramatic expansion of the spinal cord.

The only exception to this clinical pattern was the occasional patient with a nonmalignant ependymoma that had hemorrhaged. In these cases, the neurologic disability evolved over a few days or weeks and was indistinguishable from the clinical course of malignant tumors. In two of these cases, MRI disclosed the area of hemorrhage. All patients with malignant tumors died within 12 months of surgery from neuraxis dissemination. In addition, the malignant neoplasms infiltrate the spinal cord rostrally, caudally, and through the subarachnoid space, resulting in paraplegia, quadriplegia, and death. On the basis of these observations, all of these patients are treated with neuraxis radiation therapy as well as chemotherapy.

DISCUSSION

Many important observations are clearly relevant to our understanding of the biology of this group of neoplasms, as well as to the recommendations for proper surgical management. The presence of cysts that were similar in appearance to those associated with the cystic astrocytoma of the cerebellum suggests that many of these neoplasms are congenital tumors that have their inception some time during gestation. The fluid produced by the tumor extends up and down the spinal cord in the region of least resistance, that is, the central canal. In some cases, the classic symptoms of syringomyelia may in fact be a late manifestation of such a cyst, in which the tumor has either involuted or is not anatomically obvious. Perhaps the centrally located cyst may gradually expand over many years and compress the surrounding cord. In this regard, it is significant that a few patients with holocord widening had exceedingly small neoplasms, between 1.5 and 3 cm, and were mistakenly diagnosed as having syringomyelia or hydromyelia. Our experience suggests that the presence of xanthochromic cyst fluid is pathognomonic of an associated neoplasm, whereas clear fluid is diagnostic of hydromyelia.

We believe that the presence of a widened spinal cord from the cervicomedullary junction to the conus, a condition that is associated with a relatively slowly evolving neurologic deficit, is indicative of a very slowly growing neoplasm that has a good long-term prognosis and should be treated aggressively.

Nevertheless, despite a gross total tumor excision, it would be naive to assume that residual tumor fragments were not commonly left in situ. We have hypothesized that these remaining fragments may remain dormant, or involute, in a similar way to what has been noted to occur in many astrocytomas of the cerebellum.[3,4] However, whether this is reality or wish fulfillment will only be known many years from now, after long-term follow-up and retrospective analysis.

In most cases of holocord tumor, the initial complaint was a weak arm, or a mildly weak leg, and associated pain somewhere along the spinal axis. The signs and symptoms were consistently relatively minor when compared with the apparently diffuse nature of the pathologic process. It is perfectly understandable why neurosurgeons faced with this clinical dilemma have been concerned about inflicting a greater neurologic deficit as a result of extensive dissection within a well-functioning spinal cord. This rationale has been used to justify the use of a temporizing surgical approach consisting of a limited laminectomy and biopsy, and for relying on radiation therapy to control tumor growth. Unfortunately, the natural history of these tumors after radiation therapy is slow deterioration and eventual severe neurologic disability or death.

The outcome after radical resection of these tumors was directly related to the preoperative neurologic status. Although a transient increase in weakness or sensory loss was commonly present in the immediate postoperative period, only a few patients had a significant permanent increase in neurologic deficit after the operation. Patients with paraparesis or quadriparesis who were ambulatory before surgery had neurologic improvement over several weeks. The group with severe deficits preoperatively rarely made any significant improvement, although their downhill course abated.

No evidence exists that radiation will cure benign astrocytomas of the spinal cord, and abundant evidence exists that it has a deleterious effect on the immature, developing nervous and osseous systems. Spinal cord tumors should be recognized as potentially excisable lesions, and radiation therapy should be reserved for possible adjunctive use if there is a recurrence. At that time, radiation therapy might be employed after a second radical surgical resection.

SUMMARY

This chapter presented the authors' surgical experience with a large number of intramedullary spinal cord tumors in children and adults. The following concluding statements can be made.

ASTROCYTOMA

1. Holocord widening occurs in 60 percent of cases and is diagnostic of a cystic astrocytoma.
2. Despite the absence of a surgical plane of dissection, these neoplasms may be removed from inside out until a glia-tumor interface is recognized.
3. Radical tumor excision is compatible with partial or total recovery of neurologic function.
4. The efficacy and relative safety of radical surgery have been shown. Relatively little information exists to suggest the duration of remission or the likelihood of permanent cure.

EPENDYMOMA

1. Holocord widening associated with an ependymoma may be associated with rostral and caudal cysts or occasionally with solid tumor that spans the length of the spinal cord.
2. In the presence of a focal tumor of three segments or less, the likelihood of ependymoma increases.
3. The presence of a cleavage plane facilitates the surgery and makes total tumor removal technically feasible.

MALIGNANT GLIOMAS

1. The preoperative clinical evolution of neurologic dysfunction occurs over a few weeks in malignant gliomas, compared with that of "benign" neoplasms, in which disability evolves over months or even years.
2. A clear interface rarely exists between the tumor and adjacent neural tissues.
3. Surgery is only temporarily beneficial because the tumor recurs and disseminates the entire neuraxis.
4. Postoperative neuraxis radiation and chemotherapy are mandatory surgical adjuncts.

The success of surgery for all spinal tumors is directly related to the preoperative neurologic status of the patient. Paralysis or near-paralysis was never improved, whereas mild-to-moderate preoperative neurologic dysfunction often recovered. We therefore recommend surgical intervention for intramedullary spinal cord tumors before a significant neurologic deficit evolves.

REFERENCES

1. Coxe WS: Tumors of the spinal canal in children. Am J Surg 27:62–73, 1961
2. Guidetti B, Mercuri S, Vagnozzi R: Long term results of the surgical treatment of 129 intramedullary spinal gliomas. J Neurosurg 54:323–330, 1981
3. Geissinger JD, Bucy PC: Astrocytomas of the cerebellum in children. Long-term study. Arch Neurol 24:125–135, 1971
4. Bucy P, Theiman PW: Astrocytomas of the cerebellum. A study of a series of patients operated on over 28 years ago. Arch Neurol 18:14–19, 1968
5. Epstein E, Epstein N: Surgical treatment of spinal cord astrocytomas of childhood. A series of 19 patients. J Neurosurg 57:685–689, 1982
6. Epstein F, Farmer JP, Freed D: Adult intramedullary astrocytoma of the spinal cord. J Neurosurg 77:355–359, 1992
7. Epstein F, Wisoff J: Intra-axial tumors of the cervicomedullary junction. J Neurosurg 67:483–487, 1987
8. Cooper PR: Outcome after operative treatment of intramedullary spinal cord tumors in adults: Intermediate and long term results in 51 patients. Neurosurgery 25:855–859, 1989
9. Alter M: Statistical aspects of spinal cord tumors, in Vinken PJ, Bruyn GH (ed): Handbook of Clinical Neurology. Amsterdam, North Holland Publishing, 1975
10. Slooff JL, Kernohan JW, MacCarty CS: Primary Intramedullary Tumors of the Spinal Cord and Filum Terminale. Philadelphia, WB Saunders, 1964
11. Russell DS, Rubinstein LJ (eds): Pathology of Tumours of the Nervous System. Baltimore, Williams & Wilkins, 1989
12. Li MH, Holtas S: MR imaging of spinal intramedullary tumors. Acta Radiol 32(6):505–513, 1991

13. Parizel PM, Baleriaux D, Rodesch G, et al: Gd-DTPA. AJR 8:339–346, 1989
14. Shoshan Y, Constantini S, Ashkenazi E, et al: Intramedullary spinal cord renal carcinoma metastasis diagnosed by gadolinium enhanced MRI. Neuroorthopedics 11:117–123, 1991
15. Epstein F, Farmer JP, Freed D: Adult intramedullary spinal cord ependymomas: The result of surgery in 38 patients. J Neurosurg 79:204–209, 1993
16. Epstein F, Raghavendra NB, John RE, Pritchett L: Spinal cord astrocytomas of childhood: Surgical adjuncts and pitfalls, in Neurosurgery, American Society of Pediatric Neurosurgery. Basel, Munchen, Paris, London, New York, Sydney, S Karger, 1985, pp 224–237
17. Flamm ES, Ransohoff J, Wuchinich D, Broadwin A: A preliminary experience with ultrasonic aspiration in neurosurgery. Neurosurgery 2:240–245, 1978
18. Epstein F, Farmer JP, Schneider SJ: Intraoperative ultrasonography: An important adjunct for intramedullary tumors. J Neurosurg 74:729–733, 1991
19. Epstein F, Ozek M: The plated bayonet: A new instrument to facilitate surgery for intra-axial neoplasms of the spinal cord and brain stem. J Neurosurg 78:505, 1993
20. Zide BM, Wisoff JH, Epstein F: Closure of extensive and complicated laminectomy wounds. J Neurosurg 67:59–64, 1987
21. Zide BM: How to reduce the morbidity of wound closure following extensive and complicated laminectomy and tethered cord surgery. Pediatr Neurosurg 18:157–166, 1992
22. Deletis V: Intraoperative monitoring of the functional integrity of the motor pathways, in Devinsky O, Beric A, Dogali M (eds): Advances in Neurology. New York, Raven Press, 1994, pp 201–214
23. Merton PA, Morton HB: Stimulation of the cerebral cortex in the intact cerebral cortex. Nature 285:227, 1980
24. Sim FH, Svien HJ, Bickel WH, et al: Swan neck deformity following extensive laminectomy. J Bone Joint Surg 56:564–580, 1974
25. Schijman E, Zuccaro G, Monges JA: Spinal tumors and hydrocephalus. Childs Nerv Syst 8:401–405, 1981
26. Rifkinson-Mann S, Wisoff JH, Epstein F: The association of hydrocephalus with intramedullary spinal cord tumors: A series of 25 patients. Neurosurgery 27:749–754, 1990
27. Cohen AR, Wisoff JH, Allen JC, Epstein F: Malignant astrocytomas of the spinal cord. J Neurosurg 70:50–74, 1989
28. Kopelson G, Linggood RM: Intramedullary spinal cord astrocytoma versus glioblastoma. The prognostic importance of histologic grade. Cancer 50:732–735, 1982

CHAPTER 169

Management of Achondroplasia and Its Neurosurgical Complications

Benjamin S. Carson
Clair Francomano
Jeremy A. Lauer
Orest Hurko

Achondroplasia is characterized by disproportionately short stature with rhizomelic shortening of the extremities, macrocephaly, midface hypoplasia, and frontal bossing.[1,2] This skeletal dysplasia results from defective formation of endochondral bone,[3-5] the biochemical cause of which is unknown. Morbidity in achondroplasia results in large part from bony compression of the neuraxis[6-12] and respiratory system.[13,14] This chapter focuses on the three main indications for neurosurgical intervention in this condition: cervicomedullary compression, hydrocephalus, and spinal stenosis. We also address other potential causes of morbidity and recommend an approach to the expectant care of the patient with achondroplasia.

Thoracolumbar stenosis resulting in spinal compression is the commonest complication of achondroplasia, becoming symptomatic in most patients in the third decade or later.[15] Such stenosis can be accelerated in infants who develop progressive thoracolumbar kyphosis if bracing is not undertaken before vertebral wedging develops.[16] Less common problems in infancy include symptomatic airway obstruction,[17] severe cervicomedullary compression secondary to foramen magnum stenosis,[18-20] and hydrocephalus.[21,22] Rarely, swallowing difficulties and central apnea[23] may be associated with cervicomedullary compression.

Most individuals with achondroplasia have normal intelligence. Motor milestones are delayed,[24] partly because of generalized hypotonia and partly because of the mechanical disadvantage imposed by short limbs. Psychosocial problems arising from short stature include lack of acceptance by peers and a tendency for adults, including parents and teachers, to treat children with achondroplasia appropriately for their height rather than their age.[25] Involvement with other families with children of short stature, in an organization such as the Little People of America, can improve self-esteem and can assist parents in guiding their achondroplastic children through the difficulties of growing up in a culture that equates stature with status.

Respiratory complications include obstructive sleep apnea secondary to a small upper airway.[14] Many persons with achondroplasia snore, often quite loudly. Many infants sleep with their necks in a hyperextended position, a position that functionally increases the size of the upper airway, relieving intermittent obstruction. Unfortunately, the hyperextended neck position may exacerbate neurologic sequelae of a small foramen magnum and cervicomedullary compression.[26] A small thoracic cage may result in restrictive pulmonary disease in infancy. Respiration may be further compromised by aspiration secondary to gastroesophageal reflux, or swallowing dysfunction, or both, resulting in recurrent pneumonia.

Reproductive difficulties have not been conclusively documented,[27] but evidence of reduced fertility, frequent fibroid cysts, and early menopause have been reported. Women with achondroplasia must deliver their infants by cesarean section because of cephalopelvic disproportion, and administration of spinal anesthesia is strongly discouraged.[27]

Although life expectancy was formerly thought to be normal in achondroplasia, age-specific mortality has recently been estimated to be increased at all ages, with the highest increase occurring in children.[28] Moreover, cardiovascular causes of death were estimated to be increased in the adult group (25 to 54 years of age).[28] The increased mortality in childhood is likely related to severe cervicomedullary compression.

As a result of the disease, the person with achondroplasia is likelier than others to seek treatment from a neurosurgical service for one of the three potentially debilitating problems mentioned earlier, and to face the prospect of surgical correction. Often, presenting symptoms do not have strictly neurosurgical resolutions. For that reason, a comprehensive treatment plan involving a multidisciplinary team of physicians is useful.

ETIOLOGY AND PATHOPHYSIOLOGY

CLINICAL GENETICS AND GROWTH PLATE ULTRASTRUCTURE

Achondroplasia is an autosomal dominant disorder; most estimates of its frequency cluster between one in 25,000 and one in 35,000 live births[29, 30]; however, the true frequency may be slightly higher.[31] New mutations account for about 80 percent[31] of children born with achondroplasia. As in many autosomal dominant conditions, a positive correlation exists between advanced paternal age and the occurrence of new mutations.[32] Offspring of couples who are both affected by achondroplasia have a 25-percent chance of inheriting both parental achondroplasia alleles, resulting in homozygous achondroplasia, which is almost universally fatal within the first year of life.[33] The skeletal features of achondroplasia are highly exaggerated in the homozygous condition, resulting in significantly shorter limbs, a smaller chest size, and a smaller foramen magnum. Death is usually secondary to respiratory complications, and some cases of foramen magnum decompression have been reported in individuals thus affected.[34]

Achondroplasia results from impaired formation of endochondral bone. The locus of the genetic defect is not known. The histochemical features of the endochondral growth plates of achondroplastic bone have been interpreted in several ways. Some researchers[35] have suggested that although endochondral bone ossification is qualitatively intact in achondroplasia, the growth plates of achondroplastic bone are thinner and exemplify a quantitative reduction of chondrocytes. Other investigators[36] suggest that mitotic abnormalities indicate cessation of normal cell function and arrest of cell division in the chondrocytes. This impaired formation of bone from cartilage is seen in the growth of the diaphyses of long bones.[5] In addition, an enlargement of the epiphyses occurs.[5] Analogously, cartilaginous synchondroses in the spine and skull seem to fuse prematurely,[5] and hypertrophy of spinal articular surfaces occurs. The three problems seen by the neurosurgeon result from these bony malformations. Hydrocephalus and cervicomedullary compression are typically pediatric concerns, whereas spinal stenosis is usually seen in adults.

CERVICOMEDULLARY COMPRESSION

Cervicomedullary compression stems primarily from a reduction in the diameter of the foramen magnum in both the sagittal and coronal dimensions that is sometimes more than five standard deviations less than normal.[37] The cranial base (chondrocranium) derives from endochondral ossification. In achondroplasia, the base is stunted, shorter, and narrower than normal.[38] The basioccipital bone, which forms the anterior border of the foramen magnum, is narrow and angulated.[38] The lateral and posterior parts, consisting of the exoccipitalis bone, are similarly deformed,[38] resulting in the diamond, triangular, or teardrop shape of the achondroplastic foramen magnum. Additionally, the articular surfaces of the occipital bone (between the lateral occipital and the basioccipital bones, and between the lateral occipital bones and the planum nuchale of the squama) are hypertrophic[38] and can encroach on neural elements within the foramen. The pathology of the achondroplastic skull is further complicated by the small size of the posterior fossa, resulting from stunting of the endochondrally derived planum nuchale, and the resultant horizontalization[38] of both squamous portions of the occipital bone. This constricted arrangement of the skull base displaces the brainstem upward and the foramen magnum anteriorly, resulting in posterior tilting of the brainstem and further impingement on the neuraxis posteriorly.[26]

HYDROCEPHALUS

In contrast to the skull base, cranial elements that form by membranous ossification (frontal, parietal, the squama of the temporal, and the planum occipitalis of the occipital bones) appear normal, except for enlargement concomitant to the hydrocephalus that is commonly associated with achondroplasia.[9, 21, 39] Some investigators have reported that cerebrospinal fluid (CSF) dynamics are frequently abnormal, and achondroplastic patients have the potential to develop clinically significant hydrocephalus. Hydrocephalus in the achondroplastic patient is likely secondary to deformation of the cranial base.[41] Constriction of the basal foramina, particularly the jugular foramina, reduces venous drainage and potentially raises intracranial venous pressure. In theory, absorption of CSF into the sagittal venous sinus is thus reduced, resulting in hydrocephalus.[42] Identifying patients at high risk for hydrocephalus is not currently possible. Apparently, the predisposition to hydrocephalus resolves in some patients through continued growth of the cranial base during puberty.[21]

SPINAL STENOSIS

Spinal stenosis is the third reason the achondroplastic patient may seek a neurosurgical consultation.[43, 44] The anatomy of the achondroplastic spine is distinctive in several respects, all of which can contribute to compromise of the cord or to nerve root compression. The hypertrophy of epiphyseal articular processes in the long bones is mirrored at the caudal and cephalic surfaces of the vertebral bodies, resulting in a "mushroom" shape at each end and concomitant scalloping along the posterior surface that is appreciable on a contrast myelogram.[45] Abbreviated and thickened pedicles of the vertebral arches result from premature fusion of synchondroses between the laminae and vertebral bodies,[5] and the laminae are also thickened.[5] Intravertebral discs tend to bulge prominently,[45] further aggravating neural encroachment by the enlarged vertebral body articular surfaces. The interpediculate distance decreases in the lumbar region of the spine, resulting in a canal that tapers caudally,[46] the opposite of normal (the canal normally widens caudally). The overall picture is one of dramatic stenosis in every dimension of the spine, a stenosis sometimes aggravated by osteoarthritic changes or disc rupture.[47] Consequently, a generalized constriction of the spinal neural elements occurs.

EVALUATION AND DIAGNOSIS

REFERRAL CRITERIA

Recently, primary care physicians have recognized the need for comprehensive prospective management of achondroplastic patients for sleep, respiratory, and central nervous system disorders.[14, 17, 48] To aid this effort, we present our recommendations for evaluation of the achondroplastic patient for cervicomedullary compression, hydrocephalus, and spinal stenosis. Achondroplastic patients referred to our institution are usually evaluated according to a standardized protocol that involves a multidisciplinary team. This team is composed of a neurosurgeon, neurologist, pulmonary and sleep specialist, geneticist, anesthesiologist, neuroradiologist, orthopedic surgeon, and otolaryngologist. Because these patients are at risk for brainstem compression, comprehensive testing is directed toward detection of central and obstructive apnea and cervicomedullary compression, all of which contribute to the risk of sudden death.

CERVICOMEDULLARY COMPRESSION

Clinical Pathology and Presentation

Cervicomedullary compression warrants early and aggressive treatment. Results of recent studies[49, 50] suggest such compression is progressive and potentially fatal because it increases the risk of sudden death by central respiratory failure. This condition has therefore gained increasing attention[51-53] as a cause of respiratory and neurologic impairment in children with achondroplastia. In our prospective evaluation of achondroplastic infants, we found radiographic evidence of craniocervical stenosis in 58 percent of the patients studied, and a diagnosis of cervicomedullary compression was made in 35 percent.[53] Although these figures are for a selected population and are therefore certainly higher than the proportion in the general population, they are nonetheless a strong argument for the careful evaluation and treatment of achondroplastic children. A recent retrospective study[28] found excess mortality in achondroplastic children aged less than 4 years, with sudden death resulting from brainstem compression identified as the cause of half of the excess deaths. The same study also found a 7.5-percent risk of sudden death in the first year of life.

Chronic medullary and upper cervical cord compression may exist as a neurologically asymptomatic lesion,[54] exhibiting neither signs of root compression in the arms nor symptoms of cranial nerve impairment. Nonetheless, microcystic histopathologic changes,[20] cervical syringomyelia,[18] and necrosis and gliosis[50] have been reported in autopsies of achondroplastic children who died unexpectedly. Presumably, lesions of this type interrupt neural respiratory pathways from the nucleus tractus solitarius to the phrenic nerve nucleus—arresting the muscles of inspiration and resulting in sudden death in some cases. We therefore consider infants with a history of sleep apnea or other severe respiratory or neurologic abnormalities to be at increased risk for respiratory complications resulting from occult cervicomedullary compression.[53] Some authors[48] have recommended performing sleep and imaging studies on all children with achondroplastia. We feel that a careful history and neurologic examination should precede costlier and more uncomfortable diagnostics. A composite profile of the patient with cervicomedullary compression would include upper- or lower-extremity paresis, apnea or cyanosis, hyperreflexia or hypertonia, and delay in motor milestones beyond achondroplastic standards. These patients can present a striking contrast to the usual floppy, hypotonic achondroplastic infant.[55]

Evaluation

Once a high-risk patient with respiratory or neurologic symptoms or signs has been identified, we advise comprehensive testing. Parents should be carefully interviewed about the health and medical history of their child, with emphasis on respiratory symptoms, and a general physical examination, including chest measurements, should be performed. Respiratory evaluation should include the evaluation of blood pH, a chest radiograph, and overnight polysomnography. Electrocardiograms and echocardiograms should be performed to see if there is cardiac evidence of chronic oxygen deprivation during sleep. A neurologic examination for signs of brainstem compression, such as hyperreflexia, hypertonia, paresis, asymmetry of movement or strength, or abnormal plantar responses, is essential. Brainstem auditory evoked potential and upper extremity somatosensory evoked potential evaluation[56] should be considered as an adjunct, especially in patients with normal results on neurologic examination. Imaging studies of the craniocervical junction are necessary, particularly magnetic resonance imaging (MRI) in the sagittal plane. We also strongly recommend MRI flow studies of the CSF at the foramen magnum, using the new technique of synchronizing with the heart beat the succession of images. Some of these procedures have been described elsewhere.[53]

Indications for Operation

The underlying principle must be to identify patients who are at risk for neurologic damage or sudden death. We recommend that patients with cervicomedullary compression be identified and treated prophylactically, before abrupt and irreversible changes occur. For the purpose of diagnosis, we define clinically significant cervicomedullary compression to be (1) neurologic evidence of upper cervical myelopathy; (2) evidence of stenosis on imaging studies, including the absence of flow above and below the foramen magnum; and frequently (3) an otherwise unexplained respiratory or developmental abnormality. It is possible, therefore, to see a patient with both brainstem compression and obstructive apnea who nonetheless meets these criteria. Having discovered these indications, one should also ask whether the patient's status is stable or deteriorating before undertaking operative decompression, and one should also evaluate the probability for catastrophic deterioration if decompression is not performed.

HYDROCEPHALUS

Clinical Pathology and Presentation

Hydrocephalus is suspected in most patients with achondroplasia, and the suspicion of hydrocephalus was originally thought to result from the macrocrania that is a morphologic hallmark of the disease. Hydrocephalus more recently has been found also to result from enlarged ventricles[22, 40] in the achondroplastic population, but the condition generally resolves through growth and maturation of the cranial bones. Some concerns about hydrocephalus are usually present from the birth of the achondroplastic newborn. Although initially these concerns arise from the size of the achondroplastic skull or ventricles, the delayed acquisition of gross motor skills[9, 22] may subsequently contribute. Both the size and the growth rate of the achondroplastic upper cranium are greater than normal; the growth rate eventually flattens, but at a larger absolute size.[26, 57] The achondroplastic child typically displays transient hypotonia, but the papilledema that would be expected with symptomatic hydrocephalus is rare.[26] Radiographically, mild-to-moderate ventricular enlargement, prominent cortical sulci, and an increased frontal subarachnoid space are apparent, in contrast to the isolated ventricular enlargement seen in the child with obstructive hydrocephalus.[22, 26] Craniocervical decompression, however, introduces an additional variable to the CSF flow equation, and hydrocephalus severe enough to require shunting is often discovered through CSF leaks that complicate wound healing after this procedure.

Evaluation

Although we recognize that some degree of abnormal CSF dynamics is common in achondroplasia, we believe that routine surveillance of achondroplastic infants for hydrocephalus is best limited to noninvasive measures that are easily incorporated into the pediatric examination and should not require referral to special centers and complex diagnostic procedures. Longitudinally evaluating head circumference and tracking the acquisition of developmental milestones with comparison to published standards is usually sufficient. Imaging studies can be reserved for patients whose head circumference crosses percentiles on the achondroplastic chart, or those who manifest unexplained neurologic signs or developmental retardation.

Indications for Operation

Recent work[42] has demonstrated that stenosis of the jugular foramina contributes to the altered CSF dynamics in achondroplasia. We believe, however, that jugular foramen decompression[58] should be used only for the child with severe jugular stenosis and debilitating hydrocephalus for whom conventional ventriculoperitoneal shunting is contraindicated. Given the high percentage of complications, shunting is best reserved for those in whom symptoms are severe and threatening.[26] If sustained or intermittent elevations of intracranial pressure (ICP) are demonstrated and are large enough to cause permanent impairment, shunting should be considered. CSF pressure profiles can be determined with an external transducer attached to an open fontanelle, with an epidural pressure monitor, or with an intraventricular catheter in older patients.[26] If no critical pressure elevations are detected during a 48-hour period, then shunt placement is not required, ventriculomegaly notwithstanding. However, the presence of severe clinical stigmata for hydrocephalus would obviate such demonstrations.

For patients who have undergone craniocervical decompression, we expect sustained ICP to be less than 20 mm Hg during the immediate postoperative period. Transient increases above this level can be associated with activity or irritation in normal individuals. In situations in which ICP is abnormally elevated, we proceed with shunting. In situations in which the interpretation is equivocal, we extend the period of monitoring for 1 or 2 days. Occasionally, even in situations in which no elevation of ICP is documented, a persistent CSF leak or subgaleal collections of CSF develop soon after the ventriculostomy is removed. It is sometimes difficult to tell if shunting should be carried out on the basis of a developing subgaleal CSF collection. One certainly does not want to place a shunt if the fluid collection is likely to resolve on its own. For this reason, we usually wait several days while observing for resolution or an increase in the amount of scalp swelling. We have a more aggressive approach to shunting, however, if subcutaneous collections develop over the site of craniocervical decompression. The dura in this area should have been closed in a watertight fashion and checked with a sustained Valsalva maneuver of 40 mm Hg intraoperatively; therefore, the development of a fluid collection in this area most likely represents elevated ICP. Collections in this region delay wound healing. Furthermore, because this is a high-contact area (i.e., an area with a significant risk of infection due to contact transmission of microbes), there is a proclivity toward subsequent infection. For these reasons, in situations in which postoperative cervicomedullary CSF collections occur, we generally proceed with shunting much more rapidly than for scalp collections.

SPINAL STENOSIS

Clinical Pathology and Presentation

The third neurologic complication for which neurosurgery may be considered is stenosis of the vertebral canal. Whereas the problems relating to hydrocephalus and cervicomedullary compression are frequently identified in infancy and childhood, neurologic problems below the foramen magnum frequently present in late adolescence and adulthood, perhaps as a result of postural or degenerative changes superimposed on congenital stenosis. In one series of patients treated at our institution,[60] however, 35 percent became symptomatic before age 15. Moreover, estimates of the incidence of symptomatic spinal stenosis range from 37 to 89 percent,[8, 59, 61, 62] suggesting that a significant proportion will eventually have this problem. Because the achondroplastic spinal canal tends to have severe congenital constriction, more intensive early screening might reveal substantial numbers of young achondroplastic patients with occult symptoms of spinal stenosis. Some studies[61] support this hypothesis, and thorough urologic and neurologic testing[60] play a useful part in the prospective evaluation for occult stenosis.

Although symptomatic stenosis can warrant neurosurgical intervention, it is generally possible to distinguish between the neurosurgical and orthopedic aspects of the management of the achondroplastic spine,[63, 64] inasmuch as some of the neurologic complaints requiring surgical intervention are a secondary result of orthopedic deterioration. The hypotonia that the achondroplastic infant typically exhibits suggests that muscular tone may be insufficient for adequate protection of pediatric skeletal structures in weight-bearing postures.[65] Achondroplastic children are in fact developmentally delayed[24] in supporting their heads independently, as well as in upright sitting and walking, and in our opinion, parents should not encourage early sitting, because of the potential for aggravation of thoracolumbar kyphosis in this posture. Sitting and standing postures affect the curvature of the spine, and in achondroplastic children, muscular weakness, short vertebral pedicles, and lax spinal ligaments[66] complicate these mechanics. Attention has also been drawn to the dynamic effect of a small chest and a globulous abdomen[67] in the formation of a progressive kyphosis. Moreover, delayed standing predisposes to development of a gibbus, with wedging of one or more vertebral elements. These wedged deformities are both debilitating and preventable. Because surgical repair has risks, effort is well spent on prevention. The prophylactic use of orthopedic bracing[63, 64, 66, 67] can be used in cases in which formation of a wedged gibbus seems likely. Parents should also be urged not to use any infant carriers, strollers, or baby seats that exaggerate the thoracolumbar kyphosis.

In the adult, compromise can result from such abnormalities as hyperlordosis, minor disc bulging, hypertrophic osteoarthritis, or ligamentous hypertrophy.[59] The presence of a thoracolumbar kyphosis is also positively correlated with symptomatic spinal stenosis.[67] Although lower back pain is a common complaint among achondroplastic patients, those with severe stenosis can develop symptomatic neurogenic claudication. Prolonged walking first produces paresthesias, and later, weakness of the lower extremities, which is usually bilateral. These symptoms are promptly relieved by rest, squatting, or leaning forward, which straighten the lordosis and increase the transverse diameter[65] of the lumbosacral canal. With progressive stenosis, the distance walked before claudication ensues decreases, making this symptom a useful clinical parameter.

Evaluation

In more advanced cases of stenosis, neurologic abnormalities, such as weakness of the lower extremities (particularly dorsiflexors of the toes and foot) and hypesthesia, often at a truncal level, persist at rest. Occasionally, a partial Brown-Séquard syndrome is seen. Spasticity and hyperreflexia of the legs typically indicate compression of the thoracic cord but may indicate coexistent cervical compression. The results of neurologic examinations of patients with claudication often remain otherwise normal until late in the disease process. Straight-leg-raising and reverse straight-leg-raising test results are usually normal unless a superimposed disc problem is present. Therefore, the thoracolumbar spine must be evaluated in all symptomatic achondroplastic patients, even in the absence of neurologic findings. If the patient has urinary incontinence or hesitancy, such investigation is performed as an emergency. The traditional study is myelography followed by computed tomographic (CT) scanning; however, MRI techniques are becoming increasingly reliable. Because of the stenotic lumbar canal, it is advisable to inject contrast via a lateral C1, C2 puncture. Lumbar puncture is less advisable as the likelihood of herniation of the nerve roots is greater in the narrow lumbar canal.

Indications for Operation

We recommend decompressive laminectomies for achondroplastic patients whose ambulation is severely limited by claudication, who show significant weakness (other than mild extensor hallucis longus weakness) at rest, or who have urinary incontinence or urgency that is attributable to compression of the cauda equina or spinal cord. There is a high incidence of urologic complications after laminectomy, and a high correlation between preoperative urologic abnormalities and postoperative complaints.[60] We therefore recommend thorough urologic testing as part of the preoperative evaluation for patients undergoing laminectomy.

OPERATIVE MANAGEMENT

GENERAL PRINCIPLES

At our institution, we use a common high-speed drill technique for both craniocervical and spinal decompressions. Although laminectomy is a widely practiced spinal procedure, we believe that modifications that address several of its shortcomings,[15, 62] including inadequate decompression and secondary spinal instability, are necessary for its use in the achondroplastic patient.

CERVICOMEDULLARY COMPRESSION

Craniocervical surgical decompression for cervicomedullary compression in children with achondroplasia[68] has been used at several centers and most recently has yielded generally good results.[12, 23, 69] Decompression of the cervicomedullary junction has been shown to bring about dramatic and sustained improvement in neurologic and respiratory function when it is combined with other therapy as needed for respiratory compromise.[53, 55] The procedure has not received as wide currency as it might, however, because its successful performance relies on careful management of the anatomic difficulties presented by the achondroplastic patient. Clinical evaluation, moreover, is frequently difficult because achondroplastic patients can have respiratory difficulties for many reasons, some of which are unrelated to neurologic compromise. Long-term follow-up data that would allow a definitive assessment of craniocervical decompression have also been lacking. As with any surgical procedure, detailed prior consultation must be conducted with the parents to inform them of the potential risks and expected benefits for their achondroplastic child.

A large operating room is used to accommodate all the equipment and personnel necessary to decompress the craniocervical junction. Before coming to the operating room, the patient is sedated, and antibiotics are administered. Patients also receive steroids preoperatively to protect the spinal cord and brainstem from local trauma. Patients are positioned prone on the operating table with the head and neck carefully supported in slight flexion by use of a padded pediatric horseshoe headrest. Upper-extremity somatosensory evoked potentials are assessed routinely during positioning as well as during the decompression procedure itself. The anesthesiologist is situated to have easy access to the patient and is also in close proximity to the evoked potential monitoring equipment.

After some untoward experience with postoperative CSF leakage from the surgical wound, we have begun to perform a ventriculostomy before craniocervical decompression. We hypothesized that duraplasty and wound healing were compromised as a result of the raised ICP typically found in achondroplastic children. Nonetheless, not all of these children's preoperative symptoms necessarily resulted from hydrocephalus. We implemented a solution, therefore, that would address the postoperative problem without necessitating permanent shunt placement. An external ventricular drain is inserted via a right frontal approach into the anterior horn of the right lateral ventricle. The external ventricular drain is left in place (closed) throughout the subsequent decompression and is opened postoperatively to allow continuous drainage at an ICP of greater than 10 cm H_2O. ICP is monitored for 48 hours with drainage gradually increased to 15 to 20 cm H_2O. The standard protocol is to record ICP, mean arterial pressure, cerebral perfusion pressure, and the amount of CSF drainage, along with hourly vital signs. Ultimately, some of these patients will require shunting, and the ability to monitor ICP postoperatively yields important information for this determination, as discussed earlier. Thus, the benefits of perioperative ventriculostomy appear to outweigh the risks associated with this procedure in this group of patients.

For the decompression (Fig. 169–1), a midline suboccipital incision is made, and the ligaments and musculature are dissected subperiosteally, to expose the occiput and the spinous processes and laminae of C1 and C2. The arch of C1 is then removed with a high-speed drill and small curettes. One frequently sees a thick, fibrous band or pannus above the level of C1 that should be left in place during the bony dissection to protect the underlying dura and cord from incidental injury. Compression of the cervical cord occasionally necessitates removal of the arch of C2, or carrying of the decompression even further in a caudal direction. The posterior rim of the foramen magnum is thinned gradually with a high-speed drill and removed with small, straight and angled curettes. Invariably, the bone of the foramen magnum is thickened and oriented more horizontally than usual, severely indenting the underlying dura. The most delicate part of the dissection occurs as the drill approaches the posterior rim of the foramen magnum. Once the bony decompression is complete, the fibrous pannus is removed as well, often revealing a transverse dural channel that offers dramatic evidence of the extent of dural constriction; consequently, adequate attention must be paid to the soft tissue aspects of the decompression. Duraplasty, by opening the dura in the midline along the area of constriction, is performed to relieve any persistent dural constriction. Adequate cord pulsations and CSF flow can be confirmed, and a dural patch graft can be performed, using paraspinous fascia, pericranium, or commercially available human cadaveric dura. A watertight seal is confirmed, and the wound is copiously irrigated and closed in several layers but not drained so as not to potentiate the development of a CSF fistula. Somatosensory evoked potentials are evaluated before the patient is undraped, in case a decision is made to re-explore the wound. Once movement is confirmed in all four extremities, the patient is sent to the pediatric intensive care unit. Extubation is often performed immediately postoperatively; however, in some cases, facial and laryngeal edema make this procedure inadvisable for 12 to

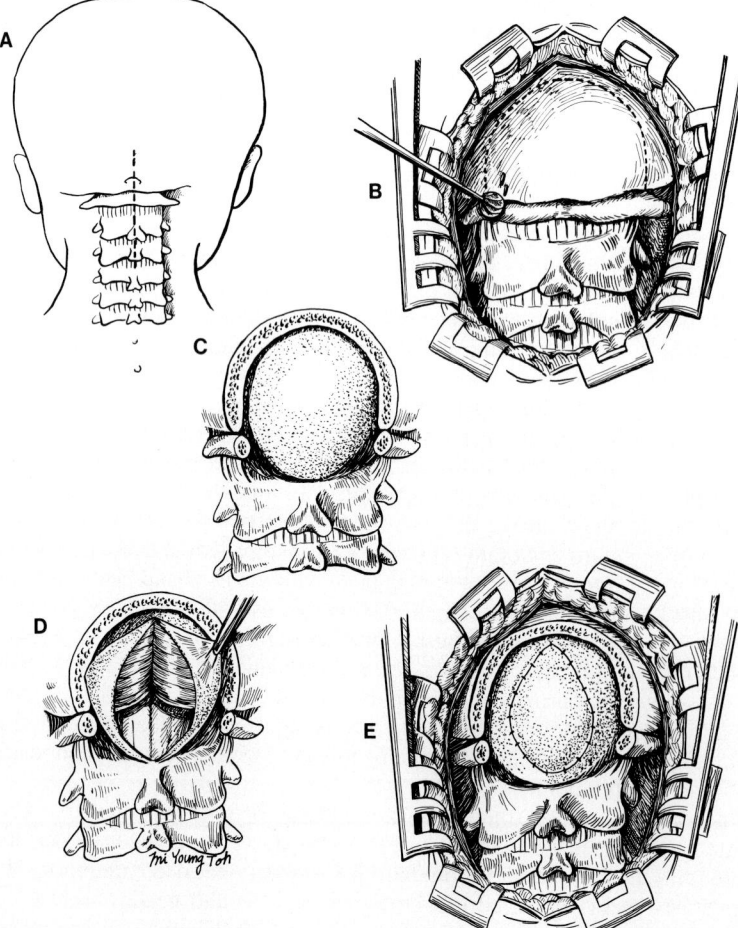

FIGURE 169–1. The surgical procedure for craniocervical decompression. (A) View of the surgical site and underlying anatomy. (B) The bony structures have been exposed. (C) The bone is removed from the arch of C1 and the posterior fossa, revealing the underlying dura. (D) A dural incision, which must be parasagittal rather than midline, is made to relieve soft tissue compression. (E) Duraplasty is performed.

24 hours. After surgery, primary attention is directed toward monitoring ICP as a part of postoperative nursing care.

The surgeon should bear in mind several important pitfalls when undertaking cervicomedullary decompression in achondroplastic patients. First, the patient's head must not be overflexed during positioning, because such a position often reduces the subarachnoid space at the cervicomedullary junction. Second, the surgeon should avoid placing any instruments beneath the posterior arch of C1 or beneath the rim of the foramen magnum, even though these patients are pretreated with steroids. The surgeon must remember that the cervicomedullary junction is already under tremendous constrictive pressure, and even the brief introduction of instruments into the already compromised space can be disastrous. The surgeon must recognize that the spinal cords and brainstems of children are small; therefore, the decompression should be correspondingly small. The surgeon must have in mind an accurate conception of the size of the spinal cord and brainstem to perform an appropriate decompression. This information can be gained by careful study of the preoperative MR images. Moreover, the decompression must be extended not only along the dorsal surface of the cervicomedullary junction but also sufficiently along the lateral dimensions of the medulla to adequately decompress the stenosis at the level of the foramen magnum.

Frequently, engorged veins exist beneath the ligamentum flavum, located dorsally and laterally, and sometimes insinuating through the ligamentum flavum. These can create enormous bleeding and must be controlled rapidly if they are compromised. The possibility of air embolization also exists through these veins, and the surgeon should ensure that the patient is not in any degree of reverse Trendelenburg's position. Finally, once the bony decompression is complete, the underlying dura, which in many cases is itself severely constricted, must be carefully checked. The dura is often fused with the ligamentum, and this soft tissue band serves to constrict the underlying neural tissues, even without the presence of the overlying bone. When this situation occurs, the band must be divided and a dural patch placed. When the band is divided, a significantly engorged annular sinus is commonly present beneath the foramen magnum; therefore, the band should be slowly divided, and measures should be taken to control the annular sinus as it is encountered.

SPINAL STENOSIS

Decompression of the achondroplastic spinal canal is difficult because of the extent and severity of the stenosis. The quantitative magnitude of this stenosis has been well documented.[70, 71] Moreover, poor postoperative results were relatively common[15, 62, 72] for spinal decompressions in achondroplastic patients. Before the era of CT and MRI, the degree and extent of spinal compression were often not appreciated with conventional myelography because of the lack of adequate contrast medium diffusion.[6, 45] Insertion of bulky instruments under the laminae during the conventional techniques also frequently traumatized neural tissue. Other sources of poor results were postoperative instability[59, 61, 72] resulting from overly wide laminectomies.

The following procedure[71] (Fig. 169–2) has been used at our institution with good results.[60, 73] Adequate anatomic de-

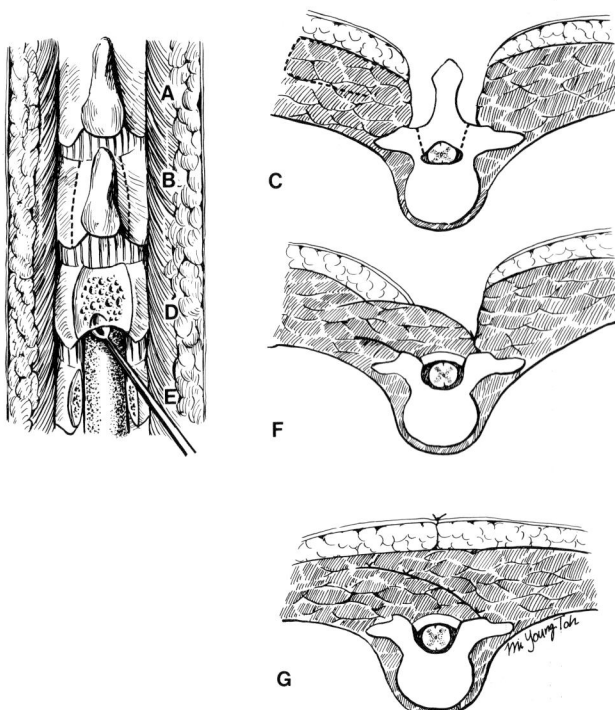

FIGURE 169–2. The surgical procedure for lumbar laminectomy. (A) View of an intact lumbar spinous process. (B) The extent of decompression is visualized. (C) Axial view of the same stage, with a split-thickness incision of the paraspinal muscle visualized. (D) The laminectomy is completed by carefully flicking away the dural mantle. (E) Adequate decompression is ascertained. (F) The paraspinal muscle flap is reflected to the opposite side, sealing the dead space over the Gelfoam. (G) The incision is closed in layers.

lineation is obtained by MRI and intrathecally enhanced CT, but myelography is sometimes useful as an adjunct. Based on the results of these studies, the surgeon can devise an operative plan for adequate decompression that includes at least three segments above the level of demonstrated block and three segments below (or to S2). The incision is midline, and dissection is carried subperiosteally to expose the spinous processes, laminae, and facet joints over the extent of the area to be decompressed. When adequate exposure is achieved, the laminae immediately medial to the facet joints are gradually thinned with a high-speed drill, forming a groove approximately parallel to the longitudinal axis of the spinal column. The drill head is held at an attitude of about 45 degrees to the laminal surface rather than 90 degrees; this angle offers the surgeon the control necessary to avoid accidental perforation of the laminae. The groove is deepened until the dura can be seen through the thinned laminal mantle. Drilling is then concluded in this area and is continued on the opposite side in a similar fashion. An opening is made at the caudal part of the groove on the first side, a thin surgical punch is inserted into the epidural space, and the laminectomy is carried along the groove. A small Leksell rongeur is inserted through this opening to complete the laminectomy by lifting off the laminae in a piecemeal fashion. This technique minimizes dural tearing, preserves the facet joints, and protects the neural structures from injury. If the facet joints are violated on both sides, spinal fusion is necessary.[71] In our experience, because the primary compressive dimension in the achondroplastic spine is cephalocaudal, not lateral, undermining of the facets is not recommended.

Removal of the spinous processes and detachment of the paraspinal soft tissues create a large and deep void, particularly at the lumbosacral junction. To minimize the risk of pseudomeningocele formation, an overlapping closure using paraspinal muscle was developed,[71] whereby muscle masses are brought in to fill the dead space. First, a paraspinal muscle encased in fascia is partially detached from the iliac spine and the lumbosacral laminae by use of a split-thickness incision, if necessary, to mobilize the required tissue, which is then reflected around its pedicle. The edge of the flap is brought down to the opposite lateral end of the lamina and is attached with heavy sutures to the inferior part of the paraspinal muscle mass on that side. The superior part of the muscle mass on that side is then retracted over the first flap, thereby completing the muscle closure and collapsing the void. As with craniocervical decompression, somatosensory evoked potentials are monitored intraoperatively. Postoperative care is generally routine, but because of the high incidence of urologic complications, the nursing staff should be advised to help the patient be prepared for this possibility.

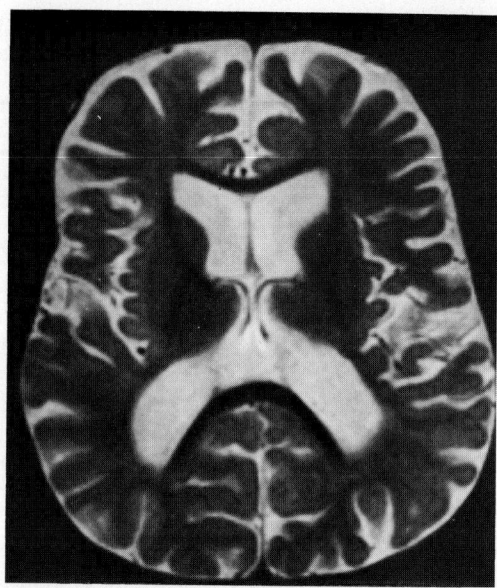

FIGURE 169-3. Axial MRI (Case Report 1) showing the typical ventriculomegaly and generous subarachnoid space seen in achondroplastic patients.

Case Reports

CASE REPORT 1

A 19-month-old white female with achondroplasia was admitted to our institution for evaluation of sleep apnea. On examination, she was found to be developmentally delayed. Sleep studies revealed severe obstructive apnea, with baseline oxygen saturations of 60 to 80 percent and some dips to 40 to 50 percent. An echocardiogram showed evidence of cor pulmonale, with a dilated main stem pulmonary artery and right ventricular enlargement. An otolaryngology consultation revealed severe tonsilloadenoid hypertrophy. Based on these findings, a tracheostomy was performed.

Her neurologic findings were remarkable for positive Babinski's reflexes bilaterally and ankle clonus. Sagittal MRIs revealed severe compression at the level of the foramen magnum. An axial MRI revealed the ventricular configuration typical even in achondroplastic patients who are asymptomatic for hydrocephalus (Fig. 169-3). A diagnosis of clinically significant cervicomedullary compression was made, and the patient underwent craniocervical decompression. Immediately after surgery her ankle clonus resolved, but the bilateral extensor response persisted. She was discharged in good condition and underwent tonsillectomy and adenoidectomy at another institution 2 months later. After this procedure, she gradually became irritable and began to vomit frequently. She was readmitted to our institution for evaluation of ICP 3 months after her first discharge. Seventy-two hours of monitoring revealed elevated ICP, and a ventriculoperitoneal shunt was placed. She has made significant growth and developmental strides since her procedures. Repeated sleep studies have revealed moderately abnormal breathing that is remarkable for frequent central apneas without severe desaturation. Results of her follow-up neurologic examinations have been normal, with the exception of a mild hypotonia.

CASE REPORT 2

A 10.5-month-old white male with achondroplasia was admitted to our institution for evaluation of cervicomedullary compression after initially being seen in our outpatient genetics clinic, where a rapidly increasing head circumference and mild cervical myelopathy were noted. His parents reported two recent episodes of otitis media, an increase in hyperextension posturing of the neck, venous engorgement of the scalp, and night awakening with crying. No frank episodes of apnea had been observed. On examination, the anterior fontanelle was found to be full and slightly tense, and there was marked engorgement of cephalic veins. Head circumference was stable at the twenty-fifth percentile on the achondroplastic chart. The child rolled over independently and sat with support. He was able to crawl and had good head control. Pupils were equal, round, and reactive to light, and extraocular movements were intact. Deep tendon reflexes were 3+ bilaterally. No ankle clonus was elicited, and tone was slightly decreased. Plantar responses were extensor. Although a sleep study revealed brief central apneas and occasional obstructive apneas, these were not deemed clinically significant.

The neurologic impression was that the child had a mild upper cervical myelopathy. Developmentally, he displayed moderate delay relative to achondroplastic standards. We examined him by MRI, which revealed dramatic compression at the foramen magnum, and a pinched, "hourglass" configuration of the cord at that level (Fig. 169-4). MRI flow studies showed complete CSF obstruction, confirming the functional significance of the stenosis.

Our usual approach for a child with moderate neurologic or developmental findings would be to observe him at 3-month intervals, looking for evidence of disease progression. In this case, however, the combination of clinical symptoms and the findings in the MRI studies warranted a diagnosis of severe cervicomedullary compression. Our opinion was that prophylactic decompression of the craniocervical junction was indicated, and surgery was performed the following week. The patient's ICP was monitored postoperatively. On the second postoperative day, his ICP readings were between 7 and 22 cm H_2O. On the third day, the ventriculostomy was removed, and the patient was transferred from pediatric intensive care. On the fifth day, however, a pseudomeningocele was noted in the incisional line, and a left-sided frontal ventriculoperitoneal shunt was placed on the sixth postoperative day. Shunt placement was without complications, and on the first day after the shunt was placed, the pseudomeningocele started to resolve. A routine tap performed after shunt placement revealed an ICP of 10 cm H_2O, when the patient was crying. The patient remained fussy and pulled at his ears, so an otolaryngology consultation was obtained that revealed a right middle ear effusion, which was treated conservatively. The remainder of the postoperative course was benign, and he was discharged on the fourth day after shunt placement. Six weeks after discharge, the patient was seen in neurosurgical clinic for follow-up. His parents reported that he was doing extremely well, and for the first time he was pulling to stand and maintaining an upright position for sustained periods. He could be placed in a seated position and independently maintain that position. He had a variety of words in his vocabulary and a social wave, and he clapped his hands appropriately. All of these actions represented significant gains over his preoperative status. Cranial nerves were intact throughout, and tone was excellent in all extremities. Deep tendon reflexes were 2+, and there was no evidence of clonus.

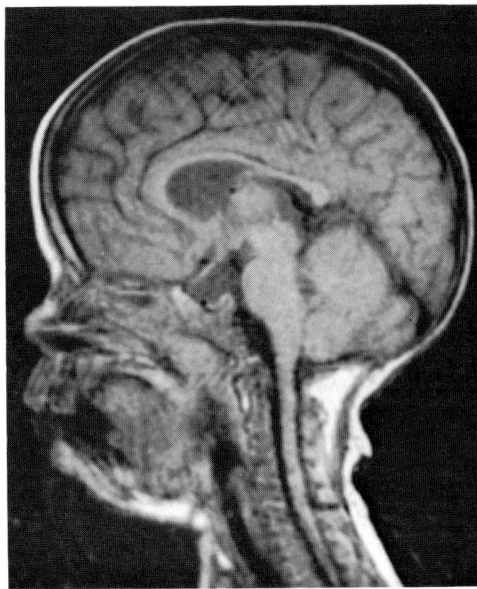

FIGURE 169–5. Sagittal MRI (Case Report 3) showing no cervicomedullary compression at the level of the foramen magnum.

CASE REPORT 3

A 15-month-old black male with achondroplasia was seen by our genetics clinic for developmental delay and history of an apneic event. Upper and lower extremity weakness, ankle clonus, and very loud breathing and snoring prompted an inpatient evaluation. The child had the typical stigmata of achondroplasia, but his usual resting posture involved severe hyperextension of the neck. A neurologic examination revealed hypotonia and three to five beats of ankle clonus bilaterally. The plantar responses were equivocal, and deep tendon reflexes were 3+. Developmental evaluation revealed mild expressive language delay, moderate fine motor delay, and severe gross motor delay. Blood gases on room air were studied initially, revealing a pH of 7.38, a PCO_2 of 44, and a PO_2 of 62. Sleep studies revealed severe obstructive apnea, with desaturation to 40 and 30 percent on a quarter liter of oxygen by nasal cannula. Apneic events lasted up to 30 seconds and occurred 6 times or more an hour. Echocardiography and electrocardiography revealed right ventricular hypertrophy, right ventricular dilatation, and pulmonary dilatation. Tracheostomy, with simultaneous tonsillectomy and adenoidectomy, was performed. No postoperative oxygen was required.

Somatosensory evoked potentials of the upper extremities revealed normal responses at Erb's point and at the craniocervical junction, but no cortical responses were obtained. A MRI revealed no evidence of compression at the foramen magnum, however (Fig. 169–5), and a CT myelogram confirmed these findings. No craniocervical decompression was performed. Within 2 weeks after his tracheostomy, ankle clonus had resolved on the right side, although two beats persisted on the left. We hypothesized that this neurologic improvement resulted from the patient's holding his head in a more neutral position. He was seen again 10 weeks after his discharge, when an MRI again revealed no compression at the level of the foramen magnum. Repeated sleep studies revealed no significant desaturation. Growth was normal, and improvement in his development was noted.

RESULTS

CRANIOCERVICAL DECOMPRESSION

Over the past decade, a total of 90 children younger than 5 years of age with achondroplasia have been evaluated at our institution for cervicomedullary compression secondary to foramen magnum stenosis. Of these, 34 were found to have clinically significant stenosis and underwent craniocervical decompression. The commonest extent of decompression was to C1 and the posterior fossa. A substantial percentage of patients subsequently required ventriculoperitoneal shunting for clinically significant hydrocephalus. In the

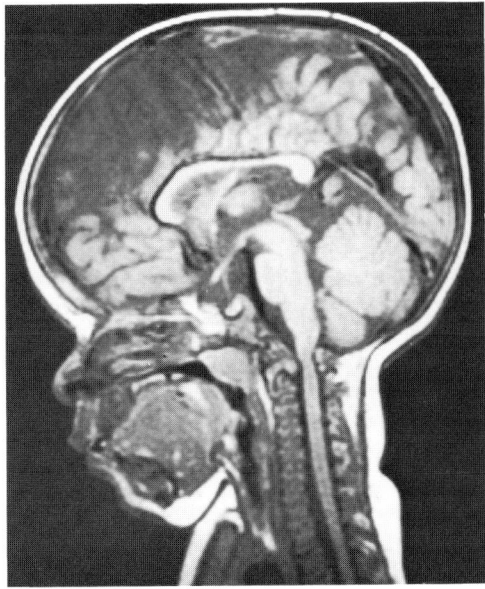

FIGURE 169–4. Sagittal MRI (Case Report 2) showing severe cervicomedullary compression at the level of the foramen magnum.

group that underwent craniocervical decompression, there has been one postoperative death, occurring suddenly at the patient's home 2 weeks after discharge from the hospital. The family declined autopsy, and a cause of death was never determined. No deaths have occurred in the shunt only and nonoperated groups, after 468 person-years of patient follow-up. Detailed follow-up data for this series will be forthcoming, but we can say that improvements in neurologic and respiratory function, as well as treatment morbidity, have been similar to those in the partial series[53,55] already reported on from our institution.

SPINAL DECOMPRESSION

Over the past 10 years at our institution, Uematsu has performed spinal decompressive laminectomies on 67 individuals who ranged in age from 10 to 66 years. The mean age at time of surgery was 37 years, and the mean duration of symptoms before operation was 5 years. Of these patients, 44 had laminectomies confined to the lower thoracic, lumbar, or sacral spine, whereas others required laminectomies in the upper thoracic and/or cervical spine as well. In the former group, the average number of segments decompressed was 11. The commonest extent of decompression was from T8 to S1. Outcome was judged by comparison of functional assessments performed preoperatively and at the time of the latest follow-up examination (mean follow-up, 29 months). Outcome was quantified by a functional rating scale that included consideration of arm strength, ambulation, urinary function, and pain. By this scale, 70 percent of patients with thoracolumbar decompressions improved, 22 percent deteriorated, and the remainder showed no change. The best predictor of improvement was the duration of symptoms before operation. Those who had been symptomatic for less than 1 year showed an average improvement of 40 percent on our functional ratings scale, whereas those who had been symptomatic for longer than 1 year had an average improvement of only 15 percent. The commonest complication of surgery was urinary retention, which developed in 38 percent of patients; however, in most patients, this was a transient problem. Forty-three percent of patients experienced either single or multiple dural tears during the procedure, and 10 percent of patients developed a pseudomeningocele that required repair. Wound infection developed in 13.5 percent. Three patients developed a gastrointestinal bleed or pseudomembranous colitis, and one patient had a deep venous thrombosis.

DISCUSSION

Several areas of controversy surround the treatment of achondroplastic patients. Some clinicians[74] dispute whether, given the risks inherent in operation, the mortality due to cervicomedullary compression in the achondroplastic population is sufficient to warrant prophylactic surgical intervention. This criticism implicitly questions whether or not the indications for cervicomedullary compression identify a population at higher-than-average mortality risk. If the indications do identify such a population, however, the criticism is unjustified. We believe that the increased mortality seen in achondroplastic children is primarily due to severe cervicomedullary compression, and that identifying and operating on the high-risk group significantly lowers this mortality. The mortality rate in the operated series at this institution is about 3 percent, and in those evaluated but not operated on, mortality is zero. The total mortality of the selected population we have evaluated is therefore about 1 percent. Other criticisms[74] that question published mortality data or suggest that cervicomedullary compression is a minor, temporary problem are unsupported by evidence or understate the demonstrated severity of the disease, respectively. Another criticism[75] emphasizes the obstructive etiology of respiratory difficulties in achondroplastic patients. We do not dispute this observation but maintain nonetheless that central compression can be both a primary cause and a secondary aggravating factor in respiratory difficulties, particularly in achondroplastic children. Moreover, our preoperative evaluation is designed to systematically elicit these distinct etiologies.

Some[74] argue that significant morbidity exists in the relatively high number of patients with cervicomedullary compression who undergo this procedure and go on to require shunts. Our feeling, however, is that this hydrocephalus is not a complication of the operation but rather is discovered as a result of the violation of the dural layer, a situation that allows a much more sensitive picture of the ICP dynamics than is otherwise possible. This view receives additional support from research that suggests a strong predisposition to hydrocephalus in achondroplastic children and a higher-than-normal ICP as a result of the bony anatomy.* In light of these findings, the morbidity and mortality of our reported craniocervical decompression series is not only low for a procedure of this delicacy but is also low relative to the general morbidity and mortality of achondroplastic disease. This argument is strengthened by the fact that a large number of the patients we diagnose have a combination of severe respiratory and neurologic disease, and that after their procedures, they go on to make developmental strides at a rapid pace, with resolution of their symptoms. Although we believe that our treatment of achondroplastic hydrocephalus is uncontroversial, our understanding of it does rest on some unproven assumptions. First, the current understanding of ICP dynamics is neither comprehensive nor general. Although evidence is strongly in favor of the theory that raised ICP in achondroplastic patients is secondary to venous hypertension, one must nonetheless admit that this view has not been conclusively proved. The balance of evidence however, both published and experiential, favors this view, and we will continue to use it as a working theory until a better understanding of ICP in general, and hydrocephalus in achondroplasia in particular, are offered.

Some surgeons[64] take a different viewpoint concerning the ideal strategy for spinal laminectomy, recommending a wide decompression with foraminotomies and mandatory undermining of the facets. The rationale for this strategy is that compression is lateral as well as longitudinal in the achondroplastic spinal canal.[68] Our experience, however, simply does not bear this out, despite the hypothesized impact of small lateral recesses in the achondroplastic vertebral foramen. Moreover, the stabilization problems encountered with wide laminectomies can be more debilitating than the initial disease. In fact, there is no reason why every spinal level

---

*See references 12, 26, 41, 42, 55, 58, and 76–80.

could not be subjected to the laminectomy we describe without the need for concomitant spinal stabilization. Therefore, in light of the results obtained at our institution with spinal decompressions, we feel that a narrow, extensive laminectomy must be the spinal decompression of choice for achondroplastic patients. Some of our surgeons have adopted this operative technique for their nonachondroplastic patients as well. The goal is adequate decompression of neural elements and not simply enlargement of bony canals.

SUMMARY

Controversies in diagnosis and treatment notwithstanding, one cannot deny that our understanding of, and the medical prospects for the patient with, achondroplasia have improved over the past decade. Achondroplasia is a complex disease whose treatment requires several disciplines and strategies. Moreover, although delicate procedures performed on children naturally involve risks, these risks can be minimized through knowledge, experience, and a well-trained support staff. Furthermore, the resilience of the child treated appropriately for his or her disease is one of the most satisfying events for a surgeon to witness.

Although spinal stenosis is more frequently encountered than cervicomedullary compression, a modified technique for laminectomy offers a better prospect for patients than the conventional technique. Craniocervical decompression, however, is a potentially life-saving procedure that appears to improve significantly the natural history of achondroplasia and allow these young patients to make developmental strides without debilitating neurologic impairment. The objective is always to identify more accurately the subpopulation of achondroplastic patients at risk, and we welcome reasoned insights to this end. Craniocervical decompression is often associated with the discovery of hydrocephalus, but this is best viewed as a pre-existing condition that surgical intervention reveals and renders treatable. Achondroplastic patients are generally predisposed to hydrocephalus as a result of their anatomy, but most of them tolerate the symptoms they experience relatively well; accordingly, those who do not undergo craniocervical decompression can be treated by a more conservative protocol. Notwithstanding the relatively low frequency of achondroplasia, if the goal of the neurosurgeon is relief of debilitating symptoms, the high incidence of central nervous system disease in this population offers several compelling opportunities to effect a satisfying and dramatic change in a patient's condition and prospects.

Acknowledgment

We would like to thank Carmen Roig, BSN, RN for helpful suggestions and careful review of the manuscript for clinical accuracy.

REFERENCES

1. Oberklaid F, Denks DM, Jensen F, et al: Achondroplasia and hypochondroplasia. J Med Genet 16:140–146, 1979
2. Cohen MM Jr, Walker GF, Phillips C: A morphometric analysis of the craniofacial configuration in achondroplasia. J Craniofac Genet Dev Biol suppl 1:139–165, 1985
3. Vogl A, Osborne BL: Lesion of the spinal cord (transverse myelopathy) in achondroplasia. Arch Neurol Psychiatry 61:644–662, 1949
4. Spillane JD: Three cases of achondroplasia with neurosurgical complications. J Neurol Neurosurg Psychiatry 15:246–252, 1952
5. Duvoisin RC, Yahr MD: Compressive spinal cord and root syndromes in achondroplastic dwarves. Neurology 12:202–207, 1962
6. Epstein JA, Malis LI: Compression of the spinal cord and cauda equina in achondroplastic dwarves. Neurology 5:875–881, 1955
7. Bergstrom K, Laurent V, Lundberg PO: Neurological symptoms in achondroplasia. Acta Neurol Scand 47:59–70, 1971
8. Nelson MA: Spinal stenosis in achondroplasia. Proc R Soc Med 65:18–19, 1972
9. Cohen ME, Rosenthal AD, Matson DD: Neurological abnormalities in achondroplastic children. J Pediatr 71:367–376, 1967
10. Galanski M, Herrman R, Knoche U: Neurological complications and myelographic features of achondroplasia. Neuroradiology 17:59–63, 1978
11. Hancock DW, Phillips DG: Spinal compression in achondroplasia. Paraplegia 3:23–33, 1965
12. Yamada H, Nakamura S, Tajima M, Kageyama N: Neurological manifestations of pediatric achondroplasia. J Neurosurg 54:49–57, 1981
13. Nelson FW, Hecht JT, Horton WA, et al: Neurological basis of respiratory complications in achondroplasia. Ann Neurol 24:89–93, 1988
14. Stokes DC, Phillips JA, Leonard CA, et al: Respiratory complications of achondroplasia. J Pediatr 102:534–541, 1983
15. Lutter LD, Langer LO: Neurological symptoms in achondroplastic dwarfs: Surgical treatment. J Bone Joint Surg Am 59A:87–92, 1977
16. Eulert J: Scoliosis and kyphosis in dwarfing conditions. Arch Orthop Trauma Surg 102:45–47, 1983
17. Goldstein SJ, Shprintzen RJ, Wu RHK, et al: Achondroplasia and obstructive sleep apnea: Correction of apnea and abnormal sleep-entrained growth hormone release by tracheostomy. Birth Defects 21:93–101, 1985
18. Hecht JT, Butler IJ, Scott CI: Long-term neurological sequelae in achondroplasia. Eur J Pediatr 143:58–60, 1984
19. Thomas IT, Frias JL, Williams JL, Friedman WA: Magnetic resonance imaging in the assessment of medullary compression in achondroplasia. Am J Dis Child 142:989–992, 1988
20. Yang SS, Corbett DP, Brough AJ, et al: Upper cervical myelopathy in achondroplasia. Am J Clin Pathol 68:68–72, 1977
21. Dandy WE: Hydrocephalus in chondrodystrophy. Johns Hopkins Hosp Bull 32:5–10, 1921
22. Mueller SM, Bell W, Cornell S, et al: Achondroplasia and hydrocephalus. A computerized tomographic, roentgenographic, and psychometric study. Neurology 27:430–434, 1977
23. Fremion AS, Garg BP, Kalsbeck J: Apnea as the sole manifestation of cord compression in achondroplasia. J Pediatr 104:398–401, 1984
24. Todorov AB, Scott CI, Warren AE, Leeper JD: Developmental screening tests in achondroplastic children. Am J Med Genet 9:19–23, 1981
25. Scott CI: Medical and social adaptation in dwarfing conditions. Birth Defects 13:29–43, 1977
26. Hurko O, Pyeritz R, Uematsu S: Neurological considerations in achondroplasia, in Nicoletti B, Kopits SE, Ascani E, McKusick VA (eds): Human Achondroplasia. New York, Plenum Press, 1988, pp 153–162
27. Allanson JE, Hall JG: Obstetric and gynecologic problems in women with chondrodystrophies. Obstet Gynecol 67:74–78, 1986
28. Hecht JT, Francomano CA, Horton WA, Annegers JF: Mortality in achondroplasia. Am J Hum Genet 41:454–464, 1987
29. Camera G, Mastroiacovo P: Birth prevalence and mutation rate of achondroplasia in the Italian multicentre monitoring system for birth defects, in Nicoletti B, Kopits SE, Ascani E, McKusick VA (eds): Human Achondroplasia. New York, Plenum Press, 1988, pp 11–15
30. Gardner RJM: A new estimate of the achondroplasia mutation rate. Clin Genet 11:31–38, 1977
31. Opitz JM: Premutation in achondroplasia, in Nicoletti B, Kopits SE, Ascani E, McKusick VA (eds): Human Achondroplasia. New York, Plenum Press, 1988, pp 17–25
32. Murdoch JL, Walker BA, Hall JG, et al: Achondroplasia—A genetic and statistical survey. Ann Hum Genet 33:227–244, 1970
33. Pauli RM, Conroy MM, Langer LO Jr, et al: Homozygous achondroplasia with survival beyond infancy. Am J Hum Genet 16:459–473, 1983
34. Moskowitz N, Carson B, Kopits S, et al: Foramen magnum decompression in an infant with homozygous achondroplasia. J Neurosurg 70:126–128, 1989

35. Horton WA, Hood OJ, Machado MA, Campbell D: Growth plate cartilage studies in achondroplasia, in Nicoletti B, Kopits SE, Ascani E, McKusick VA (eds): Human Achondroplasia. New York, Plenum Press, 1988, pp 81–89
36. Ippolito E, Maynard JA, Mickelson MR, Ponseti IV: Histochemical and ultrastructural study of the growth plate in achondroplasia, in Nicoletti B, Kopits SE, Ascani E, McKusick VA (eds): Human Achondroplasia. New York, Plenum Press, 1988, pp 61–71
37. Marin-Padilla M, Marin-Padilla TM: Developmental abnormalities of the occipital bone in human chondrodystrophies (achondroplasia and thanatophoric dwarfism). Birth Defects 13:7–23, 1977
38. Hecht JT, Nelson FW, Butler IJ, et al: Computerized tomography of the foramen magnum: Achondroplastic values compared to normal standards. Am J Med Genet 20:355–360, 1985
39. Dennis JP, Rosenberg HS, Alvord EC Jr: Megalencephaly, internal hydrocephalus and other neurological aspects of achondroplasia. Brain 84:427–445, 1961
40. Pierre-Kahn A, Hirsch JF, Renier D, et al: Hydrocephalus and achondroplasia: A study of 25 observations. Childs Nerv Sys 7:205–219, 1980
41. Friedman WA, Mickle JP: Hydrocephalus in achondroplasia: A possible mechanism. Neurosurgery 7:150–153, 1980
42. Steinbok P, Hall J, Flodmark O: Hydrocephalus in achondroplasia: The possible role of intracranial venous hypertension. J Neurosurg 71:42–48, 1989
43. Alexander E: Significance of the small lumbar spinal canal: Cauda equina compression syndromes due to spondylosis: Part 5. Achondroplasia. J Neurosurg 31:513–519, 1969
44. Bailey JA: Orthopaedic aspects of achondroplasia. J Bone Joint Surg Am 52A:1285–1301, 1970
45. Vogl A: The fate of the achondroplastic dwarf: Neurological complications of achondroplasia. Exp Med Surg 20:108–117, 1962
46. Langer LO, Bauman PA, Gorlin RJ: Achondroplasia. AJR Am J Roentgenol 100:12–26, 1967
47. Schreiber F, Rosenthal H: Paraplegia from ruptured lumbar discs in achondroplastic dwarfs. J Neurosurg 9:648–651, 1952
48. Thomas IT, Frias JL: The prospective management of cervicomedullary compression in achondroplasia. Birth Defects 25:83–90, 1990
49. Pauli RM, Scott CI, Wassman ER, et al: Apnea and sudden unexpected death in infants with achondroplasia. J Pediatr 104:342–348, 1984
50. Bland JD, Emery JL: Unexpected death of children with achondroplasia after the perinatal period. Dev Med Child Neurol 24:489–492, 1982
51. Mador MJ, Tobin MJ: Apneustic breathing: A characteristic feature of brainstem compression in achondroplasia? Chest 97:877–883, 1990
52. Wang H, Rosenbaum AE, Reid CS, et al: Pediatric patients with achondroplasia: CT evaluation of the craniocervical junction. Radiology 164:515–519, 1987
53. Reid CS, Pyeritz RE, Kopits SE, et al: Cervicomedullary compression in young patients with achondroplasia: Value of comprehensive neurologic and respiratory evaluation. J Pediatr 110:522–530, 1987
54. Blom S, Ekbom KA: Early clinical signs of meningiomas of the foramen magnum. J Neurosurg 19:661–664, 1962
55. Aryanpur J, Hurko O, Francomano C, et al: Craniocervical decompression for cervicomedullary compression in pediatric patients with achondroplasia. J Neurosurg 73:375–382, 1990
56. Nelson FW, Goldie WD, Hecht JT, et al: Short-latency somatosensory evoked potentials in the management of patients with achondroplasia. Neurology 34:1053–1058, 1984
57. Horton WA, Rotter JI, Rimoin DL, et al: Standard growth curves for achondroplasia. J Pediatr 93:435–438, 1978
58. Lundar T, Bakke SJ, Nornes H: Hydrocephalus in an achondroplastic child treated by venous decompression at the jugular foramen. J Neurosurg 73:138–140, 1990
59. Bethem D, Winter RB, Lutter L, et al: Spinal disorders of dwarfism. J Bone Joint Surg Am 63A:1412–1425, 1981
60. Streeten E, Uematsu S, Hurko O, et al: Extended laminectomy for spinal stenosis in achondroplasia, in Nicoletti B, Kopits SE, Ascani E, McKusick VA (eds): Human Achondroplasia. New York, Plenum Press, 1988, pp 261–273
61. Wynne-Davies R, Walsh WK, Gormley J: Achondroplasia and hypochondroplasia: Clinical variations and spinal stenosis. J Bone Joint Surg Br 63B:508–515, 1981
62. Morgan DF, Young RF: Spinal neurological complications of achondroplasia: Results of surgical treatment. J Neurosurg 52:463–472, 1980
63. O'Brien JP, Mehdian H: Relevant principles in the management of spinal disorders in achondroplasia, in Nicoletti B, Kopits SE, Ascani E, McKusick VA (eds): Human Achondroplasia. New York, Plenum Press, 1988, pp 293–298
64. Lonstein JE: Treatment of kyphosis and lumbar stenosis in achondroplasia, in Nicoletti B, Kopits SE, Ascani E, McKusick VA (eds): Human Achondroplasia. New York, Plenum Press, 1988, pp 283–292
65. Siebens AA, Hungerford DS, Kirby NA: Curves of the achondroplastic spine: A new hypothesis. Johns Hopkins Med J 142:205–210, 1978
66. Siebens AA, Kirby N, Hungerford D: Orthotic correction of sitting abnormality in achondroplastic children, in Nicoletti B, Kopits SE, Ascani E, McKusick VA (eds): Human Achondroplasia. New York, Plenum Press, 1988, pp 313–317
67. Kopits SE: Thoracolumbar kyphosis and lumbosacral lordosis, in Nicoletti B, Kopits SE, Ascani E, McKusick VA (eds): Human Achondroplasia. New York, Plenum Press, 1988, pp 241–255
68. Carson B, Winfield J, Wang H, et al: Surgical management of cervicomedullary compression in achondroplastic patients, in Nicoletti B, Kopits SE, Ascani E, McKusick VA (eds): Human Achondroplasia. New York, Plenum Press, 1988, pp 207–217
69. Luyendijk W, Matricali B, Thomeer RTWM: Basilar impression in an achondroplastic dwarf: Causative role in tetraparesis. Acta Neurochir (Wien) 41:243–253, 1978
70. Lutter LD, Lonstein JE, Winter RB, Langer LO: Anatomy of the achondroplastic lumbar canal. Clin Orthop 26:139–142, 1977
71. Uematsu S, Wang H, Hurko O, Kopits SE: The subarachnoid fluid space in achondroplastic spinal stenosis: The surgical implication, in Nicoletti B, Kopits SE, Ascani E, McKusick VA (eds): Human Achondroplasia. New York, Plenum Press, 1988, pp 275–281
72. Shikata J, Yamamuro T, Lida H, et al: Surgical treatment of achondroplastic dwarfs with paraplegia. Surg Neurol 29:125–130, 1988
73. O'Donnell HD, Uematsu S, Hurko O, et al: Craniospinal Stenosis in Achondroplasia. A 10 Year Surgical Experience with 64 Cases. Presented at the American Association of Neurological Surgeons Annual Meeting, Plenary Session, abstract 734, April 12–16, 1992 (San Francisco)
74. Wassman ER, Rimoin DL: Cervicomedullary compression with achondroplasia (letter). J Pediatr 113:411, 1988
75. Larsen PD, Snyder EW, Matsuo F, et al: Achondroplasia associated with obstructive sleep apnea (letter). Arch Neurol 40:769, 1983
76. Kinal ME: Hydrocephalus and the dural venous sinuses. J Neurosurg 19:195–201, 1962
77. Mueller SM, Reinertson JE: Reversal of emissary vein blood flow in achondroplastic dwarfs. Neurology 30:769–772, 1980
78. Norrell H, Wilson C, Howieson J, et al: Venous factors in infantile hydrocephalus. J Neurosurg 31:561–569, 1969
79. Sainte-Rose C, LaCombe J, Pierre-Kahn A, et al: Intracranial venous sinus hypertension: Cause or consequence of hydrocephalus in infants? J Neurosurg 60:727–736, 1984
80. Shulman K, Ransohoff J: Sagittal sinus venous pressure in hydrocephalus. J Neurosurg 23:169–173, 1965

CHAPTER 170

Surgical Management of Non–Hindbrain-Related and Posttraumatic Syringomyelia

Bernard Williams

Syringomyelia is the occurrence of longitudinally disposed cystic cavities within the spinal cord. Sizeable cavities that extend up and down the cord and result in significant neurologic deficits are less common than small cysts, which are sometimes found after trauma to the cord. The commonest abnormality associated with such big cysts is an abnormality at the hindbrain. This type of syringomyelia almost always contains cerebrospinal fluid (CSF), as do most of the symptomatic forms of syringomyelia. Tumorous cysts usually contain proteinaceous fluid but are sometimes classified as syringomyelias. Although the clinical presentation of these cases may be similar to other kinds of syringomyelia, their treatment is the same as that for tumors. For the hindbrain-related varieties of syringomyelia, the terms *hydrosyringomyelia* or *syringohydromyelia* and even *hydromyelia* have been used. In the absence of established usage, authors should make clear what manifestations they include in the terms they use. I use *syringomyelia* as a generic term to cover all intracord cavities beyond a minimum length of two segments.[1] This is a pathologic or radiologic rather than a clinical definition, and for the purpose of this chapter, it excludes tumor-related cysts and syringomyelia related to dysraphism.

The occurrence of minor cystic changes in the spinal cord after spinal injury is common. For posttraumatic cystic changes, some authors prefer the term *cystic myelopathy* rather than syringomyelia. Cystic myelopathy could be reserved for the smaller type of cyst.

CLASSIFICATION

It is not useful to classify syringomyelia by the clinical presentation, the rate of progression, the fluid it contains, or the size or level of the cavities.[2, 3] Classification by the associated lesions is preferable because they are often amenable to treatment, usually with improvement of the associated syrinx. My classification is given in Table 170–1, along with the incidence of each manifestation based on my practice.

Syringomyelia in patients made paraplegic by trauma is associated with meningeal fibrosis and is thus subsumed under this heading in Table 170–1. When meningeal fibrosis exists without a fracture, it may be diffuse or localized, depending on the cause. The interesting localized idiopathic variety with webs of meningeal fibrosis that provides a temporary obstruction to the passage of CSF in the subarachnoid space is called "pouched arachnoid webs."

INCIDENCE

The overall prevalence of syringomyelia is not known but is probably around 10 cases per 100,000. The figures given in Table 170–1 are from the Syringomyelia Clinic at the Midland Centre for Neurosurgery and Neurology. The cases were referred to an adult center with a longstanding interest in this condition. Thus, a bias exists against children and toward difficult or recurrent cases in the selection. An increased proportion of cases may be related to meningeal fibrosis because spinal injury centers are aware of difficulties in management and may tend to refer their cases to a specialist center.

The vertebral level of injury seems to be irrelevant. The time of onset may be within weeks of the injury or up to 30 years later. No safe period or level exists, and vigilance must be maintained over any patient with cord damage. The incidence of syringomyelia after paraplegia is unclear; however, syringomyelia, which demands treatment, occurs in around 3 to 5 percent of spinal cord–injured patients. Watson[4] suggested a figure of 1.1 percent in 1972, and Barnett and Jousse[5] gave an incidence of 2.3 percent for their paraplegic patients in 1976 and suggested that the condition was commoner in patients with partial spinal cord injury. Rossier and colleagues,[6] in 1985, reported a 3.2 percent incidence, and this progressive rise in incidence probably reflects a greater awareness of the disorder. With the use of routine magnetic resonance imaging (MRI) in paraplegic patients, an incidence of over 50 percent is seen if all types of cyst are included.[7, 8] Most of these, however, are small cysts, which may be called primary cysts.

Diffuse meningeal fibrosis is less common than that resulting from fracture. Localized meningeal fibrosis causing pouched arachnoid webs resulting from nontraumatic lesions is rare but is of interest because a search for it in cases of unknown etiology will reduce the number of cases categorized as idiopathic.[3, 9]

In the Midland Centre for Neurosurgery and Neurology, 99 cases of spinal meningeal fibrosis appearing to cause syringomyelia have been seen. Of these, there were 68 cases

Table 170–1. CLASSIFICATION OF SYRINGOMYELIA BY ASSOCIATED LESIONS

Classification	Incidence (%)*
Hindbrain-related syringomyelia	73
Hindbrain herniation	
Secondary to intracranial tumors	2
Brain or meningeal tumors of the posterior fossa	<1
Tumors forming the hindbrain hernia	<1
Intrinsic brain tumors	<1
Idiopathic (Chiari type 1)	32
Secondary to birth injury	39
Secondary to head injury (nonperinatal)	5
Basilar invagination, all causes	10
Associated with other cerebrospinal fluid disorders	
Hydrocephalus	10
Intracranial arachnoid pouches	2
Dandy-Walker–type cysts	<1
Early-onset hydrocephalus (aqueduct stenosis)	<1
Spina bifida (Chiari type 2)	4
Meningeal fibrosis at the foramen magnum	
Birth injury related	9
Posttraumatic (postnatal)	5
Infections	<1
Non–hindbrain-related syringomyelia	24
Spinal tumors	5
Intramedullary tumors	4
Extramedullary intradural tumors	<1
Extradural tumors, including disc disease	<1
Dysraphism without hindbrain hernia (lipoma, tethered cord)	1
Meningeal fibrosis of the spinal subarachnoid space	
Postinflammatory	
Meningitis	1
Iophendylate (Myodil, Pantopaque)	<1
Posttraumatic	11
Secondary to bony deformities	
Tuberculous bone disease	<1
Idiopathic scoliosis	<1
Posttraumatic	11
Unknown (no associated lesion found)	<1

*Percentages are derived from an unpublished database of 862 cases of syringomyelia and related diseases. They do not add up to 100% because of interventions. Such disorders as intersections and posttraumatic cases are included under both bony deformity and meningeal fibrosis because it is not possible to decide which factor is the more important. Some factors, e.g., perinatal or postnatal head injury, are difficult to evaluate. Some associated abnormalities, hydrocephalus or basilar impression, occur to varying degrees.

of traumatic paraplegia, 41 of complete paraplegia, and 27 of incomplete lesions. Twelve cases resulted from infection, one from pyogenic bone, two from tuberculous bone infections, four from pyogenic epidural infections, and eight from meningitis, two pyogenic and six tuberculous. (Case 7, discussed later, had both meningitis and tuberculous bone disease.) There were 14 idiopathic cases of meningeal fibrosis.

CLINICAL PRESENTATION

The presentation of clamant syringomyelia is variable, and the condition is often not diagnosed for many years after the symptoms start.[3, 5, 9–14]

PAIN

Pain is the commonest symptom in posttraumatic syringomyelia,[14–16] although many patients have no pain at any stage of their illness. Any paraplegic referred to a pain clinic should be suspected of having syringomyelia, although many other causes of pain exist in a paraplegic patient.

Pain due to syringomyelia may be felt around the level of the neurologic damage, below the level, or any level corresponding to the ascent of the syrinx above the level of the sensory loss. As with the sensory or motor losses, the ascending symptoms are often unilateral. Perhaps the most distinctive feature of the pain with syringomyelia is exacerbation by coughing, sneezing, or straining. The association of pain with straining may be more common in syringomyelia than in the hindbrain-related cases. The pain that accompanies coughing is often confined to a zone of the body but not usually to one dermatome and may travel through the patient's sensorium in an orderly way, going up the side of the trunk, down the inside of the arm to the hand, then back up the outside of the arm to the side of the neck. Alternatively, it may jump into the arm or the side of the neck, sparing the trunk above the level of the lesion. Such pain is often not discussed by the patient because it may have lasted for a few days or even only for a few impulse-related events, and the patient may not think to associate it with the paraplegia. Patients often remember the pain clearly because of its severity. Its replacement by numbness or dysesthetic sensory loss may be rapid. In an intermediate stage, it may be referred to as an itchiness. Not all of the pain in the region of the fracture or above it abates as it is replaced by dysesthesia: some patients may have longstanding pain that is difficult to treat.

Pain around the trunk or the abdomen in the region of the fracture is difficult to analyze and is common when no suggestion of a syrinx exists. Unsuccessful abdominal investigations are often initiated. Headaches are also common.

SENSORY LOSS

The classically described dissociated loss of the gross syringomyelia is not often seen in either hindbrain- or non–hindbrain related syringomyelia. Most of these patients should be diagnosed before they develop neuropathic joints.[17] The only case of bilateral neuropathic joints I have seen resulted from posttraumatic syringomyelia. The patients are often vague about the nature of their sensory loss, which characteristically involves the entire upper limb. The arm tends to be involved early, and the advance of the sensory loss occurs more by increase in the severity of the sensory loss rather than by extension of the area. Different examiners on different days may obtain dissimilar maps of sensory loss. The description that the hand feels as if it has a glove on or is tingly or clumsy is commoner than the patient's losing the ability to discriminate temperature.

MOTOR LOSS

Motor loss is often of later onset than sensory change. As with the sensory loss, the motor deficits are often vague and vary in severity from one day to another. Many patients feel strong until they exercise, when the arms, or one arm, suddenly becomes weak. This weakness may be diffuse and lack a discernible myotomal value. As with sensory losses, violent exercise, such as competitive sports, may cause temporary deterioration. Sudden and permanent deterioration in both motor and sensory function may result from a violent strain (Case 6).

Classic syringomyelic motor changes involve the cervical enlargement, which is susceptible to broadening of the cavity. They may start with the small muscles of the hand and present with wasting or fasciculations of the first dorsal interosseous. In fully developed cases, the hand develops a claw deformity, followed by progressive loss of forearm and upper arm musculature. As with sensory losses, a segmental level is often not definable, and a generalized thinning of the upper limb musculature and nonspecific weakness, including loss of ability to transfer, may represent the extent of the patient's motor complaints.

TENDON REFLEXES

Careful scrutiny of the arm for loss of tendon reflexes may confirm the diagnosis in the early stages of the disease. Triceps jerks in particular are easy to test. There may be an asymmetry only, but all the tendon reflexes should be carefully noted.

AUTONOMIC DYSFUNCTION

More autonomic disturbances may occur in posttraumatic patients with syringomyelia than in hindbrain-related patients. Horner's syndrome is also commoner in posttraumatic patients than in hindbrain-related ones. The manifestations are often incomplete and can consist of anisocoria without sweating disturbance. Horner's syndrome, which changes side with the patient's change of position, is also occasionally seen.

The sweating disturbances in posttraumatic syringomyelia are often gross.[18] The lower body may be affected and the disturbance is likely to be symmetrical. Upper limb manifestations are often asymmetrical and may be associated with differences in skin color. Hyperhidrosis may be followed by dryness of the skin, which may extend upward to the face.

Asymmetry of vascular reactions on one side are common: emotional reddening from blushing or anger may affect one side only, and the erythematous reaction to sunburn may affect one side more than the other.

CHANGES BELOW THE LEVEL OF INJURY

Most patients with syringomyelia lesions below the level of injury and not extending above probably remain undiagnosed. Few such cases have been seen in this clinic. In patients with paraplegia some of the changes may be beneficial; for instance, reflex spasms may be lessened by the syrinx. The changes are generally disadvantageous and include sweating disturbances and deteriorating bladder function, with impairment of reflex emptying of the bladder. This symptom may improve after treatment. Impaired bowel function may also sometimes result from syringomyelia affecting the distal cord (Case 3). Clinical evidence of a descending syrinx includes absence of leg tendon reflexes, and as with reflexes in the arms, the pattern may reflect destruction in the cord enlargement rather than in the intervening zone. The ankle jerks may disappear, whereas one or both the knee jerks may be preserved.

DETERIORATION IN NEUROLOGIC FUNCTION IN PARAPARETIC PATIENTS

If a syrinx can be destructive to the normal cord above or below the site of a fracture, the damaged section of cord in a paraparetic patient is probably also vulnerable to the depredations of a syrinx. In such cases, primary cysts are common. In a small proportion of cases, cavities that look like primary cysts and not like clamant syringomyelia extend beyond two segments. The part they play in the deterioration of such cases is speculative, and Rossier and associates[7] may be correct in opining that treatment of small cysts has no value.

RADIOLOGIC INVESTIGATIONS

Radiologic confirmation has been achieved by water-soluble contrast myelography,* endomyelography,[20] postmyelography, computed tomographic (CT) examinations,[3, 9, 10, 12, 19–21] and MRI.[3, 8, 9, 14, 15, 22–27]

PLAIN RADIOGRAPHY

An analysis of the radiologic aspects of acute spinal injury indicates that no correlation exists between the type of bony injury, the level, whether the bony canal is large or small, or whether or not a subluxation exists, and posttraumatic syringomyelia. In nontraumatic cases, evidence of bony changes, such as osteitis or kyphoscoliosis, may be found. Only rarely are there signs of longstanding enlargement of the spinal canal. Such changes are commoner in hindbrain-related syringomyelia but are sometimes found in association with an arachnoid pouch that has been present for a long while,[28] or when tumor is associated with the disorder.[29]

MYELOGRAPHY

Myelography is carried out with water-soluble, nonionic contrast media. This imaging method shows localized meningeal fibrosis at the site of injury better than MRI. Injections in the cervical spine are probably more informative than lumbar puncture. Partial obstructions of the subarachnoid space may exist because of septa and dilated, webbed, pouch-like structures formed by thin membranes that are not well seen on MRI. Some contrast agent usually travels past the level of the obstruction. This investigation is useful in the evaluation of idiopathic syringomyelia—the filmy meningeal adhesions of pouched arachnoid webs are not well seen on MRI, and a brief delay in the flow of contrast may be all there is to see radiographically. The diameters of the cord above or below the fibrosis may show enlargement. The patient may have an enlarged cord with no symptoms or may have egregious symptoms with normal cord diameters. The radiologic confirmation of a syrinx is better performed by demonstration of the cavity than by visualization of the external diameter.

POSTMYELOGRAPHY COMPUTED TOMOGRAPHY

Contrast in the syrinx cavity is best shown by postmyelographic CT scans, which almost always demonstrate that the contrast has passed the obstruction in the subarachnoid space. The region of the filling mechanism (in posttraumatic cases, the region of the fracture) should be viewed in detail about 1 hour after myelography has been performed. Contrast uncommonly enters the syrinx immediately after injection of contrast below the injury[14, 19] and suggests a wide communication. If the myelogram is performed in the morning, the next scan can be performed 4 to 6 hours after the first. At this time, axial cuts should be visualized from the site of the cord damage to the areas of clinical suspicion, rostrally to the medulla and caudally to the conus. In some cases, intracord cavities are unclear at 6 hours, and repeat scans the morning after myelography, 22 to 24 hours later, may show a cavity clearly compared with the subarachnoid space that has largely cleared of contrast.

The technique also well illustrates dilatations of the subarachnoid space and, sometimes, consequent displacement of the cord and any contained cord cavity. It is also effective at showing the postoperative collapse of a treated syrinx.

Where an intrinsic spinal cord tumor is present, the filling may partly result from secretion of proteinaceous fluid from the tumor. Postcontrast opacification may be as striking as that seen in cases in which the fluid is thought to be forced in by the local anatomic variations at the site of the injury. Thus, the secretory qualities of the tumor alone may not cause the syrinx.

ENDOMYELOGRAPHY

Endomyelography is the injection of contrast medium into the syrinx cavity by direct puncture.[20] This method is conveniently combined with fluid analysis. Endomyelography helps address the questions Do all the cavities communicate with each other? Does the patient have a primary cyst that is separated by a septum from the upper syrinx? Are other septa close to the site of proposed insertion of the drain? Although answers to these questions are useful, they can be obtained at operation, and in practice, endomyelography is seldom used.

Extensive radiologic studies have limited value in posttraumatic cases because surgical exploration gives more information, including the extent and severity of local meningeal fibrosis, which is difficult to assess radiologically.

MAGNETIC RESONANCE IMAGING

MRI provides the quickest and most complete images of the syringomyelic cavities and indicates the tension in the cyst and the presence and numbers of septa.† Imaging all parts of the syrinx on one picture is often difficult when scoliosis or malalignment of a fracture is present; therefore, the syrinx must be imaged on several pictures. Also, although the septa may be seen and may be imaged on axial cuts, determining whether they are intact or perforated is not possible because the septations almost certainly move even with minor pulsations. The bone lesions are less easy to see than on x-ray–generated images, and current MRI resolution does not adequately show sheets of minor meningeal fibrosis or pouched arachnoid webs.

IDIOPATHIC SYRINGOMYELIA

Idiopathic syringomyelia is rare because radiographic studies usually reveal the cause of the syrinx. One common error

---

*See references 3, 5, 6, 9, 11, 12, 14, and 19.

†See references 3, 8, 14, 15, 22–24, 28, 29, and 30.

is the belief that tonsillar descent is required for the syrinx to be hindbrain related. There are other causes of hindbrain-related syringomyelia than hindbrain herniation, including meningeal fibrosis around the foramen magnum, often associated with arachnoid pouches.[3, 9, 28, 31] Often, the surgeon does not appreciate how little descent of the tonsils is necessary for craniospinal pressure dissociation to occur. The idea that 5 mm of descent is necessary for the hindbrain hernia to be significant[32] is not true. The features to observe at the hindbrain are

1. Absence of cisterna magna
2. Elongation of the midline outflow tract of the fourth ventricle
3. Packing of the tonsils around the sides as well as the back of the medulla at the foramen magnum
4. Visible indentation of the sides of the medulla or pons by vascular loops, which may cause bulbar clinical features and indicates that the hindbrain is impacting energetically[33, 34]

In addition, evidence that hindbrain herniation is likely to be symptomatic includes the observation of CSF-related abnormalities, such as syringomyelia, CSF-containing pouches, or hydrocephalus.

Spinal tumor may be missed diagnostically, especially when there is a ragged cavity or difficulty in imaging because of such features as kyphoscoliosis. Results of gadolinium-enhanced MRI with careful axial cuts are usually diagnostic. CSF protein may be helpful in suspected tumor cases, as may endomyelography supplemented by analysis of syrinx fluid.

Minor degrees of meningeal fibrosis, especially the pouched arachnoid webs, are difficult to find. They may occur without any antecedent features in the history. The formation of a partial block to the free flow of CSF is the usual finding and multiple areas of obstruction may be present. Postmyelography CT may show eclipse-like displacement of the spinal cord. MRI often does not show the fibrosis directly, and the areas are easily missed on myelography because the obstruction is transient and is only effective during high-speed movements that the radiologist cannot observe. Deformation of the syrinx is an important clue. If the syrinx is not symmetrical, circular, and central in the spinal canal at one or other end, it may be the site of transient intermittent distension of the subarachnoid space.

MORPHOLOGY

LATERALITY

One striking feature about syringomyelia is that when the cavities are sizable, the cavity appears to be almost in the middle of the cord when viewed in live patients. This rule applies to many cases in which the symptoms are asymmetrical. Symmetrical symptoms in syringomyelia are unusual, and this fact is one of the principal clinical and morphologic features in favor of the hydrodynamic theories. If the disease is a degeneration, and some still think it is, then symmetry could be expected to be the norm.

HEMATOMYELIA

One mechanism that may initiate a cavity in the cord opposite the site of injury is the formation of an acute cavity resulting from liquefied cord contents, edema, and effusion of blood.[35] Such accumulation of fluid after injury has been known since the observations of Holmes.[36] The finding of a primary cyst, sometimes with blood staining in the wall, may support this theory. Greenfield pointed out that overt bleeding within the substance of the spinal cord after injury is uncommon.[1] The same findings were stressed by Kakoulas,[37] who also stated that ascending epidural hematomata and ascending spinal artery thrombosis are rare. Kakoulas wrote that the central traumatic hemorrhagic necrosis of the cord is not a space-taking lesion. Liquefaction and the formation of a cavity without overt bleeding is usual: such cavities may be multicompartmental and be crossed by astrocytic webs of residual tissue and vascular structures. This phenomenon might explain some cases in which the protein level is high or is different in differing loculi of the syrinx. Hemorrhagic liquefaction is probably responsible for primary cysts, which are usually less than one segment in length, are found in about 50 percent of cases, and when present in conjunction with a syringomyelia, are often separated from the main cavities by an intact septum. The response of such primary cysts to treatment also differs from the response of a well-developed syringomyelia.

MAINTENANCE AND ENLARGEMENT OF CYSTIC SPACES

The spinal canal is subject to continual pressure swings that are mainly mediated by the venous channels. Large veins partly occupy the epidural space, and they are in free, valveless communication with the plexuses of veins around the vertebral bodies. These veins may transmit large volumes of blood, from the azygos, hemiazygos, and other abdominothoracic veins. The intraspinal compartments, particularly the intradural fluids, are therefore subject to relatively violent pressure swings in response to such activities as lifting, coughing, sneezing, and shouting. Under normal conditions, the result of transient high pressure in the spine, such as that produced by a cough, is movement of the CSF up the subarachnoid spaces into the head and then a return of the fluid to the resting distribution. The head end of the neuraxis provides a relatively compliant closure to the top of the spinal canal. The elevation of venous pressure may produce venous engorgement in the head at the same time as that in the spine. The capacitance of the veins, especially in the neck, provides a reservoir for the venous blood, and veins all over the body are available to accommodate the volume of blood. Conversely, the CSF, when compressed in the spine, can go nowhere but rapidly up and down the neuraxis. A volume of about 12 ml passes into the head with a cough.[38, 39] The pressures involved in a cough often exceed 100 mm Hg, and the upward movement of the event is over in about one tenth of second, providing a destructive force.[9, 35, 40, 41]

In hindbrain-related syringomyelia, a transient pressure difference is often demonstrable across the site of hindbrain obstruction. Such a difference may force fluid down a presumed communication from the floor of the fourth ventricle along the central canal to the syrinx.[41] This possibility is not the only or the main explanation of hindbrain-related syringomyelia.[3, 9] An analogous pressure difference may act across the site of fracture in patients with partial obstructions down the spine. Such a pressure difference may force fluid through a communication or a porous area of the syrinx wall.

The fracture site is probably where the fluid enters the syrinx, perhaps augmented by transfer of fluid through the cavity walls once the syrinx has developed. The wall of the spinal cord is not waterproof: potential channels along the sides of the vessels of the cord have been described by Virchow and Robin. They are potential sites of weakness, and fluid may seep through them in either direction. On inspection at operation, the walls of a big syrinx may be so thin that they weep CSF, and the cavity may flatten during the exposure. The energy of the pulsation probably sets up pressure gradients across the walls or through the walls during the propagation of waves.

Ball and Dayan[42] proposed that fluid might be forced across the walls of the cord in hindbrain-related syringomyelia. This suggestion was not enthusiastically received, because it seemed improbable that the hindbrain abnormality could be causing such pressure differences between the inside and the outside of the cord so low down. However, as an explanation for posttraumatic syringomyelia and for the maintenance of existing cavities, this hypothesis has more appeal, particularly when it is considered in conjunction with ideas about wave propagation.

It is not reasonable to regard the impulsive forces that act on any intracord collection of fluid as the only mechanism. In patients with pial-arachnoid meningeal adhesions, such as those occurring after meningitis, no likelihood exists of a primary syrinx formation resulting from a hematoma or a liquefied core. The cord may be pulled open by the adhesions to the dura, both at the front and the back, and shearing stresses may play a part.

If acute liquefactive changes plus a variable amount of hemorrhage are discounted, then the mechanisms of syringomyelia are probably similar in both the posttraumatic and the postinflammatory types of meningeal fibrosis. The important similarities include the blockage of the CSF pathways around the cord; the tendency to upward extension of the syrinx cavities, particularly in association with straining; and the tendency of the disorder to progress, sometimes many years after the causative lesions. The main clinical difference between them seems to be that in some posttraumatic cases, the condition becomes evident early, only a few months after the initial cord involvement. This manifestation may result from liquefaction or a hematoma at the site of injury, as discussed earlier. Silberstein and coworkers[26] suggest that early MRI appearances may indicate the need for surgery. At present, the pathogenesis of syringomyelia is not understood, and further speculation is of limited value.

INDICATIONS FOR TREATMENT

The principles of treatment apply to both posttraumatic and postarachnoidal types. Rossier and colleagues[6] wrote that operating on a patient with a small syrinx was of no benefit. All large syrinxes were small at some stage, if they were competently treated when they were small, or if primary cysts were treated before syringomyelia developed, then such patients would not develop large syrinxes. Clinical and experimental observations suggest that a syrinx may spread rapidly and then be stable for a while. Unfortunately, a small cystic cavity cannot be observed while it grows into a big syrinx. Ideally, such cases would be treated when they are enlarging but before they become symptomatic. If small primary cysts or intermediate-sized syrinxes could be shown to resolve or to remain asymptomatic, then a waiting policy might be justifiable with cavities that are silent or are causing only minimal problems. The state of the remaining cord function below the injury affects the timing of, or the necessity for, operation. A partial paraplegic with normal bladder and sexual function who can walk well enough to get around is only likely to be interested in an operation with no complication rate. This view deserves sympathy.

REMOVAL OF METALWORK

All imaging modalities are impaired by metallic fixation performed in the early stage of acute injury. The metal work should probably be removed after the fracture has healed, and the syrinx imaging should be repeated while the patient is recovering.

PRINCIPLES OF TREATMENT

LOWERING OF CEREBROSPINAL FLUID PRESSURE

When patients with hindbrain-related syringomyelia have hydrocephalus, good reason exists for preliminary shunting: the ventricular enlargement may progress after hindbrain operations. If the patient's arachnoiditis has a generalized cause, such as tuberculous meningitis, then prior treatment of associated hydrocephalus is a reasonable option.

The deliberate lowering of the CSF pressure by shunting the fluid away to an extrathecal site from outside the syrinx is a respectable strategy in the treatment of CSF-filled syringomyelia.[43–46] The theoretical basis for this practice is that lowering of the CSF pressure allows prefilling of the veins and thus de-energizes the thrust of the venous impulses. At the same time, the diminished volume and pressure of the CSF means that it is less able to inflict damage on the tissues.[35] However, lowering of the CSF pressure in the spinal compartment may aggravate hindbrain impactation and under such circumstances, may appear to cause syringomyelia.[47]

Lowering of the CSF pressure should never be performed by thecal shunting from below the hindbrain. Such operations have been recommended[44–46] and they may indeed work well, but the price to be paid if the hindbrain impacts with a thecoperitoneal or thecopleural shunt in position is severe disability and sometimes death.[48–52] If such an impaction occurs, the shunt should be removed, and consideration should be given to craniovertebral decompression or shunting of hydrocephalus as a surgical emergency. If the hindbrain becomes impacted with a drain below the foramen magnum, long-acting and severe pressure differences can be initiated across the foramen magnum, causing bulbar dysfunction, then respiratory arrest and death.

EXPLORATION

The high frequency of idiopathic syringomyelia sometimes necessitates surgical exploration in non–hindbrain related cases as well as in some patients in whom the hindbrain may be thought to be at fault. Radiologic clues to the relevant level include delay in the passage of the contrast medium and change in the shape of the syrinx wall by accumulation of pressure intermittently on one or the other side of an arachnoid web. If a small zone of meningeal fibrosis is the cause, then it is usually at one end of the syrinx and not in the middle. Biopsy of the syrinx wall in idiopathic syringomyelia is almost never justifiable, and drainage has a questionable role in such cases.

DRAINAGE

The idea that a cavity should be drained has appeal as well as the advantage of immediate success both radiologically and clinically. Such an obvious step was taken over 100 years ago.[53] Drainage, by whatever route, may be insufficient. Removal of the cause is preferable to drainage of the resulting abnormality. If a syrinx cavity is drained forcefully to the pleura or peritoneum, it will flatten, and parts of the wall may adhere internally. Flattening the cavity almost certainly blocks the draining catheter, and gliosis will occur around the tip, and it may become buried in the wall (Fig. 170–1). If a filling mechanism is still active, or even if a sizeable residual syrinx exists in another part of the cord, a new cavity may excavate alongside the flattened syrinx. Healing of the syrinx does not prevent another cavity from developing alongside it and affecting another part of the cord. Treatment should therefore be directed to the cause, specifically, to the disablement of the filling mechanism.

SYRINGOSUBARACHNOID SHUNTING

The use of syrinx-to-subarachnoid shunting is frequently successful.[5, 6, 11–13, 16, 54–58] Residual elasticity may be present in the cord that allows a myelotomy to deflate a syrinx, but such a hole in the cord may allow a cavity to fill as well as to empty. Such filling is occasionally the apparent cause of the intracord cavity.[19, 57, 58]

Clinical evidence suggests that if an attempt is made to maintain a patent syringostomy by the use of a drainage tube, the tubing commonly becomes walled off. Even if the tubing did provide drainage so that the cavity became collapsed, this collapse might then occlude the drain (Fig. 170–1). Wicks have been recommended to counteract this effect.[59] Wicks work by using surface tension; when one end of a multi-stranded fiber is left in a syrinx cavity and the other in the subarachnoid space, once the area is once more bathed in fluid, the change has no effect other than to block up the hole, as does a nerve root.[60]

Syrinx-to-Extrathecal Drainage

If the cavity is to be effectively drained, then a shunt to a low-pressure area, such as the pleura or the peritoneum, may

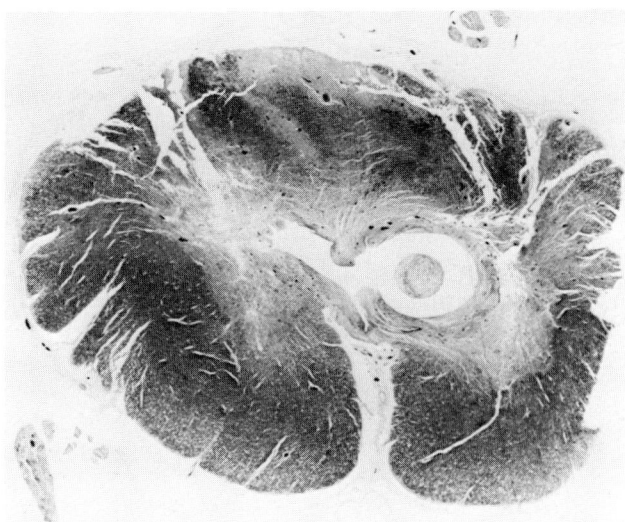

FIGURE 170–1. Histology section from a patient with a syrinx treated by drainage. The cavity has partly closed around the drain. At other levels there was complete immurement of the drain and at some other levels the syrinx remained sizeable. (Editorial Note: The word immurement is well chosen.)

be preferred to a myelotomy. This view has been shared by Barbaro and colleagues,[61, 62] Suzuki and colleagues,[63] Williams and Page,[64] Peerless and Durward,[65] and La Haye and Batzdorf.[66] Effective drainage has the additional advantage that the space-occupying qualities of the enlarged cord are lessened. The subarachnoid spaces are opened after the collapse of the swollen syrinx. Such drainage probably occurs only for a few seconds. Thus, a temporary drain attached to an external reservoir for a few days is all that may be required.

The author's present policy is to avoid intrasyrinx drains whenever possible. At present, this policy seems to be working and has the advantages of avoiding the complication rate associated with myelotomy.

Valves

In the treatment of hydrocephalus the purpose of valves as used in ventriculoatrial or ventriculoperitoneal shunting of CSF from the ventricles is not only to prevent reflux but also to minimize over-shunting, with resultant collapse of the ventricular system. The advantage of valves is that they can sometimes be pumped, and sometimes CSF can be aspirated or the patency of the lower end investigated to establish the patency of different parts of the system. None of these factors favor the use of valves when the inside of a syrinx is drained. The point of a hydrocephalus shunt is to lower the pressure to normal, and in most non–hindbrain related syringomyelia patients, the CSF pressure is normal because the absorptive mechanism is normal. A hydrocephalus valve complicates the system, and if it keeps CSF pressure up in the normal range, the valve may stop the system from working. The walls of the cord offer so little resistance that the pressure inside the most tense-looking syrinx is almost equal to that outside the cord, and the two pressures fluctuate together with changes in pulsatile conditions.

Decompression

I now believe that the creation of a free access of the fluid to traverse the site of the injury in an upward or downward direction is the key step in the management of syringomyelia. If the energy of the pulsation can be conveyed easily in the subarachnoid space, a mechanism driving the fluid into the cord is unlikely to be present.

Closure of the dura enables the fluid in the spinal canal that travels into the cord to be propelled upward under the influence of violent pressure changes, such as those induced by coughing, and to excavate new cavities in the gray matter. Nonclosure of the dura may be the most important surgical prophylaxis against this group of disorders. The best results follow a free communication from the subarachnoid spaces both above and below to a depulsating surgical meningocele.

Drainage of the syrinx is subsidiary to the above-mentioned aims; however, the maneuver may be worth performing because it helps to open up the subarachnoid spaces and encourages the syrinx cavity to heal.

Division of the Cord

The most effective disablement of the filling mechanism is excision of the area of damaged cord, as was recommended by Durward and associates.[67] The thinned cord, through which most of the CSF almost certainly enters, and the zone of arachnoiditis are thereby removed; the funnel-shaped lower end of the upper syrinx is closed, and if a drainage tube is used, it is conveniently placed. Maximal access from the subarachnoid space to the surgical meningocele of surging fluid is thereby attained. Of the cases with cord transection in this series, none has deteriorated after operation. This technique is limited to complete lesions, and determining lesion completeness is not always easy on clinical grounds. Removal of the damaged area of cord may also be indicated for the removal of dysfunctional tissue that may be responsible for the pain.[67, 68]

WHEN TO TREAT

The onset of symptoms may be sudden and involve loss of function that never returns. The complication rate of laminectomy and production of an artificial meningocele should suffice for small syrinxes in partial paraplegics or patients with injuries of the cervical or lumbar enlargements, in whom drainage via a myelotomy might be hazardous. Early treatment has its advantages, but surveillance by repeated MRI scanning is used for many cases of primary cysts, small syrinxes, or syrinxes that appear to be expanding downward only. Heavy exertion or vigorous sports probably should be avoided by patients with these lesions. One patient claimed that he recovered part of his cord function by "cutting down all physical activity by 90 percent."

SURGICAL TECHNIQUE

LOWERING CEREBROSPINAL FLUID PRESSURE

The methods for treating hydrocephalus are discussed elsewhere in this book. The author favors the use of Medos adjustable valves (Codman). The aim of treatment is to lower the pressure as far as is safe for the patient; therefore, slit ventricles are tolerated or even desired.

If the ventricles are already normal-sized or small, the surgeon may choose to drain CSF spaces outside the brain. Drainage from the lumbar theca must be practiced only if no possibility exists of impacting the hindbrain. Drainage of the lumbar theca should also be avoided if obstruction exists in the subarachnoid space. No complications from this procedure have been observed by the author in his practice or have been found in the literature, but the theoretical danger is clear. If the pressure is low below an obstruction, the pressure differences aggravated by a drain may force fluid into a syrinx or exaggerate other abnormalities, such as arachnoid pouches. Therefore, passing a drainage catheter into the subarachnoid spaces proximal to the site of meningeal fibrosis is preferable, when possible. This method may involve passing a drainage catheter up into the head, ventral to the pons and medulla (Case 1).

OPENING CEREBROSPINAL FLUID PATHWAYS

If there is no obstruction to the free passage of CSF along the subarachnoid pathways, syringomyelia is unlikely to be present. The preferred method of treating syringomyelia is to open up those pathways and to change the balance of forces that affect the disposition of the fluid. The problem of opening up the CSF pathways in the face of meningeal fibrosis is tedious and sometimes impossible, and when a lengthy zone of meningeal fibrosis is known to exist, this procedure is probably best not attempted.

The laminectomy opening should be adequate in length. If a comminuted vertebral fracture has occurred, then two bones have commonly healed together by the time the patient presents with syringomyelia. A four-segment laminectomy is usually sufficient, but if the area of damage is greater, then a five- or six-level laminectomy is best. For cases with a web of arachnoid adherence, a smaller laminectomy may suffice. If patients have an extensive length of meningeal fibrosis, the longest laminectomy may not be sufficient to treat the problem (Case 1), and the surgeon may have to settle for exposure at the top of the affected area. Because dampening of pulsation achieved by the laminectomy is presumably greater the bigger the cut, a five- to eight-lamina exposure is not unreasonable.

The dura should be opened over the length of the laminectomy and then sutured back. A V-shaped ending to the dural incision allows the end of the surgical meningocele to be square rather than tapered. If the end of the dural incision is straight, suturing back of the sides may narrow the dural tube at the ends of the incision.

If the arachnoid is adherent to the dura, which tends to happen close to the fracture site, then the two membranes may be taken back together. The arachnoid tends to be adherent to the cord in the midline, sometimes constituting a membrane that is nearly intact along the length of the cord. The arachnoid may also become adherent to the posterior nerve roots. If the nerve roots are functionless, they may be sutured back with the arachnoid and used to hold the spaces alongside the cord open. This method cannot be recommended for use above a fracture when the roots may be intact.

One of the problems after any laminectomy when the dura is deliberately left open is that blood exudes from the muscle, bone, and epidural veins and accumulates around the cord and the arachnoid. The arachnoid tissues and the repair process tend to organize the blood clot into more fibrous tissue, and a walling off of the anterior surface of the surgical meningocele and partial or complete isolation of a cystic space posterior to the cord may eventually occur. This phenomenon may compress the cord (Case 8). Such walling off impairs the purpose of the surgical meningocele, which is to depulsate the movements of the CSF around the cord and to allow free access of the CSF between all the cavities.

The method presently used by the author to hold open compromised spaces is to leave in position plastic stents to allow CSF ready access to the surgical meningocele; however, the stent must be removed. Its purpose in syringomyelia resulting from meningeal fibrosis is to keep a hole in the blood clot until the blood clot begins to contract and to keep the arachnoid pressed laterally against the dura, where it will adhere. A convenient tube to use as a stent is a No. 10 F pediatric chest drain (Portex). The tube may be a little large, and the part that will lie alongside the cord may be cut in half longitudinally if it seems likely that the cord or roots may be compressed. The outer ends of these drains are blocked off, and the drains are convenient for pulling through the skin from the inside out. If a piece of suction catheter is pulled through with a suction drain introducer, the obturator of the chest drain may be pushed into the end of the suction catheter, sutured into position, and then drawn out through a small puncture in the skin, which remains watertight. Extra holes may be cut in the wall of the drain to facilitate access of the CSF to the surgical meningocele. The obturator should be left in the end of the drain to prevent CSF from escaping.

The tubes may be removed 48 to 72 hours after the operation, and if a temporary syrinx drain has been used, this may be taken out at the same time. If they are left in for too long, CSF may escape along the track through the skin. Placement of a temporary lumbar external drain by use of a gravity bag for about 5 days may stop such leakage and help diminish protein levels in the remaining CSF. If persisting blockage of the CSF pathways exists, such as would have occurred with Case 1, lumbar drainage should be avoided if possible. Routine lumbar drainage is not advocated because a small amount of positive CSF pressure helps to hold open the surgical meningocele and to dilute and disseminate the blood products as the clots break down.

The use of a permanently implanted tube to hold open the subarachnoid space, as the author once advocated,[57] is not advisable. Re-exploration (Case 7) or necropsy examination indicates that the tubes provoke meningeal fibrosis and do not remain useful for long.

Care must also be taken when stents are placed, particularly in quadriplegic patients, when the length of the functional roots above the fracture may be short and make the nerves susceptible to damage by the stent tubing.

The dentate ligament is a useful structure to assist in the opening of the subarachnoid space. This ligament may be divided laterally on both sides in any syringomyelia, and a loose suture between the tips holds the spaces open. In post-arachnoidal cases, however, the problems tend to be greater because of the narrowness of the confines and the intensity of the fibrosis. In these causes, it is probably better to hold open the space on one side (the side in which the stent will go) only. The dentate ligament may be divided close to the cord and sutured outward, that is, to the dura, at the same time, which may hold the arachnoid out of the way.

Of course, using stents or drains is not necessary, and the decision to leave them out depends on the assessment of the risks and benefits in each case.

WOUND CLOSURE

The aim of wound closure is not only to make the CSF spaces watertight but also to maintain a sizeable space under the muscle, which is in free communication with the other parts of the CSF pathways. The author is opposed to the use of grafts in this situation, because of experiences with patients such as Case 8. Pulsatile energy is better dissipated if a big space exists. However, some surgeons object to leaving the dura open.

Dural closure may lessen the chance of leakage, but the best opportunity to make the whole wound leak proof is to close the muscle well. The stents and drains should leave the surgical meningocele well away from the skin incision. Closure usually takes place in two muscle layers, and the outer layer is the deep fascial layer, which should have been well defined on the way in. It is possible to define a layer of muscle deep to the deep fascia and to carry out a careful closure of the fascial layer with absorbable sutures. Ordinarily, the subcutaneous tissues can be satisfactorily closed with one suture layer, unless the patient is obese. If approximately every third suture is taken down to include the deep fascia, less potential space is left under the skin in which fluid may collect. Particular problems occur when previous efforts have been made to deal with a syringomyelia. Relaxing incisions in the deep fascia, excision of devitalized tissues, and supplementation of the midline tissues by fascia lata may be tried, and CSF is likely to collect in the subcutaneous spaces; the use of a subcutaneous suction drain for many days may be helpful. A drain from the CSF pathways to an outside reservoir stops leaks, but the collapse of the artificial meningocele that this method produces is unwanted.

Case Reports

CASE REPORT 1

A 35-year-old woman had an epidural anesthetic for low back pain. The catheter was left in for 26 hours to allow repeated reinjection. She returned to the hospital 5 days later with exacerbation of back pain. Ten days after that, she was admitted with fever, neck stiffness, leucocytosis, and a swollen tender back, with pus exuding from the site of the epidural catheter. She had no paralysis. Extralaminar drainage was performed. The patient was seriously ill for many days, with continuing fever, meningism, psychotic features, and total amnesia. Within 2 years, difficulty walking and balancing, severe sensory losses, absent knee and ankle jerks, and failing bladder function had developed. Syringomyelia was not diagnosed for 11 years and was then noted to extend from T3 to the conus (Fig. 170–2). A syrinx-to-pleural shunt was followed by no improvement. Within months the syrinx symptoms extended upward to involve the neck. The next MRIs showed the syrinx extending to the foramen magnum (Fig. 170–3).

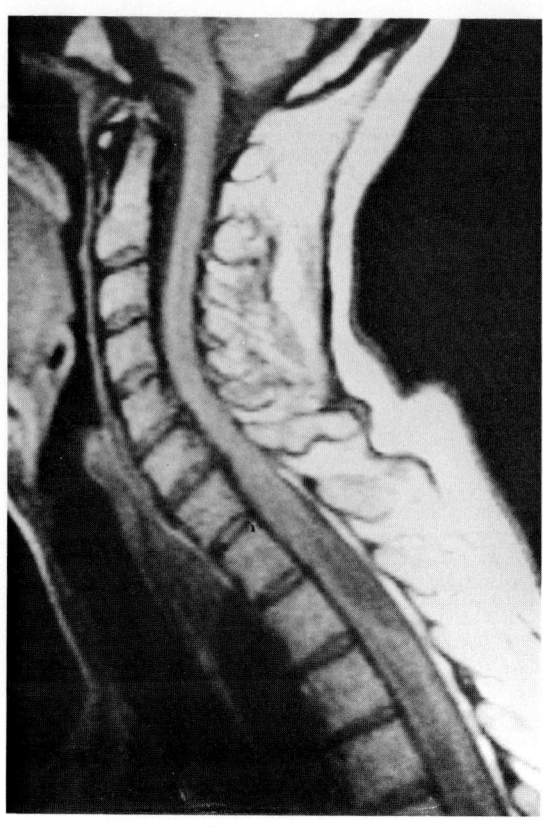

FIGURE 170–2. Case Report 1: The lower MRI scan shows a septated syrinx reaching to the conus. The cavity is visible from T3 downward. Opposite the center of T2 is a dilatation of the subarachnoid space with enlargement and distortion of the upper thoracic cord. Note that the cervical cord is normal.

A syringopleural shunt was repeated at a higher level 8 months after the first operation. After the next 3 years, the patient was paraplegic and had an extensively anesthetic left arm and a permanent indwelling Foley catheter. MRIs obtained at this time are shown in Figure 170–4. Myelography showed a severely fibrosed subarachnoid space with subarachnoid pouches as well as a gross syringomyelia that produced an increase in both the width and the length of the lower cord (Figs. 170–5 to 170–7).

The operative exploration showed no possibility of lys-

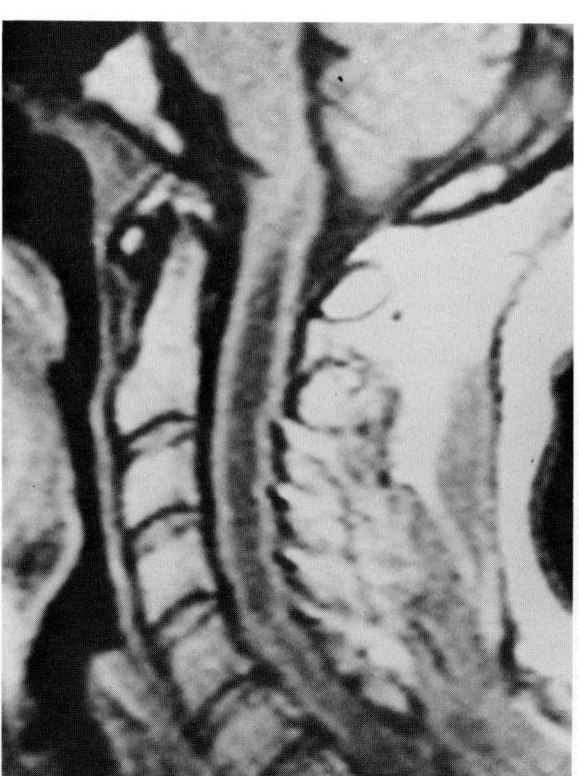

FIGURE 170–3. Case Report 1: After the syrinx was drained, which was performed in the thoracic region, the upper cord has become invaded by an extension of the syrinx.

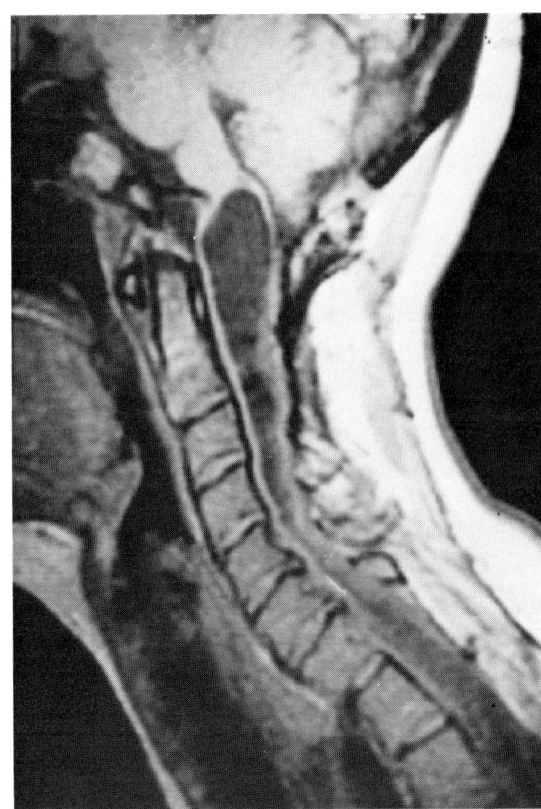

FIGURE 170–4. Case Report 1: After the patient's second high cervical drainage operation, the syrinx had advanced to the extent that patient's left arm had become useless and diaphragmatic function was threatened.

ing adhesions. The upper drain in the syrinx was immured in the wall and was removed. A subarachnoid-to-peritoneal drain was placed, and the upper end was passed ventral to the medulla and pons in the belief that there would be good

access to CSF in the cisterns and a small chance of blockage. After a stormy postoperative course, the patient made a partial recovery but did not regain the ability to walk. The left arm and hand remained severely affected by motor and

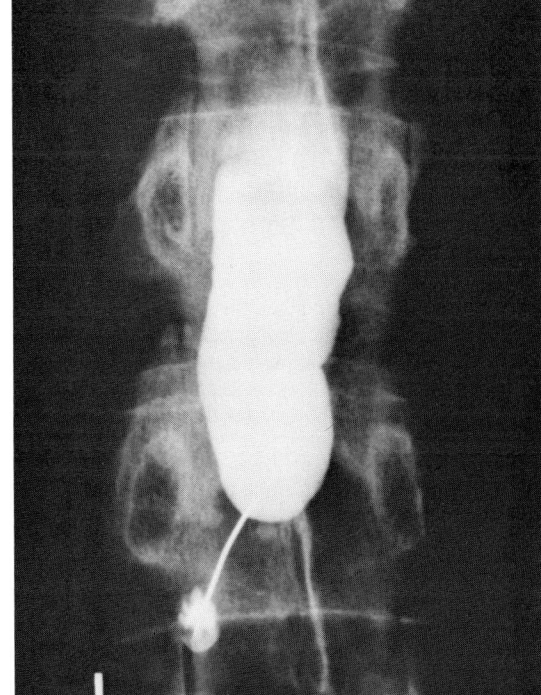

FIGURE 170–5. Case Report 1: The lower end of the spinal cord has been injected with contrast. The end of the cord is widened and lengthened, reaching down to the body of L3. Notice the featureless walls; this is a cyst of the filum terminale rather than syringomyelia.

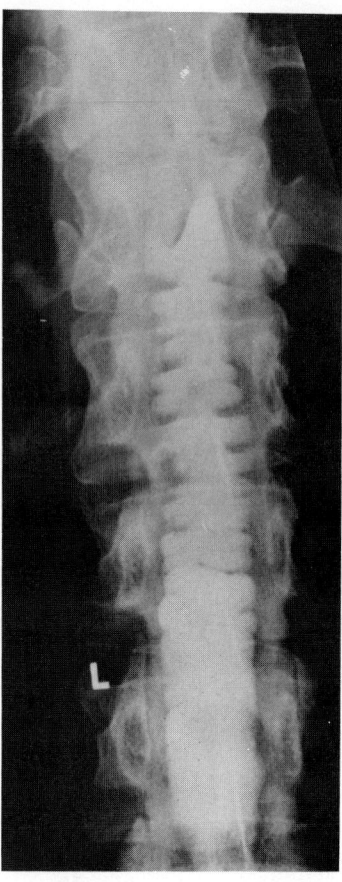

FIGURE 170-6. Case Report 1: As contrast was run upward, the morphology of the walls could be seen to change. The wall opposite L1 showed morphology suggestive of short wavelength perturbation. These irregularities may be called Haustra, they are not necessarily due to the same mechanisms as the more common septations. There was a separate outpouching opposite the lowest rib, and flow of contrast upward was delayed.

sensory losses. The right arm was almost normal. The postoperative appearance indicated that the syrinx was flattened, and the prognosis for her right hand and her diaphragm may have improved (Fig. 170-8).

CASE REPORT 2

A previously well 23-year-old man suffered multiple injuries, including a head injury that produced a right hemiplegia and mental impairment. Sternal fracturing and a fracture of T3 with paraplegia occurred. His left arm was initially normal, but he claimed that a claw deformity developed in the left hand within a week. His ulnar nerve was explored. He later developed problems with the bladder, and the neurologic problem was immediately attributed to syringomyelia. On examination, the patient was a cheerful man with slurred speech. No other bulbar feature was present in the palate or the tongue, and the speech problem appeared to reflect the extent of the head injury rather than to correlate with the extensive syrinx seen on MRI. Severe wasting of the intrinsic musculature of the left hand existed, and the entire upper limb was thinned and weakened with absent biceps and supinator jerks. The sensory loss was greatest to protopathic sensibility and extended into the trigeminal distribution. MRI showed an upwardly extending syrinx that ended within the medulla, constituting the ascending form of syringobulbia. At operation, the cord was transected and a syringopleural shunt inserted.

The patient was unchanged clinically and lived as a quadriplegic. His MRI appearance, however, was improved. Timely surgery would have probably saved his left arm function.

CASE REPORT 3

A 15-year-old girl was in a motorcycle accident that left her paraplegic from a T6 fracture. She had difficulties with bowel function, necessitating a colostomy. At her examination 2 years later, she was noted to have a sensory loss of dissociated type in the right forequarter. She was reassured by the neurologist that cysts within the cord did not progress to motor loss and that they did not require treatment. After some years, she sought further advice about the persisting numbness, although pain and motor loss were not present. At age 25, she had no motor loss and no gross autonomic features, although she had unusual "goosebumps" and sweating.

MRI examination showed the syrinx to extend from C1 to the conus. The upper part of the syrinx was not tight (Fig. 170-9), but the lower part of the cord was tightly filled with some septations, and longitudinal marking was

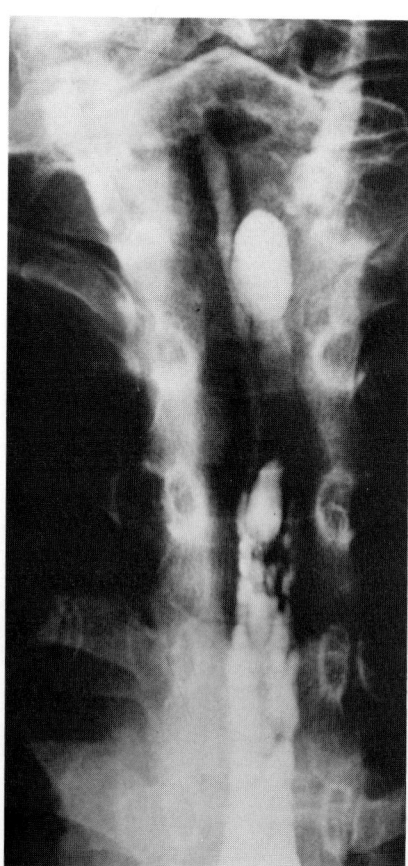

FIGURE 170-7. Case Report 1: As the contrast slowly ascended into the upper thoracic region, it showed multiple small chinks and cavities in both the subarachnoid spaces and probably also the syrinx cavity itself. It would not be surprising if sizeable holes existed in the wall of the thoracic syrinx. The configurations in the subarachnoid space are sometimes called candle gutterings.

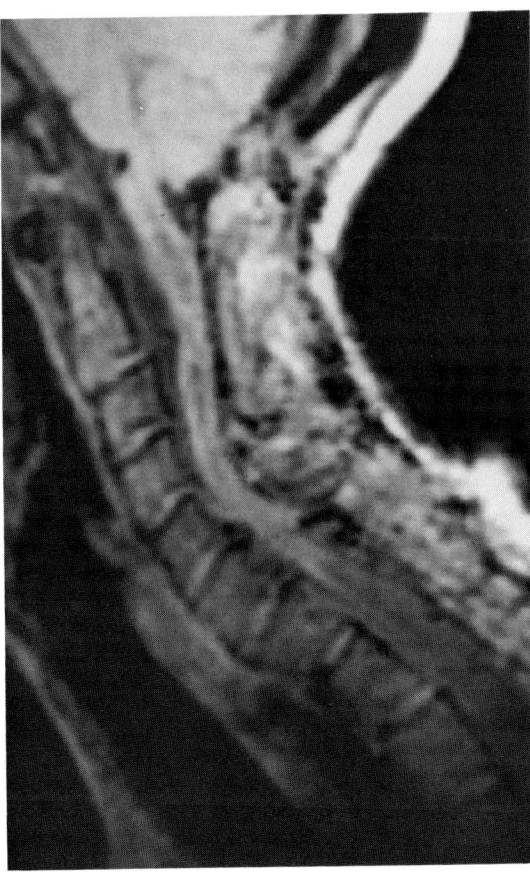

FIGURE 170–8. Case Report 1: The postoperative appearance after the patient's most recent syrinx operation, in which the subarachnoid space was drained to the peritoneal cavity. The top end of the drain was in the cisterna ambiens of the midbrain, and there was a low pressure valve in the system. No syrinx drainage was performed. The appearance of the syrinx has improved. Permanent improvement cannot be guaranteed, but MRI appearances were unchanged at 1 year.

present (Fig. 170–10). This finding suggested that the two parts of the syrinx were not in communication but that if they were to communicate in the future, the top syrinx might then be subjected to a higher pressure.

At operation, a 1.5-cm-long section of damaged spinal cord was removed. A complete septum was discovered 1 cm above the site of cord transection. A drain was passed through this septum and the lower end inserted into the right pleural cavity. No drain was used in the lower syrinx. Sensory loss was immediately reduced, and in the left side, which she had previously thought of as normal, she felt a deep and unpleasant itching. She developed an intermittent and variable pupillary inequality without ptosis. She suffered a marked change in the autonomic responses of the skin such that the left side flushed more strongly than the right in response to anger or embarrassment; however, reddening due to sunburn was symmetrical.

Three weeks after discharge from the hospital, the patient developed sudden severe headache, which was eased slightly by her lying down. At the time of her readmission, slight improvement had occurred, but the pain was still exaggerated by either sitting up or lying with the right side down. No signs of infection were present, and MRI showed an excellent result (Figs. 170–11 and 170–12). CSF pressure was unrecordably low, and it seemed the drainage tube had become dislodged and that low CSF pressure resulting from over-shunting caused her problem. The shunt was removed without reopening of the laminectomy. Recovery from the headache was immediate. MRI 1 year after shunt removal showed an unchanged appearance, with the lower syrinx still collapsed and the upper syrinx almost obliterated. Sensation had improved, although slight residual sensory loss remained along the inner border of the right forearm and palm. No change occurred in her other signs. The patient thought her hands were more nimble than before operation, and their power remained full. Her intermittent anisocoria, presumably resulting from a partial right Horner's syndrome, remained.

CASE REPORT 4

A 42-year-old man presented with weakness, clumsiness, minor sensory impairment of the left leg, and dysesthetic pain around the left side of the trunk. There was no relevant past history. On examination, dissociated sensory loss was present on the affected parts of the trunk from T8 downward, and reflexes were absent in the left leg. Myelography showed a midthoracic delay in passage of contrast, with temporary obstruction at two levels. Postmyelography CT showed the cord to contain a contrast-outlined cavity. The cord was distorted in an eclipsed manner, that is, it was partly obliterated by a shape with a circular outline, suggesting encroachment by a cystic pouch or other localized dilatation of the CSF pathways. MRI indicated a syrinx from T8 almost to the conus. Exploratory laminectomy at the level of T7 showed two pouched arachnoid webs across

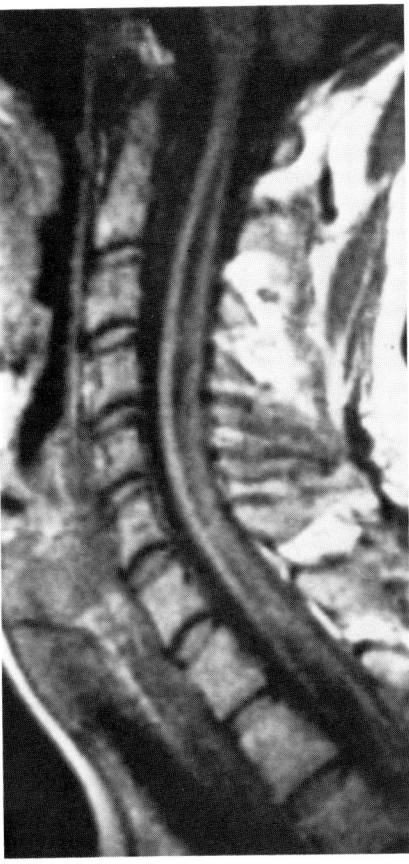

FIGURE 170–9. Case Report 3. Here, the upper syrinx does not look tense, the rate of neurologic advance was not detectable, and there were no motor losses. It might be thought reasonable to leave this syrinx alone or to keep it under observation.

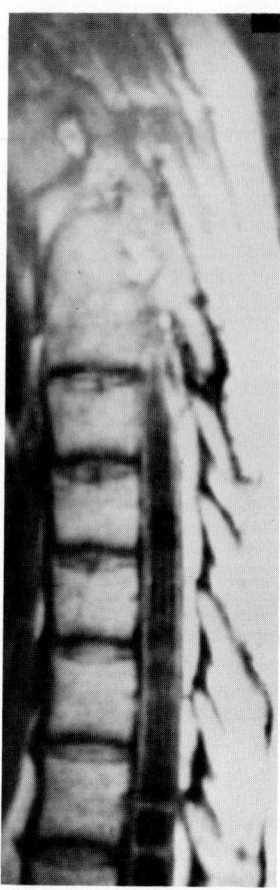

FIGURE 170–10. Case Report 3: The lower part of the syrinx shows a tight fullness with septations. Thus, it is unlikely that the two cavities communicate. The tension in the lower cavity is an uncertain indication for operation.

the entire subarachnoid space posteriorly. The configuration of the webs was such that they formed transitory pouches during upward movement and caught the CSF temporarily. The syrinx did not seem to extend cephalad to the bigger and uppermost pouched arachnoid webs of meningeal fibrosis. The distension of the pouch during such an event looked as though it would press the cord forward and possibly damage it. In addition, there would presumably be a competition between the fluid within the syrinx and the fluid in the subarachnoid space at the same level. The webs were partially removed and a surgical meningocele was formed. After operation, there was a detectable improvement in walking but little change in sensation. MRI results were improved. This case illustrates an important problem in an apparently idiopathic syrinx. Such cases are prone to deteriorate to the point of incontinence or paraplegia, and the underlying mechanisms are mysterious.

CASE REPORT 5

A 40-year-old man was thrown off a wall and suffered paraplegia from a T6-T7 fracture. A left-sided syringomyelia was diagnosed within 2 years of the assault. The sensory features were of "a painful tingly numbness," with dissociated loss and an interscapular pain. No weakness was present, the power was full, the left triceps jerk was depressed, and the biceps and supinator jerks were absent. The patient had noted increased sweating of the right leg

and had had a difficult time with his bladder, which had been treated by sphincterotomy.

MRI scanning showed a tight, multiseptated, syrinx from C1 to the upper dorsal region (Figs. 170–13 and 170–14). Below the fracture, the syrinx was slim and three segments long. At operation, the cord was divided above what seemed to be a complete septum, and a neat, almost complete septum, with a small round hole in the center, was identified above the level of transection. A drain was inserted upward and the cord sutured around it and to the posterior longitudinal ligament to prevent ascent, such as seemed to have occurred in Case 3.

Postoperatively, the patient reported immediate marked sensory improvement and further improvement for many weeks, as well as some bladder improvement. Postoperative MRI confirmed the flattening of the syrinx (Fig. 170–15), with a neat surgical meningocele.

CASE REPORT 6

A 21-year-old girl was involved in a traffic accident in 1970 with a crush fracture of T5 and paraplegia. Two years later, the patient noted numbness of the left side of the face that went down to the level of the paraplegia sensory loss. The tendon reflexes were depressed in the patient's left arm. No motor features were present. The patient curtailed her physical activity but remained able to transfer, drive, dress herself, and perform her own toilet functions until a second

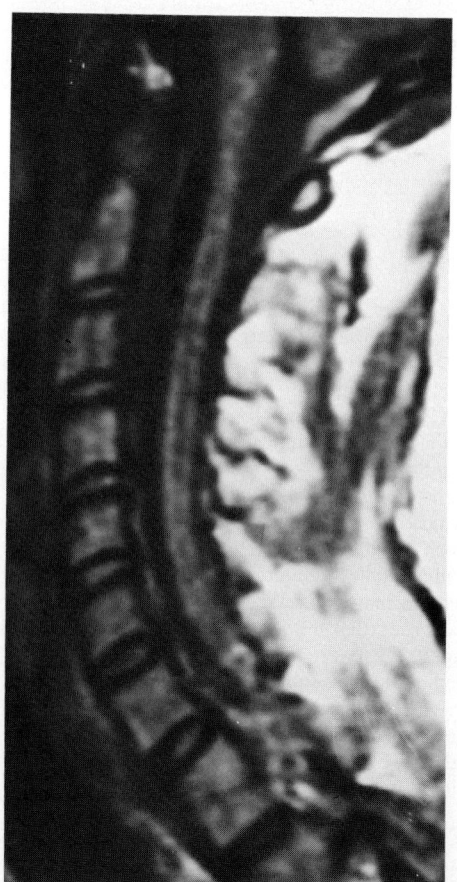

FIGURE 170–11. Case Report 3: The patient's sensation returned. She was reassured by the appearance of the upper syrinx and the knowledge that it is now less likely to advance.

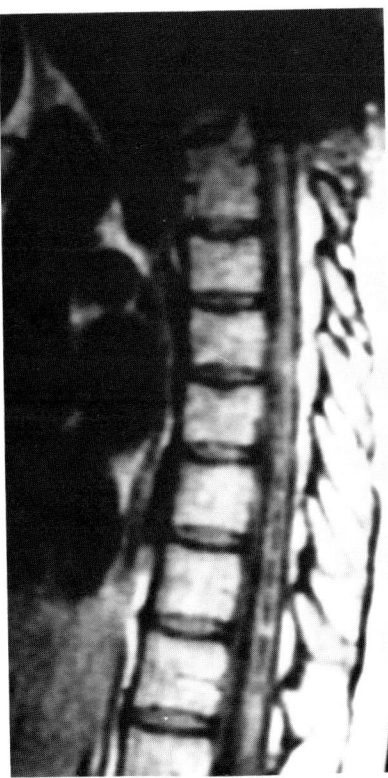

FIGURE 170-12. Case Report 3: The appearance of the lower syrinx has improved. No drain was used to effect this emptying. Only cord transection and an artificial meningocele were used.

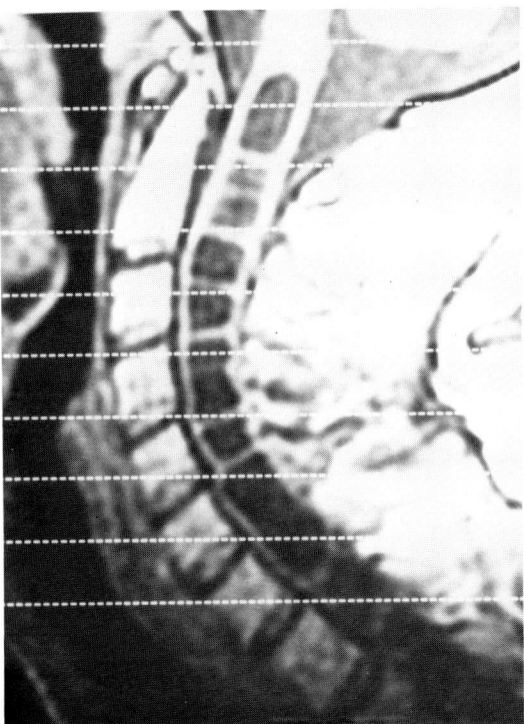

FIGURE 170-13. Case Report 5: The upper syrinx is tense, with septations close together, suggesting a short wavelength phenomenon. Note the thickness of the septae, some of which may be intact.

road traffic accident in 1985, in which the patient was severely jolted.

Immediately after the injury, she had severe neck pain and marked increase in leg spasms. She lost the ability to transfer and had to stop working. She thought these symptoms resulted from the spasms rather than weakness. There was loss of dexterity and general stiffening up of the hand and the arm, which was clinically assessed as slightly weakened. Sensory loss was bilateral at this stage, but the left side was worse than the right. MRI confirmed a tense syrinx from the medulla to T7, with a constriction at T5.

At age 38, the patient consented to an operation. Dorsal laminectomy was performed, as was resection and ligation of a severely damaged part of the cord that did not seem to be functional. A syringopleural drain was inserted from the upper syrinx to the right pleural cavity.

Rapid clinical improvement ensued. The patient could immediately make a fist, which was not possible previously. Six weeks later, the arms were stronger and the hands more nimble. Sensation improved on both sides, with the left remaining worse than the right. The pain went from the neck and arms. Spasms in the legs seemed immediately worse but improved after 3 or 4 months to become markedly better. Bladder function was unchanged. A postoperative MRI showed marked diminution in all aspects of syrinx size. The result in this case could almost certainly have been improved if operation had been undertaken at the time of diagnosis.

CASE REPORT 7

A 12-year-old boy had tuberculous meningitis and tuberculous infection of the eighth and ninth thoracic vertebrae with a paravertebral abscess. The abscess was treated by costotransversectomy and bone grafting, after which he had a weak right leg and could not walk. After 18 months of antituberculous treatment, he recovered to be neurologically normal. Five years later, he had intermittent swelling, pain, and tenderness around the left hip and developed a limp.

Myelography with follow-up CT showed the cord to be deformed, with a central cavity, but not compressed. The spinal fluid showed evidence of infection, and antituberculous treatment was restarted.

Six years after the initial illness, the patient developed hyperhidrosis and pain over the left side of the trunk and

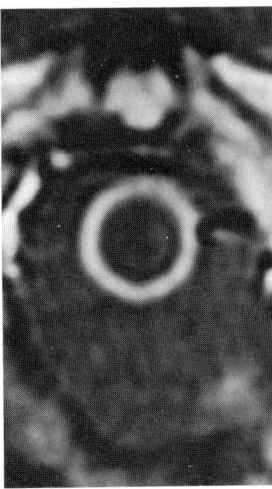

FIGURE 170-14. Case Report 5: The tension of the syrinx is indicated by the roundness of the cavity. Despite its size and centrality, the patient had sensory symptoms only on one side.

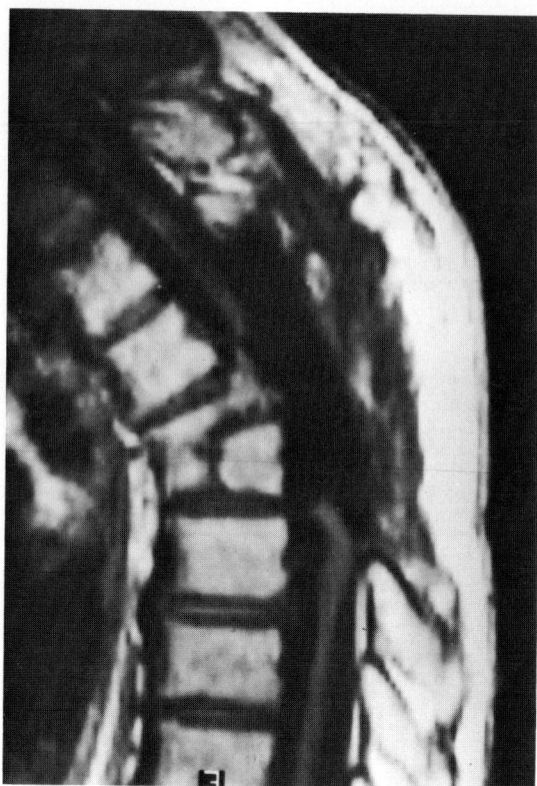

FIGURE 170–15. Case Report 5: Sagittal MRI appearances after resection of a small zone of damaged cord. Observe that because the bottom end was not sutured down to dura, it floats away. If that happens at the top, it may dislodge the drain if a drain is used. The upper syrinx (the one with the drain) has flattened impressively.

weakness of the left hand. The left biceps and supinator jerks had gone, and a left Horner's syndrome was present. The syrinx reached to C1 and had septations. The cord was exposed at laminectomy, and a typical appearance of spinal pial-arachnoid adhesions with a big syrinx cavity was seen. The CSF was slightly turbid, and when it was aspirated, the entire cyst collapsed. Tubes were inserted to hold open the subarachnoid spaces above and below the zone of maximum pathology so that the fluid would be able to enter the area of the artificial meningocele easily. The CSF showed live tubercle bacilli, and antituberculous therapy was restarted. The syringomyelia collapsed down well, and the patient's autonomic symptoms and pain disappeared, his gait improved. Five months after the first laminectomy, MRI showed that the cord above the vertebral body disease remained collapsed, and the surgical meningocele was apparently under tension. The cord was apparently distended below the gibbus. At re-operation, the surgical meningocele was not under tension, and the rounded cavity that resembled a syrinx was found to be outside the cord. The tubes were removed because they were entirely surrounded by pial-arachnoid adhesions and were apparently contributing to the problems rather than helping.

At the age of 22, the patient's neurologic state remained good. He could hop on either foot, walk any distance he wanted, and had normal bladder and hand functions. MRI appearances continued to suggest a full cavity below the gibbus but a collapsed syrinx above. The poor state of the subarachnoid drainage tubes and the gross meningeal fibrosis helped to initiate the present policy of putting in such tubes for a few days only.

CASE REPORT 8

A 22-year-old man fell from a height and sustained a fracture of L1 with a severe conus lesion. He had good dorsiflexion but no useful calf muscle power, the buttock area and posterior perineum were substantially numb, but the bladder and bowel control and sexual functions were claimed to be normal.

Syringomyelic features started 2 years after injury, with a burning sensation in the left side of the abdomen that ascended slowly over a year to affect the thorax and the arm. His bladder control worsened so that he was occasionally incontinent.

At age 25, the motor power of the arms was normal. Tendon reflexes were markedly depressed in the arms and the left knee, and left abdominal reflexes and left gluteal reflex were absent. Sensation showed the most intense loss on the ulnar border of the left arm. Generalized depression of sensitivity existed over the left side up to the face, but the front of the left thigh was spared.

Endomyelography was unrevealing. Myelography showed a complete blockage of the subarachnoid space, but the cord was not discernibly enlarged. Because of the good function in the conus and the severe increase in deficit that might be expected if the neurologic level were to ascend even one level, the laminectomy and dissection of the conus were cautiously performed. The damaged area was not fully exposed. Four attempts to obtain fluid by needle were unsuccessful. A terminal ventriculostomy was then performed. It was hoped that the laminectomy itself might also have been effective through alteration of the pulsatile dynamics of the situation.[69]

Initial improvement of the sensation in the left hand and the backs of both legs occurred. The patient needed intermittent catheterization for 5 days but then improved to his normal standard. The tendon jerks returned, although those on the left were less brisk than those on the right. The patient thought that his legs were stronger, but this effect was difficult to verify objectively. His condition stabilized over several months, and thermal sensation improved over part of the left arm and the fingertips.

Three months after the operation, the patient noticed a stabbing back pain followed by numbness ascending from the iliac crest to the sternum, left side only, with no further involvement of the leg. This sensation was similar to the original sensations and slowly spread again to reinvolve the arm. During a bout of influenza in which he had a cough, the symptoms spread to involve the previous area, and hot and cold again became indistinguishable over the entire left arm. The sensory loss spread into the back of the scalp, and hyperhidrosis developed over the left side. The left arm became mildly weak. The condition slowly progressed, and 9 months after the operation, he became incontinent of urine. The tendon reflexes had again gone.

Three years after the initial operation, his condition was worse than preoperatively. He observed that if he sneezed while standing up it made him feel ill, but that if he lay down to sneeze, it was not troublesome.

Myelography with follow-up CT confirmed a cavity from the medulla to T5. A low cervical laminectomy was performed with a syrinx-to-pleural shunt. The improvement was once again impressive and affected all modalities of cord function. Although the legs had not seemed to be much affected, the improvement in sensation was greater than after the first operation. The improvements persisted without relapse for 2 years.

Symptoms then started in the right upper limb. The patient was readmitted at the age of 30. The residual signs in the left arm were much as before: there were no motor, reflex, or gross sensory signs in the right arm. A complete block still existed at L1, and follow-up CT scans showed three syrinx cavities. One was above the fracture, which dwindled in the upper thoracic cord, and one small syrinx was on each side in the cervical region. These three cavities were likely communicating with each other.

None of these cavities seemed big enough to drain, and the issue of reoperating at the original site was again discussed. Five years later, the situation was deteriorating unrelentingly. The left hand was developing weakness, with wasting and claw deformity, and the sensory picture was worsening. MRI showed one big syrinx with an odd appearance above the laminectomy site. The cervical syringopleural shunt was not working. Re-exploration of the lumbar enlargement was carried out with an upward extension of the previous laminectomy. The area of the silicone sheeting graft showed dense fibrosis on both the front of the graft, thus involving the back of the cord, and behind the graft. The syrinx was the zone of meningeal fibrosis. This area was partly cut away, and the arachnoid was dissected above the zone of arachnoiditis. A midline myelotomy was performed and a drain inserted, brought through the skin, and drained into a bile bag. Stents were used to open the arachnoid spaces into the surgical meningocele. The improvements were again striking but varied greatly from day to day in the immediate postoperative period. The results in this patient remain satisfactory: the scans of November 1992 showed a slack, walled cyst visible at the level of the laminectomy.

The delay in gaining a good result in this case seems to be the result of surgical apprehension plus a diligent policy of warning the patient about the possibility of losing more conus function. The adoption of a more robust attitude might have produced a good result earlier.

RESULTS

Many of the patients have initially severe deficits, and objectivity in assessing improvement is difficult. Because sensory deficits, including pain, are subjective, the emotional state of the patient affects whether they claim to be improved after a procedure. Objective features, such as return of tendon reflexes, do not provide an excellent objective baseline. Likewise, motor power is often affected by the patient's morale or desire to please. Frequently, patients present a balance sheet with improvements and worsening. It is difficult for the surgeon not to distort the results upward through optimism or downward through a wish not to be thought to be making excessive claims. The results given in Table 170–2 are on the optimistic side: if some feature was definitely better, including MRI assessment as well as clinical evaluation, the patient was considered improved. If the balance sheet was about equal, they were considered unchanged. If the patient's condition definitely deteriorated and the patient regretted having had the operation, they were scored as worse. Only one death occurred that was related to a pedicled omental graft.

The results are disappointing in terms of recovery of function. Distinct improvement is often seen, but no severe weakness was reversed. However, no deaths occurred after subarachnoid bypass operations, and no major morbidity occurred in the cases operated on in this clinic. One patient had deterioration of arm power directly after resuturing of a wound that broke down. One patient broke down a pre-existing bedsore, one posttraumatic patient went into status epilepticus, and another had a severe transient metabolic disturbance, the nature of which was not determined. This is a

Table 170–2. 99 CASES OF SYRINGOMYELIA APPARENTLY DUE TO SPINAL MENINGEAL FIBROSIS FROM 112 CASES OF SPINAL ARACHNOIDITIS

	Totals	Postoperative				Unoperated	Deaths	
		IMP	UNCH	WORSE	REL		Postoperative	Late
Spinal cord injury								
Complete								
Cervical	5	1	2	—	—	2	—	—
Thoracic (2, 3, 5, 6)*	32	24	1	1	3	3	—	—
Lumbar (8)	4	2	—	—	—	2	—	—
Incomplete								
Cervical	5	1	2	2	—	—	—	—
Thoracic	16	8	3	1	1	3	—	—
Lumbar (8)	6	3	1	—	2	—	—	—
Total spinal cord injured	68	39	9	4	6	10	0	0
Meningeal fibrosis								
Known cause								
Tuberculosis (7)	6	3	—	1	1	1	1	1
Iophendylate (Myodil, Pantopaque)	6	2	3	—	1	—	—	—
Epidural sepsis (1)	4	1	1	1	—	1	—	—
Pyogenic meningitis	2	1	—	—	—	1	—	—
Unknown cause								
Widespread	8	2	1	—	1	4	—	1
Pouched arachnoid webs (4)	6	3	2	—	—	1	—	—
Total nontraumatic meningeal fibrosis	32	12	7	2	3	8	1	2

*Numbers in parentheses refer to case report numbers, as presented in text.
IMP—improved; UNCH—unchanged; REL—late relapse.

fragile set of patients, and the elderly paraplegic and those with multiple deficits may endure a difficult postoperative course.

Failure to control the pain is a disappointing feature, despite encouraging reports from Shannon and colleagues[11] and Suzuki and colleagues.[13] Some patients have reported an exacerbation of pain in an area that was previously numb but not painful. Most such patients find that the pain eases with time.

Several cases have required reoperation for the progression of symptoms. One case's course was similar to that of posttraumatic Case 2 in the development of symptoms on the opposite side after apparently successful drainage but has declined further investigation. Two have had change of sides on relapse (Table 170–2).

Another disappointing feature has been the progression of deterioration after the performance of surgery and apparently good syrinx control (Case Report 8). In typical hindbrain-related cases without any inflammatory changes around the outside of the cord, the progression of neurologic symptoms with age is common, either because of progressive gliosis or other varieties of aging being exaggerated in the damaged cord.

MRI results encourage the belief that early and thorough surgery for these lesions is worthwhile. Occasionally sections of cord do not collapse as fully as others (Case 2). However, none of these has been so egregious as to invite separate drainage. The primary cyst at the site of injury may not flatten as much as other, more remote, parts of the syrinx. The pathology of the primary cyst may be different from the main syrinx, or the decompression may be harmful to the parts of the cord immediately opposite the laminectomy. Failure of the primary cyst to collapse could result from the occurrence of meningeal adhesions despite the care of the surgeon. It could also result from altered CSF dynamics.

The author's experience of pedicled omental grafting in the treatment of syringomyelia with progressive neurologic deterioration affecting the cord was dismal. One death occurred in a fragile, 74-year-old woman, two patients were markedly worse because their partial or incomplete paraplegia deteriorated, and three more had ascent of neurologic loss after grafting. Two cases have reported slight improvements. In only one case has improvement been attributable to the grafting, and the benefits might have resulted from the decompression and the lysis of adhesions. Pedicled omental grafting is no longer recommended by the author.

Case 8 is the only patient initially operated on at this clinic to have merited three operations. No case has required reoperation after transection of the cord, and only one has required reoperation after the principle of widely opening the dura and leaving it open has been followed.

Patients who have been operated on in other centers have sometimes required numerous drainage operations. If putting in a drainage tube and closing the dura does not work the first few times, little likelihood exists of the procedure working the next time, and the policy should be changed. In patients in whom multiple interventions have been performed at different levels, the operation of extramedullary-to-extrathecal drainage to lower the CSF pressure may be preferred (see Case Report 1).

FUTURE WORK

The value of MRI in analyzing fluid movement and morphology is in its infancy. Analysis of the surgical material in series such as that discussed in this chapter must continue to advance, particularly the correlation of morphologic variants, such as the type of local cyst, the existence of septations, and the odd occurrence of a completely blocked zone at the site of injury with separate cysts below and above. The differing morphology may be correlated with the possibly bimodal distribution of the time of onset of the syrinx after the trauma in posttraumatic cases. Researchers must determine how many paraplegic cases get small syrinxes, at what age they arise, how many of them enlarge or become symptomatic, if any prognostic features can be identified from the morphology, and whether early ones may heal. Serial MRI from a sizeable population starting at an early stage may identify what proportion of cases have an early hematoma and what fraction of these then become a clear fluid–containing primary cyst. How many of these then develop a syrinx? In how many cases will a syrinx form without any seminal cavity? Some recent publications point the way for these investigations.[7, 8, 15, 22, 23, 26]

Routine MRI in patients with conservatively managed paraplegia and in those treated by cord exploration and myelotomy may well yield interesting information. Evacuation of a hematoma followed by leaving the dura open will likely minimize the chances of a syrinx developing. Closure of the dura enables the fluid that travels into the cord to be violently propelled upward along the inside of the soft gray matter under the influence of pressure changes, such as that produced by coughing, and to excavate new cavities. Nonclosure of the dura may be the most important surgical prophylaxis against this group of disorders. The likelihood of syringomyelia does not constitute an indication for cord exploration in the acute stage. The management of a large surgical meningocele in an acutely injured patient with an unstable, newly fractured spine would be hazardous.

SUMMARY

Non–hindbrain related, nontumorous syringomyelia includes a heterogenous collection of disorders that may appear to cause the syringomyelia. Meningeal fibrosis is the feature almost all have in common. Drains into the syrinx cavity have a likelihood of failure unless they are combined with improvement of the anatomic situation at the site of the pia arachnoid adhesions. The syringomyelia may be controlled in most instances by decompression of the zone of meningeal fibrosis or by lowering of the overall CSF pressure.

Acknowledgment

This work has been supported by Ann's Neurological Trust Society, a self-help group and fundraising charity. Contact via the author.

REFERENCES

1. Greenfield JG: Syringomyelia and syringobulbia, in Greenfield JG (ed): Neuropathology. London, Arnold, 1958, pp 306–309
2. Schleip G: Syringomyelia and syringobulbia, in Vinken PJ, Bruyn GW (eds): Handbook of Clinical Neurology, vol 32. Congenital Malformations of the Brain and Spinal Cord. Amsterdam, North Holland, 1978, pp 255–327
3. Williams B: Syringomyelia. Neurosurg Clin North Am 1(3):653–685, 1990
4. Watson N: Ascending cystic degeneration of the cord after spinal cord injury. Paraplegia 19:89–95, 1981
5. Barnett HJM, Jousse AT: Post-traumatic syringomyelia (cystic myelopathy), in Handbook of Clinical Neurology, vol 26. Vinken PJ, Bruyn GW (eds): Amsterdam. North Holland, 1976, pp 113–157
6. Rossier AB, Foo D, Shillito J, Dyro FM: Posttraumatic cervical syringomyelia. Brain 108:439–461, 1985
7. Silberstein M, Hennessy O: Implications of focal cord lesions following trauma: Evaluation with magnetic resonance imaging. Paraplegia 31:160–167, 1993
8. Backe HA, Betz RR, Mezgarzadeh M, et al: Post-traumatic spinal cord cysts evaluated by magnetic resonance imaging. Paraplegia 29:607–612, 1991
9. Williams B: Pathogenesis of syringomyelia, in Batzdorf U (ed): Syringomyelia: Current Concepts in Diagnosis and Treatment. Baltimore, Williams & Wilkins, 1991, pp 59–90
10. Lacert P, Trottier S, Durand J, et al: Syndromes syringomyéliques tardifs chez la paraplegiques. Rev Neurol (Paris) 133:5, 325–338, 1977
11. Shannon N, Symon L, Logue V, et al: Clinical features, investigation and treatment of post-traumatic syringomyelia. J Neurol Neurosurg Psychiatry 44:35–42, 1981
12. Lyons BM, Brown DJ, Calvert JM, et al: The diagnosis and management of post traumatic syringomyelia. Paraplegia 25:340–350, 1987
13. Vernon JD, Silver JR, Symon L: Post-traumatic syringomyelia: The results of surgery. Paraplegia 21:37–46, 1983
14. Williams B: Post-traumatic syringomyelia (cystic myelopathy), in Vinken PJ, Bruyn GW (eds): Handbook of Clinical Neurology, vol (61). Spinal Cord Trauma. Amsterdam, North Holland, 1992, pp 375–398
15. Sett P, Crockard HA: The value of magnetic resonance imaging (MRI) in the follow up management of spinal injury. Paraplegia 29:396–410, 1991
16. Barnett HJM, Jousse AT: Syringomyelia after paraplegia and quadriplegia, in Barnett HJM, Foster JB, Hudgson P (eds): Syringomyelia. Major Problems in Neurology, vol 1. Philadelphia, WB Saunders, 1973, pp 129–153
17. Foster JB: Neurology of syringomyelia, in Batzdorf U (ed): Syringomyelia: Current Concepts in Diagnosis and Treatment. Baltimore, Williams & Wilkins, 1991, pp 91–115
18. Stanworth PA: The significance of hyperhidrosis in patients with post-traumatic syringomyelia. Paraplegia 20:282–287, 1982
19. Savoiardo M: Syringomyelia associated with post-meningitic spinal arachnoiditis. Filling of the syrinx through a communication with the subarachnoid space. Neurology 26:551–554, 1976
20. Stevens JM, Olney JS, Kendall BE: Post-traumatic cystic and non-cystic myelopathy. Neuroradiology 27:48–56, 1985
21. Stanley P, Senac MO, Segall HD, Park TS: Syringohydromyelia following meningomyelocele surgery—Role of metrizamide myelography and computed tomography. Pediatr Radiol 14:278–283, 1984
22. Quencer RM: The injured spinal cord, evaluation with magnetic resonance and intraoperative sonography. Radiol Clin North Am 26:1025–1045, 1988
23. Enzmann DR: Imaging of syringomyelia, in Batzdorf U (ed): Syringomyelia: Current Concepts in Diagnosis and Treatment. Baltimore, Williams & Wilkins, 1991, pp 116–139
24. Pillay PK, Awad IA, Little JR, Hahn JF: Surgical management of syringomyelia: A five year experience in the era of magnetic resonance imaging. Neurol Res 13:3–9, 1991
25. Gebarski SS, Maynard FW, Gabrielsen TO, et al: Posttraumatic progressive myelopathy. Radiology 157:379–385, 1985
26. Silberstein M, Brown D, Tress BM, Hennessy O: Suggested MRI criteria for surgical decompression in acute spinal cord injury. Preliminary observations. Paraplegia 30:704–710, 1992
27. Heinz R, Curnes J, Friedman A, Oakes J: Exophytic syrinx, an extreme form of syringomyelia: CT, myelographic, and MR imaging features. Radiology 183:243–246, 1992
28. Andrews BT, Weinstein PR, Rosenblum ML, Barbaro NM: Intradural arachnoid cysts of the spinal canal associated with intramedullary cysts. J Neurosurg 68:544–549, 1988
29. Castillo M, Quencer RM, Green BA, Montalvo BM: Syringomyelia as a consequence of compressive extramedullary lesions: Postoperative clinical and radiological manifestations. Am J Neuroradiol 150:391–396, 1988
30. Wilberger JE, Maroon JC, Prostko ER, et al: Magnetic resonance imaging and intraoperative neurosonography in syringomyelia. Neurosurgery 20:599–605, 1987
31. Williams B: Subarachnoid pouches of the posterior fossa with syringomyelia. Acta Neurochir (Wien) 47:187–217, 1979
32. Barkovitch AJ, Wippold FJ, Sherman JL, Citrin CM: Significance of cerebellar tonsillar position on MR. Am J Neuroradiol 7:795–799, 1986
33. Morgan DW, Williams B: Syringobulbia, a surgical appraisal. J Neurol Neurosurg Psychiatry 55:1132–1141, 1992
34. Williams B: Surgery for hindbrain related syringomyelia, in Symon L (ed): Advances and Technical Standards in Neurosurgery, vol 20. Wien-New York, 1993, pp 107–164
35. Wozniewicz B, Filipowicz K, Swiderska SK, et al: Pathophysiological mechanisms of traumatic cavitation of the spinal cord. Paraplegia 21:312–317, 1983
36. Holmes G: The Goulstonian lectures on spinal injuries of warfare. BMJ 2:769, 815–821, 855–861, 1915
37. Kakoulas B: Pathology of spinal injuries. J Neurotrauma 1:117–129, 1984
38. Du Boulay G, Shah SH, Currie JC, Logue V: The mechanism of hydromyelia in Chiari type 1 malformations. Br J Radiol 47:579–587, 1978
39. Reitan H: On movements of fluid inside the cerebro-spinal space. Acta Radiol Scand 22:762–779, 1941
40. Williams B: Simultaneous cerebral and spinal fluid pressure recordings: 1. Technique physiology and normal results. Acta Neurochir (Wien) 58:167–185, 1981
41. Williams B: Simultaneous cerebral and spinal fluid pressure recordings: 2. Cerebrospinal dissociation with lesions at the foramen magnum. Acta Neurochir (Wien) 59:123–142, 1981
42. Ball MJ, Dayan AD: Pathogenesis of syringomyelia. Lancet ii:799–801, 1972
43. Krayenbühl H: Evaluation of the different surgical approaches in the treatment of syringomyelia. Clin Neurol Neurosurg 77:110–128, 1974
44. Park TS, Cail WS, Broadus WC, Walker MG: Lumbo-peritoneal shunt combined with myelotomy for treatment of syringohydromyelia. J Neurosurg 70:721–727, 1989
45. Vassilouthis J, Papandreou A, Anagnostaras S, et al: Thecoperitoneal shunt for syringomyelia: Report of three cases. Neurosurgery 33:324–328, 1993
46. Vengsarkar US, Panchal VG, Tripathi PD, et al: Percutaneous thecoperitoneal shunt for syringomyelia. J Neurosurg 74:827–831, 1991
47. Fischer EG, Welch K, Shillito J: Syringomyelia after lumboureteral shunting for communicating hydrocephalus. J Neurosurg 47:96–100, 1977
48. Chumas PD, Armstrong DC, Drake JM, et al: Tonsillar herniation—The rule rather than the exception after lumboperitoneal shunting in the paediatric population. J Neurosurg 78:568–573, 1993
49. Chumas PD, Drake JM, Del Bigio MR: Death from chronic tonsillar herniation in a patient with lumboperitoneal shunt and Crouzon's disease. Br J Neurosurg 6:595–599, 1992
50. Welch K, Shillito J, Strand R, et al: Chiari 1 ''malformation''—An acquired disorder? J Neurosurg 55:604–609, 1981
51. Aoki N: Lumbo-peritoneal shunting in cases of Chiari malformation. J Neurosurg 71:953, 1989
52. Williams B: Lumbo-peritoneal shunting in cases of Chiari malformation. J Neurosurg 71:950–951, 1989
53. Abbe R, Coley WB: Syringomyelia, operation-exploration of cord, withdrawal of fluid exhibition of patient. J Nerv Ment Dis 19:512–515, 1892
54. Tator CH, Meguro K, Rowed DW: Favourable results with syringosubarachnoid shunts for treatment of syringomyelia. J Neurosurg 56:517–523, 1982
55. Huewel ER, Perneczky A, Urban V, Fries G: Neuroendoscopic technique for the operative treatment of septated syringomyelia. Acta Neurochir Suppl (Wien) 54:59–62, 1992

56. Padovani R, Cavallo M, Gaist G: Surgical treatment of syringomyelia, favourable results with syringosubarachnoid shunting. Surg Neurol 32:173–180, 1989
57. Williams B, Terry AH, Jones HWF, McSweeney T: Syringomyelia as a sequel to traumatic paraplegia. Paraplegia 19:67–80, 1981
58. McLean DR, Miller JDR, Allen PBR, Ezzedin SA: Post-traumatic syringomyelia. J Neurosurg 39:485–492, 1973
59. Rhoton AL: Microsurgery of Arnold Chiari malformation in adults with and without syringomyelia. J Neurosurg 45:473–483, 1976
60. Irger IM, Paramonov FB: New method of draining a syringomyelic cyst. Zh Vopr Neirokhir 3:3–9, 1979
61. Barbaro NM, Wilson CB, Gutin PH: Surgical treatment of syringomyelia: Favourable results with syringoperitoneal shunting. J Neurosurg 61:531–538, 1984
62. Barbaro NM: Surgery for primarily spinal syringomyelia, in Batzdorf U (ed): Syringomyelia: Current Concepts in Diagnosis and Treatment. Baltimore, Williams & Wilkins, 1991, pp 183–198
63. Suzuki M, Davis C, Symon L, Gentili F: Syringoperitoneal shunt for treatment of cord cavitation. J Neurol Neurosurg Psychiatry 48:620–627, 1985
64. Williams B, Page N: Surgical treatment of syringomyelia with syringopleural shunting. Br J Neurosurg 1:63–80, 1987
65. Peerless SJ, Durward QJ: Management of syringomyelia: A pathophysiological approach. Clin Neurosurg 30:531–576, 1988
66. La Haye PA, Batzdorf U: Post traumatic syringomyelia. West J Med 148:657–663, 1988
67. Durward QJ, Rice GP, Ball MJK: Selective spinal cordectomy: Clinicopathological correlation. J Neurosurg 56:359–367, 1982
68. Jefferson AA: Cordectomy for intractable pain in paraplegia, in Lipton S, Miles JB (eds): Persistent Pain, vol 4. London, Academic Press, 1983, pp 115–132
69. Gardner WJ, Bell HS, Poolos PN, et al: Terminal ventriculostomy for syringomyelia. J Neurosurg 46:609–617, 1977

SELECTED READINGS

Payner TD, Prenger E, Berger TS, Crone KR: Acquired Chiari malformations: Incidence, diagnosis, and management. Neurosurgery 34:429–434, 1994

Rossier AB, Foo D, Shillito J, Dyro FM: Posttraumatic cervical syringomyelia. Brain 108:439–461, 1985

Williams B: Post-traumatic syringomyelia, an update. Paraplegia 28:296–313, 1990

Williams B: Post-traumatic syringomyelia (cystic myelopathy), in Handbook of Clinical Neurology, vol (61) Spinal Cord Trauma. Amsterdam, North Holland, 1992, pp 375–398

Williams B: Surgery for hindbrain related syringomyelia, in Simon L (ed): Advances and Technical Standards in Neurosurgery, vol 20. Vienna, Springer Verlag, 1993, pp 107–163

Editorial Commentary

William H. Sweet

The editors have devoted more time to an appraisal of the contribution of Mr. Williams than to any other chapter in either volume. As far as we have determined, he has analyzed more critically than anyone else the mechanisms involved in the development of syringomyelia of either the posttraumatic or idiopathic varieties, or those related to the hindbrain. Although his concept of creating deliberately an extensive posterior meningocele to absorb the energy of pulsation in cerebrospinal fluid and extending dorsally to the ventral aspect of the posterior muscles has no published supporters that we know of, we conclude that his thoughts and recorded results warrant presentation to a major segment of the neurosurgical fraternity. The opening of cerebrospinal fluid pathways is gaining acceptance as a treatment for hindbrain-related syringomyelia, and it is a reasonable prospect that similar surgery will become the norm for non–hindbrain-related syringomyelia in the future.

CHAPTER 171

Neurosurgical Management of Sclerosteosis

Jacquez Charl de Villiers
Jacques J. du Plessis

The craniotubular hyperostoses are a group of genetic disorders in which skeletal deformity results from bone overgrowth. Sclerosteosis is an entity within this group of disorders, in which gross skull thickening is associated with gigantism and syndactyly. It is inherited as an autosomal recessive condition, with a minimum prevalence of one in 60,000 in the Afrikaner community in South Africa and a gene frequency in excess of one in 100.[1,2] The condition has also been encountered in isolated families or sporadically in the United States, Switzerland, Brazil, and Japan.[3-5]

Sclerosteosis differs in many respects from the better-known disorder osteopetrosis (Albers-Schönberg disease),[6] and unlike osteopetrosis, which is attributed to abnormal osteoclast function, sclerosteosis appears to be primarily a disorder of osteoblast hyperactivity.[5] The term *osteopetrosis* should be reserved for the condition in which generalized skeletal sclerosis predominates in the absence of bony overgrowth.[7]

Clinically, sclerosteosis is very similar to the condition described by Van Buchem,[8,9] which seems to be a milder variant but lacks such features as syndactyly, gigantism, and severe cranial hyperostosis.[7] Van Buchem's disease is also inherited as an autosomal recessive trait, and it is common in Holland, where most of the Afrikaner population originated.

Although a clinical rarity, sclerosteosis is of considerable practical importance because the common complications of facial palsy and deafness require attention from an early age. Raised intracranial pressure develops in adulthood, and death due to medullary compression at the craniocervical outlet is a constant threat. Because of the neurologic complications of this condition, it has acquired considerable significance for the neurosurgeon.

Frontal decompression for raised intracranial pressure was the first neurosurgical operation undertaken to alleviate this problem, but despite this procedure, many patients subsequently died in episodes suggestive of medullary coning. Decompression of the posterior fossa and craniocervical junction seemed to be a logical method to relieve crowding at the cranial outlet, and promising results were obtained in a small published series.[10,11]

This chapter draws on the combined experience of the two authors in the neurosurgical management of 19 patients with this condition over the past 15 years.

CLINICAL FEATURES

Affected individuals may be recognized at birth by the presence of variable degrees of syndactyly, most commonly of the second and third fingers, with radial deviation of the terminal phalanges and nail dysplasia. The generalized bony overgrowth, particularly of the jaw and forehead, becomes apparent after the age of about 4 years and is well established by the age of 10. Gigantism becomes evident in childhood, and in adults, height may exceed 200 cm in males and 180 cm in females, with proportionate weight gain due to increased skeletal mass. The tall stature has caused some confusion with acromegaly, but endocrine abnormalities have not been detected in patients with sclerosteosis.[12] Proptosis is common, and in association with bilateral facial nerve palsy and deformity of the face and mandible, it gives a facial appearance that is characteristic, if at times grotesque (Fig. 171–1).

NEUROLOGIC FEATURES

Because of their early presentation with facial palsy and deafness, most of our patients were referred for neurosurgical attention by an ear, nose, and throat surgeon. The neurologic features of the condition are described in the light of our experience with these patients as well as information derived from the rest of these families in South Africa.[13]

Facial Palsy

Facial palsy is the earliest neurologic manifestation of this disorder. Unilateral facial palsy may be present at birth or may develop during the first year in about half the patients. Affected children suffer frequent attacks of facial paralysis that is clinically identical to Bell's palsy, but it progresses to complete, permanent facial paralysis in late childhood. This sequence of events is virtually characteristic of sclerosteosis. The disturbed facial nerve function may occur before hyperostosis of the petrous temporal bone is radiographically evident.

In adults, facial paralysis almost always occurs and is bilateral in about two thirds of patients. Decompression of

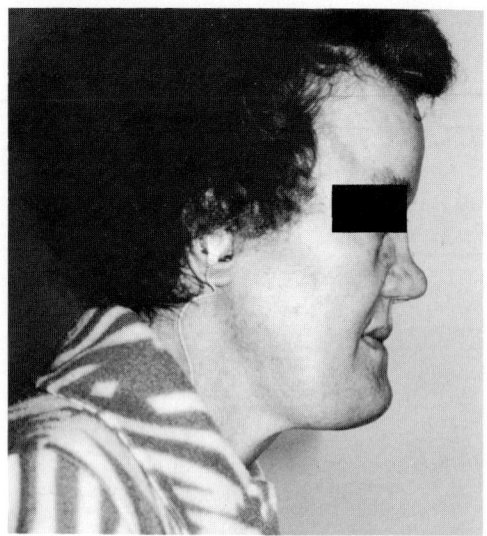

FIGURE 171–1. (Patient 18.) Note sulcus in frontotemporal region indicating edge of the prosthesis, which has reduced the prominence of the forehead. Mandibular prognathism, proptosis, and relative underdevelopment of central face is evident.

the facial nerve is carried out by the ear, nose, and throat surgeon and yields satisfactory results and may be of even greater value when undertaken prophylactically in young patients (Hamersma: Personal communication, 1993).

Deafness

Deafness is usually of a mixed conductive and perceptive type. Conductive hearing loss commences in childhood and results from impaired mobility of the middle ear ossicles and narrowing of the external auditory meatus. The use of a hearing aid is almost universal in adult patients. Deafness due to immobilization of the ossicular chain in the middle ear with bilateral conductive deafness was present in all 16 adults reported on by Beighton and colleagues.[2]

The perceptive hearing loss usually develops in the third decade but may occur much earlier and even concomitantly with the conductive hearing loss. The perceptive hearing loss results from compression of the vestibulocochlear nerve within the internal auditory canal or from interference with cochlear function at the oval or round windows. Operation for mobilization of the ossicles or opening of the oval or round window has now been abandoned because of rapidity of bone regrowth (Hamersma: Personal communication, 1993).

Optic Nerve Dysfunction

Optic nerve compression occurs late in sclerosteosis, in contrast to that occurring in patients with the autosomal recessive or malignant infantile form of osteopetrosis (Albers-Schönberg disease), in whom it is an early manifestation.

In our 19 neurosurgical patients, changes in the optic fundi included papilledema (in seven patients), optic atrophy (in two patients) and the presence of optociliary venous shunts (in five patients). Only one (patient 13) had severe visual loss (light perception only) at the time of her first operation at the age of 47.

Long-standing papilledema followed by consecutive atrophy, with or without added severe proptosis and optic nerve stretching, is undoubtedly a more potent cause of visual impairment than compression of the optic nerve in a narrowed optic canal. The complete relief of visual disturbances associated with papilledema by adequate decompressive craniotomy in our patients supports this view.

Blindness is uncommon in the South African families with sclerosteosis except as a complication of attempts at optic canal decompression for presumed but unproven compression—which occurred in two patients who were not included in this series. With magnetic resonance imaging (MRI), optic canal narrowing can be assessed more adequately than was possible in the past (Fig. 171–2).

Fifth Cranial Nerve Dysfunction

Impairment of sensation in the area of distribution of the first and second divisions of the trigeminal nerve was found in six of 25 patients in Beighton and colleagues' series[2] but was not of special concern to the patients. One middle-aged man did, however, have severe unilateral pain in the jaw that was suggestive of symptomatic trigeminal neuralgia. One of the patients in our series (patient 17) also had neuralgic trigeminal pain. Each of Klintworth's five patients with sclerosteosis had trigeminal sensory loss, and one patient had neuralgic unilateral facial pain.[14]

Olfactory Nerve Dysfunction

Olfactory nerve involvement was detected in one of the patients in our surgical group. Other South African patients did, however, have anosmia, a feature that two of Klintworth's five patients also demonstrated. At postmortem, bone

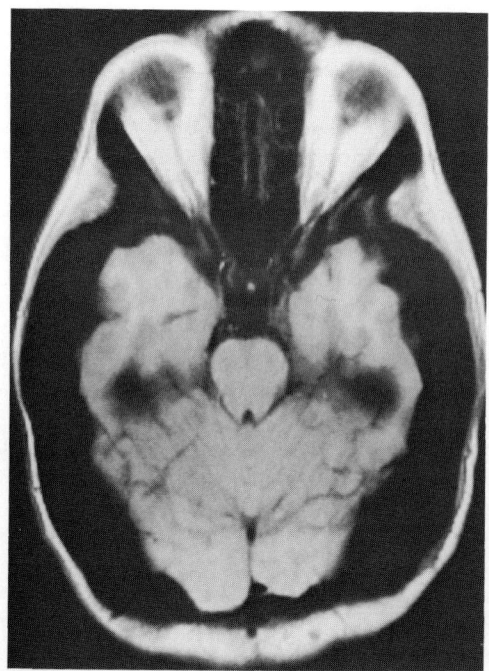

FIGURE 171–2. (Patient 16, Age 31.) MRI showing optic canal narrowing. Note surgical thinning of skull posteriorly immediately above the site of posterior fossa decompression.

overgrowth at the margin of the olfactory groove is often marked.

Dysfunction of Other Cranial Nerves

The lower cranial nerves (IX to XII) were not found to be affected in patients with sclerosteosis, probably indicating that their exits in the foramina are not involved in this condition, whereas deformity of the petrous bones occurs early and is gross; hence the early VIIth and VIIIth nerve involvement.

OTHER NEUROLOGIC FEATURES

Headache is a common complaint in young adults with sclerosteosis, and when it is associated with papilledema, it indicates the presence of raised intracranial pressure. Tonsillar impaction at the foramen magnum may be associated with episodes of severe occipital headache related to alterations in posture. Many individuals are known to have died suddenly in early adult life in a manner suggestive of acute medullary coning, and this finding has been substantiated at autopsy in several instances (patient 15).[5]

Intermittent cerebrospinal fluid (CSF) rhinorrhea may occur spontaneously and continue for years, thus serving to control the raised intracranial pressure. This situation occurred in our patient 15 and has also been observed in other patients in South Africa (personal communication). It may lead to meningitis and death, as in a patient documented by Stein and coworkers,[5] but this complication is uncommon.

Because many patients used to die from medullary compression in the second and third decades of life, the long-term sequelae of sclerosteosis are not well documented. Survival into old age without neurosurgical intervention is unusual, but a few cases have been reported.[15] The speed of progression of the disease is not of equal severity in all patients, which may explain these clinical variations.

Intellectually, affected persons are normal, but psychological problems are understandably common. Some of these patients are deeply disturbed by their grotesque appearance and shun the company of others, showing features of the Quasimodo complex. Most of them are, however, remarkably well adapted and have very pleasant personalities.

Spinal Nerve Root Compression

It used to be believed that the spine is relatively spared in this disease, but with cranial decompression lengthening survival, more patients may develop symptomatic spinal root compression. Two patients in the authors' series presented with spinal root compression. Bilateral pain and paresis in the arms attributed to cervical plexus involvement incapacitated one patient. In this individual (patient 17), operative decompression of the intervertebral foramina, where bone overgrowth had caused nerve root compression, partially relieved the symptoms.

Recurrent lumbar and cervical nerve root compression was successfully treated by repeated surgical decompression in one patient (patient 18) who also needed three craniocervical decompressions because of bone regrowth in the posterior fossa.

SURGICAL PATHOLOGY AND ANATOMY

On the basis of limited autopsy material, surgical observations, and radiologic studies, the surgical anatomy and pathology have been elucidated.

Hyperostosis may cause the vault to reach a thickness of more than 3 cm, with a loss of diploic structure and a marked increase in the external dimensions of the skull. The volume of the cranial cavity is progressively decreased as a result of internal encroachment of the thickened cranium, and the intracranial pressure consequently becomes elevated. The volume of the posterior fossa is gradually reduced by the thickening occipital squame, the foramen magnum is constricted, and chronic tonsillar herniation eventually occurs.[16]

The outer layer of the dura is densely adherent to the vault, which is deeply grooved by the small dural blood vessels (Fig. 171–3), with the intervening areas forming irregular nodular excrescences. The optic canals and lower cranial nerve exit foramina are not markedly involved in this process of bone encroachment.

The base of the skull shares in this bone overgrowth, and consequently, irregularity and deformity occur, particularly of the petrous bones. Early involvement of the petrous temporal bone may explain the sequence of the seventh, eighth and fifth cranial nerve involvement encountered clinically. A marked decrease in the dimensions of the foramen magnum also occurs.[16] The mandible increases in size and presents clinically as progressive asymmetric prognathism and dental malocclusion.

NEURORADIOLOGIC INVESTIGATION

Obtaining adequate-quality radiographs of a grossly thickened and extremely dense skull is very difficult (Fig. 171–4).[17] The patient may be exposed to massive doses of radiation with little hope of adequately demonstrating the required detail.

The increase in thickness and density of the vault and the

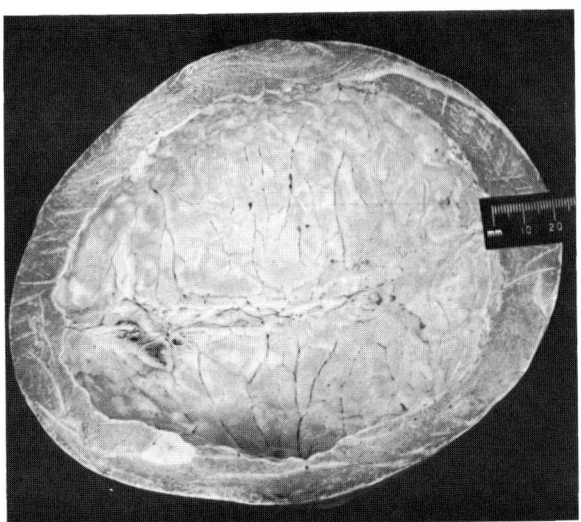

FIGURE 171–3. Inner aspect of a postmortem specimen of the vault of the skull. Note the deep grooving by meningeal vessels and bony protuberances between vessels.

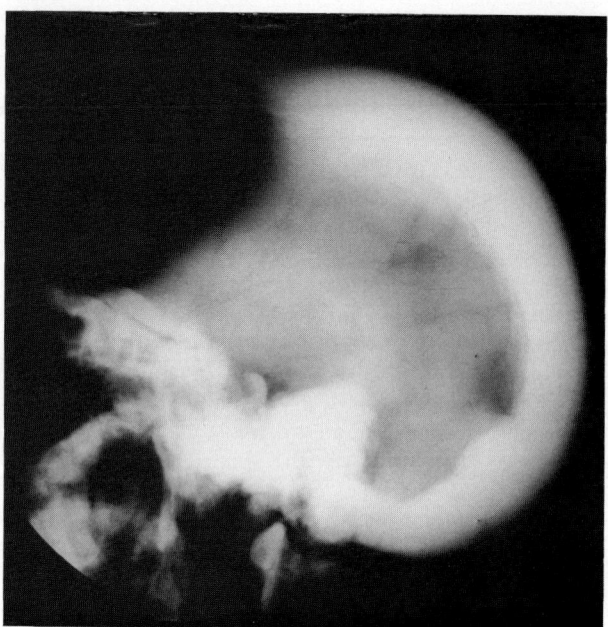

FIGURE 171–4. (Patient 18.) Skull x-ray study, lateral view. Note frontal craniotomy. Clear vascular markings are apparent despite density of skull. There is marked sclerosis and irregularity of the petrous bone.

thickening of the occipital squame and encroachment into the posterior fossa are not difficult to demonstrate. However, little information is gained about the size of the foramen magnum, except in younger patients with lesser skull density, in whom a basal view proves useful. Tomography was used to demonstrate detail in younger patients in the past, but this technology has been superseded by computed tomography (CT) and MRI.

COMPUTED TOMOGRAPHY

Skull views show an increase in cranial thickness, and bone windows demonstrate an increase in bone density. The ventricles and basal cisterns appear compressed, and the CSF spaces over the convexities are obliterated (Fig. 171–5). The prominent crista frontalis, bony overgrowth in the posterior fossa, and distortion of the foramen magnum are significant diagnostic features for the surgeon. The bony thickening in the posterior fossa may, however, produce too much artifact to allow clear definition of the cranial outlet. Regrowth of bone after frontal or posterior fossa decompressive surgery is best shown by CT (Fig. 171–6).

MAGNETIC RESONANCE IMAGING

MRI is the investigation of choice in patients with sclerosteosis because the thickened bone does not interfere with the soft tissue image. Bone thickness, size of the optic foramina, dimensions of the cranial outlet, and tonsillar herniation can be demonstrated with ease with MRI (Fig. 171–7). The deformation of the compressed cortex and the size of the ventricles and basal cisterns are also clearly shown. The slight degree of optic canal narrowing present in sclerosteosis has been demonstrated for the first time by means of MRI (see Fig. 171–2).

In the infant presenting with facial paralysis, a plain radiograph of the skull shows increased density of the base. The diagnostic investigation of choice is MRI, but early bone regrowth at the site of the decompression is best shown by CT.

PATIENT SELECTION

The 19 patients included in this study were selected for surgical management from the families described by Beighton and associates,[7] de Villiers and colleagues,[10] and du Plessis.[11] Fourteen patients were treated at the H.F. Verwoerd Hospital in Pretoria, South Africa between 1977 and 1991, and six were treated at Groote Schuur Hospital in Cape Town between 1977 and 1992. One (patient 2) was treated at both institutions. Only one (patient 1) was lost to follow-up 7 years after his last operation. Sixty-four neurosurgical procedures were performed on these 19 patients (Table 171–1).

No ancestral history of the disease could be obtained, and it is assumed that all affected persons were the offspring of asymptomatic heterozygous carriers of the faulty gene.

Eleven females and eight males were in the series, and the mean age was 24 years (range, 14 to 47 years) at the time of their first neurosurgical procedure (Table 171–2). Most patients were referred by ear, nose, and throat surgeons who had treated them for unilateral or bilateral peripheral facial nerve palsy and hearing loss.

All patients were taller than 1.8 m and had generalized bony overgrowth, mainly of the calvarium and mandible, with proptosis, malalignment of the teeth, and craniomegaly (see Fig. 171–1). Examination revealed cutaneous or bony syndactyly of the index and middle fingers with radial devia-

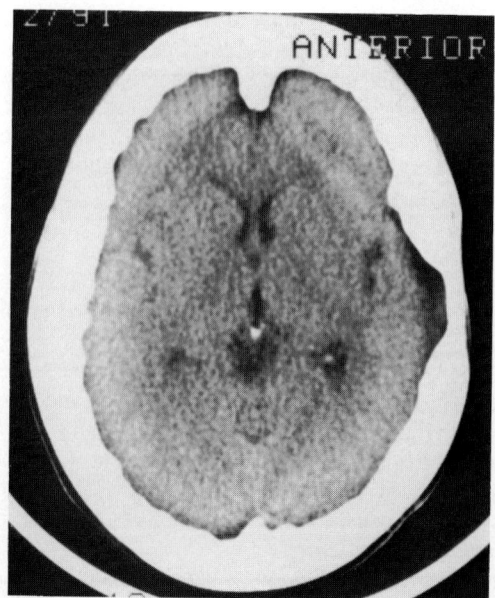

FIGURE 171–5. (Patient 5.) CT showing increased thickness of the skull with irregularity of the inner surface closely applied to the brain, obliteration of surface CSF spaces, and ventricular compression. Note prominent crista frontalis.

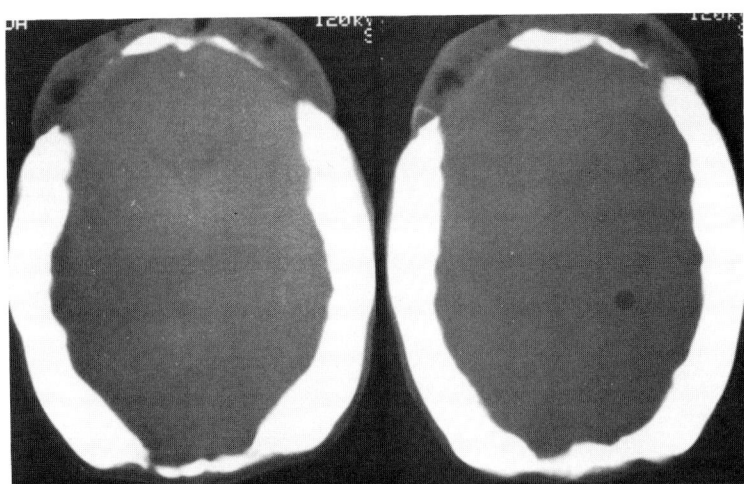

FIGURE 171-6. (Patient 16.) CT scan at two levels showing bone regrowth at sites of frontal and posterior fossa decompressions.

tion in 10 patients and some form of nail dystrophy of the fingers or toes in all of them.

CHOICE OF SURGICAL APPROACH

Surgery for this condition has mostly been directed at the temporal bone. Decompression of the facial nerve is the operation most commonly performed and is very effective in the management of facial paralysis, particularly if performed prophylactically in young patients. Mobilization of the auditory ossicles has been abandoned as a fruitless exercise because of bone regrowth (Hamersma: Personal communication, 1993).

Very few reports regarding the neurosurgical management of sclerosteosis and related disorders have been published.[5, 10, 11, 17] Unilateral parietal craniectomy to relieve raised intracranial pressure in a patient with Van Buchem's disease was performed by Dott in 1929.[18]

Klintworth[15] reported the difficulties encountered in performing a craniotomy on an extremely dense skull (2 to 3 cm thick) in a patient with Albers-Schönberg disease. These problems and surgical methods employed in the similar condition of craniometaphyseal dysplasia are well described by Millard and colleagues[19] and Faconi and colleagues.[20] Millard and colleagues[19] suggested that foramen magnum decompression should be performed as a first procedure if any degree of tonsillar herniation exists in a patient with metaphyseal dysplasia.

Decompression of the optic canal has been described fairly frequently in patients suffering from craniotubular bone disorders that produce optic nerve compression.[17] In the South African patients with sclerosteosis, proven optic nerve compression is rare, and when decompression of the nerve has been attempted, complete loss of vision on the operated side has ensued. Optic nerve decompression was not undertaken in any patient in the present series.

Bifrontal craniotomy, with removal of the bone flap to create a decompression, has the beneficial effect of relieving headache and reducing papilledema, particularly in younger patients. This operation was first performed in Pretoria, where sclerosteosis was first investigated extensively. Because some patients still died as a result of medullary coning despite a frontal decompression, the need for a craniocervical decompressive procedure became obvious, and this procedure was first performed in Cape Town in 1977.[10]

Which operation should be performed, for whom, and which operation should be performed first? In our experience, patients with severe headache, particularly in the occipital region, should be considered for decompression. If papilledema is present, operation is imperative. In adults with marked bony encroachment into the posterior fossa, a craniocervical decompression is indicated to prevent medullary

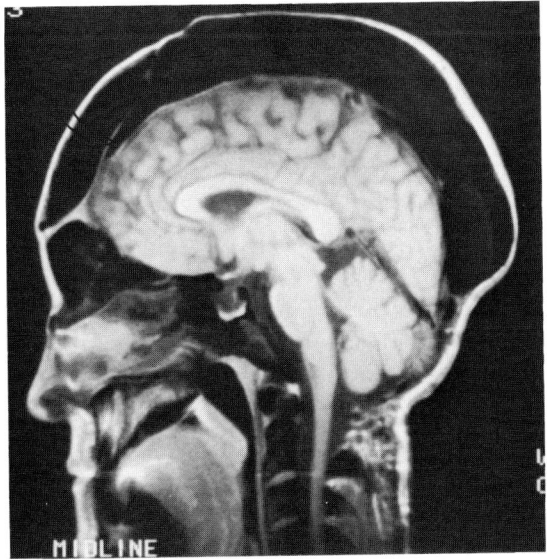

FIGURE 171-7. (Patient 16.) Sagittal MRI showing cerebral anatomic detail. Note relationships at foramen magnum and bone regrowth under frontal prosthesis (arrow).

Table 171-1. NEUROSURGICAL PROCEDURES PERFORMED ON 19 PATIENTS

Bifrontal decompressive craniotomy	15
Bifrontal-temporal decompressive craniotomy	5
Craniocervical decompressive craniectomy	26
Decompressive lumbar laminectomy	5
Decompressive cervical laminectomy	5
Cerebrospinal fluid diversions	8
Total	64

Table 171–2. SUMMARY CHARACTERISTICS, TREATMENT, AND OUTCOME OF 19 PATIENTS WITH SCLEROSTEOSIS

Case No.	Sex	Age at First Operation (yr)	Present Age (yr)	Surgical Procedure/Month + Year		Complications	Clinical Outcome
1	F	18	—	Ant fossa dec	6/77		
				Post fossa dec	8/77		
				L5-S1 laminectomy	4/82		
				L1-L5 laminectomy	2/86		Lost to follow-up
2	M	14	29	Post fossa dec	2/78		
				Ant fossa dec	11/78	Subcutaneous CSF	
				LP shunt	4/84	Postural headaches	LP shunt removed
				Bifrontotemporal dec	4/91		Asymptomatic after last operation
3	F	15	0	Ant fossa dec	6/81		
				Post fossa dec	6/82	Pseudomeningocele	Shunt removed 8/82
				LP shunt	6/82	Postural headaches	Sudden death 8/91 at age 25, 1 day postoperatively
				Post fossa dec	8/91		
4	M	18	29	Post fossa dec	7/82		
				Ant fossa dec	11/86		
				LP shunt	12/86	Postural headaches	Shunt removed Good outcome
5	M	9	20	Post fossa dec	7/82		
				Ant fossa dec	1/86	Subcutaneous CSF	
				LP shunt	12/86	Postural headaches	
				Bifrontotemporal dec	12/91		Good outcome
6	F	16	0	Post fossa dec	7/82	Fatal cardiac arrest 1 day postoperatively	Died at age 16
7	F	19	29	Ant fossa dec	4/83	Subcutaneous CSF	
				Post fossa dec	7/83		
				LP shunt	1/84	Postural headaches Shunt removed	Good outcome
8	M	22	31	Post fossa dec	3/84		
				Ant fossa dec	10/84		
				Bifrontotemporal dec	11/91		
				Post fossa dec	12/91		Good outcome
9	F	21	29	Ant fossa dec	2/85	Subcutaneous CSF	
				Post fossa dec	7/85		
				Bifrontotemporal dec	2/89		
				Post fossa dec	8/91		Emotional disturbances
10	M	19	26	Post fossa dec	6/85	CSF leak	
				LP shunt	5/86		Good outcome
11	F	20	25	Ant fossa dec	7/88	Osteitis	Prosthesis removed
				Post fossa dec	11/88	Difficult laryngeal intubation	
				Bifrontotemporal dec	7/91		Good outcome
12	F	33	38	Ant fossa dec	2/88		
				Post fossa dec + cisternoatrial shunt	4/88	Persistent headaches	Intellect subnormal
13	F	47	49	Ant fossa dec	9/91	Sagittal sinus laceration Bacterial meningitis Intracerebral hematoma	Blind and deaf
14	M	16	18	Ant fossa dec	4/91		
				Post fossa dec	5/91		Good outcome
15	M	33	0	Post fossa dec	3/77	CSF rhinorrhea	Complete relief of headache and papilledema. Bone regrowth. Died of medullary coning at 3 ½ years postoperatively

Table 171–2. SUMMARY CHARACTERISTICS, TREATMENT, AND OUTCOME OF 19 PATIENTS WITH SCLEROSTEOSIS *(Continued)*

Case No.	Sex	Age at First Operation (yr)	Present Age (yr)	Surgical Procedure/Month + Year		Complications	Clinical Outcome
16	F	16	31	Post fossa dec	2/78	Persistent papilledema	Socially well adapted
				Ant fossa dec	11/81	Subcutaneous CSF	
				LP shunt	10/82		Married, 2 children
				Post fossa dec	1/86		
				Reduce mandible	10/89		
				Reduce nasal bridge	2/90		Vision normal
17	M	33	54	Cervical laminectomy	/72	Arm pain	Persistent right arm pain
				Jaw reduction	/73	Persistent pain in right arm	
				Cervical laminectomy	10/79		
				Cervical laminectomy C5–C6	3/86		
18	F	37	56	Ant fossa dec	/74	Posttraumatic epilepsy	Hearing impaired
				Jaw reduction			Bilateral facial palsy
				Post fossa dec	8/79		Gross skeletal deformity
				Lumbar laminectomy for spinal stenosis	6/81	Bony regrowth	Lives independent life
				Lumbar laminectomy for spinal stenosis	7/83		
				Post fossa dec	1/84	Bony regrowth	
				Post fossa dec	10/88	Bony regrowth	
				C4–C5 laminectomy	8/90		
				Lumbar stenosis laminectomy	8/91		
19	F	40	51	Post fossa dec	9/82	Wound breakdown and resuture	Slight hearing loss Minimal facial weakness
				Post fossa dec	9/88	Bony regrowth	Fully employed

Ant fossa dec = anterior fossa decompressive craniotomy and placement of acrylic prosthesis; Bifrontotemporal dec = bifrontotemporal decompressive craniotomy; CSF = cerebrospinal fluid; D = dead; LP shunt = lumbar peritoneal shunt; Post fossa dec = posterior fossa decompressive craniectomy; Subcut CSF = subcutaneous cerebrospinal fluid collection.

coning, and to a lesser extent, it may reduce generalized raised intracranial pressure. In younger patients, a frontal decompression may not only be more effective in reducing raised intracranial pressure but may also be safer and easier to undertake than in adults. Indeed, frontal decompression may be indicated prophylactically in younger patients with this disorder, but craniocervical decompression, sooner rather than later, is essential to prevent medullary coning.

A posterior fossa decompressive craniectomy, combined with a C1 laminectomy and opening of the dura mater, is performed prophylactically, preferably after the supratentorial compartment has been adequately decompressed, even in asymptomatic young patients. In older patients, the posterior fossa decompression may be undertaken without prior frontal craniectomy, particularly if they do not have papilledema.

Because patients with sclerosteosis are not encountered frequently, they may be denied the benefit of surgical relief of a condition that may be life threatening. Surgical decompression of the craniocervical region is a lengthy and tedious procedure that yields very gratifying results but may have to be repeated as bone regrowth causes recurrent problems in later years.

ANESTHETIC CONSIDERATIONS

Anesthetic management poses unique problems because overgrowth of the mandible and inability to open the mouth widely may make laryngeal intubation difficult, if not impossible. A fiber optic laryngoscope has been used successfully in these patients.[21] The heavy, broadened ribs, scapulae, and claviculae in these patients cause decreased pulmonary compliance, and appropriate ventilator adjustments are necessary to ensure satisfactory intraoperative ventilation.[22]

Because these patients are of above-average height, an extension to the operating table may have to be devised to accommodate them. Because of their massive build, the risks of pressure sores developing as a result of immobilization during a lengthy operation demand special attention to pressure points, particularly of the scalp on a standard skull support. Most affected persons have proptosis and facial palsy; therefore, protection of the eyes against exposure keratitis and cleaning agents used on the scalp is mandatory.

Most adult patients have hearing difficulty without their hearing aids, and if this fact is not kept in mind, it may cause concern when the patients' level of consciousness is assessed in the recovery room.

AIDS TO SURGERY

INSTRUMENTATION

A three-pronged head support is used routinely to prevent pressure necrosis of the scalp. A Hall air drill with a rotary rasp is indispensable. Because of the increased bone density in these patients, bone-cutting instruments are rapidly blunted; therefore, replacements should be immediately available.

SURGICAL TECHNIQUE

Eventually, most patients with sclerosteosis require otologic procedures for facial palsy. These procedures are usually very successful, particularly if performed early or electively, and after the age of 20, the risks of bone regrowth and recurrent facial palsy are reduced. Surgery of the auditory ossicles and oval window has been abandoned, but opening of the narrowed external auditory meatus is useful (Hamersma: Personal communication, 1993). Cosmetic surgery for facial and mandibular deformity provides some improvement in facial appearance and can be of great psychological benefit.

FRONTAL DECOMPRESSION

A generous bifrontal decompressive craniotomy has yielded the best results as the initial procedure to control progressively rising intracranial pressure resulting from bony overgrowth of the calvarium and skull base. The frontal sinus is preferably not included in the flap, and the large bony defect is covered with a thin acrylic prosthesis.

The use of standard neurosurgical power instruments calls for adjustments of technique because the thickness of the bone is such that ordinary drill bits are too short to reach the dura at the first attempt at bone perforation. Problems are experienced with standard craniotomes because the density of the bone tends to damage power-driven instruments. One of the authors (du Plessis) has used a Hudson brace and bits for the craniotomy.

Two large burr holes adjacent to one another without any intervening bone make the angle through which the saw guide must pass less acute and decrease the chance of dural laceration and harmful compression of the underlying brain. The crista frontalis, which is often large and space occupying (see Fig. 171–5), is drilled away, and care is taken not to enter the paranasal sinuses. Fortunately, these structures were not prominent in any patient in this series.

With power tools, the burr holes are made to the maximum depth of the bit. The superficial bone is smoothed away with a rotary rasp to the depth of the burr holes, and new burr holes are sunk from this level to the dura. The normal procedure is then followed in a young patient.

Dural hitching sutures are no longer used because their use was associated with subcutaneous CSF collections. Because the dura mater is invariably tightly adherent to the bone, such sutures are superfluous; as proof of this, postoperative extradural hematomas were not encountered when these sutures were no longer used.

The tight adherence of the dura to the bone carries with it the risk of dural transgression when the bone is perforated. Because the cortex is tightly applied to the dura, dural transgression results in cortical damage, with a consequent risk of posttraumatic epilepsy.

Intraoperative complications were related to the thickness and density of the bone. Patient 13 had the thickest bone (38 mm) and at 47 was the oldest patient who came to frontal surgery. She developed numerous complications: laceration of a venous lacuna, which necessitated blood transfusion; postoperative meningitis, which was treated successfully; and a postdecompression intracerebral hematoma, which was managed conservatively.

Postoperative CSF leakage or accumulation is a constant risk because of the poor dural tissues, particularly in older patients.

Results

Frontal craniotomy relieves raised intracranial pressure effectively, as demonstrated by loss of headache and papilledema. Loss of optociliary shunts has also been demonstrated, as in the cases of Stein and coworkers.[5]

POSTERIOR FOSSA DECOMPRESSION

Posterior fossa decompressions are prolonged, tedious, and arduous and can take a heavy toll on surgical instruments.

Scalp Incision

A high, cross-bow incision is made with the horizontal part almost at the lambdoid suture to safeguard the blood supply to the flap and to allow shelving of the upper margin of the decompression, which reduces the prominent ridge left after removing 3 to 4 cm of bone. The vertical limb extends downward in the midline to the spinous process of C3. Superficial scalp flaps are raised from the horizontal incision downward and turned laterally. The superior nuchal line is exposed, and a horizontal incision is made through the cervical fascia just below it, leaving a fringe of fascia attached to the pericranium to facilitate wound closure. Pericranium is then elevated above the superior nuchal line and held laterally. The midline incision is extended downward, between the occipital muscle attachments to the upper two cervical spinous processes, and muscle is cleared from these structures. In this way, a wide exposure of the occipital bone and craniocervical junction is obtained.

Perforation of the Bone

As many burr holes as possible are made to the maximum depth allowed by the craniotome bits (Fig. 171–8). Using a craniotome with a rotary rasp, the bridges of bone between the burr holes are smoothed away until a new plane is created at the level of the maximum depth of the burr holes. The edges of the decompression are shelved so that a smooth junction is formed with the normal bone. This process of sinking burr holes and smoothing away the intervening bridges of bone is repeated until a burr hole encounters the dura; this event usually occurs when the third series of burr holes is made. At the occipital protuberance, where the bone is at its thickest and hardest, more burr holes are necessary.

At the dural level, troublesome hemorrhage may occur from small dural vessels that deeply groove the bone. This dense adherence of the dura is a very real problem, except in younger patients. Careful use of the rotary rasp, as well as

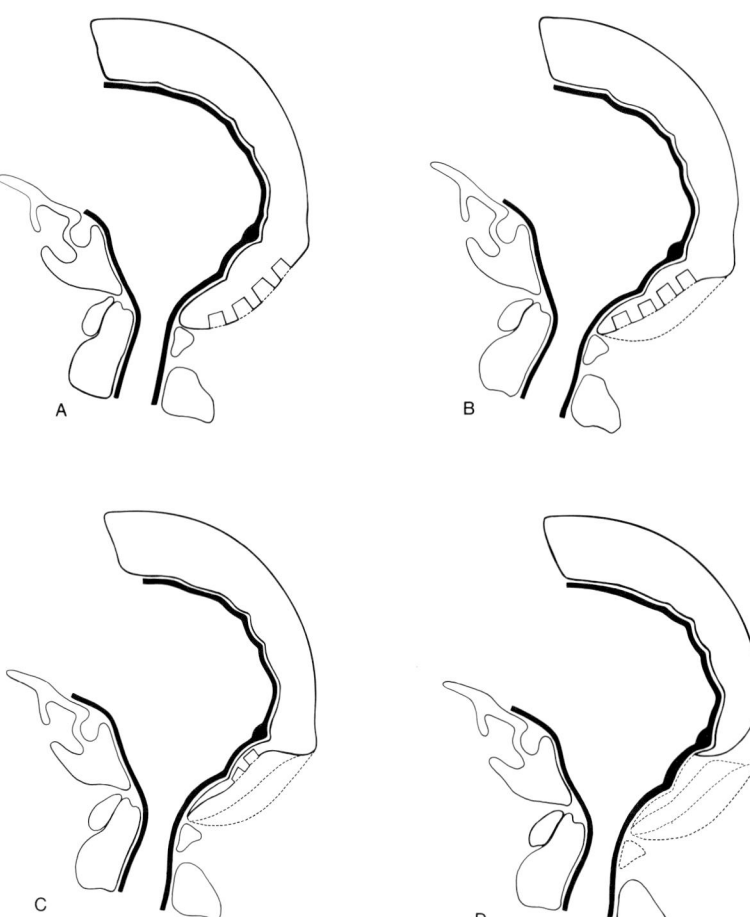

FIGURE 171–8. Posterior fossa decompression. (A) First series of burr holes in occipital squama. (B) Removal of bone bridges, and sinking of the second series of burr holes from the new plane obtained. (C) Repetition of step (B), and third set of burr holes have been sunk. (D) Removal of remaining bone to expose the dura and open the foramen magnum. Arch of atlas is removed, and bone at edges of decompression is shelved.

diamond drills of various sizes, allows fragments of bone to be removed by use of small Kerrison punches. Bone is removed meticulously, fragment by fragment, until a wide decompression of the posterior fossa is obtained. A chisel must not be employed to smooth away bone, because of the risk of a concussive effect on the compromised medulla in the foramen magnum.

Two points require emphasis:

1. A wide removal of the rim of the foramen magnum and arch of the atlas to decompress the underlying dural sac must be obtained. A diamond drill is indispensable for this purpose. In our first patient (patient 15) treated in Cape Town, the arch of the atlas was not removed, and the patient died of medullary coning three and a half years later, with bone regrowth in the posterior fossa dura.

2. The upper part of the posterior fossa decompression should not extend above the lateral sinus, because backward displacement of the sinus, with kinking and compression, could have disastrous results.

Intraoperative Problems

Hemorrhage from the dura is easily controlled with bipolar diathermy, and in cases in which a CSF leak has occurred through torn dura, it has never proved troublesome postoperatively if superficial wound closure was performed meticulously.

Closure of the lower half of the wound offers no great difficulty, but the gap between the bone and the upper ridge of the muscle has posed a problem. Because about 3 cm of bone thickness has been lost in the decompression and the margin has been bevelled, the muscle tends to fall inward postoperatively, leaving a horizontal sulcus at the nuchal line. This sulcus can be adequately covered if the patient's hair is long, but it poses a cosmetic problem that has no easy solution.

Postoperative care does not demand anything more than is required after any posterior fossa exploration.

Postoperative Complications

There was no postoperative morbidity, and patients experienced little discomfort from the large scalp incision. Only in one (patient 19) did wound breakdown that required resuture occur.

Symptoms and signs suggestive of medullary "slumping" occurred postoperatively in two patients after posterior fossa decompression with removal of the arch of the atlas; both patients died. Patient 3 had had a bifrontal decompression years earlier but redeveloped raised intracranial pressure. In patient 6, the posterior fossa decompression was performed before bifrontal decompressive surgery. Both of these patients died within 24 hours after operation, having been alert and neurologically intact immediately on recovery from the anesthetic. They developed sudden cardiovascular collapse after endotracheal suction in the intensive care unit before extubation. Postmortem examination confirmed downward displacement of the brainstem and signs of pressure necrosis in the lower medulla oblongata.

One of the earlier patients (patient 18) developed an area of pressure necrosis of the scalp in the frontal region, but this problem healed without difficulty. A three-pronged head support has been used for all posterior fossa decompression ever since.

One patient (patient 17) developed persistent arm pain and the features of craniocervical junction compression or syringomyelia. Myelography showed the cerebellar tonsils to be displaced downward to the level of C3. Reoperation was carried out, and an adequate craniocervical decompression was undertaken, particularly of the arch of the atlas. The patient improved for a time, but he later had a first-rib excision for a suspected thoracic outlet compression at another institution.

CSF fistula or pseudomeningocele after posterior fossa surgery might be expected because of dural laceration, but in adults, if wound closure is adequate, this complication is rare. Patient 10 (aged 19 years) developed a CSF fistula through the posterior fossa incision, but this condition resolved after a lumboperitoneal shunt was inserted. It became evident that once raised intracranial pressure was relieved by bifrontal craniotomy, posterior fossa surgery could be performed safely and with little risk of postoperative CSF accumulation or fistula formation. All new patients operated on since 1985 have had a bifrontal decompression as an initial procedure.

Results

The two adult patients with marked papilledema completely lost this feature within weeks of a wide posterior fossa decompression. One of these individuals had had a frontal decompression years earlier. Two young patients (aged 2 and 16 years) required bifrontal craniotomies after their posterior fossa decompression to relieve their headache and papilledema. Older patients were dramatically relieved of headache by craniocervical decompression.

One patient (patient 15) who lived about 300 km from Cape Town died suddenly 3 years after surgery in an episode that suggested medullary coning. He had repeated spells of headache and decline in consciousness associated with difficulty in breathing, from which he would recover as soon as he was placed in a sitting position. He died during such a manifestation. At postmortem, bone was found to have regrown in the dura at the foramen magnum. He was the first patient on whom a posterior fossa decompression had been performed, and the arch of the atlas had not been removed.

RECURRENT BONE OVERGROWTH

Recurrent bone overgrowth is a constant postoperative risk in this proliferative bone disorder and follows frontal or posterior fossa decompression. In adults who have had transotic decompression of the seventh nerve, bone regeneration does not seem to occur, but in children, some regrowth of the abnormal bone has been encountered.[15] Some investigators have suggested that osteoblastic activity decreases after the third decade of life, but this seems not to be the case in all patients, because bone regrowth is extremely active in some adults. Patients who developed recurrent raised intracranial pressure after previous decompressive surgery invariably showed signs of bony regrowth in the dura under the frontal prosthesis and in the posterior fossa dura (see Figs. 171–6 and 171–7). Patient 18 had to undergo three posterior fossa decompressions and three lumbar laminectomies between the ages of 42 and 55 years.

Nine of our patients developed symptoms of progressive elevation of intracranial pressure after bifrontal and posterior fossa decompressions as a result of continuous bone proliferation. This process took between 3 and 13 years to occur (average, 6.6 years), indicating that the tendency for bone proliferation varies widely from patient to patient.

Another patient (patient 19) suffered recurrence of headache and vertigo 4 years after her craniocervical decompression. Tomography showed reformation of bone at the level of the arch of C1, which was confirmed at re-exploration. After removal of the new bone, she was greatly improved.

If the posterior fossa dura ossifies after surgery, the surgeon must ascertain whether or not the condition is associated with raised pressure in the supratentorial compartment before reoperating. Failure to follow this procedure was probably the cause of death in patient 3. Relief of the raised pressure by first carrying out a frontal decompression may have averted this mishap.

Where bone has regrown, it must be surgically removed at the site of previous frontal or posterior decompressions. The new bone tends to be thinner and somewhat softer than the surrounding bone, and the dura has usually thickened in the interim.

Reoperation was performed in the frontal region in five patients. The frontal prosthesis was easily separated from the underlying new bone, which was then removed without difficulty, after which the prosthesis could be replaced. Bitemporal craniectomies have been added to create extra intracranial space in five patients; satisfactory results have been achieved, but the follow-up period is short. Unilateral subtemporal decompression should be avoided because it may lead to midline shift.

CEREBROSPINAL FLUID DIVERSIONARY PROCEDURES

Early in our series of patients, CSF diversionary procedures were used in the management of CSF collection that followed frontal decompressive operations. Ventriculoperitoneal shunting could not be employed because of the small size of the ventricles. Seven patients had lumboperitoneal shunts, and one had a cisternoatrial shunt. Four shunts had to be removed because of complaints of postural headaches, and it is uncertain whether the shunts in the asymptomatic patients are still functional. No CSF diversionary procedures have been performed since 1986, and none were performed on patients who have had posterior decompression.

DECOMPRESSIVE LAMINECTOMY

Three patients presented with symptoms and signs of nerve root compression due to bone overgrowth (patients 1,

17, and 18). One had cervical problems only (patient 17), one had lumbar problems (patient 1), and one had cervical and lumbar symptoms and signs. Despite adequate and effective decompression in the first instance, all three patients had recurrence of bone overgrowth at the site of operation that necessitated repeated surgery.

The thickness and density of the bone render the standard laminectomy instruments inadequate for the task. The bone has to be drilled away with cutting burrs, and the individual nerve root exposure is performed with diamond drills.

No operative or postoperative complications were encountered. Bone regrowth is the major problem, but reoperation is no more difficult than the primary operation.

Results

The root compression symptoms and signs, whether cervical or lumbar, were relieved by decompression. Recurrence of symptoms, even as early as 1 year postoperatively, required repeated surgery in the few patients subjected to laminectomy.

DISCUSSION

No medical treatment exists for sclerosteosis. Surgical decompression of the facial nerves alleviates symptoms in some patients,[13] but middle ear surgery for conductive deafness does not seem to provide any benefit (Hamersma: Personal communication, 1993).

The risk of sudden death, even at a young age, due to medullary compression at the cranial outlet during episodes of acute rises in intracranial pressure, such as that caused by coughing or straining, is present in all these patients.[23] The major cause of morbidity and mortality in this condition is a progressive elevation of intracranial pressure, of which the more obvious effects are a deterioration in vision and, at times, intellectual impairment.

From our experience, we believe that frontal decompression should be routinely performed in all patients, preferably shortly after puberty, even if they are asymptomatic. The advantage of early surgical intervention is that the cranial bone is still relatively soft and not yet at its maximum thickness. Furthermore, the dura mater has not become atrophic and involved in the newly formed bone. Thus, it is easier to keep the dura intact, and the risks of brain injury, postoperative brain swelling, intracerebral hemorrhage, and subcutaneous CSF accumulation are reduced. Reduction in operating time also reduces the risk of sepsis.

Posterior fossa decompression for generalized raised intracranial pressure is still a controversial topic, about which the neurosurgical literature provides little information. It is a common neurosurgical observation that patients who suffer recurrence of a posterior fossa tumor will develop headache and papilledema only at a relatively late stage, even if the dura is closed at the time of the first operation. Horsley[24] showed that removal of the occipital squame, leaving the dura intact, could relieve intracranial pressure for prolonged periods. Cushing[25] disputed this point, but Spiller and Frazier[26] confirmed Horsley's findings. More recently, this procedure has been performed, but infrequently, for severe benign intracranial hypertension.[27]

In our experience, posterior fossa decompression should be performed in patients with sclerosteosis to relieve crowding at the cranial outlet and thus reduce the risk of medullary coning. Although papilledema was relieved in a few of our adult patients, this is not its main indication—it is a prophylactic operation. However, the early postoperative deaths of two of our patients indicate that craniocervical decompression as the first procedure in patients with raised intracranial pressure may result in downward herniation of the lower brainstem and tonsils. We therefore advocate bifrontal craniectomy as the first operation in all patients.

We considered the application of sclerosing agents to the dura to prevent regrowth of bone, but this method is not practicable, because the dura is so diaphanous and fenestrated after bone removal.

A maximum postoperative follow-up period of 15 years in the management of patients with sclerosteosis has shown the value of these operative procedures. In particular, survival of patients into the fifth decade strongly supports the impression that medullary coning is prevented by craniocervical decompression. The disappearance of papilledema and the apparent prevention of consecutive atrophy and visual failure speak for the success of decompressive craniotomy.

SUMMARY

Cranial surgery for sclerosteosis should be performed early in adolescence and should commence with frontal decompression to relieve raised intracranial pressure and provide space at the cranial outlet. Careful follow-up is essential for detection of bone regrowth in the dura at the sites of decompression, the existence of which is an indication for reoperation.

The neurologic effects of vertebral overgrowth may also require decompression, and this procedure may also have to be repeated after bone regrowth.

Patients with sclerosteosis have many surgical encounters—at times, of a serious nature—and to guide them through their surgical vicissitudes, a relationship of trust and understanding must be established between surgeon, patient, and relatives. The surgery is demanding, but the processes of patient management are rewarding.

Acknowledgments

The authors would like to thank Dr. P. Beighton for advice, instruction, education, and help with this manuscript; Dr. H. Hamersma for his enthusiasm for operating on these patients, his referral of patients, and his encouragement; and Dr. N. Legg for advice and constructive criticism in the preparation of this manuscript. We would also like to thank Miss C. Small for patiently typing and retyping the manuscript, and the Medical Graphics Unit for photographic and art work.

REFERENCES

1. Beighton P: Sclerosteosis. J Med Genet 25:200–203, 1988
2. Beighton P, Cremin BJ, Hamersma H: The radiology of sclerosteosis. Br J Radiol 49:934–939, 1976

3. Higinbotham NL, Alexander SF: Osteopetrosis, four cases in one family. Am J Surg 53:444–454, 1941
4. Siguira Y, Yasuhara T: Sclerosteosis. J Bone Joint Surg Br 40B:208–218, 1975
5. Stein SA, Witkop C, Hills S, et al: Sclerosteosis: Neurogenetic and pathophysiological analysis of an American kinship. Neurology 33:267–277, 1983
6. McCleary L, Rovit RL, Murali R: Case report: Myelopathy secondary to congenital osteopetrosis of the cervical spine. Neurosurgery 20:487–489, 1987
7. Beighton P, Hamersma H: Sclerosteosis in South Africa. S Afr Med J 55:783–788, 1979
8. Van Buchem FSP, Haddens HN, Ubbens R: An uncommon familial systemic disease of the skeleton: Hyperostosis corticalis generalisata familiaris. Acta Radiol 41:109–119, 1955
9. Van Buchem FSP: The pathogenesis of hyperostosis corticalis generalisata and calcitonin. Koninkl Ned Akad Wetenschappen 73(3):243–253, 1970
10. de Villiers JC, Barnard AH, Beighton PH, Hamersma H: Craniocervical decompression for cranio-tubular bone dysplasias. Neurochirurgia (Stuttg) (suppl):118, 1981
11. du Plessis JJ: Sclerosteosis: Neurosurgical experience with fourteen cases. J Neurosurg 78:388–392, 1993
12. Epstein S, Hamersma H, Beighton P: Endocrine function in sclerosteosis. S Afr Med J 55:1105–1110, 1979
13. Beighton P, Durr L, Hamersma H: The clinical features of sclerosteosis: A review of the manifestations in twenty-five affected individuals. Ann Intern Med 84:393–397, 1976
14. Klintworth GK: The neurologic manifestations of osteopetrosis (Albers-Schönberg's disease). Neurology 13:512–519, 1963
15. Barnard AH, Hamersma H, Kretzmar JH, Beighton P: Sclerosteosis in old age. S Afr Med J 58:401–403, 1980
16. Hamersma H: Osteopetrosis (marble bone disease) of the temporal bone. Laryngoscope 80:1518–1539, 1970
17. Kirkpatrick DB, Rimoin DL, Kaitila I, Gordon SJ: The craniotubular bone modeling disorders: A neurosurgical introduction to rare skeletal dysplasias with cranial nerve compression. Surg Neurol 7:221–232, 1977
18. Dixon JM, Cull RE, Gamble P: Two cases of Van Buchem's disease. J Neurol Neurosurg Psychiatry 45:913–918, 1982
19. Millard DR, Maisel DO, Batstone JHF, Yates BW: Craniofacial surgery in craniometaphyseal dysplasia. Am J Surg 113:615–621, 1967
20. Faconi S, Fischer J, Wieland P, et al: Craniometaphyseal dysplasia with increased bone turnovers and secondary hyperparathyroidism: Therapeutic effect of calcitonin. J Pediatr 112:587–591, 1988
21. Geyser PG, Hugo JM, Ingram H: Anaesthetic management in sclerosteosis. A case report. S Afr Med J 61:488, 1982
22. Siguira Y, Yasuhara T: Sclerosteosis. J Bone Joint Surg Am 57A:273–276, 1975
23. Beighton P, Davidson J, Durr L, Hamersma H: Sclerosteosis—An autosomal recessive disorder. Clin Genet 11:1–7, 1977
24. Horsley V: Discussion on the treatment of cerebral tumours. BMJ 2:1365–1369, 1893
25. Cushing H: The establishment of cerebral hernia as a decompressive measure for inaccessible brain tumours; with the description of intermuscular methods of making the bone defect in temporal and occipital regions. Surg Gynecol Obstet 1:297–314, 1905
26. Spiller WG, Frazier CH: Cerebral decompression. Palliative operations in the treatment of tumors of the brain, based on the observation of fourteen cases. JAMA 47:679–926, 1906
27. Greer M: Management of benign intracranial hypertension (pseudotumour cerebri). Clin Neurosurg 15:161–174, 1968

SECTION XX

Cranial and Peripheral Nerves

CHAPTER 172

Surgical Correction of Facial Nerve Palsy

David W. Leitner

The surgical correction of facial nerve palsy, particularly after intracranial surgery for acoustic neuromas, is a difficult task. The harmonious interaction of the muscles contributing to normal facial expression is such that surgical restoration of these qualities can only be approximated by the techniques presently available. The goal of treatment is to achieve a static balance of these muscles, closure of the eyelids, and symmetry during voluntary and involuntary emotion.

Numerous procedures have been used to reanimate paralyzed facial muscles. These procedures involve (1) the use of a peripheral nerve other than the injured ipsilateral seventh nerve to provide innervation for the denervated musculature; (2) transfer of a local or distant muscle, with or without nerve grafting, to provide the motor power for animation; or (3) static procedures to achieve balance. Aside from the selection of the appropriate procedures for a given case, perhaps the most vexing problem is the timing of any reanimation surgery. If a person has a facial paralysis of 1 or 2 years' duration, spontaneous animation will probably not return.[1] In such a case, surgical intervention would be the only means of reanimation. If the paralysis has existed for less than 1 year, however, some function may return.[2]

In this situation, surgical intervention may be further delayed until it can be determined clinically and electromyographically whether or not facial nerve regeneration is occurring.[3]

The timing of surgery involves assessing the status of the injured facial nerve and the functional capabilities of its denervated musculature. Employing a reanimation technique that provides direct innervation to the facial muscles of the injured side requires muscle units that are capable of regaining their function after such reinnervation. The recuperative power of denervated muscle varies widely in the period of time that can elapse beyond which muscle units no longer regain their contractile capability. Although studies have demonstrated that the longer the period of denervation the less complete the recovery of muscle function, to date no specific limits have been determined.[4,5] Sunderland showed that good or complete functional recovery could occur up to 12 months after denervation.[5] Measurements of the chronaxy of the facial muscles or electromyography can be of assistance in establishing whether or not recovery or deterioration of muscles has occurred.[6,7]

METHODS OF SURGICAL TREATMENT

PERIPHERAL NERVE SURGERY

Cross-Facial Nerve Graft

Cross-facial nerve grafting, in which a nerve graft (usually the sural nerve) is routed from normal facial nerve funiculi to the affected funiculi on the contralateral side of the face, has been advocated by several authors.[8-11] This procedure depends on the potential of the denervated muscle on the affected side to regain its contractile capacity. The procedure is recommended in situations in which the facial paralysis has been present for less than 12 to 18 months. The theoretic advantage of this type of procedure is that successful reinnervation of the existing facial muscles results in the same natural directions of contracture as seen on the nonparalyzed side. In addition, the use of the contralateral facial nerve may allow the patient to regain spontaneous, emotionally induced movements as well as conscious, premeditated facial animation.[12-14] Despite these potential benefits, the procedure has not met with uniform success, particularly in older patients or in those with long-standing facial paralysis.[15,16] Although some loss of contractability of the contralateral musculature innervated by the donor seventh nerve funiculi may occur, the effects of this type of neurectomy are minimal.

Nerve Transfers

If the hypoglossal nerve is intact and functional, it can be transferred to the ipsilateral facial nerve trunk or its branches to innervate the facial muscles.[17,18] The phrenic nerve and the descending cervicalis nerve also have been used for nerve transfer but to a much lesser extent than the hypoglossal nerves.[3,19] Hypoglossal facial nerve anastomosis provides a reliable means of establishing successful dynamic reconstruction. Conley and Baker reported that in 137 patients, they had a 95 percent rate of return of facial muscle contraction.[20] The results depend on the availability of potentially functioning facial muscles.

Among the drawbacks to the hypoglossal facial nerve transfer are moderate-to-severe tongue atrophy, which occurred in 78 percent of the patients in this series.[20] There is also the problem of mass movement of the facial muscles during chewing, deglutition, and talking.[20] As in the case of cross-facial nerve grafting, the question of whether or not emotional expression can be retained is debatable.

DYNAMIC MUSCLE RECONSTRUCTION

Local Muscle Transfers

For facial paralysis in which little chance exists of reestablishing contraction of the in situ facial muscles (e.g., longstanding paralysis) and in which either the mandibular branch of the trigeminal nerve or the hypoglossi are intact, local muscle transfers can be used. The ipsilateral masseter muscle, which is innervated by the trigeminal nerve, can be used for a transfer to the region of the affected orbicularis oris. The muscle is detached from its insertion on the mandible while its origin at the zygoma is maintained. The neurovascular pedicle is maintained, and the muscle is split longitudinally, rotated anteriorly, and tunneled toward the orbicularis oris region beneath the skin, where it is attached to the orbicularis of the upper and lower lip to provide support and dynamic retraction of the oral commissure. Alternatively, because the size and arc of rotation of the masseter limit its applicability for reanimation to the oral commissure, the larger ipsilateral temporalis muscle can be used at the commissure of the mouth and to reanimate the upper and lower eyelid.[21] The temporalis muscle can be detached from its origin, elevated down to its insertion, and divided into four separate slips, which are then interdigitated with the fibers of the orbicularis oris and orbicularis oculi.

Another local muscle transfer that can be used for facial reanimation is that in which portions of the omohyoid, sternohyoid, and sternothyroid muscles are harvested with branches of the ansa cervicalis. These small muscle-nerve units are then transferred and imbedded into the substance of the musculature at the oral commissure.[22] Any subsequent muscular contraction at the commissure is the result of myoneurotization rather than the transfer of a contractile unit, such as occurs with the other muscle transfers.

Transfer of the larger muscles (e.g., masseter and temporalis) can provide good facial animation, but as with the peripheral nerve transfers, persistence and motivation are required of the patient to obtain facial movement by contraction of the appropriate muscles of mastication. The movement is a mass movement. In addition, some mastication power is lost when these transfers are used.

Distant Muscle Transfers

If local muscle transfers are not available or desirable, distant muscles or muscle groups can be transferred. Thompson suggested using a nonvascularized transfer of the extensor digitorum brevis muscle of the foot to the paralyzed side of the face.[23] The harvested muscle is placed on denervated facial musculature without any direct arterial or venous anastomosis. The nerve supply to the muscle, a branch of the anterior tibial nerve, is then sutured to a branch of the contralateral facial nerve. The muscle is then theoretically revascularized from the surrounding soft tissue. Freilinger used the same concept but preceded muscle transfer by a cross-facial nerve graft several months before the transfer so that the transplanted muscle would be innervated more rapidly.[24] The procedure produced very weak muscular activity.

With the development of microsurgical small vessel anastomosis the immediate revascularization of a transplanted muscle to the face became possible.[25, 26] Harii first demonstrated this by transferring a portion of the gracilis muscle to the face after a cross-facial nerve graft.[27] This transfer subsequently was performed using the pectoralis minor,[28] the latissimus dorsi,[29] or a portion of the serratus anterior muscle[30] as the muscle unit to be transferred to supply reanimation.

A vascularized distant muscle transfer for unilateral facial paralysis is performed in two stages. A cross-facial nerve graft is performed, and the distal end of the graft is positioned in the preauricular region on the paralyzed side (Fig. 172–1A). No attempt is made to connect the nerve to the existing facial musculature. Six to 10 months after Tinel's sign has reached the distal stump of the nerve graft, the vascularized muscle transfer can be performed (Figure 172–1B). A modification of a face lift–parotid incision is made on the paralyzed side of the face, and the recipient vessels and the distal stump of the cross-facial nerve graft are identified. The cheek is then undermined to provide space for the transferred muscle. The donor muscle and its neurovascular pedicle are simultaneously harvested. The muscle is then transferred to the face, and the microvascular repair of the vessels and nerves is completed. The muscle is anchored to the preauricular and mastoid regions, and the slips of the muscle are split and attached to the designated anatomic areas (e.g., oral commissure). Active contraction is usually seen in the transplanted muscle between 6 months and 1 year after the transfer.

The results of cross-facial nerve grafting and distant vascularized muscle transfer have varied. Reports of weak contraction, excessive contraction, bulkiness of the muscle, and mass movement have been made.[28, 29, 31, 32] Despite these possible problems, the technique is becoming more widely accepted because no facial motor re-education is needed, as is the case with local transfers. With microvascular free tissue transfers there is no loss of intact facial reanimation on the treated side.

Static Procedures

Various static techniques have been attempted to recreate facial symmetry. These procedures have been used to complement dynamic methods of reconstruction or as definitive treatment. Neurectomy or myomectomy on the contralateral side of the face have been advocated to produce balance with the paralyzed side of the face.[33, 34] Facial and dermal slings have been used to elevate specific areas of the paralyzed face, but these frequently stretched over time.[35] Wedge resections of the lower eyelids, lateral canthoplasty, lid magnets, loading the lid with weights, and various forms of palpebral springs all have had varying levels of success in protecting exposed cornea.[36–39]

SUMMARY

It has been said that "in facial paralysis, joy, happiness, sorrow, shock, surprise, and all emotions have for their common expression the same blank stare."[40] The need to correct this blank stare has prompted generations of surgeons to

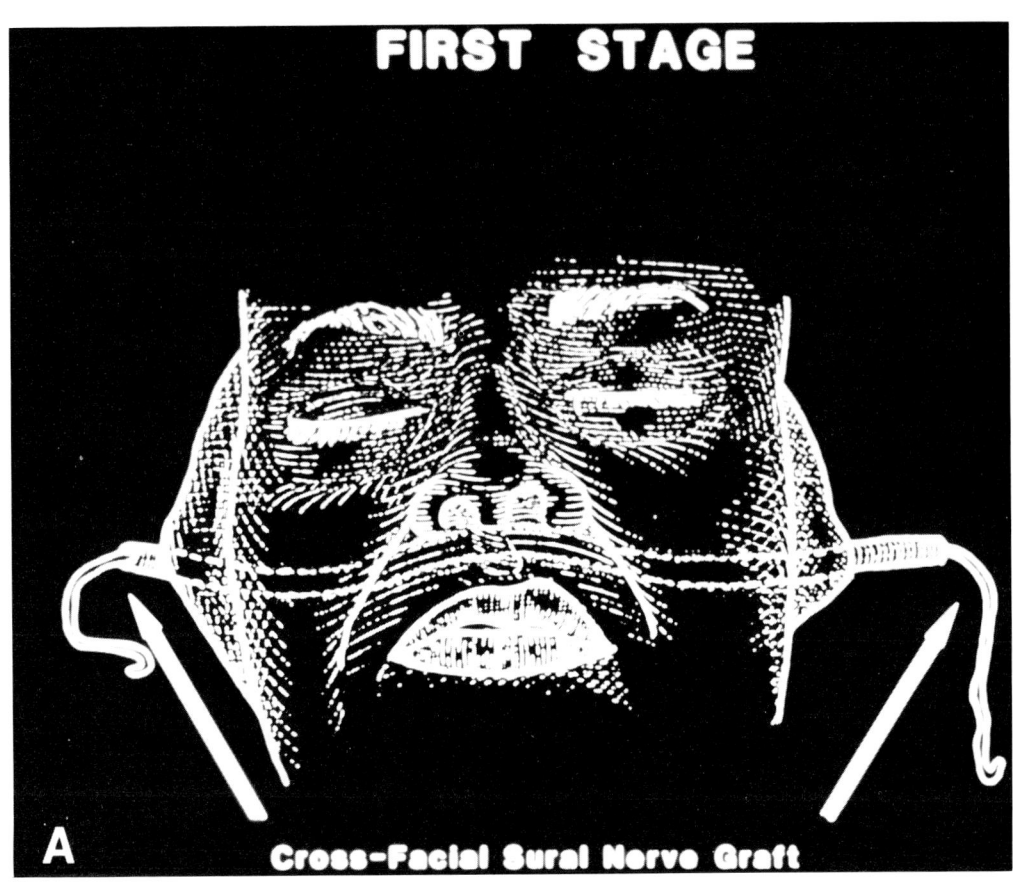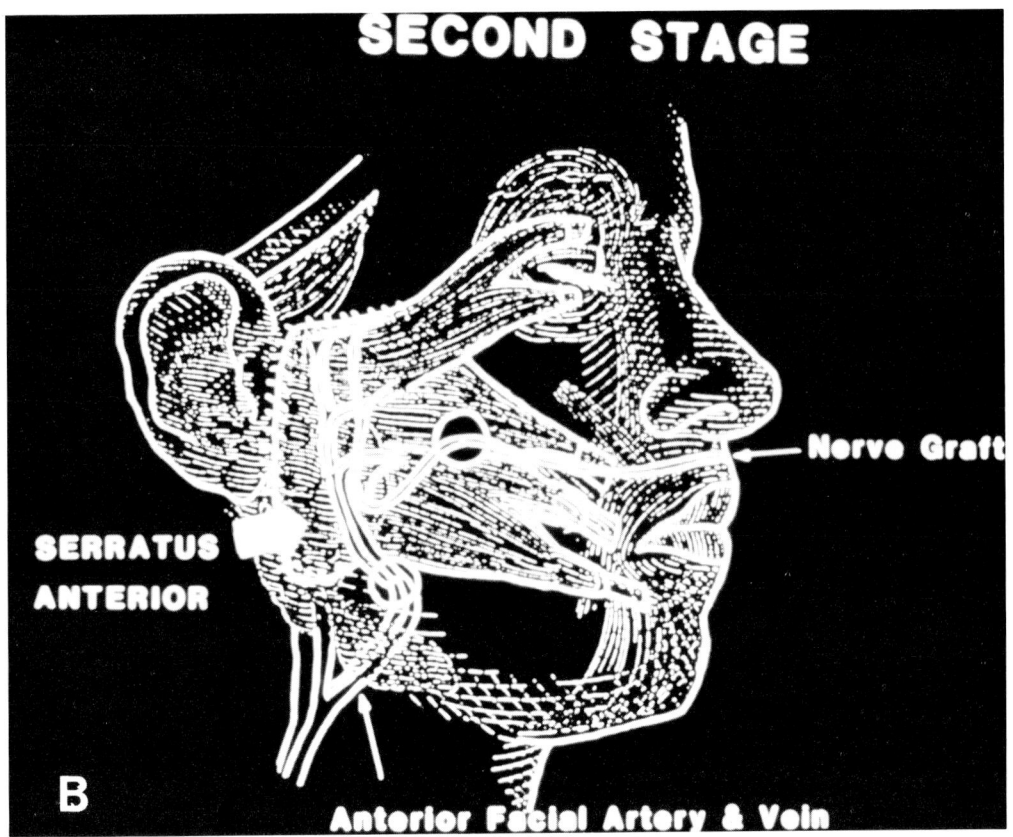

FIGURE 172–1. (A) First stage cross-facial nerve graft. (B) Second stage microneurovascular muscle transplantation. (Courtesy of H. J. Buncke, M.D.)

pursue this goal by alternative methods. Although a single procedure to recreate the natural harmony of emotion and the protective function produced by the facial musculature remains elusive, options are now available to patients with unilateral facial paralysis. These surgical options can help to break the monotony of the blank stare and by doing so, provide an affect where once there was none.

REFERENCES

1. Seddon H: Three types of nerve injury. Brain 66:237, 1943
2. Sunderland S: Nerve and Nerve Injuries. Edinburgh, Churchill-Livingstone, 1972, Chapter 9
3. Freeman B: Facial palsy, in Converse J (ed): Reconstructive Plastic Surgery, ed 2, vol 3. Philadelphia, WB Saunders, 1977, Chapter 36
4. Gutmann E, Young J: The reinnervation of muscle after various periods of atrophy. J Anat 78:15, 1944
5. Sunderland S: Capacity of reinnervated muscles to function efficiently after prolonged denervation. Arch Neurol Psychiatry 64:755, 1950
6. May M, Hardin W: Facial palsy: Interpretation of neurological findings. Laryngoscope 8:1352, 1978
7. Hughes G: Electroneurography: Objective prognostic assessment of facial paralysis. Am J Otol 4:73, 1982
8. Smith J: A new technique of facial animation, in Hueston J (ed): Transactions of the Fifth International Congress of Plastic and Reconstructive Surgery. Australia, Butterworth, 1971, p 83
9. Scarmella L: L'Anastomosi Tra I Due Nervi Facciali. Arch Otol 82:209, 1971
10. Andrel H: Reconstruction of the face through cross facial nerve transplantation in facial paralysis. Chir Plast 2:17, 1973
11. Fisch U: Facial nerve grafting. Otolaryngol Clin North Am 7:517, 1974
12. Andrel H: Cross face nerve grafting—Up to 12 months of seventh nerve disruption, in Rubin L (ed): Reanimation of the Paralyzed Face. St. Louis, CV Mosby, 1977
13. Fisch U: Current surgical treatment of intratemporal facial palsy. Clin Plast Surg 6:377, 1979
14. Conley J: Myths and misconceptions in the rehabilitation of facial paralysis. Plast Reconstr Surg 71:538, 1983
15. Delbeke J, Thauloy C: Electrophysiologic evaluation of cross-facial nerve graft and treatment of facial palsy. Acta Neurochir (Wien) 65:111, 1982
16. Tolhurst D, Bos K: Free revascularized muscle grafts in facial paralysis. Plast Reconstr Surg 69:760, 1982
17. Korte W: Ein Fall von Nervenpropfung des Nervus Fascialis auf den Nervus Hypoglossus. Dtsch Med Wochenschr 29:2, 1903
18. Sargent P: Four cases of facial paralysis treated by hypoglossal facial anastomosis. Proc R Soc Med 12:69, 1911
19. Perret G: Results of phrenicofacial nerve anastomosis for facial paralysis. Arch Surg 94:505, 1967
20. Conley J, Baker D: Hypoglossal-facial nerve anastomosis for reinnervation of the paralyzed face. Plast Reconstr Surg 63:63, 1979
21. Rubin L: Reanimation of the Paralyzed Face. St. Louis, CV Mosby, 1977
22. Tucker H: Restoration of selective facial nerve function by the nerve-muscle pedicle technique. Clin Plast Surg 6:293, 1979
23. Thompson N: Autogenous free grafts of skeletal muscle. A preliminary experimental and clinical study. Plast Reconstr Surg 48:11, 1971
24. Freilinger G: A new technique to correct facial paralysis. Plast Reconstr Surg 56:44, 1975
25. Jacobson J, Suarez E: Microsurgery in anastomosis of small vessels. Surg Forum 9:243, 1960
26. Tamai S: Free muscle transplants in dogs with microsurgical neurovascular anastomosis. Plast Reconstr Surg 46:219, 1970
27. Mayou B, Watson J, Harrison D, et al: Free microvascular and microneural transfer of the extensor digitorum brevis muscle for the treatment of unilateral facial palsy. Br J Plast Surg 34:362, 1981
28. Harrison D: The pectoralis minor vascularized muscle graft for the treatment of unilateral facial palsy. Plast Reconstr Surg 75:206, 1985
29. Harii K: Treatment of long standing facial paralysis by combining vascularized muscle transplantation with crossface nerve grafting, in Buncke H, Furnas D (eds): Symposium on Clinical Frontiers in Reconstructive Microsurgery. St. Louis, CV Mosby, 1984, pp 159–171
30. Buncke H, Alpert B, Gordon L, et al: Free serratus anterior muscle transplantation for unilateral facial nerve paralysis. Presented at the American Association of Plastic Surgeons Meeting, Chicago, 1984
31. Harii K, Ohmori K, Torm S: Free gracilis muscle transplantation with microvascular anastomosis for the treatment of facial paralysis. Plast Reconstr Surg 57:133, 1976
32. Harrison D, Mayou B: Extensor digitorum brevis and pectoralis major and minor muscles in the treatment of unilateral facial palsy, in Buncke H, Furnas D (eds): Symposium on Clinical Frontiers in Reconstructive Microsurgery. St. Louis, CV Mosby, 1984, pp 177–187
33. Niklison J: Contribution to the subject of facial paralysis. Plast Reconstr Surg 17:276, 1956
34. Rubin L, Lee G, Simpson S: Reanimation of the long-standing partial facial paralysis. Plast Reconstr Surg 77:41, 1986
35. Edgerton M, Wolfort F: The dermal flap canthal lift for lower eyelid support. Plast Reconstr Surg 43:42, 1969
36. Jelks G, Smith B, Bosniak S: The evaluation and management of the eye in facial palsy. Clin Plast Surg 6:397, 1979
37. Muhlbauer W, Sageth H, Viessman H: Restoration of lid function in facial palsy with permanent magnets. Chir Plast 1:295, 1973
38. Smellie G: Restoration of the blinking reflex in facial palsy by a simple lid load operation. Br J Plast Surg 19:279, 1966
39. Morel-Fatio D, Laladrie J: Palliative surgical treatment of facial paralysis. The palpebral spring. Plast Reconstr Surg 23:446, 1964
40. Bunnell S: Suture of the facial nerve within the temporal bone with a report of the first successful case. Surg Gynecol Obstet 45:7, 1927

CHAPTER 173

Surgical Management of Lesions of the Peripheral Nerves and Brachial Plexus

H. Millesi

ANATOMY OF PERIPHERAL NERVES

Peripheral nerves derive segmentally from the spinal cord by the joining of the ventral and the dorsal roots. The ventral roots carry motor fibers from neurons of the ventral horn. The dorsal roots contain afferent nerve fibers, emerging from the pseudounipolar neurons of the spinal ganglion and enter the dorsal horn. The spinal ganglia are collections of neurons on the dorsal roots that are located immediately lateral to the sites where the nerve roots perforate the dura mater. Each root is covered by the pia mater and is loosely invested by the arachnoid mater[1] at the level of the penetration of the dura and the arachnoidea; both roots carry with them an elongation of these tissues that elongation envelop the nerve fibers and ends at the dorsal root at the level of the spinal ganglion. The subarachnoidal space reaches to the spinal ganglion.[2–5] At the entrance of the intervertebral canal, the two roots unite to form the spinal nerve. At this level, the motor nerve fibers are located on the ventral side. The dorsal side contains afferent nerve fibers from sensory end organs to the pseudounipolar ganglion cells of the spinal ganglions. Because these nerve fibers transmit in the direction of the neurons of the ganglions, they are functionally elongated dendrites, but they have all the characteristics of peripheral axons and are usually termed as such. The dural sheathes of the spinal nerves continue with their connective tissue sheath in the intervertebral foramina.[1]

NERVE FIBER

The nerve root complex is movable, within the intervertebral canal[2, 3] which means that it can easily adapt to the movements, however, the suspension is not safe, and longitudinal traction will lead to a root avulsion. In the cranial part of the neck and at the trunk (C1, C2, and intercostal nerves 2 to 12), the spinal nerves divide into a ventral and a dorsal part. The dorsal trunk supplies the autochthonal musculature of the neck with motor fibers, and the dorsal skin, with sensory fibers. The ventral branch innervates segmental zones with motor and sensory fibers. Between C3 and C4, the nerve fibers of the spinal nerves form the cervical plexus for the neck. From C5 to T1, they merge with each other (brachial plexus) and give rise to the peripheral nerves of the upper extremity. The spinal nerves from L1 to S3 form the lumbosacral plexus and the nerve for the pelvis and the lower extremity.

The microscopic unit of a nerve is the axon with the axolemma. The axon is an elongation of a neuron, as described earlier. Unmyelinated fibers are embedded in the protoplasma of a Schwann cell, which produces trophic factors, without which the axons could not survive. Around larger axons, Schwann cells are arranged in a segmental way and produce a myelin sheath, which makes a saltatory conduction possible, leading to a much higher conduction velocity. The axon–Schwann cell complex is enveloped by a basal membrane and supported by a framework of thin collagen fibers. The outer plasma membranes of the Schwann cell and its adjacent basement membrane correspond to the neurolemma.[1]

FASCICLE

Many nerve fibers are suspended in a delicate endoneural framework of fine collagen fibrils that has a diameter of between 40 and 65 nm. This tissue contains Schwann cells and endoneurial fibroblasts in a ratio of 9:1. The nerve fibers of a fascicle are surrounded by the perineurium, which is separated from the nerve fibers by the subperineurial space. The perineurium consists of an inner layer of flat mesothelial cells with a basal membrane. These cells form a barrier against the outer environment. Collagen microfibrils are also present that have a diameter of 40 to 65 nm. The middle layer consists of several lamellae of mesothelial cells, and the outer layer contains collagen neurofibrils with a larger diameter. The perineurium separates the neural environment that is within the fascicle from the outside. It has several barrier functions.[6–8] The perineurium in the composition mentioned earlier contributes much to the tensile strength of a nerve. Its elasticity maintains the undulated course of the nerve fibers within the fascicle, which was described by Fontana.[9] It is, therefore, responsible for the relaxed state of the nerve fibers.

NERVE TRUNK

The nerve trunk is formed by fascicles in the following basic patterns:

MONOFASCICULAR PATTERN. The nerve consists of one large fascicle, which, of course, is the simplest structure. If transverse compression is exerted, the intrafascicular pressure rapidly rises, and the tissue is damaged because the monofascicular nerve segments cannot adapt to compression.

OLIGOFASCICULAR PATTERN. If two to five large, manageable fascicles are in a nerve trunk, these fascicles are able to move against each other because of the loose interfascicular epineurium that surrounds them. All fascicles are kept together by an epifascicular epineurium. The movement of the fascicles against each other allows the nerve trunk to change its shape under transverse compression thereby avoiding compression of the fascicles, even if the nerve is squeezed.

If there are five to 12 individual fascicles, the possibility of the adaption of these lesions to transverse compression is even better. They move against each other, which also allows adaptation to flexion and avoids kinking. In a nerve trunk, five to 12 fascicles can be managed by fascicular dissection.

POLYFASCICULAR PATTERN. If there are more than 12 fascicles, the possibility for adaptation is even better; however, under these conditions, the fascicles are less manageable, and in contrast to an oligofascicular pattern manipulation of the individual fascicles, this does not make sense. However, some of the polyfascicular segments show an arrangement of the fascicles in fascicle groups, and under these circumstances, surgery can follow the individual fascicle groups.

The epineurium is a dense connective tissue with collagen fibrils of between 60 and 110 nm in diameter. We may differentiate the interfascicular epineurium, which has a gliding tissue function and provides the ability of the fascicles to glide against each other, from the epifascicular epineurium, which envelopes all the fascicles of the whole nerve trunk.

The epineurium is linked to the surrounding tissue by layers of a loose connective tissue, which was studied very carefully by Lang,[10] who termed it *conjunctiva nervorum*. The conjunctiva nervorum corresponds to the adventitia of the vessels, which was termed by Lang *conjunctiva vasorum*. Others use the term *paraneurium*, which to me seems to be the proper term. If a neurovascular bundle exists, the outer layers of the adventitia of the vessels and the outer layers of the gliding tissue around the nerve may fuse and form a common layer around nerves and vessels, which then can be called adventitia. The task of the adventitia is to provide the possibility for a nerve to undergo passive motion, which is important especially for longitudinal movements.

PASSIVE NERVE MOVEMENTS

In flexion and extension, the only structures that do not move are located in the plane of motion that corresponds to a plane across the joint axis. All other tissues that are located in a certain distance to the plane of motion have to be able to move because the distance within such a plane gets shorter with flexion if a tissue is located on the flexion site and longer with flexion if the tissue is located at the extension site. The amount of motion corresponds to the distance to the plane of motion, therefore, the tissues of different planes must be able to move against each other. Zöch and coworkers[11, 12] showed that the median nerve in flexion is reduced by about 15 percent of its original length. The nerve had to be elongated again to adapt to extension. If, in addition, the wrist and the finger joints were extended, the nerve had to become elongated above the length that was measured after excision for about 4 percent. This corresponds to a real elongation.

In summary, the median nerve has a zero length after excision that corresponds to the length of the bed in extended position of the elbow joint and zero position of wrist and fingers. If elbow and wrist joints are flexed, the nerve has to reduce by 15 percent. If the elbow joint is extended again, the reduction has to be reversed. If the nerve is fixed in a flexed position by adhesions, the remaining movable segments of the nerve have to be elongated more than normal to meet full extension. But even in normal conditions, if wrist and finger joints are extended, the nerve becomes elongated beyond its zero length. A stress-strain diagram shows the forces involved in this process. These measurements have been performed with an excised nerve. Completely different values are achieved if measurements are performed in situ (Figs. 173–1 and 173–2). We realize that much less force is necessary to elongate the median nerve at the upper arm than if the total length, including the forearm, is investigated. We assume that this effect results from the presence of the branches, which leave the nerve in the distal upper arm and forearm segment. If we cut these branches, we achieve approximately the same stress-strain curve as with the segment without branches of the upper arm. If the nerve is excised and a stress-strain study performed, we again need much less force to elongate the nerve, indicating that excised nerves

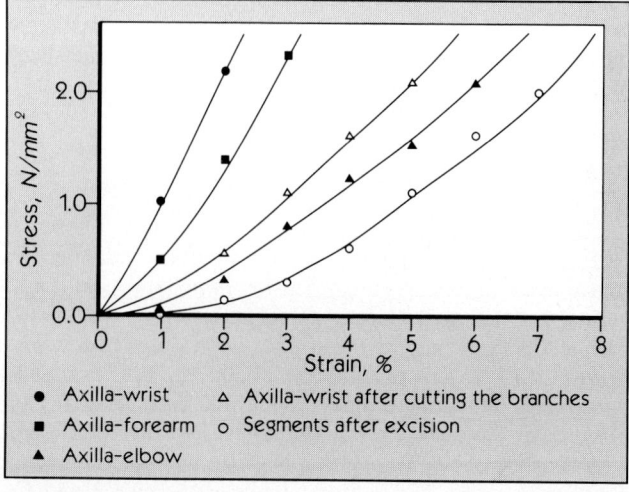

FIGURE 173–1. Stress-strain diagram of the ulnar nerve. (From Millesi H: Peripheral nerve reconstruction, in Salcman M [ed]: Current Technique in Neurosurgery, Current Medicine. Phila., PA, Current Science. 1993.)

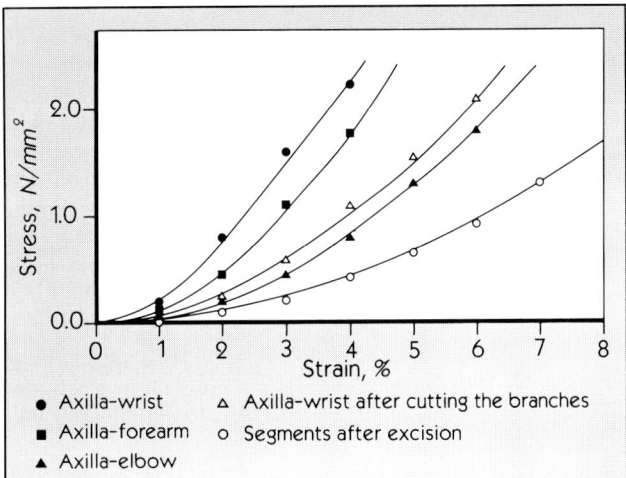

FIGURE 173-2. Stress-strain diagram of the median nerve. (From Millesi H: Peripheral nerve reconstruction, in Saloman M [ed]: Current Technique in Neurosurgery, Current Medicine. Phila., PA, Current Science, 1993.)

can be extended much easier than those in situ, even after transection of the branches, because the in situ nerve is linked to the performed after excision of the nerve, surrounding tissue by the paraneurium. Stress-strain studies, which formed the basis for surgical considerations in the past, do not correspond to reality. In situ, the forces necessary to elongate the nerve are much higher. In addition, the force necessary to elongate a nerve segment with and without branches is different. These studies are extremely important and have to take into consideration the question of whether an eventual forced end-to-end neurorrhaphy is discussed.

CLASSIFICATION OF NERVE LESIONS

A nerve can be transected by a sharp instrument, it can be damaged by a blunt instrument, it can be exposed to compression, or it can come under traction.

In clean transection, such as that achieved with a knife, the amount of damaged nerve tissue is minimal, but a loss of continuity exists, and regeneration can occur only if the two ends are approximated in a proper way.

If the nerve is hit by a blunt agent, a larger segment of nerve tissue is damaged to a different degree. Continuity may be lost or preserved. In the latter case, however, one has to consider a rather poor regeneration across the damaged section that corresponds to the degrees of damage. In cases of a loss of continuity, the two stumps suffer degrees of damage ranging from normal to mortally damaged.

Seddon[13] classified the nerve lesions into three types: neurapraxia, axonotmesis, and neurotmesis.

NEURAPRAXIA. In this situation the nerve has lost its conductivity but is not damaged on macroscopy and light microscope. The damage is rather a functional one, having to do with the ion pump, and spontaneous regeneration is possible. No further treatment is necessary.

AXONOTMESIS. Axonotmesis is the second degree of damage. In this case, the axons are transected, but the framework of the nerve is not damaged. Regeneration within the preserved nerve fibers is possible. If regeneration is not prevented by external reasons, full recovery results.

NEUROTMESIS. In these cases the nerve has suffered a more pronounced damage, and spontaneous recovery is unlikely to occur.

Sunderland[14] differentiates between five degrees of nerve lesions. The first degree corresponds to neuropraxia. The second degree corresponds to axonotmesis. The innermost part of the nerves, the axons, have lost continuity, but the other tissues are normal. In the third degree, the framework within the fascicle has been damaged, but the perineurium and, consequently, the fascicular pattern, are intact. Regeneration may occur within the fascicles if it is not prevented by compression or fibrosis; however, not all the axons reach the distal destination and, therefore, recovery is incomplete. In the fourth degree, the perineurium has also lost continuity, which means that the fascicular pattern has been lost; however, continuity is still preserved by epineurial connective tissue. In the fifth degree, a complete loss of continuity occurs.

The classification proposed by Sunderland[14] describes a traction lesion with loss of continuity at different levels. It does not take into account the reaction of the nerve tissue, which usually consists of fibrosis.

Millesi and Kovac[15-18] developed an additional classification based on the location of fibrosis. Fibrosis mainly located in the epifascicular epineurium is called type A fibrosis. If type A fibrosis develops in a first-degree lesion, according to Sunderland (IA) or in a second-degree (IIA) lesion, spontaneous recovery may be prevented. Under these circumstances, neurolysis may help.

A more extensive fibrosis, type B fibrosis, may include the interfascicular epineurium. Type B fibrosis may also prevent spontaneous recovery in a first- or second-degree lesion (IB, IIB). The same is true for a third-degree lesion, which may be combined with an epifascicular (IIIA) or an interfascicular fibrosis (IIIB).

If fibrosis develops within the endoneural space, regeneration within the fascicle may become impossible because of collagenization. This situation can be called type C fibrosis. Type C fibrosis can be combined only with a third-degree lesion (IIIC). In this case, resection and restoration of continuity, as in a type IV lesion, is indicated.

In a fourth-degree lesion proposed by Sunderland, continuity is still preserved by epineurial tissue. It may become fibrotic like a scar (IVS). This situation prevents regeneration completely, and such a segment has to be resected and the defect bridged by nerve grafts. In other cases, axon sprouts may penetrate the damaged segment like a neuroma, and some fibers may even reach the distal stumps (IVN). Even if some fibers regenerate, satisfactory functional recovery is not likely to occur, and these cases should be treated like cases with lost continuity.

Transitions between third- and fourth-degree lesions are possible (III/IV). In this situation, the better-preserved fascicle or fascicle groups can be separated from the more severely damaged part by interfascicular dissection.

HEALING OF NERVES

Immediately after the transection, the normal process of wound healing develops at the site of transection with formation of an exudate, diapedesis of leukocytes, and proliferation of fibroblasts and Schwann cells. Fibroblasts originate from the epifascicular and interfascicular epineurium, as well as from the perineurial and endoneurial tissue. As was discussed earlier, a difference exists between epineurial fibroblasts on one side and perineurial and endoneurial fibroblasts on the other side. We have also seen that the ratio of Schwann cells to fibroblasts in the endoneurium is 9:1, and we can assume that in the space between the two stumps, a similar relationship will be favorable. However, Schwann cells multiply less frequently, and, therefore, Schwann cell proliferation starts with some delay. The space between the two stumps may fill with many more epineurial fibroblasts than Schwann cells, which may create unfavorable circumstances for the axon sprouts. Proliferation of Schwann cells and proliferation of axons may be enhanced by different nerve growth factors, neurite-promoting factors, and other factors that are not completely understood.

WALLERIAN DEGENERATION

After an axon has been transected, the distal stump, being deprived from its connection with the neuron, degenerates. The myelin sheath is removed, and the Schwann cells form rows of cells at the spot where the nerve fiber had been. Degeneration occurs until the proximal node of Ranvier in the proximal stump is reached, but the degeneration in proximal direction is sometimes much longer. If the lesion is close to the neuron, the degeneration may even reach the neuron and cause degeneration of the neuron itself.

NERVE REGENERATION

Because of metabolic changes induced by the transection of the axon, the neurons are stimulated to produce axon sprouts at the distal end of each transected axon. Many sprouts may originate from the distal end of one axon. If the proximal stump of the nerve has been damaged, the axons have to travel along damaged tissue of the proximal stump until they reach the distal end. This action means loss of time. The same unfavorable conditions are present if the distal stump is damaged. Proper resection of the damaged segments provides favorable conditions for nerve healing. If the axon sprouts reach the distal cross section of the proximal stump quickly, they are able to traverse the space between the proximal and the distal stump rapidly. If they reach the distal stump, they meet Schwann cells, which provide an optimal milieu for the axon sprouts to travel along the distal stump to reach the proper target organ.

The main goal seems to be to enhance the axon sprouts to cross over from the proximal to the distal stump, therefore, attempts have been made to achieve an optimal coaption of corresponding fascicular tissues. Since the work of Lundborg and Hansson,[19,20] we know that axons are able to travel along an empty space, bringing along their own Schwann cells, provided that interference from fibroblasts from the surrounding tissue is prevented. Along a mesothelial chamber, these axon sprouts can proceed to reach the distal stump. With time, nerve tissue is produced between the two stumps that is reminiscent of a normal nerve structure. Under neuromatous neurotization, Schröder and Seiffert[21] determined the outgrowth of axon sprouts, which brought along their own Schwann cells, capillaries, and fibroblasts, to penetrate a given structure. Because of the protection against external influences by the mesothelial chamber, this type of regeneration is undisturbed and leads to beautifully arranged parallel structures.

If the nerve stump is not in contact with a distal stump by a chamber or a tube, neuroma formation also occurs, which means outgrowth of axon sprouts, Schwann cells, fibroblasts, and capillaries; however, this outgrowth is irregular, and a neuroma is formed. This process is similar to that of the axon proceeding along a preformed space.

Does the regenerated segment within a chamber or a tube represent a well-organized neuroma or a true neuroticized nerve segment, like a distal stump? In this case, the delicate structure of the endoneurium would also be imitated. In neuroma-like advancement, the connective tissue framework gives the impression of compartmentation-like minifascicles.

If the axon sprouts have reached a distal stump, the local Schwann cells take over the trophic function and produce myelin sheath. If several axon sprouts enter the same endoneurial structure, only one of them is maintained by the neurotrophic efforts of the Schwann cells, and the others degenerate. The work of Brushart[22–25] showed that there is a specificity: if a motor and a sensory axon enter a motor pathway, the motor axon will be maintained by the neurotrophic effort of the Schwann cells, and the sensory axon will degenerate. A consequent neurotropism occurs, which means that a higher number of motor axons will reach the correct distal motor pathway than expected by random chance. Brushart[25] also showed that the stimulating factor for this neurotrophic effect is located in the distal stump and not in the end organ because it acts also if the distal stump is separated from the target organ. The favorable effect results from neurotrophism rather than to neurotropism.

This question is extremely important. If a neurotopic effect exists and is able to act over a longer range, a close coaptation of the two stumps would be harmful. Leaving a distance between the two stumps would allow the axon sprouts to arrange themselves, as a result of the influence of neurotropic factors, like in a mesothelial chamber. This issue was thoroughly discussed in a symposium held in Vienna in November 1991. We have no proof that neurotropic factors act over a wider range. Therefore, we should still try to obtain as accurate an alignment as possible between fascicles and fascicle groups. Neurotropic factors are helping to arrange the fibers between the two stumps of a transected fascicle group or a proximal, respectively a distal stump and the proximal, respectively the distal end of a nerve graft with a different number and size of fascicles.[26]

If the coaptation site is under tension, a separation of the nerve tissue might develop, and the axon sprouts have to cross a wider distance. If tension is applied at a later date when continuity is already re-established, a distraction of the connective tissue might occur between the two nerve stumps, leading to distension. The connective tissue might undergo hypertrophy and excert compression. Axon sprouts that have already reached the distal stump may suffer a second damage and degenerate.[27, 28] It could be proved that healing under tension jeopardizes the result significantly.[29, 30] However, it could be demonstrated that two optimal sites of coaptation achieved by healing under optimal conditions without tension yield better conditions for regeneration than one side of coaptation performed under bad conditions. Therefore, the decision to avoid coaptation under tension and to use a nerve graft is justified. The unfavorable influence of external compression has been already discussed.

DIAGNOSIS, INDICATIONS, AND TIMING

The diagnosis is established according to the motor and sensory loss observed in clinical examination. If necessary, the diagnosis is confirmed by electrophysiologic studies.

POSTTRAUMATIC CONDITIONS

Emergency

Open Injury

In cases of a clean transection by a sharp instrument, the diagnosis is established by the location of the wound and the clinical examination. If a clinical study is not possible because the patient is unconscious, careful anatomic exploration has to be performed to confirm or rule out a nerve involvement. A primary neurorrhaphy is performed.

If blunt trauma with extensive tissue damage has occurred, the surgeon must decide whether the nerve lesion should be repaired as a primary or delayed primary neurorrhaphy, with all other damaged structures, like vessels, bone, tendons, and skin, so that a global reconstruction can be performed or should an early secondary repair be performed 3 to 6 weeks after trauma and the emergency repair be restricted to vessels, bones, tendons, and skin.

The big disadvantage of this solution is the necessity of a second operation. However, there are advantages to a two-stage procedure. At the time of the injury, the amount of damage of the two stumps can not be estimated very well. The primary repair of the damaged nerve may be performed with damaged nerve stumps, which will develop fibrosis and impede nerve regeneration. At the early secondary repair, the damaged segment has already developed fibrosis and can be easily recognized as such. A proper resection can then be performed. This advantage includes another disadvantage that usually at secondary repairs, a larger defect is created and end-to-end neurorrhaphy becomes more difficult and more often necessitates the use of nerve grafts. Because of the fibrosis of the two stumps, the nerve tissue is less extensible, a quality that favors the use of nerve grafts in secondary procedures.

Another advantage of the two-stage procedure is the fact that the repair can be performed as elective surgery with ideal personnel and material. Nerves and tendons are repaired at different times, and the danger of adhesions between them is reduced. The risk of complications, like breakdown of the skin cover, hematoma, and infection, is much reduced if the repair is performed as a secondary surgery. This advantage is especially important in cases of nerve defects, if nerve grafts have to be used. If complications occur in these cases, the nerve grafts are definitely lost.

The decision of whether a primary or early secondary repair should be performed is extremely difficult and depends very much of the experience of the surgeon. If the primary nerve repair is a failure, nothing is lost, provided that a secondary repair is performed within 6 months. However, frequently the patient is treated for a much longer period that regeneration will occur; therefore precious time for a secondary repair is lost. In this case, the decision to perform a primary repair provides a disadvantage to the patient. The surgeon who decides to perform a primary repair accepts the responsibility to perform a secondary repair in a timely fashion if the primary repair fails.

Closed Injury

In a patient with a trauma without an open wound, a peripheral nerve can be exposed to traction or compression, especially in patients with a fracture. Typical examples are the radial nerve (with humerus fractures) or the sciatic nerve (with pelvic fractures). The brachial plexus can be exposed to compression between the clavicle and the first rib, it can be damaged along with a fracture of the clavicle, or it can suffer a traction lesion. In addition to the different degrees of damage (see Classification) a peripheral nerve can suffer in a brachial plexus lesion: the rootlets may be avulsed from the spinal cord. A measure such as surgery is indicated if signs of an acute compression exist or if a large hematoma due to a vascular injury has developed. The nerve repair is performed as a secondary procedure.

Delayed Nerve Injuries

The decision of whether to perform primary or early secondary nerve repair after an open injury was discussed earlier. In cases in which the primary operation revealed a preserved continuity, and in cases of blunt trauma, in which there is the possibility of preserved continuity, the patient will receive physiotherapy and will be followed up for about 3 months. A first-degree lesion can be recognized easily by the fact that in spite of motor palsy, the conductivity of the motor fibers is preserved. In a second-degree lesion, the conductivity has been lost as a result of wallerian degeneration; however, early signs of regeneration, like the advancement of the Tinel Hoffmann sign, may be noticed. After 3 months, the surgeon should decided whether conservative treatment should be continued or whether exploration is indicated. This decision may be extremely difficult in cases of partial lesions. The clinical picture of a partial lesion may result from two different conditions: (1) irreversible damage of a part of the nerve that needs exploration, or (2) reversible damage of the whole nerve, of which only part has recovered, but full recovery may be expected with time. Observation of the clinical course, assisted by a sequence of electrophysiologic studies, helps to differentiate between these two conditions. In any case, if some part of the nerve does not show recovery, an exploration is indicated.

In brachial plexus lesions, if the diagnosis of avulsion of several roots is established by magnetic resonance imaging computed tomography plus myelography, an early operation is justified. In other cases, the observation allows differentiation between reversible or irreversible damage. The exploration is indicated if initial signs of regeneration do not occur between 3 to 6 months after the trauma. The differential diagnosis between preganglionic and postganglionic lesion is not as important as it was years ago, because all brachial plexus lesions that do not show signs of recovery have to be explored regardless of the pathology.

NONTRAUMATIC CONDITIONS

Nontraumatic lesions of peripheral nerves result from compression or chronic irritation at an anatomic site that leads to an entrapment syndrome. The diagnosis is established by a clinical estimation of an eventual motor or sensory loss, and patients usually present such symptoms as pain and paresthesia. The diagnosis is confirmed by electrophysiologic studies. We have good reason to believe that the pathology of entrapment syndromes is not always compression alone but also traction if the paraneurium at the site of entrapment has become fibrotic and the nerve is not able to follow the movement of the limb passively.

INCISIONS AND APPROACH

At primary repair, the existent wound is enlarged, if necessary, according to the rules of plastic surgery. In secondary repairs, incisions distant to the nerve are used that provide a sufficient approach for an extended exploration and that can be lengthened, if necessary. If the incision crosses the course of the nerve, constriction might develop and jeopardize the result. The nerve is exposed proximally and distally to the lesion in normal tissue. From there, the dissection starts in the direction of the lesion. Wide exposure is the key to success.

The brachial plexus may be approached with the patient in half-sitting position from in front. A zig-zag-shaped incision is used, starting behind the sternocleidomastoideus muscle, following the clavicle, traversing the pectoral region, and extending by zig-zag incisions from there to the medial midlateral line of the upper arm. We prefer to have the patient lying on his or her back, and we approach the brachial plexus from the cranial angle, using the same incision or, increasingly in recent years, using a sagittal incision following the lines of Langer across the supraclavicular fossa. A second transverse incision is performed at the trigonum colli laterale, and a third incision is started at the processus coracoideus following the Langer line to the anterior axillary fold and then continuing, as mentioned earlier, to the midlateral area of the upper arm. The skin between these incisions is elevated, providing an optimal exposure with minimal scarring.

For the suprascapular nerve, a sagittal incision is made about 2-cm more laterally than the sagittal incision for the plexus.

For the axillary nerve, we use the sagittal incision for the plexus and an oblique incision following the Langer line at the dorsal aspect of the shoulder joint and crossing the sulcus deltoideus posterior at the borderline between the cranial and middle third to explore the hiatus quadrangularis from behind. Sometimes, a curved incision underneath the axillary groove is necessary to provide access to the middle third of the nerve. A midlateral incision on the median aspect of the humerus gives access to the median, the ulnar, the musculocutaneous, and the proximal segment of the radial nerve.

The distal segments of the radial nerve are exposed by a midlateral incision on the lateral aspect of the upper arm and the radial aspect of the forearm. We prefer this midlateral incision to a spiral incision paralleling the sulcus bicipitalis lateralis.

For the ulnar and median nerve at the level of the forearm, we prefer to use a midlateral incision on the medial aspect of the forearm. If we have to treat a median and ulnar nerve lesion at the wrist, we do not use the usual transverse or oblique scars from the injury, which cross the course of the nerve, but rather a long, midlateral incision of the median aspect of the forearm that might be extended to the ulnar aspect of the middle hand.

The best incision to explore the palm is the Y-shaped incision, which starts in the center of the palm and looks like a Mercedes star. This incision causes minimal damage to the cutaneous vessels of the palmar skin because these vessels are coming from all sides toward the center of the palm.

On the finger, midlateral incisions are optimal. An alternative is a bayonet-shaped incision, starting in the midlateral line of the basal phalanx, crossing along the flexion crease to the opposite midlateral line, and continuing distally. The cutaneous nerves of the arm and forearm are exposed by small transverse incisions, as are the cutaneous nerves of the lower extremity, including the sural nerve, which is harvested as a graft.

For the exploration of the lumbal plexus, an incision is made along the iliac crest and the inguinal ligament, and the abdominal muscles are detached from their origin. The peritoneum is pushed aside, and the femoral nerve is exposed between the iliac and psoas muscles. It is then followed in cranial direction to define the other branches of the lumbar plexus. For a more distal lesion of the femoral nerve, the same incision may be used to define the nerve within the pelvis, and a more distally located parallel incision on the ventral aspect of the thigh is then made to explore the division of the nerve outside the lacuna musculorum.

The sciatic nerve is exposed by a semicircular incision on the cranial, lateral, and caudal aspect of the gluteal area. After the skin is elevated, the nerve is met by a transmuscular approach at the level of the suprapiriform and infrapiriform foramen. This incision can be extended in zig-zagged shape along the dorsal aspect of the thigh to expose the sciatic nerve at this level and its division.

For the tibial nerve, we use a zig-zag-shaped incision in the fossa poplitea that is extended distally at the mid lateral aspect of the leg. The usual incision for the tarsal tunnel syndrome starts in the sulcus retromalleolaris medialis and continues at the midlateral level of the medial aspect of the foot to the base of the big toe. We believe that this incision can cause problems if the scar after exploration of the tarsal tunnel and the external scar of the skin fuse together. Therefore, we now prefer to use an incision that passes ventrally to the malleolus internus to the lateral aspect of the foot and elevate the skin toward the tarsal tunnel to avoid a coincidence of the cutaneous scar and the tarsal tunnel.

For the plantar area of the foot, we use a dorsally convex incision, which starts at the medial aspect of the base of the big toe and ends at the medial aspect of the heel. The peroneal nerve is exposed by a series of transverse incisions, and the skin is elevated between these incisions. Transverse incisions are also used for the nerves of the dorsal aspect of the foot.

LESIONS IN CONTINUITY

The nerve is defined in normal tissue proximal and distal to the site of the lesion. When approaching the site of the lesion, the surgeon meets fibrosis between the nerve and the surrounding tissue that results in fibrosis of the paraneurium. By external neurolysis, the nerve is liberated.

The nerve is then carefully inspected and palpated. If it appears normal, the neurolysis procedure is finished. The surgeon now must consider whether the nerve should be transferred. This is especially true for the ulnar nerve, which might be transferred to the ventral aspect of the elbow joint or submuscularly after desinsertion of the flexor muscle from the humerus and the ulna so that the ulnar nerve can be placed parallel to the median nerve.

If the nerve is indurated, type A fibrosis may be present. A longitudinal epineuriotomy is performed to transect the fibrotic layer that constricts the nerve. If it is a type A fibrosis (lesion IA, IIA, IIIA) the fascicular tissue will pop out from this epineuriotomy site because of the relief of constriction. The epineuriotomy may be repeated on the other side of the nerve trunk until full decompression is achieved.

If the epineuriotomy has not achieved decompression, the interfascicular epineurium may be fibrotic. In this case, the whole epifascicular epineurium is resected (epifascicular epineuriectomy), and, if this maneuver is not sufficient, the fibrotic parts of the interfascicular epineurium is removed (interfascicular epineuriectomy). Only the fibrotic parts should be removed, and all individual fascicles need not be separated, as is described in many papers and textbooks. Such an extensive, complete interfascicular epineuriectomy may impair the blood supply of the fascicles and transect connections that carrying nerve fibers from one fascicle to another. If only the fibrotic part is resected, the blood supply is not impaired, and only a minimum of nerve fibers between the fascicles are damaged. Therefore, the interfascicular epineuriectomy has always been performed partially.

If the fasicles still do not expand and give the impression of induration after this procedure, a type C lesion is diagnosed, meaning that the content of the fascicles has become fibrotic and that chances of regeneration are minimal. Fascicles that are changed in this way are removed. At this point, the neurolysis becomes a resection, with consecutive restoration of continuity by a nerve graft.

If the epifascicular epineuriectomy shows that a fascicular pattern is no longer present, a damage of the fourth degree is diagnosed. Regardless whether the damage of IVS or IVN, such segments are resected, and, again, the neurolysis becomes a resection, with restoration of continuity.

Special attention is necessary for transient lesions between third and fourth degrees. In these cases, by interfascicular dissection, the part of the nerve that has suffered a third-degree lesion is separated from parts that no longer show a fascicular pattern.

Any neurolysis procedure has common aspects with the correction of severe scars. In both cases the goal is to improve a situation caused by fibrotic tissue by performing surgery and creating new scars, in the hope that the new scar will be better than the old one. The frequent success of neurolysis procedures results from the fact that the gliding tissue around the nerve has good potential for regeneration. If extensive scarring around the nerve can be avoided, the neurolysis procedure produces a good result. However, in some areas, the conditions for regeneration are not sufficiently good, as is the case in the tarsal tunnel and in the carpal tunnel, especially if an inflammatory process or if several operations have preceded. A limited number of patients with a thoracic outlet syndrome develop a recurrent fibrosis at the site of the operation that becomes a pathologic process on its own and develops a pain syndrome that has only marginal relations to the original thoracic outlet syndrome. In such cases, the only way to get control of the pain syndrome in some of the patients is to envelop the nerve segment in a gliding tissue flap after the neurolysis. Such a gliding tissue flap can be provided from the gliding tissue underneath the scapula, which derives its blood supply from the thoracodorsal artery and vein.[31] Alternatively, a subpectoral gliding tissue may be used that is based on the ramus pectoralis on the arteria thoracoacromialis.[32] This tissue which allows the surgeon to envelop the supraclavicular and infraclavicular brachial plexus. The flap based on the thoracodorsal artery can be transferred as a free flap.

LOSS OF CONTINUITY

An agent that damages a nerve can cause different situations of lost continuity.

1. In a relatively clean transection, continuity is lost. The adjacent segments of a nerve are damaged, but no defect exists.
2. The causal agent destroys a segment of the nerve and provokes a definite defect.
3. The distal stump of a nerve close to its target organ is damaged, and no distal stump is available.
4. The proximal segment of a nerve is avulsed from the spinal cord, as happens in a traction lesion of the brachial plexus, and no proximal stump is available.

As far as the motor axons are concerned, wallerian regeneration occurs distal to the lesion and the distal stumps, and the supplied muscles become denervated. The same is true for sensory axons, with the exception of the avulsion lesion of the brachial plexus, in which the spinal ganglion is avulsed with the spinal nerve, therefore, the sensory fibers in the distal stump do not undergo wallerian degeneration.

The aim of all surgical efforts is to achieve neurotization of the denervated distal area. In a relatively clean transection, the proximal and the distal stump are coapted (neurorrhaphy). The denervated distal stump and the target organs are neurotized from the proximal stump (nerve-to-nerve neurotization).

In case of a defect, under certain circumstances, an end-to-end neurorrhaphy can be achieved, which would involve the same nerve-to-nerve neurotization as is performed in relatively clean transections. If this is not possible, a nerve graft is carried out. An alternative to nerve grafting has to be used. The neurotization occurs either nerve (proximal stump) to nerve graft to nerve (distal stump), or nerve proximal stump, neuromatous neurotization of the interposed substitute nerve distal stump.

If there is no distal stump, the proximal stump of a motor nerve can be inserted into the muscle tissue (nerve-muscle neurotization). Alternatives are muscle-to-muscle neurotization if an innervated muscle is brought into direct contact with a denervated muscle, or muscle-nerve-muscle neurotization if an innervated muscle is connected by nerve grafts with a denervated muscle.

In cases of root avulsion, the neurotization is achieved by transferring of axons from a proximal stump of a donor nerve to the denervated distal stump.

GAP BETWEEN STUMPS

If continuity is lost, a gap exists between the two stumps. In a relatively clean transection, the gap between the two stumps is enlarged by the elastic retraction that acts on the proximal and the distal stump. To approximate the two stumps, the force of this elastic retraction has to be overcome by elongation of the adjacent segments at the proximal and distal stumps.

In cases of a secondary repair after a very clean transection, the adjacent segments of the proximal and the distal stumps, which had been exposed to the trauma, have developed a certain fibrosis and have lost their extensibility. The gap is maintained not only by the elastic retraction but also by a certain amount of a fibrotic retraction. End-to-end coaptation can be achieved by overcoming the elastic retraction by elongating the adjacent normal segments of the proximal and distal stumps. These normal segments have to be further elongated to compensate for the loss of extensibility in the directly adjacent fibrotic segments. It is, therefore, more difficult in secondary repair to achieve end-to-end coaptation, even if no defect was present.

If the transection was not very clean, the adjacent segments of the two nerve stumps have been damaged themselves and react with fibrosis in the same way that fibrosis is provoked in cases with preserved continuity. At the very distal end of the proximal stump, there might be only scar tissue, like damage occurring in IVS. The more proximal segment has developed a neuroma (IVN). More proximally, all the different damage as occur in lesions with preserved continuity may be encountered, such as IIIC, IIIB, IIIA, IIB, IIA, IB and IA. A segment with a second- and third-degree damage may be penetrated by neuromatous tissue (IIIN, respectively IIN). In operative reports, resection of the proximal stump usually occurs until normal nerve tissue is encountered. What is normal nerve tissue? There is no question that a segment showing IVS, IVN, and IIIC should be resected. Is IIIN also to be resected? The resection certainly should proceed until normal axons are encountered, which means until a morphologic structure is present. Is IA or IB also to be resected, or can we accept the fibroses? We really do not know, because no objective study exists that defines the necessary amount of resection.

These remarks may lead to a better understanding of the statement made previously that in primary repair, the estimation of the necessary dissection is nearly impossible because a grading of the damage cannot be obtained due to the fact that wallerian degeneration and fibrotic reaction have not yet commenced. In early secondary repair, the amount of damage can be estimated exactly, however, the surgeon now has to face the fibrotic retraction also. The amount of resection of damaged tissue of the proximal and distal stumps increases the distance between the two stumps that has to be overcome to achieve end-to-end approximation. With increasing distance, the distance will become too long to be managed without tension and nerve grafting, or an alternative to nerve grafting may need to be considered.

If no distal stump is available, all the considerations considered under relatively clean transections are valid. In addition, the defect of nerve tissue produced by the trauma exists. The gap between the two stumps consists of the distance created by elastic retraction, the fibers' retraction in cases of secondary nerve repair, the defect created by the proper resection of the proximal and distal stumps, and the original defect caused by the trauma.

In root avulsions, the same considerations as those for relatively clean transections and defects apply.

TECHNIQUE

Relatively Sharp Transection

If the distance between the two stumps remains under a tolerable limit, a neurorrhaphy is performed. The discussion of whether epineurial or fascicular neurorrhaphy should be preferred is endless, as is the discussion of whether suturing or gluing is the better technique. Most of these discussions do not address the issue.

A neurorrhaphy is performed in four basic steps. Each step can be carried out in different ways, and the technique applied may be a mixture of different basic techniques. The actual fascicular pattern is the decisive factor that influences the decision of which basic technique is elected.

The basic steps of a neurorrhaphy are:

PREPARATION OF THE STUMPS TO ACHIEVE PROPER RESECTION, WHICH CAN OCCUR IN TWO WAYS: segmental resection until normal tissue is met, and interfascicular dissection. The resection for each fascicle is performed individually exactly at the limit between normal and damaged tissue.

It is evident that in a monofascicular pattern or in an oligofascicular pattern with few fascicles (4 to 5), resection is the method of choice. In an oligofascicular pattern with five to 12 fascicles of manageable size, the interfascicular dissection is preferable. In a polyfascicular pattern with a group arrangement, the individual fascicle groups can be isolated. In a polyfascicular pattern without a group arrangement, the interfascicular dissection would be too traumatic for the nerve and, again, a segmental resection is preferable.

APPROXIMATION. The two nerve stumps have to be approximated, and the distance between the two stumps has to be overcome. This process can be made easier by mobilization and, of course, by flexing of the adjacent joints. However, the problem is only postponed by this action.

COAPTATION OF THE FASCICULAR TISSUE. This step is the most important one. Very often, the second and the third steps are referred to as one, but this does not really describe the situation. To achieve optimal fascicular coaptation, the two stumps must already be approximated. In a clean transection without a defect and without resection, the fascicular pattern of the two stumps corresponds very well, and trunk-to-trunk coaptation achieves fascicular coaptation if a rotational deformity is avoided. With a monofascicular pattern, trunk-to-trunk coaptation is the same as fascicle-to-fascicle coaptation because there is only one fascicle and an epineurial repair is the optimal solution.

If the cross section consists of a maximum of five large fascicles, fascicular coaptation is also to be achieved by trunk-to-trunk coaptation because the location of the fascicles can be influenced ab externo. Here, again, trunk-to-trunk coaptation (epineurial repair) is the treatment of choice.

If there are six, seven, or eight fascicles, only the externally located fascicles can be coapted well by external management, but we have no influence whatsoever on the coaptation of the central fascicle. In this situation, fascicular coaptation after the few large manageable fascicles are separated offers better chances, especially if there are pure motor and pure sensory fascicles. In this situation, motor-sensory differentiation by staining of the motor axons as a result of their higher content of acetylcholinesterase[33,34] offers an advantage. The same is true if the nerve consists of a limited number of fascicle groups with separated motor and sensory nerve fibers.

An alternative to coaptation is putting the stump into a tube, leaving a small gap between the two stumps to permit neurotropic factors to attract axons of different kind into the proper direction.

MAINTENANCE OF THE COAPTATION. Once achieved, coaptation has to be maintained by very fine, atraumatic stitches (8-0 or 10-0), or glue, or a combination of stitches and glue. If a tube is used, stitches between the tube and the nerve trunk in a distance from the end of the nerve stumps avoid separation. The surgeon must remember that only a minimal amount of stitches is necessary if the expected tension at the site of coaptation is zero and increases with a rise of tension. Glue is not able to resist tension and can be applied only if a tensionless repair is expected.

Management of Nerve Defect

There are four ways to manage nerve defects: elongation, short cut, nerve graft, and other, substitute grafts.

Elongation

ELONGATION OF THE ADJACENT NERVE SEGMENTS. This procedure can be performed preoperatively by application of an expander for the proximal or the distal segment.[35] So far, the reports of successes of these techniques are limited.

POSTOPERATIVE ELONGATION. This procedure is the usual way to manage a larger distance by end-to-end nerve repair. For nerves located at the flexor side, like the median nerve, the adjacent joints are flexed, and the bed of the nerve can be shortened by 15 percent. It is therefore possible to achieve tensionless repair after a defect of 15 percent of the median nerve as long as the limb remains in a flexed position. If the limb is immobilized after 3 to 6 weeks, the adjacent segments of the nerve have to be elongated to allow the limb to achieve full extension again. If the whole length of the nerve would be available for equal distribution of the amount of elongation over the total length of a nerve, each segment should not be elongated too much. However, the nerve becomes adherent at the site of trauma; therefore, the free length of nerve tissue available for elongation is limited. The distribution of the necessary elongation is also influenced in a negative way if the site of the injury is close to a joint or if the site of the injury is close to branches leaving the nerve. Under favorable conditions, even a neurorrhaphy under tension may lead to a useful recovery; however, the chance for this result is significantly reduced. In 1957, Nicholson and Seddon[36] demonstrated that useful recovery in median nerve lesions near the wrist joint was 70 percent if the defect was below 2.5 cm and dropped to 50 percent if the defect was between 2.5 and 5 cm. This deterioration of the prognosis cannot be accepted if an alternative with better chances is available, such as nerve grafting. Before the 1960s, the results of nerve grafts were poor, and all surgeons attempted to force an end-to-end neurorrhaphy. Since the significant improvement of nerve grafting, the situation has completely changed, and everybody agrees that beyond a certain defect, nerve grafting offers better chances than forced neurorrhaphy. Between these extremes, a gray zone remains in which some surgeons would already decide to use a graft and others still would attempt to preform an end-to-end neurorrhaphy. This decision will be influenced by the laxity or rigidity of the tissues of a particular patient, the site of the lesion, the question of whether a primary (more proper for neurorrhaphy) or a secondary (more proper for grafting) repair must be performed, and the question of whether branches are in the close neighborhood.

Animal experiments are of no help in the making of this decision. In a recent paper, Hentz and coworkers[37] claimed that in defects up to 3 or 4 cm in adults, epineurial repair seems to have advantages over the use of an autograft. I have performed experiments with macaque monkeys,[38] in which longitudinal incisions were made from the fingertip to the palm across all the flexion creases of the finger. Because of the laxity of the tissues, none of the monkeys developed a flexion contracture. By multiple excisions creating a heavy tension of the skin on the palmar aspect of the fingers, a slight contracture was produced. From these experiments, I could have made the statements that in a primate model it became apparent that longitudinal incisions along the palmar aspect of the fingers would never produce a flexion contracture. Every experienced surgeon can easily realize that such a conclusion from this primate model experience would be wrong. I would, therefore, warn against the drawing of similar conclusions from primate models as far as nerve repair is concerned.

Short Cut

If the bed of a certain nerve is longer than the direct line between two points, some gain in length can be achieved by transposition. The classic example is the ulnar nerve because of its location on the dorsal side of the elbow joint. The course of the ulnar nerve has to be longer than the short-cut connection from the medial aspect of the upper arm along the palmar side of the elbow joint to the palmar side of the forearm. If the nerve is transposed to the palmar aspect of the elbow joint, the nerve is located in a shorter bed, an effect that can be used to manage a defect of the ulnar nerve in this segment. The difference between the length of the dorsal and the palmar bed, about 2 cm, is not too important. If flexion of the elbow joint is avoided, a defect of 2 cm can be overcome. A longer defect can be managed only if the elbow joint is flexed, which means that all the problems discussed under elongation come into play.

Nerve Grafting

CLASSIFICATION OF NERVE GRAFTS. There are different ways to perform nerve grafting; therefore, an exact description is necessary if the results are to be evaluated. Comparing nerve grafts versus neurorrhaphy without giving these details is not sufficient.

ORIGIN. Usually nerve grafts are harvested from donor nerves of the same patients (autografts). In this way, immunologic problems are avoided. However, the patient has to accept some loss of function and must undergo additional surgical procedures to harvest the grafts.

A fresh allograft from another human being behaves at first like an autograft; however, an immunologic reaction is provoked that leads to the rejection of the graft. This rejection can be prevented by administration of immunosuppressive medication such as cyclosporine.[39] Even if the immunoreaction is prevented, the regeneration is less complete than that obtained with autologic nerve grafts.[40] At present, allografting is justified only in cases that need immunosuppressive therapy for other reasons, such as in patients who have had an organ transplant. Xenografts derive from an individual of another species and cause even more immunologic problems.

Preserved allografts consist only of a connective tissue framework without vital cells. They serve as a rail for a neuroma growing along the preserved allograft.[41] The results for such procedures are poor. In theory, an allogenic connective tissue framework could be popularized by Schwann cells of the recipient that are multiplied by cell culture.[42, 43]

DONOR NERVES. Cutaneous nerves like the sural nerve, the cutaneous antebrachii medialis, the cutaneous femoris lateralis, and the saphenous nerve can be excised without significant loss of function. They are of proper size to survive free grafting, which means that the spontaneous revascularization in the recipient site happens sufficiently fast to avoid tissue damage in the center of the graft.

Nerve trunks are usually not available as donors, except in cases of amputation, in brachial plexus lesions with multiple root avulsion, or if it is decided to repair one nerve, usually the median nerve, at the expense of another one. Nerve trunks are too thick to survive free grafting and spontaneous revascularization takes too long. Until revascularization reaches the center of the nerve trunk, ischemic tissue damage has happened, and fibrosis develops. Nerve trunks can be used as grafts only if circulation is maintained or immediately restored by microvascular anastomosis. If a trunk graft is available and cannot be used as a vascularized graft, the nerve trunk can be split into minor units by microscopic dissection that consists of dividing it into minor units of the proper size to survive free grafting. A successful series of split nerve grafts was reported on recently.[44] The use of cutaneous nerve grafts or split nerve grafts has another advantage: these nerve grafts can be connected with fascicles or fascicle groups of the same size of the proximal and distal stumps to areas of the distal stump. If a trunk graft is applied, the course of the axons along the graft cannot be predicted because of the plexiform structure of the nerve trunks.

In the 1940s and 1950s investigators attempted to combine several segments of cutaneous nerves to form a cable graft of the same size as the nerve to be repaired.[45] In this procedure, the cutaneous nerve segments lose a great part of their surface for contact with the surrounding tissue because it is in contact with another free graft and cannot survive well. This is one of the reasons why free cutaneous grafts did not work well in the past. Strange[46] and Shelden and associates[47] transplanted nerves as pedicled grafts with a preserved blood supply. In this procedure, one of two parallel running nerves (e.g., the median nerve) is repaired at the expense of another nerve (e.g., the ulnar nerve). The results were not convincing.[48, 49]

Taylor and Ham[50] and Taylor[51] developed a vascularized nerve graft technique. A nerve trunk is transferred, and the circulation re-established, by microvascular anastomosis of a dominant vessel, which supplies the whole nerve segment.

Breidenbach and Terzis[52, 53] studied the vascular anatomy of different nerves and described proper donor sites for vascularized nerve grafts. In brachial plexus cases, it is possible to use the ulnar nerve as a vascularized graft, thereby preserving the superior collateral ulnar artery as a vascular pedicle that supplies the whole length of the nerve. The great expectations related to this type of nerve grafting did not come true. The results of vascularized nerve grafts used under comparable conditions are not necessarily superior to free grafts. We compared the neurotization of the musculocutaneous nerve by vascularized nerve graft with the neurotization of the muscle branches to the triceps by free nerve grafts and could not find significant differences.

MECHANICS. In the past, cases with nerve defects were treated by approximation of the two stumps as much as possible to decrease the distance between the two stumps. The remaining distance was then bridged by nerve grafts. In this situation, the unfavorable circumstances of a nerve graft (having two sites of coaptation) were combined with the unfavorable situation of nerve coaptation under tension. Free nerve grafts survive by spontaneous revascularization across adhesions between the nerve graft and the surrounding tissue. They lose the necessary motility. Free nerve grafts are therefore extremely sensitive to longitudinal traction; hence, everything that leads to longitudinal traction has to be avoided. It is, therefore, important to select the length of the nerve graft to correspond to the maximal distance between the two stumps in extended position of the limb. The nerve grafting procedure is performed in this way, and the limb is immobilized in this position. After 10 days, the limb can be flexed, which means that the adherent nerve graft can slacken without being tracted in longitudinal direction. If the length of the nerve graft was defined in flexed position with minimal distance between the two stumps, the graft is exposed to longitudinal traction if the mobilization of the limb starts. The two sites of coaptation come under tension with all the deteriorating effects on the nerve regeneration. It is wrong to define the length of the nerve graft with the limb in extended position and to immobilize the limb in flexed position. In this case, the graft becomes adherent in slackened position, and in spite of the fact that the graft was originally long enough, the two sites of coaptation come under tension if the limb is mobilized.

NERVE GRAFTING TECHNIQUE. A nerve grafting procedure that uses segments of cutaneous nerve, is performed under the same rules as a neurorrhaphy at both extremities of the grafts.

STUMP PREPARATION. The preparation is carried out in a similar way. If there is a monofascicular pattern or an oligofascicular pattern with very few fascicles, the stumps are prepared by serial resections, and a sufficiently high number of cutaneous nerve segments is used to satisfy the cross section of the one or the few large fascicles. Narakas[54] suggested that the epineurium be resected at the extremities of the nerve grafts and that these extremities be glued together, using tissue coll to bring as many nerve segments as possible in close contact with the fascicular surface of the proximal or distal stump.

If the nerve stumps consist of a limited number of manageable fascicles, these fascicles are separated by microsurgical dissection, and each fascicle end is coapted with a cutaneous nerve segment.

If a polyfascicular structure with group arrangement is present, the individual groups are isolated by microsurgical dissection, and each group is connected to a cutaneous nerve graft. If polyfascicular structure without group arrangement exists, nerve grafts are coapted to certain sectors of the cross section without individualization of the large number of small fascicles.

APPROXIMATION. The nerve grafts have to be approximated to the proximal, respectively to the distal stump without damaging the tissue by mechanical manipulation. The best way to achieve this approximation is to use a 10-0 nylon stitch that is anchored in the graft and in the fascicle, respectively the fascicle group of the stumps and used to manipulate the graft to achieve optimal approximation. Because the grafts are longer than the distance between the two stumps in extended position, the approximation poses no problem.

COAPTATION. Every attempt is made to coapt the fascicular cross sections of the cutaneous nerve graft with the fascicular coaptation of the fascicles, respectively groups of fascicles of the proximal and distal stump. Especially if a group arrangement exists, an optimal coaptation cannot be achieved, because of the different number and different sizes of the fascicles within the group, respectively within the graft. In spite of this fact, optimal regeneration can be achieved.[26] I am sure that in this situation, neurotropic and neurotrophic factors help to achieve a good result.

In most cases, the one stitch used for approximation is also used to achieve optimal coaptation. Sometimes, the extremity of the graft rotates away from the cross section of the fascicle, respectively the fascicle group of the proximal and the distal stump. Under these circumstances, a second or even a third stitch may be necessary.

COAPTATION MAINTENANCE. Because no longitudinal traction exists, the few stitches needed to achieve approximation and proper coaptation are sufficient to maintain the coaptation. Extreme care is necessary to avoid shearing forces during wound closure, and the limb has to be immobilized in the exact position it was in during the operation to avoid dislocation or disrupture. We also do not use suction drainage in these cases.

The safety of the coaptation may be increased by the application of glue (fibrinogen concentrate and thrombin to produce a fibrin coagulum). However, it is not necessary.

Substitutes for Nerve Grafts

Schwann cells, capillaries, and fibroblast from the proximal stump proceed in a distal direction. To protect these efforts of regeneration against the ingrowth of fibroblasts from the surrounding tissue and to direct regeneration in the proper direction, a tissue chamber;[19] a polyglycolic acid tube,[55] which offers the additional advantage that the tube is resorbable and disappears; or a vein can be used[56] to connect the two nerve stumps. Hems and Glasby[57] suggest the use of the connective tissue framework of a muscle after freeze thawing. Recently, vein grafts were combined with freeze-thawed muscle that was stuffed into the vein.[58] Some positive results can be achieved with all these techniques; they remain, however, always inferior to an autologous nerve graft. These techniques are still reserved for less important nerves.

NO DISTAL STUMP

Neurotization by Nerve to Muscle

If no distal stump is available, motor branches of a peripheral nerve can be brought directly into contact with the denervated muscle. The nerve is split into its individual fascicles, and these fascicles are introduced into the muscle substance between the bundles of the muscle. This insertion of the distal end of the nerve, respectively its individual fascicles, is performed at the level at which most endplates can be expected (close to the muscle hilus). The connection of the nerve to the muscle is maintained by a few stitches between the epineurium of the nerve trunk and the permisium.

NO PROXIMAL STUMP (ROOT AVULSION)

Neurotization by Nerve Transfer

In cases of root avulsion of more than two roots, other nerves are transected and connected to distal stumps, either directly or by use of nerve grafts. The following nerves are used as axon donors:

Accessory nerve
Motor branches of the cervical plexus

Supraclavicular nerve for sensory fibers
Intercostal brachial nerve for sensory fibers
Hypoglossus nerve[59]
Phrenic nerve[60, 61]
Intercostal nerves[45, 62]
Root C7 of the contralateral side[63, 64]

In cases of avulsion of either four or five roots, we use transfers as indicated in Table 173–1. We have used the C7 transfer in three cases. It is too early to discuss the results; however, in none of these three cases has permanent loss of function been produced at the contralateral arm. The technical aspects are the same as those in management of a nerve defect.

Sometimes, the rootlets are avulsed but the spinal nerve remains in the intervertebral canal. In this case, the diagnosis of root avulsion cannot be established directly. For several years, we have used the central stimulation technique to get information, regardless of whether a motor stimulus travels along the ventral roots to the distal stump.[65]

POSTOPERATIVE CARE

Accurate immobilization is extremely important for the first few days after the procedure. After 8 days all splints can be removed, and the patient can start to move because the sites of coaptation are strong enough to resist the traction. This traction is low because during mobilization, the graft is relaxed rather than extended. Postoperatively, the patient undergoes physiotherapy and electric stimulation of the muscles with exponential current.

In rare cases of nerve grafting, the axons cannot cross from the distal end of the graft to the distal stump because of scar formation at this level. This situation can be recognized by the arrest of the advancement of the Tinel sign at the distal extremity of the graft. In this case, the distal end of the graft has to be explored, and eventually scarred segment in this area must be resected and a new coaptation performed.

PALLIATIVE SURGERY

Very often, surgery at the peripheral nerves does not completely solve the problem.

In cases of irreparable nerve lesion, typical tendon transfers have been developed to restore hand function to some degree (tendon transfers for radial nerve, median nerve-low and high-, ulnar nerve-low and high-, combined median and ulnar nerve). With these techniques, normal, noninvolved muscles are transferred to replace muscles that are paralyzed as a result of an irreversible nerve lesion. In brachial plexus cases, similar transfers are possible.

One such transfer is transposition of the origin of the flexor muscle from the epicondylus medialis humeri to the humerus shaft to give them additional efficiency for the flexion of the elbow joint[66] in cases of upper brachial plexus lesions. The major pectoralis muscle can be transferred for replacement of the biceps as well as the latissimus dorsi muscle. Typical tendon transfers can be performed in partial brachial plexus lesions for the forearm muscles and the hand.

In a complete brachial plexus lesion, tendon transfers, eventually combined with an arthrodesis, play an important role. In these cases, originally paralyzed muscles that have regenerated are used to replace the missing function of another muscle.

A useful procedure is the arthrodesis of the shoulder joint in peripheral brachial plexus lesions in which the serratus anterior muscle has remained intact. This muscle then moves the arm by moving the scapula. If the serratus anterior muscle is not functioning very well, arthrodesis of the shoulder joint is not indicated.

Very often, external rotation does not return, and patients with useful recovery of the elbow joint cannot use this function in space because external rotation is lacking. In these cases, we perform a rotational osteotomy of about 70 degrees and transfer either the minor or the major pectoralis muscle for active external rotation.

The trapezius muscle can be transferred, including its bony insertion at the acromion to the neck of the humerus, to stabilize the shoulder joint and eventually achieve some abduction. Because the triceps muscle regenerates sometimes better than the biceps muscle, we usually neurotize also the triceps in spite of the fact that it is an antagonist of the biceps muscle. If both achieve useful function and can be innervated independently, a good result has been achieved. Unfortunately, this is the exception. Usually, both muscles are innervated simultaneously, and one muscle impedes the function of the other muscle. This fact is taken into account at the beginning because the neurotization of both muscles has been performed in a second stage with the intention to transfer the triceps to the biceps tendon and to have both acting as flexors. A weak biceps can be replaced by a strong triceps. A weak biceps combined with a weak triceps may increase the force of elbow flexion to achieve useful function. If the

Table 173–1. FUNCTIONAL RESULTS AFTER PERONEAL NERVE LESIONS II NERVE GRAFTING ($n = 30$)

Result	Cases	NG Only (First Series)	NG Only (Second Series)	Same Patients (Second Series) After TPTT	NG + Simultaneous TPTT (Third Series)
Good	14	—	1	6	7
Satisfactory	8	—	1	1	6
Fair	1	—	—	1	—
Poor	7	5	8	—	—
Partial nerve regeneration					
No nerve regeneration	0	—	2	—	—
Total	30	5	12	8	13

NG = nerve grafting.

use of one, two, or three forearm muscles has returned in cases of complete brachial plexus lesions, a primitive grip function can be reconstructed, by use of tenodesis of the wrist joint, the interphalangeal joint of the thumb, and eventually other joints.

It is possible to replace an important function, such as elbow flexion or wrist and finger flexion, by use of a free muscle graft. Terzis (Personal communication, 1991) plans free muscle grafting at the brachial plexus reconstruction and leaves proximally connected nerve grafts distally free to attach free muscle grafts in a later stage.

Under certain instances, palliative surgery has a stimulating effect on nerve regeneration. A typical example is the peroneal nerve. This nerve has a bad reputation, and useful recoveries are rare if there is a longer defect and if more than 3 months have elapsed since the injury. The postoperative nerve regeneration can be significantly enhanced if simultaneously with the nerve repair or a short time later a tibialis posterior transfer to the dorsum of the foot is performed to correct the foot drop. This procedure achieves better equilibrium between dorsiflexion and plantar flexion and protects the anterior muscles against overextension (Table 173-1).

REFERENCES

1. Williams PL, Warwick R (eds): Gray's anatomy, 36th ed. Edinburgh, London, Melbourne, New York, Churchill Livingstone, 1980
2. Sunderland S: Meningeal-neural relations in the intervertebral foramen. J Neurosurg 40:756–763, 1974
3. Sunderland S: Mechanism of cervical nerve root avulsion in injuries of the neck and shoulder. J Neurosurg 41:705–714, 1974
4. Sunderland S: Anatomical perivertebral influences on the intervertebral foramen, in The Research Status of Spinal Manipulative Therapy. NINCDS Monograph, US Department of Health, Education, and Welfare. Bethesda, Maryland, 1975, no 15, p 129
5. Sunderland S: Avulsion of nerve roots, in Braakman R (ed): Handbook of Clinical Neurology, vol 25, Part I: Injuries of the Spinal Cord and Column. Amsterdam, North Holland Publishing Company, 1976, pp 393–435
6. Lundborg G, Nordberg C, Rydevik B, Olsson Y: The effect of ischemia on the permeability of the perineurium to protein tracers in rabbit tibial nerve. Acta Neurol Scand 49:287–294
7. Röhlich P, Weiss M: Studies on the histology and permeability of the peripheral nervous barrier. Acta Morpho Hung 5:335, 1955
8. Shanthaveerappa TR, Bourne GH: The "perineural epithelium," a metabolically active continuous, protoplasmatic cell barrier surrounding peripheral nerve fasciculi. J Anat 96:527, 1962
9. Fontana F: Traité sur le Venin de la Vipère et sur les Poissons Américains. Firenze 1781
10. Lang J: Über die Bindegewebe und die Gefäße der Nerven. Anat Embryol (Berl) 123:61–79, 1962
11. Zöch G, Reihsner R, Beer R, Millesi H: Stress and strain in peripheral nerves. Neuro-orthopedics 10:371–382, 1991
12. Zöch G: Über die Anpassung peripherer Nerven an die Bewegungen der Extremitäten durch Gleiten und Dehnung. Untersuchungen am Nervus medianus. Acta Chir Aust 96(suppl):1–16, 1992
13. Seddon HJ: Three types of nerve injury. Brain 66:237, 1943
14. Sunderland S: A classification of peripheral nerve injuries producing loss of function. Brain 74:491, 1951
15. Millesi H: Microsurgery of peripheral nerves, neurolysis, nerve grafts, brachial plexus injuries, in Buncke HJ, Furnas DW (eds): Proceedings on Clinical Frontiers in Reconstructive Microsurgery, St. Louis, CV Mosby, 1984, pp 353–373
16. Millesi H, Kovac W: Histologic observation after peripheral nerve injury and after nerve repair. Paper held at the Meeting of the Sunderland Society, Durham, NC, June 24–28, 1988
17. Millesi H: Eingriffe an peripheren Nerven, in Gschnitzer F, Kern E, Schweiberer L (eds): Chirurgische Operationslehre V. München, Wien, Baltimore, Urban & Schwarzenberg, 1986, pp 1–88
18. Millesi H, Kovac W: Morphologic classification of nerve stumps. Paper held at the symposium Peripheral Nerve Surgery Today—Turning Point or Continuous Development? Vienna, Austria, Nov 23–26, 1991
19. Lundborg G, Hansson HA: Regeneration of a peripheral nerve through a preformed tissue space. Brain Res 178:573–576, 1979
20. Lundborg G, Hansson HA: Nerve lesions with interruption of continuity. Studies on the growth pattern of regenerating in the gap between the proximal and distal nerve ends, in Gorio A, Millesi H, Mingrino S (eds): Posttraumatic Peripheral Nerve Regeneration—Experimental Basis and Clinical Implications. New York, Raven Press, 1981, pp 229–239
21. Schröder JM, Seiffert KE: Die Feinstruktur der neuromatösen Neurotisation von Nerventransplantaten. Virchows Arch B Cell Pathol B5:219, 1970
22. Brushart TM: Preferential reinnervation of motor nerves by regenerating motor axons. J Neurosci 8:1026–1031, 1988
23. Brushart TM: Preferential motor reinnervation. Pathway regulation. (abstract). Soc Neurosci 15:533, 1989
24. Brushart TM: Preferential motor reinnervation. A sequential double labelling study. Restor Neurol Neurosci 1:281–287, 1990
25. Brushart TM: Motor axons preferentially reinnervated motor pathway. J Neurosci 13:2730–2738, 1993
26. Millesi H: How exact should coaptation be? in Gorio A, Millesi H, Mingrino S (eds): Posttraumatic Peripheral Nerve Regeneration—Experimental Basis and Clinical Implications. New York, Raven Press, 1981, pp 301–306
27. Millesi H: Clinical aspects of nerve healing, in Gibson T, van der Meulen JC (eds): Wound Healing. Montreux, Foundation International Corporation on the Medical Sciences, 1975, pp 301–306
28. Millesi H: Healing of nerves. Clin Plast Surg 4:459–473, 1977
29. Millesi H, Berger A, Meissl G: Razvoj Reparatorno-Operativnih Postupaka kod Ozljeda Periferinih Zivaca. Drugi Simpozij Bolestima o Ozljedama Sake. Zagreb, Medicinska Knjga, 1970, pp 161–175
30. Millesi H, Berger A, Meissl G: Experimentelle Untersuchungen zur Heilung Durchtrenner Peripherer Nerven. Chir Plast 1:174–206, 1972
31. Wintsch K: Free flap of gliding tissue. J Reconstr Microsurg 2:143–150, 1986
32. Millesi W, Schobel G, Bochdansky H: Subpectoral gliding tissue flap. J Plastic Reconstr Surg 1994, in press
33. Gruber H, Zenker W: Acetylcholinesterase: Histochemical differentiation between motor and sensory nerve fibres. Brain Res 51:207, 1973
34. Freilinger G, Gruber H, Holle J, Mandl H: Zur Methodik der "sensomotorisch" differenzierten Faszikelnaht peripherer Nerven. Handchir Mikrochir Plast Chir 7:133, 1975
35. Wood RJ, Adson MH, Van Beek AL, et al: Controlled expansion of peripheral nerves: Comparison of nerve grafting and nerve expansion/repair for canine sciatic nerve defects. J Trauma 31:686–690, 1991
36. Nicholson OR, Seddon J: Nerve practice: Results of treatment of median and ulnar nerve lesions. BMJ 2:1065–1071, 1957
37. Hentz VR, Rosen RM, Ciao HY, McGill KC: The nerve gap dilemma: Comparison of nerves repaired end-to-end under tension with nerve grafts to the primate model. J Hand Surg [Am] 18A:417–425, 1993
38. Walzer LR, Millesi H, Kovac W, Mallinger R: Experimental flexion contractures in Rhesus monkeys, in Williams HB (ed): Transactions VIII International Congress of Plastic and Reconstructive Surgery. Montreal, 1983, pp 20–22
39. Mackinnon SE, Hudson AR, Falk RE, Hunter DA: The nerve allograft response—An experimental model in the rat. Ann Plast Surg 14:334–339, 1985
40. Schaller E, Mailänder P, Becker M, et al: Nerve regeneration im im autologen und allogenen Transplantat des Nervus ischiadicus der Ratte mit und ohne Suppression durch Cyclosporin A. Handchir Mikrochir Plast Chir 20:7–10, 1988
41. Schröder JM, Seiffert KE: Die Feinstruktur der neuromatösen Neurotisation von Nerventransplantaten. Virchows Arch B Cell Pathol B5:219–222, 1970
42. Aguayo A: Construction of graft, in Gorio A, Millesi H, Mingrino S, (eds): Post-traumatic Peripheral Nerve Regeneration—Experimental Basis and Clinical Implications. New York, Raven Press, 1981, p 365
43. Bunge RP: Contributions of tissue culture to our understanding of basic processes in peripheral nerve regeneration, in Gorio A, Millesi H, Mingrino S, (eds): Posttraumatic Peripheral Nerve Regeneration—Experimental Basis and Clinical Implications. New York, Raven Press, 1981, p 105
44. Millesi H, Eberhard D: Das Spaltnerventransplantat. Paper presented at

the Thirty-first Annual Meeting of the Austrian Society for Plastic, Aesthetic and Reconstructive Surgery, Zell am See, Oct 14–16, 1993
45. Seddon HJ: The use of autogenous grafts for the repair of large gaps in peripheral nerves. Br J Surg 35:151–167, 1947
46. Strange FGStC: An operation for nerve pedicle grafting. Preliminary communication. Br J Surg 34:423–425, 1947
47. Shelden CH, Pudenz C, McCarthy S: Two stage autograft for repair of extensive median and ulnar nerve defect. J Neurosurg 4:492–496, 1947
48. Brooks D: The place of nerve grafting in orthopaedic surgery. J Bone Joint Surg Am 37:299–305, 1955
49. Strange FGStC: Case report on pedicled nerve graft. Br J Surg 37:331, 1950
50. Taylor GI, Ham FJ. The free vascularized nerve graft. Plast Reconstr Surg 57:413–426, 1976
51. Taylor GI: Nerve grafting with simultaneous microvascular reconstruction. Clin Orthop 133:56, 1978
52. Breidenbach WB, Terzis JK: Vascularized nerve grafts. Scholarship Context American Society for Plastic and Reconstructive Surgery, 1983
53. Breidenbach WB, Terzis JK: The anatomy of free vascularized nerve grafts. Clin Plast Surg 11:65–71, 1984
54. Narakas A: Ten years of experience with tissucol in the repair of plexus brachialis. Paper present at the Symposium Update and Future Trends in Fibrin Sealing in Surgical and Non-Surgical Fields. Vienna, 1992
55. Mackinnon SE, Dellon AL: Clinical reconstruction with a bioabsorbable polyglycolic acid tube. Plast Reconstr Surg 85:419–424, 1990
56. Chiu DT, Strauch B: A prospective clinical evaluation of autogenous vein grafts used as a nerve conduit for distal sensory nerve defects of 3 cm or less. Plast Reconstr Surg 85:928–934, 1990
57. Hems TEJ, Glasby MA: Comparison of different methods of repair of long peripheral nerve defects: An experimental study. Br J Plast Surg 45:497–502, 1992
58. Battiston B, Vigasio A, Mattiuzzo V, et al: Nerve regeneration throughout vein grafts filled with muscle. First Meeting of the European Federation of Microsurgical Societies, Rome, September 26–29, 1992, abstract no. 32
59. Romana MC, Masquelet AC: Neurotisation of the musculocutaneous nerve by the hypoglossal nerve to restore elbow flexion in brachial plexus avulsed. First Meeting of the European Federation of Microsurgical Societies. Rome, September 26–29, 1992, Abstract no. 120
60. Narakas A: Remark at Panel Brachial plexus. Eleventh Symposium of the International Society of Reconstructive Microsurgery, Vienna, June 5–8, 1993
61. Gu YD, Zheng MM: Phrenic nerve transfer for brachial plexus motor neurotization. Microsurgery 10:1–3, 1989
62. Yeoman PM: quotation in Seddon HJ: Surgical Disorders of the Peripheral Nerves, 2nd ed. Edinburgh, Churchill Livingstone, 1975, p 197
63. Gu YD, Zhang GM, Chen DS, et al: Seventh cervical root transfer from the contralateral healthy side for treatment. J Hand Surg [Br] 17B:518–521, 1992
64. Chuang ChCh, Wei FC, Noordhoff MS: Cross-chest C7 nerve grafting followed by free muscle transplantations for the treatment of avulsed brachial plexus injuries: A preliminary report. Plast Reconstr Surg 92:717–727, 1993
65. Turkof E, Mayer N, Deecke L, Millesi H: Central stimulation to prove conductivity of spinal motor roots in brachial plexus surgery. Paper presented at the fourth International Congress of International Federation of Societies for Surgery of the Hand, Jerusalem, April 9–14, 1989
66. Steindler A: Tendon transplantation in the upper extremity. Am J Surg 44:260–271, 1939

CHAPTER 174

Surgical Management of Thoracic Outlet Syndrome and of Peripheral Entrapment Neuropathies

Suzie C. Tindall

This chapter outlines and illustrates the important principles of surgery of the most commonly encountered peripheral entrapment neuropathies. A brief discussion of the clinical presentation of each entity is given, but for more thorough information in this regard, one should consult the references listed, as well as several general references.[1-3]

THORACIC OUTLET SYNDROME

Thoracic outlet syndrome is one of the most controversial topics in entrapment neuropathies. Opinions differ widely as to whether or not it even exists, and if it does, its incidence; what constitutes the clinical syndrome; how it should be treated; and if it is treated surgically, what approach should be taken.[4] The diagnosis is relatively easy to make in the patient with end-stage wasting of the thenar and intrinsic muscles of the so-called Gilliatt hand as well as radiographic evidence of a cervical rib.[5] At the other end of the spectrum are patients who present with aching discomfort in the shoulder and arm, ulnar-sided paresthesias, and no abnormalities on physical, radiographic, or electrical examination. Within the latter category are many people who first experience their symptoms after an automobile accident or an on-the-job injury.

Factors important to the author in making the diagnosis of thoracic outlet syndrome are

1. A typical clinical syndrome with complaints of aching discomfort in the lateral neck, shoulder, and arm and paresthesias along the medial side of the forearm and hand
2. Symptoms made worse with activities of the arm, particularly working overhead
3. Radiographic evidence of a cervical rib, an abnormally prominent C7 transverse process, or an abnormal first thoracic rib configuration
4. Weakness or wasting of thenar and intrinsic muscles of the hand (other muscles can be involved)
5. Tenderness to palpation in the region of the thoracic outlet out of proportion to tenderness elsewhere
6. A positive Adson's maneuver
7. A prolonged ulnar sensory potential on nerve conduction testing

8. Little potential secondary gain

There are three possible surgical approaches to the thoracic outlet: supraclavicular, transaxillary first-rib resection, and posterior. The supraclavicular approach generally provides the most direct access to the area.

THORACIC OUTLET EXPLORATION: SUPRACLAVICULAR APPROACH

The incision for the supraclavicular approach is placed about 1 cm above the clavicle and extends medially from the lateral attachment of the sternal head of the sternocleidomastoid muscle laterally to the junction between the middle and lateral thirds of the clavicle (Fig. 174–1). The underlying platysma muscle, which varies in thickness, is incised in the same plane. The clavicular head of the sternocleidomastoid muscle is then resected off of the clavicle, and a small fringe of the muscle is left attached to the clavicle for later reap-

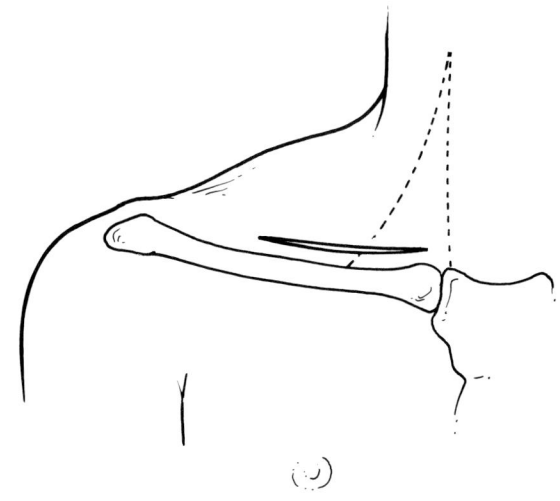

FIGURE 174–1. Skin incision for a supraclavicular exploration of the thoracic outlet. It is placed about one fingerbreadth above the clavicle, and extends from the lateral border of the sternal head of the sternocleidomastoid muscle to the junction of the middle and lateral thirds of the clavicle.

proximation at closure. Care must be taken to dissect carefully under this muscle before sectioning it because many small veins are hidden under it. This muscle is retracted upward and medially to gain exposure to the supraclavicular fat pad. Within the fat pad, the omohyoid muscle runs transversely across the exposure. This small tendinous band is sectioned, and both ends are tagged and retracted back. Likewise, the transverse cervical artery and vein are usually encountered in the more inferior part of the dissection just above the clavicle; these can be tied off and sectioned if necessary for exposure. Dissecting through the supraclavicular fat pad can be tedious because no definite planes exist, and many small vessels must be coagulated. Particularly on the left side, the surgeon must watch for lymphatic channels and tie them off to prevent postoperative difficulties of chylothorax or accumulation of chyle in the wound.

As the supraclavicular fat pad is mobilized and turned back, the scalenus anticus muscle is identified. This is a very important landmark. Over its surface runs the phrenic nerve, coursing from lateral to medial (the only nerve in this part of the neck that does so). This nerve should be mobilized and protected. Following it upward leads to its attachment to the upper trunk of the brachial plexus, which can be seen as a large nerve exiting beneath the lateral border of the scalenus anticus muscle (Fig. 174–2).

At this point, one of the most important parts of the exposure is undertaken. About 3 to 4 cm of the scalenus anticus muscle is resected to gain entrance to the thoracic outlet. The attachment of this muscle to the first rib is sectioned. Care must be taken to protect the phrenic nerve medially, the subclavian vein above, and the subclavian artery below the muscle while the muscle attachment is sectioned. The muscle attachment can be sectioned in layers while it is gently mobilized with a right-angled dissector. Care must be taken to avoid significant injury to the artery or vein or their branches in this location, which can be difficult to repair. Once the

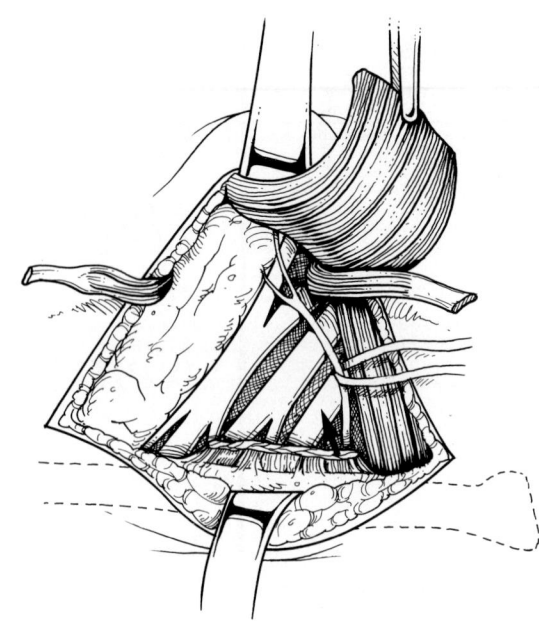

FIGURE 174–3. Final exposure of the region of the thoracic outlet after resection of the lower portion of the scalenus anticus muscle. The phrenic nerve is protected medially by a vascular loop. The three trunks of the plexus are identified in a configuration of descending stairsteps, and the subclavian artery generally has to be retracted downward so the lower trunk can be identified (single arrow).

attachment of the muscle to the first rib is sectioned, the muscle is mobilized by sectioning its attachments to the transverse processes and resecting the muscle just above the origin of the fifth root contribution to the upper trunk of the plexus.

With this muscle resected, one can identify the C5 and the C6 contributions to the upper trunk of the plexus. If the surgeon remembers that the trunks of the plexus are not laid out in a flat plane but are situated more like descending stairsteps in this area, finding the middle trunk and the C7 root just below and slightly under the C6 root is not difficult. To visualize the lower trunk, the surgeon should gently retract the subclavian artery anteroinferiorly (Fig. 174–3). Occasionally, a branch of the thyrocervical trunk needs to be sectioned between ties to mobilize the subclavian artery. As the lower trunk is followed medially, Sibson's fascia over the dome of the lung is released to identify the C8 and the T1 roots as they straddle the head of the first rib. The T1 root is often very deep in the dissection medially and behind the pleura. If a small hole is inadvertently placed in the pleura, it can be repaired around a small catheter, which is extracted under negative pressure during closure. If a sizable pneumothorax persists on a chest x-ray study postoperatively, a chest tube can be inserted.

A thorough exploration of the lower trunk from medially to laterally, and of the middle trunk as well, is necessary to ensure that all bands or offending structures are found and decompressed. Such tethering structures may be found at the level of the spinal nerve in conjunction with Sibson's fascia or the transverse process of C7 all the way out to the infraclavicular area. Tethering structures are usually anomalous white fibrous bands, but arteries and anomalous muscle fibers are also possible offenders. When a cervical rib is present, it may protrude into the plexus from behind, but the usual

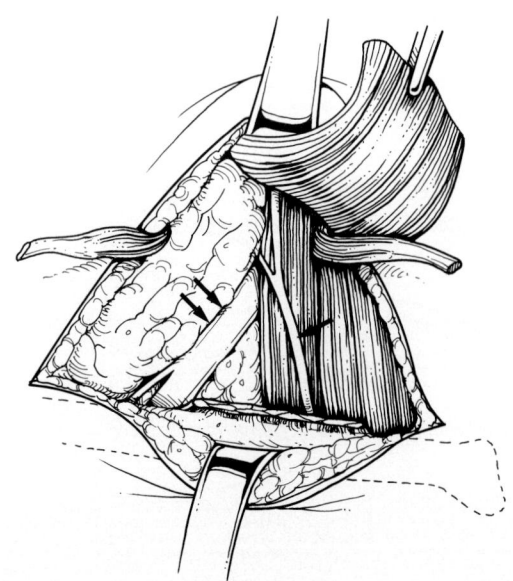

FIGURE 174–2. Halfway through the exposure of the thoracic outlet, the surgeon has sectioned the clavicular head of the sternocleidomastoid muscle and the omohyoid muscle, identified the phrenic nerve (single arrow) and the scalenus anticus muscle below it, and begun to free up the upper trunk of the brachial plexus (double arrow).

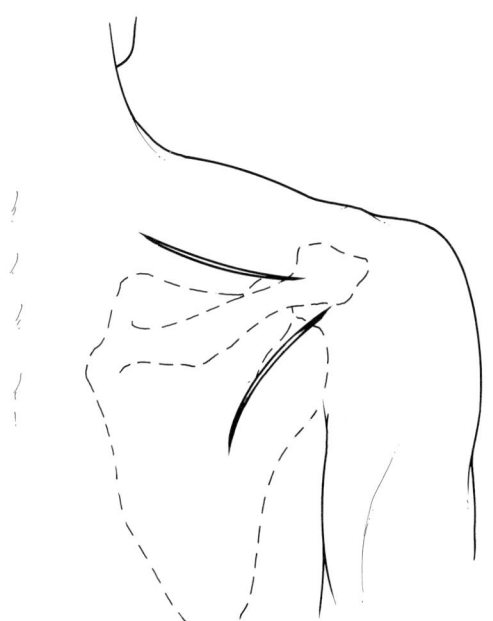

FIGURE 174-4. Skin incisions for exposure of the suprascapular nerve in the suprascapular notch and for exploration of the branch to the infraspinatus muscle.

major compressive problem is a fibrous band coming off of the cervical rib and extending down to the first rib.

A frequent quandary is the question of what constitutes the endpoint of the procedure. How much rib must be removed? Does any of the first rib need to come out? The author believes that the surgeon should remove anything that is an obvious compressive element. In most instances, the anomalous bands and muscle fibers can be removed completely. A cervical rib should be sectioned back so that it is not compressing any plexal element. This process may require considerable mobilization of the plexus elements. There is no need to remove the rib completely. Often, the patient with a cervical rib may have a prefixed plexus, and the patient with an anomalous first rib may have a postfixed plexus. Under such circumstances, the surgeon will have encountered abnormalities in the location of elements of the plexus during the original dissection. In the author's opinion, very rarely is there a need to remove part of the first rib, although this procedure can be performed. It is probable that the benefits of the transaxillary first-rib resection are derived from release of bands directly connected to the rib itself.

Closure of the wound is in anatomic layers. The scalenus anticus need not be reconstructed.

Complications of the procedure include pneumothorax, chylothorax, phrenic nerve paralysis, and pain secondary to manipulation of neural elements. If the patient fails to improve, the cause can usually be attributed to misdiagnosis preoperatively with failure to find a compressive element at the time of surgery, or to end-stage disease preoperatively (i.e., in the patient with an atrophic Gilliatt hand).

When extensive surgery has already been performed in the supraclavicular area, or when the compressive difficulty seems to be associated with an anomalous first rib, a posterior approach to the plexus may be preferred over the supraclavicular approach.[6]

SUPRASCAPULAR NERVE ENTRAPMENT

Suprascapular nerve entrapment may occur spontaneously but may be seen in weightlifters, gymnasts, and others who place a lot of stress on their shoulders. Most patients complain of pain in the posterior shoulder. Clinical examination reveals weakness isolated to supraspinatus and infraspinatus muscles; this status should be confirmed by electromyographic demonstration of denervation changes isolated to these muscles.[7]

Two exposures to this entrapment have been described, one from the front[8] and one from behind. The author prefers the latter.

POSTERIOR APPROACH

The patient is placed in the lateral position with the ipsilateral arm supported on an armrest. A small, 5- to 8-cm incision is placed over the superior scapula above the scapular spine (Fig. 174-4). Dissection is carried parallel to and through the trapezius fibers to the superior border of the scapula. In muscular individuals, this hole may be deep. The surgeon's forefinger is then placed on the top of the scapula and runs laterally until a depression in the bone is felt; this is usually the notch where the entrapment is located. After a retractor is placed to expose the notch, the suprascapular artery is dissected out. Immediately beneath it should be the suprascapular ligament (Fig. 174-5). It is usually possible to place a right-angled dissector beneath this ligament and to section it. However, if it is calcified, a Kerrison rongeur may be required. The nerve can be identified beneath the ligament within the notch. The nerve must be traced up under the supraspinatus muscle because ganglion cysts can lurk in this area and can be the source of entrapment. Rarely, patients can present with denervation in the infraspinatus muscle and may require only exposure of the nerve as it comes around the lateral aspect of the scapular spine. This procedure requires a separate incision.

Complications of this procedure are few. The surgeon may

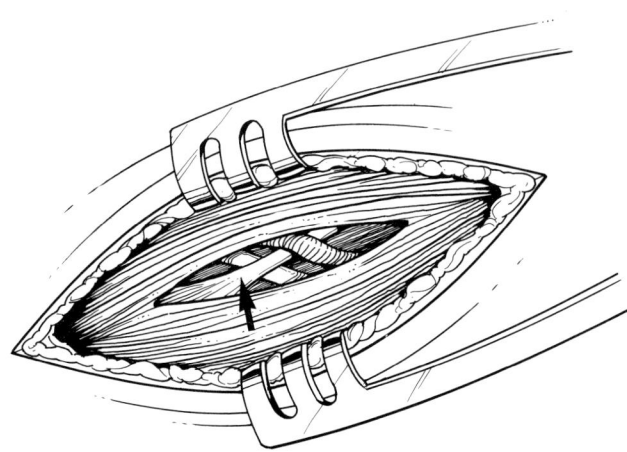

FIGURE 174-5. In this exposure of the scapular notch, the suprascapular artery passes over the ligament of the notch (single arrow) and the nerve passes under it.

ENTRAPMENTS OF THE RADIAL NERVE

The radial nerve is vulnerable to entrapment at several points along its course. The three commonest points are at the spiral groove of the humerus under the lateral head of the triceps muscle, in which case denervation and weakness are present in the brachioradialis muscle; in the proximal forearm at the supinator arcade of Frohse, which results in weakness of muscles innervated by the posterior interosseous nerve[9]; and at the proximal wrist between the tendons of the brachioradialis and the extensor carpi radialis longus, which results in a painful sensory neuropathy of the dorsal sensory branch.

With entrapment of the posterior interosseous nerve, weakness occurs in the extensors of the thumb, fingers, and the ulnar extensor of the wrist. The entrapment is usually at the fibrous arcade of Frohse in the supinator muscle, but lipomas, ganglions, and other lesions may occur in the area and may predispose to entrapment.

POSTERIOR INTEROSSEOUS NERVE PALSY: DECOMPRESSION AT THE ARCADE OF FROHSE

The skin incision for this dissection should begin about 8 cm above the flexor crease of the elbow at the anterolateral surface of the distal arm. It should then extend downward, follow the flexor crease halfway across the forearm, and then extend 10 cm down the mid–upper forearm (Fig. 174–6). The radial nerve is easily located in the distal arm if the surgeon places one thumb on the lateral surface of the biceps and brachialis muscle and the other thumb on the medial surface of the proximal brachioradialis muscle and develops this plane. It is then easily traced into the forearm, and the branches to the brachioradialis and the extensor carpi radialis are identified along the way. The superficial sensory branch originates just before the posterior interosseous nerve dives

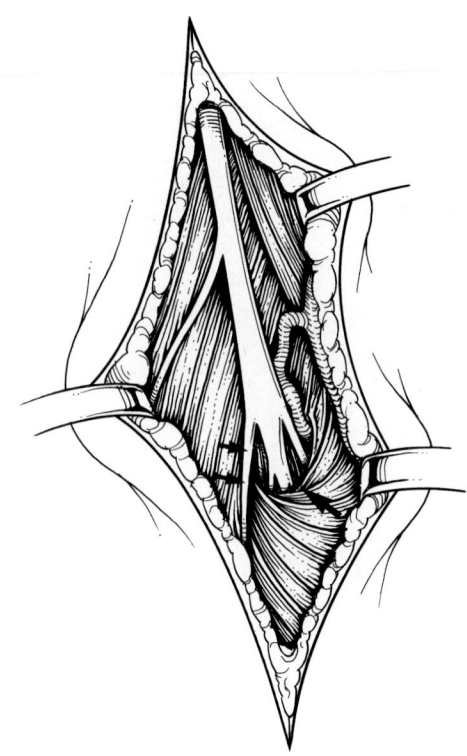

FIGURE 174–7. Exposure of the radial nerve in the forearm depicts the posterior interosseous nerve passing beneath the arcade of Frohse (single arrow) and the sensory branch (double arrow).

deep beneath the arcade (Fig. 174–7). Dissection around the arcade can prove tedious because of the presence of the recurrent radial artery and multiple small veins.

Sometimes, to achieve adequate decompression of the posterior interosseous nerve in the forearm, the nerve must be explored on the dorsal surface of the interosseous membrane. This process requires a short incision over the dorsal surface of the upper forearm (Fig. 174–8) between the extensor carpi radialis brevis and the extensor digitorum muscles. If a hemostat is passed behind the arcade into the forearm, the point of exit of the nerve beneath the supinator muscle is easily localized (Fig. 174–9). Notably, the posterior interosseous nerve has many fine branches at this point. In cases of trauma involving this nerve in the dorsal forearm, reconstruction can

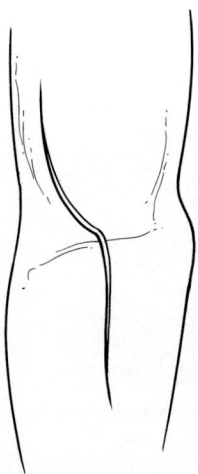

FIGURE 174–6. Skin incision for exposure of the radial nerve in the distal arm and forearm.

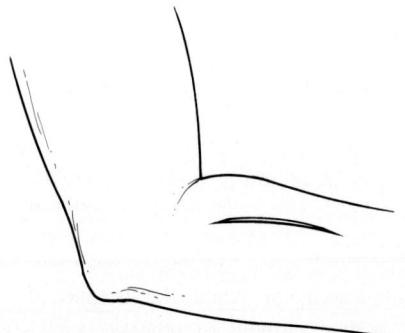

FIGURE 174–8. Skin incision for exposure of the posterior interosseous nerve and its branches from the dorsum of the forearm.

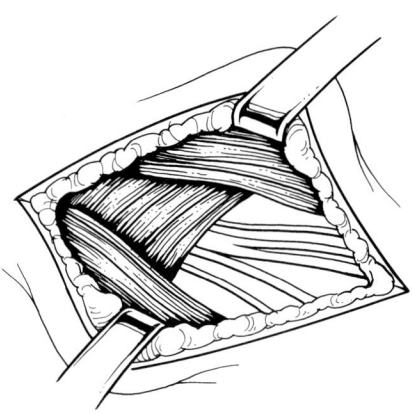

FIGURE 174-9. Exposure of the posterior interosseous nerve and its multiple branches as they exit under the suppinator muscle in the dorsal forearm.

be extremely difficult because of the presence of these many small branches.

ENTRAPMENTS OF THE MEDIAN NERVE

Median nerve entrapments are best discussed in two categories: entrapments at the elbow and entrapments at the carpal tunnel. Several possible points of entrapment exist at the elbow, including compression by a ligament from an anomalous supracondylar process of the humerus (Struthers' ligament); entrapment beneath the lacertus fibrosus, between the two heads of the pronator teres muscle or within the substance of the muscle itself; or entrapment beneath the tendinous origin of the flexor superficialis muscle. The clinical syndromes vary widely and may range from mild symptoms referable to the entire distal median nerve distribution to severe weakness in the specific distribution of the anterior interosseous nerve (long flexors of the thumb, index and middle fingers, and pronator quadratus).[10]

MEDIAN NERVE AT THE ELBOW

In entrapments of the median nerve at the elbow, the surgeon should explore the nerve from well above the elbow to a point below the tendinous origin of the flexor superficialis muscle. If radiographic evidence of a supracondylar process of the humerus exists, the surgeon would concentrate the exploration more proximally, and if the clinical syndrome is that of a pure anterior interosseous nerve entrapment, the emphasis would be more distal. A curvilinear incision is made beginning on the anteromedial side of the arm 8 to 10 cm above the elbow and is carried across the flexor crease to the midforearm and then down (Fig. 174-10). The median nerve is easily localized proximally just medial to the brachial artery and is then followed into the forearm. Dissection at the origin of the anterior interosseous nerve may be a little difficult because of the presence of multiple small arteries and veins that tend to congregate in the area of the origin of the flexor superficialis muscle (Fig. 174-11). In a pure anterior interosseous syndrome, care must be taken to follow the nerve far enough distally to release the entrapment completely.

CARPAL TUNNEL SYNDROME: ENTRAPMENT OF THE MEDIAN NERVE AT THE WRIST

Entrapment of the median nerve at the carpal tunnel is the most frequently encountered entrapment neuropathy. The

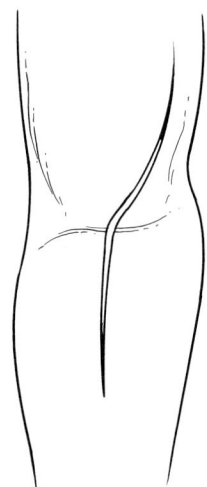

FIGURE 174-10. Skin incision for exposure of the median nerve in the distal arm and forearm.

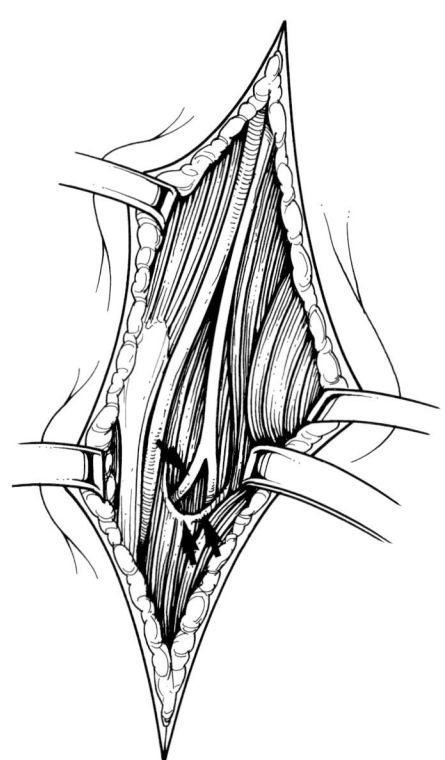

FIGURE 174-11. Exposure of the median nerve in the forearm and the anterior interosseous nerve (single arrow) as it passes beneath the sublimis bridge (double arrow).

symptoms of sometimes painful numbness in the median sensory distribution in the hand, nocturnal awakening with pain and numbness in the hand and forearm, and weakness of the thenar muscle group are legendary. In addition, the findings of decreased two-point discrimination and pin sensation in the median distribution, positive Tinel's and Phalen's signs, and weakness in the distribution of the abductor pollicis brevis muscle are well recognized. In contrast to many other entrapment neuropathies, nerve conduction studies are very specific and sensitive in this entity. A patient should not be operated on unless nerve conduction testing shows a prolonged digital sensory potential, or even more reliably, prolonged motor distal latency. Associated conditions include pregnancy, acromegaly, hypothyroidism, rheumatoid arthritis, and previous wrist fracture. Diabetes and renal failure make the median nerve more vulnerable to symptomatic carpal tunnel entrapment.

RELEASE OF THE MEDIAN NERVE WITHIN THE CARPAL TUNNEL

Although some surgeons advocate performing this procedure through a small transverse incision and employing a Paine retinaculatome[11] or an endoscope, the author prefers to use a procedure in which the entire extent of the transverse carpal ligament can be visualized and the motor branch identified and protected. The procedure is performed in an outpatient setting with the patient under local anesthesia. A slightly curved incision is outlined just ulnar to the palmar crease (Fig. 174–12), and the planned incision is injected with 8 to 10 ml of local anesthetic. After the skin is opened and the subcutaneous fat is spread, the fibers of the palmaris longus tendon are split, and the proximal transverse carpal ligament is located at the level of the distal wrist crease. The palmar cutaneous branch of the median nerve must be protected if it is seen during this part of the procedure. This small cutaneous nerve usually exits the median nerve 4 to 6 cm above the distal wrist crease and passes radially to innervate the skin of the palmar surface of the thenar eminence; however, in some cases, this median nerve comes off more distally and may pass through the proximal part of the incision outlined. If it is injured or tied up in a suture at closure, the patient may develop a painful cutaneous neuroma in the proximal part of the surgical incision.

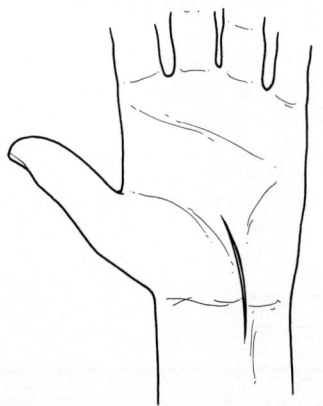

FIGURE 174–12. Skin incision for standard release of the median nerve at the carpal tunnel.

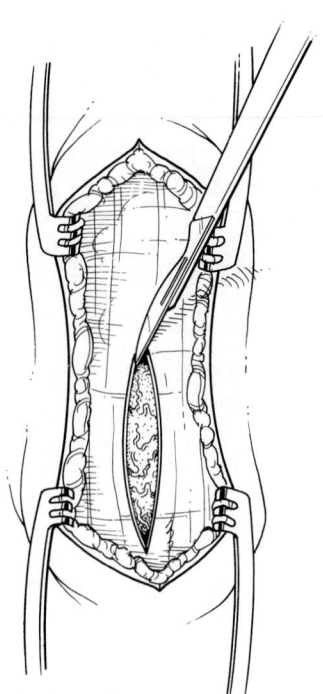

FIGURE 174–13. Sectioning the transverse carpal ligament.

Once the transverse carpal ligament is identified, it is carefully split using a No. 15 knife blade (Fig. 174–13). As the dissection is carried into the palm, fibers of the palmaris brevis muscle may be encountered and are sectioned simultaneously. As the ligament is sectioned, the surgeon should look for the motor branch to the thenar musculature and be prepared to protect it if it is seen. Although it usually leaves the nerve from its radial side and wraps around the distal ligament, variations in this anatomy are frequent. The motor branch may leave the middle or ulnar side of the nerve and come straight up through the ligament. Sectioning the distal ligament results in extrusion of a small fat pad (Fig. 174–14). The skin at the proximal part of the incision is elevated, and the ligament is sectioned back into the forearm to its junction with the forearm fascia.

Identifying or following out the motor branch is usually not necessary, except when atrophy and weakness of the abductor pollicis muscle is out of proportion to the complaints of painful paresthesias, in which case the motor branch itself may be entrapped within fibers of the retinaculum.

The author closes the wound with one superficial layer of interrupted inverted mattress sutures of 3–0 nylon. It is important for good healing that the everted epidermal skin edges abut each other and that fat is not interposed between them.

A small bandage is applied and removed 3 days after surgery. The patient is encouraged to use the hand during the recovery period, and the sutures are removed 3 weeks after the surgery.

The commonest cause for persistence of symptoms after carpal tunnel release is improper diagnosis at the outset. This problem can be avoided by not only relying on the clinical presentation but also insisting on the presence of abnormalities in nerve conduction studies as a criterion for operation.

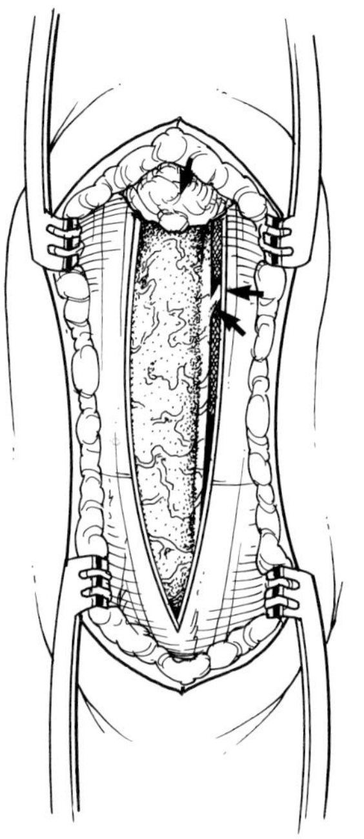

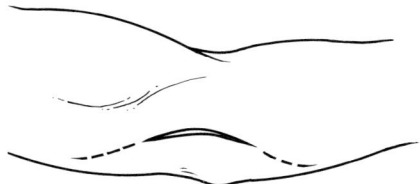

FIGURE 174-15. Skin incision for simple release (solid line) and transposition (solid plus dotted line) of the ulnar nerve at the elbow.

FIGURE 174-14. Satisfactory distal section of the transverse carpal ligament is usually greeted by herniation of a little fat (single arrow). Work still must be completed on the proximal ligament. The motor branch is shown (double arrow).

Another cause is incomplete section of the ligament either proximally or distally. Complications include painful neuroma of the palmar cutaneous nerve, section of the motor branch, postoperative fibrosis and scarring, tender or hypertrophic scars, wound infections, and bow stringing of the flexor tendons.

ENTRAPMENTS OF THE ULNAR NERVE

The two commonest locations for ulnar nerve entrapment are within the cubital tunnel at the elbow and within Guyon's canal at the wrist. With entrapment of the nerve at the elbow, patients complain of pain in the medial hand and forearm, paresthesias of the small and ring fingers, and weakness of the hand. Signs include decreased two-point discrimination and pin sensation in the small and ring fingers and over the ulnar side of the hand and weakness and wasting of the intrinsic muscles of the hand. A positive Tinel's sign may be present with palpation of the nerve at the elbow. Electrical studies are less reliable than they are in carpal tunnel entrapment, but nerve conduction studies may show a block or slowing of motor conduction across the elbow.

In the case of entrapment of the nerve at Guyon's canal, the clinical picture may vary. Most commonly, a pure motor syndrome with weakness and atrophy of the lateral intrinsic muscles of the hand occurs as a result of compression of the deep motor branch of the ulnar nerve at the hook of the hamate. Less commonly, sensory loss on the palmar surface of the hypothenar eminence and the small and ring fingers may occur with or without motor deficit. If sensory loss occurs over the dorsum of the hand, the difficulty is more proximal than Guyon's canal because the dorsal cutaneous branch arises off the ulnar nerve well above the wrist.

SURGICAL TREATMENT OF ULNAR NERVE ENTRAPMENT AT THE ELBOW

The surgical treatment of ulnar nerve entrapment at the elbow is one of the most controversial areas in the surgery for entrapment neuropathies, and the specific procedure that should be employed and under what circumstances are much debated. Procedures include simple decompression, medial epicondylectomy, and various forms of transposition of the ulnar nerve. The author prefers to use simple decompression in newly diagnosed uncomplicated cases and reserves transposition for cases in which associated pathology exists at the elbow that might make simple decompression less effective, or in cases in which reoperation is necessary.

Simple decompression can be performed with the patient under local anesthesia with a small amount of supplemental sedation. A curvilinear incision is made anterior to the medial epicondyle to keep the incision off of the dorsal surface of the elbow (Fig. 174-15). The nerve is localized by palpation and gently exposed above and below the elbow (Fig. 174-16). It is then followed through the cubital tunnel by use of a small mosquito hemostat, and the aponeurosis of the flexor carpi ulnaris is sectioned sharply (Fig. 174-17). Once the entire nerve is exposed, it is lifted out of the cubital tunnel, but all branches and blood vessels associated with it are preserved. Sometimes, the aponeurosis is closed below the nerve to prevent it from returning to the cubital tunnel. The nerve is left free in the subcutaneous tissues, and the skin and subcutaneous tissues are closed. Many recognized authorities believe this method to be a satisfactory and successful way to surgically treat ulnar nerve entrapment at the elbow.[12]

The transposition procedure is a much more involved undertaking. Several types of transpositions, including subcutaneous, intramuscular, and submuscular, and many variations have been described. The author prefers to use the submuscular procedure. General anesthesia is preferred for this operation because the operation may be lengthier than

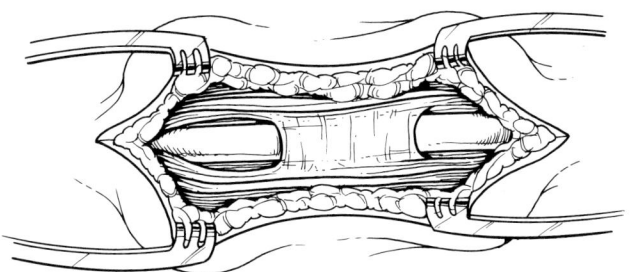

FIGURE 174-16. The ulnar nerve is located above and below the aponeurosis, between the two heads of the flexor carpi ulnaris muscle.

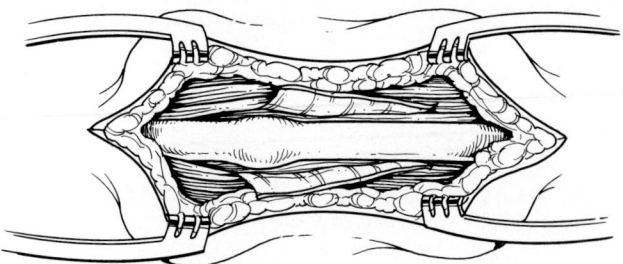

FIGURE 174–17. The cubital tunnel has been opened by section of the aponeurosis, and the ulnar nerve is decompressed.

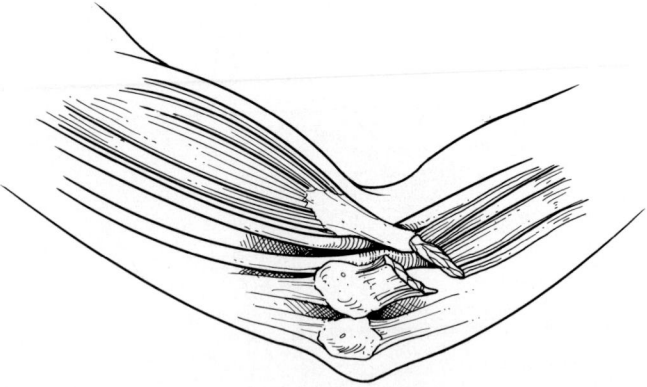

FIGURE 174–19. After section of the flexor muscle mass distal to the medial epicondyle, the ulnar nerve is transposed to the fascial plane adjacent to the median nerve, ensuring that it is without kinks, and the flexor muscle mass is repaired over it.

initially predicted and because a good deal of tissue dissection is required. The skin incision is similar to that for simple decompression but is lengthened on each end because a larger segment of the nerve needs to be exposed (see Fig. 174–15). Care should be taken to isolate and preserve cutaneous nerves in the region to prevent the development of painful neuromas or areas of skin sensitivity or anesthesia. The nerve is decompressed as outlined earlier. The median nerve is then identified at the antecubital fossa (Fig. 174–18). The flexor muscle mass just below the medial epicondyle is sectioned down to the fascial plane (some surgeons prefer to use a Z-type incision to ease the repair). The medial intermuscular septum is sectioned above the elbow, and the ulnar nerve is transposed to lie adjacent to the median nerve, (Fig. 174–19) which requires the sacrifice of several small nerve branches and nutrient blood vessels. The nerve is checked to ensure that it is not kinked or compressed and that it moves freely with elbow flexion and extension. The flexor muscle mass is repaired over the transposed nerve.

Complications of this procedure relate mostly to kinking or compression of the nerve by the intermuscular septum or elsewhere, or to the development of scarring and fibrosis, some of which may relate to devascularization of the nerve.

SURGICAL TREATMENT OF ULNAR NERVE ENTRAPMENT AT THE WRIST

A surgical incision is made beginning above the wrist crease over the ulnar artery, extending between the pisiform and the hamate bones, and curving into the palm (Fig. 174–20). The distal ulnar nerve is located next to the artery and is traced down into the wrist. It usually splits into three branches (Fig. 174–21). The motor branch should be followed deep into the palm around the hook of the hamate, and any constricting bands should be sectioned. Occasionally a ganglion is found to cause the compression and should be removed.

LATERAL FEMORAL CUTANEOUS NERVE AND MERALGIA PARESTHETICA

Constriction of the lateral femoral cutaneous nerve in the lateral inguinal ligament causes a clinical syndrome characterized by painful paresthesias and hypesthesia over the lateral thigh. Sometimes, skin changes occur in the area as well. The patient usually has tenderness during palpation of the nerve over its exit at the inguinal ligament. The syndrome may be brought on by wearing of tight pants, belts, or camping equipment, but the usual precipitating factor is obesity with poor abdominal muscle tone and a pannus overlying and everting the inguinal ligament.

The surgeon must be very careful in making this diagnosis.

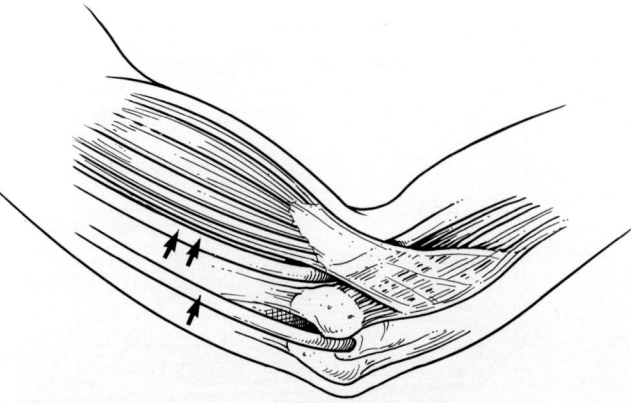

FIGURE 174–18. In preparation for transposition of the ulnar nerve, the ulnar nerve (single arrow) is located behind the medial epicondyle and decompressed in the cubital tunnel, and the median nerve (double arrow) is located medial to the pronator teres and the flexor carpi radialis muscles.

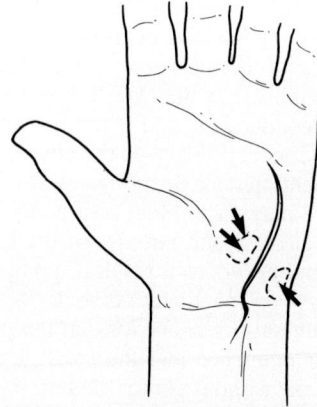

FIGURE 174–20. Skin incision for exploration of the ulnar nerve at the wrist within Guyon's canal. The nerve is located between the pisiform bone (single arrow) and the hook of the hamate bone (double arrow).

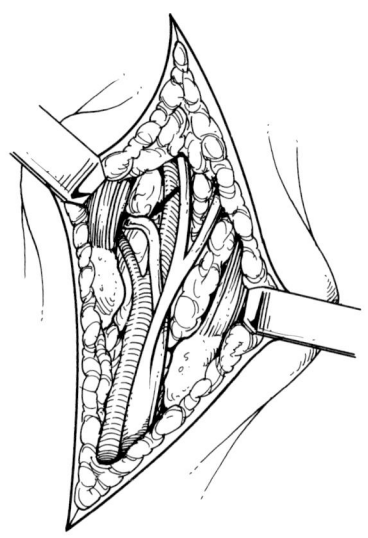

FIGURE 174–21. Exposure of the ulnar nerve in the wrist. In cases in which there is weakness of the intrinsic muscles, the deep motor branch (single arrow) should be followed deep into the palm beneath the hook of the hamate.

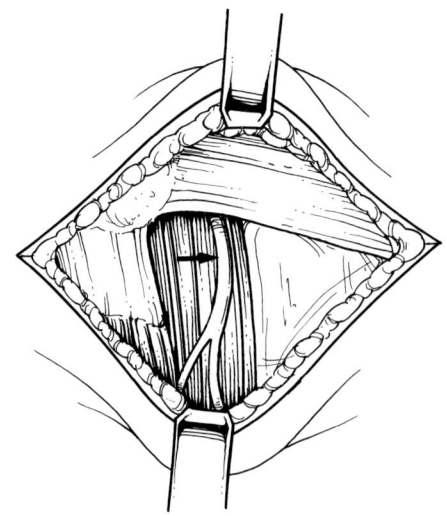

FIGURE 174–23. The lateral femoral cutaneous nerve (single arrow) has been located over the fascia of the proximal sartorius muscle, and has been traced up, under, and into the inguinal ligament.

Electrical studies are unreliable, and similar symptoms may be seen in patients with far lateral disc herniations or pelvic pathology.

SURGICAL TREATMENT OF MERALGIA PARESTHETICA

The major challenge of surgery for meralgia paresthetica is finding the lateral femoral cutaneous nerve; searching for this nerve can prove quite frustrating. A small, 4- to 6-cm incision is made about 2 cm below the attachment of the lateral inguinal ligament to the anterior superior iliac spine (Fig. 174–22). Dissection is carried through the subcutaneous fat to the fascia overlying the proximal sartorius muscle. It is often best to search for a branch of the nerve lying on the fascia and then trace it up to the main nerve trunk and then to the inguinal ligament (Fig. 174–23). Alternatively, the surgeon may look for the main nerve trunk among the fibers of the fascia. The trunk generally exits the inguinal ligament about 1 cm medial to the anterior superior iliac spine. In the rare event that the nerve cannot be found below the ligament, a small, curvilinear incision can be made above the iliac crest, the abdominal muscles can be split, and the nerve can be localized in the retroperitoneal space as it wraps over the iliacus muscle.

Two options are available once the nerve is found. Some surgeons advocate decompressing the nerve by sectioning the deeper part of the ligamentous tunnel through which it travels. If this method is tried, the author recommends that a metallic clip be placed adjacent to the nerve so that if the patient fails to obtain symptomatic relief, it will be easier to relocate the nerve within the scar tissue with radiographic assistance. Having had several patients not respond to decompression surgery for meralgia paresthetica, the author prefers to apply traction to the nerve as it exits the inguinal ligament and to sharply section it, letting it fall back into the pelvis. After this procedure, the patient will have anesthesia in the lateral thigh, but most prefer this to painful dysesthesias.

ENTRAPMENT OF THE POSTERIOR TIBIAL NERVE: TARSAL TUNNEL SYNDROME

Most patients who suffer from the tarsal tunnel syndrome complain of burning pain in the plantar aspect of the foot, either in the region of the metatarsal heads or along the medial or lateral aspect of the foot. Sometimes, pain may radiate up the calf. Standing and walking cause the pain or make it worse. Usually, patients have a positive Tinel's sign over the point of greatest entrapment. The syndrome is uncommon, and so many alternative diagnostic possibilities exist that electrical studies provide very important information for the diagnosis. Prolonged motor distal latencies in the

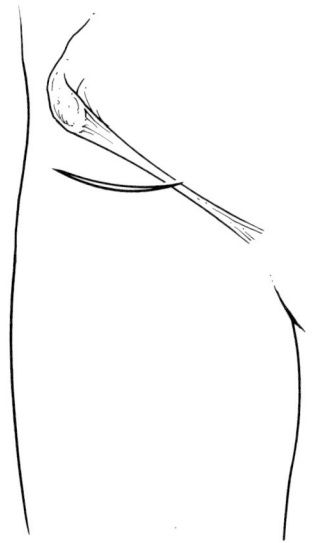

FIGURE 174–22. Skin incision for exploration, decompression, and section of the lateral femoral cutaneous nerve.

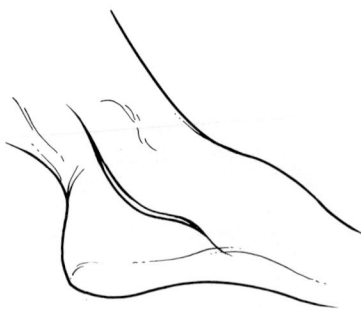

FIGURE 174–24. Skin incision for release of the posterior tibial nerve in the tarsal tunnel.

medial plantar nerves, or lateral plantar nerves, or both, are the best supporting evidence, but an earlier finding may be a prolonged or dispersed sensory potential from these nerves.

DECOMPRESSION OF THE POSTERIOR TIBIAL NERVE

Decompression of the posterior tibial nerve generally requires enough tedious dissection that the surgeon chooses

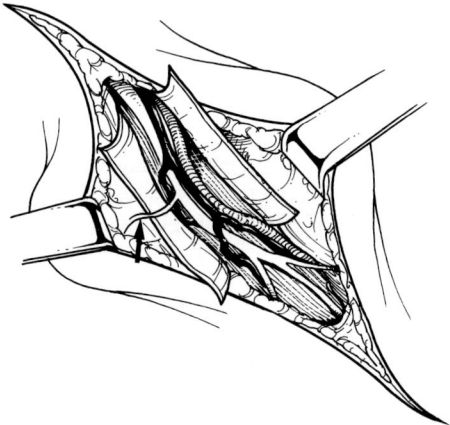

FIGURE 174–25. The flexor retinaculum (laciniate ligament) has been sectioned to expose the contents of the tarsal tunnel, including the posterior tibial artery, veins, and nerve. The calcaneal branch of the nerve may pierce the ligament (single arrow). It is important to release the medial and lateral plantar nerves deep into the foot even though this dissection may prove difficult due to veins in the vicinity.

either general anesthesia or a regional block. The incision (Fig. 174–24) is located midway between the medial malleolus and the Achilles tendon, and it curves down into the medial foot. The retinaculum is easily located immediately below the subcutaneous tissue, and opening it sharply in the proximal part of the wound reveals the neurovascular bundle. The surgeon then simply follows the nerve, sectioning the ligament along the way. The calcaneal branch, which often pierces the ligament, must be protected because injuring it can result in a numb heel or a painful neuroma. As the surgeon works more distally, dissection may be complicated by multiple small veins in the field that weave in and out between the nerve branches. The medial and lateral plantar nerves must be traced well into the medial foot to ensure that they are free of entrapment (Fig. 174–25).

REFERENCES

1. Tindall SC: Chronic injuries of peripheral nerves by entrapment, in Youmans JR (ed): Neurological Surgery, 3rd ed. Philadelphia, WB Saunders, 1988, pp 2511–2542
2. Rengachary SS: Entrapment neuropathies, in Wilkins RH, Rengachary SS (eds): Neurosurgery. New York, McGraw-Hill Book Company, 1985, pp 1771–1795
3. Mackinnon SE, Dellon AL: Surgery of the Peripheral Nerve. New York, Thieme Medical Publishers, 1988
4. Pang D, Wessel HB: Thoracic outlet syndrome. Neurosurgery 22:105–121, 1988
5. Gilliatt RW, LeQuesne PM, Logue V, Sumner AJ: Wasting of the hand associated with a cervical rib or band. J Neurol Neurosurg Psychiatry 33:615–624, 1970
6. Dubuisson AS, Kline DG, Weinshel SS: Posterior subscapular approach to the brachial plexus. Report of 102 Patients. J Neurosurg 79:319–330, 1993
7. Callahan JD, Scully TB, Shapiro SA, et al: Suprascapular nerve entrapment. A series of 27 cases. J Neurosurg 74:893–896, 1991
8. Shupeck M, Onofrio BM: An anterior approach for decompression of the suprascapular nerve. J Neurosurg 73:53–56, 1990
9. Cravens G, Kline DG: Posterior interosseous nerve palsies. Neurosurgery 27:397–402, 1990
10. Spinner M: The anterior interosseous nerve syndrome. J Bone Joint Surg Am 52A:84–95, 1970
11. Pagnanelli DM, Barrer SJ: Carpal tunnel syndrome: Surgical treatment using the Paine retinaculatome. J Neurosurg 75:77–81, 1991
12. Rengachary SS: Cubital tunnel syndrome, in Rengachary SS, Wilkins RH (eds): Neurosurgical Operative Atlas, vol 2. Baltimore, Williams & Wilkins, 1992, pp 255–259

CHAPTER 175

Surgical Management of Peripheral Nerve Tumors

David G. Kline
Alan R. Hudson

The incidence of tumors originating in nerve or extrinsic and compressing nerve is far less than that of entrapments or nerve injuries.[1] These lesions, which can be vexatious to manage, are however by no means rare.[2,3] Every neurosurgeon should have an understanding of the pathogenesis of these lesions, and those undertaking their management need experience with the surgical anatomy of the area involved by the tumor as well as the internal structure of the involved nerve itself.[4,5] Surgical removal of a neural tumor can be difficult, as can its pathologic diagnosis. As a result, these are not cases for the occasional surgeon. Significant neurologic loss can occur, and thus inadequate surgery or misinterpreted histology can result in serious disability. When in doubt, the physician should refer at least the more difficult nerve tumors to a center with surgeons and pathologists specializing in such cases.

DIAGNOSIS

The cellular pathology of nerve tumors has immense range and complexity, but the commonly encountered neoplasms, such as schwannomas, neurofibromas, plexiform neurofibromas, and neurogenic sarcomas, have characteristic gross and microscopic features.[6] Study of a few of the texts delineating these differences is of great help to the surgeon attempting to manage these lesions.[7,8]

The clinical diagnosis may present significant difficulty insofar as a nerve tumor is frequently not considered in the differential diagnosis of a mass or of pain. The classic clinical feature is that the mass can be displaced at right angles to the course of the peripheral nerve, but not in a longitudinal manner.[9] While the surgeon is palpating the mass, the patient may complain of induced paresthesias in a distribution appropriate to that particular peripheral nerve. Tapping the mass may likewise cause appropriate sensory phenomena. If a peripheral nerve tumor is suspected, evidence of other nerve tumors and von Recklinghausen's disease (VRD) is sought (Fig. 175–1). Computed tomographic (CT) scanning and magnetic resonance imaging may be useful in delineating the true extent of a tumor or VRD, and occasionally, angiography and myelography are required (Fig. 175–2).[10] Although MRI studies are not particularly helpful in managing patients with nerve injuries, it is of inestimable benefit in evaluating nerve tumors. Any suspected nerve tumor situated close to the spine should have the medial extent of the tumor carefully defined by such studies. Unfortunately, no scan or other imaging study is capable of differentiating schwannoma from neurofibroma or of diagnosing a neurogenic sarcoma with certainty. A precise diagnosis requires histologic study of tumor tissue and preferably as much of the lesion as possible.

If the diagnosis of a peripheral nerve tumor is made on clinical grounds, the surgeon must appreciate that he or she cannot ascertain at that stage whether the diagnosis is a schwannoma, neurofibroma, or even a malignant nerve tumor. Depending on the surgeon's experience with nerve tumors, it may be best to refer such a patient to an appropriate center where a definitive diagnosis can be made, and, if necessary, definitive surgery can be performed.

Nerve tumors can conveniently be divided into those that are benign and of neural sheath origin and those that, although benign and involving nerve, are not of neural sheath origin. Malignant tumors can be categorized as those of neural sheath origin, including the neurogenic sarcomas, and malignancies of nonneural origin compressing or directly involving nerve by either direct extension or metastasis.

Table 175–1 lists the peripheral nerve tumors commonly encountered but is by no means an exhaustive list of the various diagnostic possibilities.

SURGICAL MANAGEMENT

BENIGN NEURAL SHEATH TUMORS

Schwannomas

Neural sheath tumors are the commonest subset of tumors affecting nerve and include the commonest specific tumor of nerve—the schwannoma. The usual presentation of a schwannoma is as a painless but palpable mass. Rarely, an unoperated schwannoma presents with neurologic deficit or causes abnormal electromyographic results.[11] If biopsy or prior attempt at removal has been performed, presenting symptoms are more likely to be pain, paresthesias, deficit, or all of these. Tapping over the lesion, if superficial, almost always gives paresthesias in the distribution of the nerve. If the tumor is symptomatic, our practice has been to remove such lesions, providing that the general risks of an anesthetic are not considerable.

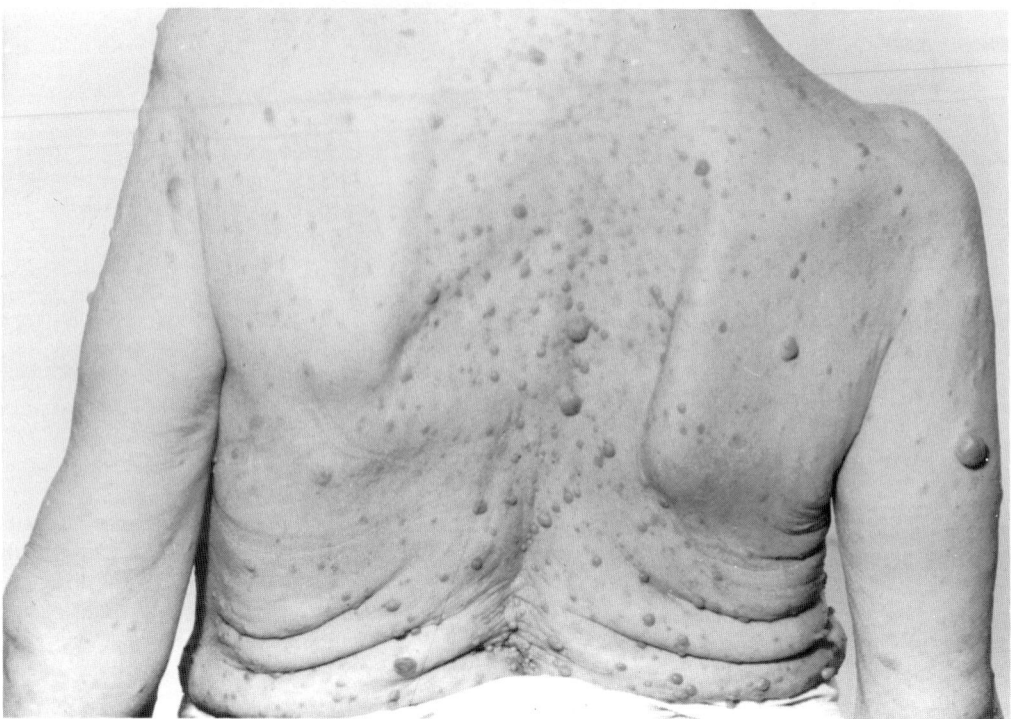

FIGURE 175–1. Von Recklinghausen's disease. The patient was referred for management of a brachial plexus tumor. In fact, the initial symptoms and signs were related to cervical syringomyelia. Thus, the central manifestations of this disease must always be kept in mind when planning therapy for more peripheral tumors.

Procedure

After induction of anesthesia, the patient is positioned so that the involved limb's response to stimulation can be observed. Surgical exposure includes nerve and related structures both proximal and distal to the lesion itself (Fig. 175–3). Exceptions may be schwannomas involving the pelvic plexus or the proximal spinal nerve level of the brachial plexus, where exposure either proximal or distal to the lesion may be difficult. The tumor is usually found nestled within nerve, with the nerve's fascicles "basketted" around the mass (Fig. 175–4).[12] As a schwannoma grows larger, it may bulge out from the nerve in an eccentric manner, leaving fascicles less symmetrically arrayed around the mass itself. Schwannomas have a capsule, and by dissecting longitudinally along the mass and splitting apart the fascicles, the surgeon can dissect them off the capsule. These fascicles can then be gently dissected away from the tumor capsule, much like pulling down a bucket or basket handle. Further dissection at the proximal and distal poles of the tumor usually reveals a relatively small fascicle entering and leaving the tumor (Table 175–2). Nerve action potential recording across such a lesion by stimulating and recording from the entering and exiting fascicle produces a flat trace, and no nerve action potential is conducted (Fig. 175–5). Stimulation alone of the proximal and, less frequently, the distal tumor fascicle sometimes gives muscle contraction in the distribution of the nerve, but the contraction results from retrograde stimulation of more healthy peripheral fascicles. Division of the entering and exiting fascicle usually permits removal of the tumor and its capsule as a single, solitary mass. Alternatively, the capsule of the schwannoma can be opened longitudinally, and its relatively soft, usually homogeneous, and sometimes cystic contents can be evacuated. Then, the capsule can be gently dissected away from the fascicles to which it is usually mildly adherent.

Most schwannomas can be totally removed as a single mass, but some large tumors involving pelvic or brachial plexus are best removed piecemeal. Several very large pelvic tumors in our series had to have a subtotal but almost complete resection, particularly when the sacral plexus was involved. Some brachial plexus tumors involving both spinal

Table 175–1. COMMONLY ENCOUNTERED PERIPHERAL NERVE TUMORS

Benign neural sheath tumors
   Schwannomas
   Solitary neurofibromas
   von Recklinghausen's disease–associated neurofibromas
   Plexiform neurofibromas
Benign nonneural sheath tumors or masses involving nerve
   Desmoids and myositis ossificans
   Myoblastomas and lymphangiomas
   Hemangiomas, venous aneurysms, fistulae, and hemangiopericytomas
   Ganglions and epidermoid cysts
   Lipomas and lipohamartomas
   Hypertrophic neuropathy, or onion whorl disease
Malignant neural sheath tumors
   Neurogenic sarcomas
   Fibrosarcomas
Malignant nonneural sheath tumors
   Carcinomas
      Lung (Pancoast)
      Breast
      Other
Sarcomas of joint origin

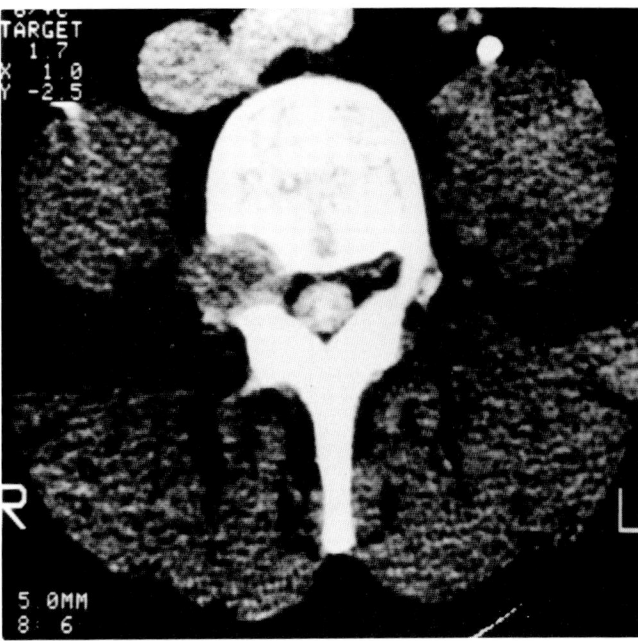

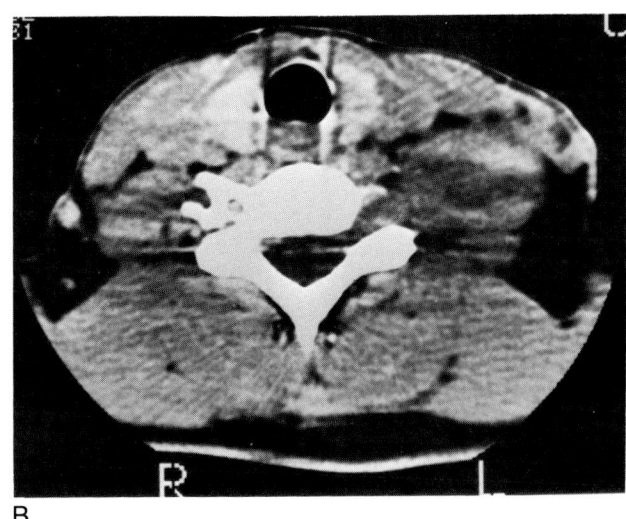

FIGURE 175-2. (A) This scan clearly delineates the position of a schwannoma within the intervertebral foramen (on patient's right side.) This patient presented with pain and neurologic disability. The myelogram was normal. (B) The figure shows a larger tumor involving not only intraforaminal spinal nerve but also a good deal of the extraforaminal plexus (on patient's left side).

Table 175-2. OPERATIVE STEPS FOR REMOVAL OF SOLITARY BENIGN NEURAL SHEATH TUMORS

1. Expose nerve well proximal and distal to the mass itself, whenever possible.
2. Dissect away and preserve other nerves or plexus elements and major vessels.
3. Dissect down to capsule in a longitudinal direction, splitting away fascicles surrounding the mass.
4. Work fascicles over mass of tumor, mobilizing them to the inferior aspect of the mass.
5. Dissect out fascicles at both poles of the tumor. Fascicles exterior to or entering leaves of the capsule need to be dissected away from the mass of the tumor and preserved. Any fascicles entering and exiting the mass of the lesion should be tested by stimulation and recording across the fascicle(s). If nonfunctional, these fascicles can be sectioned at one end or the other, and then, by working under the tumor mass, they can be dissected away from surrounding fascicles. Finally, the fascicle at the opposite pole is sectioned.
6. In some large tumors or previously operated lesions, opening any capsule, enucleating the contents, and then gently dissecting the capsule away from preserved fascicles may be necessary.

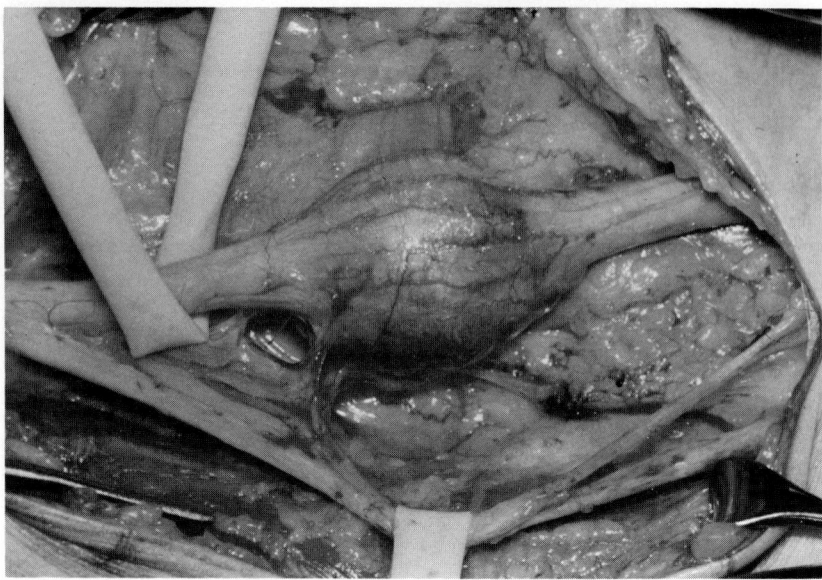

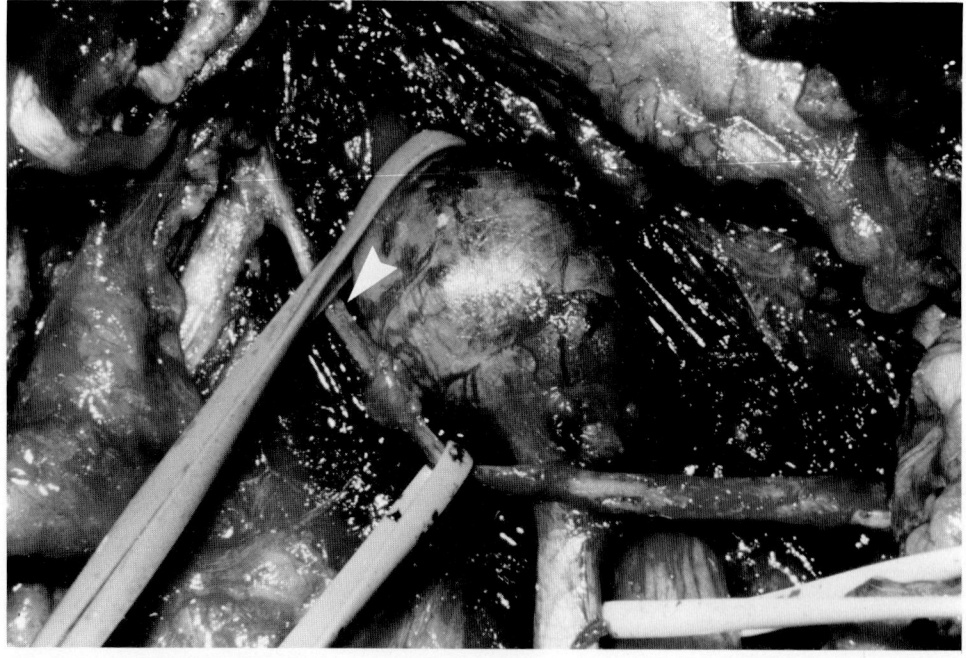

FIGURE 175-3. Typical operative appearance of a benign neural sheath tumor. (A) Note fascicles displaced to the periphery of the lesion. (Reprinted with permission, J. of Neurosurgery, 1993.) (B) Brachial plexus neural sheath tumor arising from the C6 to upper trunk region. The macroscopic dissection of the region clearly defined the adjacent structures, and these are identified and maneuvered with the aid of Silastic slings. (Arrow: phrenic nerve.)

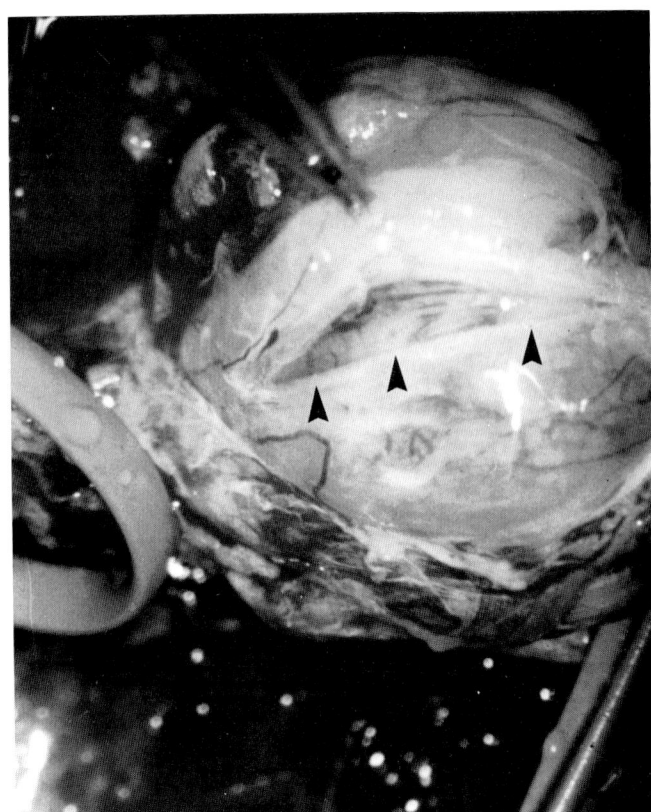

FIGURE 175–4. Schwannoma. A fascicular group is being mobilized (arrows). A few individual fascicles will be dissected subsequently and slide around the periphery of the underlying schwannoma.

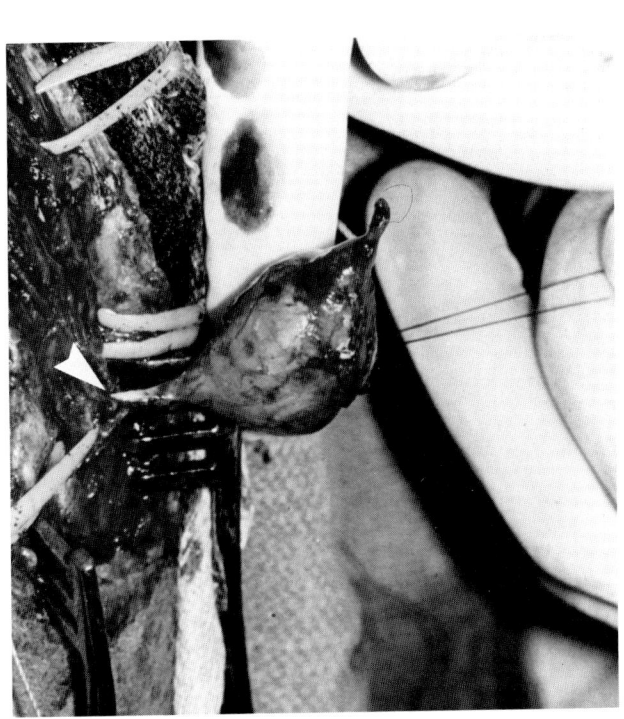

FIGURE 175–5. Schwannoma of the peroneal nerve. The schwannoma is being removed. A single fascicle has been transected proximally, and a single fascicle continuous with the distal pole of the tumor is about to be divided (arrow). These fascicular inputs and outputs for schwannomas and most neurofibromas do not transmit a NAP and can be sacrificed to permit complete tumor removal.

nerves and more proximal plexus elements have been removed through a posterior subscapular approach after resection of the first rib (Fig. 175-6).

Most investigators agree that the schwannoma's cell of origin has a basement membrane, and that the tumor most likely originates from a Schwann cell. The compact Antoni type A tissue differs from the less compact and more myxomatous matrix of a neurofibroma. Sometimes, an Antoni type B tissue with a somewhat loose stroma is present in the schwannoma, but the matrix does not stain positive with a mucopolysaccharide stain like it does for a neurofibroma.

Solitary Neurofibromas Not Associated with von Recklinghausen's Disease

Solitary neurofibromas are, as mass lesions, likelier to be associated with either local or radicular pain than schwannomas.[12] A neurologic deficit at the time of presentation is slightly more likely than with schwannomas but is also greatly increased in patients who have had prior biopsy or attempted but incomplete removal.

The cell of origin for a neurofibroma is probably more primitive than a Schwann cell. Histologically, the tumor background is less compact and more myxomatous, has more axons, and stains more positively with a mucopolysaccharide stain, such as Alcian blue, than does the schwannoma. No histologic difference exists between a neurofibroma associated with VRD and one that is not.

Procedure

Surgical approach is much the same as that for a schwannoma. In most cases, the nerve fascicles are "basketted" around the main mass and must be dissected and levered away from the main tumor mass (Fig. 175-7). These tumors usually have a capsule, even though it is more adherent to the central mass of the tumor than in a schwannoma. Some of these peripheral fascicles may be ensheathed or encapsulated by this capsule-like layer. The key steps for removal of a neurofibroma include dissecting out the fascicles at both poles or ends of the tumor. If solitary, the fascicle entering and leaving a neurofibroma is larger than that seen in a comparable-sized schwannoma. In other lesions, several fascicles approach and leave the tumor. Despite these findings, nerve action potential recording obtained across the tumor by stimulating the entering fascicle(s) and recording from the leaving fascicle(s) is usually flat, and these fascicles can be sectioned just as in a schwannoma.[13] Nerve action potential recording after the mass is removed confirms maintenance of most function just as in a schwannoma (Fig. 175-8). However, great care must be taken to determine the fascicular anatomy at each pole. Sometimes, it is more efficacious to section an entering or leaving fascicle or fascicles at one or the other pole, and then gently elevate the mass of the tumor and dissect beneath it to clear the mass away from fascicles and, at times, the capsule left on the underside. Nonetheless, occasionally, the neurofibroma requires partial graft repair after resection.

Neurofibromas Associated with von Recklinghausen's Disease

Even though it sometimes requires a more difficult dissection, the solitary and somewhat globular neurofibroma associated with VRD can, in most cases, also be excised without serious deficit (Fig. 175-9), even when the tumor involves a major nerve. The approach is the same as that for a neurofibroma unassociated with VRD. Peripherally located fascicles are dissected away. Then, the proximal and distal poles of the tumor are dissected at a fascicular level, and nonconducting fascicles are sectioned. If functioning fascicles are found entering the tumor, they must be dissected through the tumor or replaced by grafts once the mass is removed. The latter method is less likely to be efficacious if separate but smaller neurofibromas involve fascicles proximal or distal to the main tumor mass and do so in a plexiform fashion.

Plexiform Neurofibromas

Plexiform neurofibromas are histologically identical to solitary neurofibromas but involve a length of nerve in an interweaving fashion.[13] Tumor masses are both intrafascicular and extrafascicular. Operation on these plexiform lesions is difficult but possible when the indications are good (Table 175-3). Complete removal is, however, not usually possible without loss of function. When such a tumor gets quite large or when severe pain is a dominant symptom, decompression with partial removal of some of the tumorous bulk may be helpful to the patient. The lesion cannot, however, be completely resected without total or near-total loss of function. At times, even an attempt at subtotal removal of a plexiform tumor may lead to some loss of function. Section of nerve both proximal and distal to such a lesion and repair of the gap, which is lengthy, does not usually restore function. Such tumors involving less important sensory nerves or branches, such as antebrachial cutaneous, superficial sensory radial, sural, or saphenous nerves, can be removed in toto, along with the nerve of origin (Fig. 175-10).

Plexiform neurofibromas are more likely to be associated with VRD, especially its regionalized form, but surprisingly can also be encountered as solitary non-VRD–associated lesions. Sometimes, a sizable plexiform tumor is accompanied by hundreds of smaller neurofibromas involving the nerve of origin of the larger lesion. These associated tumors involve

---

Table 175-3. OPERATIVE STEPS FOR DECOMPRESSION OF PLEXIFORM TUMORS

1. Expose, if possible, involved nerve or plexus element and related structures proximal, distal, and circumferential to the lesion.
2. Plexiform tumors that are symptomatic and involve only sensory nerves or branches, e.g., saphenous, sural, superficial sensory radial, and antebrachial cutaneous, can be resected en masse along with nerve of origin.
3. An attempt can be made to decompress the bulk of the tumor when it involves major nerves or a plexus element by dissecting it out between fascicles and important branches. This process may require opening the capsule, if present, and debulking the interior of multiple interlacing and interconnecting, but interweaving masses.
4. Unfortunately, a capsule may not be present, and much of the nerve or element often interweaves within the tumor mass. Even an attempt at partial removal may lead to reduction or complete loss of function, but such a procedure may be necessary in cases in which size of the mass threatens function of adjacent, compressed nerves, or those in which significant pain is a problem or massive size may predispose to malignant change.

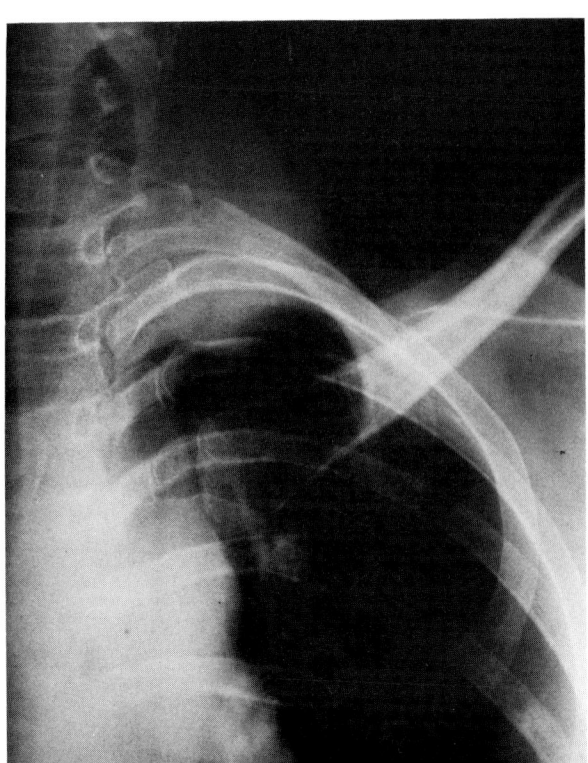

FIGURE 175-6. A large schwannoma seen at apex of lung on a chest x-ray study. This lesion, which involved the T1 spinal nerve and the lower trunk of the plexus, was removed by a posterior subscapular approach and resection of the posterior and lateral portion of the 1st rib.

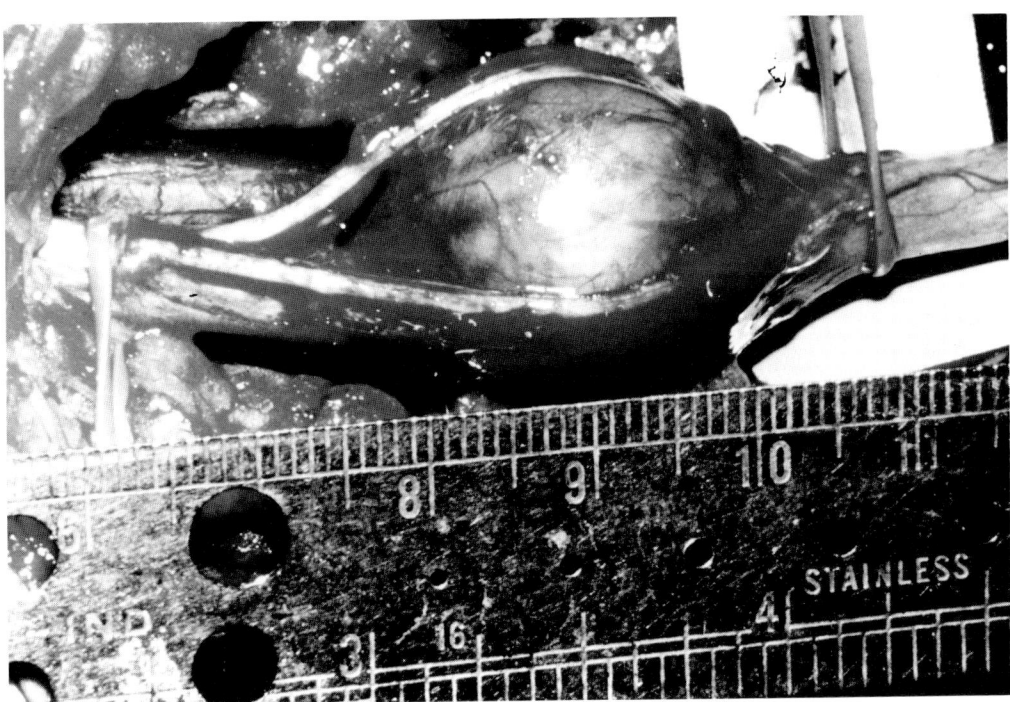

FIGURE 175-7. It was possible to isolate surface fascicular bundles and dissect them from around the mass of this neural sheath tumor. The mass proved to be a neurofibroma and was resected. Entering and exiting fascicles at each pole were tested and found not to transmit a NAP.

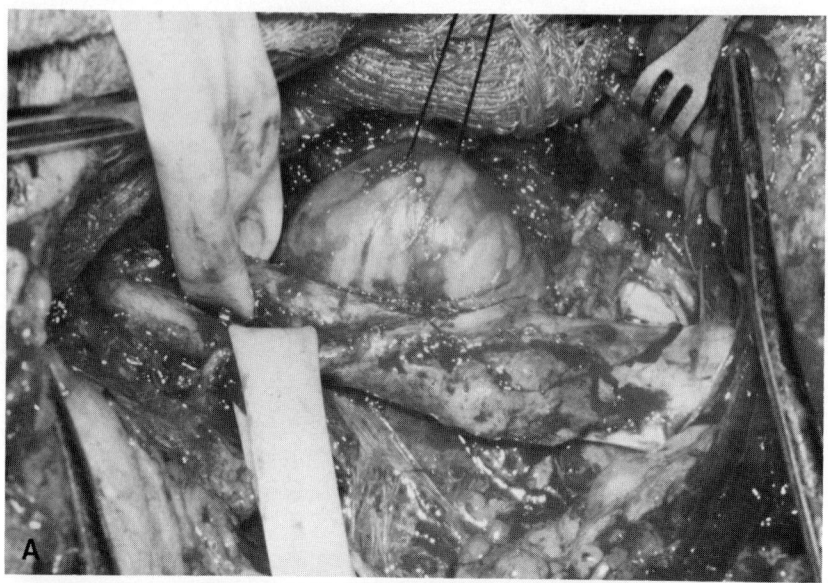
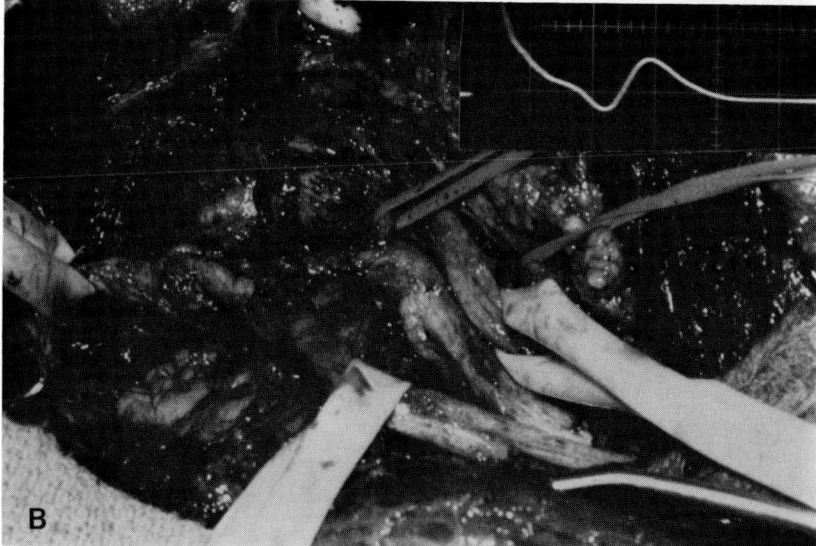

FIGURE 175–8. (A) Large benign neural sheath tumor involving the middle trunk of plexus. Upper Penrose drain is around C6, and the lower one is around C5 and the area of take-off of the subclavius branch. (B) Exposure of a neurofibroma involving plexus (see arrow) involving C8 and T1 to medial cord. Recording of NAP at top was made by stimulation of T1 and recording from the medial cor similar response was recorded after excision of the tumor. (From Craviato H: Neoplasms of peripheral nerve, in Wilkins R, Rengachary E [eds]: Neurosurgery. Baltimore, Williams and Wilkins, 1988.)

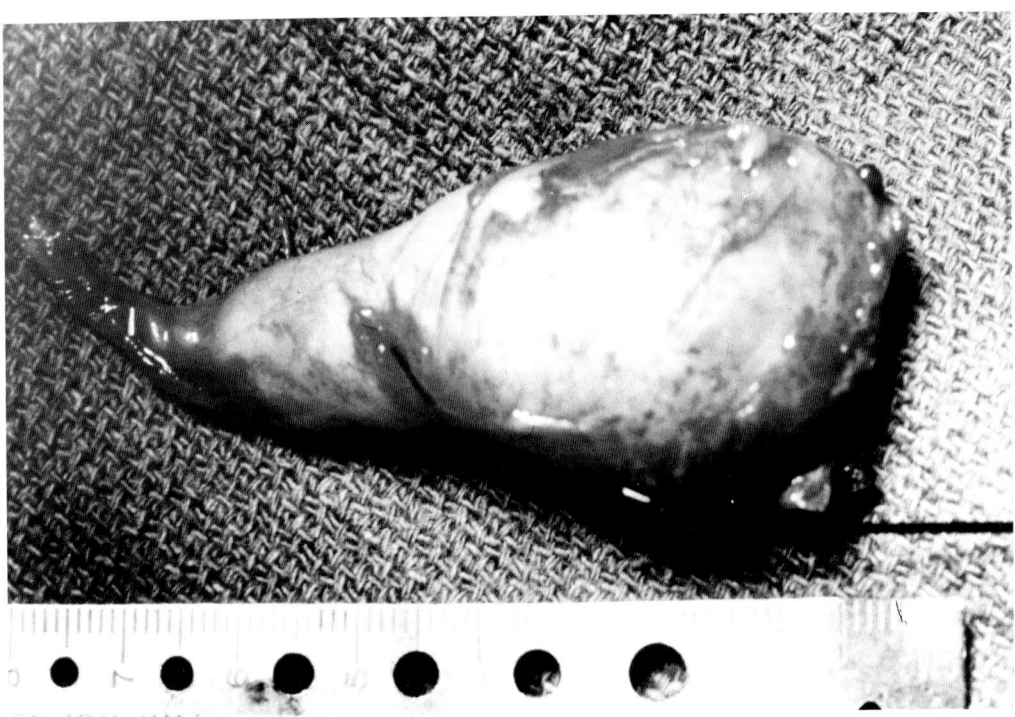

FIGURE 175-9. Neurofibroma. This operative specimen is an example of what sometimes can be achieved. Only a minor neurologic deficit followed resection of this mass from the parent trunk.

nerve well proximal and distal to the large lesion and occasionally are present in other nerves in the same limb. This phenomenon is called regionalized VRD, or neurofibromatosis type 5.[14] Under these circumstances, only a palliative operative procedure can be performed. If the plexiform tumor is quite large, and especially if it is firm, then removal may be performed to ensure that neurogenic sarcoma has not occurred or will not occur. Secondary operations for neural sheath tumors for which repair is necessary require frozen section biopsy of nerves or elements of origin to ensure that residual tumor is not incorporated in the repair (Fig. 175–11).

BENIGN NONNEURAL SHEATH TUMORS OR MASSES INVOLVING NERVE

These types of tumors occur less frequently than lesions of neural sheath origin. Nonetheless, these lesions can be responsible for pain, and in some instances, loss of nerve function. A few examples of such lesions follow.

Desmoids and Myositis Ossificans

Desmoids and myositis ossificans are felt to arise from muscle, and although they are commoner on the abdominal wall than elsewhere, they can be present in the neck, shoulder, or upper or lower extremity. When located at extraabdominal sites, they tend to involve soft tissue and can compress, incorporate, or be adherent to major nerves. They are benign in the sense that they do not metastasize to other parts of the body, but they are quite difficult to cure. Recurrence after a presumed gross total resection is common.[3]

Operation requires a relatively wide exposure of the lesion and early identification of any nerve or nerves involved. Tumor usually needs to be sharply dissected away from nerve, and involved epineurium usually requires resection. Both the firmness of these lesions and their adherence to nerves and vessels make removal without deficit difficult unless great care is taken during the dissection.

Myositis ossificans is a poorly defined disorder that may be related to previous trauma or surgery. It usually produces a very firm-to-hard mass of tissue with calcification and, like a desmoid, can envelop contiguous soft tissues, including bone. If it is symptomatic because of neural involvement, vascular involvement, or both, removal of such masses can be technically quite demanding. Again, no substitute exists for performing wide exposure, dissecting out neural elements and displacing them away from the pathologic mass, and preserving as many major vessels as possible. Complete removal is not only seldom possible, it is usually not indicated.

Myoblastomas and Lymphangiomas

These two unusual lesions are grouped together because when they involve nerve, they have similar behavior and somewhat similar appearance at the operating table. Myoblastomas are formed of plump and somewhat angular cells with acidophilic granules, whereas lymphangiomas have cells of a lymphoid nature. These tumors tend to spread as a sheet of tumorous tissue and are less likely to form a globular mass than are a desmoid tumor or a hemangioma.[3,14] Both tumors can also become adherent to nerves and, in some cases, envelop them. If care is not taken in skeletonizing the involved nerve or nerves, severe deficits can occur. As a result, it is best to plan a wide as well as a lengthy exposure and to determine normal anatomy distal and proximal to the lesion, if possible.

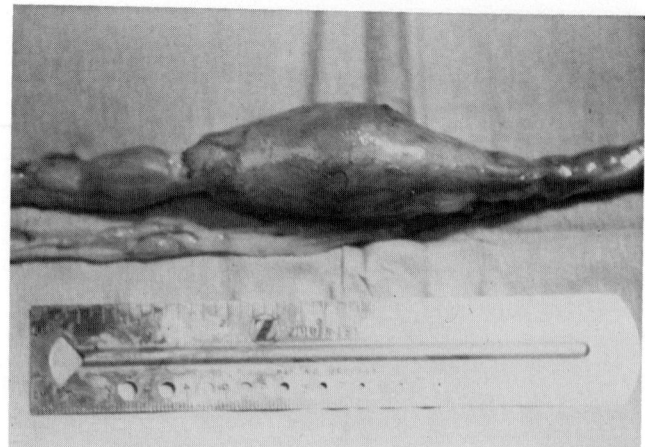

FIGURE 175–10. Surgical specimen typical of a plexiform neurofibroma. This lesion involved a sensory nerve as well as a less involved branch and was totally resected.

Lipomas and Lipohamartomas

Lipomas do not usually involve major nerves, because they are mostly subcutaneous. Exceptions occur when a large lipoma envelops or compresses nerve, or where one originates at a deeper level in the limb and compresses or entraps nerve and produces symptoms.[3] The latter behavior can occur at forearm or popliteal levels, with resultant posterior interosseous or peroneal palsy. Larger lipomas in the supraclavicular fossa can involve the brachial plexus. Large lipomas in the buttocks or leg or arm can less frequently involve median, sciatic, or ulnar nerves.

Lipohamartomas are intrinsic to nerve and usually involve median nerve at wrist or palmar levels (Fig. 175–12).[14] When pain and paresthesias occur, decompression, including section of both the transverse carpal ligament in the palm and its extension covering the nerve and the lipomatous mass at the wrist level, is necessary. When serious loss of median function occurs, more extensive surgery is required. An internal neurolysis with reduction of the bulk of the tumor from around individual fascicles can be performed or for a more focal lipohamartoma, resection and repair.

Hemangiomas and Hemangiopericytomas

Hemangiomas and hemangiopericytomas, as well as aneurysms and arteriovenous fistulae, originate close to nerves and compress or envelop them.[15] Operation for these lesions, especially if nerve is involved, is never easy. Preoperative angiography is of some help in planning surgery, but the key surgical steps include isolating vessels on the periphery of the lesion and ligating or clipping them if they are not the major supply to an extremity, and once again, dissecting nerves away from the lesion while protecting them as much as possible. Occasionally, a hemangioma, hemangioblastoma, venous aneurysm, or fistula directly involves nerve or appears to originate in it. Then, if symptoms warrant, a careful interfascicular dissection is necessary for removal. Each fascicle or group of fascicles need be stripped of the abnormal vascular tissue.

The hemangiopericytoma, which usually arises in mediastinum and secondarily involves brachial plexus, can behave in a malignant fashion and metastasize to other sites, including, rarely, the brain. It cannot usually be removed entirely, and the surgeon must be content with a subtotal but hopefully decompressive procedure for the plexus.

GANGLIONS AND EPIDERMOID CYSTS

Most ganglions arise from joints and at sites that do not usually involve nerves, such as the dorsum or the side of the wrist.[16] Less frequently, this cystic tumor arises from an area of the wrist joint that compresses the thenar sensory branch of the median or whole median nerve itself. Other sites where these ganglions are clearly of joint origin include the forearm, where they arise from radioulnar joints and compress the posterior interosseous nerve, the knee, involving the peroneal nerve; the ankle, involving the posterior tibial nerve; and the hip, involving the sciatic nerve. Ganglions at the elbow level can involve radial, and, less frequently, median or ulnar nerves, whereas those in the shoulder can involve the brachial plexus, particularly its suprascapular branch in the region of the scapular notch.

The other type of ganglion does not appear to have a connection with a joint, such as those found in the peroneal nerve over the head of the fibula (Fig. 175–13).[17] At one time, these lesions may have had a connection with the joint and the connection was then obliterated. Ganglions are not always benign in their behavior in the sense that they may extend great distances along the course of a nerve, such as the peroneal and its sciatic division, and gradually produce paralysis of eversion as well as dorsiflexion of the foot.[3] Most less extensive lesions are resectable without serious loss of function, but exceptions exist.

For ganglions extrinsic to nerve but compressing it, the surgeon must dissect around such lesions after dissecting

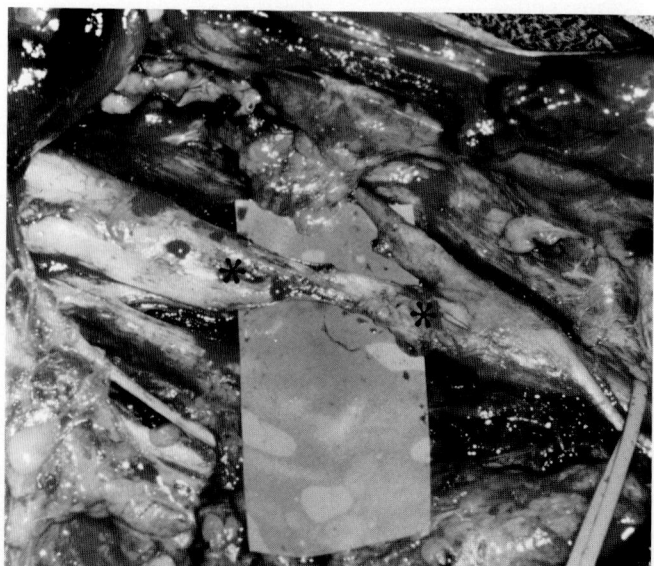

FIGURE 175–11. Brachial plexus, upper trunk. Resection of an unidentified mass resulted in almost complete destruction of the upper trunk of the plexus. Advice based on the result of quick sections and expert neuropathologic input are required to distinguish between scarring of the proximal and distal stumps (stars) and tumor prior to reconstructive grafting.

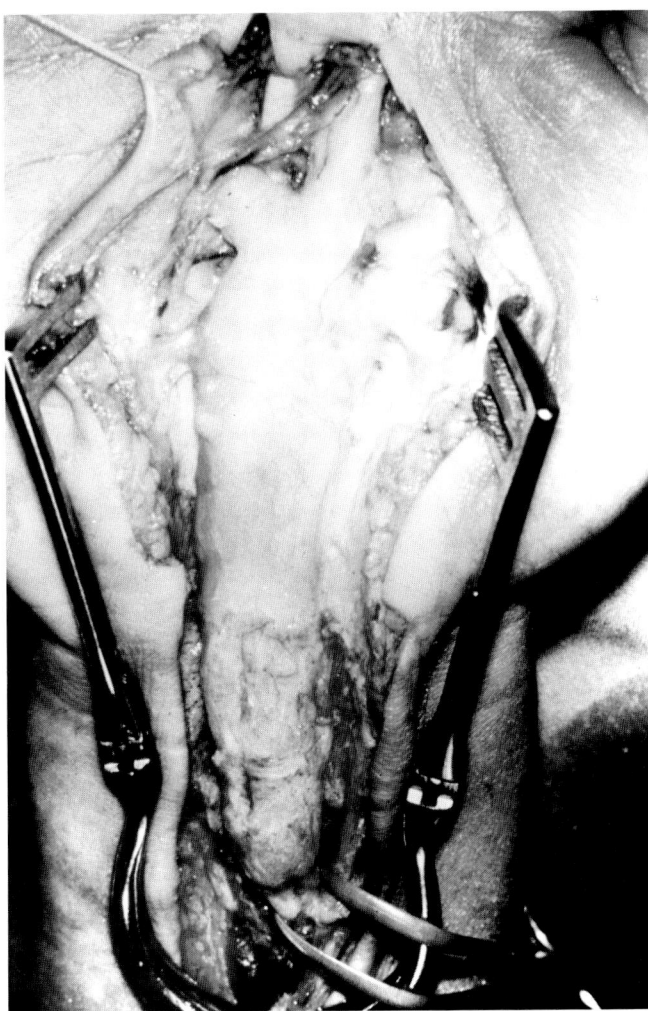

FIGURE 175–12. Median nerve. The patient had carpal tunnel syndrome. Operation revealed diffuse fatty infiltration of the median nerve. The symptoms were helped by the division of the transverse carpal ligament (lipofibromatous hamartoma).

evacuation initially and then dissection of the capsule away from adjacent tissues, including nerves.

Other benign lesions, such as those arising from bone, may involve a nerve secondarily. Although benign, such tumors may incorporate or severely deform nerve, making tumor removal without deficit difficult (Fig. 175–14).

HYPERTROPHIC NEUROPATHY, OR ONION WHORL DISEASE

This unusual disease is of unknown etiology and pathogenesis. Fascicles and individual nerve fibers become encased by connective tissue in a circular fashion, as if the endoneurium has proliferated. This phenomenon results in a hypertrophic nerve with, on microscopy, an "onion-whorl" appearance to its nerve fibers. These strange, tumor-like lesions tend to affect children or young adults and have some preference for the peroneal nerve in the leg or the median nerve in the arm.[18] Nonetheless, in our clinics, the disease has also been found in the brachial plexus as well as the ulnar, radial, and sciatic nerves.[3, 19] The lesion results in a progressive loss of function and tends to involve a fairly lengthy segment of nerve. It does not spread to other nerves or metastasize elsewhere in the body. Some of its histologic features seem to suggest either a contusive-stretch injury or a chronically compressive etiology, but a history of significant trauma is usually missing, and no obvious entrapment or irritative environment is found on surgical exploration.

Pain or progressive loss of function leads to exploration. Function is usually partially spared distal to the lesion, and, as a result, nerve action potential conduction across the lesion is present. Based on these observations, surgeons have tended to perform either an external or an external and internal neurolysis on these lesions. Unfortunately, function usually continues to deteriorate. Manipulation of the lesion, particularly by internal neurolysis, may produce additional and even complete loss, despite the fact that neurolysis is less invasive than resection. An alternative is to proceed with resection of the lesion, despite the attendant loss, and to

away and protecting the involved nerve. The origin of the cystic lesion should be ligated or secured in some other fashion close to the joint to reduce recurrence. For ganglions within a nerve, interfascicular dissection seems to work best because fascicles are cleared of the cyst and then its capsule. In a patient with the usual intraneural ganglion involving the peroneal nerve, a connection with the knee joint should always be sought and isolated and ligated, if present. In some large lesions, it may be necessary to evacuate the synovial-like contents of the cyst and then dissect the capsule away from the decompressed and split fascicles. Recurrence is a possibility, and some larger lesions require several operations before they are obliterated.

Epidermoid cysts can also compress nerve, although unlike ganglions, they usually do not arise within a nerve itself. These extraneural lesions may involve the sciatic nerve close to the sciatic notch or may be behind the knee, involving the posterior tibial nerve.[3] The surgeon can usually dissect these out and deliver them as a solitary mass after performing neurolysis on and gently retracting involved nerves. Occasionally, a large lesion at the hip or pelvic level requires

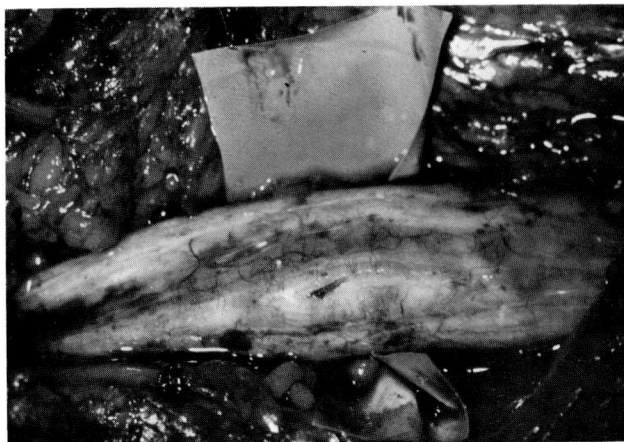

FIGURE 175–13. Typical appearance of a ganglion cyst involving the peroneal nerve. Interfascicular dissection is necessary to remove this type of tumor. Although function was maintained in this patient, this is not always the case when the lesion is large and extends up and down the nerve.

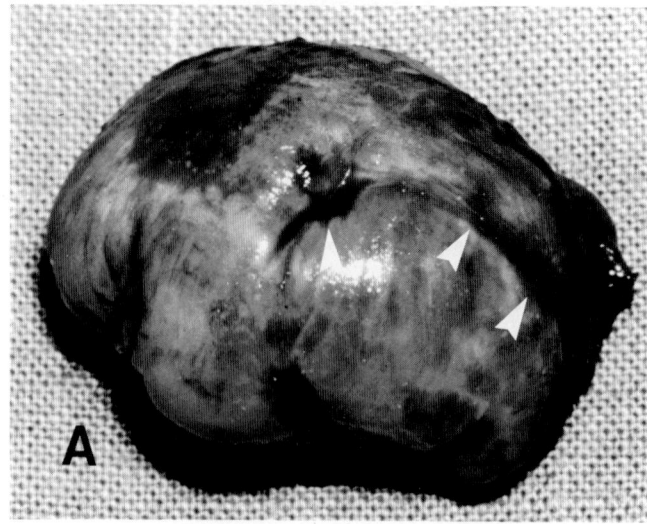
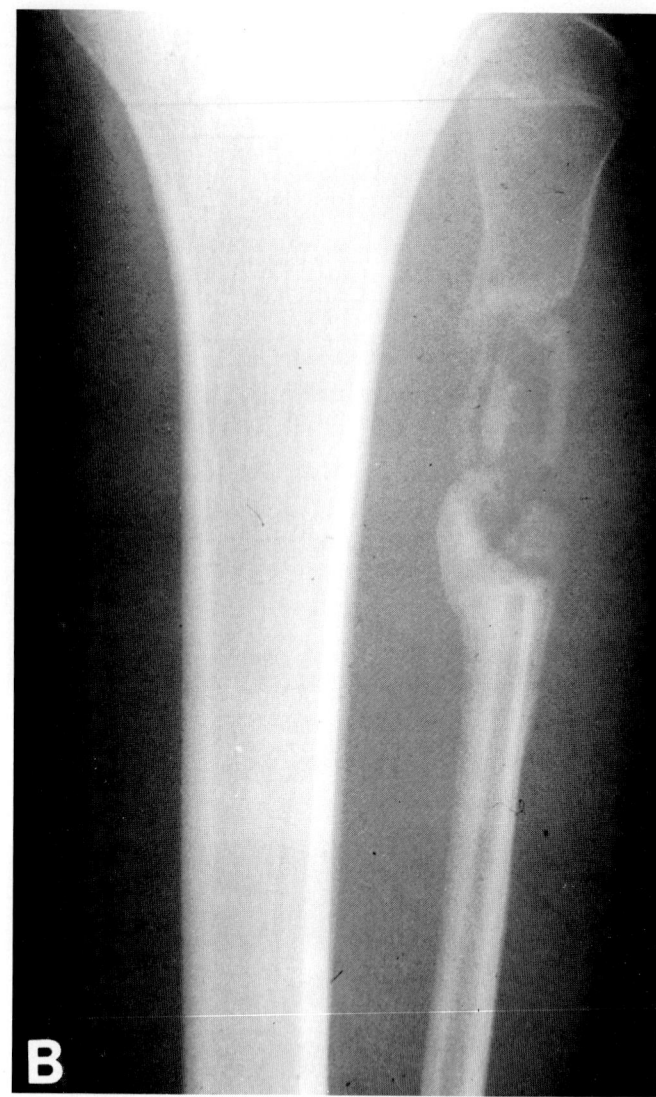

FIGURE 175–14. (A) Osteoma of the neck of the radius. The patient had a posterior interosseous nerve syndrome, and at surgery, the nerve was found to occupy a groove on the surface of this benign bone tumor (arrow). Removal required extensive mobilization of PIN well proximal and distal to the tumor site as well as over the top of the tumor. (B) Benign tumor of the proximal fibula. Patient had a normal preoperative neurologic examination. Postoperative footdrop was found to be the result of a total division of the peroneal nerve, which occurred during surgery of the bone.

replace the lost segment by grafts. This procedure has been performed in three of the 12 cases encountered on the Louisiana State University Medical School in more recent years. As a result, some degree of recovery has occurred in two of the three cases.

MALIGNANT NEURAL SHEATH TUMORS

Neurogenic sarcoma or fibrosarcoma arising from or involving nerve can be suspected if a mass increases rapidly in size, and especially if it is associated with a progressive loss of function.[20, 21] These lesions tend to be firmer than benign neural sheath tumors and are also relatively adherent to surrounding structures. They are often quite painful but not always (Table 175–4). Neurogenic malignancies have an increased incidence in patients with VRD, but can occur more frequently as solitary lesions in patients without VRD.[22]

Even though malignancy may be suggested by the preoperative symptoms and findings, the clinician cannot be certain of the diagnosis without a thorough biopsy, which usually requires an operation. If prior biopsy or operation has been performed and a diagnosis of neurogenic sarcoma or malignant schwannoma is in hand, the options are to:

1. Make certain that metastasis has not already occurred by chest x-ray study, chest CT scan, liver and spleen scan, and bone scan.

2. Perform wide local resection, including removal of adjacent as well as adherent soft tissues. Resection should include a several-centimeter margin of entering and exiting nerve shown to be free of malignant changes on frozen and

Table 175–4. CLINICAL PRESENTATION OF PATIENTS HARBORING MALIGNANT PERIPHERAL NERVE TUMORS AS REPORTED TO UNIVERSITY OF TORONTO PATHOLOGY REGISTRY (N = 37)

Clinical Presentation	Number of Patients	Percentage
Painless mass	24	55
Painful mass	12	28
Nerve dysfunction	12	28
History of previous lump excision	12	28
Associated with neurofibromatosis	12	28

Aneurysm(s) *(Continued)*
   management after, 1147
   results of, 1134–1135, 1147–1148, 1147t, 1148t, *1149*
   techniques of, 1139–1147, *1140–1146*
   symptoms of, 1134–1135
 intracavernous segment, 975–979, *977–978*
   algorithm for, *978*
   common carotid artery ligation for, 976
   direct clipping for, 979
   endovascular coils for, 979
   internal carotid artery ligation for, 976–979, *977–978*
 intraoperative rupture of, 985–990
   at aneurysm clip application, 987–988
   at aneurysm dissection, 986–987
   at presubarachnoid dissection, 985–986
   blunt dissection in, 986
   brain retraction in, 986
   coagulation for, 989–990
   distal sac clip application for, 989
   from proximal internal carotid artery, 987
   hypotension for, 986
   incidence of, 985
   location and, 985
   power instruments in, 986
   prevention of, 986, 987, 989
   sharp dissection in, 986–987
   suction for, 988
   systemic hypotension for, 989
   temporary arterial occlusion for, 988–989
 large, 1041
 lateral sellar compartment, 975–981, *977–978, 980*, 1044, 1050
 multiple, 1155–1160
   age and, 1155
   hypertension and, 1155
   incidence of, 1155
   number of, 1155–1156
   rupture of, 1156–1157
   sex and, 1155
   site of, 1156, 1156t, *1157–1159*
   size of, 1156
   surgery for, 1157–1160
 multiple clips for, 1123
 mycotic, 1133–1221. See also *Aneurysm(s), infected.*
 obliteration of, in brain revascularization, 925
 ophthalmic artery. See also *Aneurysm(s), paraclinoid.*
   case report of, 996, *997, 1000*, 1001
   surgery for, 964, 1044–1045, 1050
 paraclinoid, 993–1001
   cerebral angiography of, 993–994
   computed tomography of, 994
   giant, *1120*
   global-type, case report of, 996–998, *999, 1000*
   incidence of, 993, 993t
   magnetic resonance imaging of, 994
   preoperative evaluation of, 993–994
   surgery for, 994–996, 1122
     aneurysm decompression in, 995
     aneurysm dissection in, 994–995
     bypass in, 995–996
     carotid occlusion in, 995
     case reports of, 996–1001, *997–1000*
     clip application in, 995
     craniotomy in, 994
     positioning for, 994
     results of, 996
 serpentine, 1118, *1121*
 surgery for, anesthesia emergence phase of, 963–964
   anesthesia for, 959–960
   angiography during, 963

Aneurysm(s) *(Continued)*
   antifibrinolytics in, 959
   blood pressure control in, 961
   brain protection in, 962–963
   brain relaxation in, 959
   calcium channel blockers in, 959
   cardiopulmonary bypass in, 1123
   complications of, 964
   early, 957–958
   electrocardiographic abnormalities and, 959
   electrophysiologic monitoring in, 961–962, *963*
   endovascular techniques in, 967–974, *969–971*
     balloon catheter and, 967–968, 971, 973
     case reports of, 969–971, *969, 971*
     complications of, 972
     digital subtraction angiography in, 971–973
     outcomes of, 968t, 972
     patient selection for, 967, 968t
     results of, 971–972
     retrograde suction decompression in, 970–974, *970, 972*
   fluid management in, 958–959, 961
   hemodynamic monitoring in, 960
   hypertension in, 959
   hypocapnia, in 960
   lumbar CSF drainage in, 960–961
   management after, 964
   mannitol administration in, 961
   MAP manipulation in, 960
   neurologic deficit after, 964
   perfusion pressure in, 959–960
   pneumocephalus after, 964
   preoperative evaluation for, 958–959, *958*
   temporary proximal occlusion in, 1120–1122
   thrombosis in, 1123
   timing of, 957–958
 tandem clips for, 1123
 thrombosed, 1050
 traumatic, 102, 1050, 1127–1131
   angiography of, 1127, *1128*, 1130–1131, *1130, 1131*
   definition of, 1127
   of internal carotid artery, 981
   pathologic anatomy of, 1042
   signs of, 1127, *1128*
   surgery for, 1043, 1050, 1127, *1129, 1130*
   symptoms of, 1127, *1128*
   true, 1127
 ultralong clips for, 1123
 unclippable, 1113–1124
   configuration of, 1118, *1119–1121*
   deep hypotension in, 1118–1120
   location of, 1113–1114, 1114t
   size and, 1114–1118, *1115–1117*
 vein of Galen, 1213–1218. See also *Vein of Galen malformation.*
 vertebral artery complex, 1103–1110
   anatomy of, 1106–1107
   clinical features of, 1104–1105
   dissecting, 1105–1106, *1106*
   imaging of, 1105
   location of, 1103, *1103*
   morphology of, 1103–1104, *1104*
   preoperative evaluation of, 1105–1106
   saccular, 1105
   surgery for, 1107–1110
     anesthesia in, 1107
     clip selection in, 1110
     distal control in, 1110
     ELITE approach in, 1109
     extreme lateral inferior transcondylar exposure in, 1109

Aneurysm(s) *(Continued)*
     microsurgical techniques in, 1109–1110
     proximal control in, 1110
     retrolabyrinthine-transsigmoid approach in, 1108–1109
     suboccipital approach in, 1107–1108
 vertebrobasilar, 1071–1086, 1118
   anterior-projecting, 1072t, 1084
   bilobed, 1084
   giant, 1116
   multiple, 1156, *1159*
   posterior-projecting, 1072t, 1083
   sites of, *1072*
   surgery for, 964–965, 1074–1079, *1076–1081*
     anesthesia for, 1071, 1074
     approaches to, *1072*
     patient position for, 1074, *1075*
     results of, 1072t, 1073t, 1074t, 1085–1086
   upward-projecting, 1072t
 wrapping of, 1122
Aneurysmal subarachnoid hemorrhage, 937–953
 antifibrinolytic agents in, 948, 959
 arrhythmias in, 952–953
 AT877 (HA1077) in, 945
 atrial natriuretic factor in, 951
 calcitonin gene–related peptide in, 945, 947
 calcium channel antagonists in, 945, 947t, 959
 cardiovascular disorders with, 952–953
 cerebral angiography of, 939
 cerebral salt wasting syndrome in, 958
 clinical features of, 937–938, 938t
 computed tomography in, 938, 944, 1004
 diabetes insipidus in, 951–952
 diagnosis of, 938–939
 Doppler ultrasound in, 944
 electrocardiogram in, 959
 electrolyte disorders with, 951–952, 951t
 etiology of, 937
 evaluation of, 1012–1013, *1013*
 fluid disorders with, 951–952, 951t
 grading systems for, 937–938, 938t
 headache in, 937
 hydrocephalus with, 949–950
 hypernatremia in, 951
 hypertension in, 943t, 944–945, 958
 hypervolemia in, 943t, 944–945, 958
 hyponatremia in, 951–952, 951t, 958
 incidence of, 937
 lumbar puncture in, 938–939
 magnetic resonance imaging in, 938
 mortality from, 942t
 natural history of, 939, 940t
 neurologic impairment with, 937–938, 938t
 nicardipine in, 945
 nimodipine in, 945, 947t, 959
 onset of, 937
 papaverine in, 947
 preoperative management after, 1005
 prognosis for, 939, 941t
 pulmonary disorders with, 952
 rebleeding with, 948–949, 948t
 seizures with, 950–951, 950t
 surgery for, 943t
   age and, 941
   complications of, 942t
   early, 938–939
   indications for, 941
   outcome of, 938
   perioperative treatment in, 939–940, 942t
   timing of, 940–941, 943t
 syndrome of inappropriate secretion of antidiuretic hormone in, 951–952, 951t
 tissue plasminogen activator in, 947–948
 transluminal angioplasty in, 947

Aneurysmal subarachnoid hemorrhage *(Continued)*
  treatment of, 939–941
  vasospasm with, 941, 942t, 944–948, 944t, 958, *958*
    calcium channel antagonists for, 945, 947t
    diagnosis of, 944
    hypertension for, 944–945, 946t
    hypervolemia for, 944–945, 946t
    treatment of, 944–948, 944t
  ventricular drainage in, 949
  ventriculostomy in, 949–950
Aneurysmorrhaphy, 1122–1123
Angina, Prinzmetal's, sympathectomy for, 1575. See also *Sympathectomy*.
Angiography, in aneurysmal subarachnoid hemorrhage, 939
  in arteriovenous malformation, 1486, *1497*, 2028, 2041
  in carotid atherosclerosis, 878, *878*, 879
  in cavernous angioma, 1184
  in corpus callosotomy, 1351
  in craniopharyngioma, 358, 372, 384–385, *385*
  in depth electrode placement, 1275–1276, *1275*
  in dural arteriovenous malformation, 1219–1220, *1220*, *1221*
  in frontoethmoidal encephalomeningocele, 161
  in hemangioblastoma, 2028
  in infected aneurysm, 1150
  in intracranial aneurysm surgery, 963
  in jugular foramen schwannoma, 867–868, *867*
  in medial sphenoid ridge meningioma, 409
  in middle cerebral artery aneurysm, 1056, *1057*
  in paraclinoid aneurysm, 993–994
  in pediatric arteriovenous malformation, 1198
  in penetrating head injury, 85, 91
  in primary intracerebral hemorrhage, 929–930
  in spinal tumors, 1983
  in supraclinoid carotid aneurysm, 1004–1005
  in traumatic aneurysm, 1130–1131, *1130*, *1131*
  in tuberculum sellae meningioma, 404
Angioma, cavernous, 1183–1195
  brainstem, 1189, 1191–1192, *1191*, 1191t, *1192*
  cerebellar, 1189, *1190*, 1190t
  cerebral, 1186–1189
    headache in, 1187, *1188*
    neurologic deficit with, 1187–1188, *1189*
    surgery for, 1188–1189, 1189t
    with seizures, 1186–1187, *1187*, 1187t, *1188*
  clinical presentation of, 1184
  familial occurrence of, 1184
  Gamma Knife surgery for, 678, *678*
  natural history of, 1185
  observation for, 1186
  of cranial nerves, 1193, 1193t
  of spinal cord, 1193–1195, *1194*, 1194t
  pathologic features of, 1183
  pregnancy and, 1185, *1186*
  radiologic features of, 1183–1184, *1184*
  radiosurgery for, 1185–1186
  surgery for, 678, 1185–1186, *1906*
    results of, 1192
  third ventricle, subchoroidal trans–velum interpositum approach to, *721*
  venous, Gamma Knife surgery for, 678
Angiopathy, amyloid, primary intracerebral hemorrhage and, 928, 930
Angioplasty, transluminal, for aneurysmal subarachnoid hemorrhage–associated vasospasm, 947
Angiosarcoma, of scalp, 17, *17*

Angle closure glaucoma, optic nerve sheath fenestration and, 249
Ankylosing spondylitis, 515–523, 535–541
  bamboo appearance of, 1766, *1768*
  calcification in, 1767–1768, *1767*, *1768*
  case reports of, 1778–1779, *1778*, *1779*
  cauda equina syndrome in, 1780
  cerebrovascular disease in, 1766
  cervicothoracic, 1765–1773
    atlantoaxial subluxation in, 1772–1773
    clinical features of, 1765
    halo vest in, 1771
    hematoma in, 1772
    osteotomy in, 1772
    pseudoarthroses in, 1771–1772
    radiologic features of, 1766–1768, *1766–1768*
    stress fracture in, 1771–1772
    surgery for, complications of, 1768–1771, *1769*, *1770*
      indications for, 1765–1766, 1771
      results of, 1771
    traction in, 1771, 1773
  closing wedge osteotomy in, 1777
  colitis in, 1775
  fibrosis in, 1766, 1775
  fixed spinal deformities in, 1776–1777
  fractures in, 1776
  HLA-B27 in, 1766
  ileus in, 1777
  intubation in, 1777
  myocardial fibrosis in, 1775
  patient position in, 1769, *1769*
  postoperative ileus in, 1777
  radiation therapy in, 1766
  radiologic evaluation of, 516–518, *516–518*, 1776
  railway line appearance of, 1766, *1767*
  sacroiliitis in, 1775
  spinal stenosis in, 1780
  spondylodiscitis in, 1780
  thoracolumbar fracture in, 1777–1778, *1778*, *1779*
    treatment of, 1779–1780
  traction in, *1770*
  transpedicular fixation in, 1777
  vertebral squaring in, 1766, *1767*
Annulus of Zinn (annulus tendineus), anatomy of, 196, *198*, 206
  in intraorbital tumors, 185, *185*
Anosmia, in cerebrospinal fluid leak, 119
  in craniosynostosis, 137
  in olfactory groove meningioma, 393
  in sclerosteosis, 2142–2143
Antacids, after closed head injury, 63–64
Anterior triangle, of lateral sellar compartment, 494, *495*, 496t, 508
Anteroinferior triangle, of lateral sellar compartment, 508
Anterolateral triangle, of lateral sellar compartment, *495*, 496, 496t, 508
Antibiotics, in cerebrospinal fluid leaks, 122
  in penetrating head injury, 84, 102, 107
  in transcranial skull base tumor resection, 168, 172
Antibody, to octreotide, 308
Anticoagulation, in carotid atherosclerosis, 878, *878*
  in endocarditis, 1138
  in pregnancy, 1169
Anticonvulsants, in aneurysmal subarachnoid hemorrhage–associated seizures, 950–951, 950t
  in fetal mesencephalic tissue transplantation, 1366
  in penetrating head injuries, 84

Anticonvulsants *(Continued)*
  in pregnancy, 1169
Antifibrinolytic agents, in aneurysmal subarachnoid hemorrhage, 948, 959
Anxiety disorders, anterior capsulotomy for, 1443–1454
  anatomy for, 1444
  cognitive functions and, 1452–1453
  complications of, 1447
  contraindications to, 1444
  creativity and, 1453
  critique of, 1448–1449, 1448t
  efficacy of, 1449–1450, 1450t, 1452
  electrical stimulation in, 1446–1447
  gamma, 1449
  indications for, 1443–1444
  personality and, 1453
  preoperative evaluation for, 1444
  radiosurgical, 1447
  repeat, 1451–1452
  results of, 1447–1448, 1450–1451, *1451*, *1452*
  risks of, 1452–1453
  target localization for, 1444, *1444*, *1445*
  technique of, 1444–1445, *1445*
  vs. nonintervention, 1453–1454
  Gamma Knife surgery for, 691–692
Apert's syndrome, 142
  intelligence in, 136
  lumboperitoneal shunt in, *1967*
  proptosis in, 137
  psychomotor development in, 136
Apex, orbital, *216*
Aplasia, congenital, of scalp, 7–8
Aplasia cutis congenita, 7–8
Apnea, sleep, after open cordotomy, 1564–1565
Arachnoid cyst(s), 586–589, *587–589*
  diagnosis of, 579–580
  glial portion of, 579, *580*
  in children, 581
  in hydrocephalus, 1246
  intracranial, 579–581, *580*
  intracranial pressure measurement in, 586, *588*
  of cerebellopontine angle, 581
  of cerebral convexity, 581
  of posterior fossa, 796
  sella repair in, 337, *338*, 343
  stereotactic catheter implantation in, 455, *457*
  subdural hematoma and, 589, *589*
  suprasellar, 581–582, *582*
  wall of, 579, *580*
Arachnoidal gliomatosis, perineural, in optic nerve glioma, 255
Arachnoiditis, after lumbar disc surgery, 1936
Arachnoidocele, pituitary ademona and, 335, 337, *337*, *338*
Arc quadrant, for computer-assisted volumetric stereotactic resection, 620, *621*
Archicerebellum, 802
Arrhythmias, in aneurysmal subarachnoid hemorrhage, 952–953
Arterioles, radiation effects on, 1205
Arteriovenous malformation, 1177–1182, *1180*, *1181*
  brainstem, 1485–1498
    anatomy for, 1486
    aspiration of, 1493, 1496
    classification of, 1485
    clinical features of, 1485–1486
    natural history of, 1485
    preoperative embolization for, 1488
    preoperative evaluation for, 1486–1488, *1487*, *1488*
    rostral, 1490, *1497*, *1498*
    surgery for, 1486–1487, *1487*, *1488*
      adjuncts to, 1487–1488

Arteriovenous malformation *(Continued)*
    anesthesia for, 1487
    complications of, 1496–1497
    electrophysiologic monitoring in, 1487–1488
    management after, 1497–1498
    results of, 1498
    technique in, 1488–1493, *1489–1498*
  cerebellopontine angle, 1486, 1490
  computer-assisted volumetric stereotactic resection of, 632, *632*
  detection of, 1177
  dural, 1219–1228
    angiography of, 1219, *1220*
    arterial supply of, 1227, 1227t
    diagnosis of, 1227
    embolization for, 1219–1220, *1220*
    hemorrhage in, 1227, 1227t
    pathogenesis of, 1226–1227
    pathophysiology of, 1226–1227
    surgery for, 1220–1223
      closure in, 1223
      complications of, 1223, 1223t
      craniotomy in, 1222, *1223*, *1224*
      patient position in, 1220, *1221*, 1222, *1224*, 1228
      resection in, 1222–1223, *1225–1226*
      results of, 1223, 1223t
      scalp flap in, 1222
      sinus ligation in, 1222, *1224*
      soft-tissue dissection in, 1222
      vein of Labbé in, 1223
    symptoms of, 1226, 1226t
    venous drainage of, 1227–1228, 1228t
  Gamma Knife surgery for, 668, 670–676, 1206, 1207t
    arteriography in, 671–674, *672–675*, 674t
    decision-making in, 670
    follow-up for, 671
    neurologic outcome of, 674
    patient population for, 670–671
    peritreatment preparation for, 671
    pretreatment preparation for, 671
    rebleeding after, 674–675
    results of, 671–674, *672–675*, 674t
    target identification in, 670
    treatment variables in, 671
    undue effects of, 675–676, *676*, 676t, *677*
  in pregnancy, 1168
  pediatric, 1197–1202. See also *Vein of Galen malformation.*
    choroidal system in, 1201
    classification of, 1197
    clinical features of, 1197–1198, 1198t
    epilepsy in, 1197–1198
    mortality from, 1199, 1202
    natural history of, 1198–1199
    occult, 1201
    preoperative evaluation of, 1198
    preoperative management of, 1198
    surgery for, anatomy in, 1199
      anesthesia in, 1200
      approach selection in, 1199–1200
      care after, 1201–1202
      complications of, 1201
      mortality after, 1202
      results of, 1202
      staging of, 1201–1202
      techniques in, 1200–1201
      venous preservation in, 1201
  pontomedullary, 1486
  radiosurgery for, 668, 670–676, 1205–1211, 1206, 1207t. See also *Arteriovenous malformation, Gamma Knife surgery for.*
    Bragg peak in, 1206
    complications of, 1206–1207, 1207t

Arteriovenous malformation *(Continued)*
    hemorrhage risk and, 1206
    linear accelerator in, 1206
    patient selection for, 1205–1206
    planning for, 1207–1211, *1208*, *1209*
      dose calculations in, 1210–1211
      image acquisition in, 1208
      image registration in, 1208–1209, *1209*
      image segmentation in, 1209
      parameters of, 1209–1210
    rehemorrhage after, 1207, 1207t
    results of, 1206
    techniques for, 1206–1207, 1207t
  spinal cord, 2038–2047
    anatomy of, 2038–2040, *2039–2040*
    angiography in, 2028
    classification of, 2038–2039, *2039–2041*
    clinical presentation of, 2040–2041, *2042*
    diagnosis of, 2041–2042, *2042*
    embolization of, 2043
    juvenile, 2044
    meningeal, 2047
    natural history of, 2040–2041
    parameningeal, 2047
    surgery for, 2043–2045, *2043*, *2044*
  stereotactic biopsy and, 640
  stereotactic radiation for, 1177–1178, *1178*
  surgery for, 1178, *1180*, *1181*, 1182
    bleeding during, 1178
    embolization in, 1178, *1181*
    hemorrhage after, 1178
  thalamic–basal ganglia, 1501–1520
    anatomy of, 1501–1502, 1502t
    evaluation of, 1501–1502, 1502t
    management of, 1502–1503
    presentation of, 1501, 1501t, 1502t
    size of, 1502
    surgery for, 1504–1518
      adjuncts to, 1504
      anesthesia for, 1504
      electrophysiologic monitoring in, 1504
      management after, 1518
      principles of, 1504
      results of, 1518, 1520, 1520t
      retractor for, 1504
      stereotactic craniotomy approach to, 1503, 1518, *1519*
      transcallosal-transventricular approach to, 1503, 1504–1505, *1505–1507*
      transcortical-transventricular approach to, 1503, 1505, 1508–1513, *1509–1513*
      transsylvian approach to, 1503, 1513–1518, *1514–1518*
Artery (arteries), of lateral sellar compartment, 480, 481–483, *482*, *484*
  of scalp, 3
  radiation effects on, 1205
  sulcus-like impression of, *559*
  to pineal region, 744–745, 745t, *746*
Arthrodesis, C3-T1, 1843–1847, *1845*, *1846*
  occipito–C1-C2, 1842–1843, *1843*, *1844*
Aseptic meningitis, after glycerol rhizolysis, 1532, 1532t
Aspergillosis, *1701*
Aspergillus, 1699–1702, 1699t, 1702t
Aspiration, of brainstem vascular malformation, 1493, 1496
Astrocytoma, 549. See also *Glioma; Spinal cord tumors, intramedullary.*
  anaplastic, 517
  brainstem, curietherapy for, *464*
  cerebellar, pediatric, 801, *804*, *805*, 807–809, *809*
    surgery for, 796
  cerebral, cystic, 517–518
  computer-assisted volumetric stereotactic resection of, 631

Astrocytoma *(Continued)*
  fibrillar, stereotactic biopsy of, *454*
  giant cell, subependymal, 574
  interstitial brachytherapy for, 665
  intracavitary brachytherapy for, 664
  intramedullary, 2028, *2031–2032*, 2095–2105, *2099*. See also *Spinal cord tumors, intramedullary.*
    resection of, 2100–2101, *2100*
    vs. ependymoma, 2096–2097, *2098*, 2100
  intraventricular, computer-assisted volumetric stereotactic resection of, 632, *633*
  labeling index of, 551
  low-grade, 592, *593*
    Gamma Knife surgery for, 685, *686*
    supratentorial, 517
  optic nerve, 187, 257–265, *259–261*, *265*
  $p53$ gene in, 266
  pilocytic, 549
    computer-assisted volumetric stereotactic resection of, *627*, 631
    CT-guided stereotactic biopsy of, *451*
    juvenile, 269
  pineal region, 762
  posterior fossa, 792t
  presentation of, 518t
  radiotherapy in, 566
  S phase of, 551
  stereotactic volumetric resection of, *627*, 631, 632, *633*, 649
  telangiectatic, 271
  thalamic, curietherapy for, *464*
AT877 (HA1077), for aneurysmal subarachnoid hemorrhage–associated vasospasm, 945
Ataxia, in pediatric cerebellar tumor, 803
Atlantoaxial facets, screw fixation of, 1864–1867, *1865–1868*
Atlantoaxial joints, 1720
Atlantoaxial subluxation, in ankylosing spondylitis, 1772–1773
Atlas, 1719
Atrial natriuretic factor, in aneurysmal subarachnoid hemorrhage, 951
Atrial shunt, in pediatric hydrocephalus, 1235
Attentional disorder, after corpus callosotomy, 1355
Auditory meatus, extradural middle fossa approach to, 824
Auricular artery, 76
Auriculotemporal nerve, 76
Autonomic system, in syringomyelia, 2121
Axillary nerve, lesions of, 2164
Axis, 1719
Axon, 2159
  regeneration of, 2162–2163
Axonotmesis, 2161

Back pain. See *Lumbar disc, herniation of; Sciatica.*
Baclofen, in spasticity, 1661
Ballistics, 81–82, 89
Balloon catheter, in neuroendoscopy, 696, *698*
  intracranial aneurysm treatment with, 967–974
    case reports of, 969–971, *969*, *971*
    complications of, 972, *973*
    embolism after, 973
    outcomes of, 968t, 972
    patient selection for, 967, 968t
    results of, 971
    retrograde suction decompression in, 970–971, *970*, 972, *972*
    technique of, 967–971, *969–971*
Balloon compression, retrogasserian, in trigeminal neuralgia, 1478, 1479t, 1480t

Balloon distension pressure, in percutaneous trigeminal nerve compression, 1539–1540
Barbiturates, in closed head injury, 61
  in intracranial aneurysm surgery, 962
Basal ganglia. See also *Thalamic–basal ganglia*.
  hematomas in, 75
  postirradiation calcifications of, 254
Basilar artery, *1077, 1088*
  aneurysm of, intraoperative rupture of, 988
    surgery for, endovascular balloon catheter techniques in, 967–974, 968t
  bifurcation of, aneurysm of, 1073t, 1084
    surgery for, 1079, *1081*, 1082–1083
      clip selection in, 1082
      results of, 1072t, 1073t
    height of, 1083
  lower, aneurysm of, 1087–1100, 1087t
    surgery for, 1088–1100
      anatomy in, 1088
      case reports of, 1097–1100, *1099, 1100*
      closure for, 1091
      combined approaches in, 1091–1094, *1092–1094*
        closure for, 1094
        complications of, 1094
        intradural exposure in, 1093–1094, *1093, 1094*
        selection of, 1094
        sigmoid sinus sacrifice in, 1093, *1093*
      combined-combined approach in, 1097, *1098*
      far lateral approach in, 1095–1097, *1096, 1097*
        patient position for, 1095, *1095*
      hypothermic cardiac standstill in, 1088
      intradural exposure in, 1089
      retrolabyrinthine approach in, 1089, *1090*, 1091
      transcochlear approach in, 1089, *1090*, 1091, *1091*
      translabyrinthine approach in, 1089, *1090*, 1091
      transpetrosal approach in, 1088t, 1089–1091, *1090, 1091*
  terminal, anatomy of, *1077*
    aneurysm of, 1071–1086
      sites of, *1072*
      surgery for, 1074–1079, *1076–1081*
        anesthesia for, 1071, 1074
        approaches to, *1072*
        patient position for, 1074, *1075*
        results of, 1072t, 1073t
Beam's-eye view treatment planning, 1210
Behavior disorder, hemispherectomy and, 1342
Bernoulli principle, in optic nerve sheath fenestration, 250
Bicoronal craniosynostosis, 141–145, *144, 145*
Bilateral cleft syndrome, 157, *157*
Biopsy, brain, 615–618
  complications of, 615, 616t, 617–618, 618t
  in intracranial glioma, 521
  in metastasis, 611
  indications for, 615, 615t
  results of, 615, 616t
  sites for, 616, 616t
  slice size in, 616, *617*
  specimen handling after, 616–617, *617*
  techniques of, 616–617, 616t, *617*
  in AIDS, 1683–1684, 1684t, 1685, *1685*, 1685t
  stereotactic, 446, 450, 451–452, *451–454*, 455, 637–651
    arc quadrant positioning for, 641, *642*
    complications of, 648, 648t, 650t
    consecutive procedures after, 455, *456, 457*

Biopsy *(Continued)*
  contraindications to, 640
  Cosman-Roberts-Wells system for, 640–641, *640–643*
  direct method of, 452
  endoscopic, 704, *704, 705*
    results of, 707, *708*
  ex-post method of, 452
  frameless, 650–651, *651*
  histopathologic method for, 642–643
  histopathologic results of, 648–650, 650t, 651t
  in human immunodeficiency virus–associated lesions, 639–640
  in infratentorial lesions, 638
  in pineal region tumors, 744, 757
  indications for, 637–640, *638*, 638t, *639*
  indirect method of, 451–452
  magnetic resonance imaging–guided, 638–639, *638, 639*
  patient position for, 641, *641*
  plan for, 641, *642*
  results of, 455, 455t, 651t
  sites of, 648t
  skull opening for, 641, *642*
Bitemporal syndrome, 1272–1273, *1273*
Bladder dysfunction, after intramedullary spinal cord tumor surgery, 2103
  after open cordotomy, 1565, 1567
Blast injury, in penetrating head injury, 83
Bleeding. See also *Hemorrhage*.
  in glomus jugulare tumor surgery, 873
  in lateral orbitotomy, 225
  in optic nerve sheath fenestration, 246
  in orbital surgery, 234
Bleomycin, for craniopharyngioma, 388
Blindness, after percutaneous trigeminal rhizotomy, 1544
  in craniosynostosis, 136
  in frontoethmoidal encephalomeningocele, 164
Blood loss, in craniosynostosis treatment, 146–147
  in encephalocele treatment, 158
  in infant, 575
Blood pressure, after carotid endarterectomy, 885
  in intracranial aneurysm surgery, 960, 961
Bobble-head syndrome, 581
Bone chips, in penetrating head injury, 83
Bone cranioplasty, 21, *22*, 25, *25*
Bone fragments, in penetrating head injury, 85, 86, 101–102, 102t
Bourneville's disease, subependymal giant cell astrocytoma in, 574
Bowel function, after intramedullary spinal cord tumor surgery, 2103
  after pediatric spinal injury, 2093
Brachial plexus, avulsion injury to, DREZotomy in, 1617–1618, 1620, 1625, *1626*, 1629–1631, *1630*
  meningoceles after, 1629–1630, *1630*
  lesions of, 2163–2164
    complete, 2170–2171
    pain with, deep brain stimulation for, 1395, 1396
    surgery for, 2164
    treatment of, 2164
  neural sheath tumor of, *2186*
Brachycephaly, 141–142
Brachytherapy, 455, 457–458, 457t
  in glioblastoma, 538
  in neoplastic spinal cord compression, 2003
  indications for, 463–465, *465*, 465t
  interstitial, 655–665
    approach angle for, 657
    catheter implantation in, 658–660, *659, 660*
    catheter spacing for, 657–658

Brachytherapy *(Continued)*
    complications of, 664–665
    follow-up for, 663
    housekeeping staff information on, 663
    ^{192}Ir seeds for, 658
      afterloading of, 661–662, *662*
      postloading surveys of, 662
      postremoval surveys for, 663
      removal of, 663
      return of, 663
    isodose curves for, 660–661
    nursing staff information on, 662
    patient information on, 662
    patient selection for, 655–656
    postoperative treatment planning for, 660–661, *660*
    preoperative planning for, 656–658, *657, 658*
    preplanning for, 657–658, *658*
    radiation precautions for, 662–663
    results of, 663–665
    seed spacing for, 657–658
    target contours for, 656–657, *657*
    tumor selection for, 656
    volumetric reconstruction for, 657, *657*
    x-ray catheter identification for, 660
  radiation necrosis after, 536
  results of, 463, 463t
  technique of, 458, *460*
Bragg peak therapy, in arteriovenous malformation radiosurgery, 1206
Brain, abscess of, 1674–1676, *1675, 1677*
  computed tomography of, 1675, *1675*
  endoscopic surgery for, 706, *706*
    results of, 707, 710, *711*
  removal of, 1676, *1677*
  wall of, 1675, *1675*
  biopsy of, 615–618
    complications of, 615, 616t, 617–618, 618t
    in intracranial glioma, 521
    in metastasis, 611
    indications for, 615, 615t
    results of, 615, 616t
    sites for, 616, 616t
    slice size in, 616, *617*
    specimen handling after, 616–617, *617*
    techniques of, 616–617, 616t, *617*
  cavitation of, in penetrating head injury, 90
  damage to, in frontoethmoidal encephalomeningocele, 161, *163*, 164
  fungus of, in penetrating head injury, 103
  herniation of, after cerebral hemispherectomy, 1349
  metastases to, 599–613
    characteristics of, 599, 603
    diagnosis of, 603, 607, *607, 608*, 612
    distribution of, 599, 603, *604*
    from breast carcinoma, 689
    from bronchogenic carcinoma, 606, *607*
    from hypernephroma, 604, *608*
    Gamma Knife surgery for, 686–689, *687*, 687t, *688, 689*
      outcome of, 687t
    latent interval of, 603
    management of, 607–613, 608t
      hydrocephalus shunt in, 612
      radiation therapy in, 609, 609–610
      radiotherapy in, 610–611
      stereotactic radiosurgery in, 609–610
      steroid therapy in, 608–609, 608t
      surgical, 610–612
        biopsy in, 611
        life expectancy and, 612
        mortality of, 611
        patient selection for, 612
        stereotactic guidance in, 611–612

Brain *(Continued)*
    technique of, 611–612
        whole-brain radiotherapy in, 609, *609*
    metachronous, 603
    multiple, *603*
    single, 599, 612
    solitary, 599, *600–602*
    sources of, 599, *600–602*
    survival with, 607–613, 608t
    synchronous, 603
  protection of, in intracranial aneurysm surgery, 962–963
  radiation to, 1205
    intelligence and, 276–277
  relaxation of, in intracranial aneurysm surgery, 959
  revascularization of, 909–926
    aneurysm obliteration after, 925
    angiography in, 910
    balloon occlusion in, 911
    blood flow after, 925
    bypass patency after, 925
    complications of, 925–926
    encephaloduroarteriosynangiosis in, 923–924
    evaluation for, 910–911
    external carotid artery–saphenous vein–middle cerebral artery bypass in, 921–923, *922, 923*
    external carotid artery–saphenous vein–posterior cerebral artery bypass for, 924, *925*
    indications for, 909–910
    intracranial arterial replantation in, 923
    intraoperative angiography in, 911
    occipital artery–middle cerebral artery bypass in, 921
    occipital artery–posterior internal cerebellar artery bypass in, 924–925, *926*
    omental grafting for, 924
    protocol for, 911, 911t, 912t
    results of, 925
    subclavian artery–saphenous vein–middle cerebral artery bypass in, 923
    superficial temporal artery–middle cerebral artery bypass in, 920, *921*
    superficial temporal artery–saphenous vein–middle cerebral artery bypass for, 911–920, *913–920*
    superficial temporal artery–saphenous vein–posterior cerebral artery bypass for, 924
    tolerance test occlusion in, 910–911
    tumor surgery and, 910
    vascular complications of, 926
    venous reconstruction in, 925
    warfarin therapy in, 911
  stimulation of, 23–31. See also *Deep brain stimulation.*
  swelling of, in closed head injury, 53–54
    in craniotomy, 79
    in difficult aneurysm, 1051–1052
    in penetrating head injury, 83
  tumors of. See specific tumors, e.g., *Glioma,* and *Brain, metastases to.*
Brainstem, arteriovenous malformation of, 1485–1498
  anatomy for, 1486
  aspiration of, 1493, 1496
  classification of, 1485
  clinical features of, 1485–1486
  natural history of, 1485
  preoperative embolization for, 1488
  preoperative evaluation for, 1486–1488, *1487, 1488*
  surgery for, 1486–1487, *1487, 1488*

Brainstem *(Continued)*
    adjuncts to, 1487–1488
    anesthesia for, 1487
    complications of, 1496–1497
    electrophysiologic monitoring in, 1487–1488
    management after, 1497–1498
    results of, 1498
    technique for, 1488–1493, *1489–1498*
  astrocytoma of, curietherapy for, *464*
    stereotactic biopsy of, *454*
  cavernous angioma of, 1189, 1191–1192, *1191,* 1191t, *1192*
  glioma of, 792t
    stereotactic biopsy of, 448, 704, *704*
  mass lesions of, stereotactic biopsy of, 638
  tuberculoma of, 1697
  tumors of, 775–782, *776–780*
    clinical manifestations of, 779, 780t
    diagnosis of, 777, *777–779*
    diffuse, 777, *777*
    exophytic component of, 781
    focal, *779*
    focal-diffuse, 777, *778*
    intrinsic component of, 781
    locations of, 780
    metastatic, *606,* 611, 792t
    pseudofocal, *779*
    surgery for, 779–781, 780t
      approach for, 780, *780*
      indications for, 779
      neurologic status after, 781–782, 781t, 782t
      results of, 781–782, 781t, 782t
      technique of, 780–781
  venous anatomy of, cranial nerve relationships to, 1457
Breast carcinoma, brachial plexus injury in, DREZotomy in, 1627
  brain metastasis from, *605*
  Gamma Knife surgery for, *689*
Broca's area, *532*
Bromocriptine, complications of, 311
  in Cushing's disease, 303
  in growth hormone–secreting pituitary adenoma, 308
  in nonfunctioning pituitary adenoma, *295*
  in pregnancy, 311
  in prolactin-secreting pituitary adenoma, 310–311
  in recurrent prolactinemia, 319
  side effects of, 308
Brown-Séquard syndrome, 1595
  in spinal cord compression, 1999
Bruit, spinal, in arteriovenous malformation, 2041
Bullet, 81–82
  exploding, in penetrating head injuries, 85–86
Bullet track, in penetrating head injury, 82–83
Burn, scalp, 8, 9
Burr holes, about middle meningeal artery, *76*
  in closed head trauma, 49–50, *50*
Burst temporal lobe, 74
Buserelin, in recurrent adenoma, 319
Buttresses, of midface, 28
Butyl 2-cyanoacrylate (Histoacryl Blue), for dural defects, 234

Calcification(s), in ankylosing spondylitis, 1767–1768, *1767, 1768*
  in craniopharyngioma, 358, 376
  in oligodendroglioma, 549
  in optic nerve glioma, 253–254
  in pediatric cerebellar ependymoma, 803–804, *805*

Calcification(s) *(Continued)*
  in pineal region tumor, 743
  in tuberculoma, 1691
  postirradiation, of basal ganglia, 254
Calcitonin gene–related peptide, for aneurysmal subarachnoid hemorrhage–associated vasospasm, 945, 947
Calcium channel blockers, in aneurysmal subarachnoid hemorrhage, 945, 947t, 959
Calcospherites, in optic nerve glioma, 253–254
Callosal artery, traumatic aneurysm of, *1128*
Calvarium. See *Skull.*
Camera systems, in neuroendoscopy, 699, *700*
Canal of Vesalius, 1543–1544
Caniculus of Arnold, 1544
Cancer. See *Tumors.*
Cancer pain. See *Pain, cancer.*
Candida, 1699–1702, 1699t, 1702t
Canthal ligament, disengagement of, 221
  in anterior orbitotomy, *230*
Canthotomy, 221, 227–228
CAPIT (Core Assessment Program for Intracerebral Transplantation), in Parkinson's disease, 1362–1363, 1380, *1381,* 1382
Capsule, internal, 1444
Capsulotomy, anterior, 1443–1454
  anatomy for, 1444
  cognitive functions and, 1452–1453
  complications of, 1447
  contraindications to, 1444
  creativity and, 1453
  critique of, 1448–1449, 1448t
  development of, 1444
  efficacy of, 1449–1450, 1450t, 1452
  electrical stimulation in, 1446–1447
  gamma, 1449
  indications for, 1443–1444
  personality and, 1453
  preoperative evaluation for, 1444
  radiosurgical, 1447
  repeat, 1451–1452
  results of, 1447–1448, 1450–1451, *1451, 1452*
  risks of, 1452–1453
  target localization for, 1444, *1444, 1445*
  technique of, 1444–1445, *1445*
  vs. nonintervention, 1453–1454
Carbamazepine, in multiple sclerosis, 1533
  in myelomeningoceles, 2055
  in pregnancy, 1169
  in tuberculoma, 1695
  metabolic effects of, 386
Carbon dioxide laser. See *Laser.*
Carcinomatosis, meningeal, 613
Cardiac arrest, hypothermic, in basilar artery aneurysm, 1088
Cardiac dysrhythmia, optic nerve sheath fenestration and, 249
Carotico-oculomotor membrane, 494
Carotid artery (arteries), aneurysm of, 887–888, 1156, *1157*
  common, ligation of, in intracavernous aneurysm, 976
  dissection of, in closed head injury, 61
  exposure of, in carotid endarterectomy, 880–881, *881*
  extracranial, stenosis of, surgical therapy for, 877–885. See also *Carotid enarterectomy.*
  fibromuscular dysplasia of, 888
  fusiform dilatation of, craniopharyngioma removal and, 384–385, *385*
  infarction of, in difficult aneurysm, 1052
  internal, anatomy of, 1005, *1008*
    aneurysm of, 1003–1010, *1008*
      anatomy of, 1005

Carotid artery (arteries) *(Continued)*
    blood blister, 973
    diagnostic evaluation of, 1004–1005
    preoperative management of, 1005
    surgery for, *1006*, 1007–1010, *1007–1009*
        balloon occlusion in, 1113–1114
        carotid stump pressure in, 973–974
        endovascular balloon catheter techniques in, 967–974, 968t, *969–971*
        proximal occlusion in, 1113–1114
        results of, 1010, 1010t
        traumatic, *1130*
    bifurcation of, aneurysm of, 1115–1116, *1116*
    bypass procedure for, in lateral sellar compartment tumor surgery, 508–509
    cavernous segment of, aneurysm of, 1113
    clinoid segment of, 975
        anatomy of, 975, *978*
        aneurysms of, 979–981, *980*
    distal, ligation of, 891
        surgical exposure of, 891–895, 891t, *892, 893, 895*
    in glomus jugulare tumor surgery, 873
    in tuberculum sellae meningioma, 404
    intracavernous segment of, anatomy of, 975, *978*
        aneurysms of, 975–979, *977, 978*
            algorithm for, *978*
            infectious, 981
            traumatic, 981
        fistulae of, 981–983, *982*
    intraoperative injury to, 322
    ligation of, in clinoidal segment aneurysm, 981
    in intracavernous aneurysm, 976–979, *977–978*
    nomenclature for, 494, *495*
    occlusion of, 908, *908*
        in paraclinoid aneurysm surgery, 995
    paraclinoid, aneurysm of, endovascular balloon catheter techniques for, 967–974, 968t
    proximal, aneurysm of, rupture of, 987
    supraclinoid segment of, 1005
    kinking of, 887
    of lateral sellar compartment, *480*, 481–483, *484*, 494
    penetration of, in percutaneous trigeminal rhizotomy, 1472, *1474*
    supraclinoid, aneurysm of, 1003–1010, *1006–1009*, 1010t
    traumatic injuries of, 886–887
    trigeminal ganglion relation to, *1474*
Carotid artery bypass, in lateral sellar compartment tumor surgery, 508–509
Carotid duplex ultrasonography, in carotid atherosclerosis, 877–878
Carotid endarterectomy, 877–879
    anesthesia for, 879
    bilateral, 884
    bleeding during, 881–882
    cerebral angiography in, 879
    closure for, 883–884
    complications of, 885–886, 885t
    diagnosis of, 877–879, *878*
    distal internal carotid artery exposure in, 891–895, 891t, *892, 893, 895*
        anesthesia in, 892
        mandibular subluxation in, 892, *894*
    indications for, 877–879, *878*
    intraoperative shunt placement in, 881–882
    patch graft in, 884
    patient position for, 879, *880*
    patient selection for, 877–879, *878*
    postoperative care in, 885

Carotid endarterectomy *(Continued)*
    preoperative preparation for, 879
    restenosis after, 884–885
    results of, 886
    technique for, 879–885, *880–884*
Carotid stump pressure, in internal carotid artery aneurysm treatment, 973–974
Carotid-cavernous fistulae, 981–983, *982*
Carpal tunnel syndrome, 2177–2179, *2178, 2179*
Catecholamines, glomus jugulare tumor secretion of, 866, 874
Category Test, in intracranial glioma, 520
Catheter, balloon, 696, *698*, 967–974. See also *Balloon catheter.*
    implantation of, in arachnoidal cyst, 455, *457*
    in brachytherapy, 658–660, *659, 660*
Cauda equina, ependymoma of, 2101
    lesions of, in penetrating injury, 1974–1975
Cauda equina syndrome, in ankylosing spondylitis, 1780
Caudate, head of, subependymal giant cell astrocytoma of, 574
Caudate nucleus, 1371
    adrenal medullary autografts in, 1372–1373
    adrenal medullary cell implantation in, 1372
    fetal adrenal medulla transplantation in, 1373–1374
Causalgia, lumbar sympathectomy for, 1644–1645, *1644, 1645*
    spinal cord stimulation in, 1407
    sympathectomy for, 1574. See also *Sympathectomy.*
    upper thoracic ganglionectomy for, 1637–1641
        anatomy for, 1637–1638
        approaches to, 1638
        complications of, 1641
        results of, 1640–1641
        technique for, 1639–1640, *1639, 1640*
Cavernoma, stereotactic volumetric resection of, 648, *649*
Cavernous angioma, 1183–1195
    brainstem, 1189, 1191–1192, *1191*, 1191t, *1192*
    cerebellar, 1189, *1190*, 1190t
    cerebral, 1186–1189, *1187*, 1187t, *1188, 1189*, 1189t
        headache in, 1187, *1188*
        neurologic deficit with, 1187–1188, *1189*
        surgery for, 1188–1189, 1189t
        with seizures, 1186–1187, *1187*, 1187t, *1188*
    clinical presentation of, 1184
    familial occurrence of, 1184
    Gamma Knife surgery for, 678, *678*
    natural history of, 1185
    observation for, 1186
    of cranial nerves, 1193, 1193t
    of spinal cord, 1193–1195, *1194*, 1194t
    pathologic features of, 1183
    pregnancy and, 1185, *1186*
    radiologic features of, 1183–1184, *1184*
    radiosurgery for, 678, *678*, 1185–1186
    third ventricle, subchoroidal trans–velum interpositum approach to, *721*
Cavernous sinus. See *Lateral sellar compartment.*
Cavitation, in penetrating head injury, 90
Cavitron ultrasonic surgical aspirator, in optic nerve glioma removal, 270
    in spinal cord tumor surgery, 2097
Cellulitis, after pedicled rhinotomy, 474
    orbital, 178t, 179t
Central area, depth electrode implantation for, 1279–1282, *1280, 1282*
Central nervous system transplantation, 1371–1383
    adrenal medullary cells in, 1371–1373

Central nervous system transplantation *(Continued)*
    fetal adrenal medullary cells in, 1373–1374
    fetal mesencephalic tissue in, 1361–1367, *1362*, 1374–1383
        clinical data on, 1376–1379
        donor age and, 1375
        donor tissue preparation for, 1363–1364, *1364*
        immunosuppression and, 1376
        implantation site for, 1375–1376
        in Parkinson's disease, 1361–1363, *1362*
        management after use of, 1366
        positron-emission tomography and, 1376
        results of use of, 1367
        technique of use of, 1364–1366, *1365, 1366, 1378*, 1379–1383, *1380–1382*
        tissue viability and, 1375
Central retinal artery, 240, *241*
    occlusion of, optic nerve sheath fenestration and, 248, 248t
Central retinal vein, 241
Centrum ovale, glioma of, 560
Cerebellar artery, inferior, in acoustic neuroma, 814, 834
    posteroinferior, anatomy of, 1106–1107
        aneurysm of, 1103–1110
            anatomy of, 1106–1107
            clinical features of, 1104–1105
            dissecting, 1105–1106, *1106*
            fusiform, 1106
            imaging of, 1105
            location of, 1103, *1103*
            morphology of, 1103–1104, *1104*
            preoperative evaluation of, 1105–1106
            saccular, 1105
            surgery for, 1107–1110
                anesthesia in, 1107
                clip selection in, 1110
                distal control in, 1110
                ELITE approach in, 1109
                extreme lateral inferior transcondylar exposure in, 1109
                microsurgical techniques in, 1109–1110
                proximal control in, 1110
                retrolabyrinthine-transsigmoid approach in, 1108–1109
                suboccipital approach in, 1107–1108
    superior, aneurysm of, infected, 1141, 1143, *1145*
        surgery for, 1073t, 1084–1085, *1085*
Cerebellopontine angle, arachnoid cysts of, 581
    arteriovenous malformation of, 1486, 1490. See also *Brainstem, arteriovenous malformation of.*
    petrosal approach to, 824
    surgery at, cerebrospinal fluid leak in, 126
    translabyrinthine approach to, 813, *814*, 824
    tumors of, surgery for, 799, *799*
    venous anatomy of, cranial nerve relationships to, 1457
Cerebellum, abscess of, endoscopic evacuation of, 706, *706*
    anatomy of, 802
    astrocytoma of, 796
    cavernous angioma of, 1189, *1190*, 1190t
    hemangioblastoma of, 797, *798*
    metastases to, 792t, 796–797
    pediatric, astrocytoma of, 801, *804, 805*, 808–809, *809*
        ependymoma of, 801, 803–804, *805*
        medulloblastoma of, 801, 803, *805*, 808, 809–810, *809*
        primitive neuroectodermal tumor of, 801
Cerebral artery, anterior, anatomy of, 1014–1015, *1016–1018*

Cerebral artery *(Continued)*
   aneurysm of, 1014–1021
      morphology of, 1015
      neck of, 1015, *1019*
      sac of, 1018, *1020*
      surgery for, 1018, 1020–1021, *1020*
         anesthesia for, 1021–1022
         aneurysm dissection in, 1025–1026, *1026*
         brain tension in, 1024
         case reports of, 1029–1032, *1030, 1031*
         complications of, 1028–1029
         craniotomy for, 1022, *1023*, 1024
         discussion of, 1032
         dural opening in, 1024
         incision for, 1023–1024, *1024*
         internal carotid artery exposure in, 1024–1025, *1024, 1025*
         neck clipping in, 1026–1027, *1026*
         optic nerve exposure in, 1024–1025, *1024, 1025*
         patient position for, 1022–1023, *1023*
         postoperative management in, 1027
         results of, 1027–1028, 1028t
         scalp flap for, 1023–1024, *1024*
         technical aids for, 1021
   anomalies of, 1014–1015, *1016–1018*
   distal, aneurysm of, *1035*, 1035–1039
      surgery for, 1036–1039, *1036–1038*
         basal frontal interhemispheric approach in, 1036–1037, *1036, 1037*
         complications of, 1039
         direct interhemispheric approach in, 1037–1038, *1038*
         patient position for, 1036, *1036, 1038*
   proximal, aneurysm of, 1032–1033, *1032, 1033*
   type I, 1015, *1016*
   type II, 1015, *1017*
   type III, 1015, *1017, 1018*
   type IV, 1015, *1018*
   in subependymal giant cell astrocytoma, 574
   middle, aneurysm of, 1055–1070
      computed tomography in, 1055–1056
      evaluation of, 1055–1056, *1056*
      giant, surgery for, 1045–1046, 1064–1068, *1064–1069*, 1116, *1117*
      grade 5, surgery for, 1062, 1064
      infected, 1140, *1140*, 1141, *1144*, 1146–1147, *1146*
      magnetic resonance imaging in, 1056, *1056*
      multiple, 1156, *1158*
      preoperative medication in, 1056–1057, 1056t
      surgery for, *1121*, 1122
         approach planning for, 1058, *1058, 1059*
         at trifurcation, 1060–1064, *1061–1063*
         patient position for, 1059–1060, *1060*
         postoperative care after, 1067–1068
         results of, 1068, 1070
         timing of, 1057–1058
   Doppler ultrasound of, in aneurysmal subarachnoid hemorrhage, 944
   in superficial temporal artery–saphenous vein–middle cerebral artery bypass, 916
   trifurcation of, aneurysm of, 1060–1064, *1061–1063*
   posterior, aneurysm of, 1084–1085, *1085*
      fusiform, *1119*
      giant, 1073t

Cerebral artery *(Continued)*
      surgery for, endovascular balloon catheter techniques in, 967–974, 968t
         results of, 1073t
   in amygdalohippocampectomy, 1299
   in calcarine fissure, *532*
Cerebral blood flow, in aneurysmal subarachnoid hemorrhage, 958, *958*
   in closed head injury, 59
   in intracranial aneurysm surgery, 959–960
   postcordotomy, 1596
Cerebral contusion, in craniopharyngioma removal, 364–365
Cerebral hemispherectomy, 1341–1350
   anatomic, 1343
      Oxford-Adams modification of, 1343–1344
      white matter preservation in, 1344
   case reports of, 1347–1348, *1348*
   complications of, 1348–1349
   computed tomography for, 1342, *1342*
   electroencephalography for, 1342–1343
   functional, 1344–1346, *1344, 1345*
   indications for, 1341–1343, *1342*, 1343t
   intellectual effects of, 1349
   neurologic examination for, 1341–1342
   results of, 1349
   seizure control after, 1349
   seizure etiology and, 1343, 1343t
   seizure patterns and, 1341
   social effects of, 1349
   surgical findings at, 1343
   techniques of, 1343–1348, 1343t
Cerebral hernia, 152, *152*
Cerebral ischemia, after closed head injury, 58
Cerebral perfusion pressure, after closed head injury, 58–59, 59t, 60
   autoregulation of, impairment of, 58
Cerebral salt wasting syndrome, in aneurysmal subarachnoid hemorrhage, 958
Cerebritis, herpes simplex, *1685*
Cerebrospinal fluid (CSF). See also *Hydrocephalus.*
   absorption of, in hydrocephalus, 1247, 1247t
   circulation of, in suprasellar cyst, 581
   drainage of, after lateral ventricle tumor resection, 737
      meningitis and, 124
      volume-regulated, 123–124
   evaluation of, in AIDS, 1683
      in hydrocephalus, 1246–1247, 1247t
      in pineal region tumors, 740
      in tuberculous meningitis, 1697
   in craniosynostosis, 137
   leakage of, cranial, 117–129
      anosmia in, 119
      antibiotics in, 122
      classification of, 118
      clinical evidence of, 119
      complications of, 124
      computed tomography of, 120
      confirmation of, 119
      contrast localization of, 121
      drainage of, 123–124
      epidemiology of, 118–119
      etiology of, 118–119
      external ventricular drainage of, 123–124
      glucose in, 119
      headache in, 119
      high pressure, 122
      imaging of, 119–121, 120t
      immunologic localization of, 121
      infection prevention in, 123
      intensive care for, 122–123
      low pressure, 122
      management of, 122–123
      meningitis in, 119

Cerebrospinal fluid (CSF) *(Continued)*
      nontraumatic, 121–122
      operative management of, 124–129, 125t
         craniotomy in, 125–127
         endoscopic approaches in, 128
         extracranial approaches in, 127
         facial fracture reduction in, 127
         in anterior cranial fossa, 125–126
         in middle cranial fossa, 126
         in posterior cranial fossa, 126–127
         lumbar drainage in, 128
         polymethyl methacrylate in, 127
         shunting in, 128
         timing of, 124–125
         tissue adhesives in, 128
      patient position in, 123
      pharmacologic agents in, 124
      plain radiography of, 120
      pneumocephalus in, 119
      postoperative, 118–119
      reservoir sign in, 119
      spontaneous, 118–119, 121–122
      target sign in, 119
      tracer localization of, 120–121, 120t
      traumatic, 118, 121
   epiduro-trans-ethmoidal rhinosurgical approach for, 32–33, *33, 34*
   in children, 118
   in craniopharyngioma removal, 377, *377, 378*
   in craniosynostosis treatment, 147
   in dorsal root ganglionectomy, 1589
   in facial fracture, 127
   in frontal skull base fracture, 31, *31*
   in jugular foramen schwannoma, 870
   in lumbar disc surgery, 1938–1939, 1952
   in penetrating head injury, 86, 100–101, 102, 102t
   in pituitary adenoma removal, 288–289, 296, 297
   in recurrent adenoma removal, 322
   in sclerosteosis, 2143
   in transbasal skull base tumor removal, 427
   in transcranial skull base tumor resection, 168
   infection and, 101, 102, 102t, 123
   intraoperative, 2050
   isotope cisternography in, 120–121
   meningitis and, 124
   meningomyelocele repair and, 122
   postoperative, 125, 2049–2053
      after cerebellopontine angle surgery, 126
      after glomus jugulare tumor surgery, 873
      after suboccipital transmeatal acoustic neuroma removal, 836
      bone spicule in, 2049
      cyanoacrylates in, 2052
      diagnosis of, 2050–2051, *2050*
      dural closure techniques in, 2051–2053, *2051–2053*
      etiology of, 2049
      fibrin glue in, 2052, *2053*
      in difficult aneurysm, 1052
      in OPLL surgery, 2050
      in sclerosteosis, 2150
      localization of, *2050*, 2051
      lumbar drainage in, 2052–2053
      muscle pledget repair of, 2052, *2052*
      nerve rootlet herniation in, 2053, *2053*
      nonoperative treatment of, 2051
      prevention of, 2049
      translabyrinthine approach and, 825
      treatment of, 2051–2053, *2051–2053*
   sella repair in, 331, *332*, 339–341, 344
   spinal, 118, 128–129
   tobacco-pouch technique for, 33, *34*

Cerebrospinal fluid (CSF) *(Continued)*
  vestibular nerve section and, 1554
  lumbar drainage of, in intracranial aneurysm surgery, 960–961
    postoperative, 2052–2053
  monitoring of, in choroid plexus tumor surgery, 573
  morphine injection into, 1432–1440, *1433*, 1434t–1435t
    case reports of, 1433, 1434t–1435t
    patient selection for, 1433, 1438
    pump for, 1438–1440, *1439*
    results of, 1436t–1437t, 1437–1438
    side effects of, 1438
    vs. cordotomy, 1596
  overdrainage of, 124
  pressure of, reduction of, 124
  pressure-volume index of, in hydrocephalus, 1247, 1247t
  protein concentrations of, drainage and, 124
  shunt of, in syringomyelia, 2124
    in syringomyelic cord syndrome, *1762*, 1764
  subarachnoid, loculation of, in intramedullary spinal cord tumor surgery, 2103–2104
  volume-regulated drainage of, 123–124
Cerebrum, cavernous angioma of, 1186–1189, *1187*, 1187t, *1188*, *1189*, 1189t
  headache in, 1187, *1188*
  neurologic deficit with, 1187–1188, *1189*
  surgery for, 1188–1189, 1189t
  with seizures, 1186–1187, *1187*, 1187t, *1188*
Cervical disc, lateral herniation of, 1805–1809
  air embolism in, 1809
  clinical manifestations of, 1805–1806
  diagnosis of, 1806, *1806*
  incidence of, 1805
  neurologic deficits in, 1809
  nonsurgical treatment of, 1806
  surgery for, 1806–1809, *1807–1809*
    complications of, 1809
    patient selection for, 1806
    results of, 1809
Cervical fusion, in craniovertebral junction abnormalities, 1722–1724, *1723*, *1724*
Cervical myelopathy, 1783–1784, 1789–1790. See also *Spondylosis, cervical.*
Cervical radiculopathy, disc excision in, 1783–1790. See also *Spondylosis, cervical.*
Cervical rhizotomy, in spasmodic torticollis, 1650–1651
Cervical spine, injury to, 1831–1837
  blunt trauma and, 1834
  cardiovascular system in, 1833–1834
  C3-T1 arthrodesis in, 1843–1847, *1845*, *1846*
  diagnostic imaging of, 1834, 1837–1839, *1837–1841*
  epidemiology of, 1831
  occipito-C1-C2 arthrodesis in, 1842–1843, *1843*, *1844*
  orthotic devices in, 1842
  prehospital evaluation of, 1831–1832
  surgery in, 1842–1847, *1843–1846*
  therapy for, 1840, 1842
  traction in, 1832–1833
  pediatric, injury to, 2081–2094
    case reports of, 2087–2091, *2088–2091*
    classification of, 2081–2082
    clinical features of, 2082
    computed tomography in, 2082
    incidence of, 2081
    Larsen's syndrome and, 2091, *2091*
    magnetic resonance imaging in, 2082, *2083*
    mechanism of, 2083

Cervical spine *(Continued)*
  radiologic studies in, 2082, *2083*
  surgery for, 2085–2091, *2086*, *2088–2091*
    anatomy for, 2083–2084
    anesthesia for, 2084
    bleeding in, 2092
    bone graft site in, 2085
    candidates for, 2082–2083
    case reports of, 2087–2091, *2088–2091*
    evoked responses in, 2084–2085
    external fixation in, 2092–2093
    intraoperative complications of, 2091–2093
    metal fixation in, 2085
    pain control after, 2093
    patient position for, 2084
    retraction injury in, 2092
    spinal cord injury in, 2092
    wire-related injury in, 2092
  postlaminectomy deformity of, 1965, *1966*, *1967*
  rheumatoid, 1731–1741
    classification of, 1731–1732
    clinical features of, 1733–1734
    clinical grading of, 1734
    cranial nerve deficits in, 1734
    intubation in, 1735–1736
    myelopathy in, 1733–1734
    pathology of, 1731–1732
    pulmonary function in, 1735
    radiologic investigation of, 1732–1733, *1732*, *1733*
    spinal cord diameter in, 1734
    staircase appearance of, *1732*, 1733
    suboccipital root pain in, 1734
    surgery for, 1733–1741
      anesthesia for, 1735–1736
      anterior subaxial access for, 1737
      anterior subaxial decompression in, 1738
      anterior subaxial stabilization in, 1739–1740, *1739*
      complications of, 1741
      patient selection for, 1733–1734
      posterior access for, 1737–1738
      posterior decompression in, 1739
      posterior stabilization in, 1740–1741
      technique of, 1736–1741
      transoral access for, 1737
      transoral decompression in, 1738–1739
      ventilation in, 1736
      vertebral artery position in, 1736
  stabilization of, 1849–1872
    approaches to, 1849–1851, 1850t, *1851*
    bone graft techniques in, 1852–1853, *1853*
    indications for, 1849
    Mageral hook-plate in, 1871, *1871*
    screw fixation in, 1862–1871
      anterior atlantoaxial facet, 1864–1866, *1865*, *1866*
      C2-pedicle screws in, 1869, 1871, *1871*
      holding power of, 1864
      lateral mass screws in, 1869, *1870*
      odontoid, 1864–1866, *1865*, *1866*
      posterior atlantoaxial facet, 1866–1867, *1867*, *1868*
      principles of, 1862
    screw-plate fixation in, 1867–1868, *1868*
      anterior, 1868, *1869*
      posterior, 1868–1869
      Y-shaped, 1871, *1871*
    wiring techniques in, 1853–1856, *1853–1856*
      atlantoaxial, 1856–1862, *1857–1862*
  syringomyelia of, endoscopic surgery for, 712
Cervical spondylotic myelopathy, anterior cervical disc excision in, 1783–1784, 1789–1790. See also *Spondylosis, cervical.*

Cervical stimulation, in spasmodic torticollis, 1650
Cervicomedullary compression, in achondroplasia, 2109, 2111–2113, *2112*, 2115–2116
Cervicomedullary junction. See *Craniovertebral junction.*
Cervicothoracic junction, 1875–1886
  lesions of, clinical features of, 1875–1876, 1876t
    differential diagnosis of, 1875, 1875t
    metabolic evaluation of, 1876
    radiologic evaluation of, 1876
    surgery for, 1885t
      anesthesia for, 1881
      anterolateral thoracotomy approach in, 1876–1879, *1877–1879*
      anterolateral transthoracic approach in, *1882*, 1883, *1884*, 1885
      lateral parascapular extrapleural approach in, 1876–1879, *1877–1879*, 1881–1883, *1882*, 1885
      parascapular anatomy in, 1877, *1877*
      retromediastinal space in, 1878–1879, 1880
      scapular anatomy in, 1877, *1877*
      spinal anatomy in, 1878–1879
      superior mediastinum anatomy in, 1880
      thoracic cage anatomy in, 1877–1878, *1878*, *1879*
      thoracic inlet anatomy in, 1879–1880
      transmanubrial approach in, 1879–1880
      transmanubrial-transclavicular approach in, 1883–1884, 1885, *1885*
Cesarean section, aneurysm and, 1167, 1168
Chamberlain's line, *1720*, 1721
Chemical meningitis, 591–592, *592*
  Rathke's cleft cyst and, 596
Chemosis, optic nerve sheath fenestration and, 249
Chemotherapy, in anterior skull base tumor resection, 424
  in brain metastasis, 612
  in craniopharyngioma, 388
  in neoplastic spinal cord compression, 2002
  in pediatric brain tumor, 572, 575
  in pediatric posterior fossa ependymoma, 810
  in pineal region tumors, 741, 762
  in recurrent glioma, 537, 539, *539*
Chiari malformation, 1746, *1746*
  hydromyelia and, surgery for, 1755–1764, *1756–1763*
  in hydrocephalus, 1245–1246
  in neonate, 1260–1262, *1261*
Chiasm, cysticercosis of, 1713
  edema of, in optic nerve glioma, 270
  glioma growth into, 271–277, *271–274*
Chiasmal syndrome, in tuberculum sellae meningioma, 404
Children, arachnoid cysts in, 581
  arteriovenous malformations in, 1197–1202. See also *Arteriovenous malformation(s), pediatric.*
  cerebral aneurysm in, 1003
  cerebrospinal fluid leak in, 118
  choroid plexus tumor in, 572–573
  hydrocephalus in, 1231–1240. See also *Hydrocephalus, pediatric.*
  intracranial hematoma in, 75
  low-grade glioma in, 571–572
  myelomeningoceles in, 2055–2067. See also *Myelomeningoceles.*
  penetrating head injury in, 86–87, 95–96, *95–98*
  pleomorphic xanthoastrocytoma in, 574–575

Children *(Continued)*
  postoperative spinal deformities in, 1965–1968, *1966, 1967*
    cervical, 1965, *1966, 1967*
    in myelomeningocele patients, 1966
    lumbar, 1966, *1967*, 1968
    prevention of, 1966
    radiation therapy and, 1965
    radiologic evaluation of, 1965
    thoracic, 1966, 1968
  radiation therapy in, 389
  spasticity in, 1668–1669, 1669t
  spinal injury in, 2081–2094. See also *Cervical spine, pediatric; Lumbar spine, pediatric; Thoracic spine, pediatric.*
  subependymal giant cell astrocytoma in, 574
  supratentorial tumors in, 571–576. See also *Supratentorial tumors, pediatric.*
  vein of Galen malformation in, 1213–1218. See also *Vein of Galen malformation.*
Cholelithiasis, octreotide and, 307
Chondroma, Gamma Knife surgery in, 685
Chondrosarcoma, Gamma Knife surgery in, 685, *685*
  of jugular foramen, 872
Chordoma, of cervicomedullary junction, 1722, *1722*
  of clivus, 469–474, *470, 472, 474*, 787
  of ethmoidosphenoid, *3*
  of jugular foramen, 871
Choriocarcinoma, in pregnancy, 1167
Choroid, venous drainage of, 241
Choroid plexus, carcinoma of, 573
  papilloma of, 572–573, 726, *727*
Choroidal artery, anterior, aneurysm of, 1006–1007, *1008*
  craniopharyngioma adhesion to, 359
  in amygdalohippocampectomy, 1299
  to pineal region, 744–745, 745t, *746*
Chromaffin cells, CNS transplantation of, 1372
Ciliary artery, 240–241, *241*
Ciliary ganglion, ectopic, 483
  injury to, orbital surgery and, 234
Cimetidine, after closed head injury, 63–64
Cingulate gyri, anatomy of, 1423–1424, *1424*
Cingulotomy, 1420
  stereotactic, 1423–1430
    contraindications to, 1425
    convulsions after, 1429
    efficacy of, 1429–1430, 1429t
    in chronic pain syndrome, 1425, 1428–1430, 1429t
    management after, 1428–1429
    MRI target localization in, 1426–1428, *1427*
    patient selection for, 1424–1425
    psychiatric management after, 1428
    repeat, 1426
    safety of, 1429
    ventriculographic target localization in, 1425–1426, *1426, 1427*
Cistern(s), anatomy of, 1299
Cisternography, in cerebrospinal fluid leak localization, 120–121
  in jugular foramen schwannoma, 867
  in normal-pressure hydrocephalus, 1247–1248
  trigeminal, 1525–1526, *1525, 1526*
Claudication, neurogenic, 1957–1964. See also *Lumbar spine, stenosis of.*
  vascular, 1958
Clivus, chordoma of, 469, *470*, 787
  pedicled rhinotomy for, 469–474, *472, 474*
  closure of, after pedicled rhinotomy, 473
  exposure of, pedicled rhinotomy for, 469–475, *470–474*

Clivus *(Continued)*
  tumors of, 786–788
    classification of, 786
    computed tomography in, *784*
    diagnosis of, 786
    removal of, in transbasal tumor resection, 433, *434*, 436–437, *437*
    retraction techniques in, 786
    surgical approaches to, 786–788, *787*
Clover-leaf skull anomaly, in craniosynostosis, 136
Cluster headache, cranial nerve decompression for, 1464
  glycerol rhizolysis in, 1534–1535
  retrogasserian glycerol rhizolysis in, 1534–1535
Coagulation, bipolar, in intraoperative aneurysm rupture, 989–990
  in neuroendoscopy, 698, *699, 700*
  disorders of, in epidural hematoma, 77
  in intracerebral hemorrhage, 928
  in closed head injury, 51, 61
Coccidioides immitis, 1699–1702, 1699t, 1702t
Coccidioides neoformans, 1699–1702, 1699t, 1702t
Cochlear nerve, after suboccipital transmeatal acoustic neuroma removal, 838–839
  anatomy of, 1552, *1552*
Cognition, after temporal lobectomy, 1313
  capsulotomy and, 1452–1453
  in intracranial glioma, 519–521
  transcallosal approach and, 734
Colitis, in ankylosing spondylitis, 1775
Colloid cyst, intraventricular, computer-assisted volumetric stereotactic resection of, 632, *634*
  third ventricle, 584, 590–591, *591*
  transcallosal approach to, *719*
Coma, barbiturate, in closed head injury, 61
  in pregnancy, 1170
Communicating artery, anterior, aneurysm of, 1011–1014
  anatomy of, 1014
  clinical presentation of, 1012
  giant, surgery for, 1045
    Logue procedure in, 1115–1116
  medical therapy for, 1014
  natural history of, 1011
  pathophysiology of, 1011–1012
  rupture of, 987
  surgery for, 1045, 1115–1116, 1122
    patient selection for, 1012–1013, *1013*
    timing of, 1013
  vasospasm in, 1013
  craniopharyngioma adhesion to, 359
  posterior, anatomy of, 1005, *1008*
    aneurysm of, 1005–1006, *1008*
    surgery for, 1114–1115, *1115*
    craniopharyngioma adhesion to, 359
    craniopharyngioma erosion of, 387
COMPASS stereotactic system, 619, *620, 621*, 644–648, *644–650*
Computed tomography, in aneurysmal subarachnoid hemorrhage, 938, 944, 1004
  in arteriovenous malformation, 1227
  in brachytherapy planning, 656–657, *657*
  in brain metastasis, 603, 607, *607, 608*
  in cavernous angioma, 1183–1184
  in cerebral hemispherectomy, 1342, *1342*
  in cerebrospinal fluid leak, 120
  in cervical spondylosis, 1786
  in clivus tumor, *784*, 786
  in closed head trauma, 48, 49, 51
  in cysticercosis, 1706–1707, *1707–1709*
  in DREZotomy, 1628–1629
  in intracranial glioma, 518, 518t

Computed tomography *(Continued)*
  in intramedullary spinal cord tumors, 2096, *2097*
  in intramedullary tumor, 2028
  in jugular foramen cyst, 871
  in jugular foramen meningioma, 871
  in jugular foramen schwannoma, 868, *868*
  in lumbar disc herniation, 1944
  in lumbar spine stenosis, 1958, *1959*
  in middle cerebral artery aneurysm, 1055–1056
  in multisegmental cervical spondylosis, 1792
  in olfactory groove meningioma, *395*
  in optic nerve glioma, 254–256
  in orbital diagnosis, 219
  in paraclinoid aneurysm, 994
  in pediatric arteriovenous malformation, 1198
  in pediatric cerebellar tumor, 803
  in pediatric hydrocephalus, 1232, *1232*
  in pediatric spinal injury, 2082
  in penetrating head injury, 91, 102
  in pineal region tumors, 740
  in posterior fossa tumors, 791–792
  in sclerosteosis, 2144, *2144, 2145*
  in spinal cord compression, 1998, 1998–1999
  in stereotactic resection, 621–622, *622*. See also *Stereotactic volumetric resection.*
  in syringomyelia, 2122
  in tentorial tumors, 783, *784*
  in tuberculoma, *1692*, 1692–1694, *1693*
  in tuberculum sellae meningioma, 404
  stereotactic instruments for, 449, *450, 451*
Computer system, for volumetric stereotactic resection, 620
Conjunctiva, swelling of, optic nerve sheath fenestration and, 249
Contact radiation devices, 461–463, *461, 462*
Continuous lumbar drainage, in cerebrospinal fluid leaks, 123–124, 128
Contusion, in penetrating head injury, 83
Conus medullaris, avulsion injury to, DREZotomy for, 1625–1626, 1631
  dermoid tumor at, *2072*
  in spinal dysraphism, 2069, *2073*
  lipoma fixation to, 2071
Cordotomy, 1557–1570, 1595–1610
  open, 1557–1570
    anesthesia for, 1560
    bilateral, 1557–1558
      alternatives to, 1558
      technique of, 1564
    bladder dysfunction after, 1567
    cervical, 1563
    complications of, 1567–1568
    corticospinal tract anatomy in, 1559
    dentate ligament anatomy in, 1559
    dysesthesias after, 1567–1568
    electrophysiologic monitoring in, 1560
    failures of, 1566
    hypotension after, 1565, 1567
    indications for, 1557–1558
    Jacobsen ball in, 1562–1563, *1565, 1566*
    motor weakness after, 1565, 1567
    pain recurrence after, 1566–1567
    patient position for, 1560
    postoperative precautions with, 1564–1565
    preoperative preparation for, 1560
    respiratory complications of, 1567
    results of, 1565–1566
    sexual dysfunction after, 1567
    sleep apnea after, 1564–1565
    spinal cord anatomy in, 1558–1560, *1559*
    spinal cord width in, 1559–1560
    spinothalamic tract anatomy in, 1558–1559, *1559*
    unilateral, 1557

Cordotomy *(Continued)*
    technique of, 1560–1564, *1561–1565*
    urinary retention after, 1565
    vs. percutaneous cordotomy, 1597–1598, 1598t
  percutaneous, 1595–1610
    alternatives to, 1600, 1600t
    anesthesia for, 1600, 1606
    bilateral, 1606, 1609
    care after, 1605–1606
    complications of, 1608–1609, 1609t
    contraindications to, 1598, *1599*, 1600, 1600t
    dysesthesias after, 1608, 1609t
    electrical stimulation in, 1603–1604, 1603t, *1604*, 1604t, *1605*
    equipment for, 1601, *1601*
    history of, 1596
    impedance changes in, *1605*
    in nonmalignant disease, 1606–1607, 1607t
    indications for, 1596, 1597, 1597t
    ipsilateral pain after, 1608
    lesion making in, 1605, *1605*
    mirror pain after, 1608
    pain recurrence after, 1607, 1608
    patient position for, 1600–1601, *1600*
    penetration depth in, 1602–1603, *1603*
    physiologic localization for, 1603–1604, 1603t, *1604*, 1604t
    preoperative preparation for, 1600
    radiologic localization for, 1601–1603, *1602*, *1603*
    results of, 1607–1608
    technique of, 1598, 1600–1607
    vs. cervical commissurotomy, 1597
    vs. infusion, 1596
    vs. open cordotomy, 1597–1598, 1598t
    vs. periventricular gray stimulation, 1596
Core Assessment Program for Intracerebral Transplantation (CAPIT), in Parkinson's disease, 1362–1363, 1380, *1381*, 1382
Cornea, anesthesia of, after percutaneous rhizotomy, 1477, 1477t
  injury to, optic nerve sheath fenestration and, 249
  orbital surgery and, 234
Corpora cavernosa, vs. cavernous sinus, 484–485, *490*
Corpus callosotomy, 1350–1355
  approach to, 1351, *1352*
  complications of, 1354–1355
  patient selection for, 1350–1351
  results of, 1353–1355, 1354t, 1355t
  technique of, 1351–1353, *1351–1353*
  vs. temporal lobectomy, 1354
Corpus callosum, in depth electrode placement, 1277, *1277*
Cortex, ischemia of, fetal neuron transplantation in, 1383
Corticospinal tract, *1599*
  in open cordotomy, 1559, *1559*
Corticosteroids, in brain metastasis, 608–609, 608t
  in intracranial glioma, 521
  in neoplastic spinal cord compression, 2002–2003
  in orbital diagnosis, 220
  in tuberculosis, 1695
Cortisone, metabolic effects of, 386
Cosman-Roberts-Wells system, *639*, 640–644, *640–643*
  for stereotactic craniotomy, 643–644
  in fetal mesencephalic tissue transplantation, 1364, *1365*
Cotrel-Dobousset system, in pediatric spinal deformities, 1968

Cranial fossa, anterior, cerebrospinal fluid leaks of, 125–126
  tumors of, craniofacial resection for, 415–424, *415*, 418t, *419–423*
  middle, cerebrospinal fluid leaks of, 122, 126
  posterior. See *Posterior cranial fossa.*
Cranial nerve(s), 865–866
  cavernous angioma of, 1193, 1193t
  demyelination of, 1457
  during carotid endarterectomy, *880*, 886
  eighth, anatomy of, 1551–1553, *1551*, *1552*
    histologic morphology of, 1553
  fifth. See *Trigeminal nerve.*
  first, in craniopharyngioma removal, 364
    in olfactory groove meningioma, 393, *399*
    in sclerosteosis, 2142–2143
  fourth, anatomy of, 186, *186*, *197*
    in Gamma Knife surgery, 680
    of lateral sellar compartment, 479, *480*, *481*
    in acoustic neuroma, 833, *833–835*
    in glomus jugulare tumor, 866
    in jugular foramen schwannoma, 865–866, 866t, 870–871
    in sclerosteosis, 2141–2143, *2142*
    injury to, in difficult aneurysm surgery, 1052
    in Gamma Knife surgery, 680
    in glomus jugulare tumor surgery, 872–873
  ninth, anatomy of, 1107
    neurovascular decompression of, 1464–1466
    percutaneous rhizotomy of, *1481*, 1481–1483, *1482*
  of lateral sellar compartment, 479, *480*, 481
  second. See *Optic nerve.*
  seventh. See *Facial nerve.*
  sixth, of lateral sellar compartment, 479, *480*, 481
    paralysis of, optic nerve sheath fenestration and, 249
    vascular relationships of, 1457
  tenth, anatomy of, 1107
    in carotid endarterectomy, *880*, 880
    neurovascular decompression of, 1464–1466
    paralysis of, after glomus jugulare tumor surgery, 858–859
  third, anatomy of, 186, *186*, *197*
    of lateral sellar compartment, 479, *480*, *481*
    paralysis of, optic nerve sheath fenestration and, 249
    supraclinoid carotid artery aneurysm and, 1003, 1004
    vascular relationships of, 1457
  twelfth, transfer of, in facial nerve palsy, 2155
  vascular compression of, 1457–1459
  vascular relationships of, 1457
Cranial vault, in sclerosteosis, 2143, *2143*
Cranialization, of frontal sinus, 19, 35–36, *35*, *36*
Craniofacial dysostosis, 142
Craniopharyngioma, 357–369, 382–389
  atypical, 357
  calcifications of, 376
  capsule of, exposure of, 375–376, *376*
    pathology of, 382–384, *384*
  chemotherapy for, 388
  classification of, 357, *358*
  clinical features of, 358, 368t
  curietherapy in, *460*
  cystic, 591–592, *592*
    colloidal yttrium-90 injection in, 351, 351t, *352*
    computed tomography of, 352
    CT-guided stereotactic puncture of, 455, *456*
  drainage of, 290, 292
  endoscopic surgery for, 707, *709*
  intracavitary brachytherapy for, 664

Craniopharyngioma *(Continued)*
  puncture of, 375
  rupture of, 586, 591–592, *592*
  sella repair in, 337, 339, *339*
  stereotactic methods in, 350–352
    complications of, 351
    results of, 351t
  tube drainage of, 377
  differential diagnosis of, 372
  endocrinologic abnormalities with, 358, 365, 367–368, 385–386, 386t
  endoscopic exploration of, 704, *705*
  Gamma Knife surgery for, 682, *683*
  giant, 368, 368t
  glial layer of, 382–384, *384*
  horizontal extension in, 357
  hydrocephalus in, 365
  intraventricular, 359
  multimodality approach to, 350–352, 351t, *352*
  neural tissue in, 389
  observation for, 386
  pathology of, 382–384
  patient selection for, 358
  pituitary gland compression by, 373, 375, *375*
  postoperative management of, 365–367
  preoperative evaluation of, 358, 371–372
    endocrinologic, 371, 385–386, 386t
    neuroradiologic, 371–372
    ophthalmologic, 371, 386
    radiologic, 384–385, *385*
  recurrence of, 365–367, 378, 389
  retrochiasmatic, 359
  stereotactic radiosurgery for, 349–353, 351t, *352*
  subchiasmatic, 359
  surgical anatomy for, 358–359
  surgical approach to, 386–388, 388t
    bilateral, 359–360
    carotid artery fusiform dilatation and, 384–385, *385*
    case reports of, 363–364, *365*
    complications of, 364–365
    hormonal disturbances after, 365, 367–368
    in children, 367
    philosophy of, 388–389, 389t
    pterional, 361
    results of, 367–368, 368t, 388–389, 389t
    selection of, 359–360, *359*
    stereotactic, 349–353, 351t, *352*, 387
    subfrontal, *359*, 360–361, *360–364*
      bilateral, 360, *360*, *362*, *363*
      complications of, 364–365
      frontal sinus exenteration in, 364
      hypothalamic disturbances in, 365
      iatrogenic cerebral contusion in, 364–365
      olfactory nerve in, 364
      postfixed chiasm in, 360–361, *361*
      prefixed chiasm in, 361, *362–364*
      unilateral, 360, *360*, *361*
    subtemporal, *359*
    subtotal, 388
    survival after, 367
    transcallosal, *359*, 361, 363
    trans-lamina terminalis, 368
    transpetrosal, *359*
    transsphenoidal, 289–292, *289*, *290*, 291t, *359*, 371–378, 386–387
      cerebrospinal fluid leak after, 377, *377*, 378
      closure for, 377, *377*
      complications of, 377–378
      endocrinologic results of, 378
      indications for, 372
      management after, 378
      ophthalmologic results of, 378

Craniopharyngioma *(Continued)*
    patient position for, 372, 373
    results of, 378
    secondary, 372
    technique for, 372–377, *373–377*
    transventricular, *359*
    unilateral, 359–360
    visual outcome in, 367
  third ventricle, endoscopic biopsy of, *708*
    transcallosal approach to, *722*
  transsphenoidal approach to, 289–292, *289, 290*
  types of, *289, 290*
  vascular adhesion of, 359, 389
  vertical extension of, 357, *358*
  visual disturbances with, 386
  vs. nonfunctioning pituitary adenoma, 293
  vs. optic nerve glioma, 254, 270
Cranioplasty, 21, *22*, 25
  after meningioma, 15, *16*
  for frontotemporal fracture, *22*
  for parietal bone defect, 22, *24*
  for skull fracture, 20–22, *22, 24*, 25, *25*
  in penetrating missile injuries of head, 84
  indications for, 20
  infection and, 20
  methyl methacrylate, 21, *24*
  technique of, 21, *22, 24, 25*
  timing of, 20–21
Craniosynostosis, 135–147
  anesthesiologic care in, 138t
  anterior, 139, 141–145
    surgical indications for, 143
    surgical technique for, 143–145, *144, 145*
  bicoronal, 141–142
  classification of, 138–139, 138t
  clinical manifestations of, 136–138
  complications of, 146–147
  coronal, 142
  coronal-sphenoethmoidal ring, 139
  craniofacial, 142
  evaluation of, 138
  genetic factors in, 136
  hydrocephalus in, 137–138
  intrauterine pressure in, 136
  lambdoid, 139, 146, *146*
  metabolic disorders in, 136
  metopic, 142–143
  multiple, 145–146, *146*
  pathogenesis of, 135–136
  primary, 135, 138, 138t
  sagittal, 139–141
    surgical technique in, 139–141, *140, 141*
    transposition technique for, 141, *141*
  secondary, 135
  skull base in, 135–136
  teratogenic, 136
Craniotomy, awake, in epilepsy, 1317–1318
  complications of, 79
  in cerebrospinal fluid leaks, 125–127
  in closed head trauma, 51–53, *52–55*
  in epidural intracranial hematoma, 77
  in intracerebral intracranial hematoma, 78
  in intracranial hematoma, 75–80, *76*
  in pituitary adenoma, 297
  in posterior fossa hematoma, 70
  in sclerosteosis, 2145
  in subdural intracranial hematoma, 77–78
  intermittent positive-pressure ventilation after, 79
  stereotactic, Cosman-Roberts-Wells system for, 643–644
Craniotubular hyperostoses, 2141. See also *Sclerosteosis.*
Craniovertebral junction, abnormalities of, 1719–1729, 1720t, 1728t
  anatomy of, 1719–1721, *1720*

Craniovertebral junction *(Continued)*
  anterior transoral-transpharyngeal approach to, 1724–1728, *1726–1728*
  diagnosis of, 1721–1722, *1722*
  embryology of, 1719–1721
  immobilization for, 1722
  irreducible, *1722*, 1728t
  posterior cervical fusion for, 1722–1724, *1723, 1724*
  posterior decompression for, 1724, *1725*
  reducible, 1722–1724, *1722, 1723, 1724*, 1728t
  signs of, 1721
  symptoms of, 1721
Cranium bifidum, 149
Creatine phosphokinase MB, in aneurysmal subarachnoid hemorrhage, 952
Creativity, capsulotomy and, 1453
Cribriform fossa, CSF leak from, 127
Cricothyroidotomy, in closed head injury, 48
Crista galli, *215*
Cross-facial nerve graft, in facial nerve palsy, 2155, 2156, *2157*
Crouzon's syndrome, 142
  proptosis in, 137
  psychomotor development in, 136
Crown-rump length, fetal, in CNS transplanation donor, 1363
C3–T1 arthrodesis, 1843–1847, *1845, 1846*
Curietherapy, 455, 457–458, 457t
  indications for, 463–465, *464*, 464t
  technique of, 458, *458–460*
Currarino triad, 2065
Cushing's disease, 301–303
  adrenalectomy in, 303
  endocrine evaluation of, 301–302
  Gamma Knife surgery in, 684–685
  in pregnancy, 1166
  magnetic resonance imaging in, 302
  medical treatment of, 302–303
  radiation therapy in, 303
  recurrence of, 302
  stereotactic radiosurgery in, 347–349, 348t
  transsphenoidal surgery in, *298*, 302
Cutaneous nerves, lesions of, treatment of, 2164
Cyanoacrylates, in cerebrospinal fluid leak, 128, 2052
Cyproheptadine, in Cushing's disease, 303
Cyst(s), 579–596
  arachnoid, 579–581, *580*, 586–589, *587–589*, 792t
    in hydrocephalus, 1246
    posterior fossa, 796
    sella repair in, 337, *338, 343*
    stereotactic catheter implantation in, 455, *457*
  colloid, computer-assisted volumetric stereotactic resection of, 632, *634*
    endoscopic surgery for, 704, 706, *707*
    of third ventricle, 584, 590–591, *591, 719*
Dandy-Walker, 796, 1246
  dermoid, 796
  epidermoid, 871, 2193
  ganglion, 2192–2193, *2193*
  glioependymal, 579, *580*
  in optic nerve glioma, 270–271
  intracranial, 579–596, 580t
    clinical features of, 583–584
    colloid, 590–591, *591*
    dumbbell, 584
    endoscopic surgery for, 586–595, *587–595*, 704–706, *705*
      results of, 707, *709*
    epithelial, 589–590, *590*
    headache in, 583
    lesions associated with, 584

Cyst(s) *(Continued)*
    locations of, 580
    of septum pellucidum, 594–595, *594*
    recurrence of, 583, 584
    subchiasmatic, 585
    supratentorial, 590, *590*
    surgical excision of, 583
    toxin-leaking, 585–586
    transsphenoidal drainage of, 583
  intraspinal, *580*
  of pineal region, 595, *595*
  of septum pellucidum, 594–595, *594*
  of spinal cord. See *Syringomyelia; Syringomyelic cord syndrome.*
  posterior fossa, 796
  Rathke's cleft, 582–583, 592, *593*, 594
    chemical meningitis and, 585, 596
    excision of, 584
    foreign body reaction to, 586
  septum pellucidum, 594–595, *594*
  suprasellar, 581–582, *582*
    chemical meningitis and, 585–586
    toxin-leaking, 585–586
Cystic cerebral astrocytoma, 517–518. See also *Glioma.*
Cystic fluid, in optic nerve glioma, 270–271
Cystic myelopathy. See *Syringomyelia, non-hindbrain-related.*
Cysticercosis, 1705–1715
  acquisition of, 1705
  chiasmatic, 1713
  clinical features of, 1706
  cyst wall in, 1711
  cystic stage of, 1706, 1706t
    treatment of, 1709–1713, *1711, 1712*
  degenerated stage of, 1713–1714, *1714*
  diagnosis of, 1706–1707, *1707–1709*
  encephalitic stage of, 1705, *1711*
    treatment of, 1709
  hydrocephalus in, 1712–1713
  pathophysiology of, 1705–1706
  prognosis of, 1707–1708
  racemose stage of, 1706, *1711*
    treatment of, 1710–1711, *1712*
  spinal, 1713
  third ventricle, transforaminal transcallosal approach to, *719*
  treatment of, 1708–1714, *1710–1714*
    results of, 1714, *1714*
  ventricular, 1711–1712, *1712, 1713*
Cystoventriculostomy, endoscopic, 590, *590*
Cytotoxic edema, in neoplastic spinal cord compression, 1999–2000

Dandy-Walker malformation, 796, 1246, 1260
Deafferentation pain, 1615–1636. See also *Pain, deafferentation.*
Deafness, after vestibular nerve section, 1554
  in craniosynostosis, 137
  in Ménière's disease, 1548
  in sclerosteosis, 2142
  prevention of, in acoustic neuroma removal, 831–833, *833*
    in suboccipital transmeatal acoustic neuroma removal, 838–839
Debridement, in penetrating head injuries, 85
Deep brain stimulation, 1389–1397
  complications of, 1397, 1401
  electrode configuration in, 1395, 1400
  in amputation, 1395–1396, *1395*
  in anesthesia dolorosa, *1395*, 1396
  in brachial plexus lesions, *1395*, 1396
  in cancer, *1395*, 1396
  in failed low back surgery syndrome, *1395*, 1396

Deep brain stimulation *(Continued)*
   in neuropathy, 1396–1397
   in peripheral nerve lesions, *1395,* 1396
   in spinal cord lesions, *1395,* 1396
   in thalamic lesions, *1395,* 1396
   patient selection for, 1390–1391, 1395, 1399
   postcordotomy, *1395,* 1396
   postherpetic, *1395,* 1396
   results of, 1393–1397, 1394t, *1395,* 1400–1401
   stimulation parameters in, 1395
   target localization in, 1395
   technique of, 1391–1393, *1392, 1393,* 1399–1400
Deep vein thrombosis, after closed head injury, 64
Dellen, optic nerve sheath fenestration and, 249
Dementia, in normal-pressure hydrocephalus, 1247
Dens, 1719, 1720
Dentate ligament, in open cordotomy, 1559
   in syringomyelia surgery, 2125
Depth electrodes, 1271–1283
   complications of, 1283
   contraindications to, 1272t
   head dressing with, 1283
   historical review of, 1271–1272
   indications for, 1272–1273, 1272t
   patient monitoring of, 1282–1283
   placement of, 1273–1282
      brain mapping in, 1276
      computer work station for, 1276
      control x-rays in, 1275
      electrode implantation (stage II) in, 1280–1282, *1280, 1282*
      in central area, 1279–1280, *1280*
      in frontal lobe, 1279, *1279*
      in occipitoparietal area, 1280
      in temporal lobe, 1277, 1279, *1279*
      positron-emission tomography in, 1277
      proportional callosal grid in, 1276–1277, *1277*
      stereoscopic arteriovenous angiography in, *1275,* 1276
      stereotactic digital angiography in, 1275–1276, *1275*
      stereotactic localization (stage I) in, 1274–1280
      stereotactic magnetic resonance imaging in, 1276, *1276*
      stereotactic system for, 1273–1274, *1273–1275*
      target selection in, 1277, *1278, 1279*
      with frameless stereotaxy, 1282
   removal of, 1283
   results of, 1283, 1283t
   stimulation of, 1282–1283
Dermal sinus, 2071. See also *Spinal dysraphism.*
Dermatofibrosarcoma protuberans carcinoma, scalp, reconstruction after, 17–18, *18*
Dermoid cyst, posterior fossa, 792t, 796
Dermoid tumor, at conus, *2072*
   intramedullary, 2028. See also *Spinal cord tumors, intramedullary.*
   surgery for, 2075
Descending cranial nociceptive tract, tractotomy of, 1568–1570
Desmoid, 2191
Dexamethasone, in intracranial glioma, 521
   in neoplastic spinal cord compression, 2000–2001
Dexamethasone suppression test, in Cushing's disease, 301
Diabetes insipidus, aneurysmal subarachnoid hemorrhage–associated, 951–952
   in craniopharyngioma, 371, 378

Diabetes insipidus *(Continued)*
   in hypothalamic tumors, 774
   in pineal region tumors, 740
   in pituitary adenoma removal, 299
   in pregnancy, 1166–1167
   in suprasellar germinoma, 739
   in tuberculum sellae meningioma, 405–407, *406–407*
Diastematomyelia, 2062, 2071. See also *Spinal dysraphism.*
   imaging of, 2074, *2074*
   surgery for, 2075
Diencephalon. See *Brainstem; Hypothalamus; Thalamus.*
Digital subtraction angiography, in intracranial aneurysm treatment, 971–973
Dinorphin, 1432
Diphenylhydantoin (Dilantin), in intracranial glioma, 521
Diplegia, symmetrical, 1668–1669, 1669t
Diploë, drill holes in, for scalp defect, 14–15
Diplopia, after optic nerve sheath fenestration, 248, 249
   after percutaneous rhizotomy, 1477, 1477t
   after vestibular nerve section, 1554
Disconnection syndrome, after lateral ventricle tumor resection, 737
Dish-face deformity, prevention of, 40
Diuretics, in penetrating head injury, 91
Dopaminergic analogues, in growth hormone–secreting pituitary adenoma, 308
   in prolactin-secreting pituitary adenoma, 310–311
Doppler study, in aneurysmal subarachnoid hemorrhage, 944
   in closed head injury, 59–60
Dorsal horn, 1614
   electrode recordings from, 1615, *1615*
Dorsal root entry zone (DREZ), 1613–1616, *1613, 1614, 1616.* See also *DREZotomy.*
   anatomy of, 1623–1625, *1624, 1625*
   neuropharmacology of, *1625*
Dorsal root ganglionectomy, 1585–1592. See also *Ganglionectomy, dorsal root.*
Dorsal rootlets, 1613, *1614,* 1615–1616, *1616*
Dorsal roots, 1613, 1615–1616, *1616*
Doxorubicin, in recurrent adenoma, 319
DREZotomy, 1613–1621, *1614*
   complications of, 1635–1636
   deafferentation pain treatment by, 1615–1636
   anatomy in, 1623–1625, *1624, 1625*
   impedance measurement in, 1635
   indications for, 1625–1628, *1626–1628*
   intraoperative evoked potential recording in, 1635
   management after, 1634
   patient selection for, 1625–1628, *1626–1628*
   preoperative evaluation in, 1628–1629
   results of, 1635
   technique of, 1629–1634, *1630, 1632–1634*
   in atypical facial pain, 1633–1634, *1633, 1634*
   in brachial plexus avulsion, 1625, *1626,* 1629–1631, *1630*
   in cancer pain, 1619–1620
   in conus medullaris avulsion, 1625–1626, 1631
   in hyperspasticity, 1620
   in paraplegia, 1626, 1631, *1632*
   in peripheral nerve injuries, 1626–1628, *1629*
   in phantom limb, 1631
   in postherpetic pain, 1626, *1627,* 1631–1632
   in postrhizotomy pain, 1632
   in pure neurogenic pain, 1620
   in quadriplegia, 1626
   in reflex sympathetic dystrophy, 1632
   in spasticity, 1665–1666, *1666*

DREZotomy *(Continued)*
   in syringomyelia, 1631, *1632*
   neurophysiologic monitoring during, 1619
   of trigeminal nerve nucleus caudalis, 1633–1634, *1633, 1634*
   surgical anatomy for, 1615–1616, *1616*
   technique of, *1616,* 1616–1619
      at cervical level, 1616–1618, *1617*
      at lumbosacral level, 1618–1619, *1618, 1619*
Dura, injury to, in craniosynostosis treatment, 147
   in orbital surgery, 234
Dural sinuses, anatomy of, 112, *112*
   arteriovenous malformation of, 1219–1228
      angiography of, 1219, *1220*
      arterial supply of, 1227, 1227t
      diagnosis of, 1227
      embolization for, 1219–1220, *1220*
      Gamma Knife surgery for, 676–677, *677*
      hemorrhage in, 1227, 1227t
      pathogenesis of, 1226–1227
      pathophysiology of, 1226–1227
      surgery for, 1220–1223
         closure in, 1223
         complications of, 1223, 1223t
         craniotomy in, 1222, *1223, 1224*
         patient position in, 1220, *1221,* 1222, *1224,* 1228
         resection in, 1222–1223, *1225–1226*
         results of, 1223, 1223t
         scalp flap in, 1222
         sinus ligation in, 1222, *1224*
         soft-tissue dissection in, 1222
         vein of Labbé in, 1223
      symptoms of, 1226, 1226t
      venous drainage of, 1227–1228, 1228t
   laceration of, 111–115
      bleeding control in, 112–113, *113*
      diagnosis of, 111
      in penetrating head injuries, 86
      repair of, 112–115, *113–115*
         patient position for, 111
         saphenous vein graft in, 111, 114–115, *114, 115*
   occlusion of, 112, *113*
   shunt within, 112, *113*
   stenosis of, 113, *114*
   transverse, 112
Dysesthesias, after cordotomy, 1561, 1567–1568, 1608, 1609t
   after dorsal rhizotomy, 1586
   after ganglionectomy, 1590–1591, 1592
   after glycerol rhizolysis, 1531, 1531t
   after percutaneous trigeminal nerve compression, 1540
Dysgerminoma, 269–270
Dysphagia, in cervical spondylosis, 1784–1785, *1784*
Dysplasia, fibromuscular, of internal carotid artery, 888
   fibrous, skull base, transbasal surgical approach to, *434,* 438, *438–441*
Dysraphism, spinal, 2069–2079. See also *Spinal dysraphism.*
Dystonia, adult-onset, 1649, 1657

Edema, in difficult aneurysm, 1051–1052
   in neoplastic spinal cord compression, 1999–2000
   in penetrating head injury, 83
   optic disc, in pseudotumor cerebri, 238, *238*
   orbital, orbital surgery and, 235
   pulmonary, in aneurysmal subarachnoid hemorrhage, 952

Edema (Continued)
  vasogenic, interstitial brachytherapy and, 665
Elbow, median nerve entrapment at, 2177, *2177*
  ulnar nerve entrapment at, 2179–2180, *2179, 2180*
Electrical stimulation mapping, 1318–1320, *1319*
  current in, 1320
  extraoperative, 1321
  intraoperative, 1319–1320
  of eloquent cortex, 1318–1319, *1319*
  train duration in, 1320
Electrocardiogram, in aneurysmal subarachnoid hemorrhage, 959
Electrocochleography, in suboccipital transmeatal acoustic neuroma removal, 838
Electrocorticography, in epilepsy, 1320–1321
  in temporal lobectomy, 1289
Electrode(s), depth, 1271–1283
  complications of, 1283
  contraindications to, 1272t
  head dressing with, 1283
  historical review of, 1271–1272
  indications for, 1272–1273, 1272t
  patient monitoring of, 1282–1283
  placement of, 1273–1282
    brain mapping in, 1276
    computer work station for, 1276
    control x-rays in, 1275
    electrode implantation (stage II) in, 1280–1282, *1280, 1282*
    in central area, 1279–1280, *1280*
    in frontal lobe, 1279, *1279*
    in occipitoparietal area, 1280
    in temporal lobe, 1277, 1279, *1279*
    positron-emission tomography in, 1277
    proportional callosal grid in, 1276–1277, *1277*
    stereoscopic arteriovenous angiography in, *1275*, 1276
    stereotactic digital angiography in, 1275–1276, *1275*
    stereotactic localization (stage I) in, 1274–1280
    stereotactic magnetic resonance imaging in, 1276, *1276*
    stereotactic system for, 1273–1274, *1273–1275*
    target selection in, 1277, *1278, 1279*
    with frameless stereotaxy, 1282
  removal of, 1283
  results of, 1283, 1283t
  stimulation of, 1282–1283
  in spinal cord stimulation, 1403, 1404, *1404*, 1405, *1405*
  strip, 1265–1268
    complications of, 1267–1268
    electroencephalographic monitoring of, 1267
    indications for, 1265
    positioning of, 1266–1267
    technique for, 1265–1266, *1265*
Electroencephalography, in aneurysm surgery, 961–962, 988
  in cerebral hemispherectomy, 1342–1343
  in strip electrode monitoring, 1267
Electrolytes, in aneurysmal subarachnoid hemorrhage, 951–952, 951t
Electromyelography, in open cordotomy, 1560
Eloquent cortex, mapping of, 1317–1321, *1319*
Embolism, air, in cervical disc herniation, 1809
  pulmonary, in aneurysmal subarachnoid hemorrhage, 952
  in closed head injury, 64
  optic nerve sheath fenestration and, 249
Embolization, of arteriovenous malformation, 1219–1220, *1220*, 2043

Embolization (Continued)
  of glomus jugulare tumor, 869, 873
Embolus, in brain abscess, 1674
  in infected intracranial aneurysm, 1133
Empty sella, correction of, 335, 337, *337, 338*, 344
Empty sella syndrome, in tumor debulking, 321
Encephalocele(s), 149–158
  anesthesia in, 150
  case reports of, 150–158, *150–157*
  clinical features of, 149
  computed tomography in, 150, *150*
  decision management for, 150
  evaluation of, 150
  frontonasal, 1259–1260
  in utero, 150, *150*
  intraorbital, 187
  nasal, 152, *155*, 156, 157, *157*
  nasoethmoidal, 150, *150*, 152, *153*, 155, *156*
  naso-orbital, 152, *153, 154*
  occipital, 150–151, *151, 152*, 1258–1259, *1259*
  pathophysiology of, 149
  sincipital, 1260
  sphenoid, 155, *156*
  surgical approach to, 150
Encephaloduroarteriosynangiosis, 923–924
Encephalomeningocele(s), frontoethmoidal, 159–165
  blindness in, 164
  bony defect of, 160–161, *161–163*
  brain damage in, 161, *163*, 164
  classification of, 159, *160*
  computed tomography in, 161, *161–163*
  covering of, 159–160
  craniofacial reconstruction in, 165, *165*
  extracranial repair of, 164, *164*
  intracranial repair of, 164–165, *164*
  nasoethmoidal, 159, *160*, 162
    extracranial repair of, 164
    intracranial repair of, 164–165, *164*
  nasofrontal, 159, *160*, 161
    extracranial repair of, 164, *164*
  nasolacrimal duct obstruction in, 164
  naso-orbital, 159, *160*, 162
    intracranial repair of, 164–165, *164, 165*
  preoperative assessment of, 159–164, *161–163*
  rupture of, 160
  squints in, 164
  surgical repair of, 164–165, *164, 165*
Encephalorrhagia, apoplectic, stereotactic evacuation of, 455, *456*
Endocarditis, in infected aneurysm, 1136–1138. See also *Aneurysm(s), infected.*
Endocurie therapy, 664
Endolymphatic shunt, in Ménière's disease, 1549
Endomyelography, in syringomyelia, 2122
Endoneurosurgery. See *Neuroendoscopy.*
β-Endorphin, 1432
Endoscopes, 695–700, *696–700*, 696t
Endoscopy, 695–713. See also *Neuroendoscopy.*
Endotracheal intubation, in closed head injury, 48
Endovascular coils, in intracavernous segment aneurysm, 979
Energy, ballistic, 82
Enkephalins, 1432
Enophthalmos, after orbital surgery, 235
Ependymoma. See also *Spinal cord tumors, intramedullary.*
  cerebellar, 801, 803–804, *805*
  Gamma Knife surgery for, 686
  in infant, 576, 801, 803–804, *805*
  interstitial brachytherapy for, 664
  intramedullary, 2028, *2029–2030*, 2095–2105, *2098*. See also *Spinal cord tumors, intramedullary.*

Ependymoma (Continued)
  of fourth ventricle, 796
  of lateral ventricle, 726, *729*
  of lateral ventricle temporal horn, *732*, 733
  of posterior fossa, 792t, *805*, 808
Epidermoid cyst, nerve compression by, 2193
  of jugular foramen, 871
Epidural blood patching, 124
Epidural cervical stimulation, in spasmodic torticollis, 1650
Epidural scar, in lumbar disc surgery, 1935, 1936–1937
Epidural tumors, 1997–2023
  biologic activity of, 2000
  dexamethasone administration in, 2000–2001
  location of, 1998–1999, *1998*, 2001
  spinal cord compression by, 1997–2023, *2002*
    algorithm for, *2002*
    analgesia in, 2003
    brachytherapy in, 2003
    chemotherapy in, 2002
    corticosteroids in, 2002–2003
    diagnostic imaging of, *1998*, 1998–1999
    incidence of, 1997
    level of, 1997–1998
    neurologic status in, 2001
    pathophysiology in, 1999–2000, *1999*
    pharmacotherapy of, 2002–2003
    radiation exposure and, 2006
    radiation therapy in, 2003, 2003t
    spinal instability in, *2005*, 2005t, 2006, 2006t
    surgery for, 2003–2023, 2004t
      anterior decompression in, 2012–2019
        cervical, 2019, 2021–2023, *2021–2023*
        cervicothoracic stabilization in, 2021, 2023
        lumbar, *2017*, 2018–2019, *2020*
        thoracic, 2012–2013, *2013*
        thoracolumbar, 2018
        vertebral body replacement in, 2014–2015, *2016, 2017*
      approaches to, 2002t, 2006–2007
      bleeding in, 2008, 2012, 2014
      complications of, 2023
      indications for, 2004–2006, *2005*, 2005t, 2006t
      Isola system in, 2014–2015, *2016*
      morbidity after, 2023
      mortality after, 2023
      posterior decompression in, 2007–2012, *2007–2012*
        bone grafting in, 2010–2012
        care after, 2012
      survival after, 2000
      symptoms of, 1999
        progression of, 2001
      x-ray location of, 2008
Epilepsy, 1265–1269
  after capsulotomy, 1447
  Ammon's horn sclerosis in, 1288, 1288t, 1292, 1294
  amygdalohippocampectomy in, 1295–1303
    anatomy in, 1298–1299
    anesthesia for, 1299
    case report of, 1296, 1297–1298, *1297*
    cognitive function after, 1302
    complications of, 1301, 1302
    contraindications to, 1303
    exposure for, 1300
    indications for, 1303
    management after, 1301
    management decisions in, 1298
    patient selection for, 1295
    phase IA investigation in, 1296
    phase IB investigation in, 1296–1297

Epilepsy *(Continued)*
　　phase II investigation in, 1298
　　preoperative investigation for, 1295–1298, 1296t
　　results of, 1301
　　seizure relief after, 1302, 1302t
　　technique of, 1299–1301, *1300*
　　transcortical approach to, 1300, *1300*
　　transsylvian approach to, 1300, *1300*
　　unilateral, 1307
aneurysmal subarachnoid hemorrhage–associated, 950–951, 950t
awake craniotomy in, 1317–1318
bitemporal, *1273*
　　depth electrode in, 1272–1273, 1272t
　　presentation of, 1283t
cerebral hemispherectomy in, 1341–1350
　　anatomic, 1343
　　　　Oxford-Adams modification of, 1343–1344
　　　　white matter preservation in, 1344
　　case reports of, 1347–1348, *1348*
　　complications of, 1348–1349
　　computed tomography for, 1342, *1342*
　　electroencephalography for, 1342–1343
　　functional, 1344–1346, *1344*, *1345*
　　　　variations of, 1346
　　indications for, 1341–1343, *1342*, 1343t
　　intellectual effects of, 1349
　　neurologic examination for, 1341–1342
　　results of, 1349
　　seizure control after, 1349
　　seizure etiology and, 1343, 1343t
　　seizure patterns and, 1341
　　social effects of, 1349
　　surgical findings at, 1343
　　techniques of, 1343–1348, 1343t
characteristics of, 1324, 1324t
corpus callosotomy in, 1350–1355
　　approach to, 1351, *1352*
　　complications of, 1354–1355
　　patient selection for, 1350–1351
　　results of, 1353–1355, 1354t, 1355t
　　technique of, 1351–1353, *1351–1353*
　　vs. temporal lobectomy, 1354
depth electrodes in, 1271–1283
　　complications of, 1283
　　contraindications to, 1272t
　　head dressing with, 1283
　　historical review of, 1271–1272
　　indications for, 1272–1273, 1272t
　　patient monitoring of, 1282–1283
　　placement of, 1273–1282
　　　　brain mapping in, 1276
　　　　computer work station for, 1276
　　　　control x-rays in, 1275
　　　　electrode implantation (stage II) in, 1280–1282, *1280*, *1282*
　　　　in central area, 1279–1280, *1280*
　　　　in frontal lobe, 1279, *1279*
　　　　in occipitoparietal area, 1280
　　　　in temporal lobe, 1277, 1279, *1279*
　　　　positron-emission tomography in, 1277
　　　　proportional callosal grid in, 1276–1277, *1277*
　　　　stereoscopic arteriovenous angiography in, *1275*, 1276
　　　　stereotactic digital angiography in, 1275–1276, *1275*
　　　　stereotactic localization (stage I) in, 1274–1280
　　　　stereotactic magnetic resonance imaging in, 1276, *1276*
　　　　stereotactic system for, 1273–1274, *1273–1275*
　　　　target selection in, 1277, *1278*, *1279*

Epilepsy *(Continued)*
　　with frameless stereotaxy, 1282
　　removal of, 1283
　　results of, 1283, 1283t
　　stimulation of, 1282–1283
diagnosis of, 1265–1269, 1271–1283, *1325*
　　depth electrodes in, 1509–1521. See also *Epilepsy, depth electrodes in.*
　　grid arrays in, 1268–1269, *1268*
　　invasive, 1325, *1325–1331*
　　noninvasive, 1324–1325
　　phased, 1296–1298, 1296t
　　stereo-EEG in, 1325, *1326–1331*
　　　　central, *1331*
　　　　frontotemporal, *1329*
　　　　occipitoparietotemporal, *1330*
　　　　temporal, *1326*
　　　　temporoperisylvian, *1327*, *1328*
　　strip electrodes in, 1265–1268, *1265*
electrical stimulation mapping in, extraoperative, 1321
　　intraoperative, 1317–1321, *1319*
electrocorticography in, intraoperative, 1321
eloquent area mapping in, 1318–1319, *1319*
　　extraoperative, 1321
　　intraoperative, 1319–1320
epileptogenic area in, identification of, 1272–1273, 1272t, 1306, 1323–1324, 1337–1338
　　intraoperative mapping of, 1320–1321
etiology of, 1306
extratemporal, depth electrodes in, 1272t, 1273
Gamma Knife surgery for, 692–693
grid arrays in, 1268–1269
　　complications of, 1269
　　cortical mapping in, 1269
　　grid removal after, 1269
　　indications for, 1268
　　recordings of, 1268–1269
　　technique for, 1268, *1268*
hemispheric localization of, depth electrodes in, 1272–1273, 1272t
hemispherotomy in, 1346–1347, *1347*
in craniosynostosis, 137
in low-grade glioma, 551
in pediatric arteriovenous malformation, 1197–1198
intrahemispheric localization of, depth electrodes in, 1272t, 1273
medial temporal pathology in, 1306–1307
multilobar resection in, 1323–1338
　　anesthesia in, 1333
　　clinical management for, 1325–1326
　　complications of, 1334, 1337
　　management after, 1337
　　patient selection for, 1326, 1331, 1332t
　　preoperative evaluation for, 1324–1326, *1325–1331*
　　results of, 1337
　　surgical approach in, 1333
　　technique of, 1333–1334, *1335*, *1336*
radical hippocampectomy in, 1305–1314
　　failures of, 1312
　　findings of, 1310–1311
　　outcome of, 1311
　　patient selection for, 1308–1309, 1308t
　　reoperation after, 1312
　　seizures after, 1311–1312
　　sequelae of, 1312–1313
　　technique of, 1309–1310
recurrence of, 1312
residual interictal epileptiform activity in, intraoperative recording of, 1320–1321
strip electrodes in, 1265–1268
　　advantages of, 1268

Epilepsy *(Continued)*
　　complications of, 1267–1268
　　disadvantages of, 1268
　　electroencephalographic monitoring in, 1267
　　indications for, 1265
　　positioning of, 1266–1267
　　technique for, 1265–1266, *1265*
temporal lobectomy in, 1287–1294
　　anesthesia for, 1288–1289
　　anterior, amygdala resection in, 1291–1292, *1293*
　　closure in, 1292
　　craniotomy in, 1289–1290, *1290*, *1291*
　　fast echo planar functional imaging in, 1313–1314
　　hippocampal resection in, 1291–1292
　　history of, 1305–1306
　　outcome of, 1288t
　　parahippocampal gyrus resection in, 1291–1292
complications of, 1292
electrocorticography in, 1289
failure of, 1337–1338
medial, 1305–1314
　　anterior, 1307–1310
　　　　failures of, 1312
　　　　findings of, 1310–1311
　　　　outcome of, 1311
　　　　patient selection for, 1308–1309, 1308t
　　　　reoperation after, 1312
　　　　seizures after, 1311–1312
　　　　sequelae of, 1312–1313
　　　　technique of, 1309–1310
metabolic imaging in, 1313
neuropsychological outcome of, 1294
outcome of, 1292, 1294
patient positioning for, 1289
patient selection for, 1287
preoperative preparation for, 1288
resection extent in, 1287–1288, 1288t
seizure control after, 1292, 1294
stereotactic, 1307
subtemporal approach to, 1307
technique for, 1289–1292, *1290*, *1291*, *1293*
transsylvian approach to, 1307
vs. corpus callosotomy, 1354
transventricular amygdalectomy in, 1307
Epileptogenic area, identification of, 1272–1273, 1272t, 1323–1324, 1337–1338
　　intraoperative mapping of, 1320–1321
Escher classification, of frontal skull base fractures, 28, *30*
Esmolol, after intracranial aneurysm surgery, 964
Esthesioneuroblastoma, diagnosis of, 417
　　staging of, 418, 418t
Estrogen, in prolactin-secreting pituitary adenoma, 309
Ethambutol, in tuberculosis, 1695t
Ethics, in AIDS-related surgery, 1686–1687
Ethionamide, in tuberculosis, 1695t
Ethmoid bone, *215*
　　orbital plate of, *214*, *215*
　　orbital process of, *217*
　　reconstruction of, after transbasal tumor resection, 435, *435*
　　schwannoma of, 469, *472*
Ethmoid foramen, *214*, *216*, *217*
Ethmoid sinuses, meningioma invasion of, 398
　　tumors of, craniofacial resection for, 415–417, 415–424, 418t, *419–423*
Ethmoidal cells, anatomy of, 27–28
　　drainage of, 36
Etomidate, in intracranial aneurysm surgery, 962
Eustachian tube, dysfunction of, after glomus jugulare tumor surgery, 859

Exophthalmos, 177–181, 179t
  diagnosis of, 177–181, 178t, 179t
  in Apert's syndrome, 142
  in children, 177–181, 178t
  in craniosynostosis, 136
Exorbitism, in craniosynostosis, 136–137
Explosives, 89
Extensor digitorum brevis muscle, transfer of, in facial nerve palsy, 2156
External carotid artery–saphenous vein–middle cerebral artery bypass, 921–923, 922, 923
External carotid artery–saphenous vein–posterior cerebral artery bypass, 924, 925
Extraocular muscles, 185, 185
Extrathoracic common carotid–subclavian bypass, in subclavian steal syndrome, 902, 906, 907
Eyes, disorders of, in craniosynostosis, 136–137
  innervation of, 241
  protruding. See *Exophthalmos.*

Facial nerve, after suboccipital transmeatal acoustic neuroma removal, 837–838, 837t
  anatomy of, 814–815, 815, 1551–1553, 1551, 1552, 1552
  in acoustic neuroma, 814, 815, 819–821, 820, 822–823, 833, 833, 834
  in Gamma Knife surgery, 681
  neurovascular decompression of, 1463–1464
  paralysis of, 2155–2158
    cross-facial nerve graft for, 2155, 2157
    in sclerosteosis, 2141–2142
    muscle transfers for, 2156, 2157
    nerve transfers for, 2155–2156
    neurectomy in, 2156
    postoperative, after glomus jugulare tumor surgery, 858–859
      after suboccipital transmeatal acoustic neuroma removal, 837
      translabyrinthine approach and, 824–825, 826
    static procedures for, 2156
    vascular compression of, 1458
Facial pain. See also *Trigeminal neuralgia.*
  atypical, DREZotomy in, 1627–1628, 1628, 1633–1634, 1633, 1634
  percutaneous rhizotomy in, 1480–1481
Failed back surgery syndrome, dorsal root ganglionectomy in, 1591
  spinal cord stimulation in, 1406–1407. See also *Spinal cord stimulation.*
Falx, tumor of, 513–515
  presentation of, 513
  radiology of, 513
  surgical approach to, 513–515, 514
Fascia lata, for dural defects, 234
Fascicle, 2159
Fat plug, in cerebrospinal fluid leak, 129
Fawn's tail, in spinal dysraphism, 2072
Femoral cutaneous nerve, lateral, constriction of, 2180–2181, 2181
Fetal adrenal cells, CNS transplantation of, 1373–1374
Fetal hydantoin syndrome, craniosynostosis in, 136
Fetal mesencephalic tissue, CNS transplantation with, 1361–1364, 1362, 1364, 1374–1383
  clinical data on, 1376–1377, 1379
  disease screening in, 1379
  donor age for, 1375
  ethical protocols for, 1379
  facial flushing after, 1377
  first-trimester material in, 1379–1380
  immunosuppression in, 1376

Fetal mesencephalic tissue *(Continued)*
  implantation site in, 1375–1376
  patient assessment for, 1380, 1381, 1382
  patient selection for, 1379
  positron-emission tomography in, 1376
  second-trimester material in, 1380, 1380
  strategy for, 1378
  technique of, 1382–1383, 1382
  tissue viability in, 1375
  transplantation window in, 1375
  trials of, 1377, 1379
  unilateral, 1379
culture maintenance of, 1364
dissection of, 1363–1364, 1364
implantation of, 1363–1366, 1365, 1366
viability of, 1364
Fetus, hydrocephalus in, 1240
  monitoring of, 1170
Fever, after cerebral hemispherectomy, 1349
Fibrin clot adhesives, in cerebrospinal fluid leak repair, 128
Fibrin glue, in CSF postoperative leakage, 2052, 2053
Fibroma, ossifying, intracranial extension of, 431
Fibromuscular dysplasia, of internal carotid artery, 888
Fibrosarcoma, neurogenic, 2194–2195, 2194t, 2195
Fibrosis, in ankylosing spondylitis, 1766, 1775
  in dorsal root ganglionectomy, 1589
  in peripheral nerve lesions, 2165
Fifth cranial nerve. See *Trigeminal nerve.*
Filum terminale, 2070, 2071, 2073
  in intramedullary spinal cord tumors, 2101
  in occult spinal dysraphism, 2070
Finger tapping test, in intracranial glioma, 520
Fishgold's digastric line, 1721
Fissures, cerebellar, 802
Fistula (fistulae), carotid-cavernous, 981–983, 982
  classification of, 981
  CSF. See *Cerebrospinal fluid (CSF), leakage of.*
  dural. See *Arteriovenous malformation, dural.*
  of middle meningeal artery, 1129
  of parasellar carotid arteries, 482, 483
Flap, 3–11, 15, 16, 17
  failure of, 6
  free, 15, 17
  rotation, 5–7, 6, 7
  theory of, 5–7, 6, 7
Flocculonodular lobe, 802
Flow cytometry, of low-grade glioma, 551
Flucytosine, in fungal infection, 1700–1701
Fluids, in closed head injury, 60
  in intracranial aneurysm surgery, 961
Fluorescein, in cerebrospinal fluid leak localization, 120
Folia, cerebellar, 802
Folic acid, in myelomeningoceles, 2055
Foot drop, after dorsal root ganglionectomy, 1590
Foramen lacerum, 1544
Foramen magnum, in achondroplasia, 2108
Foramen spinosum, hemorrhage from, 77
Foraminotomy, after lumbar disc surgery, 1937–1938
Foreign body granuloma, after orbital surgery, 235
Foreign body reaction, to Rathke's cleft cyst, 586
Foster Kennedy syndrome, in medial sphenoid ridge meningioma, 408
Fourth ventricle, ependymoma of, 796
  floor of, 1489
Fracture(s), frontal bone, reconstruction for, 19–25, 20, 22–25

Fracture(s) *(Continued)*
  frontobasal, cerebrospinal fluid leaks with, 31, 31
    combined transfrontal approach to, 33, 35–36, 35
    computed tomography of, 31
    defect size in, 31, 31t
    Escher classification of, 28, 30
    ionomer cement treatment in, 43
    localization of, 31, 31t
    management of, 31
    osteosynthesis for, 36, 38–43, 38–43
    rhinosurgical approach to, 32–33, 33, 34
  frontobasilar, bicoronal incision in, 19
    cranioplasty for, 20–25, 22–25
    exposure for, 19
    management of, 19
    reconstruction for, 19–20, 20
  frontotemporal, cranioplasty for, 22
  glabellar, 39–40, 40
  in ankylosing spondylitis, 1776
  in penetrating head injury, 83
  midfacial, anatomy of, 27–28, 29, 30
    central, 28, 29
    cerebrospinal fluid leak and, 127
    classification of, 27–28, 29, 30
    mechanisms of, 27
    parietotemporofrontal, 36
    rhinobase, 28, 30
  skull, cranial bone cranioplasty for, 22, 25, 25
    occipital, 69
    reconstruction for, 19–25, 22–25
    traumatic nonfistulous aneurysm with, 981
  skull base, cerebrospinal fluid leaks with, 31, 31
    computed tomography of, 31
    defect size in, 31, 31t
    Escher classification of, 28, 30
    ionomer cement treatment in, 43
    localization of, 31, 31t
    management of, 31
    operative treatment of, 31–36
      combined transfrontal approach in, 33, 35–36, 35
      epiduro-trans-ethmoidal rhinosurgical approach in, 32–33, 33, 34
      osteosynthesis in, 36, 38–43, 38–43
      timing of, 31–32
  stress, in ankylosing spondylitis, 1771–1772, 1777–1778, 1778, 1779
  thoracolumbar, in ankylosing spondylitis, 1777–1778, 1778, 1779
Frameless stereotaxy, 650–651, 651
Frontal bone, 18–19
  advancement of, in craniosynostosis, 143–145, 144, 145
  anatomy of, 18–19
  fractures of, 19–25, 20, 22–25
  reconstruction of, 19–20, 20, 23
  tumor excision from, polytetrafluoroethylene implant for, 21, 22
Frontal horn, lateral ventricle, glioma of, 731, 732
Frontal lobe, abscess of, 1673
  depth electrode implantation for, 1279, 1279
  disconnection of, in functional hemispherectomy, 1345–1346
  function of, capsulotomy and, 1452–1453
  lesions of, for pain treatment, 1420
Frontal lobotomy, 1423
Frontal sinus, anatomy of, 27
  cerebrospinal fluid leak from, 127
  cranialization of, 19, 35–36, 35, 36
  defunctionalization of, 19
  drainage of, 36
  exenteration of, in craniopharyngioma removal, 364

Frontal sinus *(Continued)*
　fracture of, 28
　　miniplate fixation of, 21–22, *23*
　　injury to, management of, 19
　　posterior wall of, crush defects of, 35–36, *35, 36*
　　thickness of, 38, *38*
Frontal vein, in orbital venography, 218
Frontalis nerve, anatomy of, 185–186, *186*, 196, *197*
Frontobasilar fracture, bicoronal incision in, 19
　cranioplasty for, 20–25, *22–25*
　exposure for, 19
　management of, 19
　reconstruction for, 19–20, *20*
Frontoethmoidal encephalomeningoceles, 159–165. See also *Encephalomeningocele(s), frontoethmoidal.*
Frontoethmoidal vomerine pillar, 28
Frontopolar artery, in frontal lobectomy, 524, *526*
　in olfactory groove meningioma, 7, *397*
Frontotemporal fracture, cranioplasty for, *22*
Full-scale intelligence quotient, radiation therapy and, 276–277
Fungal infections, 1699–1702, 1699t
　diagnosis of, 1700, 1700t, *1701, 1702*
　in penetrating head injury, 103
　medical treatment of, 1700–1702
　pathologic features of, 1699–1700, 1700t
　surgery for, 1702, 1702t
Fusiform aneurysm, endovascular operations for, 1049–1050, *1049, 1050*
　pathologic anatomy of, 1041
　surgery for, 1047, 1049–1050, *1049, 1050*
Fusion, after lumbar disc surgery, 1939
　in pediatric spinal deformities, 1968

Gaab neuroendoscope system, 695, *696*
Gait, after medullary tractotomy, 1570
　in normal-pressure hydrocephalus, 1247
Galeal scoring, of scalp defect, 13, *14*
Gallstones, octreotide and, 307
Gamma capsulotomy, 1447
　prospective study of, 1449
Gamma Knife, 347
Gamma Knife surgery, 667–693
　definition of, 667–668
　dose calculations for, 1210–1211
　functional, 689–693
　history of, 667
　in acoustic neuroma, 681–682, *681*, 681t, *682*
　in arteriovenous malformation, 668, 670–676, 1177–1178, *1178*, 1205–1211, 1206, 1207t, 1502–1503. See also *Arteriovenous malformation, Gamma Knife surgery for.*
　in brain metastasis, 609–610
　in cavernous angioma, 1185–1186
　in cavernous hemangioma, 678, *678*
　in chondrosarcoma, 685, *685*
　in craniopharyngioma, 349–353, 351t, *352*, 387, 682, *683*
　in Cushing's disease, 684–685
　in dural arteriovenous fistulae, 983
　in dural malformations, 676–677
　in epilepsy, 692–693
　in meningioma, 493, 679–681, *680*, 680t
　in Nelson's syndrome, 684
　in pituitary adenoma, 347–349, *348*, 348t, *349*, 349t, *350*, 682–683, 684t
　in prolactinoma, 684
　in psychosurgery, 691–692
　in recurrent adenoma, 319

Gamma Knife surgery *(Continued)*
　in subependymal giant cell astrocytoma, 574
　in thalamic–basal ganglia arteriovenous malformation, 1502–1503
　in tremor, 691
　in trigeminal neuralgia, 690–691
　in venous angioma, 678–679
　indications for, 667, 668t
　low-grade glioma, 685, *686*
　method of, 668, *669*
　radiation necrosis after, 536
　tools for, 668, *669*
GammaMed iridium 192 contact radiation device, *461*
Gammathalamotomy, for cancer pain, 690
Ganglion, 2192–2193, *2193*
Ganglionectomy, dorsal root, 1585–1592
　complications of, 1590–1591
　contraindications to, 1587
　dysesthesias after, 1590–1591, 1592
　history of, 1585–1586
　patient selection for, 1586–1587
　radicular neurologic deficits after, 1590
　results of, 1589–1590, 1591–1592
　technical complications of, 1590
　technical difficulties with, 1589
　technique of, 1587–1589, *1588–1590*
　upper thoracic, 1637–1641
　　anatomy for, 1637–1638
　　approaches to, 1638
　　complications of, 1641
　　indications for, 1638–1639
　　results of, 1640–1641
　　technique for, 1639–1640, *1639, 1640*
Gastrointestinal system, hemorrhage from, after closed head injury, 64
　penetrating injury to, 1972–1973, 1976
Gate control theory, 1389
Geniculate neuralgia, neurovascular decompression of, 1463–1464
Geniculocalcarine tract, 519
Germinoma, pineal region, 762
　suprasellar, 739
Gerstmann's syndrome, 733
Ghost sella, repair of, 337, *338*
Gigantism, 305–306
　in sclerosteosis, 2141
Gill-Thomas-Cosman repeat stereotactic localizer, 651, *651*
Glabellar area, fractures of, 39–40, *40*
Glaucoma, angle closure, optic nerve sheath fenestration and, 249
Glial tumor, computer-assisted volumetric stereotactic resection of, 631
　of eloquent brain, 628, *630*
　spatial types of, 626–627, *627–629*
Glioblastoma, endocurie therapy for, 664
　interstitial brachytherapy for, 664
　intramedullary, 2028. See also *Spinal cord tumors, intramedullary.*
　intraoperative brachycurietherapy in, *459*
　stereotactic volumetric resection of, 649
Glioblastoma multiforme, 517. See also *Glioma.*
　recurrence of, 541
Glioependymal cyst, 579, *580*
Glioma, anaplastic, brachycurietherapy in, *460*
　curietherapy for, *465*
　brainstem, 792t
　　endoscopic-stereotactic biopsy of, 704, *704*
　　stereotactic biopsy of, *448*
　chiasmal invasion by, 271–277, *271–274*
　diencephalic, 765–772, 765–775, *774*, 774t
　grade IV, computer-assisted volumetric resection of, 628
　hypothalamic, 765–775, 765–770
　　clinical features of, 769, 771t

Glioma *(Continued)*
　　computed tomography in, 771, *771*, 772
　　histology of, 769, 771
　　magnetic resonance imaging in, 771, *772*
　　surgery for, 771, 773–775, *774*, 774t
　in pregnancy, 1167
　intracavitary brachytherapy for, 664
　intracranial, 517–534, 549–567
　　high-grade, Gamma Knife surgery for, 685–686
　　intramedullary, 2095–2105. See also *Spinal cord tumors, intramedullary.*
　　low-grade, 549–567
　　　biologic features of, 551–552, *552*
　　　classification of, 549–551, *550*
　　　clinical features of, 551–552
　　　doubling time of, 552
　　　flow cytometry of, 551
　　　Gamma Knife surgery for, 685, *686*
　　　growth fraction of, 551
　　　in children, 571–572, 576
　　　in infants, 575–576
　　　infiltration patterns of, *564*
　　　malignant degeneration of, 552, 553
　　　MRI-guided stereotactic biopsy of, *639*
　　　positron-emission tomography of, 551, 553
　　　radiotherapy in, 553, 566
　　　regrowth of, 566
　　　spread of, *550*
　　　surgical management of, 549–567
　　　　anesthesia for, 555
　　　　carbon dioxide laser in, 560
　　　　cerebral blood flow in, 565
　　　　closure in, 563
　　　　complications of, 565
　　　　cortical approach in, 556–558, *557–562*
　　　　craniotomy in, 555–556
　　　　display system for, 563
　　　　hemostasis in, 563
　　　　indications for, 552–553, 552t
　　　　intracranial pressure after, 566
　　　　neuronavigator in, 563, *565*
　　　　patient selection for, 553
　　　　postoperative management in, 565–566
　　　　preoperative evaluation for, 553–555, *554, 555*
　　　　results of, 566–567, *567*, 567t
　　　　somatosensory evoked potentials in, 563
　　　　stereomarkers in, 563, *565*
　　　　stereotactic, 553, 556, *556*
　　　　transsulcal, 557–559, *558–563*
　　　　tumor resection in, 558, 560, 563, *564, 565*
　　　　ultrasonic aspirator in, 560
　　　　ultrasound in, 563
　mixed, of lateral ventricle, 726, *729*
　nasal, 157, *157*
　of lateral ventricular body, 731, *731*
　of optic chiasm, 765–769, *766, 767, 768, 770, 771, 773*
　of third ventricle floor, 769
　oligoastrocytic, 549. See also *Glioma, intracranial, low-grade.*
　optic nerve, 253–277. See also *Optic nerve glioma.*
　optic tract, *771*, 773
　stereotactic volumetric resection of, 628, 649
　supratentorial, 517–534
　　anticonvulsant therapy in, 521
　　biopsy of, 521
　　corticosteroids in, 521
　　decompression in, 527, 529

Index | XIX

Glioma (Continued)
    frontal lobectomy in, 522–525, *522–526*
        deficits after, 524–525
    internal decompression of, 521–522
    intraoperative management of, 521
    manifestations of, 517–518, 518t
    neuropsychological assessment of, 519–521
    occipital lobectomy in, 526–527, *530–532*
    ophthalmologic assessment of, 519
    positron-emission tomography in, 519
    postoperative care for, 529
    preoperative assessment of, 518–521
    preoperative management of, 521
    prognosis for, 537–538
    radiographic assessment of, 518–519, 518t
    recurrence of, 519, 533, 535–543, *536*
        age at, 541
        brachytherapy for, 538, 541
        chemotherapy failure and, 537
        chemotherapy for, 539, *539*
        differential diagnosis of, 535
        interval to, 541
        Karnofsky rating in, 533, *541*
        malignant progression of, 535
        multimodality therapy for, *536*, 538–539, *540*
        patterns of, 538, *539*
        postoperative, 536–537
        prognosis for, 541–542, 542t
        radiation therapy failure and, 537
        reoperation for, 539–541, *541*
            closure for, 543
            exposure for, 542–543
            patient selection for, 541–542, 542t
            preparation for, 542
            rationale for, 539–541, *540*
        vs. radiation necrosis, 536
    reoperation for, 533
    residual, 537–538
    survival with, 533–534
    temporal lobectomy in, 525–526, *527–529*
    Wada intra-arterial sodium amytal test in, 519
  thalamic, 775, *776*
  third ventricle, 769, *772*, *773*, 775
  lateral ventricle, 726, *728*
  stereotactic volumetric resection of, 623–626, *624–626*
Gliomatosis, arachnoidal, perineural, in optic nerve glioma, 255
Gliosis, in craniopharyngioma, 382–384, *384*
Globe, innervation of, 241
  traction on, in optic nerve sheath fenestration, 245
Glomus bodies, of temporal bone, 851, *852*
Glomus jugulare tumors, 851–863, *852*
  arteriography of, 855
  bilateral, 852, *853*
  blood supply of, 859
  catecholamine secretion by, 852, 860
  clinical presentation of, 852
  cranial nerves in, 852
  embolization of, 855
  epidemiology of, 851–852, *853*
  extension of, 857
  hearing dysfunction in, 852
  radiation therapy for, 857–858
  surgery for, 855–857, *856*
    bleeding in, 859
    case reports of, 860–863, *861*, 861t, *862*
    cerebrospinal fluid leakage in, 859
    complications of, 858–860

Glomus jugulare tumors (Continued)
    cranial nerve injury in, 858–859
    facial nerve paralysis after, 858–859
    infection in, 859
    infratemporal fossa approach to, 857, *858*
    lateral skull-base approach to, 855–857, *856*, *857*
    meningitis after, 859
    results of, 860–863, *861*, 861t, *862*
    vagus nerve paralysis after, 858–859
    vascular injury in, 859
    wound healing in, 859
  surgical anatomy for, 852–853, *854*
Glossopharyngeal nerve, anatomy of, 1107
  neurovascular decompression of, 1464–1466, *1465*
  percutaneous rhizotomy of, *1481*, 1481–1483, *1482*
Glossopharyngeal neuralgia, neurovascular decompression for, 1464–1466, *1465*
  treatment options for, 1465
Glucose, in cerebrospinal fluid leak, 119
Glycerol, neurolytic activity of, 1533–1534
Glycerol rhizolysis. See *Retrogasserian glycerol rhizolysis.*
Goserelin, in recurrent adenoma, 319
Gracilis muscle, transfer of, in facial nerve palsy, 2156
Granuloma, cryptococcal, 1702, *1702*
Graves' orbitopathy, computed tomography in, 219
  misdiagnosis of, 219
Gray matter, penetrating injury to, 96, 97, *99*
Greenberg retracting system, in fronto-orbital temporal (transcranial) approach, 198–199
Grid arrays, 1268–1269
  cortical mapping in, 1269
  grid removal after, 1269
  in epilepsy, 1268–1269, *1268*
  indications for, 1268
  recordings of, 1268–1269
  technique for, 1268, *1268*
Growth fraction, of tumor, 315–316
Growth hormone–secreting pituitary adenoma, 305–309
Growth plate, endochondral, in achondroplasia, 2108
Guns, 81–82
Gunshot wounds. See *Head, penetrating missile injuries of.*

Hallpike's maneuver, 1548
Halo ring, in craniovertebral junction abnormalities, 1722
Halo vest, in ankylosing spondylitis, 1771
Halstead-Reitan neuropsychological test battery, in intracranial glioma, 520
Hamartoma, definition of, 259–260
  optic nerve glioma as, 227, 256–258
Harrington rods, in pediatric spinal deformities, 1968
Head. See also *Scalp; Skull.*
  impalement injury to, 87
  penetrating missile injuries of, 81–87
    angiography in, 84–85, 106
    antibiotics in, 84
    anticonvulsants in, 84, 106–107
    ballistics of, 81–82, 89
    blast, 83
    bone chips in, 83, 85
    bone fragment replacement in, 86
    bone fragments in, 101–102, 102t
    bullet track in, 82–83
    case reports of, 93–95, *93–95*

Head (Continued)
    cerebral edema in, 83
    cerebrospinal fluid leak in, 86, 100–101
    civilian, 105–108, 105t
        evaluation of, 106, *106*, 106t
        intracranial pressure monitoring in, 108
        medical treatment of, 106–107
        outcome of, 108
        surgical treatment of, indications for, 107
        technique of, 107–108
        transfacial, 108
    computed tomography in, 106
    contusion in, 83
    cranioplasty in, 84
    debridement of, 85
    deep, 96
    diagonal, 96–97, *98*, *99*
    dural sinus repair in, 86
    evaluation of, 106, *106*, 106t
    exploding bullets in, 85–86
    fractures in, 83
    Glasgow Coma Scale in, 106
    hematoma in, 83
    high-velocity, 93, *93*, *94*
    hydrocephalus in, 86
    impalement and, 87
    in children, 86–87, 95–96, *95–98*
    incidence of, 105
    infection in, 93–95, *94*, *95*, 101–102, 102t
    intracranial pressure in, 83
    intracranial pressure monitoring in, 84–85, 108
    intraventricular, 108
    low-velocity, 87, 105
    magnetic resonance imaging in, 106
    medical treatment of, 106–107
    metallic fragments in, 85
    migrating fragments in, 85
    outcome of, 108
    pathology of, 89–90
    pathophysiology of, 82–83
    postoperative management of, 84–87
    prophylactic antibiotics in, 107
    pulsating boots in, 107
    seizures in, 106–107
    spent bullet in, 95–96, *95–98*
    steroids in, 84
    surgical management of, 89–103
        dural closure in, 92
        hemorrhage control in, 92
        irrigation debridement in, 91–92
        postoperative care in, 102–103
        preoperative evaluation in, 90–91
        principles of, 83–84
        technique for, 91–95, *93–96*
    tangential, 83, 97, 100, *100*, *101*, 108
    transportation for, 87
    transventricular, 97, *99*
    triage for, 87
    vascular, 108
    ventriculostomy in, 86
  trauma to, 47–64
    airway management in, 48
    barbiturate therapy in, 61
    diagnosis of, 49–50
    epidemiology of, 47
    exploratory burr holes in, 49–50, *50*
    hematoma evacuation in, 50–64
        barbiturate coma after, 61
        care after, 58–63
        cerebral ischemia after, 58
        cerebral perfusion pressure after, 58–59, 59t
            management of, 60
        coagulopathy and, 51
        craniotomy and, 51–53, *52–55*

Head *(Continued)*
    deep vein thrombosis after, 64
    delayed neurologic deficit after, 61
    epidural, 55–56, *56, 57*
    gastrointestinal hemorrhage after, 64
    hematocrit after, 63
    hematoma recurrence after, 61
    hemorrhage after, 64
    hyperglycemia after, 63
    hyperthermia and, 63
    hyperventilation after, 59
    hyponatremia after, 63
    imaging in, 51
    indications for, 50–51
    infection after, 62
    intracerebral, 57–58
    intracranial hypertension after, management of, 60–61
        refractory, 61
    intracranial pressure monitoring after, 62
    intraoperative brain swelling in, 53–54
    magnesium levels after, 63
    outcome of, 64
    physiologic monitoring after, 59–60
    pneumonia after, 63–64
    preoperative preparation for, 51
    pulmonary embolism after, 64
    seizures after, 62–63
    subdural, 56–57
    ventriculostomy-related complications with, 62
  imaging in, 49
  in neonate, 1258
  ligamentous injury in, 48–49
  mannitol in, 60–61
  neurologic assessment in, 48
  patient assessment in, 47–49
  patient stabilization in, 47–49
  radiographic spine evaluation in, 48–49
  sedation in, 60
  seizure prophylaxis in, 60
  ventricular drainage in, 60
Head holder, for computer-assisted volumetric stereotactic resection, 619–620, *620*
Headache, after carotid endarterectomy, 886
  after suboccipital transmeatal acoustic neuroma removal, 837
  cerebral cavernous angioma with, 1187, *1188*
  cluster, cranial nerve decompression for, 1464
    retrogasserian glycerol rhizolysis in, 1534–1535
  in aneurysmal subarachnoid hemorrhage, 937
  in cerebrospinal fluid leak, 119
  in pediatric cerebellar tumor, 802
  in pseudotumor cerebri, 237, 247, 250
  in sclerosteosis, 2143
  in tuberculum sellae meningioma, 404
Hearing, loss of, after vestibular nerve section, 1554
  in craniosynostosis, 137
  in Ménière's disease, 1548
  in sclerosteosis, 2142
  preservation of, in acoustic neuroma removal, 831–833, *833*
    in suboccipital transmeatal acoustic neuroma removal, 838–839
Hemangioblastoma, angiography in, 2028
  cerebellar, 797, *798*
  in pregnancy, 1164–1165
  intramedullary, *2028*, 2036. See also *Spinal cord tumors, intramedullary.*
  posterior fossa, 792t
Hemangioma, capillary, orbital, 178t
  cavernous, orbital, 179t
    computed tomography of, *207*
    supraorbital approach to, 209–211, *209–211*

Hemangioma *(Continued)*
    nerve involvement of, 2192
    vertebral, in pregnancy, 1164
Hemangiopericytoma, nerve involvement of, 2192
Hematocrit, after closed head injury, 63
Hematoma. See also *Hemorrhage.*
    after carotid endarterectomy, 885
    after cerebral hemispherectomy, 1349
    after suboccipital transmeatal acoustic neuroma removal, 836
    epidural, 73–74, 77
      in ankylosing spondylitis, 1772
      traumatic, diagnosis of, 49–50
        evacuation of, 50–51, 55–56, *56, 57*. See also *Head, trauma to, hematoma evacuation in.*
    in ankylosing spondylitis, 1772
    in basal ganglia area, 75
    in penetrating head injury, 83
    intracerebral, 75, 78
      endoscopic surgery for, 706, 707, *709*
      reaccumulation of, in closed head injury, 61
      traumatic, diagnosis of, 49–50
        evacuation of, 50–51, 57–58. See also *Head, trauma to, hematoma evacuation in.*
    intracranial, 73–80
      classification of, 73–76
      clinical features of, 73–76
      operative management of, anatomy in, 75–76, *76*
        anesthesia for, 76–77
        complications of, 79
        indications for, 75
        intracranial pressure monitoring in, 78–79
        outcome of, 79–80
        postoperative management of, 79–80
        preoperative evaluation of, 75
      reaccumulation of, in closed head injury, 61
    posterior fossa, 69–71
      diagnosis of, 69
      operative management of, 69–70
      outcome of, 71
      skull fracture and, 70–71
    stereotactic-directed aspiration of, 650t
    subdural, 74–75, 77–78
      after lateral ventricle tumor resection, 736
      arachnoid cyst and, 589, *589*
      chronic, endoscopic surgery for, 706, 707, *709*
      in ankylosing spondylitis, 1772
      reaccumulation of, in closed head injury, 61
      traumatic, diagnosis of, 49–50
        evacuation of, 50–52, *54, 55, 56–57*. See also *Head, trauma to, hematoma evacuation in.*
    translabyrinthine approach and, 825
Hematomyelia, 2123
  in syringomyelia, 2123
Hemicorticectomy, in cerebral hemispherectomy, 1344
Hemidecortication, in cerebral hemispherectomy, 1344
Hemiplegia, 1667–1669, 1668t. See also *Spasticity.*
  after temporal lobectomy, 1313
  contralateral, sphenoid wind meningioma excision and, 212
Hemispherectomy, functional, central convexity tissue in, 1346, *1346*
  central region excision in, 1345, *1345*
  frontal lobe disconnection in, 1345–1346
  insulectomy in, 1346, *1346*
  parasagittal tissue in, 1346
  parieto-occipital lobe disconnection in, 1345

Hemispherectomy *(Continued)*
    temporal lobectomy in, 1344–1345
    total, 1323–1338. See also *Multilobar resection.*
Hemispherotomy, 1346–1347, *1347*
    peri-insular, 1346–1347, *1347*
    transvertex, 1346
Hemorrhage. See also *Aneurysm(s), intraoperative rupture of; Aneurysmal subarachnoid hemorrhage; Hematoma.*
  after closed head injury, 64
  after percutaneous trigeminal rhizotomy, 1544
  gastrointestinal, after closed head injury, 64
  in arteriovenous malformation, 1227, 1227t, 1486, 1497
  in brainstem arteriovenous malformation, 1497
  in dural arteriovenous malformation, 1227, 1227t
  in optic nerve glioma, 271
  in pregnancy, 1167
  in sclerosteosis, 2149
  in thalamic–basal ganglia arteriovenous malformation, 1502
  into optic nerve glioma, 255–256
  intracerebral, primary, 928–932
    angiography in, 929–930
    cerebellar, 929, 931, *932*
    classification of, 928
    clinical features of, 928–929
    computed tomography of, 929
    diagnosis of, 929–930
    intraventricular, 928–929
    lobar, 928–929, 930
    magnetic resonance imaging in, 929
    medical management of, 930
    prognosis for, 930–931
    risk factors for, 928
    surgical management of, 930–932, *932*
    thrombolytic therapy in, 931
    ultra-early surgery for, 930–931
  intraoperative, in craniotomy, 79
  intraventricular, in premature infant, 1257–1258
  orbital, optic nerve sheath fenestration and, 248
  percutaneous trigeminal rhizotomy and, 1543
  postoperative, in hypothalamic tumors, 774, 774t
    in pineal region tumors, 760, 762
  subarachnoid, aneurysmal, 937–953. See also *Aneurysmal subarachnoid hemorrhage.*
    classification of, 957t, *958*
    pediatric, 1197
Hemosiderin, in Rathke's cleft cyst, 584
Hemostasis, in lateral orbitotomy, 225
  in neuroendoscopy, 696–697, *698, 699*
  in orbital surgery, 234
  in translabyrinthine surgery, 823
Heparin, in pregnancy, 1169
Hernia, cerebral, 152, *152*
Herpes simplex, after glycerol rhizolysis, 1532, 1532t
  after percutaneous rhizotomy, 1477
Herpes simplex cerebritis, *1685*
Hippocampus, in epilepsy, 1306–1307
Histamine type 2 antagonists, after closed head injury, 63–64
Histoacryl Blue (butyl 2-cyanoacrylate), for dural defects, 234
HLA-B27, in ankylosing spondylitis, 1766
Horner's syndrome, *486*
  in parasellar artery injury, 483
  in vertebrectomy, 1800
Horsley-Clarke apparatus, 443, *444*
Human chorionic gonadotropin, in pineal region tumor, 743–744

Index | XXI

Human immunodeficiency virus (HIV),
    1681–1687. See also *Acquired
    immunodeficiency syndrome (AIDS).*
  transmission of, brain biopsy and, 617–618
Hunt-Hess classification, of subarachnoid
    hemorrhage, 957t, *958*
Huntington's disease, fetal mesencephalic tissue
    CNS transplantation in, 1383
Hydrocephalus, 1245–1253
  after cerebral hemispherectomy, 1349
  after intramedullary spinal cord tumor surgery,
    2104
  after lateral ventricle tumor resection, 736,
    737
  after suboccipital transmeatal acoustic neu-
    roma removal, 836
  aneurysmal subarachnoid hemorrhage–
    associated, 949–950
  cerebrospinal fluid absorption in, 1247, 1247t
  cerebrospinal fluid dynamic testing in, 1246–
    1247, 1247t
  choroid plexus tumor and, 573
  etiology of, 1245–1246
  fetal, 1240
  in achondroplasia, 2108, 2109–2110, 2116
  in acoustic neuroma, 830
  in brain metastasis, 612
  in cerebellar tumor removal, 806–807
  in craniopharyngioma, 358
  in craniosynostosis, 137–138
  in cysticercosis, 1712–1713
  in frontoethmoidal encephalomeningocele, 161
  in myelomeningocele, 2062
  in penetrating head injuries, 86
  in pineal region tumors, 757–758
  in posterior fossa tumors, 792, 793, *794*
  in syringomyelia, 2124–2126
  in tuberculum sellae meningioma, 404
  intracranial pressure in, 1246, 1247t
  normal-pressure, 1247–1248
  pathophysiology of, 1245–1246
  pediatric, 1231–1240, 1257
    anatomy of, 5, 1233
    atrial shunts for, 1235
    computed tomography of, 1232, *1232*
    diagnosis of, 1232–1233, 1232t, *1233*
    endoscopic third ventriculostomy for, 1236
    epidemiology of, 1231
    etiology of, 1231–1232, *1232*
    extracranial ventricular shunts for, 1233–
      1235
    frontal horn in, 1233
    intracranial pressure in, 1233
    magnetic resonance imaging of, 1232, *1233*
    occipital horn in, 1233
    peritoneal shunts for, 1235
    precocious puberty and, 1240, *1240*
    shunt infection in, 1236–1238, *1237*, 1237t
    shunt lengthening for, 1235
    shunt malfunction in, 1238–1240, *1239,
      1240*
    shunt revision for, 1236, *1236*
    stereotactic third ventriculostomy for, 1236
    symptoms of, 1232, 1232t
    transcranial Doppler in, 1233
    ultrasound in, 1232
    ventriculoatrial shunt for, 1234–1235
    ventriculoperitoneal shunt for, 1233–1234
    ventriculopleural shunt for, 1235
  pressure-volume index in, 1247, 1247t
  shunt infection in, 1252–1253
  shunt malfunction in, 1249, 1252, 1252t
  stereotactic catheter implantation in, 455
  third ventricle pathology in, 703
  tumor-associated, 1246
  vascular etiologies of, 1246

Hydrocephalus *(Continued)*
  ventricular shunt for, 1248–1249, *1249–1251*
    patient position for, 1248, *1249*
  ventriculoatrial shunt for, 1249
Hydrocortisone, in craniopharyngioma, 378, 386
Hydroencephalomeningocele, 149
Hydromyelia, 2119
  Chiari malformation and, 1746, *1746.* See also
    Syringomyelic cord syndrome.
  surgery for, 1755–1764, *1756–1763*
    results of, 1758
Hydrosyringomyelia, 2119
Hygroma, subdural, computer-assisted
    volumetric stereotactic resection and, 631
  in olfactory groove meningioma removal,
    400
Hyperalimentation, in penetrating head injuries,
    84
Hyperbaric oxygen, in myelomeningoceles, 2062
Hyperglycemia, after closed head injury, 63
Hyperhidrosis, compensatory, 1647
  incidence of, 1647
  sympathectomy for, 1573–1582. See also *Sym-
    pathectomy.*
  upper thoracic ganglionectomy for, 1637–1641
    anatomy for, 1637–1638
    approaches to, 1638
    complications of, 1641
    results of, 1640–1641
    technique of, 1639–1640, *1639, 1640*
Hypernatremia, in aneurysmal subarachnoid
    hemorrhage, 951
Hypernephroma, brain metastasis from, *604,
    608,* 688
Hyperostosis, craniotubular, 2141. See also
    Sclerosteosis.
  of sphenoid bone, 203
Hyperspasticity, DREZotomy in, 1620
Hypertelorism, in craniosynostosis, 137
Hypertension, after carotid endarterectomy, 885
  after intracranial aneurysm surgery, 963–964
  idiopathic. See *Pseudotumor cerebri.*
  in aneurysmal subarachnoid hemorrhage, 944–
    945, 946t, 958
  in closed head injury, 60–61
  in intracranial aneurysm surgery, 959
  primary intracerebral hemorrhage and, 928
Hyperthermia, after closed head injury, 63
Hypertrophic neuropathy, 2193–2194
Hyperventilation, in transcranial skull base
    tumor resection, 168
Hypervolemia, in aneurysmal subarachnoid
    hemorrhage, 944–945, 946t, 958
Hypesthesia, after glycerol rhizolysis, 1531,
    1531t
Hypocapnia, in intracranial aneurysm surgery,
    960
Hypoglossal nerve, transfer of, in facial nerve
    palsy, 2155
Hypomagnesemia, in closed head injury, 63
Hyponatremia, in aneurysmal subarachnoid
    hemorrhage, 951–952, 951t, 958
  in closed head injury, 63
Hypophyseal artery, superior, aneurysm of, 996,
    998
Hypophysectomy, 287–288
  functional, sella repair in, 339, *339*
Hypotension, after open cordotomy, 1565, 1567
  in aneurysm surgery, 959–960, 961, 1118–
    1120
  in craniosynostosis treatment, 147
  in intraoperative aneurysm rupture, 989
Hypothalamus, glioma of, 765–775, *765–770*
  clinical features of, 769, 771t
  computed tomography in, 771, *771, 772*
  growth of, 275, *275*

Hypothalamus *(Continued)*
  histology of, 769, 771
  surgery for, 771, 773–775, *774*, 774t
  topography of, *765*
  operative trauma to, in craniopharyngioma,
    385–386
  stimulation of, in pain treatment, 1390
Hypothermia, in intracranial aneurysm surgery,
    962–963
  in lower basilar artery aneurysm, 1088
  in neonatal surgery, 1255
Hypothyroidism, in craniopharyngioma, 371

Idiopathic intracranial hypertension. See
    Pseudotumor cerebri.
Ileus, postoperative, in ankylosing spondylitis,
    1777
Iliac artery, rupture of, in lumbar disc surgery,
    1951
Iliac vein, injury to, in lumbar disc surgery,
    1951
Imidazoles, in fungal infection, 1701
Immobilization, after peripheral nerve surgery,
    2170
  in craniovertebral junction abnormalities, 1722
Immune complexes, in infected aneurysm, 1133
Immunofixation method, in cerebrospinal fluid
    leak localization, 121
Immunosuppression, in fetal mesencephalic
    tissue CNS transplantation, 1366, 1376
Immunotherapy, in brain metastasis, 612
Impalement, head injury by, 87
Impotence, in prolactin-secreting pituitary
    adenoma, 309
Inappropriate secretion of arginine vasopressin,
    in pituitary adenoma removal, 299
Indigo carmine, in cerebrospinal fluid leak
    localization, 120
Infant. See *Children; Neonate.*
Infarction, after percutaneous trigeminal
    rhizotomy, 1544
  after suboccipital transmeatal acoustic neu-
    roma removal, 836
  vs. brain tumor, 518–519
Infection, 1673–1679, *1673.* See also *Abscess;
    Osteomyelitis.*
  fungal, 1699–1702, 1699t
    diagnosis of, 1700, 1700t, *1701, 1702*
    in penetrating head injury, 103
    medical treatment of, 1700–1702
    pathologic features of, 1699–1700, 1700t
    surgery for, 1702, 1702t
  in cerebral hemispherectomy, 1349
  in cerebrospinal fluid leaks, 101, 102, 102t,
    122, 123
  in closed head injury, 62
  in craniofacial resection, 424
  in cranioplasty, 20
  in craniosynostosis treatment, 147
  in difficult aneurysm, 1052
  in dorsal root ganglionectomy, 1590
  in glomus jugulare tumor surgery, 859
  in glycerol rhizolysis, 1531–1532, 1532t
  in hydrocephalus, 1236–1238, *1237,* 1237t
  in lumbar disc surgery, 1935
  in meningocele, 2065
  in orbital surgery, 235
  in penetrating head injury, 93–95, *94, 95,*
    101–102, 102t
  in suboccipital transmeatal acoustic neuroma
    removal, 837
  meningocerebral, retained bone fragments and,
    101–102, 102t
  of aneurysm. See *Aneurysm(s), infected.*

Infection *(Continued)*
  of cranial bones, 1673–1674
  of vertebral column, 1677–1679, *1678*
  osteosynthesis and, 40, 42
  parasitic, 1705–1715. See also *Cysticercosis.*
  tuberculous, 1689–1699. See also *Tuberculoma.*
Informed consent, in brain biopsy, 615
Infraorbital foramen, *215, 216*
Infraorbital groove, *214, 215, 216*
Infratentorial lesions, stereotactic biopsy of, 638
Innominate foramen, 1544
Insulectomy, in functional hemispherectomy, 1346, *1346*
Insulin, in craniopharyngioma, 386
  octreotide inhibition of, 307
Intelligence, radiation therapy effects on, 276
Intelligence quotient, after cerebral hemispherectomy, 1349
  after temporal lobectomy, 1313
  after tractotomy, 1417
  in intracranial glioma, 520
Interforniceal corridor, in third ventricle transcallosal approach, *718, 722, 722*
Interhemispheric sensory dissociation, after corpus callosotomy, 1355
Intermittent positive-pressure ventilation, postcraniotomy, 79
Interosseous nerve, posterior, paralysis of, 2176–2177, *2176, 2177*
  radial osteoma compression of, *2194*
Interpeduncular fossa, *1077*
Intracerebral hemorrhage, primary, 928–932. See also *Hemorrhage, intracerebral, primary.*
Intracranial arterial replantation, 923
Intracranial hematoma, 73–80. See also *Hematoma, intracranial.*
Intracranial hypertension, idiopathic. See *Pseudotumor cerebri.*
Intracranial pressure, head injury–associated, 60–61, 62, 83
  control of, 50
  monitoring of, 53
  in craniosynostosis, 137
  in hydrocephalus, 1246, 1247t
  increase in, cerebrospinal fluid leak and, 122
  in difficult aneurysm, 1051
  monitoring of, after craniotomy, 78–79
  in arachnoid cysts, 586, *588*
  in choroid plexus tumor surgery, 573
  in head injury, 62, 84–85
  reduction of, postcraniotomy, 79
Intracranial volume, in craniosynostosis, 137
Intraluminal ultrasound, in neuroendoscopy, 698–699, *700*
Intraocular pressure, increase of, optic nerve sheath fenestration and, 248–249
Intraorbital foramen, *214*
Intraorbital tumors, 183–193
  computed tomography of, 186–187
  diagnosis of, 186–187
  magnetic resonance imaging of, 187
  surgical anatomy of, 183–187, *183–186*
  surgical removal of, 188–192, *188–191*
    care after, 192
    closure after, 190–191, *191*
    complications of, 192
    lateral approach for, 190, *191*
    medial approach for, 189–190, *189, 190*
    tarsorrhaphy in, 191–192, *192*
Intrasellar abscess, 585
Intubation, in closed head injury, 48
Iodinated contrast, in orbital diagnosis, 217–218
Iodine-125, implantation of, in recurrent adenoma, 319
Ionomer cement, in frontal skull base fracture, 43

Iophendylate (Pantopaque), in cerebrospinal fluid leak localization, 121
Iridium 192 (^{192}Ir) seeds, 656t. See also *Brachytherapy, interstitial.*
  acquisition of, 658
  afterloading of, 661–662, *662*
  postoperative computed tomography of, 660, *660*
  quality assurance for, 658
  removal of, 663
  return of, 663
  spacing of, 657–658, *658*
Iridoplegia, orbital surgery and, 234
Ischemia, cerebral, after closed head injury, 58
  aneurysmal subarachnoid hemorrhage and, 941, 944–948, 944t
  cortical, fetal neuron transplantation in, 1383
  in multisegmental cervical spondylosis, 1792
  intraoperative, during carotid endarterectomy, 885–886
  lower extremity, spinal cord stimulation in, 1407
  subendocardial, in aneurysmal subarachnoid hemorrhage, 952
ISG Viewing Wand, 637
Isocenter, 1210
Isoflurane, in intracranial aneurysm surgery, 962
Isola system, in tumor-associated thoracic spinal cord compression, 2014–2015, *2016*
Isoniazid, in tuberculosis, 1695t
Isotopes, in interstitial radiation therapy, 457–458, 457t, 463t

Jacobsen ball, in medullary tractotomy, 1569
  in open cordotomy, 1562–1563, *1565, 1566*
Jakob-Creutzfeldt disease, stereotactic biopsy and, 640
Jugular bulb catheterization, in closed head injury, 59
Jugular foramen, anatomy of, 852–853, *854*
  chondrosarcoma of, 872
  chordoma of, 871
  cross section of, *854*
  epidermoid cyst of, 871
  meningioma of, 871
  myxoma of, 871–872, *872*
  schwannoma of, 865–871
    anatomy of, 865–866
    angiography of, 867–868, *867*
    cerebrospinal fluid leak in, 870
    computed tomography of, 868, *868*
    cranial nerve disturbances in, 866, 866t, 870–871
    diagnosis of, 866–867
    extracranial type of, 866
    growth patterns of, 866, *867*
    incidence of, 865
    intracranial type of, 866
    intraosseous type of, 866
    iophendylate cisternography of, 867
    magnetic resonance imaging of, 868, *869*
    mixed type of, 866, *867*
    plain film radiography of, 867
    pneumoencephalography of, 867
    surgery for, 868–871, *869, 870*
      patient position for, 869, *869*
    symptoms of, 866, 866t
    tumors of. See also *Glomus jugulare tumors.*
      nonglomus, 865–872, *866–872,* 866t
Jugular vein, in ventriculoatrial shunt placement, 1235

Karnofsky rating, 546t

Karnofsky rating *(Continued)*
  in recurrent intracranial glioma, 533, *541*
Karolinska Scales of Personality, 1453, *1453*
Katzman infusion test, in normal-pressure hydrocephalus, 1247
Keratitis, neurogenic, after percutaneous rhizotomy, 1477, 1477t
  neuroparalytic, orbital surgery and, 234
Keratopathy, optic nerve sheath fenestration and, 249
Kernohan's notch, in subdural hematoma, 74
Ketoconazole, in Cushing's disease, 303, 319
  in fungal infection, 1701
Kinking, of carotid artery, 887
Klippel-Feil syndrome, 1721
Kölliker-Fuse nucleus, 1389
Kyphoscoliosis, after intramedullary spinal cord tumor surgery, 2104
  in myelomeningocele patient, 1965, 1966
Kyphosis, after intramedullary spinal cord tumor surgery, 2104
  pediatric laminectomy and, 1965

Labetalol, after intracranial aneurysm surgery, 964
Labyrinthectomy, in acoustic neuroma, 818
Labyrinthitis, chronic, vs. Ménière's disease, 1548
Laceration, of scalp, 8
Lacrimal bone, *214*
Lacrimal canal, *215*
Lacrimal fossa, *216*
Lacrimal gland, *215*
  adenoid cystic carcinoma of, 233
  injury to, orbital surgery and, 234
  mixed tumor of, 233
  orbital process of, *217*
  tumors of, 179t, 232–233
Lacrimal nerve, *197*
Lambdoid craniosynostosis, 146, *146*
Laminectomy, 1887–1888
  after lumbar disc surgery, 1938
  decompressive, in sclerosteosis, 2150–2151
  for spinal tumors, 1985
  pediatric spinal deformities and, 1965
Laminotomy, in lumbar spine stenosis, 1961-1964, *1962, 1963*
Language, after corpus callosotomy, 1355
  after hemispherectomy, 1342
  localization of, 555, 556–557, *557*
    by electrical stimulation mapping, 1318–1319, *1319*
  measures of, in electrical eloquent cortex mapping, 1318–1319, *1319*
Larsen's syndrome, pediatric cervical spine injury and, 2091, *2091*
Laryngeal nerve, recurrent, 1787
  in vertebrectomy, 1800
Laser, in computer-assisted volumetric stereotactic resection, 621
  in low-grade glioma, 560
  in neuroendoscopy, 696, *698*
  in pediatric cerebellar tumor removal, 806
  in percutaneous lumbar discectomy, 1930–1932, *1930,* 1930t, 1931t
  in spinal cord tumor surgery, 2097, 2099, *2099*
  thermal effects of, *698,* 699
Lateral cleft syndrome, 156, *157*
Lateral Dominance Examination, in intracranial glioma, 521
Lateral loop, of lateral sellar compartment, *495,* 496, 496t
Lateral sellar compartment (cavernous sinus), 479–490, *976*

Lateral sellar compartment (cavernous sinus) (Continued)
 anatomic triangles of, 495–497, 496t
 aneurysms of, 975–981, *977–978, 980,* 1044
 angiography of, 487
 anterior tip of, 496
 anterior triangle of, 494
  packing of, 508
 anterolateral, packing of, 508
 arteries of, 481–483, *482, 484*
 arteriosclerotic, 975–981, *977, 978, 980*
 back of, 496
 congenital, 975–981, *977, 978, 980*
 coverings of, 479, *480*
 fistulae of, 981–983, *982*
 frontotemporal approach to, 497–504, *499–503*
 lateral triangle of, 495, *496*
 medial triangle of, 494
  packing of, 508
 meningioma of, 493, 507
 nerves of, 479, *480,* 481
 nonfistulous arterial aneurysms of, 975–981, *977, 978, 980*
 posteroinferior triangle of, 496
  hemostasis for, 508
 posterolateral triangle of, 495–496
  hemostasis for, 508
 posteromedial triangle of, 496
 postmeatal triangle of, 496–497
 premeatal triangle of, 496
 shape of, 479, *480,* 494
 superior triangle of, 494–495
 sympathetic pathways of, 483, *484, 486*
 tumors of, 493–509
  metastatic, 493
  surgical approach to, anatomy for, 493–497, *495,* 496t
   anesthesia for, 497
   carotid artery bypass in, 508–509
   closure for, 508
   frontotemporal, 497–504, *499–503*
    anterior clinoid process removal in, 502
    arachnoid dissection in, 503
    closure for, 503–504
    craniotomy for, 500–501, *500–502*
    extradural bone removal for, 501–504, *503*
    frontotemporal craniotomy in, 500
    half-and-half technique in, 499
    incision for, 498–500, *499*
    intradural transcavernous dissection in, 502–503
    optical canal unroofing in, 502
    orbitozygomatic craniotomy in, 500–501, *501, 502*
    positioning for, 498, *499*
    single-layer technique in, 498–499
    transzygomatic craniotomy in, 500, *500*
    two-layer technique in, *499,* 499–500
   hemostasis in, 507–508
   indications for, 493
   intracavernous tumor resection in, 507
   neurophysiologic monitoring for, 497
   propofol in, 497
   rhomboid, 505–507, *506*
   skull base carotid bypass procedures for, 508–509
   transcavernous, 504–505, *504, 505*
 veins of, 483–490, *486–490*
  embryology of, *484, 488*
  trabeculae of, 486–487, *487, 488*
Lateral triangle, of lateral sellar compartment, 495, *495,* 496t

Lateral ventricle. See *Ventricle(s), lateral.*
Le Fort fractures, 28, *29*
 osteosynthesis in, 39, *39*
Leptomeninges, metastasis to, 613
Leptomyelolipoma, 2071. See also *Spinal dysraphism.*
Leu-enkephalin, 1432
Levator palpebrae, 185, *185*
 sectioning of, for optic nerve glioma excision, 190, *190*
 transient palsy of, in intraorbital tumor excision, 192
Levodopa, in Parkinson's disease, 1361
Levophed (norepinephrine), in closed head injury, 60
Libido, in prolactin-secreting pituitary adenoma, 309
Lidocaine, after intracranial aneurysm surgery, 963–964
Limbic system, 1423–1424, *1424*
Linear accelerator, in arteriovenous malformation radiosurgery, 1206
Linear sebaceous nevus syndrome, craniosynostosis in, 136
Lipohamartoma, nerve involvement of, 2192, *2193*
Lipoma, intraspinal, 2069–2079, *2070*
 caudal, *2077*
  surgery for, 2075, *2077*
 computed tomography of, *2076*
 conus fixation to, 2071
 dorsal, *2076*
  surgery for, 2075, *2076*
 imaging of, 2074, *2074, 2075*
 surgery for, 2075–2079, *2076–2079*
  results of, 2079
 transitional, *2078*
  surgery for, 2075, *2078*
Lipomyelomeningocele. See *Lipoma, intraspinal.*
Lissauer's tract, 1613, 1615
Lomustine, in recurrent adenoma, 319
Longitudinal ligament, anterior, 1787
 posterior, ossification of, 1817–1828. See also *Ossification of posterior longitudinal ligament (OPLL).*
Longitudinal myelotomy, in spasticity, 1665
Lumbar disc, herniation of, 1905–1923
 anatomic changes in, 1905, *1906*
 computed tomography in, 1944
 crossed Lasègue sign in, 1907
 diagnosis of, 1943–1945, *1944*
 extraforaminal, 1951
 grading of, 1925, 1944, *1944*
 imaging of, 1941, 1944–1945, *1944*
  indications for, 1943–1944
 leg-raising test of Fajersztajn in, *1909*
 location of, 1905, *1905*
 magnetic resonance imaging of, *1943,* 1944
 mechanism of, 1941–1943, *1942, 1943,* 1943t
 myelography in, 1944
 natural history of, 1941–1943, *1942, 1943,* 1943t
 paracentral, 1950–1951
 position of, *1945*
 posterolateral, 1947, 1950
 preoperative evaluation of, 1905–1906, *1905, 1906,* 1925
 radiologic studies of, 1906, 1926
 surgery for, 1925–1926, 1941–1956, *1945–1950*
  anesthesia for, 1911
  arachnoiditis after, 1936
  arterial rupture during, 1951
  care after, 1952
  cerebrospinal fluid leak during, 1938–1939, 1952

Lumbar disc *(Continued)*
  complications of, 1951–1952
  contraindications to, 1909, 1926
  disc excision in, 1920–1921, *1921, 1922*
  dural tear in, 1919
  epidural fat in, 1917–1920
  epidural scar after, 1935
  errors in, 1950
  exploratory, 1909
  free disc fragments in, 1921
  historical development of, 1910
  incisions for, 1913–1914
  indications for, 1943–1944
  infection after, 1935
  interlaminar, 1920
  interspace in, 1917, *1917, 1918*
  intradiscal, 1951
  nerve root anomalies in, 1921–1922
  nerve root damage in, 1917–1920, *1919, 1920*
  nerve root tension in, 1920
  outcome of, 1952–1956, *1953–1955*
  patient position for, 1911, *1911–1913,* 1926, 1945–1947, *1946*
  patient selection for, 1905
  percutaneous, 1951
  precautions in, 1910–1911
  predictive score card for, 1906–1907, *1908,* 1925–1926
  repetition of, 1951
  root compression after, 1935
  root injury during, 1935
  spinal instability after, 1935
  subperiosteal dissection in, 1914–1917, *1915, 1916*
  surface landmarks for, 1911, 1913, *1913*
  symptoms after, 1935–1939
   foraminotomy for, 1937–1938
   fusion for, 1939
   laminectomy for, 1938
   patient examination for, 1936
   reoperation for, 1936–1937
   surgery for, 1936–1939
  timing of, 1926, 1945
  ventral perforation in, 1951
  wound closure in, 1923, *1923*
 temporal changes in, 1906
 percutaneous discectomy of, 1927–1933
  indications for, 1927–1928
  laser-assisted, 1930–1932, *1930,* 1930t, 1931t
   results of, 1931–1932
  mechanical, 1928–1929, *1929*
  patient position for, 1928, *1928*
  results of, 1932–1933
  stereotactic techniques for, 1930
  suction techniques for, 1929–1930, *1929*
Lumbar Disc Surgery Predictive Score Card, 1906–1907, *1908*
Lumbar puncture, in aneurysmal subarachnoid hemorrhage, 938–939
 in normal-pressure hydrocephalus, 1248
Lumbar shunt, in children, 1966, *1967*
Lumbar spine, pediatric, injury to, 2083
 stenosis of, 1957–1964
  central, 1957
  classification of, 1957, 1957t
  clinical features of, 1957–1958
  computed tomography in, 1958, *1959*
  conservative management of, 1958, 1960
  evaluation of, 1958, *1959, 1960*
  lateral, 1958
  magnetic resonance imaging in, 1958, *1959, 1960*
  pathophysiology of, 1957
  surgery for, anatomy for, 1961

Lumbar spine *(Continued)*
  approaches to, 1961–1962
  complications of, 1962–1963
  laminectomy in, 1961
  laminotomy in, 1961–1964, *1962, 1963*
  patient selection for, 1958, 1960–1961
  results of, 1963–1964
  risk factors in, 1961
Lumbar subarachnoid spinal drain, in transcranial skull base tumor resection, 168, 172
Lumbar sympathectomy, 1644–1645, *1644, 1645*
Lumboperitoneal shunting, in pseudotumor cerebri, 237
Lungs, carcinoma of, brain metastasis from, *606, 607*
  disorders of, in aneurysmal subarachnoid hemorrhage, 952
Luque rods, in pediatric spinal deformities, 1968
Lymphangioma, nerve involvement in, 2191
  orbital, 178t
Lymphocytic adenohypophysitis, in pregnancy, 1166
Lymphoma, cerebral, endoscopic-stereotactic biopsy of, 704, *705*
  Gamma Knife surgery for, *687*
  in AIDS, 1685
  of lacrimal gland, 233

M-16 rifle, 89
Macroadenoma, in pregnancy, 1166
  mortality and morbidity in, 297t
Mageral hook-plate, 1871, *1871*
Magnesium, serum, after closed head injury, 63
Magnetic resonance angiography, in aneurysmal subarachnoid hemorrhage, 939
  in carotid atherosclerosis, 878
  in pineal region tumors, 740
Magnetic resonance imaging, after amygdalohippocampectomy, 1296, *1297*
  for depth electrode placement, 1276, *1276*
  in aneurysmal subarachnoid hemorrhage, 938
  in arteriovenous malformation, 1227, 1486
  in brain metastasis, 603, *604, 607, 607*
  in cavernous angioma, 1183–1184, *1184*
  in cervical spondylosis, 1786, 1791, *1791*
  in clivus tumor, 786
  in closed head trauma, 49
  in craniopharyngioma, 358, 371–372
  in Cushing's disease, 302
  in epilepsy, 1313–1314
  in intracranial glioma, 518
  in intramedullary spinal cord tumors, 2096, *2098*
  in intramedullary tumor, 2028, *2029*
  in jugular foramen cyst, 871
  in jugular foramen meningioma, 871
  in jugular foramen schwannoma, 868, *869*
  in lumbar disc herniation, 1944
  in lumbar spine stenosis, 1958, *1959, 1960*
  in medial sphenoid ridge meningioma, 409, *409*
  in middle cerebral artery aneurysm, 1056, *1056*
  in multisegmental cervical spondylosis, 1792
  in neurofibromatosis type I, 255
  in nonfunctioning pituitary adenoma, 293, *294, 295*
  in olfactory groove meningioma, 394, *394, 395*
  in optic nerve glioma, 254–256
  in orbital diagnosis, 219–220
  in paraclinoid aneurysm, 994
  in Parkinson's disease, 1363
  in pediatric arteriovenous malformation, 1198

Magnetic resonance imaging *(Continued)*
  in pediatric brain tumors, 576
  in pediatric cerebellar tumor, 803, *804, 805*
  in pediatric spinal injury, 2082, *2083*
  in pineal region tumors, 740, 757, *758*
  in pituitary adenoma, 306
  in primary intracerebral hemorrhage, 929
  in sclerosteosis, 2144, *2145*
  in spinal cord compression, *1998,* 1998–1999
  in stereotactic biopsy, 638–639, *638, 639*
  in stereotactic resection, 621–622, *622.* See also *Stereotactic volumetric resection.*
  in syringomyelia, 2122, 2136
  in tentorial tumors, 783, 784
  in tuberculum sellae meningioma, 404, *405*
  of choroid plexus tumor, 573
  of craniopharyngioma, 384–385, *385*
  of parasagittal tumor, 513
  of pediatric hydrocephalus, 1232, *1233*
  of recurrent adenoma, 318, *318*
  of tuberculoma, 1693–1694, *1694–1696*
  stereotactic instruments for, 452, 453
Mamillary bodies, *703*
Mandible, subluxation of, in carotid endarterectomy, 892, *894*
Mannitol, after craniotomy, 79
  in cerebrospinal fluid leak, 129
  in closed head injury, 60–61
  in intracranial aneurysm surgery, 961
  in postoperative intracranial pressure reduction, 79
  in pregnancy, 1169
  in transcranial skull base tumor resection, 168
Manwaring saline torch, in neuroendoscopy, 698
Marburg neuroendoscopy guiding system, 695, *696*
Masseter muscle, transfer of, in facial nerve palsy, 2156
Maxillary bones, 27
Maxillary fracture, 28
Maxillary sinus, 27
McConnell's (capsular) artery, 482, 483, 494
McRae's line, 1721
Mean arterial pressure, in intracranial aneurysm surgery, 958, 960, 961
Meckel's cave, 481
  compartments of, *1526*
Medial sphenoid ridge, meningioma of, 410
Medial triangle, of lateral sellar compartment, 494, *495,* 496t, 508
Median nerve, entrapment of, 2177–2179, *2177–2179*
  at elbow, 2177, *2177*
  at wrist, 2177–2179, *2178, 2179*
  lesions of, treatment of, 2164
Medical Outcome Study, in lumbar disc surgery, 1952–1956, *1953–1955*
Medulla oblongata, expanding tumor of, *776, 777*
  focal-diffuse tumor of, *778*
Medullary slumping, postoperative, in sclerosteosis, 2149–2150
Medullary tractotomy, 1568–1570
Medulloblastoma, cerebellar, pediatric, 801, 803, 805, 808, 809–810, *809*
  Gamma Knife surgery for, 686
  posterior fossa, 792t
  surgery for, 795–796
Mega-cerebro-arterio-media, 1041–1042
Melanoma, metastatic, Gamma Knife surgery for, 688
  intraoperative brachycurietherapy for, *462*
Memory, after corpus callosotomy, 1355
  after temporal lobectomy, 1313
  after transcallosal surgery, 734
  electrical stimulation mapping of, 1319

Ménière's disease, 1547–1549. See also *Vertigo.*
Meningeal artery, arteriovenous fistula of, *1129*
  arteriovenous malformation of, 2047
  burr holes about, 76
Meningeal fibrosis, in syringomyelia, 2119–2120, 2123, 2124, 2135t
Meningioma, during pregnancy, 1164
  Gamma Knife surgery in, 679–681, *680,* 680t
  intraorbital, in children, 185
  of falx, 513–515, *514*
  of jugular foramen, 871
  of lateral sellar compartment, 493, 507
  of lateral ventricle, 726, *727*
  of medial sphenoid ridge, 408–412. See also *Sphenoid ridge, meningioma of.*
  of olfactory groove, 393–401. See also *Olfactory groove, meningioma of.*
  of optic nerve, 187, 190
  of optic nerve sheath, 185, 190, *207, 208*
  of orbit, 178t, 179t, 185, 254
  of right lateral ventricle trigone, *730*
  of scalp, 15, *16*
  of skull base, 437–438
  of sphenoid wing, 201, 203, 211, 212
  of tuberculum sellae, 403–408. See also *Tuberculum sellae, meningioma of.*
  parasagittal, 513–515
  perioptic, suction removal of, 227
  vs. nonfunctioning pituitary adenoma, 293
Meningitis, after glomus jugulare tumor surgery, 859
  after glycerol rhizolysis, 1532, 1532t
  after suboccipital transmeatal acoustic neuroma removal, 836–837
  cerebrospinal fluid leaks and, 119, 124
  chemical, 585–586, 591–592, *592*
  Rathke's cleft cyst and, 596
  in transbasal skull base tumor removal, 427
  translabyrinthine approach and, 825
  tuberculous, 1697–1699
    computed tomography of, 1697–1698
    diagnosis of, 1697
    incidence of, 1697
    magnetic resonance imaging of, 1698, *1698*
    medical treatment of, 1698
    surgery for, 1698–1699
      results of, 1699
    tuberculoma and, 1690
Meningocele, 149
  after brachial plexus avulsion injury, 1629–1630, *1630*
  anterolateral, 2063
  basioccipital, 2063
  cervical, 2063
  diagnosis of, 2065
  intrasacral, 2065–2067
    diagnosis of, 2065, 2067
    pathologic anatomy of, 2065
    symptoms of, 2065
  lumbar, 2063–2065
    anterior, 2063
  lumbosacral, 2063
  posterior, 2063
  sacral, anterior, 2065–2067, *2066*
    diagnosis of, 2065–2067, *2066*
    pathologic anatomy of, 2065
    symptoms of, 2065
    treatment of, 2067
  thoracic, 2063–2065, *2064*
  treatment of, 2065
Meningocele manqué, 2071, 2074–2075
Meningohypophysial artery, of lateral sellar compartment, 483
Meningomyelocele, repair of, cerebrospinal fluid leak and, 122, 128–129
Mental retardation, aggressive conduct disorders with, psychosurgery for, 1417–1420, *1418, 1419, 1420*

Mental retardation *(Continued)*
  hemispherectomy and, 1342
  in craniosynostosis, 136
  in frontoethmoidal encephalomeningocele, 161, *163*
Meralgia paresthetica, 2180–2181, *2181*
Mesencephalon, arteriovenous malformation of, 1486, *1498*. See also *Brainstem, arteriovenous malformation of.*
Meshed skin graft, for scalp defect, 14, *14*
Mesoloviotomy, in schizophrenia, 1414
Metal fragments, in penetrating head injuries, 85
Met-enkephalin, 1432
Methylmethacrylate cranioplasty, 21, *24*
Metopic craniosynostosis, 142–143
Metyrapone, in Cushing's disease, 303, 319
Miconazole, in fungal infection, 1701
Microadenoma, pituitary, growth hormone–secreting, 306
  prolactin-secreting, 309–311
  sellar repair in, 331–333, *332, 333*
  transsphenoidal approach to, 287
Microcephaly, 146
Microforceps, in neuroendoscopy, 696, *697, 698*
Microsurgical DREZotomy, 1613–1621. See also *DREZotomy.*
Midbasilar artery, aneurysm of, 469, *471*
  pedicled rhinotomy for, 469–474, *472, 474*
Middle cerebral artery. See *Cerebral artery, middle.*
Migrainous neuralgia, cranial nerve decompression for, 1464
Mitotane, in Cushing's disease, 303
Momentum, ballistic, 82
Mondini malformation, 122
Morphine, analgesic mechanisms of, 1431–1432
  intraventricular, 1431–1440, 1432–1440, *1433*, 1434t–1435t
    case reports of, 1433, 1434t–1435t
    patient selection for, 1433, 1438
    pump for, 1438–1440, *1439*
    results of, 1436t–1437t, 1437–1438
    side effects of, 1438
Motor evoked potentials, in intramedullary spinal cord tumor surgery, 2101–2102
Motor function, after corpus callosotomy, 1355
  after open cordotomy, 1565, 1567
  in syringomyelia, 2121
Mucocele, of frontal sinus, 19
  of orbit, 179t
Multilobar resection, 1323–1338
  anesthesia in, 1333
  clinical management for, 1325–1326
  complications of, 1334, 1337
  management after, 1337
  patient selection for, 1326, 1331, 1332t, 1337–1338
  preoperative evaluation for, 1324–1326, *1325–1331*
Multiple sclerosis, retrogasserian glycerol rhizolysis in, 1523, 1532–1533
  trigeminal neuralgia in, percutaneous rhizotomy in, 1480
Multiple suture craniosynostoses, 145–146, *146*
Muscle(s), after percutaneous trigeminal nerve compression, 1540
  extraocular, injury to, orbital surgery and, 234
  paralysis of, after percutaneous rhizotomy, 1477, 1477t
  resection of, in spasmodic torticollis, 1651
  transfer of, in facial nerve palsy, 2156, *2157*
  Muscle cone, orbital, 185, 186, 217
    dissection of, in anteronasal approach, 228
    in lateral orbitotomy, 226
    palpation of, 221
    visualization of, 218–219

Mutism, akinetic, postoperative, in difficult aneurysm, 1052
Mycobacterium tuberculosis, 1689–1702. See also *Tuberculoma.*
Myeloencephalocele, 149
Myelography, in arteriovenous malformation, 2041
  in intramedullary tumor, 2028
  in lumbar spinal stenosis, 1958
  in spinal metastases, 1982
  in syringomyelia, 2122
Myelomeningoceles, 2055–2063
  in neonate, 1258
  kyphoscoliosis in, 1965, 1966
  late tethering in, 2063
  placode of, 2057, *2059*
  postnatal care in, 2056
  preoperative configurations of, *2058*
  surgery for, 2057–2061
    care after, 2062
    dissection in, 2057, *2058–2060*
    skin closure in, 2057, *2059, 2061*, 2062, *2062*
  survival with, 2055–2056
  triage of, 2056
Myelopathy, cystic. See *Syringomyelia, non–hindbrain-related.*
  spondylotic, 1810–1815
    cervical, disc excision in, 1783–1784, 1789–1790. See also *Spondylosis, cervical.*
    clinical manifestations of, 1810
    diagnosis of, 1810–1811
    incidence of, 1810
    pathogenesis of, 1810
    surgery for, posterior approach to, *1785–1814*, 1811–1813
      complications of, 1813–1814
      results of, 1814–1815
Myelotomy, longitudinal, in spasticity, 1665
Myoblastoma, nerve involvement in, 2191
Myomectomy, in facial nerve palsy, 2156
Myositis ossificans, 2191
Myxoma, of jugular foramen, 871–872, *872*
  vs. neurinoma, 872

Naming, in electrical eloquent cortex mapping, 1318–1319, *1319*, 1320
Nasal bone, 214
  thickness of, 38, *38*
Nasal encephalocele, 152, *155*, 156, 157, *157*
Nasal glioma, 157, *157*
Nasociliary nerve, 186, *186*, 197
Nasoethmoidal encephalocele, 150, *150*, 152, *153, 155, 156*
Nasoethmoidal encephalomeningocele, 159, *160*, *162*. See also *Encephalomeningocele(s), frontoethmoidal.*
Nasofrontal encephalomeningocele, 159, *160*, 161. See also *Encephalomeningocele(s), frontoethmoidal.*
Nasolacrimal ducts, obstruction of, in frontoethmoidal encephalomeningocele, 164
Nasomaxillary buttress, 28
Naso-orbital encephalocele, 152, *153, 154*
Naso-orbital encephalomeningocele, 159, *160*, *162*. See also *Encephalomeningocele(s), frontoethmoidal.*
Nelson's syndrome, 303, 319
  Gamma Knife surgery for, 684
  stereotactic radiosurgery in, 349, *349*
Neocerebellum, 802
Neonate. See also *Children.*
  Chiari II malformation in, 1260–1262, *1261*

Neonate *(Continued)*
  craniotomy in, 1255, 1257
  Dandy-Walker malformation in, 1260
  ependymoma in, 576
  frontonasal encephalocele in, 1259–1260
  head trauma in, 1258
  hydrocephalus in, 1257, 1258
  hypothermia in, 1255
  intraventricular hemorrhage in, 1257–1258
  low-grade glioma in, 575–576
  myelomeningocele in, 1258
  neurosurgical procedures in, 1255–1262
    intraoperative considerations in, 1255, 1257
    patient position for, 1255, *1256*
  occipital encephalocele in, 1258–1259, *1259*
  supratentorial tumors in, 575–576
  vein of Galen malformation in, 1258
  venipuncture sites in, 1255
Nephritis, shunt, 1253
Nerve(s), anatomy of, 2159–2161
  cranial. See *Cranial nerve(s).*
  epidermoid cyst compression of, 2193
  glycerol effects on, 1533–1534
  hemangioma involvement of, 2192
  hemangiopericytoma involvement of, 2192
  injury to, orbital surgery and, 234
  lipohamartoma involvement of, 2192, *2193*
  lipoma involvement of, 2192
  lymphangioma involvement of, 2191
  myoblastoma involvement of, 2191
  of scalp, 3
  peripheral, adrenal medullary tissue grafting with, 1372
    anatomy of, 2159–2161
    elongation of, 2166
    grafting of, 2168–2169
    healing of, 2162–2163
    lesions of, classification of, 2161
      closed, 2163
      continuity loss in, 2165–2166
      delayed, 2163–2164
      diagnosis of, 2163–2164
      DREZotomy in, 1626–1628, *1629*
      fibrosis in, 2165
      in continuity, 2165
      neuroma formation in, 2166
      nontraumatic, 2164
      open, 2163
    surgery for, 2166–2170
      care after, 2170
      elongation in, 2167
      nerve grafting in, 2168–2169
      neurorrhaphy in, 2166–2167
      neurotization in, 2169–2170
      palliative, 2170–2171, 2170t
      short cut in, 2167–2168
      substitute grafting in, 2169
      treatment of, 2164–2165
    monofascicular pattern of, 2160
    oligofascicular pattern of, 2160
    passive movements of, 2160–2161, *2160, 2161*
    polyfascicular pattern of, 2160
    regeneration of, 2162–2163
    wallerian degeneration of, 2162
  radial osteoma compression of, *2194*
  regeneration of, 2162–2163
Nerve growth factor, in CNS chromaffin cell transplantation, 1372
Nerve root, in lumbar disc surgery, 1917–1922, *1919, 1920*, 1935
Nerve root block, diagnostic, in sciatica, 1587
Nerve trunk, 2160
Nervus intermedius, 1464, *1551*, 1552
Neural sheath, tumors of, 2183–2188, *2186, 2187, 2189*

Neural sheath *(Continued)*
  malignant, 2194–2195, 2194t, *2195*
Neurapraxia, 2161
Neurinoma, orbital, computed tomography of, 207
  supraorbital approach to, 209–211, *209–211*
  vs. myxoma, 872
Neurocranial capsule, growth of, 135
Neurocysticercosis. See *Cysticercosis.*
Neuroendoscopy, anesthesia for, 703
  bipolar coagulation in, 698, *700*
  camera systems in, 699, *700*
  coronal approach for, 700–701, 701t, 703, *703*
  documentation for, *702*
  hemostasis in, 696–697, *698, 699*
  in brain abscess, 706, *706, 707*, 710, *711*
  in cerebral hematoma, 707, *707*
  in cerebrospinal fluid leak repair, 128
  in chronic subdural hematoma, 707, *710*
  in cystic intracerebral lesions, 704–706, *705, 707, 709*
  in intracerebral hematoma, 706
  in septated chronic subdural hematoma, 706
  in stereotactic brain biopsy, 704, *704, 705, 707, 708*
  in stereotactic exploration, 706
  in syringomyelia, 706–707, 710, *712*
  in third ventriculostomy, 703–704, *703*, 707
  instrumentation for, 695–700, *696*, 696t, *697–701*
  intraluminal ultrasound in, 698–699, *700*
  lasers in, 696–697, *698*
  microforceps in, 696, *697, 698*
  team positions for, *701*
  ventriculoscopic technique for, 700–701, 701t, 703, *703*
Neurofibroma, dumbbell, in myelomeningocele, 2065
  in von Recklinghausen's disease, 2184, *2184*, 2188, *2191*
  orbital, 178t, 179t, 187
    excision of, 190, *191*
  plexiform, 2188, 2188t, 2191, *2192*
  solitary, 2188, *2189*
Neurofibromatosis, magnetic resonance imaging in, 255
  perineural arachnoidal gliomatosis in, 255
  thoracic meningoceles in, 2063
  vs. optic nerve glioma, 262–263
Neurogenic claudication, 1957–1958. See also *Lumbar spine, stenosis of.*
Neurologic function, after brainstem tumor surgery, 781–782, 781t, 782t
  after lateral ventricle tumor resection, 736
  after suboccipital transmeatal acoustic neuroma removal, 837
  in cervical disc herniation, 1809
  in closed head injury, 48
  in difficult aneurysm, 1052
Neuroma, acoustic, 813–826, 829–830
    arachnoid in, 814–815
    bilateral, 839–840
    facial nerve in, 814, *815*
    Gamma Knife surgery for, 681–682, *681*, 681t, *682*
    hydrocephalus in, 830
    in elderly patients, 839
    in only-hearing ear, 839
    recurrence of, 835–836, 838–839
    suboccipital transmeatal approach to, 829–840
      cerebrospinal fluid leak after, 836
      closure for, 834–835
      cochlear nerve function in, 838–839
      complications of, 836–837
      electrocochleography in, 838

Neuroma *(Continued)*
    facial nerve in, 833, *833, 834*, 837–838, 837t
    headache after, 837
    hearing preservation in, 831–833, *833*
    hematoma after, 836
    hydrocephalus after, 836
    incision for, 831, *831, 832*
    large tumor removal in, 833–834, *833, 834*
    medical complications of, 837
    meningitis after, 836–837
    monitoring during, 830, *831*
    neurologic disability after, 837
    patient position in, 830–831, *832*
    perioperative medical therapy in, 830
    plan for, 829
    preoperative hydrocephalus in, 830
    results of, 835–836
    small tumor removal in, 831–833, *833*
    subtotal removal with, 835–836
    wound infection after, 837
  translabyrinthine approach to, 813–826
    advantages of, 813–814, *814*
    anatomy for, 814–815, *815*
    anesthesia for, 815–816
    anterior quadrant dissection in, 822
    arachnoid incision for, *818*, 819
    cerebrospinal fluid rhinorrhea after, 825
    closure for, 823
    complications of, 825
    disadvantages of, 813
    extension of, 824
    facial nerve in, 819–821, *820*, 822–823, *826*
    facial paralysis after, 825
    goals of, 826
    gutting technique of, 821
    hematoma after, 825
    hemostasis in, 823
    lower quadrant dissection in, 821
    meningitis after, 825
    mortality of, 826
    patient position for, 816, *816*
    posterior quadrant dissection in, 822
    postoperative management of, 824–825
    results of, 825–826
    scalp incision for, 816, *817*
    translabyrinthine dissection in, 817–818, *819*
    tumor removal in, *818–820*, 818–821
    upper quadrant dissection in, 821, *822*
    vs. posterior fossa operation, 826
  unilateral, 839
  formation of, 2162
  in peripheral nerve injury, 2166
  glycerol effects on, 1534
Neuronavigator, in low-grade glioma, 563, *565*
Neuronitis, vestibular, vs. Ménière's disease, 1548
Neuroparalytic edema, after temporal lobectomy, 1313
Neuroparalytic keratitis, orbital surgery and, 234
Neuropsychological testing, in intracranial glioma, 519–521
  in lateral ventricle tumors, 726
Neurorrhaphy, 2166–2167
Neurostimulation, in spasticity, 1661
Neurotization, by nerve to muscle, 2169
  by nerve transfer, 2169–2170
Neurotmesis, 2161
Neurotomy, in spasticity, 1662, *1663–1665*
Neurotropism, of Schwann cells, 2162
Neurovascular decompression, 1457–1466
  in fifth cranial nerve dysfunction, 1459–1463, *1461*

Neurovascular decompression *(Continued)*
  in ninth cranial nerve dysfunction, 1464–1466, *1465*
  in seventh cranial nerve dysfunction, 1463–1464
Nicardipine, in aneurysmal subarachnoid hemorrhage–associated vasospasm, 945
Nimodipine, in aneurysmal subarachnoid hemorrhage, 945, 947t, 959
Nitrosourea therapy, for recurrent glioma, 539
Norepinephrine (Levophed), in closed head injury, 60
Normal-pressure hydrocephalus, 1247–1248
Normothermia, after closed head injury, 63
Nose, in Apert's syndrome, 142
  reconstruction of, in sella repair, 329
Nystagmus, after vestibular nerve section, 1554

Obsessive-compulsive disorder, capsulotomy in, 1443–1454, 1450t, *1451–1453*
  clinical criteria for, 1414
  subcaudate tractotomy in, 1415–1417, *1416*
Occipital artery, 76
  in scalp replantation, 11
Occipital artery–middle cerebral artery bypass, 921
Occipital artery–posterior inferior cerebellar artery bypass, 924–925, *926*
Occipital artery–posterior internal cerebellar artery bypass, 924–925, *926*
Occipital encephalocele, 150–151, *151, 152*
Occipital lobe, disconnection of, in functional hemispherectomy, 1345
Occipital nerve, 76
Occipital vertebra, 1720
Occipitoatlantoaxial joints, 1720
Occipito–C1-C2 arthrodesis, 1842–1843, *1843, 1844*
Occipitoparietal area, depth electrode implantation for, 1280
Octreotide (Sandostatin), in growth hormone–secreting pituitary adenoma, 306–308
  in recurrent adenoma, 319
  side effects of, 307–308
Oculomotor foramen, 185, *185, 186*, 206, *206*
Oculomotor nerve, 186, *186*, 197
  of lateral sellar compartment, 479, *480*, 481
  paralysis of, optic nerve sheath fenestration and, 249
  supraclinoid carotid artery aneurysm and, 1003, 1004
  vascular relationships of, 1457
Odontoid process, dysgenesis of, 1719
  screw fixation of, 1864–1866, *1865, 1866*
Olfactory groove, meningioma of, 393–401
  asymptomatic, 400
  blood supply of, 393
  clinical presentation of, 393
  ethmoid sinus invasion by, 398
  olfactory nerve in, 393, *399*
  radiologic evaluation of, 393–394, *394, 395*
  recurrence of, 400
  surgical anatomy of, 393
  surgical approach to, bifrontal, 395–398, *396–398*
    complications of, 400
    general aspects of, 394–395
    results of, 400
    unilateral, 398–400, *399*
Olfactory nerve, in craniopharyngioma removal, 364
  in olfactory groove meningioma, 393, *399*
  in sclerosteosis, 2142–2143

Oligodendroglioma, 518, 549. See also *Glioma, intracranial, low-grade.*
  interstitial brachytherapy for, 664
  lateral ventricle, 726, *728*
  presentation of, 518t
  volumetric stereotactic resection of, *629, 630,* 631
Omental grafting, for brain revascularization, 924
Omohyoid muscle, transfer of, in facial nerve palsy, 2156
Onion whorl disease, 2193–2194
o,p'-DDD (Mitotane), in Cushing's disease, 319
Ophthalmic artery, anatomy of, 185, 196, *197,* 206, *206,* 240–241, *241*
  aneurysm of. See also *Aneurysm(s), paraclinoid.*
    case report of, 996, *997, 1000,* 1001
    surgery for, 964, 1044–1045, 1050
Ophthalmic nerve, 206, *206*
Ophthalmic vein, 185, 196, *197,* 206–207, *206*
  visualization of, 218
Ophthalmoplegia, postoperative, orbital tumor excision and, 212
Opiates, receptors for, 1431–1432
OPLL. See *Ossification of posterior longitudinal ligament (OPLL).*
Optic canal, 196, 206
  decompression of, in sclerosteosis, 2145
Optic chiasm, glioma of, 765–769, *766–770*
Optic disc, swelling of, 238, *238*
Optic foramen, *214*
Optic nerve, anatomy of, 183–184, *184, 197,* 206, *206,* 239–241, *241*
  astrocytoma of, 187, 257–265, *259–261, 265*
  glioma of, 153–277. See also *Optic nerve glioma.*
  in craniosynostosis, 136
  in Gamma Knife surgery, 680
  in sclerosteosis, 2142
  in tuberculum sellae meningioma, 403
  intraoperative injury to, 322
  intratumor resection between, 432–433, *432, 433*
  lesions of, after percutaneous trigeminal rhizotomy, 1544
  medial approach to, for intraorbital tumor excision, 189–190, *189, 190*
  medial superior approach to, 186, *186*
  membranes of, 184, *184*
  meningioma of, 187, 190
  tumor of, fronto-orbital temporal approach to, 197–199, *198*
    lateral microsurgical approach to, 199–200, *200*
    pterional approach for, 201–202, *202*
    surgical excision of, 188–190, *188–190*
  vascular relationships of, 240–241, *241,* 1457
Optic nerve glioma, 253–277
  as hamartoma, 227, 256–258
  as neoplasm, 256–258
  bilateral, 255
    in von Recklinghausen's disease, 263
  calcifications with, 253–254
  case reports of, 256–258, *257–260*
  computed tomography of, *207,* 254–256
  cystic fluids in, 270–271
  excision of, 187
  growth of, 253, 269
    case reports of, 256–258, *257–260*
    exophytic, surgical management of, 271–275, *271–274*
    silver impregnation of nucleolar organizing regions in, 261–262
    variability in, 258–262, 262t
  hemorrhage into, 255–256

Optic nerve glioma *(Continued)*
  hypothalamic invasion of, surgical management of, 275, *275*
  in children, 178t
  magnetic resonance imaging of, 254–256
  multicentric, 187
  perineural arachnoidal gliomatosis in, 255
  progression of, 267t, 268t, 269t
  radiation therapy for, 260, *262,* 276–277
  recurrence of, 260, *262,* 267t, 268t, 269t
  regression of, 263, 265–266
  supraorbital approach to, 209–211, *209–211*
  surgical excision of, 188–190, *188–190*
  surgical management of, 227, 269–276, *271–275*
    cystic component in, 270–271
    edema in, 270
    exophytic tumor growth in, 271–275, *271–274*
    hemorrhagic component in, 270–271
    hypothalamic invasion in, 275, *275*
    pitfalls of, 270
  survival with, 260, *262*
  unilateral, 266–270, 267t, 268t, 269t
  visual evoked potentials in, 256, 277
  vs. craniopharyngioma, 270
  vs. meningioma, 254
  vs. neurofibromatosis type I, 262–263
Optic nerve sheath, fenestration of, pseudotumor cerebri management with, 242–250
  anesthesia for, 241
  case reports of, 247–248
  central retinal artery occlusion with, 248, 248t
  complications of, 248–249, 248t
  instrumentation for, 241–242, *242*
  lateral approach in, *244,* 246–247
    bone flap with, 247
  medial approach in, 242–246, *243*
  patient selection for, 238–239, *240*
  results of, 249–250, 250t
  lateral approach to, for fenestration, 242–246, *243*
  medial approach to, for fenestration, 242–246, *243*
  meningioma of, 185
    computed tomography of, *207*
    excision of, 190
    magnetic resonance imaging of, *208*
    supraorbital approach to, 209–211, *209–211*
Optic strut, 196
Optic tract, glioma of, *771, 773*
Orbit, anatomy of, 183, *183,* 196–197, *196–198,* 213–217, *214–217*
  anterior approach to, 220, 220t
  anteroinferior approach to, 216
  apex of, 213–214, *216*
  arteriovenous shunt of, 179t
  central surgical space (intraconal space) of, 215, 226, *227, 227*
  computed tomography of, 219
  cystic lesions of, 226
  edema of, orbital surgery and, 235
  exenteration of, in anterior skull base tumor resection, 423, 424
  floor of, 213, *215*
  lateral approach to, 215–216, 220, 220t
    for neurofibroma excision, 190, *191*
  lateral wall of, 214, *217*
  magnetic resonance imaging of, 219–220
  medial wall of, 216–217
  meningioma of, suction removal of, 227
    vs. optic nerve glioma, 254
  muscle cone of, 217
    dissection of, in anteronasal approach, 228
    in lateral orbitotomy, 226

Orbit *(Continued)*
  palpation of, 221
  visualization of, 218–219
  penetrating injury to, cerebrospinal fluid leak and, 100–101
  periorbita of, 214
  peripheral surgical space of, 214–215, 226
  rims of, 213
  roof of, 213
    in anterior orbitotomy, 231
    intraoperative plastic reconstruction of, 211, *212*
  soft tissue of, 205
  subperiosteal space of, 214
  superior approach to, 220, 220t
  surgical anatomy of, 196–197, *197, 198,* 206–207, *206,* 213–217, *214–217*
  surgical approaches to, 220–223, 220t
  surgical spaces of, 214–215
  Tenon's space of, 215
  tumors of, 179t, 195–202, 205–212
    classification of, 195–196
    clinical features of, 195–196
    debulking of, 227
    diagnosis of, 207–208, *207, 208*
      complications of, 217
      computed tomography in, 219
      contrast dyes in, 217–218
      contrast orbitography in, 218–219
      conventional radiography in, 218
      corticosteroids in, 220
      magnetic resonance imaging in, 219–220
      orbital venography in, 218
    extraconal, 196
    intracanalicular, 196
    intraconal, 196
    preoperative evaluation of, 196
    recurrence of, 235
    surgery for, 195–202, 220–223, 220t
      anterior approach in, 220, 220t, 229–232, *229–233*
        closure for, 232
        inferior incision for, 231, *232*
        superior incision for, 229, *229*
      anteromedial micro-orbitotomy approach in, 200–201, *201*
      anteronasal approach in, 227–228, *228*
      bone incisions in, 233–234
      complications of, 233–235
      contraindications to, 221
      dural injury in, 234
      enophthalmos in, 235
      foreign body reaction in, 235
      fronto-orbital temporal (transcranial) approach in, 197–199, *198,* 208–209, 208t, 209t, 211
      indications for, 221
      infection in, 235
      instrumentation for, 221
      lacrimal gland injury in, 234
      lateral approach in, 220, 220t, 221, *222*
      lateral canthotomy in, 221
      lateral microsurgical approach in, 199–200, *200*
      lateral orbitotomy in, 221, 223–229, *223–228*
      muscle injury in, 234
      nerve injury in, 234
      pterional approach in, 201–202, *202*
      skin incisions in, 233
      superior approach in, 220, 220t
      supraorbital approach in, 209–211, *209–211*
      tissue reaction in, 235
      transcranial approach in, 197–199, *198,* 208–209, 208t, 209t, 211–213, *212*

Orbit *(Continued)*
vascular damage in, 235
visual loss in, 235
surgical anatomy for, 196–197, *197, 198,* 206–207, *206*
unroofing of, for intraorbital tumor excision, 189, *189*
veins of, visualization of, 218
Orbital fissures, 206, *214–216*
Orbital venography, 218
Orbitography, contrast, 218–219
Orbitotomy, anterior, 229–232, *229–233*
lateral, 221, *222,* 223–229, *223–229*
Orotracheal intubation, in closed head injury, 48
Orthopedic surgery, in spasticity, 1666–1667
Os odontoideum, 1719–1720
Ossiculum terminale, 1719, 1721
Ossification of posterior longitudinal ligament (OPLL), 1817–1828
classification of, 1819, *1819*
clinical features of, 1817–1818
computed tomography of, 1819, *1823*
conservative treatment for, 1820
diagnosis of, 1819–1820, *1819*
electrophysiologic investigation of, 1819–1820
laboratory examinations in, 1818–1819
magnetic resonance imaging of, 1819, *1820, 1823*
neurologic status in, 1820
pathology of, 1817, *1818*
prevalence of, 1817
surgery for, 1820–1831
anterior approach to, 1820–1825, *1822, 1823*
bone extrusion after, 1824
complications of, 1824
indications for, 1824–1825
results of, 1822, 1824, 1824t
cerebrospinal fluid leakage after, 2050
patient selection for, 1820–1821
posterior approach to, 1825
tension-band laminoplasty in, 1825–1827, *1825, 1826*
results of, 1827, *1827*
Osteoma, ethmoidosphenoidal, *428*
intraorbital, 187
of radius, *2194*
Osteomyelitis, cranial, 1673–1674
postoperative, orbital surgery and, 235
spinal, 1677–1679, *1678*
Osteopetrosis, 2141. See also *Sclerosteosis.*
Osteosynthesis, bone thickness in, 38–39, *38*
complications of, 40, 42–43, *42, 43*
follow-up for, 42
in frontal skull base fractures, 36, 38–43, *38–43*
in glabellar area fracture, 39–40, *40*
in Le Fort III fracture, 39, *39*
infection and, 40, 42
maxillofacial, 38–43, *38–43*
Osteotomy, in ankylosing spondylitis, 1772
Osteotropism, of tumors, 1981
Otorrhea, 118, 122. See also *Cerebrospinal fluid (CSF), leakage of.*
Oxford-Adams hemispherectomy, 1343–1344
Oxycephaly, 139, 145
Oxytocin, in pregnancy, 1169

p53 gene, in astrocytoma, 266
Pachycephaly, posterior, 139
Pain, amputation, deep brain stimulation in, 1395–1396, *1395*
spinal cord stimulation in, 1407
brachial plexus, deep brain stimulation in, *1395,* 1396

Pain *(Continued)*
cancer, deep brain stimulation in, *1395,* 1396
DREZotomy in, 1619–1620
Gamma Knife surgery in, 690
intraventricular morphine in, 1431–1440, *1433,* 1434t–1435t, 1436t–1437t, *1439*
medullary tractotomy in, 1568–1570
open cordotomy in, 1557–1568. See also *Cordotomy, open.*
percutaneous cordotomy in, 1595–1610. See also *Cordotomy, percutaneous.*
cingulotomy for, 1420, 1425, 1428–1429
efficacy of, 1429–1430, 1429t
classification of, 1595–1596, 1595t
CNS modulation of, 1389–1390
cranial nerve decompression for, 1457–1466
fifth, 1459–1463, *1461*
ninth, 1464–1466, *1465*
seventh, 1463–1464
tenth, 1464–1466, *1465*
deafferentation, 1623
DREZotomy for, 1623–1636
anatomy in, 1623–1625, *1624, 1625*
impedance measurement in, 1635
indications for, 1625–1628, *1626–1628*
intraoperative evoked potential recording in, 1635
management after, 1634
patient selection for, 1625–1628, *1626–1628*
preoperative evaluation in, 1628–1629
results of, 1635
technique of, 1629–1634, *1630, 1632–1634*
deep brain stimulation for, 1389–1397
complications of, 1397, 1401
electrode configuration in, 1400
in amputation, 1395–1396, *1395*
in anesthesia dolorosa, *1395,* 1396
in brachial plexus lesions, *1395,* 1396
in cancer, *1395,* 1396
in failed low back surgery syndrome, *1395,* 1396
in neuropathy, 1396–1397
in peripheral nerve lesions, *1395,* 1396
in spinal cord lesions, *1395,* 1396
in thalamic lesions, *1395,* 1396
patient selection for, 1390–1391, 1399
postcordotomy, *1395,* 1396
postherpetic, *1395,* 1396
results of, 1393–1397, 1394t, *1395,* 1400–1401
technique of, 1391–1393, *1392, 1393,* 1399–1400
DREZotomy for, 1613–1621, 1623–1636
anatomy for, 1615–1616, *1616*
indications for, 1619–1620
rationale for, 1613, 1613–1614
technique of, 1616–1618, *1616–1618*
facial. See also *Trigeminal neuralgia.*
atypical, DREZotomy in, 1633–1634, *1633, 1634*
percutaneous rhizotomy in, 1480–1481
frontal lobe lesions for, 1420
hypothalamic stimulation in, 1390
in syringomyelia, 2120–2121, 2136
lancinating, 1597
lumbar sympathectomy for, *1644,* 1644–1645, *1645*
medullary tractotomy for, 1568–1570
neuropathic, deep brain stimulation for, 1391, 1396–1397
nociceptive, deep brain stimulation for, 1391
open cordotomy for, 1557–1570. See also *Cordotomy, open.*
percutaneous cordotomy for, 1595–1610. See also *Cordotomy, percutaneous.*

Pain *(Continued)*
phantom limb, DREZotomy in, 1631
postcordotomy, deep brain stimulation for, *1395,* 1396
postherpetic, abdominal, *1627*
deep brain stimulation for, *1395,* 1396
DREZotomy in, 1626, *1627,* 1631–1632
facial, *1628*
postrhizotomy, DREZotomy in, 1626–1627
post-thoracotomy, DREZotomy in, 1626–1627
recurrence of, after open cordotomy, 1566–1567
septal area stimulation in, 1390
spinal cord, deep brain stimulation for, *1395,* 1396
spinal cord stimulation for, 1403–1409
background of, 1403–1404
computerized methods for, 1407, 1409, *1409*
electrode design for, 1404, *1404, 1405*
implanted pulse generator for, 1405, *1405*
indications for, 1406–1407
results of, 1407, *1407,* 1408t
screening protocols for, 1405–1406
splanchnicectomy for, 1641–1644, *1641–1644*
sympathectomy for, 1573–1582, 1637–1645. See also *Sympathectomy.*
thalamic, deep brain stimulation in, *1395,* 1396
thoracic ganglionectomy for, 1637–1641, *1639, 1640*
Pain reflex, atropine elimination of, 1540
Painful disc syndrome, anterior cervical disc excision in, 1783–1784. See also *Spondylosis, cervical.*
Palatine bone, orbital process of, *214, 216*
pyramidal process of, *217*
Paleocerebellum, 802
Pancoast's syndrome, cordotomy in, 1598, *1599*
Pancreas, autonomic innervation to, 1641
cancer of, pain from, splanchnicectomy for, 1641–1644, *1641–1644*
Pannus, 1731
Papaverine, for aneurysmal subarachnoid hemorrhage–associated vasospasm, 947
Papilledema, in pseudotumor cerebri, 238, *238*
Papilloma, of choroid plexus, 572–573, 726, *727*
Paraclinoid aneurysm, 993–1001
cerebral angiography of, 993–994
computed tomography of, 994
global-type, case report of, 996–1000, *999*
incidence of, 993, 993t
magnetic resonance imaging of, 994
preoperative evaluation of, 993–994
surgery for, 994–996, *1120,* 1122
aneurysm decompression in, 995
aneurysm dissection in, 994–995
bypass in, 995–996
carotid occlusion in, 995
case reports of, 996–1001, *997–1000*
clip application in, 995
craniotomy for, 994
positioning for, 994
results of, 996
Parameningeal arteriovenous malformation, 2047
Paranasal sinuses. See also specific sinuses, e.g., *Frontal sinus.*
anatomy of, 27–28
tumors of, clinical presentation of, 417–418
craniofacial resection for, 415–424, *415,* 418t, *419–423*
radiologic evaluation of, *416,* 417
soft-tissue extension of, *416,* 417
TNM staging of, 418, 418t
Paraplegia, 1667–1669, 1667t, 1668t. See also *Spasticity.*

Paraplegia *(Continued)*
  DREZotomy in, 1626, 1631, *1632*
Parasellar carotid arteries, *480*, 481–483, *482*, *484*
Parasellar osteodural chamber. See *Lateral sellar compartment (cavernous sinus)*.
Paresthesias, after percutaneous trigeminal nerve compression, 1540
Parietal bone, tumor resection from, cranioplasty for, 22, *24*
Parietal lobe, disconnection of, in functional hemispherectomy, 1345
Parietotemporofrontal bone, fracture of, 36
Parinaud's sign, in pineal region tumor, 743
Parinaud's syndrome, 739
  in pineal region tumor, 757
Parkinson's disease, adrenal medullary autografts in, 1372–1373
  central nervous system transplantation in, fetal mesencephalic tissue in, 1361–1367. See also *Fetal mesencephalic tissue, CNS transplantation with.*
  CAPIT evaluation for, 1362–1363
  patient selection for, 1361–1362
  Gamma Knife surgery for, 691
  pharmacologic treatment of, 1361
  symptoms of, 1361
Pedicled rhinotomy, advantages of, 475
  care after, 474
  closure after, 473
  complications of, 474
  for clivus exposure, 469–475, *470–474*
  preparation for, 469, *471*
  results of, 474, *474*
Peduncles, cerebellar, 802
Penis, corpora cavernosa of, *490*
Percutaneous lumbar discectomy, 1927–1933
  indications for, 1927–1928
  laser-assisted, 1930–1932, *1930*, 1930t, 1931t
    results of, 1931–1932
  mechanical, 1928–1929, *1929*
  patient position for, 1928, *1928*
  results of, 1932–1933
  stereotactic techniques for, 1930
  suction techniques for, 1929–1930, *1929*
Percutaneous needling, in syringomyelic cord syndrome, 1761, *1762*
Perfusion pressure, in intracranial aneurysm surgery, 959–960
Pergolide, in growth hormone–secreting pituitary adenoma, 308
Periaqueductal and periventricular gray (PAG-PVG) area, stimulation of, in pain treatment, 1389–1390, 1391–1392, *1392*. See also *Deep brain stimulation.*
Peri-insular hemispherotomy, 1346–1347, *1347*
Perineurium, 2159
Periorbita, 184–185, *184*, *185*
Peripheral nerve(s), adrenal medullary tissue grafting with, 1372
  anatomy of, 2159–2161
  elongation of, 2166
  grafting of, 2168–2169
  healing of, 2162–2163
  lesions of, classification of, 2161
    closed, 2163
    continuity loss in, 2165–2166
    delayed, 2163–2164
    diagnosis of, 2163–2164
    DREZotomy in, 1620, 1632–1633
    fibrosis in, 2165
    in continuity, 2165
    neuroma formation in, 2166
    nontraumatic, 2164
    open, 2163
    pain with, deep brain stimulation for, *1395*, 1396

Peripheral nerve(s) *(Continued)*
    surgery for, 2166–2170
      care after, 2170
      elongation in, 2167
      nerve grafting in, 2168–2169
      neurorrhaphy in, 2166–2167
      neurotization in, 2169–2170
      palliative, 2170–2171, 2170t
      short cut in, 2167–2168
      substitute grafting in, 2169
      treatment of, 2164–2165
  metastatic carcinoma to, 2195–2196, *2195*
  monofascicular pattern of, 2160
  oligofascicular pattern of, 2160
  passive movements of, 2160–2161, *2160*, *2161*
  polyfascicular pattern of, 2160
  regeneration of, 2162–2163
  selective denervation of, in spasmodic torticollis, 1651–1654, *1653*
    technique of, 1652–1654, *1653*
  tumors of, 2183–2196, 2185t, *2186*, *2187*, *2189*
    diagnosis of, 2183, *2184*, 2184t, *2185*
  wallerian degeneration of, 2162
Peritoneal shunt, in pediatric hydrocephalus, 1235
Periventricular gray stimulation, vs. cordotomy, 1596
Peroneal nerve, lesions of, nerve grafting in, 2170t, 2171
  treatment of, 2164–2165
  schwannoma of, *2187*
Personality, capsulotomy and, 1453, *1453*
Petroclival region, transcochlear approach to, 824
Petrosal sinus, inferior, 853
Petrosal venous sinus catheterization, in Cushing's disease, 302
Petrous bone, 814–815, *815*
Phantom limb pain, deep brain stimulation for, 1395–1396, *1395*
  DREZotomy in, 1620, 1631
  spinal cord stimulation in, 1407
Phenobarbital, in pregnancy, 1169
Phenylephrine, in intracranial aneurysm surgery, 961
Phenytoin, in closed head injury, 60
  in pregnancy, 1169
  in transcranial skull base tumor resection, 168
  in tuberculoma, 1695
  metabolic effects of, 386
Physical therapy, in pediatric spinal injury, 2093
Physiotherapy, in spasmodic torticollis, 1650, 1654
Pineal apoplexy, 760
Pineal region, blood supply of, 744–746, 745t, *746*, 747t
  cyst of, 595, *595*
  tumors of, 755–762
    arterial anatomy in, 744–745, 745t, *746*
    biopsy of, 757
    cerebrospinal fluid assay in, 740
    classification of, 756–757, 756t, *757*
    clinical features of, 756–757
    CSF seeding of, 760–761, *761*
    endocrine evaluation in, 740
    Gamma Knife surgery for, 686
    management of, 739–741, *745*
    neuro-ophthalmologic examination in, 740
    pathology of, 756t
    patient evaluation in, 740–741
    preoperative evaluation of, 740, 757, *758*
    radiation therapy for, 741
    stereotactic biopsy of, 757
    surgery for, 743–754

Pineal region *(Continued)*
    anatomy in, 744–746, 745t, *746*, 747t
    anterior transcallosal transventricular trans–velum interpositum approach in, *744*, 750–754, *751–754*
    historical perspectives on, 747
    indications for, 741
    lateral-paramedian infratentorial approach in, *744*, 749–750, *750*, *751*, 751t
    occipital transtentorial approach in, *744*, 747–749, *748*, *749*, 750t
    parietal transcallosal approach in, *748*
    principles of, 743–744, *745*
    supracerebellar approach in, *744*, 755–762, *758–761*
      air embolism in, 760
      arachnoid dissection in, 759
      complications of, 760
      dural opening for, 759, *759*
      hemorrhage after, 760
      history of, 755–756
      instruments for, 759, *761*
      patient position for, *758*
      postoperative management in, 760–762, *761*
      results of, 762, 762t
    symptoms of, 739, 757
    systemic chemotherapy for, 741
    venous anatomy in, 745, *746*, 747t
Pinealoma, ectopic, 269–270
Pineocytoma, Gamma Knife surgery for, 686
  subarachnoid metastases from, 760–761, *761*
Pituitary fossa, enlargement of, in craniopharyngioma, 372
  packing of, in sella repair, 327, *327*–331, *328*, *330–332*
Pituitary gland. See also *Cushing's disease.*
  adenoma of, arachnoidocele and, 335, 337, *337*, *338*
    craniotomy for, 299, 321
    follow-up of, 317–318, 317t
    Gamma Knife surgery for, 682–684, 684t
    growth hormone–secreting, 305–309
      diagnosis of, 306
      dopaminergic analogues in, 308
      follow-up for, 309
      pharmacotherapy of, 306–308
      preoperative octreotide for, 307
      radiation therapy in, 308–309
      somatostatin analogues in, 306–308
      somatostatin-binding sites of, 307
    in Cushing's disease, 301–303
    intrasellar, sellar repair in, 333, *333*, *334*, *343*
    invasive, 285
    magnetic resonance imaging in, 306
    metastatic spread of, 316
    mortality and morbidity of, 297t
    nonfunctioning, 293–299
      diagnosis of, 293–295, *294*, *296*
      medical treatment of, 295
    radiation therapy for, 297
    recurrence of, 297
    transcranial approach to, 295
    transsphenoidal approach to, 295–296, *296*
      complications of, 296–297, 298–299
    prolactin-secreting, 309–311
      diagnosis of, 309–310
      follow-up for, 311
      pharmacotherapy in, 310–311
      radiation therapy in, 311
    recurrent, 315–323
      adrenalectomy in, 319
      biologic aspects of, 315–316, *317*
      endocrinologic examination of, 318
      incidence of, 315, 316t
      magnetic resonance imaging of, 318, *318*

Pituitary gland *(Continued)*
    medical therapy in, 319
    preoperative evaluation of, 318–319, *318*
    radiotherapy in, 319
    surgical treatment of, 320–322, *320–322,* 323t
        results of, 322–323, 323t
    symptoms of, 318
    tumor growth and, 315–316
    stereotactic radiosurgery for, 347–349, *348,* 348t, *349,* 349t, *350*
    suprasellar, sellar repair in, 333–335, *334–336*
    transsphenoidal approach to, 283–289, *285–289*
        cerebrospinal fluid leak in, 288–289
        closure after, 288–289, *288, 289*
        dural window in, 287, *287*
        endonasal approach in, 283–284, *285*
        hemitransfixion incision in, 283, *285*
        hypophysectomy in, 287–288
        sella exposure in, 285
        sellar repair after, 327–344. See also *Sella turcica, repair of.*
        sublabial approach in, 284, *285*
        tumor removal in, 287, *288*
    vs. craniopharyngioma, 372
    craniopharyngioma compression of, 373, *375,* 375
    metastatic carcinoma to, from breast carcinoma, 295
    vs. nonfunctioning pituitary adenoma, 295
    microadenoma of, growth hormone–secreting, 306
        sellar repair in, 331–333, *332, 333*
        transsphenoidal approach to, 287
    tumors of, in pregnancy, 1166–1167
Placode, 2057, *2059*
Plagiocephaly, anterior, 142, 143, 144
    posterior, 139
Planum sphenoidale, tumors of, vs. tuberculum sellae meningioma, 404
Platelet count, stereotactic biopsy and, 640
Pleomorphic xanthoastrocytoma, 574–575
Pneumatocele, in transbasal skull base tumor removal, 427
Pneumocephalus, after intracranial aneurysm surgery, 964
    in cerebrospinal fluid leak, 119
Pneumocephaly, after transcranial skull base tumor resection, 172
Pneumoencephalography, in jugular foramen schwannoma, 867
Pneumonia, after closed head injury, 63–64
    in aneurysmal subarachnoid hemorrhage, 952
Polymethyl methacrylate, in cerebrospinal fluid leak repair, 127
Polytetrafluoroethylene (Medpor), for skull reconstruction, 21, *22*
Pons, diffuse-growing tumor of, 776, 777, *777*
    focal tumor of, *779*
    focal-diffuse tumor of, *778*
    primitive neuroepithelial tumor of, *779*
    pseudofocal tumor of, *779*
Positioning slide, for computer-assisted volumetric stereotactic resection, 620, *621*
Positron-emission tomography, in depth electrode placement, 1277
    in epilepsy, 1313
    in intracranial glioma, 519
    in low-grade glioma, 551
Postamputation pain, deep brain stimulation in, 1395–1396, *1395*
    spinal cord stimulation in, 1407
Postauricular artery, in scalp replantation, 11
Postcordotomy pain, deep brain stimulation for, *1395,* 1396

Posterior cranial fossa, arachnoid cyst of, 792t, 796
    astrocytoma of, 792t, 808–809, *809*
    cerebrospinal fluid leaks of, 126–127
    cysts of, 792t, 796
    Dandy-Walker cyst of, 796
    decompression of, in sclerosteosis, 2148–2150, *2149,* 2151
    dermoid of, 792t, 796
    ependymoma of, 792t, 796, *805,* 808, 810, *810*
    exploration of, in trigeminal neuralgia, 1478, 1479t, 1480t
    glioma of, 792t
    hemangioblastoma of, 792t, 797, *798*
    hematoma of, 69–71
        computed tomography of, 69
        depressed skull fracture with, 70–71
        epidural, 70, 71
        intracerebellar, 70, 71
        operative management of, 69–70
        outcome of, 71
        signs of, 69
        subdural, 70, 71
        symptoms of, 69
    mass lesions of, stereotactic biopsy of, 638
    medulloblastoma of, 792t, 795–796, 809–810, *809*
    transtemporal approaches to, 843–850
        case reports of, 847–849, *848*
        infralabyrinthine, 846
        infratemporal fossa, 847, 850
        middle fossa, *843,* 844, *844,* 849
        middle fossa–infratemporal fossa, 847, *848,* 850
        retrolabyrinthine, *843,* 844–845, *845*
        skull base, *843,* 845–846, *845,* 849
        suboccipital, 843, *843,* 849
        suboccipital-translabyrinthine, 846, *846*
        transcanal, *843,* 845
        transcochlear, *843,* 846–847, *847*
        transcochlear-transotic, 849–850
        transcranial, 849
        translabyrinthine, *843,* 843–844, *844,* 849
        translabyrinthine-suboccipital, 849
    tumors of, adult, 791–799
        diagnosis of, 791–792
        pathology of, 791, 792t
        surgery for, 792–799, *794*
            midline craniectomy in, 793–796, *794, 795*
            patient position for, 792–793, *793, 794*
            supratentorial-infratentorial approach for, 799, *799*
            unilateral craniectomy in, 796–799, *797, 798*
        computed tomography of, 791–792
        differential diagnosis of, 791, 792t
        hydrocephalus in, 792, 793, *794*
        metastatic, 792t, 796–797
        pediatric, 801–811, *809, 810*
            clinical features of, 802–803
            diagnosis of, 803–804, *804, 805*
            hemispheric, 808
            hydrocephalus in, 806–807
            management of, 804–806
            neuroanatomy of, 802
            surgery for, 804–808, *806–808*
                complications of, 810–811
                monitoring during, 806
                patient positioning for, 806, *806*
                technical adjuncts to, 806
            vermian, 808, *808*
Posteroinferior cerebellar artery. See *Cerebellar artery, posteroinferior.*
Posteroinferior triangle, of lateral sellar compartment, *495,* 496, 496t, 508

Posterolateral triangle, of lateral sellar compartment, 495–496, *495,* 496t
Posteromedial triangle, of lateral sellar compartment, *495,* 496, 496t
Postherpetic pain, deep brain stimulation for, *1395,* 1396
    DREZotomy in, 1620, 1626, *1627*
Postmeatal triangle, of lateral sellar compartment, *495,* 496, 496t
Postural headache, in cerebrospinal fluid leak, 119
Prechiasmal syndrome, in tuberculum sellae meningioma, 404
Precocious puberty, pediatric hydrocephalus and, 1240, *1240*
Pregnancy, 1163–1170
    acoustic neuroma in, 1165
    acromegaly in, 1166
    anesthesia in, 1169–1170
    aneurysms in, 1167–1168
    anticoagulants in, 1169
    anticonvulsants in, 1169
    arteriovenous malformations in, 1168
    cavernous angioma and, 1185, *1186*
    choriocarcinoma in, 1167
    coma in, 1170
    Cushing's disease in, 1166
    diabetes insipidus in, 1166–1167
    diagnostic examinations during, 1163
    fetal monitoring in, 1170
    glioma in, 1167
    hemangioblastoma during, 1164–1165
    hyperosmolar therapy in, 1169
    lymphocytic adenohypophysitis in, 1166
    macroadenoma in, 1166
    meningioma during, 1164
    microprolactinoma in, 311
    oxytocin in, 1169
    pituitary tumors in, 1166–1167
    prolactinoma in, 1166
    schwannoma in, 1165
    steroids in, 1169
    tuberculum sellae meningioma during, 404
    tuberous sclerosis in, 1165–1166, 1165t
    tumors during, 1163–1167
    vascular lesions in, 1167–1168
    vegetative state in, 1170
    ventriculoperitoneal shunts in, 1169
    vertebral hemangioma during, 1164
    von Hippel-Lindau disease in, 1165
    von Recklinghausen's neurofibromatosis in, 1165–1166, 1165t
Premature infant, intraventricular hemorrhage in, 1257–1258
Prematurity, hydrocephalus and, 1246
Premeatal triangle, of lateral sellar compartment, *495,* 496, 496t
Pressure-volume index, in hydrocephalus, 1247, 1247t
Primitive neuroectodermal tumors (PNETs), of cerebellum, 801
Primitive neuroepithelial tumors (PNETs), of brainstem, 777
    of pons, *779*
Prinzmetal's angina, sympathectomy for, 1575. See also *Sympathectomy.*
Proatlas, 1719
Proenkephalin A, 1432
Proenkephalin B, 1432
Progesterone, in meningioma, 1164
Prolactin, in craniopharyngioma, 385
    secretion of, in growth hormone–secreting pituitary adenoma, 308
Prolactinoma, follow-up for, 317, 317t
    Gamma Knife surgery for, 684
    in pregnancy, 1166

Prolactinoma *(Continued)*
　transsphenoidal approach to, results of, *297*
　vs. nonfunctioning pituitary adenoma, 293
Pro-opio-melano-cortin, 1432
Propofol, in awake craniotomy, 1317
　in intracranial aneurysm surgery, 964
　in lateral sellar compartment surgery, 497
Proportional callosal grid, for depth electrode placement, 1276–1277
Proptosis, decision tree for, *195*
　in craniosynostosis, 137
　in sclerosteosis, 2141
Prostaglandins, in neoplastic spinal cord compression, 1999
Protein, CSF, after intramedullary spinal cord tumor surgery, 2104
ProtonKnife, 1208–1209, *1209*
Pseudoarthrosis, in ankylosing spondylitis, 1771–1772
Pseudomeningocele, postoperative, in sclerosteosis, 2150
Pseudotumor, orbital, 178t, 179t
Pseudotumor cerebri, 237–250
　diagnosis of, 237–238, *238, 239*, 239t
　evaluation of, 238–239, *240*
　headache in, 250
　incidence of, 237
　optic nerve sheath fenestration for, 242–250
　　anesthesia for, 241
　　case reports of, 247–248
　　central retinal artery occlusion with, 248, 248t
　　complications of, 248–249, 248t
　　instrumentation for, 241–242, *242*
　　lateral approach in, *244*, 246–247
　　medial approach in, 242–246, *243*
　　patient selection for, 238–239, *240*
　　results of, 249–250, 250t
　papilledema in, 238, *238*
　preoperative evaluation of, 239, *240*
　surgical anatomy in, 239–241, *241*
　thirty-degree test in, 239
　visual field perimetry in, 238, 239t
　visual function in, 237–238, *239*, 249–250, 250t
　visual loss in, 237–238, 239t, 249–250, 250t
Psychiatric disorders, 1413–1420, 1423–1430
　amygdalotomy for, 1418–1420, *1419, 1420*
　anterior capsulotomy for, 1443–1454, *1445, 1446*, 1448t, 1450t, *1452, 1453*
　frontal lobe lesions for, 1420
　psychosurgery for, 1413–1420
　　patient selection for, 1413–1415
　stereotactic cingulotomy for, 1424–1426, *1426–1428*, 1429t
　subcaudate tractotomy for, 1415–1417, *1416*
　thalamotomy for, 1418, *1418*
Psychomotor retardation, in craniosynostosis, 136
Psychosurgery, 1413–1420, 1423–1430, 1443. *See also* specific surgeries, e.g., *Capsulotomy, anterior.*
　contraindications to, 1414
　frequency of, 1415
　Gamma Knife, 691–692
　in aggressive conduct disorders, 1416–1420, *1418, 1419, 1420*
　in anxiety disorders, 1443–1454, *1445, 1446*, 1450t, *1451–1453*
　in obsessive-compulsive disorders, 1415–1417, *1416*, 1443–1454, 1450t, *1451–1453*
　in sexual aggression, 1413
　informed consent for, 1414
　patient selection for, 1413–1415
Pterygomaxillary buttress, 28
Pterygopalatine fissure, 217

Ptosis, orbital surgery and, 212, 234
Pulmonary edema, in aneurysmal subarachnoid hemorrhage, 952
Pulmonary embolism, in aneurysmal subarachnoid hemorrhage, 952
　in closed head injury, 64
　optic nerve sheath fenestration and, 249
Pulmonary embolization, computer-assisted volumetric stereotactic resection and, 631
Pulsating boots, in penetrating head injury, 107
Pulse generator, in spinal cord stimulation, 1405, *1405*
Pump, for CSF morphine injections, 1438–1440, *1439*
Pupil, in optic nerve sheath fenestration, 246, 249
　sympathetic fibers of, 1637
Putamen, 1371
　adrenal medullary autografts in, 1372–1373
　fetal mesencephalic tissue transplantation in, 1364–1366, *1365, 1366*
Pyrazinamide, in tuberculosis, 1695t

Quadrantanopsia, after temporal lobectomy, 1313
Quadriplegia, DREZotomy in, 1626
　in ankylosing spondylitis, 1768–1769
Quasimodo complex, in sclerosteosis, 2143
Quinagolide, in recurrent prolactinemia, 319

Radial nerve, entrapment of, 2176–2177, *2176, 2177*
　lesions of, treatment of, 2164
Radiation, vascular effects of, 1205
Radiation necrosis, interstitial brachytherapy and, 665
　vs. recurrent glioma, 519, 536
Radiation therapy. *See also Brachytherapy; Curietherapy.*
　CSF fistula after, 2050
　in anaplastic tumors, 463
　in ankylosing spondylitis, 1766
　in anterior skull base tumor resection, 424
　in arteriovenous malformation, 1177–1178, *1178*
　in brain metastasis, 609, *609*, 611–612
　in children, 389
　in craniopharyngioma, 388–389, 388t
　in Cushing's disease, 303
　in fourth ventricle ependymoma, 796
　in glomus jugulare tumors, 857–858
　in growth hormone–secreting pituitary adenoma, 308–309
　in hypothalamic tumors, 774–775
　in low-grade glioma, 566
　in neoplastic spinal cord compression, 2003, 2003t
　in pediatric brain tumor, 572, 575
　in pediatric cerebellar medulloblastoma, 810
　in pediatric posterior fossa ependymoma, 810
　in pineal region tumor, 741, 744, 761
　in pituitary adenoma, 296, 297
　in posterior fossa medulloblastoma, 795
　in recurrent adenoma, 319
　pediatric spinal deformities and, 1965
　recurrent glioma after, 537
　side effects of, 276–277
　stereotactic, 387
Radicular block, diagnostic, in sciatica, 1587
Radicular pain syndrome, in penetrating injury, 1976, *1977*
Radiculopathy, cervical, disc excision in, 1783–1790, 1788. *See also Spondylosis, cervical.*

Radioisotope, in brachytherapy, 655, 656t
　in interstitial radiation therapy, 457–458, 457t, 463t
Radioisotope cisternography, in normal-pressure hydrocephalus, 1247–1248
Radiosurgery, 667. *See also Gamma Knife surgery.*
　vs. microsurgery, 678–679
Radius, osteoma of, nerve involvement in, *2194*
Ranitidine, after closed head injury, 63–64
Rathke's cleft cyst, 582–583, 592, *593*, 594
　chemical meningitis with, 585, 596
　excision of, 584
　foreign body reaction to, 586
　vs. craniopharyngioma, 372
Raynaud's syndrome, sympathectomy for, 1574. *See also Sympathectomy.*
Rebleeding, after aneurysmal subarachnoid hemorrhage, 948–949, 948t
Receptors, opiate, 1431–1432
Rectus muscle, horizontal, 241
　lateral, 185, *185*
　　in lateral orbitotomy, 221, *223*, 226, 234
　medial, 185, *185*
　superior, 185, *185*, 196
　　transient palsy of, in intraorbital tumor excision, 192
　vertical, 241
Reflex sympathetic dystrophy, DREZotomy in, 1627, 1632
　spinal cord stimulation in, 1407
Reservoir sign, in cerebrospinal fluid leak, 119
Residual interictal epileptiform activity, intraoperative recording of, 1320–1321
Respiration, after carotid endarterectomy, 885
　after cordotomy, 1567, 1598, *1599*
Respiratory failure, in aneurysmal subarachnoid hemorrhage, 952
Reticulospinal tract, *1599*
　ventrolateral, in open cordotomy, 1567
Retina, injury to, optic nerve sheath fenestration and, 249
　venous drainage of, 241
Retinal artery, central, 196
Retractors, for computer-assisted volumetric stereotactic resection, 621
Retrogasserian balloon compression, in trigeminal neuralgia, 1478, 1479t, 1480t
Retrogasserian glycerol rhizolysis, trigeminal nerve, 1478, 1478t, 1480t, 1523–1541
　anatomy for, 1524–1525
　anesthesia for, 1524
　aseptic meningitis after, 1532
　bacterial meningitis after, 1532
　branch selectivity in, 1527–1528
　cistern marking in, 1528, *1528*
　cisternography in, 1525–1526, *1525, 1526*
　complications of, 1530–1532, 1531t, 1532t
　contrast evacuation in, 1527
　CSF drainage in, 1526
　dysesthesia after, 1531, 1531t
　facial sensory disturbance after, 1531
　glycerol injection in, 1527–1528
　herpes activation after, 1532
　history of, 1523
　hypesthesia after, 1531, 1531t
　in multiple sclerosis, 1532–1533
　indications for, 1523–1524
　infectious complications of, 1531–1532, 1532t
　management after, 1528–1529
　mechanisms of, 1533–1534
　morphologic effects of, 1533–1534
　neurophysiologic effects of, 1534
　patient positioning for, 1524
　preoperative evaluation for, 1524

Retrogasserian glycerol rhizolysis *(Continued)*
  reinjection in, 1528
  results of, 1529–1530, *1529t, 1530t*
  technique of, 1524–1528
Retrograde balloon catheter suction decompression, in intracranial aneurysm treatment, 970–971, *970,* 972, *972,* 973–974
Rexed's lamination, 1613, *1613*
Rhabdomyosarcoma, orbital, *178t*
Rheumatoid arthritis, cervical spine abnormalities in, 1731–1741, *1732, 1733, 1739.* See also *Cervical spine, rheumatoid.*
  craniovertebral abnormalities in, 1719–1729, *1720, 1722–1728*
Rhinopharyngeal mucosae, preservation of, in transbasal skull base tumor removal, 427–428, *430*
Rhinopharyngeal tumors, transbasal removal of, 438, 441
Rhinorrhea, 122, 188, 825. See also *Cerebrospinal fluid (CSF), leakage of.*
Rhinotomy, pedicled, advantages of, 475
  care after, 474
  closure after, 473
  complications of, 474
  for clivus exposure, 469–475, *470–474*
  nasal exposure for, 471–472, *473, 474*
  preparation for, 469, 471
  results of, 474, *474*
Rhizotomy, cervical, in spasmodic torticollis, 1650–1651, 1653–1654
  chemical, in spasticity, 1665
  dorsal, in sciatica, 1585–1586
  pain after, DREZotomy in, 1626–1627, 1632
  percutaneous, abscess after, 1544
    complications of, 1543–1546
    hemorrhage after, 1544
    infarction after, 1544
    optic nerve lesions with, 1544
    trigeminal neuralgia treatment with, 1469–1480
      alternatives to, 1477–1480, *1478t, 1479t, 1480t*
      electrode localization for, 1472, 1474, *1475*
      electrode placement for, *1471,* 1472, *1472, 1473*
      herpes simplex after, 1477
      in atypical facial pain, 1480–1481
      in multiple sclerosis, 1480
      lesion production in, 1474, 1476
      motor paresis after, 1477
      needle placement for, *1471*
      ocular side effects of, 1477, *1477t*
      patient selection for, 1469–1470
      recurrence after, 1477
      results of, 1476, *1476t*
      sensory side effects of, 1476–1477, *1476t*
      side effects of, 1476–1477, 1477, *1477t*
      technique of, *1470–1475,* 1470–1476
      vagoglossopharyngeal neuralgia treatment with, 1481–1483, *1481, 1482*
  posterior, in spasticity, 1662, 1664–1665, *1665*
Rib graft, after transbasal tumor resection, 433–435, *434, 435*
Riechert-Mundinger stereotactic instrument, 445–446, *446–451*
Rifampicin, in tuberculosis, *1695t*
Rolandic fissure, 554
Rotation flap, for scalp defect, 5–7, *6, 7*

Sacroiliitis, in ankylosing spondylitis, 1775
Sacrum, agenesis of, *2066,* 2067
Saddle-nose deformity, in frontomaxillary fracture, 38

Sagittal sinus, reconstruction of, 515
  tumor of, 513–515
    classification of, 513
    presentation of, 513
    radiology of, 513
    surgical approach to, 513–515
Sagittal suture, premature fusion of, 139–141, *140, 141*
Saphenous vein bypass, in intracavernous segment aneurysm, 977–979, *978*
  in paraclinoid aneurysm surgery, 996
Saphenous vein graft, in carotid endarterectomy, 884
  in dural sinus laceration repair, 111, 114–115, *114, 115*
  in giant middle cerebral aneurysm, 1116, *1117*
  in superficial temporal artery–saphenous vein–middle cerebral artery bypass, *914,* 915–917, *916*
Sarcoma, neurogenic, 2194–2195, *2194t, 2195*
Scalp, 3, 13
  angiosarcoma of, 17, *17*
  arteries of, 3, 76
  avulsion of, anatomy of, 9
    replantation after, 9–11, *10*
    vessel evaluation in, 11
  congenital aplasia of, 7–8
  defect of, assessment of, 4
    bed of, 4
    free skin grafts for, 4–5, *5*
    reconstruction techniques for, 4–7, *5–7*
    rotation flap for, 5–6, *6, 7*
    size of, 4
    tissue expansion in, 7
    vascularity of, 4
  dermatofibrosarcoma protuberans carcinoma of, 17–18, *18*
  electrical burns of, 9
  expansion of, in scalp reconstruction, 7, *7, 8*
  flaps of, 5–7, *6, 7,* 15, *16, 17*
  innervation of, 3
  laceration of, 8, 13
    diploë drill holes for, 14–15
    flaps for, 15, *16, 17*
    galeal scoring for, 13, *14*
    meshed skin graft for, 14, *14*
    skin grafts for, 13–15, *14*
    tissue expansion for, 15, 17–18, *17, 18*
  meningioma of, 15, *16*
  nerves of, 76
  replantation of, 9–11, *10*
  thermal burns of, 8
Scar, epidural, in lumbar disc surgery, 1935, 1936–1937
Schizophrenia, capsulotomy in, 1447
  psychosurgery in, 1414
Schwannoma, 2183–2188, *2185t, 2186, 2187, 2189*
  ethmoid-sphenoid, 469, *472*
  jugular foramen, 865–872. See also *Jugular foramen, schwannoma of.*
  vestibular. See *Neuroma, acoustic.*
Sciatic nerve, lesions of, treatment of, 2164
Sciatica, diagnosis of, 1587
  dorsal rhizotomy for, 1585–1586
  dorsal root ganglionectomy for, 1585–1592
    complications of, 1590–1591
    contraindications to, 1587
    dysesthesias after, 1590–1591, 1592
    history of, 1585–1586
    patient selection for, 1586–1587
    radicular neurologic deficits after, 1590
    results of, 1589–1590, 1591–1592
    technical complications of, 1590
    technical difficulties with, 1589
    technique of, 1587–1589, *1588–1590*

Sciatica *(Continued)*
  pathophysiology of, 1585
  surgery for, 1941–1956. See also at *Lumbar disc, herniation of.*
Scimitar sacrum, *2066*
Sclerosteosis, 2141–2151
  case studies of, *2146t—2147t*
  clinical features of, 2141–2143, *2142*
  computed tomography in, 2144, *2144, 2145*
  cranial anatomy in, 2143, *2143*
  cranial nerve dysfunction in, 2142–2143, *2142*
  CSF rhinorrhea in, 2143
  deafness in, 2142
  facial palsy in, 2141–2142
  headache in, 2143
  magnetic resonance imaging in, 2144, *2145*
  neurologic features of, 2141–2143
  olfactory nerve dysfunction in, 2142
  optic nerve dysfunction in, 2142, *2142*
  postoperative decompressive laminectomy in, 2150–2151
  Quasimodo complex in, 2143
  radiologic evaluation of, 2143–2144, *2144, 2145*
  spinal root compression in, 2143
  surgery for, 2147–2150
    anesthesia for, 2147
    approaches to, selection of, 2145, 2147
    bone overgrowth after, 2150–2151
    CSF diversion in, 2150
    decompressive laminectomy in, 2150–2151
    frontal decompression in, 2141, 2148, 2151
    instrumentation for, 2147–2148
    patient selection for, 2144–2145, *2145t, 2146t—2147t*
    posterior fossa decompression in, 2148–2150, *2149,* 2151
      bone perforation in, 2148–2149, *2149*
      complications of, 2149–2150
      hemorrhage during, 2149
      results of, 2150
      scalp incision in, 2148
    results of, *2146t–2147t*
  trigeminal nerve dysfunction in, 2142
  vs. osteopetrosis, 2141
Scoliosis, after intramedullary spinal cord tumor surgery, 2104
  pediatric laminectomy and, 1965
Screw fixation, in cervical spine stabilization, 1862–1871. See also *Cervical spine, stabilization of.*
Screw-plate fixation, in cervical spine stabilization, 1867–1868, *1868*
Seashore Rhythm Test, in intracranial glioma, 520
Sedan-Nashold cannula, *643*
Sedation, in closed head injury, 60
Seizures. See also *Epilepsy.*
  after closed head injury, 62–63
  after lateral ventricle tumor resection, 736
  after sphenoid wing meningioma excision, 212
  aneurysmal subarachnoid hemorrhage–associated, 950–951, *950t*
  cerebral cavernous angioma with, 1186–1187, *1187,* 1187t, *1188*
  Gamma Knife surgery for, 692–693
  in intracranial glioma, 518, 551
  in penetrating head injury, 106–107
  in transcranial skull base tumor resection, 168
Selective peripheral denervation, in spasmodic torticollis, 1651–1652
Selegiline (Deprenyl), in Parkinson's disease, 1361
Sella turcica, cerebrospinal fluid leak from, 127
  empty, correction of, 335, 337, *337, 338,* 343
  floor of, closure of, in sella repair, 328, *328, 329*

Sella turcica (Continued)
  ghost, repair of, 337, *338*
  overpacking of, 341, *341*
  repair of, 327–344
    complications of, 340–341, *340*, *341*
    extradural packing in, 330–331, *331*
    extradural-intradural packing in, 331, *332*
    general principles of, 327–329, *327–329*
    in arachnoidal cysts, 337, *338*
    in cerebrospinal fluid leakage, 331, *332*, 339–340
    in cystic craniopharyngioma, 337, 339, *339*
    in empty sella, 335, 337, *337*, *338*
    in functional hypophysectomy, 339, *339*
    in ghost sella, 337, *338*
    in intrasellar adenoma, 333, *333*, *334*
    in pituitary microadenoma, 331–333, *332*, *333*
    in suprasellar adenoma, 333–335, *334–336*
    intradural packing in, 330, *330*
    nasal reconstruction in, 329
    pituitary fossa packing in, *327*, 327–328, *328*
    pituitary fossa reconstruction in, 329–331, *330–332*
    results of, 341–344, 341t, 342t, *343*, *344*
    sellar floor closure in, 328, *328*, *329*
    sphenoidal sinus packing in, 328–329
    transsphenoidal approach to, 283–292, 291t, 292t
      in craniopharyngioma, 289–292, *289*, *290*
      in pituitary adenoma, 283–289, *285–289*
Semicircular canals, 814, *815*
Sendai cocktail, 1122
  in aneurysm surgery, 988
Sensory dissociation, interhemispheric, after corpus callosotomy, 1355
Sensory loss, in syringomyelia, 2121
Sensory-Perceptual Examination, in intracranial glioma, 521
Septal area, stimulation of, in pain treatment, 1390
Septum pellucidum cyst, 594–595, *594*
Sexual dysfunction, after open cordotomy, 1567
Shock waves, in penetrating head injury, 90
Shunt, antisiphon devices of, 1239
  atrial, in pediatric hydrocephalus, 1235
  cerebrospinal fluid, in cerebrospinal fluid leak repair, 128
  CSF, in sclerosteosis, 2150
  infection of, in pediatric hydrocephalus, 1236–1238, *1237*, 1237t
    risk factors for, 1238
    treatment of, 1238
  lengthening of, 1249
  lumbar, spinal complications of, 1966, *1967*
  malfunction of, 1238–1240, *1239*, *1240*
  obstructions of, 1239, *1239*
  peritoneal, in pediatric hydrocephalus, 1235
  valves of, malfunction of, 1239
  ventricular, in neonate, 1257
    malfunction of, 1252, 1252t
    obstruction of, 1252
  ventriculoatrial, in adult hydrocephalus, 1249
    in pediatric hydrocephalus, 1234–1235
    infection of, 1253
  ventriculoperitoneal, in pediatric hydrocephalus, 1233–1234
  ventriculopleural, in pediatric hydrocephalus, 1235
  visual complications of, 1239–1240
Shunt nephritis, 1253
Shunt tap, 1237, *1237*
Shunt tape, 1239
Sigmoid sinus, depressed fracture over, 71
  sacrifice of, in lower basilar aneurysm surgery, 1093, *1093*

Silver impregnation of nucleolar organizing regions, in optic nerve glioma growth, 261–262
Siphon segment, of intracavernous carotid artery, 494
Skin graft, for scalp defect, 4–5, *5*, 13–15, *14*
Skin pore, midline, in spinal dysraphism, 2072
Skull. See also *Head; Scalp.*
  anatomy of, 18–19
  copper-beaten pattern of, in craniosynostosis, 137
  deformity of, craniosynostosis and, 136. See also *Craniosynostosis.*
  fracture of, 19–25
    cranial bone cranioplasty for, 22, 25, *25*
    depressed, posterior fossa hematoma with, 70–71
    in penetrating head injury, 90
    reconstruction in, 19–25, *22–25*
      indications for, 19
    traumatic nonfistulous aneurysm with, 981
  in sclerosteosis, 2143, *2143*
  layers of, 18
  osteomyelitis of, 1673–1674
  skull base growth and, 135
  thickness of, 38–39, *38*
Skull base. See also *Clivus; Olfactory groove; Sphenoid ridge; Tuberculum sellae.*
  anatomy of, 28
  anterior, fractures of, 27–43
    classification of, 28, *30*
    diagnosis of, 28, 31, *31*
    locations of, 31, *31*
    surgery for, 31–36
      complications of, 40, 42–43, *42*, *43*
      ethmoidal cell system in, 36, *37*
      osteosynthesis in, 36, 38–39
      rhinosurgical approach to, 32–34, *33*, *34*
      transfrontal approach to, 33, 35–36, *35*
  tumors of, 415–424
    preoperative evaluation of, 418, 418t
    recurrence of, 173
    surgical approach to, 418–423, *419–423*
      complications of, 424
      management after, 423
      results of, 424
    transcranial resection of, 167–173, *167*
      closure after, 171–172, *172*
      craniotomy of, 169–170
      dissection of, 168–169
      dura dissection of, 170, *170*
      ethmoidal artery coagulation in, 170
      ethmoidectomy of, 170
      management after, 172–173
      patient position for, 168, *169*
      periorbita dissection of, 170–171, *171*
      pneumocephaly after, 172
      preparation for, 168
      technique for, 168–172, *169–172*
      tissue release of, 171, *171*
  fibrous dysplasia of, transbasal approach to, 434, 438, *438–441*
  growth of, calvarial growth and, 135
  in craniosynostosis, 135–136
  meningioma of, transbasal approach to, 437–438
  reconstruction of, after craniofacial resection, 423, *425*
    after transbasal tumor resection, 433–435, *434–436*
  rhinopharyngeal tumors of, transbasal removal of, 438, 441
  tumors of, invasive, transbasal approach to, 427–441

Skull base (Continued)
  closure for, 435–436
  dermal autograft in, 430, *431*, *432*
  dural defect repair in, 428, 430, *430–432*
  exposure for, 428
  goals of, 427
  hazards of, 427, *428*, *429*
  in bone tumors, 438, *438–441*
  in ethmoidal area, 432
  in meningiomas, 437–438
  in rhinopharyngeal tumors, 438, 441
  in sphenoidal area, 432–433, *432*, *433*
  indications for, 437–441, 437t
  limits of, 436–437, *437*
  meningeal repair in, 428, 430, *430–432*
  pericranial autograft in, 430, *431*
  preoperative preparation for, 427
  rhinopharyngeal mucosae preservation in, *4*, 427–428
  skull base reconstruction in, 433–435, *434–436*
  tumor removal in, 432–433, *432–434*
Sleep apnea, after open cordotomy, 1564–1565
Slow virus disease, transmission of, brain biopsy and, 617
Sniper fire, ballistics of, 82
Sodium, serum, after closed head injury, 63
Sodium nitroprusside, in intracranial aneurysm surgery, 961
Somatosensory evoked potentials, in intramedullary spinal cord tumor surgery, 2101–2102
  in low-grade glioma, 563, *565*
Somatostatin, analogues of, in growth hormone–secreting pituitary adenoma, 306–308
Spasmodic torticollis, 1649–1657. See also *Torticollis, spasmodic.*
Spasticity, 1661–1669
  asymmetrical, 1649
  dorsal root entry zone surgery for, 1665–1666, *1666*
  functional posterior rhizotomy for, 1664–1665, *1665*
  in adults, 1667–1668, 1667t, 1668t
  in children, 1649, 1668–1669, 1669t
  intrathecal baclofen for, 1661
  intrathecal chemical rhizotomy for, 1665
  longitudinal myelotomy for, 1665
  lumbosacral posterior rhizotomy for, 1664–1665, *1665*
  neuroablative procedures in, 1662–1666, *1662–1664*
  neurostimulation for, 1661
  operative indications in, 1667–1669, 1667t, 1668t
  orthopedic surgery for, 1666–1667
  partial posterior rhizotomy for, 1664
  pathophysiology of, 1661
  percutaneous thermorhizotomy for, 1665
  peripheral neurotomies for, 1662, *1662–1664*
  posterior rhizotomies for, 1662, 1664–1665, *1665*
  posterior selective rhizotomy for, 1664
  sectorial posterior rhizotomy for, 1664
SPECT, in epilepsy, 1313
Speech, after temporal lobectomy, 1312
Speech deficit, after transcallosal surgery, 734
Speech Sound Perception Test, in intracranial glioma, 520
S-phase fraction, of tumor, 315–316
Sphenoid bone, greater wing of, *214*, *215*, *217*
  hyperostosis of, 203
  lesser wing of, 214, *214*
  pterygoid process of, *217*

Sphenoid bone *(Continued)*
  reconstruction of, after transbasal tumor resection, 435, *435*
  schwannoma of, 469, *472*
  tumor of, transbasal approach to, 432–433, *432, 433*
Sphenoid ridge, meningioma of, 408–412
  angiography of, 409
  classification of, 408
  clinical presentation of, 408–409
  magnetic resonance imaging of, 409, *409*
  pathologic anatomy of, 408
  surgical approach to, complications of, 412
    patient selection for, 410–411, *411*
    results of, 411–412
Sphenoid sinus, anatomy of, 28
  cerebrospinal fluid leak from, 127
  packing of, in sella repair, 328–329
Sphenoid wing, meningioma of, 201, 203, 211, 212
  tumor of, pterional approach to, 201–202, *202*
Spina bifida. See *Myelomeningoceles.*
Spina bifida occulta, 2069–2079. See also *Spinal dysraphism, occult.*
Spinal accessory nerve, 1107
  branches of, *1653*
Spinal accessory nerve roots, microvascular lysis of, in spasmodic torticollis, 1650
Spinal artery, injury to, in intramedullary spinal cord tumor surgery, 2103
Spinal cord, abscess of, 1677
  arterial systems of, 2038
  arteriovenous malformation of, 2038–2047
    anatomy of, 2038–2040, *2039–2040*
    classification of, 2038–2039, *2039–2041*
    clinical presentation of, 2040–2041, *2042*
    diagnosis of, 2041–2042, *2042*
    diffuse, 2046
    dorsal, long, 2045–2046
    embolization of, 2043
    glomus, 2046
    juvenile, 2044, 2046
    meningeal, 2047
    natural history of, 2040–2041
    parameningeal, 2047
    surgical excision of, 2043–2045, *2043, 2044*
      evoked potentials in, 2041
      results of, 2046–2047
  cavernous angioma of, 1193–1195, *1194*, 1194t
  cervical, hemisection of, 1595
  in open cordotomy, 1558–1560, *1559*
  lesions of, 1831–1837
    blunt trauma and, 1834
    cardiovascular system in, 1833–1834
    diagnostic imaging of, 1834, 1837–1839, *1837–1841*
    DREZotomy in, 1620
    epidemiology of, 1831
    orthotic devices in, 1842
    pain with, deep brain stimulation in, *1395*, 1396
      spinal cord stimulation in, 1407. See also *Spinal cord stimulation.*
    prehospital evaluation of, 1831–1832
    surgery in, 1842–1847, *1843–1846*
    therapy for, 1840, 1842
    traction in, 1832–1833
  tethered, 2069–2079. See also *Spinal dysraphism.*
  tumors of. See *Spinal cord tumors.*
  width of, in open cordotomy, 1559–1560
Spinal cord stimulation, 1403–1409
  advantages of, 1405–1406
  background of, 1403–1404

Spinal cord stimulation *(Continued)*
  computerized methods for, 1407, 1409, *1409*
  disadvantages of, 1406
  electrode configuration in, 1403
  electrode design for, 1404, *1404, 1405*
  implanted pulse generator for, 1405, *1405*
  indications for, 1406–1407
  neurochemical mechanisms of, 1403–1404
  patient evaluation for, 1406
  percutaneous techniques in, 1404, *1404*
  results of, 1407, *1407*, 1408t
  screening protocols for, 1405–1406
Spinal cord tumors, intramedullary, 2027–2038
  case report of, 2037
  clinical presentation of, 2027–2028, 2095–2096, 2105
  computed tomography of, 2096, *2097*
  diagnosis of, 2096–2097, *2097, 2098*
  epidemiology of, 2095
  filum terminale expansion in, 2101
  laser in, 2097, 2099, *2099*
  lower extremity weakness in, 2095
  magnetic resonance imaging of, 2096, *2098*
  myelography of, 1754, *1755*
  radicular pain in, 2095
  scoliosis in, 2096
  segmental location of, 2103
  sensory abnormalities in, 2096
  spasticity in, 2096
  sphincter laxity in, 2096
  surgery for, 1761, *1762, 1763*, 2032–2036, *2034, 2035*, 2097–2102, *2099, 2100*
    anterior spinal artery injury in, 2103
    case report of, 2037
    Cavitron ultrasonic surgical aspirator in, 2035
    closure after, 2101, *2101*
    complications of, 2102–2104
    cystic collections in, 2035–2036
    evoked potentials in, 2101–2102
    hemorrhage after, 2104
    hydrocephalus after, 2104
    incompleteness of, 2103
    instrumentation for, 2097, *2099*
    myelotomy in, *2034–2035*, 2035
    neurologic dysfunction after, 2102–2103
    paraplegia and, 2102–2103
    patient position for, 2033
    radicular pain after, 2037
    results of, 2036–2038, 2037t
    spinal deformity after, 2104
    subarachnoid spinal fluid loculation in, 2103–2104
    technique of, 2097, *2099, 2100*
    treatment after, 2036
    ultrasound during, 2103
    wound dehiscence in, 2101
  surgical pathology of, 2028, *2031–2033*
  upper extremity symptoms in, 2096
  total vs. astrocytoma, 2096–2097, *2098*, 2100
Spinal deformity, pediatric, postoperative, 1965–1968, *1966, 1967*
  cervical, 1965, *1966, 1967*
  in myelomeningocele patients, 1966
  lumbar, 1966, *1967*, 1968
  prevention of, 1966
  radiation therapy and, 1965
  radiologic evaluation of, 1965
  thoracic, 1966, 1968
Spinal dysraphism, conus in, 2069, *2073*
  fawn's tail in, 2072
  incidence of, 2072
  midline skin pore in, 2072
  occult, 2069–2079
    clinical presentation of, 2072–2073

Spinal dysraphism *(Continued)*
  cutaneous abnormalities in, 2072
  diagnosis of, 2073–2074, *2074, 2075*
  filum terminale in, *2070*, 2073, *2073*
  neurologic impairment in, *2070*, 2071–2072
  pathology of, 2069–2072, *2070, 2072*
  radiographic studies in, 2073–2074, *2074, 2075*
  spina bifida occulta in, 2072
  surgery in, 2074–2079, *2076–2079*
    complications of, 2079
    indications for, 2073–2074
    results of, 2079
  vascular impairment in, 2072
  surgical repair of, cerebrospinal fluid leak and, 128–129
Spine. See also *Cervical spine; Lumbar spine; Thoracic spine; Thoracolumbar spine.*
  abscess of, extradural, 1676, *1677*
    intramedullary, 1677
    subdural, 1676–1677
  cysticercosis of, 1713
  in closed head injury, 48–49
  instability of, in neoplastic spinal cord compression, 2004–2006, *2005*, 2005t, 2006t
  neoplastic zones of, 2006–2007, *2007*
  osteomyelitis of, 1677–1679, *1678*
  pediatric, injury to, 2081–2094. See also *Cervical spine, pediatric.*
  penetrating injury to, 1971–1979
    cauda equina injury with, 1974–1975, 1979
    chest injury with, 1973
    classification of, 1971–1972, 1972t
    clinical features of, 1972–1973
    complete deficits with, 1974, *1975, 1976*, 1978–1979
    computed tomography of, 1973, *1973, 1974*
    evaluation of, 1973, *1973, 1974*
    incidence of, 1971
    injury associated with, 1972–1973
    location of, 1972
    missile, 1971, 1972t
    nonmissile, 1971, 1972t
    perioperative considerations in, 1973–1974
    progressive deficit with, 1976
    radicular pain syndrome with, 1976, *1977*
    surgery for, *1975*
      anterolateral approach to, 1978, *1978*
      complications of, 1971, 1979
      dorsal approach to, 1977–1978, *1977*
      indications for, 1974–1976, *1975, 1976*
      instrumentation for, 1977
      lateral extracavitary approach to, 1978, *1978*
      management after, 1978
      neurophysiologic monitoring in, 1977
      results of, 1978–1979
      timing of, 1976–1977
      wound closure in, 1978
    visceral penetration with, 1976
    without radiographic abnormality, 1975–1976
  stability of, in neoplastic spinal cord compression, 2004–2006, *2005*, 2005t, 2006t
  stenosis of. See also *Lumbar spine, stenosis of.*
    in achondroplasia, 2107, 2108, 2110–2111, 2113–2116, *2113–2115*. See also *Achondroplasia.*
    in ankylosing spondylitis, 1780
  three-column concept of, 2004–2005, *2005*
  tuberculosis of, 1678
  tumors of, 1981–1995, 1997–2023, *2002*
    algorithm for, *2002*
    analgesia in, 2003

Spine (Continued)
  brachytherapy in, 2003
  chemotherapy in, 2002
  clinical presentation of, 1981–1982, 1982t
  computed tomography of, *1987*
  corticosteroids in, 2002–2003
  diagnostic imaging of, *1998,* 1998–1999
  grades of, 1982–1983
  in children, 1965
  incidence of, 1981, 1997
  level of, 1997–1998
  neurologic status in, 2001
  pathophysiology of, 1999–2000, *1999*
  pharmacotherapy of, 2002–2003
  radiation exposure and, 2006
  radiation therapy in, 2003, 2003t
  radiologic evaluation of, 1982–1983
  spinal instability in, *2005,* 2005t, 2006, 2006t
  surgery for, 1984–1995, *1984,* 2003–2023, 2004t
    anterior decompression in, 2012–2019
      cervical, 2019, 2021–2023, *2021–2023*
      cervicothoracic stabilization in, 2021, 2023
      lumbar, *2017,* 2018–2019, *2020*
      thoracic, 2012–2013, *2013*
      thoracolumbar, 2018
      vertebral body replacement in, 2014–2015, *2016, 2017*
    approaches to, 2002t, 2006–2007
    bleeding in, 2008, 2012, 2014
    complications of, 2023
    for neurologic salvage, 1983
    for pain relief, 1984
    for stabilization, 1983
    for tissue diagnosis, 1984
    in cancer therapy, 1983
    indications for, 1983–1984, 2004–2006, *2005,* 2005t, 2006t
    Isola system in, 2014–2015, *2016*
    laminectomy in, 1985
    morbidity after, 2023
    mortality after, 2023
    posterior decompression in, 2007–2012, *2007–2012*
      bone grafting in, 2010–2012
      care after, 2012
    preoperative evaluation for, 1984
    transthoracic approach to, 1985–1992, *1986–1993*
    vertebral body resection in, 1985–1992, *1986–1993*
  survival after, 2000
  symptoms of, 1999
    progression of, 2001
  x-ray location of, 2008
Spinothalamic tracts, *1599*
  in open cordotomy, 1558–1559, *1559*
  neuron of, VPL-VPM stimulation inhibition of, 1390
Splanchnicectomy, 1575, 1580, *1581,* 1641–1644
  anatomy for, 1641
  complications of, 1644
  indications for, 1641
  results of, 1644
  technique for, 1641–1644, *1641–1644*
Split notochord syndrome, 2062
Spondylitis, ankylosing, 515–523, 535–541, 1765–1773. See also *Ankylosing spondylitis.*
Spondylodiscitis, in ankylosing spondylitis, 1780
Spondylosis, cervical, 1745–1752, 1791–1802, 1805–1815
  anatomy of, 1786–1787, *1786, 1787*
  anterior cervical disc excision in, 1783–1790

Spondylosis (Continued)
  anatomy for, 1786–1787, *1786, 1787*
  bleeding in, 1788
  Cloward blade position in, 1787, 1788
  complications of, 1788
  esophageal perforation in, 1788
  graft complications in, 1788
  incision for, 1786–1787, *1786, 1787*
  indications for, 1783–1785, *1784*
  retraction-related complications of, 1788
  technique of, 1787–1788
  tracheal perforation in, 1788
  anterolateral cervical disc excision in, 1788–1790
  biomechanical studies in, 1785–1786, *1786*
  computed tomography in, 1786
  diagnostic evaluation of, 1785–1786, *1785, 1786*
  dysphagia in, 1784–1785, *1784*
  magnetic resonance imaging in, 1786
  multisegmental, 1791–1802
    computed tomography in, 1792
    diagnosis of, 1792
    ischemia in, 1792
    magnetic resonance imaging in, 1791, *1791,* 1792
    pathology of, 1791–1792, *1791*
    vertebrectomy in, 1791–1802, *1793, 1794, 1796*
      case reports of, 1796–1798, *1796–1799*
      complications of, 1798–1800
      graft in, 1801
      graft-related problems in, 1800
      Horner's syndrome after, 1800
      indications for, 1792–1793, 1800–1802
      laryngeal nerve palsy after, 1800
      plate selection in, 1801–1802
      posterior longitudinal ligament in, 1801
      results of, 1794–1796, *1796*
      technique of, 1793–1794, *1793, 1794*
      upper airway obstruction in, 1801
  myelopathy in, 1810–1815
    clinical manifestations of, 1810
    diagnosis of, 1810–1811
    differential diagnosis of, 1810
    incidence of, 1810
    nonsurgical treatment for, 1811
    pathogenesis of, 1810
    surgery for, 1811–1815, *1812–1814*
      complications of, 1813–1814
      failure of, 1815
      instability after, 1814
      laminectomy in, 1811–1815, *1812–1814*
      posterior approach to, 1811–1815, *1812–1814*
      results of, 1814–1815
  posterior cervical disc excision in, 1805–1815
    complications of, 1809
    patient selection for, 1806
    results of, 1809
    technique of, 1806–1809, *1807–1809*
  posterior cervical laminectomy in, 1789–1790
  vertebral artery compression in, 1785
Spongioblastoma, polar, 269, 276
Squints, in frontoethmoidal encephalomeningocele, 164
Staphylococcus epidermidis, in chemical meningitis, 585
Steatorrhea, octreotide and, 307
Stellate ganglion block, 1575
Stenosis, aqueductal, in pediatric hydrocephalus, 1245

Stenosis (Continued)
  spinal. See *Lumbar spine, stenosis of.*
Stereoelectroencephalography (stereo-EEG), 1271. See also *Depth electrodes.*
  central, *1331*
  frontotemporal, *1329*
  in drug-resistant epilepsy, 1325, *1325–1331*
  occipitoparietotemporal, *1330*
  temporal, *1326*
  temporoperisylvian, *1327, 1328*
Stereoencephalotome, 443, *444*
Stereomarkers, in low-grade glioma, 563, *565*
Stereotactic biopsy, 446, 451–457, 637–651. See also *Biopsy, stereotactic.*
Stereotactic frame, COMPASS, 619, *620, 621*
Stereotactic instruments, 443–446, *444–451,* 446t
  for computed tomography, 449, *450, 451*
  for magnetic resonance imaging, 452, *453*
  of Hayne and Meyers, 445
  of Horsley-Clarke, 443, *444*
  of Leksell, 445, *445*
  of Lorimer, 445
  of Talairach, 443, *444*
  phantom device of, *448*
  polar coordinate principle of, *447*
  Riechert-Mundinger, 445–446, *446–451*
Stereotactic radiosurgery. See *Gamma Knife surgery.*
Stereotactic radiotherapy, 387, 443–446, *444–451,* 455, 457–465. See also *Brachytherapy; Curietherapy.*
Stereotactic volumetric resection, 619–634, 644–648
  COMPASS system for, 644–648, *644–650*
  computer-assisted, 619–634, 644–648
    accessory instruments for, 621
    arc quadrant for, 620, *621*
    computer system for, 620
    data acquisition in, 621–622, *622*
    fiducial system for, 644, *644*
    hardware for, 620
    head holder for, 619–620, *620*
    heads-up display for, 621
    in cavernoma, 648, *649*
    in contrast-enhancing lesions, 627–628
    in deep lesions, 624–626, *625, 626*
    in glial tumors, 626–627, *627–629,* 631
    in intraventricular lesions, 632, *633, 634*
    in large tumors, 626, *626*
    in low-grade astrocytoma, 631
    in metastatic tumors, 631–632
    in nonenhancing lesions, 628, *629, 630*
    in superficial lesions, 623–624, *624*
    in temporal sclerosis, 648, *650*
    in vascular malformations, 632, *632*
    instrumentation for, 619–621, *620*
    laser for, 621
    methods of, 621–628, *622–630*
    morbidity with, 630–631
    mortality with, 630–631
    patient rotation in, 622–623, *623*
    patient selection for, 626
    planning for, 622
    results of, 628, 630, 630t
    retractor system for, 621, 644, *645*
    software for, 620–621
    stereotactic frame for, 619, *620*
    surgical trajectory in, 622
    three-dimensional positioning slide for, 620, *621*
    viewing image for, *647,* 648
    volume reconstruction in, 622, 645, *645–647*
Stereotaxy, frameless, 650–651, *651*
Sternocleidomastoid muscle, denervation of, in spasmodic torticollis, 1652, *1653*

XXXVI | Index

Sternohyoid muscle, transfer of, in facial nerve palsy, 2156
Sternothyroid muscle, transfer of, in facial nerve palsy, 2156
Sternotomy, median, 1892
Steroids, in brain metastasis, 608–609, 608t
　in penetrating head injuries, 84
　in pregnancy, 1169
Stimulation-produced analgesia, 1389. See also *Deep brain stimulation.*
Strabismus, in craniosynostosis, 137
Streptomycin, in tuberculosis, 1695t
Stress fracture, in ankylosing spondylitis, 1771–1772
Stridor, in myelomeningoceles, 2062
Strip electrodes, 1265–1268
　complications of, 1267–1268
　electroencephalographic monitoring of, 1267
　indications for, 1265
　positioning of, 1266–1267
　technique for, 1265–1266, *1265*
Stryker saw, bone incision with, 233–234
Sturge-Weber syndrome, cerebral hemispherectomy in, 1341, 1342, *1342*
　hemispheric atrophy in, 1342, *1342*
Subarachnoid space, cervical, cerebrospinal fluid drainage from, 129
　dilatations of, in craniosynostosis, 137
　glioma growth in, 271–277, *271–274*
Subchoroidal corridor, in third ventricle transcallosal approach, 717, *718*, *721*
Subclavian artery, stenosis of, 898, 900, *900*
Subclavian artery–saphenous vein–middle cerebral artery bypass, 923
Subclavian steal syndrome, extrathoracic common carotid–subclavian bypass for, *906*, *907*
　extrathoracic common carotid-to-subclavian bypass for, *902*, *906*
　subtraction arch study of, *901*
Subclavian-carotid stenosis, *906*, 907–908
Subependymal giant cell astrocytoma, 574
Subependymoma, of lateral ventricle, 726
Substance P, 1432
Substantia nigra, 1371
Suction, in intraoperative aneurysm rupture, 988
Sulcus (sulci), central, goniometric identification of, 554, *554*, *555*
　cortical, *558*
　vs. arterial impression, *559*
Superficial temporal artery–middle cerebral artery bypass, 909–926, *920*, *921*
　evaluation for, 910–911
　indications for, 909–910
　protocol for, 911, 911t, 912t
　tumor surgery and, 910
Superficial temporal artery–saphenous vein–middle cerebral artery bypass, 911–920, *913–920*
　anesthesia for, 912
　brain protection during, 918
　closure for, 920
　craniotomy for, 913–915, *913*
　distal anastomosis of, *917*, 918
　instrumentation for, 912
　middle cerebral artery branch preparation for, 916
　patient position for, 912
　proximal anastomosis of, 918–920, *919*
　superficial temporal artery preparation for, 912–913, *913*
　vein graft preparation for, *914*, 915–916, *916*, *916*–917
Superficial temporal artery–saphenous vein–posterior cerebral artery bypass, 924
Superior triangle, of lateral sellar compartment, 494–495, *495*, 496t

Supraorbital artery, 3, *76*
　in scalp replantation, 11
Supraorbital nerve, *76*
Supraorbital notch, *214*, *217*
Supraorbital ridge, *214*
Suprascapular nerve, entrapment of, 2175–2176, *2175*
　exposure of, *2175*
　lesions of, treatment of, 2164
Suprasellar abscess, 585
Suprasellar cyst, 581–582, *582*
　chemical meningitis and, 585–586
Suprasylvian region, aneurysm of, 1140–1141, *1142–1143*
Supratentorial tumors, pediatric, 571–576
　benign, 571
　biology of, 571–572
　chemotherapy for, 572
　craniotomy for, 572
　differential diagnosis of, 572
　histology of, 571
　malignant, 571
　radiotherapy for, 572
　resection of, 571
Supratrochlear artery, *76*
Supratrochlear nerve, *76*
Sutures, cranial, fusion of, 135
　premature. See *Craniosynostosis.*
　in penetrating missile injuries of head, 84
Sweating, in syringomyelia, 2121
Sympathectomy, 1573–1582, 1573t. See also *Ganglionectomy; Splanchnicectomy.*
　alcohol, 1578, 1580
　bilateral, 1577
　evaluation of, 1573
　in hyperhidrosis, 1638
　indications for, 1574–1575, 1574t
　interscapular approach to, 1566–1577, *1576*
　lumbar, 1577–1578, *1579*, 1580, 1644–1645, *1644*, *1645*
　　complications of, 1645
　　indications for, 1644
　　results of, 1645
　　technique of, 1644–1645, *1644*, *1645*
　outcome of, 1573, 1581–1582
　phenol, 1578, 1580
　splanchnic, 1580, *1581*
　　indications for, 1575
　supraclavicular approach to, 1577
　thoracic, 1576–1578, *1576*, *1578*
　　indications for, 1574, 1574t
　transaxillary transcostal approach to, 1577
Syndactyly, in Apert's syndrome, 142
　in sclerosteosis, 2141
Syndrome of inappropriate secretion of antidiuretic hormone, in aneurysmal subarachnoid hemorrhage, 951–952, 951t, 958
Syringohydromyelia, 2119
Syringomyelia, 1745–1764, 2119–2136
　classification of, 2119, 2120t
　DREZotomy in, 1631, *1632*
　endoscopic surgery for, 706–707
　　results of, 710, *712*
　non–hindbrain-related, 2119–2136, 2120t
　　autonomic dysfunction in, 2121
　　clinical presentation of, 2120–2122
　　computed tomography in, 2122
　　endomyelography in, 2122
　　hematomyelia in, 2123
　　idiopathic, 2122–2123
　　incidence of, 2119–2120
　　magnetic resonance imaging in, 2122, 2136
　　meningeal fibrosis in, 2119–2120, 2123, 2124, 2135t
　　morphology of, 2123–2124

Syringomyelia *(Continued)*
　　motor loss in, 2121
　　myelography in, 2122
　　neurologic deterioration in, 2121, 2136
　　pain in, 2120–2121
　　radiologic investigations in, 2122
　　sensory loss in, 2121
　　surgery for, case reports of, 2127–2135, *2128–2134*, 2135t
　　　cerebrospinal fluid drainage in, 2126–2127
　　　cerebrospinal fluid shunt in, 2124
　　　cord division in, 2126
　　　decompression in, 2126
　　　drainage in, 2125, *2125*
　　　exploration in, 2125
　　　hydrocephalus valves in, 2125
　　　indications for, 2124
　　　lumbar external drain in, 2127
　　　principles of, 2124–2126
　　　results of, 2135–2136, 2135t
　　　syringosubarachnoid shunt in, 2125–2126
　　　syrinx-to-extrathecal drainage in, 2125
　　　technique of, 2126–2135, *2128–2134*
　　　wound closure in, 2127
　　sweating in, 2121
　　tendon reflexes in, 2121
　　venous pressure in, 2123–2124
Syringomyelic cord syndrome, 1745–1764
　cerebrospinal fluid shunt in, *1762*, 1764
　clinical factors in, 1747
　computed tomography in, *1751–1752*
　diagnosis of, 1747–1755, *1748–1755*
　fourth ventriculostomy for, *1762*
　hydrodynamic theory of, 1745
　magnetic resonance imaging in, *1748–1749*
　myelography in, *1750*, *1753*, *1754*
　pathology of, 1745, *1746*
　percutaneous needling in, 1761, *1762*
　surgery for, 1755–1764, *1756–1763*
　terminal ventriculostomy for, 1761, *1762*, *1764*
　venous pressure in, 2123–2124
Syrinx, DREZotomy in, 1631, *1632*
Syrinx-to-subarachnoid shunt, 2125–2126

Tachycardia, after intracranial aneurysm surgery, 963–964
Tactile Performance Test, in intracranial glioma, 520
Tangential injury, in penetrating head injury, 83
Target sign, in cerebrospinal fluid leak, 119
Tarsal tunnel syndrome, 2181–2182, *2182*
Tarsorrhaphy, in intraorbital tumor removal, 191–192, *192*
Temperature, body, after closed head injury, 63
Temporal artery, posterior, aneurysm of, 1143, *1145*, 1146
　superficial, *76*
　　in scalp replantation, 11
Temporal artery–middle cerebral artery bypass, 909–926
　evaluation for, 910–911
　indications for, 909–910
　protocol for, 911, 911t, 912t
　tumor surgery and, 910
Temporal artery–saphenous vein–middle cerebral artery bypass, 911–920, *913–920*
　anesthesia for, 912
　brain protection during, 918
　closure for, 920
　craniotomy for, 913–915, *913*
　distal anastomosis of, *917*, 918
　instrumentation for, 912

Temporal artery–saphenous vein–middle cerebral artery bypass *(Continued)*
  middle cerebral artery branch preparation for, 916
  patient position for, 912
  proximal anastomosis of, 918–920, *919*
  superficial temporal artery preparation for, 912–913, *913*
  vein graft preparation for, *914*, 915–917, *916*
Temporal artery–saphenous vein–posterior cerebral artery bypass, 924
Temporal bone, *217*
  cerebrospinal fluid leak through, 122
  glomus bodies of, 851, *852*
  posterior cranial fossa approach by, 843–850. See also *Posterior cranial fossa, transtemporal approaches to.*
Temporal horn, lateral ventricle, ependymoma of, *732*, 733
Temporal lobe, depth electrode implantation for, 1277, *1278*, 1279, *1279*
  frontotemporal approach to, 1279
  occipitotemporal approach to, 1277, 1279
  pathology of, in epilepsy, 1305–1306
Temporal lobectomy, in epilepsy, 1287–1294, 1307–1314. See also *Epilepsy, temporal lobectomy in.*
  in functional hemispherectomy, 1344–1345
  vs. corpus callosotomy, 1354
Temporalis muscle, in lateral orbitotomy, 223, 225
Temporoparietal area, tangential penetrating injury to, 97, 100, *100*, *101*
Tendon reflexes, in syringomyelia, 2121
Tenon's capsule, 241
Tenon's space, of orbit, 215
Tension-band laminoplasty, in ossification of posterior longitudinal ligament, 1825–1827, *1825*, *1826*
Tentorial artery, of lateral sellar compartment, 494
Tentorial hiatus, tumors of, 799, *799*
Tentorium, tumor of, 783–786, *784*, *785*
  diagnosis of, 783, *784*
  retraction techniques in, 786
  surgery for, approaches for, 784–786, *785*
    instruments for, 786
    position for, 783–784, *785*
Teratoma, intramedullary, 2028, 2036. See also *Spinal cord tumors, intramedullary.*
  lateral ventricle, 726
Terminal ventriculostomy, for syringomyelic cord syndrome, 1761, *1762*, *1764*
Testosterone, in prolactin-secreting pituitary adenoma, 309, 311
Tethering, in myelomeningoceles, 2063
Tetraplegia, 1667–1669, 1668t. See also *Spasticity.*
Texas-Scottish-Rite-Hospital system, in pediatric spinal injury, 2087
Thalamic–basal ganglia, vascular malformations of, 1501–1520
  anatomy of, 1501–1502, 1502t
  evaluation of, 1501–1502, 1502t
  management of, 1502–1503
  presentation of, 1501, 1501t, 1502t
  size of, 1502
  surgery for, 1504–1518
    adjuncts to, 1504
    anesthesia for, 1504
    electrophysiologic monitoring in, 1504
    management after, 1518
    principles of, 1504
    results of, 1518, 1520, 1520t
    retractor for, 1504
    stereotactic craniotomy approach to, 1503, 1518, *1519*

Thalamic–basal ganglia *(Continued)*
    transcallosal-transventricular approach to, 1503, 1504–1505, *1505–1507*
    transcortical-transventricular approach to, 1503, 1508–1513, *1509–1513*
    transsylvian approach to, 1503, 1513–1518, *1514–1518*
Thalamotomy, dorsomedial, in aggressive conduct disorders, 1418
  for tremor, 691
  in adult-onset dystonia, 1657
  intralaminar, in aggressive conduct disorders, 1418, *1418*
Thalamus, astrocytoma of, curietherapy for, *464*
  glioma of, 775, *776*
  lesions of, pain with, deep brain stimulation in, *1395*, 1396
Thermocapsulotomy. See *Capsulotomy.*
Thermorhizotomy, percutaneous, in spasticity, 1665
Third ventricle. See *Ventricle(s), third.*
Thirty-degree test, in pseudotumor cerebri, 239
Thoracic disc, herniation of, 1895–1904
  clinical features of, 1895
  preoperative evaluation of, 1895
  surgery for, anterolateral approach in, *1896*, 1896t
    anterolateral extrapleural approach in, *1896*, 1900–1902, *1900*, *1901*
    approach selection for, 1895–1897, *1896*, 1896t
    costotransversectomy in, *1896*, 1898, *1898–1900*
    laminectomy in, *1896*
    lateral extracavitary approach in, 1898, 1900
    patient selection for, 1895
    posterolateral approach in, *1896*, 1896t
    transpedicular approach in, *1896*, 1897–1898, *1898*
    transthoracic transpleural approach in, *1896*, 1902, *1902–1904*
Thoracic outlet syndrome, 2173–2175, *2173*, *2174*
  supraclavicular exploration of, 2173–2175, *2173*, *2174*
Thoracic spine, pediatric, injury to, 2083, 2084, 2090–2091, *2090*
  surgical approach to, 1887–1893, 1887t
    anterior, 1892
    anterolateral, 1890–1892
    extracavitary, lateral, 1889
    posterior, 1887–1888
    posterolateral, 1888–1890
    thoracoabdominal, 1892
    transpedicular, 1889–1890
  syringomyelia of, endoscopic surgery for, *712*
  tumor-associated compression of, 1997–2023. See also *Spine, tumors of.*
Thoracolumbar spine, fracture of, in ankylosing spondylitis, 1777–1778, *1778*, *1779*
  surgical approach to, 1887–1893, 1887t
    anterior, 1892
    anterolateral, 1890–1892
    extracavitary, lateral, 1889
    posterior, 1887–1888
    posterolateral, 1888–1890
    thoracoabdominal, 1892
    transpedicular, 1889–1890
  tumors of, surgery for, 1992–1995, *1994*
    lateral osteotomy approach in, 1995
Thoracotomy, 1890–1892
Thrombosis, after closed head injury, 64
Thyroid eye disease, 178t, 179t
Thyroxin, in craniopharyngioma, 386
Tibial nerve, lesions of, treatment of, 2164

Tibial nerve *(Continued)*
  posterior, entrapment of, 2181–2182, *2182*
Tic convulsif, 1463
Tic douloureux, clinical features of, 1459
  diagnosis of, 1459
  magnetic resonance imaging in, 1459–1460
  neurovascular decompression for, 1459–1463, *1461*
    care after, 1462
    complications of, 1462–1463
    patient position for, 1460
    preparation for, 1460
    results of, 1462
    technique of, 1460–1462, *1461*
  preoperative evaluation of, 1459
  treatment of, 1459–1460
Tissue expansion, in scalp defect, 7, *7*, *8*, 15, 17–18, *18*
Tissue plasminogen activator, for aneurysmal subarachnoid hemorrhage–associated vasospasm, 947–948
Tissue reaction, orbital surgery and, 235
Titan oxide, allergic reaction to, 43, *43*
  osteosynthetic, removal of, 42–43
Titanium miniplates, 39, *39*
Tobacco-pouch technique, for cerebrospinal fluid leaks, 33, *34*
Tolerance test occlusion, in brain revascularization evaluation, 910–911
Torticollis, spasmodic, 1649–1657
  accessory nerve root lysis for, 1650
  anterior cervical rhizotomy for, 1650–1651
  conservative management of, 1649–1650
  epidural cervical stimulation for, 1650
  management of, 1656–1657
  muscle resection for, 1651
  peripheral cervical rhizotomy for, 1653–1654
  physiotherapy for, 1654
  posterior ramisectomy for, 1653–1654, *1654*
  selective peripheral denervation for, 1651–1652
    results of, 1654–1656, 1654t
    technique of, 1652–1654, *1653*
  sternocleidomastoid muscle denervation for, 1652, *1653*
Toxin-leaking CNS cyst, 585–586
Toxoplasmosis, cerebral, in AIDS, 1681, 1681t, 1684, 1684t
Tracers, in cerebrospinal fluid leak localization, 120, 120t
Tract of Lissauer, 1613, 1615
Traction, in ankylosing spondylitis, *1770*, 1771
Tractotomy, medullary, 1568–1570
  anatomy of, 1568
  anesthesia for, 1569
  complications of, 1570
  indications for, 1568–1569
  instrumentation for, 1569
  patient position for, 1569–1570
  technique of, 1569–1570
  subcaudate, complications of, 1416
    in obsessive-compulsive disorders, 1415–1417, *1416*
    results of, 1417
Trailmaking test, in intracranial glioma, 521
Transforaminal corridor, in third ventricle transcallosal approach, 717, *718*, *720*
Transsphenoidal surgery, 283–292, 291t, 292t
  complications of, 291t
  for craniopharyngioma, 289–292, *289*, *290*
  for nonfunctioning pituitary adenoma, 295–297, *296*, *298–299*
  for pituitary adenoma, 283–289, *285–289*
  in Cushing's disease, 302
  operating room setup for, *284*

Transsphenoidal surgery *(Continued)*
  patient position for, 283, *284*
  results of, 292t
  sella repair after, 327–344. See also *Sella turcica, repair of.*
Transverse sinus, depressed fracture over, 71
Trauma. See at *Head; Fracture(s).*
Tremor, Gamma Knife surgery for, 691
Triage, for penetrating head injury, 87
Triangles, of lateral sellar compartment, 494–497, *495*, 496t
Trigeminal cephalgia, in pseudotumor cerebri, 250
Trigeminal cistern, anatomy of, 1524–1525
Trigeminal cisternography, 1525–1526, *1525, 1526*
Trigeminal nerve, *1474*
  at cerebellopontine angle, 1458
  carotid artery relation to, *1474*
  decompression of, 1459–1463, *1461*
    complications of, 1545t, 1546
  glycerol effects on, 1533–1534
  in Gamma Knife surgery, 680, 681
  in sclerosteosis, 2142
  nucleus caudalis of, 1627–1628, *1628*
    DREZotomy of, 1633–1634, *1633, 1634*
  of lateral sellar compartment, 479, *480*
  percutaneous rhizotomy of, ocular side effects of, 1477
  vascular compression of, 1458
Trigeminal neuralgia, atypical, 1463
  bilateral, 1541
    percutaneous trigeminal nerve compression for, 1541
  Gamma Knife surgery for, 690–691
  glossopharyngeal neuralgia with, 1464
  in multiple sclerosis, 1532–1533, 1541
  microvascular decompression for, complications of, 1545t, 1546
  percutaneous rhizotomy for, 1469–1480
    complications of, 1543–1546
    disease recurrence after, 1477
    electrode localization for, 1472, 1474, *1475*
    herpes simplex after, 1477
    in atypical facial pain, 1480–1481
    in multiple sclerosis, 1480
    lesion production in, 1474, 1476
    motor paresis after, 1477
    ocular side effects of, 1477
    patient selection for, 1469–1470
    results of, 1476, 1476t
    sensory side effects of, 1476–1477, 1476t
    side effects of, 1476–1477, 1476t, 1477t
    technique of, 1470–1476, *1470–1475*
    vs. peripheral neurectomy, 1478
    vs. posterior fossa exploration, 1478, 1479t, 1480t
    vs. retrogasserian balloon compression, 1478, 1479t, 1480t
  percutaneous trigeminal ganglion compression for, 1537–1546
    balloon distension pressure in, 1539–1540
    in multiple sclerosis, 1541
    motor weakness after, 1540
    pain reflex in, 1540
    paresthesia after, 1540
    sensation after, 1540
    technique of, 1537–1539, *1538, 1539*
    trochar in, 1539
  retrogasserian glycerol rhizolysis in, 1523–1541
    anatomy for, 1524–1525
    anesthesia for, 1524
    aseptic meningitis after, 1532
    bacterial meningitis after, 1532
    branch selectivity in, 1527–1528

Trigeminal neuralgia *(Continued)*
  cerebrospinal fluid drainage in, 1526
  cistern marking in, 1528, *1528*
  cisternography in, 1525–1526, *1525, 1526*
  complications of, 1530–1532, 1531t, 1532t
  contrast evacuation in, 1527
  dysesthesia after, 1531, 1531t
  facial sensory disturbance after, 1531
  glycerol injection in, 1527–1528
  herpes activation after, 1532
  history of, 1523
  hypesthesia after, 1531, 1531t
  in multiple sclerosis, 1532–1533
  indications for, 1523–1524, 1535
  infectious complications of, 1531–1532, 1532t
  management after, 1528–1529
  mechanisms of, 1533–1534
  morphologic effects of, 1533–1534
  neurophysiologic effects of, 1534
  patient positioning for, 1524
  preoperative evaluation for, 1524
  reinjection in, 1528
  results of, 1529–1530, 1529t, 1530t
  technique of, 1524–1528
Trigone, tumors of, 726, *730*, 731
Trigonocephaly, 142–143, 145
Trochar, in percutaneous trigeminal nerve compression, 1539
Trochlea, in anterior orbitotomy, 231
Trochlear nerve, 186, *186*, 197
  in Gamma Knife surgery, 680
  of lateral sellar compartment, 479, *480*, 481
Tuberculoma, 1689–1697, 1689t
  anticonvulsant medications in, 1695
  antituberculous drugs in, 1694–1695, 1695t
  calcification in, 1691
  clinical features of, 1690
  computed tomography of, 1692–1694, *1692–1696*
  corticosteroids in, 1695
  forms of, 1691
  immunohistochemistry of, 1691
  incidence of, 1689–1690
  location of, 1690, 1690t
  magnetic resonance imaging of, 1693–1694, *1694–1696*
  medical treatment of, 1694–1695, 1695t
  pathologic features of, 1691, *1691*
  radiologic features of, 1691–1692
  surgery for, 1695–1697
  tuberculous meningitis and, 1690
  ultrastructural characteristics of, 1691
Tuberculosis, 1689–1699, 1689t
  in AIDS, 1690
Tuberculous meningitis, 1697–1699, *1698*
Tuberculum sellae, meningioma of, 403–408
  classification of, 403–404
  clinical presentation of, 404
  pathologic anatomy in, 403–404
  preoperative evaluation of, 404, *405*
  recurrence of, 407–408
  surgical approach to, 405–407, *406, 407*
    patient selection for, 404–405
  results of, 407–408
Tuberous sclerosis, subependymal giant cell astrocytoma in, 574
Tumors. See also at specific structures and tumors, e.g., *Brainstem; Glioma.*
  during pregnancy, 1163–1167
  hydrocephalus with, 1246
  metastatic, cerebellar, 796–797
    computer-assisted volumetric stereotactic resection of, 631–632
    extracranial, 612
    leptomeningeal, 599, *605*

Tumors *(Continued)*
  orbital, 178t, 179t
  pituitary, vs. nonfunctioning pituitary adenoma, 295
  spinal, 1981–1995. See also *Spine, tumors of.*
  subarachnoid, from pineocytoma, 760–761, *761*
  to brain, 599–613. See also *Brain, metastases to.*
  to peripheral nerves, 2195–2196, *2195*
  to posterior fossa, 792t, 796–797
  osteotropism of, 1981
Turbinate bone, middle, rotating flap with, 37

Ulnar nerve, entrapment of, 2179–2180, *2179, 2180*
  at elbow, 2179–2180, *2179, 2180*
  at wrist, 2180, *2180, 2181*
  lesions of, treatment of, 2164
Ultrasonic aspirator, in low-grade glioma, 560
Ultrasonography, intraoperative, in intracranial glioma, 519
  of vein of Galen malformation, 1214, *1214, 1216*
Ultrasound, intraluminal, in neuroendoscopy, 698–699, *700*
Urea, after closed head injury, 63
Urinary incontinence, in normal-pressure hydrocephalus, 1247
Urinary retention, after open cordotomy, 1565

Vacuum phenomenon, 1941–1943, *1942, 1943,* 1943t
Vagoglossopharyngeal neuralgia, percutaneous rhizotomy for, 1481–1483, *1481, 1482*
Vagus nerve, 1107
  in carotid endarterectomy, 880, *880*
  neurovascular decompression of, 1464–1466
  paralysis of, after glomus jugulare tumor surgery, 858–859
Valproate, in pregnancy, 1169
Valproic acid, in myelomeningoceles, 2055
Valsalva maneuver, intraoperative, 128
Vasogenic edema, in neoplastic spinal cord compression, 1999
  interstitial brachytherapy and, 665
Vasospasm, aneurysmal subarachnoid hemorrhage–associated, 941, 944–948, 944t, 958, *958*
  AT877 (HA1077) for, 945
  calcitonin gene–related peptide in, 945, 947
  calcium channel antagonists for, 945, 947t
  diagnosis of, 944
  hypertension for, 943t, 944–945
  hypervolemia for, 943t, 944–945
  nicardipine for, 945
  nimodipine for, 945, 947t
  papaverine for, 947
  tissue plasminogen activator for, 947–948
  transluminal angioplasty for, 947
  treatment of, 943t, 944–948
  in anterior communicating artery aneurysm, 1013
  in closed head injury, 61
Vecuronium, in closed head injury, 60
Vegetative state, in pregnancy, 1170
Vein(s), from pineal region, 745, *746,* 747t
  of lateral sellar compartment, 483–490, *486–490*
  orbital, visualization of, 218
Vein of Galen malformation, 1213–1218, 1258

Vein of Galen malformation *(Continued)*
 classification of, 1213–1214
 clinical features of, 1213–1215, *1214*
 preoperative evaluation of, 1215
 surgery for, anesthesia for, 1215
  care after, 1217
  hemorrhage after, 1217
  mortality after, 1217–1218
  patient selection for, 1215, *1215*
  results of, 1217–1218
  techniques for, 1215–1217, *1216, 1217*
 type I, 1214, *1214*
 type II, 1214–1215
 ultrasound of, 1214, *1214,* 1216
 venography in, 1215, *1215*
Vein of Labbé, in arteriovenous fistula, 1223
Velum interpositum, 753
Venography, in vein of Galen malformation, 1215, *1215*
 orbital, 218
Ventricle(s), cerebrospinal fluid accumulation in. See *Hydrocephalus.*
 cysticercosis of, 1711–1712, *1712, 1713*
 fourth, ependymoma of, 796
  floor of, anatomy of, *1489*
 lateral, body of, tumors of, 731, *731*
  ependymoma of, 726, *729*
  frontal horn of, glioma of, 731, *732*
  glioma of, 726, *728,* 731, *732, 732*
  hematoma of, endoscopic surgery for, *709*
  horn of, tumors of, 731, *732*
  meningioma of, 726, *727*
  metastases to, 726, *730*
  mixed glioma of, 726, *729*
  oligodendroglioma of, 726, *728*
  subependymoma of, 726
  temporal horn of, ependymoma of, *732,* 733
   tumors of, *732,* 733
  teratoma of, 726
  tumors of, 725–737
   anterior temporal lobectomy for, 733
   approach selection for, 735
   complications of, 736
   intraoperative management of, 735–736
   lateral temporal parietal incision for, 733
   middle frontal gyrus approach for, 734
   middle temporal gyrus incision for, 733
   neuropsychological testing in, 726
   occipital lobectomy for, 733
   pathology of, 726, *727–730*
   postoperative care in, 736–737
   postoperative focal neurologic deficits in, 736
   postoperative hydrocephalus in, 736
   postoperative seizures in, 736
   postoperative subdural hematoma in, 736
   subtotal resection of, 736
   superior parietal occipital incision for, 734
   surgical mortality in, 736
   transcallosal approach for, 734–735
 third, cavernous angioma of, subchoroidal trans–velum interpositum approach to, *721*
  colloid cyst of, 584, 590–591, *591,* 715
   endoscopic surgery for, 704, 706, *709*
   transcallosal approach to, *719*
  craniopharyngioma of, 359, 382–383, 715
   endoscopic biopsy of, *708*
   transcallosal approach to, *722*
  cysticercosis of, transforaminal transcallosal approach to, *719*
  floor of, glioma of, *769*
  glioma of, *769, 772,* 773
  hydrocephalus effects on, 703
  lesions of, computer-assisted volumetric stereotactic resection of, 632, *633, 634*

Ventricle(s) *(Continued)*
 posterior. See *Pineal region.*
  transcallosal approach to, 715–722
   incision for, *716*
   indications for, 715, 717
   interforniceal corridor in, *718,* 722, *722*
   subchoroidal corridor in, 717, *718, 721*
   technique of, *716,* 717–722, *718–722*
   transforaminal corridor in, 717, *718, 720*
  upper part of, glioma of, 775
Ventricular body, tumors of, 731, *731*
Ventricular drainage, in aneurysmal subarachnoid hemorrhage, 949
 in closed head injury, 60
Ventricular shunt, in neonate, 1257
 malfunction of, 1252, 1252t
 obstruction of, 1252
Ventricular system, penetrating injury to, 97, *99*
Ventriculoatrial shunt, in adult hydrocephalus, 1249
 in pediatric hydrocephalus, 1234–1235
 infection of, 1253
Ventriculoperitoneal shunt, in pediatric hydrocephalus, 1233–1234
 in tuberculoma, 1697
 in tuberculous meningitis, 1698
Ventriculopleural shunt, in pediatric hydrocephalus, 1235
Ventriculostomy, fourth, in syringomyelic cord syndrome, 1762
 in aneurysmal subarachnoid hemorrhage–associated hydrocephalus, 949–950
 in closed head injury, 62
 in penetrating head injuries, 86
 in posterior fossa hematoma, 70
 terminal, in syringomyelic cord syndrome, 1761, *1762, 1764*
 third, 703–704, *703*
  coronal approach to, 700–701, 701t, 703, *703*
  in pediatric hydrocephalus, 1236
  positioning of, 703, *703*
  results of, 707
Ventrolateral reticulospinal tract, in open cordotomy, 1567
Ventroposterolateral and ventroposteromedial (VPL-VPM) thalamic nulcei, stimulation of, in pain treatment, 1390, 1392–1393, *1393.* See also *Deep brain stimulation.*
Vermis, 802
 cerebellar, pediatric, tumors of, 808, *808*
Vertebral artery, bilateral stenosis of, extraluminal decompression for, 898, *899*
 collateral branches of, *1654*
 compression of, in cervical spondylosis, 1785
 extracranial, lesions of, 897–908, *898–905*
 occlusion of, 897–908
 scalenotomy for, 898, *898*
 subtotal, *907,* 908, *908*
 second portion of, bilateral stenosis of, 898, *899*
 stenosis of, subclavian artery stenosis and, 898, *900*
  vertebral artery amputation for, 898, *900, 901*
Vertebral artery complex, aneurysm of, 1103–1110
 anatomy of, 1106–1107
 clinical features of, 1104–1105
 dissecting, 1105–1106, *1106*
 fusiform, 1106
 imaging of, 1105
 location of, 1103, *1103*
 morphology of, 1103–1104, *1104*
 preoperative evaluation of, 1105–1106
 saccular, 1105

Vertebral artery complex *(Continued)*
 surgery for, 1107–1110
  anesthesia in, 1107
  clip selection in, 1110
  distal control in, 1110
  ELITE approach in, 1109
  endovascular balloon catheter techniques in, 967–974, 968t
  extreme lateral inferior transcondylar exposure in, 1109
  microsurgical techniques in, 1109–1110
  proximal control in, 1110
  retrolabyrinthine-transsigmoid approach in, 1108–1109
  suboccipital approach in, 1107–1108
Vertebral artery insufficiency, vertigo with, 1549
Vertebral body, replacement of, in neoplastic spinal cord compression, 2012–2019, *2016, 2017*
 resection of, for spinal tumors, 1985–1992, *1986–1993*
Vertebral endarterectomy, 900, 902–907, *902–905*
 closure for, 904–905, *905*
 exposure for, *903*
 skin incision for, *902*
 subclavian artery incision in, *904*
Vertebrectomy, in multisegmental cervical spondylosis, 1792–1800, *1793, 1794, 1796–1799*
Vertebrobasilar artery, anatomy of, *1076*
 aneurysm of, 964–965, 1071–1086
  giant, 1116
  sites of, *1072*
  surgery for, anesthesia for, 1071, 1074
   approaches to, *1072*
   results of, 1072t, 1073t, 1074t, 1085–1086
Vertebrobasilar insufficiency, 897–908
 clinical features of, 897–900, *898–902*
 vertebral endarterectomy for, 900, 902–907, *902–905*
Vertebrobasilar junction, aneurysm of, 1118
Vertigo, 1547–1554
 after suboccipital transmeatal acoustic neuroma removal, 837
 central, 1548
 differential diagnosis of, 1548–1549
 nonsurgical treatment for, 1548
 peripheral, 1548
 positional, benign, 1548
 vestibular nerve section for, 1547–1554
  care after, 1554
  complications of, 1554
  cranial nerve anatomy in, 1551–1553, *1551, 1552*
  history of, 1547–1548
  results of, 1554
  retrolabyrinthine exposure in, 1547–1548, 1550–1551, *1550*
  retrolabyrinthine-retrosigmoid exposure in, 1551
  technique of, 1553–1554, *1553*
Vestibular nerve, 1551–1553, *1551, 1552*
 section of, 1547–1554
  care after, 1554
  complications of, 1554
  cranial nerve anatomy in, 1551–1553, *1551, 1552*
  patient position for, 1550
  patient preparation for, 1549
  results of, 1554
  retrolabyrinthine exposure for, 1547–1548, 1550–1551, *1550*
  retrolabyrinthine-retrosigmoid exposure for, 1551

Vestibular nerve *(Continued)*
    technique of, 1553–1554, *1553*
    vascular cross compression of, 1549
Vestibular schwannoma. See *Neuroma, acoustic.*
Vestibulocochlear nerve, 1551–1553, *1551, 1552*
    histologic morphology of, 1553
Vision, after orbital surgery, 235
    in craniopharyngioma, 358, 371, 386
    in hypothalamic tumors, 774
    in intracranial glioma, 519
    in medial sphenoid ridge meningioma, 408–409, 412
    in pediatric cerebellar tumor, 803
    in pseudotumor cerebri, 237–238, 239t, 247–250, 250t
    in suprasellar germinoma, 739–740
    in tuberculum sellae meningioma, 404, 407–408
Visual evoked potentials, in lateral orbitotomy, 226, 227
    in optic nerve glioma, 256, 277

Visual field perimetry, in pseudotumor cerebri, 238, 239t
Vomiting, in pediatric cerebellar tumor, 802–803
Von Recklinghausen's disease, 2184, *2184*
    bilateral optic nerve gliomas in, 263
    neurofibromas in, 2184, *2184,* 2188, *2191*
    thoracic meningoceles in, 2063

Wackenheim's clivus-canal line, *1720,* 1721
Wada intra-arterial sodium amytal test, in intracranial glioma, 519
Walking, after medullary tractotomy, 1570
Wallerian degeneration, 2162
Wechsler Adult Intelligence Scale, in intracranial glioma, 520
Wernicke's area, *532*
Wound healing, after glomus jugulare tumor surgery, 859
Wrapping, aneurysmal, 1122
Wrist, median nerve entrapment at, 2177–2179, *2178, 2179*
    ulnar nerve entrapment at, 2180, *2180, 2181*

Xanthoastrocytoma, pleomorphic, in children, 574–575
XURF-P2-40 (A7955) endoscope, 695, 696t
Xylohypha bantiana, 1699–1702, 1699t, *1701,* 1702t

Yttrium-90 injection, in cystic craniopharyngioma, 351, 351t, *352*

Zygomatic bone, *215, 216, 217*
    fracture of, 28
    in lateral orbitotomy, 223, *223–225*
    osteosynthesis of, 38